CLINICAL AND PATHOGENIC MICROBIOLOGY

MCLINICAL AND PATHOGENIC MICROBIOLOGY

BARBARA J. HOWARD, D.A., M.T. (ASCP)

Associate Professor, Department of Biology
Director, Medical Technology Programs
The Catholic University of America
Washington, D.C.

JOHN KLAAS II, Ph.D.,
  Diplomate (Parasitology), ABMM

Former Assistant Professor
Medical Laboratory Science
Northeastern University
Boston, Massachusetts

SALLY JO RUBIN, Ph.D.,
  Diplomate, ABMM

Former Director, Microbiology Division
Saint Francis Hospital and Medical Center
Hartford, Connecticut;
Former Associate Professor
Department of Laboratory Medicine
University of Connecticut School of Medicine
Farmington, Connecticut
(Deceased)

ALICE S. WEISSFELD, Ph.D.,
  Diplomate, ABMM

Director, Microbiology Specialists, Inc.;
Adjunct Assistant Professor
Department of Microbiology and Immunology
Baylor College of Medicine
Houston, Texas

RICHARD C. TILTON, Ph.D.,
  Diplomate, ABMM

Professor of Laboratory Medicine;
Director of Microbiology Division
Department of Laboratory Medicine
University of Connecticut School of Medicine
Farmington, Connecticut

With 355 illustrations and 32 color plates

The C.V. Mosby Company

St. Louis • Washington, D.C. • Toronto   1987

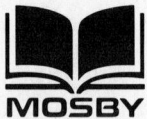

MOSBY

A TRADITION OF PUBLISHING EXCELLENCE

Editors: Dennis Carson, Stephanie Bircher
Assistant Editors: Elizabeth Raven, Anne Gunter
Project Manager: Patricia Tannian
Production Editors: Celeste Clingan, Steven Dierkes, Kathy Lumpkin
Designer: Susan E. Lane

Printed in the United States of America

The C.V. Mosby Company
11830 Westline Industrial Drive, St. Louis, Missouri 63146

Library of Congress Cataloging-in-Publications Data

Clinical and pathogenic microbiology.

   Includes bibliographies and index.
   1. Medical microbiology. 2. Diagnostic
microbiology. I. Howard, Barbara J.
[DNLM: 1. Mycology—methods. 2. Parasitology
—methods. 3. Virology—methods. QY 110 C641]
QR46.C57   1987   616′.01   87-18560
ISBN 0-8016-2287-5

TS/VH/VH   9 8 7 6 5 4 3 2 1   03/B/340

Contributors

Rebecca D. Almazan, B.S., MT (ASCP) SM
Supervisor, Clinical Microbiology Laboratory
Walter Reed Army Medical Center
Washington, D.C.

Raymond C. Bartlett, M.D.
Director, Division of Microbiology
Hartford Hospital
Hartford, Connecticut;
Professor of Laboratory Medicine
University of Connecticut School of Medicine
Farmington, Connecticut

Edward J. Bottone, Ph.D., Diplomate, ABMM
Professor of Clinical Microbiology
Mount Sinai School of Medicine;
Director, Department of Microbiology
The Mount Sinai Hospital
New York, New York

Jill E. Clarridge, Ph.D., Diplomate, ABMM
Chief, Microbiology Section, Veterans Administration
    Medical Center;
Assistant Professor, Department of Pathology and
    Microbiology and Immunology
Baylor College of Medicine
Houston, Texas

James J. Damato, Ph.D., SM(AAM)
Lieutenant Colonel, United States Army;
Human Immunodeficiency Virus Clinical Project Manager
Walter Reed Army Institute of Research
Washington, D.C.

Madeline J. Ducate, M.S., M.P.H., MT(ASCP)SM
Scientific Associate
G.H. Besselaar Associates
Princeton, New Jersey

J.J. Farmer III, Ph.D.
Chief, Enteric Identification Laboratories
Enteric Bacteriology Section
Center for Infectious Diseases
Centers for Disease Control
Atlanta, Georgia

Bruce A. Gunn, Ph.D., SM(AAM)
Lieutenant Colonel, United States Army;
Chief, Microbiology Branch
Laboratory Sciences Division
Academy of Health Sciences
Fort Sam Houston, Texas

Joyce S. Hayes, R.N., M.P.H., C.I.C.
Infection Control Practitioner
Jewish Hospital
St. Louis, Missouri

J. Michael Janda, Ph.D., Diplomate, ABMM
Research Microbiologist
Microbial Diseases Laboratory
California Department of Health Services
Berkeley, California

John L. Johnson, Ph.D.
Professor of Microbiology
Department of Anaerobic Microbiology
Virginia Polytechnic Institute and State University
Blacksburg, Virginia

Russell C. Johnson, Ph.D.
Professor, Department of Microbiology
University of Minnesota
Minneapolis, Minnesota

Raymond L. Kaplan, Ph.D.
Associate Professor, Department of
    Immunology/Microbiology;
Unit Director, Section of Clinical Microbiology, OCLS
Rush Presbyterian St. Luke's Medical Center
Chicago, Illinois

John F. Keiser, M.D., Ph.D.
Medical Director, Clinical Microbiology;
Assistant Professor, Department of Pathology
George Washington University
Washington, D.C.

Wesley E. Kloos, Ph.D.
Professor of Genetics and Microbiology
North Carolina State University
Raleigh, North Carolina

Mark T. LaRocco, Ph.D., M(ASCP)
Assistant Professor, Department of Pathology and Laboratory
    Medicine;
Associate Director, Clinical Microbiology Laboratory
Hermann Hospital and the University of Texas Health Science
    Center
University of Texas Health Science Center
Houston, Texas

Mary Ellen Mangum, Dr.P.H., MT(ASCP)
Clinical Immunology and Microbiology Laboratories
North Carolina Memorial Hospital
Chapel Hill, North Carolina

Michael R. McGinnis, Ph.D., Diplomate, ABMM
Director, Clinical Mycology and Mycobacteriology Laboratory
North Carolina Memorial Hospital;
Associate Professor, Department of Microbiology and
    Immunology
University of North Carolina at Chapel Hill
Chapel Hill, North Carolina

J. Michael Mullins, Ph.D.
Associate Professor, Department of Biology
The Catholic University of America
Washington, D.C.

Thomas R. Oberhofer, Dr.P.H.
U.S. Army (Retired);
Formerly Chief, Microbiology Section
Madigan Army Medical Center
Tacoma, Washington

A. William Pasculle, Sc.D.
Assistant Director of Microbiology
Presbyterian-University Hospital;
Associate Professor of Pathology
University of Pittsburgh School of Medicine
Pittsburgh, Pennsylvania

John C. Rees, Ph.D., MT(ASCP)
Director, Clinical Immunology and Serology
Washington Hospital Center
Washington, D.C.

Thomas F. Smith, Ph.D., Diplomate, ABMM
Director, Virology Laboratory;
Professor of Microbiology and Laboratory Medicine
Mayo Clinic
Rochester, Minnesota

Barbara M. Soule, R.N., B.S., C.I.C.
Nurse Epidemiologist
St. Peter Hospital
Olympia, Washington

Alexander von Graevenitz, M.D., Diplomate, ABMM
Professor of Medical Microbiology;
Director, Department of Medical Microbiology
University of Zurich
Zurich, Switzerland

Sonia Zighelboim-Daum, Ph.D.
Scientific Associate
New England Deaconess Hospital/Harvard Medical School
Boston, Massachusetts

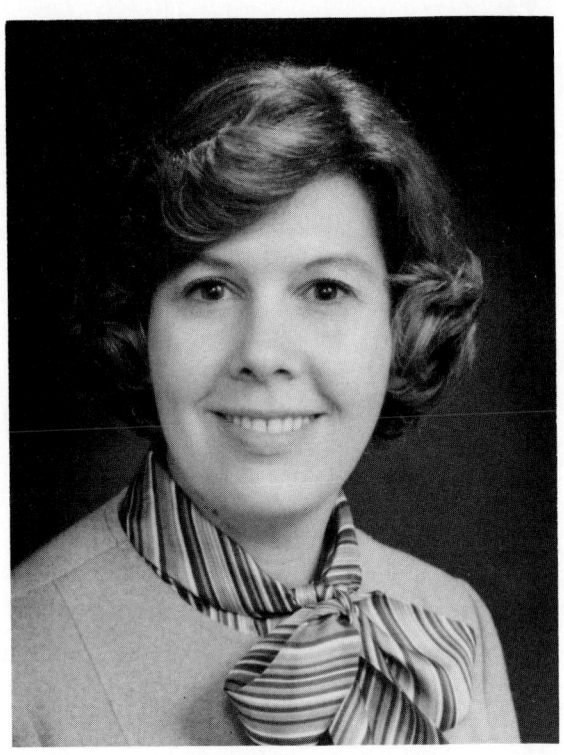

This book is dedicated to Dr. Sally Jo Rubin
(1943-1985)

We were devastated to learn of Sally Jo's illness shortly after we started this book. She gave her disease no quarter and was a tireless colleague in spite of it. She was an inspiration and an example to all of us. We will never forget her. In some way, we hope that this book, *Clinical and Pathogenic Microbiology*, stands as a lasting tribute to Dr. Rubin's quest for excellence, her uncompromising standards, and her love for microbiology.

Preface

Although separate treatments of clinical and pathogenic microbiology abound, no previous work has satisfactorily integrated these two subject areas. *Clinical and Pathogenic Microbiology* combines in one volume the study of the materials and methods used for the identification of pathogenic organisms and the study of these organisms in relation to their disease processes in humans. The authors have striven to create a comprehensive book that strikes a balance between theory and practice.

Clinical and Pathogenic Microbiology is intended as a text for medical technology students and students in pathogenic and diagnostic microbiology courses at advanced undergraduate and graduate levels. In addition, clinical laboratories will find the book to be a well-documented reference tool.

The reader will find comprehensive coverage of mycology, parasitology, and virology, which should obviate the need for supplementary texts in these areas. The use of consistent subheadings throughout the text makes all material readily accessible.

The student can easily assimilate complex material in *Clinical and Pathogenic Microbiology* because the text has not neglected extensive explanatory information and coverage of basic science. The reader is led through difficult material in a logical fashion. Basic concepts that are presented early in the text are carefully followed and given enhanced treatment through the remainder of the text.

I acknowledge gratefully the assistance of many individuals in the preparation of this book. Invaluable suggestions and reviews of chapters were made by Dean (Ike) Armstrong, Marilyn S. Bartlett, Don Brenner, William J. Brown, Elizabeth P. Cato, Patricia Charache, Marie B. Coyle, Cecil S. Cummins, Madeline Ducate, Richard R. Facklam, James C. Feely, Lynn S. Garcia, G.L. Gilardi, Patricia Greenup, Dieter H.M. Groschel, George R. Healy, Dannie G. Hollis, Marguerite M. Jackson, J. Michael Janda, William M. Janda, Samuel W. Joseph, Raymond L. Kaplan, John F. Keiser, Michael T. Kelly, Mogens Kilian, Wesley E. Kloos, James T. Kvach, Jean F. MacFaddin, Abe Macher, J. Kenneth McClatchy, Michael R. McGinnis, Cedric A. Mims, Linda Minnich, Josephine A. Morello, David Power, Eileen L. Randall, Alan M. Rauch, Arthur L. Reingold, Morrison Rogosa, Louis DS. Smith, Walter E. Stamm, Thomas F. Smith, A. von Graevenitz, and Robert E. Weaver. I am also most appreciative of the skill of Jack P. Tandy in preparing our illustrations and for the photographs supplied by Leon J. LeBeau, Carol A. Ormes, and many others cited in the text. The work would never have been realized without the expert typing and retyping of the manuscript by numerous individuals including Diane Haddick, Grace Cannata, Judy Smith, Pansy Palmer, Adrianne Lucke, and Gloria Condit. A very special thanks goes to Thu-Thao Trinh, Maria Finelli, Joanne Comerford, and Eugene P. Kennedy who assisted in checking references, renumbering references, proofreading galleys, and perhaps most important, keeping up my spirits. And finally I extend my deepest gratitude to my family for their unending patience and support.

Barbara J. Howard

Contents

†Deceased.

PART ONE

GENERAL

CHAPTER 1

Classification

John L. Johnson

Many different types of organisms, including viruses, bacteria, fungi, protozoa, helminths, and arthropods, are able to parasitize humans and animals. The correct identification of these organisms is important because of their impact on the health of humans and animals. Identification is based on the biologic classification, the purpose of which is to characterize, group, and name organisms in a manner that will promote accurate scientific communication. Although identification and classification are among the oldest of scientific exercises, they are dynamic as a result of the continual introduction of new methods and information. This chapter applies mostly to the classification of bacteria, although the principles are the same for all groups of organisms.

Classification is the orderly arrangement of organisms into groups on the basis of their relationship to one another. *Taxonomy*, as defined by Simpson, is "the theoretical study of classification, including its basis, principles, procedures, and rules."[9] *Nomenclature* is the applying of names to the groups delineated in the classification step. *Identification* is the allocation or assignment of an unidentified organism to the correct classified and named group.

CLASSIFICATION

The basis for classification is the characteristics of the organisms. The classification of large animals and plants has been going on for thousands of years. However, microbial classification began with the invention of the microscope and viral classification with the electron microscope. Because of microbes' small size and lack of complex structures, advances in their classification have been dependent on comparisons at the physiologic and molecular levels of organization.

In 1773 the German scientist Müller[7] could recognize only two genera of bacteria, *Vibrio* and *Monas*. One hundred years later, probably because of improved microscopes, Cohn[3] recognized 10 genera. The introduction of pure culture techniques and the germ theory of disease by Koch in the 1880s provided a means for the comparison of physiologic properties, and classification began to assume increasing importance. During the early to mid-1900s, antigenic properties of organisms were analyzed, metabolic pathways were discovered, and additional compounds that could be tested as substrates were purified. These factors all contributed to more accurate comparisons and the recognition of increased numbers of bacterial groups. Watson and Crick proposed the structure of deoxyribonucleic acid (DNA) in 1953. The current understanding of DNA structure allows us to compare organisms at the level of genetic information. As a result of these advances and current and ongoing research, new properties for comparisons are continually being discovered.

It should be noted that there are no firm rules for classification. Neither correct nor incorrect classifications exist. If one wishes to classify bacteria only on the basis of the Gram stain reaction or on the basis of cell shape, these are valid classifications. Usually a classification is judged as good or poor on the basis of how useful it is to the greatest number of people.

One of the more comprehensive bacterial classification manuals has been *Bergey's Manual of Determinative Bacteriology*. Through the efforts of D. Bergey and R.E. Buchanan, the manual was first published in 1923. The eighth edition was published in 1974.[2] Recently the format of this manual has been enlarged and the name changed to *Bergey's Manual of Systematic Bacteriology*. This new edition is being published in four volumes. Volume 1, which includes gram-negative organisms, was published in 1984, and volume 2 on gram-positive organisms was published in 1986. The discussion of bacterial classification in this book is based on *Bergey's Manual of Systematic Bacteriology*. However, because of ongoing taxonomic studies, new species are continually being described and changes in nomenclature being made. Thus in some cases even *Bergey's Manual of Systematic Bacteriology* will be out of date. Students interested in the most current information on classification should first consult *Bergey's Manual of Systematic Bacteriology* and then the *International Journal of Systematic Bacteriology*. All proposed new species must be published in that journal, and once published there, the species name is considered official unless it is challenged. Details concerning the challenge procedure are discussed by Brenner.[1]

TAXONOMY

The properties used for classification are of major concern for taxonomists. The two types of properties are *phenotypic* and *phylogenetic*. Phenotypic classification is based on the observed physical and chemical properties (gene products) of the organisms, whereas phylogenetic classification is based on evolutionary relationships between organisms. For higher organisms the phylogenetic data have come primarily from fossil records. However, since bacteria have left almost no fossil records, properties with phylogenetic significance have in some cases been determined rather subjectively. More objectivity in classifying organisms has been sought through *numerical taxonomy*, a statistical method for grouping organisms into taxa dependent on characteristic similarities. The general philosophy of numerical taxonomy is that the phylogenetic significance of a given phenotypic trait (that is, whether the trait represents differences between very closely related organisms or characterizes a broad group of organisms) is difficult to judge. Therefore a large number of traits are analyzed and given equal weight in the statistical analysis. Numerical taxonomy has contributed to the recognition, at least regarding bacteria, that it is difficult to assign particular traits as characteristic of specific taxonomic levels. As a result, many of the older, hierarchically arranged microbial taxonomies have been replaced in recent years by classification schemes that emphasize the species and to a lesser extent the genus levels of classification. With increases in understanding of the structures of nucleic acids and other macromolecules of the cell, however, taxonomists are now in a position to more accurately measure phylogenetic relationships. This has resulted in a renewed interest in phylogenetic relationships at the kingdom, superfamily, and family levels, and these are again being emphasized in microbial classification.

Below are the more common types of properties used in classification. Following the example of Norris, these properties are grouped as levels of expression*:

Level 1: Genome
1. DNA (in the case of some viruses, RNA): base composition, nucleotide sequence similarity, genome size
2. Cytoplasmic DNA, phage and plasmid DNA: base composition, nucleotide sequence similarity, genome size
3. Ribosomal RNA: nucleotide sequence similarities

Level 2: Cell components
1. Cell wall composition
2. Lipid composition
3. Antigens: proteins, lipoproteins, polysaccharides, lipopolysaccharides
4. Proteins: charge and size, amino acid sequence

Level 3: Morphology and behavior
1. Morphology: macroscopic and/or microscopic structure
2. Motility: the presence, morphology, and arrangements of flagella
3. Substrate utilization tests
4. Enzyme activity tests
5. Physiology: temperature optimum, aerobic or anaerobic growth, toxin production, antimicrobial resistance, bacteriocin production
6. Nutritional requirements: vitamin, amino acid, or ion requirements

The group of organisms being investigated will dictate which properties are applicable. Of major importance are the cellular complexity of the organisms and whether they can be cultivated in pure culture. The levels of expression along with some examples are discussed in the following sections.

LEVEL 1

Level 1 represents the most basic information level in the cell. All the information required for the growth and replication of an organism resides in the nucleic acids. For most organisms the information storage material is double-stranded DNA, although for some viruses it may be single-stranded DNA or single- or double-stranded ribonucleic acid (RNA). The double-stranded DNA exists in a helical structure referred to as native DNA. The strands consist of a backbone of alternating

---

*From Norris, J.R.: Introduction. In Goodfellow, M., and Board, R.G., editors: Microbial classification and identification, The Society for Applied Bacteriology Symposium Series No. 8, London, 1980, Academic Press.

phosphate and deoxyribose molecules, with a purine or pyrimidine base linked to the 1-position of each sugar molecule. The two strands are held together by hydrogen bonds between the purine and pyrimidine bases. There are four major bases occurring as two base pairs, adenine-thymine (AT) and guanine-cytosine (GC). The two strands are complementary; if there is an adenine on one strand, a thymine is directly across from it on the other strand. The genetic information is coded by the linear arrangement of the bases on the DNA strands. Therefore two organisms that are identical have DNA with identical linear base arrangements.

The base compositions of DNA from bacteria range from about 25 to 75 moles percent guanine plus cytosine (mol% G+C). The mol% G+C values of DNA from viruses are also variable, but for most eukaryotic organisms the mol% G+C values are in the low to middle 40 mol% G+C range. If the DNAs of two organisms differ by several mol% G+C, that is good evidence that the two organisms do not belong to the same species. On the other hand, if the DNAs of two organisms have the same mol% G+C, this indicates one of two possibilities: that the organisms are very similar or simply that two very distinct organisms have DNA with similar mol% G+C. All animals, for example, have DNA with about 45 mol% G+C.

DNA has some unique properties that enable us to determine both the mol% G+C values and similarities in the linear base arrangements. These properties are schematically demonstrated in Figure 1-1. The helical structures at the left of the figure represent fragments of double-stranded or native DNA with the connecting lines representing either AT or GC base pairs held together by hydrogen bonds. The 260 nm absorbance of this preparation is given as 1.0 on the strip chart shown in the upper part of the figure. As the temperature of the sample is increased, the base pairs begin to dissociate (the high AT base pair regions first), which results in an increase in the absorbancy until all of the complementary strands have separated. At this time the absorbance of the DNA sample has increased by about 40%, to 1.4. The curve is called the melting curve, and the midpoint of the curve (the temperature at which half of the base pairs have dissociated) is called the T_m. The T_m is a function of the mol% G+C content of the DNA and represents the most common way of estimating the G+C content of a given DNA. When a high concentration of salt (for example 0.4 to 1 M NaCl) is included in the DNA sample and after denaturation, lowering the temperature to about 25° C below the T_m, the single-strand fragments will reassociate (renature) with complementary fragments of DNA to form duplex structures that are nearly identical to the original fragments. These reactions are diagrammed at the right in Figure 1-1 by the decrease in absorbance and the reformation of the helical structures (duplexes). The duplexes are not even at the ends; this is because the fragmentation of the DNA preparation was random, so the complementary fragments are not exactly the same lengths. This physical ability of DNA to reassociate allows us to test whether the DNAs from organisms A and B have similar enough sequences to reassociate with each other.

Experiments measuring the reassociation of DNA are usually referred to as DNA homology or hybridization experiments, and the results are expressed variously as percent homology, percent hybridization, percent reassociation, percent similarity,

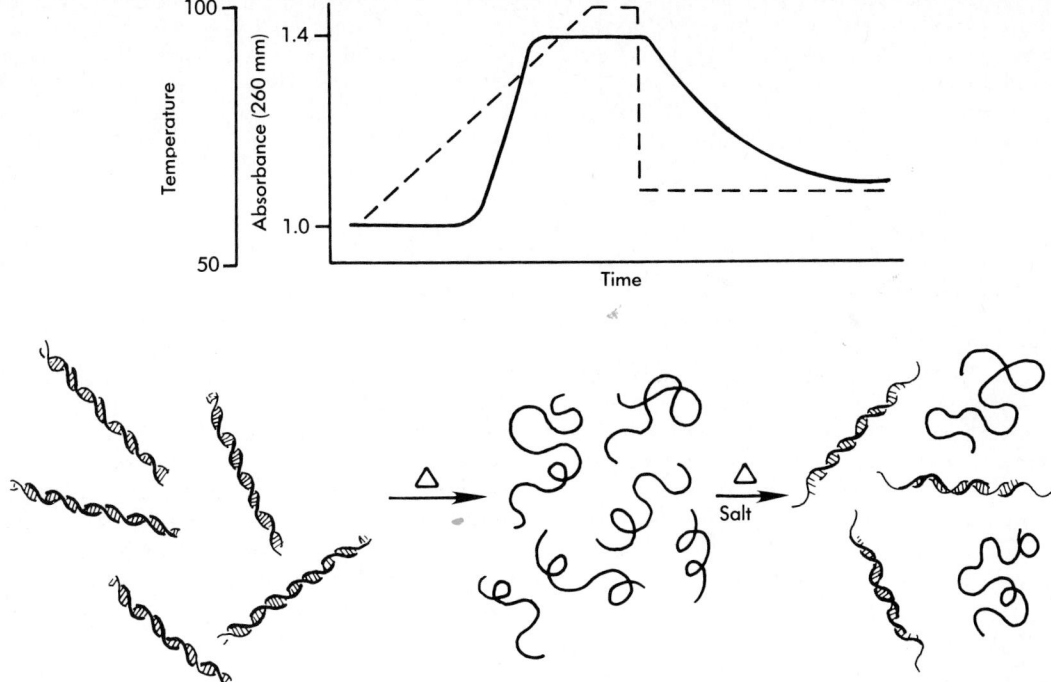

FIGURE 1-1. Schematic representation of DNA denaturation and reassociation. (Modified and reprinted by permission of the publisher from "Schematic Representation of labeled DNA reassociating with unlabeled homologous or unrelated heterologous DNA preparation" by John L. Johnson, Clin. Microbiol. Newsletter **2**:1-3, 1980, by Elsevier Science Publishing Co., Inc.)

percent relatedness, D values, and others. These percent values all refer to the genomic fraction of DNA from one organism that can reassociate with DNA from another organism under specific experimental conditions.

The DNA homology experiments can be performed in several ways. Relative reassociation rates for DNA preparations from organism A, those from organism B, and an equal mixture of DNA from the two organisms can be measured spectrophotometrically. By comparing these rates, one can determine if reassociation has occurred between the DNAs from the two organisms. The more commonly used procedures involve the use of radioactively labeled DNA. The use of labeled DNA is shown schematically in Figure 1-2. In this example the labeled probe DNA is present at a very low concentration so that only a negligible amount of reassociation occurs during the reassociation time period. On the other hand, a high concentration of unlabeled test DNA is included, such that reassociation of these fragments will approach completion during the same time period. As a result, if the labeled DNA is identical to the unlabeled DNA, it will reassociate with the unlabeled DNA at the rate at which the unlabeled DNA is reassociating. If the two DNAs are unrelated, they will reassociate independently of each other. Thus, because of the low concentration of the labeled DNA, it will remain single stranded. There are several ways to separate the single- and double-stranded DNA fragments and determine the amount of probe DNA that has duplexed with the unlabeled DNA. Double-stranded DNA can be selectively adsorbed to hydroxyapatite and separated from the single-stranded DNA by column chromatography. Also, single-stranded DNA can be

degraded by single-strand-specific nuclease, and the amount of labeled DNA present in intact duplex structures can be measured in a scintillation counter either as an acid precipitate collected on a filter or after absorbing the duplexes to DEAE paper. Another method, in fact the oldest, is to immobilize the unlabeled DNA on a nitrocellulose membrane (at a high salt concentration, single-stranded DNA will bind tightly to the membrane, after which the rest of the binding sites can be covered by other compounds) and then incubate the membrane in the presence of labeled DNA fragments. The labeled fragments will be able to bind to the membrane only if they form duplexes with the immobilized DNA. All of these methods can be used to determine the fraction of one organism's genome that is similar enough to reassociate with the genome of another.

The DNA homology experiments provide an overall measurement of genetic similarity between organisms, which reflects their past history. Thus the similarity values represent phylogenetic relationships. Since these experiments are physical measurements, independent of growth media or other growth conditions, they provide sets of measurements that have similar meanings for all groups of organisms. For example, two groups of *Propionibacterium* that have 50% intergroup similarity probably have the same degree of relatedness as two groups of *Bacteroides* or *Clostridium* with 50% intergroup similarity. Organisms are usually considered to belong to a homology group if they have 60% or more DNA similarity to the reference strain of that group, although the homogeneity of the DNA homology groups varies from one group of organisms to the next. Therefore it is probably unwise to be too dogmatic in the

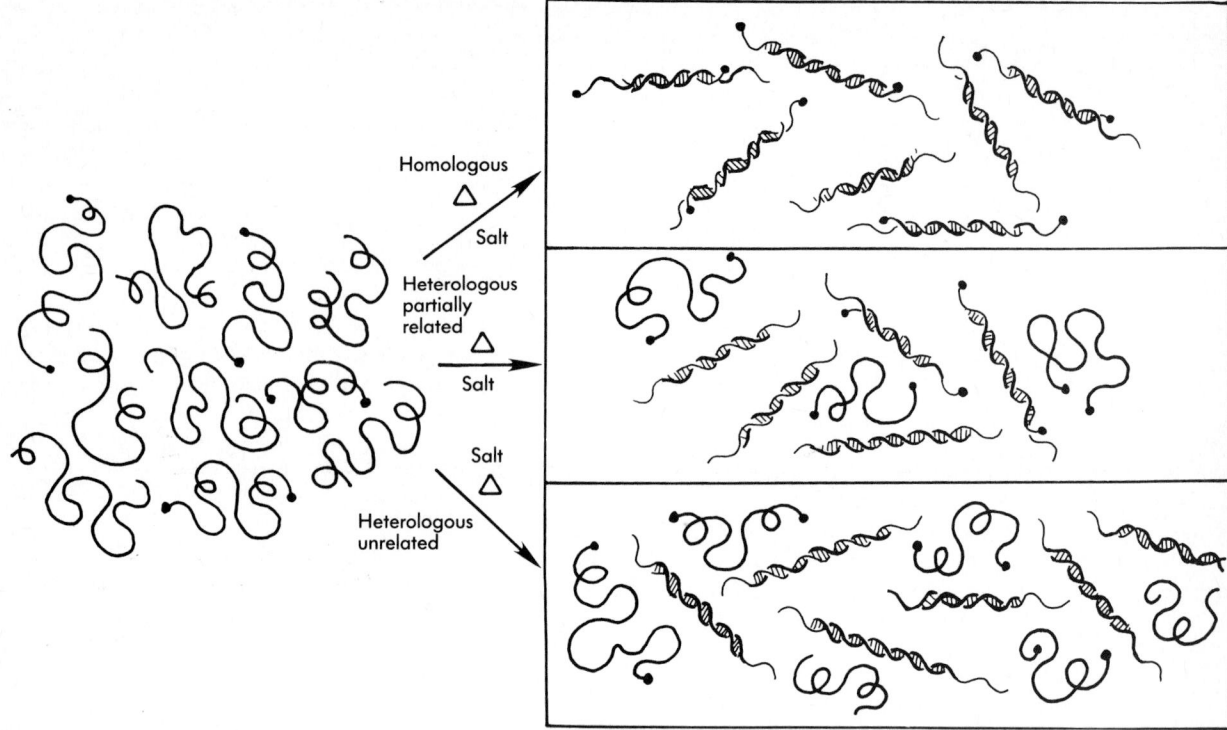

FIGURE 1-2. Schematic representation of labeled DNA reassociating with unlabeled homologous, partially related heterologous, or unrelated heterologous DNA preparation. (Modified and reprinted by permission of the publisher from ''Schematic Representation of labeled DNA reassociating with unlabeled homologous or unrelated heterologous DNA preparation'' by John L. Johnson, Clin. Microbiol. Newsletter **2**:1-3, 1980, by Elsevier Science Publishing Co., Inc.)

interpretation of these relationships. It is also common to find intergroup DNA relatedness values in the 50%, 35%, and 20% ranges, which represent closely related species. The DNA homology studies have provided a more unifying concept for a bacterial species and also for the species of other microorganisms.

Many organisms have extrachromosomal or cytoplasmic DNA, usually called plasmids. These small circular elements are not essential for the growth of the organism but may exert a great influence on an organism by containing important genes such as ones for antimicrobial resistance, toxin production, and bacteriocin production. DNA from bacteriophages may also behave as plasmids or may be inserted into the host genome. These elements may be readily transferred from one organism to another and thus do not represent phylogenetic traits of the host organism; however, one can measure phylogenetic relationships among the plasmid or phage genomes.

More distant phylogenetic relationships have been determined by comparing the ribosomal ribonucleic acid (rRNA) genes. These genes have been found to be more conserved (have experienced less change in base sequence) than the bulk of the genes in all organisms that have been investigated. Comparisons can be made by rRNA hybridization experiments (which are similar to DNA homology experiments described previously but involve hybrid duplexes containing one DNA and one RNA fragment), by oligonucleotide mapping, or by nucleotide sequencing of the gene. Woese and his collaborators[4,6,10] have contributed greatly to these studies, which enable us to measure phylogenetic relationships at higher taxonomic levels.

LEVEL 2

Many of the cell components are translation products of the nucleic acids, and as a result, their properties often correlate with the nucleic acid similarities. This is particularly true of the cell wall compositions, although the cellular lipid compositions may at times be medium dependent. The whole cell antigenic properties of an organism commonly used for comparison may be dependent on only a few surface components. There is often antigenic heterogeneity among these surface components, and thus considerable antigenic variation may be observed among closely related organisms. An example of this is the large number of serovars found among the *Salmonella*. Recent advances in immunology may enable investigators to select antigens that will be unique for specific groups of organisms. The electrophoresis of soluble cellular proteins has been extensively developed in recent years as a rapid identification method. The migration of proteins in an electrical field is a function of the protein's ionic charge and size, which results in a pattern of protein bands characteristic for that organism. By correlating the protein band patterns with DNA similarity values, one can identify specific bands or patterns of bands that are most useful in identification. Specific proteins can also be isolated and the amino acid sequence in them determined. Comparisons of the amino acid sequences of homologous proteins have shown that they may be more conserved than the DNA sequences from which they were transcribed and translated. This is due to the redundancy of the genetic code (that is, more than one three-nucleotide codon can code for the same amino acid). Thus comparisons of amino acid sequences can be used for determining distant relationships that cannot be measured by DNA homology.

LEVEL 3

Level 3 represents most of the classical tests that have been used for microbial classification and identification. These include cell morphology, motility, Gram stain reaction, optimal growth temperatures, fermentation tests, oxidation tests, growth of single carbon or nitrogen sources, expression of specific enzymatic activities, nutritional requirements, and many others. Whether a particular trait is considered to have phylogenetic significance is often dependent on the group of organisms for which it is used. In one case the utilization of a particular carbohydrate may correlate with two distinct but closely related groups as determined by DNA relatedness, whereas in another case it may be common to two very different organisms such as a bacterium and a yeast. A property may also vary among very closely related organisms, either because of mutation or because the gene coding for that property is located on plasmid or virus DNA, which may or may not be present in a given isolate.

NOMENCLATURE

The applying of names to the groups, called taxa, that are generated in the classification process is subject to a set of rules. These rules and recommendations, referred to as a code, are agreed to by the societies of researchers studying a particular group of organisms. For example, bacteriologists use the International Code of Bacterial Nomenclature.[5] By tradition, Latin or latinized Greek names are given to taxa, and taxa representing different hierarchic levels have different specific endings. The rules maintain an order in naming organisms and guarantee that all scientists form the names in the same way so that each name has the same meaning to everyone.

IDENTIFICATION

Identification of organisms represents the practical use of classification and nomenclature, the correct assignment of an unidentified organism to a taxon. Identification is usually done with the aid of keys or tables. A key consists of a set of contrasting statements designed to lead the user to the correct identification (see p. 612), whereas a table lists the major discriminatory features. A problem with keys is that variability among strains for a specific trait (either real or owing to technical error) may result in an incorrect identification. The problems are greatest when an error is made early in a key because it affects all of the subsequent steps. Although tables may be more difficult to use, they do allow for some trait variation. Where good classification systems have been developed and the variability of the specific traits is known, the probabilities of correct identification can be calculated. These calculations are usually made by a computer and form the basis for many of the commercial identification systems.

REFERENCES

1. Brenner, D.J.: Taxonomy, classification, and nomenclature of bacteria. In Lennette, E.H., et al., editors: Manual of clinical microbiology, ed. 4, Washington, D.C., 1985, American Society for Microbiology.
2. Buchanan, R.E., and Gibbons, N.E., editors: Bergey's manual of determinative bacteriology, ed. 8, Baltimore, 1974, The Williams & Wilkins Co.
3. Cohn, F.: Untersuchugen uber Bacterien II, Beitr. Biol. Pfl., Heft 3, **1**:141, 1875.
4. Fox, G.E., et al.: The phylogeny of prokaryotes, Science **209**:457, 1980.
5. Lapage, S.P., et al., editors: International code of nomenclature of bacteria, Washington, D.C., 1975, American Society for Microbiology.
6. Ludwig, W., et al.: The phylogenetic position of *Streptococcus* and *Enterococcus,* J. Gen. Microbiol. **131**:543, 1985.
7. Müller, O.F.: Vermium terrestrium et fluviatilium, seu animalium infusorium, helminthicorum et testaceorum, non marionum, Succincta Historia 1 (pt. 1):1, 1773.
8. Norris, J.R.: Introduction. In Goodfellow, M., and Board, R.G., editors: Microbial classification and identification, The Society for Applied Bacteriology Symposium Series No. 8, London, 1980, Academic Press.
9. Simpson, G.G.: Principles of animal taxonomy, New York, 1961, Columbia University Press.
10. Weisburg, W.G., et al.: Natural relationship between *Bacteroides* and flavobacteria, J. Bacteriol. **164**:230, 1985.

ADDITIONAL READINGS

Carlile, M.J., Collins, M.J., and Moseley, B.E.B., editors: Molecular and cellular aspects of microbiol evolution, Cambridge, Eng., 1981, Cambridge University Press.

Colwell, R.R.: Genetic and phenetic classification of bacteria, Adv. Appl. Microbiol. **16**:137, 1973.

Goodfellow, M., and Board, R.G., editors: Microbial classification and identification, The Society for Applied Bacteriology Symposium Series No. 8, London, 1980, Academic Press.

Johnson, J.L.: Nucleic acids in bacterial classification. In Krieg, N.R., editor (Holt, J.G., editor-in-chief): Bergey's manual of systematic bacteriology, vol. 1, Baltimore, 1984, Williams & Wilkins Co.

Sneath, P.H.A., and Sokal, R.R.: Numerical taxonomy, San Francisco, 1973, W.H. Freeman & Co.

CHAPTER 2

Host-Parasite Interactions: Mechanisms of Pathogenicity

Barbara J. Howard
John C. Rees

Host-parasite relationships are fundamental in any discussion of clinical microbiology; indeed the entire field of clinical microbiology is founded on attempts to clarify these relationships. A variety of terms have been used to describe such relationships and their eventual outcome. The relationships can be beneficial to both members; such relationships are called symbiotic. The relationships that are of benefit to one member and cause little effect on the other are considered commensal. Relationships in which one member is benefited at the expense of the other are considered parasitic.

Factors that affect the final outcome of the host-parasite relationship determine health or disease. The relationships are dynamic, and isolation of a single factor responsible for the final disposition of the relationship is an impossibility. It is far more appropriate to consider the establishment of the relationship as a mechanism with several stages. This suggests constant change in both the organism and the host. The term "parasitic" therefore must be viewed as describing a relationship in which one member has the potential to damage the tissues or cells of another.

A pathogen is defined as an organism that has the potential to cause disease. This ability depends on several factors, including infectious dose of the organism, portal of entry of the organism, and most important, the host. These factors are discussed later in the chapter. Microorganisms that have a greater probability of causing disease when introduced are considered virulent. Predisposing conditions such as the following may lead to infection with the indicated organisms*:

Foreign body implantation (for example, indwelling intravenous catheters, prosthetic heart valves, ventriculoatrial shunt)—*Staphylococcus aureus* and *epidermidis, Propionibacterium acnes, Aspergillus* spp., *Candida albicans, Mycobacterium chelonae*
Indwelling urinary catheters—*Serratia marcescens, Pseudomonas aeruginosa*
Splenectomy—*Streptococcus pneumoniae*
Hematoproliferative disorders—*Cryptococcus neoformans,* varicella-zoster virus, *Listeria monocytogenes*
Diabetes—*S. aureus, C. albicans, P. aeruginosa,* phycomycetes
Alcoholism—*S. pneumoniae, Klebsiella pneumoniae*
Burns—*P. aeruginosa*
Cortisone—*S. aureus, S. epidermidis, Mycobacterium tuberculosis,* fungi

Immunosuppression—*Nocardia asteroides,* mycobacteria, *Aspergillus* spp., *C. albicans, Toxoplasma gondii, Pneumocystis carinii,* herpes simplex virus, varicella-zoster virus, cytomegalovirus, diphtheroids

Those organisms that induce disease only when the host's defense mechanisms are compromised or weakened are considered opportunistic.

The most successful pathogen is not the one that can inflict extensive damage or even death on the host, but the one that can establish a state of balanced pathogenicity.[80] Parasites that kill all infected cells eventually lead to their own extinction.[41] The successful parasite must utilize nutrients provided by the host without causing more damage than is necessary to maintain its physiology, metabolism, and growth.

For several reasons many parasites have not achieved this state of balanced pathogenicity.[80] One reason concerns the natural host of the parasite. Some of the most severe infections in terms of morbidity (number of cases) or mortality (number of deaths) are those that are probably acquired from animals. Examples are Lassa fever, caused by the arenavirus found in rodents, and bubonic plague, caused by *Yersinia pestis* found in rodents and transmitted by fleas. Among the many others are rabies, leptospirosis, psittacosis, anthrax, and brucellosis. The etiologic agents of these diseases have not evolved toward less pathogenic forms in humans because humans are irrelevant for their survival; humans simply serve as accidental hosts.[80]

HOW DISEASES ARE TRANSMITTED

Diseases may be transmitted directly from person to person, or they may be transmitted via other animate or inanimate vectors. Table 2-1 summarizes the primary mechanisms of direct and indirect transmission.

CONGENITAL TRANSFER

Direct congenital transfer may occur transplacentally or as the child passes through the birth canal. The child may contract group B beta-hemolytic streptococci (*S. agalactiae*), *Neisseria gonorrhoeae,* cytomegalovirus, and herpes simplex virus (HSV) from the mother at birth, and many virus infections such as rubella are transmitted transplacentally. With the latter infections the severity of the child's disease is related to the stage of pregnancy in which the mother became infected; infections early in pregnancy usually have more serious effects.

CONTACT

Numerous diseases are spread by direct contact with an infected individual or source. The contact may be sexual, hand to hand, or by contact with infected respiratory secretions (droplet). The sexually transmitted diseases—syphilis, gonor-

*Modified from Albini, B., and van Oss, C.J.: Microbial pathogenicity and host parasite relationships. In Milgrom, F., and Flanagan, T.D., editors: Medical microbiology, New York, 1982, Churchill Livingstone. By permission.

TABLE 2-1. Transmission of Disease

Mechanism	Organisms	Disease
DIRECT TRANSMISSION		
Congenital transfer[a]	Bacteria	
	Streptococcus agalactiae (group B beta-hemolytic streptococcus)	Neonatal meningitis
	Neisseria gonorrhoeae	Ophthalmia
	Listeria monocytogenes	Neonatal meningitis
	Treponema pallidum	Stillbirth, abortion
	Protozoa	
	Toxoplasma gondii	Stillbirth, mental retardation, hydrocephalus
	Viruses	
	Cytomegalovirus	Malformations, mental retardation, congenital heart disease
	Rubella	Malformation, abortion, heart defects, encephalitis
	Herpes simplex virus (type 2)	Brain damage, hepatoadrenal necrosis with jaundice, abortion
	Hepatitis B	Abortion, stillbirth, neonatal hepatitis
Contact		
Sexual	Bacteria	
	T. pallidum	Syphilis
	N. gonorrhoeae	Gonorrhea
	Viruses	
	Herpes simplex virus	Herpes
	HIV	Acquired immunodeficiency syndrome (AIDS)
Hand to hand	Bacteria	
	Salmonella typhi	Typhoid fever
	Shigella spp.	Shigellosis
	Viruses	
	Rhinovirus	Common cold
Via respiratory secretions	Bacteria	
	Streptococcus pneumoniae	Pneumococcal pneumonia
	Corynebacterium diphtheriae	Diphtheria
	Viruses	
	Epstein-Barr virus	Infectious mononucleosis
	Influenza A and B virus	Influenza
INDIRECT TRANSMISSION		
Fomites	Bacteria	
	Serratia marcescens	Urinary tract infection
	Staphylococcus aureus	Endocarditis
	Fungi	
	Candida albicans	Candidiasis
	Viruses	
	Hepatitis A virus	Viral hepatitis
Food and water	Bacteria	
	S. typhi	Typhoid fever
	Salmonella enteritidis	Salmonellosis
	Shigella spp.	Shigellosis, dysentery
	Vibrio parahaemolyticus	Gastroenteritis
	Vibrio cholerae	Cholera
	Clostridium botulinum	Botulism
	Leptospira spp.	Leptospirosis
	Helminths	
	Trichinella spiralis	Trichinosis
	Protozoa	
	Giardia lamblia	Giardiasis
	Viruses	
	Poliovirus	Poliomyelitis
	Hepatitis A	Hepatitis

TABLE 2-1. Transmission of Disease—cont'd

Mechanism	Organisms	Disease
Airborne	Bacteria	
	Bacillus anthracis	Anthrax
	Mycobacterium tuberculosis	Tuberculosis
	Fungi	
	Blastomyces dermatitidis	Blastomycosis
	Coccidioides immitis	Coccidioidomycosis
	Histoplasma capsulatum	Histoplasmosis
	Paracoccidioides brasiliensis	Paracoccidioidomycosis
Animals		
Vertebrates	Bacteria	
	Francisella tularensis	Tularemia
	Spirillum minus	Rat-bite fever
	Brucella spp.	Brucellosis
	Viruses	
	Rabies virus	Rabies
Arthropods	Bacteria	
	Rickettsia prowazekii	Epidemic typhus
	Rickettsia rickettsii	Rocky Mountain spotted fever
	Protozoa	
	Plasmodium vivax	Malaria

[a]The diseases listed for congenital transfer represent the effects seen in the child.

rhea, acquired immunodeficiency syndrome (AIDS), and herpes—are transmitted by sexual intercourse. Rhinovirus, the etiologic agent of the common cold, is most commonly transmitted by shaking the hand of an infected individual; typhoid fever may be spread by feces-soiled hands. Contaminated respiratory secretions, which become aerosolized and are inhaled by individuals, may be transmitted by coughing, sneezing, singing, and kissing.

FOMITES

Fomites are inanimate vehicles of infection. Examples include eating utensils, intrauterine devices (IUDs), tampons, hospital instruments (such as catheters) and equipment, clothing, door handles, and money. Nosocomial (hospital-acquired) infections are commonly spread by contaminated patient-care equipment, instruments, or therapeutic agents such as intravenous solutions (see Chapter 4).

FOOD AND WATER

Food and water are the most frequent vehicles for dissemination of microbial diseases. They are often responsible for the development of epidemics, or widespread occurrences of disease in many individuals within a short period of time. Contamination of improperly treated water or the introduction of microorganisms after treatment may result in outbreaks of typhoid fever, shigellosis, salmonellosis, gastroenteritis, giardiasis, dysentery, cholera, and infectious hepatitis. Improperly prepared, preserved, or stored food can be a significant factor in the transmission of disease. Uncooked or undercooked meats and fish,[20] raw milk, and food containing contaminated seasoning have all been associated with outbreaks of disease. Incriminated organisms have included *Salmonella, Shigella, Campylobacter, Vibrio, Staphylococcus aureus,* mycobacteria, and

viruses. Improperly refrigerated food may support the growth of organisms that were introduced during preparation. Examples are foods containing dairy products such as eggs, milk, and cream, which support the growth of *Staphylococcus, Salmonella,* and *Listeria* organisms.

The organisms capable of causing foodborne or waterborne epidemics may be excreted from patients with active infections or in some cases from carriers, individuals who harbor infecting organisms but do not display signs of clinical disease. These persons may have recovered from clinical disease or may have had a subclinical infection. In any event, infecting organisms lodge in some organ or tissue of the body and continue to be excreted, increasing the potential for transmission. The importance of carriers in the transmission of typhoid fever is illustrated by the notorious Mary Mallon, better known as Typhoid Mary, a cook in New York City and Long Island in the early part of this century. She was a carrier of *Salmonella typhi.* Her employment in a number of households and institutions resulted in over 200 cases of typhoid fever. It should be noted that some foodborne diseases such as botulism are not infectious but result from ingestion of microbial toxins.

AIRBORNE TRANSMISSION

Indirect transmission via the airborne route is commonly seen with the systemic fungi, an example of which is *Coccidioides immitis,* the etiologic agent of coccidioidomycosis. This fungus grows in soil of the southwestern United States and northern Mexico. It produces arthroconidia (arthric conidia that result from the fragmentation of a hypha; see Chapter 28) that become aerosolized by duststorms and windstorms or during construction work, farming, or archaeologic digs.[94] Inhalation of the arthroconidia by humans may lead to inapparent to moderately severe pulmonary disease or to severe disseminated pulmonary disease characterized by burrowing abscesses in meninges, bones, joints, and subcutaneous and cutaneous tissues (see Chapter 34). The severity is related to sex, race, and the adequacy of host defense mechanisms.

Viral hepatitis, often thought of as transmitted by the fecal-to-oral route, can also be acquired by way of aerosols created during centrifugation. This is a major source of laboratory-acquired hepatitis.

ANIMALS

Several diseases occur primarily in animals but occasionally are accidentally transmitted to humans. These zoonoses include rabies, which is transmitted through the bite of infected animals such as dogs or raccoons, and tularemia, which is contracted through contact with an infected rabbit.

Vertebrates are not the only animals capable of transmitting disease; arthropods are also important vectors of human infection. The primary arthropod vectors are flies, ticks, mites, lice, and mosquitoes. Flies are responsible for the spread of shigellosis and typhoid fever; ticks, mites, and lice transmit rickettsial diseases; and mosquitoes transmit malaria.

FACTORS INFLUENCING HOST SUSCEPTIBILITY

The adequacy of the host defense mechanisms (host susceptibility) determines whether an encounter with an organism will result in the production of disease. Host susceptibility is, in turn, influenced by numerous environmental and genetic factors.

ENVIRONMENTAL FACTORS

The initial exposure to an organism may depend on the host's socioeconomic class, behavioral patterns, and occupation. Sexually promiscuous individuals are most likely to contract the sexually transmitted diseases. Dairy farmers, veterinarians, and workers in meat packing plants are more frequently exposed to *Brucella* organisms, which are responsible for brucellosis, a disease transmitted to humans by infected tissue from goats, dairy cattle, swine, and sheep. Occupational hazards affect not only exposure but also host defenses. Coal miners, for example, inhale fine particles of silica, resulting in a lung condition known as silicosis; this may lead to damage of the alveolar macrophages, inhibition of phagocytosis, and increased susceptibility to infectious diseases of the lung. Environmental lung disease is not limited to coal miners. There is a clear relationship between inhalation of many organic substances and infectious pulmonary disease.[128]

The host's overall health (both immunologic and physiologic) at the time of initial exposure is inversely related to susceptibility to infection. Infection is much less likely to develop in well-nourished, healthy, immunologically competent individuals than in malnourished, immunologically weakened ones. Host defenses are impaired by advancing age, preexisting infection, hormonal imbalances, alcoholism, nutritional status, and other factors.

Other environmental factors, such as infectious dose and portal of entry, also affect the eventual outcome of the host-parasite encounter. The infectious dose is the number of organisms required to establish an infection. For humans the infectious dose of *Salmonella* organisms is 10^5 and that of *Shigella* is 10^1 to 10^2. The route or portal of entry by which an organism gains access to the body is a major factor in determining the success of the parasite. Organisms with receptors for particular cells cannot establish themselves if introduced into an environment unsuitable for attachment. For example, *Neisseria gonorrhoeae* binds to columnar epithelial cells but not to squamous epithelial cells.

Another example of the importance of infectious dose and portal of entry is seen with *Streptococcus pneumoniae*. When encapsulated *S. pneumoniae* is introduced into the lung, only two or three organisms may ultimately lead to disease. A hundredfold more organisms are required to produce disease if these organisms are injected into healthy muscle. The susceptibility of the hosts is not different in these two cases, nor has the virulence of the microbe increased; the outcome is determined by the portal of entry.

An often overlooked factor markedly affecting host-microbe interactions involves the mixed biotic environment of most tissues. Some indigenous organisms establish a microecology that hinders the colonization of other organisms. The importance of indigenous microorganisms in the host-parasite relationship is indicated by the following list of mechanisms by which indigenous microorganisms inhibit potential pathogens*:

Direct effects
  Bacteriocin production
  Production of toxic metabolic end products
  Induction of low oxidation-reduction potential
  Depletion of essential nutrients
  Suppression of adherence
  Inhibition of translocation
  Degradation of toxins
Indirect effects
  Enhancement of antibody production
  Phagocyte stimulation
  Stimulation of clearance mechanisms
  Augmentation of interferon production
  Bile acid deconjugation

However, previous establishment of one organism may also enhance subsequent colonization of other organisms.[69] This is especially important with viruses. The establishment of numerous viruses in the respiratory tract may predispose to bacterial invasion.[78] Infection with respiratory syncytial virus, influenza virus (A or B), and adenovirus predisposes to the development of otitis media by *S. pneumoniae* and *Haemophilus influenzae* that are present in the nasopharnyx.[43] In fact, these viruses appear to induce the pathophysiologic alterations necessary for otitis media to occur.

Antecedent influenza A infections may actually potentiate the growth of numerous organisms, including *H. influenzae*, *S. pneumoniae*, *Staphylococcus aureus*, and *Streptococcus agalactiae* (group B beta-streptococcus).[78] Cytomegalovirus infections are another example of microbial synergism between viruses and bacteria. Although rarely fatal themselves, these infections are a major cause of increased mortality resulting from other microorganisms,[78] such as the genera *Pseudomonas*, *Escherichia*, *Klebsiella*, *Candida*, and *Pneumocystis*. The

---

*From Mackowiak, P.A. Reprinted by permission of the New England Journal of Medicine **307:**83, 1982; modified from Savage, D.C.: Colonization by and survival of pathogenic bacteria on intestinal mucosal surfaces. In Britton, G., and Marshall, K.C., editors: Adsorption of microorganisms to surfaces, New York, 1980, John Wiley & Sons, Inc.

ability of viruses to predispose to bacterial infections may be related to induced dysfunctions of phagocytes, immunosuppressive actions, and effects on T suppressor/cytotoxic cells.[101] These are discussed later in the chapter.

GENETIC FACTORS

The development of the immune response is under genetic control. Certain genes, designated immune responses (Ir) genes, control the responses to specific antigens.[98] Ir genes are linked to human leukocyte antigen (HLA) genes located on chromosome 6 of the major histocompatibility complex (MHC) (see definitions, p. 17). Because of the linkage of HLA and Ir genes, researchers are investigating the association of certain HLA haplotypes with susceptibility to various infections.[57,111]

The innate resistance to certain parasitic diseases is also genetically based. Individuals who do not possess the Duffy antigen on their erythrocytes apparently do not acquire *Plasmodium vivax* malaria. Evidence suggests that the Duffy antigen or an antigen closely related to it serves as a receptor for the parasite; red blood cells without the receptor are spared.[79] Another example has to do with hemoglobin S (Hgb S). When present in the heterozygous state, this abnormal hemoglobin is responsible for sickle cell trait; however, it also protects against *Plasmodium falciparum* malaria. The resistance can probably be attributed to interference with development of the parasite in cells containing Hgb S. Unfortunately, individuals who are homozygous for Hgb S do not share this protection. They suffer more severely from both malaria and sickle cell anemia. Perhaps their impaired reticuloendothelial system increases their susceptibility to infection and the infection exacerbates the anemia.[79]

HOST DEFENSE MECHANISMS

As stated previously, disease is the exception rather than the rule in most parasite-host encounters. This implies the need for an active role by the host to remain disease free. The host has a variety of mechanisms to resist attachment, colonization, and the growth of microorganisms. These systems can be grouped loosely into those an individual is born with and possesses *ab inito,* those that are inducible but not entirely specific, and those that are inducible and highly specific.

The inborn, nonspecific factors are considered native or natural mechanisms. Among the many examples are the intactness and fatty acid content of the skin, the low pH of the stomach, and the enzyme content of tears or other body fluids. Substances contained in tissues also contribute to this natural resistance. Transferrin and lactoferrin, for example, firmly bind growth-essential iron and thereby severely restrict its availability to potential pathogens for growth.[61] Host barriers such as pleural, pericardial, and synovial membranes are also included here. The importance of any of these factors is demonstrated by the increased risk of disease that results from their impairment.

The mechanisms that are inducible yet not entirely specific in their actions include activation of complement (see p. 15), production of interferon, and the processes of inflammation and phagocytosis.

The immune response is the inducible, highly specific host defense system. This system is comprised of humoral components called immunoglobulins and cellular components that include specifically activated lymphocytes and their products. The immunologic responses are directed against specific organisms or even specific molecules on individual organisms, such as the M protein of *Streptococcus pyogenes*. All of these systems are considered in the following sections.

NATURAL OR NATIVE MECHANISMS
Skin

The normal flora of the skin is an important deterrent to infection. These organisms, which include coagulase-negative staphylococci, propionibacteria, corynebacteria, and diphtheroids, produce free fatty acids from the secretions of the numerous sebaceous glands. These fatty acids and the resulting low pH of the skin are inhibitory to most other organisms. Constant washing or prolonged dietary restrictions and hormonal imbalances such as diabetes often lead to alterations of the normal cutaneous flora and subsequent disease of the skin and scalp.

With a few exceptions, skin infections occur only when the continuity of the skin is broken and organisms gain entrance into hair follicles and sweat gland openings. The skin's continuity may be broken by bites, wounds, or various manipulations such as the use of needles and sutures. Rabies virus enters the skin through the bite of an infected animal. *Plasmodium* spp., the etiologic agents of malaria, enter through the bite of an infected mosquito. Fungi may cause infections in moist, soft areas of the skin. For example, the moist environment and absence of sebaceous glands between the toes make this area particularly susceptible to the fungi causing athlete's foot.

Respiratory Tract

The average person inhales at least eight microorganisms a minute, or 10,000 each day.[80] The mucociliary linings of the upper and lower respiratory tract efficiently inhibit establishment of these organisms. Particles entrapped in the nasal cavity, often by the nasal hairs, are swept by the beating action of the cilia along the mucous stream to the back of the throat where they are swallowed and destroyed by the low pH of the stomach.

In a healthy individual probably less than 5% of inhaled bacteria pass beyond the upper respiratory tract.[36] Those particles that reach the bronchi or bronchioles are carried by the mucociliary stream to the pharynx where they are swallowed. The few particles small enough to reach the alveoli of the lungs are usually phagocytized and destroyed by alveolar macrophages.

Other nonspecific defense mechanisms of the healthy respiratory tract are the coughing and sneezing reflexes. Furthermore, nasal secretions often contain lysozyme, an enzyme that lyses the cell wall of certain bacteria.

The respiratory and digestive tracts are the most common portals of entry for microorganisms. Numerous viruses, including influenza and parainfluenza, as well as bacteria such as *S. pneumoniae, H. influenzae, Mycobacterium tuberculosis, Bordetella pertussis,* and *Mycoplasma pneumoniae,* enter the body through the respiratory tract. In some cases these organisms produce substances that inhibit mucociliary activity or in some other way decrease host defenses. These organisms also possess structures enabling them to attach to epithelial surface receptors.

Gastrointestinal Tract

The production of hydrochloric acid and the resulting low pH in the stomach is a first line of defense for the gastrointestinal tract. In fact, the low pH renders the stomach virtually sterile. Conditions that predispose to achlorhydria (absence of hydrochloric acid), such as pernicious anemia, greatly increase the risk of gastric infection.

The normal peristalsis of the small intestine rapidly sweeps microorganisms to the large intestine, allowing little time for attachment and multiplication. The mucosal epithelium, the normal flora of the small intestine, the presence of secretory IgA, bile acids, and enzymes, and the low pH also limit the establishment of infection in the intestine. The normal intestinal flora, present in numbers as high as 10^{11} in the large intestine, includes both anaerobic and facultative organisms. The anaerobic organisms produce volatile fatty acids and the facultative organisms produce bacteriocins, both of which inhibit the growth of potential pathogens. Futhermore, exogenous organisms may have to compete with the normal flora for nutrients or attachment sites.

Urogenital Tract

The normal flushing action and bacteriostatic pH of the urine inhibit establishment and growth of microorganisms in the urogenital tract. As might be expected, interference with urine flow by structural abnormalities, an enlarged prostate, or pregnancy disrupts the homeostasis and increases the potential for attachment, growth, and possibly disease. Because of anatomic differences, bladder infections occur more frequently in women than in men. The urethra of men is approximately 20 cm long and is rarely traversed by organisms unless they are introduced by instrumentation. On the other hand, the short urethra (5 cm) of women provides easy access to the bladder for microorganisms normally found in the intestine or vagina.

The normal flora of the vagina, predominantly lactobacilli, inhibits the growth of most other bacteria. The lactobacilli metabolize the glycogen of the vaginal epithelium to produce lactic acid, resulting in a low pH that limits some potential pathogens. Hormonal changes may disrupt this ecosystem and predispose postmenopausal women to different infections from premenopausal women.

Conjunctiva

Organisms are most commonly deposited in the eye from the fingers. Usually the flushing action of the tears carries the microorganisms through the lacrimal duct to the mucociliary blanket of the nasopharynx. Lysozyme, present in the tears, also helps to limit the number of viable microorganisms available for establishment of infection.

INDUCIBLE BUT NOT ENTIRELY SPECIFIC MECHANISMS
Inflammatory Response

Microorganisms that are able to attach to the host epithelial cells through the mechanisms discussed later in the chapter initiate an inflammatory response. Inflammation is a series of closely regulated events considered part of wound healing. It is a primitive host response to external trauma. Inflammation sets the stage for wound repair by release of chemical substances that affect vessels and other cells. The inflammatory response occurs after any trauma, and the steps are essentially identical in sterile trauma and in septic trauma.[123]

The characteristic features of inflammation are hemodynamic changes of the microvasculature, especially increased vascular permeability, and chemotaxis and migration of phagocytic cells to the injured site. These changes are mediated through histamine and kinins released from lymphocytes and tissue macrophages and from inflammatory materials released from the multiplying organisms.

Hemodynamic changes[95]

On invasion of the subepithelial spaces, numerous changes occur in the microvasculature. The arterioles and the capillaries become dilated, the blood flow increases, and the permeability of the microvasculature also increases. These result in outpouring of numerous plasma proteins, including complement, properdin, interferon, and previously formed antibody. The increased permeability also results in the packing of the red blood cells in the small blood vessels. Phagocytic cells, polymorphonuclear neutrophils (PMNs) and macrophages, begin to adhere to the vascular endothelium and then migrate across the vessels in a process known as diapedesis. PMNs arrive first, and their metabolism reduces the pH locally. Later macrophages arrive and aid in healing. Specific characteristics of these phagocytic cells are discussed in the following sections.

The clinical manifestations of inflammation—redness, warmth, swelling, and pain—reflect these hemodynamic changes. The affected site appears red because of dilation of the blood vessels and increased blood flow. The inflamed area is warm owing to increased dilation. Swelling results from the accumulation of fluid and cells, and pain is caused by the pressure of the fluid on the nerve endings and the release of prostaglandins. In some cases pus forms because of an accumulation of phagocytes, microorganisms, and body fluid.

Chemotaxis

The PMNs and macrophages that leave the bloodstream reach the injured area by both a directed motion called chemotaxis and random movement called chemokinesis. Chemotaxis is thought to be directed by the effect of substances generated or released at the infected site. These chemotactic factors include bacterial products and components of the complement system. Examples of the former are endotoxin, cell wall components, and several bacterial enzymes.[127] Some of these factors act directly in the absence of serum, whereas others act indirectly by activating complement.[127] Chemotactic factors are produced by *S. aureus*, *S. pyogenes*, *S. pneumoniae*, *Escherichia coli*, *M. tuberculosis*, and *Corynebacterium parvum*.[127] The major host-derived chemotactic factors come from complement and include C3a, C5a, C567, and C3b. These can be generated by immunologic reactions, by bacterial products, and by proteolytic enzymes (trypsin, plasmin, and other tissue proteases) in plasma and tissue.

Phagocytosis

As mentioned previously, the major classes of phagocytic cells are PMNs and macrophages. Both are produced in the bone marrow, but they differ in several ways. Neutrophils have a short life; they circulate in the blood for 6 to 7 hours before migrating through endothelial cell junctions into tissues, where they live for only a few days. Neutrophils contain granules (lysosomes) with numerous antimicrobial enzymes and substances such as lactoferrin.

Macrophages live in the tissues for weeks or months. Monocytes are the precursors of macrophages. Once monocytes leave the bloodstream and enter the tissue, they become known as macrophages. The two types of macrophages are those that wander in the numerous body tissues and spaces and those that are fixed to the vascular endothelium of the liver, spleen, lymph nodes, and other tissues. Macrophages in the tissues are referred to as histiocytes, those in the liver as Kupffer cells, and those in the lungs and peritoneal cavities as alveolar and peritoneal macrophages, respectively. Macrophages produce various antimicrobial substances depending on the species and site of localization.[22] However, unlike the neutrophils, they produce these substances only on activation. Macrophages play an active role in initiating inflammation by release of factors that affect vascular integrity and by attracting other cell types to areas of inflammation. Macrophages are also pivotal cells in the generation and regulation of specific acquired immune responses.[75]

Two steps are involved in phagocytosis: attachment and ingestion.[48] Most organisms, especially encapsulated ones, do not attach to the phagocytic cell unless they are coated with serum factors known as opsonins. The best-characterized opsonins are IgG and a component of C3. These substances facilitate phagocytosis by acting as ligands between the organism and the phagocyte surface. Both PMNs and macrophages possess receptors for C3b and the Fc component of immunoglobulin.

Invagination of the phagocyte to form a phagosome follows attachment of the organism. Phagosome formation then triggers the respiratory burst and the fusion of lysosomes with the plasma membrane of the phagosome to form phagolysosomes. The respiratory burst is a coordinated series of metabolic events including increased oxygen uptake, increased activity of the hexose monophosphate pathway, and increased production of several oxygen-derived antimicrobial substances such as hydrogen peroxide and superoxide anion. The formation of phagolysosomes results in the exposure of the phagocytized microbes to the antimicrobial substances of the lysosomes. The respiratory burst and the formation of phagolysosomes both effect killing of microorganisms. The microbicidal mechanisms of the respiratory burst are termed oxygen-dependent mechanisms, while those of phagolysosome formation are termed oxygen independent.

Both oxygen-dependent and oxygen-independent microbicidal mechanisms appear to be operative in neutrophils.[5,12,60] These polymorphonuclear phagocytes possess two types of granules or lysosomes. The primary or azurophilic granules release acid hydrolases, lysozyme, neutral proteases, cationic antibacterial proteins, and myeloperoxidase, and the specific or secondary granules release lactoferrin, lysozyme, and phospholipase. The precise role of these granules' contents in killing has not been clearly defined,[12] although the role of myeloperoxidase has been more clearly defined than that of the other substances.

The enzyme myeloperoxidase actually augments the microbicidal effects of the respiratory burst, which as stated previously, results in the generation of various antimicrobial oxygen metabolites, including hydrogen peroxide (H_2O_2), superoxide anion (O_2^-), singlet oxygen ($^1O_2$), and hydroxyl radicals ($OH \cdot$). In the presence of myeloperoxidase and halide ions (iodide chloride, and bromide) H_2O_2 causes bacterial death. The pre-

cise mechanism of action of the H_2O_2-halide-myeloperoxidase system is unknown; the various theories that have been proposed are discussed by Beaman and Beaman.[12]

Macrophages also appear to effect killing by oxygen-dependent and oxygen-independent mechanisms, although these mechanisms are not as clearly defined as those in neutrophils.[12] The lysosomes of macrophages include several hydrolases such as acid phosphatase and beta-glucuronidase. These hydrolases and other enzymes (such as lysozyme) secreted by the macrophage may function primarily to digest damaged organisms.[12] The respiratory burst of macrophages is not as dramatic as that of PMNs, although correlations have been observed between the killing of *Leishmania donovani*, *Trypanosoma cruzi*, *Toxoplasma gondii*, and *Candida albicans* by activated macrophages and the ability of the macrophage to produce O_2^- and H_2O_2 in the respiratory burst.[12] Both oxygen-dependent and oxygen-independent mechanisms are thought to be important to the killing of *Entamoeba histolytica*.[99] The role of the H_2O_2-halide-myeloperoxidase system in the killing effects of macrophages is not clear.[12]

Complement

Complement is a system of several serum proteins that may be activated by immune (classical) or nonimmune (alternate) pathways. The classical pathway is activated by specific antigen-antibody complexes. The alternate pathway does not require the presence of antibody and may be activated by the polysaccharide or lipopolysaccharide components of certain bacteria. The alternate pathway is especially important in nonspecific resistance, since it provides a more rapid method for the activation of complement. Through a series of cleavage steps both pathways result in the generation of numerous biologically active complement components and fragments that ultimately bind to the cell membrane and cause lysis or death (Figure 2-1).[97]

Complement plays an important role in host protection. As mentioned previously, the C3b component is an opsonically active protein that coats the bacterial or viral surface. C3a and C5a components are anaphylactic, resulting in vasodilation and increased leakage of plasma proteins into extravascular tissues; they are also chemotactic, attracting additional white blood cells to the inflamed area. Complement-depleted animals show increased morbidity or mortality when they are infected with a variety of bacterial species, certain fungi (*Candida albicans*), and a number of viruses (such as measles and influenza). Patients with C3 deficiencies have more frequent infections with pyogenic (pus-producing) bacteria, whereas patients with deficiencies of complements C5 through C9 appear to be more at risk for disseminated meningococcal and gonococcal infections.[73,91,92]

Other Inducible Nonspecific Defense Mechanisms

The production of interferon is a nonspecific defense mechanism that occurs during viral infection. Interferon is a glycoprotein that is synthesized by infected cells in response to the presence of double-stranded RNA. After release, interferon rapidly enters uninfected cells where it induces a state of resistance to viral replication. The exact mechanism of action of interferon is unknown, but this substance seems to interfere with transcription of viral RNA or the translation of viral protein.

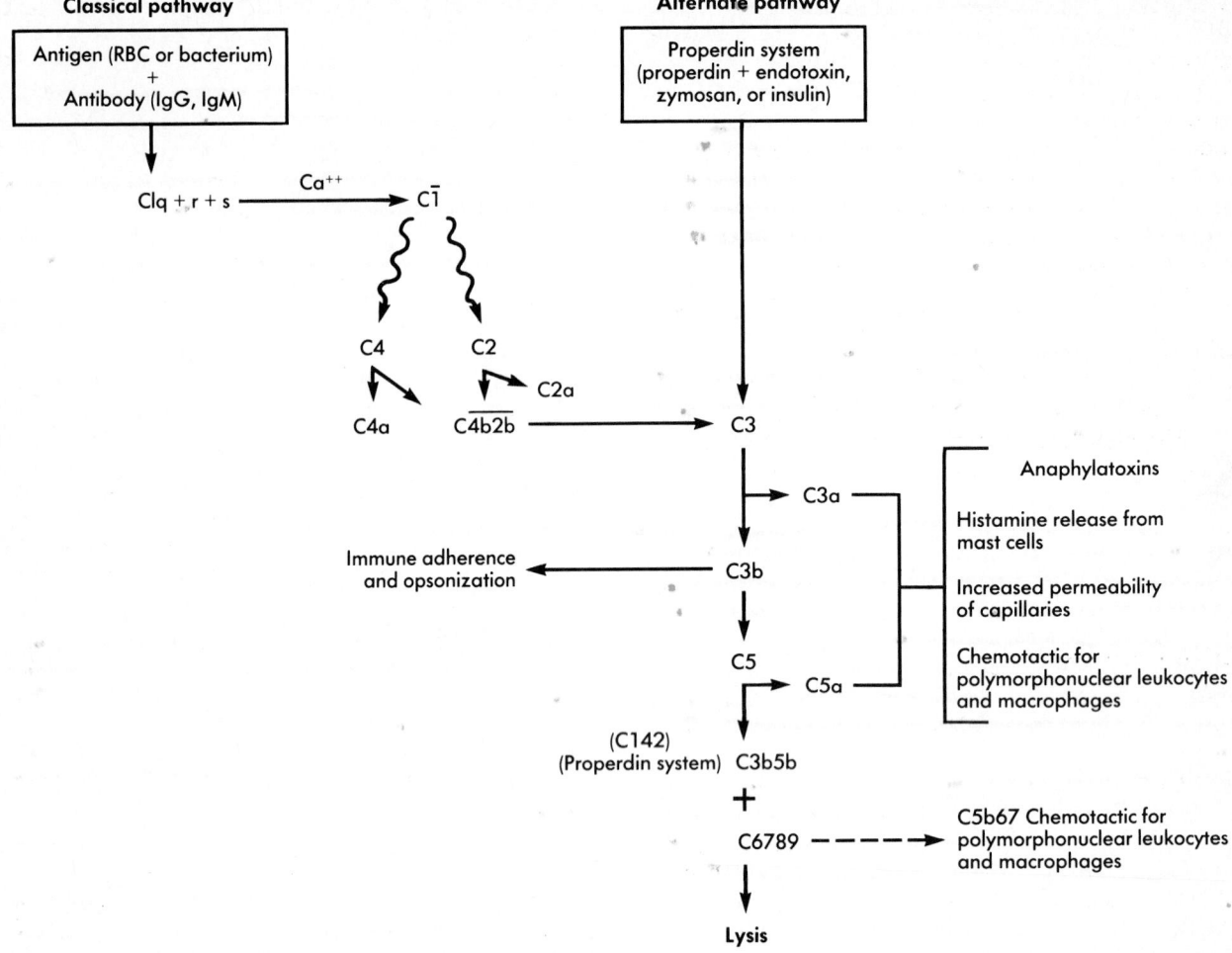

FIGURE 2-1. Major steps in classical and alternate pathways of complement and biologic activities generated at different steps. (Modified from Root, R.K., and Ryan, J.L.: Humoral immunity and complement. In Mandell, G.L., Douglas, R.J., Jr., and Bennett, J.E., editors: Principles and practice of infectious diseases, ed. 2. Copyright © 1985, John Wiley & Sons, Inc., New York. Reprinted by permission of John Wiley & Sons, Inc.)

IMMUNE RESPONSE

The specific acquired immune response is manifest in three ways: the production of immunoglobulins, cell-mediated immunity, and the establishment of a tolerant state, that is, a specific state of unresponsiveness.

Organisms that reach the subepithelial tissues are carried by the peripheral lymphatics to local draining lymph nodes. Microbes that traverse the mucosal surfaces of the respiratory and gastrointestinal tracts are also exposed to large accumulations of lymphoid tissue. This mucosal-associated lymphoid tissue (MALT)[96] includes the appendix and the Peyer's patches in the lamina propria of the small intestine. A few organisms that invade the submucosal surfaces enter subepithelial blood vessels directly or are introduced directly into the blood and carried to the spleen. All of these lymphoid structures (the lymph nodes, MALT, and spleen and peripheral blood) are known as secondary lymphoid tissues. In these structures the organisms are exposed to macrophages that ingest and process the antigen and present it to the lymphocytes involved in the immune response. The lymphocytes involved in antibody pro-

duction or humoral immunity are B cells and T cells. T cells are also responsible for cell-mediated immunity and control of all specific immune responses.

B cells and T cells are named for the primary lymphoid organs in which they mature or develop into immunologically competent cells. B cells mature in the bursa of Fabricius in chickens. The structures with equivalent function in humans are the bone marrow and the lymph nodes. T cells mature in the thymus under the influence of thymic epithelium. After maturation the T and B lymphocytes leave the primary lymphoid organs and migrate to specific locations within the secondary lymphoid organs. T cells also migrate from the lymph nodes and recirculate throughout the body via the blood and lymph. The recirculation provides the opportunity to encounter antigen that may be present in peripheral tissue. Most B cells do not circulate but remain in germinal centers in spleen and lymph nodes. Both B cells and T cells carry surface receptors that confer on the cells their antigenic specificity.

The T cells have been divided into subtypes of cells including inducer cells, transducer cells, and effector cells.[19] These cells are distinguished according to antigenic determinants and function. Inducer cells may be functionally divided into helper-inducer and suppressor-inducer cells.

Inducer cells bear the T_4 (CD4/Leu 3)* determinants in humans (Ly 1 in mice). These cells are equipped to respond to signals from macrophage-processed antigen and to release a signal that assists B cells in the differentiation into plasma cells. Inducer (T_4) cells cannot respond to free antigen; their responses are limited to antigens on the membranes of macrophages and in close association with class II histocompatibility antigens.† The process by which inducer cells are triggered by macrophage-processed antigen is complex and not clearly understood but involves the release of interleukin-1 (IL-1) by the macrophage. IL-1 in association with antigen induces a new receptor, interleukin-2 (IL-2), on the helper-inducer cell. When IL-2 receptor binds to IL-2 the helper-inducer cell proliferates and activates several classes of effector cells (Figure 2-2). The majority of cells induced by antigen are helper-inducer cells, but a smaller number are considered suppressor-inducer cells. These latter cells, as discussed in the following section, are involved in the suppression of both humoral and cell-mediated immune responses.

Cell-Mediated Immunity

The term "cell-mediated immunity" (CMI) was originally reserved for localized reactions to microorganisms that did not involve the participation of immunoglobulin. This is indeed one manifestation of CMI but not the only aspect of the process. In fact, CMI may be manifest in different ways depending on the antigen and the group of T cells involved. Manifestations of CMI include delayed hypersensitivity and cytotoxicity reactions. Cytotoxicity may be mediated by a variety of cells including cytotoxic T lymphocytes and natural killer (NK) cells.

Delayed hypersensitivity

One group of effector T cells that is generated (activated) by the antigen-stimulated helper-inducer cells responds by releasing substances termed lymphokines (Table 2-2). Some of these products attract macrophages to the site, others increase the efficiency of intracellular killing by macrophages, and still others increase vascular permeability, which allows the influx of more T cells and macrophages into the tissue site. These events

---

*T_4, CD4, and Leu 3 are all types of nomenclature used to describe the antigenic determinants on T cells. CD stands for clusters of differentiation or cell-defined antigens and is the nomenclature recommended by the World Health Organization. Leu stands for leukocyte and is the terminology used by the Becton, Dickinson Company (Mountain View, Calif.). T stands for T cells; this nomenclature is used by several investigators. Thus a helper-inducer cell bears determinants identified as T_4 or CD4 or Leu 3.

†Histocompatibility antigens are cell surface determinants that allow the immune system to distinguish "self" from "nonself." These cell surface determinants are coded for by gene clusters on the major histocompatibility complex (MHC). There are two structurally distinct classes of histocompatibility antigens. Class I determinants are glycoproteins with alpha-chains and are associated with a beta$_2$-microglobulin; in humans they are called HLA-A, HLA-B, and HLA-C. Class II antigens consist of two nonidentical membrane-associated proteins and are called HLA-D.[132]

TABLE 2-2. Types of Lymphokines

Cells Affected	Lymphokine
Macrophages or monocytes	Migration inhibitory factor (MIF) Macrophage activating factor (MAF) Chemotactic factor
Lymphocytes	Mitogenic factors Suppressor factors Chemotactic factor Transfer factor Lymphocyte activating factor
Polymorphonuclear leukocytes	Chemotactic factors for neutrophils, eosinophils, and basophils Eosinophil stimulation promoter Histamine releasing factor Leukocyte inhibitory factor (LIF)
Other cells	Cytotoxic factors—lymphotoxin (LT) Osteoclast activating factor (OAF) Collagen producing factor Colony stimulating factor Gamma-interferon[a] Immunoglobulin binding factor (IBF)

[a]This immune interferon differs from the interferons produced in response to viral infection.

lead to the development of a hard, red, indurated area in the skin.[54,96] This phenomenon was observed as early as 1882 following the injection of certain proteins into the skin of animals infected with microorganisms such as *Mycobacterium tuberculosis* or *Listeria monocytogenes*. Because this cutaneous reaction was in contrast to the immediate reaction seen in animals with circulating antibody, it was called delayed-type hypersensitivity. Histologically the lesions are comprised of macrophages and lymphocytes. This unique reaction is due to T cells and their effect on macrophages and other T cells; antibody plays no role. Delayed hypersensitivity reactions offer protection against several facultative or obligate intracellular bacteria, viruses, fungi, and protozoa. Examples include the bacteria *L. monocytogenes*, *Salmonella typhi*, *M. tuberculosis*, *Brucella* spp., and *Nocardia* spp.; the fungi *Cryptococcus neoformans*, *C. albicans*, and *Histoplasma capsulatum;* the viruses herpes simplex, varicella-zoster, mumps, measles, influenza, rubella, and vaccinia; the protozoa *Toxoplasma gondii*, *Trypanosoma cruzi*, and *Leishmania* spp.; and the helminth *Schistosoma mansoni*.

Cytotoxicity reactions

The antigen-activated helper-inducer cells can also convert precytotoxic cells to cytotoxic cells, which are designated as T_8 (CD8/Leu 2) cells (Figure 2-2). These cells are important effector cells in cell-mediated resistance to enveloped viruses such

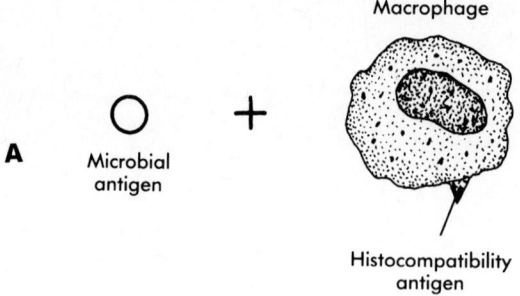

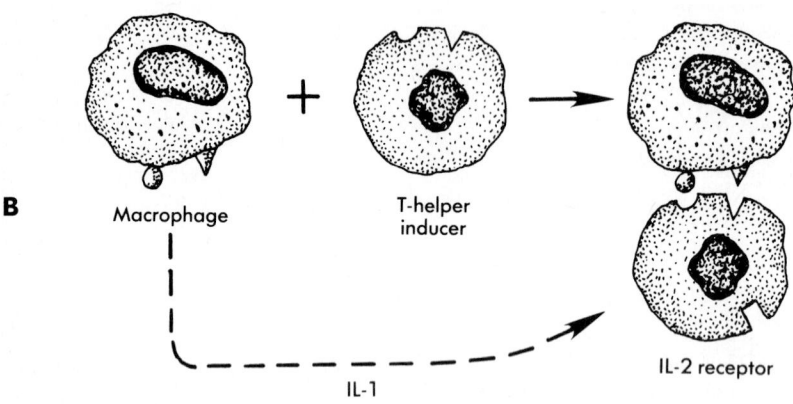

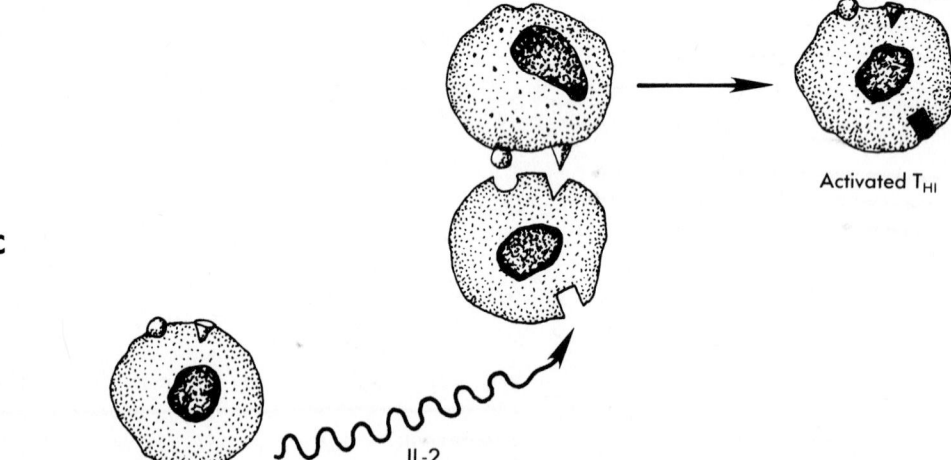

FIGURE 2-2. T cell interactions. **A,** Macrophages, which possess class II histocompatibility antigens, process microbial antigen. **B,** Processed antigen binds to receptors on T helper-inducer (T_{HI}) cells. Activated T_{HI} cells release soluble factors. This induces macrophages to release interleukin-1 (IL-1). Binding of IL-1 to other T_{HI} cells causes formation of interleukin-2 (IL-2) receptors. **C,** Binding of IL-2 to activated T_{HI} cell induces its proliferation. (NOTE: IL-2 acts only on T_{HI} cells to induce proliferation.)

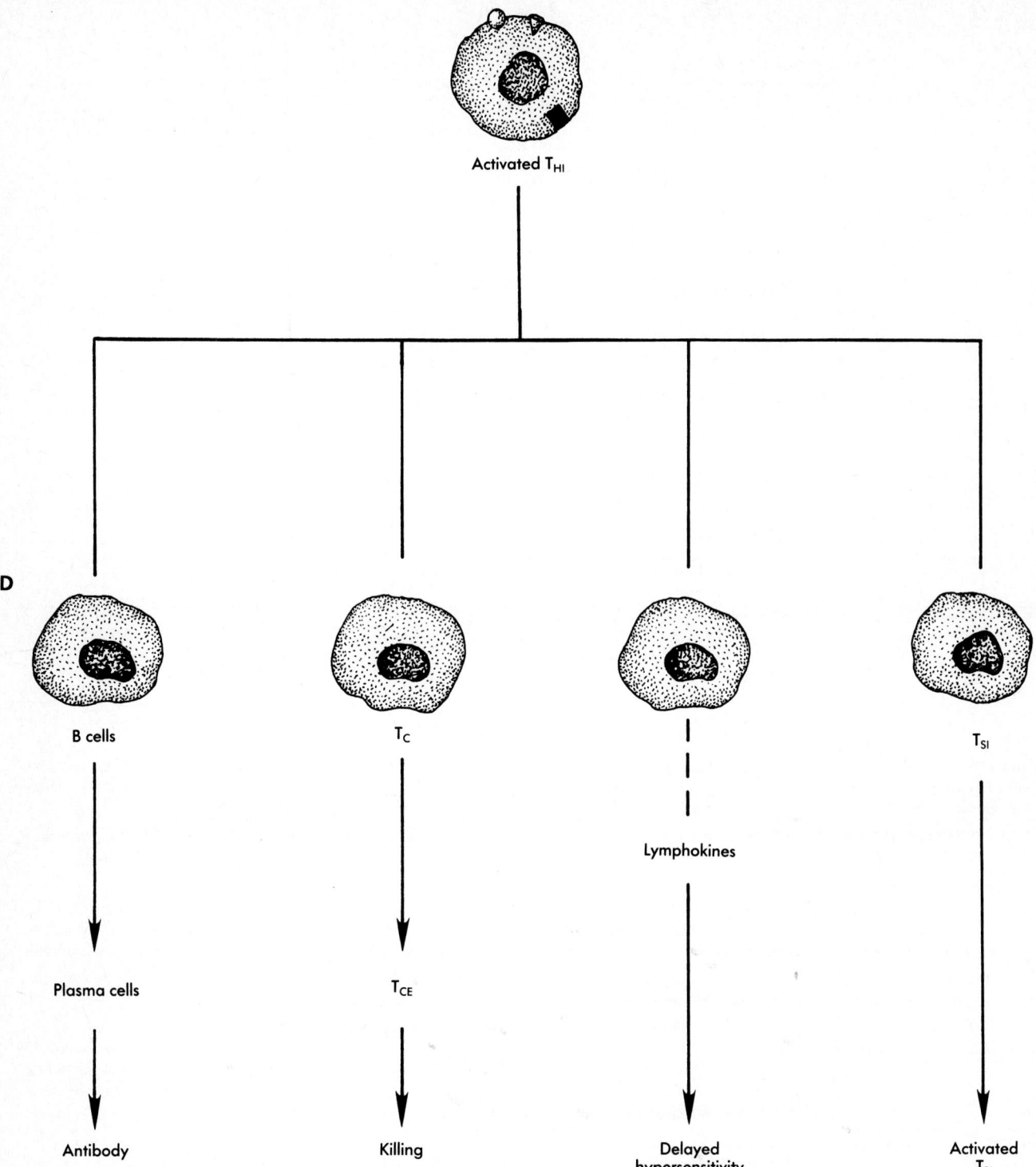

D

Activated T_{HI}

B cells

T_C

Lymphokines

T_{SI}

Plasma cells

T_{CE}

Antibody

Killing

Delayed
hypersensitivity

Activated
T_{SI}

FIGURE 2-2, cont'd. D, Activated T_{HI} cells, which express IL-2 receptors and bind IL-2, act on resting B cells to induce them to become antibody-producing plasma cells. They also induce resting T cytotoxic (T_C) cells to become effector cytotoxic (T_{CE}) cells, which react to class I histocompatibility antigens and promote killing. Another group of effector cells responds by releasing lymphokines, leading to delayed hypersensitivity. T suppressor-inducer (T_{SI}) cells are also activated.   *Continued.*

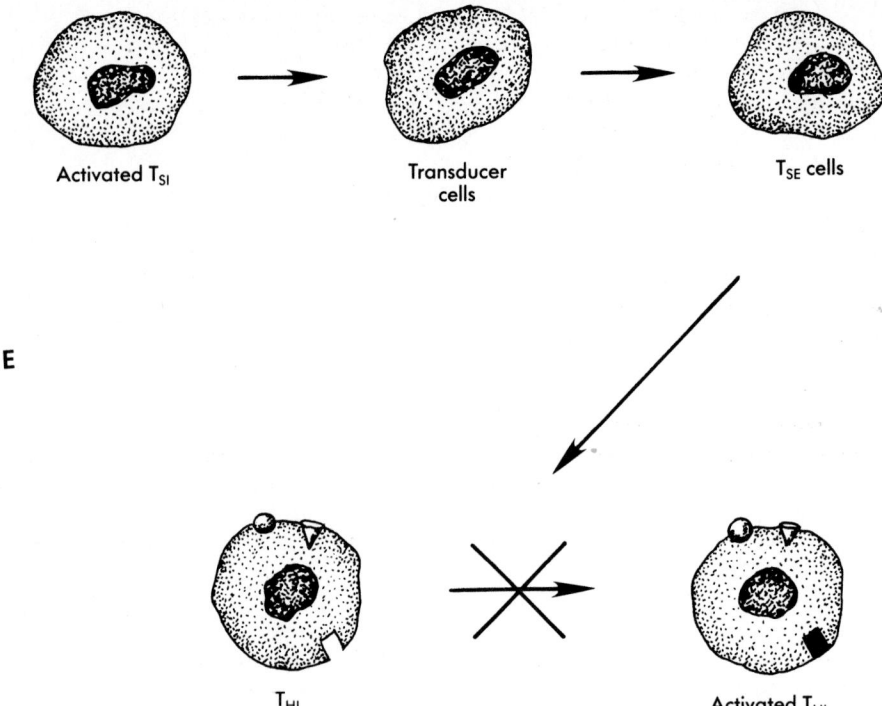

E

Activated T$_{SI}$ Transducer   T$_{SE}$ cells
                              cells

T$_{HI}$ Activated T$_{HI}$

FIGURE 2-2, cont'd. **E,** These activated T$_{SI}$ cells act on a population of transducer cells. When properly activated, transducer cells signal resting T suppressor-effector (T$_{SE}$) cells to become active. Target of T$_{SE}$ cells is T$_{HI}$ cells.

as rubella, measles, and influenza. Cytotoxic T lymphocytes (CTLs) recognize the virus-specified antigen in combination with a class I MHC antigen on the infected target cells, and respond by lysing the infected cell. If this occurs before mature virions (infectious viral particles; see Chapter 46) are formed, the spread of virus to other cells is inhibited.

Two additional cell-mediated cytotoxic reactions may protect the host from microbial infections. These are antibody-dependent cell-mediated cytotoxicity (ADCC) and cytotoxicity from natural killer cells (NK cells). ADCC is mediated by several types of cells, including macrophages, neutrophils, eosinophils, and null cells (also called K cells), all of which can bind specific antibody via Fc receptors. These ADCC effector cells recognize and attach to the Fc region of antibody-coated target cells (microorganisms) and in so doing kill the target cells. ADCC is involved in protection against a wide variety of parasitic and viral infections.

NK cells include a subpopulation of cells, called third population cells, present in most normal mammalian and avian species. The cell lineage of NK cells is unresolved. Various laboratories have suggested a T cell lineage, a monocyte lineage, or an independent cell lineage.[34] NK cells have direct cytotoxic effects against tumor cells; they can also produce and are activated by soluble factors such as interferon. Increasing evidence suggests that these cells play a role in the defense against microbial infections. Various studies have suggested their involvement in resistance against herpes simplex type I virus, cytomegalovirus, influenza virus, vaccinia virus, *Babesia microti, Trichinella spiralis,* and *Cryptococcus neofor-*

mans,[13,45,65,81,110] as well as other agents discussed by Herberman[44] and Lotzová and Herberman.[68] (The comprehensive review by Lotsová and Herberman also discusses the role of NK cells in defense against neoplasia and several other biologic phenomena.)

Humoral Response

The triggering of the humoral response involves the cooperation of the T helper-inducer (T$_4$) cells, the B cells, and the macrophages. T$_4$ cells recognize the foreign antigen in combination with the class II MHC antigen and through a series of events act by triggering B cells.

When activated the B cells undergo several cell divisions to produce memory cells and plasma cells, the antibody-producing cells. During the primary antibody response or the first encounter with an antigen, it takes several days for antibody to be detected in the serum. This lag time represents the time required for processing, selection, and transformation of enough plasma cells for production of antibody. During the secondary antibody response, also known as the anamnestic response, antibody appears more quickly because of the presence of memory cells.

Antibodies of different classes and types as well as different specificities and avidities are produced to different microbial antigens and to microbial products (for example, enzymes, toxins, and metabolites). Specific properties of the five classes of antibodies are outlined in Table 7-1. The antibodies (as well as the memory cells) enter the circulation and tissues where they are able to react with antigens at distant sites.

Antibodies are generally important against extracellular organisms. In the case of viruses, they are most effective against those (such as polio, measles, mumps, and chickenpox) that must pass into and through the bloodstream to reach their target organ. Antibodies in conjunction with complement neutralize these viruses, preventing their attachment to target cells. Viruses that pass contiguously from cell to cell are not influenced by the presence of antibody. Antibodies can also neutralize the effects of various bacterial toxins and enzymes.

In combination with complement, antibodies can lyse selected bacteria and viruses. This occurs more efficiently with gram-negative bacteria.[38] Antibody- and complement-mediated lysis has been demonstrated in vitro for the viruses herpes simplex, vaccinia, influenza, mumps, and measles.[32]

Secretory IgA antibodies prevent the adherence of bacteria and viruses to mucosal surfaces and neutralize viruses.[77] The latter activity is especially important in protection against viruses that replicate locally and do not disseminate, such as influenza virus, parainfluenza virus, rhinovirus, and respiratory syncytial virus. In fact, there is a correlation between the level of secretory IgA and the immunity to infection by these viruses.

Antibodies also act as effective opsonins, thus enhancing phagocytosis. Perhaps the most important way that antibody offers protection from infectious disease is through the cooperative effects of complement and phagocytes.

The clinical presentation of a disease is often completely different in the presence of antibody. For example, varicella-zoster virus gives rise to an exanthem and febrile illness (chickenpox) in immunologically naive children. In individuals with circulating antibody, however, the disease is localized and called zoster or shingles.

Role of the Immune Response in Various Infections

Although humoral and cell-mediated responses are induced in most infections, the magnitude and quality of these responses vary greatly depending on the infection.[80] The role of each of these responses in immunity or resistance to reinfection also varies greatly depending on the organism. Humoral and cell-mediated responses are important in immunity to bacterial and viral infections. With fungi the cell-mediated response appears to be primarily responsible for resistance,[86,94] although some studies have suggested that the humoral response may be equally important in protecting against systemic invasion by *Candida albicans*.[86] Some studies support a role for antibodies in protection against disease caused by *Cryptococcus neoformans,* although others refute it.[86] Helminths and protozoa also elicit the production of antibodies, as well as cell-mediated reactions, but their precise role in immunity has been defined in only a few cases.[122]

Control of the Immune Response and Infection

As mentioned previously, some T cells are involved in the overall control of immune responses. Each of the cell-mediated reactions discussed previously must also be controlled. This control is accomplished by suppressor-inducer cells that bear the T_4 (CD4, Leu 3) determinants. Following proper activation these cells send signals to another group of cells that in turn activate suppressor-effector cells bearing the T_8 (CD8, Leu 2) determinants. The major function of these suppressor-effector cells is to interact with helper-inducer cells to prevent the B cells from differentiating into antibody-producing plasma cells. Such cells also interfere with the maturation of precursor T cytotoxic cells into T cytotoxic cells.

Errors in receipt or in transmission of signals by T lymphocytes at any stage affect overall control of the immune response. Cytomegalovirus infections are associated with alterations in T lymphocyte subsets, specifically a decrease in the T_4 (helper-inducer) population and an increase in the T_8 (cytotoxic suppressor-effector) population.[101] This inverted T_4/T_8 ratio, which is also seen in AIDS,[67] appears to be a marker for an increased risk of opportunistic infections and may also be an important pathogenetic factor.[101] Epstein-Barr virus infects human B cells; this initial infection is followed by a proliferation of T cells, which suppress subsequent T cell proliferation to specific antigen and immunoglobulin production.[42,58] Systemic rheumatic diseases such as rheumatoid arthritis or systemic lupus erythematosus are also often cited examples of regulation imbalance–mediated diseases. These disorders involve the inability to generate suppressor-effector cells.

MECHANISMS OF PATHOGENICITY[80]

Although humans have developed numerous effective systems to protect them from the organisms to which they are continuously exposed, these organisms have developed a variety of mechanisms to circumvent the defenses. Before discussing these mechanisms, here and throughout the book, we must stress that it is the host and not the microbe that determines the eventual outcome of the host-parasite relationship. These mechanisms are discussed in terms of the parasite so readers will recognize the potential capability of these organisms.

Mechanisms of pathogenicity are best understood when examined in context of the host defenses they exploit. As such they are divided into the following groups: (1) those that allow attachment and multiplication, (2) those that permit the acquisition of nutrients from the host, (3) those that inhibit the phagocytic process, (4) those that permit evasion of the immune response, (5) those that inflict direct damage on the host, and (6) those that inflict indirect damage via immunopathologic processes. As discussed in the following sections, many organisms owe their virulence to a complex interplay of several pathogenic factors and not to a single mechanism.

Most mechanisms of pathogenicity have been proposed based on in vitro data. In only a few instances are they known to operate in vivo. One cannot automatically assume a direct correlation between in vitro data and the in vivo situation because reproducing the environmental conditions that occur within the host during infection is extremely difficult (if not impossible).[113] The in vivo conditions are dynamic and remain largely undefined. As Emil Golschlich stated, "The host-parasite relationship is more profitably described as a long-standing adaptism."[41]

MECHANISMS ALLOWING ATTACHMENT AND MULTIPLICATION

Adherence to host epithelial cells may be the essential first step in the pathogenesis of many infectious diseases,[10,93,130] and in fact the ability to adhere may explain why some species are able to cause disease whereas others are not.[93] Adherence allows the organisms to colonize and multiply at a rate faster than their removal, offers access to the body's tissues and cells, and provides a focus for elaboration of enzymes and toxins.

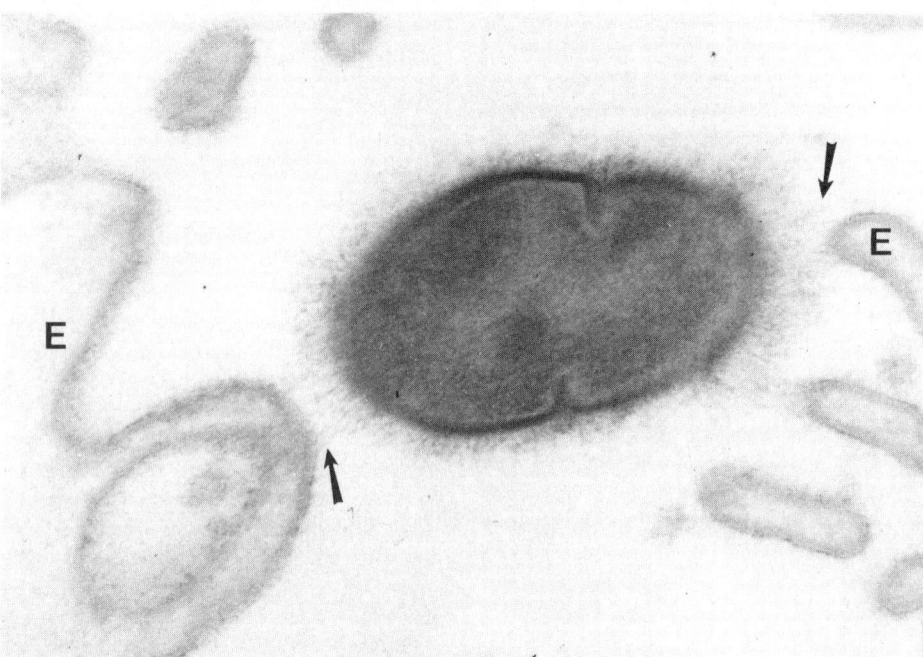

FIGURE 2-3. Fimbriae radiating from group A streptococcus to membrane *(arrows)* of human oral epithelial cell (*E*). (Reproduced from Beachey, E.H., and Ofek, I.: The Journal of Experimental Medicine, **143**:759, 1976, by copyright permission of The Rockefeller University Press.)

Adherence may also be nutritionally important, since nutrient materials tend to concentrate at the solid-liquid interfaces of the body.[74]

Adherence has been studied most extensively among the bacteria and viruses. Bacterial or viral adhesive structures are called adhesins, whereas complementary adhesive structures on the surfaces of host cells are called receptors. The binding between adhesin and receptor involves many forces and is virtually irreversible at constant pH. This binding is also very specific and determines to some degree both the species and tissue specificity of many infectious agents.[2]

The structural components of specific adhesins and receptors have been reported for several organisms.[10] *Streptococcus pyogenes*, one etiologic agent of pharyngitis, attaches to pharyngeal epithelial cells via the lipoteichoic acid present in the surface fimbriae (Figure 2-3), the fine filamentous appendages that surround the organism. Certain membrane proteins of *M. pneumoniae*, the etiologic agent of primary atypical pneumonia, attach to sialic acid residues on the ciliated epithelia of the respiratory tract. Mannan, a polysaccharide present in the cell wall of *Candida albicans*, appears to mediate the attachment of this organism to epithelial cells.[93] Numerous other structural components including the pili of *Neisseria gonorrhoeae* and the fimbriae (or pili) of *Escherichia coli* are involved in attachment and are discussed throughout the text.

Following attachment, organisms must resist both nonspecific and specific host defenses long enough to multiply to sufficient numbers to cause damage to underlying cells and tissues. Many organisms multiply in the epithelial surface at the site of entry into the body, produce a spreading infection in the epithelium, and are shed directly to the exterior.[80,81] The spread of infection may occur rapidly when the epithelium is covered with a layer of liquid as in the respiratory tract or alimentary tract.[80,81] Several respiratory viruses, such as rhinovirus, influenza virus, and parainfluenza virus, are generally confined to the epithelial surfaces. The spread of these viruses to subepithelial tissues is inhibited by the inflammatory response and other nonimmunologic resistance factors such as interferon and perhaps by growth characteristics of the virus.[80] Influenza and parainfluenza viruses, for example, bud only from the free (external) surface of the epithelial cells. Rhinoviruses replicate well at 33° C, the temperature of the nasal epithelium, but poorly at 37° C, the internal body temperature.[80]

Other organisms also multiply only on epithelial surfaces. *Corynebacterium diphtheriae*, the etiologic agent of diphtheria, multiplies only on the mucosal surfaces of the upper respiratory tract; however, the potent toxin that is elaborated by this organism does have systemic action. It is absorbed through the mucous membranes into the circulation and transported to the heart, kidneys, and nervous system. *Shigella* organisms penetrate the epithelial cells and pass laterally through them but do not invade deeper tissues; they cause disease by destroying the epithelial cell layer.

The organisms in Table 2-3 commonly traverse epithelial cell surfaces and invade the basement membrane and subepithelial tissues. From here (provided they circumvent the host's acquired defenses), they may spread systemically via the lymphatics and blood. A few organisms, such as herpes simplex virus and rabies virus, are spread along the nerve cells.

Circulating organisms selectively localize in numerous body sites. The molecular or biochemical basis for this localization or organotropism is unknown except for a few noted exceptions. The presence of erythritol in the placenta of cows, sheep, and pigs makes this the target organ of *Brucella abortus*. This

TABLE 2-3. Organisms and Diseases Associated with Crossing of Epithelial Surfaces and Subsequent Spread through the Body

Microbe	Respiratory Tract or Conjunctiva	Urogenital Tract	Skin	Intestinal Tract
Viruses	Measles, smallpox, rubella, varicella	Herpes simplex 2	Arboviruses	Enteroviruses, certain adenoviruses
Chlamydiae	Psittacosis	Lymphogranuloma venereum	—	—
Bacteria	*Mycobacterium tuberculosis, Yersinia pestis*	*Treponema pallidum*	*Bacillus anthracis*	*Salmonella typhi*
Rickettsiae	Q fever	—	Typhus	Q fever(?)
Fungi	Cryptococcosis, histoplasmosis	—	Maduromycosis	Blastomycosis
Protozoa	Toxoplasmosis	—	Malaria, trypanosomiasis	*Entamoeba histolytica*

From Mims, C.A.: The pathogenesis of infectious disease, ed. 2, New York, 1982, Academic Press, Inc.

organism is responsible for abortions in these animals. Human placentas do not contain this nutritive substance and thus are affected differently by the organism. Brucellosis in humans is a systemic disease, whereas it is a localized disease in cattle. The propensity of *Staphylococcus aureus* to localize in sebaceous glands because of the production of lipase may also be considered a form of organotropism.

MECHANISMS PERMITTING THE ACQUISITION OF NUTRIENTS

Other factors possessed by microorganisms that influence the eventual outcome of the host-parasite relationship include unique mechanisms to acquire nutrients. Some better-investigated mechanisms involve substances known as siderophores.[62,124] These are ligands secreted by bacteria in inverse proportion to the availability of iron. Siderophores can remove transferrin- (or lactoferrin-) bound iron and deliver it to the microbial cells via receptors on the surface of the cells. Iron, not generally available in adequate concentration, is therefore now available for growth and the elaboration of toxins. Mycobactin, a siderophore produced by *Mycobacterium tuberculosis,* remains associated with the surface of the bacteria. Another siderophore produced by *Escherichia coli* is formed extracellularly. Both have been associated with pathogenicity.

MECHANISMS INHIBITING THE PHAGOCYTIC PROCESS[25,29]

Microorganisms have managed to develop a mechanism for inhibiting every step in the normal phagocytic process (Table 2-4).

Inhibition of Chemotaxis[127]

Microbial surface components appear to be responsible for several mechanisms of pathogenicity[112] considered in this chapter, including the inhibition of chemotaxis. Among the specific structural components inhibiting the migration of phagocytic cells are the hyaluronic acid of *Streptococcus pyogenes,* type III–specific antigens of *Streptococcus agalactiae,* and cord factor, a lipid present in the cell wall of *Mycobacterium tuberculosis.*

Toxins are also able to inhibit the chemotaxis of leukocytes. Examples are the cholera toxin of *Vibrio cholerae,* enterotoxin of *Escherichia coli,* alpha-toxin of *Staphylococcus aureus,* streptolysin O of *S. pyogenes,* and theta-toxin of *Clostridium perfringens.*

Inhibition of Attachment of Phagocytes

The bacterial capsule is by far the most important and ubiquitous antiphagocytic substance.[48] Encapsulation of a large variety of organisms, including *Streptococcus pneumoniae, S. aureus, E. coli, Haemophilus influenzae, Streptococcus pneumoniae, Salmonella typhi, Klebsiella pneumoniae,* and *Neisseria meningitidis,* has been associated with virulence.

Recent studies with encapsulated and unencapsulated strains of *E. coli* have helped to delineate the antiphagocytic properties of capsules.[49] Capsules prevent the phagocyte from interacting with subcapsular bacterial determinants that allow engulfment of the organism. In addition, capsules are not able to fix complement; consequently, complement is unavailable for interaction with the C3 receptors on the phagocyte. The presence of anticapsular antibody overcomes the antiphagocytic effect of the capsule. The antibody is able to fix complement, thus rendering the organism susceptible to Fc or C3 receptor–mediated phagocytosis.

Numerous other structural components are antiphagocytic.[48] Examples include pili, the protein A of *S. aureus,* the M proteins of streptococci, the Vi antigen of *Salmonella typhi,* and the outer membrane proteins of *Neisseria gonorrhoeae.* These are discussed throughout the text.

Inhibition of Lysosome Fusion

Exposure to the lysosomal hydrolytic granules can be circumvented by inhibiting the fusion of the lysosome with the phagosome, thus offering an advantage to the engulfed microorganism. Studies with *Toxoplasma gondii* and *Mycobacterium tuberculosis* suggest that this may be accomplished in different ways. The sulfatides (glycolipids) present in the cell wall of *M. tuberculosis* may prevent or delay phagosome-lysosome fusion in macrophages infected with this organism.[40] The inhibition of fusion of macrophages infected with *T. gondii* may be due to

TABLE 2-4. Microbial Mechanisms that Inhibit the Phagocytic Process[a]

Mechanism	Bacteria	Fungi	Protozoa	Viruses
Inhibition of chemotaxis	*Capnocytophaga* spp. *Clostridium perfringens* *Escherichia coli* *Mycobacterium tuberculosis* *Staphylococcus aureus* *Streptococcus agalactiae* *Streptococcus pyogenes* *Vibrio cholerae*	Area for further research	Area for further research	Influenza
Inhibition of attachment and ingestion[b]	*Bacteroides fragilis* *E. coli* *Haemophilus influenzae* *Klebsiella pneumoniae* *Listeria monocytogenes* *Neisseria gonorrhoeae* *Neisseria meningitidis* *Pasteurella multocida* *Salmonella typhi* *S. aureus* *Streptococcus pneumoniae* *S. pyogenes* *Yersinia* spp.	*Cryptococcus neoformans*	*Trypanosoma cruzi*	Area for further research
Inhibition of lysosome fusion	*Chlamydia* spp. *Legionella pneumophila* *M. tuberculosis*	*Aspergillus flavus* *Histoplasma capsulatum*	*Leishmania donovani* *Leishmania mexicana* *Toxoplasma gondii*	Influenza
Resistance to killing in phagolysosome	*Brucella abortus* *Coxiella burnetti* *E. coli* *Mycobacterium leprae* *M. tuberculosis* *Salmonella typhimurium*		*T. gondii*	Reovirus
Escape from phagosome into cytoplasm	*Mycobacterium bovis*	Area for further research	*Trypanosoma cruzi*	Vaccinia
Killing of phagocyte	*P. aeruginosa* *S. aureus* *S. pyogenes*	Area for further research	*Entamoeba histolytica*	LDV[c]

Modified from Mims, C.A.: The pathogenesis of infectious disease, ed. 2, New York, 1982, Academic Press, Inc., and Densen, P., and Mandell, G.L.: Rev. Infect. Dis. **2**:817, 1980.
[a]Organisms listed are examples.
[b]Some of these organisms can resist phagocytosis only in the absence of antibody.
[c]Lactate dehydrogenase elevating virus of mice.

the secretion of a substance that alters the phagosome membrane in such a way that fusion cannot occur.[56]

In either of the above cases, the inhibition of fusion is an active process requiring living organisms. Opsonization of *M. tuberculosis* and *T. gondii* with antibody induces phagolysosome formation. This facilitates the killing of *T. gondii;* however, *M. tuberculosis* remains viable. The activation of macrophages by lymphokines enables the macrophages to destroy both organisms, once again demonstrating the delicate balance between host and parasite in infectious processes. The genus *Legionella* is also thought to inhibit fusion of the lysosome and the phagosome.

Influenza virus inhibits fusion of lysosomes with phagosomes containing staphylococci and inhibits release of myeloperoxidase.[1] This may explain the pathogenesis of secondary infections in patients with influenza virus infections.

Resistance to Killing in Phagolysosome

Facultative or obligate intracellular parasites must be able to resist killing and to increase in numbers in the phagocyte. They may do this by inhibiting lysosome fusion as discussed previously or by developing the ability to resist either the oxygen-dependent or oxygen-independent antimicrobial actions of the phagolysosome enzymes. Resistance to oxygen-independent microbicidal activities may be mediated by surface properties of the organism. For example, in vitro studies suggest that the lipopolysaccharide (see p. 30) of *Salmonella typhimurium* sterically hinders the binding of granular extracts.

The way in which organisms avoid the lethal effects of the toxic metabolites produced during the respiratory burst is unknown.[12] Because these toxic substances are also produced during normal aerobic metabolism of all organisms, most organisms synthesize enzymes (superoxide dismutase, catalase, and peroxidase) to convert these toxic substances to nontoxic products (see Chapter 20 for mechanisms of action of these enzymes). Interestingly, despite the possession of these enzymes, most organisms are killed by PMNs.[12] Recent studies suggest why other organisms may not be killed. *Nocardia asteroides*, for example, appears resistant to the superoxide anion and H_2O_2 because of the production of high levels of catalase and a unique superoxide dismutase.[11,12] Similar mechanisms may exist in *Mycobacterium tuberculosis* and *Legionella pneumophila*.

Other mechanisms may also render the organism resistant to phagolysosome killing. *Toxoplasma gondii* appears not to stimulate the respiratory burst, and as a result the reactive oxygen metabolites are not generated.[129] The ability of *Coxiella burnetii*, the obligate intracellular parasite responsible for Q fever, to reside within the phagolysosome appears to be related to its acidophilic biochemistry and enzymatic activities.[6] Active metabolism of *C. burnetii* appears to occur at low pH, specifically at 4.5 to 4.8, the pH of the phagolysosome. The production of superoxide dismutase and catalase may also help protect the organism from the toxic oxygenated products of the host.

Escape from Phagolysosome into Cytoplasm

Fascinating electron micrograph studies of the interaction of the trypomastigotes (see Chapter 43 for definition) of *Trypanosoma cruzi* with mouse peritoneal macrophages illustrate the potential importance of this mechanism. These organisms are taken into the macrophage by formation of phagosomes; however, after approximately 1 hour no evidence of the phagosome can be found and free trypomastigotes are observed in the cytoplasm. The way in which the trypomastigotes promote the disappearance of the phagosome is unknown, but suggested mechanisms include lysis by a parasite-released factor or a direct membrane-membrane interaction.[82]

Several viruses enter the host cells in phagocytic vacuoles, but they manage to escape from the vacuoles before fusion with lysosomes.[108] Vaccinia virus is an example. This virus enters host cells within a phagocytic vacuole; however, the viral lipoprotein envelope interacts with the vacuolar membrane resulting in the dissolution of both membranes and the release of DNA-containing viral cores into the cytoplasm. However, if the virus is opsonized by IgG, it cannot escape from the phagosome and is sequestered by lysosomes.[109]

Killing of the Phagocyte

Several organisms kill phagocytic cells. Most of these produce toxins that depolarize the phagocytic cell membrane with subsequent massive degranulation and cell death. *Entamoeba histolytica* appears to kill cells merely through contact.[53]

Streptolysins O and S are responsible for some of the cytolytic activity of *Streptococcus pyogenes*.[46] These enzymes differ in their mechanism of action. Streptolysin O initially binds to cholesterol in the phagocyte membrane and through the mechanisms discussed in Chapter 13 eventually leads to the formation of membrane-penetrating channels that create large membrane defects and subsequent lysis. Streptolysin S appears to exert its cytolytic effect by altering membrane permeability.[119] Staphylococcal leukocidin, anthrax toxin, and toxin A from *Pseudomonas aeruginosa* also appear to be toxic for phagocytes.[25]

MECHANISMS INHIBITING THE IMMUNE RESPONSE

Table 2-5 includes examples of mechanisms that allow organisms to inhibit the effects of the immune response.[114]

Residing in Locations Protected from Host Defense

Organisms that are able to reside intracellularly are shielded from some effects of the immune response. *Brucella, Listeria*, and *Mycobacterium* spp. survive in macrophages, whereas herpes simplex virus and herpes varicella-zoster virus reside in dorsal root ganglia cells.[80] Residence in such sites may result in a state of latency,[71] but reactivation and disease may occur when the host's immunocompetence is compromised. The occurrence of these phenomena, of which viruses are undoubtedly the masters, involves a complex interplay of many of the mechanisms included under "Mechanisms Inhibiting the Immune Response." Although latency is well recognized, little is known in regard to its molecular basis.[72] The reader is referred to Mahy,[72] Mackowiak,[71] Huang,[52] Wildy and Gell,[126] and Mims[81] for discussions of the mechanisms of latency.

Other immunologically privileged sites include the inner eye, tissues of the cerebrum, testicles, thymus, and liver.[8] These structures and the organisms that lodge within them are sequestered from the lymphoid system. The liver protects the invasive forms of *Entamoeba histolytica* and the flukes of *Fasciola hepatica*.[23] Encystment of various parasites may also serve as a barrier against immune attack.[9]

Antigen Shedding

Some organisms such as *Entamoeba histolytica*,[18] *Trypanosoma cruzi*,[100] *Toxoplasma gondii*, and *Leishmania* spp. shed their antigens through a process called capping. The binding of antibody to these organisms induces structural changes in the membrane and movement of cell surface antigens toward one pole. The antigens are then spontaneously released. Although this phenomenon has been observed only in vitro, it may possibly enable the organism to evade host antibodies in vivo.

Several organisms are able to liberate their surface antigens in soluble form during systemic infections. Examples include *Candida albicans* and *Streptococcus pneumoniae*. Although the in vivo significance of this phenomenon is unknown, possibly it promotes the pathogenic potential of the organism by binding specific antibody to nonviable substances or by inactivating T cells.[80]

Variation of Antigens

Organisms may evade the immune response by modifying their surface antigens. This may occur during a single infection or over a period of time with different infections.[41]

Perhaps the best example of antigenic variation is that of the trypanosomes, the parasites responsible for African trypanosomiasis.[26,27] This disease is characterized by repeated episodes of bloodstream invasion and remission. Although trypano-

TABLE 2-5. Mechanisms that Inhibit the Immune Response[a]

Mechanism	Bacteria	Helminths	Protozoa	Fungi	Viruses
Hiding in protected locations	*Brucella* spp. *Listeria monocytogenes* *Mycobacterium* spp.	*Fasciola hepatica* *Taenia solium* *Trichinella spiralis*	*Entamoeba histolytica* *Plasmodium* spp.	*Histoplasma capsulatum* Agents of mycetoma	Herpes simplex Varicella-zoster
Shedding of antigens	*Streptococcus pneumoniae*	*Schistosoma mansoni*	*Entamoeba histolytica* *Leishmania* spp. *Plasmodium* spp. *Toxoplasma gondii* *Trypanosoma cruzi*	*Candida albicans* *Cryptococcus neoformans*	Measles
Variation of antigens	*Borrelia recurrentis* *Neisseria gonorrhoeae*	*S. mansoni*	*Plasmodium* spp. *Trypanosoma brucei*	Area for further research	HIV Influenza A
Immunosuppression	*Fusobacterium nucleatum* *Klebsiella pneumoniae* *Mycoplasma pneumoniae*	*Onchocerca volvulus* *S. mansoni* *Trichinella* spp. *Wuchereria bancrofti*	*Leishmania* spp. *Plasmodium* spp. *T. brucei*	Area for further research	Cytomegalovirus Epstein-Barr HIV Mumps Measles
Antibody cleavage	*Haemophilus influenzae* *Neisseria meningitidis* *S. pneumoniae*		*T. cruzi*		

Modified from Mims, C.A.: The pathogenesis of infectious disease, ed. 2, New York, 1982, Academic Press, Inc.
[a]Organisms listed are examples.

somes are continually exposed to antibodies present in the bloodstream, they are able to circumvent the effects of these antibodies by changing the antigens present on their surface coat. These antigens are glycoprotein in nature and are designated variable surface glycoproteins (VSGs). Antibodies are initially produced to the VSGs on the invading parasites. These antibodies are able to kill the majority of these trypanosomes, but a few organisms are able to escape by producing a new coat of VSGs to which the early antibodies cannot bind. This antigenic variation occurs with each episode of bloodstream invasion, leaving the immune system of the host unable to cope with the infection.

Production of various VSGs is dependent on VSG genes. A single trypanosome possesses at least a few hundred and perhaps as many as a thousand of these genes.[26,27] Only one gene is expressed at a time. Expression of the VSG genes is controlled by complex gene rearrangements, the mechanism of which is slowly being unraveled although much remains unknown. It appears that the genes must be located near a telomere (the end of a chromosome) to be expressed.[26,27] Genes in the interior of a chromosome need to be duplicated and translocated (as an expression-linked copy) to an expression site near a telomere to be transcribed.[26,27] Genes already located near a telomere can be transcribed and expressed without being duplicated. The precise mechanism that triggers the

switch from one gene to another remains unknown.[27]

Antigenic variation is also seen in malaria.[120,122] The life cycle of *Plasmodium* spp., the cause of malaria, is complex. These parasites go through several developmental stages, including one as an infective sporozoite, which is injected by the mosquito into the bloodstream of humans. Within 20 minutes the sporozoites enter the liver and undergo schizogony, resulting in the merozoite stage (see Chapter 43). The merozoites, which differ antigenically from the sporozoites, are released and invade red blood cells to undergo a second cycle of schizogony. Again they are released and invade other red blood cells. This cycle is repeated several times with each recurrent parasitemia consisting of a population of organisms that is antigenically distinct from the preceding one and thus resistant to previously produced antibodies. Unlike trypanosomiasis, however, the malarial recrudescences are eventually controlled by the host, probably because of cross-immunity between variants.[122]

The incorporation of host antigens into its surface membrane may help *Schistosoma mansoni*, a lumen-dwelling helminth discussed in Chapter 41, avoid the effects of the immune response. Adult schistosomes survive in the bloodstream where they are able to acquire A, B, H, and Lewis blood group antigens.[21,39] It has been hypothesized that acquisition of these antigens protects the adult worms by masking susceptible parasite antigens. Other studies have suggested that the acquisition of host substances alters the susceptibility of the organism to complement or cell-mediated damage and thus has a stabilizing rather than an antigen-masking effect.[115]

Viruses may also demonstrate antigenic variation. Influenza virus undergoes minor and major antigenic changes in some of its surface antigens, specifically the hemagglutinin (HA) and neuraminidase (NA) antigens. When the virus changes from one HA or NA to another, this is considered a major change and is called antigenic shift. Antigenic shift occurs about every 10 years and often results in an influenza pandemic, since immunity to the original virus is not protective against the modified virus. This is discussed more thoroughly in Chapter 51.

Like African trypanosomiasis, relapsing fever associated with the spirochete *Borrelia* is characterized by repeated episodes of bloodstream invasion and remission. Different serotypes of *Borrelia* are recovered from each relapse. In fact, each relapse population may consist of several serotypes, each differing in certain protein surface antigens[7,118] and each able to avoid the effects of antibody to previous serotypes.

Human immunodeficiency virus (HIV)* may also demonstrate some antigenic variation,[31] which may partially explain the lack of immunity in patients with antibody to HIV.

Immunosuppression

A state of immunosuppression may develop in the host during infection with bacteria, viruses, fungi, protozoa, and helminths (Table 2-5).[15,23,69,81,102] This immunosuppression may be manifested as a depressed response to organisms unrelated to the infecting organism, or it may be specific and directed only against the antigens on the invading organism. Both types of immunosuppression have been observed with some infections. General and specific immunosuppression may involve both the humoral and cell-mediated responses.[103]

An organism that is able to suppress the specific acquired immune response is able to promote its own survival. The inducement of a state of general immunosuppression is significant in that it may predispose individuals to secondary infections[15,125] and affect the pathogenesis of many diseases.[106,107] Cytomegalovirus, for example, appears to suppress both cell-mediated and humoral immunity[47,78] and in so doing predisposes the host to severe infections by several other organisms. *Fusobacterium nucleatum* is another example. This organism, which is found as part of many microbiotic infections including trench mouth, periodontal disease, and even malignancy, has been shown to be immunosuppressive for T cell–mediated events.[106] This has been proposed as a mechanism by which an infection with *F. nucleatum* can lead to local immunosuppression, subsequent establishment of other organisms, and eventual disease.[106] It has also been suggested that the impaired immune responses observed in patients with systemic mycotic diseases could be the factor predisposing to disease rather than the result of disease.[24,86,117]

In some cases selected products of organisms such as cell membrane components, enzymes, and toxins are thought to be responsible for the induction of immunosuppression.[33,103,125] In other instances it is not known whether the organism itself is responsible for the immunosuppression or induces the production of a suppressive factor.

For the most part it is not known whether the suppressive substances act directly on B and T cells or act on intermediary cells. Some studies have suggested that macrophages may be the pivotal cell in immunosuppression and in fact may provide a common pathway for induction of general immunosuppression in a variety of infections.[3,4] The generation of specific suppressor T cells may mediate specific suppression in certain parasitic and fungal infections.[50,51,85]

Immunosuppression by Alteration of Receptors on Immune Cells[66]

As discussed in Chapter 10, HIV, a member of the retrovirus family, is responsible for AIDS. This retrovirus is capable of interfering with the immune response. However, this immunosuppression is considered separately because it appears to be unique in its involvement of the alteration of receptors on immune cells.

HIV infects T_4 (CD4, Leu 3) cells. As discussed previously, T lymphocytes are critical in all immune responses. A normal T_4 cell reacts to foreign antigen in association with class II histocompatibility antigens on the surface of a macrophage and differentiates and divides. This requires not only the antigen signal but also the binding of interleukin 1. When a T_4 cell is infected with HIV, the ability of the cell to express the T_4 determinant is diminished or altered. These infected cells are therefore incapable of reacting with class II determinants or with foreign antigen on the surface of antigen-presenting cells. This block or alteration could essentially stop any release of interleukin 2 from these T cells, as well as maturation of T cytotoxic cells (T_8 cells). Thus a drastic and rapid decline would occur in the host's ability to kill other virus-infected cells or to eliminate those T_4 cells infected with HIV. Indeed some evidence suggests that the infection with HIV may actually alter the expression of class I antigens on the T_4 cell surface, thus protecting the cell from immune elimination early in the infectious process. The immunosuppression following viral infection is not unique to human retroviruses, but the manner in which the virus induces such immunosuppression is restricted to these viruses and may be restricted to the human retroviruses alone.

Antibody Cleavage

Neisseria meningitidis,[84] *Streptococcus pneumoniae*, and *Haemophilus influenzae*[59,83] produce protease enzymes that specifically cleave certain subclasses of IgA. As previously discussed, the production of secretory IgA is responsible for the local immunity of the respiratory and gastrointestinal tracts.[87] It has been suggested that the production of IgA protease by *H. influenzae* and *S. pneumoniae* could inactivate this defense system, allow colonization, and predispose the host to respiratory infections.[83] Furthermore, since the three organisms that produce the protease are the major etiologic agents of bacterial meningitis, the protease has been suggested as an important virulence factor in the pathogenesis of this disease.[59]

Certain stages of *T. cruzi* also produce an antibody-cleaving

---

*This is the virus responsible for AIDS. The virus was named HTLV-III by Robert Gallo and his co-workers at the National Institutes of Health and lymphadenopathy associated virus (LAV) by L. Montagnier at the Institut Pasteur. The Human Retrovirus Subcommittee empowered by the International Committee on the Taxonomy of Viruses has recently proposed that the AIDS virus be officially designated as the human immunodeficiency virus (HIV).[53a]

protease. This enzyme splits attached antibody, leaving bound Fab fragments that are unable to activate complement.[63] The protease thus protects the organism from complement-mediated lysis and phagocytosis.

Induction of Ineffective Antibodies

Antibodies that are nonprotective, or alternatively enhance the growth of organisms, are ineffective antibodies. Although high levels of antibodies are formed in malaria and trypanosomiasis, for example, many of these antibodies are not parasite specific and therefore are ineffective.

Ineffective blocking antibodies may be formed in response to certain strains of *N. gonorrhoeae,* also known as gonococci. These antibodies are able to bind to specific receptors on the surface of gonococci and in so doing sterically "block" access to the antigen that binds the effective antibacterial antibody. Gonococci that possess receptors for the blocking antibody are resistant to killing by antibody and complement in normal human serum and are able to invade the blood to produce disseminated infection. However, those gonococci that do not possess the receptor for the blocking antibody are readily killed by human serum and cause only localized genital infections.[76]

DIRECT DAMAGE VIA TOXINS AND ENZYMES

Microbial toxins may be classified as exotoxins or endotoxins. Exotoxins are produced by metabolizing bacteria and are secreted into the surrounding environment. Endotoxins form part of the cell membrane of gram-negative bacteria and are released in large quantities only when the cell is lysed.

Exotoxins

Exotoxins are produced primarily by gram-positive bacteria and occasionally by gram-negative bacteria. They are immunogenic proteins that often behave as enzymes. Their effects may be manifested either locally or systemically depending on the toxin.

Exotoxins may be classified according to their site of action or biologic effect. Neurotoxins such as tetanus toxin and botulinum toxin exert their primary activity on the nervous system. Enterotoxins act on the intestinal tract. Numerous bacteria including *Shigella dysenteriae, Escherichia coli,* and *Staphylococcus aureus* produce enterotoxins. Cytotoxins, such as diphtheria toxin, destroy cells.

Examples of exotoxins that have been suggested to play a role in disease are indicated in Table 2-8. Three of these toxins—diphtheria, tetanus, and botulinum—act as the sole determinants of disease.[17] Antibody developed to these proteins is protective for the toxic effects but does not affect the attachment or colonization of the microorganism.

Special mention should be made of the fungal exotoxins produced by *Aspergillus flavus* and *Claviceps purpurae.* Neither of these fungi invade humans, but they may be indirectly responsible for human disease through their contamination of various foods. *C. purpurae* infects wheat and rye and produces a toxin known as ergotamine; humans are poisoned by eating contaminated grain. Aflatoxin, produced by *A. flavus,* has been detected in nuts, oilseeds, grains, and the derived products of all of these. Ingestion of these contaminated goods has caused hepatocellular damage and carcinoma of the liver in a variety of animals. Although a direct cause-and-effect relationship has not been firmly established, aflatoxin has been strongly associated with liver cell damage and liver cancer in humans.[89,121]

The mechanisms of action of the toxins in Table 2-6 and other exotoxins will be discussed throughout the book.

Endotoxins

Endotoxin is the lipopolysaccharide component of the outer membrane of gram-negative bacteria (Figure 2-4). The toxicity of endotoxin resides in the lipid A portion. The potency of endotoxins varies greatly among the gram-negative organisms; some are extremely toxic, whereas others are not toxic at all.

Experimental animal studies have revealed the numerous biologic activities of endotoxin.[30] This substance stimulates the liberation of endogenous pyrogen from blood leukocytes and other cells, producing fever. It produces thrombocytopenia and a transient leukopenia followed by marked granulocytosis. It is also capable of activating the complement system by both the classical and alternate pathways. When injected in large quantities into the bloodstream, endotoxin may result in shock and even death. Endotoxin also exerts several metabolic effects, notably a decrease in both gluconeogenesis and glycogen synthesis.[14] Furthermore, endotoxin is a potent activator of macrophages and can induce them to release factors important for inflammation.[75]

Although endotoxin is capable of producing these pathologic processes in experimental animals, its role in human infections remains largely unresolved.[105] Most likely endotoxin participates in host damage when bacterial invasion of blood and tissues is extensive, since cell lysis and endotoxin liberation probably occur more readily under these conditions.[112]

Genetic determinants of toxin production

The production of toxins by bacteria may be mediated by the possession of a plasmid or a bacteriophage, and not necessarily by the bacterial chromosome. As mentioned in Chapter 1, plasmids are extrachromosomal pieces of DNA that are capable of autonomous replication. Some plasmids can be transferred between bacterial cells by a process known as conjugation (see Chapter 8 for explanation). These are transmissible or conjugative plasmids. The enterotoxins of *Escherichia coli* and the exfoliatin toxin of *Staphylococcus aureus* are coded for by transmissible plasmids. The exfoliatin toxin of *S. aureus* is responsible for scalded skin syndrome, a disease characterized by the formation of bullae and the peeling off of large sheets of epidermis (see Chapter 12 and Plate 6, *A*).

Bacteriophages may be classified as temperate or virulent. Virulent bacteriophages lyse the cells they infect. Temperate bacteriophages may exhibit two actions: they may lyse the infected cells as do virulent bacteriophages, or they may establish a persistent infection and continue to replicate within the bacterial cell. The latter condition is termed lysogeny. Toxins that are coded for by lysogenic phages include diphtheria toxin, botulinum toxins C and D, *Clostridium novyi* toxins, and streptococcal erythrogenic toxin.[116] The specific actions of these toxins are discussed later in the book.

Enzymes

Bacterial invasion of tissues is often facilitated by the possession of enzymes. Among these are hyaluronidase, collagenase, coagulase, and fibrinolysin. The role and mechanisms of

TABLE 2-6. Exotoxins

Species	Disease	Toxin
Aspergillus flavus	Liver cancer (?)	Aflatoxin
Bacillus anthracis	Anthrax	Anthrax toxins (lethal factor, protective factor, edema factor)
Claviceps purpurae	Ergot poisoning	Ergotamine
Clostridium botulinum	Botulism	Neurotoxins A, B, E, and F[a]
Clostridium difficile	Antibiotic-associated pseudomembranous colitis	Toxin A, toxin B
Clostridium perfringens	Gas gangrene Food poisoning	Alpha-toxin, kappa-toxin, lambda-toxin Enterotoxin
Clostridium tetani	Tetanus	Tetanospasmin (tetanolysin may be involved)
Corynebacterium diphtheriae	Diphtheria	Diphtheria toxin
Escherichia coli	Traveler's diarrhea	Enterotoxin
Shigella dysenteriae	Dysentery	Shiga toxin (possesses enterotoxic, cytotoxic, and neurotoxic activities)
Staphylococcus aureus	Pyogenic infections Scalded skin syndrome Food poisoning Toxic shock syndrome	Alpha-toxin Exfoliatin toxin Enterotoxin Toxic shock syndrome toxin-1
Streptococcus pyogenes	Scarlet fever	Erythrogenic toxin
Vibrio cholerae	Cholera	Enterotoxin (choleragen)

[a]Eight neurotoxins are produced, but these four are most commonly associated with human infections.

these enzymes are discussed throughout the book. Fungi may also elaborate enzymes. The dermatophytes, for example, produce keratinase, which provides them with the ability to invade keratinized tissue such as hair, skin, and nails (see Chapter 32).

INDIRECT DAMAGE VIA IMMUNOPATHOLOGIC REACTIONS

Organisms may cause tissue damage directly by producing toxins or indirectly by eliciting immune-mediated destruction or immunopathologic reactions. Although the immunopathologic damage is minimal in most infections, in others it is severe and forms the major part of the disease. Immunopathologic reactions may be divided into four categories based on the classification of Coombs and Gell.[35]

Anaphylactic Reactions (Type I Reactions)

IgE antibodies are associated with anaphylactic reactions in humans. Large amounts of these antibodies are produced by allergic individuals in response to certain antigens called allergens. The IgE antibodies are homocytotropic; this means that they bind nonspecifically to human mast cells and basophils via their Fc regions. Allergens, on reexposure, bind to the IgE antibodies on the cells and precipitate a series of reactions resulting in cellular degranulation. The products released, histamine, eosinophilic chemotactic factor of anaphylaxis (ECF-A), slow-reacting substance of anaphylaxis (SRS-A), and others, are responsible for the clinical manifestations and immunopathologic results.

Histamine and the SRS-A cause contraction of smooth muscle and increased vascular permeability. ECF-A attracts eosinophils to the site, enhances complement reactions, and destroys histamines. Specific symptoms depend on the portal of entry and site of binding of the antigen. For example, allergens that enter the respiratory tract bind to sensitized mast cells in that site. The release of histamine causes contraction of the smooth muscles surrounding the bronchioles, leading to respiratory distress and edema. Clinically this is hay fever or asthma. If the antigens bind to cells in the circulation, the reaction may be systemic, leading to anaphylactic shock.

Although type I reactions are not commonly associated with bacterial disease, evidence suggests that they may be associated with the disease resulting from fungal and parasitic infections.[88] Large quantities of IgE are produced in response to helminth infestations. Although these antibodies are protective in that they participate with eosinophils and macrophages in ADCC reactions against the parasite, they may also contribute to anaphylactic reactions. *Ascaris lumbricoides,* a helminth, is the etiologic agent of ascariasis, an infestation that appears in the tropics and the southern United States. The clinical manifestations of ascariasis include asthmatic breathing, coughing spasms, bronchial rales, and in more severe cases a pneumonia-like syndrome known as Loeffler's syndrome. These symptoms are assumed to be the result of an allergic reaction to the larvae

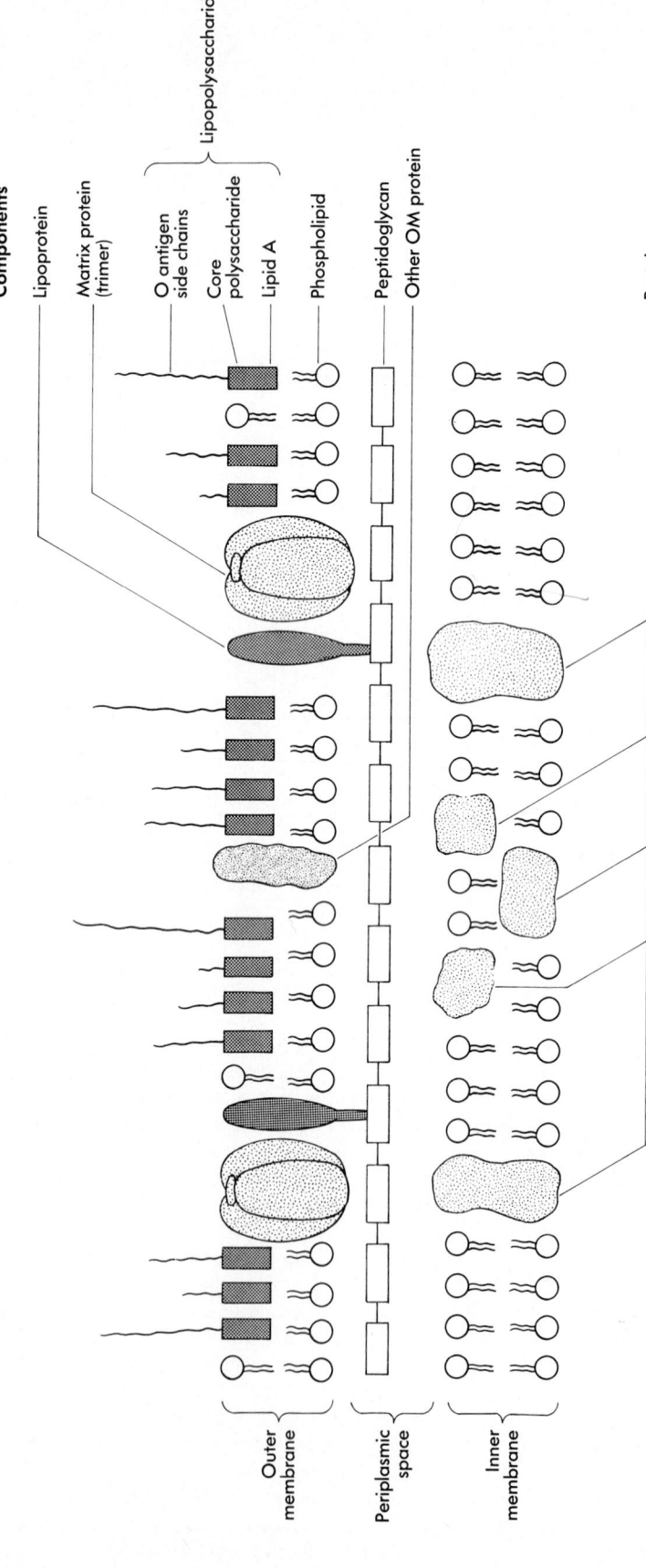

FIGURE 2-4. Diagram of gram-negative cell envelope. Components are listed on right. Trimers of matrix protein of outer membrane are associated with lipoprotein and with lipopolysaccharide (LPS) (of variable polysaccharide length), and lipoprotein is covalently bound to peptidoglycan. Phospholipid molecules are illustrated with circle for polar groups and line for each fatty acid acyl moiety. (From Davis, B.D., et al.: Microbiology, ed. 3, Hagerstown, Md., 1980, Harper & Row, Publishers, Inc.)

that migrate through the lungs. *A. lumbricoides* may also invoke anaphylactic reactions in the absence of actual infection. This occurs among laboratory workers who have become sensitized to the volatile allergens produced by the worm.[90]

A much more severe anaphylactic reaction is associated with the parasite *Echinococcus granulosus*. The infective stage of this organism for humans is the egg, and these are usually acquired from infected dogs. The eggs hatch in the small intestine and migrate most frequently to the liver and lungs. Here they develop into hydatid cysts that may reach considerable size. Leakage of the hydatid fluid from the cyst may produce sensitization in the patient. If extensive leakage subsequently occurs spontaneously or at surgery, a severe or fatal anaphylactic reaction may follow.

Anaphylactic reactions have also been suggested in the immunopathology of allergic bronchopulmonary aspergillosis associated with members of the genus *Aspergillus*.[37] This condition is discussed in detail in Chapter 37.

Cytotoxic Reactions (Type II Reactions)

Cytotoxic or cytolytic reactions involve the combination of IgG and IgM antibodies with antigens on the target cell surface or antigens that have attached to cell membranes, such as drugs or microorganisms. These reactions include those that are complement dependent as well as those that are complement independent, that is, ADCC reactions. In either case the result is lysis and death of the target cell. If the target cell is a red blood cell, a platelet, or an endothelial cell of the glomeruli, tissue injury results and is amplified by the indirect effects of the released complement components (Figure 2-1) or the products liberated from the inflammatory cells.

It has been suggested that cytotoxic reactions may be involved in the pathogenesis of American trypanosomiasis, also known as Chagas' disease. This disease occurs in the southern parts of the United States, Mexico, and Central and South America. It is caused by *Trypanosoma cruzi,* a parasite that infects rodents, opossums, armadillos, and reduviid bugs that feed on these animals. Humans become infected from the bite of the reduviid bug. The organism is carried by the lymphatic system to lymph nodes and the bloodstream. Numerous tissues and organs may become infected as the organism is carried throughout the body; however, the liver, spleen, and heart are preferentially invaded. The severe heart damage and myocardial lesions that develop may be due to the binding of the parasitic antigens to the heart and the subsequent attack of the anti–*T. cruzi* antibodies.[104]

The bacterium, *M. pneumoniae*, induces antibodies that bind to the I antigens on human red blood cells. These antibodies may be important in the pathogenesis of primary atypical pneumonia.

Immune Complex Reactions (Type III Reactions)

The damage in several infectious diseases is attributed to the deposition of antigen-antibody complexes in various body tissues. These immune complexes may be formed initially in the bloodstream and then deposited in the tissues, or they may be formed by the combination of antibody with antigen that has previously lodged in or attached to the tissue.[55]

The fate of antigen-antibody complexes formed in the bloodstream depends on the relative proportions of antigen and antibody and the size of the complex. Complexes that are formed in antibody excess or at equivalance are removed by the macrophage-monocyte-phagocyte system; however, soluble complexes that are formed in slight antigen excess are not removed by this system. These complexes continue to circulate in the blood and localize in small blood vessels such as the cutaneous vasculature or the glomeruli. Some deposited immune complexes can activate complement, resulting in the generation of several biologically active components (Figure 2-1). Several of these components are chemotactic for neutrophils. Neutrophils accumulate at the site of localization of the complexes and on degranulation release several lysosomal enzymes that hydrolyze collagen, elastin, and other proteins, resulting in extensive injury. Recent evidence suggests that tissue injury is also mediated by the release of toxic oxygen products including H_2O_2, the hydroxyl radical, and singlet oxygen.[55]

Extensive tissue injury in the kidneys may lead to immune complex glomerulonephritis. This condition may be seen following malaria, syphilis, schistosomiasis, streptococcal pyoderma and pharyngitis, and serum hepatitis. In the first three infections the glomerulonephritis is manifested clinically as the nephrotic syndrome. The evidence of immune mechanisms in these diseases is supported by the demonstration of immunoglobulin and complement in the damaged tissue.

Extensive tissue injury in the blood vessels results in vasculitis. The vasculitis may be manifested clinically in several different forms depending on the extent of injury and the affected vessels. Erythema nodosum is characterized by the presence of tender red nodules in the skin caused by the deposition of antigen, antibody, and complement in the superficial capillaries. This condition is seen after streptococcal infection or during treatment of patients with leprosy. In serum hepatitis, small arteries may be affected, leading to polyarteritis nodosa.

Immune complex–mediated disease has been associated with a wide variety of microorganisms. An example is farmer's lung disease, a clinical pneumonitis (allergic alveolitis) following repeated inhalation of spores from *Micropolyspora faeri,* an actinomycete found in wet hay. In addition to the anaphylactic disorder previously described, *Aspergillus* spores may induce immune complex–mediated lung diseases.

Cell-Mediated Reactions (Type IV Reactions)

As previously discussed, the response of cytotoxic T lymphocytes (CTLs) is important in controlling the invasion of several viruses. However, in some situations this response may cause more tissue damage than the virus itself. This is best exemplified by the action of CTLs in lymphocytic choriomeningitis (LCM) virus infection in mice. When mice are infected intracerebrally with the virus, it grows in the meninges and ependyma, but no signs of damage or dysfunction can be seen in the infected cells. After 7 to 10 days, however, the mouse dies as the result of severe meningitis with submeningeal and subependymal edema.[80] Death is not due to the effects of the virus but rather to the effects of the CTLs.

The conditions of viral infection determine whether the effects of the CTLs will be beneficial or detrimental to the host. With a highly cytopathic virus the CTL is beneficial to the host, since either the CTLs destroy the virus-infected cells or the virus destroys the infected organ or tissue. However, under conditions of low viral cytopathogenicity or extensive spread of the virus to a critical organ, the CTLs may cause more tissue damage than the virus itself.[131]

Delayed hypersensitivity reactions are also responsible for immunopathologic effects. The lymphokines involved in these reactions may directly or indirectly cause tissue damage. The macrophages that are activated by the lymphokines are able to destroy invading organisms, but they also simultaneously and indiscriminately destroy autologous tissue.

The granuloma formation and subsequent lung damage that occurs in tuberculosis is also attributed to delayed hypersensitivity reactions. Granulomas form around the *Mycobacterium tuberculosis* organisms as a result of the accumulation of macrophages and other cell types in response to substances in the cell walls of these organisms. These granulomas and other surrounding host cells gradually undergo caseation necrosis, disintegrating to form a coagulated, cheeselike mass that may persist in the lungs for years. Caseation has been attributed to the harmful effects of the lymphokines and the release of numerous toxic products from the activated macrophages. The intracellular growth of *M. tuberculosis* in macrophages is uncontrolled until the host demonstrates evidence of cell-mediated immunity or delayed hypersensitivity, at which time isolated macrophages arrest these organisms' intracellular growth.

The tuberculin skin test is also an example of a delayed hypersensitivity reaction. It represents on a smaller scale what is occurring focally in tuberculosis. In this test certain prepared antigens of the *M. tuberculosis* organism known as tuberculins are injected into the skin of the patient. The tuberculin may be prepared and injected in different ways. In the standard intracutaneous or Mantoux test, 0.1 ml of a purified protein derivative (PPD) of tuberculin containing 5 tuberculin units is injected intracutaneously into the forearm. After 24 to 48 hours those patients who have become sensitized to *M. tuberculosis* produce an area of induration approximately 16 to 17 mm in diameter. These changes reflect the development of delayed hypersensitivity and indicate that the patient is currently infected or has been previously infected with *M. tuberculosis* or related mycobacteria. Delayed hypersensitivity skin tests may be used to determine present or previous infection with several organisms.

The major symptoms of schistosomiasis are also attributed to cell-mediated immunopathologic reactions. The organisms associated with this disease, *Schistosoma mansoni, S. japonicum,* and *S. haematobium,* live in snails. The larvae of these parasites are shed into fresh water and are able to penetrate the skin of humans. The schistosome larvae or cercariae invade the bloodstream, are carried to the lungs, and eventually come to live in the small mesenteric or pelvic veins. Here the females lay as many as 100 eggs per day. These eggs become lodged in various body tissues such as the liver where they induce formation of inflammatory granulomas or pseudotubercles. These granulomas, and not the eggs per se, are probably responsible for the hepatosplenomegaly, portal hypertension, and esophageal varices that frequently occur.[115]

REFERENCES

1. Abramson, J.S., et al.: Inhibition of neutrophil lysosome-phagosome fusion associated with influenza virus infection in vitro: role in depressed bactericidal activity, J. Clin. Invest. **69:**1393, 1982.
2. Albini, B., and van Oss, C.J.: Microbial pathogenicity and host-parasite relationships. In Milgrom, F., and Flanagan, T.D., editors: Medical microbiology, New York, 1982, Churchill Livingston.
3. Askonas, B.A.: Interference in general immune function by parasite infections: African trypanosomiasis as a model system, Parasitology **88:**633, 1984.
4. Askonas, B.A.: Macrophages as mediators of immunosuppression in murine African trypanosomiasis, Curr. Top. Microbiol. Immunol. **117:**119, 1985.
5. Babior, B.M.: Oxygen-dependent microbial killing by phagocytes, N. Engl. J. Med. **298:**659, 1978.
6. Baca, O.G., and Paretsky, D.: Q fever and *Coxiella burnetti:* a model for host-parasite interactions, Microbiol. Rev. **47:**127, 1983.
7. Barbour, A.G., Tessier, S.L., and Stoenner, H.G.: Variable major proteins of *Borrelia hermsii,* J. Exp. Med. **156:**1312, 1982.
8. Barker, C.F., and Billingham, R.E.: Immunologically privileged sites, Adv. Immunol. **25:**1, 1977.
9. Barriga, O.O.: The immunology of parasitic infections, Baltimore, 1981, University Park Press.
10. Beachey, E.H.: Bacterial adherence: adhesion-receptor interactions mediating the attachment of bacteria to mucosal surfaces, J. Infect. Dis. **143:**325, 1981.
11. Beaman, B.L., et al.: Role of superoxide dismutase and catalase as determinants of pathogenicity of *Nocardia asteroides:* importance in resistance to microbicidal activities of human polymorphonuclear neutrophils, Infect. Immun. **47:**135, 1985.
12. Beaman, L., and Beaman, B.L.: The role of oxygen and its derivatives in microbial pathogenesis and host disease, Annu. Rev. Microbiol. **38:**27, 1984.
13. Bell, R.G., Adams, L.S., and Ogden, R.W.: Intestinal mucus trapping in the rapid expulsion of *T. spiralis* by rats: induction and expression analyzed by quantitative worm recovery, Infect. Immun. **45:**267, 1984.
14. Berry, L.J.: Metabolic effects of endotoxin. In Schlessinger, D., editor: Microbiology—1975, Washington, D.C., 1975, American Society for Microbiology.
15. Bloom, B.: Games parasites play: how parasites evade immune surveillance, Nature **279:**21, 1979.
16. Boral, L.I., and Cheung, K.W.K.: The HLA antigens in organ grafting. I. Pretransplantation tests, Lab. Management, January 1986, p. 45.
17. Boyd, R.F.: Host-parasite relationship. In Boyd, R.F., and Marr, J.J., editors: Medical microbiology, Boston, 1980, Little, Brown & Co.
18. Calderón, J., de Lourdes Muñoz, M.A., and Acosta, H.M.: Surface redistribution and release of antibody-induced caps in entamoebae, J. Exp. Med. **151:**184, 1980.
19. Canter, H., and Gershon, R.K.: Immunological circuits: cellular composition, Fed. Proc. **38:**2058, 1979.
20. Centers for Disease Control: Enteric illness associated with raw clam consumption—New York, MMWR **31:**449, 1982.
21. Clegg, J.A., Smithers, S.R., and Terry, R.J.: Acquisition of human antigens by *Schistosoma mansoni* during cultivation in vitro, Nature **232:**653, 1971.
22. Cline, M.J., et al.: Monocytes and macrophages: functions and diseases, Ann. Intern. Med. **88:**78, 1978.
23. Cohen, S.: Survival of parasites in the immunocompetent host. In Cohen, S., and Warren, K.S., editors: Immunology of parasitic infections, ed. 2, Oxford, Eng., 1982, Blackwell Scientific Publications.
24. Cox, R.A.: Cell-mediated immunity. In Howard, D., editor: Fungi pathogenic for humans and animals. Part B. Pathogenicity and detection, New York, 1983, Marcel Dekker.
25. Densen, P., and Mandell, G.L.: Phagocyte strategy vs. microbial tactics, Rev. Infect. Dis. **2:**817, 1980.
26. Donelson, J.E., and Rice-Ficht, A.C.: Molecular biology of trypanosome antigenic variation, Microbiol. Rev. **49:**107, 1985.
27. Donelson, J.E., and Turner, M.J.: How the trypanosome changes its coat, Sci. Am. **252:**44, 1985.
28. Dwyer, S.M.: The cell-mediated immune system. In Dwyer, S.M., et al., editors: Management of the immune-compromised patient, Berkeley, Calif., 1983, Cutler Biological.
29. Edelson, P.J.: Intracellular parasites and phagocytic cells: cell biology and pathophysiology, Rev. Infect. Dis. **4:**124, 1982.

30. Elin, R.J., and Wolff, S.M.: Biology of endotoxin, Annu. Rev. Med. **27:**127, 1976.

31. Essex, M.: H.T.L.V. immunosuppression and immunodiagnosis (round table discussion), Annual Meeting of the American Society for Microbiology, Las Vegas, Nevada, March 3-7, 1985.

32. Ewan, P.W., and Lachmann, P.J.: Immunology and virus infection. In Lachmann, P.J., and Peters, D.K., editors: Clinical aspects of immunology, vol. 2, ed. 4, London, 1982, Blackwell Scientific Publications.

33. Falconi, G., and Campa, A.: Bacterial interferences with immune responses. In O'Grady, F., and Smith, H.P., editors: Microbial perturbations of host defenses, London, 1981, Academic Press.

34. Fitzgerald, P.A., et al.: Heterogeneity of human NK cells: comparison of effectors that lyse HSV-1-infected fibroblasts and K562 erythroleukemia targets, J. Immunol. **130:**1663, 1983.

35. Gell, P.G.H., and Coombs, R.R.A.: Clinical aspects of immunology, Oxford, Eng., 1968, Oxford Scientific Publications.

36. Gillies, R.R.: Lecture notes on medical microbiology, ed. 2, Oxford, Eng., 1978, Blackwell Scientific Publications.

37. Glimpf, R.A., and Bangen, A.S.: Fungal pneumonias. Part 3. Allergic bronchopulmonary aspergillosis, Chest **80:**85, 1981.

38. Glynn, A.A.: Immunity to bacterial infection. In Lachmann, R.J., and Peters, D.K., editors: Clinical aspects of immunology, vol. 2, ed. 4, London, 1982, Blackwell Scientific Publications.

39. Goldring, O.L., et al.: Acquisition of human blood group antigens by *Schistosoma mansoni*, Clin. Exp. Immunol. **26:**181, 1976.

40. Goren, M.B., et al.: Prevention of phagosome-lysosome fusion in cultured macrophages by sulfatides of *Mycobacterium tuberculosis*, Proc. Natl. Acad. Sci. **73:**2510, 1976.

41. Gotschlich, E.C.: Thoughts on the evolution of strategies used by bacteria for evasion of host defenses, Rev. Infect. Dis. **5**(suppl. 4):S778, 1983.

42. Hamblin, T.J., et al.: Immunological reasons for chronic ill health after infectious mononucleosis, Br. Med. J. **287:**85, 1983.

43. Henderson, F.W., et al.: A longitudinal study of respiratory viruses and bacteria in the etiology of acute otitis media with effusion, N. Engl. J. Med. **306:**1377, 1982.

44. Herberman, R.B., editor: NK cells and other natural effector cells, New York, 1982, Academic Press.

45. Herberman, R.B., and Ortaldo, J.R.: Natural killer cells: their role in defenses against disease, Science **214:**24, 1981.

46. Hirsch, J.G., Bernteimer, A.W., and Weissman, G.: Motion picture study of the toxic actions of streptolysins on leukocytes, J. Exp. Med. **118:**223, 1963.

47. Ho, M.: Cytomegalovirus: biology and infection, New York, 1981, Plenum Medical Book Co.

48. Horwitz, M.A.: Phagocytosis of microorganisms, Rev. Infect. Dis. **4:**104, 1982.

49. Horwitz, M.A., and Silverstein, S.C.: Influence of the *Escherichia coli* capsule on complement fixation and on phagocytosis and killing by human phagocytes, J. Clin. Invest. **65:**82, 1980.

50. Howard, J.G.: Manipulation of the immune responses in parasitic infections, Parasitology **88:**665, 1984.

51. Howard, J.G., Hale, C., and Lieu, F.Y.: Immunological regulation of experimental cutaneous leishmaniasis. III. Nature and significance of specific suppression of cell-mediated immunity in mice highly susceptible to *Leishmania tropica*, J. Exp. Med. **152:**594, 1980.

52. Huang, A.S.: Persistent viral infections: introduction, Rev. Infect. Dis. **4:**998, 1982.

53. Hudler, H., et al.: *Entaemoeba histolytica*. II. Einfluβ humoraler immunmechanismen auf die zytotoxische Aktion, Tropenmed. Parasitol. **35:**5, 1984.

53a. Human Retrovirus Subcommittee: Human immunodeficiency viruses (letter), Science **232:**697, 1986.

54. Humphrey, J.H., and White, R.G.: Immunology for students of medicine, ed. 3, Philadelphia, 1970, F.A. Davis Co.

55. Johnson, K.J., and Ward, P.A.: Newer concepts in the pathogenesis of immune complex-induced tissue injury, Lab. Invest. **47:**218, 1982.

56. Jones, T.C., and Hirsch, J.G.: The interaction between *Toxoplasma gondii* and mammalian cells. II. The absence of lysosomal fusion with phagocytic vacuoles containing living parasites, J. Exp. Med. **136:**1173, 1972.

57. Keesey, J.: M.H.C. simplified, Boehringer-Manneheim, B.M. Biochemica **2:**6, 1985.

58. Kieff, E., et al.: The biology and chemistry of Epstein-Barr virus, J. Infect. Dis. **146:**506, 1982.

59. Kilian, M., Mestecky, J., and Schrohenloher, R.E.: Pathogenic species of the genus *Haemophilus* and *Streptococcus pneumoniae* produce immunoglobulin Al protease, Infect. Immun. **26:**143, 1979.

60. Klebanoff, S.J.: Antimicrobial mechanisms in neutrophilic polymorphonuclear leukocytes, Semin. Hematol. **12:**117, 1975.

61. Kochan, I.: Nutritional regulation of antibacterial resistance. In Schlessinger, D., editor: Microbiology—1974, Washington, D.C., 1975, American Society for Microbiology.

62. Kochan, I.: Role of siderophores in nutritional immunity and bacterial parasitism. In Weinberg, E.D., editor: Microorganisms and minerals, New York, 1977, Marcel Dekker.

63. Krettli, A.U., and Eisen, H.: Escape mechanisms of *Trypanosoma cruzi* from the host immune system, Semaine Inserm Seillac, France; cited by Cohen, S., and Warren, K.S., editors: Immunology of parasitic infections, ed. 2, Oxford, Eng., 1982, Blackwell Scientific Publications.

64. Lalonde, R.G., and Holbein, B.E.: Role of iron in *Trypanosoma cruzi* infection of mice, J. Clin. Invest. **73:**470, 1984.

65. Lanier, L.L., et al.: Subpopulations of human and natural killer cells defined by expression of the Leu-7 (HNK-1) and Leu-11 (NK-15) antigens, J. Immunol. **131:**1789, 1983.

66. Lawrence, J.: The immune system in AIDS, Sci. Am. **253:**84, 1985.

67. Lewis, D.L., et al.: Disporportionate expansion of a minor T cell subset in patients with lymphadenopathy syndrome and acquired immunodeficiency syndrome, J. Infect. Dis. **151:**555, 1985.

68. Lotzová, E., and Herberman, R.B.: Immunology of natural killer cells, Boca Raton, Fla., 1986, CRC Press.

69. Mackowiak, P.A.: Microbial synergism in human infections, N. Engl. J. Med. **298:**21, 1978.

70. Mackowiak, P.A.: The normal microbial flora, N. Engl. J. Med. **307:**83, 1982.

71. Mackowiak, P.A.: Microbial latency, Rev. Infect. Dis. **6:**649, 1984.

72. Mahy, B.W.J.: Strategies of viral persistence, Br. Med. Bull. **41:**50, 1985.

73. Makela, P.H., et al.: Evasion of host defenses. In Smith, H., Skehel, J.J., and Turner, M.J., editors: The molecular basis of microbial pathogenicity, Weinheim, Ger. 1980, Verlag Chemie.

74. Marshall, K.C., and Bitton, G.: Microbial adhesion in perspective. In Bitton, G., and Marshall, C., editors: Absorption of microorganisms on surfaces, New York, 1980, John Wiley & Sons, Inc.

75. McCarthy, J.B., et al.: Mediation of macrophage collagenase production by 3'-5' cyclic adenosine monophosphate, J. Immunol. **124:**2405, 1980.

76. McCutchan, J.A., et al.: Role of blocking antibody in disseminated gonococcal infection, J. Immunol. **121:**1884, 1978.

77. McNabb, P.C., and Tomasi, T.B.: Host defense mechanisms at mucosal surfaces, Annu. Rev. Microbiol. **35:**477, 1981.

78. Mills, E.L.: Viral infections predisposing to bacterial infections, Annu. Rev. Med. **35:**469, 1984.

79. Mims, C.A.: Innate immunity to parasitic infections. In Cohen, S., and Warren, K.S., editors: Immunology of parasitic infections, ed. 2, Oxford, Eng., 1982, Blackwell Scientific Publications.

80. Mims, C.A.: The pathogenesis of infectious disease, ed. 2, New York, 1982, Academic Press.

81. Mims, C.A., and White, D.O.: Viral pathogenesis and immunology, Oxford, Eng., 1984, Blackwell Scientific Publications.

82. Mogueira, N., and Cohn, Z.: *Trypanosoma cruzi:* mechanisms of entry and intracellular fate in mammalian cells, J. Exp. Med. **143:**1402, 1976.

83. Mulks, M.H., Kornfeld, S.J., and Plaut, A.G.: Specific proteolysis of human IgA by *Streptococcus pneumoniae* and *Haemophilus influenzae,* J. Infect. Dis. **141:**450, 1980.

84. Mulks, M.H., and Plaut, A.G.: IgA protease production as a characteristic distinguishing pathogenic from harmless *Neisseriaceae,* N. Engl. J. Med. **299:**973, 1978.

85. Murphy, J.W.: Effects of first-order *Cryptococcus*-specific T-suppressor cells on induction of cells responsible for delayed-type hypersensitivity, Infect. Immun. **48:**439, 1985.

86. Murphy, J.W.: Host defenses against pathogenic fungi, Clin. Immunol. Newsletter **7:**17, 1986.

87. Okabe, T.: Protective effects of antibody against intestinal invasion by *Escherichia coli,* Microbiol. Immunol. **27:**303, 1983.

88. Parrish, W.E.: Host damage resulting from hypersensitivity to bacteria, Symp. Soc. Gen. Microbiol. **22:**157, 1972.

89. Patten, R.C.: Aflatoxins and disease, Am. J. Trop. Med. Hyg. **30:**422, 1981.

90. Pawlowski, Z.S.: Ascariasis, Clin. Gastroenterol. **7:**157, 1978.

91. Petersen, B.H., Graham, J.A., and Brooks, G.F.: Human deficiency of the eighth component of complement, J. Clin. Invest. **57:**283, 1976.

92. Petersen, B.H., et al.: *Neisseria meningitidis* and *Neisseria gonorrhoeae* bacteremia associated with C6, C7, and C8 deficiencies, Ann. Intern. Med. **90:**917, 1979.

93. Ray, T.L., Digre, K.B., and Payne, C.D.: Adherence of *Candida* species to human epidermal corneocytes and buccal mucosal cells: correlation with cutaneous pathogenicity, J. Invest. Dermatol. **83:**37, 1984.

94. Rippon, J.W.: Medical mycology, ed. 2, Philadelphia, 1982, W.B. Saunders Co.

95. Robbins, S.L., and Cotran, R.S.: Inflammation and repair. In Robbins, S.L., and Cotran, R.S., editors: Pathologic basis of disease, ed. 2, Philadelphia, 1979, W.B. Saunders Co.

96. Roitt, I.M., Brostoff, J., and Male, D.K.: Immunology, St. Louis, 1985, The C.V. Mosby Co.

97. Root, R.K., and Ryan, J.L.: Humoral immunity and complement. In Mandell, G.L., Douglas, R.J., Jr., and Bennett, J.E., editors: Principles and practice of infectious diseases, ed. 2, New York, 1985, John Wiley & Sons, Inc.

98. Rosenstreich, D.L., Weinblott, A.C., and O'Brien, A.: Genetic control of resistance to infection in mice, CRC Crit. Rev. Immunol. **3:**263, 1982.

99. Salata, R.A., Pearson, R.D., and Ravdin, J.I.: Interaction of human leukocytes and *Entamoeba histolytica:* killing of virulent amoebae by the activated macrophage, J. Clin. Invest. **76:**491, 1985.

100. Schmunis, G.A., et al.: *Trypanosoma cruzi:* antibody-induced mobility of surface antigens, Exp. Parasitol. **50:**90, 1980.

101. Schooley, R.T., et al.: Association of herpesvirus infections with T-lymphocyte-subset alterations, glomerulopathy, and opportunistic infections after renal transplantation, N. Engl. J. Med. **308:**307, 1983.

102. Schwab, J.H.: Suppression of the immune response by microorganisms, Bacteriol. Rev. **39:**121, 1975.

103. Schwab, J.H.: Bacterial interference with immunospecific defences, Philos. Trans. R. Soc. Lond. (Biol.) **303:**123, 1983.

104. Scott, M.T., and Snary, D.: American trypanosomiasis. In Cohen, S., and Warren, K.S., editors: Immunology of parasitic infections, ed. 2, Oxford, Eng., 1982, Blackwell Scientific Publications.

105. Shands, J.W., Jr.: Endotoxin as a pathogenic mediator of gram-negative infection. In Schlessinger, D., editor: Microbiology—1975, Washington, D.C., 1975, American Society for Microbiology.

106. Shenker, B.J., and DiRienzo, J.M.: Suppression of human peripheral blood lymphocytes by *Fusobacterium nucleatum,* J. Immunol. **132:**2357, 1984.

107. Shenker, B.J., Listgarten, M.A., and Taichman, N.S.: Suppression of human lymphocyte responses by oral spirochetes: a monocyte-dependent phenomenon, J. Immunol. **132:**2039, 1984.

108. Silverstein, S.C.: The reovirus replicative cycle, Annu. Rev. Biochem. **45:**375, 1976.

109. Silverstein, S.C.: The role of mononuclear phagocytes in viral immunity. In Van Furth, R., editor: Mononuclear phagocytes in immunity, infection, and pathology, Oxford, Eng., 1973, Blackwell Scientific Publications.

110. Sissons, J.G.P., and Oldstone, M.B.A.: Antibody-mediated destruction of virus-infected cells, Adv. Immunol. **29:**209, 1980.

111. Skamene, E.: Genetic regulation of host resistance to bacterial infection, Rev. Infect. Dis. 5(suppl. 4):S823, 1983.

112. Smith, H.: Microbial surfaces in relation to pathogenicity, Bacteriol. Rev. **41:**475, 1977.

113. Smith, H.: The effect of environmental conditions in vivo and in vitro on the determinants of microbial pathogenicity. In Smith, H., Skehel, J.J., and Turner, M.J., editors: The molecular basis of microbial pathogenicity, Weinheim, Federal Republic of Germany, 1980, Verlag Chemie.

114. Smith, H.: The biochemical challenge of microbial pathogenicity, J. Appl. Bacteriol. **57:**395, 1984.

115. Smithers, S.R., and Doenhoff, M.J.: Shistosomiasis. In Cohen, S., and Warren, K.S., editors: Immunology of parasitic infections, ed. 2, Oxford, Eng., 1982, Blackwell Scientific Publications.

116. Stephen, J., and Pietrowski, R.A.: Bacterial toxins, Washington, D.C., 1981, American Society for Microbiology.

117. Stobo, J.D., et al.: Suppressor thymus-derived lymphocytes in fungal infection, J. Clin. Invest. **57:**319, 1976.

118. Stoenner, H.G., Dodd, T., and Larsen, C.: Antigenic variation of *Borrelia hermsii,* J. Exp. Med. **156:**1297, 1982.

119. Sullivan, G.W., Sullivan, J.A., and Mandell, G.L.: Leukotoxic streptococci and neutrophil degranulation (abstract), Clin. Res. **26:**407A, 1978.

120. Turner, M.J.: Antigenic variation in parasites, Parasitology **88:**613, 1984.

121. Uray, B.B.: Aflatoxin and Reye's syndrome: a case control study, Pediatrics **68:**473, 1981.

122. Wabelin, D.: Immunity to parasites: how animals control parasite infections, London, 1984, Edward Arnold.

123. Ward. P.A., and Kunkel, S.: Bacterial virulence and the inflammatory system, Rev. Infect. Dis. 5(suppl. 4):S793, 1983.

124. Weinberg, E.D.: Iron and infection, Microbiol. Rev. **42:**45, 1978.

125. Weir, D.M., and Blackwell, C.C.: Interaction of bacteria with the immune system, J. Clin. Lab. Immunol. **10:**1, 1983.

126. Wildy, P., and Gell, P.G.H.: The host response to herpes simplex virus, Br. Med. Bull. **41:**86, 1985.

127. Wilkinson, P.C.: Leukocyte locomotion and chemotaxis: effects of bacteria and viruses, Rev. Infect. Dis. **2:**293, 1980.

128. Willoughby, W.F., and Willoughby, J.B.: Immunologic mechanisms of parenchymal lung injury, Environ. Health Perspect. **55:**239, 1983.

129. Wilson, C.B., Tsai, V., and Remington, J.S.: Failure to trigger the oxidative metabolic burst by normal macrophages, J. Exp. Med. **151:**328, 1980.

130. Yayoshi, M.: Association between *M. pneumoniae* hemolysis, attachment and pulmonary pathogenicity, Yale J. Biol. Med. **56:**685, 1983.

131. Zinkernagel, R.M.: Major transplantation antigens in host responses to infection, Hosp. Pract. **13:**83, 1978.

132. Zinkernagel, R.M., and Doherty, P.C.: MHC-restricted cytotoxic T-cells: studies on the biological role of polymorphic major transplantation antigens determining T cell restriction—specificity, function and responsiveness, Adv. Immunol. **27:**51, 1979.

CHAPTER 3

Quality Control

Alice S. Weissfeld
Raymond C. Bartlett

The Centers for Disease Control (CDC) developed and published the first guidelines for systematic quality control in clinical microbiology to implement the Clinical Laboratory Improvement Act (CLIA) of 1967 (Federal Register, vol. 33, October 15, 1968). These regulations established quality control standards for laboratories licensed by the CDC to engage in interstate commerce and have been adopted since by the Health Care Financing Administration (HCFA), the College of American Pathologists (CAP) Inspection and Accreditation Committee, and the Joint Commission on Accreditation of Hospitals (JCAH).

IMPORTANCE

Quality control helps to ensure that data generated by personnel performing laboratory work are accurate, reproducible, and reliable. Each laboratory monitors all aspects of its performance through the establishment of multifaceted programs; these programs involve continuing education, proficiency testing, review and updating of procedure manuals (at least annually), and maintenance of records of performance tests of equipment, media, and reagents.[7,9]

Although quality control is undeniably an important part of a laboratory's work, several authors have recently questioned the cost effectiveness of certain procedures.[2,3,14] Undoubtedly, quality assurance regulations will be revised in the coming years as laboratories and accrediting agencies struggle to maintain the highest level of patient care in the face of dwindling reimbursements.

ELEMENTS OF A QUALITY CONTROL PROGRAM

Every laboratory should have written instructions for each procedure that the laboratory performs, which should be compiled in a standard operating procedure manual. This manual includes specific instructions for maintaining laboratory equipment and validating individual test results, as well as details of specific procedures to follow when results do not fall within acceptable limits (often called tolerance limits).

Quality control forms are usually developed for recording data. Figure 3-1 is an example of a form that can be used for charting the performance of incubators. The form is designed for ease of use and includes a space for recording corrective action (such as adjustments of temperature) if necessary. Some laboratories also maintain a separate problem log (Figure 3-2), which summarizes daily problems and corrective action. Quality control records should be reviewed regularly by supervisory personnel.

RECOMMENDED PROCEDURES
SPECIMENS

Guidelines for specimen quality control must be established as part of an overall quality control program because the clinical relevance of culture results depends on proper specimen collection and transport.[17] Laboratory costs are also reduced if unacceptable specimens are not cultured.[1]

The specimen quality control program begins with a detailed instruction guide for physicians and nurses; in-service training regarding proper specimen collection is also important. Specimen rejection criteria should then be established. The individual responsible for specimen setup should notify the physician, nurse, or ward clerk if a specimen is unacceptable; no specimen should be discarded. Agreement should be established with the medical staff that such specimens will be held for a limited period of time (such as 5 days) pending a call from a physician regarding processing.

Specimens are unacceptable if the patient identification on the requisition and that on the specimen container differ, or if the specimen container is leaking. Information that should be included in the requisition is noted in Table 11-1. Foley catheter tips, specimens (except stool) received in nonsterile containers, material received in fixative, dry swabs, and more than one specimen on the same day from the same source are unacceptable for culture except blood for culture. Specimens (throat, nose, mouth, lower respiratory secretions except transtracheal aspirate, vaginal and cervical swabs, urine, stool, or skin) likely to be contaminated with normal flora should not be cultured anaerobically.

As a general rule, specimens (except those of urine and sputum) should be received within 60 minutes of collection unless an appropriate transport medium is used[13]; urine and sputum should be refrigerated if not received (or processed) within 60 minutes of collection (see Chapter 11). Transport media should be performance tested, as indicated in Table 3-1.

Sputum specimens for bacterial culture should be screened by Gram stain for suitability for culture[18] by examining a grossly purulent portion of the sample under low-power magnification for the presence of squamous epithelial cells, polymorphonuclear leukocytes, alveolar macrophages, and columnar cells. Urine specimens may be screened in a similar manner by exam-

Permission to use portions of M22-T (Quality Assurance for Commercially Prepared Microbiological Culture Media; Tentative Standard) has been granted by the National Committee for Clinical Laboratory Standards. The complete current standard may be obtained from NCCLS, 771 E. Lancaster Ave., Villanova, PA 19085.

Month _____ Year _____

INCUBATOR

Unit No. _____

Temperature, Humidity, CO$_2$ Record

Date	Range 34-36 Temp °C	Range 30%-50% Humidity	H$_2$O Level*	Range 4%-6% CO$_2$	Init.	Corrective action
1						
2						
3						
4						
5						
6						
7						
8						
9						
10						
11						
12						
13						
14						
15						
16						
17						
18						
19						
20						
21						
22						
23						
24						
25						
26						
27						
28						
29						
30						
31						

*Water level adequate in humidity pan (fill with sterile deionized water)

Date	Reviewed by	Comments/Action

FIGURE 3-1. Sample quality control equipment form.

Problem Log

Problem	Date	Tech. Init.	Action taken	Reviewed by	Date	Comments

FIGURE 3-2. Sample problem log.

TABLE 3-1. Performance Standards for Transport Media and Systems

Medium	Test Organisms[a]	Incubation Conditions	Expected Results
Culturette swab	*Haemophilus influenzae* 10211	Pick one colony on swab. Reinsert swab into tube and crush vial. Hold tube at room temperature for 24 hr. Use swab to inoculate chocolate agar. Incubate plate at 35° C in CO_2 for 24 hr.	Good growth
	Streptococcus pneumoniae 6305	Pick one colony on swab. Reinsert swab into tube and crush vial. Hold tube at room temperature for 24 hr. Use swab to inoculate sheep blood agar. Incubate plate at 35° C aerobically for 24 hr.	Good growth
Cary-Blair medium	*Campylobacter jejuni* 33292	Pick one colony on swab. Place swab in medium. Hold tube at 4° C for 24 hr. Use swab to inoculate Campy blood agar. Incubate plate at 42° C under microaerophilic conditions for 24 hr.	Good growth
Jembec plate	See Selective media for pathogenic *Neisseria* in Table 3-3		
Anaerobic transport swabs	*Bacteroides fragilis* 25285	Pick one colony on swab. Reinsert swab in tube. Hold tube at room temperature for 4 hr. Use swab to inoculate anaerobic blood agar plate. Incubate plate at 35° C anaerobically for 24 hr.	Good growth
Anaerobic transport vials	*B. fragilis* 25285	Pick one colony into tube of enriched thioglycolate broth. Aseptically inject 3-5 ml of fluid into vial. Hold vial at room temperature for 4 hr. Remove 2-3 drops, and inoculate anaerobic blood agar plate. Incubate plate at 35° C anaerobically for 24 hr.	Good growth

[a]Numbers are American Type Culture Collection (ATCC) numbers. The NCCLS standard M22-T[23] recommends that manufacturers of laboratory media and users who perform quality control procedures on their own media use the ATCC strains that are indicated in this table and the following tables. These strains are also available from commercial sources.

ining a drop of uncentrifuged urine. A specimen containing a preponderance of squamous epithelial cells and few, if any, polymorphonuclear leukocytes is probably contaminated with material from the skin or mucous membranes, and a second specimen should be requested (see Chapter 11). Specimens for fungal or mycobacterial culture should be set up regardless of the cellular constituents. Specimens from patients known to be leukopenic, or from hospital locations where such patients are cared for, should be processed without regard to the presence of neutrophils unless squamous cells are seen, in which case a second specimen should be requested.

CULTURE AND BIOCHEMICAL MEDIA

Quality control testing is required for all laboratory-prepared media and for some kinds of commercially prepared, ready-to-use media. A worksheet is prepared for each lot of media used in the laboratory. Sample worksheets for commercial and laboratory-prepared media are shown in Figures 3-3 and 3-4, respectively. The worksheet for each lot of medium should be retained on file for a minimum of 2 years.

Laboratory-Prepared Media

General procedures for media preparation, including formulations, should be available for each medium prepared in the laboratory. Dehydrated media received from commercial manufacturers should be dated on receipt and again when opened; the manufacturer's expiration date should also be noted. The amount, source, lot number, and method of sterilizing all components, the date of preparation, the expiration date, the quantity prepared, and the initials of the preparer should be carefully recorded. Autoclave temperature recording charts should be saved and monitored, since excessive heating is a common source of error.

A representative sample of each lot of laboratory-prepared media should then be sterility tested. For lots of 100 or fewer plates or tubes, a 5% sample (but not fewer than two plates or tubes) is tested.[7] For larger lots, 10 randomly selected plates or tubes are incubated. Media should be incubated at the temperature at which they will be used. Bacteriologic media are incubated 48 hours, and media used for mycology and mycobacteriology are incubated for 5 days. If more than 10% of the plates or tubes are contaminated, the entire lot of medium must be incubated at 35° C for 24 hours. If more than 3% of the entire lot is contaminated, the media should be discarded. If less than 3% of the entire lot is contaminated, the contaminated plates or tubes should be discarded, and the expiration date should be changed to one half of the usual dating—for example, 4 weeks instead of 8 for plates sealed in bags and 3 months instead of 6 for screw-capped tubed media. Blood and other supplements are also sterility tested before use.

Each lot of medium must be tested to determine if it is suitable for laboratory use. Samples of commercial or laboratory-prepared media should be inoculated with stock organisms of known physiologic and biochemical properties. Maintenance

I. Identification
    A. Name: D. Date rec'd:
    B. Lot no.:   E. Expir. date:
    C. Source: F. Storage conditions:

II. Appearance of medium
    A. Packaging damage?
    B. Medium color?
            clarity?
            excess moisture or drying?
    C. Visible contamination?
    D. Date checked: By:

III. Performance test
      Test organism   Expected result   Observed result

      Date checked: By:

IV. Corrective action:

V. Final action:

FIGURE 3-3. Quality control worksheet for commercial media. If medium does not need to be retested, a stamp with words ''N/A. This medium has been tested by the manufacturer and conforms to the standards outlined in NCCLS publication M22-T'' may be used in part III.

of stock organisms is discussed below. Reference organisms should demonstrate the selectivity, inhibitory effects, colonial morphology, and growth characteristics or biochemical reactions for which the medium is intended. Suggested performance standards for commonly used media are given in Tables 3-2 to 3-11. Media that fail to perform satisfactorily after repeat testing must be discarded.

Commercially Prepared Media

Until recently, requirements for quality control testing of commercially prepared, ready-to-use culture media placed a substantial burden on the clinical microbiology laboratory. Some of this testing was considered to be unnecessary because quality control was being carried out by manufacturers. A subcommittee of the National Committee for Clinical Laboratory Standards (NCCLS) reviewed the status of the quality of commercially prepared, ready-to-use media and developed a standard for quality control practices that would apply to companies selling media to clinical laboratories and to the laboratories themselves.[23] When the NCCLS document was formulated, it was anticipated that regulatory agencies would accept the standard, but it must be understood that the standard constitutes only a recommendation and does not have the force of regulation. Nonetheless, JCAH, CAP, and HCFA have adopted the NCCLS standard.

The following paragraphs include recommendations from the NCCLS standard.[23] Readers should be sure to obtain the entire document to be aware of all of the details that cannot be covered in this chapter. The NCCLS standard applies to bacte-

riologic, mycologic, and mycobacteriologic media but does not include media used for isolation of parasites, viruses, mycoplasmas, and chlamydiae, Mueller-Hinton medium used for antimicrobial susceptibility testing, or media commercially prepared and packaged in kits consisting of two or more different substrates (primarily used for microbial identification).

The NCCLS standard recommends that the following commercially prepared, ready-to-use media need not be retested by purchasers provided that the media are obtained from commercial sources that employ the quality control criteria recommended by the NCCLS and assure the purchaser that the criteria have been met*:

1. Solid media
    a. Blood, aerobic and anaerobic
    b. MacConkey
    c. Eosin–methylene blue
    d. Colistin–nalidixic acid (aerobic)
    e. Lowenstein-Jensen
    f. Phenylethyl alcohol (aerobic)
    g. Hektoen enteric
    h. Sabouraud dextrose
    i. Xylose lysine deoxycholate
    j. Mannitol salt
    k. Middlebrook
    l. Mycology, selective
    m. Salmonella-Shigella

---

*Users must retest any medium not in this list even if it has been tested by the manufacturer.

Text continued on p. 53.

I.   Identification
     A.   Name: D.   Expir. date:
     B.   Lot no.:   E.   Storage conditions:
     C.   Date prep.:   F.   Prepared by:

II. Preparation
     A.   Ingredients
          Name   Source   Lot no.   Amount

     B.   Sterilization
                                    Base   Supplements

          Method(s):
          Time:
          Temp.:
     C.   Final pH of medium:
     D.   Total no. of plates/tubes prepared:

III. Sterility test
     A.   No. of units tested:
     B.   Time and temp. of incubation:
     C.   Results:

     D.   Date checked: By:

IV. Performance test
          Test organism   Expected result   Observed result

     Date checked: By:

V.   Corrective action:

VI. Final action:

FIGURE 3-4. Quality control worksheet for laboratory-prepared media.

TABLE 3-2. Performance Standards for Blood Culture Broths

Medium	Test Organisms[a]	Incubation Conditions	Expected Results
Blood culture bottles— aerobic[b,c]	*Streptococcus pneumoniae* 6305 *Pseudomonas aeruginosa* 27853	35° C/vented/7 days	Visible turbidity; good growth on subculture to blood agar at 35° C; Gram stain of uninoculated media should show no bacteria
Blood culture bottles— anaerobic[c,d]	*Bacteroides fragilis* 25285 *Clostridium perfringens* 13124	35° C/unvented/7 days	Visible turbidity; good growth on subculture to anaerobic blood agar at 35° C in anaerobic atmosphere; Gram stain of uninoculated media should show no bacteria
Blood culture bottles—bi- phasic for fungus[c,e]	*Cryptococcus neoformans*[f]	30° C/vented/48 hr	Good growth on agar and in broth after 48 hr; Gram stain of uninoculated media should show no bacteria or fungi

[a]Number given is ATCC number.
[b]Suspend three to five colonies in a small volume of tryptic digest casein soy broth (TSB) and incubate 4 to 5 hours to obtain exponential growth phase. Adjust turbidity to match that of McFarland no. 0.5 standard. Inoculate medium to be tested with 0.01 ml of this suspension using a calibrated loop. Incubate vented for 7 days at 35° C.[23]
[c]User testing not required if tested by manufacturer according to NCCLS standard.[23]
[d]Same as note b, but use enriched thioglycolate broth instead of TSB. Incubate unvented.[23]
[e]Inoculate one colony into 10 ml brain heart infusion (BHI) broth; mix and remove 0.001 ml (use calibrated loop) and inoculate another 10 ml BHI. Mix and remove 1 ml with sterile syringe and inoculate blood culture bottle; wash broth over agar slant. Check number of colonies in inoculum (should be fewer than 200) by removing 0.5 ml with sterile syringe and inoculating Sabouraud dextrose agar; spread inoculum for plate count and incubate for 48 hr at 30° C.
[f]Standardized reference strains have not been established.

TABLE 3-3. Performance Standards for Media Used for Aerobic, Microaerophilic, and Facultatively Anaerobic Bacteria[a]

Medium	Test Organisms[b]	Incubation Conditions	Expected Results
Sheep blood agar[c]	*Streptococcus pyogenes* 19615	35° C/aerobic or CO_2/24 hr	Good growth, beta-hemolysis
	Staphylococcus aureus 25923		Good growth
	Streptococcus pneumoniae 6305		Good growth, alpha-hemolysis
	Escherichia coli 25922		Good growth
Rabbit or horse blood agar	*Haemophilus influenzae* 10211	35° C/CO_2/24 hr	Good growth, no hemolysis
	Haemophilus haemolyti-cus[d]		Good growth, beta-hemolysis
Phenylethyl alcohol (PEA) agar[c] or colis- tin–nalidixic acid (CNA) agar[c]	*Proteus mirabilis* 12453 *S. pneumoniae* 6305 *S. pyogenes* 19615 *S. aureus* 25923	35° C/CO_2/24 hr	Inhibition, partial Good growth, alpha-hemolysis Good growth, beta-hemolysis Good growth
Chocolate agar[e]	*Neisseria gonorrhoeae* 43069, 43070	35° C/CO_2/18-48 hr	Good growth
	H. influenzae 10211		Good growth
Selective media for pathogenic *Neisseria* (including Thayer- Martin)[e]	*N. gonorrhoeae* 43069, 43070	35° C/CO_2/24-48 hr	Good growth
	P. mirabilis 43071; not to be used with media containing trimethoprim lactate		Inhibition, partial
	Staphylococcus epidermid- is 12228		Inhibition, partial

Continued.

TABLE 3-3. Performance Standards for Media Used for Aerobic, Microaerophilic, and Facultatively Anaerobic Bacteria[a]—cont'd

Medium	Test Organisms[b]	Incubation Conditions	Expected Results
MacConkey agar[c]	E. coli 25922	Aerobic, 24 hr	Good growth, rose-red colonies
	P. mirabilis 12453		Good growth, colorless colonies, inhibition of swarming
	Salmonella typhimurium 14028		Good growth, colorless colonies
	Enterococcus faecalis 29212		Inhibition, partial
Eosin–methylene blue (EMB) agars (Levine EMB agar, EMB agar, modified[c])	E. coli 25922	Aerobic, 24 hr	Good growth, blue-black colonies with green metallic sheen
	S. typhimurium 14028		Good growth, colorless to amber colonies
	E. faecalis 29212		Inhibition, partial
Xylose lysine deoxy-cholate (XLD) agar[e]	S. typhimurium 14028	Aerobic, 24 hr	Good growth, colonies red with black center
	Shigella flexneri 12022		Good growth, colonies red
	E. faecalis 29212		Inhibition, partial
	E. coli 25922		Inhibition, partial; colonies yellow, yellow red
Hektoen enteric agar[c]	S. typhimurium 14028	Aerobic, 24 hr	Good growth, colonies blue to green-blue with black centers
	S. flexneri 12022		Good growth, colonies green to blue-green
	E. faecalis 29212		Inhibition, partial; colonies yellow
	E. coli 25922		Inhibition, partial; colonies yellow to salmon colored
Salmonella-Shigella (SS) agar[c]	S. typhimurium 14028	Aerobic, 24 hr	Good growth, colonies colorless with or without black centers
	S. flexneri 12011		Good growth, colorless colonies
	E. faecalis 29212		Inhibition, complete
	E. coli 25922		Inhibition, partial; colonies pink to rose-red with precipitate
Bismuth sulfite agar	E. coli 25922	35° C/aerobic/48 hr	No growth or few colonies; pale green colonies
	S. typhi[d]		Good growth; black colonies with metallic sheen
Brilliant green agar	E. coli 25922	35° C/aerobic/24 hr	No growth or few colonies; yellow-green colonies with yellow-green zone in medium
	S. typhimurium 14028		Good growth; pink-white colonies with red zone in medium
DNAse agar	Serratia marcescens[d]	35° C/aerobic/24 hr	Clear zone after addition of 1 N HCl; DNA positive
	Enterobacter cloacae[d]		No zone after addition of 1 N HCl; DNA negative
Mannitol salt agar[c]	S. aureus 25923	35° C/aerobic/24 and 48 hr	Growth, yellow zones around colonies at 48 hr
	S. epidermidis 12228		Growth, red zone around colonies at 48 hr
Tryptic digest casein agar	S. pyogenes 19615	35° C/aerobic/24 hr	Good growth
	E. coli 25922		Good growth
Bordet-Gengou agar	Bordetella pertussis[d]	35° C/aerobic/moist jar/6 days	Good growth

TABLE 3-3. Performance Standards for Media Used for Aerobic, Microaerophilic, and Facultatively Anaerobic Bacteria[a]—cont'd

Medium	Test Organisms[b]	Incubation Conditions	Expected Results
Tinsdale agar	*Corynebacterium diphtheriae*[d]	35° C/aerobic/24-48 hr	Good growth, black colonies with brown halos
	Corynebacterium pseudodiphtheriticum[d]		Light growth, black colonies with no halos
	S. aureus 25923		No growth or few colonies; black colonies without halos
Loeffler agar	*C. diphtheriae*[d]	35° C/aerobic/24-48 hr	Good growth
Feeley-Gorman (FG) agar	*Legionella pneumophila*[d]	35° C/CO_2/moist jar/3-5 days	Good growth, browning of medium
Charcoal–yeast extract (CYE) agar	*L. pneumophila*[d]	35° C/CO_2/moist jar/3-5 days	Good growth
Thiosulfate–citrate–bile salts–sucrose (TCBS) agar	*Vibrio parahaemolyticus*[d]	35° C/aerobic/24 hr	Good growth, blue-green colonies
	Vibrio alginolyticus[d]		Good growth, yellow colonies
	E. coli 25922		No growth
Campylobacter agar[e]	*Campylobacter jejuni* 33291	Reduced O_2/42° C/48 hr	Growth
	E. coli 25922		Inhibition, partial
Tryptic digest casein soy broth (TSB)[c]	*S. pneumoniae* 6305	35° C/aerobic/24 hr	Growth
	Pseudomonas aeruginosa 27853		Good growth
Mueller-Hinton (MH) broth	*S. aureus* 25923	35° C/aerobic/24 hr	Good growth
	E. coli 25922		Good growth
Brain heart infusion (BHI) broth[c]	*S. pneumoniae* 6305	35° C/aerobic/24 hr	Good growth
	P. aeruginosa 27853		Good growth
	Candida albicans 10231	30° C/aerobic/24 hr	Good growth
Todd-Hewitt broth	*S. pyogenes* 19615	35° C/aerobic/24 hr	Good growth
	S. typhimurium 14028	35° C/aerobic/18 hr	Good growth on subculture to an enteric medium
Enrichment broths for enterics (GN broth, selenite F broth)	*S. typhimurium* 14028	Aerobic/24 hr	Good growth on subculture
	Shigella sonnei 9290		Inhibition (partial to complete) on subculture; growth on subculture from GN broth
	E. coli 25922		Inhibition (partial to complete)
Campy thioglycolate	*C. jejuni* 33291	4° C/aerobic/24 hr	Good growth on subculture to Campy blood agar at 42° C in microaerophilic atmosphere
	E. coli 25922		No growth or few colonies on subculture to Campy blood agar at 42° C in microaerophilic atmosphere

[a]To test nutrient capacity, suspend three to five colonies in small volume of tryptic digest casein soy broth (TSB) and incubate 4 to 5 hours. Adjust turbidity to MacFarland no. 0.5 standard. Dilute suspension 1:100 in normal saline, and inoculate plate with 0.01 to 0.001 ml to provide 10^3 to 10^4 CFU per plate. Isolated colonies must be produced.[23] To test inhibitory capacity, do the preceding but dilute suspension 1:10 in saline. Inoculate 0.01 to 0.001 ml to provide 10^4 to 10^5 CFU per plate. Use lighter inoculum if confluent growth occurs.[23]

[b]Numbers are ATCC numbers.

[c]User testing not required if tested by manufacturer according to NCCLS standard.[23]

[d]Standardized reference strains have not been established.

[e]User testing required of these media even when tested by manufacturer.

TABLE 3-4. Performance Standards of Media Used for Anaerobic Bacteria[a]

Medium	Test Organisms[b]	Incubation Conditions	Expected Results
Anaerobic blood agar[c]	*Clostridium perfringens* 13124	35° C/anaerobic/48 hr	Good growth (double zone of beta-hemolysis around colonies)
	Bacteroides fragilis 25285	35° C/anaerobic/48 hr	Good growth
Egg yolk agar	*C. perfringens* 13124	35° C/anaerobic/48 hr	Good growth, lecithinase positive (colonies surrounded by opaque zone), lipase negative
	Clostridium sporogenes[d]	35° C/anaerobic/48 hr	Good growth, lipase positive (iridescent sheen on surface of colonies), lecithinase negative
Brucella agar with laked blood, vitamin K₁, hemin, kanamycin, and vancomycin (LKV)	*B. fragilis* 25285	35° C/anaerobic/48 hr	Good growth
	Escherichia coli 25922	35° C/anaerobic/48 hr	No growth or few colonies
Neomycin blood agar	*C. perfringens* 13124	35° C/anaerobic/48 hr	Good growth, double-zone beta-hemolysis
	E. coli 25922	35° C/anaerobic/48 hr	No growth or few colonies
Phenylethyl alcohol (PEA) agar	*Peptostreptococcus prevotii*[d]	35° C/anaerobic/48 hr	Good growth
	E. coli 25922	35° C/anaerobic/48 hr	No growth or few colonies
Bacteroides bile esculin (BBE) agar	*B. fragilis* 25285	35° C/anaerobic/48 hr	Good growth with black colonies
	Bacteroides melaninogenicus[d]	35° C/anaerobic/48 hr	No growth
	Fusobacterium varium	35° C/anaerobic/48 hr	Good growth without black colonies
Cooked meat broth (with or without carbohydrate)	*B. fragilis* 25285	35° C/anaerobic/48 hr	Good growth
	C. perfringens 13124	35° C/anaerobic/48 hr	Good growth
Peptone-yeast-glucose (PYG) broth	*B. fragilis* 25285	35° C/anaerobic/48 hr	Good growth with pH < 5.7 after 48 hr
Anaerobic broths			
Thioglycolate medium without indicator	*Clostridium novyi* A 7659	35° C/aerobic[e]/48 hr	Good growth
	Bacteroides vulgatus 8482	35° C/aerobic/48 hr	Good growth
	Staphylococcus aureus 25923	35° C/aerobic/48 hr	Good growth
Thioglycolate medium enriched	*Bacteroides levii* 29147	35° C/aerobic/48 hr	Good growth
	C. perfringens 13124	35° C/aerobic/48 hr	Good growth

[a]Lightly touch one colony for performance testing.
[b]Number is ATCC number. See comment in Table 3-1.
[c]User testing not required if tested by manufacturer according to NCCLS standard.[23]
[d]Standardized reference strains have not been established.
[e]Caps should be tightened.

TABLE 3-5. Performance Standards for Media Used for Mycology[a]

Medium	Test Organisms[b]	Incubation Conditions	Expected Results
Sabouraud dextrose agar[c]	*Trichophyton mentagrophytes* 9533	25° C[d]/aerobic/7 days	Good growth
	Candida albicans 60193	25° C/aerobic/7 days	Good growth
Sabouraud dextrose agar with chloramphenicol and cycloheximide[c]	*Trichophyton menta-grophytes* 9533	25° C/aerobic/7 days	Good growth
	Aspergillus niger 16404		Inhibition, partial to complete
	Escherichia coli 25922		Inhibition, partial to complete
	C. albicans 10231		Good growth
Brain heart infusion	*Sporothrix schenckii*[e]	25° C/aerobic/5-7 days	Good growth

[a]Lightly touch one colony for performance testing.
[b]Number is ATCC number.
[c]User testing not required if tested by manufacturer according to NCCLS standard.[23]
[d]Incubation at 30° C may also be used.
[e]Standardized reference strains have not been established.

TABLE 3-6. Performance Standards for Media Used for Mycobacteriology[a]

Medium	Test Organisms[b]	Incubation Conditions	Expected Results
Lowenstein-Jensen (LJ) agar[c]	*Mycobacterium tuberculosis* H37a 25177	35° C/CO$_2$/up to 21 days	Good growth
Middlebrook 7H10 agar[c]	*Mycobacterium kansasii* 12478		Good growth
7H-9 broth	*Mycobacterium scrofula-ceum* 19901		Good growth

[a]Use a spadeful of growth from 4-week-old control to test broth media; use 2 to 3 drops from a broth culture of a 4-week-old control to test solid media.
[b]Number is ATCC number.
[c]User testing not required if tested by manufacturer according to NCCLS standard.[23]

TABLE 3-7. Performance Standards of Biochemical Differential Media Used for Aerobic, Microaerophilic, and Facultatively Anaerobic Bacteria[a]

Medium	Test Organisms	Incubation Conditions	Expected Results
Bile esculin (BE) agar	*Enterococcus faecalis*[b]	35° C/aerobic/24 hr	Growth (black color)
	Streptococcus, "viridans" group	35° C/aerobic/24 hr	No growth
6.5% NaCl	*E. faecalis*	35° C/aerobic/24 hr	Growth
	Streptococcus, "viridans" group	35° C/aerobic/24 hr	No growth
Hippurate hydrolysis	Group B streptococci	35° C/aerobic/4 hr	Color with ninhydrin (hydrolysis)
	Group A streptococci	35° C/aerobic/4 hr	No color with ninhydrin
Acetate agar	*Escherichia coli*	35° C/aerobic/24 hr	Growth, blue color
	Shigella flexneri	35° C/aerobic/24 hr	No growth
Acetamide agar	*Pseudomonas aeruginosa*	35° C/aerobic/24 hr	Positive = blue color
	Pseudomonas maltophila	35° C/aerobic/24 hr	Negative = no color change

Continued.

TABLE 3-7. Performance Standards of Biochemical Differential Media Used for Aerobic, Microaerophilic, and Facultatively Anaerobic Bacteria[a]—cont'd

Medium	Test Organisms	Incubation Conditions	Expected Results
Cetrimide agar	*P. aeruginosa*	35° C/aerobic/24 hr	Growth
	E. coli	35° C/aerobic/24 hr	No growth
Citrate agar (Simmons)	*Klebsiella pneumoniae*	35° C/aerobic/24 hr	Positive = blue color
	E. coli	35° C/aerobic/24 hr	Negative = no color change
Decarboxylase media Arginine	*Enterobacter cloacae*	35° C/aerobic (overlay with oil)/24 hr	Positive/alkaline = purple
	K. pneumoniae	35° C/aerobic (overlay with oil)/24 hr	Negative/acid = yellow
	E. faecalis	35° C/aerobic (overlay with oil)/24 hr	Positive/alkaline = purple
	Streptococcus bovis	35° C/aerobic (overlay with oil)/24 hr	Negative/acid = yellow
Lysine	*K. pneumoniae*	35° C/aerobic (overlay with oil)/24 hr	Positive/alkaline = purple
	E. cloacae	35° C/aerobic (overlay with oil)/24 hr	Negative/acid = yellow
Ornithine	*E. cloacae*	35° C/aerobic (overlay with oil)/24 hr	Positive/alkaline = purple
	K. pneumoniae	35° C/aerobic (overlay with oil)/24 hr	Negative/acid = yellow
Control	*E. cloacae*	35° C/aerobic (overlay with oil)/24 hr	Negative/acid = yellow
	K. pneumoniae	35° C/aerobic (overlay with oil)/24 hr	Negative/acid = yellow
	S. faecalis	35° C/aerobic (overlay with oil)/24 hr	Negative/acid = yellow
	S. bovis	35° C/aerobic (overlay with oil)/24 hr	Negative/acid = yellow
Enteric esculin agar	*K. pneumoniae*	35° C/aerobic/24 hr	Positive = black color
	S. flexneri	35° C/aerobic/24 hr	Negative = no black color
Gelatin	*Proteus vulgaris*	25° C/aerobic/24 hr	Positive = liquefaction
	Enterobacter aerogenes	25° C/aerobic/24 hr	Negative = no liquefaction
Indole broth	*E. coli*	35° C/aerobic/48 hr	Positive = red ring
	E. cloacae	35° C/aerobic/48 hr	Negative = no red color
10% dextrose slants	*P. aeruginosa*	35° C/aerobic/24 hr	Positive = acid
	Alcaligenes faecalis	35° C/aerobic/24 hr	Negative = alkaline
10% lactose slants	*Pseudomonas cepacia*	35° C/aerobic/24 hr	Positive = acid
	P. aeruginosa	35° C/aerobic/24 hr	Negative = alkaline
Lysine iron agar (LIA)	*Salmonella typhimurium*	35° C/aerobic/24 hr	Alkaline slant and butt, H_2S positive
	S. flexneri	35° C/aerobic/24 hr	Alkaline slant, acid butt
	P. vulgaris	35° C/aerobic/24 hr	Red slant, acid butt
Malonate broth	*E. cloacae*	35° C/aerobic/24 hr	Positive = blue color
	E. coli	35° C/aerobic/24 hr	Negative = no color change
Methyl red–Voges-Proskauer (MR-VP) broth	*E. coli*	35° C/aerobic/48 hr	MR positive (red color); VP negative (no red color)
	E. cloacae	35° C/aerobic/48 hr	MR negative (no red color); VP positive (red color)
Motility agar	*E. coli*	35° C/aerobic/24 hr	Motile
	K. pneumoniae	35° C/aerobic/24 hr	Nonmotile

TABLE 3-7. Performance Standards of Biochemical Differential Media Used for Aerobic, Microaerophilic, and Facultatively Anaerobic Bacteria[a]—cont'd

Medium	Test Organisms	Incubation Conditions	Expected Results
KCN broth	*P. vulgaris*	35° C/aerobic/24 hr	Growth
	E. coli	35° C/aerobic/24 hr	No growth
Nitrate broth	*E. coli*	35° C/aerobic/48 hr	Positive for nitrite
	P. aeruginosa	35° C/aerobic/48 hr	Positive for nitrite and gas
	Acinetobacter anitratus	35° C/aerobic/48 hr	Negative for nitrite and gas
Phenylalanine deaminase agar	*P. vulgaris*	35° C/aerobic/24 hr	Positive = green color after addition of ferric chloride
	E. coli	35° C/aerobic/24 hr	Negative = no color change after addition of ferric chloride
Pigment P agar	*P. aeruginosa*	35° C/aerobic/24 hr	Positive = blue or green pigment
	A. faecalis	35° C/aerobic/24 hr	Negative = no pigment production
Pigment F agar	*Pseudomonas fluorescens*	35° C/aerobic/24 hr	Positive = yellow or green pigment; fluorescence with UV light
	A. faecalis	35° C/aerobic/24 hr	Negative = no pigment production
Urea agar (Christensen's)	*P. vulgaris*	35° C/aerobic/24 hr	Positive = pink color
	E. coli	35° C/aerobic/24 hr	Negative = no color change
Triple sugar iron agar (TSI)	*S. typhimurium*	35° C/aerobic/24 hr	Alkaline slant, acid butt, with gas, H_2S positive
	S. flexneri	35° C/aerobic/24 hr	Alkaline slant, acid butt
	P. aeruginosa	35° C/aerobic/24 hr	Alkaline slant, no change in butt
	E. coli	35° C/aerobic/24 hr	Acid slant, acid butt, with gas
Jordan's tartrate	*S. typhimurium*	35° C/aerobic/24 hr	Positive = acid
	E. cloacae	35° C/aerobic/24 hr	Negative = no change
Mucate	*E. coli*	35° C/aerobic/24 hr	Positive = yellow color
	S. flexneri	35° C/aerobic/24 hr	Negative = no color change
Litmus milk	*A. faecalis*	35° C/aerobic/24 hr	Alkaline (blue)
	P. cepacia	35° C/aerobic/24 hr	Peptonization
	Enterococcus faecium[b]	35° C/aerobic/24 hr	Acid (curd or clot)
Tetrazolium agar	*E. faecalis*	35° C/aerobic/24 hr	Colonies with brick-red centers
	S. bovis	35° C/aerobic/24 hr	No growth or clear colonies
5% sucrose broth	*Streptococcus morbillorum*	35° C/aerobic/24 hr	No gelling
	Streptococcus sanguis I	35° C/aerobic/24 hr	Partial gelling
Starch agar	*S. bovis*	35° C/aerobic/24 hr	Positive = hydrolysis of starch
	E. faecalis	35° C/aerobic/24 hr	Negative = no hydrolysis
Pyruvate broth	*E. faecalis*	35° C/aerobic/24 hr	Positive = yellow
	S. bovis	35° C/aerobic/24 hr	Negative = green
Brucella broth	*Campylobacter jejuni*	42° C/microaerophilic/24 hr	Good growth as evidenced by many organisms with darting motility on darkfield examination
Carbohydrate fermentation broth (Andrade's)			
Adonitol	*K. pneumoniae*	35° C/aerobic/24 hr	Positive = yellow color[c]
	E. coli	35° C/aerobic/24 hr	Negative = no color change
Arabinose	*K. pneumoniae*	35° C/aerobic/24 hr	Positive
	P. vulgaris	35° C/aerobic/24 hr	Negative

Continued.

TABLE 3-7. Performance Standards of Biochemical Differential Media Used for Aerobic, Microaerophilic, and Facultatively Anaerobic Bacteria[a]—cont'd

Medium	Test Organisms	Incubation Conditions	Expected Results
Dulcitol	*E. coli*	35° C/aerobic/24 hr	Positive
	P. vulgaris	35° C/aerobic/24 hr	Negative
Glucose	*E. coli*	35° C/aerobic/24 hr	Positive with gas
	S. flexneri	35° C/aerobic/24 hr	Positive no gas
Inositol	*K. pneumoniae*	35° C/aerobic/24 hr	Positive
	E. coli	35° C/aerobic/24 hr	Negative
Lactose	*E. coli*	35° C/aerobic/24 hr	Positive
	P. vulgaris	35° C/aerobic/24 hr	Negative
Maltose	*E. coli*	35° C/aerobic/24 hr	Positive
	Providencia rettgeri	35° C/aerobic/24 hr	Negative
Mannitol	*E. coli*	35° C/aerobic/24 hr	Positive
	P. vulgaris	35° C/aerobic/24 hr	Negative
Mannose	*E. coli*	35° C/aerobic/24 hr	Positive
	P. vulgaris	35° C/aerobic/24 hr	Negative
Cellobiose	*K. pneumoniae*	35° C/aerobic/24 hr	Positive
	E. coli	35° C/aerobic/24 hr	Negative
Glycerol	*K. pneumoniae*	35° C/aerobic/24 hr	Positive
	P. vulgaris	35° C/aerobic/24 hr	Negative
Raffinose	*K. pneumoniae*	35° C/aerobic/24 hr	Positive
	E. coli	35° C/aerobic/24 hr	Negative
Rhamnose	*E. coli*	35° C/aerobic/24 hr	Positive
	P. vulgaris	35° C/aerobic/24 hr	Negative
Salicin	*K. pneumoniae*	35° C/aerobic/24 hr	Positive
	P. vulgaris	35° C/aerobic/24 hr	Negative
Sorbitol	*E. coli*	35° C/aerobic/24 hr	Positive
	P. vulgaris	35° C/aerobic/24 hr	Negative
Sucrose	*K. pneumoniae*	35° C/aerobic/24 hr	Positive
	E. coli	35° C/aerobic/24 hr	Negative
Trehalose	*E. coli*	35° C/aerobic/24 hr	Positive
	Edwardsiella tarda	35° C/aerobic/24 hr	Negative
Xylose	*K. pneumoniae*	35° C/aerobic/24 hr	Positive
	Serratia marcescens	35° C/aerobic/24 hr	Negative
Carbohydrate utilization media for *Neisseria*			
Glucose	*Neisseria gonorrhoeae*	35° C/aerobic/4 hr	Positive = yellow color[c]
	Branhamella catarrhalis	35° C/aerobic/4 hr	Negative = no color change
Lactose	*Neisseria lactamica*	35° C/aerobic/4 hr	Positive
	Neisseria meningitidis	35° C/aerobic/4 hr	Negative
Maltose	*N. meningitidis*	35° C/aerobic/4 hr	Positive
	N. gonorrhoeae	35° C/aerobic/4 hr	Negative
Sucrose	*Neisseria sicca*	35° C/aerobic/4 hr	Positive
	N. gonorrhoeae	35° C/aerobic/4 hr	Negative
Carbohydrate fermentation broth (bromcresol purple indicator)			
Lactose	*Streptococcus mutans*	35° C/aerobic/24 hr	Positive = yellow color[c]
	S. morbillorum	35° C/aerobic/24 hr	Negative = no color change

TABLE 3-7. Performance Standards of Biochemical Differential Media Used for Aerobic, Microaerophilic, and Facultatively Anaerobic Bacteria[a]—cont'd

Medium	Test Organisms	Incubation Conditions	Expected Results
Mannitol	S. mutans	35° C/aerobic/24 hr	Positive
	S. morbillorum	35° C/aerobic/24 hr	Negative
Inulin	S. sanguis I	35° C/aerobic/24 hr	Positive
	E. faecalis	35° C/aerobic/24 hr	Negative
Raffinose	S. mutans	35° C/aerobic/24 hr	Positive
	S. morbillorum	35° C/aerobic/24 hr	Negative
Oxidation-fermentation (OF) media			
Fructose	P. aeruginosa	35° C/aerobic/24 hr	Positive = acid[c]
	A. faecalis	35° C/aerobic/24 hr	Negative = alkaline
Glucose	P. cepacia	35° C/aerobic/24 hr	Positive
	A. faecalis	35° C/aerobic/24 hr	Negative
Lactose	P. cepacia	35° C/aerobic/24 hr	Positive
	A. faecalis	35° C/aerobic/24 hr	Negative
Maltose	P. cepacia	35° C/aerobic/24 hr	Positive
	A. faecalis	35° C/aerobic/24 hr	Negative
Mannitol	P. cepacia	35° C/aerobic/24 hr	Positive
	A. faecalis	35° C/aerobic/24 hr	Negative
Sucrose	P. cepacia	35° C/aerobic/24 hr	Positive
	A. faecalis	35° C/aerobic/24 hr	Negative
Xylose	P. aeruginosa	35° C/aerobic/24 hr	Positive
	A. faecalis	35° C/aerobic/24 hr	Negative

[a]Lightly touch four or five isolated colonies. Standardized reference strains have not been established.
[b]*Enterococcus faecalis* and *Enterococcus faecium* were previously known as *Streptococcus faecalis* and *Streptococcus faecium*. See Chapter 13.
[c]The positive and negative reactions are the same for all the carbohydrates cited for this medium.

TABLE 3-8. Performance Standards of Biochemical Differential Media Used for Anaerobic Bacteria[a]

Medium	Test Organisms	Incubation Conditions	Expected Results
Carbohydrate fermentations			
Arabinose	Bacteroides vulgatus	35° C/anaerobic/48 hr	Positive
	Veillonella parvula	35° C/anaerobic/48 hr	Negative
Cellobiose	Bifidobacterium eriksonii	35° C/anaerobic/48 hr	Positive
	V. parvula	35° C/anaerobic/48 hr	Negative
Fructose	B. vulgatus	35° C/anaerobic/48 hr	Positive
	V. parvula	35° C/anaerobic/48 hr	Negative
Glucose	B. vulgatus	35° C/anaerobic/48 hr	Positive
	V. parvula	35° C/anaerobic/48 hr	Negative
Inositol	Clostridium perfringens	35° C/anaerobic/48 hr	Positive
	V. parvula	35° C/anaerobic/48 hr	Negative
Lactose	B. vulgatus	35° C/anaerobic/48 hr	Positive
	V. parvula	35° C/anaerobic/48 hr	Negative
Maltose	B. vulgatus	35° C/anaerobic/48 hr	Positive
	V. parvula	35° C/anaerobic/48 hr	Negative
Mannitol	B. eriksonii	35° C/anaerobic/48 hr	Positive
	V. parvula	35° C/anaerobic/48 hr	Negative

Continued.

TABLE 3-8. Performance Standards of Biochemical Differential Media Used for Anaerobic Bacteria[a]—cont'd

Medium	Test Organisms	Incubation Conditions	Expected Results
Mannose	B. vulgatus	35° C/anaerobic/48 hr	Positive
	V. parvula	35° C/anaerobic/48 hr	Negative
Raffinose	B. vulgatus	35° C/anaerobic/48 hr	Positive
	V. parvula	35° C/anaerobic/48 hr	Negative
Rhamnose	B. vulgatus	35° C/anaerobic/48 hr	Positive
	V. parvula	35° C/anaerobic/48 hr	Negative
Sorbitol	B. eriksonii	35° C/anaerobic/48 hr	Positive
	V. parvula	35° C/anaerobic/48 hr	Negative
Starch	B. vulgatus	35° C/anaerobic/48 hr	Positive
	V. parvula	35° C/anaerobic/48 hr	Negative
Sucrose	B. vulgatus	35° C/anaerobic/48 hr	Positive
	V. parvula	35° C/anaerobic/48 hr	Negative
Trehalose	Bacteroides thetaiotaomicron	35° C/anaerobic/48 hr	Positive
	V. parvula	35° C/anaerobic/48 hr	Negative
Xylose	B. vulgatus	35° C/anaerobic/48 hr	Positive
	V. parvula	35° C/anaerobic/48 hr	Negative
Esculin broth	B. vulgatus	35° C/anaerobic/48 hr	Black color after addition of ferric ammonium citrate
	Fusobacterium nucleatum	35° C/anaerobic/48 hr	No color after addition of ferric ammonium citrate
Indole-nitrate broth	F. nucleatum	35° C/anaerobic/48 hr	Indole positive, nitrate negative
	V. parvula	35° C/anaerobic/48 hr	Indole negative, nitrate positive
Urease	Clostridium sordellii	35° C/anaerobic/48 hr	Positive = pink color
	C. perfringens	35° C/anaerobic/48 hr	Negative = no color change

[a]Lightly touch four or five isolated colonies. Standardized reference strains have not been established.

TABLE 3-9. Performance Standards of Biochemical Differential Media Used for Mycology[a]

Medium	Test Organisms	Incubation Conditions	Expected Results
Germ tube medium	Candida albicans	35° C/aerobic/2 hr	Positive = germ tube formed
	Candida tropicalis	35° C/aerobic/2 hr	Negative = no germ tube formed
Urea agar (Christensen's)	Cryptococcus neoformans	30° C/aerobic/3 days	Positive = pink color
	C. albicans	30° C/aerobic/3 days	Negative = no color change
Yeast fermentation sugars[b]			
Glucose	C. tropicalis	30° C/aerobic/24 days	Positive = gas produced[c]
	Cryptococcus laurentii	30° C/aerobic/24 days	Negative = no gas produced

TABLE 3-9. Performance Standards of Biochemical Differential Media Used for Mycology[a]—cont'd

Medium	Test Organisms	Incubation Conditions	Expected Results
Galactose	*Candida pseudotropicalis*	30° C/aerobic/24 days	Positive
	C. laurentii	30° C/aerobic/24 days	Negative
Lactose	*C. pseudotropicalis*	30° C/aerobic/24 days	Positive
	C. laurentii	30° C/aerobic/24 days	Negative
Maltose	*C. tropicalis*	30° C/aerobic/24 days	Positive
	C. laurentii	30° C/aerobic/24 days	Negative
Sucrose	*C. pseudotropicalis*	30° C/aerobic/24 days	Positive
	C. laurentii	30° C/aerobic/24 days	Negative
Trehalose	*C. tropicalis*	30° C/aerobic/24 days	Positive
	C. laurentii	30° C/aerobic/24 days	Negative
Yeast assimilation sugars[b]			
Glucose	*Cryptococcus laurentii*	30° C/aerobic/24 days	Positive = growth
Maltose	*C. laurentii*	30° C/aerobic/24 days	Positive = growth[c]
	C. krusei	30° C/aerobic/24 days	Negative = no growth
Sucrose	*C. laurentii*	30° C/aerobic/24 days	Positive
	C. krusei	30° C/aerobic/24 days	Negative
Lactose	*C. laurentii*	30° C/aerobic/24 days	Positive
	C. krusei	30° C/aerobic/24 days	Negative
Galactose	*C. laurentii*	30° C/aerobic/24 days	Positive
	C. krusei	30° C/aerobic/24 days	Negative
Melibiose	*C. laurentii*	30° C/aerobic/24 days	Positive
	C. krusei	30° C/aerobic/24 days	Negative
Cellobiose	*C. laurentii*	30° C/aerobic/24 days	Positive
	C. krusei	30° C/aerobic/24 days	Negative
Inositol	*C. laurentii*	30° C/aerobic/24 days	Positive
	C. krusei	30° C/aerobic/24 days	Negative
Xylose	*C. laurentii*	30° C/aerobic/24 days	Positive
	C. krusei	30° C/aerobic/24 days	Negative
Raffinose	*C. laurentii*	30° C/aerobic/24 days	Positive
	C. krusei	30° C/aerobic/24 days	Negative
Trehalose	*C. laurentii*	30° C/aerobic/24 days	Positive
	C. krusei	30° C/aerobic/24 days	Negative
Galactitol	*C. laurentii*	30° C/aerobic/24 days	Positive
	C. krusei	30° C/aerobic/24 days	Negative
Nitrate broth[b]	*Cryptococcus albidus*	30° C/aerobic/21 days	Positive
	C. neoformans	30° C/aerobic/21 days	Negative
Casein agar	*Streptomyces* spp.	30° C/aerobic/14 days	Hydrolysis
	Nocardia asteroides	30° C/aerobic/14 days	No hydrolysis
Tyrosine agar	*Streptomyces* spp.	30° C/aerobic/28 days	Hydrolysis
	N. asteroides	30° C/aerobic/28 days	No hydrolysis
Xanthine agar	*Streptomyces* spp.	30° C/aerobic/21 days	Hydrolysis
	N. asteroides	30° C/aerobic/21 days	No hydrolysis
Cornmeal agar with Tween 80	*C. albicans*	22°-26° C/aerobic/18-24 hr	Pseudohyphae, blastoconidia, and chlamydospores formed

Continued.

TABLE 3-9. Performance Standards of Biochemical Differential Media Used for Mycology[a]—cont'd

Medium	Test Organisms	Incubation Conditions	Expected Results
Potato glucose agar	*Trichophyton rubrum*	25° C/aerobic/7 days	Good growth, red pigment
	Trichophyton mentagrophytes	25° C/aerobic/7 days	Good growth, no pigment
Trichophyton agars Nos. 1, 2, 3, 4	*Trichophyton tonsurans*	25° C/aerobic/7-10 days	Enhanced growth on Nos. 3 and 4
	T. rubrum	25° C/aerobic/7-10 days	Good growth on all four media

[a]Lightly touch four or five isolated colonies. Standardized reference strains have not been established.
[b]Wickerham method.
[c]Positive and negative reactions are the same for all of the following carbohydrates.

TABLE 3-10. Performance Standards of Biochemical Differential Media Used for Mycobacteriology[a]

Medium	Test Organisms	Incubation Conditions	Expected Results
Niacin	*M. tuberculosis*	35° C/CO_2/3-4 wk	Positive = yellow color
	M. avium complex	35° C/CO_2/3-4 wk	Negative = no color change
Nitrate	*M. tuberculosis*	35° C/CO_2/3-4 wk	Positive = red color
	M. avium complex	35° C/CO_2/3-4 wk	Negative = no color change
Catalase, 45 mm	*M. fortuitum*	35° C/CO_2/2 wk	Positive = bubbles > 45 mm in tube
	M. tuberculosis	35° C/CO_2/2 wk	Negative = bubbles < 45 mm in tube
Catalase, 68° C	*M. fortuitum*	35° C/CO_2/2 wk	Positive = bubbles
	M. tuberculosis	35° C/CO_2/2 wk	Negative = no bubbles
Pigment production	*M. kansasii*	35° C/CO_2/2 wk	Positive = yellow after light exposure
	M. tuberculosis	35° C/CO_2/2 wk	Negative = buff after light exposure
Arylsulfatase, 3 days	*M. fortuitum*	35° C/CO_2/2 wk	Positive = pink color
	M. phlei	35° C/CO_2/2 wk	Negative = no color change
Growth on MacConkey agar	*M. fortuitum*	35° C/CO_2/2 wk	Positive = growth
	M. phlei	35° C/CO_2/2 wk	Negative = no growth
Iron uptake	*M. fortuitum*	35° C/CO_2/2 wk	Positive = rusty brown color in colonies
	M. chelonae	35° C/CO_2/2 wk	Negative = no color change
Sodium chloride tolerance	*M. fortuitum*	35° C/CO_2/4 wk	Positive = growth
	M. tuberculosis	35° C/CO_2/4 wk	Negative = no growth
Tellurite reduction	*M. avium* complex	35° C/CO_2/7 days	Positive = jet black precipitate
	M. kansasii	35° C/CO_2/7 days	Negative = no precipitate
Tween 80 hydrolysis	*M. kansasii*	35° C/CO_2/2 wk	Positive = red color
	M. avium complex	35° C/CO_2/2 wk	Negative = no red color
Urease	*M. kansasii*	35° C/CO_2/2 wk	Positive = pink color
	M. avium complex	35° C/CO_2/2 wk	Negative = no color change
Thiophen-2-carboxylic acid hydrazide (TCH) susceptibility	*M. bovis*	35° C/CO_2/3-4 wk	No growth at ≤ 1 µg/ml
	M. tuberculosis	35° C/CO_2/3-4 wk	Growth at ≤ 1 µg/ml

[a]Perform tests according to standard protocol. Standardized reference strains have not been established.

TABLE 3-11. Performance Tests of Media and Cell Cultures Used for the Isolation of Chlamydiae, Mycoplasmas, and Viruses[a]

Medium or Cell Culture	Test Organism	Incubation Conditions	Expected Result
Mycoplasma isolation			
SP-4 agar	*Mycoplasma pneumoniae*[b]	35° C/anaerobic/3 days	Good growth, with typical fried-egg colonies
A7 agar	*Ureaplasma urealyticum*[c]	35° C/anaerobic/2 days	Good growth, with typical brown accretion colonies
Chlamydia isolation			
McCoy cells[d]	*Chlamydia trachomatis*[e]	35° C/aerobic/48 hr	Good growth, with at least 30% of cells containing inclusions
Virus isolation			
MRC-5[d]	Herpes simplex virus[f]	35° C/aerobic/48 hr	Characteristic cytopathic effects
HEp-2[d]	Adenovirus[f]	35° C/aerobic/48 hr	Characteristic cytopathic effects
Primary rhesus monkey kidney (PMK)[d]	Parainfluenza virus[f]	35° C/aerobic/48 hr	Characteristic hemadsorption

[a]Standardized reference strains have not been established.

[b]Low passage (fewer than 20 broth passages), freshly isolated *M. pneumoniae* should be used. Organism is grown in 30 to 40 ml of SP-4 broth until turbidity and slight acidic pH are noted. Approximately 1 ml aliquots of this culture are then frozen at −70° C in small screw-capped glass vials. This stock *M. pneumoniae* should be titrated in SP-4 broth using a series of nine 10-fold dilutions; dilution series is incubated for 2 weeks at 35° C. Endpoint is read as last vial in series that shows acid pH; this becomes standard number of color-changing units to be used as test inoculum; 0.1 ml is used.

[c]Low passage (fewer than 20 broth passages), freshly isolated *U. urealyticum* should be used. Organism is grown in 30 to 40 ml of urea broth until turbidity and slight alkaline pH are noted. Approximately 1 ml aliquots of this culture are then frozen at −70° C in small screw-capped glass vials. This stock *U. urealyticum* should be titrated in urea broth using a series of nine 10-fold dilutions; dilution series is incubated at 35° C for 1 to 2 days. Endpoint is read as last vial in series that shows alkaline pH; this becomes standard number of color-changing units to be used as test inoculum; 0.1 ml is used.

[d]Continuous cell lines maintained in laboratory should be checked monthly for evidence of *Mycoplasma* contamination; this is most easily accomplished with a fluorescent dye that stains DNA. Hoechst stain kit is available from Flow Laboratories (McLean, Va.) and can be used for this purpose.

[e]Low passage (fewer than 20 passages), freshly isolated *C. trachomatis* should be used. Scrape monolayer and prepare series of four 10-fold dilutions. Inoculate 0.1 ml of cell suspension to fresh vials of McCoy cells; spin for 1 hour at 3000 rpm at 25° to 37° C, add fresh culture medium with cycloheximide, and incubate at 35° C for 48 hr. Read endpoint as last vial that shows 30% infected cells; 0.2 ml aliquots of this dilution are frozen in small screw-capped glass vials.

[f]Low passage (fewer than 20 passages), freshly isolated herpes simplex virus, adenovirus, or parainfluenza virus should be used. Monolayers are frozen and thawed in acetone–dry ice bath (16 times), and cells are scraped. Cells are pelleted, and six 10-fold dilutions are prepared using growth medium; 0.2 ml of each supernatant is added to tubes containing fresh monolayers and adsorbed for 1 hr at 35° C. Growth medium (1.8 ml) is then added, and tubes are incubated at 35° C; endpoint is read as last tube that shows 30% infected cells (by cytopathic effect or hemadsorption); 0.2 ml aliquots of this dilution are frozen in small screw-capped glass vials.

    2. Liquid media
      a. Thioglycolate
      b. Tryptic digest casein soy
      c. Gram-negative (GN)
      d. Enterococcus, selective
      e. Thiol
      f. Brain heart infusion
      g. Selenite

The manufacturers complete necessary performance testing on these media and apply criteria to testing of each medium to establish that the contamination rate is below 5%.

The user must retest certain media because they have displayed higher than acceptable failure rates; these are:
    1. Campylobacter agar
    2. Chocolate agar
    3. Any medium used for isolation of pathogenic *Neisseria* spp.

Furthermore, insufficient data have been collected to justify elimination of the need for retesting of any commercially prepared, ready-to-use medium not listed in the outline above. Tables 3-2 through 3-6 provide recommended criteria for testing of these media.

Regardless of whether additional testing is required, all laboratories must examine new lots of media from commercial suppliers for signs of damage to the packaging, which can lead to possible contamination or leakage of liquid media, difference in color or clarity as compared with previous lots, visible contamination, and evidence of dehydration or excess moisture in agar media. In the absence of specific manufacturer's guidelines, plates and tubes of media should be stored at 4° C. One exception is thioglycolate broth, which is stored in the dark at room temperature. Thioglycolate broth and other anaerobic media should not be stored at 4° C because the water condensing on the inside walls of refrigerators retains oxygen.

STOCK CULTURES

All laboratories must maintain a positive and negative control for each culture medium, biochemical reaction, and serologic determination performed. Strains chosen as quality control test organisms must exhibit predictable and reproducible reactions. Reference strains are available from several sources, including the American Type Culture Collection (ATCC) of Rockville, Md., and several other commercial suppliers. The ATCC markets freeze-dried vials of recommended reference strains for quality control of media and rapid identification systems (Preceptrol Cultures) and for Kirby-Bauer and dilution antimicrobial susceptibility testing (Susceptol Kits). Cultures dried on paper disks are supplied by Remel, Lenexa, Kan. (Bacti-Disks) and Difco Laboratories, Detroit, Mich. (Bactrol Disks). These disks are advantageous because they are stable at 4° C for up to 1 year, require no maintenance, and are inexpensive. Single disks can be removed from a vial, grown in broth for 4 to 6 hours, and plated on solid medium for use in quality-control tests. Well-characterized clinical isolates or organisms received from proficiency test programs or local or state health departments may also be used as stock cultures.

Bacterial Stock Cultures

Control strains of bacteria may be obtained from the American Type Culture Collection (ATCC), 12301 Parklawn Drive, Rockville, MD 20852, or from other commercial sources. Frozen stock cultures may be prepared but should be checked at least annually for viability and performance. These cultures may be prepared by suspending organisms in a cryoprotective medium consisting of defibrinated sheep or rabbit blood or soybean casein digest broth containing glycerol in a final concentration of 10% to 15% (vol/vol). This suspension may be frozen in a large number of small vials. When needed, these vials can be thawed and used to initiate testing of media or transferred to a solid medium for isolation of colonies. Up to two serial subcultures may be prepared to constitute primary working control cultures. In turn, three serial subcultures of the primary working control cultures may be made to provide secondary working control cultures. For testing the nutritive capacity of a medium, a suspension of the control culture adjusted to a turbidity matching a McFarland no. 0.5 standard should be diluted 1:100 in saline to result in the inoculation of 10^2 to 10^4 colony-forming units (CFU) per plate. For testing the inhibitory capacity of a medium, the cell suspension is diluted only 1:10 in saline and inoculated onto the medium to be tested using a 10 μl calibrated loop to provide 10^3 to 10^5 CFU/plate. Tube media may be tested by inoculating 10 μl of the undiluted suspension of the control culture. The incubation period varies from 18 to 48 hours depending on the medium to be tested.

Fungal Stock Cultures

Yeasts may be stored in sterile distilled water at room temperature or 4° C for long periods. A 72- to 96-hour culture on Sabouraud dextrose agar is covered with 4 ml of sterile water and agitated gently, and the yeast suspension is drawn off with a capillary pipette into a small screw-capped vial. The same technique may be used to preserve mycelial cultures. When the culture begins to sporulate, 5 ml of sterile water is added to the slant, and all surface growth is gently scraped into the water; care should be taken to prevent agar from getting into the suspension. Organisms are recovered from stock by streaking approximately 0.1 ml onto Sabouraud dextrose agar. The remainder of the stock can then be resealed and stored. Well-sporulated cultures of molds can also be maintained by the oil overlay technique just described.

Stock Cultures for Mycobacteriology

Reference cultures for mycobacteriology (the Trudeau Mycobacterial Culture Collection) may be obtained from The National Jewish Center for Immunology and Respiratory Medicine, Denver, Colo. Cultures should be grown in Middlebrook 7H9 broth, dispensed into small screw-capped tubes, and stored at −70° C.[15] Working stocks can be maintained for 3 months on Lowenstein-Jensen slants stored in the dark at room temperature.

Quality Control Material for Parasitology

Reference slides and PVA- and formalin-fixed material can be purchased from Trend Scientific, Inc., Minneapolis, Minn.

Mycoplasmal, Chlamydial, and Viral Stock Cultures

Reference strains of mycoplasmas, chlamydiae, and viruses are maintained at −70° C. The passage history of all organisms should be well documented. Reference strains are available from the American Type Culture Collection.

LABORATORY EQUIPMENT

Routine preventive maintenance is required for all laboratory equipment, and checks are scheduled according to the manufacturer's recommendations. Preventive maintenance is usually performed (1) under service contract with the instrument manufacturer or an independent company of specialists or (2) by on-site biomedical engineers. Performance standards for each unit of equipment are based on the manufacturer's performance specifications and should take into account the tolerance limits for the procedure(s) for which the unit is used. A sticker listing these performance standards, the telephone number to call for emergency service, the date of last service, and the initials of the individual who performed the maintenance is posted on each instrument. Table 3-12 lists general guidelines for various pieces of laboratory equipment; suggested monitoring procedures for laboratory equipment are shown in Table 3-13.

TEMPERATURE

Temperature measurements are made only with calibrated thermometers. The sensing section (mercury bulb) of a thermometer used to monitor temperatures between 0° and 100° C is immersed in a flask of water. Thermometers used to monitor temperatures above 100° C are immersed in mineral oil, and those used to monitor temperatures below 0° C are immersed in ethyl alcohol or a similar solution that does not freeze at this temperature. Temperature charts attached to autoclaves, freezers, and refrigerators are maintained for 2 years.

CO₂ CONTENT OF INCUBATORS

A Fyrite CO_2 measuring device (American Scientific Products, McGaw Park, Ill.; Arthur H. Thomas Co., Philadelphia, Penn.) is used to check the CO_2 content of appropriate incubators.

pH METER CALIBRATION

A set of certified buffers is used to calibrate pH meters. The recommended set includes pH 4.0, 7.0, and 10.0 buffers.

WEIGHT CALIBRATION

A set of National Bureau of Standards certified weights is used to calibrate analytic balances. These weights are stored in a cool, dry place away from any corrosive fumes. The weights should never be handled with bare hands.

STERILITY

Spore strips (Amsco, Erie, Penn.) or spore suspensions (Attest, 3M Co., St. Paul, Minn.; Proof, Amsco) are used to check

TABLE 3-12. Suggested Tolerance Limits for Common Laboratory Equipment

Equipment	Acceptable Range
Incubators	
Temperature	Stated temperature, ± 1° C
Humidity	30%-50%
CO_2 content	4%-6%
Water baths/heating blocks	Stated temperature, ± 0.5° C
Refrigerators	4°-8° C
Freezer compartments	−5° to −1° C
Freezers	−20° ±5° C
Ultradeep freezers	≤ −60° C
Hot-air sterilizers	15° to 165° C
Steam sterilizers	121° to 122° C
Bacterial count of distilled water	≤ 10 colonies/ml
Safety cabinets:	
UV lamps	≥ 70% of rated output
Air flow velocity	≥ 50 linear ft/min
Filter pressure	10 to 15 mm H_2O
Settling plates	1 colony per plate
Calibrated inoculating loops	0.01 ml ± 20% or 0.001 ml ± 20%
Automatic pipettors	± 1% of expected value
Microliter pipettes	10-200 μl ±1% 200-1000 μl ±0.5%

TABLE 3-13. Performance Monitoring Schedules for General Laboratory Equipment

Item	Frequency	Action
Incubators	Daily	1. Temperature is measured and recorded each morning.
		2. CO_2 content, if applicable, is measured and recorded each morning.
		3. Humidity, if applicable, is measured each morning.
	Semiannually	1. Thermometers used to record the temperature are recalibrated.
		2. Continuous recorders are recalibrated.
Refrigerators	Daily	1. Temperature is measured and recorded each morning.
	Quarterly	1. Refrigerator is cleaned thoroughly.
		2. Freezer compartment, if present, is defrosted and cleaned thoroughly.
	Semiannually	1. Thermometers used to record the temperature are recalibrated.
		2. Continuous recorders are recalibrated.
Freezers	Daily	1. Temperature is measured and recorded each morning.
	Quarterly	1. Freezer is defrosted and cleaned thoroughly.
	Semiannually	1. Thermometers used to record the temperature are recalibrated.
		2. Continuous recorders are recalibrated.
Water bath	Daily before use	1. Water level is checked. Level should be one half to two thirds as high as column of liquid in vessels that are being heated. Add only distilled or deionized water if level is low.
		2. Temperature is measured and recorded.
	Monthly	1. Thorough cleaning is done. Add only distilled or deionized water.
	Semiannually	1. Thermometers used to record the temperature are recalibrated.
Heating blocks	Daily before use	1. Temperature is measured and recorded.
	Monthly	1. Block is cleaned thoroughly.
	Semiannually	1. Thermometers used to record temperature are recalibrated.
Steam sterilizers	With each load	1. Temperature and duration of sterilizing cycle are checked and recorded.
		2. Temperature-sensitive indicator tape is attached to each separate item in the load that is to be sterilized.

Continued.

TABLE 3-13. Performance Monitoring Schedules for General Laboratory Equipment—cont'd

Item	Frequency	Action
	Weekly	1. Biologic indicators (spore strips or spore suspensions) are run, and results are recorded. 2. Peak temperature is measured and recorded.
	Semiannually	1. Temperature and pressure gauges are checked and recalibrated.
Hot air sterilizers	With each load Weekly	1. Temperature and duration of sterilizing cycle are checked and recorded. 1. Biologic indicators (spore strips or spore suspensions) are run, and the results are recorded.
	Semiannually	1. Thermometer used to record temperature is recalibrated.
Biologic safety cabinets	Daily before use	1. Air flow pattern is checked with an air current detector. 2. Air pressure across filter is checked.
	Every 2 weeks	1. Air flow velocity across cabinet opening is measured with air flow meter. 2. UV lights are cleaned.
	Monthly	1. Output of UV lights is measured and recorded. 2. Sterility of air flow is checked by exposure of six blood agar plates in cabinet for 1 hour. Record results.
GasPak jars	Before each use	1. Catalyst is changed in jar lid. 2. Anaerobic indicator is placed in each jar.
	Daily	1. All jars in use are checked for proper indicator change.
	Semiannually	1. Old catalyst is discarded and replaced with new catalyst.
Anaerobic glove box	Daily Monthly Semiannually	1. Anaerobic indicator is checked each morning. 1. Catalyst used in glove box is changed. 1. Old catalyst is discarded and replaced with new catalyst.
pH meters	Daily	1. Check is made to make sure that tips of electrodes are immersed in buffer or distilled water.
	Before each use	1. Temperature compensation is set if it is not automatic. 2. Meter is standardized against a certified buffer whose pH is not more than ± 2 pH units from the desired pH of the test solution. 3. Check is made to ensure that electrodes are filled. 4. Filling side arm of reference electrode is opened to atmosphere before any standardization or measurements are attempted. Close side arm when measurements are completed.
Analytic balances	Each use	1. Check is made to ensure that balance is level. 2. Weighing papers or boats are used in preference to beakers or other heavy vessels for weighing. 3. Soft brush is used to clean pan and base of balance after each use.
	Quarterly	1. Accuracy of balance is checked with set of certified weights, and results are recorded.
Spectrophotometer	Each use	1. Transmittance is checked at a specified wavelength with a suitable standard. Record results.
Water stills and deionizers	Daily	1. The pH of distilled and deionized water is checked and recorded.
	Weekly	1. Electrical conductivity of distilled and deionized water is checked and recorded.
	Monthly	1. Distilled water from spigots is cultured with Millipore Total Count Sampler. Record results.
Microscopes	Each use	1. Eyepiece and objectives are cleaned after each use. 2. Microscope is covered with plastic or similar cover at end of day.
Centrifuges	Each use	1. All loads are balanced before being centrifuged. Add 70% ethanol to carrier if load must be balanced. Be sure rubber disks are in bottom of carrier if glass tubes are centrifuged. 2. Run is monitored with tachometer if speed is critical.
	Quarterly	1. Rheostat control settings are calibrated against tachometer while typical load is being run in centrifuge.
Calibrated inoculating loops	Daily	1. Check is made for signs of corrosion, buildup, or incinerated material. 2. Check is made to ensure that loop is still round and weld has not parted.

TABLE 3-13. Performance Monitoring Schedules for General Laboratory Equipment—cont'd

Item	Frequency	Action
	Every 2 weeks	1. Used loop is replaced with newly calibrated loop.
		2. Old loop is saved for recalibration.
	As necessary	1. Calibration of old loops is checked. Those not meeting the standard are discarded.
Automatic pipettors	Daily	1. Check is made to ascertain whether pipettor is clean and operates smoothly.
		2. Check is made to ensure that dispensor is set at proper volume mark.
		3. If used for dispensing antimicrobial media, volume dispensed is checked.
	Monthly	1. All used tubing is replaced.
	Quarterly	1. Dispensor is recalibrated.
Microliter pipettors	Each use	1. Check is made for appearance and cleanliness.
		2. Check is made for leakage, inaccurate sampling, and abnormal strokes.
	Quarterly	1. Shaft, O-ring, and seal are cleaned with distilled water.
		2. Volume return level is checked (five times) on a marked pipette tip.
	Semiannually	1. Calibration is checked gravimetrically.

the sterility of autoclaves, gas sterilizers and dry heat ovens. Spores of *Bacillus stearothermophilus* are used to check autoclaves; *Bacillus subtilis* var. *niger* (see Chapter 5) spores are used to check gas sterilizers and dry heat ovens.

BACTERIAL COUNT OF TYPE 1 WATER

Reagent grade water is classified into three types based on purity.[8,19] In general, type 1 water is used for procedures requiring minimal impurities. Tissue culture methods, for example, require type 1 quality water. The bacterial count of type 1 water can be checked using a Millipore Total Count Sampler (Millipore Corp., Bedford, Mass.).

GLASSWARE

Glassware is inspected regularly, and chipped or etched glassware discarded. Glassware must also be free of residual detergent. Bromsulphthalein (BSP) solution (Hynson, Westcott & Dunning, Baltimore, Md.) may be used to detect residual detergent[11]; one randomly chosen piece of glassware from each load is tested. A small amount of detergent should be added to one piece of glassware as a positive control. Sterile glassware should not be stored more than 3 weeks before use.

CALIBRATED INOCULATING LOOPS

Inoculating loops are calibrated in a colorimetric dye-dilution procedure.[5]

UV LAMP OUTPUT

The output of UV lamps is measured with a UV lamp meter (Westinghouse SM-600 meter, Westinghouse Electric Corp., Bloomfield, N.J.; Ultraviolet Products, San Gabriel, Calif.). The UV lamp is dusted frequently so that rays are not absorbed by the dust that has accumulated on the bulb.

THERMOMETERS

All thermometers are calibrated against a reference thermometer from the National Bureau of Standards. The water in which they are calibrated must be within ($\pm$) 5° C of the temperature at which the thermometer is ordinarily used. For example, a thermometer used in a 37° C water bath must be tested in water at a temperature between 32° and 42° C. Thermometers used below 0° C may be checked at 4° C, and those used above 100° C may be checked at 90° C. Each thermometer should be tagged with the date of calibration, the calibration temperature, and the initials of the technologist who performed the check.

GAS-LIQUID CHROMATOGRAPH

Retention times of both volatile and nonvolatile products are checked once each day of use against known standards. Each new batch of medium is also checked for the presence of fatty acids to determine baseline levels.

OCULAR MICROMETER

The ocular micrometer must be calibrated for each microscope and combination of objectives used for parasitology. Ocular micrometer units are compared with a scale of known dimensions.[16] Calibration figures for the ocular micrometer are posted on each microscope for easy reference.

AIR FLOW

Air flow velocity in biologic safety cabinets is measured with an air flow meter (Gelman Instrument Co., Ann Arbor, Mich.); air flow patterns are measured with an air current detector (Safety, Inc., St. Louis, Mo.).

MICROLITER PIPETTES

Microliter pipettes are calibrated using a gravimetric procedure.[6]

CENTRIFUGE SPEED

Centrifuge speeds are calibrated with a tachometer (Pioneer Electric and Research, Forest Park, Ill.) or stroboscope (Power Instruments Corp., Skokie, Ill.)

AUTOMATIC DILUTORS

Automatic pipettors and dilutors may be calibrated in either a spectrophotometric method or a gravimetric procedure or by measuring the amount of liquid delivered into a precalibrated graduated cylinder.[12]

TABLE 3-14. Performance Test Procedures and Standards for Stains

Stain	Test	Test Interval	Expected Results
Gram stain	*Escherichia coli* *Staphylococcus aureus*	Each lot and weekly thereafter	Gram-negative rods Gram-positive cocci
Methylene blue	*Corynebacterium diphtheriae*	Each lot and each use thereafter	Metachromatic granules from Loeffler agar
Spore stain	*Bacillus* spp. *E. coli*	Each lot and each use thereafter	Positive = green spherules in red-stained rods Negative
Flagellar stain	*Proteus mirabilis* *Klebsiella pneumoniae*	Each lot and each use thereafter	Postive = peritrichous flagella Negative
Acid-fast stain (Kinyoun)	*Nocardia asteroides* *Streptomyces* spp.	Each lot and each use thereafter	Positive = red bacilli or branching forms Negative = blue bacilli or branching forms
Acid-fast stain (Ziehl-Neelsen)	Sputum with *Mycobacterium tuberculosis*[a] Sputum without acid-fast bacilli	Each lot and each use thereafter	Red bacilli No red bacilli
Auramine-rhodamine stain	Sputum with *M. tuberculosis*[a] Sputum without acid-fast bacilli	Each lot and each use thereafter	Fluorescence No fluorescence
Giemsa stain	Routine thin film blood smear	Each lot and weekly thereafter	Clear and distinct staining of white blood cells and red blood cells
Iodine solution	Formalin-treated specimen with protozoan cysts	Each lot	Cyst nuclei should stain and become clearly visible
Trichrome stain	Smear of PVA-fixed specimen with protozoan cysts	Each lot and each use thereafter	Nuclear characteristics clearly stained

[a]Positive control slides may be prepared from digestates of clinical specimens containing numerous acid-fast bacilli. Alternately, negative sputum concentrates may be seeded with an equal volume of a 7H9 broth culture containing acid-fast bacilli; the seeded concentrate should be vortexed vigorously to obtain a homogeneous suspension that contains individually occurring bacilli and not clumps of rods.[24]

STAINING PROCEDURES

Stains are checked before each batch is used with known positive and negative control cultures. Performance standards and testing intervals for common stains are shown in Table 3-14.[25] Methods of monitoring the accuracy and reproducibility of Gram-stained smears have been developed[4] and include multiple examinations of the same smear by independent observers and the preparation of suspensions of cellular constituents and bacteria to yield identical smears for subsequent examinations as unknowns.

ANTIMICROBIAL SUSCEPTIBILITY TESTING

Quality control guidelines for antimicrobial susceptibility tests have been published by the National Committee for Clinical Laboratory Standards (NCCLS).[22] Reference strains used to monitor the accuracy and precision of antimicrobial susceptibility tests are shown in Table 3-15. New lots of disks or media are tested in parallel with old lots before routine use. Moreover, weekly (rather than daily) testing of quality control reference organisms is permitted once test proficiency has been repeatedly demonstrated by daily testing. This change is based

TABLE 3-15. Performance Standards of Media Used for Susceptibility Testing

Medium	Test Organisms[a]	Incubation Conditions	Expected Results
Mueller-Hinton agar (plain)	*Escherichia coli* 25922 *Staphylococcus aureus* 25923 *Pseudomonas aeruginosa* 27853 *Enterococcus faecalis* 33186	Run new lot in parallel with lot in use. Use same standardized inoculum. Incubate at 35° C, aerobically, for 24 hr.	Zone sizes of new lot should be within ±2 mm of old lot and must fall within limits specified by NCCLS. Zone of 24-32 mm with trimethoprim-sulfamethoxazole, no colonies inside zone of inhibition.
Mueller-Hinton agar (5% sheep blood)	*Streptococcus pneumoniae*	Run new lot in parallel with lot in use. Use same standardized inoculum. Incubate at 35° C, aerobically, for 24 hr. Test oxacillin disk only.	Zone sizes of new lot should be within ±2 mm of old lot and must fall within limits specified by NCCLS.
"Chocolate" Mueller-Hinton agar	*Haemophilus influenzae*	Run new lot in parallel with lot in use. Use same standardized inoculum. Incubate at 35° C, aerobically, for 24 hr. Test ampicillin, chloramphenicol, tetracycline, and trimethoprim-sulfamethoxazole disks only.	Zone sizes of new lot should be within ±2 mm of old lot and must fall within limits specified by NCCLS.
GC agar base	*Neisseria gonorrhoeae*	Run new lot in parallel with lot in use. Use same standardized inoculum. Incubate at 35° C in CO_2 for 24 hr. Test penicillin disk only.	Zone sizes of new lot should be within ±2 mm of old lot and must fall within limits specified by NCCLS.
Macrodilution tubes, microdilution trays, or agar-dilution plates containing appropriate medium and drug	*E. coli* 25922 *P. aeruginosa* 27853 *S. aureus* 29213 *E. faecalis* 29212	Run new lot in parallel with lot in use. Use same standardized inoculum. Incubate at 35° C, aerobically, for 24 hr.	Minimum inhibitory concentrations (MICs) of new lot should be within ±1 $\log_2$ dilution of expected MIC and must fall within limits specified by NCCLS.
Wilkins-Chalgren agar	*Bacteroides fragilis* 25285 *Bacteroides vulgatus* 29327 *Clostridium perfringens* 13124 *Peptostreptococcus magnus* 29328 *Bacteroides thetaiotaomicron* 29741 *B. thetaiotaomicron* 29742 *Peptostreptococcus asaccharolyticus* 29743	Run new lot in parallel with lot in use. Use same standardized inoculum. Incubate at 35° C, anaerobically for 48 hr.	Good growth
Wilkins-Chalgren agar plates with antimicrobial agents	*C. perfringens* 13124 *B. fragilis* 25285 *B. thetaiotaomicron* 29741	Incubate at 35° C, anaerobically, for 48 hr.	Mode MICs must fall within limits specified by NCCLS.

[a]Numbers are ATCC numbers.

on the observation that the interval of quality control testing did not influence the outcome of the results on proficiency test samples sent out by the College of American Pathologists.[14]

DISK AGAR DIFFUSION TEST[22]

Disks are allowed to equilibrate to room temperature after removal from the freezer or refrigerator; exposure of cold disks to warm and humid room air causes moisture to condense in the vial and the antimicrobial agent to leach out of the disk. Disks must not be used after the manufacturer's expiration date. Standardization of bacterial suspensions must be carefully performed, and the depth of the medium must be checked routinely. Mueller-Hinton agar is monitored in regard to cation concentration, dextrose content, and pH. Reference strains may be stored on soybean casein digest agar slants at 4° C and subcultured to fresh slants every 2 weeks. Organisms may be used as long as there are no significant changes in mean inhibition zone diameters.

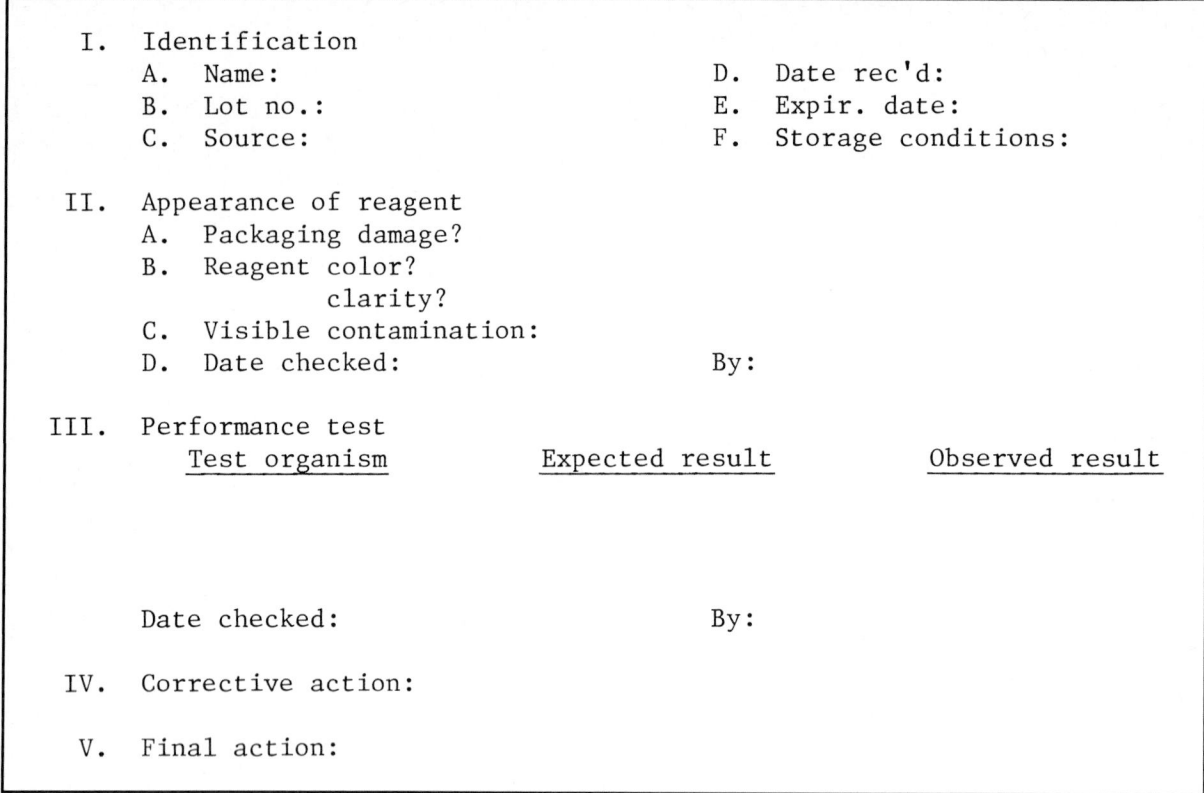

I.   Identification
      A. Name: D. Date rec'd:
      B. Lot no.:   E. Expir. date:
      C. Source: F. Storage conditions:

II.   Appearance of reagent
      A. Packaging damage?
      B. Reagent color?
                clarity?
      C. Visible contamination:
      D. Date checked: By:

III. Performance test
         Test organism   Expected result   Observed result

         Date checked: By:

IV.   Corrective action:

V.   Final action:

FIGURE 3-5. Quality control worksheet for commercial reagents.

DILUTION TESTS FOR AEROBIC AND FACULTATIVELY ANAEROBIC BACTERIA[21]

The cation content of new lots of Mueller-Hinton broth or agar is monitored. A growth control (basal medium without antimicrobial agent) is included with each test to assess the viability of the test organism, and a sample of each inoculum is streaked onto a suitable agar plate as a purity control. Additionally, the laboratory should periodically perform plate counts on representative inocula to ensure that standardization procedures are accurate.

DILUTION TESTS FOR ANAEROBIC BACTERIA[20]

The NCCLS has published proposed guidelines for an agar-dilution procedure. This technique, one of several used in the clinical laboratory, is intended as a reference method for comparison with other procedures. One or more reference strains are tested each time a test is performed.

REAGENTS AND ANTISERA

Quality control testing is required for all commercial and laboratory-prepared reagents and antisera used for diagnostic purposes. Lots of commercial reagents or antisera that do not meet the manufacturer's claims should be reported to the U.S. Pharmacopeia (12601 Twinbrook Parkway, Rockville, MD 20852).

Reagents

A worksheet is prepared for each lot of reagent used in the laboratory. Sample reagent worksheets for commercial and lab-oratory-prepared reagents are shown in Figures 3-5 and 3-6, respectively; these worksheets should be retained on file for a minimum of 2 years.

New lots of reagents from commercial suppliers are examined for signs of damage to the packaging, differences in color or clarity as compared with previous lots, and visible contamination. Chemicals should be dated on receipt, labeled with the proper expiration date, and stored in a cool, dry area; bottles should be dated when opened.

The amount, source, all the components' lot numbers, date of preparation, expiration date, initials of the preparer, and storage conditions should be carefully recorded for all laboratory-prepared reagents. Most reagents are stored in lightproof, tightly stoppered bottles at either 4° C or room temperature. The performance standards for commonly used reagents and the frequency of their testing are given in Tables 3-16 to 3-19.[10] A stock culture of each organism to be used in the test procedure should be removed from storage and streaked for purity before use; reagents are then evaluated in standard laboratory procedures. The pH of all buffers used for parasitology, myco-bacteriology, and virology is checked each time a new reagent is prepared and periodically thereafter. Reagents that fail to perform satisfactorily should not be used.

Antisera

Antisera are dated on receipt and again when opened and rehydrated. They should be stored at 4° C and should be examined for clarity and evidence of contamination or deterioration each time they are used. The reactivity of new lots of antiserum

```
  I.  Identification
      A.  Name:                    D.  Expir. date:
      B.  Lot no.:                 E.  Storage conditions:
      C.  Date prepared:           F.  Prepared by:

 II.  Preparation
      A.  Ingredients
          Name         Source        Lot no.         Amount




      B.  Special procedures (sterilization, filtration, etc.):




III.  Performance test
          Test organism      Expected result        Observed result




      Date checked:                    By:

 IV.  Corrective action:

  V.  Final action:
```

FIGURE 3-6. Quality control worksheet for laboratory-prepared reagents.

TABLE 3-16. Performance Test Procedures and Standards of Reagents for Aerobic, Microaerophilic, and Facultatively Anaerobic Bacteria

Reagent	Test Organisms	Test Interval	Expected Result
A disk (bacitracin)	Group A streptococci Group B streptococci	Each lot and weekly thereafter	Inhibition No inhibition
P disk (Optochin)	*Streptococcus pneumoniae* *Enterococcus faecalis*	Each lot and weekly thereafter	Inhibition (zone $\geq$ 16 mm) No inhibition
X, V, and XV strips	*Haemophilus influenzae*	Each lot and each use thereafter	Growth around XV strip only
Coagulase plasma	*Staphylococcus aureus* *Staphylococcus epidermidis*	Each lot and each use thereafter	Positive at 4 hr, 37° C Negative at 4 hr, 37° C and overnight at 22° C
3% H_2O_2 (catalase)	*S. aureus* *E. faecalis*	Each lot and daily thereafter	Positive = bubbles Negative = no bubbles
10% sodium deoxy-cholate	*S. pneumoniae* *E. faecalis*	Each lot and monthly thereafter	Positive = lysis Negative = no lysis
Ninhydrin	Group B streptococci Group A streptococci	Each lot and monthly thereafter	Positive = purple color Negative = no color change

Continued.

TABLE 3-16. Performance Test Procedures and Standards of Reagents for Aerobic, Microaerophilic, and Facultatively Anaerobic Bacteria—cont'd

Reagent	Test Organisms	Test Interval	Expected Result
ONPG (beta-galacto-sidase)	*Escherichia coli* *Salmonella typhimurium*	Each lot and each use thereafter	Positive = yellow color Negative = no color change
Spot indole reagent	*E. coli* *Proteus mirabilis*	Each lot and monthly thereafter	Positive (color depends on reagent) Negative
Nitrate reagents	*E. coli* *Acinetobacter anitratus*	Each lot and monthly thereafter	Positive = red color for nitrite Negative = no color change
Substrate for porphyrin test (delta-aminolevulinic acid)	*Haemophilus parainfluenzae* *H. influenzae*	Each lot and weekly thereafter	Positive = red fluorescence Negative = no fluorescence
Beta-lactamase disks	*H. influenzae* (Enzyme +) *H. influenzae* (Enzyme −)	Each lot and each use thereafter	Positive = red color Negative = no color change
Lead acetate strips for H$_2$S	*Campylobacter jejuni*	Each lot and monthly thereafter	Positive (over) TSI at 42° C, under microaerophilic conditions
CampyPak II envelope (BBL)	*C. jejuni*	Each lot	Good growth on Campy blood agar incubated at 42° C under microaerophilic conditions for 48 hr
Methyl red indicator	*E. coli* *Enterobacter cloacae*	Each lot and monthly thereafter	Positive = red color Negative = no color change
Voges-Proskauer (VP) reagents	*E. cloacae* *E. coli*	Each lot and monthly thereafter	Positive = red color Negative = no color change
Indole reagent (Kovac's)	*E. coli* *E. cloacae*	Each lot and monthly thereafter	Positive = red color Negative = no red color
FeCl$_3$ (phenylalanine deaminase)	*Proteus vulgaris* *E. coli*	Each lot and monthly thereafter	Positive = green color Negative = no color change
Oxidase Dimethyl	*Neisseria lactamica* *E. coli*	Each lot and daily thereafter	Positive = blue-black color Negative = no color change
Tetramethyl	*Pseudomonas aeruginosa* *E. coli*		Positive = blue-black color Negative = no color change
Cytochrome	*P. aeruginosa* *E. coli*	Each lot and each use thereafter	Positive = blue-black color Negative = no color change

TABLE 3-17. Performance Test Procedures and Standards of Reagents for Anaerobic Bacteria

Reagent	Test Organisms	Test Interval	Expected Results
SPS disks	*Peptostreptococcus anaerobius* *Peptococcus* spp.	Each lot and weekly thereafter	Positive = inhibition Negative = no inhibition
Nitrate reagents	*Clostridium perfringens* *Bacteroides fragilis*	Each lot and monthly thereafter	Positive = red color Negative = no red color
Indole reagents (Ehrlich's)	*Bacteroides asaccharolyticus* *B. fragilis*	Each lot and monthly thereafter	Positive = red color Negative = no red color

TABLE 3-17. Performance Test Procedures and Standards of Reagents for Anaerobic Bacteria—cont'd

Reagent	Test Organisms	Test Interval	Expected Results
C. perfringens antitoxin type A (Nagler reaction)	*C. perfringens* (with antitoxin) *C. perfringens* (without antitoxin)	Each lot and each use thereafter	Positive = inhibition of lecithinase production Negative = lecithinase production
1% ferric ammonium citrate (indicator for liquid esculin)	*B. fragilis* *B. asaccharolyticus*	Each lot of reagent and each lot of liquid esculin	Positive = brown color Negative = no color change
GasPak envelope	*Clostridium novyi*	Each lot	Good growth on anaerobic blood agar in 48 hr
Disk identification tests for *B. fragilis* Bile	*Bacteroides vulgatus* *Fusobacterium nucleatum*	Each lot Each lot	Growth up to disk Inhibition of growth around disk
Colistin (10 μg[a])	*B. vulgatus* *F. nucleatum*	Each lot Each lot	Resistant (< 10 mm) Sensitive (≥ 10 mm)
Kanamycin (1000 μg[a])	*B. vulgatus* *F. nucleatum*	Each lot Each lot	Resistant Sensitive
Vancomycin (5 μg[a])	*B. vulgatus* *F. nucleatum*	Each lot Each lot	Resistant Resistant or sensitive

[a]Disk content.

TABLE 3-18. Performance Test Procedures and Standards for Reagents Used for Mycobacteriology

Reagent	Test Organisms	Test Interval	Expected Results
Nitrate reagents	*M. tuberculosis* *M. avium* complex	Each lot and each use thereafter	Positive = red color Negative = no color change
0.2% potassium tellurite	*M. avium* complex *M. kansasii*	Each lot and each use thereafter	Positive = jet black precipitate Negative = no precipitate
Tween 80 hydrolysis reagents	*M. kansasii* *M. avium* complex	Each lot and each use thereafter	Positive = red color Negative = no red color
Urea disk	*M. kansasii* *M. avium* complex	Each lot and each use thereafter	Positive = pink color Negative = no color change
Arylsulfatase reagents	*M. fortuitum* *M. phlei*	Each lot and each use thereafter	Positive = pink color Negative = no color change
30% H_2O_2 with 10% Tween 80 (catalase)	*M. fortuitum* *M. tuberculosis*	Each lot and each use thereafter	Positive is > 45 mm Negative is < 45 mm
20% ferric ammonium citrate (iron uptake)	*M. fortuitum* *M. chelonei*	Each lot and each use thereafter	Positive = rusty brown color in colonies Negative = no color change
Niacin strips	*M. tuberculosis* *M. avium* complex	Each lot and each use thereafter	Positive = yellow color Negative = no color change

TABLE 3-19. Performance Test Procedures and Standards for Reagents Used for Parasitology

Reagent	Test Organisms	Test Interval	Expected Results
Zinc sulfate	Check specific gravity with hydrometer	Each lot and daily thereafter	Specific gravity is 1.18 (fresh specimens) and 1.20 (formalinized specimens)
Polyvinyl alcohol (PVA) fixative	Smear of stool mixed with buffy coat cells[a]	Each lot	White blood cells are well fixed; typical morphology is visible after staining

[a]Mix approximately 2 g soft, fresh stool with 10 ml PVA. Collect fresh lavender-top (EDTA anticoagulant) tube of blood; centrifuge blood and remove buffy coat (which contains white blood cells). Add several drops of buffy coat cells to PVA-stool mixture and fix for 30 minutes. Pour stool-PVA-cell mixture onto paper towels to absorb excess PVA, prepare slides, and allow them to dry thoroughly (60 minutes at room temperature) before staining.[10]

should be established before use in parallel tests with the current lot. Positive and negative controls are run with each test. Smooth, homogeneous bacterial suspensions that are stable for up to 5 months at 4° C may be prepared in-house[25] or purchased commercially; diagnostic *Salmonella*- and *Shigella*-grouping sera controls are available—for example, from Fisher Diagnostics (Orangeburg, N.Y.). Antisera quality control results are recorded, and logs are maintained for a minimum of 2 years.

AUTOMATED INSTRUMENTS AND COMMERCIAL IDENTIFICATION KITS

The large number of automated instruments and commercial identification kits precludes a separate discussion of each in this chapter. However, the package insert that accompanies the disposable items for each instrument or kit contains the manufacturer's recommendations for quality control testing. Generally, each new lot of media or reagents is tested before use; additionally, reagents for serologic detection of microbial antigens should be tested each day of use.

CHECK SAMPLES AND BLIND UNKNOWNS

Check samples and blind unknowns test both the skill of the staff and the adequacy of testing procedures. Used properly, they serve as a source of continuing education, since laboratories are often challenged to identify organisms they rarely isolate and to perform tests they may not use routinely. Critiques that are returned with the proficiency testing results contain useful, up-to-date information and should be reviewed by all staff members and discussed at general laboratory meetings. Two types of proficiency testing programs, external and internal, are available. All accredited clinical and public health laboratories are required to participate in some external program to maintain their licensure; many also choose to run their own internal surveys.

External Programs

Check samples and external unknowns are available from the College of American Pathologists (CAP), the American Society of Clinical Pathologists (ASCP), the American Association of Bioanalysts (AAB), and numerous city, county, and state health departments. Specimens are usually received on a quarterly basis, and results must be returned within a specified time. Generally, external proficiency specimens are acknowledged to receive special handling and more critical attention than routine patient cultures because they are viewed as a test of a labora-

tory's abilities. Critics of external testing programs therefore argue that this is not a valid method for assessing a laboratory's performance. These programs do have several advantages. Chief among these is that errors point up deficiencies that can then be corrected by appropriate training or changes in methodology. In addition, laboratory personnel have a chance to compare their procedures with a variety of methods used by other participants.

Internal Programs

Internal programs are administered as an adjunct to external programs. Simulated clinical specimens may be seeded with unknown bacteria, or randomly selected routine specimens may be reprocessed for analysis by different technologists. Simulated specimens might be labeled as autopsy cultures to prevent a technologist from having to search for a nonexistent patient with a reportable pathogen.

REFERENCES

1. Bartlett, R.C.: Medical microbiology: quality, cost, and clinical relevance, New York, 1974, John Wiley & Sons, Inc.
2. Bartlett, R.C.: Cost-effective quality control in microbiology, Clin. Microbiol. Newsletter 7:3, 1985.
3. Bartlett, R.C., Rutz, C.A., and Konopacki, N.: Cost effectiveness of quality control in bacteriology, Am. J. Clin. Pathol. 77:184, 1982.
4. Bartlett, R.C., et al.: Quality assurance of Gram-stained direct smears, Am. J. Clin. Pathol. 72:984, 1979.
5. Barry, A.L., Smith, P.B., and Turck, M.: Laboratory diagnosis of urinary tract infections. In Gavan, T.L., editor: Cumitech 2, Washington, D.C., 1975, American Society for Microbiology.
6. Bermes, E.W., and Forman, D.T.: Basic laboratory principles and procedures. In Tietz, N.W., editor: Fundamentals of clinical chemistry, Philadelphia, 1976, W.B. Saunders Co.
7. Blazevic, D.J., Hall, C.T., and Wilson, M.E.; Practical quality control procedures for the clinical microbiology laboratory. In Balows, A., editor: Cumitech 3, Washington, D.C., 1976, American Society for Microbiology.
8. Commission on Laboratory Inspection and Accreditation: Reagent water specifications, Skokie, Ill., 1978, College of American Pathologists.
9. Ellis, R.J.: Quality control procedures for microbiological laboratories, ed. 3, Atlanta, 1981, Department of Health and Human Services, Centers for Disease Control.
10. Garcia, L.S., and Ash, L.R.: Diagnostic parasitology clinical laboratory manual, ed. 2, St. Louis, 1979, The C.V. Mosby Co.
11. Glassware detergent check, Lab. Med. 8:113, 1977.

12. Hamlin, W.B., et al.: Laboratory instrument maintenance and function verification, Danville, Ill., 1974, College of American Pathologists.

13. Isenberg, H.D., Schoenknecht, F.D., and von Graevenitz, A.: Cumitech 9: Collection and processing of bacteriological specimens, Washington, D.C., 1979, American Society for Microbiology.

14. Jones, R.N., Edson, D.C., and Marymont, J.V.: Evaluations of antimicrobial susceptibility test proficiency by the College of American Pathology Survey Program: a clarification of quality control recommendations, Am. J. Clin. Pathol. **78:**168, 1982.

15. Kim, T.H., and Kubica, G.P.: Preservation of mycobacteria: 100% viability of suspensions stored at −70° C, Appl. Microbiol. **25:**956, 1973.

16. Melvin, D.M., and Brooke, M.M.: Laboratory procedures for the diagnosis of intestinal parasites, HHS No. (CDC)80-8282, Atlanta, 1980, Department of Health and Human Services, Centers for Disease Control.

17. Merrick, T.A.: Specimen quality assurance for the microbiology laboratory, Lab. Med. **13:**498, 1982.

18. Murray, P.R., and Washington, J.A., II: Microscopic and bacteriologic analysis of expectorated sputum, Mayo Clin. Proc. **50:**339, 1975.

19. National Committee for Clinical Laboratory Standards: Specifications for reagent water used in the clinical laboratory (Approved standard: C3-A, February, 1980), Villanova, Penn., 1980, The Committee.

20. National Committee for Clinical Laboratory Standards: Reference agar dilution procedure for antimicrobial susceptibility testing of anaerobic bacteria (Tentative standard: M11-T, April, 1982), Villanova, Penn., 1982, The Committee.

21. National Committee for Clinical Laboratory Standards: Standard methods for dilution antimicrobial susceptibility tests for bacteria which grow aerobically (Tentative standard: M7-T, January, 1983), Villanova, Penn., 1983, The Committee.

22. National Committee for Clinical Laboratory Standards: Performance standards for antimicrobial disc susceptibility tests, ed. 3 (Approved standard: M2-A3, December, 1984), Villanova, Penn., 1984, The Committee.

23. National Committee for Clinical Laboratory Standards: Quality assurance standards for commercially prepared microbiological culture media (Tentative standard), NCCLS publication M22-T, Villanova, Penn., 1987, The Committee.

24. Smithwick, R.W., and Stratigos, C.B.: Preparation of acid-fast microscopy smears for proficiency testing and quality control, J. Clin. Microbiol. **8:**110, 1978.

25. Wright, D.N., Welch, D.F., and Matsen, J.M.: Use of preserved organisms for individual test-use quality control of bacterial typing antisera, J. Clin. Microbiol. **11:**305, 1980.

CHAPTER 4

Nosocomial Infections: An Overview

Joyce S. Hayes
Barbara M. Soule
Mark T. LaRocco

Nosocomial infections represent a major hazard in health care facilities; their effects are felt by the infected patients, their families, and the health care system. Despite the many advances in modern medicine, nosocomial infections still pose a significant risk to patients and result in numerous adverse outcomes. The best current estimates place the added length of hospital stay for each nosocomial infection between 4 to 10 days depending on the type of infection.[42] Based on charges to patients and third-party payors, the estimated annual cost of nosocomial infections is about $4 billion nationwide with an average cost of $1833 per infection. The number of deaths truly attributable to nosocomial infections is staggering. Of the more than 2 million nosocomial infections that occur in U.S. hospitals annually, more than 20,000 (1 in 10) contribute directly to death and another 60,000 (3 in 10) are believed to play a significant role in the death of the patient.[42] If the 20,000 deaths were counted as part of mortality statistics, nosocomial infections would rank just below the tenth leading cause of death in the United States, and if all 80,000 deaths that are in part attributable were counted, nosocomial infections would rank as the fourth leading cause of death, just behind heart disease, cancer, and stroke.[42]

The term "nosocomial" comes from the word *nosocome* pertaining to a hospital, which is derived from the Greek word *nosos* meaning disease. Therefore a nosocomial infection is an infection associated with a hospital or a health care facility.

Nosocomial infections occur after hospitalization; they are not present or incubating at the time a patient is admitted to the health care facility.[15,51] A postoperative wound infection or pneumonia, or a bacteremia related to intravenous therapy, would be classified as a nosocomial infection. Classification of an infection as nosocomial does not mean the infection is always preventable nor that it was caused by improper technique or by an error in practice. Preventable and nonpreventable infections are discussed later in the chapter.

An infection can also be classified as community acquired, meaning that it was present or incubating at the time of admission to the health care facility. Patients admitted with a urinary tract infection, pneumonia, or hepatitis B have community-acquired infections.

CLASSIFICATION OF NOSOCOMIAL INFECTIONS

Organisms that are associated with nosocomial infections can originate from endogenous or exogenous sources.[10] Those organisms present as part of the patient's normal flora (for example, in the gastrointestinal tract) may cause endogenous infections. Exogenous infections result from transmission of organisms from external sources to the patients. Common sources are hands of health care personnel, contaminated biomedical devices, and occasionally the inanimate hospital environment.

Colonization is the presence, growth, and multiplication of microorganisms in or on a host with no clinical manifestations or detectable immune response. Infection indicates the replication of microorganisms in the tissues of the host, the response to which is variable, depending on the numerous factors discussed in Chapter 2. When the host and microorganisms interact to cause a detectable immune response but no overt signs or symptoms, the infection is subclinical, or inapparent.[10] The clinical expression of infection is known as disease and indicates that sufficient damage is being done to result in clinical signs and symptoms.[10] (It should be noted that these terms are frequently used much less precisely in clinical medicine and in the literature.) Whether patients or personnel are colonized *or* infected, they can serve as reservoirs for organisms that may cause disease if transmitted to others. Transmission of microorganisms occurs continually and is partially responsible for the endemic level of infections (that is, the "expected or usual" occurrence of disease in the health care facility).[10] An epidemic (outbreak) occurs when the level of disease exceeds the "expected or usual" frequency.[10] During investigation of an epidemic, culture studies of patients or staff may be necessary to determine colonization. These findings are used to evaluate the extent of the reservoir and design interventions to reduce infection risk or stop the epidemic. Microbiologic characterization of organisms colonizing or infecting patients (for example, by morphology, staining characteristics, growth requirements, and other attributes) can be helpful in determining their source. Methods used for epidemiologic typing, such as antibiograms, biotyping, plasmid profiles, and bacteriophage typing, are valuable as well. These methods are discussed throughout the text.

The term "nosocomial" implies a temporal relationship between admission to the health care facility and onset of symptoms. Provided an infection meets the criterion that it was not present or incubating on admission, it is classified as nosocomial regardless of the origin of the causative organisms and whether it is potentially preventable. A preventable infection is one that could have been avoided if an event related to the

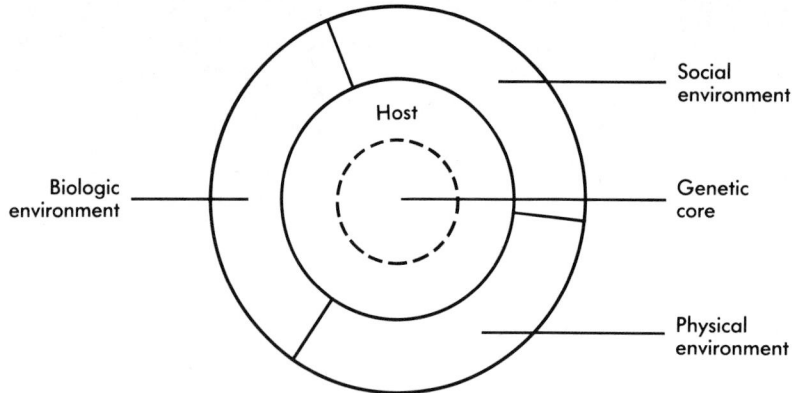

FIGURE 4-1. "Wheel" model of human-environment interactions in disease causation. (From Mausner, J.S., and Bahn, A.K.: Epidemiology: an introductory text, Philadelphia, 1974, W.B. Saunders Co.)

infection had been altered.[10] For example, handwashing before handling an intravenous device may prevent transmission of gram-negative organisms from the hands of personnel to the intravenous insertion site. The nosocomial infections that are most preventable are caused primarily by medical devices used for patient care, improper handwashing practices, and breach of surgical technique.[43,47,102] A nonpreventable infection is one that occurs regardless of all prevention strategies. An immunocompromised patient who develops a gram-negative septicemia from his normal flora (an endogenous source) has a nonpreventable infection.[10] In the 1970s the Centers for Disease Control (CDC) conducted a large study to determine the efficacy of infection control programs. In this study it was estimated that about one third of infections classified as nosocomial were potentially preventable.[47] The investigators determined that the greatest likelihood for prevention was for surgical wound infections, followed by urinary tract infections, bacteremias, and pneumonias. This prevention was achieved in hospitals that established "very effective" infection control programs, including adequate numbers of qualified staff and particular types of surveillance, reporting, and control methods.

To classify infections as nosocomial or community acquired, each health care facility must use a consistent set of definitions or criteria. Several options for definitions are available,[15,17,23] but only institutions using the same definitions and having comparable patient populations, hospital type, and size can compare their data directly. Definitions are discussed in the surveillance section later in the chapter.

EPIDEMIOLOGY OF NOSOCOMIAL INFECTIONS

Many factors influence the risk of nosocomial infection. The "wheel" model of disease causation[79] is useful for discussing the complex and dynamic interrelationship of factors specific to nosocomial infections (Figure 4-1). This model places the host with his genetic makeup at the center of activities and emphasizes the interaction between the host and the surrounding biologic, social, and physical environments.

HOST

Each patient brings to the health care setting a unique set of characteristics that influence his susceptibility to infection and the severity of infection. For example, patients with severe burns or patients receiving chronic hemodialysis, bone marrow transplants, or antineoplastic therapy have specific physiologic or immunologic defects that considerably increase their risk of infection.[12,34,72,94] The following are examples of host factors that may predispose to nosocomial infections:

1. Age
2. Sex
3. Heredity
4. Disease history or underlying disease
5. Altered immune status
6. Nutritional status (severe malnutrition, obesity)
7. Immunization status
8. Subjection to diagnostic and therapeutic procedures
9. Anatomic and physiologic alterations
10. Treatment with antimicrobial agents, chemotherapeutic agents, steroids

Other events, such as trauma, may allow entry of organisms into body areas that are normally sterile or may permit organisms that reside as normal flora in one part of the body to move to another part where they can cause disease; a ruptured bowel is an example. Congenital abnormalities, neoplasms, foreign bodies, clots, or emboli may cause obstruction and provide an opportunity for bacterial growth. All of these factors disrupt the normal host defense mechanisms (discussed in Chapter 2) and increase the potential for infection.

BIOLOGIC ENVIRONMENT

The biologic environment includes the many organisms that are potential agents of disease. The interrelationship of the host and parasite in the hospital setting involves the numerous factors discussed in Chapter 2, as well as some unique factors. Studies have shown that during the first few hours to days of hospitalization, the patient's flora (primarily pharyngeal and intestinal flora) begins to change and becomes colonized with organisms that are present in the hospital environment.[58,59,92] These organisms are frequently the major nosocomial pathogens. The characteristics of these organisms have changed over the last few years because of the advent of new therapies and technologies and the intensive and sometimes indiscriminate use of antimicrobial agents.[80] The multitude of new therapies and technologies have prolonged the life of patients, the purpose for which they were designed. At the same time, however, they have created a situation in which many patients have decreased immunocompetence.[80] Consequently, opportunistic organisms such as *Serratia* and *Pseudomonas* have emerged as important causes of nosocomial infections. Moreover, the widespread use of broad-spectrum antimicrobial agents in hospitals has resulted in the emergence of resistant strains. As a result, many of the opportunistic organisms that are responsible for nosocomial infections are also resistant to antimicrobial agents.

As discussed in Chapter 8, R factors or transposons are frequently responsible for antimicrobial resistance, and transfer of these resistance determinants can occur widely and rapidly.

In recent years methicillin-resistant *Staphylococcus aureus* (MRSA) have become important hospital pathogens (see Chapter 12). They have caused serious outbreaks,[9,29,32,91] and as early as 1972 they were reported to cause as much as 80% of staphylococcal disease (most of which was nosocomial) in European hospitals.[61] Gram-negative organisms such as *Escherichia coli, Klebsiella, Enterobacter, Serratia, Proteus,* and *Pseudomonas* have progressively become less susceptible to common antimicrobial agents. These organisms most commonly colonize patients who are very ill and in high-risk areas such as intensive care units and burn units.

PHYSICAL ENVIRONMENT
Biomedical Devices and Invasive Procedures

In addition to exposure to hazards from the biologic environment, patients undergo a staggering array of diagnostic and therapeutic procedures that may be critical for their care but also bypass natural host defenses and thus place them at increased risk of nosocomial infection.[109] In 1978, Stamm[102] estimated that about 850,000 device-related infections occur each year; this number represents approximately 45% of all nosocomial infections.

The risk associated with a device or procedure depends on the skill with which the device is used or the procedure is performed, the persistent or transient nature of contamination introduced, and the resistance of the host to the presence or manipulation of a foreign body. Biomedical devices should be used only when necessary and as briefly as possible to place the patient at the least risk of infection. Those who perform invasive procedures such as surgery, intravenous therapy, and urinary instrumentation should be well trained and competent. Biomedical devices and equipment used for invasive procedures should be sterile.[24] An overview of sterilization procedures is presented in Chapter 5. Details of the procedures for sterilization of various medical devices are discussed by Favero.[35]

Handwashing, Gloves, and Aseptic Techniques

Handwashing is the most important procedure for preventing nosocomial infection.[24] Both resident and transient flora are found on normal skin. Resident microorganisms can be repeatedly cultured from the skin where they live and multiply in superficial or deep epidermal skin layers. Transient flora are acquired during care of patients and contact with their body substances, specimens, or soiled equipment and supplies used in their care. Transient organisms can be transmitted from person to person (patients or personnel) and are most often responsible for nosocomial infection. Studies have demonstrated per-

sistent carriage of aerobic gram-negative bacteria on hands of health care personnel,[63] and epidemiologic evidence has implicated hands of personnel as a major mechanism for transmission of organisms.[14,62]

The optimal frequency and indications for handwashing have not been defined in well-controlled studies; however, the CDC has developed the following general guidelines to assist patients, staff, and personnel in the health care setting.[24] According to these guidelines, handwashing should be performed:

1. Before prolonged and intense contact with any patient
2. Before performing invasive procedures
3. Before caring for particularly susceptible patients (such as severely immunocompromised patients, newborns)
4. Before and after touching wounds
5. After microbial contamination of hands
6. After handling any body substances (such as blood, urine, feces, and sputum)
7. After touching inanimate contaminated sources (such as urine measuring devices)
8. Anytime contamination is a possibility
9. Anytime for personal hygiene

If contact with any patient's mucous membranes, nonintact skin, or moist body substances is anticipated, gloves should be worn.[24,26,52,55,111]

Transient organisms and some resident flora can be removed by handwashing using running water, friction, and soap for at least 10 seconds. Waterless combinations of various chemicals (for example, alcohol plus chlorhexidine) have also been demonstrated to be effective in reducing microbial counts of certain organisms and can be used when handwashing facilities are unavailable.[103] In some high-risk areas or for high-risk populations or procedures, antimicrobial soaps may be appropriate.[24] Antimicrobial soaps are usually indicated for clinical microbiology laboratories. Gloves should be readily accessible to personnel in patient care areas, laboratories, and departments handling soiled material.

Adherence to aseptic techniques is of critical importance in reducing the risk of nosocomial infection. Asepsis is implemented on a continuum. The least rigorous asepsis includes routine handwashing and cleaning instruments to reduce the number of organisms present. This may be called medical asepsis or clean technique.[71] The other end of the continuum is called surgical asepsis. It includes surgical scrub technique before invasive procedures and sterilization of equipment to eliminate all organisms. The degree of asepsis required for a particular situation is determined by the possibility of transmitting potentially infectious agents and by an assessment of the risk of an adverse outcome to the patient should transmission occur. The use of aseptic technique in patient care practices is discussed thoroughly in various texts.[69,71]

Inanimate Environment

Humans interact constantly with the nonliving or inanimate environment. Organisms reside in water, food, and the air and on virtually all surfaces. In a health care facility, organisms can be cultured from water faucets, bedside tables, carpets, or ventilation systems. Although organisms from these sources have occasionally been implicated in nosocomial infections, conclusively establishing their role in disease is often difficult.[96]

Organisms that proliferate in water reservoirs are potential sources of pathogenic organisms for patients. *Pseudomonas cepacia, Pseudomonas aeruginosa, Acinetobacter calcoaceticus,* and *Legionella pneumophila,* for example, have been implicated in infections related to humidifiers, air cooling towers, dialysis fluid, physical therapy tanks, intravenous infusates, and other environmental sources.[8,76,83,84,90]

Organisms such as respiratory syncytial virus (RSV) and hepatitis B are present on many hospital articles (such as blood tubes, dialysis machines, and patient care furniture).[34,50] Transmission to patients or personnel from these environmental sources has been demonstrated in some cases.[50] Even though organisms are always present in carpets and flower vases, nosocomial transmission has not been established, and infection hazard to personnel or patients from soiled linen is extremely rare.[96]

Air has been a concern as a vehicle for transmission of nosocomial disease throughout history.[56] Organisms such as *Mycobacterium tuberculosis,* varicella-zoster virus, and influenza virus are transmitted by the airborne route.[96] *L. pneumophila* and *Aspergillus* have been implicated in several airborne epidemics,[2,4,5,40,85] and *Staphylococcus aureus* is probably transmitted occasionally by air,[38] but airborne transmission is extremely rare for gram-negative bacteria. However, gram-negative organisms are responsible for the majority of nosocomial infections.[16,51]

A landmark study by Maki and associates[77] suggests that people are the primary source of the organisms that contaminate the environment. They found that floors, walls, water faucets, and sink drains in a new, uninhabited facility were relatively free from growth before occupancy. After 6 months of occupancy, however, a second set of cultures revealed organisms similar to those in the "old" facility from which the patients were transferred. The nosocomial infection rate, pathogens, and sites were not different in the new and old hospitals, suggesting that the inanimate environment contributes very little to nosocomial infection risk.

Social Environment

"People risk factors" are often difficult to distinguish from infection hazards in the biologic and physical environments. Nevertheless, certain variables particularly related to the social environment of a health care setting influence risk of nosocomial infection.

Since removal of transient organisms from hands of personnel is acknowledged to be critical for reducing risk of cross-transmission of microorganisms, an environment that promotes handwashing is important in prevention of nosocomial infections. Yet many people do not wash their hands even when they care for patients who are probably heavily colonized with microorganisms or are at significant risk for becoming infected.[3] Larson and Larson[65] found that when a physician role model washed his hands between patient contacts, medical students and house staff followed suit 48% of the time, but when no role model was present, these persons washed their hands only 24% of the times indicated. In another study the reasons for noncompliance with isolation procedures were explored. Personnel did not follow isolation guidelines because they were often unaware they had become contaminated or did not perceive that patients were infectious.[64]

The preceding are examples of social behavior that may significantly affect infection risk. Education about infection prevention and control as a student and the influence of this edu-

cation on behavior later in practice may also contribute to an individual's perception of the importance of handwashing, aseptic technique, and other strategies to reduce infection risk for patients.

Other factors that shape the social environment include administrative and financial support for the infection control program, norms and values of the staff, rewards for desirable activities, communication systems, and most important, the infection control practitioner's ability to influence behavior that will lead to practices reducing risk and incidence of nosocomial infections.

NATIONAL NOSOCOMIAL INFECTION STATISTICS

Efforts to understand the epidemiology of nosocomial infections and to estimate rates of occurrence have led to surveillance studies that began in hospitals and are now being conducted in long-term and chronic care facilities as well. Since only 2% to 4% of nosocomial infections occur as part of an epidemic,[46,110] most surveillance studies have focused on endemic infections.

Since 1970 the CDC has prospectively collected and analyzed data on the frequency of nosocomial infections in the United States through the National Nosocomial Infections Surveillance System (NNIS).[16] Approximately 50 to 75 volunteer hospitals (depending on the year) conduct active hospital-wide surveillance, using uniform definitions of nosocomial infections, and report their data monthly to the CDC. A summary of these data is published annually. The participating hospitals range in size from 80 to over 1200 beds and include hospitals owned by state and local governments and by for-profit and nonprofit organizations.[51] The NNIS hospitals are geographically representative of all U.S. hospitals. The overall infection rates reported by NNIS remained relatively constant (average of about 3%) from 1980 through 1984. This rate is probably an underestimation of true incidence of nosocomial infection because of differences in the intensity of surveillance and availability of diagnostic laboratory support.[51] By adjusting for the percent of the infections detected during this surveillance one can derive an estimate of a nationwide rate in the range of 5%.[41]

Although the hospitals enrolled in NNIS are not representative in size of all U.S. hospitals (the majority are larger, teaching hospitals), the data collected can be usefully interpreted by stratifying the reporting hospitals into nonteaching, small teaching, and large teaching categories. The nosocomial infection rate varies by category of hospital, with nonteaching hospitals having consistently lower rates than large teaching hospitals. This difference probably reflects severity of underlying illness (patient mix) and the extent to which invasive diagnostic and therapeutic procedures are performed in these hospitals.[51]

The CDC performed an extensive study of nosocomial infection programs in 1975-1976 and compared that data to information from 1970.[47] This study, known as the Study on the Efficacy of Nosocomial Infection Control (SENIC), was a retrospective chart review conducted in a representative sample of U.S. hospitals. Parts of the study were repeated again in 1983.[48] In the SENIC study the definitions used to classify the major types of associated infections were more clearly defined than in previous NNIS studies, and specially trained reviewers analyzed charts in a consistent manner. SENIC estimated that at least 2.1 million nosocomial infections occurred among the 37.7 million admissions to 6449 acute care U.S. hospitals during the 12-month period studied. The nationwide estimate was 5.7 nosocomial infections per 100 admissions, with 4.5% of hospitalized patients experiencing at least one nosocomial infection during their stay. Nosocomial infection rates appeared to increase by about 10% from 1970 to 1976. Therefore it has been suggested that infection rates are probably higher in the 1980s than in the 1970s unless the factors that increase nosocomial infection risks have changed.[42] There is no indication that such a change has occurred.[42]

The CDC has not conducted similar nationwide studies in long-term and chronic care facilities, although some investigators have performed such studies.[37,73,100] Unfortunately, these researchers used different methods to calculate infection rates and different study designs, so rates cannot be directly compared.[54] By extrapolation one expert estimates a current rate of as many as 1.5 million infections in nursing homes per year.[41] When results from systematic, observational surveillance studies in these facilities are eventually reported, infections from this older population may significantly increase the nationwide nosocomial infection rates.

The NNIS, SENIC, and other studies have generated a wealth of information about the specific characteristics and epidemiology of nosocomial infections. According to the NNIS data from 1984, the most recent study, urinary tract infections are the most frequent nosocomial infections. These are followed by lower respiratory infections, surgical wound infections, primary bacteremia, and cutaneous infections.[51] These data vary to some degree by size and type of hospital. For example, primary bacteremia accounted for a higher percentage of infections in large teaching hospitals than in either nonteaching or small teaching hospitals.

Cultures were obtained in 90% of infections reported by NNIS in 1984, and of these infections, 64% were caused by single pathogens and 20% by multiple pathogens. No pathogen was identified in 6% of the infections.[51] When a pathogen was identified, 86% of infections were caused by aerobic bacteria, only 2% by anaerobic bacteria, and 8% by fungi.[51] Together, viruses, protozoa, and parasites accounted for 5% of the infections.[51] In general, infection rates were reported to be highest on the surgery and medicine services.* This was true for all three hospital categories and suggests that the patients at highest risk of acquiring nosocomial infection are found on these services.

Escherichia coli, Pseudomonas aeruginosa, enterococci (*Enterococcus* spp.), and *Staphylococcus aureus* were the most frequently reported pathogens overall. For all services, *E. coli* was the most common pathogen causing urinary tract infections. It was followed by *P. aeruginosa* on surgery and pediatrics services and enterococci (*Enterococcus* spp.) on obstetrics, gynecology, and medicine services. *S. aureus* was most often isolated from surgical wound infections and cutaneous infections on all services except gynecology and obstetrics where *E. coli* predominated in wounds and cutaneous lesions. *P. aeruginosa* was the most common pathogen causing lower respiratory infections on all services. For primary bacteremia, coagulase-negative staphylococci predominated in patients on the newborn, pediatric, and surgical services. On the medical

and obstetrics services, the most common pathogen causing primary bacteremia was *S. aureus,* whereas on gynecology it was *E. coli.* Additional NNIS data are presented in Tables 4-1 and 4-2.

VIRAL NOSOCOMIAL INFECTIONS

From studies conducted by Valenti, Hall, and their co-workers[50,106] it is apparent that nosocomial viral infections have been greatly underreported. This has probably been due to lack of access to laboratory support for identifying viruses in most hospitals and to the absence of uniform criteria for classifying viral infections as nosocomial or community acquired. Recent developments in rapid viral diagnostic techniques and the increase in the number of clinical laboratories offering diagnostic virology services have resulted in a more accurate estimate of the incidence and importance of nosocomial viral infections. In 1980, Valenti[49,106] estimated that viruses caused over 5.3% of nosocomial infections in his facility, which led him to suggest that over 75,000 nosocomial viral infections may occur in the United States each year.

The epidemiology of viral nosocomial infections differs somewhat from that of bacterial nosocomial infection. The anatomic sites most frequently involved in nosocomial viral infections are the respiratory and gastrointestinal tracts. Over 90% of all nosocomial viral infections, but less than 15% of bacterial nosocomial infections, occur at these sites. Nosocomial viral infections occur most frequently in patients on the newborn and pediatric services (where the number of nosocomial upper and lower respiratory tract infections caused by viruses far exceeds those caused by bacteria).[106] Elderly and chronically ill adults and patients in closed or semiclosed populations (psychiatric units, nursing homes) are also at risk.[78,107,108] Viruses of primary concern in nosocomial infections include influenza viruses A and B, parainfluenza virus, respiratory syncytial virus, adenovirus, and rhinovirus. The hepatitis viruses (A, B, and non-A, non-B), some herpes viruses (cytomegalovirus, herpes simplex virus, varicella-zoster virus), and rotavirus are also well established as pathogens. Studies of over 1000 health-care workers who have been stuck with needles from acquired immunodeficiency syndrome (AIDS) patients have identified only four people who have developed HIV infection*; therefore the risk of nosocomial transmission of HIV appears low.[67a,87,88,104]

FUNGAL AND PARASITIC NOSOCOMIAL INFECTIONS

Individuals who have chronic underlying diseases or are immunosuppressed are at high risk for infections caused by fungi, as well as by bacteria and viruses. Jarvis[57] reported that over 12,000 (6%) of the nosocomial infections reported by NNIS hospitals between 1980 and 1984 were caused by fungi. The organisms most frequently identified were in the genera *Candida* (76%) and *Torulopsis* (7%). The rate of *Candida* infections doubled from 1980 to 1984. This upward trend was noted at medical school–affiliated hospitals but did not occur at nonteaching hospitals. The increase in reported rates is probably due to an increasing pool of susceptible patients, a heightened awareness in surveillance personnel, and to a lesser degree, improved diagnostic techniques (serology, open lung

---

*A service is a classification system based on similar diagnoses or treatment.

*The CDC recently reported HIV infection in three additional health-care workers following skin or mucous membrane (non-needle-stick) exposure to blood from infected patients.[26b]

TABLE 4-1. The 15 Most Frequently Isolated Pathogens and Their Percentage Distribution on Each Service, 1984

Pathogen	Service (%)						Total Isolates	%
	MED	SURG	OB	GYN	PED	NEW		
Escherichia coli	19.6	16.2	21.2	29.8	11.4	9.3	5266	17.8
Pseudomonas aeruginosa	11.4	13.0	1.3	4.3	9.7	6.7	3366	11.4
Enterococci	9.6	10.5	16.6	18.1	5.3	5.7	3063	10.4
Staphylococcus aureus	9.2	10.4	8.0	5.8	16.6	24.8	3059	10.3
Klebsiella spp.	9.0	6.9	2.1	4.8	6.6	6.7	2193	7.4
Coagulase-negative staphylococci	5.6	6.1	5.7	5.2	13.2	15.3	1868	6.3
Enterobacter spp.	4.7	7.5	2.1	3.7	4.2	3.7	1748	5.9
Candida spp.	7.0	4.9	1.1	2.2	7.6	3.8	1620	5.5
Proteus spp.	5.6	5.4	3.4	5.3	0.3	1.0	1522	5.1
Serratia spp.	2.1	2.9	0.2	0.3	1.4	1.3	691	2.3
Other fungi	2.3	1.5	0.1	0.1	1.2	1.0	496	1.7
Citrobacter spp.	1.5	1.5	1.1	0.8	1.0	0.8	414	1.4
Bacteroides spp.	0.6	1.4	4.6	2.8	0.3	0.2	355	1.2
Group B *Streptococcus*	0.8	0.5	7.9	3.8	1.2	6.2	348	1.2
Other anaerobes	0.9	0.9	4.8	2.0	0.3	0.2	300	1.0
All others[a]	10.1	10.4	19.8	11.0	19.7	13.3	3253	11.1
Number of isolates	11304	14596	1024	1016	590	1032	29562	100.0

SYMBOLS: MED, Medicine   GYN, Gynecology
SURG, Surgery   PED, Pediatrics
OB, Obstetrics   NEW, Newborn

From Horan, T.C., et al.: MMWR **35**(1SS):17, 1986.
[a]No other pathogen accounted for more than 3% of the isolates on any service.

biopsy, and fiberoptic bronchoscopy).[57] Fungal infections are often difficult to diagnose clinically and frequently are not identified until autopsy. Furthermore, the accuracy of rapid diagnostic tests has not been well assessed. For these reasons the NNIS data probably greatly underestimate the incidence of nosocomial fungal infections.

Nosocomial parasitic infections are few in number relative to bacterial, viral, and fungal infections. The exact incidence is unknown. Organisms such as *Toxoplasma gondii, Strongyloides stercoralis,* and *Pneumocystis carinii* have caused infections primarily in immunocompromised hosts with cancer, AIDS, and transplants.[12,94,98] Parasitic infections in these patients occur as reactivation of endogenous flora or from contaminated tissue organs that are transplanted from donor to patient.[12] Institutional spread of parasitic microorganisms has never been convincingly demonstrated in the United States, but scabies and other parasitic infestations have been reported in many nosocomial outbreaks.[66,67]

INCIDENCE, RISK, BACTERIOLOGIC CHARACTERISTICS, AND PREVENTION OF MAJOR TYPES OF NOSOCOMIAL INFECTIONS

The incidence, risk factors, bacteriologic factors, and prevention strategies of four major types of nosocomial infections are discussed in this section. Guidelines for prevention and control of nosocomial infections from the Centers for Disease Control,[18,21,22,24-26] data from NNIS,[16,51] SENIC,[47] and research by investigators are used as major sources of data.

URINARY TRACT INFECTIONS

The urinary tract is the most frequent site of nosocomial infection, accounting for 35% to 45% of all nosocomial infections reported by acute care hospitals each year.[18] Urinary tract infections (UTIs) are also the most common device-related infections.[18]

The majority (66% to 86%) of nosocomial urinary tract infections follow catheterization or urologic instrumentation

TABLE 4-2. The 15 Most Frequently Isolated Pathogens and Their Percentage Distribution on Each Site of Infection, 1984

Pathogen	UTI	SWI	LRI	BACT	CUT	Other	Total Isolates	%
Escherichia coli	30.7	11.5	6.4	10.1	7.0	7.4	5266	17.8
Pseudomonas aeruginosa	12.7	8.9	16.9	7.6	9.2	6.7	3366	11.4
Enterococci	14.7	12.1	1.5	7.1	8.8	7.0	3063	10.4
Staphylococcus aureus	1.6	18.6	12.9	12.3	28.9	14.6	3059	10.3
Klebsiella spp.	8.0	5.2	11.6	7.8	3.8	4.6	2193	7.4
Coagulase-negative staphylococci	3.4	8.3	1.5	14.9	11.5	11.6	1868	6.3
Enterobacter spp.	4.8	7.0	9.4	6.3	4.5	3.9	1748	5.9
Candida spp.	5.4	1.7	4.0	5.6	5.8	14.1	1620	5.5
Proteus spp.	7.4	5.2	4.2	0.8	3.3	2.1	1522	5.1
Serratia spp.	1.2	2.1	5.8	3.0	2.2	1.5	691	2.3
Other fungi	2.2	0.4	1.4	1.3	0.9	2.8	496	1.7
Citrobacter spp.	1.8	1.4	1.4	0.7	0.7	0.9	414	1.4
Bacteroides spp.	0.0	3.7	0.2	3.4	1.2	1.4	355	1.2
Group B *Streptococcus*	0.9	1.3	0.7	2.3	1.1	1.9	348	1.2
Other anaerobes	0.0	1.7	0.1	1.8	0.8	4.4	300	1.0
All others[a]	5.2	10.9	22.0	15.0	10.3	15.1	3253	11.1
Number of isolates	12218	5500	4567	2264	1690	3323	29562	100.0

> **Symbols:** UTI, Urinary tract infection
> SWI, Surgical wound infection
> LRI, Lower respiratory infection
> BACT, Primary bacteremia
> CUT, Cutaneous

From Horan, T.C., et al.: MMWR **35**(1SS):17, 1986.
[a] No other pathogen accounted for more than 3% of the isolates at any site.

such as cystoscopy.[18] About 10% of hospitalized patients are catheterized, and catheter-associated UTI develops in 20% to 25% of these.

Specific host factors associated with increased risk of UTI include female sex, older age, and increasing severity of underlying illness.[36] For the most part these factors are unalterable, and therefore many UTIs are not preventable. The factors that can be influenced include duration and type of catheterization, catheter care techniques, and the type of drainage system. Long-term indwelling catheterization is generally associated with a higher infection rate than short-term, intermittent, or single procedures.[18,36]

Escherichia coli, *Enterococcus* spp., and *Pseudomonas aeruginosa* account for the vast majority of catheter-associated UTIs.[51] Microorganisms causing UTIs can originate from endogenous sources such as the patient's bowel flora or from exogenous sources such as hands of personnel and contaminated equipment or solutions. The microorganisms may reach the bladder in several ways: (1) from the distal urethra at the time of catheterization, (2) through the lumen of the catheter (intraluminal route), or (3) along the external surface of the catheter in the mucous sheath between the catheter and urethral mucosa (extraluminal route). The last is thought to be the most common route when a closed drainage system is used.[13]

Procedures that have been shown to be most effective in reducing UTIs include using closed urinary catheter systems, employing aseptic technique for insertion and care of urinary devices, and minimizing the duration of indwelling catheterization.[18,36]

SURGICAL WOUND INFECTIONS

Surgical wound infections (SWIs) comprise about one fourth of all nosocomial infections. They are an important cause of morbidity and mortality, as well as additional hospital costs.[11,25,30]

Most nosocomial SWIs (60% to 80%) occur in the incision,

but some involve deep soft tissue or adjacent sites.[45] The three most important factors determining risk of infection are the degree of bacterial contamination of the wound, the condition of the wound at the completion of the procedure (related to surgical techniques and disease process), and the resistance of the host.[25] Patients who are very young or very old or who have infection in another body site or an underlying condition such as diabetes or severe malnutrition at the time of surgery are predisposed to infection. The presence of a foreign body, inadequate blood supply, or devitalized tissue places the patient at additional risk.

Gram-negative aerobic bacilli comprise approximately 40% of the pathogens isolated from surgical wounds, but *Staphylococcus aureus* is the single most frequently isolated species.[51] Fungi and viruses are not common isolates. Organisms responsible for SWIs appear to be commonly acquired from the patient's endogenous flora; organisms from the gastrointestinal tract are frequent isolates.[99] Exogenous contamination can come from personnel or environmental sources. Regardless of the source, most SWIs appear to result from contamination occurring during the surgical procedure.[25]

Control of bacterial contamination is the goal of a myriad of surgery-related procedures. Special methods for processing, wrapping, and storing surgical equipment, for scrubbing and gowning, and for ventilation and traffic patterns are a few examples. These and other procedures have been part of operating room practice for many years. In the past decade, research data have helped clarify those procedures that are truly effective as infection prevention control strategies.

Measures that have been associated with a reduction in infection rates include preoperative treatment of active infections, a brief preoperative hospital stay, eliminating or reducing shaving of the operative site, thorough cleansing of the skin of both the surgical team and the patients, and the use of prophylactic antimicrobial agents for certain high-risk procedures.[25] Ultimately, however, skillful surgical technique with careful intraoperative management of the patient is the key to minimizing infection risk. Infection prevention and control efforts should be directed toward achieving this goal.[25]

Nosocomial Pneumonia

Nosocomial pneumonia accounts for 10% to 20% of all hospital-associated infections. Nosocomial pneumonias have the highest case-fatality rate of any of the nosocomial infections.[22,39]

Aerobic gram-negative bacilli are the primary group of pathogens causing pneumonias. *Pseudomonas* spp., *Klebsiella* spp., and *Staphylococcus aureus* were most often reported in the 1984 NNIS study.[51] *Enterobacter* spp. also represented a significant number of cases. Fungi were reported less often and anaerobes only occasionally.[51] A study published in 1980 by Valenti and others[106] established that viruses were responsible for 20% of nosocomial pneumonias in their hospital, with respiratory syncytial, parainfluenza, and influenza viruses predominating in a large number of cases.

Organisms are believed to gain access to the lower respiratory tract primarily through aspiration from secretions of colonized upper airway tracts. The oropharyngeal region of the majority of healthy individuals does not support the growth of aerobic gram-negative bacilli; however, chronically or severely ill hospitalized patients rapidly become colonized with these bacteria.[58,59,92] The organisms may be acquired from exogenous sources, such as the hands of medical personnel, contaminated respiratory equipment, or contaminated fluids and medications introduced into the respiratory system,[95] or they may spread from the patient's endogenous flora, most likely in the gastrointestinal tract.[98]

Patients at greatest risk for nosocomial pneumonia are those who have abnormal swallowing or other conditions predisposing to aspiration, have had recent surgery, are colonized with gram-negative bacilli, have impaired immunologic functions, or are using respiratory therapy equipment for prolonged periods.[22] The SENIC study reported that 75% of cases of nosocomial pneumonia occur in patients who have had surgery, particularly thoracoabdominal operations.

Control measures are extensive and include care of the patient before and after surgical procedures, care of the respiratory therapy and anesthesia equipment, handwashing precautions or use of gloves during direct care procedures such as suctioning and care of tracheostomies, and where possible, reduction of colonization and enhancement of host defenses (for example, with vaccines or cessation of smoking).[22]

Nosocomial Bacteremias Resulting from Infusion Therapy

About 20 million patients, or over 50% of patients hospitalized in the United States each year, receive infusion therapy.[74] This therapy allows direct access to a patient's vascular system for hemodynamic monitoring and administration of medications, blood products, electrolytes, and other therapeutic agents. However, cannulas (catheters) inserted into the cardiovascular system bypass the normal defenses of the skin and provide a potential route for microorganisms to enter and cause infection. A fibrin sheath forms around the intravenous portion of the cannula soon after insertion. This sheath provides a site for replication of organisms that may be introduced from the patient's own skin flora or from the hands of hospital personnel during insertion of the cannula.[74] Intravenous therapy–related infections may also follow the infusion of contaminated fluids.

At least one third of all epidemics of nosocomial bacteremia and another one third of endemic bacteremias result from infusion therapy.[74] Generally, infections associated with contaminated cannulas are endemic in nature, whereas infusate-related infections are more commonly associated with epidemics.[74]

Gram-positive and gram-negative aerobic bacteria, as well as *Candida* spp., are responsible for bacteremia in cannula-associated infections. Coagulase-negative staphylococci that are introduced from the skin cause over 50% of these infections.[74] Bacteremia resulting from the infusion of contaminated fluid is most frequently associated with members of the genera *Klebsiella, Enterobacter,* and *Serratia.* Organisms such as *Pseudomonas cepacia, Enterobacter cloacae,* and *Enterobacter agglomerans* have also been reported in epidemics.[76] Isolation of these organisms from the blood of patients with infusion devices and no other site of infection should prompt an immediate investigation of the infusate as a potential source of infection.[60]

In general, infection hazards appear greater with plastic catheters, long catheters, and catheters inserted into the central circulation (for example, Hickman-Broviac catheters). The risk appears to be less with steel needles, short catheters, and peripheral venous catheters.[74] Catheters placed by surgical cutdown (that is, incisions made through the skin) are more hazardous than those inserted percutaneously through the skin. With every type of cannula in a peripheral vessel, the risk of bacteremia increases the longer the device is left in place.[21,74]

A number of host factors increase the risk of infection from intravascular devices: trauma near the site of insertion, immunosuppression, cardiovascular implants or structural defects, remote sites of infection, and severe malnutrition.[21]

The risk of infection from intravenous devices can be significantly reduced by meticulous attention to aseptic technique during insertion and care of any intravenous device. Equipment should be sterile; strict aseptic technique should be used at all times. Guidelines for appropriate selection of the type of cannula, area of placement, and method of insertion have been published. Duration of cannulation is an important risk factor. Although removal of the cannula after 48 to 72 hours and tubing changes at 48 hours have been recommended to reduce infection risk, ongoing studies are reevaluating these recommendations.[21,86]

Strategies for reducing infection risk and guidelines and recommendations for patient care are reevaluated as new data become available. Nosocomial infections will never be eliminated entirely, but efforts to achieve the maximal number of preventable infections continue.

INFECTION CONTROL PROGRAM
INFECTION CONTROL COMMITTEE

Although the American Hospital Association recommended the establishment of infection control committees as early as 1958, only in the last 15 years have hospitals established structured programs aimed at the surveillance and control of nosocomial infections.[44] The infection control committee in today's hospital setting is the central decision- and policy-making body for infection control in the hospital. This is a multidisciplinary committee whose membership may include an infectious disease physician, infection control practitioner, microbiologist, hospital epidemiologist, surgeon, hospital administrator, employee health nurse, pharmacist, and personnel representing various support services such as housekeeping and central services. Several accrediting bodies, government agencies, and national organizations outline and define the primary activities of an infection control committee. The Joint Commission on the Accreditation of Hospitals (JCAH) provides minimum standards for an infection control program in an institution.[60] Compliance with these standards is mandatory for accreditation of the hospital by JCAH.

The CDC, an agency of the U.S. Department of Health and Human Services, has an organizational unit, the Hospital Infections Program (HIP) in the Center for Infectious Diseases, that is involved exclusively with prevention of nosocomial infections. HIP personnel evaluate methods for the prevention and control of nosocomial infections and, based on these studies, publish recommendations for use by hospital infection control committees.

INFECTION CONTROL PRACTITIONER

The infection control practitioner (ICP) occupies a key position in the infection control program. The practitioner must have knowledge of infection prevention and control and the ability to influence their practice at all levels in the health care setting. In the past, over 95% of the individuals holding this position have been nurses. Now professionals from other disciplines such as microbiology, public health, and epidemiology are entering the field in greater numbers.[70] The Association for Practitioners in Infection Control (APIC), founded in 1972, is the professional organization for ICPs and offers support at the local and national levels. ICPs have similar responsibilities regardless of the size and type of the hospital in which they work. These include surveillance, education, consultation, research, and epidemiologic investigation.[33]

Surveillance

Surveillance is a systematic method of collecting, recording, and analyzing data about patients with infections so proper measures can be instituted.

Data sources for nosocomial infection surveillance in health care facilities include the following[53]:
1. Admission records
2. Autopsy reports
3. Interviews and ward rounds
4. Medical records (physician and nurses' notes, progress notes, therapy records)
5. Microbiology data (culture results, antimicrobial susceptibility tests)
6. Operating room records
7. Patient care plans (Kardex)
8. Pharmacy
9. Radiographic data
10. Temperature records

Several surveillance methods can be used.[70] Use of standard criteria to classify nosocomial infections is essential to have consistent and comparable data. Health care facilities use definitions for classification of infections developed by the CDC or NNIS or develop their own criteria. The major purpose and benefits of surveillance in infection control programs are to establish a system to evaluate the incidence of nosocomial infections and the factors that influence their development, to identify hospital practices that may result in nosocomial infections, to meet national and local accreditation standards, to use an epidemiologic approach to evaluate infections and other events, and to provide direction for the infection control committee.[70]

The microbiology laboratory plays a major role in surveillance by providing the ICP with the microbiologic data needed for an infection surveillance system.

Education

Education of hospital personnel, patients, and the community about nosocomial infections is an important function of the ICP. The ICP is responsible for providing information regarding disease entities and the use and rationale of policies and procedures. A strong education program can help achieve the goals of the infection control program.

Consultation

The ICP is a person with specialized knowledge who functions as a consultant on infection prevention and control issues for various departments within the institution. The ICP acts as a resource in finding solutions to infection control problems and assists in the planning to minimize infection risks. In this role the ICP helps develop policies and procedures, evaluate products, and manage patient care. For example, the employee health department can consult with the ICP on issues such as vaccines for employees, treatment after exposure to an infectious agent, and development of policies.

Research

Most published infection control research has been conducted by physicians and microbiologists. In the past few years, however, ICPs have made valuable contributions to the study of infection control. Research performed by ICPs will become more predominant in this field in the future.

Epidemiologic Investigations

A classic epidemic is marked by an unusual, statistically significant increase in the incidence of a particular disease; it usually occurs during a brief interval, involves a specific patient population with defined susceptibility factors, and is caused by a single microbial strain.[31] Any cluster of infections that might fall into this category needs to be evaluated. When outbreaks of nosocomial infections are identified, they should be dealt with as rapidly as possible. The ICP and laboratory personnel work collaboratively in handling the epidemic situation. This may require the laboratory staff to process and evaluate large numbers of cultures, not only from patients but also from personnel who may be colonized with the epidemic strain.

TRAINING AND STANDARDS

To meet all of the responsibilities and expectations, an ICP must be well trained. APIC recognized the need for a uniform approach to infection control practice and the necessity of providing educational resources for professionals working in the field. In 1981, APIC identified the following eight educational standards that represent the knowledge base necessary for the effective practice of infection control:
1. Epidemiology and statistics
2. Microbiology
3. Infectious diseases
4. Sterilization, disinfection, and sanitation
5. Patient care practices
6. Education
7. Management and communication skills
8. Employee health

Information for all standards was consolidated into a single publication, *The APIC Curriculum for Infection Control Practice*,[101] published in 1983.

ROLE OF THE MICROBIOLOGY LABORATORY

An essential feature of a successful infection control program is the optimum utilization of the clinical microbiology laboratory. Close cooperation between the laboratory and the ICP is of key importance. The laboratory can help the ICP understand what constitutes an appropriate specimen for microbiologic evaluation, the characteristics of specific pathogenic organisms, the organisms that comprise the normal flora of certain anatomic sites, and how antimicrobial susceptibility tests are performed and interpreted.

In many hospitals the laboratory representative brings to the infection control committee the necessary expertise for determining the significance of laboratory data and how the data

may influence surveillance, cluster or outbreak investigations, or special studies. The laboratory performs several functions that contribute to effective nosocomial infection prevention and control.[81]

ACCURATE IDENTIFICATION OF ORGANISMS

The laboratory must be able to identify microorganisms in positive cultures regardless of whether the cultures represent true infection or colonization. This helps the ICP track the source or movement of organisms in the health care facility. The laboratory should closely monitor the quality of specimens so the information presented to the ICP reflects organisms actually associated with the patient's site of culture rather than contaminants. Quality of a specimen should be assessed at the time the laboratory receives it. The examination of Gram stains of sputa and wounds is an excellent method for determining the quality of these specimens.[7] An aggressive approach by the laboratory in processing only good-quality specimens not only provides more accurate infection control data but also promotes optimum patient care, reduces cost, and minimizes diagnostic errors and unnecessary antimicrobial therapy.

At present the majority of nosocomial infections involve gram-negative bacilli such as *Escherichia coli* and *Pseudomonas* spp. and the gram-positive cocci *Staphylococcus aureus* and enterococci (*Enterococcus* spp.).[51] These organisms are easily identified by most clinical microbiology laboratories. In recent years, however, an increasing number of more fastidious organisms have been implicated in nosocomial infections, and the laboratory must maintain or have ready access to diagnostic and culture techniques that will pinpoint these pathogens. Included in this group are *Legionella* spp., viral agents (particularly rotavirus), anaerobes, fungi (particularly *Candida* spp.), and parasites such as *Pneumocystis carinii*.[81] Variants of nosocomial pathogens such as methicillin-resistant *S. aureus* (MRSA) also require special procedures to ensure the interpretation of accurate antimicrobial susceptibility patterns.

TIMELY REPORTING OF LABORATORY DATA

The ICP combines data from the microbiology laboratory with clinical information obtained on patient rounds to accurately estimate the rate of occurrence of nosocomial infections. As problems arise, the ICP must quickly and effectively implement control measures, and this necessitates frequent communication and sharing of information between laboratory and infection control personnel. Results from Gram stains, cultures, and special tests should be reported promptly to the ICP when intervention will make a difference in quality of care or infection risk. The ICP should share clinical information that may help the microbiologist select special tests.

The microbiology personnel and ICP in each health care facility can develop guidelines regarding culture or smear results that should be reported immediately to the ICP. This system helps the ICP act quickly to implement appropriate precautions or investigation. Examples include multiply resistant organisms, such as MRSA, positive acid-fast smears, reportable organisms or diseases,* and organisms that may con-

---

*The isolation of certain organisms such as *Salmonella*, *Shigella*, and *Mycobacterium* spp. and *Neisseria gonorrhoeae* must be reported to public health institutions with the names and addresses of individuals from whom these organisms are recovered.

stitute employee exposure or employee or patient risk. The microbiology laboratory should assist the ICP and the medical staff by preparing and distributing regular reports analyzing institutional antimicrobial susceptibility trends. The most commonly isolated organisms are listed with the percent susceptibility to each antimicrobial agent. These reports are extremely valuable for prescribing appropriate empiric therapy and may also be used to monitor the emergence of resistant isolates.

PROVIDING SUPPORT FOR INVESTIGATIONS

Surveys of patients, personnel, or the hospital environment may be useful during the investigation of specific problems within a hospital. These measures should be instituted only as a means of addressing specific epidemiologic findings; otherwise, a plethora of worthless and misleading information may be generated. This is especially true regarding environmental sampling. Requests for such sampling should be approached with caution, and the way in which the results will benefit patient care or infection control measures should be clearly defined. Environmental sampling on a routine basis is not recommended.[81]

During investigation of specific infection problems, certain items may be cultured. Samples of blood products implicated in a transfusion reaction should be collected and cultured for both aerobic and anaerobic organisms. Bacteremia associated with parenteral therapy may require culture of the fluid being administered, as well as the intravascular therapy equipment. A membrane filtration technique[68] is well suited for culturing parenteral fluids. Catheters and needles should be cultured using semiquantitative methods,[75] since these lead to more clinically useful information. Simultaneous blood cultures should always be obtained.

Tubes and containers may be cultured by filling them with a suitable quantity of brain heart infusion broth. The filled items are agitated vigorously, and a sample of the rinse broth is aseptically collected. The broth is serially diluted and plated onto 5% sheep blood agar. The plates are incubated at 35° C, and colony counts are determined at 24 and 48 hours.

Although contamination of disinfectants and antiseptics has been implicated in nosocomial infections,[81] bacterial analysis of these compounds requires specialized media not routinely found in most clinical microbiology laboratories. Such analysis is best handled by industrial laboratories.

Although airborne spread of infectious agents can occur, it is an uncommon event. Therefore air sampling for microbiologic evaluation should not be routinely performed.[1] When sampling is required, it may be accomplished with either settling plates or more sophisticated techniques using volumetric air samplers, slit samplers, or centrifugal samplers.[81] Uniform agreement on the standards for levels of air contamination is lacking because of the poor correlation between such levels and the occurrence of nosocomial infections.[81]

A variety of methods have been described for the laboratory evaluation of environmental samples such as floor surfaces, water, and ice.[28,81,82] However, the clinical usefulness of the data generated from such studies is suspect, and it is ill advised for clinical microbiology laboratories to routinely engage in these activities.

Certain microbiologic studies of hospital personnel and environment should be performed as a routine part of the infection

control program. All steam and ethylene oxide gas sterilization systems should be checked at least once a week with a suitable live spore preparation.[24,82] The procedures for checking the proper functioning of these sterilization systems are discussed in Chapters 3 and 5. Results that indicate the possibility of faulty sterilization equipment or procedures should be reported to the appropriate personnel, including the ICP.

At least once a month the water used in the preparation of dialysis fluid and the fluid obtained at the end of treatment should be tested by colony count.[81] The dialysis water should contain fewer than 200 colony-forming units (CFU)/ml, and the fluid at the end of treatment should contain fewer than 2000 CFU/ml.[6] Recommendations for routine and periodic sampling of the personnel and environment in hospitals follow[83]:

I. Routine monitoring recommended
  A. Sterilizers
    1. Steam
    2. Ethylene oxide
    3. Dry heat
  B. Blood components prepared in open systems
  C. Infant formula prepared in hospital
  D. Other high-risk products prepared in hospital
  E. Dialysis fluid
II. Routine monitoring not recommended
  A. Hospital personnel
  B. Patients (culture surveys)
  C. Sterile commercial products
  D. Antiseptics and disinfectants
  E. Blood culture units
  F. Respiratory therapy equipment
III. Periodic environmental monitoring recommended
  A. For investigation of specific problem
  B. For educational purposes

Finally, periodic sampling of items such as disinfected (rather than sterilized) equipment, blood components, and infant formula may be performed but is not mandatory. Performance standards and the frequency of monitoring these and related materials should be determined by the infection control committees of individual hospitals.[81]

ADHERENCE TO SAFETY PRECAUTIONS

Individuals working in clinical laboratories are at risk of nosocomial laboratory-associated infections. This is especially true in the clinical microbiology laboratory where infectious agents and contaminated materials are routinely handled. Certain pathogens, however, such as hepatitis B virus and HIV, pose a threat to all laboratory workers who come in contact with blood or serum samples. Thus all laboratories should establish and maintain a comprehensive safety program to minimize the threat of exposure to biologic hazards.

The incidence of clinical laboratory–acquired infections is unknown because many are unrecognized and most are probably never recorded.[27] In Pike's summary[93] of almost 4000 cases of laboratory-associated infections, less than 20% resulted from known overt exposures or accidents. Self-inoculation with a needle and syringe and aspiration while pipetting by mouth accounted for over one third of the known accidents but only about 9% of all laboratory-associated infections.

The most common mechanisms of acquisition of laboratory infections involve the inhalation of aerosols produced during routine laboratory manipulation and the ingestion of pathogenic

TABLE 4-3. Summary of Recommended Biosafety Levels for Infectious Agents

Safety Level	Practices and Techniques	Safety Equipment	Facilities
1	Standard microbiologic practices	None: primary containment provided by adherence to standard laboratory practices during open bench operations	Basic
2	Level 1 practices plus: laboratory coats; decontamination of all infectious wastes; limited access; protective gloves and biohazard warning signs as indicated	Partial containment equipment (i.e., Class I or II biologic safety cabinets) used to conduct mechanical and manipulative procedures having high aerosol potential that may increase the risk of exposure to personnel	Basic
3	Level 2 practices plus: special laboratory clothing; controlled access	Partial containment equipment used for all manipulation of infectious material	Containment
4	Level 3 practices plus: entrance through change room where street clothing is removed and laboratory clothing is put on; shower on exit; all wastes are decontaminated on exit from facility	Maximum containment equipment (i.e., Class III biologic safety cabinet or partial containment equipment in combination with full-body, air-supplied, positive-pressure personnel suit) used for all procedures and activities	Maximum containment

From Centers for Disease Control and National Institutes of Health: Biosafety in microbiological and biomedical laboratories, DHHS Pub. No. (CDC) 84-8345, Washington, D.C., 1984, U.S. Public Health Service.

microorganisms.[27,97] Not surprisingly, therefore, recommended safety procedures emphasize methods and techniques that minimize the production of infectious aerosols. Recommended "biosafety levels" for specific microbiologic agents have been published[105] and are summarized in Table 4-3. According to these guidelines, the majority of conventional clinical microbiology laboratories dealing with moderate-risk agents are in biosafety level 2, which allows routine work to be conducted on an open benchtop but requires the use of a biologic safety cabinet for procedures with high aerosol potential. Biosafety level 3 is recommended for any manipulation of cultures of high-risk organisms such as *Coccidioides immitis, Mycobacterium tuberculosis, Mycobacterium bovis, Francisella tularensis,* and *Brucella* spp. Some authors advise more stringent guidelines in the application of biosafety levels, particularly in regard to the handling of routine clinical specimens.[27,97] They suggest that the initial processing of all specimens should be conducted in a biologic safety cabinet. The ideal safety cabinet for the clinical microbiology laboratory is a class II, vertical laminar flow type that uses high-efficiency particulate air (HEPA) filters. The routine use of a biologic safety cabinet for the initial processing of patient specimens provides maximum protection for personnel and eliminates the need for numerous decisions regarding the relative hazard of unusual specimens submitted to the laboratory.[26]

General Precautions[26,79]

A combination of good microbiologic technique, appropriate safety equipment, and awareness on the part of the laboratory worker is essential in the prevention of laboratory infections.

The following general safety precautions must always be followed:

1. Pipetting by mouth of all solutions should be prohibited.
2. During pipetting, bubble production should be avoided.
3. Needles and syringes should never be used as a substitute for a pipette.
4. Inoculating loops should be cooled before use.
5. Cylindric electric burners should be used when culturing specimens from patients with tuberculosis.
6. When rubber stoppers are being removed from test tubes, the tops should be covered with an alcohol pad.
7. All hazardous procedures should be carried out in a biologic safety cabinet.
8. Centrifugation should be conducted in a well-ventilated room that can be closed off in case of an accident. Careful balancing is critical, and only sturdy plastic screwtop tubes should be used.
9. For parenteral injections or aspiration of fluids, only syringes with locking hubs should be used. An alcohol pad should be placed around the stopper and needle when withdrawing the needle from a rubber-stoppered vial. Excess air and bubbles should be expelled into an alcohol pad.
10. Used needles and syringes should not be bent, sheared, or resheathed but rather placed directly into a narrow-mouthed, puncture-proof container for disposal.
11. All contaminated materials should be autoclaved before discarding.

12. All contaminated slides and pipettes should be placed in a jar of disinfectant until they are autoclaved.
13. All specimens should be autoclaved before discarding.
14. No eating, drinking, or smoking should be permitted in the laboratory.
15. Personnel should wash hands and remove laboratory coats before leaving the laboratory.
16. No food should be stored in refrigerators that contain specimens or serum products.

Laboratories working with infectious agents should develop emergency plans in anticipation of the type of accident or emergency that is most likely to develop within the facility. The laboratory supervisor is responsible for instructing personnel in applicable procedures and conducting drills in the use of emergency procedures and equipment.[97]

The possibility of spills of infectious materials exists in almost every clinical laboratory. In the case of minor spills of moderate-risk agents, a wash bottle of disinfectant containing a phenolic compound for bacteria and fungi or a hypochlorite for viruses should be sufficient for adequate decontamination.[26] Spills outside of a biologic safety cabinet involving *M. tuberculosis, C. immitis, F. tularensis,* or *Brucella* spp. are considered major hazards and require special procedures for handling.[26,89]

Special Precautions (Hepatitis B and HIV)

Laboratory workers, particularly those working with blood or serum specimens, are at increased risk of infection with hepatitis B virus. Infection can be acquired by the alimentary, conjunctival, or respiratory route, as well as by transdermal inoculation through cuts and needle puncture. Transmission of the HIV virus appears to have a pattern similar to that of hepatitis B. The CDC has recommended biosafety level 2 standards and practices, as described in the CDC-NIH biosafety manual, for handling clinical specimens that may contain HIV or hepatitis B virus.[26a,105] These are essentially the same practices recommended for handling all clinical specimens, with emphasis on the wearing of gloves and the use of a biologic safety cabinet when there is a potential for aerosolization. The CDC has also recommended that all health care workers who have contact with tissues or mucous membranes while performing or assisting in invasive procedures should wear gloves.[26] Procedures involving extensive contact with blood or other body fluids potentially infective with HIV may require gloves, gowns, masks, and eye coverings.[26b] Hands and other contaminated skin surfaces should be washed thoroughly and immediately if accidentally contaminated with blood.[26b]

Some authors[52,56] have questioned the practice in many clinical laboratories of handling with special precautions, such as flagging, only known positive specimens or specimens from patients at high risk of harboring hepatitis B or HIV. Their rationale is that flagging provides a false sense of security for laboratory workers because hepatitis B or AIDS may not be diagnosed until after specimens have been analyzed.

Other precautions that should be followed include:
1. Laboratory workers who have frequent contact with blood or serum should receive hepatitis B virus vaccine.[19]
2. All accidents must be documented. An employee who sustains any cut or needle-puncture wound or who swal-

lows any blood or blood product should report it to the supervisor immediately. Appropriate hospital protocols should be followed.

Additional guidelines for handling specimens from AIDS patients are discussed in Chapter 10.

REFERENCES

1. Air sampling in operating theaters (editorial), J. Hosp. Infect. **5:**1, 1984.
2. Aisner, J., et al.: *Aspergillus* infections in cancer patients: association with fireproofing materials in a new hospital, JAMA **235:**411, 1976.
3. Albert, R.K., and Condie, F.: Handwashing patterns in medical intensive care units, N. Engl. J. Med. **304:**1465, 1981.
4. Arnow, P.M., et al.: Pulmonary aspergillosis during hospital renovation, Am. Rev. Respir. Dis. **118:**49, 1978.
5. Arnow, P.M., et al.: Nosocomial Legionnaire's disease caused by aerosolized tap water from respiratory devices, J. Infect. Dis. **146:**460, 1982.
6. Association for the Advancement of Medical Instrumentation: American national standard for hemodialysis systems, Arlington, Va, 1981, The Association.
7. Bartlett, R.C.: Medical microbiology: quality, cost, and clinical relevance, New York, 1974, John Wiley & Sons, Inc.
8. Berkelman, R.L., et al.: *Pseudomonas cepacia* peritonitis associated with contamination of automated peritoneal dialysis machines, Ann. Intern. Med. **96:**456, 1982.
9. Boyce, J.M., White, R.L., and Spruill, E.Y.: Impact of methicillin-resistant *Staphylococcus aureus* on the incidence of nosocomial staphylococcal infections, J. Infect. Dis. **148:**763, 1983.
10. Brachman, P.S.: Epidemiology of nosocomial infections. In Bennett, J.V., and Brachman, P.S., editors: Hospital infections, ed. 2, Boston, 1986, Little, Brown & Co.
11. Brachman, P.S., et al.: Nosocomial surgical infections: incidence and cost, Surg. Clin. North Am. **60:**15, 1980.
12. Brooks, R.G., and Remington, J.S.: Transplant-related infections. In Bennett, J.V., and Brachman, P.S., editors: Hospital infections, ed. 2, Boston, 1986, Little, Brown & Co.
13. Burke, J.P., Larsen, R.A., and Stevens, L.E.: Nosocomial bacteriuria: estimating the potential for prevention by closed sterile urinary drainage, Infect. Control **7:**96, 1986.
14. Casewell, M., and Phillips, I.: Hands as a route of transmission for *Klebsiella* species, Br. Med. J. **2:**1315, 1977.
15. Centers for Disease Control: National nosocomial infections study site definitions manual, Atlanta, U.S. Department of Health and Human Services, unpublished.
16. Centers for Disease Control: National nosocomial infection study reports, Altanta, 1970-1984 (published annually), U.S. Department of Health and Human Services.
17. Centers for Disease Control: Algorithms for diagnosing infections used in the Study on the Efficacy of Nosocomial Infection Control (SENIC), published as Appendix E, Am. J. Epidemiol. **111:**635, 1980.
18. Centers for Disease Control: Guideline for prevention of catheter-associated urinary tract infections, Guidelines Activity, Hospital Infections Branch, Center for Infectious Diseases, Atlanta, 1981, U.S. Department of Health and Human Services.
19. Centers for Disease Control: Recommendations of the Immunization Practices Advisory Committee: inactivated hepatitis B virus vaccine, MMWR **31:**317, 1982.
20. Centers for Disease Control: Acquired immune deficiency syndrome (AIDS): precautions for clinical and laboratory staffs, MMWR **31:**577, 1982.
21. Centers for Disease Control: Guideline for prevention of intravenous therapy–related infections, Guidelines Activity, Hospital Infections

Branch, Center for Infectious Diseases, Altanta, 1982, U.S. Department of Health and Human Services.

22. Centers for Disease Control: Guideline for prevention of nosocomial pneumonia, Guidelines Activity, Hospital Infections Branch, Atlanta, 1982, U.S. Department of Health and Human Services.

23. Centers for Disease Control: Outline for surveillance and control of nosocomial infections, Atlanta, 1972. U.S. Department of Health and Human Services, 1972. (Reprinted in Soule B.M., editor: The APIC curriculum for infection control practice, Dubuque, Iowa, 1983, Kendall/Hunt.)

24. Centers for Disease Control: Guideline for handwashing and hospital environmental control. Sect. I. Handwashing, Guidelines Activity, Hospital Infections Branch, Center for Infectious Diseases, Centers for Disease Control, Atlanta, 1985, U.S. Department of Health and Human Services.

25. Centers for Disease Control: Guideline for prevention of surgical wound infections, Guidelines Activity, Hospital Infections Branch, Center for Infectious Diseases, Atlanta, 1985, U.S. Department of Health and Human Services.

26. Centers for Disease Control: Recommendations for preventing transmission of infection with human T-lymphotropic virus type III/lymphadenopathy-associated virus during invasive procedures, MMWR **35:**22, 1986.

26a. Centers for Disease Control: Human T-lymphocyte virus type III/lymphadenopathy associated virus: agent summary statement, MMWR **36:**540, 1986.

26b. Centers for Disease Control: Update: human immunodeficiency virus infections in health-care workers exposed to blood of infected patients, MMWR **36:**285, 1987.

27. Coyle, M.B., and Schoenknecht, F.D.: The clinical laboratory. In Bennett, J.V., and Brachman, P.S., editors: Hospital infections, ed. 2, Boston, 1986, Little, Brown & Co.

28. Craythorn, J.M., et al.: Membrane filter contact technique for bacteriological sampling of moist surfaces, J. Clin. Microbiol. **12:**250, 1980.

29. Crossley, K., Landesman, B., and Saske, D.: An outbreak of infections caused by strains of Staphylococcus aureus resistant to methicillin and aminoglycosides. II. Epidemiologic studies, J. Infect. Dis. **139:**280, 1979.

30. Cruse, P.J.E., and Foord, R.: The epidemiology of wound infection: a ten-year prospective study of 62,939 wounds, Surg. Clin. North Am. **60:**27, 1980.

31. Dixon, R.E.: Investigation of endemic and epidemic nosocomial infections. In Bennett, J.V., and Brachman, P.S., editors: Hospital infections, ed. 2, Boston, 1986, Little Brown & Co.

32. Dunkle, L.M., et al.: Eradication of epidemic methicillin-gentamicin-resistant Staphylococcus aureus in an intensive care nursery, Am. J. Med. **70:**455, 1981.

33. Emori, T.G., Haley, R.W., and Stanley, R.C.: The infection control nurse in U.S. hospitals, 1976-1977: characteristics of the position and its occupant, Am. J. Epidemiol. **111:**592, 1980.

34. Favero, M.S.: Dialysis-associated diseases and their control. In Bennett, J.V., and Brachman, P.S., editors: Hospital infections, ed. 2, Boston, 1986, Little, Brown & Co.

35. Favero, M.S.: Sterilization, disinfection, and antisepsis in the hospital. In Lenette, E.H., et al., editors: Manual of clinical microbiology, ed. 4, Washington, D.C., 1986, American Society for Microbiology.

36. Garibaldi, R.A.: Hospital acquired urinary tract infection. In Wenzel, R.P., editor: Handbook of hospital acquired infections, Boca Raton, Fla., 1981, CRC Press.

37. Garibaldi, R.A., Brodine, S., and Matsumiya, S.: Infections among patients in nursing homes: policies, prevalence, and problems, N. Engl. J. Med. **305:**731, 1981.

38. Goldman, D.A.: Epidemiology of Staphylococcus aureus and group-A streptococci. In Bennett, J.V., and Brachman, P.S., editors: Hospital infections, ed. 2, Boston, 1986, Little, Brown & Co.

39. Gross, P.A., et al.: Deaths from nosocomial infections: experience in a university hospital and community hospital, Am. J. Med. **68:**218, 1980.

40. Haley, C.E., et al.: Nosocomial Legionnaires' disease: a continuing common-source epidemic at Wadsworth Medical Center, Ann. Intern. Med. **90:**583, 1979.

41. Haley, R.W.: Incidence and nature of endemic and epidemic nosocomial infections. In Bennett, J.V., and Brachman, P.S., editors: Hospital infections, ed. 2, Boston, 1986, Little, Brown & Co.

42. Haley, R.W.: Managing hospital infection control for cost-effectiveness: a strategy for reducing infectious complications, Chicago, 1986, American Hospital Publishing, Inc.

43. Haley, R.W., and Garner, J.S.: Infection surveillance and control programs. In Bennett, J.V., and Brachman, P.S., editors: Hospital infections, ed. 2, Boston, 1986, Little, Brown & Co.

44. Haley, R.W., and Schachtman, R.H.: The emergence of infection surveillance and control programs in U.S. hospitals: an assessment, Am. J. Epidemiol. **111:**574, 1980.

45. Haley, R.W., et al.: Nosocomial infections in U.S. hospitals, 1975-1976: estimated frequency by selected characteristics of patients, Am. J. Med. **70:**947, 1981.

46. Haley, R.W., et al.: How frequent are outbreaks of nosocomial infection in community hospitals? Infect. Control **6:**233, 1985.

47. Haley, R.W., et al.: The efficacy of infection surveillance and control programs in preventing nosocomial infections in U.S. hospitals, Am. J. Epidemiol. **121:**182, 1985.

48. Haley, R.W., et al.: Update from the SENIC project: hospital infection control; recent progress and opportunities under prospective payment, Am. J. Infect. Control **13:**97, 1985.

49. Hall, C.B.: Nosocomial viral respiratory infections: perennial weeds on pediatric wards, Am. J. Med. **70:**670, 1981.

50. Hall, C.B., and Douglas, R.G., Jr.: Modes of transmission of respiratory syncytial virus, J. Pediatr. 99:100, 1981.

51. Horan, T.C., et al.: Nosocomial infection surveillance 1984, MMWR **35**(1SS):17, 1986.

52. Jackson, M.M.: From ritual to reason—with a rational approach for the future: an epidemiologic perspective (fifth annual Carole Demille lecture), Am. J. Infect. Control **12:**213, 1984.

53. Jackson, M.M., and Checko, P.J.: Epidemiology and statistics. In Soule, B.M., editor: The APIC curriculum for infection control practice, Dubuque, Iowa, 1983, Kendall/Hunt Co.

54. Jackson, M.M., and Fierer, J.: Infections and infection risk in residents of long-term care facilities: a review of the literature, 1970-1984, Am. J. Infect. Control **13:**63, 1985.

55. Jackson, M.M., and Lynch, P.: Infection control: too much or too little? Am J. Nurs. **84:**208, 1984.

56. Jackson, M.M., and Lynch, P.: Isolation practices: a historical perspective, Am. J. Infect. Control **13:**21, 1985.

57. Jarvis, W.R.: Surveillance of nosocomial fungal infections: current problems, read before the 85th Annual Meeting of the American Society for Microbiology, Las Vegas, March 7, 1985.

58. Johanson, W.G., Pierce, A.K., and Sanford, J.P.: Changing pharyngeal bacterial flora of hospitalized patients: emergence of gram-negative bacilli, N. Engl. J. Med. **281:**1137, 1969.

59. Johanson, W.G., et al.: Nosocomial respiratory infections with gram-negative bacilli: the significance of colonization of the respiratory tract, Ann. Intern. Med. **77:**701, 1972.

60. Joint Commission on Accreditation of Hospitals: Accreditation manual for hospital, Chicago, 1986, The Commission.

61. Kayser, F.H., and Mak, T.M.: Methicillin resistant staphylococci, Am. J. Med. Sci. **264:**197, 1972.

62. Knittle, M.A., Eitzman, D.V., and Boer, H.: Role of hand contamination of personnel in the epidemiology of gram-negative nosocomial infections, J. Pediatr. **86:**433, 1975.

63. Larson, E.: Persistent carriage of gram-negative bacteria on hands, Am. J. Infect. Control **9:**112, 1981.

64. Larson, E.: Compliance with isolation technique, Am. J. Infect. Control **11**:221, 1983.

65. Larson, E., and Larson, E.: Influence of a role model on handwashing behavior, Am. J. Infect. Control **11**:146, 1983.

66. Lempert, K.D., et al.: Pseudouremic pruritus: a scabies epidemic in a dialysis unit, Am. J. Kidney Dis. **5**:117, 1985.

67. Lerche, N.W., et al.: Atypical crusted ''Norwegian'' scabies: report of nosocomial transmission in a community hospital and an approach to control, Cutis **31**:637, 1983.

67a. Lifson, A.R., et al.: National surveillance of AIDS in health care workers, JAMA **256**:3231, 1986.

68. Longfield, J.N., et al.: Comparison of broth and filtration methods for culturing of intravenous fluids, Infect. Control **3**:397, 1982.

69. Luckmann, J., and Sorensen, K.C., editors: Basic nursing: a psychophysiologic approach, Philadelphia, 1986, W.B. Saunders Co.

70. Lynch, P.: Epidemiology and surveillance. In Axnick, K.J., and Yarbrough, M., editors: Infection control: an integrated approach, St. Louis, 1984, The C.V. Mosby Co.

71. Lynch, P., and Jackson, M.M.: Infection control: medical asepsis. In Sorensen, K.C., and Luckmann, J., editors: Basic nursing: a psychophysiologic approach, Philadelphia, 1986, W.B. Saunders Co.

72. MacMillan, B.C., Holder, I.A., and Alexander, J.W.: Infections of burn wounds. In Bennett, J.V., and Brachman, P.S., editors: Hospital infections, ed. 2, Boston, 1986, Little, Brown & Co.

73. Magnussen, M.H., and Robb, S.S.: Nosocomial infections in a long-term care facility, Am. J. Infect. Control **2**:12, 1980.

74. Maki, D.G.: Infections due to infusion therapy. In Bennett, J.V., and Brachman, P.S., editors: Hospital infections, ed. 2, Boston, 1986, Little, Brown & Co.

75. Maki, D.G., Weise, C.E., and Sarafin, H.W.: A semi-quantitative culture method for identifying intravenous catheter-related infection, N. Engl. J. Med. **296**:1305, 1977.

76. Maki, D.G., et al.: Nationwide epidemic of septicemia caused by contaminated intravenous products. I. Epidemiologic and clinical features, Am. J. Med. **60**:471, 1976.

77. Maki, D.G., et al.: Relation of the inanimate hospital environment to endemic nosocomial infection, N. Engl. J. Med. **307**:1562, 1982.

78. Mathur, U., Bentley, D.W., and Hall, C.B.: Concurrent respiratory syncytial virus and influenza A infections in the institutionalized elderly and chronically ill, Ann. Intern. Med. **93**:49, 1980.

79. Mausner, J.S., and Bahn, A.K.: Epidemiology: an introductory text, Philadelphia, 1974, W.B. Saunders Co.

80. McGowan, J.E., Jr.: Antimicrobial resistance in hospital organisms and its relation to antibiotic use, Rev. Infect. Dis. **5**:1033, 1983.

81. McGowan, J.E., Jr.: Role of the microbiology laboratory in prevention and control of nosocomial infections. In Lennette, E.H., et al., editors: Manual of clinical microbiology, ed. 4, Washington, D.C., 1985, American Society for Microbiology.

82. McGowan, J.E., Jr., Weinstein, R.A., and Mallison, G.F.: The role of the laboratory in control of nosocomial infections. In Bennett, J.V., and Brachman, P.S., editors: Hospital infections, ed. 2, Boston, 1986, Little, Brown & Co.

83. McGucken, M.B., Thorpe, P.J., and Abrutyn, E.: An outbreak of *Pseudomonas aeruginosa* wound infection related to Hubbard tank treatments, Arch. Phys. Med. Rehabil. **62**:283, 1981.

84. Meyer, R.D.: *Legionella* infection: a review of five years research, Rev. Infect. Dis. **5**:258, 1983.

85. Muder, R.R., et al.: Nosocomial Legionnaires' disease discovered in a prospective pneumonia study, JAMA **249**:3184, 1983.

86. National Intravenous Therapy Association: Intravenous nursing standards of practice, Belmont, Mass., 1981, The Association.

87. Needlestick transmission of HTLV-III from a patient infected in Africa, Lancet **2**:1376, 1984.

88. Occupational risk of the acquired immunodeficiency syndrome among health care workers (special report), N. Engl. J. Med. **314**:1127, 1986.

89. Office of Research Safety, National Cancer Institute and the Special Committee of Safety and Health Experts: Laboratory safety monograph: a supplement to the NIH guidelines for recombinant DNA research, Bethesda, Md., 1979, National Institutes of Health.

90. Parrott, P.L., et al.: *Pseudomonas aeruginosa* peritonitis associated with contaminated poloxamer-iodine solution, Lancet **2**:683, 1982.

91. Peacock, J.E., Jr., Marsik, F.J., and Wenzel, R.P.: Methicillin-resistant *Staphlococcus aureus:* introduction and spread within a hospital, Ann. Intern. Med. **93**:526, 1980.

92. Penn, R.G., Sanders, W.E., and Sanders, C.C.: Colonization of the oropharynx with gram-negative bacilli: a major antecedent to nosocomial pneumonia, Am. J. Infect. Control **9**:25, 1981.

93. Pike, R.M.: Laboratory-associated infections: summary and analysis of 3,921 cases, Health Lab. Sci. **13**:105, 1976.

94. Polsky, B., and Armstrong, D.: Infectious complications of neoplastic disease, Am. J. Infect. Control **13**:119, 1985.

95. Reinarz, J.A., et al.: The potential role of inhalation therapy equipment in nosocomial pulmonary infections, J. Clin. Invest. **44**:831, 1965.

96. Rhame, F.S.: The inanimate environment. In Bennett, J.V., and Brachman, P.S., editors: Hospital infections, ed. 2, Boston, 1986, Little, Brown & Co.

97. Richardson, J.H., and Barkley, W.E.: Biological safety in the clinical laboratory. In Lennette, E.H., et al., editors: Manual of clinical microbiology, Washington, D.C., 1985, American Society for Microbiology.

98. Sanford, J.P.: Lower respiratory tract infections. In Bennett, J.V., and Brachman, P.S., editors: Hospital infections, ed. 2, Boston, 1986, Little, Brown & Co.

99. Selden, R., et al.: Nosocomial *Klebsiella* infections: intestinal colonization as a reservoir, Ann. Intern. Med. **74**:657, 1971.

100. Setia, U., Serventi, I., and Lorenz, P.: Nosocomial infections among patients in a long-term care facility: spectrum, prevalence, and risk factors, Am. J. Infect. Control **13**:57, 1985.

101. Soule, B.M., editor: The APIC curriculum for infection control practice, Dubuque, Iowa, 1985, Kendall/Hunt Publishing Co.

102. Stamm, W.E.: Infections due to medical devices, Ann. Intern. Med. **89**(part 2):764, 1978.

103. Stratton, C.: Waterless agents for decontaminating the hands, Infect. Control **7**:186, 1986.

104. Stricof, R.L., and Morse, D.L.: HTLV III/LAV seroconversion following a deep intramuscular needlestick injury, N. Engl. J. Med. **314**:1115, 1986.

105. U.S. Public Health Service, Centers for Disease Control and National Institutes of Health: Biosafety in microbiological and biomedical laboratories, Pub. No. (CDC) 84-8345, Washington, D.C., 1984, Department of Health and Human Services.

106. Valenti, W.M., et al.: Nosocomial viral infection. I. Epidemiology and significance, Infect. Control **1**:33, 1980.

107. Valenti, W.M., et al.: Concurrent outbreaks of rhinovirus and respiratory syncytial virus in an intensive care nursery: epidemiology and associated risk factors, J. Pediatr. **100**:722, 1982.

108. Van Voris, L.P., Belshe, R.B., and Shaffer, J.L.: Nosocomial influenza B in the elderly, Ann. Intern. Med. **96**:153, 1982.

109. Weinstein, R.A.: Other procedure-related infections. In Bennett, J.V., and Brachman, P.S., editors: Hospital infections, ed. 2, Boston, 1986, Little, Brown & Co.

110. Wenzel, R.P., et al.: Hospital acquired infections in intensive care unit patients: an overview with emphasis on epidemics, Infect. Control **4**:371, 1983.

111. Williams, W.W., and Garner, J.S.: Personnel health services. In Bennett, J.V., and Brachman, P.S., editors: Hospital infections, ed. 2, Boston, 1986, Little, Brown & Co.

CHAPTER 5

Disinfection and Sterilization

Jill E. Clarridge

An understanding of the principles of sterilization and disinfection is fundamental to the microbiology laboratory. The growth of organisms must be closely controlled to prevent both environmental organisms from contaminating cultures and cultured organisms from contaminating the environment or causing infections. This requires the use of effective sterile techniques along with the disinfection of the laboratory area and the sterilization or destruction of all media and materials that were used or exposed to microorganisms before reuse or disposal. In addition, the microbiology laboratory may be required to monitor the biologic cleanliness of an institution's environment and supplies. Other areas such as the housekeeping department may seek the consultation of a microbiologist to determine the best methods for sterilization or the best products for disinfection. Although microbiologists at all levels should be aware of the basic concepts presented here, much more detailed and extensive information is available from Block,[2] Favero,[3] and Groschel.[4]

Many terms are used to express the concepts of removing or killing microbes on or in a material, area, or person. They are defined by what forms of microbes are affected, whether the microbes are killed, removed, or inhibited, and whether the process is performed on a person or inanimate object. Some of these terms and the methods used to obtain them are discussed in the following paragraphs.

Sterilization is the process of destroying or removing all life forms. However, laboratories and hospitals use the term in a more empiric sense: the process of destroying or removing only certain defined microorganisms. For each method of sterilization there are appropriate tests for sterility (Table 5-1).

Disinfection denotes a process that reduces or destroys most microbial forms but not spores. A broad definition of disinfection is the killing of pathogenic organisms by chemical or physical means applied directly. Disinfectants that can safely be topically applied to people or animals are called *antiseptics* and are regulated as drugs by the Food and Drug Administration. The term ''disinfectant'' is more properly reserved for chemicals that are to be used on inanimate objects. They are regulated and registered by the Environmental Protection Agency.

Germicide is a commonly used term associated with a chemical that can kill many types of pathogenic microorganisms but not necessarily spores. Agents that destroy bacteria, viruses, fungi, or spores are called, respectively, *bactericides, virucides, fungicides,* or *sporocides.* These terms are used to indicate the microorganisms against which a disinfectant may be effective.

METHODS OF STERILIZATION
MOIST HEAT

Steam at atmospheric pressure can attain a temperature of only 100° C. However, if steam is enclosed and put under pressure as in an autoclave or pressure cooker, the temperature at 15 pounds of pressure is increased to 121° C. Under these conditions all known pathogens and essentially all known life forms including bacterial spores and vegetative cells, viruses, and fungi are killed if the exposure is long enough for the moist heat to penetrate throughout the objects.

Because *Bacillus stearothermophilus* spores are one of the life forms most resistant to this type of killing, they are used as indicator organisms. The spore carrier should be placed in the sterilizer in the center of a large load or in an area least likely to reach sterilizing temperatures. Several commercial spore carriers are available; laboratories should carefully follow manufacturer's instructions.

DRY HEAT

Temperatures of 171° C for 1 hour, 160° C for 2 hours, or 121° C for 16 hours can sterilize. The process is useful on heat-stable materials and on substances that steam cannot penetrate, such as oil. Again, the heat must penetrate to the center of the material for the given time. Dry heat sterilization is monitored with *Bacillus subtilis* var. *niger (globigii)* spores, which should be processed according to the manufacturer's recommendations. Dry heat is the preferred method for the destruction of pyrogens, part of the bacterial cell wall. These substances are smaller than bacteria and cannot be removed by routine filtration with a 0.22 μm pore diameter filter. Pyrogens cause an adverse effect in humans and can be found in water supplies.

FILTRATION

Liquids can be sterilized by filtration. Filters for sterilizing are most commonly made from cellulose and are available with varying pore sizes. A pore size of 0.22 μm is small enough to remove bacteria. This filter would not ordinarily retain viruses, mycoplasmas, and bacterial products. The selective use of the term ''sterilization'' is obvious here; a ''filter-sterilized'' medium is not necessarily free of all life forms.

RADIATION

Sterilization by gamma rays is used for delicate supplies such as syringes and sutures, as well as increasingly for food. Radiation kills bacteria and other life forms by damaging most

TABLE 5-1. Methods of Sterilization

Method	Examples of Use	Usual Conditions	Test for Sterility	Limits and Drawbacks
Moist heat[a] (steam)	Heat-stable media and supplies, instruments, discarded contaminated media	Autoclave at 121° C for 15-30 min	*Bacillus stearothermophilus* spores killed; test spore carrier for growth; there should be none	Some materials (e.g., sugars, plastics) may be heat labile; oil-based materials not well penetrated
Dry heat[a]	Glassware, oils, instruments, powders	Oven at 160°-200° C for 1-4 hr	*Bacillus subtilis* var. *niger* spores killed; spore carrier should be tested	Dry heat takes much longer to kill spores than moist heat
Gas (ethylene oxide)	Surgical supplies, plastics, instruments, bandages	Special sterilizer, 700 mg ethylene oxide per liter chamber space at 60° C for 2 hr	*B. subtilis* var. *niger* spores killed; spore carrier should be tested	Residual gas on materials such as gloves or bandages can cause skin irritation; toxic; flammable
Filtration	Gases, heat-labile fluids, pharmacy products	0.20 μm pore filter used	Visually inspect filter and apparatus for gross leaks; test aliquot of filtrate for growth	Removes spores and most bacteria but not viruses and mycoplasmas
Ionizing radiation (gamma rays)	Bandages, sutures, large-scale use in manufacturing plastics and food	2.5 to 4.5 megarad exposure	*Enterococcus faecium*[b] killed	High equipment costs and safety requirements

[a]See Chapter 3 for performance monitoring schedules.
[b]Previously known as *Streptococcus faecium* (see Chapter 13).

cell constituents, including DNA, usually by free radical formation. Sources for the radiation are cobalt-60 and cesium-137.

GAS (ETHYLENE OXIDE)

It has been suggested that ethylene oxide sterilizes by denaturing nucleic acids or by alkylating sulfhydryl bonds of proteins; either mechanism could cause injury or death to the microbe. Sterilization can be accomplished by using 450 to 700 mg of ethylene oxide per liter of chamber space at 55° to 60° C for 2 hours. Lower concentrations or lower temperatures can be used if the time is increased. Various acceptable protocols are described by Block.[2] Ethylene oxide is useful for sterilizing plastics and other delicate or heat-labile materials. However, because it can react with many chemicals to form toxic products, appropriate safety measures during sterilization and for the sterilized materials (such as venting to be sure residual gas is removed) must be instituted.

LIQUID

Glutaraldehyde, hydrogen peroxide, and formaldehyde can be used as sterilants for such objects as instruments and medical devices. Their effectiveness depends on the concentration, the time of exposure, and the prior cleanliness and type of material to be sterilized. For example, soaking in 2% glutaraldehyde for 8 hours sterilizes most material, whereas soaking for 30 minutes only disinfects. The manufacturer's recommendations for exposure times and conditions should be followed. After sterilization is complete, objects must be rinsed with sterile water.

METHODS OF DISINFECTION
PHYSICAL METHODS

Physical disinfection processes include treatment with heat and ultraviolet light. Temperatures of 100° C, that is, boiling water, kill most bacteria in a few minutes. Even heating to 70° C for 30 minutes, a process called pasteurization, kills milkborne pathogens including *Mycobacterium* spp. and *Brucella* spp. Hot water at 75° to 100° C can be used to disinfect reusable hospital goods such as anesthesia and respiratory therapy tubings. Ultraviolet light is used extensively in biologic safety cabinets and tissue culture areas to kill airborne and surface microbes.

CHEMICAL METHODS

A variety of chemicals are used for disinfection. They are evaluated as to whether they kill vegetative bacteria, mycobacteria, fungi, or spores. Table 5-2 describes commonly used disinfectants and antiseptics. The need for handwashing with skin disinfectants in infection control is discussed in Chapter 4.

The importance of following the manufacturer's instructions for sterilization and disinfection procedures cannot be overemphasized. Autoclaves, gas sterilizers, and other mechanical equipment can be dangerous if not used correctly. The laboratory should verify that all people operating such equipment have been properly instructed in its use. Chemical sterilants and disinfectants must also be used according to the manufacturer's directions. The effect of most germicides depends on their concentration. For example, the alcohols are more effective for disinfection or antisepsis when they are diluted to 70% with

TABLE 5-2. Chemical Disinfectants and Antiseptics

Class	Name	Examples	Killing Activity[a]	Usage
Phenolic	Phenol	5% aqueous phenol solution; 2% aqueous phenol-alcohol solution with detergent	B, TB, F, V (30)	Environmental; laboratory benches; biologic safety cabinet; used swabs, pipettes, inoculators (soak overnight); spills; operating room
	Substituted phenols	Orthohydroxydiphenyl (e.g., Lysol), hexachlorophene (e.g., pHisoHex)	B (10)	Skin
Chlorine	Hypochlorite	2%-10% household bleach which has 5% hypochlorite	B, TB, F, V, S, (1)	Occasional environmental (can corrode), spills
Iodine	Povidone-iodine	Betadine	B, F, V (5)	Skin and instruments (lipid and soap soluble)
	Iodophor	Wescodyne		Environmental, skin, instruments
Quaternary ammonium compounds	Substituted ammonium chloride, cationic detergent	Many trade names and formulas	B, F, ±V (10)	Environmental, instruments, inactivated by soaps and detergents
Glutaraldehyde		2% aqueous solution of glutaraldehyde (Cidex)	B, TB, F, V, S (30)	Instruments
Formaldehyde		3%-8% aqueous solution of formaldehyde	B, F, V (10) TB, S (30)	Disinfecting buildings and rooms and preserving tissue
Alcohol	Isopropanol	50%-70% aqueous solution of propanol	B, F, V (10)	Skin
	Ethanol	70% aqueous solution of ethanol		Tops of blood culture bottles
Hydrogen peroxide	Stabilized hydrogen peroxide	3%-6% solution 6%-25% solution	B, V B, V, F, S (60)	Disinfection of medical devices Possible sterilization of medical devices

SYMBOLS: B, Bacteria   F, Fungus   S, Spore
TB, *Mycobacterium tuberculosis*   V, Virus   (), Approximate contact time in minutes necessary for disinfection

[a]Signifies type of microbe killed. Some disinfectants might be sterilants if time and conditions of exposure sufficient.

water than when used full strength. The quaternary ammonium compounds are useful as general environmental disinfectants when they are diluted to about 0.2% in water; increasing the concentration does not lead to more effective disinfection but rather is more expensive and may lead to skin irritation on the part of the user. Glutaraldehyde in a 2% aqueous solution can be used as a sterilant that kills even bacterial spores if the contact time is long enough (6 to 10 hours) and the material clean (adhering debris and altered pH decrease effectiveness). However, disinfection is accomplished with exposure times of 30 minutes. Similarly, the concentration of the active agent in iodophor compounds, the free iodine, is related to the dilution. The manufacturer indicates the aqueous dilution that provides the greatest germicidal activity.

As early as 1888 the American Public Health Association[1] recommended fire, steam under pressure, boiling in water for ½ hour, and chloride for destroying spore-containing infectious material, with the addition of 5% carbolic acid (phenol) and dry heat for infectious material without spores. These methods are valid today; the innovations have been toward gentler methods

that kill microorganisms while preserving the object. At the end of the nineteenth century, considerable work was being done on the design of sterilizing equipment, the exact times and concentrations of chemicals that would kill microorganisms, and the public utilization of these to stop the spread of foodborne and contagious disease. For many diseases such as cholera, control of spread of the disease preceded isolation of the etiologic agent.

REFERENCES

1. American Public Health Association, Committee on Disinfection: Disinfection and disinfectants, Concord, N.H., 1888, Republican Press.
2. Block, S.S., editor: Disinfection, sterilization and preservation, ed. 3, Philadelphia, 1983, Lea & Febiger.
3. Favero, M.D.: Sterilization, disinfection and antisepsis in the hospital. In Lennette, E.H., et al., editors: Manual of clinical microbiology, ed. 4, Washington, D.C., 1985, Amerian Society for Microbiology.
4. Groschel, D.M.: Sterilization, disinfection and antisepsis. In Sonnenwirth, A.C., and Jarrett. L., editors: Gradwohl's clinical laboratory methods and diagnosis, ed. 8, St. Louis, 1980, The C.V. Mosby Co.

CHAPTER 6

Microscopy and Staining

Jill E. Clarridge
J. Michael Mullins

MICROSCOPY

Microscopes are used to study structural detail too small to be observed with the unaided eye. Although magnification is an essential feature of microscope function, the critical factor that determines the smallest detail that can be observed is not the degree of magnification but rather the *resolution* provided by the microscope lenses.

The *resolution limit* of a lens (or lens system) is the smallest distance by which two points can be separated and still be observed as distinct points. Two points closer together than the resolution limit of a lens are seen as a single, blurred image, even though the points are actually separate. The unaided human eye has a resolution limit of approximately 0.1 mm. Structural detail with spacings smaller than 0.1 mm cannot be resolved by the eye. Magnifying lenses, or microscopes, must be employed to see smaller detail. These devices have a resolution limit smaller than that of the eye and magnify detail in the specimen such that its spacings appear equal to or greater than the eye's resolution limit. For example, suppose one needs to resolve two points separated by 0.5 μm (0.0005 mm). A lens system must be used that has a resolution limit no greater than 0.5 μm, or the two points will not be resolved. Furthermore, the image delivered to the eye must be magnified at least 200× so the distance between the points will be 0.1 mm or greater (200 × 0.0005 mm = 0.1 mm) and thus at or above the eye's resolution limit.

Two fundamental microscope systems are available. The compound light microscope uses visible (or ultraviolet) light to illuminate the specimen and form an image. The electron microscope uses a beam of accelerated electrons to accomplish these purposes.

COMPOUND LIGHT MICROSCOPE

Resolution limits of approximately 10 μm (0.01 mm) can be obtained with a simple microscope consisting of a single lens. To resolve structural details of individual eukaryotic cells or microorganisms, a compound microscope must be used.

The compound microscope typically employs two lens systems for image magnification (Figure 6-1). Initial magnification of the specimen is provided by the objective lens. The image from the objective lens is further magnified by the ocular, or eyepiece. Final image magnification is the product of the magnifications of the objective and ocular. A condenser lens, positioned beneath the specimen, is used to focus light on the specimen, providing a bright and evenly illuminated field.

The critical factors for determining the resolution limit of the compound microscope are the design and quality of the objective lens. The resolution limit depends on the numerical aperture (NA)* of the objective and the wavelength (λ) of light used. Mathematically, the resolution limit (d_{min}) is defined as:

$$d_{min} = \frac{\lambda}{NA}$$

Thus the best resolution (smallest d_{min}) is obtained by using the shortest possible wavelength of visible light and an objective lens of the highest possible numerical aperture. The highest numerical apertures, approximately 1.4, are obtained with oil immersion lenses. With such a lens and blue light of wavelength 0.5 μm, a compound microscope attains a resolution limit of approximately 0.2 μm.

The compound light microscope can be used without modification for brightfield microscopy, or accessories can be added to allow performance of other types of microscopy. Some of these types are discussed in the following sections.

Brightfield Microscope

Simple observation of specimens by transmitted light using the compound microscope is termed brightfield microscopy. Brightfield microscopy depends on differential absorption of light by different parts of the specimen, rendering some structures darker than others and so making structure visible.

With the exception of naturally occurring pigments, such as chlorophyll and melanin, biologic molecules do not show significant absorption of visible light. Living specimens viewed with the basic compound microscope thus provide images with little contrast. To produce contrast, dyes are used to stain biologic specimens. Dye molecules selectively absorb light. Those parts of the specimen to which dye is bound take on the color of the transmitted wavelengths of light and appear darker. The dyes, or stains, that are used in clinical microbiology are discussed in the second half of this chapter.

Brightfield microscopy is most commonly used with stained specimens, but it may also be used to examine the morphologic characteristics and especially the motility of organisms in the living unstained state. This is accomplished by preparing a hanging drop or wet mount. The hanging drop procedure uses a depression slide and is performed as follows. (1) A ring of petroleum jelly is spread around the concavity of the depression slide. (2) A loopful of bacterial culture is placed in the center of

---

*The numerical aperture reflects the light-gathering ability of a lens.

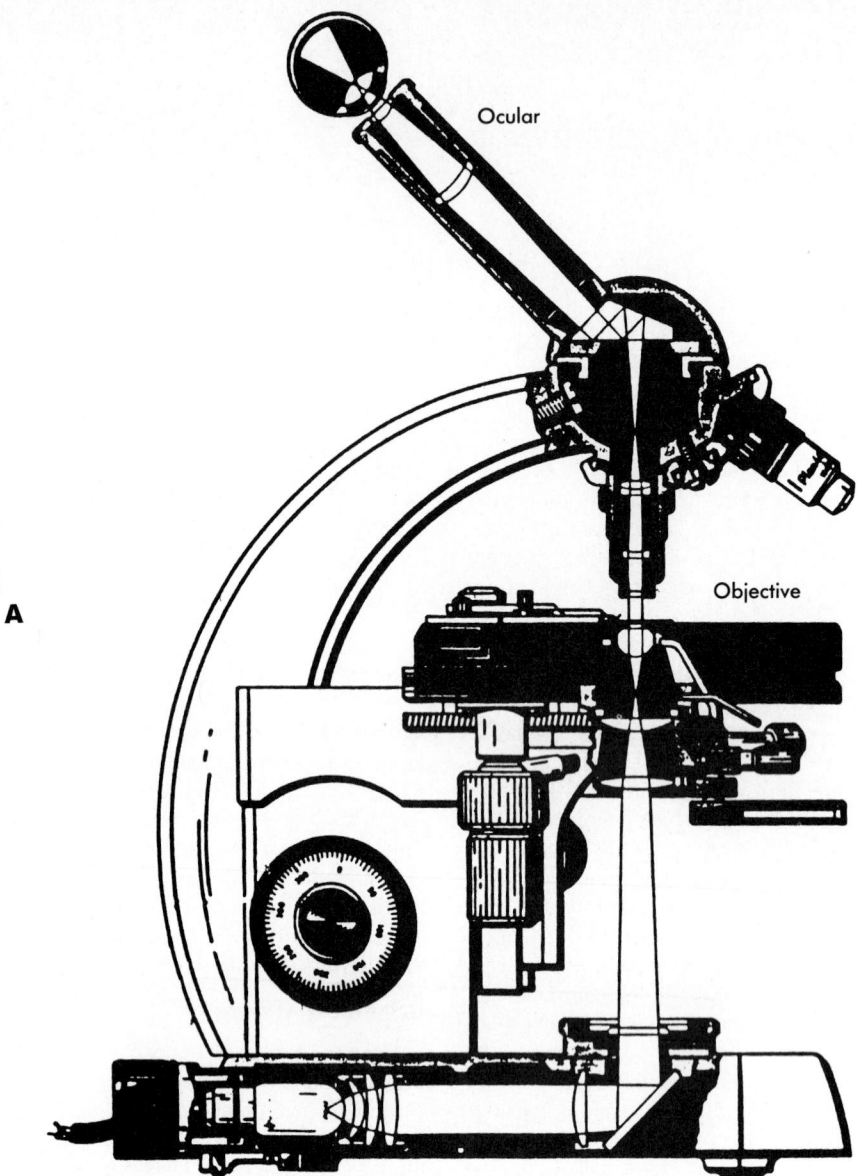

Ocular

Objective

FIGURE 6-1. A, Typical compound microscope.

a coverslip. (3) The depression slide (with the concavity facing down) is lowered onto the coverslip and pressed gently to form a seal. (4) The depression slide is turned over for examination of the "hanging drop." When observing the hanging drop the examiner should focus on the periphery to detect motility on the fluid-air interface.

Wet mounts may be prepared by placing a loopful of liquid culture on a glass slide and covering with a coverslip. Wet mounts of nonliquid material (such as bacterial colony or clinical material) are prepared by emulsifying a loopful of the material in a loopful of water and then adding the coverslip.

Darkfield Microscope

The darkfield microscope provides a means of producing contrast in the images of living or unstained specimens. In con-

trast to brightfield microscopy, in darkfield microscopy specimens are not observed by transmitted illumination. Instead a special condenser focuses a hollow cone of light onto the specimen (Figure 6-2). The specimen is illuminated at an oblique angle so any light transmitted directly through the specimen does not enter the objective lens. With no specimen in the field of view, the field appears uniformly dark. When a specimen is introduced, its various structural features act to scatter light. Some of the light is scattered at angles that allow it to enter the objective lens (Figure 6-2). Scattered light is thus used to form the image of the specimen, which appears bright against a dark background.

The extent to which a structure scatters light depends on the difference between its refractive index and that of the material surrounding it. For a structure to be observed by darkfield

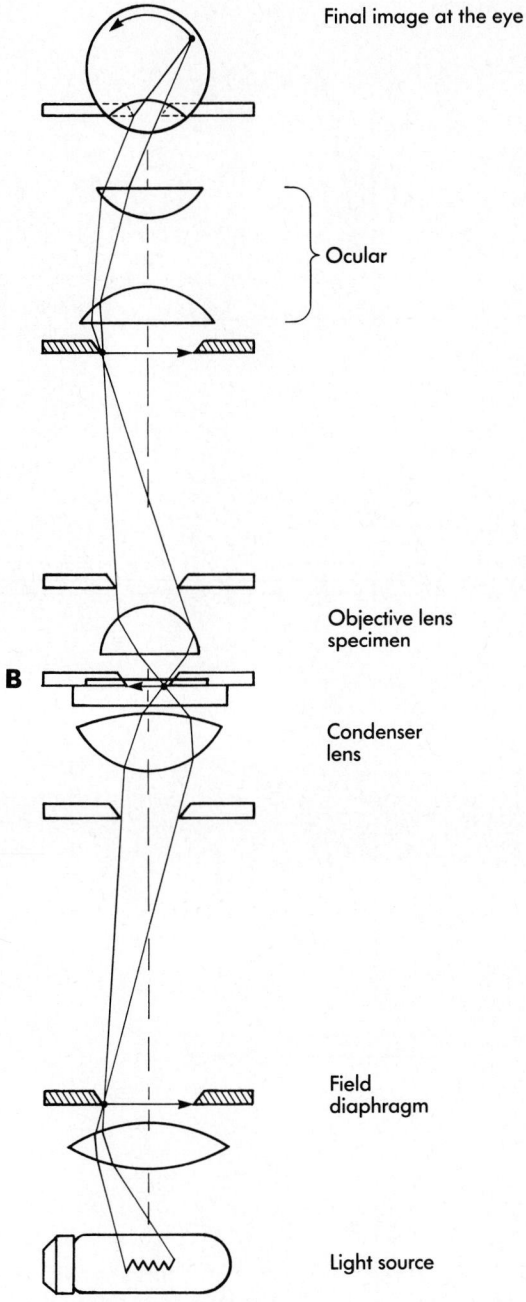

Final image at the eye

Ocular

Objective lens
specimen

B

Condenser
lens

Field
diaphragm

Light source

Imaging beam path

FIGURE 6-1, cont'd. B, Diagrammatic representation of light paths established in compound microscope. (Courtesy Carl Zeiss, Inc., Thornwood, N.Y.)

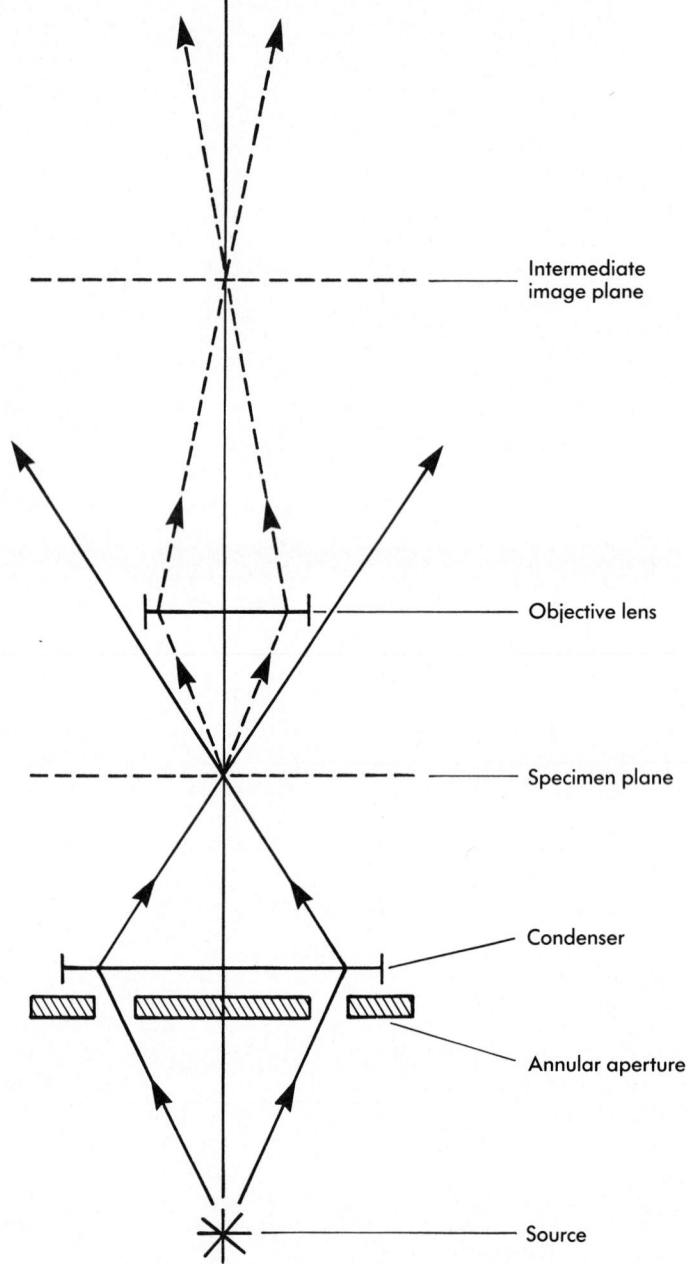

Intermediate
image plane

Objective lens

Specimen plane

Condenser

Annular aperture

Source

FIGURE 6-2. Operation of darkfield condenser to achieve darkfield microscopy. Annular aperture in condenser focuses hollow cone of light onto specimen. Only rays scattered by specimen *(dotted lines)* enter objective to form image. (Modified from Ruthman, A.: Methods in cell research, London, 1970, G. Bell & Sons, Ltd.)

microscopy, the difference in the two refractive indexes must be pronounced. Because most cell structures do not differ significantly in refractive index, considerable cellular structure cannot be observed by darkfield microscopy, although cell shapes and some features are readily discerned. Microorganisms that are not readily stained for brightfield microscopy, such as *Treponema pallidum*, may be examined with darkfield optics.

Fluorescence Microscope

Fluorescence microscopy makes use of the properties of compounds termed fluorochromes. Fluorochromes fluoresce; that is, they absorb light from the short visible to long ultraviolet portion of the spectrum, reemitting the absorbed energy in the form of longer wavelength visible light. The wavelengths absorbed and emitted are characteristic of the particular fluorochrome used.

A number of fluorochromes, each with specific staining properties, are available. Fluorochromes such as acridine orange and auramine may be used to stain organisms directly. This is especially useful for detection of organisms in blood culture or for the identification of acid-fast bacilli in smears. Alternatively, fluorochromes such as fluorescein isothiocyanate may be conjugated to antibodies. The use of fluorochrome-conjugated antibodies, also known as immunofluorescence, provides a highly sensitive and specific means for localizing and identifying particular antigens or microorganisms in a specimen. The presence of a particular type of infecting bacterium, for example, may be detected by treating a specimen with fluorochrome-labeled antibodies against the bacterium in question. Where the bacterium is present in the specimen, antibody molecules will be bound, causing the bacterium to fluoresce when viewed with the fluorescence microscope. The various techniques and uses of immunofluorescence are discussed in Chapter 7.

The basic features of a modern fluorescence microscope are illustrated in Figure 6-3. High-intensity mercury arc or xenon lamps are used to provide illumination of sufficient intensity at the required wavelengths. Light is directed through the objective lens and onto the specimen by means of a dichromatic beam splitter. The objective lens also serves as the condenser in such an epi-illumination system. Exciter filters are used to limit the incident illumination to the wavelengths that produce maximum fluorescence from the fluorochrome in use. Where fluorochrome is bound in the specimen, fluorescence occurs; the longer wavelengths produced by fluorescence pass the objective and the beam splitter to form the image. Where no fluorochrome is bound, the image is dark. Barrier filters in the light path limit transmission to the fluoresced wavelengths.

Phase Contrast Microscope

When light passes through an unstained biologic specimen, phase differences are created that, by means of special interference optics, can be used to produce contrast in the microscope image. A microscope equipped with such optics can thus be used to observe living cells and unstained specimens. The most commonly employed interference system is the phase contrast microscope. Phase contrast microscopy may be used in lieu of staining and brightfield microscopy to detect fungi, inclusion bodies in virus-infected material, and parasites in a variety of specimen types.

The basic features of the phase contrast microscope are illustrated in Figure 6-4. An annulus in the condenser provides a hollow cone of light to illuminate the specimen. Some of the light traverses the specimen without deviation *(solid lines)*, but some of the light is deviated from a straight path *(one such ray is drawn as a dotted line)*. For many biologic structures the deviated rays experience a phase shift of about 90 degrees (one fourth of a wavelength) because the light slows as it passes through the specimen. The degree of phase shift depends on the thickness and the refractive index of the particular structure. A phase plate in the objective lens is designed so the undeviated rays experience an additional phase shift of 90 degrees over the deviated rays. When the deviated and undeviated rays combine to form the image, they are out of phase by 180 degrees (one half of a wavelength), producing destructive interference and causing the structure to appear dark against a brighter background.

Ultraviolet Microscope

As noted in the discussion of brightfield microscopy, biologic specimens show little selective absorption of visible light. Ultraviolet light, however, is selectively absorbed by biologic molecules. Nucleic acids and proteins absorb ultraviolet light at wavelengths of 260 and 280 nm, respectively. Unstained specimens can thus be observed with an ultraviolet microscope.

Although some gain in resolution is obtained with the ultraviolet microscope, the system has disadvantages. Conventional glass lenses are opaque to ultraviolet light, necessitating the use of expensive quartz optics that transmit such light. Because the eye cannot detect ultraviolet wavelengths and would suffer damage from exposure to them, images from an ultraviolet microscope must be recorded photographically or by means of an ultraviolet-sensitive video system.

ELECTRON MICROSCOPE

The maximum resolution attainable with the compound light microscope is limited by the wavelengths of visible light. The shortest wavelengths, in the blue part of the visible spectrum, are approximately 400 nm. Electrons accelerated in an electrical field are associated with very short wavelengths. For example, electrons accelerated in a 100 kV field have wavelengths of approximately 0.004 nm. The use of an electron beam for illumination in a modern transmission electron microscope allows attainment of resolution limits of approximately 3 Å (1 Å = 10^{-7} mm). The principal advantage of the electron microscope over the compound light microscope is thus the considerable improvement in resolution it offers.

Electron microscopy has been used to determine bacterial ultrastructure, as well as to identify viruses (Figure 6-5). It has been particularly useful in the detection of noncultivable viruses such as hepatitis B virus and rotavirus. Types of electron microscopes include the transmission electron microscope (Figure 6-6), scanning electron microscope, and scanning transmission electron microscope. Since the transmission electron microscope has been used most frequently in clinical microbiology, it is considered here. Detailed reviews of the scanning electron microscope are available from Hayat.[11]

The essential features of a transmission electron microscope are shown in Figure 6-7. Electrons emitted from a tungsten filament are accelerated by an electrical field. Since electrons are readily scattered by air, the interior of the microscope col-

Text continued on p. 95.

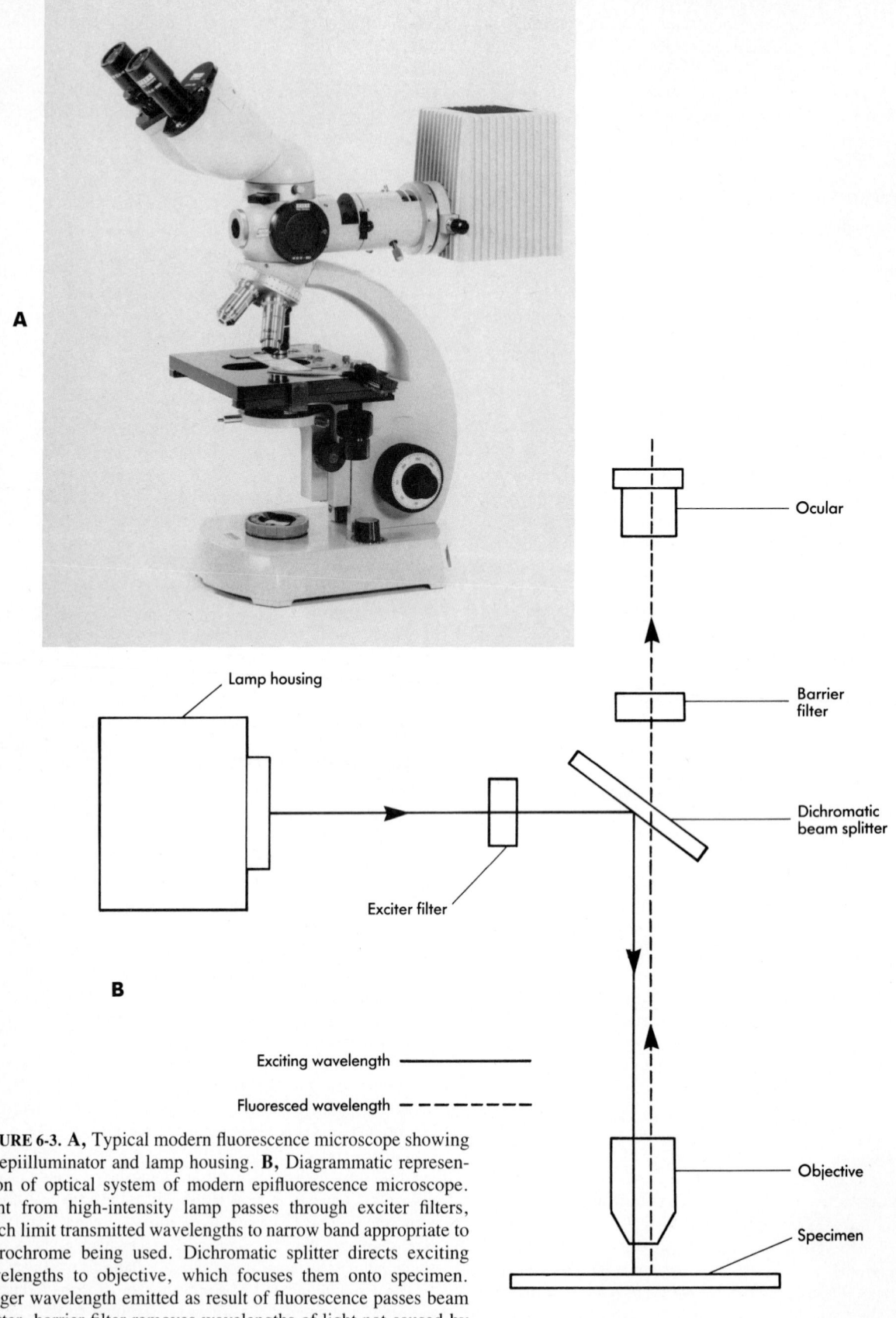

Ocular

Barrier
filter

Dichromatic
beam splitter

Lamp housing

Exciter filter

B

Objective

Specimen

Exciting wavelength ————————

Fluoresced wavelength – – – – – – –

FIGURE 6-3. A, Typical modern fluorescence microscope showing the epiilluminator and lamp housing. **B,** Diagrammatic representation of optical system of modern epifluorescence microscope. Light from high-intensity lamp passes through exciter filters, which limit transmitted wavelengths to narrow band appropriate to fluorochrome being used. Dichromatic splitter directs exciting wavelengths to objective, which focuses them onto specimen. Longer wavelength emitted as result of fluorescence passes beam splitter, barrier filter removes wavelengths of light not caused by fluorescence, and image is observed directly or photographed. (**A** courtesy Carl Zeiss, Inc., Thornwood, N.Y.)

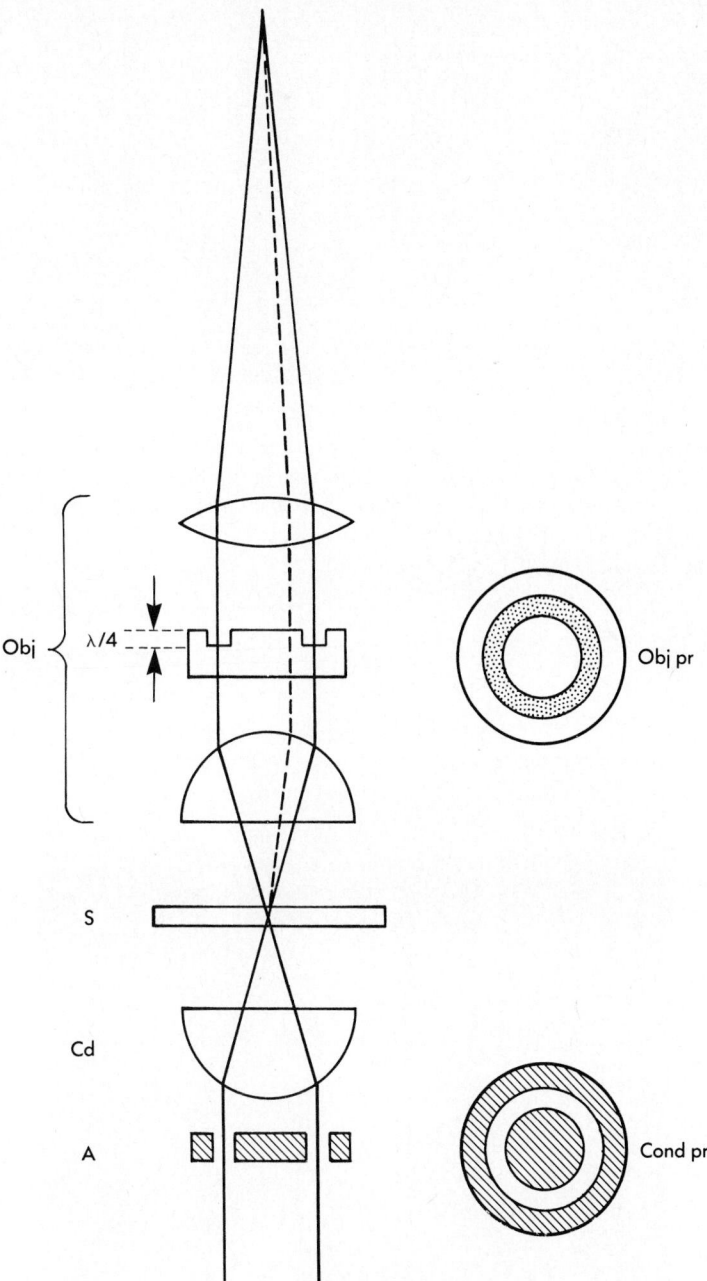

FIGURE 6-4. Basic optical features of phase contrast microscope displayed in diagram form. Comparison of pathway taken by representative deviated ray *(dotted line)* and undeviated ray *(solid line)* illustrates how phase plate retards deviated rays by additional one quarter wavelength *($\lambda/4$)*, leading to interference and production of contrast in the image. *A,* Annulus; *Cd,* condenser lens; *S,* specimen; *Obj,* phase contrast objective; *Obj pr,* phase ring; *Cond pr,* condenser phase ring. (Modified from Ruthman, A.: Methods in cell research, London, 1970, G. Bell & Sons, Ltd.)

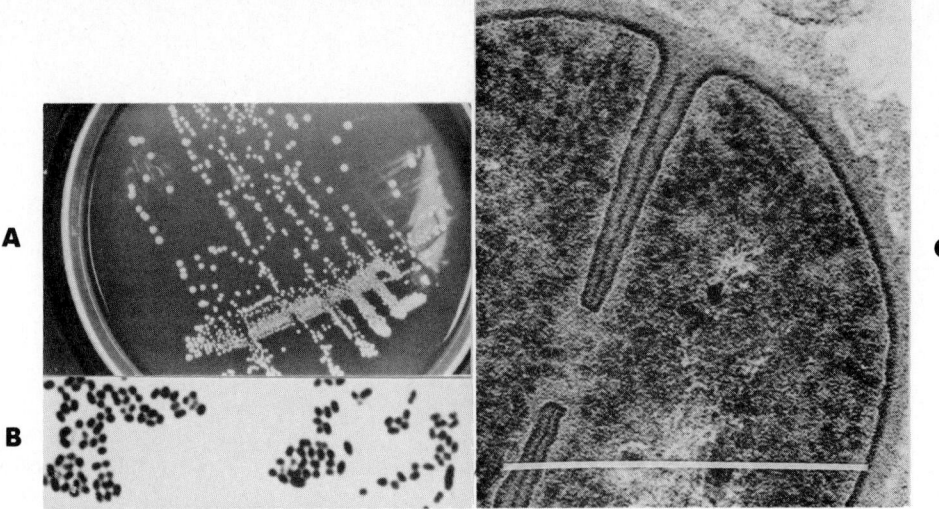

FIGURE 6-5. *Staphylococcus aureus* visualized by different microscopic techniques. **A,** Colonies visualized by unaided eye. **B,** Gram-stained organisms viewed with compound microscope by oil immersion. (×1000.) **C,** Transmission electron micrograph of thin section. (×100,000.) Each bar is 0.5 μm. (From Douglas, S.D.: Microscopy. In Lennette, E.H., et al., editors: Manual of clinical microbiology, ed. 4, Washington, D.C., 1985, American Society for Microbiology.)

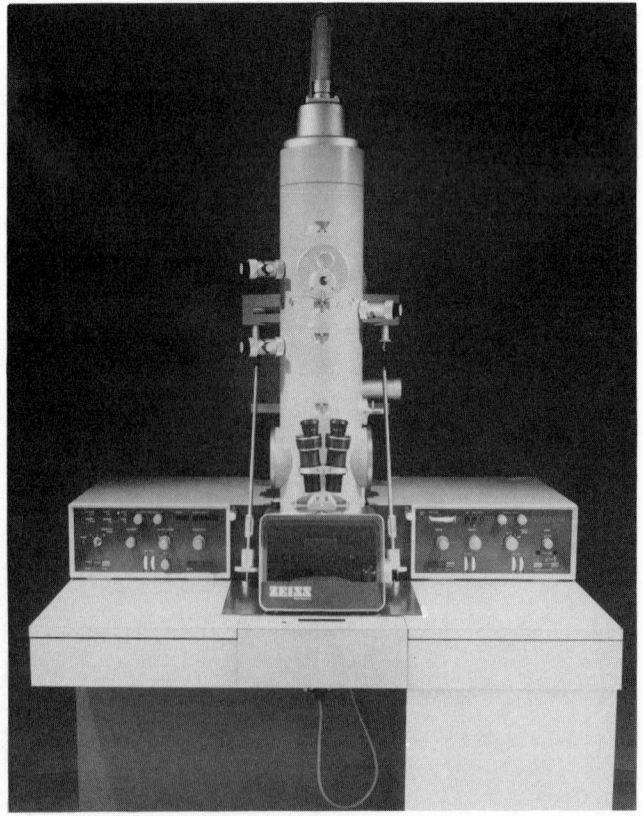

FIGURE 6-6. Transmission electron microscope. (Courtesy Carl Zeiss, Inc., Thornwood, N.Y.)

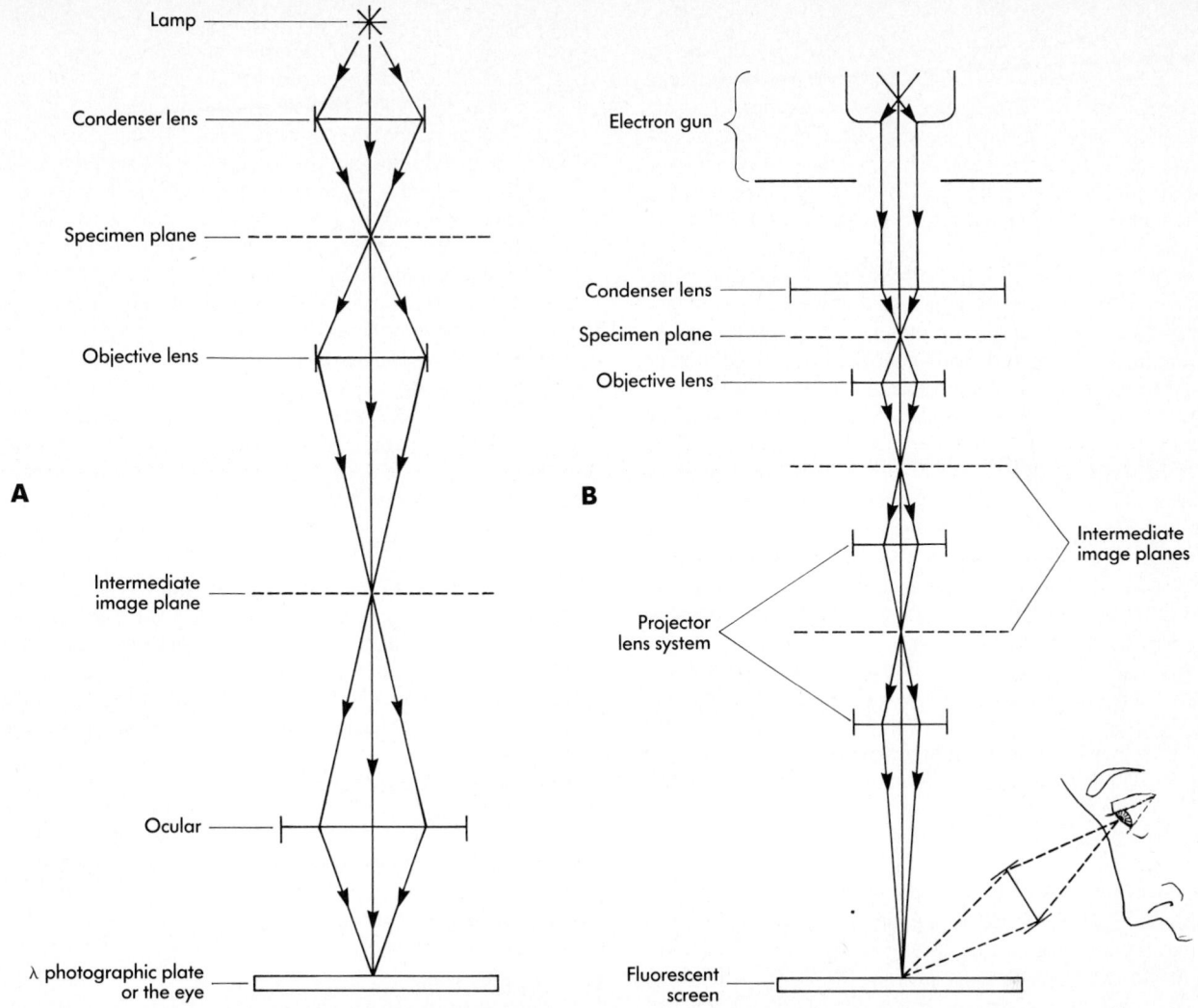

FIGURE 6-7. Comparison of optical systems of, **A,** inverted light microscope and, **B,** transmission electron microscope. Basic layouts are similar, but focusing electron beam requires electromagnetic rather than glass lenses, and electron gun instead of incandescent lamp. (Modified from Slayter, E.M.: Optical methods in biology, New York, 1970, John Wiley & Sons, Inc.)

umn must be maintained at high vacuum; live specimens thus cannot be examined. Focusing of the electron beam is accomplished by varying the magnetic field of electromagnetic lenses. The setup of these lenses is basically the same as in an inverted light microscope (Figure 6-7). One or two condenser lenses concentrate the electron beam onto the specimen; an objective lens provides initial magnification; and one or more projector lenses act to magnify the image further in the manner of the ocular of the light microscope. Since the eye is not sensitive to the electron beam, an image is formed by focusing the beam onto a fluorescent screen. Resolution on the screen is inferior to that provided in the actual image, so specimens are photographed for critical observation.

Specimen contrast is attained by staining specimens with heavy metals such as uranium, osmium, and lead. Where these dense elements are present in the specimen, electrons are scattered from the beam, causing the corresponding part of the image to appear darker on the fluorescent screen or in electron micrographs. Specimens must be very thin (typically 80 nm or less) to allow the electron beam to pass through them and form an image. Individual cells, parts of cells, viruses, or molecules may be affixed to thin electron-transparent films and stained by pooling heavy metal stain around them. Such negatively stained preparations are quickly prepared (see Figures 46-2 and 46-3). For examination of interior features of intact cells, tissue specimens must be fixed, embedded in plastic, and sectioned using diamond or glass knives on an ultramicrotome. Such sections, typically stained with osmium, uranium, and lead, provide considerable structural information. Specimen preparation is time consuming, however, and sectioning requires a reasonable amount of skill. Furthermore, the extremely thin sections (60 to 90 nm in thickness) provide what is essentially only a two-dimensional image of three-dimensional structures and require careful interpretation for many purposes.

STAINING

As previously mentioned, staining is used in conjunction with brightfield microscopy to allow better visualization of microorganisms. Staining is the artificial coloration of a substance. In microbiology, staining has several purposes: to demonstrate microorganisms and sometimes human cells in a specimen, to elucidate structures such as spores or flagella, and to differentiate organisms on the basis of a property such as cell wall chemistry.

The first step in any staining procedure is the proper preparation of the smear. Smears are typically made from colonies, from broths, or from clinical specimens. Ideally, organisms to be examined should form a monolayer that is concentrated enough for easy viewing but sufficiently sparse that the organisms are separated from one another. Smears from colonies are made by placing a small drop of bacteria-free water on a clean slide, transferring a portion of a colony with loop, stick, or needle to the drop, and gently mixing. For broths a drop is placed on a slide. Preparing adequate smears from specimens requires judgment, both in selecting the portion of the specimen to use and in spreading the specimen to the right density. For example, a purulent portion of sputum is selected and spread so there is sufficient material to be easily read with the oil immersion lens, yet not so much material that it would be lost during staining. All smears are allowed to air dry or dry with gentle heat. The smears are then fixed with heat on an electric slide warmer or by passing them rapidly two or three times through the flame of a Bunsen burner. Alternatively, the smears may be fixed with methanol. This is accomplished by placing a few drops of methanol on the air-dried smear and again allowing it to air dry. The smear is then ready for staining.

Table 6-1 lists the most commonly used stains in clinical microbiology and indicates the number of the stain as it is designated in the following discussion. The stains, such as Fites acid-fast or Dieterle stain, that are used for tissue sections and the stains for fungi and parasites are not discussed here but can be found in staining manuals[2] or in the mycology or parasitology sections of this book.

DIFFERENTIAL STAINS

Differential staining is the use of more than one stain to demonstrate differences between the chemical compositions of bacterial cells. Simple staining, on the other hand, is the use of only a single basic dye to visualize the cell. In clinical microbiology the most commonly used differential stains are the Gram stain and the acid-fast stain.

Gram Stains
Principle

There are two basic types of bacterial cell walls. Among other differences, one type is distinguished by large amounts of teichoic acids, the other by having lipopolysaccharides in the outer membrane. In 1884, Christian Gram developed a staining technique that colored some bacteria deep blue and some colorless or stained only by the counterstain. Subsequent work showed that the so-called gram-positive bacteria (those that stained deep blue) had a cell wall with teichoic acid and those that were gram negative (red) contained lipopolysaccharides. Thus, fortuitously, the Gram stain has become the most basic stain in bacteriology, delineating major structural and taxonomic groups of organisms.

The Gram stain uses four different reagents. The initial stain, crystal violet (hexamethyl-*p*-rosanaline chloride) colors all cells a deep blue. A potassium iodide–iodine solution is then added. Since the bulkier iodide replaces the chloride in the crystal violet molecule, the complex formed becomes insoluble in water. Thus far both gram-positive and gram-negative cells react in the same way. When the decolorizer is added, however, the stain is removed only from the gram-negative cells. Although a variety of reasons have been evoked for this, such as differential binding to magnesium, ribonucleates, polyamines, or nucleic acids or differential permeability,[2] recent evidence[3,7] suggests that the alcohol decolorizer damages the outer membrane of the gram-negative organisms, which allows the crystal violet–iodine complex to leak out. The undamaged gram-positive cell wall retains the stain.[3,7] The safranin counterstain makes the gram-negative cells visible. The counterstain also stains gram-positive cells that had damaged cell walls for other reasons (for example, old, dead cells).

Types of Gram stains

Hucker modification of Gram stain (stain 1)[1,13]

PRINCIPLE. Christian Gram's original stain used gentian violet, a mixture of crystal violet, which stains deep blue, and methyl violet, which has reddish hues. Hucker's modification of the Gram stain uses pure crystal violet and is recommended because it is very stable and allows better differentiation of the organisms.

REAGENTS
1. Crystal violet stain
   Stock solution

Crystal violet (90% to 95% dye content)	300 g
Ethanol (95%)	3000 g

   Working solution

Ammonium oxalate	24 g
Distilled water	2400 ml
Filtered stock crystal violet	600 ml

2. Iodine stain
   Stock solution (Lugol's iodine)

Iodine (crystal or resublimed)	25 g
Potassium iodide	50 g
Distilled water	500 ml

   Mix or let stand until dissolved.
   Working solution

Stock iodine solution	100 ml
Distilled water	1400 ml

3. Decolorizer
   General

Acetone	1500 ml
Ethanol (95%)	1500 ml

   For anaerobes and student use

Ethanol (95%)	As is

4. Safranin O counterstain
   Stock solution

Safranin O	50 g
Ethanol (95%)	2000 ml

   Working solution

Safranin stock	300 ml
Distilled water	2700 ml

In some clinical laboratories it is convenient to make stock solutions of the stable Gram stain components and mix them when needed. The solutions just given will last even a large

TABLE 6-1. Stains and Uses

Type	Recommended Procedure[a]	Use
DIFFERENTIAL STAINS		
Gram stain	1. Hucker modification	General bacterial stain
	2. Gram stain with carbol-fuchsin counterstain	Anaerobes, *Legionella* spp., *Brucella* spp.
	3. Kopeloff modification	Anaerobes
Acid-fast stains	4. Ziehl-Neelsen	Good general acid-fast stain for direct smears or confirmation of colonies of mycobacteria; may be modified for use with *Nocardia* (see Chapter 30) or for detection of spores or *Cryptosporidium* (see below)
	5. Kinyoun	Same as Ziehl-Neelsen stain
	6. Fluorochrome	Direct specimen screening
	Hank's modified acid-fast stain	*Nocardia* spp.—see Chapter 30 and Appendix B
	Fite	Mycobacteria in tissue and *Mycobacterium leprae*
STAINS FOR DEMONSTRATING STRUCTURES		
Flagella	7. Leifson	All of these stains demonstrate pattern of bacterial flagellation
	8. Silver	
	9. Ryu	
Spores	10. Malachite green (heated)	
	11. Ziehl-Neelsen modification	
Metachromatic granules	12. Albert stain	Stain a variety of organisms; especially useful for demonstrating metachromatic granules of *Corynebacterium diphtheriae*
	13, 14. Methylene blue	
Capsule	15. Anthony/Hiss method	Demonstrates capsule surrounding bacteria
	India ink, mucicarmine	See Chapter 29 and Appendix B
STAINS FOR DEMONSTRATING COLONIES		
Mycoplasma spp.	16. Dienes	All of these stains distinguish *Mycoplasma* colonies from artifacts or other bacterial colonies on a plate
	13, 14. Methylene blue	
ANTIBODY-CONJUGATED STAINS		
Immunofluorescence	Direct and indirect procedures (see specific chapters)	*Streptococcus pyogenes, Bacteroides fragilis, Bordetella pertussis, Legionella, Chlamydia trachomatis,* herpes simplex virus, influenza virus, and others
Enzyme-labeled stains	Immunoperoxidase	Several viruses

Continued.

TABLE 6-1. Stains and Uses—cont'd

Type	Recommended Procedure[a]	Use
OTHER MICROBIAL STAINS		
General stains	17. Acridine orange	Distinguishes bacteria from human cells and debris as in blood or CSF; also used for the staining of *Mycoplasma* spp. and some parasites
	13, 14. Methylene blue	
Legionella spp.	Dieterle silver Gimenez Direct fluorescent antibody (DFA) stain	See above and Chapter 24
Cryptosporidium spp.	11. Ziehl-Neelsen modification	
Spirochetes	18. Silver nitrate (Fontana)	
Pneumocystis carinii	Gomori methenamine–silver nitrate stain[5] Giemsa	See Chapter 43
Parasites	Trichrome Iron hematoxylin Giemsa	To distinguish parasites; see Chapter 40 and Appendix B
Fungi	Gomori methenamine–silver nitrate Lactophenol cotton blue Periodic acid–Schiff	To discern yeasts and fungi; see Chapter 29 and Appendix B
Viruses	Direct and indirect immunofluorescence Immunoperoxidase	See Chapter 45 for specific viruses

[a]Numbers refer to stain number in text.

hospital laboratory for months. The solutions fit in the brown chemical bottles that are often discarded after use and thus make economical stain containers. The reagents can obviously be scaled down. A single bottle of crystal violet stain can be made by mixing 5 g crystal violet, 50 ml ethanol (95%), 2 g ammonium oxalate, and 200 ml distilled water. Similarly, Gram's iodine contains 1 g iodine, 2 g potassium iodine, and 300 ml distilled water. However, mixing a large amount of stain provides efficiency and a uniform lot.

PROCEDURE. Prepare smears as discussed previously. Allow all smears to dry, and heat fix them at temperatures achieved on a slide fixer (about 55° to 65° C) or by passing through a Bunsen burner flame rapidly several times. The specimen should not be scorched. Several smears can be made on the same slide as long as they are separated and labeled. A convenient labeling method is a separate paper "slide guide" that has the same divisions as the slide and on which one can record the number or identification of each smear.

After preparing the smear, flood slides with crystal violet solution. After 30 seconds rinse with iodine solution. After another 30 seconds remove the iodine and rinse with tap water. Decolorize with acetone-alcohol for about 1 to 5 seconds (until most of the crystal violet is removed) and rinse with tap water.

A longer time is needed for destaining if ethanol is used. Counterstain with safranin for 30 seconds. Gram-negative bacteria are red, and gram-positive bacteria are dark blue (Plate 1, *A* and *B*). Most tissue cells are red.

The Gram stain has certain limitations. As mentioned previously, gram-positive bacteria may stain gram-negative when the integrity of the cell wall is disrupted. Furthermore, several gram-positive anaerobic bacteria decolorize easily and thus may be incorrectly identified as gram-negative organisms. *Streptobacillus moniliformis* may stain gram positive, although it is actually gram negative. Several alternative methods may be used to confirm the Gram reaction of questionable organisms. The potassium hydroxide (KOH) test is performed by adding a loopful of a bacterial colony to 2 drops of a 3% solution of KOH on a glass slide.[10] The bacteria are mixed continuously in the solution for 30 seconds. During this time the inoculating loop is occasionally raised 1 to 2 cm from the surface of the slide. If the test isolate is gram negative, the cell wall is broken down, releasing DNA to form a viscous mucoid solution that strings when the loop is raised from the solution. Gram-positive organisms show no stringing. A second method for distinguishing gram-positive from gram-negative organisms involves the use of the substrate L-alanine-4-nitroanilide.[4]

Gram-negative organisms produce an aminopeptidase enzyme that hydrolyzes the substrate to produce nitroaniline, a yellow product. Cotton swabs impregnated with L-alanine-4-nitroanilide are available from Remel Laboratories (Lenexa, Kan.). Finally, almost all-gram negative organisms are susceptible to colistin, and almost all gram-positive organisms are susceptible to vancomycin. Regular antimicrobial susceptibility disks may be used to determine this characteristic.

Gram stain for anaerobes and *Legionella* (stain 2)[25]

PRINCIPLE. With the usual Gram stain, *Bacteroides* spp. and *Fusobacterium* spp. may stain weakly, and *Legionella* organisms may not retain the stain at all. The carbol-fuchsin counterstain is more intense than the safranin, and the greater staining time allows better penetration into the cell. Thus these gram-negative organisms are more easily viewed. The ethanol destaining solution is weaker than that used for stain 1, which may allow the anaerobic cocci to retain the crystal violet stain more predictably.

PROCEDURE. Follow the same protocol as for the previous Gram stain except destain with 95% ethanol for about 30 seconds or until most of the crystal violet is removed and counterstain with carbol-fuchsin (a 1:5 aqueous dilution of the Ziehl-Neelsen formulation or a 0.8% wt/vol aqueous solution of basic fuchsin) for 1 minute or longer.[24]

Kopeloff modification (stain 3)[12]

PRINCIPLE. The Kopeloff modification may also be used to allow better visualization of anaerobes. It is recommended by the Virginia Polytechnic Institute.[12]

REAGENTS

1. Alkaline crystal violet stain
   Solution A: Dissolve 10 g crystal violet in 1000 ml distilled water.
   Solution B: Dissolve 50 g $NaHCO_3$ in 1000 ml distilled water.
2. Iodine
   Dissolve 4 g NaOH in 25 ml distilled water. Add 20 g of iodine and 1 g of potassium iodide. Dissolve well. Gradually add 975 ml of distilled water; mix well with each addition.
3. Decolorizer
   Mix 300 ml acetone with 700 ml of 95% ethyl alcohol.
4. Safranin counterstain
   To 20 g safranin add only enough 95% ethyl alcohol to dissolve the safranin. Add 1000 ml distilled water to the safranin solution.

PROCEDURE. Flood the slide with solution A. Add approximately 5 drops of solution B to solution A on the slide. Leave the crystal violet solution on the slide for a minimum of 1 minute. Rinse and apply iodine for a minimum of 2 minutes. Hold the slide in a tilted position, apply decolorizer, and rinse immediately. Add safranin counterstain for a minimum of 40 seconds.

Acid-Fast Stains
Principle

Certain organisms, most notably the mycobacteria, retain stains even after attempts at decolorizing with acids, acid-alcohol, or acid-acetone solutions. This property, called acid fastness, is attributed to a cell wall containing mycolic acid (a lipid) in mycobacteria and closely related organisms and to undefined impermeability factors for endospores and *Cryptosporidium*.

Since these factors make staining the organism more difficult, heat, organic solvents, or detergents are needed to facilitate stain penetration. The principle for the three acid-fast stains presented here is the same except that the rhodamine-auramine stain must be examined with fluorescence microscopy.

Types of acid-fast stains
Ziehl-Neelsen stain (stain 4)[24]
REAGENTS

1. Carbol-fuchsin stain

Basic carbol-fuchsin, saturated solution (3 g basic fuchsin in 100 ml 95% ethanol)	10 ml
Distilled water	90 ml
5% aqueous solution of phenol	3 ml

2. Decolorizer

Concentrated hydrochloric acid	3 ml
95% ethanol	97 ml

3. Counterstain

Methylene blue chloride	0.3 ml
Distilled water	100 ml

PROCEDURE. Fix smears by gentle heating over a Bunsen flame (or on an electric slide warmer at 65° C for 2 hours). Place a piece of filter paper, slightly larger than the smear, on each slide. Flood the slides with carbol-fuchsin solution and heat to steaming with a flame; allow them to stand for 5 minutes without further heating. (If an electric staining rack is used, allow the slides to stain for 15 minutes.) Remove filter paper strips and wash the slides in tap water. Decolorize in several successive portions of acid-alcohol until no more color appears in the washings (about 2 minutes; a longer time may be required for thicker smears). Wash with tap water to reduce contamination of organisms from one slide to another; use a staining rack. Do not use a common staining jar or dish. Counterstain with methylene blue for about 30 seconds. Wash with water and air dry. Acid-fast organisms appear red, and background material appears blue (Plate 1, *C*). Reading and reporting of the smear are discussed in Chapter 26.

Kinyoun stain (stain 5)[24]
REAGENTS

1. Carbol-fuchsin stain

Basic fuchsin	4 g
Ethyl alcohol (95%)	20 ml
Dissolve and add slowly while shaking.	
Distilled water	100 ml
Liquefied phenol (melted crystals)	8 g

2. Decolorizer

Ethanol (95%)	97 ml
Concentrated hydrochloric acid	3 ml

3. Counterstain

Methylene blue chloride	0.3 ml
Distilled water	100 ml

PROCEDURE. Prepare smear; fix with gentle heat. Stain with Kinyoun carbol-fuchsin for 3 minutes (do not heat), and then wash gently in running water. Decolorize with acid-alcohol until no more color appears in the washing (about 2 minutes); wash gently in running water. Counterstain with methylene blue for 30 seconds. Wash gently in running water, and dry in air. Acid-fast organisms appear red, and background material appears blue. Reading and reporting of the smear are discussed in Chapter 26.

Fluorochrome stain (stain 6)[24]

REAGENTS

1. Auramine-rhodamine stain (store in dark bottle)

Auramine	1.5 g
Rhodamine	0.75 g
Glycerol	75 ml
Phenol	10 ml
Distilled water	50 ml

2. Decolorizer

Concentrated hydrochloric acid	0.5 ml
Ethanol (70%)	100 ml

3. Counterstain (store in dark place)

Potassium permanganate	0.5 g
Distilled water	100 ml

or

Acridine orange	0.01 g
0.01% Na$_2$HPO$_4$ solution (0.01 g/dl distilled water)	100 ml

PROCEDURE. Heat fix the smear on a slide warmer or with flame as for Ziehl-Neelsen stain. Flood the smear with auramine-rhodamine stain. Let stand at room temperature for 15 minutes. Do not heat. Rinse with tap water. Decolorize with acid-alcohol for 2 minutes. Rinse with tap water. Flood the smear with one of the two counterstains for 2 and not more than 4 minutes. Rinse with tap water. Air dry. Do not blot. Read as soon as possible after staining.

Examine the slide with fluorescence microscopy equipment and techniques. Use of an exciter filter allowing light of wavelengths 510 to 560 nm to pass and a barrier filter allowing light of wavelengths 580 to 590 nm to pass is recommended. The fluorescent properties of fluorescein-isothiocyanate require the use of a different set of filters—an exciter filter allowing wavelengths of 450 nm to 490 nm to pass and a barrier filter allowing a wavelength of 520 nm to pass. Acid-fast organisms emit a bright yellow fluorescence. With the potassium permanganate counterstain, debris is usually a pale yellow and the background dark. With the acridine orange counterstain, the background is stained red or orange, which sharply contrasts with the bright yellow acid-fast organisms. Smears may be scanned rapidly with a 10× objective. Occasionally it may be necessary to use the 40× or 45× objective for confirmation of bacterial morphology. The fluorochrome smear may be confirmed by a Ziehl-Neelsen stain by overstaining without removing the rhodamine-auramine stain. If overstained with Ziehl-Neelsen stain, however, the smear is no longer satisfactory for fluorescence examination. Reading and reporting of the smear are discussed in Chapter 26.

STAINS FOR DEMONSTRATING STRUCTURES

Differentiation among various genera of bacteria (and in some cases among species) is frequently aided by demonstration of specific structures, including spores and capsules. The most commonly used stains include the following.

Flagella Stains
Principle

Flagella are the motile organelles of bacteria. The filament portion of the flagella is composed of protein subunits called flagellin molecules. It takes about 10,000 flagellin monomers polymerized together in an orderly fashion to make a single flagellum. Several problems are associated with demonstrating flagella on bacteria in a clinical laboratory. First, bacterial production of flagella is not continuous but is controlled by temperature, nutrients, and stage of growth cycle, among other factors. Unfavorable growth conditions can turn off synthesis of flagellin. Second, flagella can be sheared mechanically from the cell body by, for example, shaking or pipetting too vigorously. Third, flagella become depolymerized easily. Heat over 60° C and acid (pH 4) can cause the flagella to dissociate into flagellin monomers. Urea, organic solvents, and bases can also depolymerize flagella. Fourth, even though flagella may be present, they are too narrow (about 15 nm in diameter) to be seen with the light microscope unless their width is first increased.

Taking these points into account, an effective protocol is as follows. Bacteria are grown in brain infusion agar, blood trypticase soy agar, or trypticase soy agar for 18 hours at about 30° C (22° to 37° C has been recommended for specific organisms, but 30° C is an adequate temperature for almost all bacteria). The bacteria are gently transferred to a slide and air dried. Tannic acid or tannin, a polymer of gallic acid, is added. This attaches to the flagella, making them wider (Plate 1, D and E). The stain then attaches to the tannic acid. Unfortunately, the tannic acid also attaches to background material and the glass slide, so the major problem in flagella staining is a background that is too high. The timing is important. If staining proceeds too long, everything will be red.

Types of flagella stains

Leifson stain (stain 7)[6,16]
REAGENTS

1. Solution A

Fuchsin (certified for flagella staining)	0.5 g
Ethyl alcohol, 95%	50 ml

    Shake and let stand overnight to dissolve.

2. Solution B

Distilled water	100 ml
Sodium chloride	0.75 ml
Tannic acid	1.5 g

Combine solutions A and B and mix thoroughly. The stain is ready for use immediately and should remain satisfactory for about 1 to 2 months when stored at 4° to 5° C. The precipitate that develops during storage should not be disturbed when the stain is used.

PROCEDURE. With a loop or needle, transfer a clump of cells about the size of a pin head to 3 to 5 ml distilled water in a test tube. Touch the loop or needle to the side of the tube to resuspend the cells. Invert the tube once to mix. Place 1 drop of this suspension on a clean microscope slide and allow it to air dry. Special cleaning is not needed. Cover the slide with stain. Allow the stain to remain on for about 5 minutes until the greenish sheen that starts from the edges of the stain covers half the area. Do not allow the stain to dry on the slide. Rinse the stain off with water.

Silver stain for flagella (stain 8)[26]
REAGENTS

1. Solution A

Saturated aqueous aluminum phosphate	25 ml
10% aqueous tannic acid	50 ml
5% aqueous ferric chloride	5 ml

2. Solution B

    a. Prepare 100 ml of 5% silver nitrate solution.

b. To 90 ml of the above solution add, drop by drop, 2 to 5 ml of concentrated ammonium hydroxide. A brown precipitate forms; as more stain is added, it dissolves. Stop just as the solution clears.

c. Reverse the procedure and add the remaining 5% silver nitrate one drop at a time until the solution becomes faintly cloudy.

d. Store the solution in a dark bottle at room temperature. The solution is stable for several months.

PROCEDURE. Place the slides on a staining rack. Flood the slides with solution A. Leave 4 minutes. Rinse with distilled water. Flood them with solution B. Heat just until steam is emitted by running a burner under the slides on the rack. Stain 4 minutes. Rinse with distilled water. Slant to dry.

Ryu modification of flagella stain (stain 9)[14]

PRINCIPLE. The principle for this flagella stain is the same as for the Leifson flagella stain (stain 7) in that the tannic acid polymerizes to the flagella, making them wider. The crystal violet stains them. A major advantage is the stability of the reagents even at room temperature.[13]

REAGENTS

1. Solution A

Tannic acid	10 g
Saturated aqueous aluminum potassium sulfate	50 ml
5% aqueous phenol	50 ml

2. Solution B

Crystal violet	12 g
Ethanol (95%)	100 ml

PROCEDURE. Prepare the slides as for the Leifson stain. Mix 10 ml of solution A and 1 ml of solution B. Stain for 5 minutes with a mixture of A and B.

Spore Stains
Types of spore stains

Malachite green stain (stain 10)[1]

PRINCIPLE. The spore wall is a barrier to passage of materials in and out of the spore. Driving stain into the spore interior and rinsing it out are difficult. Therefore a long staining time and heat are used to ensure the stain penetration. Water removes most of the malachite green from vegetable cells, and a contrasting counterstain applied for a short time allows easier viewing.

REAGENTS. 5% malachite green
Safranin for Gram stain

PROCEDURE. Make a smear and heat fix it. Flood the slide with 5% malachite green solution. Steam by heating from below as for Ziehl-Neelsen stain. Let the hot stain remain for 5 minutes. Wash with water. Counterstain with safranin for 30 seconds. Wash, dry, and blot. Spores appear green, and background material appears red.

Ziehl-Neelsen stain for spores and *Cryptosporidium* spp. (stain 11)[9,22]

PRINCIPLE. The cyst form of *Cryptosporidium*, the usual stage seen in fecal specimens, is resistant to passage of materials to and from its interior as are spores. Heat facilitates the entry of the stain. *Cryptosporidium* cysts and bacterial spores retain the stain during treatment with acid-alcohol solution, whereas vegetative and tissue cells do not.

REAGENTS. As for Ziehl-Neelsen acid-fast stain.

PROCEDURE. For spores, prepare smear as discussed previously and heat fix. For *Cryptosporidium* cysts, fix specimens in 10% formalin (with 10% potassium hydroxide if mucoid) and then remove sediment by centrifugation. Place the supernatant on a slide and heat fix at 70° C for 10 minutes.[9] Flood the slide with carbol-fuchsin. Heat the slide to steaming and allow it to stain for 5 to 10 minutes. Destain with acid-alcohol solution no more than 30 seconds. Counterstain with methylene blue. Spores and *Cryptosporidium* organisms appear red; background and most cells and bacteria are blue.

Stains for Metachromatic Granules
Types of stains

Albert stain and Christensen modification for granules (stain 12)[1]

PRINCIPLE. Metachromatic granules, or as they are also called, volutin granules, are an accumulation of inorganic polyphosphorates. The term "metachromatic" is used because the granules appear reddish when stained with a basic blue dye such as methylene blue or toluidine blue. The polyphosphates, which are polymers of orthophosphate of varying chain lengths, may be a source of adenosine triphosphate (ATP). Although many microorganisms may form metachromatic granules, they are particularly characteristic of some of the species of corynebacteria.

REAGENTS

1. Solution A

Toluidine blue	0.15 g
Ethanol (95%)	2 ml
Dissolve dye in ethanol.	
Distilled water	100 ml
Glacial acetic acid	5 ml

2. Solution B
Gram stain iodine
3. Solution C
Gram stain safranin

PROCEDURE. Make a smear of *Corynebacterium diphtheriae* or other organisms and heat fix. Cover slide with solution A. After 1 minute rinse with water. Drain. Flood slide with solution B. Rinse with water. Drain. Counterstain with solution C for 1 minute. Drain. Blot. The metachromatic granules are black and the remainder of the bacterium is red. Dark green to black bands may be seen in some organisms as a result of irregular staining.

Methylene blue stain for granules and bacteria (stain 13)

PRINCIPLE. Methylene blue is an aniline dye commonly used in staining. Most bacteria absorb this stain more intensely than tissue cells do. Thus it is a useful stain for viewing, for example, spinal fluid in which discerning gram-negative bacteria against a red background would be difficult. In addition, methylene blue imparts a deeper blue or red hue to the metachromatic granules of *C. diphtheriae*.

REAGENTS. Methylene blue counterstain used in Ziehl-Neelsen stain (stain 4) (0.3% aqueous solution of methylene blue chloride) is adequate. The methylene blue chloride salt is soluble in water, eliminating the need to alkalinize.[22]

The acid methylene blue used for parasite trophozoites[19] or Loeffler alkaline methylene blue can also be used as a stain for granules and bacteria.

PROCEDURE. Prepare and fix the smear. Flood the slide with methylene blue for 1 to 2 minutes. Granules are deep blue or reddish blue, and cell bodies are light blue.

Loeffler alkaline methylene blue (stain 14)

PRINCIPLE. The Loeffler alkaline methylene blue stain is based on the same principle as the other methylene blue stain (stain 13). It is included in this chapter mainly for historical interest. Whether the methylene blue is dissolved only in water as for the Ziehl-Neelsen counterstain or with alcohol and sodium hydroxide does not affect its use as a bacterial stain.

REAGENTS

Methylene blue (C.I. 52015)	0.3	g
Ethyl alcohol, 95%	30	ml
Potassium hydroxide	0.01	g
Distilled water	100	ml

PROCEDURE. Use gentle heat to fix the smear. Flood the smear with the stain, and let it stand for 1 minute. Wash with tap water and blot dry.

Capsular Stains

Anthony/Hiss stain (stain 15)

PRINCIPLE. The capsular material of almost all bacteria is polysaccharide (the capsule of *Bacillus anthracis* is an exception; it is polypeptide) and thus does not bind to protein stains such as crystal violet. To demarcate the outer boundary of the capsule, the bacteria are suspended in a proteinaceous fluid such as milk or serum and dried on a slide. After treatment with a protein stain, the clear area around the cells marks the location of the capsule. Copper sulfate stains capsular material.

REAGENTS. 1% aqueous crystal violet
Gram stain crystal violet
20% aqueous copper sulfate

PROCEDURE. Provide a proteinaceous background for the capsule by suspending the cells on the slide in a drop of skimmed milk, litmus milk, or 10% serum solution. Air dry. Flood with crystal violet for 2 minutes. Wash with 20% copper sulfate. Air dry in a vertical position. The background is light purple, cells are deep purple, and capsules are light blue or clear.

OTHER STAINS

A variety of other stains are also used in clinical microbiology. Many of these are used to identify specific organisms.

Types of stains

Dienes stain (stain 16)[8,17,20,22]

PRINCIPLE. *Mycoplasma* agar and most artifacts that might be in media used for the isolation of *Mycoplasma* do not stain with methylene blue or azure II, but *Mycoplasma* colonies readily absorb the stain and appear as deep blue dots in the medium. Some bacterial colonies reduce the dye and appear colorless; they are not confused with *Mycoplasma* colonies.

REAGENTS

Methylene blue	2.5	g
Azure II	1.25	g
Maltose	10	g
Sodium carbonate	0.25	g
Distilled water	100	ml

Dissolve and filter before use.

PROCEDURE. Using a loop or cotton swab, place a small amount of the stain next to a suspected colony. The stain diffuses and the colony becomes blue if it is *Mycoplasma*.

Acridine orange stain (stain 17)[15,18,21,23]

PRINCIPLE. As discussed previously, acridine orange is a fluorochrome. It also binds to nucleic acids. These properties were used to develop a differential stain in which, at pH 3 to 4, bacteria and yeast appear bright red or orange and tissue cells appear yellowish green or black. The fact that hemoglobin absorbs some light so that red cells do not fluoresce makes the stain useful for screening blood cultures for growth of organisms. Acridine orange stains *Mycoplasma* cells green or orange-green[20] and *Pneumocystis carinii* trophozoites yellow to orange with a green to yellow cell background.[22] The colors observed depend on the filter system used with the fluorescence microscope.

REAGENTS

Acridine orange	0.02	g
0.2 M sodium acetate buffer (pH 3.5 to 4)	100	ml

PROCEDURE. Place sample from blood culture bottle or specimen on a slide. Dry in air or with gentle heating. Fix in absolute methanol for 2 minutes. Dry. Flood the slide with acridine orange stain for 1 minute and rinse with tap water. This stain is used to differentiate bacteria, which stain bright orange, from tissue, which is yellow to green. The procedure for *Pneumocystis carinii* trophozoites is essentially the same.[23] *Mycoplasma* colonies can be placed on agar before staining to immobilize them, making fixation unnecessary.[21]

Stain for spirochetes (Fontana) (stain 18)[1]

PRINCIPLE. Spirochetes are too narrow to be seen with the light microscope. As in the flagella stain, the tannic acid polymerizes to the bacteria, making them wider. The silver nitrate in solution attaches to the bacteria and is oxidized, forming a brown-black coating.

REAGENTS. Tannic acid, 5% solution in 1% phenol
Fontana silver solution

Dissolve 5 g of silver nitrate ($AgNO_3$) in 100 ml of distilled water. Remove a few milliliters, and to the rest of the solution add drop by drop a concentrated ammonia solution until the precipitate that forms redissolves. Then add drop by drop enough $AgNO_3$ solution back to produce a slight cloudiness that persists after shaking. The solution should remain in good condition for several months.

PROCEDURE. Prepare the smear and fix it with heat. Pour on a solution of 5% tannic acid and 1% phenol and steam 30 seconds. Wash with water. Cover the smear with 1 drop of ammoniacal silver nitrate, heat gently over a flame, and allow it to stand 20 to 30 seconds after steaming begins. Wash in water. Blot dry. Spirochetes are stained brown to black.

REFERENCES

1. Bartholomew, J.W.: Stains for microorganisms in smears. In Clark, G., editor: Staining procedures, ed. 4, Baltimore, 1981, The Williams & Wilkins Co.
2. Bartholomew, J.W., and Mittwer, T.: The Gram stain, Bacteriol. Rev. **16:**1, 1952.
3. Beveridge, T.J., and Davies, J.A.: Cellular responses of *Bacillus subtilis* and *Escherichia coli* to the Gram stain, J. Bacteriol. **156:**846, 1983.
4. Cerny, G.: Method for the distinction of gram-negative from gram-positive bacteria, Eur. J. Appl. Microbiol. **3:**223, 1976.
5. Churukian, C.T., and Schenk, E.A.: Rapid Gromott's methenamine-silver-nitrate method for fungi and *Pneumocystis carinii*, Am. J. Clin. Pathol. **68:**427, 1977.
6. Clark, W.A.: A simplified Leifson flagella stain, J. Clin. Microbiol. **3:**632, 1978.

7. Davies, J.A., et al.: Chemical mechanism of the Gram stain and synthesis of a new electron-opaque marker for electron microscopy which replaces the iodine mordant of the stain, J. Bacteriol. **156:**837, 1983.

8. Dienes, L: Permanent stained agar preparation of *Mycoplasma* and L-forms of bacteria, J. Bacteriol. **93:**689, 1967.

9. Garcia, L.S., et al.: Techniques for the recovery and identification of *Cryptosporidium* cysts from stool specimens, J. Clin. Microbiol. **18:**185, 1983.

10. Halebian, S., et al.: Rapid method that aids in distinguishing gram-positive from gram-negative anaerobic bacteria, J. Clin. Microbiol. **13:**444, 1981.

11. Hayat, M.A.: Introduction to biological scanning electron microscopy, Baltimore, 1978, University Park Press.

12. Holdeman, L.V., Cato, E.P., and Moore, W.E.C., editors: Anaerobe laboratory manual, ed. 4, Blacksburg, Va., 1977, Virginia Polytechnic Institute.

13. Hucker, G.J.: A new modification and application of the Gram stain, J. Bacteriol. **6:**395, 1921.

14. Kodata, H., et al.: Practical procedure for demonstrating bacterial flagella, J. Clin. Microbiol. **16:**948, 1982.

15. Kronvall, G., and Myhre, E.: Differential staining of bacteria in clinical specimens using acridine orange buffered at low pH, Acta Pathol. Microbiol. Scand. (Sect. B) **85:**249, 1977.

16. Leifson, E.: Staining, shape, and arrangement of bacterial flagella, J. Bacteriol. **62:**377, 1951.

17. Madoff, S.: Isolation and identification of PPLO, Ann. N.Y. Acad. Sci. **88:**390, 1960.

18. McCarthy, L.R., and Senne, J.E.: Evaluation of acridine orange stain for detection of microorganisms in blood cultures, J. Clin. Microbiol. **11:**281, 1980.

19. Nair, E.P.: Rapid staining of intestinal amoebae in wet mounts, Nature **172:**1051, 1953.

20. Paik, G.: Reagents, stains, and miscellaneous test procedures. In Lennette, E.H., et al., editors: Manual of clinical microbiology, ed. 3, Washington, D.C., 1980, American Society for Microbiology.

21. Rosendal, S., and Valdiviesco-Garcia, A.: Enumeration of mycoplasmas after acridine orange staining, Appl. Environ. Microbiol. **41:**1000, 1981.

22. Sonnenwirth, A.: Stains and staining procedures. In Sonnenwirth, A.C., and Jarrett, L., editors: Gradwohl's clinical laboratory methods and diagnosis, ed. 8, St. Louis, 1980, The C.V. Mosby Co.

23. Thomson, R.B., and Smith, T.F.: Acridine orange staining of *Pneumocystis carinii,* J. Clin. Microbiol. **16:**191, 1982.

24. Vestal, A.L.: Procedures for the isolation and identification of mycobacteria, DHEW Pub. No. (CDC) 75-8230, Atlanta, 1975, Center for Disease Control.

25. Weaver, R.E., and Feely, J.C.: Cultural and biochemical characterization of the Legionnaires' disease bacterium. In Jones, G.L., and Hébert, G.A., editors: ''Legionnaires'': the disease, the bacterium, and methodology, Atlanta, 1979, Centers for Disease Control.

26. West, M., Burdash, N.M., and Freimuth, F.: Simplified silver-plating stain for flagella, J. Clin. Microbiol. **6:**414, 1977.

ADDITIONAL READINGS

Jones, R.M.: Basic microscopic techniques, Chicago, 1966, University of Chicago Press.

Ruthmann, A.: Methods in cell research, Ithaca, N.Y., 1970, Cornell University Press.

Slayter, E.M.: Optical methods in biology, New York, 1970, John Wiley & Sons, Inc.

CHAPTER 7

Immunoserology in the Clinical Microbiology Laboratory

Richard C. Tilton

Early diagnosis and prompt institution of specific antimicrobial therapy are required for the optimal treatment of infectious disease. Traditionally the laboratory has isolated and identified the specific etiologic agent and when possible determined its antimicrobial susceptibility profile. If this approach was not successful, diagnosis could often be made by observing the appearance of a mixture of specific antibody types, such as IgG and IgM. Although the detection of these antibodies is still important in the diagnosis of infectious disease, the process is time consuming, since for optimal results an acute and a convalescent serum sample must be collected 2 to 3 weeks apart. Detection of specific IgM antibodies in serum and immunologic detection of microbial antigens in body fluids provides a much more rapid diagnosis of infectious disease.

Fundamental discoveries in immunology have influenced virtually every area of biology and medicine. Immunology is used for both diagnosis and treatment. As discussed in Chapter 2, the success of the immune response invariably depends on the immune system's ability to recognize ''foreign'' substances and mount an effective defense. The synthesis of specific antibody in response to antigen stimulus and subsequent recognition of the same foreign antigen forms the basis for immunologic tests in microbiology. A myriad of human cells also play a vital role in the immune response. They include macrophages, mononuclear phagocytes, lymphocytes, and polymorphonuclear leukocytes (see Chapter 2).

Diagnostic tests are based on the recognition of both antigens and antibodies. Antigens are molecular structures with determinant groups capable of stimulating the synthesis of specific antibodies. Antigens, especially those of microbial origin, also are effective markers for the presence of a disease-causing agent. Antigens may be protein, polysaccharide, glycolipid, or nucleoprotein. They occur as components of microbial cells such as capsules, cell wall lipopolysaccharides, teichoic acids, and both structural and secretory proteins. Toxic proteins such as diphtheria toxin and botulinum toxin are strong antigens, as are the molecular components of viruses, fungi, and parasites.

Although exciting discoveries have been made in all areas of immunology, three are particularly important for their relationship to the clinical microbiology laboratory: the discovery of five distinct classes of immunoglobulin and their associated factors, the ability to synthesize monoclonal antibody, and the development of the enzyme immunoassay.

The term ''immunoglobulin'' (Ig) designates all types of protein with antibody activity. Five distinct classes of immunoglobulin exist in humans: IgG, IgA, IgM, IgE, and IgD. Table 7-1 summarizes the properties of human immunoglobulins.[1]

As can be seen in Table 7-1, IgG crosses the placenta. Thus in infants the demonstration of antibodies to a specific microbial agent may not reflect infection but only maternal transfer of IgG. IgM does not cross the placenta and is produced as an early response to infection. Therefore its specific detection in the blood of an infant, as well as an immunologically mature individual, may be diagnostic.

A frequent criticism of immunologic diagnostic tests has been that reagents, particularly antisera, were of poor quality. Antisera were often of low titer, lacked sensitivity, and were relatively nonspecific; that is, they cross-reacted with a number of similar microbial antigens. This inability to consistently produce a sensitive, specific antibody curbed the acceptance of routine immunologic tests for antigen detection. The discovery of the hybridoma technique and the subsequent synthesis of monoclonal antibodies have solved most but not all of these problems.

Most antisera made to microorganisms or other antigens contain multiple antibodies to different antigenic sites, even if a pure antigen is used. If a single antibody-producing cell could be grown in vitro, it would provide an unlimited supply of monoclonal antibody that would bind only to a single antigenic determinant. Kohler and Milstein[39] mixed spleen cells from an immunized mouse with malignant myeloma cells. Some of the cells fused; that is, a mouse spleen cell fused to a myeloma cell. These cells were called hybridomas. Consequently, the technology is now available to produce cells that will continuously divide and synthesize a very pure monoclonal antibody.

Cell lines that secrete antibody of the desired specificity can be cloned and then maintained in tissue culture or transferred to mouse peritoneum for continuous production of monoclonal antibodies. Although the advantages of a continuous antibody synthesizing system are obvious, monoclonal antibodies have limitations. Specificity is fixed; that is, a monoclonal antibody, unlike a polyclonal one, cannot be made more specific. Also, the monoclonal antibody has fixed affinity for an antigen that may not be high enough to be diagnostically useful. Affinity cannot be altered. Furthermore, the antibody may not be multifunctional, since each cell line synthesizes only a single class or subclass of antibody. In heterogeneous antisera a number of activities such as complement fixation, cytotoxicity, agglutination, and antigen precipitation may be present. Each monoclonal antibody may have only one or two of these activities, not necessarily all.

The process of monoclonal antibody formation is shown in Figure 7-1. Monoclonal antibodies were initially used in research. Many are now available commercially and have been incorporated into kits for antigen detection of *Neisseria gonorrhoeae*, *Neisseria meningitidis* group B, herpes simplex virus 1

TABLE 7-1. The Immunoglobulins

Class	Molecular Weight	Diagnostic Importance	Biologic Properties
IgG	150,000	Binds to *Staphylococcus aureus* protein A; antibodies to most bacteria; virus neutralizing antibodies; hemagglutinins	Produced as late response to antigenic stimulus; activates complement; traverses placenta
IgM	900,000	Predominant antibody formed to gram-negative bacterial infection; Wasserman antibody, heterophil antibody, rheumatoid factor, cold agglutinins, hemolysins, isohemagglutinins	Produced as early response to antigen stimulus; does *not* traverse placenta; fixes complement
IgA	160,000	At present time, there are no diagnostic tests for specific IgA antibodies	Does *not* activate complement; secreted in saliva, mucus, colostrum; does *not* traverse placenta; may be first line of defense to infection at mucous membrane
IgD	180,000		No known biologic function but may play role in regulation of other Ig synthesis
IgE	190,000	IgE may be significantly increased in hyperallergenic persons	Also known as "reagin"; does *not* traverse placenta; sensitizes skin leukocytes; active role in hypersensitivity; may combine with invading parasites while Fc portion of molecule is still combined with mast cells; this would release histamine and destroy parasite

Modified from Alexander, J.W., and Good, R.A.: Fundamentals of clinical immunology, Philadelphia, 1977, W.B. Saunders Co.

and 2, *Chlamydia trachomatis,* and hepatitis B virus.

Yet another important advance in immunology has been the development of the enzyme immunoassay. The search for methodology that has the advantages of radioimmunoassays and few of the disadvantages culminated in the discovery of the enzyme immunoassay technique. Engvall and Perlmann[18] first used the enzyme-linked immunosorbent assay (ELISA) to measure rabbit IgG.

ELISA has wide application in clinical microbiology. The concept is similar to RIA. An antibody or an antigen is bound to a solid support, such as a plastic tube, a tray, or a polystyrene bead. The complementary substance forms an antigen-antibody complex. In the simplest procedure an anti–species enzyme–tagged antibody is added to the developing "sandwich." After separation of the bound and free enzyme-tagged antibody (or antigen), enzyme substrate is added and the resulting color formation indicates the presence of either antigen or antibody. The two major types of enzyme immunoassays, homogeneous and heterogeneous, are discussed in detail later in the chapter.

The intent of this chapter is not to exhaustively review traditional immunologic procedures but to focus on techniques that provide rapid and sensitive aids to the detection of microorganisms or their components in the clinical microbiology laboratory.

A few serologic tests are still being performed in clinical microbiology laboratories. Some, such as C-reactive protein and cold agglutinins, are nonspecific acute phase reactants, and others, such as the antistreptolysin O titer and febrile agglutinins, are specific for a particular bacterial disease. Table 7-2 summarizes these tests and the interpretation of the results. Other tests for antibody to bacterial, fungal, viral, and protozoan antigens are discussed in the appropriate chapters.

DETECTION OF MICROBIAL ANTIGENS

Nontraditional approaches to immunologic detection of antibodies and antigens have become popular in clinical microbi-

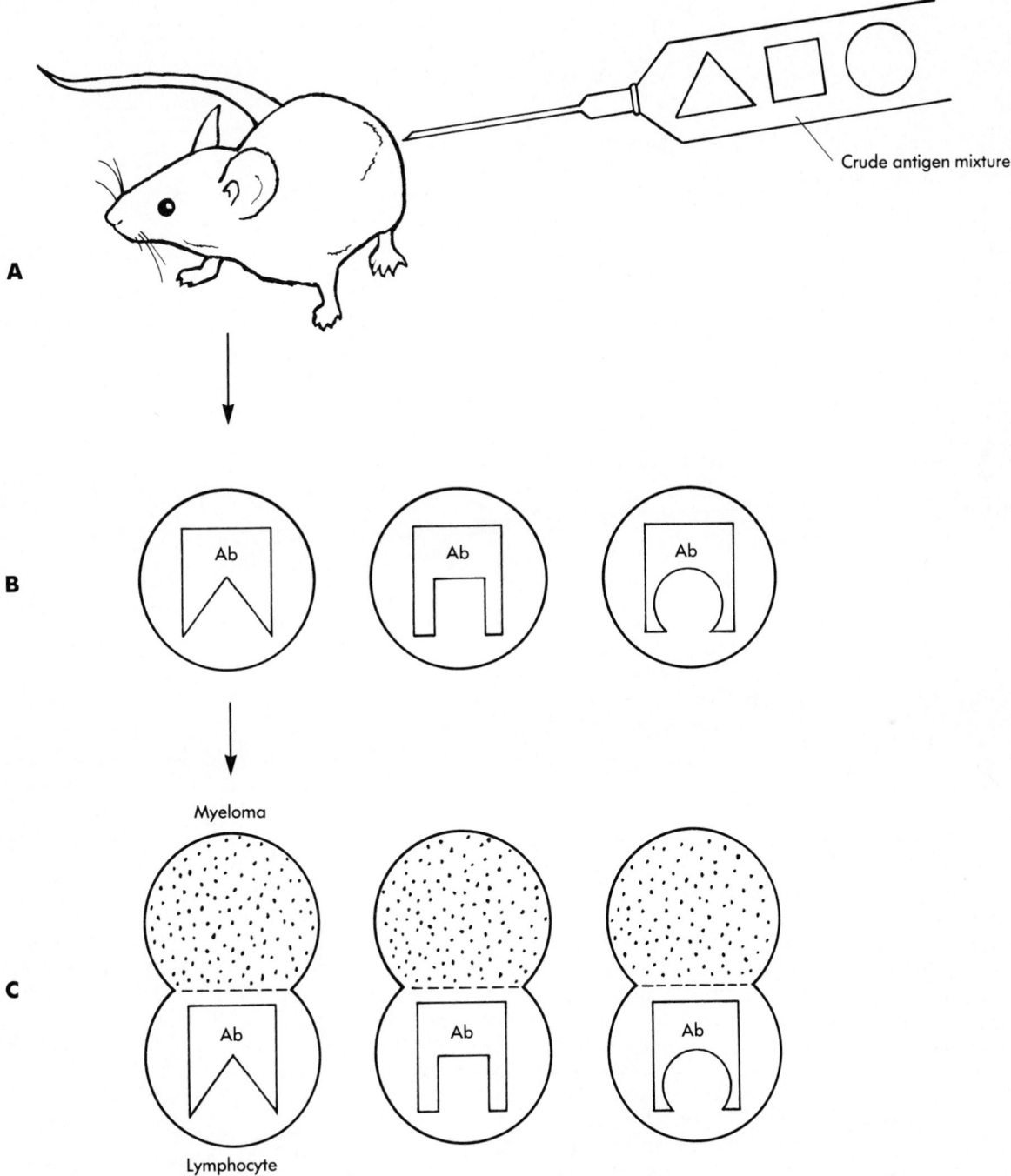

FIGURE 7-1. Monoclonal antibody formation. **A,** Immunization with antigen mixture. **B,** Harvesting of antibody-producing cells from lymph nodes or spleen. **C,** Fusion of antibody-producing cells and myeloma cells to form hybridomas.   *Continued.*

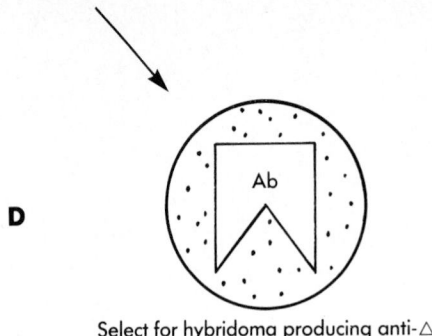

Select for hybridoma producing anti-△

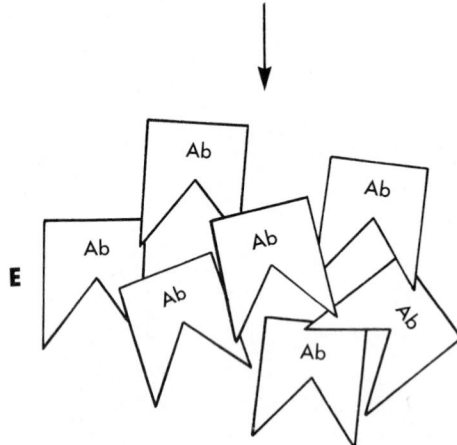

FIGURE 7-1, cont'd. D, Growth of hybridomas, screening for production of antibody specific to antigen of interest, and cloning (typically ×2) of hybridoma cells producing specific antibody. **E,** Expansion of population to form cell line for antibody production, purification, further characterization, and actual use.

ology laboratories because the techniques are relatively simple, are of moderate cost, and provide diagnostic answers quickly enough to still be of consequence to the patient's treatment. Routinely available tests include counterimmunoelectrophoresis, latex agglutination, coagglutination, radioimmunoassay, fluorescence immunoassay, enzyme immunoassay, and immunofluorescence. In all of these tests the quality of the antigen or antibody reagent is the key to success. Quality in immunologic terms can be measured by a number of factors: sensitivity, specificity, affinity of the antibody, and avidity of the antibody.

A sensitive test is one in which there are few if any false-negative results. In other words, a test that is 99% sensitive will almost certainly detect an antigen present in the body fluid. It is also customary to define sensitivity limits. For example, the sensitivity of *Haemophilus influenzae* polysaccharide detection by counterimmunoelectrophoresis is 0.1 to 0.5 μg/ml of cerebrospinal fluid (CSF). A specific test is one in which there are few if any false-positive results. That is, a positive test for *H. influenzae* polysaccharide reliability predicts the presence of *H. influenzae* antigen, not some cross-reacting or nonspecific component in the test system.

Sensitivity and specificity of a test are directly related to the affinity and avidity of the antibody. The antibody (for example, IgG) is a bifunctional molecule. One fragment known as Fab portion retains the antigen-binding properties of the molecule.

The other, the Fc portion, has the ability to adhere to neutrophils, macrophages, subpopulations of lymphocytes, and *Staphylococcus aureus* protein A (Figure 7-2).

An antibody with high affinity binds its homologous antigen strongly, structurally related but not identical antigen moderately well, and an unrelated antigen not at all. Affinity is the strength of binding of a single combining site antibody to a monovalent antigen, whereas avidity is the sum total of all of the individual affinities. Avidity is the strength of binding of the entire antibody molecule. Table 7-3 illustrates the relationship among sensitivity, specificity, and avidity.

For an immunologic test to be useful, high-quality reagents must be readily available and of consistent quality. Following are methods used for microbial antigen detection.

COUNTERIMMUNOELECTROPHORESIS

Counterimmunoelectrophoresis (CIE) was originally described in 1959 by Bussard[6] and was first used clinically for the detection of Australia antigen, now known as hepatitis B surface antigen (Hb$_s$Ag). Radioimmunoassay soon replaced CIE for Hb$_s$Ag, but CIE became a valuable immunologic tool for rapid detection of microbial antibodies and antigens.

CIE is a rapid precipitin reaction in which the reactants are driven by an electric current. The precipitin reaction is a function of the precipitation of antibody and soluble antigen at the equivalence point. CIE combines the advantages of immuno-

TABLE 7-2. Serologic Tests Commonly Performed in Clinical Microbiology Laboratories

Serologic Test	Specificity	Disease Detected	Tests Available	Interpretation	Utility
Cold agglutinins (CA) (human erythrocytes agglutinated at 0°-5° C)	CA present in 50%-90% of patients with pneumonia due to *Mycoplasma pneumoniae;* also observed in leptospirosis, leishmaniasis, hepatic disease	Primary atypical pneumonia (PAP) (*M. pneumoniae*)	Hemagglutination	Titer of ≥1:32 suggestive of PAP; fourfold rise in CA titer, peaking at 4 weeks, is diagnostic	Good screening test for PAP; should be followed by testing for *M. pneumoniae* CF antibodies
Rheumatoid factor (RF) (RF is an IgM antibody that reacts with IgG antibodies)	RF present in 95% of adult patients with rheumatoid arthritis (RA) and 10%-25% of children with juvenile RA; may occur in other inflammatory diseases such as endocarditis, tuberculosis, leprosy[53]	Rheumatoid arthritis	Latex agglutination, hemagglutination, coagglutination, precipitin tests	For latex agglutination, titers of 1:20-1:80 may not be diagnostic of RA; titers greater than 1:1280 are diagnostic (titers vary depending on method)	Good test for RA; false-positive findings may occur if complement Clq is elevated or if blood is lipemic
C-reactive protein (CRP)[61] (acute phase alphaglobulin; forms precipitate with polysaccharide of *Streptococcus pneumoniae*)	Usually present in patients with rheumatic fever, myocardial infarction, carcinoma, streptococcal infections, and pneumonia[52,56]	Indicator of acute inflammatory disease	Slide agglutination, latex agglutination, nephelometric tests	No CRP present present in patients without disease; rising titer is diagnostic	Indicates inflammation but not specific for a particular disease
Antistreptolysin O (ASO) titer[64] (streptolysin O is protein secreted by group A beta-hemolytic streptococci)	False-positive findings may be observed with elevated serum beta-lipoproteins; ASO may be produced in response to infections by other beta-hemolytic streptococci such as groups C and G	Streptococcal disease (such as rheumatic fever, acute glomerulonephritis, scarlet fever)	Micro- and macro-RBC lysis method, latex agglutination	Titer increase of ≥ 2 dilutions above reference values is significant; reference interval for children is 85-240 Todd units (TU)	Excellent test for diagnosing invasive streptococcal disease, especially when coupled with another determination of antistreptococcal antibodies
Other antistreptococcal antibodies (anti-DNAse B, anti-NADase, antihyaluronidase, antistreptokinase)	Rare strains of beta-hemolytic streptococci groups C and G produce DNAse B	Streptococcal disease (such as rheumatic fever, acute glomerulonephritis, scarlet fever)	Macro- and micro-neutralization test	Elevated anti-DNAse B titer is indicative of infection; titer increases later than ASO titer; more sensitive than ASO, particularly in patients with streptococcal glomerular nephritis; elevated serum DNAse in acute pancreatitis may cause false-negative results	Anti-DNAse B best single test for antibody response to streptococci and is especially useful for diagnosis of streptococcal pyoderma

Continued.

TABLE 7-2. Serologic Tests Commonly Performed in Clinical Microbiology Laboratories—cont'd

Serologic Test	Specificity	Disease Detected	Tests Available	Interpretation	Utility
Streptozyme[b] (polyvalent test for antibodies to ASO, DNAse B, hyaluronidase, NADase, and streptokinase)	Rare strains of beta-hemolytic streptococci groups C and G produce DNAse B	Streptococcal disease (such as rheumatic fever, acute glomerulonephritis, scarlet fever)	Slide hemagglutination	Positive test indicates acute streptococcal infection	May lack sensitivity

FEBRILE AGGLUTININS[43]

Serologic Test	Specificity	Disease Detected	Tests Available	Interpretation	Utility
Salmonella typhi group D (O [somatic] and H [flagellar] antigens)	Specificity and sensitivity affected by (1) stage of disease, (2) presence of "normal" antibodies, (3) previous immunization, (4) antibiotics[53]	Typhoid fever	Slide and tube agglutination tests	No "minimal" titer justified because of the many factors affecting disease; only fourfold rise in titer suggestive of salmonellosis	See note a
Salmonella enteritidis groups A, B, C, E (O and H antigens)		Paratyphoid fever, salmonellosis	Slide and tube agglutination tests		
Proteus OX-19, OX-2, OX-K (Weil-Felix test—*Proteus* antigens cross-react with antibodies to rickettsiae)	Lacks specificity owing to ubiquity of *Proteus* spp.; all tests should be followed up with complement fixation for *Rickettsia*	Rickettsial disease	Slide and tube agglutination	Diagnostic patterns of Weil-Felix test may be found in number of manuals[43,53]; fourfold increase in titer to ≥ 1:320 may be diagnostic; single titers ≤ 1:160 not significant	—
Brucella abortus	Cross-reactions seen with antibodies to *Francisella tularensis, Vibrio cholerae, Yersinia enterocolitica*	Brucellosis	Slide and tube agglutination	When standard techniques are used, single titer of ≥ 1:320 or fourfold increase in titer to ≥ 1:320 may be diagnostic	—
Francisella tularensis	Cross-reactions seen with antibodies to *B. abortus* and *Proteus* OX-19	Tularemia	Slide and tube agglutination	Titers of 1:40-1:80 may indicate past infection; mean peak titer seen is 1:640; fourfold rise in titer to ≥ 1:160 may be diagnostic	—

[a]Febrile agglutinins are not intended as substitutes for conventional microbiologic isolation and identification of infecting organisms. In fact, many laboratories no longer offer them. We do not suggest offering these tests as a battery for the detection of fever of unknown origin. At best, an individual test might be ordered if the clinical presentation is suggestive of that disease.
[b]Available from Wampole Diagnostics, Stamford, Conn.

TABLE 7-3. Relationship between Antibody Avidity and the Sensitivity and Specificity of an Immunologic Test

Test Quality	Avidity of Antibody A	
	To Antigen A	To Antigen C (Unrelated to A)
High sensitivity and specificity	High	Low
Low sensitivity and specificity	Low	High
High sensitivity and low specificity	High	High
Low sensitivity and high specificity	Low	Low

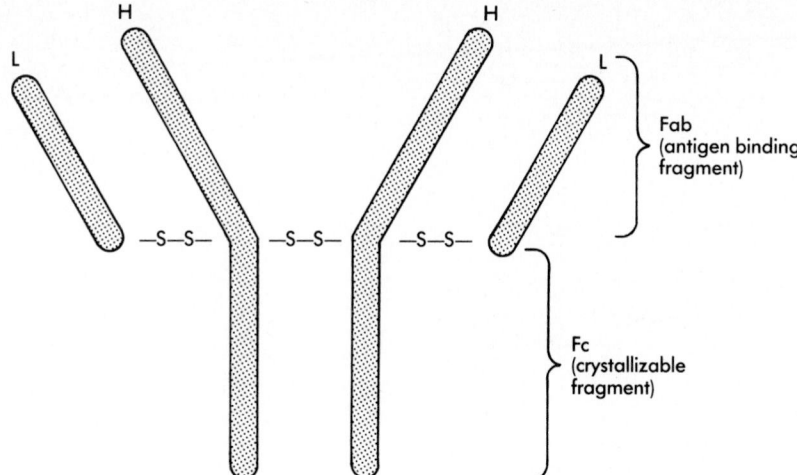

FIGURE 7-2. Immunoglobulin molecule (IgG). *L,* Light chains; *H,* heavy chains; *S–S,* disulfide bond.

diffusion and electrophoresis. The antigen (Ag) is placed in a well on the cathodic side of a solid support, and the antibody is placed on the anodic side. The antigen, if negatively charged, migrates toward the anode, and the antibody, which usually has a weak negative charge, also migrates toward the anode. Positively charged buffer ions, however, sweep the antibody molecule to the cathode. This is called endosmotic flow.[62] If conditions of voltage, current, buffer, pH, antigen/antibody concentration, and quality of antisera are optimum, a precipitin line appears between the two wells after as little as 30 minutes of electrophoresis (Figure 7-3).

A number of variables must be standardized if CIE is to be a reliable, reproducible method in the clinical laboratory. They include quality of antisera, buffer, ionic strength, pH, support systems, the electrophoresis chamber, current, and voltage. If these many variables are well controlled, a precipitin line will appear approximately equidistant between the two wells when antigen and antibody undergo electrophoresis.

Although some authors do not recommend staining, I believe staining should be performed if CIE results are negative. The staining procedure using Coomassie blue is an overnight process, but it improves the test sensitivity and provides a permanent record of the procedure.

Anhalt, Kenny, and Rytel[2] list the following applications of CIE in infectious disease:

1. Detection of antigen in body fluids
2. Determination of antibody titers
3. Prognostic assessment
4. Identification and typing of clinical isolates
5. Elucidation of the role of circulating antigens in disease pathogenesis

CIE is used primarily for the detection of microbial antigens in body fluids and the direct immunologic identification of certain bacteria such as the beta-hemolytic streptococci.[11-13,50] In some cases it may be necessary to treat the body fluid to extract the cell-associated antigen with heat, acid, or enzymes.

CIE may be used to test virtually any body fluid, including CSF, urine, serum, pleural fluid, synovial fluid, peritoneal fluid, abscess drainage, and pericardial fluid. In general, fluids that have less protein, such as CSF and urine, are easier to process because there are fewer spurious precipitin lines or areas of nonspecific precipitation of protein or lipoprotein.

Several early studies demonstrated the value of CIE in the rapid diagnosis of bacterial meningitis using CSF, serum, and urine.* The most commonly detected antigenic components are *Haemophilus influenzae, Streptococcus pneumoniae,* group B streptococci *(Streptococcus agalactiae),* and *Escherichia coli* K1. A few investigators have reported that, in groups A and C meningococcal meningitis and in *H. influenzae* meningitis, the amount of antigen detected in the CSF correlated with severity and prognosis of infection.[10,23,27] CIE has also been used for the diagnosis of both pneumococcal and *H. influenzae* pneumonia, although some limitations of these methods have been noted.[9,26] Other reported uses of CIE include the detection of *Klebsiella pneumoniae*[16,37,57] and *S. pneumoniae* in blood (again with reported limitations[5,65]), typing of streptococci,[15] and the prospective diagnosis of early-onset group B streptococcal disease in infants.[17,31] Students reading these studies will better understand the historical development of this first important departure from traditional culture techniques. Nevertheless, the newer, more sensitive methods of antigen detection such as latex agglutination, coagglutination, and immunoassay have made CIE a transitional technology.

LATEX AGGLUTINATION

Latex polystyrene beads were first used to detect rheumatoid factor in serum.[58] Either antigen or IgG antibody is nonspecifically absorbed to the surface of the latex polystyrene beads of uniform diameter, usually 0.8 μm. Addition of the specific antibody or antigen visibly agglutinates the milky-white latex suspension. Although latex agglutination (LA) tests can be done in test tubes, they are usually performed on slides.

Depending on the system, the procedure for the detection of antigen or antibody by LA may be quite simple. A drop or two of the latex reagent is mixed with a suspension of the colony or the body fluid to be tested. The suspension is incubated at room temperature with occasional rotation of the slide. Agglutination is a positive finding.

LA reagents are commercially available for identification of

---

*References 14, 19, 23, 34, 47, 54, and 62.

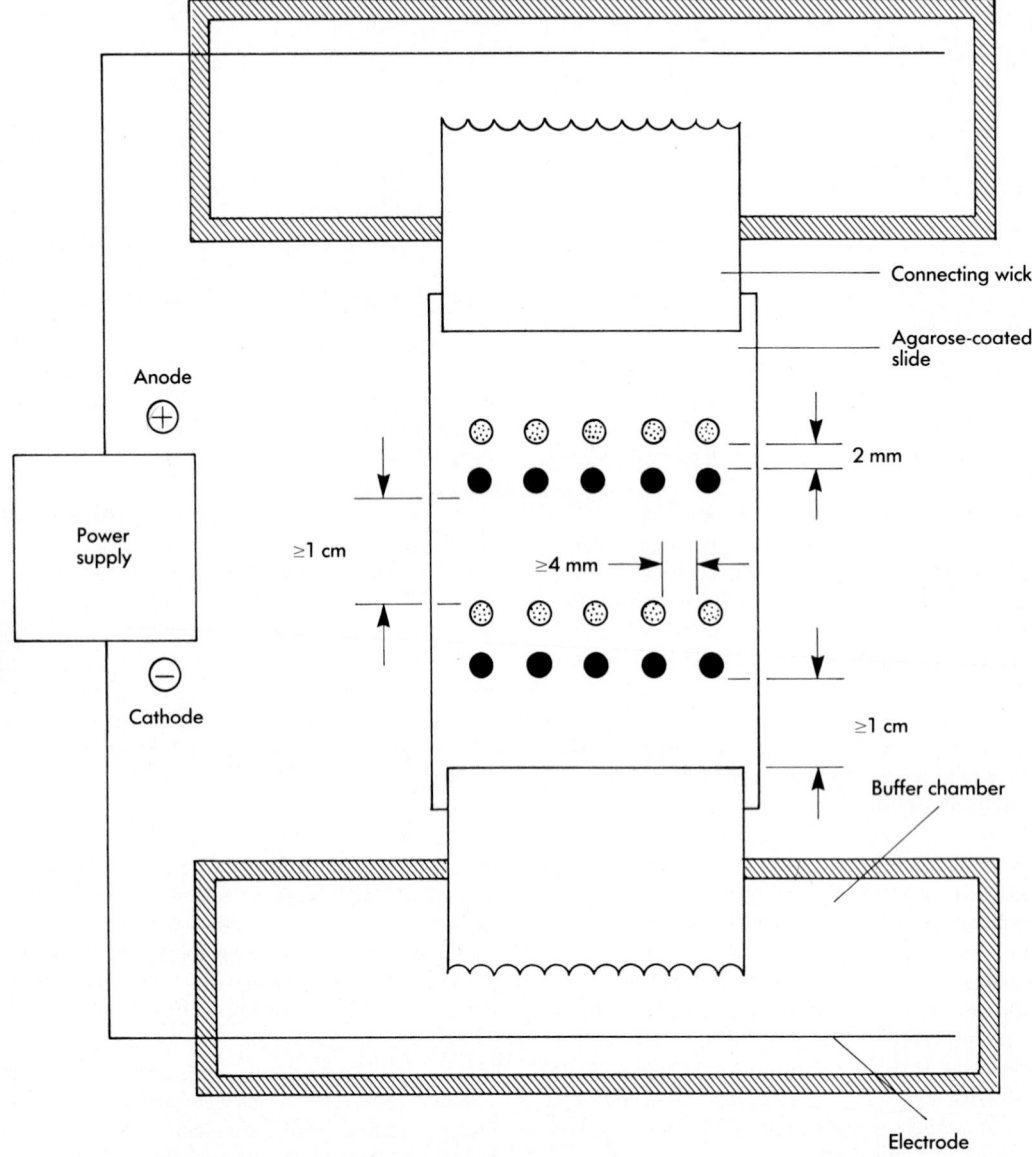

FIGURE 7-3. Diagram of basic counterimmunoelectrophoresis procedure showing two rows of pairs of wells. *Dotted circles,* Well in which antibody is placed; *black circles,* well in which fluid to be tested for antigen is placed. (From Anhalt, J.P., Kenny, G.E., and Rytel, M.W.: Detection of microbial antigens by counterimmunoelectrophoresis. In Gavan, T.L., editor: Cumitech 8, Washington, D.C., 1978, American Society for Microbiology.)

colonies or detection of antigens of the following organisms: streptococci groups A, B, C, D, F, and G; *Neisseria gonorrhoeae; Cryptococcus neoformans; Candida albicans; Haemophilus influenzae* types a to f; *Streptococcus pneumoniae* (83 serotypes); *Staphylococcus aureus;* and *Neisseria meningitidis* groups A, B, C, Y, and W135. Although several commercial reagents are available, preparation of LA reagents in the laboratory is not difficult. Sedgwick and Tilton[55] described the preparation of latex reagents for the identification of *Legionella pneumophila* colonies. Antiserum, 0.1 ml, was added to a tube containing 1 ml of 10% solution of Dow latex polystyrene and incubated at 37° C for 2 hours. The reagent was then diluted 1:20 with glycine-buffered saline containing 0.1% bovine serum albumin. The diluted latex reagent was filtered through a thin layer of absorbent cotton to remove any clumped particles.

A major drawback to LA is nonspecific reactions with specimens such as urine, sputum, serum, and synovial fluid. False-positive agglutination can sometimes be eliminated by heating the specimen to 60° C for 15 minutes[48] or to 100° C for 5 minutes.[67] In one study,[30] although CIE and latex agglutination were similarly sensitive for detection of *H. influenzae* meningitis, false-positive latex agglutination was observed in almost 20% of culture-negative CSF samples. However, in a more recent study,[63] few if any false-positive or nonspecific LA reactions were seen in CSF.

The ability of LA to detect cryptococcal polysaccharide in serum or CSF has been well documented.[46,51] It is specific and more sensitive than demonstration of the capsule of *C. neoformans* by india ink (see Chapter 29). Rheumatoid factor (RF) may invalidate the test because of a cross-reaction. An enzymatic method for elimination of RF interference has been proposed.[59]

Newman, Stevens, and Gaafar[48] detected *H. influenzae* capsular antigen by LA in 27 of 29 CSF samples positive by culture. Ingram, O'Reilly, and Pond[29] showed that both CIE and LA tests were positive in 75% of patients with *H. influenzae* meningitis. Kaldor, Asznowicz, and Buist[33] studied 95 patients with purulent meningitis and 63 control patients with other diseases. Latex reagents were available at the time for *H. influenzae* type b, *N. meningitidis* groups A and C, *S. pneumoniae*, and *C. neoformans*. With the exception of one urine specimen, none of the uninfected control patients had positive LA results, whereas 62 of 95 CSF specimens, 10 of 14 sera, and 11 of 17 urine specimens were positive by LA.[33] Although these investigators found many false-positive agglutinations initially, fractionation of antisera and the heating of urine to 100° C increased the specificity.

In a similar study Leinonen and Herva[41] tested 103 CSF samples for *H. influenzae* type b and *N. meningitidis* groups A and C by LA. They reported that LA was at least as sensitive as CIE. They had little success, however, detecting *N. meningitidis* group B antigen in CSF by either LA or CIE.

Bromberger and co-workers[4] reported in a preliminary study that group B streptococci could be detected in body fluids more sensitively by LA than by CIE, especially in urine. For type-specific antigens, however, CIE was more sensitive than LA. The authors stated that the risk of false-positive findings was greater with LA than with CIE.

An interesting variation of LA discussed in Chapter 12 involves the coating of latex particles with human plasma. This

TABLE 7-4. Sensitivity of Antigen Detection by Counterimmunoelectrophoresis, Latex Agglutination, and Radioimmunoassay

Method	Polysaccharide (μg/ml)		
	H. influenzae Type B	*N. meningitidis*	
		Group A	Group C
Counterimmuno-electrophoresis	20	50	75
Latex agglutination	5	10	25
Radioimmunoassay	0.5	2	5

From Leinonen, M., and Käyhty, H.: J. Clin. Pathol. **31:**1172, 1978.

reagent, containing fibrinogen and IgG, reacts with both the clumping factor of *S. aureus* and protein A. A modification of this test is now commercially available and used for the identification of staphylococci.

Leinonen and Käyhty[42] compared CIE, LA, and RIA for detection of *H. influenzae* b and *N. meningitidis* A and C polysaccharide. RIA was consistently the most sensitive, followed by LA and then CIE. The data in Table 7-4 present the sensitivity of the three methods.

Several other recent reports confirm the value of latex agglutination for detection of microbial antigens in body fluids.[3,8,30,63]

Of recent interest is the use of LA, coagglutination, and enzyme immunoassay for rapid detection of group A streptococci directly from throat swabs of patients with suspected pharyngitis.[16,38,49] This is discussed in Chapter 13.

COAGGLUTINATION

Kronvall[40] was the first to introduce the coagglutination (CoA) technique for the detection of pneumococcal antigens. Certain strains of *Staphylococcus aureus,* in particular Cowan strain I, contain a cell surface protein known as protein A. Antibodies of the IgG class adhere to protein A by their Fc portion, leaving the Fab ends free to complex homologous antigen (Figure 7-4). The presence of antigen results in the visible agglutination of the staphylococci.

The agglutination of sensitized protein A containing staphylococci may be less distinct than that of latex. The procedure, like latex agglutination, is subject to nonspecific agglutination in body fluids such as CSF, serum, and urine.

The preparation of CoA reagents is technically simple, and once prepared, the sensitized staphylococci are more stable than latex reagents. The procedure is as follows.

S. aureus (Cowan strain I) is grown overnight in brain heart infusion broth. The broth is centrifuged at 10,000 × g for 20 minutes to recover the cells. The cell pellet is then washed three times with phosphate-buffered saline (PBS) at pH 7.2 and resuspended in 3 ml of 0.5% formalin-PBS. The suspension is incubated at room temperature for 3 hours and then centrifuged at 10,000 × g for 20 minutes and the pellet again washed three times with PBS. The cells are adjusted to 10% (wt/vol) in PBS and heated at 80° C in a waterbath for 1 hour. Antibody, 0.1 ml, is added to 1 ml of the *S. aureus*–protein A suspension.

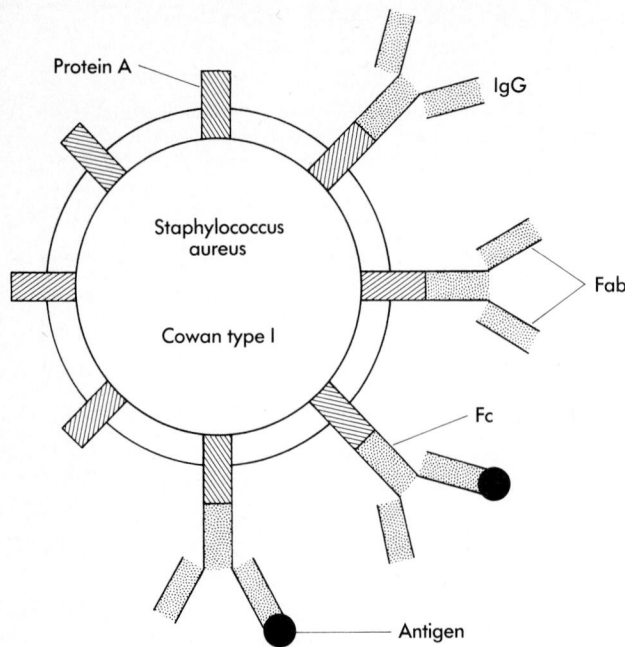

FIGURE 7-4. Coagglutination reagent.

The suspension is diluted to 10 ml with PBS. Reagents are stable at refrigerator temperatures.

CoA reagents can potentially be used to detect any antigen that can be detected by LA. At the time of writing, reagents for *N. gonorrhoeae,* streptococci groups A, B, C, D, and G, *H. influenzae* types a to f, *N. meningitidis* A, B, C, Y, and W-135, and *S. pneumoniae* are commercially available.

Early studies confirmed the utility of commercially available coagglutination tests for identification of *N. gonorrhoeae* and beta-hemolytic streptococci.[7,24,44,45] These findings were substantiated by later studies discussed in Chapters 13 and 14.

Several investigators have compared these immunoserologic procedures for bacterial antigen identification. Thirumoorthi and Dajani[60] reported that CoA was as sensitive as LA and more sensitive than CIE for *H. influenzae* antigen detection. They reported nonspecific agglutination with LA and CoA as have others. Many of these nonspecific agglutination reactions disappeared after the specimen was premixed with soluble protein A.

Wasilauskas and Hampton[66] analyzed 80 CSF specimens by CIE and CoA. Their results indicated that more culture-positive specimens were detected by the commercial CoA reagents (Pharmacia Diagnostics) than by either CIE or the laboratory-prepared CoA reagents. Tilton, Dias, and Ryan[63] confirmed the utility of commercially available CoA kits for antigen detection in CSF, although they noted that CoA appeared to be less sensitive than LA but more sensitive than CIE. Collins and Kelly[8] reported similar results, although they observed little difference in sensitivity between CoA and LA. Studies by Fung and Tilton[20a] also compared the sensitivity of CIE, CoA, and LA.

• • •

All of these test methods produce results faster than culture. As in any immunologic procedure, there are inherent problems of cross-reactions, nonspecific agglutination, sensitivity, and specificity. The appearance of monoclonal antibody may solve some but not all of these problems.

Furthermore, although these new antigen detection tests may be simple, fast, and accurate, several factors must be considered in establishing their specific use in the clinical laboratory. Each laboratory must carefully evaluate their diagnostic advantage as compared with traditional methods.[22]

RADIOIMMUNOASSAY

Radioimmunoassay (RIA) techniques use a radioisotope, usually ^{125}iodine, to detect antigen-antibody reactions. These techniques combine the specificity of immunology and the sensitivity of radiochemistry. Although the principal use of RIA is in endocrinology for the assay of hormones, all areas of laboratory medicine have found RIA to be a useful tool. RIA has many variations, but in most applications in the clinical setting a competitive protein binding assay is used to measure antigen. In this assay a known amount of radiolabeled antigen competes with an unknown quantity of antigen in a patient's serum for available binding sites on a specified amount of homologous antibody. If high concentrations of unlabeled antigen are present in the patient's serum, the amount of labeled antigen bound by antibody is reduced. After equilibrium between the bound and the unbound antigen is reached, the bound fraction is separated from the unbound fraction by precipitation or centrifugation, and the radioactivity in the bound or free phase (or both) is measured in a scintillation counter. The counts are then related to concentration with the use of a standard curve. Several other RIA techniques are discussed in Chapter 46.

Käyhty, Makila, and Ruoslahti[36] described an RIA procedure for detection of *N. meningitidis* groups A and C and *H. influenzae* antigens in CSF. RIA detected antigen in 14 of 15 patients with *H. influenzae* meningitis, 18 of 23 patients with meningitis caused by *N. meningitidis* group A, and two of four patients with *N. meningitidis* group C meningitis. No false-positive reactions were observed.

Although microbiologic research employs RIA widely, it is rarely used routinely in clinical microbiology laboratories except for the determination of hepatitis A or B antibodies and antigens (see Chapters 46 and 54). It has not been widely used in bacterial antigen detection, primarily because of the cost of equipment, paucity of standardized reagents, and rapidity with which enzyme immunoassay is replacing RIA in the clinical laboratory.

ENZYME IMMUNOASSAY

The search for methodology that was as sensitive as RIA but nonradioisotopic culminated in the discovery of the enzyme immunoassay (EIA) technique. Engvall and Perlmann[18] first used EIA to measure rabbit IgG.

The two major types of enzyme immunoassays are the homogeneous and the heterogeneous. Heterogeneous immunoassays require physical separation of bound and unbound antigen, whereas homogeneous assays do not. Enzyme-multiplied immunoassays (EMIT) are homogeneous assays, and enzyme-linked immunosorbent assays (ELISA) are heterogeneous.

EMIT is a competitive assay (Figure 7-5). The substance to be tested, usually a low–molecular weight antigen, is attached

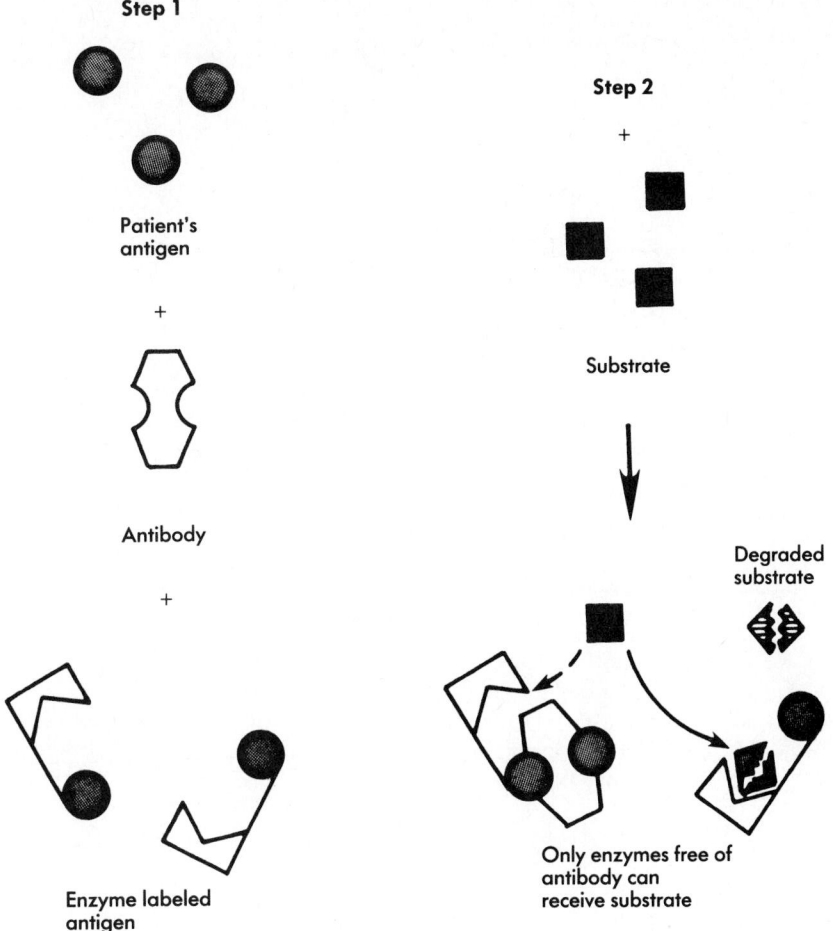

Step 1

Patient's
antigen

+

Antibody

+

Enzyme labeled
antigen

Step 2

+

Substrate

Degraded
substrate

Only enzymes free of
antibody can
receive substrate

FIGURE 7-5. Diagram of homogeneous enzyme immunoassay. (Modified from Stansfield, W.D.: Serology and immunology: a clinical approach, New York, 1981, Macmillan, Inc.)

to an enzyme. This attachment occurs in such a way that binding of antibody to the antigen sterically blocks substrate binding. In the clinical test a body fluid that purportedly contains free or unbound antigen is mixed with antibody and the enzyme-labeled or bound antigen.[21] Both free and bound antigen compete for binding sites on the antibody. The more free antigen present, the more enzyme remains unbound and catalytically active on the addition of a specific enzyme substrate. The reaction is read spectrophotometrically; the greater the enzyme activity, the greater the change in absorbance of the substrate. The absorbance change is directly correlated to the concentration of antigen in the patient's specimen.

The concept of ELISA is similar to RIA. Figure 7-6 depicts antigen measurement by the ELISA double sandwich technique. An antibody is bound to a solid support, such as a plastic tube, a tray, or polystyrene beads. The antigen-containing body fluid is layered over the sensitized solid phase. An enzyme-labeled antibody is then added to form an antibody-antigen-antibody "sandwich." After separation of the bound and free enzyme-tagged antibody, a specific chromogenic enzyme substrate is added. The bound enzyme reacts with its substrate to

produce a color change, which indicates the presence of antigen. Enzyme substrate combinations commonly used include alkaline phosphatase and nitrophenyl phosphate or horseradish peroxidase and orthophenylenediamine. A competitive ELISA (similar to the competitive RIA) may also be used to detect antigen.

An indirect ELISA may be used to determine the presence of antibody. In this procedure the antigen is bound to the solid phase. The test serum is added, and the test antibody binds to the antigen. After washing, an enzyme-labeled antiglobulin and substrate are added. If specific antibody is present, the enzyme-labeled antiglobulin combines with the antibody and hydrolysis of the substrate occurs.

In either procedure the amount of hydrolysis of the substrate is directly related to the amount of antigen or antibody present. The reaction may be read visually or spectrophotometrically. For screening tests, that is, simply determining positive or negative results, manual reading is acceptable. For most applications, however, quantitation of antigen or antibody content is desirable.

Although ELISA methodology is not conceptually difficult,

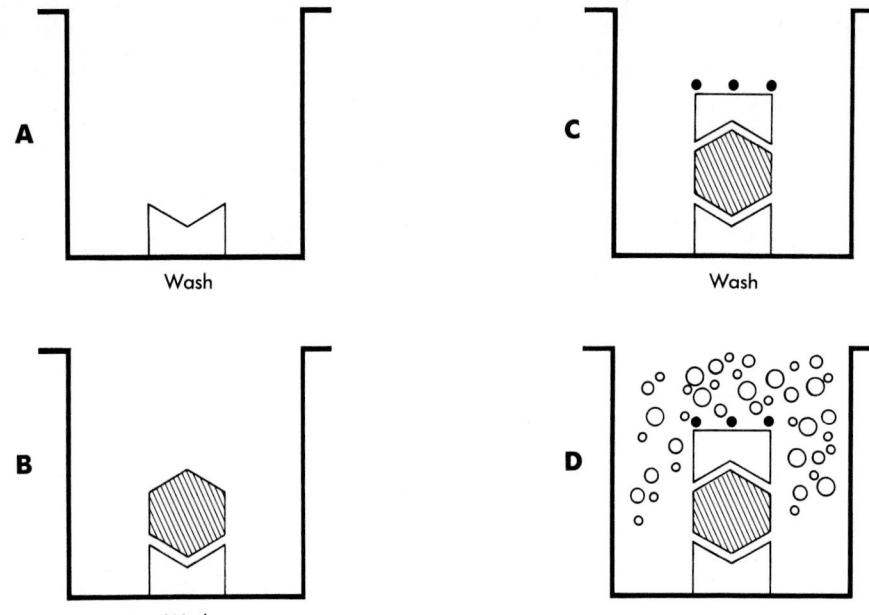

FIGURE 7-6. Double antibody sandwich method of ELISA for assay of antigen. **A,** Antibody is adsorbed to surface. **B,** Test solution containing antigen is added. **C,** Enzyme-labeled specific antibody is added. **D,** Enzyme substrate is added. Amount of hydrolysis equals amount of antigen present. (**A** to **C** show condition of well after excess, unbound reagents have been washed away.) (From Tilton, R.C.: Culture [Oxoid], Sept. 1982.)

as with CIE there are many variables to control. They include solid phase, the washing process, enzymes used, substrates, and the termination of the reaction.

EIA may be used to identify antibody to the following organisms or products of organisms:

1. Bacteria
   a. *Brucella abortus*
   b. *Corynebacterium diphtheriae* toxin
   c. *Escherichia coli* labile toxin (LT) and stable toxin (ST)
   d. *Legionella pneumophila*
   e. *Mycoplasma pneumoniae*
   f. *Neisseria meningitidis*
   g. *Salmonella* spp.
   h. *Streptococcus pyogenes* (M protein)
   i. *Streptococcus pyogenes* (C carbohydrate)
   j. Tetanus toxin
   k. *Vibrio cholerae* toxin
   l. *Mycobacterium tuberculosis*
   m. *Yersinia enterocolitica*
2. Fungi
   a. *Candida albicans*
   b. *Aspergillus fumigatus*
3. Parasites
   a. *Echinococcus granulosus*
   b. *Onchocerca volvulus*
   c. *Plasmodium falciparum*
   d. *Schistosoma mansoni*
   e. *Toxocara canis*
   f. *Toxoplasma gondii*
   g. *Trichinella spiralis*
   h. *Trypanosoma brucei*
   i. *Trypanosoma cruzi*
   j. *Trypanosoma rhodesiense*
4. Spirochetes—*Treponema pallidum*
5. Viruses and rickettsiae
   a. Adenovirus
   b. Arbovirus
   c. Coxsackie virus
   d. Cytomegalovirus
   e. Hepatitis A (IgG, IgM)
   f. Hepatitis B (antibody to HB_sAg [hepatitis B surface antigen], HB_cAg [hepatitis B core antigen], HB_eAg [hepatitis B e antigen])
   g. Herpes simplex 1 and 2
   h. Influenza A
   i. Influenza B
   j. Measles
   k. Mumps
   l. Rabies
   m. Respiratory syncytial virus
   n. *Rickettsia typhi*
   o. *Rochalimaea quintana*
   p. Rotavirus
   q. Rubella

EIA may also be used to detect the following microbial antigens:

1. Bacteria
   a. *Brucella abortus*
   b. *Clostridium difficile* toxin A and B
   c. *Clostridium difficile* antigen
   d. *Escherichia coli* toxin (LT)
   e. *Legionella pneumophila*
   f. *Mycoplasma pneumoniae*

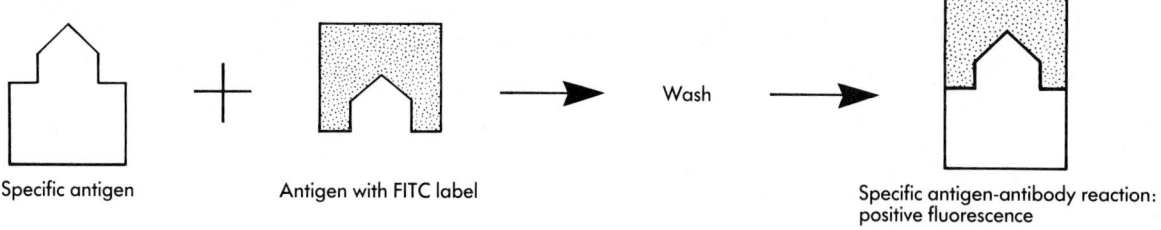

Specific antigen   Antigen with FITC label   Specific antigen-antibody reaction:
                                                                  positive fluorescence

FIGURE 7-7. Direct immunofluorescence.

g. *Salmonella typhi*
h. *Staphylococcus aureus* toxin A
i. *Staphylococcus aureus* toxin E
j. *Streptococcus pyogenes*
k. *Streptococcus agalactiae*
l. *Vibrio cholerae* (enterotoxin)
m. *Yersinia enterocolitica*
2. Fungi
   a. *Aspergillus* spp. (aflatoxin B)
   b. *Candida albicans*
   c. *Cryptococcus neoformans*
3. Parasites
   a. *Giardia lamblia*
   b. *Pneumocystis carinii*
   c. *Schistosoma mansoni*
   d. *Toxoplasma gondii*
4. Viruses and rickettsiae
   a. Adenovirus
   b. Epstein-Barr virus
   c. Hepatitis A
   d. HB_sAg, HB_eAg
   e. Herpes simplex 1 and 2
   f. Human immunodeficiency virus (HIV)
   g. Influenza virus
   h. Parainfluenza virus
   i. Respiratory syncytial virus
   j. Rotavirus (human, calf)

An example of a semiautomated EIA system is the Quantum (Abbott Labs, N. Chicago, Ill.). The system consists of EIA reagent kits for detection of a variety of antigens and antibodies directly from the patient specimen and a spectrophotometer to measure the completed reactions. The spectrophotometer can be programmed to perform all calculations automatically. Kits that are available for use with the Quantum system include those for detection of antigens of *Neisseria gonorrhoeae*, *Streptococcus pyogenes*, *Chlamydia trachomatis*, rotavirus, respiratory syncytial virus, and hepatitis B virus and others for detection of antibodies to hepatitis A and B viruses, HIV, and *Toxoplasma*.

The clinical applications of EIA are numerous. A recent application of interest is determination of antibodies to HIV. Second-generation EIAs that detect antibodies to molecular components of HIV such as p24, p41, and p120 are now being introduced to clinical laboratories.

FLUORESCENCE

The fluorescent antibody (FA) (or immunofluorescence) technique consists of an antigen-antibody reaction made visible with a fluorescent dye. The tagged antigen-antibody complex is activated by a specific light source (usually ultraviolet), and the light emitted is then detected by either a fluorescence microscope (see Chapter 6) or a fluorimeter. The method is rapid, sensitive, relatively specific, and readily applicable in clinical microbiology. The two basic fluorescence techniques in use today are immunofluorescence microscopy and fluorescence immunoassays.

Immunofluorescence Microscopy

Two basic immunofluorescence techniques are used in microscopy: direct and indirect. With direct immunofluorescence (also known as the direct fluorescent antibody test) the specimen to be stained is placed on a slide, which is then stained with specific antibody conjugated with fluorescein isothiocyanate (FITC) (Figure 7-7). This technique may be used for the detection of microorganisms. The indirect method (or indirect fluorescent antibody test) may be used to detect microorganisms and antibody to microorganisms. In this method the antigen-antibody reaction is detected with an FITC-antispecies antiserum (Figure 7-8). In the indirect method, for example, CMV-infected cells are fixed on a microscope slide, which is incubated with dilutions of serum from a patient suspected of having an antibody titer to CMV. The slide is then stained with FITC-labeled antihuman globulin. Virus-infected portions of the cell fluoresce if CMV antibody is present. The endpoint of antibody titer is determined by observing fluorescence as a function of the serum dilution.

Immunofluorescence microscopy is used in many laboratories for a number of procedures, including fluorescent treponemal antibody tests and identification of a wide variety of organisms: group A beta-streptococci, *Bacteroides fragilis*, *Bacteroides melaninogenicus*, *Bordetella pertussis*, *Legionella*, respiratory syncytial virus, herpes simplex virus, influenza virus, and *Chlamydia trachomatis*. Many specific FITC-labeled antibodies are available for immunofluorescence microscopy, and their use is limited only by the ingenuity of the microbiologist.

Fluorescence Immunoassays

The fluorescence immunoassay[35] is similar to the other assays described (RIA, ELISA) except that fluorescing compounds are used to tag antigens or antibodies instead of radioisotopes or enzymes. The assays may be competitive or noncompetitive. Plastic beads, disks, tubes, or paddles are coated with an antigen or antibody. If the tests are competitive, fluorescing labeled compounds compete with nonlabeled compounds for binding sites. As in the other systems, the bound and free components are separated by centrifugation, decanting, and most recently the use of magnetic beads.[20]

An example of a solid phase fluorescence immunoassay is the FIAX,[25] a unique paddle system available from Internation-

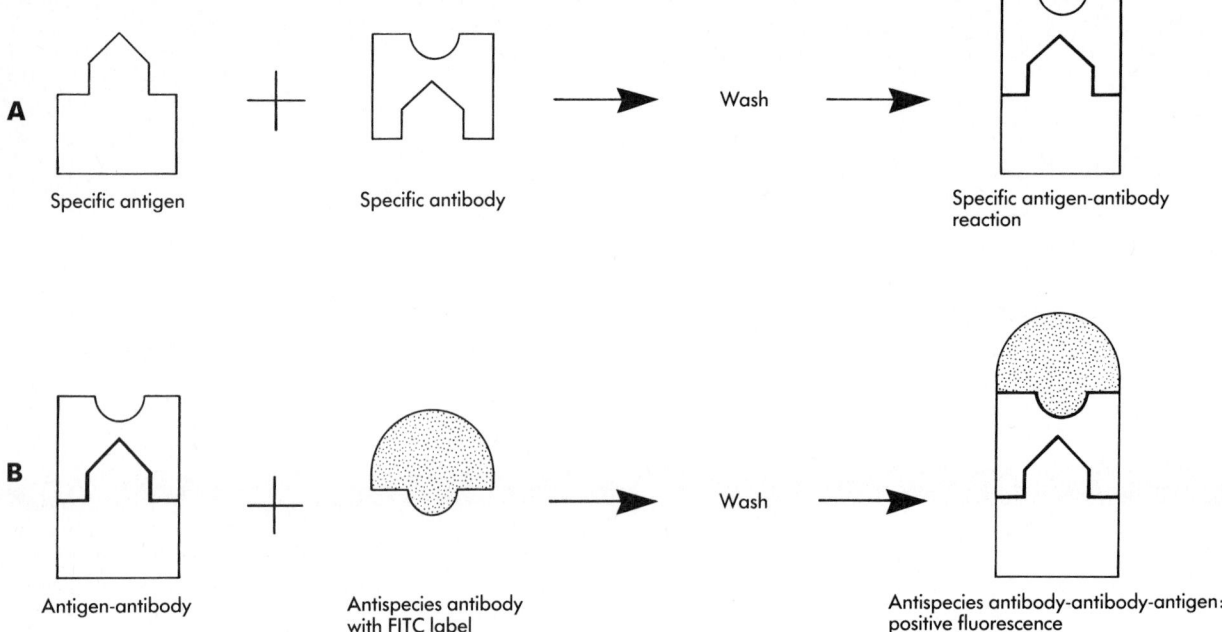

FIGURE 7-8. Indirect immunofluorescence. **A,** Step 1. **B,** Step 2.

al Diagnostic Technology Corp. (Santa Clara, Calif.). The paddle is coated with either antibody or antigen and is dipped into the specimen to be tested. The paddle is then stained with the fluorescein-labeled component, washed, and read in a fluorimeter. Assays are available for a number of viral antibodies including rubella virus, herpesvirus, and cytomegalovirus, as well as antinuclear antibodies, complement, and immunoglobulins.

An instrument (Abbott TDX, Abbott Laboratories, Chicago) based on fluorescence polarization immunoassay (FPIA)[13] has received acclaim in many laboratories. FPIA is a nonseparation immunoassay; that is, the bound and free complexes need not be separated before the test is read. FPIA is also a competitive assay in that bound and free antigen-antibody complexes generate different signals when fluorescent light is polarized in both horizontal and vertical planes. FPIA combines the specificity of an immunoassay with the speed and convenience of a homogeneous method. Methods are currently available for the measurement of aminoglycosides and vancomycin in serum, as well as other low–molecular weight substances such as digoxin, cortisol, and drugs of abuse.[32]

Time-resolved fluoroimmunoassay (TRFIA)[58a] reduces background fluorescence by selective detection of long decay fluorescing molecules such as europium and terbium. These molecules in the form of their lanthanide chelates have a high quantum yield that enables emission peaks to be discerned from background. A TRFIA instrument from Wallac (Turku, Finland) is widely used in Europe for viral antigen detection.

• • •

There is little doubt that immunoassays of one kind or another will capture a significant amount of the workload in microbiology, whether for antibody identification or for rapid detection of microbial antigens in body fluids. The laboratory of the future will rely heavily on immunoassay employing high-quality monoclonal antibodies for the rapid and specific detection of many microorganisms directly from patient specimens.

REFERENCES

1. Alexander, J.W., and Good, R.A.: Fundamentals of clinical immunology, Philadelphia, 1977, W.B. Saunders Co.
2. Anhalt, J.P., Kenny, G.E., and Rytel, M.W.: Detection of microbial antigens by counterimmunoelectrophoresis. In Gavan, T.L., editor: Cumitech 8, Washington, D.C., 1978, American Society for Microbiology.
3. Baker, C.J., and Rench, M.A.: Commercial latex agglutination for detection of group B streptococcal antigen in body fluids, J. Pediatr. **102:**393, 1983.
4. Bromberger, P.I., et al.: Rapid detection of neonatal group B streptococcal infections by latex agglutination, J. Pediatr. **96:**104, 1980.
5. Buck, L.L., and Tuttle, K.: Letter to the editor, Clin. Microbiol. Newsletter **2:**7, 1980.
6. Bussard, A.: Description d'une technique combinant simultanement l' electrophorese et la precipitation immunologique dans un gel: l' electrosynerese, Biochim. Biophys. Acta **34:**258, 1959.
7. Christensen, P., et al.: New method for the serological grouping of streptococci with specific antibodies adsorbed to protein A–containing staphylococci, Infect. Immun. **7:**882, 1973.
8. Collins, J.K., and Kelly, M.T.: Comparison of Phadebact coagglutination, Bactogen latex agglutination, and counterimmunoelectrophoresis for detection of *Haemophilus influenzae* type b antigens in cerebrospinal fluid, J. Clin. Microbiol. **17:**1005, 1983.
9. Coonrod, J.D.: Use of CIE for antigen detection in bacterial infections, Lab. Management 33, 1979.
10. Coonrod, J.D., and Rytel, M.W.: Detection of type specific pneumococcal antigens by counterimmunoelectrophoresis. II. Etiologic diagnosis of pneumococcal pneumonia, J. Lab. Clin. Med. **81:**778, 1973.
11. Croix, J.C., Bajolle, F., and Dalle, M.: Applicatrion de l' electroimmunodiffusion au groupage des streptocoques, Ann. Biol. Clin. **33:**149, 1975.

12. Dajani, A.S.: Rapid identification of beta hemolytic streptococci by counterimmunoelectrophoresis, J. Immunol. **6:**1702, 1973.

13. Dandliker, W.B., et al.: Fluorescence polarization immunoassay: theory and experimental method, Immunochemistry **10:**219, 1973.

14. Edwards, E.A.: Immunologic investigations of meningococcal disease. I. Group-specific *Neisseria meningitidis* antigens present in the serum of patients with fulminant meningococcemia, J. Immunol. **106:**314, 1971.

15. Edwards, E.A., and Larson, G.L.: Serological grouping of hemolytic streptococci by counterimmunoelectrophoresis, Appl. Microbiol. **26:**899, 1973.

16. Edwards, E.A., Phillips, I.A., and Suiter, W.C.: Diagnosis of group A streptococcal infections directly from throat secretions, J. Clin. Microbiol. **15:**481, 1982.

17. Edwards, M.S., and Baker, C.J.: Prospective diagnosis of early-onset group B streptococcal infection by countercurrent immunoelectrophoresis, J. Pediatr. **94:**286, 1979.

18. Engvall, E., and Perlmann, P.: Enzyme linked immunosorbent assay (ELISA): quantitative assay of immunoglobulin G, Immunochemistry **8:**1175, 1971.

19. Feigin, R.D., et al.: Countercurrent immunoelectrophoresis of urine as well as of CSF and blood for diagnosis of bacterial meningitis, J. Pediatr. **89:**773, 1976.

20. Friedman, H., and Specter, S.: Microbiology and serology: progress in automation, Lab. Management 37, 1981.

20a. Fung, J.C., and Tilton, R.C.: Detection of bacterial antigens. In Wicher, K., editor: Microbial antigenodiagnosis, Boca Raton, Fla., CRC Press. In press.

21. Galen, R.S., et al.: The enzyme multiplied immunoassay, Lancet **2:**852, 1976.

22. Gerber, M.A.: Critical appraisal of the clinical relevance of rapid diagnosis in pediatrics, Diagn. Microbiol. Infect. Dis. **3:**39S, 1985.

23. Greenwood, B.W., Whittle, H.C., and Dominic-Rajkovic, O.: Countercurrent immunoelectrophoresis in the diagnosis of meningococcal infection, Lancet **2:**519, 1971.

24. Hahn, G., and Nyberg, I.: Identification of streptococcal groups A, B, C, and G by slide co-agglutination of antibody-sensitized protein A-containing staphylococci, J. Clin. Microbiol. **4:**99, 1976.

25. Harte, R.A.: Fluoroimmunometry and the FIAX system, Clin. Immunol. Newsletter **1:**2, 1980.

26. Hilman, B.C.: Limitations of countercurrent immunoelectrophoresis (CCIE) in the diagnosis of empyema, Chest **78:**866, 1980.

27. Hoffman, T.A., and Edwards, E.A.: Group specific polysaccharide antigen and humoral antibody response in disease due to *Neisseria meningitidis*, J. Infect. Dis. **126:**636, 1972.

28. Holsclaw, D.S., and Schaeffer, D.A.: Counterimmunoelectrophoresis in the diagnosis of *Haemophilus influenzae* pleural effusion, Chest **78:**867, 1980.

29. Ingram, D.L., O'Reilly, R.J., and Pond, P.J.: Diagnosis of *Haemophilus influenzae* b and other meningitides: Gram stain, latex agglutination and countercurrent immunoelectrophoresis, Pediatr. Res. **9:**341, 1975.

30. Ingram, D.L., Suggs, D.M., and Pearson, A.W.: Detection of group B streptococcal antigen in early-onset and late-onset group B streptococcal disease with the Wellcogen Strep B latex agglutination test, J. Clin. Microbiol. **16:**656, 1982.

31. Jacobs, R.F., Yamauchi, T., and Eisinach, K.D.: Detection of streptococcal antigen by counterimmunoelectrophoresis, Am. J. Clin. Pathol. **75:**203, 1981.

32. Jolley, M.E., et al: An automated system for therapeutic drug determination, Clin. Chem. **27:**1575, 1981.

33. Kaldor, J., Asznowicz, R., and Buist, D.G.P.: Latex agglutination in diagnosis of bacterial infections: with special reference to patients with meningitis and septicemia, Am. J. Clin. Pathol. **68:**284, 1977.

34. Kaplan, S.L., and Feigin, R.D.: Rapid diagnosis of bacterial meningitis. In Rytel, M.W., editor: Rapid diagnosis in infectious disease, Boca Raton, Fla., 1979, CRC Press.

35. Kawamura, A.: Fluorescent antibody techniques and their applications, ed. 2, Baltimore, 1977, University Park Press.

36. Käyhty, H., Makela, P.H., and Ruoslahti, E.: Radioimmunoassay of capsular polysaccharide antigens of groups A and C meningococci and *Haemophilus influenzae* type b in cerebrospinal fluid, J. Clin. Pathol. **30:**831, 1977.

37. Kenny, J.E., et al.: Correlation of circulating capsular polysaccharide with bacteremia in pneumococcal pneumonia, Infect. Immun. **6:**431, 1972.

38. Kholy, A.E., et al.: Serological identification of group A streptococci from throat scrapings before culture, J. Clin. Microbiol. **8:**725, 1978.

39. Kohler, G., and Milstein, C.: Continuous cultures of fused cells secreting antibody of predefined specificity, Nature **256:**495, 1975.

40. Kronvall, G.: A rapid slide agglutination method for typing pneumococci by means of specific antibody absorbed to protein A–containing staphylococci, J. Med. Microbiol. **6:**187, 1973.

41. Leinonen, M., and Herva, E.: The latex agglutination test for the diagnosis of meningococcal and *Haemophilus influenzae* meningitis, Scand. J. Infect. Dis. **9:**187, 1977.

42. Leinonen, M., and Käyhty, H.: Comparison of counter-current immunoelectrophoresis, latex agglutination, and radioimmunoassay in detection of soluble capsular polysaccharide antigens of *Haemophilus influenzae* type b and *Neisseria meningitidis* of groups A or C, J. Clin. Pathol. **31:**1172, 1978.

43. Lennette, E.H., et al., editors: Manual of clinical microbiology, ed. 4, Washington, D.C., 1985, American Society for Microbiology.

44. Lim, D.V., Smith, R.D., and Day, S.: Evaluation of an improved rapid coagglutination method for the serological grouping of beta-hemolytic streptococci, Can. J. Microbiol. **25:**40, 1979.

45. Lim, D.V., and Wall, T.: Confirmatory identification of *Neisseria gonorrhoeae* by slide coagglutination, Can. J. Microbiol. **26:**218, 1980.

46. Muchmore, H.G., Felton, F.G., and Scott, E.N.: Rapid presumptive identification of *Cryptococcus neoformans*, J. Clin. Microbiol. **8:**166, 1978.

47. Naiman, H.L., and Albritton, W.L.: Counterimmunoelectrophoresis in the diagnosis of acute infection, J. Infect. Dis. **142:**524, 1980.

48. Newman, R.B., Stevens, R.W., and Gaafar, H.A.: Latex agglutination test for the diagnosis of *Haemophilus influenzae* meningitis, J. Lab. Clin. Med. **76:**107, 1970.

49. Petts, D.N.: Early detection of streptococci in swabs by latex agglutination before culture, J. Clin. Microbiol. **19:**432, 1984.

50. Portas, M.R., Hogan, N.A., and Hill, H.R.: Rapid specific identification of group D streptococci by counterimmunoelectrophoresis, J. Lab. Clin. Med. **88:**339, 1976.

51. Prevost, E., and Newell, R.: Commercial cryptococcal latex kit: clinical evaluation in a medical center hospital, J. Clin. Microbiol. **8:**529, 1978.

52. Roantree, R.J., and Rantz, L.A.: Clinical experience with the C-reactive protein test, AMA Arch. Intern. Med. **96:**674, 1955.

53. Rose, N.R., and Friedman, H.: Manual of clinical immunology, ed. 2, Washington, D.C., 1980, American Society for Microbiology.

54. Rytel, M.W.: Rapid diagnosis in infectious disease, Boca Raton, Fla., 1979, CRC Press.

55. Sedgwick, A.K. and Tilton, R.C.: Identification of *Legionella pneumophila* by latex agglutination, J. Clin. Microbiol. **17:**365, 1982.

56. Shetlar, M.R., et al.: Comparison of serum C-reactive protein, glycoprotein, and seromucoid in cancer, arthritis, tuberculosis, and pregnancy, Proc. Soc. Exp. Biol. Med. **88:**107, 1955.

57. Simpson, R.A., and Speller, D.C.E.: Detection of bacteremia by countercurrent immunoelectrophoresis, Lancet **1:**1206, 1977.

58. Soini, E.: The principle of time-resolved fluorometry. In Habermehl, K.O., editor: Rapid methods and automation in microbiology and immunology, Berlin, 1985, Springer-Verlag.

59. Stockman, L., and Roberts, G.D.: Specificity of the latex test for cryptococcal antigen: a rapid, simple method for eliminating interference factors, J. Clin. Microbiol. **16:**965, 1982. .

60. Thirumoorthi, M.C., and Dajani, A.S.: Comparison of staphylococcal coagglutination, latex agglutination, and counterimmunoelectrophoresis for bacterial antigen detection, J. Clin. Microbiol. **9:**28, 1979.

61. Tillet, W.S., and Francis, T.O., Jr.: Serological reactions in pneumonia with a non-protein somatic fraction of pneumococcus, J. Exp. Med. **52:**561, 1930.

62. Tilton, R.C.: Counterimmunoelectrophoresis in biology and medicine. In Critical reviews in laboratory medicine, Boca Raton, Fla., 1978, CRC Press.

63. Tilton, R.C., Dias, F., and Ryan, R.W.: Comparative evaluation of 3 commercial products and counterimmunoelectrophoresis for the detection of antigens in cerebrospinal fluid, J. Clin. Microbiol. **20:**231, 1984.

64. Todd, E.W.: Antihemolysin titers in hemolytic streptococcus infections and their significance in rheumatic fever, Br. J. Exp. Pathol. **12:**248, 1932.

65. Truant, A.L., et al.: Limitations of rapid identification of *Streptococcus pneumonia* from blood cultures by counterimmunoelectrophoresis, Clin. Microbiol. Newsletter **3:**53, 1981.

66. Wasilauskas, B.L. and Hampton, K.D.: Determination of bacterial meningitis: a retrospective study of 80 cerebrospinal fluid specimens evaluated by four in vitro methods, J. Clin. Microbiol. **16:**531, 1982.

67. Webb, B.J., Edwards, M.S., and Baker, C.J.: Comparison of slide coagglutination test and countercurrent immunoelectrophoresis for detection of group B streptococcal antigen in cerebrospinal fluid from infants with meningitis, J. Clin. Microbiol. **11:**263, 1980.

CHAPTER 8

Antimicrobial Susceptibility Testing

Richard C. Tilton
Barbara J. Howard

A critical facet of clinical microbiology is the determination of the antimicrobial susceptibility of an isolated microorganism. While these in vivo analyses are relatively simple in both principle and performance, the in vivo response of both host and parasite to an antimicrobial agent is a complex of interrelationships. A clinical microbiologist must have knowledge of antimicrobial agents and antimicrobial susceptibility methods to choose the most appropriate test method for the clinical and laboratory situation.

Numerous classes of antimicrobial agents are used to treat microbial infections. A general class has multiple representatives, each with its own particular properties. In this chapter the chemistry, mode of action, and mechanism of resistance are discussed for the major groups of antimicrobial agents. A summary of the pharmacokinetics of these agents may be found in comprehensive texts by Goodman and Gilman[24] and Kucers and Bennett.[36]

ANTIMICROBIAL AGENTS
PENICILLINS

The parent compound penicillin was isolated from *Penicillium notatum* by Fleming in 1924. It was introduced to clinical medicine during World War II by Chain and Florey and abruptly changed the practice of medicine. The initial penicillin was a mixture of which penicillin G was the most satisfactory component. Stable salts of penicillin G, that is, sodium or potassium penicillin G, are now widely used.

The basic formula for penicillin is depicted in Figure 8-1 and consists of a thiazolidine ring (*a*), a beta-lactam ring (*b*), and a side chain (*R*). Although penicillin was originally isolated as a natural product, many biologic and chemical alterations have been made to the basic structure (Figure 8-1). These alterations have resulted in a broader antimicrobial spectrum, more stability (especially to acid), and improved pharmacokinetics.

Penicillin G is effective against streptococci (including *S. pneumoniae, S. pyogenes, S. agalactiae,* and *S. viridans*), *Neisseria* spp., and non-penicillinase-producing staphylococci. This antibiotic was effective in treating staphylococcal infections until the emergence of the large numbers of penicillinase-producing staphylococci in the 1950s. The advent of these strains prompted the development of the so-called penicillinase-resistant penicillins, such as methicillin, nafcillin, and oxacillin. These penicillins had bulky side chains that rendered them resistant to penicillinase-producing staphylococci; however, like penicillin G, they were unable to penetrate gram-negative rods. Subsequent changes were made in the side chain structure to provide activity against this group of organisms. Ampicillin, developed by introducing an alpha-amino group

into the benzyl chain, had enhanced activity against *Escherichia coli, Proteus mirabilis,* and *Haemophilus influenzae.* The carboxypenicillins were made by introducing an alpha-carboxy group into the benzyl side chain. These penicillins, ticarcillin and carbenicillin, inhibit *E. coli, Proteus vulgaris,* some *Enterobacter* spp., *Providencia rettgeri, Providencia stuartii,* the genera *Salmonella* and *Shigella,* and some *Serratia* spp.[51] An important advantage of these penicillins is their inhibition of *Pseudomonas aeruginosa,* with ticarcillin more active than carbenicillin. The genera *Klebsiella* and *Yersinia* are resistant. The carboxypenicillins are less active than penicillin G or ampicillin against most gram-positive organisms and less active against *H. influenzae* than ampicillin. The acylaminopenicillins are the newest extended penicillins and include azlocillin, mezlocillin, and piperacillin. Azlocillin and mezlocillin have a ureido ring in their side chain (Figure 8-1) and are also referred to as ureidopenicillins. Piperacillin possesses a piperazine ring (Figure 8-1). The acylaminopenicillins have increased activity against many gram-negative organisms, especially *Klebsiella pneumoniae, Serratia marcescens,* and *P. aeruginosa,* when compared with the carboxypenicillins.[16] They are more effective than ampicillin against *H. influenzae.* Both the carboxypenicillins and the aminoacylpenicillins are susceptible to beta-lactamases with one exception. The aminoacylpenicillins are able to inhibit the beta-lactamases of *K. pneumoniae* because these penicillins readily penetrate *Klebsiella* organisms and bind to the penicillin-binding proteins before they are destroyed by the beta-lactamases of this species.[56]

With few exceptions the mode of action of penicillins is similar: they inhibit cell wall synthesis. The precise mechanism by which this is accomplished, however, is unknown.

The cell wall of both gram-positive and gram-negative organisms is composed of peptidoglycan or murein. Peptidoglycan is comprised of polysaccharide chains containing alternating residues of *N*-acetyl-glucosamine and *N*-acetyl-muramic acid. These chains are cross-linked via peptide units extending from the *N*-acetyl-muramic acid (Figure 8-2). The cross-linking peptide units are originally synthesized as pentapeptides consisting of the amino acids L-alanine-D-glutamic acid-R-D-alanine-D-alanine (R may be a variety of amino acids, depending on the bacterium). During the final stage of cell wall synthesis known as transpeptidation, a transpeptidase enzyme cleaves the peptide bond between the two terminal D-alanines on one chain and a bond is formed between the carboxyl group of the penultimate D-alanine and the free amino group of the third amino acid of the neighboring chain (Figure 8-3). In gram-negative bacteria, a direct cross-link is formed between these two amino acids, but in gram-positive bacteria a short peptide or single

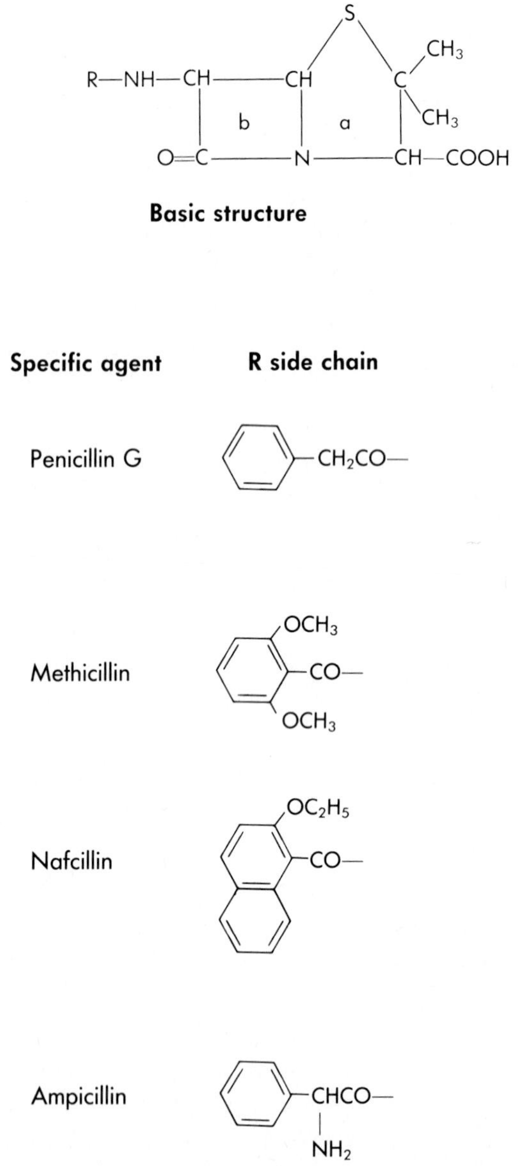

FIGURE 8-1. Chemical structure of the penicillins. Basic structure is seen at top of figure. R side chains vary according to specific agent.

Specific agent   **R side chain**

Carbenicillin

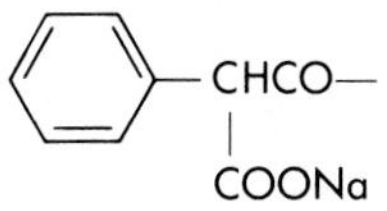

Ticarcillin

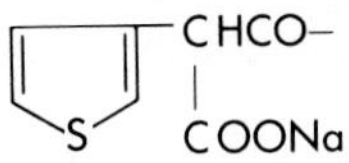

Piperacillin

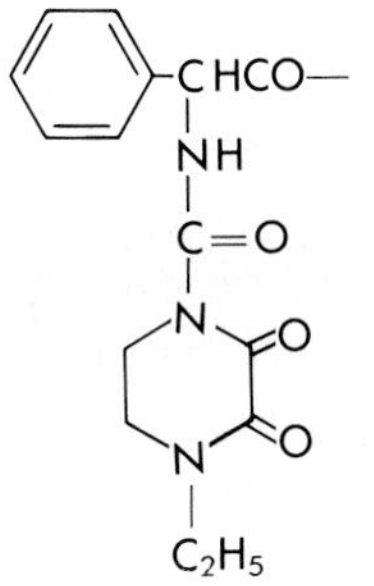

Mezlocillin

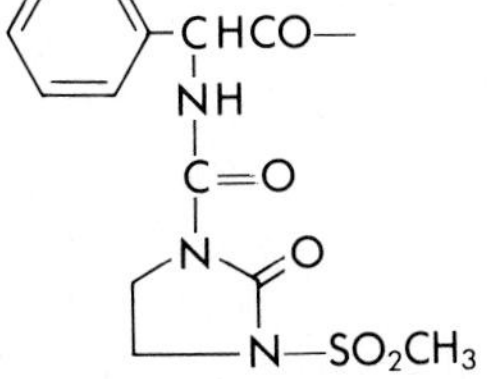

FIGURE 8-1, cont'd. For legend see opposite page.

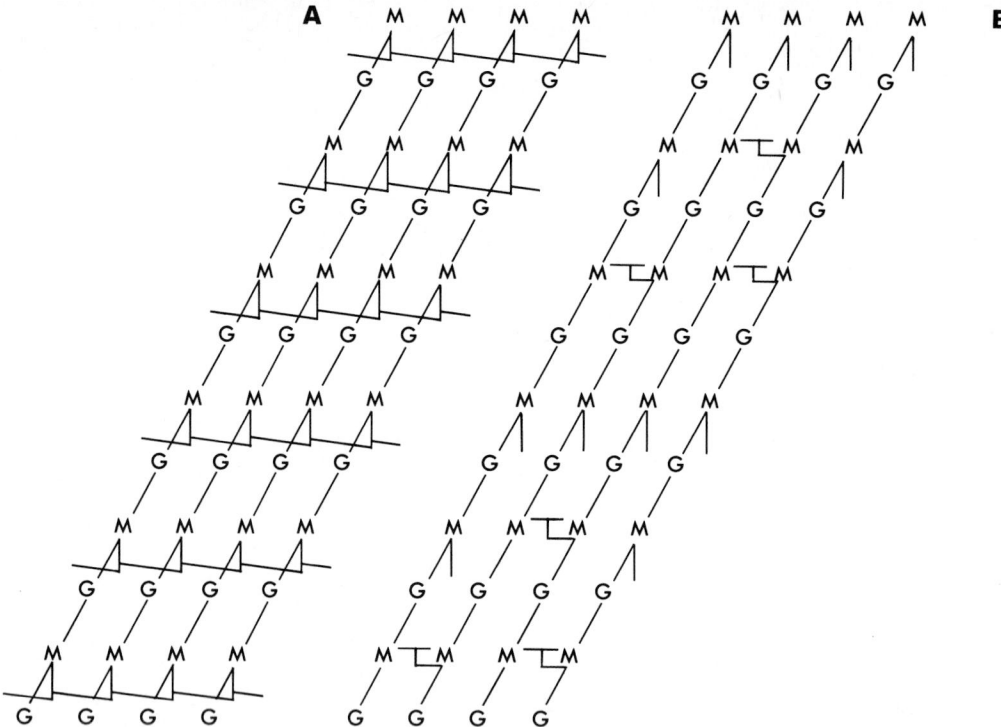

FIGURE 8-2. Diagrammatic representation of single layer of peptidoglycan from, **A,** *Staphylococcus aureus* and, **B,** *Escherichia coli. G,* N-Acetyl-glucosamine; *M,* N-acetyl-muramic acid. (Redrawn from Mandelstam, J., and McQuillen, K.: Biochemistry of bacterial growth, ed. 2, Oxford, Eng., 1973, Blackwell Scientific Publications.)

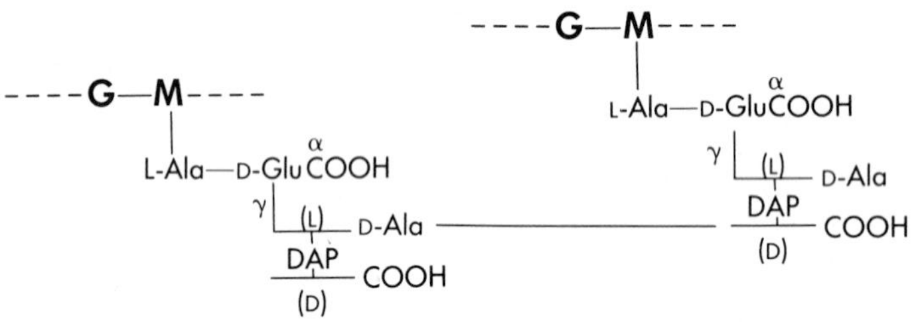

FIGURE 8-3. Peptidoglycan of *Escherichia coli.* Direct cross-link joins tetrapeptides. (From Mandelstam, J., and McQuillen, K.: Biochemistry of bacterial growth, ed. 2, Oxford, Eng., 1973, Blackwell Scientific Publications.)

amino acid links the two chains (Figure 8-4). The terminal D-alanine is removed by a carboxypeptidase enzyme.

Early studies on the mechanism of action of penicillin suggested that it inhibited the transpeptidation reaction by acting as a structural analogue of D-alanyl-D-alanine. The penicillin combined with the transpeptidase enzyme and inactivated it. More recent studies uncovering the presence of penicillin-binding proteins (PBPs) suggest that the mechanism may be more complex.

PBPs are the primary biochemical targets of beta-lactam antibiotics. (Beta-lactam antibiotics include the penicillins and cephalosporins, both of which possess a beta-lactam ring.) PBPs are probably the enzymes involved in cell wall synthesis. Numerous PBPs with different functions have been identified.

Treatment of bacteria with a beta-lactam antibiotic that targets a specific PBP results in aberrant morphology of the cell. In fact, different morphologic changes may be observed with different antibiotics. For example, cephaloridine produces lytic effects on *E. coli,* cephalexin and ampicillin cause the formation of long filaments in *E. coli,* and other agents cause *E. coli* to form ovoid cells.[72] The different morphologic changes probably reflect differences in the targeted PBP.

Researchers have also recently recognized that cell wall autolysins are necessary mediators in the bactericidal effects of the beta-lactam antibiotics.[57] Binding to PBPs and subsequent inhibition of cell wall synthesis may activate autolytic enzymes that are responsible for cell death. This observation helps to explain "penicillin tolerance," a new mechanism of bacterial

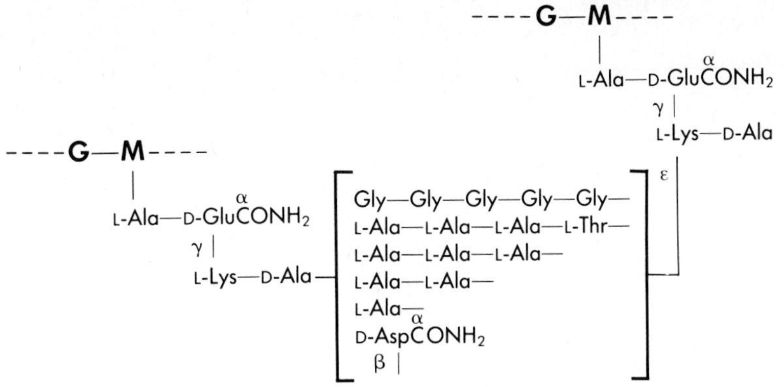

FIGURE 8-4. Peptidoglycan of many gram-positive bacteria. Short peptide chain or single amino acid links the tetrapeptides. (From Mandelstam, J., and McQuillen, K.: Biochemistry of bacterial growth, ed. 2, Oxford, Eng., 1973, Blackwell Scientific Publications.)

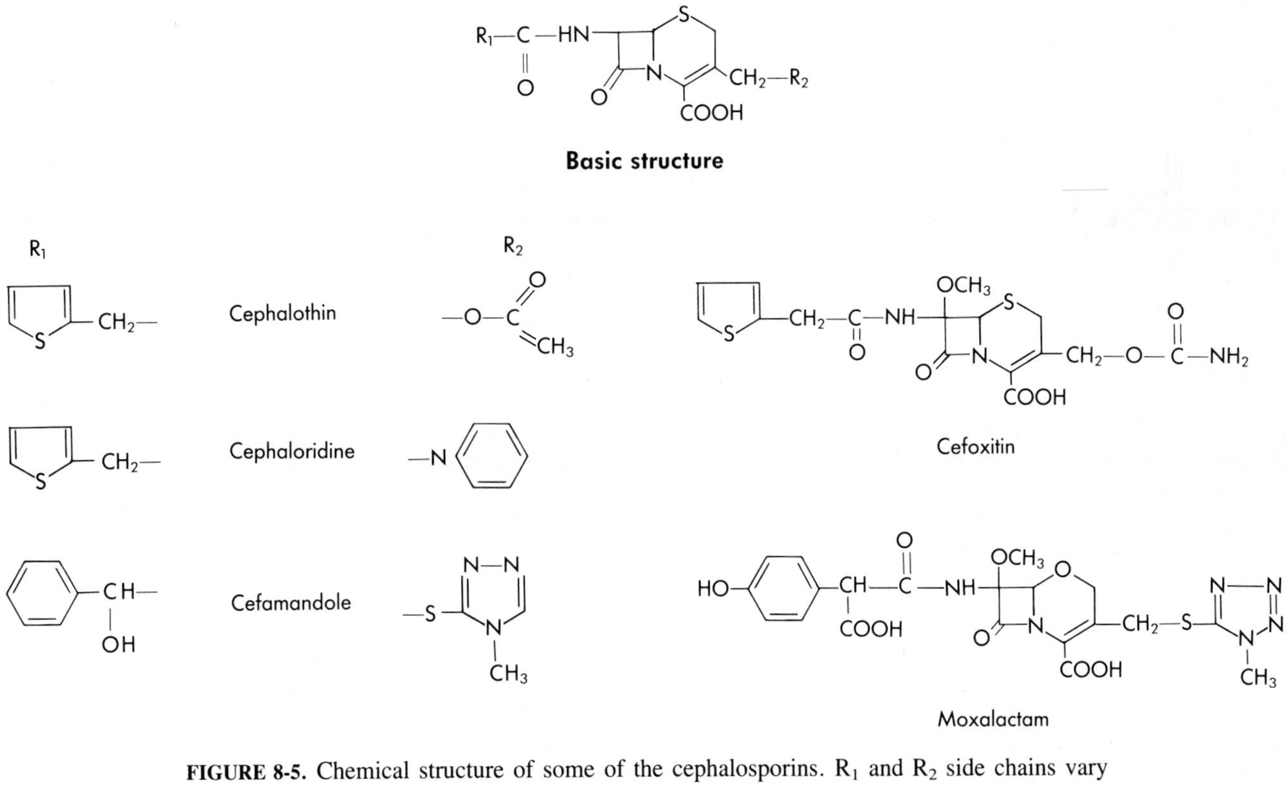

Basic structure

FIGURE 8-5. Chemical structure of some of the cephalosporins. R_1 and R_2 side chains vary according to specific agent. Note that structures for cefoxitin and moxalactam are complete structures and not R_1 and R_2 side chains.

resistance to penicillin. It was observed that some strains of staphylococci, primarily *S. aureus,* were only inhibited, not killed, by potentially lethal concentrations of penicillin. This "tolerance" has been associated with a deficiency in autolytic enzyme activity.

CEPHALOSPORINS

The first clinically useful cephalosporin, cephalosporin C, was isolated in 1948 from *Cephalosporium acremonium.* Acid modification of this antibiotic rendered 7-aminocephalospo-

ranic acid, the base structure of all subsequent cephalosporins. The cephalosporins are structurally similar to the penicillins, and they both have a beta-lactam ring; however, the cephalosporins have a six-member dihydrothiazine ring instead of the five-member thiazolidene ring (Figure 8-5).

Like penicillins, the various cephalosporins have been created by synthesis of side chains attached at positions R_1 and R_2 of 7-aminocephalosporanic acid, resulting in what have been called first-, second-, and third-generation cephalosporins:

1. First generation

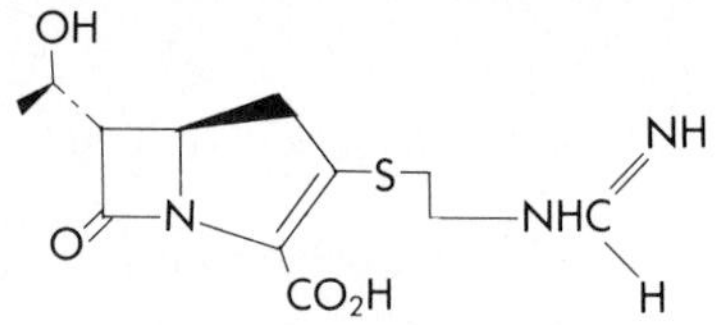

FIGURE 8-6. Imipenem (*N*-formimidoyl thienamycin).

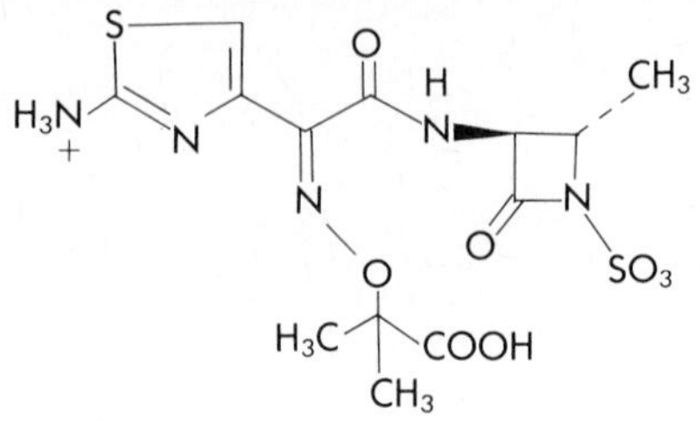

a. Cephalothin
b. Cephaloridine
c. Cefazolin
d. Cephalexin
e. Cephradine
f. Cephaloglycin
g. Cefaclor
2. Second generation
   a. Cefamandole
   b. Cefoxitin
   c. Cefonicid
   d. Ceforanide
   e. Cefuroxime
   f. Cefotetan
3. Third generation
   a. Moxalactam
   b. Cefotaxime
   c. Ceftazidime
   d. Ceftriaxone
   e. Ceftizoxime
   f. Cefmenoxime
   g. Cefoperazone
   h. Cefsulodin

One of the second-generation cephalosporins, cefoxitin, is more precisely characterized structurally as a cephamycin. Cephamycins resemble the cephalosporins but have a methoxy group (OCH_3) attached to the beta-lactam ring (Figure 8-5). Moxalactam also differs slightly in structure from the other cephalosporins; it has a methoxy group attached to the beta-lactam ring and an oxygen instead of sulfur in position 1 of the dihydrothiazine ring (Figure 8-5). The addition of the methoxy group to the beta-lactam ring renders the ring resistant to hydrolysis by most penicillinases and cephalosporinases.

The first-generation cephalosporins have good activity against gram-positive organisms (excluding enterococci, *Listeria* spp., and methicillin-resistant *Staphylococcus aureus*). They are also effective against some gram-negative bacteria including *Escherichia coli*, the genera *Klebsiella* and *Shigella*, and *Proteus mirabilis*, as well as anaerobes excluding *Bacteroides fragilis*. The gram-negative spectrum of the second-generation cephalosporins is expanded to include some *Morganella*, *Citrobacter*, and *Providencia* spp. and *B. fragilis*. The second-generation cephalosporins may be less active than the first-generation cephalosporins against *S. aureus*, *Streptococcus pneumoniae*, and *Streptococcus pyogenes*. The third-generation cephalosporins, depending on the specific agent, are effective against the same gram-negative organisms as the second-generation cephalosporins and also have increased activity against the more resistant gram-negative organisms including *Serratia* spp., *Pseudomonas aeruginosa*, and *Enterobacter* spp. (except for some strains of *E. cloacae*). The third-generation cephalosporins are also effective against *Neisseria men-

FIGURE 8-7. Aztreonam.

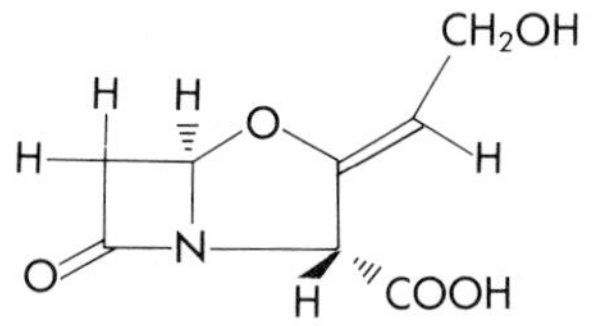

FIGURE 8-8. Clavulanic acid.

ingitidis, against beta-lactamase-producing *Neisseria gonorrhoeae* and *Haemophilus influenzae*, and against many gram-positive bacteria.

The cephalosporins bind to PBPs and inhibit cell wall synthesis. Their mechanism of action is thought to be similar to that of the penicillins.

OTHER BETA-LACTAM ANTIBIOTICS[56]

The thienamycins and monobactams are recently developed beta-lactam antibiotics. The thienamycins are derived from *Streptomyces cattleya* and the monobactams from the genera *Gluconobacter*, *Acinetobacter*, and *Chromobacterium*. Imipenem (Figure 8-6) is an example of a thienamycin, and aztreonam (Figure 8-7) is an example of a monobactam. With few exceptions these antibiotics are resistant to plasmid- and chromosomal-mediated beta-lactamases. Imipenem is active against the beta-lactamases of *Staphylococcus aureus*, *Escherichia coli*, *Enterobacter cloacae*, *Citrobacter freundii*, *Providencia rettgeri*, *Serratia marcescens*, *Proteus vulgaris*, *Klebsiella oxytoca*, *Pseudomonas aeruginosa*, *Pseudomonas cepacia*, and *Bacteroides fragilis*. It is partially hydrolyzed by the beta-lactamase of *Pseudomonas maltophilia*. Imipenem is also quite active against gram-positive species and anaerobes. Aztreonam is not effective against the latter two groups of organisms but is resistant to the beta-lactamases of most gram-negative rods except for the beta-lactamases of some strains of *Klebsiella oxytoca* and *Pseudomonas cepacia*.

Clavulanic acid (Figure 8-8), a derivative of *Streptomyces clavuligerus*, is a beta-lactamase inhibitor that acts synergistically with amoxicillin, ampicillin, piperacillin, and mezlocillin. It is commercially available in combination with amoxicillin as Augmentin. A similar product, Timentin, consists of ticarcillin and clavulanic acid. Clavulanic acid resembles penicillin in structure and binds with the beta-lactamase enzyme, allowing amoxicillin to reach its target site.

ERYTHROMYCIN

Erythromycin is a member of the macrolide group of antimicrobics, which is characterized by the presence of a large lactone ring of 12 to 22 carbon atoms attached to one or more

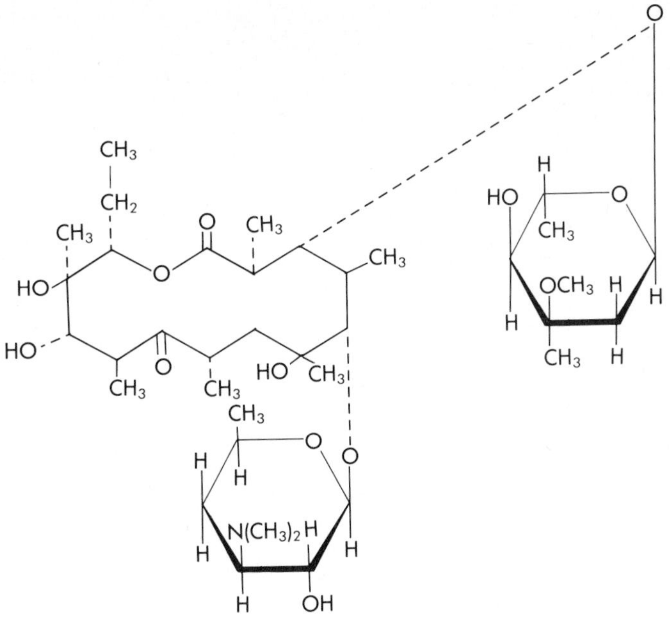

FIGURE 8-9. Erythromycin.

sugars (Figure 8-9). Macrolides are produced by species of *Streptomyces*.

The activity of erythromycin against many common clinical isolates is seen in Tables 8-1 and 8-2. In addition, erythromycin is effective against *Bordetella pertussis, Campylobacter jejuni, Legionella pneumophila, Chlamydia trachomatis, Treponema pallidum, Mycoplasma pneumoniae, Ureaplasma urealyticum,* actinomycetes, mycobacteria, and some strains of *Rickettsia*.

Erythromycin inhibits bacterial protein synthesis. After binding to the 50S ribosome, it may inhibit transpeptidation, that is, the transfer of the growing peptide chain from the P site (peptidyl or donor site) to the amino acid at the A site (aminoacyl or acceptor site) on the ribosome (Figure 8-10).[60] Subsequent translocation of the peptidyl-tRNA from the A site to the P site is also inhibited.

TETRACYCLINES

The tetracycline family of antimicrobics has numerous members. The first tetracyclines discovered were produced by *Streptomyces aureofaciens* (chlortetracycline) and *Streptomyces rimosus* (oxytetracycline). The others, including demeclocycline, methacycline, doxycycline, and minocycline, were either derived from mutants of *Streptomyces* or completely or partially synthesized in the laboratory. The basic structure of the tetracyclines consists of four fused rings; the various analogues differ in their substitutions at R_1, R_2, R_3, and R_4 (Figure 8-11).

Although many common gram-positive and gram-negative organisms may be susceptible to tetracycline (see Tables 8-1 and 8-2), plasmid-mediated resistance is common. Thus in most cases more effective agents are available for treating infections caused by these organisms. The tetracyclines are also active against mycoplasmas, rickettsiae, chlamydiae, and some yeasts and protozoa.

The tetracyclines are bacteriostatic antimicrobics, and their principal mode of action is the inhibition of protein synthesis. They bind to the 30S ribosomal subunit and inhibit the attachment of aminoacyl-tRNA to the acceptor site on the mRNA-ribosome complex (Figure 8-10).

CHLORAMPHENICOL

Chloramphenicol was isolated in 1947 from *Streptomyces venezuelae* and was the first antimicrobic that was truly "broad spectrum"; that is, it inhibited a variety of both gram-positive and gram-negative bacteria. Chloramphenicol is a derivative of dichloracetic acid and contains a nitrobenzene ring (Figure 8-12). Chloramphenicol may cause aplastic anemia, and thus, despite its broad-spectrum activity, it is used only to treat certain conditions such as typhoid fever or meningitis caused by ampicillin-resistant *Haemophilus influenzae*.

Chloramphenicol is a bacteriostatic antimicrobic, although in gram-positive bacteria, notably the streptococci, it appears to be bactericidal.[20] It is an inhibitor of protein synthesis and binds to the 50S ribosomal portion where, like erythromycin, it inhibits transpeptidation.[80] If chloramphenicol is removed from the target site, protein synthesis is reinitiated, which explains the bacteriostatic nature of the drug. Prolonged exposure of the bacterium to chloramphenicol results in cell lysis and death.[28]

AMINOGLYCOSIDES

The members of the aminoglycoside family share certain characteristics. The aminoglycosides consist of amino-sugars with glycosidic linkages to an aminocyclitol ring and should more correctly be called aminocyclitols. Included in this group are streptomycin, kanamycin, gentamicin, tobramycin, amikacin, netilmicin, sisomicin, and neomycin.

As a group, the aminoglycosides are effective against many aerobic and facultative gram-negative bacilli. The spectrum of activity does vary somewhat among the different agents. Many gram-negative bacilli are resistant to streptomycin because of the presence of inactivating enzymes; however, streptomycin is active against *Francisella tularensis, Yersinia pestis, Brucella* spp., and *Mycobacterium tuberculosis*. Gentamicin, tobramy-

TABLE 8-1. Activity of Common Antimicrobial Agents against Gram-Positive Organisms[a]

Antimicrobial Agent	Staphylococcus	Streptococcus	Enterococcus
Penicillin	+	+ + + +	+
Ampicillin	+	+ + + +	+ + + +
Carbenicillin	+	+ + + +	+ + + +[b]
Oxacillin, methicillin	+ + +[c] + + + +[d]	+ + + +	−
Piperacillin, mezlocillin	+	+ + + +	+ + + +[b]
Cephalosporins First generation	+ + + +[e,f]	+ + + +	−
Second generation	+ + + +[f]	+ + + +	−
Third generation	+	+ + + +	−
Erythromycin	+ + +[c] + + + +[d]	+ + + +	+ +
Tetracyclines	+ + +[c] + + + +[d]	+ + +	+
Chloramphenicol	+ + + +	+ + + +	+ + + +
Gentamicin, tobramycin	+ + + +	−	+
Amikacin	+ + + +	−	−
Vancomycin	+ + + +	+ + + +	+ + + +
Clindamycin	+ + +[c] + + + +[f]	+ + + +	−
Trimethoprim- sulfamethoxazole	+ + + +	+ + + +	NA

> **SYMBOLS:**   + + + +, >80% susceptible   +, 5% to 25% susceptible
>   + + +, 50% to 80% susceptible   −, Resistant
>   + +, 25% to 50% susceptible   NA, Not usually used for treatment

[a]The purpose of this table is to give an overview of the antimicrobial spectrum of these antimicrobial agents. The actual percentages may vary from institution to institution.
[b]Enterococci are susceptible to moderately high concentrations of carbenicillin, piperacillin, and mezlocillin (mean MICs = 25 μg/ml).
[c]*S. epidermidis.*
[d]*S. aureus.*
[e]Methicillin- and oxacillin-resistant *S. aureus* should be considered resistant to cephalothin.
[f]Susceptibility of beta-lactamase and *S. aureus* varies as a function of the cephalosporin tested.

TABLE 8-2. Activity of Common Antimicrobial Agents against Gram-Negative Organisms[a]

Antimicrobial Agent	Escherichia coli	Klebsiella	Enterobacter	Pseudomonas	Serratia	Proteus	Haemophilus	Neisseria gonorrhoeae
Penicillin	−	−	−	−	−	−	−[b]	++++
Ampicillin	+++	−	−	−[c]	−	−[d]	+++	++++
Carbenicillin	+++	−	+++	++++[e]	+++	+++[d]	+++	++++
Oxacillin, methicillin	−	−	−	−	−	−	−	++++
Piperacillin, mezlocillin	+++	++++	++++	++++	++++	+++	+++	++++
Cephalosporins First generation	++++	++++	−	−	−	−[d]	++	++++
Second generation	++++	++++	++++	−	−[f]	++++	+++[g]	++++
Third generation	++++	++++	+++[h]	++++[h]	++++[h]	++++	++++	++++
Erythromycin	−	−	−	−	−	−	++++	+++
Tetracyclines	+++	++++	++++	−	−	++[i]	++++	++++
Chloramphenicol	++++	++++	++++	−	+++	+++[d]	++++	+++
Gentamicin, tobramycin	++++	++++	+++[j]	++	++++[j]	++++	+++	++++
Amikacin	++++	++++	++++	+++	++++	++++	+++	++++
Vancomycin	−	−	−	−	−	−	−	−
Clindamycin	−	−	−	−	−	−	−	+++
Trimethoprim-sulfamethoxazole	++++	++++	++++	−	++++	++++	++++	+++

Symbols:	++++, >80% susceptible	++, 25% to 50% susceptible
	+++, 50% to 80% susceptible	−, Resistant

[a] The purpose of this table is to give an overview of the spectrum of these antimicrobial agents. The actual percentages may vary from institution to institution.

[b] *Haemophilus* spp. are usually regarded as resistant to penicillin, but MICs are low. Exception is beta-lactamase-producing strains, whose MICs are high.

[c] *P. pseudomallei* >80% susceptible.

[d] *P. mirabilis* >80% susceptible.

[e] *P. aeruginosa* rapidly develops resistance to carbenicillin and ticarcillin.

[f] *S. liquefaciens* >80% susceptible.

[g] *H. influenzae* may develop resistance to cefamandole.

[h] Variable susceptibility as a function of the individual antimicrobial agent.

[i] *P. mirabilis* resistant.

[j] Gentamicin- and tobramycin-resistant *Enterobacter* and *Serratia* organisms are often seen, particularly in hospital-associated infections.

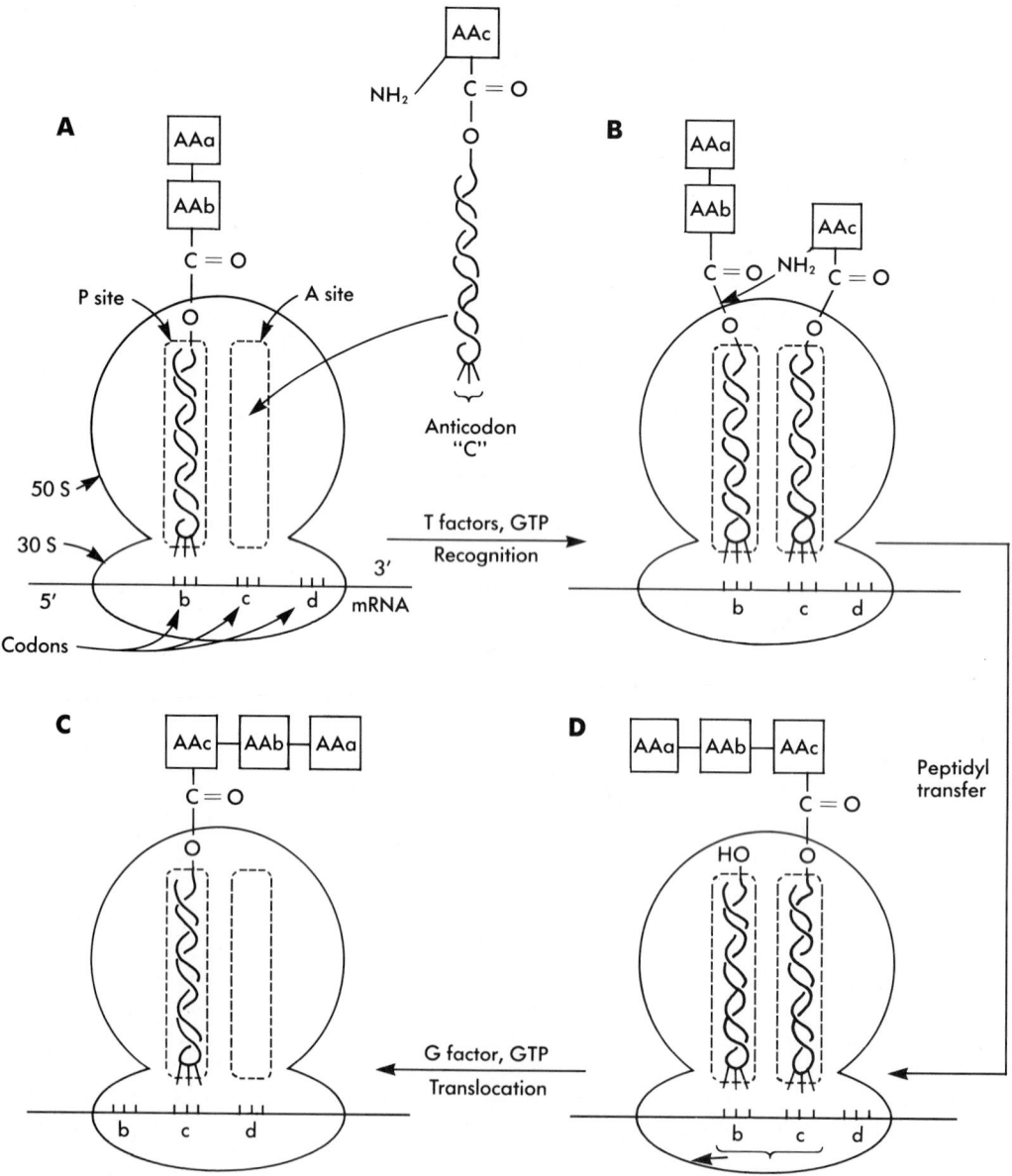

FIGURE 8-10. Protein synthesis. **A,** Peptidyl-tRNA bound to peptidyl site (P site) of ribosome. **B,** Binding of specific aa-tRNA, coded for by next free codon, to aminoacyl site (A site). **C,** Peptide chain transfer to A site by formation of peptide bond with aa-tRNA bound to that site. **D,** Movement of peptidyl-tRNA, along with corresponding region of mRNA, from A to P site, ejecting free tRNA. (From Davis, B.D., et al.: Microbiology, ed. 3, Hagerstown, Md., 1980, Harper & Row Publishers, Inc.)

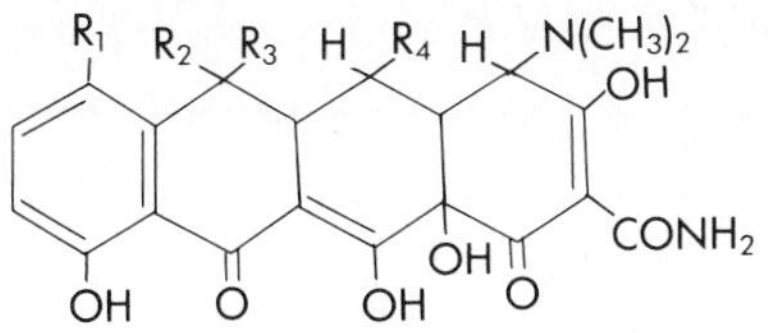

FIGURE 8-11. Structural formulas for tetracycline and some of its derivatives. (From Joklik, W.K., Willett, H.P., and Amos, B.D.: Zinsser microbiology, ed. 18, New York, 1984, Appleton-Century-Crofts.)

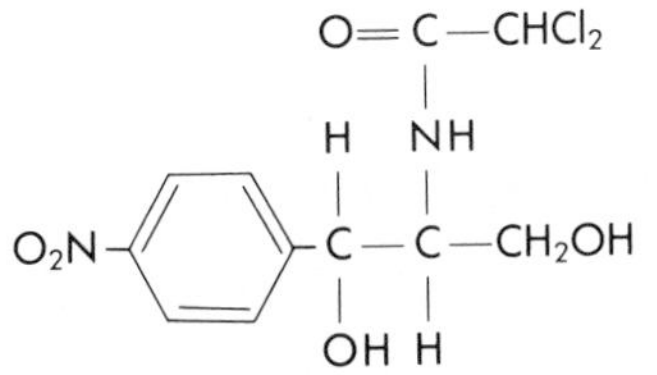

	R_1	R_2	R_3	R_4
Tetracycline	H	OH	CH_3	H
Oxytetracycline	H	OH	CH_3	OH
Chlortetracycline	Cl	OH	CH_3	H
Demethylchlortetracycline	Cl	OH	H	H
Doxycycline	H	H	CH_3	OH
Minocycline	$N(CH_3)_2$	H	H	H

FIGURE 8-12. Chloramphenicol.

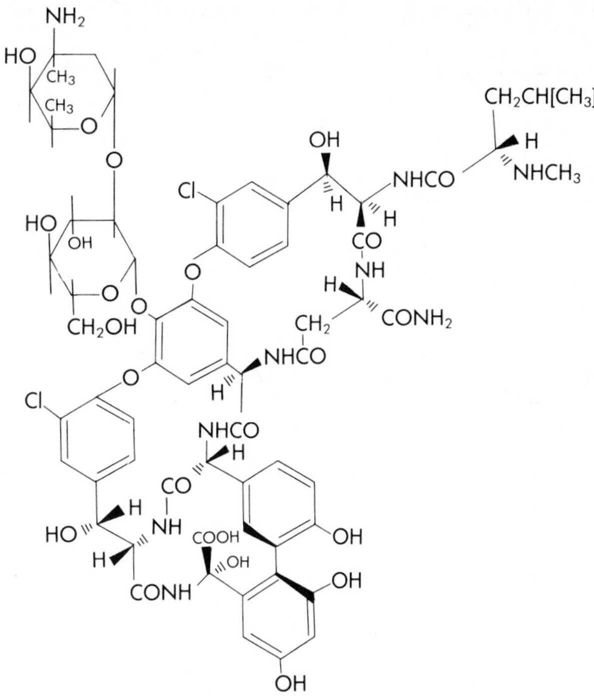

FIGURE 8-13. Vancomycin.

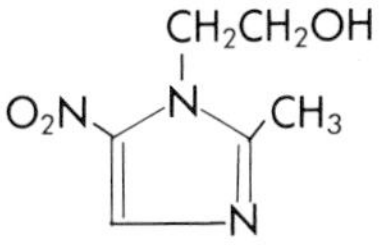

FIGURE 8-14. Metronidazole.

cin, and netilmicin are active against many *Enterobacteriaceae* and *Pseudomonas aeruginosa*; tobramycin is more active against *P. aeruginosa*, and gentamicin more potent against *Serratia* spp. Netilmicin is resistant to many inactivating enzymes and thus may be used against some gentamicin-resistant isolates. Amikacin is also active against many strains of gram-negative rods that are resistant to other aminoglycosides.

The modes of action of the various aminoglycosides are similar. They are bactericidal drugs and inhibitors of microbial protein synthesis in both gram-positive and gram-negative bacteria. They bind to a P10 protein in the 30S ribosome complex. The mRNA codon is misread, and the wrong amino acids are incorporated into protein. Misreading of proteins, however, does not explain the lethal or bactericidal effect of aminoglycosides on bacteria; this mechanism remains unclear.

VANCOMYCIN

Vancomycin is a complex polypeptide (Figure 8-13) obtained from *Streptomyces orientales*. It is active against gram-positive organisms including *Staphylococcus aureus*, *Staphylococcus epidermidis*, *Listeria monocytogenes*, the genera *Clostridium*, *Bacillus*, and *Actinomyces*, and many streptococci. It is the drug of choice for methicillin-resistant staphylococci and has been used effectively in treating conditions associated with *Clostridium difficile* (see Chapter 20). Gram-negative organisms are resistant to vancomycin.

Vancomycin inhibits cell wall synthesis by forming complexes with the terminal acyl-D-alanine-D-alanine side chains of peptidoglycan molecules.

METRONIDAZOLE[63]

Metronidazole is a nitroimidazole derivative (Figure 8-14) that is active against *Trichomonas vaginalis*, *Entamoeba histolytica*, *Giardia lamblia*, *Clostridium difficile*, and all species of anaerobes except certain nonsporeforming gram-positive bacilli (such as the genera *Actinomyces*, *Arachnia*, and *Propionibacterium*) and certain gram-positive cocci.

Metronidazole is reduced on entry into susceptible organisms. This reduction results in the generation of cytotoxic intermediates that disrupt DNA.

CLINDAMYCIN

Clindamycin is produced by chemical modification of lincomycin (7-chloro-7-deoxy-lincomycin) (Figure 8-15). This antimicrobic is active against most aerobic gram-positive cocci, including staphylococci, pneumococci, *Streptococcus pyogenes*, and viridans streptococci, and is very active against most clinically significant anaerobes, especially *Bacteroides fragilis*. Clindamycin is inactive against *Neisseria meningitidis*, *Enterobacteriaceae*, enterococci, and *Haemophilus influenzae*.

The mechanism of action of clindamycin is like that of erythromycin; it binds to the 50S ribosome and inhibits protein synthesis by interfering with transpeptidation.

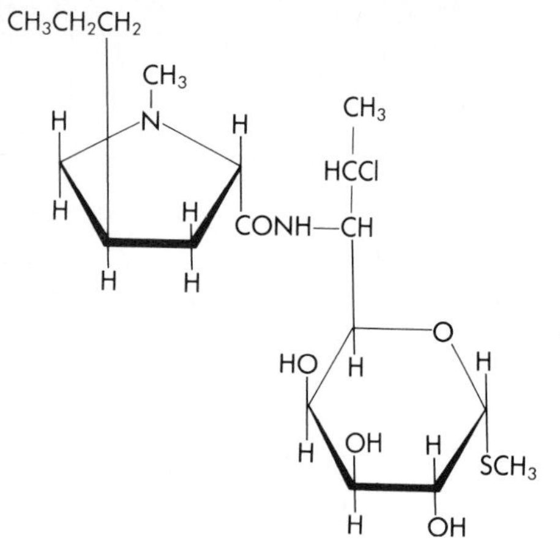

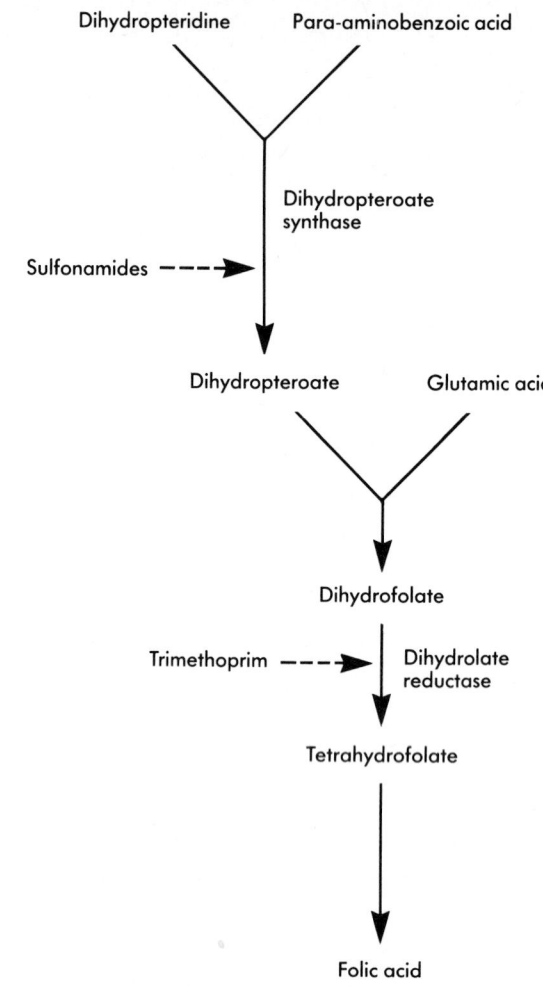

FIGURE 8-15. Clindamycin.

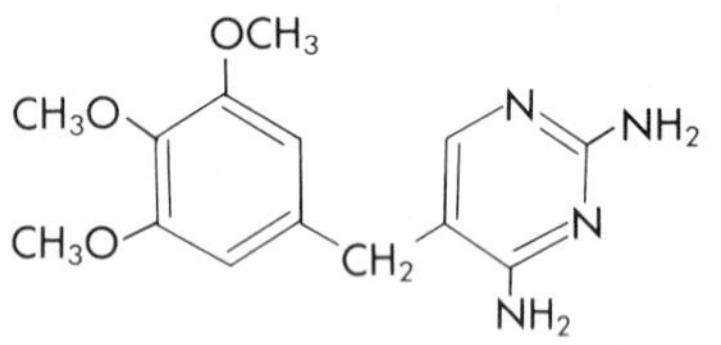

FIGURE 8-16. Trimethoprim.

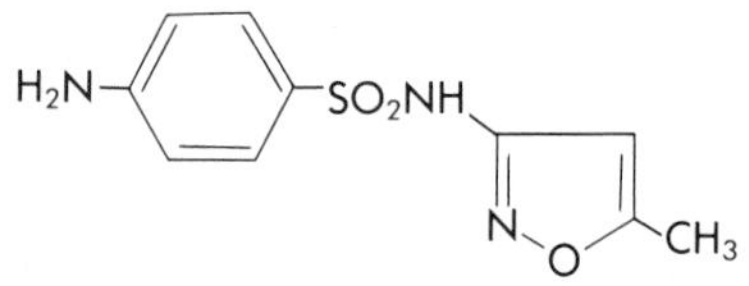

FIGURE 8-17. Sulfamethoxazole.

FIGURE 8-18. Synthesis of folic acid.

TRIMETHOPRIM-SULFAMETHOXAZOLE

Trimethoprim (TMP) is a diaminopyrimidine (Figure 8-16), and sulfamethoxazole (SXT) (Figure 8-17) is a sulfonamide derived from sulfanilamide. The combination of these two agents shows synergistic activity against most *Enterobacteriaceae* spp., *Pseudomonas cepacia, Pseudomonas pseudomallei, Neisseria gonorrhoeae, Haemophilus influenzae, Staphylococcus aureus, Streptococcus pyogenes,* and *Streptococcus pneumoniae.*

SXT and TMP inhibit the synthesis of folic acid in bacteria (Figure 8-18). Folic acid is required for DNA synthesis. The sulfonamides are similar in structure to para-aminobenzoic acid (PABA) and compete with PABA for combining sites on the enzyme dihydropteroate synthase. TMP inhibits the enzyme dihydrofolate reductase, which reduces dihydrofolate to tetrahydrofolate.

QUINOLONES[2]

The quinolones include nalidixic acid, cinoxacin, norfloxacin, ciprofloxacin, and others under development. All are synthetic derivatives of 1,8-napthyridine (Figure 8-19) and are used to treat urinary tract infections. Clinical studies indicate that these agents will be effective in treating a variety of other infections.

The quinolones are thought to inhibit DNA replication by inhibiting DNA gyrase, an enzyme responsible for the supercoiling of DNA in bacterial cells; the precise mechanism of inhibition is unknown.

Nalidixic acid is active against most members of the family *Enterobacteriaceae* but is inactive against most species of *Pseudomonas* and many gram-positive organisms including *Staphylococcus aureus, Enterococcus faecalis,* and *Streptococcus pneumoniae.* Norfloxacin and ciprofloxacin are several times more active than nalidixic acid, and their spectrum of activity also includes the genera *Staphylococcus, Enterococcus,* and *Pseudomonas.* Ciprofloxacin is the most potent quinolone. Compared with norfloxacin, it has greater activity against all organisms, such as staphylococci (including methicillin-resistant *S. aureus*), streptococci, *Listeria monocytogenes,* and *Bacteroides fragilis.*

ANTIMYCOBACTERIAL AGENTS[42]

There are at least six major antituberculous drugs: isoniazid, rifampin, para-aminosalicylic acid, ethambutol, pyrazinamide, and streptomycin. Isoniazid and rifampin are the most efficacious and are generally used to treat patients with newly diagnosed tuberculosis. Others such as cycloserine, capreomycin, kanamycin, and ethionamide are used when the other six drugs are unacceptable because of toxicity or drug resistance. As explained in Chapter 26, the resistance of mycobacteria to these

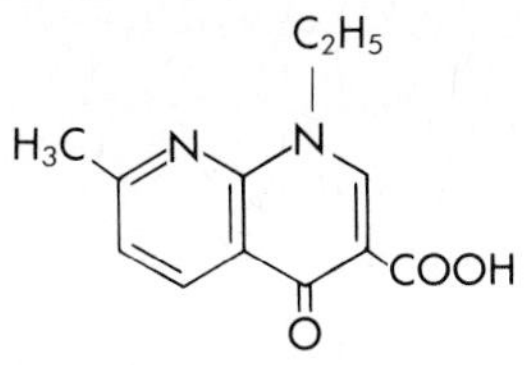

FIGURE 8-19. Nalidixic acid, cinoxacin, norfloxacin, and ciprofloxacin.

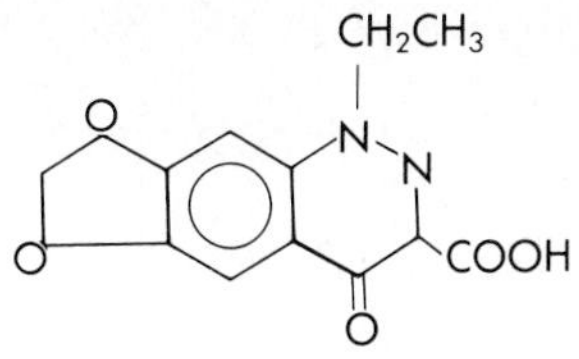

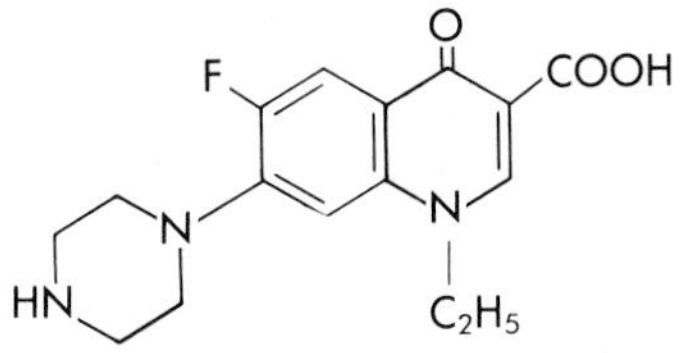

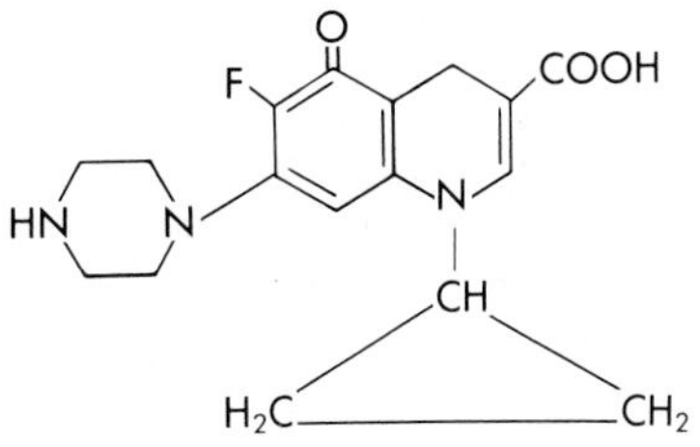

drugs is attributed to the selective emergence of naturally resistant mutant strains.

ISONIAZID

Most strains of *Mycobacterium tuberculosis* are susceptible to INH, but the majority of mycobacteria other than *M. tuberculosis* are resistant. Because *M. tuberculosis* frequently becomes resistant to isoniazid during treatment, isoniazid is always used in combination with one or two additional drugs (see Chapter 26).

The mechanism of action of isoniazid is unknown. Several investigators have speculated that INH inhibits nucleic acid synthesis in mycobacteria.[82,86] Others have suggested that mycolic acid synthesis is inhibited; mycolic acid normally comprises 40% of the mycobacterial cell wall.

RIFAMPIN[79]

Rifampin is a chemical derivative of the rifamycins, a class of antimicrobial agents that are fermentation products of *Nocardia meditteranei*. Rifampin inhibits RNA polymerase, the enzyme responsible for transcription of DNA to RNA. It is active against *Mycobacterium tuberculosis*, *M. bovis*, *M. marinum*, *M. kansasii*, and some strains of *M. avium-intracellulare*.

Resistance to rifampin is caused by alteration of the RNA polymerase. Alterations occur in the binding site for rifampin as a result of chromosomal mutation.

PARA-AMINOSALICYLIC ACID

Para-aminosalicylic acid (PAS) is synthesized chemically. Its mechanism of action is similar to that of the sulfonamides. It inhibits folic acid synthesis by acting as a structural analogue of para-aminobenzoic acid (PABA). PAS is bacteriostatic and is active against *Mycobacterium tuberculosis* only.

ETHAMBUTOL

Ethambutol is also a bacteriostatic agent that is synthesized chemically. It is similar to rifampin in activity. The mechanism of action of ethambutol is unknown, but some studies have suggested that it inhibits RNA synthesis. The mechanism of resistance is unknown.

PYRAZINAMIDE

Pyrazinamide is a synthetic derivative of niacinamide. Its mechanisms of action and resistance are unknown. Pyrazinamide is active only against *Mycobacterium tuberculosis*.

STREPTOMYCIN

The mechanism of action and resistance of streptomycin are discussed above. This aminoglycoside is active against *Mycobacterium tuberculosis*.

ANTIFUNGAL AGENTS

Compared with the many antimicrobial agents that are active against bacteria, there are relatively few antifungal agents. They include amphotericin, 5-fluorocytosine, nystatin, griseofulvin, and the imidazoles, which include cotrimazole, econazole, miconazole, and ketoconazole.

AMPHOTERICIN

Amphotericin is a polyene (heptaene) antifungal agent isolated from *Streptomyces nodosus*.[26] It is the only polyene that is routinely used, since the others discovered are either insoluble or unstable. Amphotericin B is also insoluble but is marketed as a colloidal suspension.

Amphotericin B binds to ergosterol in yeast cell membranes, interfering with transport of amino acids and other essential products. In high concentrations it is fungicidal, but in usually achievable concentrations it is fungistatic. Most fungi are susceptible to amphotericin at a concentration of <2 µg/ml, although resistance has been noted among some of the aspergilli, the zygomycetes, and the dematiaceous fungi. Merz[44] has reported amphotericin-resistant yeasts, including *Candida tropicalis*, *C. krusei*, *C. parakrusei*, and *C. lusitaneae*.

5-FLUOROCYTOSINE

The agent 5-fluorocytosine (5-FC) is a fluorinated pyrimidine and was initially synthesized as an antineoplastic drug.

Grunberg[27] noted that 5-FC had antifungal activity, albeit limited to pathogenic yeasts. Some strains of the aspergilli and the dematiaceous fungi may be susceptible, but most are resistant.

The 5-FC is taken up by an active permease system into the susceptible fungus and deaminated by cytosine deaminase to 5-fluorouracil, which is then incorporated into both ribosomal RNA and transfer RNA, resulting in defective protein synthesis. Wagner and Shadomy[77] reported that the anti-*Aspergillus* activity of 5-FC may be due to inhibition of DNA synthesis, not protein synthesis. Susceptible organisms may become resistant during therapy because of permeability alterations, enzyme modification, or the presence of competing metabolites such as purines and pyrimidines. Since human cells do not have cytosine deaminase, 5-FC is essentially nontoxic for humans.

To stem the developing resistance to 5-FC, it is usually employed in combination with another drug such as amphotericin B. Ostensibly, amphotericin B destroys membrane permeability and the uptake of 5-FC is increased. Because of the development of resistance in persons who are receiving 5-FC therapy or have a natural resistance to 5-FC, antifungal susceptibility testing should be performed on significant isolates, especially *Cryptococcus neoformans,* which is notable for its development of secondary resistance.

IMIDAZOLES

Of the imidazoles potentially available, miconazole and ketoconazole are the only ones routinely used. Miconazole is a synthetic antifungal agent developed in Belgium by Godefroi and co-workers.[25]

Miconazole is broadly fungicidal against dimorphic fungi, dematiaceous fungi, *Pseudallescheria* spp., dermatophytes, and aspergilli.[14] Miconazole decreases the activity of oxidase, peroxidase, cytochrome oxidase, and catalase and inhibits cell membrane ergosterol synthesis in susceptible fungi.[73]

GRISEOFULVIN AND NYSTATIN

The two most widely used topical antifungal agents are griseofulvin and nystatin, although other preparations are available. Griseofulvin was isolated from *Penicillium griseofulvium* in 1939. It has also been used orally, since it is absorbed from the gastrointestinal tract. Griseofulvin is employed primarily to treat fungi that cause dermatophytic infections and has little activity against other fungi. Griseofulvin inhibits fungal growth, resulting in distorted hyphae. The exact mechanism is unknown.

Nystatin is similar to amphotericin B in that it is a polyene antimicrobic isolated from a *Streptomyces* sp.; it was isolated from *S. noursei* in 1950. Nystatin cannot be used for parenteral administration because of its toxicity. It binds sterols in the cytoplasmic membrane of susceptible fungi. The architecture is destroyed, and essential metabolites leak out. Nystatin is broadly active against yeasts, the genera *Aspergillus, Trichophyton, Epidermophyton,* and *Microsporum,* and some dimorphic fungi. It is most commonly used to treat fungal infections of the skin and mucous membranes.

ANTIVIRAL AGENTS[32]

Vidarabine, acyclovir, idoxuridine, and amantadine and its structural analogue rimantadine are examples of antiviral agents that have proven therapeutic efficacy. Vidarabine inhibits DNA synthesis of herpes viruses by acting as a competitive inhibitor of DNA polymerase. Acyclovir also inhibits the DNA synthesis of herpes simplex by inhibiting viral DNA polymerase. Cytomegalovirus, another herpes virus, does not require the enzyme and hence is resistant to acyclovir. Idoxuridine inhibits the in vitro replication of herpes viruses and poxviruses by acting as a competitive inhibitor of DNA synthase. Ribavirin may act by inhibiting the synthesis of mRNA or RNA polymerase. The exact mechanism of action of amantadine and rimantadine is unknown, but these agents appear to inhibit multiplication of influenza A virus by blocking the uncoating of the virus. Azidothymidine (AZT), which is used for the treatment of AIDS (see Chapter 10), acts by inhibiting the reverse transcriptase of HIV.

ANTIPARASITIC AGENTS

Antimicrobial therapy for protozoan infections relies on the same basic principle as is used against most bacterial infections: inhibit the multiplication of the organism and the infection will be arrested or cured. In helminth infections, however, the parasites need not multiply in the host to survive and thus are usually unaffected by antimicrobics that inhibit synthesis of macromolecules such as nucleic acids and proteins. Instead, effective anthelminthic drugs usually act on the neuromuscular junction to paralyze the worm or on the worm's energy-producing processes. The mode of action for the more common antiparasitic drugs (Table 8-3) illustrates these general differences in the mode of action of antiprotozoan and anthelminthic drugs.

BACTERIAL RESISTANCE TO ANTIMICROBIAL AGENTS

Antimicrobial resistance may be intrinsic or nonintrinsic. Intrinsic resistance is present in most strains of a given species and was present long before antibiotic usage by humans. It is a fundamental property of the organism. An example is the intrinsic resistance to polymyxins (polymyxin B and colistin) of the genera *Serratia, Proteus, Providencia, Morganella, Edwardsiella,* and *Cedecea.* Most strains of these genera are resistant to polymyxins regardless of their source of isolation. This is in contrast to most other genera of *Enterobacteriaceae,* which are susceptible. Table 16-22 summarizes the well-documented intrinsic resistances in *Enterobacteriaceae.* Another example of intrinsic resistance is the resistance of *Staphylococcus epidermidis* to novobiocin (see Chapter 12). Intrinsic resistance patterns are useful characteristics in the taxonomic identification of an organism.[13]

The best way to document intrinsic resistance is to show that it was present in strains isolated before the antibiotic era. A second way is to study strains from sources that should have had minimum exposure to antimicrobial agents. This could include strains from water, soil, insects or other invertebrates, and even humans who are not taking antimicrobial agents. A third method is to study a collection of several hundred strains of a species from a wide variety of sources.

Nonintrinsic resistance is not normally found in strains of a given species unless they have had exposure to antimicrobial agents. Nonintrinsic resistance may occur as a result of spontaneous chromosomal mutations or by acquisition of extrachromosomal elements such as plasmids and transposons.

Chromosomal mutations occur spontaneously at the frequency of one gene mutation per 10^5 to 10^7 cells per cell division; these mutations can occur during treatment or in the absence of the drug against which resistance develops. Exposure to the antimicrobic exerts selective pressure, and as a result the resistant cells are able to rapidly outgrow the susceptible cells and a new population of resistant cells emerges.

The acquisition of drug-resistant factors (R factors) is a more efficient way of developing antimicrobial resistance and is probably the most important way by which resistance is acquired in clinical isolates. Of particular interest is the recently defined role of transposons in the acquisition of drug resistance. Transposons are pieces of DNA that may carry resistance genes. Transposons have helped to explain the wide distribution of resistance determinants among the plasmids and chromosomes of many different bacterial species.[23] For years it was thought that genes could be transferred between plasmids and bacterial chromosomes only as a result of classical recombination mechanisms whereby the plasmid and the chromosome recombined or exchanged pieces of DNA in areas of genetic homology. This exchange was dependent on the presence of a rec A gene. It is now known that transposons can insert into plasmids or chromosomes in areas where no homology exists and independent of the presence of a rec A gene. Thus transposons have undoubtedly facilitated the movement of resistance determinants among chromosomes, R factors, and bacteriophages.[23]

BIOCHEMICAL MECHANISMS OF BACTERIAL RESISTANCE[12,53-55]

The genetic alterations just discussed give rise to several biochemical mechanisms that allow bacteria to resist the actions of antimicrobial agents. These mechanisms may be classified into five categories: modification of the receptor or binding site of the antimicrobial agent, enzymatic inactivation of the agent, decreased membrane permeability and entry of the agent, synthesis of an alternative enzyme or pathway that bypasses the vulnerable pathway, and a combination of two or more of these mechanisms (Table 8-4).

MODIFICATION OF RECEPTOR OR BINDING SITE

As discussed previously, antimicrobial agents frequently inhibit bacteria by binding to key sites on the ribosomes, on the cell wall, or on specific enzymes. Modification of these target sites may result in a decreased affinity of the agent for the binding site or the inability of the antimicrobial agent to bind. This mechanism may be responsible for bacterial resistance to beta-lactams, streptomycin, rifampin, erythromycin, clindamycin, and nalidixic acid.

Penicillin-binding proteins (PBPs) are the primary biochemical targets of beta-lactam antibiotics. PBPs are enzymes that are involved in cell wall synthesis. When chromosomal mutations result in alterations of the PBPs, the beta-lactam antibiotics are unable to combine with these sites and consequently are unable to inhibit cell wall synthesis. Numerous PBPs with different functions have been identified. Altered PBPs have been responsible for penicillin resistance in *Streptococcus pneumoniae*[29] and *Neisseria gonorrhoeae*[15] and may be responsible for methicillin resistance in *Staphylococcus aureus*.[30]

TABLE 8-3. Mode of Action of Common Antiparasitic Drugs

Drug	Mode of Action
ANTHELMINTHICS	
Antimony potassium tartrate and related antimonials	Inhibit sulfhydryl enzymes and phosphofructokinase
Diethylcarbamizine	Unknown
Mebendazole	Inhibits glucose uptake
Niclosamide	Inhibits conversion of adenosine diphosphate (ADP) to adenosine triphosphate (ATP)
Niridazole	Inhibits inactivation of phosphorylase causing glycogen depletion
Piperazine citrate	Causes hyperpolarization and paralysis of muscles
Praziquantel	Unknown
Pyrantel pamoate	Neuromuscular blocking
Pyrivinium pamoate	Prevents uptake of exogenous carbohydrates
Thiabendazole	Inhibits fumarate reductase
ANTIPROTOZOANS	
Chloroquine phosphate	Inhibits nucleic acid synthesis
Emetine and dehydroemetine	Inhibits protein synthesis by blocking tRNA
Melarsoprol	Inhibits sulfhydryl enzymes
Metronidazole	Acts as electron acceptor and is reduced to toxic form
Pentamidine	Inhibits aerobic glycolysis and possibly nucleic acid synthesis
Primaquine	Binds to nucleoproteins(?)
Pyramethamine	Folic acid antagonist
Stibogluconate (also anthelminthic)	Inhibits sulfhydryl enzymes and phosphofructokinase
Suramin	Inhibits nucleic acid synthesis

Data from references 34, 45, 68, and 85.

TABLE 8-4. Biochemical Mechanisms of Bacterial Resistance to Antimicrobial Agents

Mechanism	Antimicrobial Agents	Representative Organisms
ALTERED RECEPTORS		
Altered penicillin-binding proteins	Penicillins	*Staphylococcus aureus, Staphylococcus epidermidis, Streptococcus pneumoniae, Enterococcus faecalis, Escherichia coli, Pseudomonas aeruginosa, Neisseria gonorrhoeae*
Altered RNA polymerase	Rifampin	*S. aureus*, pseudomonads, *Haemophilus influenzae, Neisseria meningitidis, Enterobacteriaceae*
Methylated 23s RNA	Erythromycin, clindamycin	*S. aureus*
Altered DNA gyrase	Nalidixic acid	*Enterobacteriaceae*
DECREASED ENTRY OR ACCUMULATION		
Decreased uptake and increased efflux	Tetracycline	Staphylococci, streptococci, *Enterobacteriaceae*, pseudomonads
Poor uptake owing to aminoglycoside-modifying enzymes	Aminoglycosides	Staphylococci, *Enterobacteriaceae*, pseudomonads
Altered porin channels	Aminoglycosides	*P. aeruginosa, Enterobacteriaceae*
Lack of oxidative transport system	Aminoglycosides	Anaerobes
INACTIVATION OF DRUG		
Beta-lactamase	Penicillins, cephalosporins	Staphylococci, *Enterobacteriaceae, N. gonorrhoeae, H. influenzae*
Acetyltransferase	Chloramphenicol	*H. influenzae, S. pneumoniae, S. aureus, Enterobacteriaceae*
Acetylases, adenylases, phosphorylases	Aminoglycosides	Staphylococci, *Enterobacteriaceae*, pseudomonads
SYNTHESIS OF RESISTANT METABOLIC PATHWAY		
Synthesis of resistant dihydrofolate reductase	Trimethoprim	*N. meningitidis*, streptococci, *Enterobacteriaceae, H. influenzae*
Synthesis of resistant dihydropteroate synthase	Sulfonamides	*N. meningitidis*, streptococci, *Enterobacteriaceae, Haemophilus* spp., pseudomonads

Data from references 52 to 54.

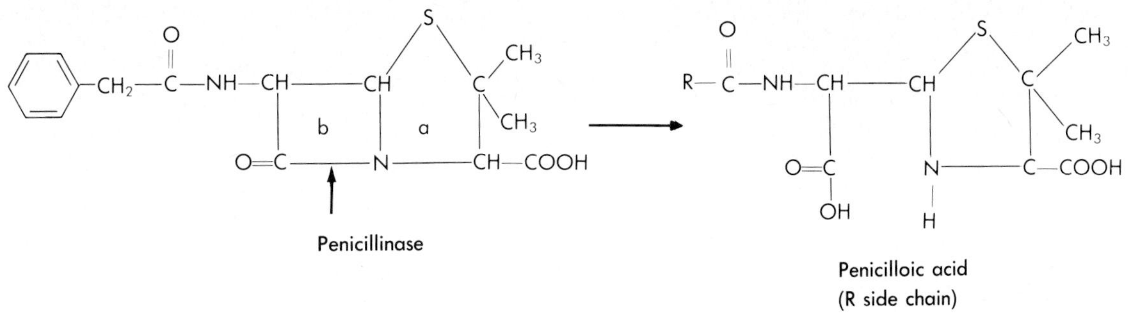

FIGURE 8-20. Hydrolysis of penicillin G by penicillinase.

A change of a single amino acid in the 30S ribosomal subunit prevents the binding of streptomycin; the change is chromosomally mediated. Resistance to erythromycin is plasmid mediated and may be present on transposons. A plasmid-induced enzyme methylates the 23S component of the 50S RNA. The methylated RNA is unable to bind the antimicrobial agent effectively.

Resistance to rifampin is caused by alteration of the targeted RNA polymerase. Alterations in the enzyme occur on the binding site for rifampin as a result of chromosomal mutation.

INACTIVATION OF THE ANTIMICROBIAL AGENT

Bacterial resistance may be mediated by the production of enzymes that are able to convert an active drug into an inactive derivative.

Several organisms, including *Neisseria gonorrhoeae*, staphylococci, *Haemophilus influenzae*, *Enterobacteriaceae*, and other gram-negative rods, produce beta-lactamases. These enzymes hydrolyze the beta-lactam ring of penicillins and cephalosporins, the beta-lactam antibiotics. Numerous beta-lactamases have been identified. They may be classified in many ways, including their specific substrate. The beta-lactamases, known as penicillinases, hydrolyze the beta-lactam ring of penicillin to the inactive penicilloic acid (Figure 8-20). The cephalosporinases hydrolyze the beta-lactam ring of cephalosporin to cephalosporanic acid, an unstable compound that spontaneously undergoes a series of degradative reactions (Figure 8-21).

Beta-lactamases may be plasmid mediated or chromosomally mediated. The most common beta-lactamase is designated TEM-1. It is encoded by a transposon and is said to be responsible for 75% to 80% of plasmid-mediated beta-lactamase resistance.[54] This enzyme has been found in the genera *Haemophilus* and *Neisseria* and in numerous species of *Enterobacteriaceae*. As discussed above, several new beta-lactam antibiotics with a variety of side chains have been developed to circumvent the action of the beta-lactamases.

In some genera, such as *Pseudomonas*, *Serratia*, *Enterobacter*, and *Citrobacter*, beta-lactamases may be inducible enzymes.[66,67] The capacity to produce the enzyme is chromosomally present but is expressed only during therapy with a beta-lactam drug.

Another example of bacterial drug resistance resulting from enzymatic inactivation is the production of chloramphenicol acetyltransferase. This enzyme, produced by both gram-negative and gram-positive organisms, acetylates the hydroxyl

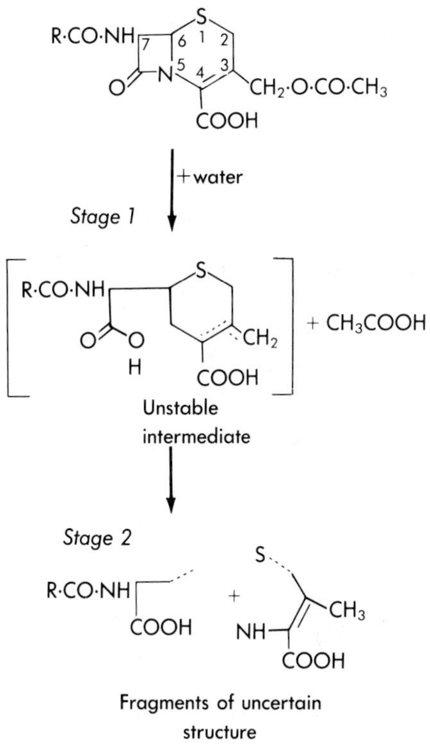

FIGURE 8-21. Diagrammatic representation of effect of beta-lactamase on cephalosporin C. Stage 1: opening of lactam and loss of acetate from position 3. Stage 2: fragmentation of nucleus R═D—alpha—aminodipyl—. (From Gale, E.F., et al.: The molecular basis of antibiotic action, ed. 2, New York, 1981, John Wiley & Sons, Inc.)

groups of chloramphenicol, destroying its antimicrobial properties. Production of chloramphenicol acetyltransferase is usually plasmid mediated and may be associated with a transposon. A few strains of *Proteus mirabilis* produce a chromosomally mediated chloramphenicol acetyltransferase.[23]

Resistance to the aminoglyosides is attributed to three types of aminoglycoside-modifying enzymes: acetylases, adenylases, and phosphorylases. The acetylases modify the amino groups on the aminoglycosides, whereas the adenylases and phosphorylases modify the hydroxyl groups. There are several different types of acetylases, adenylases, and phosphorylases; they are classified according to the target hydroxyl and amino groups. As shown in Table 8-4, aminoglycoside resistance may be classified as inactivation of the drug or as decreased entry or accumulation of the drug. Resistance is probably more correctly classified under the latter biochemical mechanism, since the primary effect of the aminoglycoside-modifying enzymes is to modify the aminoglycosides in such a way that they do not bind well to ribosomes, and as a result their uptake is poor or does not occur.

DECREASED MEMBRANE PERMEABILITY AND ENTRY OR ACCUMULATION OF ANTIMICROBIAL AGENT

Antimicrobial agents must be able to penetrate the bacterial cells to exert their action. Entry into cells may be impeded by the lack or modification of a transport system, by modification of the antimicrobic so transport cannot occur, or by the presence of permeability barriers. Gram-negative bacteria, for example, are frequently resistant to agents that are effective against gram-positive organisms because their outer membrane renders them impermeable to these drugs. Some organisms are able to "pump out" the antimicrobial agent from the cell and thus prevent it from reaching the concentration necessary for its antimicrobial effect.

Tetracycline resistance is due to decreased accumulation of the antimicrobial agent, which is thought to result from a combination of decreased uptake of the agent and increased efflux or "pumping out" of the agent, although the specific mechanism is unresolved. The synthesis of three plasma proteins appears to be associated with plasmid-encoded resistance in *Escherichia coli*. The precise mode of action of these proteins is unknown, but they appear to alter the transport system.[11] Tetracycline resistance may occur in both gram-positive and gram-negative organisms. In most cases resistance is plasmid encoded, but chromosomal resistance may also occur.

As mentioned previously, acetylases, adenylases, and phosphorylases modify the aminoglycosides in such a way that uptake is poor or does not occur. Some aminoglycoside-resistant strains of *Pseudomonas aeruginosa* and *Enterobacteriaceae* do not make aminoglycoside-modifying enzymes but appear to be resistant to aminoglycosides because of altered porin channels.[52] Porins are holes in the membranes through which the antimicrobial agents pass. Anaerobes are generally resistant to aminoglycosides; the resistance is intrinsic and is attributed to the lack of an oxidative electron transport system required for uptake of these agents.[10]

SYNTHESIS OF AN ALTERNATIVE ENZYME OR PATHWAY THAT BYPASSES THE VULNERABLE PATHWAY

Bacterial enzymes are the targets of certain antimicrobial agents such as trimethoprim and sulfamethoxazole. Resistance plasmids may provide bacteria with a replacement enzyme that is identical to the susceptible enzyme in biochemical activity but differs in being resistant to the antimicrobial agent. Resistance to trimethoprim, for example, is encoded by plasmids that specify the production of a trimethoprim-resistant dihydrofolate reductase enzyme.[59] Similarly, resistance to the sulfonamides is determined by the presence of a plasmid-encoded resistant dihydropteroate synthetase.[83]

COMBINATION OF MECHANISMS

In most cases a combination of several mechanisms renders a cell resistant to antimicrobial agents (Table 8-4). For example,

resistance of *Pseudomonas aeruginosa* to beta-lactam antibiotics may be mediated by beta-lactamase production, altered porin proteins, and altered PBPs.[54] *Neisseria gonorrhoeae* may produce beta-lactamases and altered PBPs.

ANTIMICROBIAL SUSCEPTIBILITY TESTS

As stated previously, essential roles of a clinical microbiology laboratory are the isolation of clinically significant microorganisms from clinical specimens and the assessment of their response to antimicrobial agents. As recently as the 1950s, laboratories lacked the ability to accurately predict the in vitro response of a bacterium to an antimicrobial agent. The efforts of Bauer and co-workers[8] to standardize the disk diffusion antimicrobial susceptibility test have resulted in a more reliable, more reproducible method. In the intervening two decades, moreover, considerable work has been accomplished on the disk diffusion test and a myriad of quantitative and nonquantitative manual and automated procedures for antimicrobial susceptibility testing have been developed. Susceptibility test results, however, do not always equate with patient response to therapy. Such discrepancies underline the most basic tenet of in vitro antimicrobic susceptibility; that is, the response of an infected patient to antimicrobial agents is a complex interrelationship of host response, drug dynamics, and microbial activity.

Tests for antimicrobial susceptibility of bacteria can be divided into those that are agar or broth based and those that are quantitative or broadly interpretative (specifying only whether a bacterium is resistant, indeterminate, or susceptible). The methods most commonly used are disk agar diffusion, agar dilution, broth dilution, and microbroth dilution.

DISK AGAR DIFFUSION

In principle the disk agar diffusion (DAD) test is simple. A bacterial inoculum is applied to an agar plate, and then paper disks to which antimicrobial agents have been added are placed on the agar surface. The plates are incubated at 35° C, and the zone size is examined the following day. In practice, however, if established methodology is not followed, variation in zone size occurs and the test is not reproducible. The DAD test was standardized for fast-growing aerobic and facultative bacteria, and its application to fastidious bacteria is not valid unless prior standardization and parallel testing have been accomplished.

The type of growth medium, its cation content, the antimicrobic concentration in the disk, inoculum concentration, temperature and atmosphere of incubation, and method of reading all affect the zone of inhibition around the antimicrobic disk. All of these variables must be monitored and controlled.

The DAD test currently recommended by the Food and Drug Administration (FDA) and the National Committee on Clinical Laboratory Standards (NCCLS) is a modification of the Bauer-Kirby test. The NCCLS method is as follows:

1. Colonies of bacteria to be tested for susceptibility are chosen. The colonies should be well defined and free from contaminating organisms.
2. Four or five single colonies are placed in 1 to 2 ml of Mueller-Hinton broth or trypticase soy broth (TSB) and incubated at 35° C for 4 to 6 hours or until a slight turbidity is observed. The broth is then standardized so the turbidity matches that of a McFarland 0.5 nephelometer

standard, approximately 1 x 10^8 CFU/ml.* Dilution of the inoculum may be made with sterile broth or saline.

3. Mueller-Hinton plates (150 mm diameter, 4 mm thick, pH 7.2 to 7.4) are inoculated by dipping a sterile cotton swab in broth, expressing excess broth by rotating the swab firmly against the inside of the tube, and streaking the swab evenly over the entire surface of the plate. Five percent to 10% sheep blood may be added to the medium for testing some gram-positive organisms. (Barry and co-workers[5] have proposed an alternative agar overlay method for inoculation.)

4. The antimicrobial-containing sensitivity disks are placed on the agar plates within 15 minutes of inoculation by a multiple disk dispenser. The disks are pressed on the agar surface to ensure contact and subsequent diffusion. The plates are inverted and incubated for 18 hours at 35° C in an air incubator.

5. In some cases when rapidity of results is essential, the plates may be read 6 to 8 hours after initial incubation. The plates must then be incubated overnight and the results confirmed.

6. For interpretation, the diameter of the inhibitory zone is measured with either a ruler or calipers on the underside of the plate. The endpoint is the complete inhibition of growth as determined by the unassisted eye. In the case of sulfonamides, slight growth (80% inhibition) is ignored and the margin of heavy growth is measured. The swarming of *Proteus* organisms is ignored and the obvious zone is measured. Assay plates containing blood may be read from the top of the plate. The zone sizes around the individual antimicrobial agents can be converted to susceptible, indeterminate, or resistant using tables provided in publications of the NCCLS or the *Manual of Clinical Microbiology*, ed. 4,[6] published by the American Society for Microbiology. Table 8-5 is a compilation of interpretive standards from NCCLS.[48] Quality control strains of *Escherichia coli, Staphylococcus aureus,* and *Pseudomonas aeruginosa* should be tested at frequent intervals. Procedures for quality control may be found in the NCCLS publication or the *Manual of Clinical Microbiology*.

Basic Principles of the Disk Diffusion Test
Determination of breakpoints[1]

The disk diffusion test depends on the development of a gradient of antimicrobic concentration. The antimicrobic diffuses from the disk, gradually decreasing in concentration as the distance from the disk increases. At a critical point the amount of antimicrobial agent in the medium is unable to inhibit the growth of the test organism and a zone of inhibition develops. The point at which this zone of inhibition occurs is related to the minimum inhibitory concentration (MIC), the lowest concentration of antimicrobial agent that visibly inhibits the growth of the organism.

The relationship between zone diameter and MIC has been

*The standard is made by adding 0.5 ml of 0.048M $BaCl_2 \cdot 2H_2O$ to 99.5 ml of 0.36 NH_2SO_4. It should be mixed well, stored in the dark, and vortexed before use.

used to determine the breakpoints for defining a zone of inhibition as susceptible, resistant, or intermediate, the basis for reporting in the Bauer-Kirby system. To establish these breakpoints, a sample of at least 150 to 200 organisms, representing the species for which the antimicrobial agent will be used, is tested in the disk diffusion method and in the agar dilution method. The MIC is then expressed in logarithmic form and plotted on the y axis, and the zone sizes are plotted on the x axis on an arithmetic scale. Through performance of linear regression statistics, a "line of best fit" or regression line can be determined (Figure 8-22) and specific MICs can be correlated to specific zone diameters.

The pharmokinetics of the drug must be considered before breakpoints can be confirmed by in vivo studies.

Class disk concept

Another facet of the DAD test is the "class disk" concept. The concept states that a single antimicrobial disk within the class can accurately predict susceptibility or resistance to other members of the family. The class disk concept is valid only when all antimicrobial agents in the family demonstrate a similar activity spectrum. The representative agent should be the one with the least activity, since false resistance is preferable to false susceptibility. A commonly cited example is cephalothin. Cephalothin is the class disk for all the first-generation cephalosporins, including cephalothin, cefazolin, cephaloridine, cephalexin, cephacetrile, cephradine, cefaclor, and cephapirin. Unfortunately, opinion is divided as to whether the class disk concept is valid for the new-generation cephalosporins. For example, cefoperazone is a different antimicrobial agent in vitro than moxalactam.[32]

Factors Influencing the Size of the Inhibition Zones[4,74]

Variables that may influence the inhibition zone size and thus must be carefully standardized include inoculum density, composition and depth of the agar medium, temperature of incubation, and potency of the disks.

Inoculum density

The size of the inoculum is the most important single variable in the disk diffusion test. The zone of inhibition develops at the time when a critical concentration of antimicrobic is unable to inhibit the growth of a critical mass of organisms. If the inoculum is too small, the critical density of organisms will take longer to achieve, the antimicrobic will have more time to diffuse into the medium, and a larger zone of inhibition will result. Conversely, a larger inoculum will give smaller zones. It is imperative that the inoculum be standardized to the turbidity of a McFarland 0.5 standard.

Composition and depth of the agar medium

The composition of the agar medium may influence the activity of the antimicrobial agent, the rate of diffusion of the agent, and the growth rate of the test organism.

Because lot-to-lot variation may affect the performance of Mueller-Hinton agar, each new lot must be tested with the recommended quality control strains before use.[6] Failure to maintain the pH of the medium at 7.2 to 7.4 may alter the activity of many antimicrobial agents. The pH of the medium should be checked with a surface electrode or by macerating the medium

TABLE 8-5. Zone Diameter Interpretive Standards and Approximate Minimum Inhibitory Concentration (MIC) Correlates

Antimicrobial Agent	Disk Content	Zone Diameter (Nearest Whole mm)				Approximate MIC Correlates	
		Resistant	Intermediate[a]	Moderately Susceptible[a]	Susceptible[a]	Resistant	Susceptible
Amikacin[b]	30 µg	≤14	15-16	—	≥17	≥32 µg/ml	≤16 µg/ml
Ampicillin[c]							
When testing gram-negative enteric organisms	10 µg	≤11	12-13	—	≥14	≥32 µg/ml	≤8 µg/ml
When testing staphylococci[d]	10 µg	≤28	—	—	≥29	Beta-lactamase[d]	≤0.25 µg/ml
When testing *Haemophilus* spp.[e]	10 µg	≤19	—	≥20	≥20	≥4 µg/ml	≤2 µg/ml
When testing enterococci[f,g]	10 µg	≤16	—	≥17[g]	—	≥16 µg/ml	—
When testing group D nonenterococci and *Listeria monocytogenes*[f,g]	10 µg	≤21	—	22-29	≥30	≥4 µg/ml	≤0.12 µg/ml
Augmentin							
When testing *Haemophilus* spp. and staphylococci[d,e]	20/10 µg	≤19	14-17	—	≥20	—	≤4/2 µg/ml
When testing other organisms	20/10 µg	≤13	—	—	≥18	≥32/16 µg/ml	≤8/4 µg/ml
Azlocillin when testing *Pseudomonas* spp.[d]	75 µg	≤14	15-17	—	≥18	≥256 µg/ml	≤64 µg/ml
Aztreonam[h]	30 µg	≤15	—	16-21	≥22	≥32 µg/ml	≤8 µg/ml
Carbenicillin							
When testing *Enterobacteriaceae*[d]	100 µg	≤17	18-22	—	≥23	≥32 µg/ml	≤16 µg/ml
When testing *Pseudomonas* spp.	100 µg	≤13	14-16	—	≥17	≥512 µg/ml	≤128 µg/ml
Cefamandole[h]	30 µg	≤14	15-17	—	≥18	≥32 µg/ml	≤8 µg/ml
Cefazolin[h]	30 µg	≤14	15-17	—	≥18	≥32 µg/ml	≤8 µg/ml
Cefonicid[h]	30 µg	≤14	15-17	—	≥18	≥32 µg/ml	≤8 µg/ml
Cefoperazone[h]	75 µg	≤15	—	16-20	≥21	≥64 µg/ml	≤16 µg/ml
Cefotaxime[h]	30 µg	≤14	—	15-22	≥23	≥64 µg/ml	≤8 µg/ml
Cefoxitin[h]	30 µg	≤14	15-17	—	≥18	≥32 µg/ml	≤8 µg/ml
Ceftazidime[h]	30 µg	≤14	15-17	—	≥18	≥32 µg/ml	≤8 µg/ml
Ceftizoxime[h]							
When testing urinary isolates of *Pseudomonas aeruginosa*	30 µg	≤10	—	≥11	—	≥64 µg/ml	—
When testing other organisms	30 µg	≤14	—	15-19	≥20	≥32 µg/ml	≤8 µg/ml
Ceftriaxone[h]	30 µg	≤13	—	14-20	≥21	≥64 µg/ml	≤8 µg/ml
Cefuroxime[h]	30 µg	≤14	15-17	—	≥18	≥32 µg/ml	≤8 µg/ml
Cephalothin[h]	30 µg	≤14	15-17	—	≥18	≥32 µg/ml	≤8 µg/ml
Chloramphenicol	30 µg	≤12	13-17	—	≥18	≥25 µg/ml	≤12.5 µg/ml
Cinoxacin[i]	100 µg	≤14	15-18	—	≥19	≥64 µg/ml	≤16 µg/ml
Clindamycin[j]	2 µg	≤14	15-16	—	≥17	≥2 µg/ml	≤1 µg/ml
Doxycycline[k]	30 µg	≤12	13-15	—	≥16	≥16 µg/ml	≤4 µg/ml

Antimicrobial agent	Disk content	Resistant	Intermediate	Susceptible	MIC Resistant	MIC Susceptible
Erythromycin	15 µg	≤13	14–17	≥18	≥8 µg/ml	≤2 µg/ml
Gentamicin[b]	10 µg	≤12	13–14	≥15	≥8 µg/ml	≤4 µg/ml
Imipenem	10 µg	≤13	14–15	≥16	≥16 µg/ml	≤4 µg/ml
Kanamycin	30 µg	≤13	14–17	≥18	≥25 µg/ml	≤6 µg/ml
Methicillin when testing staphylococci[l]	5 µg	≤9	10–13	≥14	—	≤3 µg/ml
Mezlocillin[d]	75 µg	≤12	13–15	≥16	≥256 µg/ml	≤64 µg/ml
Minocycline[k]	30 µg	≤14	15–18	≥19	≥16 µg/ml	≤4 µg/ml
Moxalactam[h]	30 µg	≤14	15–22	≥23	≥64 µg/ml	≤8 µg/ml
Nafcillin when testing staphylococci[l]	1 µg	≤10	11–12	≥13	—	≤1 µg/ml
Nalidixic acid[l]	30 µg	≤13	14–18	≥19	≥32 µg/ml	≤8 µg/ml
Netilmicin[b]	30 µg	≤12	13–14	≥15	≥32 µg/ml	≤12 µg/ml
Nitrofurantoin[i]	300 µg	≤14	15–16	≥17	≥100 µg/ml	≤25 µg/ml
Norfloxacin	10 µg	≤12	13–16	≥17	≥16 µg/ml	≤4 µg/ml
Oxacillin						
When testing staphylococci[l]	1 µg	≤10	11–12	≥13	—	≤1 µg/ml
When testing pneumococci for penicillin G susceptibility	1 µg	≤19	—	≥20	—	≤0.06 µg/ml
Penicillin G						
When testing staphylococci[d]	10 units	≤28	—	≥29	Beta-lactamase[d]	≤0.1 µg/ml
When testing *Neisseria gonorrhoeae*	10 units	≤19	—	≥20	Beta-lactamase	≤0.1 µg/ml
When testing enterococci[f,g]	10 units	≤14	≥15[g]	—	≥16 µg/ml	—
When testing group D nonenterococci and *L. mono-cytogenes*[f,g]	10 units	≤19	20–27	≥28	≥4 µg/ml	≤0.12 µg/ml
Piperacillin[d]	100 µg	≤14	15–17	≥18	≥256 µg/ml	≤64 µg/ml
Streptomycin	10 µg	≤11	12–14	≥15	—	—
Sulfonamides[i,m]	250 or 300 µg	≤12	13–16	≥17	≥350 µg/ml	≤100 µg/ml
Tetracycline[k]	30 µg	≤14	15–18	≥19	≥16 µg/ml	≤4 µg/ml
Ticarcillin[d]	75 µg	≤11	12–14	≥15	≥128 µg/ml	≤64 µg/ml
Tobramycin[b]	10 µg	≤12	13–14	≥15	≥8 µg/ml	≤4 µg/ml
Trimethoprim[i,m]	5 µg	≤10	11–15	≥16	≥16 µg/ml	≤4 µg/ml
Trimethoprim-sulfamethoxazole[m]	1.25/23.75 µg	≤10	11–15	≥16	≥8/152 µg/ml	≤2/38 µg/ml
Vancomycin	30 µg	≤9	10–11	≥12	—	≤5 µg/ml

Permission to reprint Table 2 from M2-A3, "Performance Standards for Antimicrobial Disk Susceptibility Tests—Third Edition; Approved Standard," has been granted by the National Committee for Clinical Laboratory Standards. NCCLS is not responsible for errors or inaccuracies. The data in the interpretive table are valid only if the methodology in M2-A3 is followed. This document and current supplements may be obtained from NCCLS, 771 E. Lancaster Avenue, Villanova, PA 19085. NOTE: NCCLS has recently published a supplement to this table. See Performance standards for antimicrobial susceptibility testing; first informational supplement (1986). NCCLS Pub. No. M100-S.

Continued.

TABLE 8-5. Zone Diameter Interpretive Standards and Approximate Minimum Inhibitory Concentration (MIC) Correlates—cont'd

[a]The category "Intermediate" should be reported. It generally indicates that the test result is equivocal. When designated in this table, a "moderately susceptible" result should be reported to indicate susceptibility under certain conditions. Other beta-lactams are currently being considered for definition of a moderately susceptible category.

[b]The zone sizes obtained with aminoglycosides, particularly when testing *P. aeruginosa*, are very medium dependent because of variations in divalent cation content. These interpretive standards are to be used only with Mueller-Hinton medium that has yielded zone diameters within the correct range when performance tests were done with *P. aeruginosa* ATCC 27853. Organisms in the intermediate category may be either susceptible or resistant when tested by dilution methods and should therefore more properly be classified as "indeterminant" in their susceptibility.

[c]Class disk for ampicillin, amoxicillin, bacampicillin, cyclacillin, and hetacillin.

[d]Resistant strains of *S. aureus* produce beta-lactamase and the testing of the 10-unit penicillin disk is preferred. Penicillin G should be used to test the susceptibility of all penicillinase-sensitive penicillins, such as ampicillin, amoxicillin, bacampicillin, azlocillin, carbenicillin, hetacillin, carbenicillin, mezlocillin, piperacillin, and ticarcillin. Results may also be applied to phenoxymethyl penicillin or phenethicillin.

[e]For testing *Haemophilus* use Mueller-Hinton agar supplemented with 1% hemoglobin (or 5% horse blood) and 1% IsoVitaleX (BBL), Supplement XV (Difco), or an equivalent synthetic supplement. Adjust pH to 7.2. Prepare the inoculum by suspending growth from a 24-hour chocolate agar plate in Mueller-Hinton broth to the density of a turbidity standard. The vast majority of ampicillin-resistant strains of *Haemophilus* produce detectable beta-lactamase.

[f]For enterococci, *Streptococcus* spp. and non-penicillinase-producing penicillin-sensitive organisms, and *Listeria monocytogenes*, the former "Intermediate" interpretation should be reported as "Moderately Susceptible." Results in this category include enterococci and *Listeria*, which for blood or serious invasive tissue infections require high dosage of penicillin or ampicillin, often combined with an aminoglycoside (gentamicin) for improved therapeutic response and bactericidal action.

[g]For streptococci, staphylococci, and other penicillin-sensitive organisms, "Susceptible" results should be regarded as "Very Susceptible." Enterococci strains (*E. faecalis, E. faecium, and E. durans*) producing zones ≥30 mm for ampicillin or ≥28 mm for penicillin are quite unusual, and the speciation procedures should be reexamined.

[h]Cefazolin, cefamandole, cefonicid, cefuroxime, cefoxitin, cefotaxime, moxalactam, ceftizoxime, ceftazidime, ceftriaxone, cefoperazone, and aztreonam are recently studied beta-lactams having a separate diagnostic disk and a wider spectrum of antimicrobial activity, especially against gram-negative bacilli, than do other previously approved cephalosporins. Therefore the 30 μg cephalothin disk cannot be used as the class representative for these drugs even though cefazolin is considered a "first-generation" drug. The cephalothin disk should be used only for testing susceptibility to cephalothin, cefaclor, cefadroxil, cephalexin, cephapirin, and cephradine. Cefazolin, cefamandole (or cefonicid or cefuroxime or cefuranide), cefoxitin, cefoperazone, cefotaxime (or aztreonam or ceftazidime or ceftizoxime or ceftriaxone or moxalactam) should be tested separately against the enteric bacilli. *S. aureus* exhibiting resistance to one of the penicillinase-resistant penicillins (MRSA) *must* be reported as resistant to cephalosporin-like antimicrobial agents, regardless of in vitro disk test results, because most cases of documented MRSA infection have responded poorly to cephalosporin chemotherapy. Methicillin-resistant, coagulase-negative *Staphylococcus* spp. also appear not to respond well to cephalosporin treatment.

[i]Susceptibility data for cinoxacin, nalidixic acid, nitrofurantoin, norfloxacin, sulfonamides, and trimethoprim apply only to organisms isolated from urinary tract infections.

[j]The clindamycin disk is used for testing susceptibility to both clindamycin and lincomycin.

[k]Tetracycline is the class disk for all tetracyclines, and the results can be applied to chlortetracycline, demeclocycline, doxycycline, methacycline, minocycline, and oxytetracycline. However, certain organisms may be more susceptible to doxycycline and minocycline than to tetracycline.

[l]Of the antistaphylococcal, beta-lactamase-resistant penicillins, oxacillin, nafcillin, or methicillin may be tested, and results can be applied to the other two of these drugs and to cloxacillin and dicloxacillin. Oxacillin is preferred because it is more resistant to degradation in storage, applicable to pneumococcal testing (methicillin also usable), and more likely to detect heteroresistant strains easily. Do not use nafcillin on blood-containing media. Cloxacillin disks should not be used because they may not detect methicillin-resistant *S. aureus*. When an Intermediate result is obtained with staphylococci, the strains should be further investigated to determine whether they are heteroresistant.

[m]The sulfisoxazole disk can be used for any of the commercially available sulfonamides. Blood-containing media, except media containing lysed horse blood, are not satisfactory for testing sulfonamides. The Mueller-Hinton agar should be as thymidine free as possible for sulfonamide and/or trimethoprim testing.

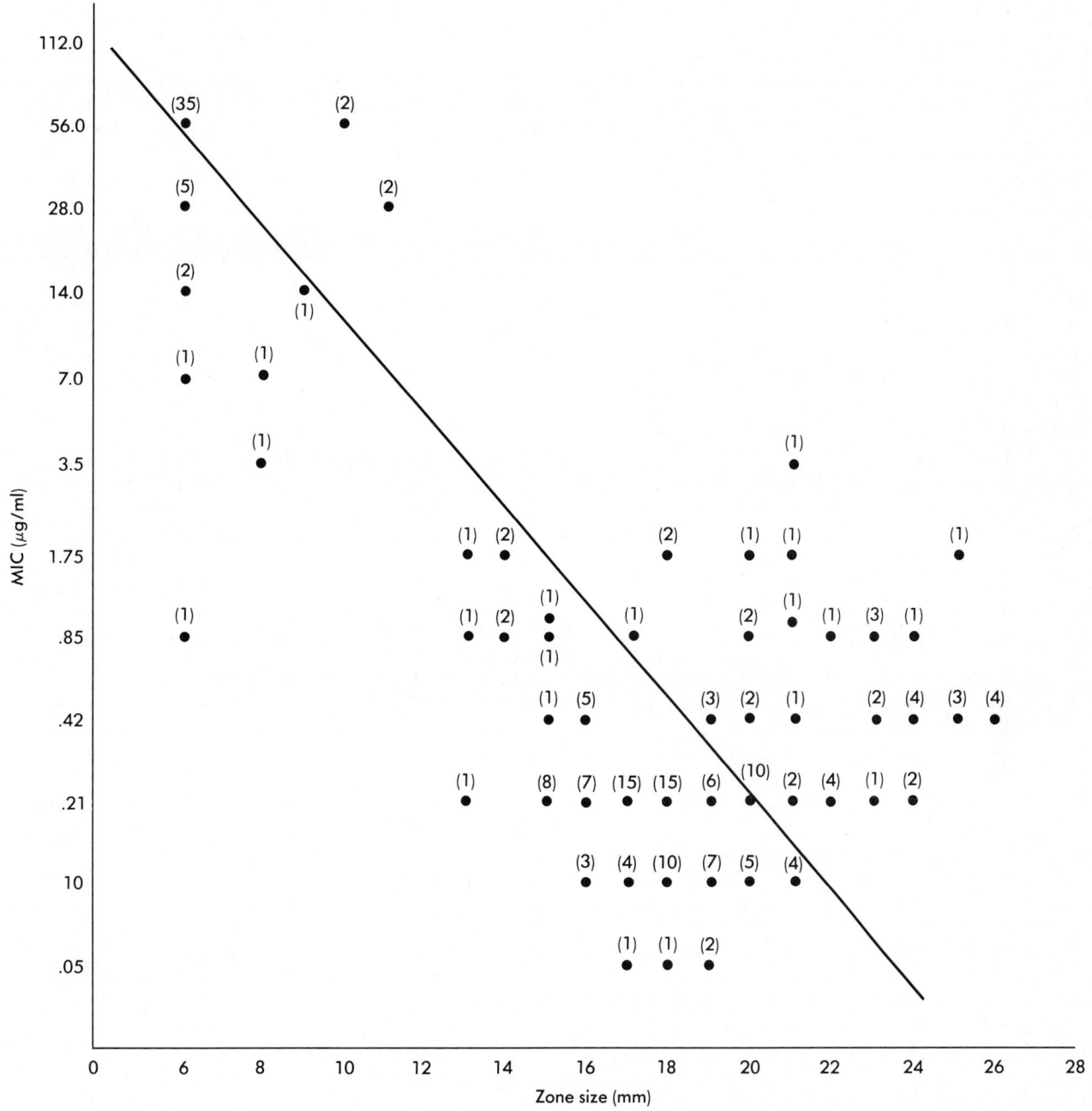

FIGURE 8-22. Scatter diagram with regression line. Numbers in parentheses indicate numbers of isolates.

in neutral distilled water after it has cooled to room temperature. Plates should be poured to a depth of 4 mm. Thicker agar plates may result in smaller zones of inhibition. Incubation in CO_2 must be avoided because the carbonic acid that is produced may cause a shift in pH.

Temperature of incubation

All antimicrobial susceptibility tests should be incubated at 35° C except when testing for methicillin-resistant staphylococci (see below). At lower temperatures the rate of growth is prolonged, antimicrobics diffuse more slowly, and zone sizes appear larger than expected. Care must be taken not to stack plates too deep during incubation, or the center plates will take much longer to reach the required temperature and zone sizes will appear larger than normal.

Potency of disks

Proper handling and storage of disks prevent deterioration of the antimicrobial agents. Cartridges of disks are purchased commercially in containers with desiccants. Containers should be stored at 2° to 8° C or if possible frozen at −14° C or below. Disks containing penicillins or cephalosporins must be stored frozen; a working supply may be stored at 2° to 8° C for 1 week.

Unopened containers of disks should be allowed to come to room temperature before opening. This minimizes the condensation that may occur on the cartridges when the warm room air reaches the cold containers.[6] Disk dispensers should be stored in containers with tightly fitting covers and refrigerated after each use; these containers should also be warmed to room temperature before opening. Antimicrobial disks should never be used after their expiration date.

Sources of Error in the DAD Test

Barry and Thornsberry[6] list the following common sources of error in the DAD test:
1. Variability of Mueller-Hinton (MH) agars
2. Failure to measure the pH of MH agar plates at the time of preparation
3. Use of outdated medium or unsatisfactorily stored plates
4. Improper storage of diffusion disks
5. Inaccurate preparation or inappropriate storage of turbidity reference standard
6. Failure to express surplus inoculum from the swab before inoculating plates
7. Excessive delay between culture standardization and plate inoculation
8. Excessive delay in applying the disks after inoculation of plates
9. Excessive delay in incubating the plates after application of disks
10. Incubation deviating from 35° C or use of an increased CO_2 atmosphere
11. Failure to measure zone borders carefully at a standardized angle and with a source of illumination
12. Application of the procedure to slow growers and to anaerobes
13. Failure to include quality control strains or to record the results of control tests
14. Transcription error in recording results of individual tests

Modifications of the DAD Test

In several situations the DAD test must be modified to ensure accurate results. The notable examples are testing for methicillin-resistant staphylococci, penicillin-resistant *Streptococcus pneumoniae,* and beta-lactamase-negative *Haemophilus influenzae.*

Methicillin-resistant staphylococci

Methicillin-resistant *Staphylococcus aureus* (MRSA) was first reported in 1961 shortly after the introduction of methicillin as a therapeutic agent for penicillin-resistant *S. aureus*. MRSA became a major gram-positive nosocomial pathogen in Europe, but was relatively rare in the United States. The failure to isolate MRSA in the United States was first attributed to inadequate laboratory methods, but appropriate techniques confirmed that MRSA was truly rare in the United States. An increase in the incidence of MRSA in the United States began in the mid-1970s.

Staphylococcal resistance to the penicillinase-resistant penicillins (PRPs)—methicillin, nafcillin, and oxacillin—is not mediated by an enzyme that modifies the drug. It is generally agreed that resistance is chromosomally mediated, and a role for penicillin-binding proteins has been reported (see Chapter 12 for further discussion).

The term "heteroresistant" has also been used to describe MRSA because of the occurrence of two subpopulations of cells within each culture; one population is intrinsically resistant to methicillin whereas the other is susceptible. Each of these subpopulations has different characteristics. The strains in the methicillin-resistant subpopulation grow more slowly than the methicillin-susceptible subpopulation and grow better at 35° C. The methicillin-resistant subpopulation also grows better if the salt content of the medium is greater than is usually used.

Reliable laboratory methods to detect MRSA include a modified disk agar diffusion test, agar screen, and the microdilution method discussed later in the chapter. The modifications in the DAD test just discussed include the following: (1) prepare the inoculum by suspending colonies from an 18- to 24-hour agar plate in MH broth to the density of a McFarland no. 0.5 standard and (2) incubate the plates a full 24 hours at 35° C in ambient air. As noted in footnote 1 of Table 8-5, use of a 1 μg oxacillin disk for determining heteroresistant staphylococci is preferred. After incubation the zone of inhibition around the oxacillin disk should be carefully observed for tiny colonies or a light haze of growth, which is indicative of heteroresistant staphylococci and thus should be reported as resistant. Oxacillin- and methicillin-resistant strains are also usually resistant to cephalosporins (although in vitro tests sometimes indicate otherwise), and physicians should be alerted to this fact.[6] Coudron and co-workers[11a] reported that the sensitivity and specificity of the disk diffusion method is increased for detection of methicillin-resistant *S. aureus* and *S. epidermidis* if 4% NaCl is added to the agar. (However, the addition of NaCl affects results of other susceptibility patterns.) Coudron and associates also found methicillin to be as good as, if not better than, oxacillin for detecting methicillin-resistant *S. epidermidis*.

To perform the agar screen, methicillin (10 μg per ml) or oxacillin (6 μg per ml) is added to sterilized and cooled (50° C) MH agar that has been supplemented with 4% NaCl. Plates are inoculated by dipping a cotton swab into a suspension of the organism prepared to the density of a McFarland no. 0.5 standard, expressing excess liquid from the swab, and touching the cotton swab to a spot on the plate. An agar spread method may also be used. After incubation of the plate at 35° C, any growth is an indication that the isolate is heteroresistant. This procedure is reportedly reliable for *S. epidermidis* and *S. aureus*.[11a]

Penicillin-resistant *Streptococcus pneumoniae*

As with methicillin-resistant *Staphylococcus aureus,* use of the routine DAD does not detect penicillin-resistant *Streptococcus pneumoniae.* An oxacillin disk should be used in addition to a penicillin disk. A zone size of ≥19 mm around an oxacillin disk usually correlates with resistant MICs.

Beta-lactamase-negative *Haemophilus influenzae*

Beta-lactamase or antimicrobial susceptibility testing or both should be performed on all clinically significant isolates of *Haemophilus influenzae.*[41] Although these tests are usually reliable for predicting resistance to beta-lactam antimicrobial agents, there are several reports of ampicillin-resistant, beta-lactamase-negative *H. influenzae.*[40,58] Thus it is recommended that a negative result of a beta-lactamase test be confirmed with an ampicillin susceptibility test.[75] Ampicillin susceptibility may be determined with a modified Bauer-Kirby method, agar dilution method, or broth dilution method. In the modified Bauer-Kirby method, Mueller-Hinton agar is supplemented with 1% IsoVitaleX (BBL, Cockeysville, Md.) or the equivalent and 1% hemoglobin. The suspension of the test organism is prepared in Mueller-Hinton broth and adjusted to the turbidity of a McFarland 0.5 standard. The plates are inoculated and incubated as for the standard DAD test. Ampicillin-susceptible strains produce zones of inhibition ≥20 mm, whereas resistant strains produce inhibition zones ≤19 mm.[75] According to McCarthy,[41] susceptibility testing of antimicrobial agents other than ampicillin should be performed by agar or broth dilution methods because disk diffusion zone size breakpoints used with the standard Bauer-Kirby method do not accurately predict susceptibility or resistance of *Haemophilus* spp.[61]

QUANTITATIVE DILUTION SUSCEPTIBILITY TESTS

The disk diffusion susceptibility test can be employed, at least theoretically, as a quantitative test by reading the y axis MIC value as a function of the zone size for a particular antimicrobic-microorganism combination. This is not routinely done. It is time consuming and may be susceptible to error in that minor variations in zone size may cause a significant error in MIC. Dilution susceptibility tests, either in agar or broth, are used when knowledge of the MIC of an antimicrobial agent is needed.

In certain instances a dilution procedure is required. These procedures include tests on slow-growing, nutritionally or environmentally fastidious microorganisms and the requirement for a quantitative result when the administration of a toxic antimicrobial agent must be strictly controlled. Quantitative susceptibility testing may also be required to evaluate treatment failure and in patients with endocarditis, meningitis, osteomyelitis, or septicemia.

Many institutions use MIC methodology as the sole test procedure. While it can be argued that quantitative data are not necessary for all relevant isolates, the MICs can be interpreted in the laboratory as susceptible, indeterminate, or resistant. Commercial MIC methods make it possible for virtually every microbiology laboratory to have this capability. In a few instances the bactericidal activity of an antimicrobial agent should be determined. (The minimum bactericidal concentration is known as the MBC.) These include patients with enterococcal endocarditis, "tolerant" staphylococcal infections, or seriously compromised immune defenses.

AGAR DILUTION TEST

The agar dilution test (ADT) is the reference standard against which other tests are evaluated. In this test, graded concentrations of a single antimicrobial agent are added to individual agar plates. Test organisms are placed on the plates, the plates incubated, and the inhibitory endpoints determined to find the MIC. The advantages of the ADT are that multiple organisms can be tested on the same set of plates and that the ADT MIC may be slightly more reproducible.[19] The ADT is readily applicable to anaerobic bacteria, fastidious organisms such as *Haemophilus* and *Neisseria,* and organisms that require special nutritional supplementation. The concentrations of antimicrobial agent are not necessarily limited to serial twofold dilutions. The disadvantages are that antimicrobic-containing agar plates must be homemade and shelf life is limited. Commercial ADT systems are not generally available from commercial sources, with the possible exception of Repliscan (Cathra International, St. Paul, Minn.). Another major disadvantage is that, while 36 organisms may be tested simultaneously, many laboratories have only one or two isolates a day that require MICs. Relatively few laboratories routinely perform ADT MICs.

The reference procedure for agar dilution susceptibility testing was published in the World Health Organization–sponsored International Collaborative Study,[19] outlined in the *Manual of Clinical Microbiology*[78] and in the NCCLS publication, M7-A.[49a] The reader is referred to these sources for detailed information.

BROTH DILUTION

With the exception of volume and tube size, the test parameters for the macrotube broth dilution method are similar to the microdilution test. The necessity for manual dilution of antimicrobial agents in large tubes limits the routine use of this method to only a few isolate-antimicrobic pairs at a time.

Microbroth Dilution Tests

The widespread availability of microtitration equipment and frozen or dried microdilution plates (see Figure 9-9) containing prediluted antimicrobial agents has created a situation in which virtually every hospital, regardless of size, can have the facilities for quantitative susceptibility testing. In the past, implementation of microdilution MICs usually meant that the laboratory produced and controlled quality of its own plates.

The principle of microdilution MICs is as follows. Antimicrobial agents are quantitatively prepared in a suitable suspending medium to a given concentration. An appropriate broth medium is selected for the microorganisms to be tested and added to a U-bottom, flat bottom, or V-bottom microdilution plate. The antimicrobic is added to the plate, and serial twofold dilutions are made using manual or semiautomated microdiluters. A standardized inoculum is added, and the plate is

TABLE 8-6. Ingredients for Wilkins-Chalgren Broth

	Source	Catalog No.	Amount (g)
Trypticase (pancreatic digest of casein)	BBL[a]	11921	10
Gelysate (pancreatic digest of gelatin)	BBL	11870	10
Yeast extract	Difco[b]	0127-01	5
Glucose	Fisher[c]	D-16 73423	1
NaCl	Fisher	S-271 78440 or 78443	5
L-Arginine–free base	Sigma[d]	A-5006	1
Pyruvic acid–sodium salt	Sigma	P-2256	1

[a]BBL, Cockeysville, Md.
[b]Difco Laboratories, Inc., Detroit.
[c]Fisher, Orangeburg, N.Y.
[d]Sigma Chemical Co., St. Louis.

incubated overnight under the appropriate conditions. On the following day (18 to 24 hours later) the MIC is determined as the lowest concentration of antimicrobial agent visibly inhibiting the growth of the organism. Alternatively, plates may be prepared by using batch dispensers such as the MIC-2000 (Dynatech, Vineland, N.J.) or the Quick Spense (Bellco, Vineland, N.J.). Commercially available microdilution systems are discussed in Chapter 9.

The broth MIC endpoints differ from agar dilution endpoints for many organism-antimicrobic combinations. Usually the broth endpoint is lower (that is, more susceptible) than the agar endpoint.

Microdilution MIC procedure

Media. Following are media used for microdilution MICs:
1. Wilkins-Chalgren (W-C) broth, used for fastidious organisms, such as anaerobes, *Campylobacter* spp., and all streptococci
2. Calcium-magnesium-adjusted Mueller-Hinton broth, used for all facultative gram-negative rods, enterococci, and staphylococci
3. Low Thymidine Eugonic Broth (Organon Teknika, Durham, N.C.), which must be used when testing sulfonamides; 10% (filtered through a 0.22 μm membrane filter)

Preparation of broth media
WILKINS-CHALGREN BROTH
1. Dispense the ingredients in Table 8-6 and dissolve in 1000 ml of water. The pH should be 7 to 7.2.
2. Add 10 ml hemin and 0.2 ml vitamin K_1 solutions to yield final concentrations of 5 μg/ml for hemin and 0.5 μg/ml for vitamin K_1. The preparation of vitamin K_1 and hemin is as follows:
   a. Vitamin K_1 stock
      Sigma Chemical Co., St. Louis, catalog no. V-3501
      Stock solution—0.05 ml of vitamin K_1 solution and 20 ml of 95% ethanol
      Filter sterilize (membrane filter, 0.22 μm).

Stock solution should be kept in a dark bottle at 4° C for 1 month and then discarded.
   b. Hemin stock
      Sigma Chemical Co., St. Louis, catalog no. H-2375, hemin, equine type III
      Stock solution—0.025 g of hemin, 0.5 ml of 1 N NaOH, 49.5 ml of water (500 μg/ml)
      Autoclave at 121° C for 12 minutes (fast exhaust).
      Stock solution should be kept frozen at −20° C for no longer than 1 month.
3. Boil for 2 minutes or until medium dissolves.
4. Autoclave at 121° C for 15 minutes (slow exhaust).

CATION-ADJUSTED MUELLER-HINTON (AMH) BROTH
1. Prepare AMH broth according to the manufacturer's directions.
2. After autoclave sterilization, assay a small portion of the AMH broth for Ca^{++} and Mg^{++}. Add appropriate amounts of Ca^{++} and Mg^{++} stock solution to the chilled MH broth to yield final concentrations of 25 mg/L of magnesium and 50 mg/L of calcium.
   a. *Magnesium stock solution.* Dissolve 836 mg of $MgCl_2 \cdot 6\ H_2O$ in 10 ml of deionized distilled water, filter sterilize, and store at 4° C. This solution contains 10 mg of Mg^{++}/ml.
   b. *Calcium stock solution.* Dissolve 367.5 mg of $CaCl_2 \cdot 2\ H_2O$ in 10 ml of deionized distilled water, filter sterilize, and store at 4° C. This solution contains 10 mg of Ca^{++}/ml.
3. After adding the Ca^{++} and Mg^{++} to the AMH broth, again assay a small sample for Mg^{++} and Ca^{++} concentrations to ensure that correct amounts were added.
4. Once this is established, note the lot number of the AMH broth and add the same amounts of Ca^{++} and Mg^{++} to future batches of AMH broth with the same lot number.
5. Make periodic checks to ensure correct Mg^{++} and Ca^{++} concentrations in the AMH broth.

Preparation of antimicrobic stock solutions. A simple formula to determine the amount of antimicrobic to be weighed

TABLE 8-7. Dilution of Antimicrobics[a] for Preparation of Stock Solutions

Antimicrobial	Solvent[b]	Diluent
Amoxicillin[c]	PO_4 buffer (0.1 M, pH 8)	PO_4 buffer (0.1 M, pH 6); H_2O
Amphotericin B	Dimethylformamide	H_2O
Ampicillin[c]	PO_4 (0.1 M, pH 8)	PO_4 buffer (0.1 M, pH 6); H_2O
Ceftazidime	1 ml Na_2CO_3 solution (5%)	H_2O
Cephalosporins	PO_4 (0.1 M, pH 6)	H_2O
Chloramphenicol	Methanol	H_2O
Erythromycin	Methanol	PO_4 buffer (0.1 M, pH 8)[d]
Imidazoles	Dimethylformamide	H_2O
Moxalactam	HC1 (0.04 M)[e]	H_2O
Nalidixic acid	1 ml NaOH (0.1 M)/10 mg drug	H_2O
Oxolinic acid	1 ml NaOH (0.1 M)/10 mg drug	H_2O
Rifampin	Methanol	H_2O
Sulfonamides	1 ml NaOH (0.1 M)/10 mg drug	H_2O
Trimethoprim	1 ml HC1 (0.05 M)/10 mg drug	H_2O

Modified from Anhalt, J.P., and Washington, J.A., II: Preparation and storage of antimicrobial solutions. In Lennette, E.H., et al.: Manual of clinical microbiology, ed. 4, Washington, D.C., 1985, American Society for Microbiology.
[a]For other antimicrobial agents, water may be used as diluent. If antimicrobial agent fails to go into solution, gentle heating (37° to 40° C) and stirring may facilitate process.
[b]Solvents are used to dissolve dry powder initially, and diluents are used to prepare stock solutions containing high concentrations (1280 μg/ml) of antimicrobial agent.
[c]Dilute with water after first 1:10 dilution with phosphate buffer at pH 6.
[d]Alcohol solutions of erythromycin are unstable because of ester formation and should be diluted immediately.
[e]For detailed preparation see Anhalt and Washington.[3]

out is as follows:

$$\frac{\mu g/ml \text{ (concentration needed*)} \times \text{Volume (in ml)}}{\text{Potency of antimicrobial agent (in } \mu g/ml)} =$$

mg of antimicrobial agent to be weighed

Antimicrobic stock solutions frozen at −20° C (1280 μg/ml) have a shelf life of at least 30 days. They should not be used beyond this time period, especially the cell wall–active antibiotics such as penicillin and the cephalosporins. The working solution of the antimicrobics is prepared from the stock solutions using the particular test broth as the diluent. All working solutions of antimicrobics are prepared by making a 1:5 dilution of the stock antimicrobic solution in liquid media, resulting

in an initial concentration of 256 μg/ml. The exceptions are carbenicillin and trimethoprim-sulfamethoxazole (SXT-TMP), which are used undiluted (1280 μg/ml). In this case the diluent for the stock solution is the broth medium to be used. Penicillin is diluted 1:10 (128 μg/ml).

PREPARATION OF MICROTITER MIC PLATES
1. Using a sterile 0.05 ml disposable pipette, dispense 1 drop of the appropriate broth into wells 1 to 11 (rows A to H), one row for each antimicrobic being tested. Dispense 1 drop in well 12 of row G and 2 drops in well 12 of row H. These will serve as the inoculum and broth controls, respectively.
2. Using another sterile 0.05 ml disposable pipette, dispense 1 drop of antimicrobic working solution into well 1 of each row for each antimicrobic being tested.
3. Dilute wells 1 to 11 horizontally, using sterile 0.05 ml microdiluters. This results in serial doubling dilutions of the antimicrobial agents, from 64 to 0.06 μg/ml. The exceptions are carbenicillin (or ticarcillin) and trimethoprim-sulfamethoxazole, which range from 320 to 0.31 μg/ml, and

---

*All antimicrobic stock solutions are initially prepared at a concentration of 1280 μg/ml in the proper diluent for that particular antimicrobial agent (Table 8-7).

penicillin, which ranges from 32 to 0.03 μg/ml.

PREPARATION OF INOCULUM. Using a fresh culture (overnight growth on the plate), standardize the inoculum. The inoculum may be standardized by (1) adjustment to match a McFarland 0.5 standard (1×10^8 CFU/ml), (2) use of a nephelometer such as that found on the Autobac system, or (3) dilution of an overnight broth culture (5×10^8 to 1×10^9 CFU/ml). The standardized inoculum is then diluted with the growth medium to 1×10^5 CFU/ml for aerobic and facultative bacteria and 1×10^6 CFU/ml for anaerobic bacteria. Care must be taken not to agitate the anaerobic inoculum.

ADDITION OF INOCULUM TO THE PLATES AND INCUBATION

1. Using another sterile 0.05 ml disposable pipette, dispense 1 drop of inoculum into wells 1 to 11 of each row. Also add 1 drop of inoculum to well 12 of row G to serve as the inoculum control. Well 12 of row H serves as the broth control.
2. Culture the inoculum tube to check for purity.
3. Seal the microdilution plate with either plate sealers or another microdilution plate, whichever is appropriate for the incubation conditions. (If the plate is to be incubated in CO_2 or an anaerobic jar, use a plate for a cover; use plate sealers for all others.) Incubate 18 to 24 hours under the proper conditions for the particular isolate. NOTE: *Campylobacter* MICs may be incubated in a GasPak anaerobic jar from which the catalyst has been removed. Care must be taken not to ignite the residual H_2 gas. Alternatively a Campy Pak (see Chapter 23) may be used. Incubation is at 42° C.
4. After 18 to 24 hours of incubation, observe the MIC plates for growth. If anaerobic MIC plates show little or no growth after 24 hours, reincubate for an additional 24 hours. Under most conditions, prereduction of the anaerobic MIC plates in an anaerobic jar is not necessary. Failure of an isolate to grow may dictate prereduction of plates.

INTERPRETATION

1. For each row (that is, each antimicrobic) the well with the lowest concentration of agent that visibly inhibits the growth of the organism (no turbidity) is the MIC of that antimicrobial agent for that microorganism. The results are reported in micrograms per milliliter (μg/ml).
2. The broth control well must be free from growth.
3. The inoculum control well should have visible growth. If the endpoint of growth is difficult to determine, 0.2% *p*-iodo-nitro-tetrazolium violet (Sigma no. 1-8577), prepared in distilled H_2O, can be used. The presence of viable organisms causes the reduction of this compound to a pink-red precipitate called formazan. The tetrazolium solution must be stored at 4° C in a dark bottle.

Reading of plates. The use of a viewer is recommended for reading microdilution plates. It provides both adequate lighting and magnification of the wells. Any moisture that has accumulated on the bottom of the plate should be removed with a tissue or gauze before reading. Reproducible MICs are a function of the rigidity with which growth is defined and the strict adherence of all microbiologists to the standard. Obvious growth results in confluent turbidity. Often, especially with gram-positive cocci, growth is granular. A single microcolony in the well of ≥ 2 mm diameter or multiple particles of any size constitute "growth." The growth control well and the sterility

control well should be routinely evaluated to determine whether nonspecific medium flocculation has occurred or whether the organism is growing in a granular pattern even in the absence of antimicrobial agents.

Microdilution procedure for NaCl supplementation for methicillin-resistant staphylococci[76]

1. Prepare a 20% NaCl solution. Aliquot the solution to sterile 1 dram vials (2.2 ml/vial).
2. Add 2 ml of NaCl to 8 ml of cation-adjusted MH broth (AMH) (see previous discussion).
3. Prepare an inoculum of 1.5 to 3×10^7 CFU/ml from an 18- to 24-hour culture on an agar plate.
4. Add 0.1 ml of this inoculum to the NaCl-supplemented AMH and 0.1 to 10 ml of AMH (no NaCl).
5. Inoculate the methicillin and cephalothin rows and one control well of the microdilution plate with the NaCl-supplemented AMH inoculum.
6. Inoculate the remaining rows with the AMH inoculum.
7. Label the time on the plate and incubate at 35° C.
8. Read at 24 hours.

INTERPRETATION

Oxacillin resistant: ≥ 4 μg/ml
Methicillin resistant: ≥ 16 μg/ml

Although the method described here detects most strains of heteroresistant staphylococci, certain results can serve as flags to alert the analyst to the possibility of heteroresistant staphylococci. These are as follows:

1. *An indeterminate result.* Almost all strains should fall within the susceptible or resistant categories; a true indeterminate will remain so.
2. *Cross-resistance between cephalothin and the three penicillins.* MRSA should be resistant to cephalothin; an MIC of 2, 4, or 8 μg/ml should be a clue that the strain is probably methicillin and cephalothin resistant.
3. *Multiple resistance.* The strain is resistant to erythromycin, clindamycin, chloramphenicol, and penicillin.

QUALITY CONTROL

Controversy exists as to how often the antimicrobial susceptibility test should receive quality control checks. If the control of reagents, media, and antimicrobial agents is the goal, once or twice a week is sufficient. However, if the total performance of the test is to be assessed, daily quality control seems mandatory. This is best achieved through the use of quality control bacteria, the MICs of which are known for the particular test system. If results are out of control for a day or period of days, more extensive search for aberrant parameters is essential.

Control strains have been chosen because the MIC values are stable and the MIC falls approximately in the middle of the range of drug concentrations tested. For example, a strain with an MIC of 0.06 μg/ml would not be satisfactory if the lowest antimicrobic concentration tested was 0.03 μg/ml. Day-to-day variation should not exceed 1 dilution interval from the expected value. Table 8-8 lists the microdilution MIC quality control strains and the anticipated MIC values.

ANTIMICROBIAL SUSCEPTIBILITY TESTING OF FASTIDIOUS BACTERIA
ANAEROBES

Routine susceptibility testing of anaerobes is usually not performed because of the long periods of time required for isola-

TABLE 8-8. MICs for Commonly Used Quality Control Strains by the Broth Microdilution Procedure

	MIC (µg/ml)			
Antimicrobial Agent	*Escherichia coli* ATCC 25922	*Enterococcus faecalis*[a] ATCC 29212	*Staphylococcus aureus* ATCC 29213	*Pseudomonas aeruginosa* ATCC 27853
PENICILLINS				
Penicillin	VR	2	0.25	VR
Ampicillin	2	1	0.5	VR
Methicillin	VR	VR	1-2	VR
Carbenicillin	4-8	32	4	32
Ticarcillin	2-4	32	4	16
Mezlocillin	4	2	4	16
Piperacillin	1	2	2	2
CEPHALOSPORINS				
Cephalothin	8	16-32	0.12-0.25	VR
Cefazolin	1	16	0.5-1	VR
Cefamandole	0.5	32	1	VR
Cefoxitin	2-4	VR	2-4	VR
Cefuroxime	2	VR	0.5	VR
Cefotaxime	<0.12	VR	2	8
Cefoperazone	0.25	16-32	1-2	2-4
Moxalactam	0.25	VR	4-8	4-8
AMINOGLYCOSIDES				
Kanamycin	2-4	32	1	VR
Gentamicin	0.5	8	0.5-1	2-4
Tobramycin	0.5	16	1	1
Amikacin	1-2	128	2	4-8
OTHERS				
Chloramphenicol	4	8	4	VR
Clindamycin	VR	8-16	0.06-0.12	VR
Erythromycin	VR	1	0.12-0.25	VR
Tetracycline	2	VR	0.5	ND
Trimethoprim-sulfamethoxazole (1/19[b])	≤9.5/0.5	X	≤9.5/0.5	ND
Vancomycin	VR	2	1	VR
Nalidixic acid	2	VR	VR	VR
Nitrofurantoin	8	8	16	VR

SYMBOLS: VR, Strain is very resistant to the antimicrobial agent.
ND, No data are available.
X, This strain can be used to detect interfering substances (thymidine etc.) in broth media. A value of ≤9.5/0.5 implies an acceptable broth lot.

From Jones, R.N., et al.: Susceptibility tests: microdilution and macrodilution broth procedures. In Lennette, E.H., et al., editors: Manual of clinical microbiology, ed. 4, Washington, D.C., 1985, American Society for Microbiology.
[a]As previously noted, *Streptococcus faecalis* is now known as *Enterococcus faecalis*.
[b]Ratio of trimethoprim to sulfamethoxazole.

tion of these organisms and execution of the susceptibility procedures. Physicians initiate empiric therapy based on probable susceptibility patterns of the organisms (Tables 8-3 and 20-23) and the site and seriousness of the infection.[21] Although this approach is usually satisfactory, antimicrobial susceptibility patterns are changing and vary among hospitals; thus laboratories should be cautious in relying totally on the results in another institution.[62] Susceptibility testing is mandatory for life-threatening conditions such as brain abscess, endocarditis, and serious intra-abdominal and pelvic conditions,[21] for infections that fail to respond to empiric therapy, and for infections that require prolonged therapy.[21,22]

The Bauer-Kirby disk diffusion technique has not been standardized with anaerobes and should not be used for susceptibility testing of these organisms. An agar dilution procedure is recommended by the NCCLS[50] as the reference method for susceptibility testing of anaerobic bacteria. With this procedure, graded dilutions of the antimicrobial agents are added to tubes of Wilkins-Chalgren agar; the agar is mixed and poured into Petri dishes. The inoculum is prepared by inoculating portions of five or more colonies (to provide a 3 mm loopful of growth) into supplemented thioglycolate medium without indicator. The thioglycolate broth is incubated 6 to 24 hours or until visible turbidity is observed. Before testing, the turbidity of the inoculum is adjusted to that of a McFarland 0.5 standard. With a replicator the inoculum is added to the antimicrobial plates beginning with the lowest concentration of antimicrobial agent and proceeding to the highest. The plates are incubated at $35° \pm 2° C$ in an anaerobic jar or other anaerobic environment for 48 hours. The MIC is the lowest concentration of antimicrobic yielding no growth, one discrete colony, or a fine, barely visible haze as determined with the unaided eye and as compared with the growth controls.

Although precise and reproducible, the agar dilution method is time consuming and impractical for routine use in clinical microbiology laboratories. It is intended as a reference for comparison of the accuracy of other methods.[62] Several other, more practical methods, including those of Wilkins and Thiel[81] and Kurzynski,[37] have been proposed for susceptibility testing of anaerobic bacteria. The NCCLS[49] has also recently proposed guidelines for the use of three alternative, more practical methods, which may be used as written or modified to meet the user's needs. These methods include limited agar dilution, broth microdilution, and broth disk elution. The limited agar dilution procedure is similar to the reference agar dilution procedure except that only two concentrations of each antimicrobial agent are tested. These concentrations represent breakpoints of susceptibility and are tested in a single divided agar plate. The MIC is determined as for the reference agar dilution method.

The broth microdilution procedure uses microdilution trays containing various concentrations of antimicrobial agents incorporated into Schaedler's, Wilkins-Chalgren, brain heart infusion, or other acceptable broths. After inoculation and incubation, the MIC is determined as the lowest concentration of antimicrobial agent that visibly inhibits the growth of the organism. The microdilution procedure outlined previously is also sufficient for testing anaerobes.[64]

The broth disk elution procedure is the simplest and most practical method, although it provides qualitative and not quantitative results. An inoculum of test organism is incubated in thioglycolate containing a specific concentration of the antimicrobic; this concentration is obtained by adding an appropriate number of commercially prepared antimicrobial disks to 5 ml of broth. Only one concentration of antimicrobic is tested, that corresponding to the achievable blood level. A growth control tube containing no antimicrobial disk is also inoculated. Susceptibility is determined as the absence of growth or as less than 50% of the growth of the control tube. The broth disk elution procedure proposed by the NCCLS is a modification of the method of Kurzynski,[37] which in turn is a modification of the original broth-disk method of Wilkins and Thiel.[81] The reader should see NCCLS publication M17-P[48] for details concerning these procedures.

OTHER ORGANISMS

The microdilution procedure as outlined previously suffices for the testing of *Haemophilus influenzae* and the nutritionally demanding streptococci. When one is testing for *Haemophilus influenzae,* the test broth should be supplemented with 5% Fildes enrichment, 1% (final concentration) Levinthal's, or 2% to 3% laked horse blood plus 10 $\mu g/ml$ NAD. If an agar dilution procedure is used for *H. influenzae,* the Mueller-Hinton test medium should be supplemented with the same ingredients.[75] Ampicillin-susceptible strains of *H. influenzae* generally have MICs of 0.5 $\mu g/ml$ or less, and ampicillin-resistant strains generally have MICs of 8 $\mu g/ml$ or greater. Strains with MICs of 2 $\mu g/ml$ or greater should be considered ampicillin resistant in cases of meningitis.[75]

USE OF MINIMUM INHIBITORY CONCENTRATIONS

In vitro quantitative antimicrobial susceptibility tests can provide useful information to the clinician treating a patient for an infectious disease. A working knowledge of the uses of such tests is of significant advantage to both clinicians and the laboratory technologists.

The MIC of an antimicrobial agent for a given antimicrobic-organism combination is a laboratory-derived value of little significance unless other parameters are known. The MICs reported routinely in the laboratory most often relate to the achievable concentration of the antimicrobic in blood. For example, the MIC of gentamicin when tested against *Pseudomonas aeruginosa* was reported as 8 $\mu g/ml$. To use this number in treating a patient, certain other information is necessary. For example, how reliable is the number? Most MIC systems are based on data achieved from doubling dilutions; that is, antimicrobic dilutions of 1:2, 1:4, 1:8, 1:16, and so on are tested with a microbial isolate. It is generally accepted that a 1 dilution error is within the expected accuracy of the MIC test. An MIC of 8 $\mu g/ml$, then, may actually be 4, 8, or 16 $\mu g/ml$. In practice, however, the mean variation is usually less than 1 doubling dilution.

The MIC is meaningless unless the achievable blood level of the antimicrobic is known. In the case of gentamicin the mean peak blood level of the antimicrobic after an accepted dose is 8 $\mu g/ml$. One might assume that an isolate of *P. aeruginosa* with an MIC of 8 $\mu g/ml$ would be susceptible to gentamicin. Such is not the case. Because of a number of factors related to both the host and the bacterium, a concentration of at least two to four times the MIC is used in determining the effective achievable blood level. The gentamicin concentration would have to be 16 to 32 $\mu g/ml$ to ensure effective treatment. Although such levels are possible pharmakinetically, concentrations above 12 μg/ml are toxic to both the kidneys and the ears. Therefore *P. aeruginosa* with an MIC of 8 μg/ml is resistant to gentamicin.

MICs are based on the blood level of the antimicrobial agent. For most infections the blood level is a reasonable approximation of the antimicrobic activity in other tissues. There are exceptions, however. Many antimicrobial agents are excreted by the kidneys, and high concentrations of the agent can be found in the urine. Based on blood levels, all *Escherichia coli* isolates are resistant to penicillin. That is, blood levels of penicillin that would cause eradication of the organism cannot be achieved with normally used dosage schedules. Because penicillin is concentrated in the urine, penicillin could be used, at least theoretically, to treat urinary tract infection (cystitis) caused by *E. coli*.

The MIC measures the bacteriostatic action of the antimicrobial agent. In some clinical situations the MIC may not reflect the agent's ability to cure the infection. An example is meningitis. Host defenses are relatively ineffective in eradication of microorganisms from the cerebrospinal fluid (CSF). Little if any bactericidal or opsonic activity takes place in the CSF. The microorganisms, then, must be killed, not just inactivated, for the antimicrobic to be successful. The activity of antimicrobics is based on a dynamic relationship between the susceptibility of the parasite; host factors such as antibody, opsonins, phagocytes, and leukokines; and the distribution and concentration of the antimicrobial agent throughout the various tissue and fluid spaces of the body.

AUTOMATED ANTIMICROBIAL SUSCEPTIBILITY TESTS

Instruments for automated antimicrobial susceptibility tests are discussed in Chapter 9.

REPORTING OF ANTIMICROBIAL SUSCEPTIBILITY TESTS

A gradual evolution has occurred in the reporting of susceptibility tests. Most laboratories have followed the traditional convention of S (susceptible), I (intermediate), and R (resistant) because the disk diffusion breakpoints were distributed around these three designations. While it is conceptually simple to believe that populations of microorganisms fall discretely into one of three groups, susceptibility to antimicrobial agents cannot be so easily defined. The point of testing is to predict the in vivo response of the microorganism to the agent based on in vitro data. Clinical response is a function of a dynamic relationship between host, drug, and microorganism. Ericsson and Sherris[19] have recommended four categories of susceptibility, based on the following concepts:

1. The relationship of the MIC of the organism to levels of antimicrobial agent attainable in the blood, tissues, or urine on particular dose schedules
2. The relationship of the susceptibility of the strain under examination to that of others of the same species
3. The relationship of the susceptibility of the strain to that of a particular standard strain
4. The relationship of the in vitro findings to clinical responsiveness.

The four categories are as follows:

Group 1. Organisms in this group have a high degree of susceptibility that makes in vivo response probable when mild to moderately severe systemic infections are treated with the usual dosage of antimicrobial agent. The agent would be administered by the oral route when applicable (for example, ampicillin). Group 1 can be defined as "susceptible" without further qualification.

Group 2. Group 2 organisms have a degree of susceptibility that makes in vivo response probable in systemic infections when the antimicrobic is given in high dosage or up to the limits of safety.

Group 3. These organisms have a degree of susceptibility that makes in vivo response probable in the treatment of localized infections at sites where the agent can be concentrated by physiologic processes or local application.

Group 4. Group 4 organisms have a degree of resistance that makes in vivo response improbable. This group can be designated "resistant."

A laboratory capable of performing quantitative tests (MICs) may easily translate the MIC data (in micrograms per milliliter) to one of the four categories.

Recently the NCCLS proposed four categories similar to those just discussed. The NCCLS categories are susceptible (group 1), moderately susceptible (group 2), resistant (group 4), and conditionally susceptible (group 3).

Ellner and Neu[18] have recommended that laboratories report an inhibitory quotient (IQ) in addition to the MIC. The IQ is derived from the MIC of the organism-antimicrobic pair and the average peak level for that drug. IQs may be calculated for any body fluid and reflect the multiple of the MIC that might be achieved with the lowest clinical dosage. For example, an antimicrobic with a serum IQ of 4 for a particular organism should approach a level of approximately four times the MIC in serum. It is assumed to be a better choice than an antimicrobial agent with an IQ of 1.

Regardless of the reporting system used, the education of the clinician is a critical factor. If a major change in method is contemplated, for example, from the disk diffusion test to the MIC, an effective educational effort is imperative. Lack of understanding will cause the clinician to become frustrated, necessitate a sharp increase in phone calls to the laboratory, and ultimately result in poor patient care.

SUSCEPTIBILITY TESTING OF FUNGI, VIRUSES, PARASITES, AND MYCOBACTERIA

The methods employed for fungal susceptibility testing are not fundamentally different from those previously outlined. The compounds to be tested, however, have different properties from most antibacterial agents and the techniques are not standardized. Certain fungi grow either as yeasts or molds, optimum temperatures for growth may be different, and many fungi are slow growers. To solve the problems of temperature, Shadomy and Espinel-Ingroff[70] suggest that all media be incubated at 30° C. The need for susceptibility testing of fungi is also controversial. Although the controversy will not be settled by this chapter, susceptibility of fungi to the available agents is not predictable, but there are instances in which susceptibility tests are critically important, particularly for patients whose immune defenses may be compromised.

A complete description of fungal susceptibility testing may be found in the *Manual of Clinical Microbiology*,[70] or the *Laboratory Handbook of Medical Mycology*.[43]

Because of the specialized nature and relative difficulty of fungal susceptibility tests and the limited numbers of situations when they are needed, only major referral centers such as departments of health, university hospitals, or large community hospitals should offer the service. Regionalization of fungal susceptibility tests is both cost and quality effective.

Viral susceptibility testing is currently not routinely performed but will undoubtedly be used more frequently in the next few years. Efficacy testing of antiparasitic drugs is totally impractical for the clinical laboratory. Susceptibility testing of mycobacteria is discussed in Chapter 26.

MISCELLANEOUS TESTS
BETA-LACTAMASE

The development of beta-lactam antibiotics over the past 40 years has resulted in a wide variety of drugs with differing spectra. Similarly, a number of enzymes that bind to or otherwise inactivate the beta-lactam antibiotics have been discovered. Although beta-lactamases are the most significant inactivating enzymes clinically, amino acid acylases, esterases, and dehydropeptidases that also inactivate beta-lactam antibiotics have been discovered.

Determination of the presence of beta-lactamase is an important laboratory test, since therapy can often be redirected if the organism contains beta-lactamase. In addition, the beta-lactamase test is often more rapid than a traditional susceptibility test. When testing staphylococci, however, it should be remembered that some beta-lactamases may be inducible. Hence the organism may need exposure to penicillin before it produces beta-lactamase. This can be accomplished by taking the growth from the edge of the inhibition zone around a methicillin or penicillin disk.

Laboratory tests for beta-lactamase include the rapid acidometric method,[75] chromogenic cephalosporin method,[35,47] and the starch-iodine (iodometric) method.[75] The principle and procedure for each method is discussed in Appendix A.

Although beta-lactamase tests are usually reliable for predicting resistance to beta-lactam antibiotics, several reports of ampicillin-resistant, beta-lactamase-negative *Haemophilus* organisms have appeared,[40,58] but such organisms are very rare. It is recommended that a negative beta-lactamase test always be confirmed by standard tests of ampicillin susceptibility.

MINIMUM BACTERICIDAL CONCENTRATION

The minimum bactericidal concentration (MBC) of an isolate can be measured after the MIC has been determined. Quantitative subcultures are made from the microdilution wells or tubes showing no visible growth. The growth control and the last well or tube showing visible growth should also be cultured for quantitative comparison. This is done by removing 0.1 ml from the macrotube or 10 µl from the microdilution well and streaking for well-separated colonies on an agar plate. The plates are incubated overnight at 35° C. The MBC is the lowest concentration of antimicrobial agent that effects a 99.9% kill, that is, a 3 log reduction in growth from the original inoculum. If the original inoculum was 1×10^5 CFU/ml, a 99.9% reduction in colony count would be equivalent to 100 colonies/ml (10^2). A 10 µl sampling of this population would result in one colony per plate. Recognizing that microbial counts may not be accurate and that there is statistical variation around a mean colony count, three to nine colonies are taken as a practical MBC endpoint. This test is difficult to perform and must be strictly controlled.

MINIMUM ANTIBIOTIC CONCENTRATION[39]

The MAC is the minimum antibiotic concentration that produces a structural change in the microorganism, detectable by light or electron microscopy, or the minimum antibiotic concentration producing a 1 log decrease in the population. The clinical significance of the MAC and its determination (which is not routinely performed) are discussed by Lorian.[39]

ANTIBIOTIC TOLERANCE

Antibiotic tolerance in *Staphylococcus aureus* has been described by Sabath and associates.[65] In tolerant strains of bacteria, the MBC of the tested drug (originally penicillin) is at least 32 times greater than the MIC. Tolerance is seen in a small portion of the microbial population and is thought to be related to the defect in cellular autolytic enzymes. The tolerance trait is not stable and, like the "paradoxic effect" in which the bactericidal action of penicillin is reduced at high concentrations, is often lost or reduced after 24 hours' incubation. Tolerance has been observed in other organisms and other antibiotics. Its clinical significance has not been proved.

SERUM BACTERICIDAL TESTS

The Schlicter test,[69] or "serum bactericidal test" (SBT), was developed to measure the effectiveness with which penicillin in serum kills bacteria associated with endocarditis. The SBT is the highest dilution of the patient's serum that kills 99.9% of the original inoculum. The test has become a favorite of many clinicians to measure the in vivo response of an isolate to an antimicrobic. The rule of thumb has been that a serum bactericidal titer of 1:8 to 1:16 is therapeutic. The test was not standardized until recently, when NCCLS proposed a standard method.* Apart from the built-in error of serial twofold dilution tests, the diluent used to dilute the serum seems to have been the prime contributor to variation. The SBT has been modified in our laboratory to include initial dilutions of 1:2 and 1:3. These initial dilutions are then diluted serially twofold. This procedure reduces the inherent error in a twofold dilution series and increases precision of the test. A review by Wolfson and Swartz[84] discusses both clinical and laboratory issues surrounding the SBT.

SYNERGY TESTS

Antimicrobial agents may be used in combination to achieve a synergistic effect, that is, greater antimicrobial activity from the combination of the individual agents than their sum would indicate. Combination therapy is commonly used for immunocompromised patients, particularly those with low white cell counts. Administration of both an aminoglycoside and a penicillin is often necessary to cure enterococcal endocarditis. However, without a laboratory test it is not always possible to predict which combination of agents will be synergistic or antagonistic for an individual isolate. Three laboratory methods are used to determine antimicrobic synergy: the microdilution checkerboard test, time-kill curves, and the synergy screen.

Microdilution Checkerboard Test

With use of a microdilution plate and diluters, it is possible to expose an isolate to multiple concentration ratios of two

---

*Methodology for the serum bactericidal test; proposed guideline (1987), NCCLS Pub. No. M21-P.

antimicrobial agents. MICs for each drug alone are determined on the same plate. After overnight incubation, examination of the growth in the plate can detect synergy, antagonism, or a neutral effect of the two agents tested.

Time-Kill Curve

Moellering, Wennerstern, and Weinberg[46] should be consulted for detail concerning methodology of time-kill curves. Simply stated, the test strain inoculum is adjusted to 1 to 5 $\times$ 10^8 CFU/ml. Antimicrobial agents are added at concentrations less than the individual MICs. The assay tubes are incubated at 35° C, and standard plate counts are performed immediately and at 4, 8, and 24 hours. Synergy is defined as a reduction of 100 times in bacterial colony count in the presence of both agents as compared with each one individually.

Synergy Screen

Enterococci are usually resistant or moderately resistant to penicillin and resistant to aminoglycosides. However, many enterococci are susceptible to the synergistic effects of penicillin (or other cell wall antibiotics) and an aminoglycoside. The presence or absence of synergism between a cell wall antibiotic and an aminoglycoside against enterococci has been shown to correlate with absence or presence of very high level resistance to the aminoglycoside. A simple screening test may be used to provide this differentiation.

Organisms exhibiting high-level ribosomal resistance to the aminoglycoside grow in the presence of 2000 μg/ml of the aminoglycoside, whereas organisms with lower-level or more moderate resistance do not. The former organisms, when exposed to both a cell wall antibiotic and the given aminoglycoside, are highly resistant to the combination of both agents, whereas the latter organisms are susceptible. The use of a 2000 μg/ml streptomycin disk predicts ribosomal resistance to streptomycin, gentamicin, and tobramycin but not kanamycin or amikacin.[46]

ASSAYS OF ANTIMICROBICS IN BODY FLUIDS

Many factors have played a role in increasing the demand for assay of antimicrobial agents in body fluids. Among them are (1) the universal use of toxic agents such as the aminoglycosides, (2) the administration of antimicrobial agents for treatment of closed space infections, such as meningitis, when the penetration kinetics of the agent may not be predictable (an example is the newer cephalosporins such as moxalactam and cefotaxime), and (3) the trend toward more precise antimicrobial therapy as evidenced by the demand for MICs, MBCs, and pharmacokinetics consultation. The provision for quantitative susceptibility data has led to a need to determine the antimicrobic concentration in a body fluid, usually serum. With such information the clinician, the pharmacist, and the microbiologist may be better able to predict clinical efficacy or understand treatment failure.

Until recently the assay of antimicrobial agents was performed microbiologically with the exception of some, such as sulfa, that could be measured chemically. One disadvantage of most microbiologic assays is the necessity of waiting until the next day for results. Contemporary pharmacokinetics requires data on trough and peak antimicrobic levels to be available before the next dose is given. This may be as short as 4 hours and is usually no longer than 8 hours. The "trough" sample is drawn just before the antimicrobic is administered and reflects the minimum concentration of antimicrobic in the serum of the patient. The "peak" specimen is drawn after the dose is given and is timed so the anticipated concentration is the highest observed during the dosing period. For most antimicrobial agents (depending on the route of administration), peak levels are observed 30 to 90 minutes after administration.

In addition to the time required for the test, a drawback of microbiologic assays is the interference of a second (or third) antimicrobial agent in the serum. Usually this interference can be overcome by removal of the interfering antimicrobial agent or judicious choice of the test organism.

Types of microbiologic assays include agar disk or well diffusion, broth dilution, microdilution, turbidometric, inhibition of pH change, and radiometric. Detailed discussion of these assays may be found in Edberg's review.[17]

NONMICROBIOLOGIC ASSAYS

The extensive use of toxic antimicrobics has dictated that methods for their assay be both rapid and precise. With the exception of some modifications of the DAD assay that allow reading in 3 to 4 hours,[17] none of the traditional microbiologic methods is suitable for contemporary demands. A wide variety of other assays, including immunologic, chromatographic, or enzymatic, have become available in recent years and offer speed, sensitivity, specificity, and precision. Most are commercially available in kit form primarily for the aminoglycosides (gentamicin, tobramycin, amikacin, netilmicin, and kanamycin) and vancomycin.

Radioimmunoassay

The principle of radioimmunoassay (RIA) is presented in Chapter 7. RIA of antimicrobics meets the criteria of rapidity, sensitivity, specificity, and precision. The major disadvantages are the necessity of handling radiolabeled compounds and the need for a gamma counter.

The procedure is summarized as follows. Both ^{125}I-gentamicin-labeled and unlabeled gentamicin (from the serum sample) are mixed with antibody to gentamicin.[38] The labeled and unlabeled gentamicins compete for binding sites on the antibody protein. The amount of radiolabeled gentamicin bound is inversely proportional to the unlabeled gentamicin in the serum. The bound antibody-antigen complex is removed from solution by one of a number of techniques and counted. The amount of bound radiolabeled gentamicin can be used to directly calculate the amount of serum gentamicin. This procedure may also be used with other aminoglycosides.

Radioenzymatic Tests

Smith, Van Otto, and Smith[71] described a rapid chemical test for gentamicin. An R factor–mediated enzyme from *Escherichia coli* W677/JR66 that adenylated both kanamycin and gentamicin was employed. ^{14}C-ATP served as a source for the adenyl group to be enzymatically transferred to gentamicin. ^{14}C-adenylated gentamicin, but not ATP, binds to negatively charged phosphocellulose paper. The radiolabeled adenylated gentamicin was eluted from the paper and counted. A standard curve was constructed and used to measure gentamicin in serum. This is the basis of the radioenzymatic tests used today, which depend on adenylation and acetylation reactions in the presence of radiolabeled products.

Immunoassays

The general principles of immunoassays are discussed in Chapter 7. The EMIT system for assay of aminoglycoside antibiotics is available from Syva (Palo Alto, Calif.). EMIT is a competitive protein-binding procedure. Serum containing an unknown concentration of gentamicin is added to antigentamicin antibody and glucose 6-phosphate dehydrogenase–labeled gentamicin. Enzyme-linked gentamicin and free gentamicin compete for binding sites on the antibody. Free, unbound, gentamicin-enzyme complex is measured by the addition of the substrate, glucose 6-phosphate. The reaction is followed by monitoring the reduction of the cofactor, NAD, at 340 nm.

The Ames Co. (Elkhart, Ind.) markets a fluorescence immunoassay (FIA) kit for aminoglycosides. The principle underlying this test is that free antimicrobic competes with antimicrobic coupled to a fluorigenic substrate for antibody binding sites. An enzyme, beta-galactosidase, cleaves the unbound fluorescent substrate. Fluorescence is measured at an excitation wavelength of 400 nm and an emission wavelength of 450 nm.

As discussed in Chapter 7, the TDX system (Abbott Laboratories, North Chicago, Ill.) may be used for detection of drugs of abuse and therapeutic drug monitoring. Included in the system are kits for gentamicin, tobramycin, amikacin, netilmycin, and vancomycin. The basis of the test is a fluorescence polarization immunoassay (FPIA). A gentamicin molecule is labeled with fluorescein. Labeled and unlabeled gentamicin compete for antibody binding sites. In FPIA the binding of fluorescein-labeled gentamicin to antibody is measured directly by determining its fluorescence polarization, which is directly proportional to the amount of labeled gentamicin bound and inversely proportional to the unlabeled gentamicin.

The FIAX (International Diagnostics Technology, Santa Clara, Calif.), also discussed in Chapter 7, is another fluorescence immunoassay for antimicrobial agents, although it is better known for determination of antibodies to infectious agents. This system depends on competition between labeled and unlabeled gentamicin for binding sites on an antibody bound to a solid-phase polymeric surface (StiQ). The solid phase resembles a paddle. In operation the paddle, or StiQ, is immersed sequentially in fluorescein-labeled gentamicin and the test serum. Labeled gentamicin bound to the StiQ is determined in a fluorimeter and is inversely proportional to the serum gentamicin concentration.

Latex Agglutination Inhibition

A latex agglutination inhibition (LAI) card test is available for gentamicin, tobramycin, and amikacin assay in serum (BBL, Cockeysville, Md.). The LAI test is based on the binding of aminoglycoside protein–activated latex particle to a rabbit antiaminoglycoside antibody. Twelve nongeometric dilutions of the test serum are made on a black cardboard card. Antiaminoglycoside antibody is added to each well and also to four standards. The aminoglycoside protein-activated latex reagent is then added. At that dilution, where there is insufficient aminoglycoside in the patient's serum to bind antibody, latex agglutination occurs with the free antiaminoglycoside antibody. The concentration of aminoglycoside is calculated by multiplying the highest reciprocal dilution in which agglutination inhibition was observed by the lowest aminoglycoside standard concentration in which agglutination was inhibited.

Chromatography

Gas-liquid, thin-layer, and paper chromatography have been used in the past for detection and measurement of antimicrobics. These methods have little practical value, and they are not widely employed. High-performance liquid chromatography (HPLC), however, is an excellent method for antimicrobic assay. In HPLC a liquid solvent carrying the substance to be separated and detected is pumped at high pressure through a particulate column. Many column packings are available, depending on the application. After separation, substances are detected spectrophotometrically, usually in the ultraviolet range at 254 or 280 nm. The major advantages of HPLC over GLC are better and faster resolution of peaks, greater reproducibility and specificity, and alleviation of the need for derivitization in many instances. The assay of certain antimicrobics lends itself to HPLC, and a number of reviews such as that of Anhalt[3] have been published.

The major advantages of HPLC appear to be for the assay of antimicrobics for which no commercial kit is available. Such drugs include chloramphenicol, the antifungal agents, and the third-generation cephalosporins.

Chemical Assays

Although many antimicrobial agents have been measured by direct chemical methods, the only one routinely measured is sulfa. Several procedures are available. They are based on the Bratton-Marshall reaction[9] in which para-aminobenzene derivatives (of which sulfa is one) react with nitrite in acid solution to form a diazonium salt. The excess nitrite is destroyed by ammonium sulfamate, and the diazonium salt couples with N-1 (naphthyl-ethylenediamine) to form a stable dye that can be read spectrophotometrically at 500 nm. The reaction is linear over a wide range of sulfa concentrations.

REFERENCES

1. Acar, J.F., and Goldstein, F.W.: Disk susceptibility. In Lorian, V., editor: Antibiotics in laboratory medicine, Baltimore, 1986, The Williams & Wilkins Co.
2. Andriole, V.T.: Urinary tract agents: quinolones, nitrofurantoin, and methenamine. In Mandell, G.L., Douglas, R.G., and Bennett, J.E., editors: Principles and practice of infectious diseases, ed. 2, New York, 1985, John Wiley & Sons, Inc.
3. Anhalt, J.P.: Clinical antibiotic assays by HPLC. In Hawk, G.L., editor: Biological/biomedical application of liquid chromatography, vol. II, New York, 1979, Marcel Dekker.
4. Barry, A.L.: The antimicrobic susceptibility test: principles and practices, Philadelphia, 1976, Lea & Febiger.
5. Barry, A.L., Garcia, F., and Thrupp, L.D.: An improved single disk method for testing the antibiotic susceptibility of rapidly growing pathogens, Am. J. Clin. Pathol. 53:149, 1970.
6. Barry, A.L., and Thornsberry, C.: Susceptibility tests: diffusion test procedures. In Lennette, E.H., et al., editors: Manual of clinical microbiology, ed. 4, Washington, D.C., 1985, American Society for Microbiology.
7. Barry, A.L., et al.: In vitro evaluation of LY127935 (6059-S) in comparison with eleven related beta-lactam compounds and two aminoglycosides. In Nelson, J.D., and Grassi, C., editors: Current chemotherapy and infectious disease, Washington, D.C., 1980, American Society for Microbiology.
8. Bauer, A.W., et al.: Antibiotic susceptibility testing by a standardized single disk method, Am. J. Clin. Pathol. 45:493, 1966.
9. Bratton, A.C., and Marshall, E.K.: A new coupling component for sulfonilamide determination, J. Biol. Chem. 128:537, 1939.

10. Bryan, L.E., Koward, S.K., and Van Den Elzen, H.M.: Mechanism of aminoglycoside antibiotic resistance in anaerobic bacteria: *Clostridium perfringens* and *Bacteroides fragilis*, Antimicrob. Agents Chemother. **15**:7, 1979.

11. Chopra, I., and Howe, T.G.B.: Bacterial resistance to the tetracyclines, Microbiol. Rev. **42**:707, 1978.

11a. Coudron, P.E., et al.: Evaluation of laboratory tests for detection of methicillin-resistant *Staphylococcus aureus* and *Staphylococcus epidermidis*, J. Clin. Microbiol. **24**:764, 1986.

12. Davies, J.: General mechanisms of antimicrobial resistance, Rev. Infect. Dis. **1**:23, 1979.

13. Davies, J.: Microbial resistance to antimicrobial agents. In Ristuccia, A.M., and Cunha, B.A., editors: Antimicrobial therapy, New York, 1984, Raven Press.

14. Dixon, D.M., et al.: "In vitro" comparison of the antifungal activities of R34,000, miconazole, and amphotericin B, Chemotherapy **24**:364, 1978.

15. Dougherty, T.J., Koller, A.E., and Tomasz, A.: Penicillin-binding proteins of penicillin-susceptible and intrinsically resistant *Neisseria gonorrhoeae*, Antimicrob. Agents Chemother. **18**:730, 1980.

16. Drusano, G.L., Schimpff, S.C., and Hewitt, W.L.: The acylampicillins: mezlocillin, piperacillin, and azlocillin, Rev. Infect. Dis. **6**:13, 1984.

17. Edberg, S.C.: The measurement of antibiotics in human body fluids: techniques and significance. In Lorian, V., editor: Antibiotics in laboratory medicine, ed. 2, Baltimore, 1986, The Williams & Wilkins Co.

18. Ellner, P.D., and Neu, H.C.: The inhibitory quotient, JAMA **246**:1575, 1981.

19. Ericsson, H.M., and Sherris, J.C.: Antibiotic sensitivity testing: report of an international collaborative study, Acta Pathol. Microbiol. Scand. Sect. B **217**(suppl.):1, 1971.

20. Fedor, H.M., Jr., Osier, C., and Maderazo, E.G.: Chloramphenicol: a review of its use in clinical practice, Rev. Infect. Dis. **3**:479, 1980.

21. Finegold, S.M.: Antimicrobial therapy for anaerobic infections, Scand. J. Gastroenterol. **91**(suppl.):61, 1984.

22. Finegold, S.M., and Rolfe, R.D.: Susceptibility testing of anaerobic bacteria, Diagn. Microbiol. Infect. Dis. **1**:33, 1983.

23. Franklin, T.J., and Snow, G.A.: Biochemistry of antimicrobial action, New York, 1981, Chapman & Hall.

24. Gilman, A.G., et al.: Goodman and Gilman's the pharmacological basis of therapeutics, ed. 7, New York, 1985, Macmillan, Inc.

25. Godefroi, E.F., et al.: The preparation and antimycotic properties of derivatives of l-phenethylimidazole, J. Med. Chem. **12**:784, 1969.

26. Gold, W., et al.: Amphotericins A and B: antifungal antibiotics produced by a streptomycete. In Welch, H., and Marti-Ibanez, F., editors: Antibiotics annual: 1955-56, New York, 1956, Medical Encyclopedia, Inc.

27. Grunberg, E., Titsworth, E., and Bennett, M.: Chemotherapeutic activity of 5-fluorocytosine, Antimicrobial Agents and Chemotherapy-1963. Proceedings of the Third Interscience Conference on Antimicrobial Agents and Chemotherapy, American Society for Microbiology.

28. Gupta, R.S.: Killing and lysis of *Escherichia coli* in the presence of chloramphenicol: relation to cellular magnesium, Antimicrob. Agents Chemother. **7**:748, 1975.

29. Hakenbeck, R., Tarpay, M., and Tomasz, A.: Multiple changes of penicillin-binding proteins in penicillin-resistant clinical isolates of *Streptococcus pneumoniae*, Antimicrob. Agents Chemother. **17**:364, 1980.

30. Harnden, M.R., editor: Approaches to antiviral agents, Houndmills, Eng., 1985, Macmillan Press, Ltd.

31. Hartman, B., and Tomasz, A.: Altered penicillin-binding proteins in methicillin-resistant strains of *Staphylococcus aureus*, Antimicrob. Agents Chemother. **19**:726, 1981.

32. Hayden, F.G., and Douglas, R.G., Jr.: Antiviral agents. In Mandell, G.L., Douglas, R.G., and Bennett, J.E., editors: Principles and practice of infectious diseases, ed. 2, New York, 1985, John Wiley & Sons, Inc.

33. Hinkle, A.M., LeBlanc, B.M., and Bodey, G.P.: "In vitro" evaluation of cefoperazone, Antimicrob. Agents Chemother. **17**:423, 1980.

34. Hoeprich, P.D.: Antimicrobics and anthelminthics for systemic therapy. In Hoeprich, P.D., editor: Infectious diseases, ed. 3, Hagerstown, Md., 1983, Harper & Row, Publishers, Inc.

35. Kammer, R.B., et al.: Rapid detection of ampicillin-resistant *Haemophilus influenzae* and their susceptibility to sixteen antibiotics, Antimicrob. Agents Chemother. **8**:91, 1974.

36. Kucers, A., and Bennett, N.: The use of antibiotics, ed. 3, London, 1979, William Heinemann Medical Books, Ltd.

37. Kurzynski, T.A., et al.: Aerobically incubated thioglycollate broth-disk method for antibiotic susceptibility testing of anaerobes, Antimicrob. Agents Chemother. **10**:727, 1976.

38. Lewis, J.E., Nelson, J.C., and Elder, H.A.: Radioimmunoassay of an antibiotic: gentamicin, Nature **239**:214, 1972.

39. Lorian, V.: Effect of low antibiotic concentrations on bacteria: effects on ultrastructure, their virulence, and susceptibility to immune defenses. In Lorian, V., editor: Antibiotics in laboratory medicine, ed. 2, Baltimore, 1986, The Williams & Wilkins Co.

40. Markowitz, S.: Isolation of an ampicillin resistant, non-beta-lactamase producing strain of *Haemophilus influenzae*, Antimicrob. Agents Chemother. **17**:80, 1980.

41. McCarthy, L.R.: Advances in the understanding of *Haemophilus* spp., Clin. Microbiol. Newsletter **5**:27, 1983.

42. McClatchy, J.K.: Antimycobacterial drugs: mechanisms of action, drug resistance, susceptibility testing, and assays of activity in biological fluids. In Lorian, V., editor: Antibiotics in laboratory medicine, ed. 2, Baltimore, 1986, The Williams & Wilkins Co.

43. McGinnis, M.: Laboratory handbook of medical mycology, New York, 1980, Academic Press, Inc.

44. Merz, W.G., and Sandford, G.R.: Isolation and characterization of a polyene-resistant variant of *Candida tropicalis*, J. Clin. Microbiol. **9**:677, 1979.

45. Meshnick, S.R., and Cerami, A.: Host-parasite interface: biochemistry. In Warren, K.S., and Hahmoud, A.A.F., editors: Tropical and geographical medicine, New York, 1984, McGraw-Hill Book Co.

46. Moellering, R.C., Jr., Wennerstern, C.B.G., and Weinberg, A.N.: Studies on antibiotic synergism against enterococci, J. Lab. Clin. Med. **77**:821, 1971.

47. Montgomery, K., Raymundo, L., Jr., and Drew, W.L.: Chromogenic cephalosporin spot test to detect beta-lactamase in clinically significant bacteria, J. Clin. Microbiol. **9**:205, 1979.

48. National Committee for Clinical Laboratory Standards: Performance standards for antimicrobial disk susceptibility tests, ed. 3, approved standard, NCCLS Pub. No. M2-A3, Villanova, Penn., 1984, The Committee.

49. National Committee for Clinical Laboratory Standards: Alternative methods for antimicrobial susceptibility testing of anaerobic bacteria: proposed guideline, NCCLS Pub. No. M17-P, Villanova, Penn., 1985, The Committee.

49a. National Committee for Clinical Laboratory Standards: Methods for dilution antimicrobial susceptibility tests for bacteria that grow aerobically, approved standard, NCCLS Pub. No. M7-A, Villanova, Penn., The Committee.

50. National Committee for Clinical Laboratory Standards: Reference agar dilution procedures for antimicrobial susceptibility testing of anaerobic bacteria, approved standard, NCCLS Pub. No. M11-A, Villanova, Penn., 1985, The Committee.

51. Neu, H.C.: Carbenicillin and ticarcillin, Med. Clin. North Am. **66**:61, 1982.

52. Neu, H.C.: Penicillins—new insights into their mechanisms of activity and clinical use, Bull. N.Y. Acad. Med. **58**:681, 1982.

53. Neu, H.C.: The emergence of bacterial resistance and its influence on empiric therapy, Rev. Infect. Dis. **5**(suppl.):S9, 1983.

54. Neu, H.C.: Changing mechanisms of bacterial resistance, Am. J. Med. **77**(1B):11, 1984.

55. Neu, H.C.: Current mechanisms of resistance to antimicrobial agents in microorganisms causing infection in the patient at risk for infection, Am. J. Med. **76**(5A):11, 1984

56. Neu, H.C.: Other beta lactam antibiotics. In Mandell, G.L., Douglas, R.G., and Bennett, J.E., editors: Principles and practice of infectious diseases, ed. 2, New York, 1985, John Wiley & Sons, Inc.

57. Nishino, T., and Nakazawa, S.: Bacteriological study on effects of beta-lactam group antibiotics in high concentrations, Antimicrob. Agents Chemother. **9**:1033, 1976.

58. Offit, P.A., Campos, J.M., and Plotkin, S.A.: Ampicillin resistant, beta-lactamase negative *Haemophilus influenzae* type b, Pediatrics **69**:230, 1982.

59. Pattishall, K.H., et al.: Two distinct types of trimethoprim-resistant dihydrofolate reductase specified by R-plasmids of different compatibility groups, J. Biol. Chem. **252**:2319, 1977.

60. Pestka, S.: Inhibitors of protein synthesis. In Weissbach, H., and Pestka, S., editors: Molecular mechanisms of protein biosynthesis, New York, 1977, Academic Press, Inc.

61. Robinson, B.E., et al.: In vitro susceptibility of *Haemophilus influenzae* to six antimicrobial drugs, Abstracts Annual Meeting, p. 315, Washington, D.C., 1982, American Society for Microbiology.

62. Rosenblatt, J.E.: Antimicrobial susceptibility testing of anaerobic bacteria, Rev. Infect. Dis. **6**(suppl. 1):S242, 1984.

63. Rosenblatt, J.E., and Edson, R.S.: Metronidazole, Mayo Clin. Proc. **58**:154, 1983.

64. Ryan, R.W., and Tilton, R.C.: Modified-microdilution antimicrobial susceptibility test for anaerobic bacteria, Curr. Microbiol. **3**:365, 1980.

65. Sabath, L.D., et al.: A new type of penicillin resistance of *Staphylococcus aureus*, Lancet **1**:443, 1977.

66. Sanders, C.C.: Novel resistance selected by the new expanded-spectrum cephalosporins: a concern, J. Infect. Dis. **147**:575, 1983.

67. Sanders, C.C., and Sanders, W.E., Jr.: Microbial resistance to newer generation β-lactam antibiotics: clinical and laboratory implications, J. Infect. Dis. **151**:399, 1985.

68. Saz, H.J.: Biochemistry of parasites: helminths. In Braude, A.I.: Medical microbiology and infectious diseases, Philadelphia, 1981, W.B. Saunders Co.

69. Schlichter, J.G., MacLean, H., and Malzer, A.: Effective penicillin therapy in subacute bacterial endocarditis with penicillin, Am. J. Med. Sci. **217**:600, 1949.

70. Shadomy, S., and Espinel-Ingroff, A.: Susceptibility testing with antifungal drugs. In Lennette, E.H., et al., editors: Manual of clinical microbiology, ed. 4, Washington, D.C., 1985, American Society for Microbiology.

71. Smith, D.H., Van Otto, B., and Smith, A.L.: A rapid chemical assay for gentamicin, N. Engl. J. Med. **286**:583, 1972.

72. Spratt, B.G.: Distinct penicillin binding proteins involved in the division, elongation, and shape of *Escherichia coli* K12, Proc. Natl. Acad. Sci. USA **72**:2999, 1975.

73. Swamy, K.H.S., Sirsi, M., and Rao, G.R.: Studies of the mechanism of action of miconazole: effect of miconazole on respiration and cell permeability of *Candida albicans,* Antimicrob. Agents Chemother. **5**:420, 1974.

74. Thornsberry, C.: The agar diffusion antimicrobial susceptibility test. In Balows, A., editor: Current techniques for antibiotic susceptibility testing, Springfield, Ill., 1974, Charles C Thomas, Publisher.

75. Thornsberry, C., Gavan, T.L., and Gerlach, E.H.: Cumitech 6: new developments in antimicrobial agent susceptibility testing, Washington, D.C., 1977, American Society for Microbiology.

76. Thornsberry, C., and McDougal, L.K.: Successful use of broth microdilution in susceptibility tests for methicillin-resistant (heteroresistant) staphylococci, J. Clin. Microbiol. **18**:1084, 1983.

77. Wagner, J.G., and Shadomy, S.: Mode of action of fluocytosine in *Aspergillus* species, Chemotherapy **3**:211, 1979.

78. Washington, J.A., II: Susceptibility tests: agar dilution. In Lennette, E.H., et al., editors: Manual of clinical microbiology, ed. 4, Washington, D.C., 1985, American Society for Microbiology.

79. Wehrli, W.: Rifampin: mechanism of action and resistance. Rev. Infect. Dis. **5**(suppl. 3):407, 1983.

80. Weisberger, A.S.: Inhibition of protein synthesis by chloramphenicol, Annu. Rev. Med. **18**:483, 1967.

81. Wilkins, T.D., and Thiel, T.: Modified broth disk method for testing the antibiotic susceptibility of anaerobic bacteria, Antimicrob. Agents Chemother. **3**:350, 1973.

82. Wimpenny, J.W.T.: Effect of isoniazid on biosynthesis in *Mycobacterium tuberculosis* var. *bovis* BCG, J. Gen. Microbiol. **47**:379, 1967.

83. Wise, E.M., and Abou-Donia, M.M.: Sulfonamide resistance mechanism in *Escherichia coli:* R plasmids can determine sulfonamide-resistant dihydropteroate synthases, Proc. Natl. Acad. Sci. USA **72**:2621, 1975.

84. Wolfson, J.S., and Swartz, M.N.: Serum bactericidal activity as a monitor of antimicrobial therapy, N. Engl. J. Med. **312**:968, 1985.

85. Yoshikawa, T.T.: Antiprotozoan drugs. In Yoshikawa, T.T., Chow, A.W., and Guze, L.B., editors: Infectious diseases: diagnosis and management, Boston, 1980, Houghton Mifflin.

86. Youatt, J.: A review of the action of isoniazid, Am. Rev. Respir. Dis. **99**:720, 1969.

ADDITIONAL READINGS

Edberg, S.C., and Berger, S.A.: Antibiotics and infection, New York, 1983, Churchill Livingstone.

Franklin, T.J., and Snow, G.A.: Biochemistry of antimicrobial action, London, 1981, Chapman & Hall.

Gale, E.F., et al.: The molecular basis of antibiotic action, ed. 2, London, 1981, John Wiley & Sons.

Joklik, W.K., Willett, H.P., and Amos, D.B.: Zinsser microbiology, ed. 18, Norwalk, Conn., 1984, Appleton-Century-Crofts.

Mandell, G.L., Douglas, R.G., Jr., and Bennett, J.E.: Principles and practice of infectious diseases, ed. 2, New York, 1985, John Wiley & Sons, Inc.

Ristuccia, A.M., and Cunha, B.A.: Antimicrobial therapy, New York, 1984, Raven Press.

CHAPTER 9

Instrumentation and Rapid Methods

Richard C. Tilton

The history of instrumentation and rapid methods in microbiology began only in the 1970s, when clinical microbiology changed to reflect a growing awareness of computerization and advanced automation technology. The fact that clinical microbiologists have lagged far behind the rest of the laboratory community in responding to technologic innovation can be attributed to the nature of specimens and microorganisms and the characteristics of microbiologic instrumentation.

Most specimens for microbiologic analysis are different from those submitted for chemical or hematologic examination. Microbiologists must analyze living organisms in these specimens, unlike other laboratory workers, who detect finite quantities of a substance or a cell type within a specimen. The microbiologic specimen is a dynamic, living thing. From the time it is taken from the patient, its biologic characteristics undergo change. Exposed to the atmosphere, organisms both grow and die at varying rates. Interaction with host factors, such as phagocytes, continues even after the specimen has been removed from the patient. Inactivation of microorganisms by drugs does not cease, even though the specimen is in a plastic container. As discussed in Chapter 11, the specimen is labile, and delay in transport may render it useless for microbiologic analysis. Even refrigeration, which halts most microbial proliferation, may harm the specimen.

There are essentially two types of specimens: a specimen that has been collected from a normally sterile body site and a specimen that has been collected from a site that has been contaminated by either trauma or invading normal flora or that is contiguous to mucous membranes. The microbiologic approach to a problem of usually sterile specimens is to identify the etiologic agent present and interpret its presence in light of the clinical situation. On the other hand, a contaminated specimen such as feces or sputum contains large numbers of normal inhabitants. The task of the microbiologist then is to sort out the offending pathogens that may be present in small numbers and isolate and identify them. These polymicrobic specimens offer the greatest challenge for the microbiologist but are the least amenable to automation and rapid-detection technology.

The microbial world consists of thousands of microorganisms, relatively few of which are pathogenic. In a single specimen, however, 10 or 15 different microorganisms are commonly present, including bacteria, fungi, protozoa, rickettsiae, chlamydiae, and viruses. Microbiologists believed for a century that for proper processing of clinical specimens the suspect microorganisms had to be isolated and purified. This strict adherence to the pure culture technique, in addition to the inherent slow growth rate of microorganisms, relegated microbiology to a confirmatory science rather than one that plays a dynamic role in disease diagnosis. With few exceptions, such as the Gram stain, immunoserologic detection systems (see Chapter 7), and nucleic acid probes, microbiology procedures are not fast enough to direct therapy. Most microbiology laboratory reports either confirm or deny the clinician's original clinical suspicion and therapy.

The question is how rapid microbiologic diagnosis must be to play an effective role in patient management. In the outpatient setting the report must be generated within the time the patient is willing to wait, probably less than an hour. Information on acute infections in inpatients should be available within the time the clinician is willing to withhold treatment. This is usually less than an hour, except in life-threatening situations in which treatment must be initiated immediately. Relatively few instruments or methods currently satisfy the time requirement for an acutely ill patient. Those that do include the Gram stain, direct fluorescent antibody stains, immunologic detection of antigen in body fluids, and nucleic acid probes.

Advances in automation and rapid methods in microbiology have been delayed by the necessity for comparing these many innovative techniques with methods that (1) have not changed for 100 years, (2) are enslaved by the pure-culture technique, and (3) are ensnared by the tyranny of the growth curve. Recently introduced techniques, however, hold promise for circumventing traditional methodology and abandoning the leisurely approach of growing microscopically distinct colonies. These techniques and examples of the numerous rapid and automated methods are discussed in this chapter. Comprehensive lists of commercial bacterial identification systems are available in an article by Fenn and Matsen.[49]

MINIATURIZED MICROBIOLOGIC METHODS

The methods of bacterial identification in the clinical laboratory have been revolutionized during the last decade. In the past, laboratories either prepared or purchased individual media or reagent-containing tubes for biochemical testing. Each laboratory had its favorite panel of tests to identify gram-negative rods, gram-positive cocci, and other bacteria that might be clinically significant. These traditional methods consumed valuable storage space and were slow and labor intensive. No laboratory had a data base more sophisticated than a set of charts showing anticipated results of a chosen set of biochemical tests. Historical studies by Lindner,[95] Hartman,[67] and Weaver, Arnold, and Hannan[152] showed that the use of large inocula significantly reduces incubation time and that "little tubes" are as sensitive as similar macrotechniques. This technology formed the basis for the number of products introduced in the marketplace during the early 1970s.

IDENTIFICATION OF *ENTEROBACTERIACEAE*

The first products to appear for the identification of members of the family *Enterobacteriaceae* included Pathotec strips (General Diagnostics), the API system (API) (Plate 2, *A*), Enterotube (Roche), the RB system (Corning), and Auxotab (Consolidated Laboratories) (Plate 2, *B*). The API and the Auxotab used a strip of plastic cupules containing dried reagents for a series of biochemical tests. The RB system was unique in that it incorporated multiple tests (up to eight) in two agar-containing tubes and an information-processing machine called the Enteric Analyzer.[22] The Enterotube consists of eight separate compartments containing eight prepared selective media that are inoculated simultaneously by drawing up the central needle. Nord and co-workers,[113] at the First International Symposium on Rapid Methods and Automation in Microbiology, described five different multitest systems: Pathotec, Enterotube, API, Auxotab, and RB. Nord reported that the commercial test systems were easy to use, accurate in the identification of unknown cultures, easily stored, and economical. Correlation of results between these miniaturized tests and traditional, large-tube tests ranged from 80% to 100%, with most tests agreeing over 90% of the time. All provided the laboratory with a simple, reliable method of genus and species identification. Table 9-1 summarizes many of the currently available systems for the identification of the family *Enterobacteriaceae*. Other systems are discussed by Fenn and Matsen.[49]

All the kits for identification of *Enterobacteriaceae* have associated data bases. The early products relied on the data base of Edwards and Ewing.[43] However, because each product used different media, pH indicators, and inoculum strengthens, a unique computerized data base was subsequently designed for each system. The data base is entered by derivation of a number, usually an octal one, determined from test results. The most extensive data base is that of API. The data bases are stored either in manuals provided for the laboratory or on disks in a computer. As new taxonomic information becomes available, these manuals or computer bases are updated for the user.

IDENTIFICATION OF NONFERMENTATIVE GRAM-NEGATIVE BACTERIA

The introduction of commercial microtest systems has provided the clinical microbiology laboratory with simple, rapid, and relatively inexpensive means to identify the nonfermentative gram-negative bacteria (NFB). The miniaturized multiple-medium kits all include computer-generated interpretation manuals for convenience and standardization of the respective identification systems. Some of them use the same test menu as used for the *Enterobacteriaceae* but with an expanded data base. The most commonly used systems, and those that have been evaluated most extensively, include the API 20E system (Analytab Products, Inc., Plainview, N.Y.), the Oxi/Ferm system (Roche Diagnostics, Nutley, N.J.), the Flow N/F system (Flow Laboratories, Roslyn, N.Y.), and the Rapid NFT (API Systems, S.A., France).

Oxi/Ferm System[114,115]

The Oxi/Ferm system is an assemblage of eight compartments in a plastic tube, each containing a specific substrate, to generate nine test results: acid from glucose (anaerobic), arginine dihydrolase, nitrate reduction, hydrogen sulfide (H_2S) production, indole production, acid from glucose and xylose (aerobic), urea hydrolysis, and citrate utilization (Plate 2, *D*). An inoculation rod traverses the media, and after an inoculum is gathered at the tip, the rod is pulled through the tube and each compartment. The tube is incubated for 48 hours at 35° C. Although with some organisms (*Acinetobacter anitratus*) completed test results are available at 24 hours, others require 48 hours for complete identification. The advantages of the Oxi/Ferm system are the rapid inoculation (does not require an initial suspension of organisms), ease of handling, and the small number of tests necessary to provide the minimum number of characteristics required for identification.

Minitek System[30,88,154]

The Minitek system consists of a plastic plate containing 12 or 20 wells to hold disks impregnated with the user's choice of substrates (Figure 9-1). A heavy suspension of the test organism is made in the manufacturer-formulated broth, which is dispensed with a pipette into the disk-containing wells. After incubation at 35° C for 48 hours, the observed reactions are interpreted with tables and the code book. An advantage of the Minitek system is its flexibility; substrates, in addition to those prescribed for proper test performance, can be selected and varied to meet the needs of the individual laboratory, such as consideration of the types of organisms most frequently encountered. Another advantage is the long shelf life of the disks (at least 2 years at 4° C).

Uni N/F System[11,26,88]

The Uni N/F system (Flow Laboratories) consists of two screening tubes and a round plate (Uni-N/F-Tek) that is divided into 12 sections (Plate 2, *E*). The first screening tube, GNF, is constricted and detects glucose fermentation in the base of the agar and denitrification and fluorescein production in the upper portion (Plate 2, *F*). The second screening tube, 42P, detects growth at 42° C with subsequent production of pyocyanin (Plate 2, *G*). The tubes are inoculated only with oxidase-positive organisms. The circular plate consists of 11 independently sealed peripheral wells and a central unsealed well. Each contains an agar medium for the determination of the following 12 biochemical reactions: acid from glucose, xylose, mannitol, lactose, and maltose; growth in acetamide; esculin hydrolysis; urea hydrolysis; DNAse production; hydrolysis of ONPG; H_2S production; and indole production. A heavy suspension of the test organism is prepared in saline, and 1 drop is added to each test well. The GNF and 42P are incubated overnight at 35° and 42° C, respectively, and the plate is incubated at 35° C for 24 to 48 hours. An advantage of the N/F system is that the two tubes allow economical identification of *P. aeruginosa* within 24 hours. Also, oxidase-negative organisms are identified rapidly with the circular plate.

Rapid NFT[6,88]

The Rapid NFT is a strip with 20 cupules that determines eight enzymatic reactions and 12 assimilation tests for the identification of the nonfermentative gram-negative organisms, as well as some fermentative organisms not belonging to the family *Enterobacteriaceae*, such as the genera *Vibrio* and *Aeromonas*. The enzymatic activities determined include nitrate reductase, tryptophanase, glucose fermentation, arginine dihydrolase, urease, esculin hydrolysis, gelatinase, and beta-galac-

TABLE 9-1. Commercially Available Kits for the Identification of *Enterobacteriaceae*

Product Name	Description	Substrate/Test	Operation	Comments
API 20E (Analytab Products; Plate 2, A)	Twenty miniature cupules containing dehydrated substrates are in plasticized strip. After addition of standardized inoculum (McFarland 0.5) and incubation, color changes are read visually. Reagents must be added to some cupules before reading.	Hydrolysis of *o*-nitrophenyl-beta-galactopyranoside (ONPG) Arginine dihydrolase Lysine decarboxylase Ornithine decarboxylase Citrate utilization Production of hydrogen sulfide (H$_2$S) Urea hydrolysis Tryptophan deaminase Formation of indole Production of acetoin (Voges-Proskauer test) Liquefaction of gelatin Fermentation of: Glucose Mannitol Inositol Sorbitol Rhamnose Sucrose Melibiose Amygdalin Arabinose	Each cupule is manually inoculated with Pasteur pipette. Some cupules are overlaid with oil to provide conditions of reduced O$_2$ tension. Strip is placed in humid chamber and incubated either 5 hr for rapid test or 18-24 hr for overnight result. Seven-digit number is derived from scoring the seven sets of three reactions each. Number is then found in code book that reveals identification of bacterium, probability of its being correct, and aberrant test results.	This is largest commercially available microbiologic data base in world. Many reports indicate >90% agreement with conventional methods for both 18-hr and 5-hr system.[68,70,112]
API Rapid E (API Systems, S.A.)	This system is essentially identical to API 20E except that substrates are not buffered and microtubes are smaller.	Hydrolysis of ONPG Lysine decarboxylase Ornithine decarboxylase Urea hydrolysis Phenylalanine deaminase Esculin Citrate utilization Malonate utilization Indole production Voges-Proskauer test Fermentation of: Arabinose Xylose Adonitol Rhamnose Cellobiose Melibiose Sucrose Trehalose Raffinose Glucose	Operation is identical to API 20E except initial incubation period is 4 hr.	Results are available in 4 or 18 hr.[9,107,117] This test is acceptable alternative to API 20E.

Continued.

TABLE 9-1. Commercially Available Kits for the Identification of *Enterobacteriaceae*—cont'd

Product Name	Description	Substrate/Test	Operation	Comments
R/B Enteric (Roche Diagnostics)	Fourteen determinations are available through use of four constricted Beckford tubes containing slanted agar media. Two tubes provide presumptive identification of *Enterobacteriaceae* based on eight tests. Remaining two tubes, called "Expanders," provide additional tests.	R/B 1 Phenylalanine deaminase Lactose fermentation H₂S production Glucose fermentation Lysine decarboxylase R/B 2 Indole production Ornithine decarboxylase R/B Expander (1) Citrate utilization Rhamnose fermentation R/B Expander (2) DNAse production Raffinose fermentation Sorbitol fermentation Arabinose fermentation	Agar tube is stabbed with long needle, and then agar surface is streaked with same needle. Tubes are loosely capped and incubated overnight at 35° C. Color changes are read visually and compared to chart provided in kit.	Results of collaborative study indicate >90% agreement with conventional methods. [73]
Entero-Set (Fisher Scientific Co.)	System is similar in appearance to API. Two cards have 10 miniature plastic cupules each. Cards are used as presumptive and confirmatory test series. Each cupule is inoculated with capillary pipette. Hourglass cupule shape provides anaerobic conditions in bottom sector.	*Entero-Set (1)* Resazurin (growth control) Malonate utilization Phenylalanine deaminase H₂S production Sucrose fermentation Hydrolysis of ONPG Lysine decarboxylase Ornithine decarboxylase Urea hydrolysis Indole production *Entero-Set (2)* Arginine dihydrolase Citrate utilization Fermentation of: Salicin Adonitol Inositol Sorbitol Arabinose Maltose Trehalose Xylose	Single colony is transferred to 5 ml of BHI and incubated for 3 to 4 hr. Growth is resuspended in 1.8 ml of H₂O, and strips are inoculated. If chambers are overfilled, significant biosafety hazard may result.	>90% agreement with conventional tests. Test results are available 3 to 4 hr after incubation at 35° C.

System	Description	Tests	Method	Comments
Micro-ID (Organon Teknika) (Plate 2, C)	Kit consists of 15 tests in plastic tray. Reaction chamber has inoculation part at top. Five of the chambers have both substrate and detection disk; other five have combination substrate-detection disk. Strip is sealed during incubation.	Voges-Proskauer (production of acetoin) Nitrate reduction Phenylalanine deaminase H₂S production Indole production Ornithine decarboxylase Lysine decarboxylase Malonate utilization Urea hydrolysis Esculin hydrolysis Hydrolysis of ONPG Fermentation of: Arabinose Adonitol Inositol Sorbitol	A heavy suspension (McFarland no. 1 standard) is prepared from the colony to be identified. Each chamber is inoculated with 0.2 ml, and strip is then incubated in upright position. Care must be taken so the substrate strips are moistened but the five separate detection strips remain dry. After 5 hr of incubation, strip is rotated 90 degrees to moisten detection strips. Color reactions are read visually.	One of first ''rapid'' identification systems. Identification is based on constitutive enzyme activity and is not growth dependent. Numerous studies indicate >90% agreement with traditional methods.[2,58]
Minitek (BBL Systems, Inc.) (Figure 9-1)	This kit contains multiwelled plastic tray, 30 reagent disks, and assorted reagents and accessories.	Thirty substrate disks are included. Manufacturer suggests following for *Enterobacteriaceae:* Arginine Citrate Esculin H₂S Indole Lysine Malonate ONPG PDA Urea Voges-Proskauer test	Operator selects substrates to be tested and adds one disk to each of the 12 wells. Inoculum is prepared to density of McFarland no. 0.5 standard, and 50 µl is added to each well. Disks are overlaid with oil, and results are read using color comparison chart after 18 to 24 hr of incubation.	>90% agreement with conventional systems. System can be used for nonfermenters and anaerobes, as well as *Enterobacteriaceae.*
Microdilution identification systems (see text for discussion)	All microdilution products have capability for identification of *Enterobacteriaceae*, as well as other organisms. Substrates are included in trays either dried or frozen. Panels for identification only or combination identification-antimicrobial susceptibility panels are available (see text).	Most microdilution products include 20 tests similar to those in API 20E strip. There are minor differences.	Standardized inoculum is added either in very small quantity (3 to 5 µl) with disposable multipronged inoculator or as 50 to 100 µl aliquot with semiautomated inoculation device.	>90% agreement with traditional methods. One advantage is combination with antimicrobial susceptibility test.

Continued.

TABLE 9-1. Commercially Available Kits for the Identification of *Enterobacteriaceae*—cont'd

Product Name	Description	Substrate/Test	Operation	Comments

Enteric-Tek (Flow Laboratories)	Unlike most kits described, Enteric-Tek is a compartmented wheel with central well and 11 surrounding wedge-shaped chambers containing agar media. Fourteen tests can be performed with one wheel.	Indole production
		Tryptophan-deaminase
		H_2S production
		Citrate utilization
		Malonate utilization
		Lysine decarboxylase
		Ornithine decarboxylase
		Urea hydrolysis
		Fermentation of:
		  Glucose
		  Lactose
		  Rhamnose
		  Adonitol
		  Sorbitol
		  Arabinose
			One drop of inoculum is added to each chamber with Pasteur pipette. To provide anaerobic conditions, medium in central well and lysine and ornithine wells should be stabbed. Wheel is incubated right side up for 18 hr at 35° C. Color changes are noted. Spot indole test can be performed from center well.	Agreement is >90% with conventional methods.

Quantum II (Abbott Labs)	This is multipurpose instrumental system using plastic cartridge containing 20 chambers and dual wavelength photometer.	Lysine decarboxylase
		Ornithine decarboxylase
		Urea hydrolysis
		Citrate utilization
		Malonate utilization
		Arginine dihydrolase
		Indole production
		Growth in acetamide
		Polymixin B susceptibility
		Fermentation of:
		  Lactose
		  Arabinose
		  Xylose
		  Adonitol
		  Rhamnose
		  Sucrose
		  Glucose
		  Inositol
		  Mannitol
		  Sorbitol
			Four or five isolated colonies are suspended in sterile H_2O and adjusted to McFarland no. 0.5 standard; 200 μl of inoculum is added to each chamber. Chamber is sealed and incubated for 4 to 5 hr before reading.	Murray and co-workers[107] indicated that Quantum II correctly identified 97% of 492 isolates of *Enterobacteriaceae* and 83.3% of 40 oxidase-positive gram-negative bacilli.

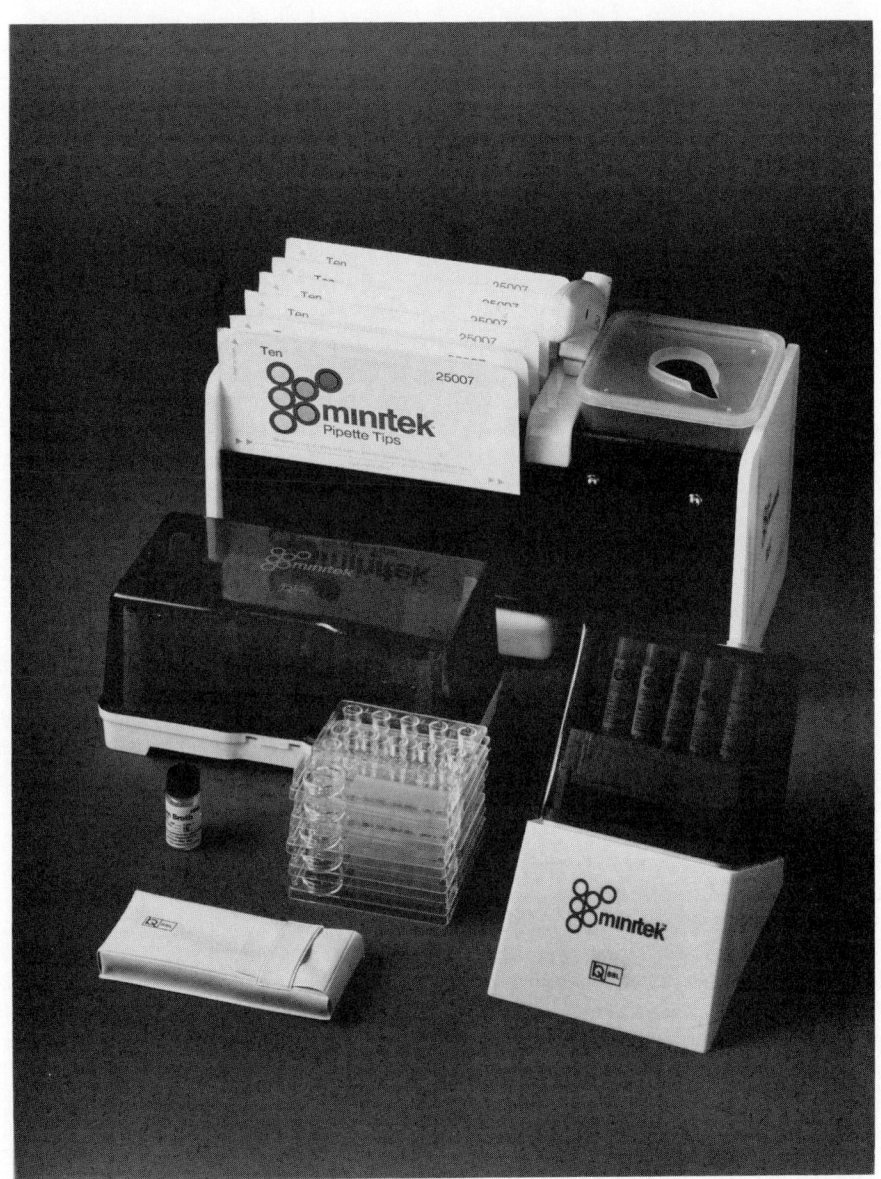

FIGURE 9-1. Minitek System. (Courtesy BBL Microbiology Systems, Division of Becton Dickinson & Co., Cockeysville, Md.)

tosidase. The assimilation tests determine the ability of the organism to grow in the presence of the following single sources of carbon: D-glucose, L-arabinose, D-mannose, D-mannitol, *N*-acetyl-D-glucosamine, maltose, D-gluconate, caprate, adipate, L-malate, citrate, and phenylacetate.

An oxidase test is performed on the test organism, and a suspension of the organism is prepared in sterile saline to yield the turbidity of a McFarland no. 0.5 standard. This suspension is used to inoculate the eight enzymatic cupules. The inoculum for the assimilation tests is prepared by adding 4 drops of the suspension to a vial of auxotrophic medium supplied by the manufacturer. After inoculation of the assimilation cupules, the strip is incubated for 24 hours at 30° C. Reagents are added to specific tests, and based on color changes in the enzymatic cupules and the presence of turbidity in the assimilation cupules, a seven-digit code number is generated. Identification is achieved with the API code book or with the extended computer service available from the company. If the isolate cannot be identified, the strip is incubated for an additional 24 hours.

IDENTIFICATION OF STREPTOCOCCI AND STAPHYLOCOCCI

Most of the commercially available systems for identifying the streptococci are immunologic; that is, they detect the Lancefield group antigens (A, B, C, D, F, and G). These systems are discussed in Chapter 13. The commercially available biochemical systems include the API 20S (Analytab Products, Inc., Plainview, N.Y.), Rapid Strep (API Systems, S.A., France), the RapID STR system (Innovative Diagnostic Systems, Inc., Atlanta, Ga.), and the Gram-Positive Identification Card, which is used with the AutoMicrobic system discussed below.

The API 20S system, a miniaturized conventional biochemical and chromogenic substrate strip, determines the following 20 parameters: hydrolysis of hippurate; hydrolysis of indoxyl acetate; hydrolysis of esculin; utilization of arginine; fermentation of mannitol, sorbitol, glycerol, sorbose, raffinose, lactose, sucrose, and trehalose; and enzymatic activities of beta-glucosidase, *N*-acetyl-beta-D-glucosaminidase, beta-galactosidase, alkaline phosphatase, pyroglutamic acid arylamidase, and leucine, arginine, and serine aminopeptidases. These 20 reactions plus hemolysis on sheep blood agar classify streptococci as *S. pyogenes* (Lancefield group A), *S. agalactiae* (Lancefield group B), beta-hemolytic streptococci groups C, F, or G, enterococci (*Enterococcus* spp.), group D nonenterococci, viridans streptococci, *S. pneumoniae, S. avium,* and *Aerococcus*. A suspension of the test organism equivalent to that of a McFarland no. 1 standard is prepared in 0.85% saline, and 2 or 3 drops is used to fill each cupule. The tray is incubated for 4 hours at 35° C in a non-CO$_2$ incubator. Based on color changes, a seven-digit number is generated by the user and the identification is determined by use of the manufacturer's code book.

Keville and Doern[85] tested 96 strains by the API 20S system compared with Streptex and Serostat, which are latex agglutination tests for the streptococcal group antigen (see Chapter 13). The results of the three tests were compared with the Lancefield precipitin test. The API 20S system correctly categorized 92.7% of the isolates as compared with 92% with the latex agglutination reagents. A disadvantage of the API 20S strip was that it had to be incubated for 4 hours, whereas the

immunologic tests could be read within a few minutes after antigen extraction.

Appelbaum[7] and Facklam[47] and their co-workers have compared the API 20S system and the AutoMicrobic Gram Positive Identification Card (GPI) for the identification of streptococci. Appelbaum and associates[7] reported that both systems provided accurate identification of groups A and B streptococci, with API providing the highest accuracy (100%), but were considerably less satisfactory for the identification of groups C, F, and G streptococci. Both systems were quite effective in identifying *Enterococcus* spp., but supplemental tests were needed for accurate identification of group D nonenterococci. The identification rate of the viridans streptococci varied depending on the species tested (that is, some species were identified more accurately than others) and the use of supplemental tests. In Facklam's study[47] the API 20S system identified 84% (190 of 226 strains) of 10 species of viridans streptococci, but supplemental tests were required to identify 49% (110 of the 226 strains). According to Facklam, the GPI system identified 79% of the same viridans streptococci without supplemental testing. Appelbaum reported that the API 20S identified 12.6% of the viridans species without the use of supplemental tests while the GPI identified 57.2% of these organisms without supplemental testing. Using the API 20S, Facklam identified 82% of 92 strains of *S. pneumoniae* with 10 strains requiring supplemental testing, and Appelbaum identified 53.9% of *S. pneumoniae* without supplemental tests. The GPI identified 80.8% of *S. pneumoniae* in one study[7] and 84% in another[47] without the use of supplemental tests.

The Rapid Strep may be used for the identification of streptococci after 4 hours or 24 hours of incubation. This system consists of a strip of 20 cupules that determine the activities of several enzymes or chromogenic substrates or the fermentation of several carbohydrates. Included are tests for the production of acetoin, hydrolysis of hippurate, determination of the enzymatic activities of beta-glucosidase, pyrrolidonyl arylamidase, alpha-galactosidase, beta-glucuronidase, beta-galactosidase, alkaline phosphatase, leucine arylamidase, and arginine dihydrolase and fermentation of ribose, L-arabinose, mannitol, sorbitol, lactose, trehalose, inulin, raffinose, starch, and glycogen. A subculture of the test organism on blood agar that has been incubated anaerobically at 35° C for 18 to 20 hours is used to prepare a dense suspension (greater than a McFarland no. 4 standard) for inoculation of the strip. After incubation for 4 hours a seven-digit profile number is generated by the user and compared with those in a code book for identification of the isolate. If the isolate cannot be identified after 4 hours' incubation, the strip is reincubated overnight. The manufacturer suggests serogrouping to confirm the identities of *S. pyogenes, S. agalactiae, S. equisimilis,* and group G streptococci. Facklam, Rhoden, and Smith[46] found the Rapid Strep system to identify accurately nearly all the beta-hemolytic streptococci found in human infections when used in conjunction with serogrouping. The system also identified 95% of group D nonenterococci, 98% of *Enterococcus* spp., 90% of *S. pneumoniae,* and 60% of aerococci. The Rapid Strep correctly identified 85% of the most frequently occurring species of viridans streptococci but only 10% of the less frequent species.

The recently introduced RapID STR system is claimed to represent a worthwhile advance in the identification of group D and viridans streptococci.[9]

The API Staph-Ident (Analytab Products, Inc.), used for the

identification of clinically significant staphylococci, determines the following 10 parameters: production of acid from mannose, mannitol, trehalose, and salicin; utilization of arginine and urea; and presence of the enzymes alkaline phosphatase, beta-glucosidase, beta-glucuronidase, and beta-galactosidase. Similarly the API Staph Trac (API Systems, S.A., France) identifies the clinically significant staphylococci and also differentiates staphylococci from micrococci on the basis of tests for acid production from glucose, fructose, mannose, maltose, lactose, trehalose, mannitol, xylitol, melibiose, raffinose, xylose, saccharose, alpha-methylglucoside, and *N*-acetylglucosamine, as well as the utilization of arginine and urea, reduction of nitrate to nitrite, and production of alkaline phosphatase and acetylmethylcarbinol. The inoculum for the Staph-Ident system is prepared in 0.85% saline to the turbidity of a McFarland no. 3 standard, whereas that of the Staph Trac is prepared in Staph Trac inoculation medium to the turbidity of a McFarland no. 0.5 standard. The Staph-Ident provides identification 5 hours after incubation at 35° C, and the Staph Trac requires 24 hours' incubation. With both systems a profile number is generated and identification is accomplished with the aid of the accompanying manufacturer's code book or the extended API computer service.

Kloos and Wolfshohl[86] found excellent agreement (greater than 90%) between Staph-Ident and conventional systems. They suggested the addition of a test for novobiocin susceptibility to increase the accuracy of identification of *S. saprophyticus*. In another study[55] the Staph Trac correctly identified 88.3% of nine species of coagulase-negative staphylococci when compared with the conventional methods of Kloos and Schleifler (see Chapter 12).

The microtitration identification systems (Sceptor, Micro-Scan, Micro Media, Sensititre) have gram-positive identification panels for staphylococci and streptococci. AutoMicrobic System (AMS, Vitek, Hazelwood, Mo.) also has a gram-positive identification card. These systems are discussed later in the chapter.

Several latex agglutination tests are available for the identification of *Staphylococcus aureus*. These kits, which provide an effective substitute for tube coagulase testing, are discussed in Chapter 12.

IDENTIFICATION OF ANAEROBIC BACTERIA

Details of anaerobic culture techniques are reviewed in Chapter 20. A variety of commercial kits are marketed for the detection and identification of anaerobic bacteria. Usually they provide both small and large laboratories with a standardized method for identification of anaerobic bacteria without resorting to homemade prereduced media. However, Gram staining of fluids or tissue potentially infected with anaerobic bacteria may yield the most rapid results; since many anaerobic bacteria have distinctive morphologies, their presence in specimens can readily be detected even though the precise identification of the organism may not yet be apparent. Commercially available fluorescent antibody reagents are also available for *Bacteroides fragilis* and *Bacteroides melaninogenicus* group. These are discussed in Chapter 20.

Allen[3] reported on rapid identification systems for anaerobic bacteria. Until recently the two commercial kits most widely used were the API 20A and the Minitek system (BBL Systems, Inc., Cockeysville, Md.). Minitek uses paper disks that are impregnated with various biochemical substrates. The user

chooses the desired substrates. The API system has 16 carbohydrate-containing cupules and four cupules containing gelatin, esculin, urea, and indole. The API cupules are inoculated with a heavy inoculum (McFarland no. 1 standard) and incubated in an anaerobic jar or chamber for 24 to 48 hours. The API system has been evaluated by a number of investigators,[65,109,141] and agreement with traditional methods has ranged from 71% to 99%. Similarly, the Minitek system has been compared with conventional methods,[56,66,140,146] and agreement has ranged from 95% to 100%. Hansen, Cassoria, and Martin[65] reported that 68% of clinical isolates were identified with API 20A using the profile index and about 50% of the isolates with the Minitek system that did not have a numerical identification manual. Most investigators have found that these kits must be supplemented with other tests. Moore, Sutter, and Finegold[104] tested 130 anaerobic isolates using the API 20A, the Virginia Polytechnic Institute PRAS system, and a conventional system that used a thioglycolate base supplemented with hemin and vitamin K_1. Agreement between all systems was 80%. API 20A agreed with the conventional system 91% of the time and with PRAS 85% of the time. The conventional system and the PRAS agreed with each other 85% of the time.

Beaucage and Onderdonk[20] tested the PRAS II system (Scott Laboratories, Fiskeville, R.I.) for the identification of anaerobic bacteria. The PRAS II system consists of prereduced tubed media, a colony picker that allows the technologist to remove a colony from the plate and directly inoculate the broth, a calibrated syringe for dispensing liquid cultures into the tubed media, and a pH microelectrode for measuring fermentation of carbohydrates as a function of acid production. No gas cannula is necessary. In Beaucage and Onderdonk's study the overall correlation with the standard prereduced tube method was 96.4%.

The AN-IDENT (Analytab Products, Plainview, N.Y.) and RapID ANA (Innovative Diagnostic Systems, Inc., Atlanta, Ga.) have recently been introduced for the identification of anaerobes. These systems provide identification in 4 hours based on the utilization of chromogenic substrates by constitutive enzymes present in heavy inocula.

The AN-IDENT determines the following 21 biochemical reactions: indole production, utilization of arginine, catalase activity, hydrolysis of indoxyl acetate, and activity of the enzymes *N*-acetyglucosaminidase, alpha-glucosidase, alpha-arabinosidase, beta-glucosidase, alpha-fucosidase, phosphatase, alpha-galactosidase, beta-galactosidase, leucine aminopeptidase, proline aminopeptidase, pyroglutamic acid arylamidase, tyrosine aminopeptidase, arginine aminopeptidase, alanine aminopeptidase, histidine aminopeptidase, phenylalanine aminopeptidase, and glycine aminopeptidase. An inoculum of the test organism is prepared in sterile distilled water to the density of a McFarland no. 5 standard. Two drops of the suspension is inoculated into each cupule, and the strip is placed in a covered plastic tray and incubated in air at 35° C for 4 hours. After appropriate reagents are added to selected cupules, a numerical profile number is generated based on color changes of the substrates and identification is determined from the AN-IDENT Analytical Profile Index.

The RapID ANA determines 18 biochemical reactions: indole production, utilization of arginine, fermentation of trehalose, reduction of triphenyltetrazolium, and activity of the enzymes phosphatase, *N*-acetyl-glucosaminidase, beta-galactosidase, alpha-glucosidase, beta-glucosidase, alpha-fucosidase, alpha-galactosidase, leucine aminopeptidase, proline aminopeptidase, serine aminopeptidase, arginine aminopeptidase, phenylalanine aminopeptidase, glycine aminopeptidase, and pyrrolidonyl aminopeptidase. A suspension of the test organism is prepared in the inoculation fluid provided by the manufacturer and adjusted to the turbidity of a McFarland no. 3 standard. The suspension is poured into the tray, which is tilted to permit distribution of the inoculum. After incubation for 4 hours at 35° C in air, appropriate reagents are added to selected tests. Based on color changes of the substrates, a six-digit biotype number is generated and used to identify the isolate from the RapID Code Compendium.

Studies of both of these systems have been favorable,[5,27,108] although one study shows the accuracy and reproducibility of RapID ANA to be laboratory dependent.[5] Both systems are able to identify the majority of isolates of *Bacteroides* and *Clostridium* spp., nonsporeforming bacilli, and anaerobic cocci.[27,108] Some of the microdilution systems discussed below may also be used for identification of anaerobic bacteria.

The API ZYM system has been used in research laboratories for the identification of anaerobic bacteria.[100]

IDENTIFICATION OF *NEISSERIA*

Commercially available identification systems for pathogenic *Neisseria* spp. include the Minitek (BBL Microbiology Systems, Cockeysville, Md.), Gonochek II (E.I. DuPont de Nemours & Co., Wilmington, Del.), RIM-N (American MicroScan, Mahwah, N.J.), and the RapID NH (Innovative Diagnostics, Atlanta, Ga.).

The Minitek system discussed previously uses the carbohydrate fermentation patterns of glucose, maltose, sucrose, and lactose to differentiate among the various *Neisseria* spp. If a heavy inoculum is used, 91% of the isolates can be identified with 98% accuracy in 4 hours.

The Gonochek II differentiates *Neisseria gonorrhoeae, Neisseria meningitidis, Neisseria lactamica,* and *Branhamella catarrhalis.* This system is a single tube containing three chromogenic substrates that permit the detection of mutually exclusive enzymes in these organisms. A suspension of the test organism is prepared in 4 drops of distilled water and then added to the Gonochek tube. The tube is incubated for 30 minutes at 37° C. *N. lactamica* produces the enzyme beta-galactosidase, which hydrolyzes the substrate beta-D-galactoside to produce a blue color. *N. meningitidis* produces the enzyme gamma-glutamyl-*p*-aminopeptidase, which hydrolyzes gamma-glutamyl-*p*-nitroanilide to produce a yellow color. The prolyl aminopeptidase enzyme produced by *N. gonorrhoeae* hydrolyzes beta-napthyl amino acid derivative to release a free beta-napthylamine derivative that forms a pink color on the addition of E-Y 20 reagent (a diazonium salt) provided with the kit. A beta-lactamase tube is also included with the kit to detect penicillinase-producing *N. gonorrhoeae* (see Chapter 14).

Several studies have found the Gonochek II system to be a rapid, reliable, easily performed procedure for the identification of pathogenic *Neisseria* organisms.[25,76,124,153] Because a small inoculum (five to 10 colonies) is required, the test can frequently be performed from the primary isolation medium, thus saving the laboratory both time and money.[76,153]

The RIM-N system differentiates *N. gonorrhoeae, N. meningitidis, N. lactamica, N. mucosa, N. sicca, N. subflava,* and *Branhamella catarrhalis* on the basis of their carbohydrate utilization patterns. The system, which depends on the presence of preformed enzymes, uses a large inoculum and a small amount of substrate. A loopful of the test organism is inoculated into microtubes containing 3 drops of 2% solutions of glucose, maltose, sucrose, or lactose plus a substrate blank containing no carbohydrate. The tubes are mixed on a Vortex for 10 seconds and incubated in air at 35° C for 1 hour. A change in the phenol red indicator from red-pink to yellow or yellow-orange indicates acid production. Provided certain precautions are followed, the RIM-N system is a rapid method for identification of *Neisseria* spp.[54,76]

The RapID NH system uses conventional and single substrate chromogenic tests for the identification of *N. gonorrhoeae, N. meningitidis,* and *N. lactamica.* The system differentiates these organisms from other *Neisseria* spp., *Moraxella* spp., *B. catarrhalis,* CDC M groups, and *Kingella* spp. As discussed in the following section, the system may also be used for the identification of *Haemophilus* spp.

This 4-hour method uses the following tests: hydrolysis of phosphate, hydrolysis of an *o*-nitrophenyl-beta-D-galactopyranoside, nitrate reduction, resazurin reduction, proline aminopeptidase activity, gamma-glutamyl aminopeptidase activity, utilization of glucose and sucrose, production of indole from tryptophan, hydrolysis of urea, and ornithine decarboxylation. The test kit includes inoculation fluid in which a heavy suspension (McFarland no. 3 standard) of test organism is prepared. The suspension is mixed and added to a designated area of the plastic test panel. The panel is tilted to distribute the inoculum to all the wells and then incubated for 4 hours at 35° C. A code book is used to identify the isolate. Studies have shown the RapID NH to be 90% to 100% accurate for the identification of *N. gonorrhoeae, N. meningitidis,* and *N. lactamica.*[124,128]

IDENTIFICATION OF *HAEMOPHILUS*

The RapID NH system includes a data base for the differentiation of *Haemophilus influenzae, H. haemolyticus, H. ducreyi, H. parainfluenzae, H. aphrophilus,* and *H. paraphrophilus. H. influenzae* and *H. parainfluenzae* may also be biotyped on the basis of the indole, urease, and ornithine decarboxylase reactions (see Chapter 15). Doern and Chapin[39] reported that this system correctly identified 89.8% of clinical isolates of *H. influenzae.* According to these investigators, however, the inoculum size required for the test invariably required an overnight subculture of isolates recovered on the primary isolation medium.

Other rapid commercially available systems for the identification of *Haemophilus* spp. include RIM-H (Austin Biological Laboratories, Inc., Austin, Tex.) and HNID (American MicroScan, Campbell, Calif.). These are discussed by Fenn and Matsen.[49]

IDENTIFICATION OF YEASTS

Several commercial products are available for the identification of yeasts. With the exception of the exoantigen tests (see Chapter 38), few methods have been developed for the rapid identification of fungi other than yeasts. Systems available for yeasts include the API 20C (Analytab Products), the Uni-Yeast Tek System (Flow Laboratories), Minitek (BBL), the Microdrop System (Clinical Sciences), Microstix (Ames Co.), AMS (Vitek), Autobac (Organon Teknika), and MS-2 (Abbott). The last three systems are discussed later in the chapter.

The API 20C consists of 20 cupules that determine the assimilation of a variety of carbohydrates. The Uni-Yeast Tek system consists of three screening tubes and a circular plate similar to that of the Uni N/F system. The screening tubes include the CN screen for *Cryptococcus neoformans,* the GBE tube for germ tube production, and the SAM tube for sucrose assimilation. The test isolate is first inoculated to the GBE tube. If the findings are positive, the SAM tube is inoculated. If they are negative, the Uni-Yeast Tek plate is inoculated; this plate determines urea hydrolysis, morphology on cornmeal agar, nitrate reduction, and assimilation of several carbohydrates. If the identity cannot be determined with the Uni-Yeast Tek plate, the CN screen is inoculated. Evaluations of the API 20C and Uni-Yeast Tek system are discussed later in the chapter.

The Minitek system with the impregnated reagent disks can also be used for carbon assimilation studies. The Minitek requires approximately 3 days for completion, compared with 24 days for the traditional Wickerham method.

Ames Microstix has been clinically evaluated by Tilton, Kenney, and Corcoran.[144] It consists of a pad of cellulose containing dehydrated Nickerson medium and alginate at the end of a clear plastic strip. The pad is moistened, and then the swab containing the specimen is rolled on the specimen. If *Candida* spp. are present, the bismuth indicator in Nickerson medium turns brown. In the study by Tilton and co-workers, 82% of patients who showed yeasts on culture also had positive results with this screening product. A positive result should be followed up by a complete mycologic examination.

The Microdrop Kit (Clinical Sciences, Whippany, N.J.) includes test reagents for the fermentation and assimilation of 12 carbohydrates, urea, and nitrate utilization. Included also in the kit are vials of yeast identification agar that are melted and distributed evenly along with the yeast inoculum in the reaction plates. One drop of a test reagent is added to each agar-filled well, and the plate is incubated at ambient temperature for 48 hours. Several studies have compared the API 20, Microdrop, and the Uni-Yeast Tek systems with conventional fermentation and assimilation methods.[21,32,36,89] Uni-Yeast Tek agreed 99% of the time, API 94%, and Microdrop 84%. Some reports suggest that the Uni-Yeast Tek system is the easiest to use and requires the least amount of a technologist's time.

An additional study evaluated 239 yeasts with the Abbott Quantum II system (distinct from the Abbott MS-2).[130] Quantum II proved to be 92% accurate in identification of common isolates such as *Candida albicans* and *Torulopsis glabrata* but only 73% effective for the less frequently encountered yeasts such as *Trichosporon beigelii.*

RAPID CONVENTIONAL TESTS

The conventional tests that have historically been used in clinical microbiology and that are discussed throughout the text and in Appendix A are based on the metabolism of a wide variety of substrates. Although many conventional tests take up to 48 hours or even longer for completion, several conventional tests may be used in combination with colonial morphology and microscopic examination to provide presumptive identification of isolates within minutes to hours. A number of these, such as catalase, oxidase, coagulase, bile solubility, and the germ tube test, are discussed throughout the text.

Several modifications have been made in other conventional

tests to provide more rapid results. As seen in Appendix A, many conventional tests are now available as reagent-impregnated paper disks or strips. Other conventional tests have been modified by increasing the inoculum, decreasing the concentration of substrate, or increasing the sensitivity of the reagents to provide more rapid results. For example, Barry[12] suggests the use of three screening tests to identify the common gram-negative bacilli (Figure 9-2). These organisms, *Escherichia coli, Klebsiella* spp., and *Enterobacter* spp., are prompt lactose fermenters and appear as pink or red colonies on MacConkey agar (see Chapter 16 and Appendix A). (Procedures for these tests are included in Appendix A.) Organisms that demonstrate the reactions in Figure 9-2 can be reported with confidence, since variations are relatively uncommon.

A rapid spot indole test may be used in conjunction with colonial morphology for the rapid identification of *E. coli.*[148] This test may be performed by rubbing a loopful of a well-isolated colony on a piece of filter paper saturated with a solution of 1% *p*-dimethylaminobenzaldehyde or *p*-dimethylaminocinnamaldehyde in 10% hydrochloric acid.[97] A positive finding with the *p*-dimethylaminobenzaldehyde reagent is a red color, whereas a bluish green color is a positive result with the *p*-dimethylaminocinnamaldehyde reagent. Studies have shown that the indole spot test can correctly identify approximately 97.5% of colonies of *E. coli,* which appear as flat, dry, rapid lactose fermenters on MacConkey agar.[69,118]

Use of screening tests such as these allows rapid and efficient identification of the most commonly isolated pathogens and permits concentration of the laboratory's resources (such as funds and technologists' time) for identification of the atypical and less common pathogens.[12] When selecting a screening test the microbiologist must weigh the advantages of speed and efficiency against the possibility of misidentification.[12] Rapid screening tests must be designed to recognize those isolates that require additional testing.[12]

SEMIAUTOMATED/AUTOMATED SYSTEMS FOR IDENTIFICATION AND ANTIMICROBIAL SUSCEPTIBILITY TESTING

During the last few years several automated systems have been developed for identification, antimicrobial susceptibility testing, and in some cases urine screening. These systems, including the Autobac (Organon Teknika, Durham, N.C.), MS-2 (Abbott Labs, Irving, Tex.), AutoMicrobic (Vitek Systems, Hazelwood, Mo.), Aladin (Analytab Products, Plainview, N.Y.), and several microdilution systems specified later in the chapter, actually represent a spectrum of automation. The AutoMicrobic and the Aladin are truly automated in that the user adds inoculum to a disposable cassette or tray and all other procedures including incubation, test reading and interpretation, and reporting are performed by the machine. The MS-2 and Autobac are more appropriately referred to as semiautomated, since the user intervenes during the test process. The microdilution systems, like the miniaturized systems previously discussed, may be read visually without an instrument or may use semiautomated readers such as the Sensititre system or the AutoScan 4. One system, MicroScan (Baxter MicroScan Division, Sacramento, Calif.), is fully automated; as with the Aladin and AMS, once the microtiter plate is placed in the machine, all subsequent processes are automatically performed without further input from the technologist.

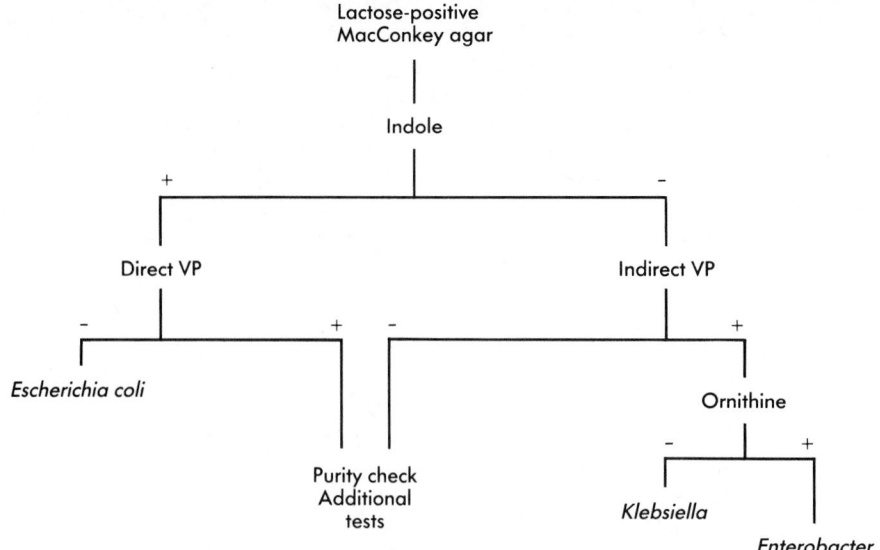

FIGURE 9-2. Flowchart for presumptive identification of prompt lactose-fermenting common gram-negative bacilli. (From Barry, A.L.: Clin. Lab. Med. **5**:3, 1985.)

TABLE 9-2. Biochemicals in MS-2 Identification Cartridges

Chamber Number	Active Substance	Reaction
1	Glucose	Fermentation
2	Lysine hydrochloride	Decarboxylation
3	Ornithine hydrochloride	Decarboxylation
4	Sodium citrate	Utilization
5	Sodium malonate	Utilization
6	Esculin	Hydrolysis
7	Urea	Hydrolysis
8	Adonitol	Fermentation
9	L-Arabinose	Fermentation
10	L-Inositol	Fermentation
11	Lactose	Fermentation
12	Mannitol	Fermentation
13	L-Rhamnose	Fermentation
14	Sorbitol	Fermentation
15	Sucrose	Fermentation
16	D-Xylose	Fermentation
17	Empty	
18	L-Tryptophan	Indole production
19	Empty	
20	Empty	

The Autobac and MS-2 systems were initially designed for rapid antimicrobial susceptibility testing and the AMS for primary urine microbiology. The work of Bauer and associates[18] in the 1960s and the subsequent development of the now classic Bauer-Kirby disk diffusion test set the stage for much of the work on both rapid and automated antimicrobial susceptibility testing. The progenitor of the present susceptibility test instruments was the Technicon TAAS system,[72] which used an electronic counter to count microbial particles. Although this instrument was never sold commercially, it was a conceptual basis for later instruments.

Although the instruments discussed in the following sections have the capabilities for both antimicrobial susceptibility and identification, laboratories frequently elect to use only one of these capabilities. Each function must be evaluated independently in terms of its accuracy, reproducibility, and ability to fit within the laboratory's workflow.

MS-2

The MS-2 instrument consists of an analysis module, a control module, and a disk dispenser-sealer. The disk dispenser-sealer is used only with the antimicrobial susceptibility function. The analysis module is an electro-optical scanning device and an incubator shaker. The electro-optical system consists of diodes and matched photo detectors that determine growth photometrically (that is, by changes in light transmission). The analysis module has eight positions; only position 8 is used for antimicrobial susceptibility testing and urine screening. The control module is essentially a computer data-processing center that receives, stores, and reports the readings from the analysis module.

The bacterial identification cartridge is a disposable plastic cassette containing 20 optically clear chambers (Table 9-2). Lyophilized biochemical substrates are incorporated in 17 of the chambers and, with one exception, include indicators that change color in response to the metabolic reactions of the bacteria.

Table 9-2 lists the biochemicals in the MS-2 identification cartridges and their reactions. The initial three-laboratory collaborative evaluation[102] of the MS-2 system for the *Enterobacteriaceae* indicated that on 150 coded organisms the system was 97%, 98%, and 93% accurate, respectively, in the three laboratories. It was 94% accurate compared with the conventional tube methods in identifying over 1000 clinical isolates of 26 species of the *Enterobacteriaceae.*

A yeast identification cartridge is also marketed for the MS-2 system.[31,33] This cartridge contains 17 substrates in individual wells for the assimilation of carbon sources using a yeast nitrogen-based medium. Urea, nitrate, and growth on *p*-hydroxybenzoic acid are also included in the cuvette. Additional tests used in conjunction with the MS-2 yeast cartridge include the germ tube test, chlamydoconidia production, presence of pseudohyphae, arthroconidia produced on cornmeal polysorbate agar, and india ink. The yeast cartridge is incubated for 24 hours. One hundred and sixty-five isolates were tested in parallel with the MS-2 and the Uni-Yeast Tek. In the initial phase of the study 95% of the isolates were correctly identified. In the second phase, in which an additional 165 clinical isolates were examined, 90% were correctly identified with the MS-2. Discrepancies were noted with some strains of *Candida albicans* and *Candida tropicalis.* The combined agreement in the two phases of the study was 93%.

For susceptibility testing the MS-2 system uses a special cuvette that consists of 11 upper growth chambers and 11 lower chambers in which the individual susceptibility tests are run (one of the lower chambers is a growth control). Filter paper disks containing antimicrobial agents are automatically dispensed and sealed into the lower chambers using the disk dispenser-sealer. Broth and a standardized inoculum of the test organism are added to the upper chambers. After appropriate specimen data are entered into the computer, the cuvettes are placed in the analysis module, which photometrically monitors the organism's growth and records it at 5-minute intervals. The inoculum in the MS-2 system is not exposed to the antimicrobial agent until the early logarithmic growth phase. This is accomplished by allowing the organism to grow in the upper part of the cartridge before being automatically distributed into the lower disk-containing chambers. When the culture shows a clean-cut increase in optical density (indicative of logarithmic growth), it is automatically transferred into the 11 lower chambers by introducing pulses of air pressure into the upper chambers.[142] The antimicrobial agents are then eluted into the broth and readings are again taken at 5-minute intervals. With the MS-2 research model these data are plated and a growth curve for the individual isolates is constructed. In the clinical model the growth curves for each isolate are stored in the computer, one curve in the presence of an antimicrobial agent and one for the control without the agent. When a growth threshold is reached, the computer calculates the susceptibility or resistance to the antimicrobial agent based on comparison of the two growth curves. The MS-2 has the capability for reporting minimum inhibitory concentrations (MICs). In actual practice, however, only the MICs of those organism-antimicrobic pairs found to be ''indeterminate'' are reported.

More recently, Abbott Labs has marketed a second-generation MS-2 instrument known as the Avantage Microbiology Center. This system has a different computer system than the MS-2 system and offers more test capabilities. It also has data management and epidemiology capabilities.

AUTOBAC

The Autobac IDX instrument consists of a light-scattering, photometer module that also serves to standardize the initial inoculum, an incubator-shaker module, a disk-dispenser (for antimicrobial susceptibility testing), and a data terminal printer (Figure 9-3). This system differs from other instruments in that identification is based on selective growth inhibition by dyes, antimicrobics, and other substances rather than traditional biochemical tests. The instrument derives profiles of growth inhibition by analyzing light-scattering indexes (LSIs) of the test organism with a two-stage quadratic discriminate analysis; the LSI represents a comparison between the extent of growth in a cuvette chamber containing inhibitory agent and a control chamber containing no agent.[134] For example, Figure 9-4 shows two populations of organisms: A and B. Each strain is located in two-dimensional space by its LSI when exposed to two different inhibitory agents: I and J. Strain A8 yielded an LSI of 0.04 when challenged with inhibitory agent I and an LSI of 0.76 when challenged with agent J. As the ellipses show, the true groups A and B tend to cluster together. The two populations of organisms A and B are distributed normally. In Figure 9-5 these normal distributions are plotted. The ellipses represent levels of equal probability. For population A the center ellipse is the .30 probability ellipse. Thus the chance that a member of population A will fall outside of that ellipse is only 30%. Likewise, the chance is only 5% that a member of population A will fall outside of the outer ellipse. The unknown falls in the 5% level for group A and the 10% level for group B. It would be placed in group B because the probability level for that group is higher.

Before the Autobac IDX system is set up, supplementary test results must be entered into the computer. These include growth on a MacConkey agar plate, lactose fermentation and bile precipitation, a blood agar plate examined for the swarming growth of *Proteus* organisms, indole production, and the presence of oxidase. The standardized Autobac broth inoculum tube is attached to an 18-chamber Autobac cuvette that has been loaded with disks containing 18 inhibitory agents. The agents are acraflavine, brilliant green, cobalt chloride, cycloserine, 3,5-dibromosalycylic acid, dodecylamine hydrochloride, floxuridine, malachite green, methylene blue, omadine disulfide, sodium azide, thallous acetate, carbenicillin, cephalothin, colistin, kanamycin, novobiocin, and cycloserine. The cuvette is incubated for 3 hours and read. The computer identifies the organism as previously described. In addition to the primary plate data and the Autobac LSI data, the first- and second-choice identifications for this organism are printed. Associated with each choice is a relative probability value, which is a degree of certainty that the organism belongs to that particular group. Sielaff, Matsen, and McKie[133] reported that of 3726 strains tested, the Autobac system agreed with the conventional biochemical identification 88.4% of the time. Barry and coworkers[16] in a multicenter study, as well as Kelly and associates,[84] compared the Autobac system with standard reference methods for identifying glucose nonfermenters and glucose fermenters. The overall accuracy of the Autobac system was 95.3% in Barry's study and 95% in Kelly's study.

A plastic cuvette containing 13 chambers is used for susceptibility testing with the Autobac system (Figure 9-6). A single-strength antimicrobial disk is added to 12 of these chambers with the disk dispenser. A colony to be tested is suspended in broth, and the concentration adjusted to 1.5 to 3×10^7 CFU/ml

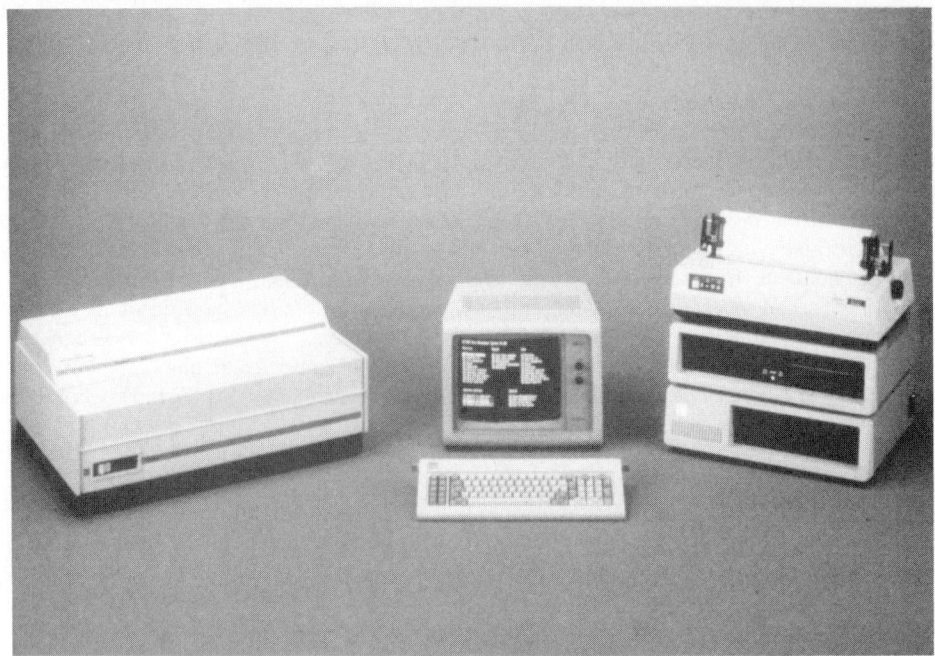

FIGURE 9-3. Autobac Series 2. (Courtesy Organon Teknika, Durham, N.C.)

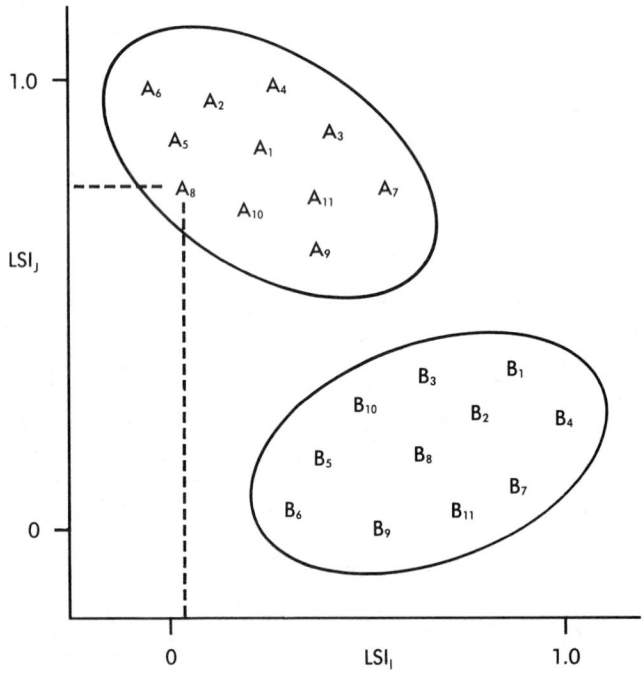

FIGURE 9-4. Bivariate representation of strains of two bacterial groups. (From Sielaff, B.H., Matsen, J.M., and McKie, J.E.: Rapid identification by use of growth inhibitor technology and nephelometry on the Autobac system. In Tilton, R.C., editor: Rapid methods and automation in microbiology, Washington, D.C., 1981, American Society for Microbiology.)

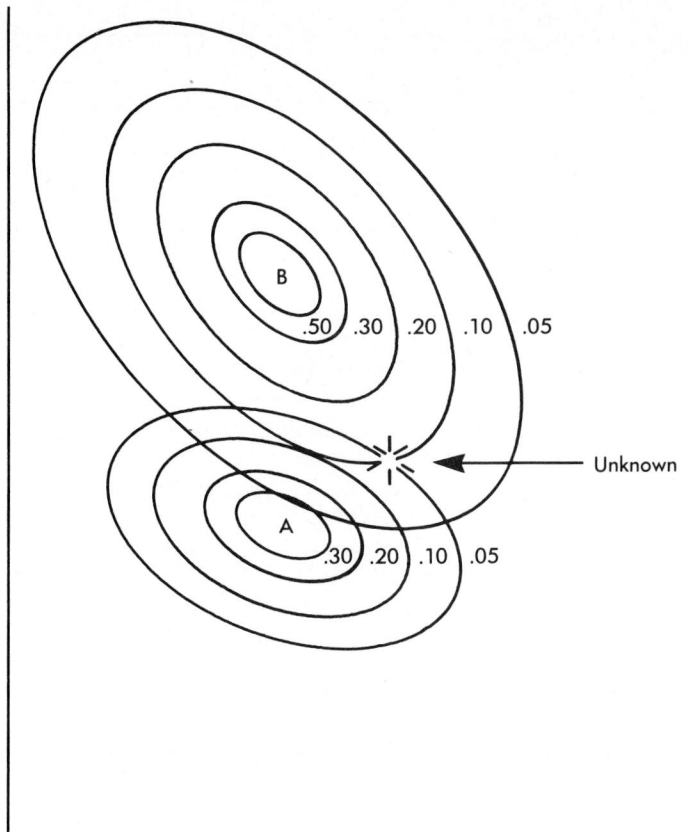

FIGURE 9-5. Equiprobability levels for two bivariate normal probability models. Unknown falls on 5% probability level for A and 10% level for B. Therefore unknown is assigned to B. (From Sielaff, B.H., Matsen, J.M., and McKie, J.E.: Rapid identification by use of growth inhibitor technology and nephelometry on the Autobac system. In Tilton, R.C., editor: Rapid methods and automation in microbiology, Washington, D.C., 1981, American Society for Microbiology.)

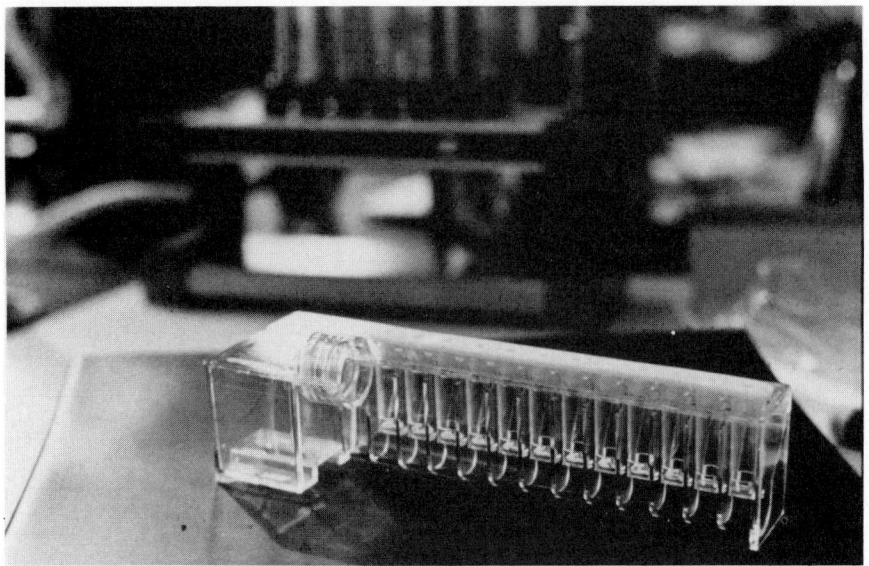

FIGURE 9-6. Cuvette used for susceptibility testing with Autobac system.

in the photometer module. After standardization the inoculum tube is screwed on to the cuvette. The inoculum is then distributed evenly in each of the 12 antimicrobic-containing chambers and the control growth chamber. The cuvette is placed in the incubator shaker for 3 hours at 35° C. The cuvette is then placed in the photometer for reading. The control well is read first. If the organisms have not undergone three division cycles, the cuvette is rejected. If they have achieved such growth, each successive chamber containing antimicrobics is read and the LSI of each chamber recorded. The LSI is compared with that of the control well, and a determination of susceptible, indeterminate, or resistant is printed out on the report ticket. The LSI scale is from 0 to 1.000: 0.5 signifies resistance, 0.5 to 0.6 indeterminate, and (with the exception of penicillin) greater than 0.6 susceptible. With penicillin an LSI of 0.9 or greater is considered susceptible.

More recently Organon Teknika has marketed the Autobac Series 2. This system has the same capabilities as the Autobac IDX, as well as data management capabilities.

AUTOMICROBIC SYSTEM

The AutoMicrobic system (AMS) is a highly automated system consisting of six modules: a diluent dispenser, vacuum card-filling module, card-sealing apparatus, reader-incubator, computer control module, and data terminal-printer. This system is capable of performing identification of gram-negative bacilli, gram-positive organisms, and yeasts; urine screening and identification; and determination of MICs.

The Enterobacteriaceae Biochemical Card (EBC) containing 30 reagents was originally used with the AMS for identification of members of the family *Enterobacteriaceae*. This card has now been replaced by the EBC+ card, which includes O-F dextrose, acetamide, and cetrimide and adds the capability of identification of some nonfermentative gram-negative rods. The EBC+ is more reproducible than the original EBC.[13] A standardized inoculum is prepared in a sample injector tube that is attached to a special strawlike holder inserted into the EBC+ card. This apparatus is placed in the vacuum card-filling module, and the substrates within the card are automatically reconstituted with the inoculum. The EBC card is then inserted into the reader-incubator module, which monitors microbial activity in the eight wells during an 8-hour incubation period. The data are accumulated and interpreted, and the organism's identification and the probability of a correct identification are printed out. A study of the EBC+ with 1743 clinical isolates in two laboratories showed the card to be quite satisfactory for the identification of the vast majority of isolates within 8 to 13 hours.[17] The investigators noted that it was difficult for the system to identify some hydrogen sulfide–negative strains of *Citrobacter freundii* and that *Pseudomonas cepacia* was often reported out nonspecifically; that is, several other organisms were misidentified as *P. cepacia*.

The use of the AutoMicrobic Gram Positive Identification Card for the identification of streptococci was discussed earlier in the chapter. Evaluations of the card for the identification of coagulase-negative staphylococci are discussed by Grasmick, Naito, and Bruckner[60] and Almeida, Jorgensen, and Johnson.[4] The AutoMicrobic Yeast Identification system is accurate and reliable and provides a substantial savings in setup and reporting time.[33,90,116]

A small, multiwelled plastic cassette is used for antimicro-

bial susceptibility testing with the AMS. Either single or multiple concentrations of antimicrobial agent are included in the small cassette. A standardized inoculum is drawn into the cassette by vacuum as discussed previously, and the cassette is placed in the reader-incubator module. The cassettes are read photometrically for growth at stated intervals. Differences between growth in the presence of antimicrobial agents and in the control wells are plotted by the computer, and an interpretive evaluation is printed as resistant, susceptible, or indeterminate. The computer in the AMS allows the user to choose whether susceptibility test results are interpreted as susceptible (S), indeterminant (I), or resistant (R); or as S, conditionally susceptible (CS), moderately resistant (MR), or R; or whether MICs are reported as serial twofold dilutions (2, 4, 8, and 16 μg/ml) or continuous values (4, 5, 6, 7, and 8 μg/ml). This MIC capability is especially useful for the aminoglycosides such as gentamicin in which the difference between toxic and therapeutic ranges is very narrow.

Cassettes for susceptibility testing of gram-positive and gram-negative organisms are available and have been evaluated.[83,110] Woolfrey, Lally, and Ederer[155] tested the AMS for its ability to detect methicillin-resistant *Staphylococcus aureus* (MRSA). The AMS failed to detect over 75% of these organisms; however, if gentamicin resistance was used as a marker for MRSA, the reliability of the AMS improved markedly. Woolfrey and co-workers[157] also evaluated the reliability of the AMS in testing resistance of *Pseudomonas aeruginosa* to aminoglycosides. They reported that the AMS does not give acceptable MIC results when compared with reference methods.

ALADIN SYSTEM

One of the newest instruments in development is the API Aladin system. Aladin is a totally automated instrument designed to read all UniScept products. UniScept is a trademark for a new group of miniaturized products from API. These products consist of microcupules of dehydrated substrates. Although the UniScept products have been reconfigured so they are physically compatible with Aladin, they may also be used as free-standing systems. The Aladin system is designed to inoculate, incubate, read, interpret, and dispose of all UniScept identification and susceptibility systems. At this time Aladin has not been approved by the Food and Drug Administration.

Aladin consists of a floor model reading device and an external IBM computer. The universal carrier promotes reliable movement of UniScept tests through the system. The universal carrier is a disposable plastic frame with dimensions of approximately 5 × 8⅝ inches.

The incubator module has a capacity of 60 universal carriers; since each carrier can contain an identification strip, susceptibility tray, and micro-MIC strip, the 60 carriers may be used for as many as 180 individual tests.

The reagent dispense station automatically dispenses up to 20 different liquid reagents into UniScept identification products. The system is preprogrammed for each UniScept product as to reagent type, volume, and cupules to be dispensed.

The Aladin disposal station is the final destination of all processed tests whose results have already been interpreted and stored in the computer's memory. Following interpretation of test results, processed tests are automatically placed into a biohazard bag for decontamination and disposal.

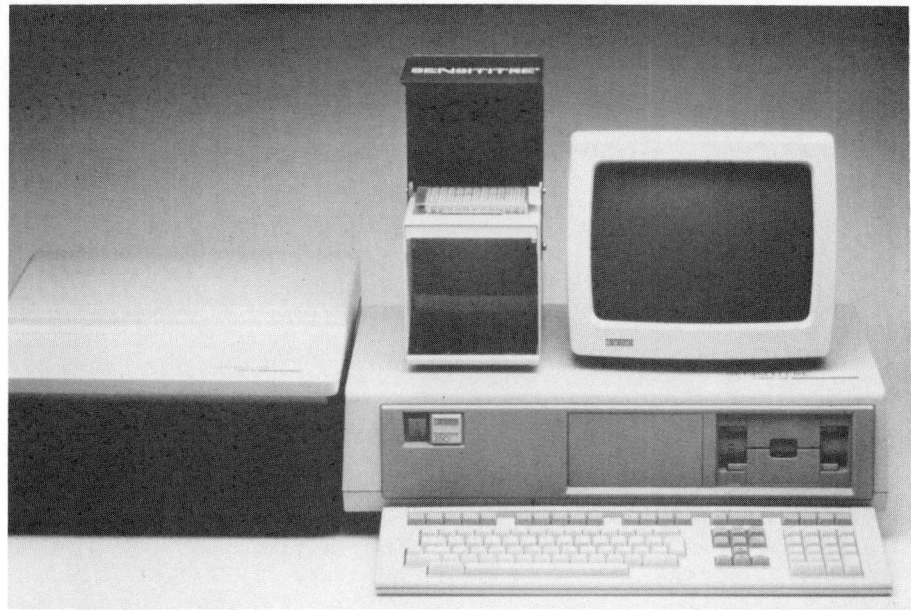

FIGURE 9-7. Sensititre microdilution system (Sensititre, Inc., Salem, N.H.).

The heart of the Aladin is its video image processor-read station. This is the first application of video image processing in the diagnostic microbiology industry; it is used to interpret colored biochemical reactions or turbidimetric growth patterns in susceptibility tests. Video image processing can be defined as a method of digitizing an image into a large matrix. Each matrix element is referred to as a pixel. Only those portions of the digital image that are of interest (such as microtiter wells and identification strip microcupules) are maintained in the image processor's memory; these are referred to as "areas of interest." Through software, areas of interest can be easily defined as to their size, shape, and position relative to one another.

• • •

The advantages of automated systems for bacterial identification include handling ease, speed of identification, and computer-stored data base. The microbiologist, however, is locked into a specific set of biochemical data. The MS-2, AMS, and Aladin base their identification on commonly used biochemical tests, but the Autobac uses an entirely different set of inhibitors not previously used in bacteriology.

Multiple evaluations, reviews, and collaborative comparisons of the AMS, MS-2, and Autobac have been reported.* The advantage of all the instruments is that they provide the laboratory with a standardized method for antimicrobial susceptibility testing and that test results are generally available 3 to 5 hours after the isolated colony is seen on an agar plate. At present the AMS is the most highly automated system available for microbiology. After initial preparation of the sample, no more of the technologist's time is required. However, AMS takes longer (4 to 10 hours) to process a specimen than either the Autobac or the MS-2 (3 to 6 hours). The Aladin promises rapid results and "hands-off" automation coupled with the capability of performing either standard MICs or "breakpoint"

MICs, that is, the testing of two or three antimicrobial agent concentrations at the breakpoints of S, I, and R.

MICRODILUTION AND AGAR DILUTION SYSTEMS[106]

Several microdilution systems are available for bacterial identification and antimicrobial susceptibility testing including MicroMedia System (MMS) (Microbiology Systems of Beckman Instruments, Carlsbad, Calif.), MicroScan (Baxter Micro-Scan Division, Sacramento, Calif.), Sensititre (Sensititre, Inc., Salem, N.H.) (Figure 9-7), Sceptor (BBL, Cockeysville, Md.) (Figure 9-8), Pasco (Difco, Detroit, Mich.), and UniScept (API, Plainview, N.Y.). These systems all use plastic disposable trays with numerous tiny wells that contain a variety of biochemical reagents or serial dilutions of antimicrobial agents for determination of MICs (Figure 9-9). These systems have varying degrees of sophistication and differ in the nature of the plastic tray, the variety of antimicrobial agents or biochemical tests used for identification, the manner in which plates are prepared (for example, frozen or dried), the manner in which plates are inoculated, and the procedure for reading and interpretation of results.

Identification or antimicrobial susceptibility panels (or both) of commercially available microdilution systems include the following:
1. MicroMedia System
   a. Gram-negative UTI MIC/ID
   b. Gram-positive Plus Panel
   c. Gram-negative UTI MIC
   d. Anaerobe MIC
   e. Twin GNI
2. Sceptor
   a. Enteric MIC
   b. Enteric MIC/ID
   c. *Pseudomonas* MIC
   d. *Pseudomonas* MIC/ID
   e. Gram-positive MIC
   f. Gram-positive MIC/ID

---

*References 1, 74, 99, 136, 143, and 145.

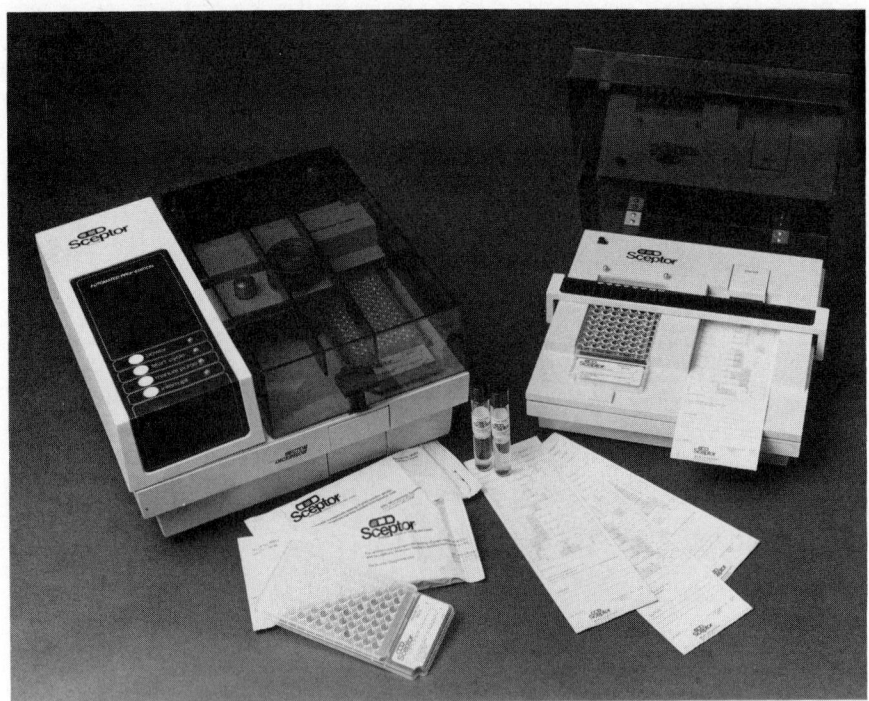

FIGURE 9-8. Sceptor system. (Courtesy Johnston Laboratories, Division of Becton Dickinson, Towson, Md.)

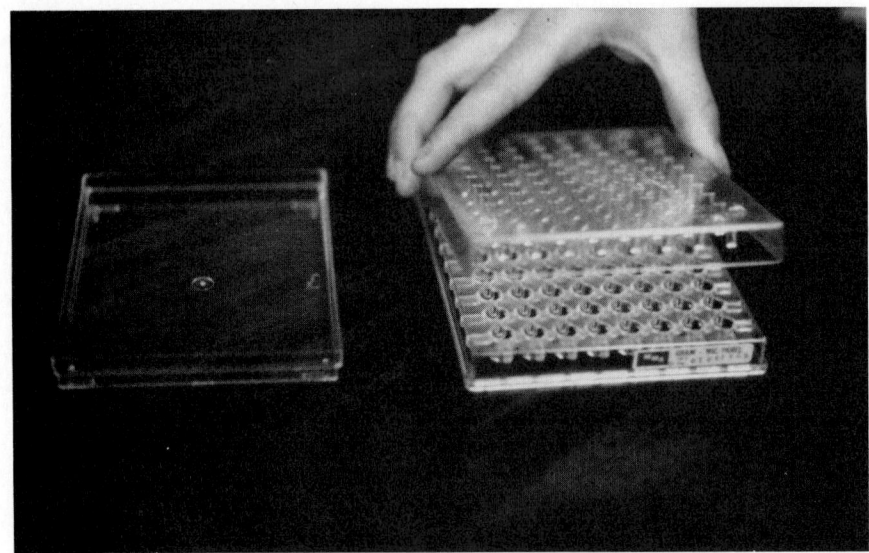

FIGURE 9-9. Typical plastic disposable tray used in microdilution systems. Note numerous tiny wells.

g. Anaerobe MIC
h. Anaerobe MIC/ID
i. Urine MIC/ID
j. Beta-lactam plus panel
k. Breakpoint panel

3. Sensititre
   a. Gram-negative enteric identification
   b. Gram-negative MIC—AGNM1,2,3
   c. Gram-positive MIC—AGPM1
   d. Urinary MIC—AGNUM
   e. Gram-negative ID—5-hour fluorogenic

4. Pasco
   a. Gram-positive D
   b. Gram-negative D
   c. Cystitis panel D
   d. RX panel
   e. MIC/ID gram-negative
   f. MIC/ID cystitis

5. Microscan
   a. Gram-negative combo
   b. POS combo
   c. Urine combo

6. UniScept
   a. UniScept 20E
   b. UniScept 20GP
   c. UniScept KB
   d. UniScept MIC

The MMS and MicroScan provide frozen microdilution panels. The MicroScan panels are all combination panels providing both identification and susceptibility. Some of the MMS panels are combination panels, and others offer these capabilities separately. Among the systems using dried panels, the Sceptor system provides four panels exclusively for antimicrobial susceptibility tests and four panels for combined identification and susceptibility. Pasco provides three panels for MICs alone, two combination panels, and one panel (RX) that includes the newer antimicrobial agents for use with appropriate organisms. Two of the UniScept panels are designed for identification and two for antimicrobial susceptibility testing; one of the latter panels provides qualitative results and the other quantitative results. The systems with frozen products provide a multi-pronged disposable inoculating device, whereas the systems with dried products have a two-stage inoculator that rehydrates the dried reagents and inoculates each well individually.

Interpretation and reporting of results of the microdilution systems may be done manually with a viewbox or with instruments that process the manually entered results and generate an identification report. These semiautomated instruments generally have a lighted viewing area on which the test panel is placed after appropriate incubation. The technologist reads the results and inserts them into the instrument by moving a bar or pressing a button on a keyboard, and the computer interprets the results and produces a report form. Three of these products may be used with a semiautomated system. The Autoscan 4 (Baxter MicroScan Division), and Autoreader (UniScept) read and interpret the test reactions automatically on the basis of turbidity for the antimicrobial susceptibility results and on the basis of color changes (colorimetry) for the biochemical reactions. Results are calculated and printed on a report form.

Sensititre also has a reader known as the AutoReader. This instrument is unique in that it does not determine growth on the basis of turbidity but rather on the basis of fluorescence liberated by bacterial enzymatic activity on fluorogenic substrates (enzyme substrates that are linked to a fluorophor to the growth medium). As the organism grows, it hydrolyzes the substrate and releases the fluorophor. Each well of the Sensititre plate is automatically scanned by a fluorometer after 5 hours' or 18 hours' incubation, and the extent of fluorescence is interpreted by the computer-controlled instrument and converted to an MIC. Staneck and co-workers[139] tested 828 isolates of gram-negative bacilli with the Sensititre AutoReader after 18 hours of incubation. Only 3.5% of the AutoReader results were greater than 1 dilution interval from the control MIC value. Studies by J.L. Staneck and R.C. Tilton indicate that the AutoReader is also very reliable for determining MICs after 5 hours' incubation with the exception of some strains of *Pseudomonas* and some *S. aureus* resistant to penicillin.

The Micur system is used for antimicrobial susceptibility testing only. This dried microdilution system includes three panels for determination of MICs: a gram-negative panel, a gram-positive panel, and a urinary tract panel. MICs are determined manually with a mirror-reader.

Many of the microdilution products have been extensively evaluated, and others are undergoing evaluation. The products that have been evaluated have generally been found to produce accurate and reproducible results.* Should laboratory technologists wish to produce their own microdilution susceptibility or identification plates, a number of mechanized methods are available. Studies have shown that plates made with the Dynatech MIC 2000 or the Sandy Springs system are comparable to the commercially produced plates.

Repliscan (Cathra International, St. Paul, Minn.) is an agar dilution identification system in which biochemical and antimicrobial agent reactions are determined on 16 agar plates. The system uses an inoculating device based on the replicator principle, allowing the inoculation of up to 36 isolates per plate. The plates are incubated overnight and then placed on a viewing table where reactions are visually interpreted and then electronically transmitted by a light pin assembly to a computer terminal that processes the information and prints the identification. Woolfrey, Quall, and Fox[156] compared the Repliscan system with the API 20E. Agreement at the genus level between the two systems was 62%. Although the initial evaluation was not satisfactory, the system is economical because a large number of isolates can be tested on one plate.

ANTIMICROBIAL SUSCEPTIBILITY TESTING AND BACTERIAL IDENTIFICATION DIRECT FROM A PATIENT SPECIMEN

The direct processing of clinical specimens provides an obvious time advantage for the clinical laboratory and thus may actually direct patient management. However, as pointed out previously, polymicrobic specimens are the least amenable to automated methods.

Wasilauskas and Ellner[151] were the first to suggest the possibility of identifying organisms directly from blood cultures. Bacteria could be removed from the blood by centrifugation, and the resulting pellet washed and then used to inoculate a series of standard biochemical tests. This same procedure may be used today for direct rapid identification or susceptibility

---

*References 14, 15, 34, 53, 75, 78-81, 108, and 125.

testing with a miniaturized system such as the API Rapid E or Micro-ID, a disk diffusion susceptibility plate, or select semi-automated systems. This technique has been shown to agree with conventional pure culture techniques greater than 90% of the time in most studies.

Other methods for direct detection of organisms in blood include those based on radiometry, infrared spectroscopy, impedance, lysis filtration and centrifugation, and photometry. The early work of Deland and Wagner[35] was the basis for the development of the first Bactec instrument,[10] which used radiometry to detect organisms in blood. The Bactec 460, one of the Bactec instruments available today, uses radiometry. Basically, radiometry is the detection of radiolabeled CO_2 produced by the organisms' metabolism of uniformly labeled glucose and amino acids in the growth medium. After inoculation into Bactec bottles containing $^{14}CO_2$-labeled substrate, the bottles are agitated on a rotator-shaker and placed in the Bactec monitoring unit where they move slowly past a sampling position. When each bottle reaches this position, a set of dual sterile needles punctures the rubber stopper of the bottles and aspirates the head gas into an ionization chamber. The bottle is then flushed with aerobic (5% CO_2) or anaerobic (85% N_2, 5% H_2, and 10% CO_2) gas depending on the type of medium, and the bottles continue to rotate (the needles are heat sterilized before insertion into the next bottle). In the ionization chamber the amount of $^{14}CO_2$ that is present (or the growth index [GI]) in the sample is measured and compared to a threshold level. If the GI is higher than the threshold level, a red warning light appears, signaling the presence of a positive culture.

The Bactec system is not inherently faster than conventional culture, but the ease of sampling allows cultures to be checked multiple times during the first 1 to 2 days of growth.

Numerous studies have been published regarding use of the Bactec 460. In general these studies agree that the instrument's findings are the same as conventional culture results almost 100% of the time,[24,44,126,135] and that it provides a significant degree of standardization and labor savings to blood processing.[121] The most recent Bactec instruments available, the Bactec 660 (Figure 9-10) and 730, are not radiometric but use infrared spectroscopy to detect CO_2 generated by the metabolism of organisms. (The difference between the 660 and the 730 is in the extent of automation.) These instruments circumvent the major disadvantage of the Bactec 460, specifically the handling and disposal of isotopes. A recent report by Jungkind and co-workers[82] indicates that no overall significant differences exist between the radiometric instrument and the infrared instruments in the ability or the time required to detect microbial growth.

The Bactec 460 has also been used successfully for the direct detection, identification, and antimicrobial susceptibility of mycobacteria from respiratory tract specimens. This is discussed in Chapter 26. This is the only example in which an automated approach has been used successfully to detect organisms directly from respiratory tract specimens, and with the exception of the Gram stain it is the only method available for direct processing of these specimens.[121]

Impedance methods detect the change in the flow of an electric current through a medium; this change parallels the growth of microorganisms.[64,146] The Bactometer is an impedance system that has been evaluated with blood cultures[63,64] but is now available only to the food industry for microbial monitoring of foodstuffs. Impedance-based instruments have recently been developed in England for detection of organisms in blood and urine and are currently undergoing trials.

The goal of both lysis filtration and centrifugation is the removal of bacteria from a hostile host environment after lysis of both red and white blood cells. In the lysis filtration method[159] the blood is lysed with a combination of nonionic detergent and an enzyme and is filtered through a 0.45 μm membrane. The lysis filtration method for blood cultures has not been commercially packaged.

Clinical studies by Dorn, Burson, and Haynes[40,41] indicate that lysis centrifugation, that is, the lysis of the blood followed by centrifugation of the lysed cells and pelleting of the bacteria, is as sensitive as inspection of the bottle for turbidity. The Isolator (Dupont, Wilmington, Del.) is a commercially available lysis centrifugation system. A pediatric Isolator (Isolator 1.5, DuPont, Wilmington, Del.) is also available. Only lysis, with no centrifugation, is recommended for the pediatric version.

The semiautomated AMS, Autobac, and MS-2 systems discussed previously may also be used for the identification and antimicrobial susceptibility testing of gram-negative bacilli directly from blood.[38,98,103,131]

Several automated methods have been developed for the direct detection of organisms in urine. These systems are discussed under "Urine Screening" later in the chapter.

Few instrument-oriented approaches with the exception of chromatography have been developed for the direct analysis of other body specimens. Rapid direct analysis of cerebrospinal fluid (CSF) or other fluids is best accomplished with the immunoserologic procedures discussed in Chapter 7. (Although these methods are not discussed in this chapter, they certainly qualify as rapid methods and in fact are the most rapid systems available in clinical microbiology.) Gas-liquid chromatography (GLC) is a powerful and versatile analytic tool capable of producing such large amounts of significant data that its invasion of the clinical microbiology laboratory should be inevitable. Unfortunately, except for the detection of metabolic end products of anaerobic bacteria, GLC has not been routinely adopted. GLC has been used to detect metabolic products of anaerobic organisms directly from specimens of pus, amniotic fluid, synovial fluid, and serous fluid.[59,61] The principles of GLC and the use of this system in anaerobic bacteriology are discussed in Chapter 20.

Several variations of GLC have been used for detection of microbial metabolites in body fluids. These methods are primarily research tools, however, and beyond the scope of most clinical microbiology laboratories. The sample may be pyrolyzed, that is, burned at temperatures of 1300° C before its passage through the gas chromatograph. A mass spectrophotometer can be used to identify products coming out of the GLC column. Brooks and co-workers[23] have used frequency pulsed, electron capture gas-liquid chromatography to detect bacterial products in body fluids. This work has suggested that the compounds detected, whether of microbial or host origin, may be present in normal body fluids but are altered in the diseased state. These changes are specific for particular agents of disease. Larsson[91] reported that GLC expedited diagnosis of blood cultures from which anaerobic bacteria eventually were recovered. Peaks corresponding to short-chain fatty acids and alcohols were seen in the blood culture medium. Moss[105] com-

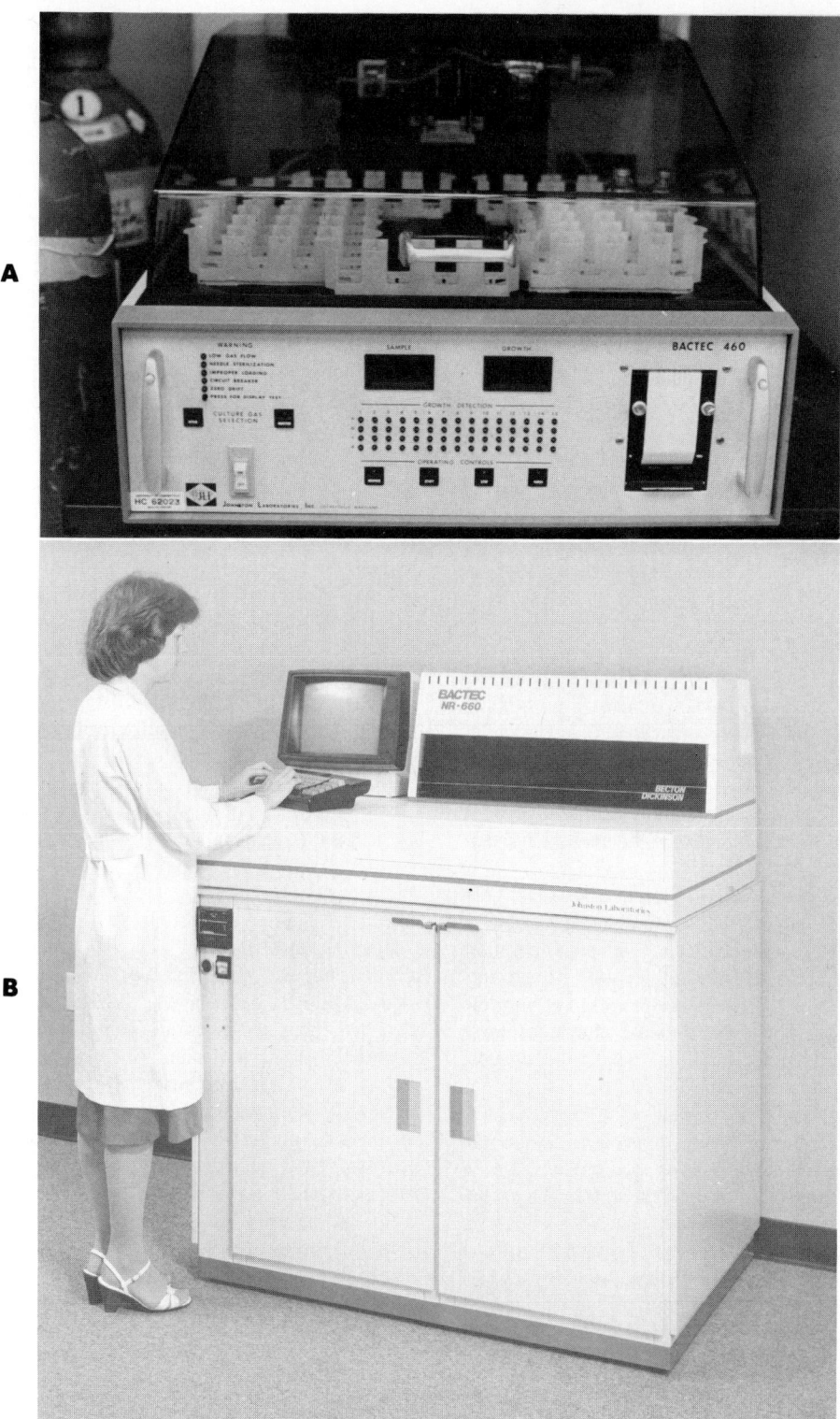

FIGURE 9-10. **A,** Bactec 460. **B,** Bactec 660. (Courtesy Johnston Laboratories, Division of Becton Dickinson, Towson, Md.)

mented that the identification and classification of bacteria have been aided by the GLC determination of cellular fatty acid composition. An example is the use of GLC to detect branched chain fatty acids of *Legionella pneumophila*. More than 300 isolates of *L. pneumophila* have shown similar fatty acid profiles, and a large percentage of the total acids that have been detected have been branched chain. Although not clinically useful, these data have been invaluable in defining the various serogroups of the genus *Legionella* as well as new species of the family *Legionellaceae*. As discussed in Chapter 26, GLC has also been used for the identification of mycobacteria.

High-performance liquid chromatography (HPLC) is a powerful tool in the clinical laboratory. HPLC is similar to gas-liquid chromatography except that liquid phases are pumped through separatory columns at extremely high pressures, partition occurs, and then the components are monitored by a detector. Although used in microbiology only for the assay of antimicrobial agents in body fluids, HPLC offers distinct possibilities for analysis of microbial products. The detection of short-chained acids and alcohols in anaerobic bacteria by HPLC has proved successful.

MICROBIOLOGIC SCREENING TESTS

The requirements for and characteristics of a microbiologic screening test follow.

1. The screening test must be rapid and provide information soon enough for expedient patient care. An overnight screening test might be appropriate if the definitive test would take 5 days to complete. On the other hand, an 8-hour screening test for beta-hemolytic streptococci in the throat offers little advantage over the traditional method.

2. The screening test must be cost effective.

3. The screening test is not usually definitive. It provides a yes or no answer. The screening test is generally a test for detection and not for precise identification of the agents of infectious disease. The primary purpose of the urine screening tests described in this chapter, for example, is to detect urine specimens that do not contain pathogens, which is true of approximately 80% of urine specimens submitted for culture.[119] By not culturing these negative specimens the laboratory saves considerable time and money, and the technologists' energies can be directed toward the specimens that are positive in screening tests.

4. The screening test must have a high sensitivity (percent of patients with positive results in the presence of disease) and a high negative predictive value (percent of patients with negative results who are nondiseased). Although the optimum screening test is both sensitive and specific, lack of specificity is not as critical as lack of sensitivity, since false-positive screening tests can be confirmed or denied by a traditional procedure.

Perhaps the most common screening test in microbiology is the Gram-stained smear. In this chapter the Gram stain is discussed in the context of urine screening for significant bacteriuria. The Gram stain provides significant information, however, for any specimen on microbial etiology, specimen quality, and inflammatory response.

DETECTION OF ENDOTOXEMIA

The *Limulus* amebocyte lysate test was proposed as an effective screening method to detect circulating endotoxin in a patient with endotoxemia. The *Limulus* lysate test is based on the observation that amebocytes from the horseshoe crab, *Limulus polyphemus,* clot in the presence of bacterial endotoxin. Extremely small concentrations of endotoxin (picogram amounts) cause gelation of lysate from *Limulus* amebocytes. Levin and Bang[94] reported satisfactory results from 98 patients in whom gram-negative sepsis was suspected. Several groups later reported that the test was of limited use clinically[48,101] because of a lack of sensitivity, as well as the rapid clearance of endotoxin from circulation. The *Limulus* test has also been used to screen urine and cerebrospinal fluid for endotoxin as an indicator of gram-negative bacteria.

URINE SCREENING

A rapid, cost-effective, and sensitive means for detecting bacteriuria is needed. Numerous methods have been proposed. Any method for urine screening, however, must take into consideration the fact that a significant/nonsignificant breakpoint of 1×10^5 CFU/ml is no longer useful for all patients. Stamm and co-workers[138] found that young symptomatic women with acute urethral syndrome (see Chapter 10) may have low colony counts (10^2 CFU/ml of urine) and still be infected.

Examination of a Gram-stained smear is a rapid, reliable, economical method of screening urine specimens for significant bacteriuria. A known quantity of uncentrifuged urine is placed on a slide, air dried, and stained. Multiple (more than 10) oil immersion fields are observed, and the average number of organisms per field can be correlated with the urine colony count. The Gram stain is reportedly sensitive and specific.[77,120,150] A recent report showed the Gram stain to be much more specific than the AutoMicrobic system or acridine orange stain, although the sensitivities of all these methods were similar.

Several dipslide or dipstick kits, among them the Microstix, Bactercult, and Uricult, are available for the detection of bacteriuria. The Microstix 3 (Ames Co., Elkhart, Ind.) is a paper dipstick with three reagent pads. The strip is moistened with urine and incubated in a sterile cellophane envelope. One pad is impregnated with *N*-2-naphthol ethylene diamine, which turns red in the presence of nitrite, a product of microbial nitrate reduction. The other two pads contain two culture media, one that detects gram-negative bacteria and one that shows total bacterial count after overnight incubation. The other dipsticks consist of small, screw-capped, plastic paddles, the surfaces of which are coated with a nonselective agar. Information on the ability of these methods to detect bacteriuria is voluminous but inconsistent. Another dipstick, the Chemostrip LN (Biodynamics, Inc., Indianapolis, Ind.) incorporates a test for leukocyte esterase (a white blood cell enzyme) with a test for bacterial nitrate reduction. This product reportedly detects 10 leukocytes/ml urine and when coupled with nitrate reduction yields acceptable sensitivity and specificity for bacteriuria screening. Clinical studies, however, have noted varying degrees of success with this product.

Currently seven instrumental systems are available for detection of bacteriuria: the AMS, MS-2, and Autobac discussed previously, the Lumac (3M Company, St. Paul, Minn.), the Monolight 2001 (Analytical Luminescence Laboratory Inc., San Diego, Calif.), the Turner Luminometer (Turner Designs, Mountain View, Calif.), and the Bac-T-Screen (Vitek, Hazelwood, Mo.).[119]

The AMS, MS-2, and Autobac systems detect changes in

light transmission that occur as the organisms grow. Each of these systems uses plastic cuvettes for urine screening. The AMS, unlike the Autobac or MS-2, not only determines the numbers of bacteria in the urine but also identifies the nine most common urinary pathogens.[111]

When detecting pure pathogens at a concentration of at least 10^5 CFU/ml, each of these three systems has a sensitivity exceeding 95% and a negative predictive value exceeding 99%.[119] The detection time for these systems ranges from 2 to 5 hours with the MS-2 offering the lowest average detection time. The AMS is the least labor-intensive system, and the Autobac is the most. The revised urinary identification card (UID) used with the AMS is more specific than earlier cards.[71]

The Lumac, Monolight 2001, and Turner Luminometer, unlike the Autobac, MS-2, and AMS, are not dependent on growth of the organism and thus provide results more rapidly (from 2 minutes to 1 hour) (Figure 9-11). These methods are based on the principle of bioluminescence or, specifically, the detection of bacterial ATP with the firefly luciferin-luciferase system. In the presence of ATP the firefly enzyme luciferase catalyzes the oxidation of the substrate luciferin to produce light, which is proportional to the amount of ATP that is present. Both host cells and bacterial cells contain ATP. Thus, when using the bioluminescence systems, one must first add reagents to the urine that cause the release and destruction of ATP from somatic cells. An ATP-releasing reagent for bacterial cells is then added followed by the luciferin-luciferase mixture. The amount of light that is formed is proportional to the amount of bacterial ATP and can be correlated with numbers of organisms.

The Bac-T-Screen (Figure 9-12) is a colorimetric filtration method. Urine is filtered through a membrane filter and then stained with safranin; the degree of staining of the microbial biomass and leukocytes on the filter is determined by the number of organisms in the urine. The major advantages of this instrument are simplicity of operation, the ability to achieve results in 2 minutes or less, and the detection of leukocytes (nonspecifically) as well as bacteria.

Evaluations of these urine screening methods are discussed by Pezzlo,[119] Wu and co-workers,[158] Bartlett, O'Neill, and McLaughlin,[19] Pfaller and associates,[123] Pfaller and Koontz,[122] and Lipsky and associates.[96] The decision to screen urine specimens and discard negatives without culture is an individual one that must be made with knowledge of the cost and reliability of the proposed test system, as well as the population of patients to be screened.

PROCESS AUTOMATION

Industrial microbiologists have been leaders in process automation or automating routine processes or functions. Several mechanized instruments are now available for process automation in clinical microbiology.

PREPARATION OF AGAR PLATES

Most clinical microbiology laboratories buy prepared agar from commercial sources. However, a number of machines are available that allow laboratory technologists to make their own agar plates. The Agarmatic, a benchtop sterilizer, is available from New Brunswick Scientific Co., New Brunswick, N.J. The ingredients are placed in a stainless steel vessel. Sterilization time and maintenance of the sterilizing and dispensing temperatures are adjustable and automatic.

Plate-pouring machines that can be coupled to agar sterilizers pour molten agar into sterilized culture dishes, stack them, and label them. One system, the Manostat Mediamatic system (Manostat Corp., New York), can fill, stack, and label approximately 1200 plates per hour. A similar instrument called the Petrimat is available from Bellco (Vineland, N.J.). It is about half as fast as the Manostat.

STREAKING OF AGAR PLATES

Several instruments are available for the automated streaking of agar plates. The spiral plater has been adopted by the Association of Official Analytical Chemists (AOAC) for food and cosmetic work. The advantage is that, when a plate is streaked in a spiral pattern, 35 μl of inoculum is diluted 10,000:1 at the end of the spiral. About 50 samples per hour can be processed.

The most sophisticated agar plate processor is the Autostreaker (TomTec, Orange, Conn.). It provides for total processing of an agar plate. By virtue of a computerized memory, it chooses the agar plates for a particular specimen, streaks them in one of two modes, either isolation or quantitation, labels the plates, and stacks them. The plates to be streaked are stored in a refrigerated compartment in the machine. The agar plates that are streaked by the TomTec have well-separated colonies, and colony counts compare favorably with those produced by manual means.

AUTOMATIC STAINING INSTRUMENTS

Available slide stainers include the Honeywell HMS 360 (Honeywell Test Instruments Division, Denver, Colo.); this instrument can process up to 360 slides per hour. An automated Gram staining machine is also available from Tomtec (Orange, Conn.). More than 100 Tomtec machines have been placed worldwide, and the results have been quite good. The Microstainer 2[50] is no longer marketed.

COLONY COUNTERS

Several automated instruments use video scanners to count colonies on a plate. They are used primarily in industry but can be used in the clinical laboratory as well, particularly for quantitative urine microbiologic tests. The disadvantage of these colony counters is that many of them cannot read colonies on opaque media such as blood agar. The machines may also have difficulty differentiating between closely adjoining colonies.

OTHER INSTRUMENTS

A variety of other instruments that are common in chemistry laboratories may also be useful in microbiology laboratories. They include automatic pipettors and dilutors, automated ELISA plate washers, and others. As yet, laboratories do not have robots that will receive specimens, log them in, streak plates, and place them in an incubator, but specimen preparation robots for clinical chemistry use are being evaluated with some degree of success.

COMPUTERS IN MICROBIOLOGY

Computers have revolutionized virtually all areas of science and medicine. In clinical laboratories the computerization of microbiology has perhaps been the most difficult to achieve for the following reasons.

Specimen processing and reporting are not discrete events

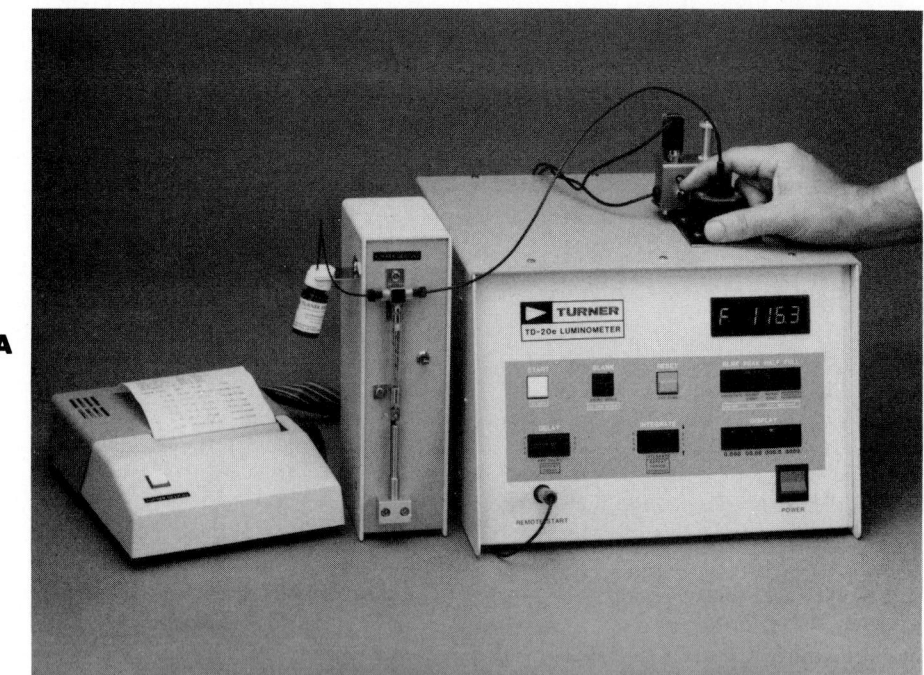

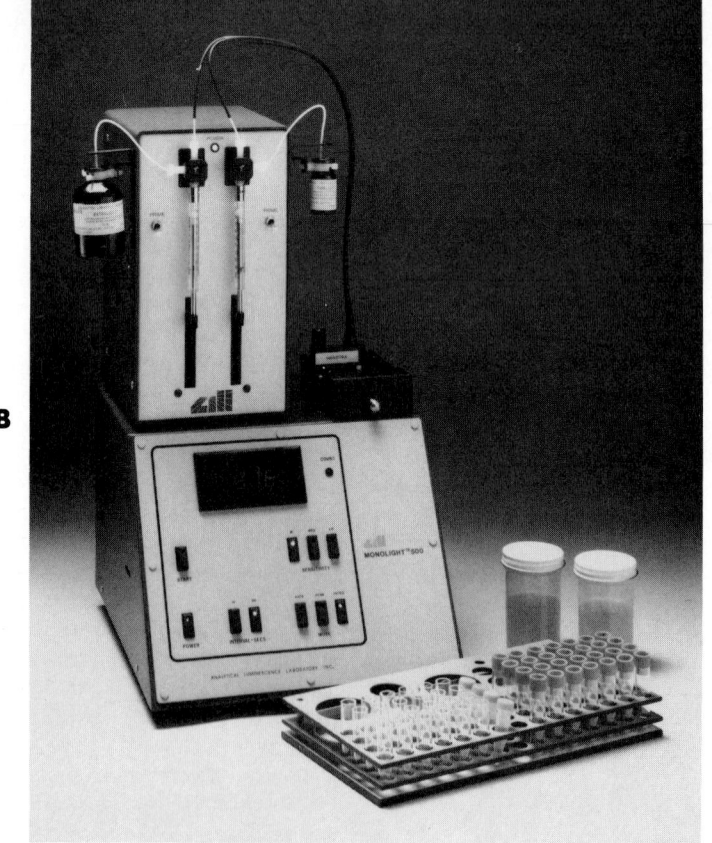

FIGURE 9-11. Bioluminescence systems for urine screening. **A,** Turner Luminometer. **B,** Monolight 500 Instruments System. (**A** courtesy Turner Designs, Mountain View, Calif. **B** courtesy Analytical Luminescence Laboratory, Inc., San Diego, Calif.)

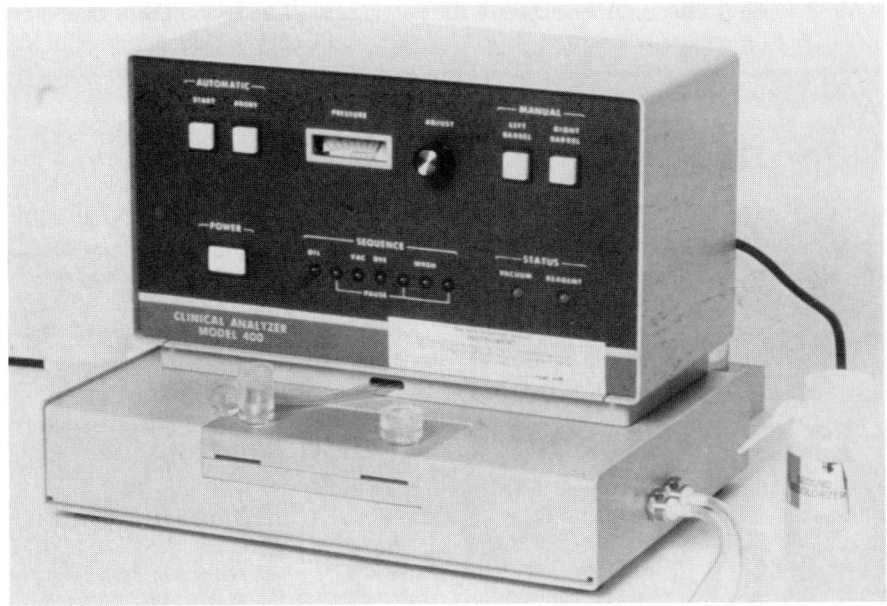

FIGURE 9-12. Bac-T-Screen. (Courtesy Marion Laboratories, Inc., Kansas City, Mo.)

that can be carried out in 1 day. Specimens received often are processed over multiple days, and partial reports are disseminated as the results of identification and susceptibility testing become available.

Microbiology, for the most part, is not numerically based. The language of microbiology is verbal. With some exceptions in immunology, descriptive reports and terminology are often arcane. Furthermore, a large number of possible organism combinations could be reported out for any one specimen.

Although the computerization of microbiology is difficult, obvious advantages exist. The processing of microbiology specimens, their logging in and reporting out, is probably the most time consuming of any task in the clinical laboratory. Microbiologic data for infection control, such as antibiograms and patterns of bacterial isolations as a function of source and site, are difficult and time consuming to retrieve manually but are quite amenable to computerized data storage and retrieval. Two of the most significant advantages are the generation of the cumulative susceptibility report and the ability to store and retrieve microbiologic data.

A computer system in microbiology can be acquired in at least three ways:

1. Most hospitals have computers for patient processing and billing. The laboratory's data terminal-printer can be appended to the main hospital computer. The advantage of this arrangement is that the laboratory does not have to buy a computer. The obvious disadvantage is that processing of laboratory data may not take precedence over accounting data.
2. The laboratory can purchase their own computer with a link to the hospital computer. This is probably the best system because it gives the laboratory a computer dedicated to its needs and appropriate types of ancillary hardware can be placed in the various laboratories.
3. Individual minicomputers or microcomputers can be placed in each laboratory to collect data and process it from instrumentation.

Many of the automated instruments in microbiology are connected to a computer. With appropriate safeguards, data from the Bactec, AMS, MS-2, Autobac, Aladin, and microdilution instruments can be channeled directly to patient floors or to data stations. Even manual data entries from the laboratory can be automatically checked by matching the results with an expected profile. The failure of a manually inputted result to agree with an expected result profile triggers an error message. With the storage of laboratory data in either small desktop computers or a central laboratory facility, laboratory workers are able to retrieve various data combinations at will. Workload recording statistics are simplified because the computer automatically generates detailed reporting of the number of tests performed and the amount of time spent on each test. Quality control results can be kept on disks within the computer itself. Maintenance logs in the machines may be entered into the computer, and individual maintenance sheets printed for each instrument.

Comprehensive discussions of the use of computers in microbiology have been presented by Gavan, Brotzman, and Smith,[52] Ryan,[129] Lawrie and co-workers,[92] and Kunz and co-workers.[87] The applications of computers in microbiology are directly related to the microbiologist's ingenuity. A computer coupled with automated instrumentation and rapid methods of identification can finally bring microbiology to a prospective instead of a retrospective discipline in laboratory medicine.

RECENT APPROACHES TO DETECTION AND IDENTIFICATION OF ORGANISMS

Recent innovative approaches to rapid and automated detection and identification of microorganisms are listed below*:
1. Molecular probes for microbe-specific nucleic acid

---

*Used and modified with permission of Robert Kreisler, Inc., New York; further information is available in references 28, 29, 45, 57, 62, 93, 127, 132, 147, and 149.

2. Flow cytometry: rapid scanning, fluorescence-activated cell sorting employing monoclonal antibodies
3. Nuclear magnetic resonance
4. Filtration and colorimetric detection of bacteria in blood cultures
5. Cross-flow filtration for separation of bacteria from whole blood
6. Detection of microorganisms by infrared spectroscopy
7. Particle concentration fluorescence immunoassay
8. Bioelectrochemistry as applied to immunoassay
9. Identification of microorganisms by circular intensity differential scattering
10. Robotics

While some of these technologies are not yet available, all potentially may contribute to "real-time" reporting of infectious disease agents. A brief summary of each follows.

Nucleic Acid Probe Technology

Recombinant DNA technology has created exciting new tools for the clinical microbiology laboratory. Medicine has already seen significant advances from these techniques, among them the synthesis of human insulin, human growth factor, and interferon. DNA and RNA probes, like monoclonal antibodies, may revolutionize the rapid identification of infectious disease.

DNA consists of a double-helical structure. Each strand is composed of alternating phosphate and sugar groups, as well as complementary pairs of the nucleotide bases adenine, guanine, cytosine, and thymine. As has been known for nearly 30 years, the series of base pairs called genes code for the synthesis of amino acids and subsequently proteins. Each genus and species of microorganisms has characteristic genes that render it genetically distinctive.

The initial stage in the construction of a DNA probe is to isolate the specific fragments of DNA that are characteristic of a particular bacterium or virus. These fragments are isolated by the use of restriction enzymes that cleave DNA at specific spots (Figure 9-13), for example, between guanine and cytosine and adenine and thymine. There are over 50 restriction endonucleases, mainly of bacterial origin. These can be purchased commercially. Once the specific DNA sequence has been isolated by restriction endonuclease activity, large quantities of the sequence must be made by cloning. Figure 9-14 shows how a piece of DNA is cloned. After the DNA has been cleaved by restriction enzymes, it is inserted into a vector molecule. This vector is usually a plasmid, although it can be a bacterial virus or a large plasmid called a cosmid. The size of the DNA to be incorporated into the vector is the deciding factor as to which vector should be used. Restriction endonucleases are used to insert the particular DNA into the plasmids as illustrated. The plasmid containing the specific DNA can then be inserted into a host organism such as *Escherichia coli*. The recombinant DNA fragment is reproduced in the host resulting in many copies of the "foreign" DNA.

Many of the studies reported in the literature concerning the use of DNA probes for diagnosis of infectious disease have used radioactive probes. However, for practical reasons, nonradioactive probes are being developed. The former limitations of DNA probes such as sensitivity, stability, and time required for processing are being conquered so that rapid development of probes for many infectious diseases is imminent.

Once the probe is made, several techniques can be applied to analysis of clinical specimens. The dot blot assay or probe filter assay has been widely used for probing specimens for the presence of specific bacteria such as *Neisseria gonorrhoeae*. Figure 9-15 depicts the dot blot assay. DNA is extracted from a patient specimen and fixed to a matrix such as a nitrocellulose filter. The trapped DNA is denatured so the double-stranded DNA becomes single stranded. Single-stranded probe DNA is added to the filter, and complementary DNA binding takes place. Unbound probe DNA is washed off the filter. The presence of the DNA complex on the filter is detected with an isotopic fluorescent or enzymatic label.

For specimens that contain viruses such as herpes simplex virus (HSV), the in situ hybridization assay may be more practical. In this assay the hybridization of the probe DNA and the viral DNA is done on a glass slide. A specific staining reagent is added and the slide examined microscopically for labeled inclusions. A study by Fung, Shanley, and Tilton[51] showed similar sensitivity and specificity of HSV probes and the direct fluorescent antibody identification of HSV. This study also reported some false-positive probe results; that is, viral DNA was found in the patient specimens and the virus was not cultured. It may be that this reflects a false-negative culture result and not a false-positive DNA probe test. However, Diegutis and co-workers[37] reported that three serum samples from healthy individuals were hepatitis B surface antigen negative but were positive when assayed by a DNA dot-hybridization probe. All other hepatitis markers were negative. These false-positive results were shown to be due to sequences in the serum that reacted with residual bacterial plasmid vector sequences. Fung, Shanley, and Tilton[51] attempted to explain false-positive HSV probe results by proposing the reaction of beta-lactamase sequences in the patient's specimens with pBr 322 plasmid sequences. However, the same specimens showed negative results when tested with a CMV DNA probe cloned also in pBr 322. Although DNA probes are theoretically highly specific, one cannot dismiss the possibility of cross-reacting genetic sequences.

Commercial DNA probe kits are currently available from two companies: Enzo Biochemical, New York, N.Y., and Gene-Probe, San Diego, Calif. Enzo has probes for HSV and cytomegalovirus. The probes are biotin-streptovidin in situ hybridization techniques.

The Gene-Probe kits are DNA probes to ribosomal RNA. At present these are radioactive probes (^{125}I) and available for detection of *M. pneumoniae* and the genus *Mycobacterium* in specimens and for culture confirmation of *M. avium-intracellulare, M. tuberculosis,* and *Legionella* spp. Other probes are currently being developed. Edelstein[42] recently evaluated the Gene-Probe DNA probe for colonies of *Legionella* organisms. He reported that it was specific for confirming colonies of suspicious organisms as the genus *Legionella.**

Flow Cytometry

Flow cytometry is a technique that adjusts the flow of a particle suspension (bacteria) through an electronic orifice so only one or a few particles pass per unit time. As the particles

---

*In a study to be published, Tilton and Dias found excellent correlation between the Gene-Probe method for *Mycoplasma pneumoniae* and culture results.

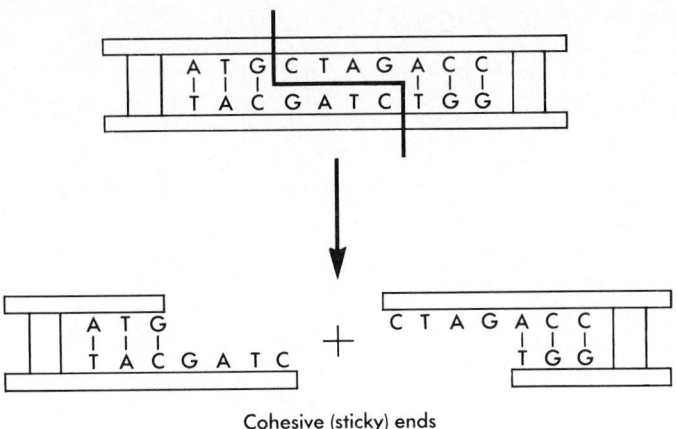

FIGURE 9-13. Cleavage by restriction endonuclease. (Used with permission of Medical Economics, Inc. From Berry, A.J., and Peter, J.D.: Diag. Med. **7**(3):62, 1984.)

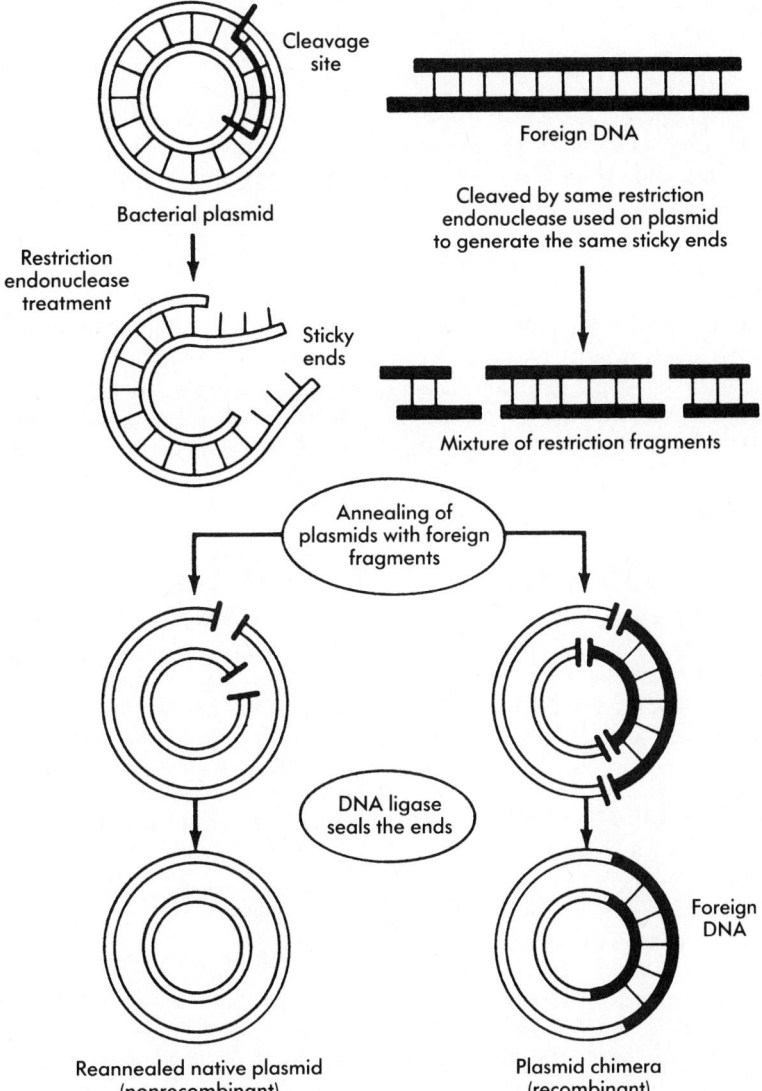

FIGURE 9-14. Construction of recombinant cloning vector. (Used with permission of Medical Economics, Inc. From Berry, A.J., and Peter, J.D.: Diag. Med. **7**(3):62, 1984.)

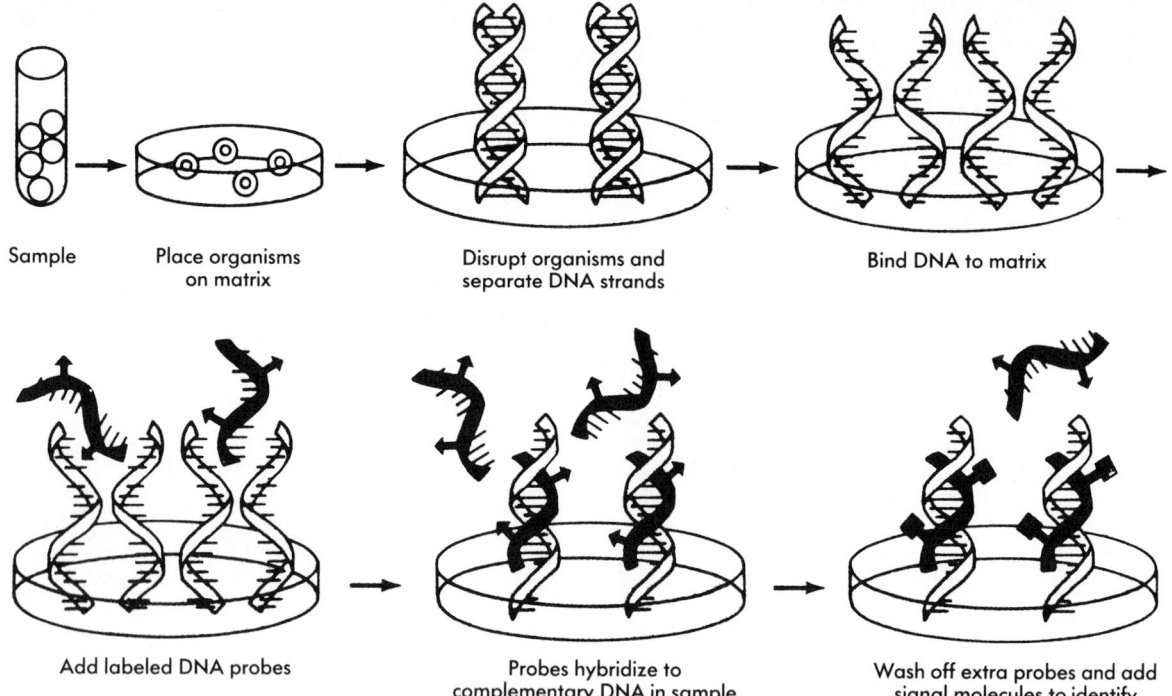

FIGURE 9-15. DNA probe filter assay. (Used with permission of Medical Economics, Inc. From Berry, A.J., and Peter, J.D.: Diag. Med. **7**(3):62, 1984.)

pass through the orifice, they are monitored in a number of ways. Light, using either an ultraviolet source or monochromatic lasers, is used to illuminate the cells, and their excitation is monitored by detectors. The signal may be altered by the inclusion of specific dyes, supravital stains, or fluorescein-conjugated monoclonal antibodies. Particles can be sized as well. This technique has the potential of directly identifying microbial particles in body fluids.

NUCLEAR MAGNETIC RESONANCE

Nuclear magnetic resonance (NMR) spectroscopy or magnetic resonance imaging (MRI) is used currently as an imaging technique. It has the capability, however, of examining the metabolic sequences of mammalian cells or a microorganism in a nondestructive manner. Although NMR at present is a relatively insensitive method, the possibility exists of detecting specific infectious processes in tissues by examining the metabolic state of the infected organ.

FILTRATION AND COLORIMETRIC DETECTION OF BACTERIA IN BLOOD CULTURES

Based on the filtration of urine and the subsequent nonspecific staining of bacteria and leukocytes trapped on the filter (Bac-T-Screen), a similar instrument has been invented for rapid detection of bacteria in blood. In principle a sample of blood is lysed and filtered. The bacteria are trapped on the filter while cellular debris flows through. Selective backwashing of the filter removes the bacteria, and they are again entrapped on a filter. The filter is stained, and the extent of color is proportional to the concentration of the bacteria in the blood. The instrument, called the Sep-T-Screen, has not yet been marketed.

CROSS-FLOW FILTRATION FOR SEPARATION OF BACTERIA FROM WHOLE BLOOD

The principle of cross-flow filtration is similar to the Sep-T-Screen and was designed to decontaminate blood. Bacteria are mechanically separated from blood by continuous flow filtration through a pleated microfiltration cartridge. Although the method was devised for the possibility of autotransfusion of autologous blood, it offers interesting possibilities for rapid identification of bacteria from septic patients.

DETECTION OF MICROORGANISMS BY FOURIER TRANSFORM INFRARED SPECTROSCOPY

Fourier transform infrared spectroscopy (FT-IS) may provide a rapid, sensitive, and specific method for detecting bacteria in body fluids. A microorganism has a characteristic Fourier transform infrared spectrum that can be recorded in less than 1 minute on microgram quantities of bacteria. The FT-IS spectrum of whole bacterial cells is complex and reflects the characteristic vibrational spectroscopic patterns of the individual cell constituents such as cell wall, membranes, and nucleic acids. These spectra are specific enough to provide bacterial "fingerprints" and hence rapid microorganism identification. This technique is still in the developmental stage.

PARTICLE CONCENTRATION FLUOROIMMUNOASSAY

Particle concentration fluoroimmunoassay (PCFIA) is an interesting modification of an immunoassay. Instead of a solid phase such as a tube or microdilution well, the ligand is bound to a latex polystyrene particle. The immunoassay is carried out on the latex particle using a fluorophore as a tag. PCFIA increases the sensitivity of FIA by providing a large number of binding sites for antigen-antibody interaction.

BIOELECTROCHEMISTRY

If an enzyme such as lactate dehydrogenase, which catalyzes an oxidation-reduction reaction, is used in an enzyme immunoassay (EIA) system, an electron acceptor such as ferrocene can be employed as an indicator of enzymatic activity. A specific electrode is used to measure the reduction of this electron transport intermediate. This results in increased sensitivity of the EIA.

IDENTIFICATION OF MICROORGANISMS BY CIRCULAR INTENSITY DIFFERENTIAL LIGHT SCATTERING

Circular intensity differential light scattering (CIDS) is a new technique for rapid microbial identification. CIDS is the differential scattering of right and left circularly polarized light. Scattering occurs throughout the whole spectrum, not just at particular absorption bands as in circular dichroism. Presumably CIDS measures the three-dimensional packaging of the microbial nucleic acids RNA and DNA. Microorganisms with different guanine-cytosine ratios or different tertiary structure should have different CIDS spectra. Early experiments seem to bear out this contention.

ROBOTICS

A laboratory robot could be designed to perform simple tasks repetitively. A robot would be particularly important if these tasks involved high-risk specimens. Robots available from several companies have been used for a number of tasks including manipulation of glassware in an aseptic environment, preparation of pharmaceutical samples, sterility testing, radioimmunoassay, and detection of endotoxin by the *Limulus* amebocyte lysate test.

• • •

In a short time those procedures that now seem innovative may be commonplace. Interest in rapid methods and automation in microbiology is great and will increase as clinical microbiologists and infectious disease practitioners demand clinically relevant and cost-effective data for patient care and treatment. The applications of new and exciting technology such as hybridomas for the production of sensitive and specific monoclonal antibodies and the routine use of molecular methods such as plasmid analysis and nucleic acid probes for rapid identification of microorganisms may revolutionize the clinical microbiology laboratory. Even now it is technically feasible for the laboratory to generate same-day results of culture and susceptibility testing on many of the isolates submitted to the clinical laboratory. Whereas in the recent past Louis Pasteur would have felt very much at home in the clinical microbiology laboratory, perhaps in the next decade Pasteur would feel like a stranger.

REFERENCES

1. Aldridge, C., et al.: Automated microbiological detection/identification system, J. Clin. Microbiol. **6:**406, 1977.
2. Aldridge, K.E., et al.: Comparison of Micro-ID, API 20E and conventional media systems in identification of *Enterobacteriaceae*, J. Clin. Microbiol. **10:**293, 1978.
3. Allen, S.D.: Systems for rapid identification of anaerobic bacteria. In Tilton, R.C., editor: Rapid methods and automation in microbiology, Washington, D.C., 1982, American Society for Microbiology.
4. Almeida, R.J., Jorgensen, J.H., and Johnson, J.E.: Evaluation of the AutoMicrobic system gram-positive identification card for species identification of coagulase-negative staphylococci, J. Clin. Microbiol. **18:**438, 1983.
5. Appelbaum, P.C., Kaufmann, C.S., and Depenbusch, J.W.: Accuracy and reproducibility of a four-hour method for anaerobic identification, J. Clin. Microbiol. **21:**894, 1985.
6. Appelbaum, P.C., and Leathers, D.J.: Evaluation of the rapid NFT system for identification of gram-negative, nonfermenting rods, J. Clin. Microbiol. **20:**730, 1984.
7. Appelbaum, P.C., et al.: Comparative evaluation of the API 20S and the automicrobic system gram-positive identification card for species identification of streptococci, J. Clin. Microbiol. **19:**164, 1984.
8. Appelbaum, P.C., et al.: Evaluation of the Micro-ID, the API 20E, and the Rapid 20E for same-day identification of *Enterobacteriaceae*, Eur. J. Clin. Microbiol. **4:**498, 1985.
9. Appelbaum, P.C., et al.: Accuracy and reproductibility of the IDS rapID STR system for species identification of streptococci, J. Clin. Microbiol. **23:**843, 1986.
10. Bannatyne, R.M., and Harnett, N.: Radiometric detection of bacteremia in neonates, Appl. Microbiol. **27:**1067, 1974.
11. Barnishan, J., and Ayers, L.W.: Rapid identificaton of nonfermentative gram negative rods by the Corning N/F system, J. Clin. Microbiol. **9:**239, 1979.
12. Barry, A.L.: Simple and rapid methods for bacterial identifications, Clin. Lab. Med. **5:**3, 1985.
13. Barry, A.L., and Badal, R.E.: Identification of *Enterobacteriaceae* by the automicrobic system: *Enterobacteriaceae* biochemical cards versus *Enterobacteriaceae*-plus biochemical cards, J. Clin. Microbiol. **15:**575, 1982.
14. Barry, A.L., Badal, R.E., and Effinger, L.J.: Identification of *Enterobacteriaceae* in frozen microdilution trays prepared by Micro-Media Systems, J. Clin. Microbiol. **10:**492, 1979.
15. Barry, A.L., Jones, R.N., and Gavan, T.L.: Evaluation of the micro-media system for quantitative antimicrobial drug susceptibility testing: a collaborative study, Antimicrob. Agents Chemother. **13:**61, 1978.
16. Barry, A.L., et al.: Accuracy and precision of the autobac system for rapid identification of gram-negative bacilli: a collaborative evaluation, J. Clin. Microbiol. **15:**1111, 1982.
17. Barry, A.L., et al.: Sensitivity, specificity, and reproducibility of the automicrobic system (with the *Enterobacteriaceae*-plus biochemical card) for identifying clinical isolates of gram negative bacilli, J. Clin. Microbiol. **15:**582, 1982.
18. Bartlett, R.C., O'Neill, D., and McLaughlin, J.C.: Detection of bacteriuria by leukocyte esterase, nitrite, and the AutoMicrobic system, Am. J. Clin. Pathol. **82:**683, 1984.
19. Bauer, A.W., et al.: Antibiotic susceptibility testing by a standardized disk diffusion method, Am. J. Clin. Pathol. **45:**493, 1966.
20. Beaucage, C.M., and Onderdonk, A.B.: Evaluation of a prereduced anaerobically sterilized medium (PRAS II) system for identification of anaerobic microorganisms, J. Clin. Microbiol. **16:**570, 1982.
21. Bowman, P.I., and Ahearn, D.G.: Evaluation of commercial systems for the identification of clinical yeast isolates, J. Clin. Microbiol. **4:**49, 1976.
22. Brenner, D.J., and Balows, A.: Evaluation of the enteric analyzer, an instrument to aid in the identification of *Enterobacteriaceae*, J. Clin. Microbiol. **2:**235, 1975.
23. Brooks, J.R., et al.: Gas chromatography as a potential means of diagnosing arthritis. I. Differentiation between staphylococcal, streptococcal, gonococcal, and traumatic arthritis, J. Infect. Dis. **129:**660, 1974.
24. Brooks, K., and Sodeman, T.: Rapid detection of bacteremia by a radiometric system: a clinical evaluation, Am. J. Clin. Pathol. **61:**859, 1974.
25. Brown, J.D., and Thomas, K.R.: Rapid enzyme system for the identification of pathogenic *Neisseria* spp., J. Clin. Microbiol. **21:**857, 1985.

26. Burdash, N.M., et al.: A comparison of four commercial systems for the identification of nonfermentative gram negative bacilli, Am. J. Clin. Pathol. **73:**564, 1980.

27. Burlage, R.S., and Ellner, P.D.: Comparison of the PRAS II, AN-Ident, and RapID-ANA systems for identification of anaerobic bacteria, J. Clin. Microbiol. **22:**32, 1985.

28. Busby, B.E., Hank, D., and Markovic, M.J.: Successful separation of bacteria from blood by cross-flow filtration, Abstracts of the Eighty-fourth Annual Meeting of the American Society for Microbiology, Q-28, 1984.

29. Chamblin, R.B., Quarles, J.M., and Hall, C.F.: Rapid identification of bacteria using methyl-umbelliferone fluorescence assay, Abstracts of the Eighty-fourth Annual Meeting of the American Society for Microbiology, March 1984, St. Louis, C-22, 1984.

30. Chester, B., and Cleary, T.J.: Evaluation of the Minitek system for identification of nonfermentative and nonenteric fermentative gram negative bacteria, J. Clin. Microbiol. **12:**509, 1980.

31. Cooper, B.H.: Rapid identification of *Enterobacteriaceae* and medically important yeasts with the MS-2 system. In Tilton, R.C., editor: Rapid methods and automation in microbiology, Washington, D.C., 1982, American Society for Microbiology.

32. Cooper, B.H., Johnson, J.B., and Thaxton, E.S.: Clinical evaluation of the Uni-Yeast-Tek system for rapid presumptive identification of medically important yeasts, J. Clin. Microbiol. **7:**349, 1978.

33. Cooper, B.H., et al.: Collaborative evaluation of the Abbott yeast identification system, J. Clin. Microbiol. **19:**853, 1984.

34. D'Amato, R.F., et al.: Collaborative evaluation of the UniScept qualitative antimicrobial susceptibility test, J. Clin. Microbiol. **21:**293, 1985.

35. Deland, F.H., and Wagner, H.N., Jr.: Early detection of bacterial growth with carbon-14-labeled glucose, Radiology **92:**154, 1969.

36. Dickgiesser, N., and Pieringer, E.: Suitability of the modified API 20 C, Mycotube and Bacto-*Candida-albicans*-Antiserum for the identification of yeasts in the routine laboratory, Zentralbl. Bakteriol. [A] **247:**132, 1980.

37. Diegutis, P.S., et al.: False positive results with hepatitis B virus: DNA dot hybridization in hepatitis B surface antigen negative specimens, J. Clin. Microbiol. **23:**797, 1986.

38. Dipersio, J.R., Ficorilli, S.M., and Vaga, F.J.: Direct identification and susceptibility testing of gram-negative bacilli from BACTEC bottles by use of the MS-2 system with updated bacterial identification software, J. Clin. Microbiol. **20:**1202, 1984.

39. Doern, G.V., and Chapin, K.C.: Laboratory identification of *Haemophilus influenzae:* effects of basal media on the results of the satellitism test and evaluation of the RapID NH system, J. Clin. Microbiol. **20:**599, 1984.

40. Dorn, G.L., Burson, G.G., and Haynes, J.: Blood culture technique based on centrifugation: clinical evaluation, J. Clin. Microbiol. **3:**258, 1976.

41. Dorn, G.L., Haynes, J.R., and Burson, G.G.: Blood culture technique based on centrifugation: development phase, J. Clin. Microbiol. **3:**251, 1976.

42. Edelstein, P.H.: Evaluation of the Gen-Probe DNA probe for the detection of *Legionellae* in culture, J. Clin. Microbiol. **23:**481, 1986.

43. Edwards, P.R., and Ewing, W.H.: Identification of *Enterobacteriaceae,* Minneapolis, Minn., 1972, Burgess Publishing Co.

44. Ellner, P.D., et al.: Critical analysis of hypertonic medium and agitation in detection of bacteremia, J. Clin. Microbiol. **4:**216, 1976.

45. Erlanger, B.F., and Wasserman, W.H.: Models of photoregulation. In Helene, C., and Laustriat, G., editors: Trends in photobiology, New York, 1982, Plenum Publishing Corp.

46. Facklam, R.R., Rhoden, D.L., and Smith, P.B.: Evaluation of the Rapid Strep system for the identification of clinical isolates of *Streptococcus* species, J. Clin. Microbiol. **20:**894, 1984.

47. Facklam, R., et al.: Comparative evaluation of the API 20S and automicrobic gram-positive identification systems for non-beta-hemolytic streptococci and aerococci, J. Clin. Microbiol. **21:**535, 1985.

48. Feldman, S., and Pearson, T.A.: The Limulus test and gram negative bacillary sepsis, Am. J. Dis. Child. **128:**172, 1974.

49. Fenn, J.P., and Matsen, J.M.: Packaged commercial bacterial identification systems, Clin. Lab. Med. **5:**19, 1985.

50. Fung, D.Y.C.: Evaluation of an automatic Gram staining machine, J. Milk Food Technol. **38:**262, 1975.

51. Fung, J.C., Shanley, J., and Tilton, R.C.: Comparison of the detection of herpes simplex virus in direct clinical specimens with herpes simplex virus-specific DNA probes and monoclonal antibodies, J. Clin. Microbiol. **22:**748, 1985.

52. Gavan, T.L., Brotzman, B., and Smith, C.: Description of a clinical information system. In Tilton, R.C., editor: Rapid methods and automation in microbiology, Washington, D.C., 1982, American Society for Microbiology.

53. Gavan, T.L., Jones, R.N., and Barry, A.L.: Evaluation of the Sensititre system for quantitative antimicrobial drug susceptibility testing: a collaborative study, Antimicrob. Agents Chemother. **17:**464, 1980.

54. Germer, J.J., and Washington, J.A., II: Evaluation of a rapid identification method for *Neisseria* spp., J. Clin. Microbiol. **21:**987, 1985.

55. Giger, O., Charilaou, C.C., and Cundy, K.R.: Comparison of the API Staph-Ident and DMS Staph-Trac systems with conventional methods used for the identification of coagulase-negative staphylococci, J. Clin. Microbiol. **19:**68, 1984.

56. Gilliland, S.E., and Speck, M.L.: Use of the Minitek system for characterizing lactobacilli, Appl. Environ. Microbiol. **33:**1289, 1977.

57. Godsey, J.H., et al.: Rapid identification of *Enterobacteriaceae* with microbial enzyme activity profiles, J. Clin. Microbiol. **13:**483, 1981.

58. Gooch, W.M., and Hill, G.A.: Comparison of Micro ID and API 20E in rapid identification of *Enterobacteriaceae,* J. Clin. Microbiol. **15:**885, 1982.

59. Gorbach, S.L., et al.: Rapid diagnosis of anaerobic infection by direct gas-liquid chromatography of clinical specimens, J. Clin. Invest. **57:**478, 1976.

60. Grasmick, A.E., Naito, N., and Bruckner, D.A.: Clinical comparison of the automicrobic system gram positive identification card, API Staph-Ident, and conventional methods in the identification of coagulase-negative *Staphylococcus* spp., J. Clin. Microbiol. **18:**1323, 1328, 1983.

61. Gravett, M.G., et al.: Rapid diagnosis of amniotic fluid infection by gas-liquid chromatography, N. Engl. J. Med. **306:**725, 1982.

62. Gress, C.T., and Salzman, G.C.: Rapid microbial identification by circular intensity differential scattering, Abstracts of the Fourth International Symposium on Rapid Methods and Automation in Microbiology and Immunology (Paper S-80), Berlin, 1984.

63. Hadley, W.K., and Kazenka, W.: Abstract of the Annual Meeting, American Society for Microbiology, Washington, D.C. C-69, 1976, The Society.

64. Hadley, W.K., and Senyk, G.: Early detection of microbial metabolism and growth by measurement of electrical impedance. In Schlessinger, D., editor: Microbiology—1975, Washington, D.C., 1975, American Society for Microbiology.

65. Hansen, S.L., Cassoria, R., and Martin, W.J.: API and Minitek systems in identification of clinical isolates of anaerobic gram negative bacilli and *Clostridium* species, J. Clin. Microbiol. **10:**14, 1979.

66. Hansen, S.L., and Stewart, B.J.: Comparison of API and Minitek to Center of Disease Control methods for the biochemical characterization of anaerobes, J. Clin. Microbiol. **4:**227, 1976.

67. Hartman, P.A.: Miniaturized microbiologic methods, New York, 1968, Academic Press, Inc.

68. Hayek, L.J., and Willis, G.W.: A comparison of two commercial methods for identification of the *Enterobacteriaceae* API 20E and the enterotube with conventional methods, J. Clin. Pathol. **29**:158, 1976.

69. Hicks, M.J., and Ryan, K.J.: Simplified scheme for identification of prompt lactose-fermenting members of the *Enterobacteriaceae*, J. Clin. Microbiol. **4**:511, 1976.

70. Holmes, B., Wilcox, W.R., and Lapage, S.P.: Identification of *Enterobacteriaceae* by the API 20E system, J. Clin. Pathol. **31**:22, 1978.

71. Huber, T.W.: The automicrobic system for detection of bacteriuria: efficacy of revised urine identification cards, Am. J. Clin. Pathol. **84**:637, 1985.

72. Isenberg, H.D., Reichler, A., and Wiseman, D.: Prototype of a fully automated device for determination of bacterial antibiotic susceptibility in the clinical laboratory, Appl. Microbiol. **22**:980, 1981.

73. Isenberg, H.D., et al.: R/B expanders: their use in identifying routinely and unusually reacting members of *Enterobacteriaceae*, Appl. Microbiol. **27**:575, 1974.

74. Isenberg, H.D., et al.: Clinical laboratory evaluation of automated microbial detection/identification system in analysis of clinical urine specimens, J. Clin. Microbiol. **10**:226, 1979.

75. Isenberg, H.D., et al.: Collaborative evaluation of the UniSept quantitative antimicrobial susceptibility test, J. Clin. Microbiol. **19**:733, 1984.

76. Janda, W.M., et al.: Evaluation of the RIM-N, Gonochek II, and Phadebact systems for the identification of pathogenic *Neisseria* spp. and *Branhamella catarrhalis*, J. Clin. Microbiol. **21**:734, 1985.

77. Johnson, H.H., Curtis, G.D.W., and Nicholas, W.W.: Current status of bioluminescence as a means of detecting significant bacteriuria. In Tilton, R.C., editor: Rapid methods and automation in microbiology, Washington, D.C., 1982, American Society for Microbiology.

78. Jones, R.N., Gavan, T.L., and Barry, A.L.: The evaluation of the Sensititre microdilution antibiotic susceptibility system against recent clinical isolates: a three-laboratory collaborative study, J. Clin. Microbiol. **11**:426, 1980.

79. Jones, R.N., et al.: Evaluation of the Sceptor microdilution antibiotic susceptibility testing system: a collaborative investigation, J. Clin. Microbiol. **13**:184, 1981.

80. Jones, R.N. et al.: Collaborative evaluation of the Micro Media systems anaerobe susceptibility panel: comparisons with reference methods and test reproductibility, J. Clin. Microbiol. **16**:245, 1982.

81. Jones, R.N., et al.: Evaluation of the MICUR system for quantitative antimicrobial susceptibility testing: a multiphasic comparison with reference methods, J. Clin. Microbiol. **16**:153, 1982.

82. Jungkind, D., et al.: Clinical comparison of a new automated infrared blood culture system with the BacTec 460 system, J. Clin. Microbiol. **23**:262, 1986.

83. Kellogg, J.A.: Inability to adequately control antimicrobial agents on AutoMicrobic system gram positive and gram negative susceptibility cards, J. Clin. Microbiol. **21**:454, 1985.

84. Kelly, M.T., et al.: Collaborative clinical evaluation of the Autobac IDX System for identification of gram negative bacilli, J. Clin. Microbiol. **19**:529, 1984.

85. Keville, M.W., and Doern, G.V.: Comparison of the API 20S *Streptococcus* identification system with an immunorheophoresis procedure and two commercial latex agglutination tests for identifying beta hemolytic streptococci, J. Clin. Microbiol. **16**:92, 1982.

86. Kloos, W.E., and Wolfshohl, J.F.: Identification of *Staphylococcus* species with the API staph IDENT system, J. Clin. Microbiol. **16**:509, 1982.

87. Kunz, L.J., et al.: The role of the computer in microbiology. In Prier, J.E., Bartola, J.T., and Friedman, H., editors: Modern methods in medical microbiology: systems and trends, Baltimore, 1976, University Park Press.

88. Lampe, A.S., and van der Reijden, T.J.K.: Evaluation of commercial test systems for the identification of nonfermenters, Eur. J. Clin. Microbiol. **3**:301, 1984.

89. Land, G.A., et al.: Evaluation of the new API 20C strip for yeast identification against a conventional method, J. Clin. Microbiol. **10**:357, 1979.

90. Land, G., et al.: Update and evaluation of the AutoMicrobic yeast identification system, J. Clin. Microbiol. **20**:649, 1984.

91. Larsson, L.: Head-space chromatography in clinical microbiology. In Tilton, R.C., editor: Rapid methods and automation in microbiology, Washington, D.C., 1982, American Society for Microbiology.

92. Lawrie, D.J., et al.: Microbiology subsystem of a total dedicated laboratory computer system, J. Clin. Microbiol. **10**:861, 1979.

93. Leland, D.S., et al.: Identification of Herpes simplex virus types 1 and 2 using flow cytometry. In Lennette, E.H., editor: Laboratory diagnosis of viral infections, New York, 1984, Marcel Dekker.

94. Levin, J., and Bang, F.B.: Clottable protein in limulus: its localization and kinetics of its coagulation by endotoxin, Thromb. Diath. Haemorrh. **19**:186, 1968.

95. Lindner, P.: Wochschr. Brau. **17**:336, 1901. Cited by Hartman, P.A.: Miniaturized microbiologic methods, New York, 1968, Academic Press, Inc.

96. Lipsky, B.A., et al.: Comparison of the automicrobic system, acridine orange-stained smears, and gram-stained smears in detecting bacteriuria, J. Clin. Microbiol. **22**:176, 1985.

97. Lowrance, B.L., Reich, P., and Traub, W.H.: Evaluation of two spot-indole reagents, Appl. Microbiol. **17**:923, 1969.

98. Malloy, P.J., Ducate, M.J., and Schreckenberger, P.C.: Comparison of our rapid methods for identification of *Enterobacteriaceae* from blood cultures, J. Clin. Microbiol. **17**:493, 1983.

99. Malloy, P.J., Miceika, B.G., and Ducata, M.J.: Automated methods in microbiology. II. Identification and susceptibility testing, Am. J. Med. Technol. **49**:313, 1983.

100. Marler, L., Allen, S., and Siders, J.: Rapid enzymatic characterization of clinically encountered anaerobic bacteria with the API ZYM system, Eur. J. Clin. Microbiol. **3**:294, 1984.

101. Martinez, L.A., Quintiliani, R., and Tilton, R.C.: Clinical experience on the detection of endotoxemia with the limulus test, J. Infect. Dis. **127**:102, 1973.

102. McCracken, A.W., et al.: Evaluation of the MS-2 system for rapid identification of the *Enterobacteriaceae*, J. Clin. Microbiol. **12**:684, 1980.

103. Moore, D.F., et al.: Rapid identification and antimicrobial susceptibility testing of gram-negative bacilli from blood cultures by the automicrobic system, J. Clin. Microbiol. **13**:934, 1981.

104. Moore, H.B., Sutter, V.L., and Finegold, S.M.: Comparison of three procedures for biochemical testing of anaerobic bacteria, J. Clin. Microbiol. **1**:15, 1975.

105. Moss, C.W.: Identification and classification of bacteria by cellular fatty acid composition. In Tilton, R.C., editor: Rapid methods and automation in microbiology, Washington, D.C., 1982, American Society for Microbiology.

106. Murray, P.R.: Microdilution and agar replica identification test systems, Clin. Lab. Med. **5**:67, 1985.

107. Murray, P.R., Gauthier, A., and Niles, A.: Evaluation of the Quantum II and Rapid E identification systems, J. Clin. Microbiol. **20**:509, 1984.

108. Murray, P.R., Weber, C.J., and Niles, A.C.: Comparative evaluation of three identification systems for anaerobes, J. Clin. Microbiol. **22**:52, 1985.

109. Nadaud, M., and Cancet, B.: Parallel study of two techniques for identification of gram negative anaerobic bacilli, Zentralbl. Bakteriol. **237**:530, 1977.

110. Nadler, H.L., et al.: Accuracy and reproducibility of the automicrobic system gram-negative general susceptibility-plus card for testing selected challenge organisms, J. Clin. Microbiol. **22**:355, 1985.

111. Nicholson, D.P., and Koepke, J.A.: The automicrobic system for urines, J. Clin. Microbiol. **10:**823, 1979.

112. Nord, C.E., Lindberg, A.A., and Dahlback, A.: Evaluation of the test kits—API, Auxotab, Enterotube, Pathotec, and R/B for identification of *Enterobacteriaceae,* Med. Microbiol. Immunol. **159:**211, 1974.

113. Nord, C.E., Wadstrom, T., and Dahlback, A.: Evaluation of different diagnostic kits for *Enterobacteriaceae.* In Heden, C.G., and Illeni, T., editors: New approaches to the identification of microorganisms, New York, 1975, John Wiley & Sons, Inc.

114. Oberhofer, T.R.: Use of the API 20E, Oxi/Ferm and Minitek systems to identify nonfermentative and oxidase-positive fermentative bacteria: seven years of experience, Diagnos. Microbiol. Infect. Dis. **1:**241, 1983.

115. Oberhofer, T.R., et al.: Evaluation of the Oxi/Ferm tube system with selected gram-negative bacteria. J. Clin. Microbiol. **6:**559, 1977.

116. Oblack, D.L., Rhodes, J.C., and Martin, W.J.: Clinical evaluation of the automicrobic system yeast biochemical card for rapid identification of medically important yeasts, J. Clin. Microbiol. **13:**351, 1981.

117. Overman, T.L., et al.: Comparison of the API Rapid E Four-hour system with the API 20E overnight system for the identification of routine clinical isolates of the family *Enterobacteriaceae,* J. Clin. Microbiol. **21:**542, 1985.

118. Peterson, W.C., Hale, D.C., and Matsen, J.M.: An evaluation of the practicality of the spot-indole test for the identification of *Escherichia coli* in the clinical microbiology laboratory, Am. J. Clin. Pathol. **78:**755, 1982.

119. Pezzlo, M.T.: Detection of bacteriuria by automated methods, Clin. Lab. Med. **15:**539, 1984.

120. Pezzlo, M.T., et al.: Screening of urine cultures by three automated systems, J. Clin. Microbiol. **15:**468, 1982.

121. Pfaller, M.A.: Automated instrument approaches to clinical microbiology, Diagn. Microbiol. Infect. Dis. **3:**15S, 1985.

122. Pfaller, M.A., and Koontz, F.P.: Use of rapid screening tests in processing urine specimens by conventional culture and the automicrobic system, J. Clin. Microbiol. **21:**783, 1985.

123. Pfaller, M.A., et al.: Improved urine screening using a combination of leukocyte esterase and the Lumac system, Diagn. Microbiol. Infect. Dis. **3:**243, 1985.

124. Philip, A., and Garton, G.C.: Comparative evaluation of five commercial systems for the rapid identification of pathogenic *Neisseria* species, J. Clin. Microbiol. **22:**101, 1985.

125. Phillips, I., Warren, C., and Waterworth, P.M.: Determination of minimum inhibitory concentrations by the Sensititre system. In Johnson, H.H., and Newsome, S.W.B., editors: Second international symposium on rapid methods and automation in microbiology, Oxford, 1976, Learned Information (Europe), Ltd.

126. Renner, E.D., Gatherdige, L.A., and Washington, J.A., II: Evaluation of radiometric system for detecting bacteremia, Appl. Microbiol. **26:**368, 1973.

127. Robinson, G., Forrest, G.C., and Philo, R.D.: The application of bioelectrochemistry to immunoassay, Abstracts of the Oak Ridge Conference on Advanced Analytical Concepts for the Clinical Laboratory (Paper 7), Charleston, S.C., April 11-12, 1985.

128. Robinson, M.J., and Oberhofer, T.R.: Identification of pathogenic *Neisseria* species with the rapID NH system, J. Clin. Microbiol. **17:**400, 1983.

129. Ryan, K.J.: The computer in microbiology: future applications in test performance and reporting, Ann. N.Y. Acad. Sci. **428:**243, 1984.

130. Salkin, I.F., et al.: Evaluation of Abbott Quantum II yeast identification system, J. Clin. Microbiol. **22:**442, 1985.

131. Schifman, R.B., and Ryan, K.J.: Rapid automated identification of gram-negative bacilli from blood cultures with the automicrobic system, J. Clin. Microbiol. **15:**260, 1982.

132. Seydel, U., and Lindner, B.: Qualitative and quantitative investigations on mycobacteria with LAMMA: Fresenius Z, Anal. Chem. **308:**253, 1981.

133. Sielaff, B.H., Matsen, J.M., and McKie, J.E.: Novel approach to bacterial identification that uses the Autobac system, J. Clin. Microbiol. **15:**1103, 1982.

134. Sielaff, B.H., Matsen, J.M., and McKie, J.E.: Rapid identification by use of growth inhibitor technology and nephelometry on the Autobac system. In Tilton, R.C., editor: Rapid methods and automation in microbiology, Washington, D.C., 1982, American Society for Microbiology.

135. Smith, A.G., and Little, R.R.: Detection of bacteremia by an automated radiometric method and a tubed broth method, Ann. Clin. Lab. Sci. **4:**448, 1974.

136. Smith, P.B., et al.: Multi-laboratory evaluation of an automated microbial detection/identification system, J. Clin. Microbiol. **8:**657, 1978.

137. Snyder, J.W.: Adaptability of the Autobac MTS for the study of yeast carbohydrate assimilation. In Tilton, R.C., editor: Rapid methods and automation in microbiology, Washington, D.C., 1982, American Society for Microbiology.

138. Stamm, W.E., et al.: Diagnosis of coliform infection in acutely dysuric women, N. Engl. J. Med. **307:**463, 1982.

139. Staneck, J.L., et al.: Automated reading of MIC microdilution trays containing fluorogenic enzyme substrates with the Sensititre autoreader, J. Clin. Microbiol. **22:**187, 1985.

140. Stargel, D., et al.: Modification of the Minitek miniaturized differentiation system for characterization of anaerobic bacteria, J. Clin. Microbiol. **3:**291, 1976.

141. Starr, S.E., et al.: Micromethod system for identification of anaerobic bacteria, Appl. Microbiol. **25:**713, 1973.

142. Thornsberry, C., et al.: Laboratory evaluation of a rapid, automated susceptibility testing system: report of a collaborative study, Antimicrob. Agents Chemother. **71:**466, 1975.

143. Thornsberry, C., et al.: Clinical laboratory evaluation of the Abbott MS-2 automated antimicrobial susceptibility testing system: report of a collaborative study, J. Clin. Microbiol. **12:**375, 1980.

144. Tilton, R.C., Kenney, H., and Corcoran, L.: A screening test for vaginal candidiasis, Health Lab. Sci. **12:**100, 1975.

145. Tilton, R.C., Kwasnik, I., and Ryan, R.: Comparison of rapid methods of antimicrobial susceptibility in *Haemophilus influenzae,* Ann. Clin. Lab. Sci. **8:**70, 1978.

146. Ur, A., and Brown, D.F.J.: Impedance monitoring of bacterial activity, J. Med. Microbiol. **8:**19, 1975.

147. Van Dilla, M.A., et al.: Bacterial characterization by flow cytometry, Science **220:**620, 1983.

148. Vracko, R., and Sherris, J.C.: Indole-spot test in bacteriology, Am. J. Clin. Pathol. **39:**429, 1963.

149. Wallis, C., and Melnick, J.L.: Rapid colorimetric method for the detection of microorganisms in blood culture, J. Clin. Microbiol. **21:**505, 1985.

150. Washington, J.A., II, et al.: Detection of significant bacteriuria by microscopic examination of urine, Lab. Med. **12:**294, 1981.

151. Wasilauskas, B.L., and Ellner, P.D.: Presumptive identification of bacteria from blood cultures in four hours, J. Infect. Dis. **124:**499, 1971.

152. Weaver, R.H., Arnold, W.M., Jr., and Hannan, J.: The development of quick microtechniques for identification of cultures, J. Bacteriol. **51:**565, 1946.

153. Welborn, P.P., Uyeda, C.T., and Ellison-Birang, N.: Evaluation of Gonocheck-II as a rapid identification system for pathogenic *Neisseria* species, J. Clin. Microbiol. **20:**680, 1984.

154. Wellstood-Nuesse, S.: Comparison of the Minitek system with conventional methods for identification of nonfermentative and oxidase-

positive fermentative gram negative bacilli, J. Clin. Microbiol. **9:**511, 1979.

155. Woolfrey, B.F., Lally, R.T., and Ederer, M.N.: Evaluation of the AutoMicrobic system for detection of resistance of *Staphylococcus aureus* to methicillin, J. Clin. Microbiol. **19:**464, 1984.

156. Woolfrey, B.F., Quall, C.O., and Fox, J.M.: Evaluation of the Repliscan system for *Enterobacteriaceae* identification, J. Clin. Microbiol. **13:**58, 1981.

157. Woolfrey, B.F., et al.: Evaluation of the AutoMicrobic system of susceptibility testing of *Pseudomonas aeruginosa* to gentamicin, tobramycin, and amikacin, J. Clin. Microbiol. **19:**502, 1984.

158. Wu, T.C., et al.: Evaluation of three bacteriuria screening methods in a clinical research hospital, J. Clin. Microbiol. **21:**796, 1985.

159. Zierdt, C.H., Kagan, R.L., and MacLowry, J.D.: Development of a lysis-filtration blood culture technique, J. Clin. Microbiol. **5:**46, 1977.

CHAPTER 10

Clinical Syndromes and Diseases of Interest to Clinical Microbiologists

Alice S. Weissfeld
Sonia Zighelboim-Daum

This chapter is a discussion of miscellaneous syndromes or diseases that are of interest to clinical microbiologists. Although the causes of not all of these illnesses are known, evidence remains strong that each of them has an infectious etiology.

ACUTE URETHRAL SYNDROME

Acute urethral syndrome (AUS) or pyuria-dysuria syndrome is the term used to describe the illness of a subset of women who have symptoms typical of lower urinary tract (bladder) infection but whose clean-voided urine specimen either is sterile or contains fewer than 10^5 organisms/ml. Studies have shown that 30% to 50% of sexually active women with lower tract symptoms may have this syndrome.[53]

EPIDEMIOLOGY

AUS affects women primarily between the ages of 21 and 25 years.[53]

CLINICAL PRESENTATION

The triad of symptoms present in women with AUS is pyuria, dysuria, and frequency. Dysuria may be a symptom of vaginitis, cystitis, or urethritis. Factors favoring a diagnosis of vaginitis include a history of recently increased or changed vaginal discharge, vaginal odor, vaginal or labial itching, or previous recurrent vaginitis. Vaginitis results from infection with *Trichomonas vaginalis, Candida albicans,* or *Gardnerella vaginalis.* To make the diagnosis the physician usually performs a pelvic examination, determines the vaginal pH, and examines vaginal secretions microscopically.

If vaginitis is excluded, women with lower urinary tract symptoms may be divided into two groups, those with cystitis and those with urethritis. More than 90% of women with either illness exhibit pyuria. Thus women with AUS cannot be distinguished from those with cystitis on the basis of clinical presentation alone.

ETIOLOGIC AGENT

Women with a low-count bacteriuria (fewer than 10^5 organisms/ml) are most likely to be infected with the gram-negative rods *Escherichia coli, Klebsiella* or *Enterobacter* spp., or *Staphylococcus saprophyticus.*[114] Patients with sterile pyuria (white cells in the urine but no growth on routine culture) are more likely to be infected with chlamydiae[112,123] or *Neisseria gonorrhoeae.*[38] The genital mycoplasmas (*Ureaplasma urealy-*

ticum and *Mycoplasma hominis*) and, rarely, herpes virus are also thought to be involved in this syndrome.

LABORATORY DIAGNOSIS

Many microbiologists and clinicians are currently reevaluating accepted criteria regarding the workup of clean-voided, midstream urine specimens, particularly from young, healthy women.[111] The presence of at least 10^5 colony-forming units (CFU)/ml in quantitative urine cultures was originally shown to differentiate specimen contamination from true bacteriuria in asymptomatic women and women with acute pyelonephritis (kidney or upper urinary tract infection).[76-78,101] Symptomatic women with acute lower urinary tract infections were not studied, since tests to differentiate between upper and lower tract disease were not readily available when these landmark studies were performed. Thus the association of fewer than 10^5 organisms/ml with lower urinary tract disease is only now being fully explored.

Factors that influence colony count include state of patient hydration, frequency of urination, urine pH, urine osmolarity, recent use of antimicrobics, and collection, transport, and culture methods employed.[111] It is important for the physician to alert the laboratory to the presence of lower urinary tract symptoms in female patients so the microbiologist can determine how far to carry identification and susceptibility testing of low numbers of *Escherichia coli, Klebsiella* spp., *Enterobacter* spp., or *S. saprophyticus,* or whether cultures of more fastidious organisms should be obtained. However, even without this valuable clinical information, the presence of pyuria may guide the microbiologic workup. The presence of white blood cells may be determined by routine urinalysis, Gram staining of unspun urine,[114] use of a hemocytometer chamber to enumerate leukocytes per cubic millimeter of unspun urine, or the leukocyte esterase dipstick technique. If abnormal numbers of leukocytes are present, 10^2 to 10^4 colonies of *E. coli* or *S. saprophyticus* are more likely to be of etiologic importance. Microbiologists should be cautious about using Gram stains or automated methods to screen urine specimens for culture, since these techniques lack sensitivity when fewer than 10^4 CFU/ml are present. Thus patients infected with 10^2 to 10^4 bacteria may be misclassified as uninfected.

TREATMENT

Treatment of patients with AUS depends on the cause of the syndrome.[113] Women with lower counts of *E. coli* or *S. sap-*

rophyticus can be treated with regimens effective against cystitis, such as sulfonamides, trimethoprim-sulfamethoxazole, or nitrofurantoins. Women with *Chlamydia trachomatis* infection should be treated with tetracycline, and women with *N. gonorrhoeae* should receive amoxicillin followed by tetracycline.

KAWASAKI SYNDROME

Kawasaki syndrome (KS), also known as Kawasaki disease and mucocutaneous lymph node syndrome, is a febrile illness of unknown origin that occurs predominantly in children less than 5 years of age. The syndrome was first described in Japan in 1967 by Kawasaki. Hallmark features include prolonged fever; conjunctival injection; oropharyngeal inflammation; extremity changes including edema, erythema, or desquamation of the skin; truncal rash; and lymphadenopathy.[6]

EPIDEMIOLOGY

KS appears to be most prevalent in Japan and Hawaii but occurs worldwide. In the United States outbreaks have occurred in New York, California, Massachusetts, Hawaii, Colorado, Illinois, Michigan, Wisconsin, North Carolina, Virginia, Tennessee, the District of Columbia, Indiana, Texas, and Washington.[33] The overall case-fatality ratio is 0.5% to 2.8%.[6] Fatal KS is more common in men and in children less than 2 years old.[88] The prevalence is highest among Orientals, intermediate for blacks, and lowest for whites. There is no evidence for direct person-to-person transmission. Although cases may occur throughout the year, most cases in the United States occur in winter and spring.

In some studies parents of patients appear to have a significantly higher level of education than controls and patients are more likely than controls to have had an antecedent respiratory illness of unknown cause within 30 days of onset.[6] Epidemiologic investigations suggest that exposure to the application of rug shampoo and sleeping on floor mats may be risk factors for acquisition of KS in the United States and Japan, respectively.[52,92] The pathogenesis of the disease remains to be determined, however.

CLINICAL PRESENTATION

KS has three phases: acute febrile, subacute, and convalescent.[88] The first phase begins abruptly with the onset of fever and is followed within 1 to 3 days by the following other diagnostic features[6]:

1. Fever lasting 5 days or more
2. Bilateral conjunctival injection (dilatation of blood vessels of ocular conjunctivae)
3. At least one of the following mucous membrane changes:
   a. Injected or fissured lips
   b. Diffuse reddening of oral and pharyngeal mucosa
   c. Protuberance of tongue papillae; also called "strawberry tongue"
4. At least one of the following extremity changes:
   a. Erythema of palms and soles
   b. Edema of the hands and feet
   c. Desquamation approximately 1 to 2 weeks from onset
5. Erythematous rash of body trunk without vesicles or crusts

6. Cervical lymphadenopathy (swelling of at least one node to 1.5 cm or more in diameter)

Aseptic meningitis, diarrhea, and hepatic dysfunction may also occur during this period. The acute febrile phase usually lasts from 7 to 14 days.

The subacute phase is characterized by persistent anorexia, irritability, thrombocytosis, and desquamation. Arthritis, arthralgia, and myocardial dysfunction may occur during this period, and the prognosis in each case depends on the extent and severity of the cardiovascular disease. This second phase lasts from approximately the tenth to the twenty-fifth day of illness.

The convalescent phase of KS lasts from the period when all signs of illness have disappeared until the sedimentation rate has returned to normal (usually 6 to 8 weeks from onset).

ETIOLOGIC AGENT

The cause of KS is unknown, although the acute febrile onset and occurrence of community-wide epidemics suggest an infectious agent. Possibly the frequently observed preceding respiratory illness triggers an abnormal host response leading to KS. Evidence suggests that the house dust mite may be involved in KS. In two studies mite antigen was detected in circulating immune complexes in patients' sera during the acute phase of illness.[50,52] In addition, patients in the acute phase of disease have increased serum levels of anti-mite-specific IgG. Alternatively, the mite may be a vector carrying the causative agent. *Rickettsia*-like bodies have been observed by electron microscopy in biopsy specimens of skin and lymph nodes of KS patients.[51,53,64] *Rickettsia*-like bodies have also been found in the digestive canals of mites collected from house dust of patients' rooms. Several investigators have recently suggested that an unusual strain of *Propionibacterium acnes* may be the cause of KS.[80] These workers reported isolating the same strain of *P. acnes* from the blood and lymph nodes of a few patients, as well as from house dust mites in their homes.

LABORATORY DIAGNOSIS

Laboratory abnormalities in KS are generally nonspecific and nondiagnostic.[88] The total white blood cell count is elevated during the acute febrile phase of illness with a shift to the left (predominance of polymorphonuclear leukocytes with both mature and band forms) in approximately half of Kawasaki syndrome patients. The erythrocyte sedimentation rate is elevated and C-reactive protein is present during the acute stage. Thrombocytosis occurs during the subacute phase and corresponds with the period of highest risk of coronary artery thrombosis. There are a marked increase in the serum IgE level in the second, third, or fourth week of illness and increased levels of circulating immune complexes.

Bacterial, viral, and leptospiral cultures of blood, urine, throat, and stool are commonly performed to rule out other infectious agents.

TREATMENT

Antimicrobial therapy for KS awaits delineation of the etiologic agent. Aspirin is usually prescribed for both its anti-inflammatory properties and its effect in inhibiting platelet aggregation.[88] Corticosteroids may be contraindicated, since in one study, when used alone, they appeared to increase the frequency of aneurysm.[79]

LYME DISEASE

Lyme disease (LD) or Lyme arthritis was initially recognized in the United States in 1975 because of the geographic clustering of cases of inflammatory arthritis in Lyme, Connecticut.[42] The disease usually begins in summer following the bite of an *Ixodes* tick. The disease has recently been shown to be caused by a new species of *Borrelia*, *B. burgdorferi*,[7,10,70,72,115] carried by the tick vector.

EPIDEMIOLOGY

Cases of LD have been reported in 24 states with the majority of cases occurring along the northeastern coast (Connecticut, Massachusetts, New York, New Jersey, and Rhode Island) and in the Midwest (Wisconsin and Minnesota). *Ixodes dammini* is the primary tick vector in these geographic areas. Fewer cases of LD have been reported in the West (California, Nevada, and Oregon) where *I. pacificus* is the tick vector.[106] Recently another tick, *Amblyoma americanum*, was implicated as a vector of LD.[107] Lyme disease is also present in Europe where it is frequently referred to as erythema migrans disease. This disease was first recognized in Sweden in 1909; the European tick vector is *I. ricinus*. Lyme disease also occurs in Australia,[115] but an arthropod vector has not been identified. Deer, the preferred host for the adult form of the *Ixodes* tick, are present in areas where LD occurs. The aggressive nymphal (immature) form of the tick most frequently transmits LD. Because of its small size (several millimeters) it is often overlooked, which probably explains why only 30% of patients with LD recall a tick bite.

Patients with the B cell alloantigen DR2 may have a more severe and prolonged illness.[41] During 1984 more than 1000 cases of LD were diagnosed in the United States.

CLINICAL PRESENTATION

LD is a systemic illness that may begin with the appearance of a red skin lesion called erythema chronicum migrans (ECM), which is often accompanied by a hot, burning, or pruritic sensation at the site. The lesion begins as a red macule or papule and expands in a circular manner, sometimes reaching a diameter of 12 inches or more. Lesions vary considerably in size and form (Plate 3, *A*). At least 30% of patients have multiple lesions. Fever, headache, stiff neck, nausea and vomiting, myalgias (muscle pain), and fatigue commonly accompany ECM. In untreated persons significant cardiac (8%), neurologic (15%), or arthritic (40% to 60%) complications develop weeks to months later; frank arthritis may develop. Attacks of arthritis may recur for several years and lead to erosion of cartilage and bone.[42]

ETIOLOGIC AGENT

The association of LD with the bite of the *Ixodes* tick and the beneficial effect of penicillin and tetracycline on the course of the disease suggested that the illness was caused by a tick-transmitted bacterium. In 1982 a previously unrecognized spirochete was isolated from *Ixodes dammini* collected from a known endemic area of LD in New York.[10] This spirochete was subsequently recovered from the blood, skin, or cerebrospinal fluid of 3 of 56 patients with LD[115] and has been identified as *Borrelia burgdorferi*.[99] In contrast to the borreliae that cause relapsing fever, *B. burgdorferi* is antigenically stable and both American and European isolates belong to the same species.

Modified Kelly medium with kanamycin and 5-fluorouracil is selective for these organisms.[71]

LABORATORY DIAGNOSIS

Diagnosis of LD is usually based on compatible clinical findings, history of a tick bite, and exposure in an endemic area. Although isolation of the spirochete permits a definitive diagnosis, it is not a high-yield procedure.[3,115] In contrast to the relapsing fever borreliae, examination of blood smears during the acute phase of LD is not a useful technique because of the low level of spirochetemia. Serologic testing is currently the best laboratory method of diagnosis. Serodiagnosis of LD is possible because the spirochete can be cultured and is antigenically stable. The serologic tests in use at state health department laboratories and at the Centers for Disease Control (CDC) are the indirect immunofluorescence assay (IFA) (Plate 3, *B*) and the enzyme-linked immunosorbent assay (ELISA).[37,86,99] Both tests are highly specific and sensitive for complicated LD in which high antibody titers are present. The CDC uses a cutoff titer of >256 for a positive result. However, diagnostic laboratories have not reached general agreement as to what constitutes a significant titer, particularly in the early phase of the disease. Early in the illness diagnosis can be made from the presence of ECM and exposure in an endemic area, and a serologic test is not required. In the absence of ECM, LD may be confused with some of the viral infections. The uncertainty as to the significance of low antibody titers (less than 256) presents a major diagnostic problem for the physician in the absence of compatible clinical findings. Sera from patients with treponemal infections (syphilis, yaws, and pinta) cross-react significantly with *B. burgdorferi*, and the sera of some patients with LD give a positive fluorescent treponemal antibody absorption (FTA-ABS) test result. These false-positive results can be resolved with the rapid plasma reagin (RPR) and microhemagglutination–*Treponema pallidum* tests for syphilis. Sera from patients with LD give negative results in these tests.[99]

Common nonspecific findings include an elevated erythrocyte sedimentation rate, increased serum IgM, the presence of serum cryoglobulins, and cerebrospinal fluid (CSF) lymphocytic pleocytosis.

TREATMENT

Tetracycline appears to be the most effective drug for treating early LD.[116] Penicillin and erythromycin also lead to attenuation or prevention of subsequent bouts of arthritis if they are started early in the course of the illness. Penicillin in high doses is being used to treat the arthritic and neurologic complications of LD.

TOXIC SHOCK SYNDROME

Toxic shock syndrome (TSS) is an acute illness that is associated primarily with *Staphylococcus aureus* phage group I and was first described in 1978.[118] Signs and symptoms include high fever, headache, confusion, conjunctival injection, a macular diffuse rash, and an abrupt onset of vomiting and watery diarrhea. Acute renal failure, hepatic abnormalities, disseminated intravascular coagulation, and severe prolonged shock may develop; death ensues in severe cases. Most patients with TSS are women of childbearing age who become ill during or shortly after menstruation.

EPIDEMIOLOGY

As of June 15, 1983, 2204 cases of TSS had been reported in the United States.[25]* Ninety-six percent of cases have occurred in women; most patients (99%) were tampon users.[1] Blood-soaked tampons appear to create a favorable milieu for growth of the organism and may also enhance toxin production.[109] Case-control studies of different tampon brands showed increased risk of TSS in women who used Rely tampons,[81,104] and Procter & Gamble voluntarily removed them from the market. Most tampon-associated cases (97%) have occurred in white, non-Hispanic women, and 5% of these patients have died. Approximately 40% of patients who continue to use tampons have recurrent episodes of TSS.[36]

The proportion of TSS cases unrelated to menstruation and tampon use seems to be increasing.[98] Many of these cases have been associated with surgical wound infections,[5] and there is also evidence of neonatal TSS[61] and of nosocomial transmission.[5]

CLINICAL PRESENTATION

TSS is an acute febrile illness that begins with the abrupt onset of vomiting or diarrhea, or both, and a precipitous drop in the systolic blood pressure.[109] A characteristic erythematous skin rash and hyperemia of the mucous membranes are seen. Desquamation (principally of the palms and soles) usually occurs during the second week of illness (Plate 3, C). The principal features of TSS are indicated in the following list[109]:

1. Fever (38.9° C)
2. Vomiting or diarrhea or both
3. Diffuse macular erythematous rash
4. Hypotension (systolic blood pressure of 90 mm Hg or less for adults)
5. Desquamation of palms and soles 1 to 2 weeks after onset of illness

Several of the following are also usually present:

1. Severe myalgia
2. Vaginal, oropharyngeal, or conjunctival injection
3. Renal insufficiency
4. Hepatic dysfunction
5. Thrombocytopenia (platelet level of 100,000/mm³ or less)
6. Central nervous system changes

TSS must be distinguished from other febrile exanthema such as Rocky Mountain spotted fever, meningococcemia, leptospirosis, erythema multiforme, scarlet fever, scalded skin syndrome, and Kawasaki syndrome. TSS most closely resembles the last two illnesses named. However, scalded skin syndrome is caused by *Staphylococcus aureus* of phage group II, and in this syndrome desquamation is limited to the distal extemities and the profound systemic toxicity and multiple organ involvement characteristic of TSS do not occur. Patients with Kawasaki syndrome are usually less than 5 years of age, do not exhibit the myalgias, abdominal pain, hypotension, prolonged shock, renal insufficiency, or thrombocytopenia seen in TSS, and have enlarged lymph nodes and characteristic cardiac abnormalities.

---

*As of August 1, 1986, a total of 2962 cases had been reported in the United States; 78.9% of these were menstruation related.[56a]

ETIOLOGIC AGENT

S. aureus is the agent of TSS; strains isolated from patients have been predominantly phage group I,[1] and all isolates have been resistant to penicillin.[36] A toxin, now referred to as toxic shock syndrome toxin-1 (TSST-1), has been isolated from incriminated strains; this toxin is also known as pyrogenic exotoxin C[105] and staphylococcal enterotoxin F.[8]

The production of TSST-1 is enhanced when the concentration of magnesium ion is low. The tampon fibers that have been epidemiologically related to TSS have been shown to bind Mg^{++} and could therefore promote toxin production.[91]

LABORATORY DIAGNOSIS

All patients with symptoms of TSS should have cultures for *S. aureus*. However, the recovery of the organism from one or more body sites cannot be considered proof that a given patient has the disease, since *S. aureus* is commonly recovered from cultures (particularly vaginal and nasopharyngeal) of healthy individuals. Attempts to demonstrate toxin in blood or urine from patients have only rarely been successful, although toxin may be demonstrated in isolates of *S. aureus*. Most patients with TSS do not exhibit a significant rise in antibodies against toxic shock syndrome toxin-1.[8] Thus no test is currently available to confirm the diagnosis of TSS.

Nonspecific laboratory findings may include an elevated creatinine phosphokinase level; a blood urea nitrogen (BUN) or creatinine level at least twice normal; the presence of sterile pyuria (at least 5 white blood cells per high-power field); elevated bilirubin, serum aspartate aminotransferase (SGOT), or serum alanine aminotransferase (SGPT); and a platelet count of 100,000/mm³ or less.

TREATMENT

Antistaphylococcal therapy with beta-lactamase-resistant antibotics is recommended for treatment of TSS, although they do not appear to alter the acute course in affected individuals.[36,40] Severe disease requires intensive supportive therapy.

PREVENTION

Women who have an episode of TSS should avoid using tampons for several months to prevent recurrence.

ACQUIRED IMMUNODEFICIENCY SYNDROME

The acquired immunodeficiency syndrome (AIDS) was first recognized in the spring of 1981 when *Pneumocystis carinii* pneumonia or Kaposi's sarcoma, or both, appeared in several previously healthy homosexual men in New York and California. It soon became apparent that other opportunistic infections were occurring along with *P. carinii* pneumonia and that groups other than homosexuals were also at risk, including intravenous drug abusers, hemophiliacs, recipients of blood transfusions, and heterosexual contacts of persons at increased risk.

By the autumn of 1981 AIDS had acquired epidemic status and the CDC created a task force to study the disorder and conduct clinical, laboratory, and epidemiologic investigations. This surveillance definition of AIDS was put forward:

a reliably diagnosed disease, at least moderately predictive of a defect in cell-mediated immunity (e.g., Kaposi's sarcoma in a person less than 60 years of age, *Pneumocystis carinii* pneumonia, or other opportunistic infections), occurring in a person with no known cause for diminished resistance to that disease (e.g., congenital immunodeficiency, immunosuppressive therapy, lymphoreticular malignancies).*

As of September 1986 over 24,000 cases had been reported from all states, the District of Columbia, and Puerto Rico,[29,34b,34d] and 559 cases from at least 10 other countries.[31,31a] The number of cases of AIDS has been doubling every 10 months, making the illness a public health problem of epidemic proportions. The prevention and cure remain to be determined.

EPIDEMIOLOGY

Several groups are at increased risk for AIDS.[23,29,34b,34d]

Population	AIDS Cases (%)†
Homosexual or bisexual men	71
Intravenous drug abusers (heterosexual)	17
Haitians	5
Hemophiliacs	1
Recipients of blood transfusions	1
Heterosexual contacts of persons at increased risk	1
Persons in none of the above groups	4

Among homosexual and bisexual men, the group at greatest risk, several factors seem to predispose an individual to AIDS: multiple sexual partners, type of sexual practices, especially behaviors that result in mucosal trauma, and use of recreational drugs such as nitrite inhalants, cocaine, and marijuana. The prevalence of AIDS among homosexual and bisexual men suggested early in the course of the epidemic that a sexually transmitted infectious agent or exposure to a common environment had an important role in the development of the disease.

Intravenous drug abusers with no history of homosexuality comprise 17% of the total number of patients with AIDS. The spread of the disease to this group reinforced the notion that AIDS was caused by a transmissible infectious agent.

Haitian immigrants to the United States represent 4% of the total number of cases of AIDS. These individuals have no admitted history of homosexuality or intravenous drug use.[15] The outbreak of AIDS in this population is unique in that it occurs within a single ethnic group of previously healthy men without any of the other risk factors. It is possible that a high proportion of Haitians with AIDS are in fact homosexuals, since for cultural reasons a Haitian national would be unlikely to admit homosexuality. Since the appearance of AIDS among Haitians in the United States, it has been determined that the disease is also found in Haiti, where 85% of affected persons reside in an area near Port-au-Prince where male and female promiscuity is high. In 1985 Haitian-born AIDS patients were placed into the "Persons in none of the above" group. The separate listing of Haitian-born patients was discontinued in light of current epidemiologic information that suggests that

both heterosexual contact and exposure to contaminated needles (not associated with intravenous drug abuse) play a role in disease transmission.[34b]

Patients with hemophilia account for 1% of the reported cases of AIDS. Therapy for the hemorrhagic complications of hemophilia involves transfusion of the coagulation factors that hemophiliacs lack. These factors are available in several forms: a cryoprecipitate, a plasma factor concentrate, and fresh-frozen plasma. The use of these preparations exposes the recipients to numerous donors. As of October 1984, 52 cases of AIDS in patients with hemophilia had been reported.[30] The risk of AIDS appears higher in patients who have received factor VIII concentrates. AIDS appeared among hemophiliacs 2 to 2½ years after it was recognized for the first time among the homosexual population. This time lag may represent latency after introduction of the AIDS agent into blood products (7 to 14 months) plus any processing time of the blood products before they reached a susceptible population (12 to 15 months).[44] With only one exception,[30] patients with hemophilia who develop AIDS have only the opportunistic infections characteristic of the syndrome but do not develop Kaposi's sarcoma or other unusual neoplasms.[24]

Unfortunately, AIDS has not remained confined to the original risk groups but has also spread to other populations, including recipients of blood transfusions and heterosexual contacts of persons at increased risk. Four percent of patients with AIDS have no known risk factors.[12,20,29,39]

Not included among the risk groups listed on this page are the recently described cases of AIDS in children.[29] Table 10-1 compares the major risk factors for AIDS in children with those in adults. Each of the pediatric patients with AIDS either has received transfusions of blood or blood products or has had exposure to one or more individuals with known risk factors (that is, the mother is an intravenous drug abuser, a Haitian, or the heterosexual contact of an AIDS patient or herself has AIDS).

AIDS is manifest in children mainly as opportunistic infection; two cases of Kaposi's sarcoma had been described as of 1983.[9] Mortality is as high as 69%. The early onset of the illness in some infants and the fact that in many cases it was the patient's mother who had the risk factor for AIDS support the hypothesis that transmission of the AIDS agent occurs in utero or shortly after birth.

As of September 1986, over 24,000 patients who meet the

TABLE 10-1. Major Risk Factors for AIDS

Major Risk Factor	Adult AIDS	Pediatric AIDS
Homosexuality	+	−
Prostitution	+	+ (mother)
Intravenous drug abuse	+	+ (mother)
Haitian	+	+ (mother)
Blood transfusions	+	+
Hemophilia	+	+

SYMBOLS, +, Present
−, Absent

---

*From Centers for Disease Control: Update on acquired immune deficiency syndrome (AIDS)—United States, MMWR **31**:507, 1982.
†These percentages have changed since the chapter was written. See reference 34e.

CDC surveillance definition of AIDS had been reported.[29,34b,34d] The cases came from all states, the District of Columbia, and Puerto Rico. The states of New York, California, Florida, and New Jersey account for 78% of all cases. Within these states most cases have been reported among residents of large cities:

Area of Residence	Percentage of Total Cases
New York City	42
San Francisco	12
Los Angeles	8
Miami	4
Newark, New Jersey	3
Houston	3
Elsewhere	28

The concentration of AIDS in these particular metropolitan areas is probably related to the presence of large homosexual communities in New York City, San Francisco, and Houston and the concentration of recent Haitian immigrants in the Miami area.

Europe has reported 559 cases. These patients belong to the same risk groups as the U.S. AIDS victims: 87.2% are male homosexuals, 3.4% are hemophiliacs, and 1.4% are drug abusers. None of the risk factors could be found for 6.9% of the patients.[31,34a]

Of particular interest is the finding of AIDS in Africa. The patients have clinical features and immunologic abnormalities similar to those reported from the United States and Europe, but an important difference is a 1:1 ratio of males to females, which implies a heterosexual transmission of AIDS. Recent data also show the disease to be increasing in the heterosexual population in the United States; 4% of the total number of cases are currently seen in this group.[34e]

Although substantiating evidence is lacking, researchers have speculated that AIDS originated in Central Africa, where it was transmitted to Haitians who were in Zaire between the early 1960s and the mid-1970s for professional training and then returned to their country. The AIDS agent may have been imported to the United States by vacationing homosexuals and quickly spread in this population by means of frequent, often anonymous, sexual encounters in bath houses and elsewhere. Homosexual drug addicts might have introduced the agent, via the parenteral route, into the heterosexual intravenous drug abusing population.[120]

Of the total number of cases of AIDS reported to the CDC, 90% have been in individuals between 20 and 49 years of age; 58% have occurred among whites, 25% among blacks, and 14% in persons of Hispanic origin. Women account for 7% of all cases.[29,34b]

CLINICAL PRESENTATION

If AIDS follows the pattern of other infectious diseases, the host response to the putative AIDS agent would be expected to range from subclinical to severe. The original surveillance definition of AIDS put forward by the CDC includes the severe cases in which "there is a reliably diagnosed disease moderate-

ly predictive of a defect in cell-mediated immunity, occurring in a person with no known cause for diminished resistance to that disease."[17] Recently the CDC[17a] expanded the definition to include the entire spectrum of AIDS manifestations, ranging from the absence of symptoms in the presence of laboratory evidence of immune deficiency, passing through nonspecific symptoms, such as fever, weight loss, and generalized lymphadenopathy, to the full-blown syndrome included in the original definition.

Underlying this devastating disease are striking defects in the patient's immune system[45,85] that include profound leukopenia, with total lymphocyte counts of less than 500 cells/mm^3; decrease in or absence of killer T cell activity; polyclonal activation of B cells, resulting in elevated levels of circulating immunoglobulins; presence of a heat-labile form of alpha-interferon; elevated alpha-1-thymosin levels; and presence in the serum of substances capable of suppressing the in vitro immune responses of normal lymphocytes. The leukopenia is due to a selective decrease in the number of the helper-inducer subset of T lymphocytes (that is, lymphocytes that have antigens called T_4 on their surface and that "help" or "induce" B lymphocytes to produce antibodies). The number of suppressor-cytotoxic T cells (which are lymphocytes that have antigens called T_8 on their surface and that "suppress" antibody production by B lymphocytes) remains normal, and as a result the ratio of helper to suppressor cells, which normally is around 2:1, is markedly reduced in AIDS patients (see Chapter 2). It is not known whether the severe immunologic dysfunction seen in AIDS is due to the imbalance between help and suppression or more directly to the depletion of T-helper cells. The consequence of this particular defect in cellular immunity is a profound alteration of in vivo and in vitro T cell function.

The end result of this severe immune deficiency is a host highly susceptible to opportunistic infections and unusual neoplasms. The clinical spectrum of AIDS includes opportunistic infections, of which the most common is *P. carinii* pneumonia; unusual malignant neoplasms, especially Kaposi's sarcoma; generalized lymphadenopathy; and wasting illness.

Opportunistic Infections

Although *P. carinii* pneumonia is by far the most common opportunistic infection in AIDS patients, several other etiologic agents cause problems in this population.

Bacterial infections

The most common bacterial infections in AIDS patients are due to *Mycobacterium avium-intracellulare* and *Mycobacterium tuberculosis*. *M. avium-intracellulare* is a common environmental saprophyte that in the past was rarely associated with disseminated human infection. However, in AIDS patients it causes a fatal fulminating disease.[60] The organism can be recovered from the bone marrow, lymph nodes, liver, and blood, suggesting that the immunologic defect in AIDS selectively predisposes the patients toward disseminated infection with this unusual pathogen.

M. tuberculosis produces infection primarily among the Haitian group of AIDS patients, probably because tuberculosis is endemic among Haitian immigrants in the United States.[94]

Salmonella and other gram-negative aerobic bacilli are frequently associated with infections. Notably absent is *Listeria monocytogenes,* an opportunistic intracellular bacterium that commonly infects other patients with cellular immune deficiencies.

Viral infections

Devastating viral infections are seen among AIDS patients. The main viral pathogens are cytomegalovirus (CMV), herpes simplex virus (HSV) type 2, and papovavirus.

CMV infections in AIDS disseminate widely in the body, and at autopsy the virus can be found in almost every organ, with greatest involvement of the lungs, central nervous system, gastrointestinal tract, and adrenal glands. Retinal involvement may be the earliest evidence of CMV dissemination. Initially the retinal lesions are asymptomatic, but they rapidly progress, causing perivascular exudates and hemorrhages and giving rise to the so-called cotton-wool spots. Eventually the infection involves the macula and the vision becomes compromised. CMV infections are so prevalent among AIDS patients that until recently it was postulated that CMV might be the causative agent of AIDS.[59] CMV causes immunosuppression in humans (see Chapter 2) and can persist in the semen for months at high titer. However, more than 90% of healthy homosexual men have antibodies against the virus, indicating previous exposure to CMV[42] and suggesting that CMV infection in AIDS may be only a reactivation of a latent infection during immunosuppression, in a manner analogous to infection in renal transplant patients. CMV is now believed to be simply another opportunistic pathogen attacking a population with a severe deficiency in cellular immunity.

Both primary and recurrent herpes simplex virus infection occur frequently in AIDS. The infection appears as vesicular lesions on erythematous bases in the oral, genital, and perianal areas. Most commonly the chronic perianal ulcerations progress to severely hemorrhagic, undermining ulcerative lesions, even in the absence of previous vesicles (Plate 3, *D*).

The papovavirus strain JC appears to be the cause of a subacute demyelinating illness called progressive multifocal leukoencephalopathy (PML). The disease, which is manifest as weakness and cerebellar dysfunction, is rare even in the case of severe immunosuppression. However, it is common in AIDS patients, in whom the diagnosis is made by computerized tomography (CT) and brain biopsy, which shows viral particles and intranuclear inclusions in different nervous tissue cells.

Varicella-zoster and adenovirus infections have also been described but with less frequency.

Fungal infections

Most of the opportunistic fungi may infect AIDS patients, but the most common species are *Candida albicans, Cryptococcus neoformans,* and *Aspergillus* spp. AIDS patients commonly develop oral thrush (oral candidiasis), often before the documentation of Kaposi's sarcoma or other opportunistic infections. The oral mucosa appears covered with patches of cream-white pseudomembranes, which are composed of yeast and pseudohyphae of *Candida* spp. The lesions are painful and debilitating, interfering with food intake (Plate 3, *E*).[59] *Candida* esophagitis is also common in AIDS. Disseminated candidiasis is rare in this population, suggesting that the functioning part of the immune system is capable of keeping the pathogen confined to the upper gastrointestinal tract.

Disseminated cryptococcosis is a common complication of AIDS, as is the presence of invasive or disseminated aspergillosis. Coccidioidomycosis and histoplasmosis have also been reported in association with AIDS.

Protozoal infections

Three genera of protozoa cause severe infection in patients with AIDS: *Pneumocystis carinii, Cryptosporidium* spp., and *Toxoplasma gondii.* Conspicuously absent from this group is *Strongyloides stercoralis,* a parasite known to cause serious infection in other patients with compromised cellular immune function, such as persons who have lymphoma or leukemia or are receiving immunosuppressive therapy.

P. carinii pneumonia (PCP) is the most common opportunistic infection in AIDS; 59% of all patients have this disease (Table 10-2).[29] In these patients PCP develops as an insidious process that unfolds over weeks or months and is characterized by dyspnea, with or without a nonproductive cough, and fever. The characteristic histologic finding is abundant honeycombed material filling the airspaces, alveoli, and bronchioles. The honeycombed appearance results from cohesion of masses of *P. carinii* cysts (Plate 3, *F*). When, instead of hematoxylin and eosin (H & E), Grocott-Gomori methenamine–silver nitrate is used to stain the tissue sections, the cyst walls can be clearly seen (Plate 4, *A* and *B*). With Giemsa stain it is possible to see the internal sporozoites on impression smears of the infected lungs (Plate 4, *C*).

P. carinii is thought to be spread by the respiratory route, and patients probably transmit the organisms to each other. However, at the present time evidence is insufficient to determine whether PCP in these patients is due to a recent infection or to a latent infection that becomes reactivated as a consequence of the immunologic lesion seen in this population.

Cryptosporidium is a parasite commonly found in AIDS patients, where its presence leads to persistent or recurrent diarrhea that may last months or even years, resulting in severe malnutrition and probably contributing to death.[119] Until recently the diagnosis of cryptosporidiosis was made by intestinal biopsy and microscopic demonstration of the endogenous stages of the parasite attached to the brush border of epithelial cells (Plate 4, *D* and *E*). With the increase in cases of cryptosporidiosis resulting from the AIDS epidemic, new methods have been developed to make the diagnosis by noninvasive techniques; these include the identification of oocysts in the stool using specific stains, such as acid-fast stains (Plate 4, *F*), and specific concentration techniques, such as the Sheather sugar flotation (Plate 5, *A*). (See Chapter 42 for further discussion of the laboratory diagnosis of *Cryptosporidium.*)

Together with lymphomas, *Toxoplasma gondii* is the most common cause of mass lesions in the central nervous system of patients with AIDS. The parasite can cause retinochoroiditis.

Unusual Malignant Neoplasms: Kaposi's Sarcoma

Kaposi's sarcoma (KS) and several types of malignant lymphomas occur with high frequency among patients with AIDS. The lymphomas include Burkitt's lymphoma, primary lymphoma of the central nervous system, Hodgkin's lymphoma, and diffuse, undifferentiated non-Hodgkin's lymphoma.

KS was described in 1872 by Moricz Kaposi as an ''idiopathic multiple pigmented sarcoma of the skin.'' Until recently

TABLE 10-2. Comparison of Classical and Epidemic Kaposi's Sarcoma

Characteristic	Classical KS	Epidemic KS
Skin lesions	Usually localized to lower extremities	Generalized
Lymphadenopathy	None	Common
Visceral involvement	Rare	Frequent
Course	Indolent	Fulminant
Associated conditions	Other malignancies (37%)	Opportunistic infections
Immune dysfunction	Rare	Profound
Survival	10 to 15 years	Short
Male/female ratio	10 to 15:1	Predominantly males
Mean age of patients	63	37
Sexual preference of patients	Primarily heterosexual	Homosexual or bisexual
Geographic distribution	Nonclustering	Predominantly in New York, San Francisco, Miami, Houston, Los Angeles
Ethnic background of patients	Mostly Italian or Eastern European Jewish origin	Mixed

most cases of classical KS have occurred in 50- to 60-year-old men of Eastern European Jewish or Italian origin. Classical KS is most often a benign, indolent disease that is manifest as a localized, nodular tumor ranging in color from blue to purple, most frequently seen on the lower extremities. The tumor is relatively sensitive to irradiation or chemotherapy, and survival has been between 8 and 13 years. In the United States the incidence is 0.02 to 0.06 per 100,000 population.

Two exceptions to this benign pattern of classical KS should be noted. First, KS occurs in the Bantu tribe of South Africa and in an endemic belt located in equatorial Africa, where it accounts for 9% of all tumors. In Africa KS is observed in black adults between the ages of 25 and 45 years, with a male/female ratio of 17:1. The disease in this population can follow three different patterns:

1. The benign nodular type seen in patients with classical KS
2. A more florid and aggressive form with local invasion of subcutaneous tissue and bone
3. The most remarkable type, seen primarily among black children between the ages of 2 to 15 years, in which there is widespread lymph node and visceral involvement but few if any cutaneous lesions. The male/female ratio is 3:1, and the mortality is very high.

Second, patients receiving renal transplants or immunosuppressive therapy have a higher incidence of KS, which may remain localized but usually shows widespread dissemination and visceral involvement.[56,67,93]

The epidemic form of KS occurring in patients with AIDS, in which there are widely disseminated, multifocal mucocutaneous and visceral lesions, closely resembles the lymphadenopathic form of KS seen in African children and in immunosuppressed transplant patients.[12,49]

Table 10-2 compares the main features of classical and epidemic KS. The mucocutaneous clinical manifestations of epidemic KS are much more varied than those in the classical form of the disease; the skin lesions are not limited to the lower extremities but may appear anywhere on the upper or lower extremities, trunk, genitals, and face, particularly behind the ear and on the earlobes (Plate 5, B). Lesions are commonly found not only on the skin but widespread in the oral mucosa, the esophagus, and the rest of the gastrointestinal tract. The disease is slowly progressive, and most deaths are due to the opportunistic infections that accompany KS in this syndrome.[48]

There seems to be a genetic predisposition for KS, as evidenced by a statistically significant incidence of HLA-DR5 among patients with both the classical and the epidemic form of the disease. Thus it appears possible that genetically predisposed persons, when immunosuppressed for various reasons, are particularly susceptible to this type of tumor.[49]

Of the total number of cases of AIDS, 53% have been reported to have PCP without KS, 24% have KS without PCP, 6% have both PCP and KS, and 17% have other opportunistic infections without either PCP or KS (Table 10-3).[29]

Early studies showed the mortality of AIDS to be approximately 73%, although more recent evidence suggests that the real mortality approaches 100%.

Symptoms

Generalized lymphadenopathy, night sweats, chills, easy fatigability, fever, anorexia, and weight loss are nonspecific symptoms that may occur months before the onset of an opportunistic infection or KS or both.

The terms "pre-AIDS," "chronic lymphadenopathy syndrome," "lymphadenopathy syndrome," and "AIDS-related

TABLE 10-3. Distribution and Mortality of AIDS by Disease Group

Disease Group	Percentage of Total Cases	Case-Mortality Ratio (%)
PCP without KS (with or without OOI)	53	47
KS without PCP (with or without OOI)	24	21
PCP with KS (with or without OOI)	6	68
OOI without KS or PCP	17	48

SYMBOLS:	PCP, *Pneumocystis carinii* pneumonia
	KS, Kaposi's sarcoma
	OOI, Other opportunistic infections

complex'' (ARC) have been coined to define the unexplained lymphadenopathy seen originally in homosexual men and now found in so many patients in whom the full-blown syndrome later develops.[16] The precise significance of the ARC syndrome is unknown. It may be a milder manifestation of AIDS or alternatively may be a prodrome of the disease, in which case patients will ultimately develop AIDS. A recent report indicates that in 83% of patients with ARC, opportunistic infections or unusual neoplasms, or both, develop within a year.[89]

The weight loss may reach 30% to 50% of body weight, even in the absence of diarrhea, and is so striking that AIDS has been referred as the "wasting syndrome."[90] Fever may be intermittent or persistent and may cause severe disability. The causes of fever and weight loss are unclear.

Patients with AIDS frequently develop a generalized encephalopathy, which includes dementia as a dominant feature. Initially depression, memory loss, and impaired concentration occur; these are followed over months by a peculiar apathy, withdrawal, and a lack of expression. Finally the patient shows severe cognitive impairment and withdraws into a near-catatonic state.[90,110]

ETIOLOGIC AGENT

Almost since the appearance of AIDS, the epidemiologic evidence has strongly suggested that the disease is caused by an infectious agent, possibly a virus, with several modes of transmission. Cytomegalovirus and herpes virus were initially implicated but were subsequently recognized as opportunistic pathogens attacking an immunologically compromised host. It now appears that a retrovirus of the human T-cell lymphoma-leukemia (HTLV) family is the causative agent of AIDS.

Members of the HTLV family of retrovirus share a pronounced tropism for helper-inducer T lymphocytes; a magnesium-dependent, high-molecular-weight reverse transcriptase; and the capacity to inhibit, transform, or kill the infected T cells.[108] Before the discovery of the AIDS virus, two types of HTLV virus had been described: HTLV-I, which is associated with T cell malignancies in adults in the United States,[95,96] Israel, the West Indies, Africa, and southern Japan,[97] and HTLV-II, which is associated with hairy cell leukemia.[73]

That a virus of the HTLV family might be implicated in the etiology of AIDS was suggested almost simultaneously by several investigators in May 1983. First, Essex and co-workers[43] showed that 25% of patients with AIDS and 26% of patients with ARC have antibodies against a cell membrane antigen of lymphocytes infected with HTLV-I. This antigen was later found to be a glycoprotein called gp61, which is related to the HTLV viral glycoprotein.[82] Second, Gallo and co-workers[57] found HTLV-I proviral DNA in the lymphocytes from two of 33 AIDS patients. Third, the same group of researchers isolated a virus related to HTLV-I from a patient with AIDS and then successfully transmitted the virus into human T cells from the umbilical cord of a newborn.[54]

The more frequent detection in AIDS patients of antibodies to a membrane protein (gp61) rather than to HTLV internal structural core proteins (p19, p24), together with the low incidence of isolation of HTLV-I and II from these patients, suggested that a new variant of HTLV might be the causative agent of AIDS. Further support for this idea came the same year from L. Montagnier and his co-workers at the Pasteur Institute in France. They isolated a retrovirus belonging to the HTLV family but clearly distinct from HTLV-I and HTLV-II, from a patient with the lymphadenopathy syndrome (LAS, ARC, Pre-AIDS). Like HTLV-I and II, the virus was a typical type C RNA tumor virus, had a high-molecular-weight reverse transcriptase that preferred magnesium ion for activity, and had an internal antigen (p25) similar to HTLV p24. Antibodies from this patient reacted with proteins from viruses of the HTLV-I group. That this newly discovered retrovirus was not the same as HTLV-I was demonstrated by the fact that type-specific antisera to HTLV-I did *not* precipitate proteins of the new virus. This new isolate was named "lymphadenopathy-associated virus" (LAV) and was successfully transmitted to cord blood lymphocytes.[4]

A year after these original obervations, R.C. Gallo and his co-workers[55] at the National Cancer Institute reported the isolation and characterization of a new member of the HTLV family, which they named HTLV-III. This virus was isolated from 18 of 21 patients with ARC (86%), 26 of 72 patients with AIDS (36%), and none of 115 normal, heterosexual individuals tested. The researchers suggested that the frequency of viral isolation was lower from patients with AIDS (36%) than from ARC patients (86%) because serum samples from patients in the later stages of the disease contained many dying cells and few viable T_4 lymphocytes.[55] However, a high proportion of patients with ARC and AIDS have circulating antibodies against HTLV-III.[102]

HTLV-III virions have a diameter of 100 to 120 nm and are produced in high numbers from infected cells by budding from the cell membrane, where mature virions appear to have a cylindric core.[55]

Numerous lines of evidence have shown that HTLV-III is indeed a member of the HTLV family of retroviruses. It now appears that HTLV-III, LAV, and the retrovirus isolated from AIDS patients in San Francisco[84] are all independent isolates of a single species of virus.

Infected individuals develop antibodies against HTLV-III. AIDS later develops in 5% to 19% of seropositive individuals, and ARC in an additional 25%.[34] Antibodies against HTLV-III[102] and LAV[50] have been found in 68% to 100% in patients with AIDS and in 84% to 100% of patients with ARC. Less than 1% of heterosexual subjects not at high risk for AIDS are seropositive.[34]

Even though the evidence implicating HTLV-III/LAV as the causative agent of AIDS is strong, the unequivocal proof of a specific etiologic relation between a given microorganism and a given disease requires the fulfillment of Koch's postulates. The first and second postulates were met by the isolation of HTLV-III/LAV from patients with AIDS or ARC and in some individuals at risk of acquiring AIDS,[55] coupled with the presence of antibodies against the virus in these populations.[102] The isolated virus can be cultured in the laboratory, is highly infectious, and can be transmitted to fresh umbilical cord blood and peripheral blood or bone marrow lymphocytes.[55] Postulates three and four were more difficult to fulfill, since experimental inoculation of the HTLV-III/LAV virus to chimpanzees causes immunologic abnormalities and prolonged lymphadenopathy, but the opportunistic infections or tumors characteristic of AIDS have not developed in these animals.[2,26,47] An experiment of nature allowed the fulfillment of these last two postulates: LAV was isolated from both a blood donor and the recipient of that donor's blood. AIDS developed in the recipient even though she had no other risk factor for AIDS; the donor died of AIDS.[46] It is now widely accepted that HTLV-III/LAV is the causative agent of AIDS. As noted in Chapter 2, the virus has been renamed human immunodeficiency virus (HIV).*

HIV is primarily transmitted through intimate sexual contact; sharing of contaminated needles; transfusion of whole blood, blood cellular components, plasma, or clotting factor concentrates that are not heat treated; or from infected mother to child before, at, or shortly after birth.[34]

HIV has now been cultured from the semen of two patients with AIDS[124] and from the semen and blood of a healthy homosexual man whose serum contained antibodies to HIV.[66] The finding of HIV in the semen supports the epidemiologic data suggesting that AIDS can be transmitted by sexual contact. The demonstration of HIV in a seropositive healthy homosexual man suggests that development of an asymptomatic, virus-positive, carrier state is possible, during which transmission of the disease may occur.

The isolation of HIV from symptom-free, seronegative individuals suggests the existence of a period between the acquisition of the virus and the development of anti-HIV antibodies, during which the person harbors infectious virus and can transmit the disease without being detected by any of the presently available screening methods.[100]

Even though there is no evidence that AIDS can be transferred by casual contact, the isolation of the virus from the saliva of people with ARC and healthy homosexuals at risk for AIDS represents a serious warning that saliva may be a vehicle of horizontal transmission of the disease.[63] Even though this is probably a rare route of spread for HIV, one case of AIDS transmitted through saliva has been reported.[100]

A recent report indicates that HIV, in addition to causing the immune defect underlying AIDS, may play a role in the pathogenesis of AIDS encephalopathy. Both DNA and RNA of HIV were detected in the brains of five of 15 AIDS patients with encephalopathy, indicating that the virus is not only present in the tissue but is expressing itself there. Since certain surface antigens are present in both lymphocytes and brain cells, possibly HIV has tropism for brain cells as well as T_4 lymphocytes.[110]

Studies to determine the origin of HIV are in progress.[75]

DIAGNOSIS

Clearly AIDS is a disease of the immune system in which there is a characteristic depletion of the T_4 helper-inducer subset of T lymphocytes, which causes the host to be extraordinarily susceptible to Kaposi's sarcoma, *Pneumocystis carinii* pneumonia, and other opportunistic infections.

Before the discovery of HIV as the etiologic agent of AIDS, the diagnosis of the disease was based solely on (1) determining the presence of KS, PCP, and other opportunistic infections, all of which can be diagnosed in the laboratory by standard methods, and (2) demonstration of a reduced T_4-helper/T_8-suppressor ratio in a person with no known cause for immunodeficiency.

A reversal of the T_4/T_8 ratio of lymphocytes in itself does not mean that a person has AIDS or is at risk of developing the full-blown syndrome. There are two ways by which the T_4/T_8 ratio can be decreased: decrease in the number of T_4 lymphocytes, or increase in the number of T_8 lymphocytes. In AIDS patients the low T_4/T_8 ratio is due to a decrease in the number of cells in the T_4-helper subset of T lymphocytes. However, as discussed in Chapter 2, a number of viral infections (such as cytomegalovirus and Epstein-Barr virus infections) can increase the T_8-suppressor subset of T lymphocytes without substantially lowering the T_4-helper subset, thus causing a reduced T_4/T_8 ratio in the absence of AIDS. Special attention should be paid to not labeling patients with these infections as having ARC or AIDS, since the social and psychologic consequences of such a mistake can be devastating.

Many other laboratory tests have been proposed for the diagnosis of AIDS, including the measuring of alpha-thymosin, beta$_2$-microglobulin, interferon levels, or immune complexes or the demonstration of inhibition of cellular immunity. However, none of these tests is useful in itself for diagnosing AIDS or identifying individuals at risk for the disease.

The establishment of HIV as the etiologic agent of AIDS has led to the development of tests for the detection of antibodies against the virus. Anti-HIV antibodies can now be detected by several methods, including radioimmunoassay (RIA), immunofluorescence (IF), enzyme-linked immunosorbent assay (ELISA), and Western blotting techniques.[43,74,102,103]

Researchers using these various techniques have now reported that 68% to 100% of patients with AIDS and 84% to 100% of patients with ARC have antibodies against HIV, compared with less than 1% seropositivity for control populations.[34,102]

Patients with ARC or newly diagnosed AIDS have a higher antibody titer than patients with advanced AIDS, and the anti-

---

*This discussion refers to HIV-I; however, other HIV viruses have recently been reported.

bodies are directed mainly against the major envelope protein of the virus.[102] Furthermore, the virus itself is isolated in 85% of cases of ARC but in only 50% of cases of AIDS.[55] This is consistent with the idea that the virus attacks a specific subset of T lymphocytes (T_4), causes an initial proliferation of the cells but eventually leads to their destruction, and thus causes a loss of T-helper functions, including stimulation of antibody production. During the ARC period, HIV is present in a high proportion of patients, and since the T-helper function has not yet been destroyed, antibody production continues, especially against the envelope proteins of the virus. As the disease progresses and ARC becomes AIDS, the target population of T_4 cells is destroyed and so is the capacity to produce antibodies in response to a new antigenic challenge; thus the antibody titers are lower.

Several U.S. companies are now producing ELISA kits for the detection of antibodies against HIV. Results indicate that the test is both highly specific and sensitive; however, in a low-prevalence population even this test with a specificity of greater than 99% results in false-positive reactions. Thus repeated positives ($\times 2$) should be confirmed with another test.

The recent finding of four seronegative, symptom-free individuals from whom it was possible to isolate HIV indicated that probably the only way to detect all infected individuals is by developing tests by which viral antigens themselves are detected.[100] Several of these antigen detection kits are currently being evaluated by the FDA.

TREATMENT

Until the discovery of the etiologic agent, the treatment of AIDS focused on treatment of opportunistic infections and malignancies and attempts to reconstitute the crippled immune system. The treatment of opportunistic infections is characterized by a slow response and a tendency for the infection to recur, probably because of the persistence of the immune defect.[45]

Trimethoprim-sulfamethoxazole is the drug of choice for *Pneumocystis carinii* infections in immunocompromised patients.[68,122] However, in patients with AIDS the frequency of adverse reactions to this drug is extraordinarily high, and pentamidine isothianate is now used with increasing frequency in this population.[58]

Toxoplasmosis has been treated with sulfadiazine and pyrimethamine, drugs that in some cases limit the progression of the disease but are immunosuppressive and therefore aggravate the underlying immune deficiency.

No effective treatment has been found for cryptosporidiosis.[14] Encouraging reports of successful treatment with spiramycin have appeared.[32] This drug is a macrolide compound used in Europe and Canada to treat infections caused by *Toxoplasma gondii;* it has an antimicrobial activity similar to those of erythromycin and clindamycin.

Candidiasis in AIDS patients is treated with conventional antifungal therapy (nystatin, orally administered ketoconazole, intravenously administered amphotericin B), but relapses are common after termination of therapy.

Cryptococcal disease is difficult to treat, and active infection is usually found at autopsy despite therapy with either amphotericin B or fluorocytosine.

At present there is no effective treatment for cytomegalovirus (CMV) and Epstein-Barr virus (EBV) infections. A new experimental drug, DHPG, is available for the treatment of systemic CMV disease. The Centers for Disease Control makes DHPG available only for treatment of patients with culture-proven CMV infection or pathologic findings consistent with CMV disease. Since in conventional cell-culture methods, cytopathic effects appear approximately 17 days after inoculation, in many cases the drug is no longer needed by the time the patient meets the criterion. A new cell-culture method for detecting CMV uses as the diagnostic endpoint, not the production of cytopathic effects, but the appearance of early virus-coded proteins in the infected cells, which can be detected by monoclonal antibodies and indirect immunofluorescence.[62] Rapid diagnosis of CMV infection would allow the use of potentially successful drugs early in the disease, increasing the chances of response.

Acyclovir is used to treat herpes simplex type 2 infections, but recurrence is the rule.[117]

Infections caused by *Mycobacterium avium-intracellulare* have not been treated successfully. The organism is resistant to all known antituberculous drugs, and trials with other medications such as ansamycin and the antileprosy drug clofazamine have been a failure.[45,61,125]

KS and other malignancies have been treated with conventional chemotherapy and radiotherapy. However, these treatment regimens only add more immunosuppression to the already devastated immune system, and patients usually die of opportunistic infections. The observation that in renal transplant patients the tumor regresses after discontinuation of immunosuppressive therapy strongly supports the view that treatment should be directed toward reversing the immune defect, rather than antineoplastic therapy.[56,67]

From the dismal results obtained by treating the opportunistic infections and malignancies in patients with AIDS, it became obvious that the cause of death ultimately stems from an immunologic dysfunction. Attempts to reconstitute the immune system have included therapy with interleukin-2, alpha- and gamma-interferon, and bone marrow transplantation. The trials in this direction have been uniformly unsuccessful, and most major hospitals are moving away from this approach.

Azidothymidine has recently been used for treatment and appears to be at least temporarily effective in decreasing mortality and morbidity in some patients with AIDS or AIDS-related complex, although bone marrow toxicity with this drug may be severe.[2a]

The cure for AIDS will probably rest on the inhibition and killing of the causative agent, HIV. This goal might be accomplished by using inhibitors of the reverse transcriptase, such as sodium suramin or ribavirin,[87] or agents that block the infection of T_4 lymphocytes by HIV.

PREVENTION

Since HIV appears to be transmitted through intimate sexual contact, sharing of contaminated needles, or transfusion of blood or blood products, the following steps to prevent the spread of the disease have been recommended by the CDC:

1. Sexual contact with persons known or suspected to have AIDS should be avoided. Members of high-risk groups should be aware that multiple sexual partners increase the probability of developing AIDS.[21]

2. Members of groups at increased risk for AIDS should refrain from donating plasma or blood.[21] With the availability of tests for the detection of antibodies to HIV, it is now possible to identify and exclude plasma and blood with any probability of transmitting the virus.[121]

3. Physicians should adhere strictly to medical indications for transfusions, and autologous blood transfusions should be encouraged.[21]

4. The National Hemophilia Foundation has issued specific recommendations for the management of patients with hemophilia.[13,30,83]

   a. Since the risk of transmission of HIV appears to be higher when factor VIII concentrates are used instead of cryoprecipitates, it is recommended that cryoprecipitate be used in factor VIII–deficient newborns, infants, and children under 4 years of age and in newly identified patients never before treated with factor VIII concentrates.

   b. Fresh-frozen plasma should be used in factor IX–deficient patients in the groups just mentioned.

   c. Desmopressin should be used whenever possible in patients with mild or moderate hemophilia A.

   d. For the majority of patients with hemophilia who do not fit in any of the groups mentioned, it is recommended that heat-treated factor concentrates be used. Preliminary evidence indicates that heat treatment (48 hours at 60° C) substantially reduces the viability of retrovirus in plasma factor concentrates and thus reduces the potential for transmission of HIV to these patients.[84]

5. Precautions discussed in Chapter 4 and reference 34c should be taken to avoid direct contact of skin and mucous membranes with blood, blood products, excretions, secretions, and tissues of persons with AIDS or suspected of having AIDS.[13,18]

Studies discussed in Chapter 4 and in references 18, 19, 22, 27, and 65 suggest that the procedures currently recommended for AIDS are adequate, that the risk of transmission within the hospital is low, and that accidental needle-stick exposure by health-care workers provides little additional risk of acquiring AIDS. It has been speculated that HIV is a virus with low infectivity, whose targets are activated T_4 lymphocytes, which are present in higher numbers in susceptible populations at high risk of acquiring AIDS, whereas the general population is less susceptible to the virus.

REFERENCES

1. Altemeier, W.A., et al.: *Staphylococcus aureus* associated with toxic-shock syndrome: phage typing and toxin capability testing, Ann. Intern. Med. **96:**978, 1982.

2. Alter, H.J., et al.: Transmission of HTLV-III infection from human plasma to chimpanzees: an animal model for AIDS, Science **226:**549, 1984.

2a. Azidothymidine for AIDS, Med. Lett. **28:**107, 1986.

3. Barbour, A.G.: Isolation and cultivation of Lyme disease spirochetes, Yale J. Biol. Med. **57:**521, 1984.

4. Barré-Sinoussi, F., et al.: Isolation of a T-lymphotropic retrovirus from a patient at risk for acquired immune deficiency syndrome (AIDS), Science **220:** 868, 1983.

5. Bartlett, P., et al.: Toxic-shock syndrome associated with surgical wound infections, JAMA **247:**1448, 1982.

6. Bell, D.M., et al.: Kawasaki syndrome: description of two outbreaks in the United States, N. Engl. J. Med. **304:**1568, 1981.

7. Benach, J.L., et al.: Spirochetes isolated from the blood of two patients with Lyme disease, N. Engl. J. Med. **308:**740, 1983.

8. Bergdoll, M.S., et al.: A new staphylococcal enterotoxin, enterotoxin F, associated with toxic-shock syndrome isolates, Lancet **1:**1017, 1981.

9. Buck, B.E., et al.: Kaposi sarcoma in two infants with acquired immune deficiency syndrome, J. Pediatr. **103:**911, 1983.

10. Burgdorfer, W., et al.: Lyme disease—a tick-borne spirochetosis? Science **216:**1317, 1982.

11. Carter, R.F., Haynes, M.E., and Morton, J.: Rickettsia-like bodies and splenitis in Kawasaki disease, Lancet **2:**1254, 1976.

12. Centers for Disease Control: A cluster of Kaposi sarcoma and *Pneumocystis carinii* pneumonia among homosexual male residents of Los Angeles and Orange Counties, California, MMWR **31:**305, 1982.

13. Centers for Disease Control: Acquired immune deficiency syndrome (AIDS): precautions for clinical and laboratory staffs, MMWR **31:**577, 1982.

14. Centers for Disease Control: Cryptosporidiosis: assessment of chemotherapy of males with acquired immune deficiency syndrome (AIDS), MMWR **31:**589, 1982.

15. Centers for Disease Control: Opportunistic infections among Haitians in the United States, MMWR **31:**353, 1982.

16. Centers for Disease Control: Persistent, generalized lymphadenopathy among homosexual males, MMWR **31:**249, 1982.

17. Centers for Disease Control: Update on acquired immune deficiency syndrome (AIDS)—United States, MMWR **31:**507, 1982.

18. Centers for Disease Control: Acquired immunodeficiency syndrome (AIDS): precautions for health-care workers and allied professionals, MMWR **32:**450, 1983.

19. Centers for Disease Control: An evaluation of the acquired immuno-deficiency syndrome (AIDS) reported in health-care personnel—United States, MMWR **32:**358, 1983.

20. Centers for Disease Control: Immunodeficiency among female sexual partners of males with acquired immunodeficiency syndrome (AIDS)—New York, MMWR **31:**697, 1983.

21. Centers for Disease Control: Prevention of acquired immunodeficiency syndrome (AIDS): report of inter-agency recommendations, MMWR **32:**101, 1983.

22. Centers for Disease Control: Update on acquired immunodeficiency syndrome (AIDS)—United States, MMWR **32:**389, 1983.

23. Centers for Disease Control: Update: acquired immunodeficiency syndrome (AIDS)—United States, MMWR **32:**465, 1983.

24. Centers for Disease Control: Update: acquired immunodeficiency syndrome (AIDS) among patients with hemophilia—United States, MMWR **32:**613, 1983.

25. Centers for Disease Control: Update: toxic-shock syndrome—United States, MMWR **32:**398, 1983.

26. Centers for Disease Control: Experimental infection of chimpanzees with lymphadenopathy-associated virus, MMWR **33:**442, 1984.

27. Centers for Disease Control: Prospective evaluation of health-care workers exposed via parenteral or mucous membrane routes to blood or body fluids of patients with acquired immunodeficiency syndrome (AIDS), MMWR **33:**181, 1984.

28. Centers for Disease Control: Update: acquired immunodeficiency syndrome (AIDS)—United States, MMWR **32:**688, 1984.

29. Centers for Disease Control: Update: acquired immunodeficiency syndrome (AIDS)—United States, MMWR **33:**337, 1984.

30. Centers for Disease Control: Update: acquired immunodeficiency syndrome (AIDS) in persons with hemophilia, MMWR **33:**589, 1984.

31. Centers for Disease Control: Update: acquired immunodeficiency syndrome—Europe, MMWR **33:**607, 1984.

32. Centers for Disease Control: Update: treatment of cryptosporidiosis in patients with acquired immunodeficiency syndrome (AIDS), MMWR **33:**117, 1984.

33. Centers for Disease Control: Multiple outbreaks of Kawasaki syndrome—United States, MMWR **34:**33, 1985.

34. Centers for Disease Control: Provisional Public Health Service interagency recommendations for screening donated blood and plasma for antibody to the virus causing acquired immunodeficiency syndrome, MMWR **34:**1, 1985.

34a. Centers for Disease Control: Update: acquired immunodeficiency syndrome—Europe, MMWR **34:**21, 1985.

34b. Centers for Disease Control: Update: acquired immunodeficiency syndrome—United States, MMWR **34:**245, 1985.

34c. Centers for Disease Control: Human T-lymphocyte virus type III/lymphadenopathy associated virus: agent summary statement, MMWR **35:**540, 1986.

34d. Centers for Disease Control: Immunization of children infected with HTLV III/LAV lymphadenopathy-associated virus, MMWR **35:**595, 1986.

34e. Centers for Disease Control: **35:**757, 1986.

35. Clumek, N., et al.: Acquired immunodeficiency syndrome in African patients, N. Engl. J. Med. **310:**492, 1984.

36. Cohen, J.I.: Toxic-shock syndrome, Johns Hopkins Med. J. **148:**14, 1981.

37. Craft, J.E., Grodzicki, R.L., and Steere, A.C.: Antibody response in Lyme disease: evaluation of diagnostic tests, J. Infect. Dis. **149:**789, 1984.

38. Curran, J.W.: Gonorrhea and the urethral syndrome, Sex. Transm. Dis. **4:**119, 1977.

39. Curran, J.W., et al.: Acquired immunodeficiency syndrome (AIDS) associated with transfusions, N. Engl. J. Med. **310:**69, 1984.

40. Davis, J.P., et al.: Toxic-shock syndrome: epidemiologic features, recurrence, risk factors, and prevention, N. Engl. J. Med. **303:**1429, 1980.

41. Dembert, M.L.: Lyme disease, Am. Fam. Phys. **25:**121, 1982.

42. Drew, W.L., et al.: Prevalence of cytomegalovirus infection in homosexual men, J. Infect. Dis. **143:**188, 1981.

43. Essex, M., et al.: Antibodies to cell membrane antigens associated with human T-cell leukemia virus in patients with AIDS, Science **220:**859, 1983.

44. Evatt, B.L., et al.: The acquired immunodeficiency syndrome in patients with hemophilia, Ann. Intern. Med. **100:**499, 1984.

45. Fauci, A.S., et al.: Acquired immunodeficiency syndrome: epidemiologic, clinical, immunologic, and therapeutic considerations, Ann. Intern. Med. **100:**92, 1984.

46. Feorino, P.M., et al.: Lymphadenopathy-associated virus infection of a blood donor recipient pair with acquired immunodeficiency syndrome, Science **225:**69, 1984.

47. Francis, D.P., et al.: Infections of chimpanzees with lymphadenopathy-associated virus, Lancet **2:**1276, 1984.

48. Friedman-Kien, A.E., and Ostreicher, R.: An overview of classical and epidemic Kaposi's sarcoma. In Friedman-Kien, A.E., and Laubenstein, A.J., editors: AIDS: the epidemic of Kaposi's sarcoma and opportunistic infections, New York, 1985, Masson Publishing Company, U.S.A., Inc.

49. Friedman-Kien, A.E., et al.: Disseminated Kaposi's sarcoma in homosexual men, Ann. Intern. Med. **96:**693, 1982.

50. Fujimoto, T., et al.: Immune complex and mite antigen in Kawasaki disease, Lancet **2:**980, 1982.

51. Fujiwara, H., et al.: Microorganism in the heart of Kawasaki disease, Lancet **2:**620, 1983.

52. Furusho, K., et al.: Possible role for mite antigen in Kawasaki disease, Lancet **2:**194, 1981.

53. Gallagher, D.J.A., Montgomerie, J.Z., and North, J.D.K.: Acute infections of the urinary tract and the urethral syndrome in general practice, Br. Med. J. **1:**622, 1965.

54. Gallo, R.C., et al.: Isolation of human T-cell leukemia virus in acquired immune deficiency syndrome (AIDS), Science **220:**865, 1983.

55. Gallo, R.C., et al.: Frequent detection and isolation of cytopathic retroviruses (HTLV-III) from patients with AIDS and at risk for AIDS, Science **224:**500, 1984.

56. Gange, R.W., and Jones, E.W.: Kaposi's sarcoma and immunosuppressive therapy: an appraisal, Clin. Exp. Dermatol. **3:**135, 1978.

56a. Gellin, B. (Meningitis and Special Pathogens Branch, Div. of Bacterial Disease, Center for Infectious Disease, Centers for Disease Control): Personal communication, March 1987.

57. Gelman, E.P., et al.: Proviral DNA of a retrovirus, human T-cell leukemia virus, in two patients with AIDS, Science **220:**862, 1983.

58. Gordin, F.M., et al.: Adverse reactions to trimethoprim-sulfamethoxazole in patients with the acquired immunodeficiency syndrome, Ann. Intern. Med. **100:**495, 1984.

59. Gottlieb, M.S., et al.: *Pneumocystis carinii* pneumonia and mucosal candidiasis in previously healthy homosexual men: evidence for a new acquired cellular immunodeficiency, N. Engl. J. Med. **305:**1425, 1981.

60. Green, J.B., Sidhu, G.S., and Lewin, S.: *Mycobacterium avium-intracellulare:* a cause of disseminated life-threatening infection in homosexuals and drug abusers, Ann. Intern. Med. **97:**539, 1982.

61. Green, S.L., and LaPeter, K.S.: Evidence for postpartum toxic-shock syndrome in a mother-infant pair, Am. J. Med. **72:**169, 1982.

62. Griffiths, P.D., et al.: Rapid detection of cytomegalovirus infection in immunocompromised patients by detection of early antigen fluorescent foci, Lancet **2:**1242, 1984.

63. Groopman, J.E., et al.: HTLV-III in saliva of people with AIDS-related complex and healthy homosexual men at risk for AIDS, Science **226:**447, 1984.

64. Hamashima, Y., Kishi, K., and Tasaka, K.: Rickettsia-like bodies in infantile acute-febrile mucocutaneous lymph-node syndrome, Lancet **2:**42, 1973.

65. Hirsh, M.S., et al.: Risk of nosocomial infection with human T-cell lymphotropic virus III (HTLV-III), N. Engl. J. Med. **312:**1, 1985.

66. Ho, D.D., et al.: HTLV-III in the semen and blood of a healthy homosexual man, Science **226:**451, 1984.

67. Horshaw, R.A., and Swartz, R.A.: Kaposi sarcoma after immunosuppression therapy with prednisone, Arch. Dermatol. **116:**1280, 1980.

68. Hughes, W.T., et al.: Efficacy of trimethoprim-sulfamethoxazole in the prevention and treatment of *Pneumocystis carinii* pneumonia, Antimicrob. Agents Chemother. **5:**289, 1974.

69. Jaffe, H.W., Bregman, D.J., and Selik, R.M.: Acquired immune deficiency syndrome in the United States: the first 1,000 cases, J. Infect. Dis. **148:**339, 1983.

70. Johnson, R.C., et al.: *Borrelia burgdorferi* sp. nov.: etiological agent of Lyme disease, Int. J. Syst. Bacteriol. **34:**496, 1984.

71. Johnson, S.E., et al.: Lyme disease: a selective medium for isolation of the suspected etiological agent, a spirochete, J. Clin. Microbiol. **19:**81, 1984.

72. Kahan, A., et al.: Spirochaetal aetiology for Lyme disease, Lancet **2:**174, 1983.

73. Kalyanaraman, V.S., et al.: A new subtype of human T-cell leukemia virus (HTLV-III) associated with a T-cell variant of hairy cell leukemia, Science **218:**571, 1982.

74. Kalyanaraman, V.S., et al.: Antibodies to the core protein of lymphadenopathy-associated virus (LAV) in patients with AIDS, Science **225:**321, 1984.

75. Kanki, P.J., Alroy, J., and Essex, M.: Isolation of T-lymphotropic retrovirus related to HTLV-III/LAV from wild-caught African green monkeys, Science **230:**951, 1985.

76. Kass, E.H.: Chemotherapeutic and antibiotic drugs in the management of infections of the urinary tract, Am. J. Med. **18:**764, 1955.

77. Kass, E.H.: Asymptomatic infections of the urinary tract, Trans. Assoc. Am. Phys. **69:**56, 1956.

78. Kass, E.H.: Bacteriuria and the diagnosis of infections of the urinary tract: with observations of the use of methionine as a urinary antiseptic, Arch. Intern. Med. **100:**709, 1957.

79. Kato, H., Koike, S., and Yokoyama, T.: Kawasaki disease: effect of treatment on coronary artery involvement, Pediatrics **63:**175, 1979.

80. Kato, H., et al.: Variant strain of *Propionibacterium acnes:* a clue to the aetiology of Kawasaki disease, Lancet **2:**1383, 1983.

81. Kehrberg, M.W., et al.: Risk factors for staphylococcal toxic-shock syndrome, Am. J. Epidemiol. **114:**873, 1981.

82. Lee, T.J., et al.: Human T-cell leukemia virus-associated membrane antigens: identity of the major antigens recognized after virus infection, Proc. Natl. Acad. Sci. U.S.A. **81:**3856, 1984.

83. Levy, J.A., Mitra, G., and Mozen, M.M.: Recovery and inactivation of infectious retroviruses from factor VIII concentrates, Lancet **2:**722, 1984.

84. Levy, J.A., et al.: Isolation of lymphocytopathic retroviruses from San Francisco patients with AIDS, Science **225:**840, 1984.

85. Lopez, C., Fitzgerald, P.A., and Siegal, F.P.: Immunologic alterations in acquired immune deficiency syndrome (AIDS). In Ma, P., and Armstrong, D., editors: The acquired immune deficiency syndrome and infections in homosexual men, New York, 1984, Yorke Medical Books.

86. Magnarelli, L.A., et al.: Comparison of an indirect fluorescent-antibody test with an enzyme-linked immunosorbent assay for serological studies of Lyme disease, J. Clin. Microbiol. **20:**181, 1984.

87. McCormick, J.B., et al.: Ribavirin suppresses replication of lymphadenopathy-associated virus in cultures of human adult T-lymphocytes, Lancet **2:**1367, 1984.

88. Melish, M.E.: Kawasaki syndrome (the mucocutaneous lymph node syndrome), Annu. Rev. Med. **33:**569, 1982.

89. Metroka, C.E.: Generalized lymphadenopathy in homosexual men. In Friedman-Kien, A.E., and Laubenstein, L.J., editors: AIDS: the epidemic of Kaposi's sarcoma and opportunistic infections, New York, 1985, Masson Publishing Co., U.S.A., Inc.

90. Mildvan, D.: Acquired immune deficiency syndrome (AIDS) or an opportunistic infection? Toward a clinical definition of AIDS. In Ma, P., and Armstrong, D., editors: The acquired immune deficiency syndrome and infections of homosexual men, New York, 1983, Yorke Medical Books.

91. Mills, J.T., et al.: Control of production of toxic-shock syndrome toxin-1 (TSST-1) by magnesium ion, J. Infect. Dis. **151:**1158, 1985.

92. Patriarca, P.A., et al.: Kawasaki syndrome: associated with the application of rug shampoo, Lancet **2:**578, 1982.

93. Penn, I.: Kaposi sarcoma in organ transplant recipients: reports of 20 cases, Transplantation **27:**8, 1979.

94. Pitchenik, A.E., et al.: The prevalence of tuberculosis and drug resistance among Haitians, N. Engl. J. Med. **307:**162, 1982.

95. Poiesz, B.J., et al.: Detection and isolation of type C retrovirus particles from fresh and cultured lymphocytes of a patient with cutaneus T-cell lymphoma, Proc. Natl. Acad. Sci. U.S.A. **77:**7415, 1980.

96. Poiesz, B.J., et al.: Isolation of a new type C retrovirus (HTLV) in primary uncultured cells of a patient with Sezary T-cell leukemia, Nature (Lond.) **294:**268, 1981.

97. Popovic, M., et al.: Isolation and transmission of human retrovirus (human T-cell leukemia virus), Science **219:**856, 1983.

98. Reingold, A.L.: Nonmenstrual toxic-shock syndrome: the growing picture, JAMA **249:**932, 1983.

99. Russell, H., et al.: Enzyme-linked immunosorbent assay and indirect immunofluorescence assay for Lyme disease, J. Infect. Dis. **149:**465, 1984.

100. Salahuddin, S.Z., et al.: HTLV-III in symptom-free seronegative persons, Lancet **2:**1418, 1984.

101. Sanford, J.P., et al.: Evaluation of the "positive" urine culture: an approach to the differentiation of significant bacteria from contaminants, Am. J. Med. **20:**88, 1956.

102. Sarngadharan, M.G., et al.: Antibodies reaction with human T-lymphotropic retroviruses (HTLV-III) in the serum of patients with AIDS, Science **224:**506, 1984.

103. Saxinger, C., and Gallo, R.C.: Application of the indirect enzyme-linked immunosorbent assay microtest for the detection and surveillance of human T-cell leukemia-lymphoma virus (HTLV), Lab. Invest. **49:**371, 1983.

104. Schlech, W.F., III, et al.: Risk factors for development of toxic-shock syndrome: associated with a tampon brand, JAMA **248:**835, 1982.

105. Schlievert, P.M., et al.: Identification and characterization of an exotoxin from *Staphylococcus aureus* associated with toxic-shock syndrome, J. Infect. Dis. **143:**509, 1981.

106. Shrock, C.G.: Lyme disease: additional evidence of widespread distribution, Am. J. Med. **72:**700, 1982.

107. Schulze, T.L., et al.: *Ambyloma americanum:* a potential vector of Lyme disease in New Jersey, Science **224:**601, 1984.

108. Schupbach, J., Serological analysis of a subgroup of human T-lymphotropic retroviruses (HTLV-III) associated with AIDS, Science **224:**503, 1984.

109. Shands, K.N., et al.: Toxic-shock syndrome in menstruating women: association with tampon use and *Staphylococcus aureus* and clinical features in 52 cases, N. Engl. J. Med. **303:**1436, 1980.

110. Shaw, G.M., et al.: HTLV-III in brains of children and adults with AIDS encephalopathy, Science **227:**177, 1985.

111. Stamm, W.E.: Interpretation of urine cultures, Clin. Microbiol. Newsletter **5:**15, 1983.

112. Stamm, W.E., et al.: Causes of the acute urethral syndrome in women, N. Engl. J. Med. **303:**409, 1980.

113. Stamm, W.E., et al.: Treatment of the acute urethral syndrome, N. Engl. J. Med. **304:**956, 1981.

114. Stamm, W.E., et al.: Diagnosis of coliform infection in acutely dysuric women, N. Engl. J. Med. **307:**463, 1982.

115. Steere, A.C., et al.: The spirochetal etiology of Lyme disease, N. Engl. J. Med. **308:**733, 1983.

116. Steere, A.C., et.al.: Treatment of the early manifestations of Lyme disease, Ann. Intern. Med. **99:**22, 1983.

117. Strauss, S.E., et al.: Oral acyclovir to suppress recurring herpes simplex virus infections in immunodeficient patients, Ann. Intern. Med. **100:**522, 1984.

118. Todd, J., et al.: Toxic-shock syndrome associated with phage-group-I staphylococci, Lancet **2:**1116, 1978.

119. Tzipori, S.: Cryptosporidiosis in animals and humans, Microbiol. Rev. **47:**84, 1983.

120. Vieira, J., et al.: Acquired immune deficiency in Haitians: opportunistic infections in previously healthy Haitian immigrants, N. Engl. J. Med. **308:**125, 1983.

121. Weiss, S.H., et al.: Screening test for HTLV-III (AIDS agent) antibodies: specificity, sensitivity, and applications, JAMA **253:**221, 1985.

122. Winston, D.J., et al.: Trimethoprim-sulfamethoxazole for the treatment of *Pneumocystis carinii* pneumonia, Ann. Intern. Med. **92:**762, 1980.

123. Wong, E.S., and Stamm, W.E.: Urethral infections in men and women, Annu. Rev. Med. **34:**337, 1983.

124. Zaguri, D., et al.: HTLV-III in cells cultured from semen of two patients with AIDS, Science **226:**449, 1984.

125. Zakowski, P., et al.: Disseminated *Mycobacterium avium-intracellulare* infection in homosexual men of acquired immunodeficiency, JAMA **248:**2980, 1982.

PART TWO

BACTERIA

CHAPTER 11

Specimen Collection and Processing

Sally Jo Rubin

SPECIMEN COLLECTION

Clinical microbiologists find working up improperly collected or transported specimens frustrating. No matter how expert the technologist, a poor specimen leads to poor results and possibly improper treatment of the patient. Although laboratory workers rarely collect specimens, they can and should provide guidelines for appropriate specimen collection. This includes defining criteria for specimen collection and the selection of containers and providing clear instructions. Consultation with an interested physician and nurse is important in establishing these guidelines.

Certain general principles apply to all specimen collection no matter what the source. Every effort should be made to collect specimens before administering antimicrobial agents. A child with bacterial meningitis previously treated with oral antimicrobics may have a negative culture, as may a patient with endocarditis. The laboratory must be informed of any antimicrobial agents given before culture collection so corrective measures, such as the use of antimicrobial-removing resins for blood cultures, can be attempted.

The specimen must be representative of the infection with as little contamination from normal flora as possible. A culture of saliva is not useful for the diagnosis of pneumonia; neither does a surface swab represent a deep wound, nor are nasal secretions appropriate specimens for sinusitis (Table 11-1).

The stage of disease must be considered because organisms may be isolated from one site during acute disease and from another as the disease progresses. *Salmonella typhi* is found in the blood early in the disease and in the stool a week or so later (see Chapter 16). Similarly, *Leptospira* organisms are usually in the blood early in infection and are later shed in the urine (see Chapter 27).

Geographic location is also important. *Vibrio cholerae* is an unlikely isolate in New England but not in Louisiana. Season can be a factor. For example, in the United States *Vibrio* spp. are usually not isolated in the winter.

An adequate amount of material must be collected for all needed smears and cultures. If insufficient material is submitted, the physician must be consulted to determine correct test priorities.

Finally the specimen must be transported promptly and maintained in a manner that allows survival of fastidious organisms and prevents overgrowth by more hardy bacteria.

Other common problems are how many, how often, and when specimens should be collected. Generally one good specimen is sufficient except for stool and blood. Repeat specimens are collected if the patient's condition changes or laboratory data indicate a lack of response to antimicrobial therapy.

Collection time may be important and varies with the specimen type. In bacteriology pooled 24-hour specimens are not recommended.

Specimen collection methods include direct passage by the patient into an appropriate container (such as that for urine or that for feces), transfer from the infected site to a swab, needle aspiration, or biopsy. Whenever feasible, attempts are made to prevent contamination with normal skin or mucosal flora. Thus when specimens are collected through the intact skin by aspiration, the site is first cleansed with 70% alcohol and then decontaminated with an iodophor (1% to 2% tincture of iodine or 10% povidone-iodine solution). The iodophor must act for at least 1 minute because antisepsis does not occur immediately.[45] Because many specimens cannot be collected by aspiration or during surgery, selective media, quantitation, and microscopic examination of material for the presence of squamous epithelial cells are used to reduce or screen for the presence of contaminating flora (see the following discussion and individual specimen types).

SPECIMEN TRANSPORT
CONTAINERS

The simplest and most accessible collection and transport device is a needle and syringe; their use should be encouraged when appropriate. If a fairly large volume is collected in a syringe (2 ml or more), anaerobic bacteria survive for 24 hours at room temperature.[6] Following collection, excess air is expressed, the needle is capped or stuck in a rubber stopper, and the syringe is labeled and delivered to the laboratory.

Specimens such as sputum or urine require a leak-proof sterile container. Many such containers are commercially available, ranging from simple screw-capped cups to complex devices.

Many specimen types are collected on swabs. Swabs consist of wooden, plastic, or wire sticks with cotton, rayon, Dacron, or calcium-alginate tips. Cotton is the least desirable material because it may be toxic. Swabs without a transport medium should not be used because most bacteria are susceptible to drying and may not survive transport.[4] A number of transport media are available including Amies and Stuart transport media for facultative bacteria, and prereduced anaerobically sterilized (PRAS) carrier media for anaerobic bacteria. The transport medium is used to maintain pH, prevent drying, and most important, preserve the organisms in the ratio collected, which is critical when specimens are collected from contaminated sites such as the throat or cervix or in a mixed infection. Many swab–transport media devices are commercially available, including those designed for preservation of anaerobic bacteria.

TABLE 11-1. Criteria for Rejection of Specimens

Criterion	Action
Mislabeled requisition or container	Call nursing station, request new specimen, consult physician if new specimen is unobtainable.
Unlabeled container	As above; if processed, write "container not labeled" on requisition.
No source or incorrect source; delay of more than 2 hours in transport	Call nursing station; see "Mislabeled requisition" above.
Dry swabs	See "Mislabeled requisition"; if processed, write "dry swab unsatisfactory for bacteriologic evaluation" on requisition.
Foley catheter tips	Do not process. Refer physician to reference 24.
Pooled 24-hour urine, feces, or sputum	Request new specimen.
Improper or unsterile container	See "Mislabeled requisition." If processed, write "improper container for _____ specimen, may invalidate results."
Nasal secretions for sinusitis	Consult physician.
Sputum with evidence of contamination	See "Mislabeled requisition."
Anaerobic culture request on unacceptable source	Do not process anaerobically; consult physician.

Most swab-transport systems for facultative bacteria consist of a dry swab and a tube containing a transport medium. The medium is sealed in some manner to prevent contact with the swab until after specimen collection. The medium may be released by inserting the swab through the seal or by the user breaking a small ampule containing the liquid medium.

Anaerobic systems provide an anaerobic atmosphere through several approaches. The Anaswab (Scott Laboratories, Inc.; Figure 11-1, *A*) consists of two rubber-stoppered tubes that contain oxygen-free CO_2. One tube has a swab attached to the stopper. The specimen is collected on the swab, the second tube is unstoppered, and the stopper with the swab is quickly inserted. Tubes are held upright so that the CO_2, which is heavier than air, does not escape.

The Port-a-Cul (BBL Microbiology Systems; Figure 11-1, *B*) contains a semisolid transport medium with a reducing agent and an oxygen-reduction (redox) indicator. The reducing agent lowers the redox potential if oxidation occurs during collection.

The Anaerobic Culturette system (Marion Scientific) consists of a plastic tube containing a swab, sealed ampules of Cary-Blair transport medium, and a hydrogen-CO_2-generating tablet. After the specimen is collected, the swab is replaced, the system sealed, and the ampules broken by hand. The tube is then placed in a sealed bag containing catalyst and desiccant.

The Bio-Bag system (Marion Scientific) (Figure 11-1, *C*) is similar, except that the specimen can be collected using any swab-tube combination desired. It is then placed in a plastic bag containing ampules of indicator, catalyst, and a hydrogen-CO_2 generator. After the bag is sealed, each ampule is crushed, subsequently producing anaerobic conditions. The Bio-Bag may also be used for transporting tissue for anaerobic culture.

Specimens should be delivered to the laboratory as soon as possible after collection and certainly within 1 to 2 hours.[31] Ideally all specimens should be processed immediately; however, this is often not practical or possible. Certain specimens such as urine[31] or sputum[59] may be held overnight in the refrigerator. Many specimens collected on a swab and placed in transport media can be held several hours at room temperature[15] and at least overnight in the refrigerator.[10,15] Exceptions are specimens that might contain temperature-sensitive organisms such as *Neisseria* spp. or anaerobic bacteria.[25,31] These should ideally be processed at once but can be held at room temperature. In fact, in a gassed-out tube with carrier medium, most anaerobic bacteria survive at least 24 hours at room temperature.[28,29]

Cerebrospinal fluid, other fluids collected by needle aspiration, and specimens obtained in the operating room always should be processed immediately. Essentially any specimen collected by an invasive procedure should be cultured promptly. They are obtained at considerable cost, discomfort, and possibly danger to the patient and must be handled with care.

TRANSPORT BY MAIL

Federal regulations govern interstate mail shipment of specimens or cultures (Figure 11-2). Packaging must protect the material during transit and prevent danger to the recipient. The specimen or culture is put in a screw-capped tube or vial and sealed with waterproof tape. The tube is then placed in a waterproof shipping can and packed with absorbent material to protect the tube from breakage and to absorb any leakage. This container is placed in a cardboard shipping container and surrounded with shock-absorbing material. The outer container is sealed and labeled appropriately (Figure 11-2). If available, a styrofoam-lined cardboard shipping container is preferred.

SPECIMEN PROCESSING
INITIAL PROCESSING

On the specimen's arrival in the laboratory, its label and the requisition are checked to make sure that the same patient information is on both and that all necessary information is present. The date and time of arrival are noted on the requisition. The following information is needed on the requisition form, specimen label, or both:

Patient name, sex, age	Both
Hospital location, room number	Both
Working diagnosis	Requisition form
Antimicrobial therapy	Requisition form
Immune status	Requisition form

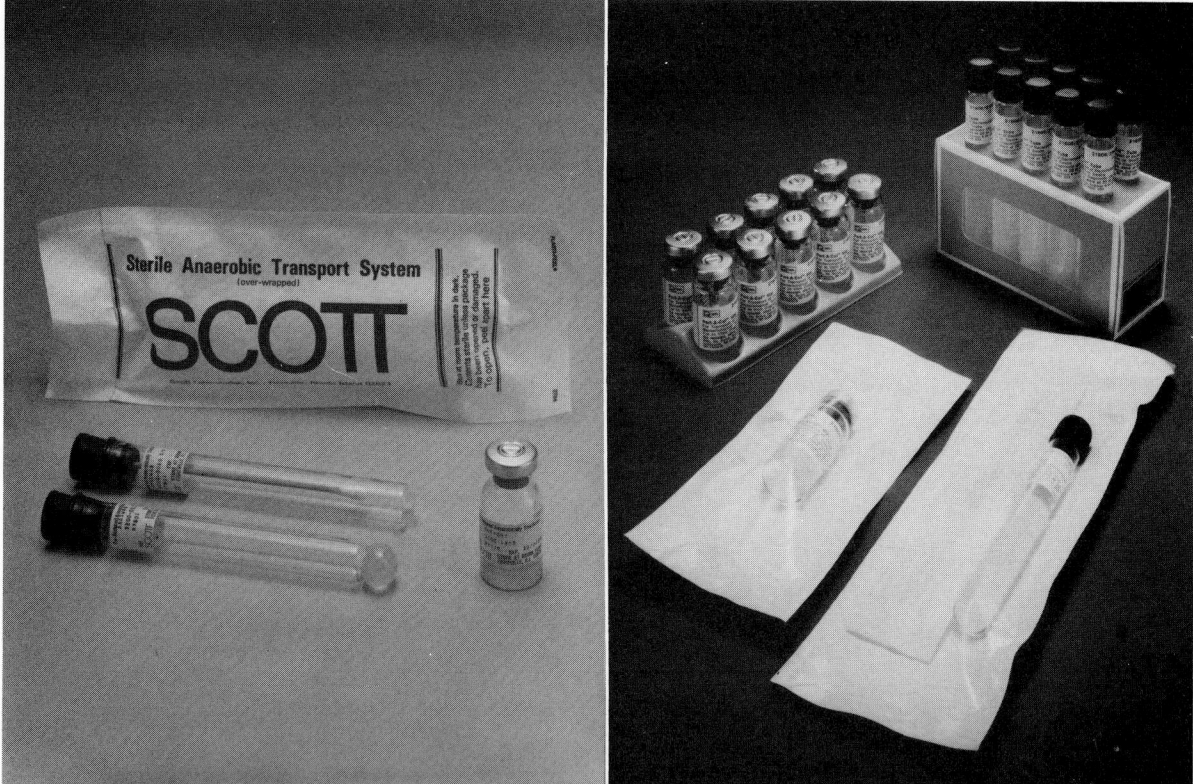

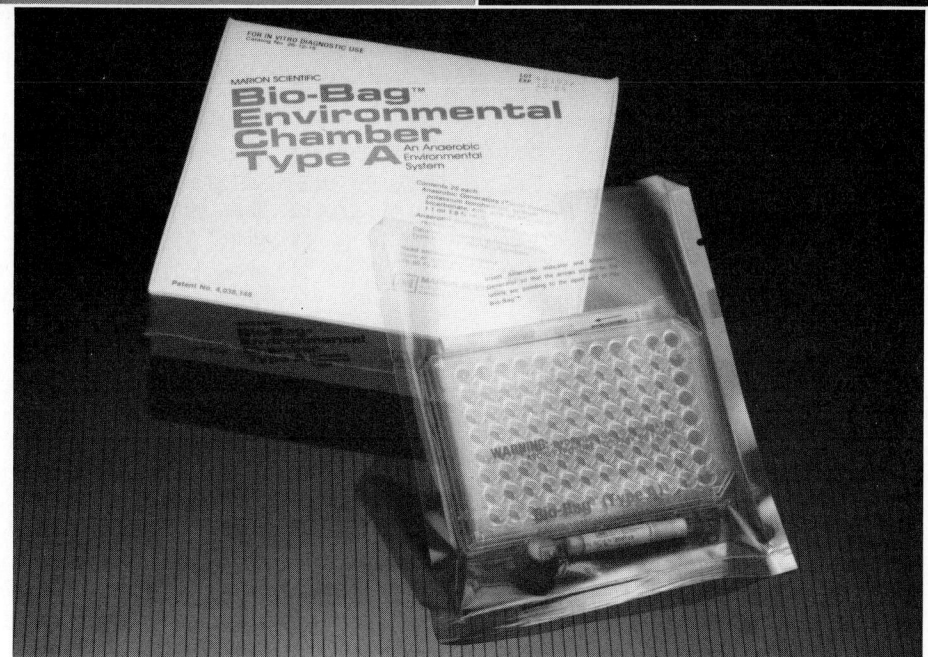

FIGURE 11-1. A, Anaswab system consisting of two rubber-stoppered tubes with oxygen-free CO_2. One tube has swab attached to stopper. **B,** Port-a-Cul tubes, vials, tube and swabs sterile pack, and vial sterile pack. Tubes and vial contain semisolid transport medium with reducing agent and redox indicator. **C,** Bio-Bag Environmental Chamber Type A. Each set contains gas-impermeable environmental chamber; gas generator with one tablet potassium borohydride and bicarbonate and 0.5 ml ampule of 1.8 N hydrochloric acid; catalyst container; and anaerobic indicator with 0.5 ml ampule of 1% resazurin. (**A** courtesy Scott Laboratories, Inc., Fiskeville, R.I.; **B** courtesy BBL Microbiology Systems, Div. of Becton Dickinson & Co., Cockeysville, Md.; **C** courtesy Marion Laboratories, Kansas City, Mo.)

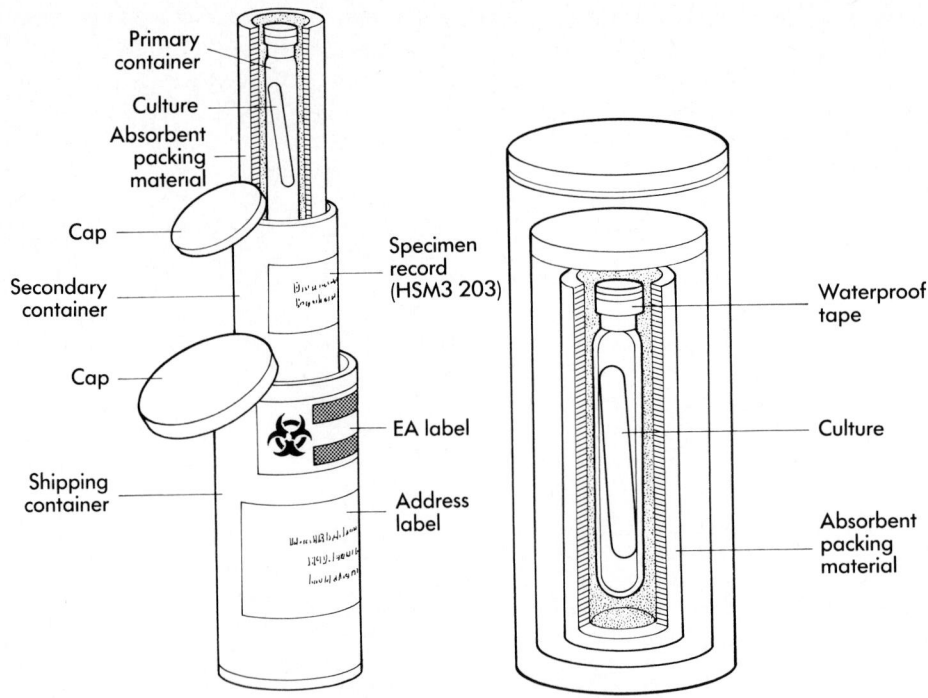

FIGURE 11-2. Packaging and labeling required for mailing microorganisms. (From Jones, G.L., and Herbert, G.A.: Legionnaires': the disease, the bacterium, and methodology, HHS Pub. No. [CDC] 79-8375, Atlanta, 1979, Center for Disease Control.)

Date and time collection	Requisition form
Source	Both
Examination requested	Requisition form
Ordering physician	Requisition form

The specimen type is examined, and if it is improper (Table 11-1), the physician is consulted directly. "An uncultured specimen should never be discarded without obtaining a new specimen or consulting with the patient's physician, or both."[31]

MICROSCOPIC EXAMINATION

The first step in a microbiologic workup is often microscopic examination. Some specimens (for example, sputum or vaginal) may be examined by light or phase microscopy.

Darkfield microscopy is used to visualize spirochetes. *Treponema pallidum* may be seen in fluid from a chancre, the genus *Leptospira* in urine, and the genus *Borrelia* in blood.

Immunoserologic techniques, such as the quellung test, immunofluorescence, latex agglutination, coagglutination, enzyme immunoassay, and others discussed in Chapter 7, may provide rapid identification of certain bacteria. Immunofluorescence is particularly helpful in diagnosing infections caused by highly virulent bacteria such as *Yersinia pestis* and *Francisella tularensis*.

Examination of a Gram-stained smear is an important step in

a microbiologic evaluation. Smears may be fixed with heat or methanol. The latter procedure prevents lysis of any red cells in the specimen. The Gram stain reveals the morphologic appearance of bacteria, determines specimen acceptability, and often guides in primary plating media selection.

Gram-stained smears are examined first under a low power (10× objective) to determine the presence and type of cells in the specimen. Generally white blood cells are easy to differentiate from squamous or ciliated epithelial cells. An abundance of squamous epithelial cells indicates contamination with mucosal or skin flora (Plate 5, *C*). An acceptable specimen (that is, one not contaminated) is then examined with the oil immersion lens, and all morphologic types of organisms and their relative numbers are recorded as either a descriptive term or approximate numbers (that is, fewer than 5 per field, or few; 5 to 10 per field, or moderate; and greater than 10 per field, or many). To see about one bacterium per oil immersion field, the specimen must contain 10^4 to 10^5 CFU/ml (a CFU is a colony-forming unit). Some organisms stain poorly or not at all with Gram stain; if their presence is suspected, the specimen must be stained with special stains, including the following:

Organism	Stain
Legionella pneumophila	Dieterle silver, Gimenez, DFA
Calymmatobacterium granulomatis	Giemsa, Wright
Borrelia spp.	Giemsa, Wright
Rickettsia spp.	Giemsa, Wright, Gimenez
Chlamydia spp.	Giemsa, Gimenez, DFA

Media Selection

Clinical microbiology requires both solid and liquid (broth) media. Solid media permit colony isolation, selection or differentiation of potential pathogens from normal flora, and determination of relative numbers of organisms present in a specimen. Broth media allow isolation of small numbers of organisms or more fastidious organisms; some enrich for a particular pathogen.

Solid Media

A nutrient agar base supplemented with 5% blood, most commonly sheep blood, supports growth of most clinical isolates and reveals patterns of bacterial hemolytic activity. More fastidious bacteria, such as *Haemophilus influenzae,* require a chocolatized agar. Blood is heated before being added to the nutrient base to release hemoglobin, or a hemoglobin suspension is added in place of blood.

Some pathogenic microorganisms such as *L. pneumophilia* and anaerobic bacteria have special growth requirements, and specific media must be inoculated for their isolation. Some of these organisms are isolated so infrequently in the United States that routine inoculation of media for their isolation is not appropriate. The clinician has the responsibility of alerting the laboratory if these bacteria are suspected. Media for their isolation (Table 11-2) were previously available only from public health laboratories but are now available from several commercial sources. The specimen may also be sent to a reference laboratory.

Clinical microbiologists also include selective and differential media for specimen inoculation. Selective media contain ingredients that inhibit the growth of some organisms but allow others to grow. For example, anaerobic blood agar containing kanamycin and vancomycin inhibits growth of most bacteria except *Bacteroides* spp. Differential media contain compounds such as a sugar and a pH indicator that allow groups of organisms to be separated. Most differential media are also selective. For example, MacConkey agar is selective for many gram-negative rods and differentiates lactose-fermenting and non-lactose-fermenting bacteria.

Many types of media are commercially available, either completely prepared or in dehydrated form. The number and types used vary from laboratory to laboratory depending on budgets, personnel, and personal bias. Media selection is governed by the specimen source. Media that allow growth of the majority of potential pathogens from a particular source are included. Some microbiologists advocate using a number of different selective media. whereas others believe that familiarity with growth patterns on a relatively small number of selective media is better.[31] The primary plating media suggested in Table 11-3 reflect the latter attitude.

Inoculation and Isolation Techniques

Traditional identification methods depend on obtaining isolated colonies. Many clinical specimens contain a mixture of bacteria; therefore specimens are diluted to produce single colonies of each organism type present. Dilution techniques include streaking with a wire loop, spreading with a glass rod, or inoculating pour plates. The choice depends on the material to be cultured, the result desired, and the laboratory's preference. Everyone in a laboratory should use the same technique.

Streak Plate

The streak plate method is practical and fast. All streak plate methods are designed to provide a continuous dilution of the specimen. Either a stainless steel or nickel and chromium (Nichrome) wire or a plastic bacteriologic loop is acceptable, although Nichrome should not be used for anaerobic bacteria. In the most common method (Figure 11-3) a portion of the specimen is deposited in one quadrant of an agar plate free of moisture.

Transferring the inoculum to the plate depends on the specimen type. Liquid specimens are usually inoculated by transfer with a sterile pipette or syringe and needle. One or 2 drops is placed in the first quadrant of the plate. Urine is an exception and must be plated quantitatively.

Specimens received on swabs can be planted directly by rolling the swab over an area about 2 cm in diameter in the first quadrant of the plate. Alternatively, if Amies transport medium is used, the swab can be placed in 1 ml of broth and blended with a vortex mixer.[31] Then the specimen can be treated as a liquid specimen.

Feces and sputum are most easily inoculated by dipping a swab into the specimen rather than attempting to use a loop.

After implantation of the inoculum, a wire loop is flamed and cooled, or a sterile plastic disposable loop is selected. The loop is held between the thumb and index finger and passed at a 90-degree angle several times through the initial inoculum into the second quadrant of the plate (streak area 1). The plate is turned 90 degrees, and the process is repeated, streaking into the third quadrant (streak area 2), and finally—after another 90-degree turn—into the fourth quadrant (streak area 3). The loop is flamed between quadrants unless the inoculum is light or the medium is selective or inhibitory. When streak plates are used, the laboratory can report relative numbers of bacteria present, which may be helpful to the clinician, particularly if different organism types are present.

Several methods of semiquantitation are used (see Figure 11-3). Some laboratories use *very few, few, moderate,* or *many;* others use *1+* to *4+*, based on the following criteria[5]:

Score	Number of Colonies in Streak Area		
	1	*2*	*3*
1+	<10		
2+	>10	<5	
3+	>10	>5	<5
4+	>10	>5	>5

Quantitative Methods

Sometimes determining the actual colony count of a specimen is necessary (one colony equals one colony-forming unit, or CFU). For a colony count the specimen must be in a liquid form. Nonliquid specimens, such as tissue, are weighed, ground, mixed with a known amount of broth, and centrifuged. The supernatant is then treated as a liquid specimen. Three quantitative methods are used: calibrated loop, broth dilution and streak, and pour plates.

If counts less than 10^2 or 10^3 CFU/ml are not desired, loops may be used to deliver either 0.01 or 0.001 ml. The flamed, cooled loop is dipped vertically into a well-mixed specimen. One loopful is streaked down the center of a plate. Without

TABLE 11-2. Isolation of Bacterial Pathogens Uncommon in the United States[a]

Organism	Sources	Isolation Media
Gram-negative bacteria		
Bordetella pertussis	Nasopharynx	Regan-Lowe[44]; Bordet-Gengou agar
Brucella spp.	Blood, tissue	Blood agar; Castañeda technique
Calymmatobacterium granulomatis	Genital lesion, aspirate	Embryonated eggs (yolk sac); Dulaney slant
Francisella tularensis	Blood, pus, biopsy material, respiratory secretions	Glucose-cysteine blood agar
Haemophilus ducreyi	Genital	Enriched chocolate agar + vancomycin and other media in Chapter 15
Pseudomonas pseudomallei	Blood, sputum	Blood agar, enteric agar
Spirillum minus	Blood	Noncultivable; examine wet mounts or Wright-Giemsa-stained blood films or lymph nodes; animal studies
Streptobacillus moniliformis	Blood, joint fluid, lesion,	Basal media enriched with ascitic fluid, blood, or serum; Rogosa medium
Vibrio spp.	Feces, wound, blood	Alkaline peptone water enrichment; thiosulfate–citrate–bile salts–sucrose (TCBS) agar
Yersinia enterocolitica	Feces, mesenteric lymph nodes	Cold or alkali enrichment; cefsulodin-irgasan-novobiocin (CIN) agar
Yersinia pestis	Blood, sputum, pus	Blood agar
Gram-positive bacteria		
Corynebacterium diphtheriae	Nasopharynx, throat, skin	Loeffler medium, cystine-tellurite agar
Bacillus anthracis	Pus, sputum, feces	Blood agar
Erysipelothrix rhusiopathiae	Wound, blood	Blood agar
Spirochetes		
Borrelia recurrentis	Blood	Darkfield examination; Giemsa or Wright stained smears; rodent inoculation
Leptospira interrogans	Blood, urine, CSF	Bovine serum albumin–Tween 80 semisolid, Fletcher semisolid
Treponema pallidum	Genital lesion, lymph node	Noncultivable; darkfield examination
Chlamydiae		
C. psittaci	Sputum, lung	McCoy cells, embryonated eggs

TABLE 11-2. Isolation of Bacterial Pathogens Uncommon in the United States[a]—cont'd

Organism	Sources	Isolation Media
C. trachomatis L$_1$-L$_3$ (lymphogranuloma venereum)	Pus (lymph node)	McCoy cells, embryonated eggs
C. trachomatis	Conjunctiva, urethra, cervix, rectum[b]	McCoy cells, embryonated eggs
Rickettsia spp. (except *Rochalimaea quintana*)	Blood	Embryonated eggs, guinea pig

[a]Other suitable media are discussed in the respective chapters.
[b]Specimen varies according to specific type (A to K) of *C. trachomatis* (see Chapter 54).

TABLE 11-3. Suggested Routine Culture Media

Source	Microscopic Examination	Agar Plates	Broth
Blood			EB (CO$_2$, ANO$_2$)
Body fluids			
Cerebrospinal	G	BA, CHOC, ABA, THIO (abscess)	EB
Pericardial, peritoneal, pleural	G	BA, CHOC, ABA	EB
Synovial	G	BA, CHOC, ABA, THIO	EB
Catheters (IV)		BA	
Ear			
Otitis media	G	BA, EA, CHOC	EB
Otitis externa	G	BA, EA, CHOC	
Eye			
Conjunctiva	G	BA, EA, CHOC	
Cornea	G	BA, CHOC	
Intraocular	G	BA, EA, CHOC, ABA, AnPEA	EB
Feces or rectal swab	MB	EA, ESAM, ESAH, CSA	EEB
Genital—male			
Urethra	G	MTM/NYC/ML	
Prostatic fluid	G	BA, EA, MTM/NYC/ML	
Aspirates	G	BA, EA, MTM/NYC/ML	EB
Genital—female			
Vagina	G	BA	
Urethra		MTM/NYC/ML	
Cervix		MTM/NYC/ML	
Endometrium	G	BA, EA, MTM/NYC/ML, ABA, PV[a]	EB
Bartholin's gland	G	BA, EA, MTM/NYC/ML, ABA, AnPEA, PV[a]	EB
Upper tract	G	BA, EA, MTM/NYC/ML, ABA, AnPEA, PV[a]	EB
Respiratory tract—upper			
Nose		BA	
Nasopharynx		BA, CHOC	
Throat		BA	
Sinus	G	BA, EA, CHOC, ABA	

Continued.

TABLE 11-3. Suggested Routine Culture Media—cont'd

Source	Microscopic Examination	Agar Plates	Broth
Respiratory tract—lower			
Sputum	G	BA, EA, CHOC	
Bronchial aspirate or brushings	G	BA, EA, CHOC	
Tracheal aspirate	G	BA, EA, CHOC	
Transtracheal aspirate	G	BA, EA, CHOC, ABA, AnPEA	EB
Lung aspirate or biopsy	G	BA, EA, CHOC, AnPEA	EB
Urine			
Clean-catch or catheterized	O	BA, EA (0.001 ml/plate)[b]	
Suprapubic bladder tap	G	BA, EA, (0.1 ml/plate)	
Wounds			
Superficial	G	BA, EA	
Burns, ulcers	G	BA, EA	
Abscess	G	BA, EA, ABA, PV,[a] BBE	EB
Tissue	G	BA, EA, ABA, PV,[a] BBE	EB

> **Symbols:** CO_2, Incubate with 5% to 10% carbon dioxide   G, Gram stain   O, Optional
> ANO_2, Incubate under anaerobic conditions   MB, Methylene blue stain   BA, Blood agar[c]
> EA, Enteric agar (MacConkey, eosin–methylene blue, deoxycholate)[d]
> CHOC, Chocolate agar (CO_2)[e]
> ESAM, Enteric selective agar of moderate selectivity (Hektoen enteric, xylose lysine deoxycholate, Salmonella-Shigella, deoxycholate citrate)[c]
> ESAH, Enteric selective agar of high selectivity (bismuth sulfite, brilliant green)[d]
> CSA, *Campylobacter*-selective agar (Skirrow, Butzler, Campy blood agar)[f]
> ML, Martin-Lewis[e]   MTM, Modified Thayer-Martin[e]   NYC, New York City medium[e]
> ABA, Anaerobic blood agar[g] (supplemented with hemin and vitamin K_1)
> EB, Enrichment broth (prereduced brain heart infusion, enriched thioglycolate, chopped meat glucose)
> EEB, Enteric enrichment broth (GN, selenite F, tetrathionate)
> PV, Paromomycin-vancomycin blood agar
> BBE, Bacteroides bile esculin agar (for use in intra-abdominal abscesses)

[a]Kanamycin-vancomycin laked blood agar may be used instead of PV agar; see Chapter 20 for further discussion.
[b]Also 0.01 ml per plate in acute urethral syndrome.
[c]Some laboratories incubate all BA with CO_2; others vary with specimen source.
[d]Incubate in air.
[e]Always CO_2.
[f]Incubate under microaerophilic conditions.
[g]Always ANO_2.

flaming, cross-streaks at a 90-degree angle are made perpendicular to the original streak. Cross-streaks should be close together and extend toward the edge of the plate (Figure 11-4).

The number of colonies growing on the agar plate times the dilution factor (10^3 if a 0.001 ml loop is used) equals the number of CFU per milliliter in the original specimen.

Broth dilution followed by streaking a known amount of each dilution is more cumbersome but more accurate, and is most useful for specimens thought to contain large numbers of different bacteria. Serial dilutions are made, and a specific amount of each dilution (usually 0.1 ml) is placed in the center of an agar plate. The inoculum is evenly distributed over the surface with a sterile, bent, glass rod. Plates with 30 to 300 colonies are counted.

An accurate count can also be determined by the pour-plate method. Known amounts of diluted and undiluted material are each thoroughly mixed with a known volume of melted, cooled (to about 50° C) agar medium. The inoculated medium is poured into a Petri plate, allowed to harden, and then incubated. Again plates with 30 to 300 colonies provide the most

accurate count. If the medium contains blood, hemolytic activity can be determined.

Pure Culture Techniques

For the identification of bacteria using traditional methods, pure cultures must be used. To obtain a pure culture, the center of a well-isolated colony is touched with a flamed, cooled loop, and the material is transferred to the first quadrant of an agar plate. Because the number of bacteria in a single colony is high, only a small amount of growth is transferred. The plate is streaked in the same manner as for primary specimens. The loop is flamed between each quadrant, and only a few cross-streaks into the previous quadrant are made.

To subculture a broth culture to an agar plate, one loopful is planted in the first quadrant. The turbidity of the broth (that is, the inoculum size) dictates whether to flame the loop in between cross-streaks and how many cross-streaks to make.

No matter what method of planting is used, technologists must always consider the expected concentration of organisms and the medium inoculated. The higher the bacterial count, the

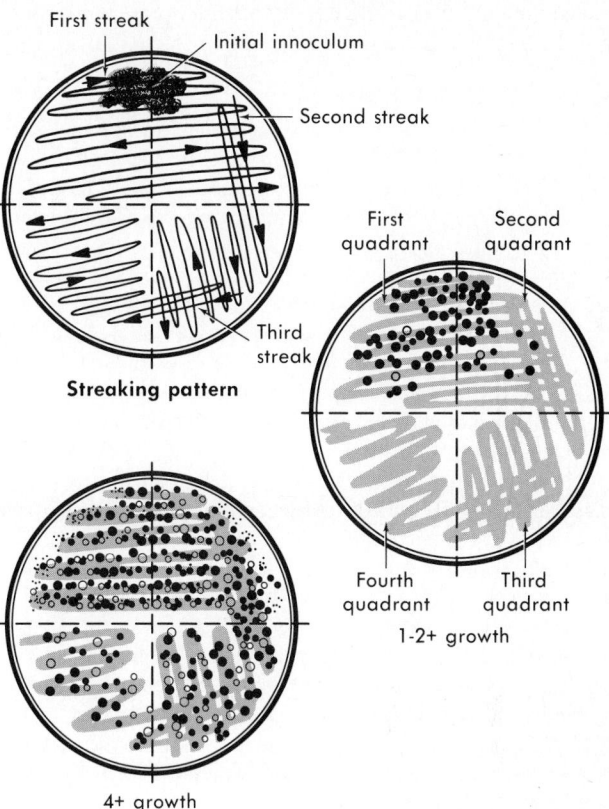

FIGURE 11-3. Streaking pattern for primary inoculation of plates to achieve isolated colonies. Growth in initial half of plate only is semiquantitated as 1+ or 2+ (sparse); growth into third quadrant is reported as 3+ (moderate); and growth into fourth quadrant is reported as 4+. If numbers of colonies can be counted, this number should be reported. (From Finegold, S.M., and Baron, E.J.: Bailey and Scott's diagnostic microbiology, ed. 7, St. Louis, 1986, The C.V. Mosby Co.)

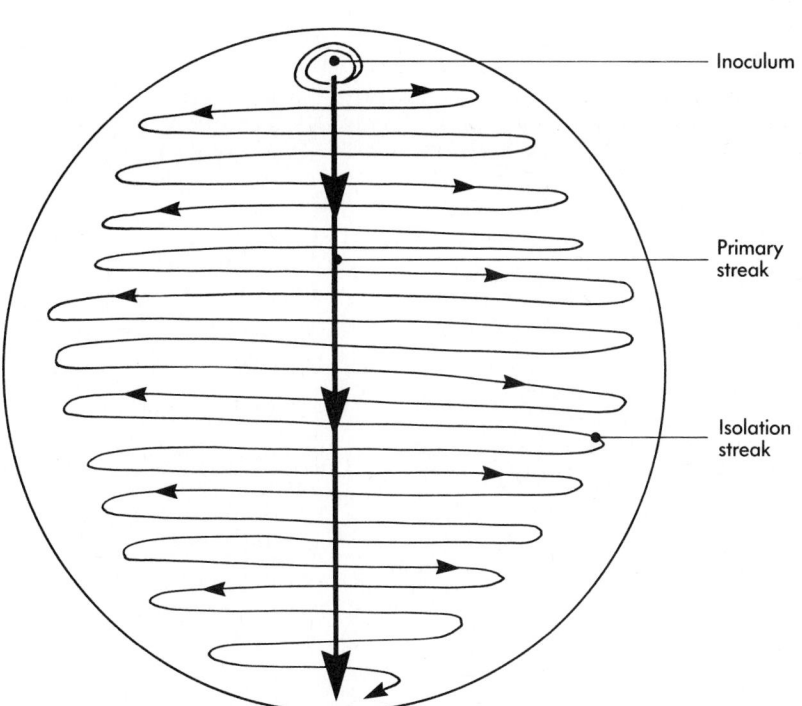

FIGURE 11-4. Quantitative streak plate method of specimen inoculation with calibrated loop.

more dilution is necessary, the more inhibitory is the medium, and the larger is the required inoculum.

CULTURE INCUBATION

Inoculated plates are incubated inverted to prevent the water of condensation from dropping onto the agar surface, which can result in the colonies coalescing and is a safety hazard.

The optimal growth temperature for most bacterial pathogens is 35° C. *Campylobacter jejuni*, which requires 42° C, is one of the few exceptions. Most bacteria produce visible colonies in about 18 hours, although some require 48 to 72 hours.

Generally bacteria require a relative humidity of 70% to 80%. Most new incubators have a water reservoir. If an incubator does not have a mechanism for humidity regulation, a pan containing water kept at a constant level can be placed on the incubator's lowest shelf.

Many bacteria grow well in air but some need either increased CO_2 (5% to 10%) (capnophilic), decreased O_2 and increased CO_2 (microaerophilic), or anaerobic conditions. Carbon dioxide may be provided by a CO_2 incubator, a candle jar, or a container with a CO_2-generating device. A candle jar is simply a wide-mouthed container with a tightly fitting top. Inoculated media are placed in the jar. A lighted candle is placed on top of the media, and the top is replaced.

Microaerophilic conditions are required for isolation of the genus *Campylobacter*. Commercial H_2- and CO_2-generating envelopes are available.[9] Other techniques such as those employing a gas tank and plastic bags or the Fortner principle are also acceptable (see Chapter 23).

Anaerobic conditions can be achieved by evacuation and replacement of gases in an anaerobe jar, a GasPak jar, or an anaerobic glove box (see Chapter 20).

CULTURE EXAMINATION

The first step in culture evaluation is visual inspection of colonial morphology on the surface of agar plates. Both the types and the numbers of each morphologic set are determined. With experience, the clinical microbiologist learns to classify colonial types visually into various groups and to distinguish potential pathogens from normal flora. This classification is aided by the presence or absence of growth on selective media and is a guide for selecting biochemical tests for further identification.

Each type of medium is examined with bright, direct illumination. A hand lens or dissecting microscope is useful if a number of colony types, spreading growth, or very small colonies are on the plates. Colonial characteristics to be noted include the following:

1. Size in millimeters
2. Form: circular, radiate, rhizoid, irregular, filamentous
3. Elevation: flat, raised, convex, dome shaped (pulvinate), umbonate, umbilicate
4. Surface: smooth, rough, fine, dull, glistening, granular
5. Margin: entire, undulate, lobate, erose, filamentous, curled
6. Opacity: transparent, translucent, opaque
7. Consistency: butyrous, mucoid, friable, membranous
8. Color: white, yellow, gray, green, black
9. Pigment: color, fluorescent, iridescent, opalescent

Some of these properties are illustrated in Figure 11-5. Some organisms have a distinctive odor, although this is a more subjective characteristic. *Pseudomonas aeruginosa* has a grapelike odor, many anaerobic bacteria are putrid, and *Streptomyces* spp. are earthy or musty.

In addition to examination of the colonial morphology, organism-induced reactions in the media are recorded. Many organisms partially (alpha-hemolysis) or completely (beta-hemolysis) hemolyze certain red blood cells; alpha-hemolysis appears as a greenish zone around the colony, whereas beta-hemolysis results in a clear zone. Some bacteria are nonhemolytic (gamma-hemolysis), and a few produce double zones of hemolysis.

Selective and differential media allow further classification of colonies seen on agar plates. For example, MacConkey agar contains the sugar lactose and the pH indicator neutral red—so lactose-fermenting bacteria produce an acid pH, and their colonies are pink, whereas non-lactose-fermenters produce colorless colonies. Examples of other reactions detected from primary agar plates include H_2S production, lysine decarboxylation, and salt tolerance.

After colonial morphology is evaluated, examination of a stained smear may be helpful to confirm the initial classification. Color reactions and arrangement of bacterial cells are not always typical in smears made from growth on agar; however, the Gram stain reaction combined with the colonial appearance can give the microbiologist a good idea of the organism's identity. For example, gram-negative rods that are gray and beta-hemolytic on blood agar and are pink (lactose fermenting), round, and umbilicate on MacConkey agar are likely to be *Escherichia coli*. Gram-positive cocci in clusters from yellow, creamy, convex beta-hemolytic colonies on blood agar are likely to be staphylococci.

If more than one colony type is present, usually a subculture must be made from a single colony of each type to ensure a pure culture for further biochemical characterization. Most biochemical tests require additional incubation. Some tests, however, can be performed directly on the growth from the agar plate. These can be helpful in determining genus and species and provide further information for a more accurate preliminary identification. These tests include the following:

1. Catalase
2. Slide coagulase
3. Cytochrome oxidase
4. Bile solubility
5. Spot indole
6. Motility
7. Serologic: quellung, agglutination, coagglutination, latex agglutination

Often these tests can result in a correct identification of genus and sometimes even of species (for instance, a positive coagulase test identifies gram-positive, catalase-positive cocci as *Staphylococcus aureus*). This preliminary information may be critical to the physician and should be reported without waiting for a final identification. In fact, the trend in clinical microbiology is to develop more rapid techniques for identification and susceptibility testing. Many of these newer methods are described in Chapter 9.

SPECIMEN COLLECTION AND PROCESSING: INDIVIDUAL SITES
BLOOD

Bacteremia may be continuous, intermittent, or transient. If infection is intravascular (for example, endocarditis), organisms are continuously in the blood, whereas in most other infec-

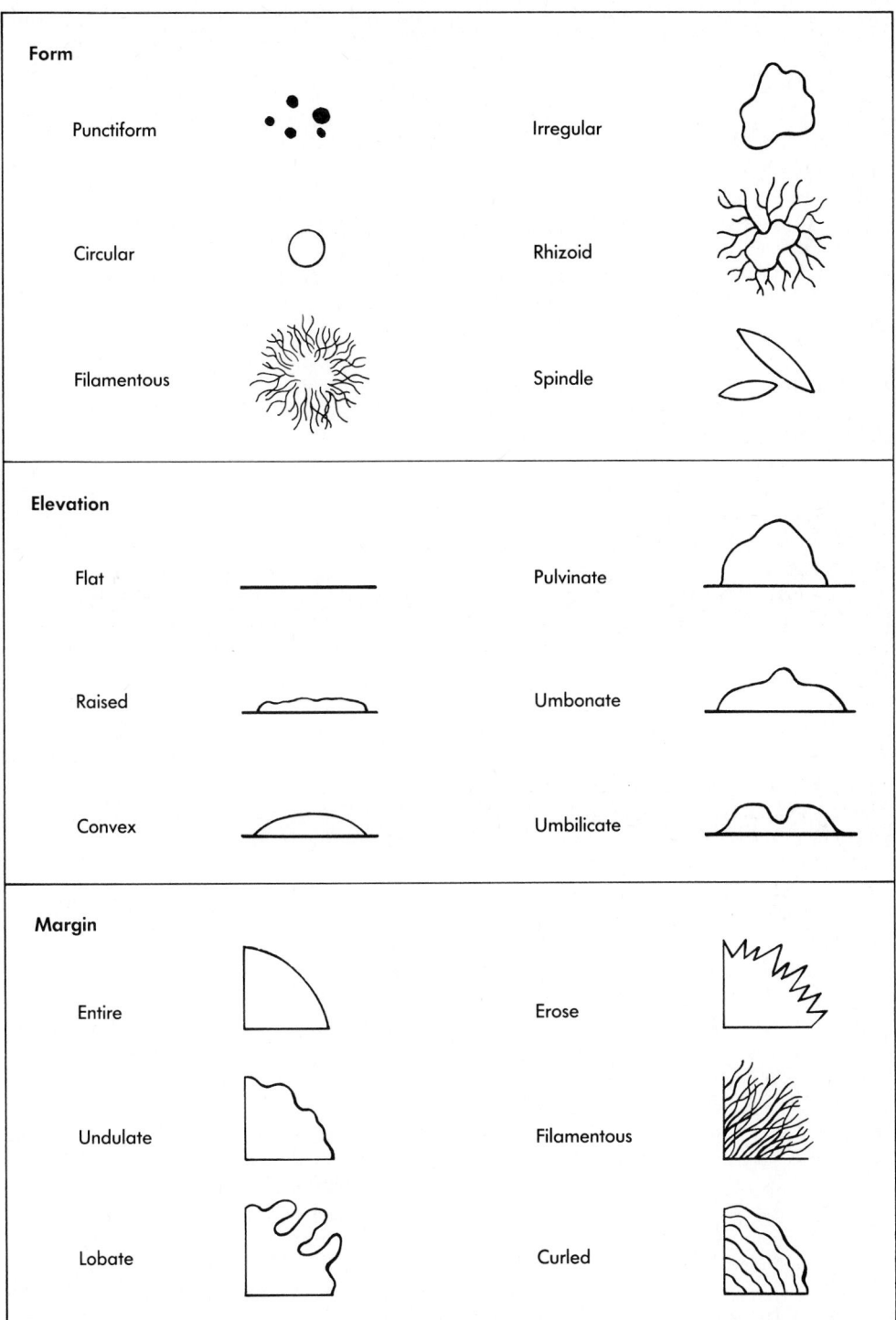

FIGURE 11-5. Characteristics of bacterial colonies on surface of agar plates. (From Dowell, V.R., Jr., and Hawkins, T.M.: Laboratory methods in anaerobic bacteriology, CDC laboratory manual, DHEW Pub. No. [CDC] 74-8272, Washington, D.C., 1974, U.S. Government Printing Office.)

TABLE 11-4. Collection of Blood Cultures

Endocarditis (intravascular infection)	Two or three cultures over 1 or 2 hours
Acute sepsis	Two or three cultures from separately prepared veins
Fever of unknown origin	Two or three cultures at least 1 hour apart; if negative at 24 hours, repeat
After antimicrobic treatment	Use antimicrobic removal systems (ARD, Marion Scientific; Bactec 16B, 17C, Johnston Laboratories); add penicillinase; collect four to six cultures over 2 days

tions bacteremia is intermittent. Bacteria from nonvascular infected sites are shed into the blood via the lymphatic system. The source of these bacteria may be urinary tract infections, respiratory infections, meningitis, abscesses, or other infections. Organisms are usually cleared from the blood in minutes to hours except in cases of overwhelming or intravascular infection. Transient bacteremia occurs if bacteria are shed directly into the blood after various manipulations of normal mucosa, such as tooth extraction, barium enema, and cystoscopy. These organisms are usually normal bacterial flora and are cleared in about 15 minutes. Under certain circumstances, such as in a patient with a damaged heart valve, transient bacteremia can result in infection.

Because most bacteremias are intermittent, blood for culture is collected at various times. After the influx of bacteria into the bloodstream the patient's temperature may rise, possibly accompanied by chills. Unfortunately, by the time the temperature is elevated, organisms may already be cleared from the blood. Generally, blood cultures are collected about an hour apart or at the time of temperature elevation, except if early treatment is imperative. Then several cultures are collected from different sites with a separate needle and syringe for each specimen (Table 11-4). The majority of bacteremias are detected with three sets of blood cultures. Rarely are more needed during a febrile episode.[45]

Before a blood culture is collected, the skin is decontaminated, and blood is obtained by venipuncture. The number of bacteria per milliliter of blood is usually small (1 to 10 CFU/ml), making the volume collected critical. At least 10 ml per culture is collected [26] but no more than 30 ml. Much less blood is required from infants (1 to 5 ml). Blood is inoculated either directly into blood culture broth or into a tube containing the anticoagulant sodium polyanethol sulfonate (SPS) and rapidly carried to the laboratory for inoculation. Other anticoagulants are inhibitory and should not be used. Conventionally blood is cultured in a liquid medium. Blood-to-medium ratios from 1:5 to 1:30 are acceptable.[47] Lower dilutions may result in bacterial inhibition by serum factors, and higher dilutions prolong detection time.

The Isolator system (E.I. DuPont de Nemours & Co., Wilmington, Del.) is a lysis centrifugation system (see Chapter 9) that may be used to concentrate bacteria (or fungi) present in blood. This system contains several agents, including saponin, which lyses the red blood cells. Organisms are pelleted during centrifugation, and the sediment is plated to solid media. This

system provides improved recovery of certain organisms, including fungi (see Chapter 29).

Conceivably any bacterium can cause bacteremia, but formulating a medium that supports the growth of all bacteria is impossible. In practice, many nutritionally enriched liquid media are suitable for culture of most organisms from the blood; they include the following:
1. Aerobic and anaerobic bacteria
   a. Trypticase soy broth
   b. Supplemented peptone broth
   c. Brucella broth
   d. Brain heart infusion broth
   e. Columbia broth
2. Anaerobic bacteria only
   a. Thiol broth
   b. Thioglycolate

Commercially prepared blood culture media are bottled under vacuum. The atmosphere in the bottle may contain CO_2 in air or an inert gas. The oxidation-reduction potential (E_h) of most unvented bottles is low enough to support the growth of most clinically significant anaerobic bacteria. Because some organisms—such as yeasts or members of the genus *Pseudomonas*—may not grow at this redox potential, two bottles are inoculated. One is left unvented (and may contain a medium that does not support the growth of all aerobic and facultative organisms). The other bottle is transiently vented by inserting a sterile, cotton-plugged needle into the rubber septum of the bottle.

Most blood culture media contain SPS. SPS not only prevents clotting but neutralizes the bactericidal effect of human serum, inhibits complement activity and phagocytosis, and inactivates aminoglycosides. The SPS concentration used (0.025% to 0.05%) is inhibitory for some strains of *Neisseria*[51] and *Peptostreptococcus anaerobius*.[58] This inhibition can be overcome by supplementing the medium with 1.2% gelatin.[16]

Reports vary as to the efficacy of supplementing blood culture media with 10% to 20% sucrose or sorbitol, probably because their effect on organism recovery is media dependent. These substances are thought to provide osmotic support to cell wall–defective organisms. Among patients who have received cell wall–acting antimicrobials for treatment of endocarditis or undefined meningitis, such supplemented media may improve bacterial isolation.[36]

Although blood for culture should be collected before any antimicrobial agents are given, this is not always possible, particularly in patients with persistent symptoms of sepsis. If treatment is with beta-lactamase-susceptible antimicrobials, penicillinase can be added to the medium. However, the penicillinase solution must be cultured with each use to test it for contamination. Alternatively, the blood can be mixed either before culture (Figure 11-6, *A*) or during culture (Figure 11-6, *B*) with various antimicrobial-adsorbing resins. These resins appear to increase bacteremia detection in patients receiving antimicrobials.[1]

In the traditional approach, inoculated bottles are incubated at 35° to 37° C for 1 week and examined at various intervals. In cases in which slow-growing or more fastidious bacteria are suspected, bottles are incubated an additional week before discarding. Bottles are examined visually (macroscopically), microscopically (Gram stain or acridine orange stain), or by subculture to agar medium.

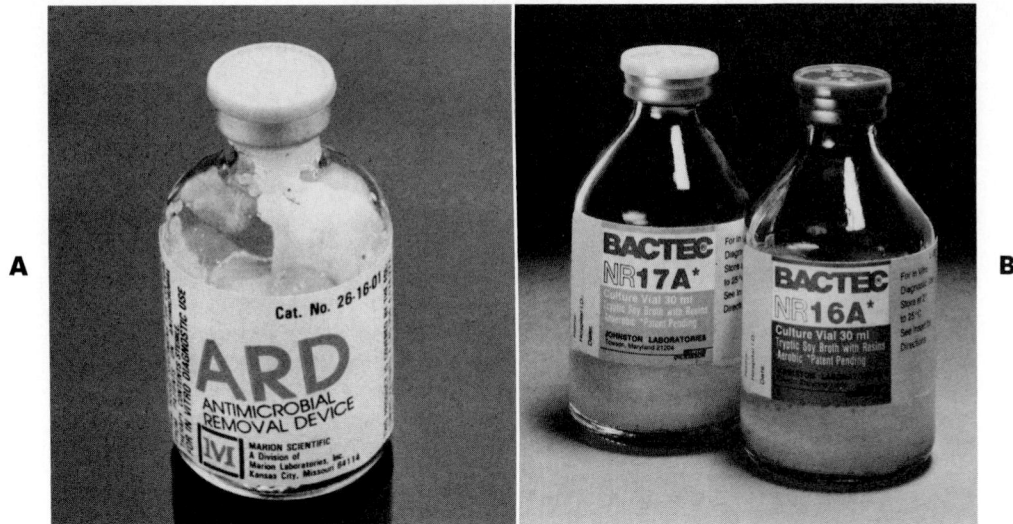

FIGURE 11-6. A, Antimicrobial Removal Device. **B,** Bactec resin vials: aerobic (NR 16A) and anaerobic (NR 17A). (**A** Courtesy Marion Laboratories, Inc., Kansas City, Mo.; **B** courtesy Johnston Laboratories, Div. of Becton Dickinson & Co., Towson, Md.)

Bottles are initially examined after 6 to 18 hours of incubation.[48] A sample is removed by needle and syringe from bottles with visual evidence of growth (turbidity, gas, hemolysis of blood, pellicle formation), and a smear is Gram stained. Media are then inoculated, based on the Gram stain results, but chocolate agar should always be included. To produce visible changes, a liquid medium must contain at least 10^7 organisms per milliliter. Because smaller numbers may be present, more sensitive examination is required. Bottles that initially are macroscopically negative may be blindly subcultured to chocolate agar that is incubated at 35° to 37° C in 5% to 10% CO_2 or examined by acridine orange stain. Subcultures are incubated 2 days. Anaerobic incubation of subcultured plates will allow maximal recovery of anaerobic organisms, although the necessity has been questioned.[41] Subsequently, visual screening is performed daily. The blind screen by acridine orange stain or subculture is repeated after 2 days' incubation. No further blind subcultures are routinely necessary.[21,45]

Positive blood culture results should be reported as rapidly as possible. Broth can be removed from macroscopically or microscopically positive bottles and, after subculturing, the remainder processed by centrifugation to concentrate the organisms. A preliminary low-speed spin pellets the blood cells leaving the bacteria in the supernatant. A higher speed spin of the supernatant pellets the bacteria. The bacteria can be resuspended to the appropriate turbidity and rapid direct tests,[13] rapid or conventional biochemical tests,[14] and susceptibility tests[39] inoculated, thus reducing identification time by at least 24 hours. Many laboratories use the Bactec instruments (see Chapter 9). The Bactec blood culture media are screened periodically for 7 days before being reported as negative. No blind subcultures are necessary.[2,38]

Almost any microorganism can cause septicemia; therefore any isolate should be reported. The most common clearly significant isolates are *Escherichia coli* and other enterics, *Staphylococcus aureus, Streptococcus pneumoniae,* and anaerobic bacteria (usually 5% to 15% of all isolates). Between 6% and 15% of positive blood cultures are polymicrobial.

During collection and processing, blood cultures may be contaminated with skin flora or environmental organisms. Common contaminating bacteria include *Staphylococcus epidermidis,* propionibacteria, corynebacteria, and *Bacillus* spp. Isolation of these organisms from a single bottle is rarely significant. Viridans streptococci and enterococci found in one bottle only are also usually not significant[52] and are probably the result of transient bacteremias. Occasionally all of these bacteria can cause significant infection. Therefore the decision of significance must be based on both the laboratory and the clinical evaluation.

In case further testing is needed (for susceptibility or bactericidal levels), all blood isolates are maintained on a slant or frozen (−70° C) for at least several weeks.

BODY FLUIDS

Body fluid specimens are all collected by needle aspiration following skin decontamination (Figure 11-7). The specimen may be delivered in the syringe or in a sterile screw-capped tube. As much fluid as possible is collected because organism numbers may be small. Bacteria are then concentrated by centrifugation or filtration. For cerebrospinal fluid (CSF), centrifugation at 1500 × g for 15 minutes is sufficient.[40] Filtration does not seem to offer any advantage and may inhibit bacteria if antimicrobial agents are in the fluid.

Cerebrospinal Fluid

Bacterial meningitis, an inflammation of the meninges, is life threatening, so CSF should be processed immediately. Smears of turbid CSF are made before and after centrifugation, and smears of clear fluid are made after concentration. Clean, sterile slides are used to make certain that dead, contaminating organisms from the slide do not confuse the diagnosis. If organisms are seen on a Gram-stained smear (Plate 5, *D*), media selection is based on smear results. Otherwise blood agar, chocolate agar, and enriched thioglycolate broth are inoculated with the sediment. Plates are incubated in 5% to 10% CO_2 and examined daily for 2 to 3 days. The broth is incubated 5 to 7

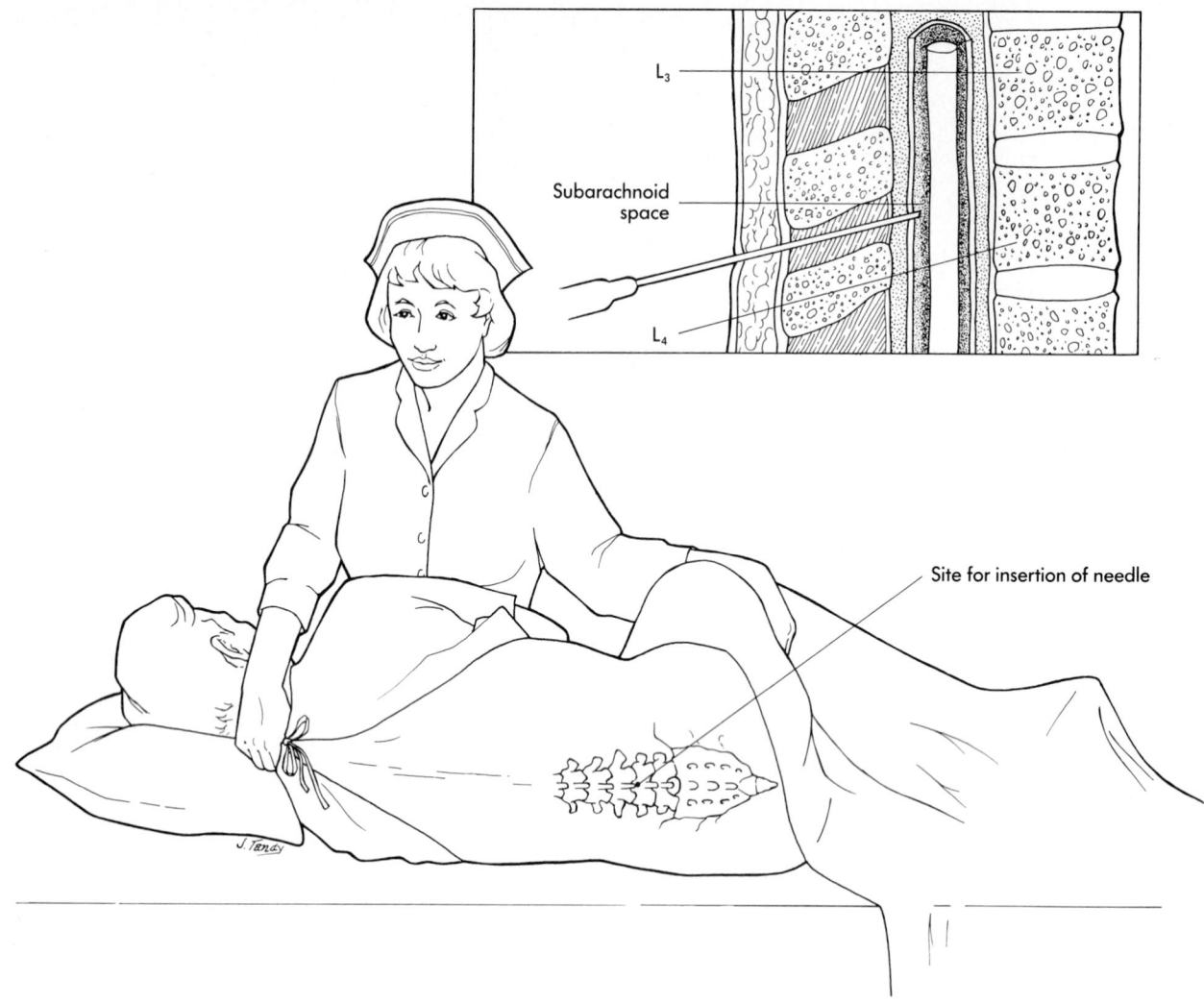

Subarachnoid
space

L₃

L₄

Site for insertion of needle

J. Tandy

FIGURE 11-7. Collection of cerebrospinal fluid.

days and examined daily for turbidity. Any sediment remaining can be incubated at 35° C and, if plates are negative after 24 hours, may be reexamined by smear. The supernatant can be held frozen (−70° C) in case further studies are ordered (such as viral cultures).

The chemical and cellular composition of CSF is determined as an aid to diagnosis (Table 11-5). In bacterial meningitis the CSF is usually purulent (more than 1000 cells/mm³), containing polymorphonuclear leukocytes (PMNs), and the glucose level is usually low. The cell count in tubercular, fungal, or viral meningitis is usually low, and cells are mostly mononuclear. However, early in viral or tuberculous meningitis, cells may be PMNs. Glucose levels are normal or somewhat reduced. Cell counts may be low in partially treated meningitis or in immunosuppressed patients; therefore all CSF should be cultured whether cells are present or not.

Practically any organism can be isolated from the CSF, but the most common causes of bacterial meningitis are *Haemophilus influenzae* (2 months to 5 years), *Neisseria meningitidis* (all ages, most common in older children and young adults), and *Streptococcus pneumoniae* (all ages) (Table 11-6). *Streptococcus agalactiae* (group B) and *E. coli* are the major causes of meningitis in the newborn. Less common agents of bacterial

meningitis include *Mycobacterium tuberculosis,* staphylococci, *Listeria monocytogenes, Leptospira interrogans, Citrobacter* spp., and other gram-negative rods. Anaerobic bacteria are rarely isolated from CSF, and unless anaerobic bacteria are highly suspected, anaerobic agar media are usually not inoculated. *Staphylococcus epidermidis* is often isolated from shunt infections. These strains are frequently multiply resistant and difficult to eradicate. Thus any bacterium isolated from CSF should be reported immediately.

Nonbacterial meningitis may be caused by viruses, fungi, or free-living amoebae. The latter two can sometimes be detected by direct examination of the CSF.

Several rapid techniques are available for the diagnosis of the most common causes of bacterial meningitis. Coagglutination, latex agglutination, or counterimmunoelectrophoresis can be performed directly on CSF. If organisms resembling *H. influenzae* or *S. pneumoniae* are seen on smear, a quellung test with specific antiserum provides an immediate identification.

Latex agglutination can detect cryptococcal antigen in CSF or serum and is more sensitive than direct detection by india ink.

The meninges are not necessarily the primary site of infection in meningitis; therefore other specimens are also collected.

TABLE 11-5. Chemical and Cellular Composition of Cerebrospinal Fluid

CSF	Cell Count	PMNs (%)	Protein (mg/100 ml)	Glucose (mg/100 ml)
Normal	<5	20	<40	>45[a]
Meningitis				
Bacterial	10-5000	>50	↑	↓
Aseptic	10-1000	<50	N or ± ↑	N
Tuberculous or fungal	10-1000	<50	↑	N or ↓

SYMBOLS:	PMNs, Polymorphonuclear leukocytes	↑, Increased
	N, Normal	↓, Decreased
	±, Variable	

[a]One half blood glucose.

TABLE 11-6. Age Distribution of Cases of Bacterial Meningitis

Age	Percent Meningitis Cases Caused by				
	Streptococcus pneumoniae	*Neisseria meningitidis*	*Haemophilus influenzae*	Other Streptococci	Staphylococci
Newborn	5	Rare	—	23	5
2-60 mo	10	20	60	2	—
5-40 yr	20	45	5	5	10
>40 yr	50	10	2	5	13

Blood cultures should always be included. Specimens may be taken from the ears or sinuses. A Gram-stained smear from the petechial rash of meningococcal disease may reveal organisms.

Other Fluids

Pleural, pericardial, peritoneal, and synovial fluids are processed in the same manner that CSF is. In addition to blood agar, chocolate agar, and an enriched broth, culture of pleural and peritoneal fluid should include anaerobic agar media. Cultures of synovial fluid are examined for *Neisseria gonorrhoeae* and other potential pathogens. Pleural and peritoneal fluid may also be cultured for mycobacteria, and pleural fluid for fungi and *Legionella* spp.

CATHETERS

Foley catheters or tips should not be cultured because they become colonized with urethral flora, and cultures do not correlate with urine culture or urinary tract infection.[24] Vascular cannulas, however, are frequently submitted for culture because they can become colonized, especially with yeasts and staphylococci, and serve as a source of fungemia or bacteremia. Before their removal the skin is decontaminated. Short catheters (2 to 3 inches) are removed and severed aseptically at a point that was just inside the skin interface. Two segments of about 2 inches each are collected from longer catheters (8 to 24 inches)—one from the skin interface and one from a section that was within the blood vessel.[37] Catheter segments are asep-

tically placed in sterile wide-mouthed containers and transported immediately to the laboratory.

Almost any organism can colonize an intravascular cannula and serve as a focus of bacteremia. The most common are staphylococci and yeasts. Catheter segments can be contaminated during collection by the same organisms that can cause infection; therefore a broth medium should not be used. Results from a semiquantitative method suggested by Maki, Weise, and Sarafin[37] are easier to interpret. A sterile forceps is used to place the catheter segment on a blood agar plate. The catheter is rolled over the agar surface in four directions and then lightly pressed into the agar. Plates are incubated in air at 35° C for 48 hours. The number of colonies is counted and the approximate number reported. More than 15 colonies of the same species is considered significant. Any number present is reported.

EAR

Laboratory diagnosis of otitis media (middle ear infection) is usually attempted only in cases of therapeutic failure or in neonates because specimens must be collected by needle aspiration through the eardrum (tympanocentesis). If the eardrum is ruptured, exudate may be collected by inserting a sterile swab through an auditory speculum.

Material from otitis externa, which is a bacterial infection of the skin of the auditory meatus, can be collected with a swab.

The major etiologic agents of otitis media are *Streptococcus pneumoniae, Haemophilus influenzae* (often nonencapsulated), and *Streptococcus pyogenes*. Less often *Branhamella catarrhalis*, *Enterobacteriaceae*, *Staphylococcus aureus*, and *Pseudomonas* spp. or anaerobic bacteria are involved.[3] Culture media for anaerobic bacteria should be included only on specimens collected by tympanocentesis. All specimens are examined by Gram-stained smear, inoculated onto blood agar and chocolate agar, and incubated in 5% to 10% CO_2 at 35° to 37° C for up to 48 hours. If gram-negative rods are seen on smear, an enteric differential medium such as MacConkey agar can also be inoculated.

Otitis externa is frequently caused by *Pseudomonas aeruginosa* ("swimmer's ear"), other gram-negative rods, and *S. aureus*. Specimens are taken from the skin of the outer ear: therefore cutaneous flora such as *Staphylococcus epidermidis* and diphtheroids may be isolated but are not considered significant.

These specimens are inoculated onto blood agar and an enteric selective medium and incubated at 35° to 37° C for a total of 48 hours.[3]

EYE

Except in cases of purulent conjunctivitis, swabs are usually inadequate for culture of ocular infections. Specimens should be collected by an ophthalmologist. With corneal infection the conjunctivae are first swabbed, and then multiple scrapings are collected and inoculated directly onto agar media. Intraocular fluid is collected by needle aspiration and should be processed immediately.[32]

Conjunctivitis may be caused by bacteria, fungi, and viruses. *S. aureus*, *H. influenzae*, *S. pneumoniae*, and *N. gonorrhoeae* are the major causes of bacterial conjunctival infection. Members of the family *Enterobacteriaceae* and other gram-negative rods are a rare cause of conjunctivitis and are usually isolated only from immunosuppressed patients. Normal bacterial flora may also be isolated from conjunctival swabs in the following order of frequency: *S. epidermidis*, diphtheroids, *S. aureus*, *Streptococcus* spp., and *B. catarrhalis*. Conjunctival swabs are inoculated onto blood agar and chocolate agar and incubated in 5% to 10% CO_2 at 35° to 37° C for 48 hours.

Almost any bacterium can infect the traumatized cornea and cause keratitis. Major isolates are *S. aureus*, *S. pneumoniae*, *Pseudomonas* spp., and members of the family *Enterobacteriaceae*. Media that are directly inoculated by the ophthalmologist should include blood agar and chocolate agar, as for conjunctival swabs. In addition, an enriched broth and possibly media for mycobacteria and fungi should be inoculated.

Endophthalmitis is a serious infection caused by a number of organisms including *S. aureus*, *S. epidermidis*, *S. pneumoniae*, *Enterobacteriaceae* spp., *H. influenzae*, *Neisseria meningitidis*, *Bacillus* spp., and *Mycobacterium fortuitum*.

Pus or intraocular fluid is examined by smear and inoculated, as for corneal specimens. Media for mycobacteria, fungi, and anaerobic bacteria may be included if such infection is suspected.

GASTROINTESTINAL TRACT

Feces, vomitus, and duodenal contents may be submitted for isolation of bacteria causing diarrhea. Feces are passed directly into a clean, leakproof container or may be collected from a bedpan. Portions containing pus, blood, or mucus are pre-

ferred; a 1 or 2 g quantity is sufficient. If passed feces are unobtainable, the specimen can be collected by passing a swab beyond the anal sphincter, rotating carefully, and withdrawing. In acute disease when large numbers of organisms are shed, a single specimen is probably enough. Most *Salmonella* and *Shigella* strains are detected in two or three specimens. To rule out the carrier state, three negative specimens in a row are necessary.[46]

Outside the body, stool temperature drops, producing a pH change that particularly affects *Shigella* spp., so ideally specimens are plated directly.[53] If the specimen cannot be plated within an hour or two of collection, it should be mixed with a transport medium and refrigerated. Buffered glycerol saline is superior to Cary-Blair medium for *Shigella*[57] but is not good for *Vibrio* spp. or *Campylobacter jejuni*. Therefore, whenever culturing will be delayed, use of Cary-Blair medium is advisable.

Infectious diarrhea can be caused by bacteria, viruses, and parasites. The most frequent isolates from bacterial diarrheas in the United States are *C. jejuni* and species of *Salmonella* and *Shigella*. *Yersinia enterocolitica*, *Vibrio* spp., *Aeromonas hydrophila*, *Plesiomonas shigelloides*, and *S. aureus* are less frequently encountered. *Bacillus cereus*, *Clostridium perfringens*, and *S. aureus* are major causes of food poisoning but are rarely diagnosed by the hospital laboratory. Generally the suspected food must be examined for organisms or their toxins, usually by public health authorities. *E. coli* is rarely a cause of gastroenteritis in the United States.

Thus the task of the clinical laboratory is to isolate and identify the three major causes of bacterial diarrhea. Laboratories should be able to isolate other pathogens on request. Because the incidence of *Y. enterocolitica* and *Vibrio* spp. varies geographically, laboratories in areas of high incidence may culture for these bacteria routinely.

Normal feces contain from 10^{11} to 10^{12} bacteria per gram. The most abundant are nonsporeforming anaerobic bacilli, but gram-negative facultative bacteria such as *E. coli* and other members of the family *Enterobacteriaceae* are also present in relatively large numbers. Thus the laboratory must use selective and differential media to isolate pathogens from normal fecal flora. Sometimes pathogenic bacteria exist in small numbers: therefore enrichment techniques are used to ensure their isolation.

Microscopic examination of feces is useful to determine if leukocytes are present. Feces are mixed on a slide with Loeffler methylene blue stain, a coverslip is applied, and the slide is examined on "high dry." A strongly positive smear suggests infection with an invasive organism.

C. jejuni is the most common bacterial pathogen isolated from feces in developed countries. Several selective media are available for *C. jejuni* isolation, including Skirrow medium, Butzler medium, and Campy BAP.[8] Plates are incubated at 42° C in a microaerophilic atmosphere for 48 to 72 hours. Some laboratory workers advocate the use of an enrichment technique. Feces are inoculated into thioglycolate broth with 0.16% agar, vancomycin, trimethoprim, polymyxin B, amphotericin B, and cephalothin (Campy Thio). The broth is held overnight in the refrigerator, and then material about ½ inch below the surface is subcultured to a *Campylobacter*-selective agar medium.

An enrichment broth, such as selenite F, tetrathionate, or

GN broth, should always be inoculated for *Salmonella* spp. *Shigella* spp. grow in GN broth but not in the other two. The broth is incubated at 35° to 37° C for varying lengths of time depending on the type and is then subcultured to the same medium used for direct plating.

No one medium is ideal for isolation of *Salmonella* and *Shigella* spp.; some isolates may grow on a particular medium, whereas others do not. Therefore several different selective and differential media are inoculated. In practice, most laboratories use one plate that is mildly selective (MacConkey agar, eosin–methylene blue agar), one that is moderately selective (xylose lysine deoxycholate, Hektoen enteric, Salmonella-Shigella, or deoxycholate agars), and one that is highly selective (bismuth sulfite or brilliant green agars). These media are designed to inhibit normal fecal flora and allow *Salmonella* spp. and, in some cases, *Shigella* spp. to grow. *Shigella* does not grow on the highly selective media. All of these selective media are also differential. Most contain lactose and a pH indicator allowing differentiation of the non-lactose-fermenting *Salmonella* and *Shigella* organisms from other fecal flora.

In acute disease *Y. enterocolitica* is usually isolated with ease on MacConkey agar. In addition, specific *Yersinia*-selective agars are available with cefsulodin-irgasan-novobiocin (CIN) agar appearing to be the best.[27] Once the acute phase is over, the number of organisms that are shed decreases, and enrichment may be necessary. One method is cold enrichment, in which feces are inoculated into phosphate-buffered saline (pH 7.6) and held at 4° to 5° C for 3 weeks. Samples are subcultured to MacConkey agar at weekly intervals.[46] A more rapid and thus clinically significant method is alkali treatment. Stool is mixed with 0.5% potassium hydroxide (KOH) at a ratio of 1:2 by a vortex mixer for 2 minutes, and 0.1 ml is inoculated onto MacConkey agar and incubated at room temperature, or 37° C, for a total of 48 hours.[56]

Vibrio spp. may also require enrichment. Alkaline peptone water incubated at 35° to 37° C for 6 to 12 hours is suitable. The agar medium of choice for isolation of *Vibrio* spp. is thiosulfate–citrate–bile salts–sucrose (TCBS) agar. TCBS agar varies with different manufacturers in its ability to support the growth of *Vibrio* spp. and to inhibit lactose-fermenting normal intestinal flora. Thus careful quality control must be maintained for TCBS agar.

Most cases of antibiotic-induced diarrhea are caused by a toxin produced by *Clostridium difficile*. Diagnosis depends on demonstration of toxin in the stool filtrate. Toxin assays are performed in cell culture. *C. difficile* can be isolated on cycloserine–cefoxitin–fructose–egg yolk (CCFA) agar incubated anaerobically for 48 to 72 hours.[20]

MALE GENITAL TRACT

The urethra is the most common male genital site cultured. The laboratory may also receive testicular or epididymal aspirates or prostatic fluid. Prostatic fluid is obtained by digital massage through the rectum and collected in a sterile tube or on a swab. If urethral exudate is present or can be "milked" from the urethra, the usual swab may be used. Otherwise a thin urethrogenital swab is inserted about 2 cm into the urethra, gently rotated, and removed. Specimens for culture of *N. gonorrhoeae* are planted directly after collection by using one of several culture-transport devices, such as Jembec plates containing either modified Thayer-Martin (MTM), Martin-Lewis (ML), or

New York City (NYC)[18] media (see Chapter 14). A CO_2-generating system (Bio-Bag, Marion Laboratories) can be used to transport inoculated standard laboratory plates containing one of these media. The CO_2 in Transgrow bottles may vary from bottle to bottle within the same lot. This variation is not a problem in transport systems in which CO_2 is generated after inoculation.[17] Jembec plates, and standard laboratory plates are all incubated in 5% to 10% CO_2 at 35° to 37° C. In areas where vancomycin-resistant *N. gonorrhoeae* has been isolated, MTM (without vancomycin) or chocolate agar may also be inoculated. Plates or bottles are examined after overnight incubation and again after 48 hours of incubation.

Prostatic secretions are sometimes collected to diagnose bacterial prostatitis. Quantitative cultures are performed. Organisms found are the same as those isolated from urinary tract infections, with facultative gram-negative rods being the most common. The significance of gram-positive isolates is difficult to assess because staphylococci are found in the normal urethra. However, this decision is made by the physician.

In men over 35 years, lactose-fermenting normal intestinal flora and *Pseudomonas* spp. are the most common isolates in epididymitis, whereas *Chlamydia trachomatis* is the major isolate in younger men. Epididymal aspirates are treated like other aspirates: examined by Gram-stained smear and cultured aerobically and anaerobically (see the later section on wounds).

FEMALE GENITAL TRACT

Although anatomic barriers are not well defined, infections of the female genital tract can be described as lower tract (vulva, vagina, cervix) or upper tract (uterus, tubes, ovaries). With suspected lower tract gonococcal infection, cervical, urethral, or anal specimens may be submitted. The cervix is visualized using a speculum moistened with water (no lubricant). The cervical mucus plug is removed, the cervix is compressed gently with the speculum, and exudate is collected on a swab. If no exudate is seen, the swab is inserted into the endocervical canal, rotated, and removed. Urethral exudate may be stimulated by massaging the urethra against the pubic symphysis through the vagina. If no discharge is expressed, a urethrogenital swab is used, as for men. Anal cultures may be collected before and after treatment because the rectum may be the only positive posttreatment site.[17] A swab is inserted about 1 inch into the anal canal just inside the anal ring, moved from side to side, and removed. No fecal material should be on the swab.[33]

Pus from Bartholin's gland abscesses can sometimes be collected from the Bartholin's ducts. Otherwise, material can be aspirated directly by needle and syringe.

Specimens from the endometrium are best collected by transabdominal aspiration. They should not be collected through the cervix with a swab because they will be contaminated by cervical and vaginal flora—the same bacteria that cause endometritis. Protected swabs may reduce such contamination.[43]

Specimens for the diagnosis of pelvic inflammatory disease (PID) are all collected by invasive techniques. Peritoneal fluid may be collected from the cul-de-sac by aspiration through the posterior vaginal vault (culdocentesis). Material taken directly from the fallopian tubes or ovaries is collected surgically.

Intrauterine devices have been associated with infection and may be submitted for culture. They should be surgically removed to prevent contamination with cervical or vaginal flora, and the entire device, including any pus or secretions, should be placed in a sterile container for transport to the laboratory.

Lower tract infection is generally caused by exogenous pathogens such as *N. gonorrhoeae* or is a result of overgrowth of organisms normally present in small numbers *(Candida albicans, Gardnerella vaginalis).* Upper tract infection is often caused by a mixture of organisms. Although *N. gonorrhoeae* may ascend through the cervix and cause upper tract infection, many of these infections are caused by both aerobic and anaerobic normal lower genital tract flora.

The predominant members of the cervical and vaginal flora are lactobacilli, *S. epidermidis,* diphtheroids, anaerobic gram-positive cocci, and anaerobic gram-negative rods. Members of the family *Enterobacteriaceae, G. vaginalis,* streptococci, and yeasts are also found but in lower concentrations.

Scrapings, aspirates, or biopsy material from vulvar lesions is rarely submitted because bacterial vulvar infections (except syphilis) are rare in the United States. The clinician should specifically indicate the suspected causative agent. Possible isolates are *Haemophilus ducreyi, Calymmatobacterium granulomatis,* and *C. trachomatis* (Table 11-2).

Vaginal cultures are rarely useful because the major causes of vaginitis *(Trichomonas vaginalis, C. albicans)* are detected by smear or wet mount. The significance of *G. vaginalis* in nonspecific vaginitis remains controversial. The organism can be isolated on several media such as colistin–nalidixic acid blood agar, V agar, or human blood bilayer medium.[22,54] In certain cases vaginal swabs may be submitted for isolation of *S. aureus* (suspected toxic shock syndrome), *Streptococcus agalactiae* (group B), or *Listeria monocytogenes.* All three are isolated on blood agar plates, although *Listeria* may require cold enrichment.

Cervical or urethral exudate is cultured for *N. gonorrhoeae,* (as described in the section on the male genital tract). Columnar epithelial cells—not exudate—are required for isolation of *C. trachomatis.*

Specimens labeled ''endometrium'' should be screened by Gram-stained smear. The presence of squamous epithelial cells indicates cervicovaginal contamination. Such specimens should be cultured only after consultation with the clinician. If possible a new specimen should be submitted.[7]

Bartholin's gland abscesses and upper tract infection may be caused by *N. gonorrhoeae* or by many aerobic and anaerobic bacteria, frequently as mixed infections. Specimens are all examined microscopically. Appropriately collected specimens are cultured for *N. gonorrhoeae* and aerobic and anaerobic bacteria. Plates are treated in the same manner as those inoculated with other tissues or aspirates (see the section on wounds).

UPPER RESPIRATORY TRACT

Specimens from the upper respiratory tract include swabs of the anterior nares, nasopharynx, and throat and aspirates from sinus cavities. Nasal swabs are used for detection of staphylococcal carriers.

Nasopharyngeal secretions are collected with a small swab on a flexible wire such as the Calgiswab Type IV (Spectrum Diagnostics, Glenwood, Ill.). The swab is gently inserted through the nose into the nasopharynx, carefully rotated, removed, and placed in an appropriate transport medium. If whooping cough is suspected, special transport media must be used, or the specimen should be processed within 3 hours.[3]

Throat cultures are obtained by first depressing the tongue with a tongue depressor or swab (Figure 11-8). A sterile swab is vigorously rubbed over both tonsillar areas, the posterior pharynx, and any inflamed or ulcerated areas. Care should be taken not to touch the cheeks, tongue, uvula, or lips.

The only appropriate specimen for laboratory diagnosis of sinusitis is material directly aspirated from a sinus cavity. Nasal or nasopharyngeal specimens are not acceptable.[3]

The predominant microflora of the upper respiratory tract are nonpathogenic *Neisseria* spp., alpha-hemolytic and nonhemolytic (gamma) streptococci, *Haemophilus* spp., diphtheroids, and anaerobic bacteria. *S. pneumoniae* and staphylococci may also be isolated. Normally small numbers of gram-negative rods or yeasts may be isolated, but they are more common among alcoholic, diabetic, and hospitalized patients. The longer the hospitalization, the greater the incidence of gram-negative rod colonization of the respiratory tract.

Usually bacterial pharyngitis is caused by *S. pyogenes* (group A beta-hemolytic streptococci). Groups C and G may be infrequent causes of pharyngitis, but their identification is not critical unless they are the predominant organisms isolated.[3] Gonococcal pharyngitis is uncommon; therefore throat swabs are processed for *N. gonorrhoeae* only when specifically requested.

Other unusual bacterial causes of upper respiratory infection are *Bordetella pertussis* (whooping cough) and *Corynebacterium diphtheriae* (diphtheria). Both require special transport and culture media (Table 11-2 and Chapters 21 and 22).

Routine nasopharyngeal swabs for bacterial culture are to be discouraged. They may be submitted to detect meningococcal carriers or to diagnose whooping cough (Table 11-2).

Unless circumstances warrant, throat swabs are examined for beta-hemolytic streptococci only. Most microbiologists do not advocate direct smears for the diagnosis of streptococcal pharyngitis.[3] Culture on sheep blood agar in a low-dextrose nutrient base such as trypticase soy or Brucella agar is the standard method of diagnosis. After one streaks the plate, the loop is stabbed into the agar in the area of heaviest inoculum to enhance hemolysis and help create the anaerobic conditions required by streptolysin O.

Several comparison studies[12,34,42] have been completed to determine the best incubation atmosphere for recovery of group A beta-hemolytic streptococci from throat cultures (additional studies are noted in Chapter 13). Anaerobic incubation is recommended for reasons discussed in Chapter 13.

Sinusitis is caused most commonly by *S. pneumoniae* and *H. influenzae.* Less often anaerobic bacteria, aerobic streptococci, *Neisseria* spp., and *Branhamella catarrhalis* are involved, and infrequently *S. aureus* and aerobic facultative gram-negative rods are the causative agents. Appropriate specimens are obtained by direct aspiration and are thus processed like other aspirates (see the section on wounds), except that chocolate agar is included for isolation of *H. influenzae.* Before culture inoculation, examination of a Gram-stained smear may provide a presumptive diagnosis.

Diagnosis of thrush (oral candidiasis) depends on visualizing yeast cells on a direct KOH preparation rather than isolating some *Candida* organisms from the oral cavity.

Acute epiglottitis is usually a disease of children 2 to 4 years old and is almost always caused by *H. influenzae.* Occasionally

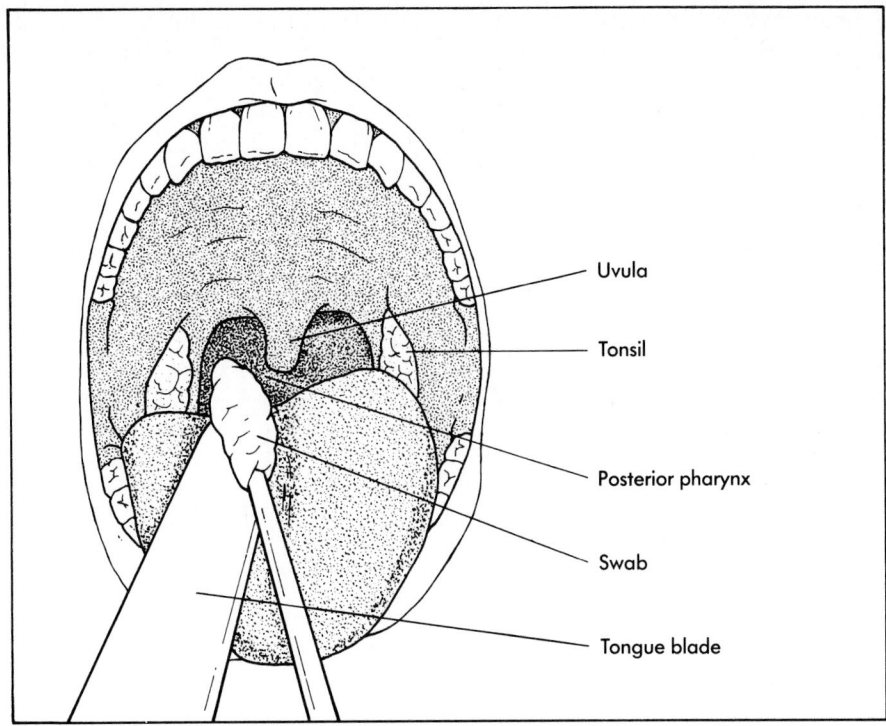

FIGURE 11-8. Collection of throat cultures.

S. pyogenes, S. aureus, or *S. pneumoniae* is involved. Cultures are not recommended because manipulation of a swollen, inflamed epiglottis can result in serious respiratory obstruction. Diagnosis is essentially clinical, although blood cultures are useful because half the patients are bacteremic.

LOWER RESPIRATORY TRACT

Expectorated sputum is the most common specimen submitted from patients with suspected pneumonia. The patient coughs deeply and expectorates into a sterile container. Sometimes sputum must be induced. If saline nebulization is used, the saline must not contain any bacteriostatic agents.

Lower respiratory secretions may also be collected by bronchoscopy, suction through tracheostomy or endotracheal tubes, transtracheal aspiration, direct lung aspiration, or biopsy.

Bronchial brushings are preferable to bronchial washings because the washings are more dilute. Specimens collected via bronchoscopy are contaminated with oral microbial flora, which can be greatly reduced by collecting secretions with a triple-lumen bronchoscope.[60]

Transtracheal aspiration is performed by a physician (Figure 11-9). The trachea below the larynx is normally sterile, except in patients with chronic pulmonary disease or endotracheal or tracheostomy tubes. A needle is inserted through the cricothyroid membrane into the trachea, a catheter is passed through the needle, and the needle is removed. Secretions are then aspirated through the catheter. Because the procedure is invasive, it is usually reserved for critically ill patients who are not producing sputum or who are suspected of having an anaerobic infection.

Lung aspirates are obtained by direct aspiration through the chest wall (pleural fluid, empyema fluid, thoracentesis fluid).

Transtracheal aspirates, lung aspirates, or lung tissue should be transported and processed without delay.[5,7]

Infections of the lower respiratory tract are caused by many microorganisms, including bacteria, mycoplasmas, fungi, viruses, and protozoa. *S. pneumoniae* remains the major cause of community-acquired acute bacterial pneumonia. Other, less common bacterial etiologic agents are *Legionella pneumophila, S. aureus,* and *H. influenzae.* The latter two are often isolated from patients with postinfluenza pneumonia. Aspiration pneumonia develops in patients with altered states of consciousness that cause abnormal gag and swallowing reflexes. Aspiration is more frequent in hospitalized patients but can occur in certain people in the community, such as alcoholics. Aspiration pneumonia is often a mixed infection caused by aspirated oropharyngeal flora. Anaerobic bacteria are almost always involved.

The upper respiratory tract of hospitalized patients who are debilitated or immunocompromised often becomes colonized with gram-negative rods. These organisms can invade the lower respiratory tract and produce disease. Hospital-acquired bacterial pneumonia may also be caused by other bacteria, such as *S. aureus* and *L. pneumophila.*

Empyema (an inflammatory exudate of the pleural cavity) is secondary to infection elsewhere, usually pneumonia or a lung abscess. About a third of these are mixed (aerobic and anaerobic) bacterial infections. Gram-negative rods and *S. aureus* are relatively common, but since the development of antimicrobial agents empyema caused by *S. pneumoniae* or *S. pyogenes* is rare.

Lung abscesses are usually secondary to aspiration and thus are usually caused by aerobic and anaerobic bacterial flora. Gram-negative rods and aerobic gram-positive cocci may be

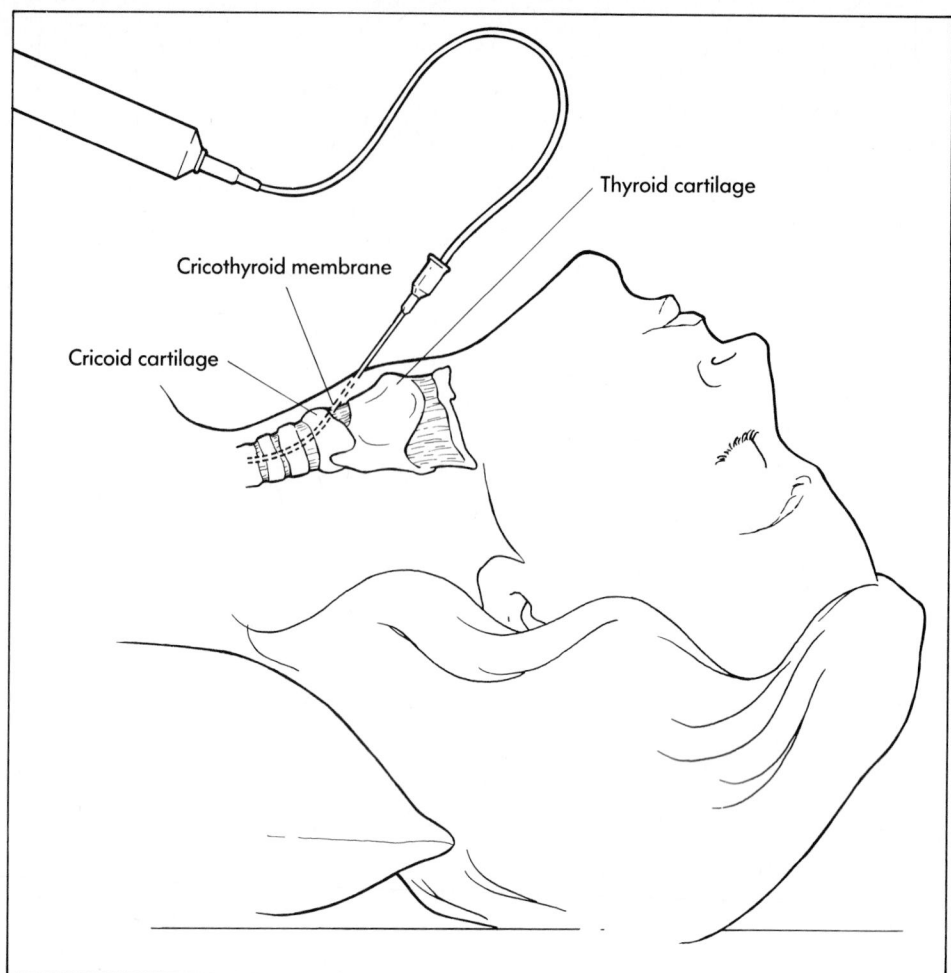

Thyroid cartilage

Cricothyroid membrane

Cricoid cartilage

FIGURE 11-9. Collection of lower respiratory secretions by transtracheal aspiration.

involved, particularly in nosocomial infection.

Chronic pneumonia can be caused by the same bacteria that cause acute pneumonia, although *S. pneumoniae* pneumonia rarely progresses to chronic disease. Other causes include mycobacteria, fungi, actinomycetes, and parasites.

Although sputum is the easiest specimen to collect, expectorated sputum cultures are among the most difficult to interpret. All expectorated sputum is contaminated to some degree by oral flora as it passes through the upper respiratory tract during collection. Virtually all sputa yield anaerobic bacteria from this contamination. Because anaerobic pulmonary infection is caused by normal oral flora, only specimens collected in a way that bypasses the oral cavity are cultured anaerobically.

A Gram-stained smear is made from a purulent portion of the specimen (1) to assess the degree of contamination and therefore the acceptability of the specimen and (2) to guide the clinician in selection of initial treatment. The smear is first examined under a low power (×100) for the numbers and types of cells present. An acceptable specimen should contain an abundance of leukocytes and few squamous epithelial cells. Several systems are used. The simplest is to consider the presence of more than 25 squamous epithelial cells per field unacceptable.[5]

Others base the evaluation on the number of leukocytes seen (specimens with more than 25 leukocytes per field are acceptable).[55] If the leukocyte count is used, the reader should remember that severely leukopenic patients may not have white cells in their sputum. Sputum screens are applicable only for specimens submitted for bacteriologic evaluation. Techniques for the isolation of mycobacteria, fungi, or viruses from sputum use decontamination methods and selective media, so the presence of oral flora is less important. If the specimen is unacceptable, the ordering physician must be notified so that a new specimen can be collected.

Acceptable specimens are examined with the oil immersion lens for the number and types of bacteria. Large numbers of similar organisms may be useful for rapid diagnosis of community-acquired pneumonias, such as pneumococcal (gram-positive diplococci), postinfluenza staphylococcal (gram-positive cocci in clumps), meningococcal (intracellular gram-negative diplococci), or *Klebsiella* (gram-negative rods).

Sputum is inoculated onto blood agar and chocolate agar (incubated in CO_2) and MacConkey or eosin–methylene blue agar (incubated in air). Plates are examined after 24 hours at 35° to 37° C. If the plates are negative and the smear was positive or if the patient is receiving antimicrobial agents, the plates should be incubated an additional 24 hours.[5]

Specimens obtained by bronchoscopy are contaminated by

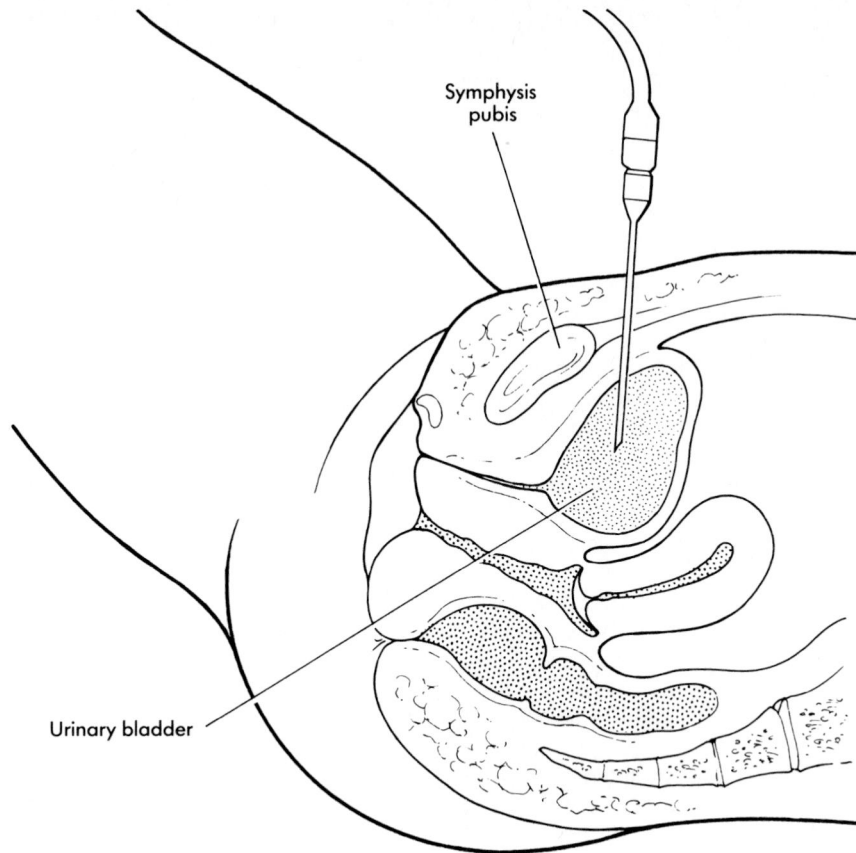

Symphysis
pubis

Urinary bladder

FIGURE 11-10. Urine collection by suprapubic bladder aspiration.

oral flora during passage of the bronchoscope and therefore are not cultured for anaerobic bacteria. The smear and culture are performed as for sputum, except that all bronchoscopically collected secretions should be cultured. Their collection entails considerable discomfort and expense for the patient.

Specimens collected through a tracheostomy or endotracheal tube are difficult to evaluate. Patients become colonized with potential pathogens within 24 hours of insertion of the tube and have an inflammatory response to it. Thus the specimen from a patient without lower respiratory disease can contain large numbers of leukocytes and bacteria. Tracheal aspirates are processed like sputa.

Transtracheal aspirates, lung aspirates, or lung tissue is processed like sputum. In addition, anaerobic agar media are inoculated. If *L. pneumophila* is suspected, the media discussed in Chapter 24 are also inoculated. The recovery of *M. pneumoniae* is considered in Chapter 25.

URINARY TRACT

In patients with symptoms of urinary tract infection (painful urination, urgency, frequency) urine is collected for culture at the onset of symptoms and may be repeated 48 to 72 hours after institution of therapy. If bacteriuria is asymptomatic, two or three specimens may be necessary to confirm an initial positive culture. In suspected renal tuberculosis three consecutive first-morning specimens should be submitted. Pooled 24-hour collection of urine is unacceptable.

Urine is collected by clean-catch, catheterization, or supra-

pubic aspiration (Figure 11-10). A midstream clean-catch specimen must be obtained in a manner that prevents contamination by organisms that colonize the distal urethra, vagina, and perineum. The patient is instructed to clean the periurethral area well with a mild detergent, followed by rinsing. The detergent may be bacteriostatic and must be completely rinsed off. The labial folds or glans penis is retracted, the patient begins to void, and then a midstream sample is collected.

To collect a specimen from a catheterized patient, the tubing is cleaned with alcohol and punctured with a 21-gauge needle, and the urine is aspirated with a syringe. Some urinary catheter systems have a special port for culture collection. The catheter is never disconnected from the drainage bag to collect a specimen, nor should urine be collected directly from the bag.

Urine is collected in a sterile screw-cap container. Most bacteria grow well in urine held at room temperature[30]; therefore specimens must be processed within 2 hours or refrigerated to prevent overgrowth by small numbers of contaminating bacteria. Alternatively, the urine may be aspirated into commercially available devices that contain a preservative fluid that maintains bacteria in the urine for at least 24 hours at room temperature.[35]

Infection of the urinary tract may involve the lower tract (cystitis, acute urethral syndrome) or upper tract (pyelonephritis). Diagnosis is based on demonstrating significant numbers of bacteria in the urine.

Because urine is frequently contaminated with small numbers of organisms during collection, quantitative cultures are mandatory. Broth culture precludes quantitation and thus is never used. Also, only urine collected by suprapubic bladder tap should be cultured anaerobically, because anaerobic bacteria are found among the urethral colonizing organisms.

Several techniques can be used for quantitating the number of bacteria in urine. Direct streaking with a calibrated loop may be used. A calibrated platinum loop (0.01 or 0.001 ml) is inserted vertically into the urine, and one loopful is inoculated, as described earlier, onto blood agar and MacConkey or eosin–methylene blue agar. Plates are examined after overnight incubation at 35° to 37° C and, if negative, after an additional 24 hours of incubation.

Urine collected by direct aspiration from the bladder is also cultured quantitatively, but a pipette is used, and 0.1 ml is dropped onto each plate. After drying, the drop is cross-streaked like other urine specimens.

Microscopic examination of unspun urine by Gram-stained smear can provide helpful information. The presence of more than one organism per oil immersion field correlates quite well (75% to 95%) with a colony count of more than 10^5/ml.

Deciding what colony count is significant is related to the clinical situation. In women with asymptomatic bacteriuria or pyelonephritis, colony counts equal to or greater than 10^5 CFU/ml correlate with infection, whereas contaminating bacteria (from the distal urethra) are usually present in numbers less than 10^3 CFU/ml.

Colony counts between 10^3 and 10^5/ml in these people can be difficult to interpret, since significant counts may be decreased because of antimicrobial therapy, frequency of urination, or dilution of the urine from excessive hydration. Counts between 10^3 and 10^5 CFU/ml are an indication for repeat culture. Most laboratories consider 10^4 CFU/ml or less in a clean-catch specimen to be insignificant.

Low counts (10^3 or more) are probably significant in specimens collected by aspiration from a catheter port. Any number greater than 10/ml of organisms isolated from suprapubic bladder tap specimens is significant.

Women with symptoms of urinary tract infection and pyuria but counts of less than 10^5 are designated as having acute urethral syndrome. Organisms associated with this syndrome are discussed in Chapter 10 and in reference 50.

Almost any bacterium can cause urinary tract infection, but the most common urinary pathogens are *E. coli* and other gram-negative rods, *Staphylococcus saprophyticus*, *S. aureus*, yeasts, enterococci, and beta-hemolytic streptococci. Common contaminants are often the same organisms that cause infection. No evidence supports the pathogenicity in the urinary tract of lactobacilli or diphtheroids even if present in numbers greater than 10^5 CFU/ml. Their isolation is more likely an indication of improper collection or transport.

Three or more different bacteria isolated from a clean-catch urine specimen is almost always caused by contamination. Patients with long-term catheterization with two or more organisms present at counts greater than 10^5 may be at risk for polymicrobial bacteremia.[23] A repeat culture is recommended whenever two or more organisms are isolated.

WOUNDS

Material from closed wounds or abscesses is best collected by needle and syringe after skin decontamination. If collection is done at surgery, a portion of the abscess wall should also be cultured. Specimens from superficial wounds are frequently collected by swab. Certain infections, such as ulcers and burns, are best sampled by biopsy because organisms isolated from surface swabs of these sites usually represent only colonization. Tissue and aspirates should be transported and processed without delay. Tissue should be submitted in a sterile container without carrier medium.

Postmortem specimens are often of limited value because of their poor correlation with antemortem cultures; however, they may be useful in selected cases. Ideally a 6 cm³ specimen with one serosal or capsular surface intact should be collected by the pathologist.

Almost any bacterium can be isolated from wounds, but certain bacteria are more commonly associated with particular skin and tissue infections. Superficial wounds cultured by a swab often yield skin flora, such as corynebacteria and *S. epidermidis*, that are not significant. *Bacillus* spp. on rare occasions cause infection in immunocompromised patients. The most frequent causes of cellulitis and other superficial infections are *S. pyogenes*, *S. aureus*, and gram-negative rods. Bites are contaminated with oral flora, and these organisms can then cause infection. *Pasteurella multocida* is often isolated from infected dog- or cat-bite wounds.

Subcutaneous infections and abscesses are most often caused by anaerobic bacteria and facultatively anaerobic gram-negative rods, but any organism isolated should be considered significant.

Any material collected from a wound should be examined with a Gram-stained smear. The smear can be extremely helpful in selecting initial antimicrobial therapy. For example, gram-positive cocci in chains seen in a specimen from cellulitis are almost always *S. pyogenes*. Early and appropriate therapy may be critical in these infections.

Specimens from superficial wounds are not acceptable for anaerobic culture. Blood agar and MacConkey agar are inoculated and incubated a total of 48 hours at 35° to 37° C.

Burns and ulcers quickly become colonized, especially with gram-negative rods. The significance of organisms isolated directly from swabs of these lesions is difficult to assess. A quantitative culture of a biopsy specimen may be more helpful. The specimen is briefly flamed to remove surface organisms, weighed, and ground by mortar and pestle with a known volume of broth to make about a 10% suspension. Serial dilutions are plated on aerobic and anaerobic media. Counts of greater than 10^5 CFU per gram are associated with a greater risk of developing wound sepsis.

Specimens from a closed wound or abscess are routinely inoculated to blood, MacConkey, and anaerobic blood agars and an enriched anaerobic broth. A selective medium for *Bacteroides* spp. increases the yield of anaerobic bacteria.[49] Aerobic plates are incubated 48 hours. Anaerobic plates are incubated under anaerobic conditions, examined at 48 hours, and reincubated an additional 48 hours (see Chapter 20). The broth is incubated 1 week.

If a large enough sample of tissue is received, a 1 cm cube is aseptically cut from the center. A smaller sample can be briefly flamed or put in boiling water for 2 to 3 minutes. The tissue is then minced with scissors and finally ground with a small amount of sterile 6-mesh aluminum oxide. Sterile broth is added to make a 10% to 20% suspension.[11] Aerobic and anaerobic media are inoculated and incubated, as for abscess specimens. Any remaining suspension is saved (at −70° C) in case further workup is necessary. The laboratory must be informed by the physician if any unusual organisms are suspected, such as *Legionella* or *Brucella* (Table 11-2).

REFERENCES

1. Appleman, M.D., Swinney, R.S., and Heseltine, P.N.R.: Evaluation of the antibiotic removal device, J. Clin. Microbiol. **15:**278, 1982.
2. Araj, G.F., et al.: Value of terminal subcultures from negative Bactec blood culture bottles, J. Clin. Microbiol. **14:**589, 1981.
3. Bannatyne, R.M., Clausen, C., and McCarthy, L.R.: Cumitech 10. In Duncan, I.B.R., editor: Laboratory diagnosis of upper respiratory tract infections, Washington, D.C., 1979, American Society for Microbiology.
4. Barry, A.L., Fay, G.D., and Sauer, R.L.: Efficiency of a transport medium for the recovery of aerobic and anaerobic bacteria from applicator swabs, Appl. Microbiol. **24:**31, 1972.
5. Bartlett, J.G., Brewer, N.S., and Ryan, K.J.: Cumitech 7. In Washington, J.A., II, editor: Laboratory diagnosis of lower respiratory tract infections, Washington, D.C., 1978, American Society for Microbiology.
6. Bartlett, J.G., et al.: Anaerobes survive in clinical specimens despite delayed processing, J. Clin. Microbiol. **3:**133, 1976.
7. Bartlett, R.C.: Making optimum use of the microbiology laboratory. II. Urine, respiratory, wound and cervicovaginal exudate, JAMA **247:**1336, 1982.
8. Blaser, M.J., and Reller, L.B.: *Campylobacter* enteritis, N. Engl. J. Med. **305:**1444, 1981.
9. Buck, G.E., et al.: Evaluation of the Campy Pak II gas generator system for isolation of *Campylobacter fetus* subsp. *jejuni*, J. Clin. Microbiol. **15:**41, 1982.
10. Christian, D.L., and Ederer, G.M.: Evaluation of bacteriological transport media, Am. J. Med. Tech. **39:**12, 1972.
11. Dolan, C.T.: Autopsy microbiology. In Ludwig, J., editor: Current methods of autopsy practice, Philadelphia, 1972, W.B. Saunders Co.
12. Dykstra, M.A., McLaughlin, J.C., and Bartlett, R.C.: Comparison of media and techniques for detection of group A streptococci in throat swab specimens, J. Clin. Microbiol. **9:**236, 1979.
13. Edberg, S.C., et al.: Direct inoculation procedure for the rapid classification of bacteria from blood culture, J. Clin. Microbiol. **2:**469, 1975.
14. Edberg, S.C., et al.: Rapid identification of *Enterobacteriaceae* from blood cultures with the Micro-ID system, J. Clin. Microbiol. **10:**693, 1979.
15. Ederer, G.M., and Christian, D.L.: Evaluation of bacteriological transport systems, Am. J. Med. Tech. **41:**299, 1975.
16. Eng, J., and Holten, E.: Gelatin neutralization of the inhibitory effect of sodium polyanethol sulfonate on *Neisseria meningitidis* in blood culture media, J. Clin. Microbiol. **6:**1, 1977.
17. Eschenbach, D., Pollock, H.M., and Schachter, J.: Cumitech 17. In Rubin, S.J., editor: Laboratory diagnosis of female genital tract infections, Washington, D.C., 1983, American Society for Microbiology.
18. Faur, Y.C., et al.: Field evaluation of New York City medium in the biological environment–CO_2 chamber in recovery of *Neisseria gonorrhoeae* and urogenital mycoplasmas, J. Clin. Microbiol. **5:**137, 1977.
19. Feeley, J.C., et al.: Charcoal-yeast extract agar: primary isolation medium for *Legionella pneumophila*, J. Clin. Microbiol. **10:**437, 1979.
20. George, W.L., et al.: Selective and differential medium for isolation of *Clostridium difficile*, J. Clin. Microbiol. **9:**214, 1979.
21. Gill, V.J.: Lack of clinical relevance in routine terminal subculturing of blood cultures, J. Clin. Microbiol. **14:**116, 1981.
22. Golberg, R.L., and Washington, J.A., II: Comparison of isolation of *Haemophilus vaginalis (Corynebacterium vaginale)* from peptone-starch-dextrose agar and Columbia colistin-nalidixic acid agar, J. Clin. Microbiol. **4:**245, 1976.
23. Gross, P.A., Flower, M., and Barden, G.: Polymicrobic bacteriuria: significant association with bacteremia, J. Clin. Microbiol. **3:**246, 1976.
24. Gross, P.A., et al.: Positive Foley catheter tip: fact or fancy? JAMA **228:**72, 1974.
25. Hagen, J.C., Wood, W.S., and Hashimoto, T.: Effect of chilling on the survival of *Bacteroides fragilis,* J. Clin. Microbiol. **4:**432, 1976.
26. Hall, M.M., Ilstrup, D.M., and Washington, J.A., II: Effect of volume of blood cultured on detection of bacteremia, J. Clin. Microbiol. **3:**643, 1976.
27. Head, C.B., Whitty, D.A., and Ratnam, S.: Comparative study of selective media for recovery of *Yersinia enterocolitica*, J. Clin. Microbiol. **16:**615, 1982.
28. Helstad, A.G., Kimball, J.L., and Maki, D.G.: Recovery of anaerobic, facultative, and aerobic bacteria from clinical specimens in three anaerobic transport systems, J. Clin. Microbiol. **5:**564, 1977.
29. Hill, G.B.: Effects of storage in an anaerobic transport system on bacteria in known polymicrobial mixtures and in clinical specimens, J. Clin. Microbiol. **8:**680, 1978.
30. Hindman, R., Tronic, B., and Bartlett, R.: Effect of delay on culture of urine, J. Clin. Microbiol. **4:**102, 1976.
31. Isenberg, H.D., Schoenknecht, F.D., and von Graevenitz, A.: Cumitech 9. In Rubin, S.J., editor: Collection and processing of bacteriological specimens, Washington, D.C., 1979, American Society for Microbiology.
32. Jones, D.B., Liesegang, T.J., and Robinson, N.M.: Cumitech 13. In Washington, J.A. II, editor: Laboratory diagnosis of ocular infections, Washington, D.C., 1981, American Society for Microbiology.
33. Kellogg, D.S., Jr., Holmes, K.K., and Hill, G.A.: Cumitech 4. In Marcus, S., and Sherris, J.C., editors: Laboratory diagnosis of gonorrhea, Washington, D.C., 1976, American Society for Microbiology.
34. Kurzynski, T.A., and van Holten, C.M.: Evaluation of techniques for isolation of group A streptococci from throat cultures, J. Clin. Microbiol. **13:**891, 1981.
35. Lauer, B.A., Reller, L.B., and Mirrett, L.: Evaluation of preservative fluid for urine collected for culture, J. Clin. Microbiol. **10:**42, 1979.
36. Louria, D.B., et al.: Study on the usefulness of hypertonic culture media, J. Clin. Microbiol. **4:**208, 1976.
37. Maki, D., Weise, C.E., and Sarafin, H.W.: A semi-quantitative culture method for identifying intravenous-catheter–related infection, N. Engl. J. Med. **296:**1305, 1977.
38. McLaughlin, J.C., Evers, J.L., and Officer, J.L.: Lack of requirement for blind subcultures of Bactec blood culture media, J. Clin. Microbiol. **14:**567, 1981.
39. Mirrett, S., and Reller, L.B.: Comparison of direct and standard antimicrobial disk susceptibility testing for bacteria isolated from blood, J. Clin. Microbiol. **10:**482, 1979.
40. Murray, P.R., and Hampton, C.M.: Recovery of pathogenic bacteria from cerebrospinal fluid, J. Clin. Microbiol. **12:**554, 1980.
41. Murray, P.R., and Sondag, J.E.: Evaluation of routine subcultures of macroscopically negative blood cultures and detection of anaerobes, J. Clin. Microbiol. **8:**427, 1978.
42. Murray, P.R., et al.: Effects of selective media and atmosphere of incubation on the isolation of group A streptococci, J. Clin. Microbiol. **4:**54, 1976.
43. Pezzlo, M.T., et al.: Improved laboratory efficiency and diagnostic accuracy with new double-lumen–protected swab for endometrial specimens, J. Clin. Microbiol. **9:**56, 1979.
44. Regan, J., and Lowe, F.: Enrichment medium for the isolation of *Bordetella,* J. Clin. Microbiol. **6:**303, 1977.

45. Reller, L.B., Murray, P.R., and MacLowry, J.D.: Cumitech 16. In Washington, J.A., II, editor: Blood cultures IA, Washington, D.C., 1982, American Society for Microbiology.

46. Sack, R.B., Tilton, R.C., and Weissfeld, A.S.: Cumitech 12. In Rubin, S.J., editor: Laboratory diagnosis of bacterial diarrhea, Washington, D.C., 1980, American Society for Microbiology.

47. Salventi, J.F., et al.: Effect of blood dilution on recovery of organisms from clinical blood cultures in medium containing sodium polyanetholsulfonate, J. Clin. Microbiol. **9:**248, 1979.

48. Silva, H.S., and Washington, J.A., II: Optimal time for routine early subculture of blood cultures, J. Clin. Microbiol. **12:**445, 1980.

49. Sondag, J.E., Ali, M., and Murray, P.R.: Relative recovery of anaerobes on different isolation media, J. Clin. Microbiol. **10:**756, 1979.

50. Stamm, W.E., et al.: Causes of the acute urethral syndrome in women, N. Engl. J. Med. **303:**409, 1980.

51. Staneck, J.L., and Vincent, S.: Inhibition of *Neisseria gonorrhoeae* by sodium polyanetholsulfonate, J. Clin. Microbiol. **13:**463, 1981.

52. Swenson, F.J., and Rubin, S.J.: Clinical significance of viridans streptococci isolated from blood cultures, J. Clin. Microbiol. **15:**725, 1982.

53. Taylor, W.I., and Schelhart, D.: Effect of temperature on transport and plating media for enteric pathogens, J. Clin. Microbiol. **2:**281, 1975.

54. Totten, P.A., et al.: Selective differential human blood bilayer media for isolation of *Gardnerella (Haemophilus vaginalis)*, J. Clin. Microbiol. **15:**141, 1982.

55. Van Scoy, R.E.: Bacterial sputum cultures: a clinician's viewpoint, Mayo Clin. Proc. **52:**39, 1971.

56. Weissfeld, A.S., and Sonnenwirth, A.C.: Rapid isolation of *Yersinia* spp. from feces, J. Clin. Microbiol. **15:**508, 1982.

57. Wells, J.G., and Morris, G.K.: Evaluation of transport methods for isolating *Shigella* spp., J. Clin. Microbiol. **13:**789, 1981.

58. Wilkins, T.D., and West, S.E.H.: Medium-dependent inhibition of *Peptostreptococcus anaerobius* by sodium polyanetholsulfonate in blood culture media, J. Clin. Microbiol. **3:**393, 1976.

59. Williams, S.G., and Kaufman, C.A.: Survival of *Streptococcus pneumoniae* in sputum from patients with pneumonia, J. Clin. Microbiol. **7:**3, 1978.

60. Wimberley, N., Faling, L.J., and Bartlett, J.G.: A fiberoptic bronchoscopy technique to obtain uncontaminated lower airway secretions for bacterial culture, Am. Rev. Respir. Dis. **119:**337, 1979.

CHAPTER 12

Staphylococci

Barbara J. Howard
Wesley E. Kloos

Staphylococci are gram-positive organisms that are primarily associated with the skin, skin glands, and mucous membranes of humans and other warm-blooded animals. Some species of staphylococci are common opportunistic pathogens in humans. *Staphylococcus aureus* is responsible for toxic shock syndrome, discussed in Chapter 10, as well as for other toxigenic diseases discussed in this chapter.

CLASSIFICATION

Bergey's Manual of Systematic Bacteriology includes the genus *Staphylococcus* together with the genera *Micrococcus* and *Planococcus* in the family *Micrococcaceae*.[99] The three genera are composed of catalase-positive, gram-positive cocci with a cell wall peptidoglycan containing L-lysine as the diamino acid; however, they are not closely related phylogenetically and are included in one family simply as a matter of historical and practical convenience. Staphylococci are most closely related to the broad *Bacillus-Lactobacillus-Streptococcus* cluster.

According to *Bergey's Manual* the genus *Staphylococcus*[70] consists of gram-positive cocci, 0.5 to 1.5 μm in diameter, occurring singly, in pairs, and in tetrads, and characteristically dividing in more than one plane to form irregular clusters. The cell wall contains peptidoglycan and teichoic acid. Most strains grow in the presence of 10% NaCl and between the temperatures of 18° and 40° C. Metabolism is respiratory and fermentative. Carbohydrates and amino acids are utilized as carbon and energy sources. For most species the main product of glucose fermentation is lactic acid, and in the presence of air the main products are acetic acid and CO_2. Most species require an organic source of nitrogen (amino acids and certain B group vitamins). Others can grow with $(NH_4)_2SO_4$ as a sole source of substrate nitrogen. Staphylococci are susceptible to lysis by lysostaphin but are resistant to lysis by lysozyme under standard conditions.

Several staphylococcal species preferentially colonize specific niches of the human body.[61,62,64,66,69] *S. aureus* prefers the anterior nares. From 10% to 40% of the general human population carry this species in their nares; up to 70% of hospitalized individuals (patients and personnel) carry this organism.[1] *S. epidermidis* is the most versatile species, producing large populations in the anterior nares, axillae, inguinal and perineal areas, and toewebs and on areas of the face. *S. epidermidis* comprises 90% to 100% of the staphylococci isolated from the nares when *S. aureus* is not present.[66]

S. hominis and *S. haemolyticus* prefer the moist axillae, the inguinal and perineal areas, which are richly supplied with apocrine glands, and the toewebs. However, they also colonize the drier regions of skin (for example, the arms and legs) more successfully than most other species. They are second to *S. epidermidis* in their extent of distribution. *S. capitis* has a strong predilection for the head, especially the scalp, forehead, and external auditory meatus, where sebaceous glands are numerous. *S. auricularis* is largely confined to the external auditory meatus. *S. saprophyticus* is only occasionally isolated from human skin, but this species appears to have a higher capacity to adhere to uroepithelial cells than to buccal or skin cells and does so better than other staphylococcal species.[22] *S. saccharolyticus*, *S. warneri*, *S. cohnii*, *S. xylosus*, and *S. simulans* are only occasionally isolated from human skin. *S. saccharolyticus* has been mainly isolated from regions of the face, especially the forehead; it is an anaerobic species that presumably colonizes deeper recesses of follicular canals.[32]

The species *S. sciuri*, *S. lentus*, *S. hyicus*, *S. intermedius*, *S. carnosus*, *S. caseolyticus*, *S. gallinarum*, *S. arlettae*, *S. equorum*, and *S. kloosii* are associated with animals.* *S. caprae* has been isolated from goat milk[27] and humans. *S. xylosus* and *S. simulans* have also been isolated from both humans and animals.[61,124] *S. warneri*, *S. haemolyticus*, *S. cohnii*, and *S. auricularis* are each subdivided into human and nonhuman primate subspecies.[64,74,76] Human and animal staphylococci are exchanged occasionally by contact, but such transfers are usually only transient.

Before the 1970s, *S. aureus* and *S. epidermidis*, or *S. albus*, were the only recognized staphylococcal species. *S. aureus* was considered a pathogen, and *S. epidermidis*, when it appeared in clinical material, was regarded as a contaminant. In the mid-1970s, Kloos and Schleifer conducted comprehensive systematic studies of staphylococci and micrococci and described seven new species of staphylococci and two new species of micrococci.[67,68,73,102] These investigators also amended the descriptions of *S. epidermidis* and the species *S. saprophyticus*, which at the time was just removed from the genus *Micrococcus*. Several other new species have been described over the past decade. It is now well known that *S. epidermidis* and *S. saprophyticus* are common opportunistic pathogens in humans.

The pathogenic potential of other staphylococcal species is summarized as follows:
1. Common pathogen
    a. *S. aureus*
    b. *S. epidermidis*
    c. *S. saprophyticus*

---

*References 26, 27, 46, 72, 100, 101, and 104.

2. Uncommon pathogen
   a. *S. haemolyticus*
   b. *S. hominis*
   c. *S. warneri*
   d. *S. saccharolyticus*
   e. *S. cohnii*
   f. *S. simulans*
3. Undetermined or rare pathogen
   a. *S. capitis*
   b. *S. auricularis*
   c. *S. xylosus*

In addition, *S. aureus, S. intermedius,* and *S. hyicus* are common opportunistic pathogens of animals.

GROWTH REQUIREMENTS
MEDIA

Most staphylococci grow on any nutrient medium containing peptone. They grow well on sheep blood agar and tryptic or trypticase soy and brain heart infusion agars or broths. The more pathogenic species also grow well in the anaerobic portions of thioglycolate broth or semisolid agar.

A selective medium can be used to isolate staphylococci from specimens that are likely to be contaminated heavily with other bacterial flora. The commonly used selective media include phenylethyl alcohol (PEA) agar, Columbia nalidixic acid (CNA) agar, and mannitol salt agar (MSA) (see Appendix A). The phenylethyl alcohol in PEA agar inhibits the growth of gram-negative organisms but supports the growth of gram-positive organisms. The nalidixic acid of CNA agar performs a similar function. The selectivity of MSA is based on its high concentrations of salt. Staphylococci are able to tolerate these high concentrations (up to 10%) and thus grow on MSA, whereas most other organisms grow poorly or not at all. *S. epidermidis* and *S. hominis* do not grow as well as most other staphylococcal species on MSA.

NUTRITIONALLY VARIANT STAPHYLOCOCCI (DWARF COLONIES)[2]

Certain strains of *S. aureus* have increased nutritional requirements, necessitating supplementation of the media with hemin, menadione, thiamine, or pantothenate. These isolates are called dwarf colonies because they appear as microcolonies on routine laboratory media that have not been supplemented with their additional growth requirements. CO_2-requiring variants of *S. aureus* can also produce dwarf colonies. These variants appear as minute (0.1 mm or less in diameter), clear colonies resembling streptococci when cultured in air but as typical *S. aureus* colonies when provided with increased CO_2.[110,114] Thiamine- or menadione-requiring strains are associated with severe human infections, such as osteomyelitis and septicemia,[2] whereas CO_2-requiring strains are associated with septicemia.[114]

It is not known why these nutritionally variant strains of *S. aureus* are selected in the host. Possibly thiamine- or menadione-requiring strains are selected in the presence of structural analogues of the essential nutrients. For example, thiamine-requiring strains have been isolated from patients being treated with trimethoprim-sulfamethoxazole or barbiturates, both of which contain a portion of thiamine.

Although these strains are isolated only rarely, laboratories should be aware of their existence. The use of enriched media, such as chocolate agar containing IsoVitaleX and menadione, is recommended for cultures that might possess thiamine- or menadione-requiring *S. aureus*. Examples include sterile cultures when *S. aureus* is observed on Gram stain, cultures obtained from patients who are known to have *S. aureus* infections and are receiving antimicrobial therapy, and cultures from patients with chronic staphylococcal infections, especially osteomyelitis.

ENVIRONMENTAL REQUIREMENTS

Most staphylococci are facultative anaerobes. *S. saccharolyticus* is an anaerobic species.

Incubation for 18 to 24 hours at 35° to 37° C will allow abundant growth of most species of *Staphylococcus* on agar. *S. auricularis* and *S. lentus* require somewhat longer incubation periods. Growth in most nonselective commercial broths is abundant within 4 to 12 hours, depending on inoculum size and the particular species.

CULTURAL CHARACTERISTICS
STAINING REACTIONS

Staphylococci, when Gram stained from solid media, appear as gram-positive cocci, usually in clusters (Plate 1, *A*). In fact, the genus name *Staphylococcus* is derived from the Greek word *staphyle,* meaning a bunch of grapes. The formation of clusters is due to the tendency of the organisms to divide in different planes.

Gram stains should be performed on young cultures because staphylococci can appear gram negative or gram variable with age. Staphylococci can also appear as short chains, usually of fewer than five members, when a Gram stain is prepared from liquid media.

COLONIAL MORPHOLOGY

After 18 to 24 hours' incubation, staphylococci appear as opaque, smooth, circular colonies with a butyrous consistency. Although the presence of golden-yellow pigmentation and alpha- and beta-hemolysins has classically been used to distinguish *S. aureus* (Plate 5, *E*), these two characteristics are not totally reliable. Several staphylococcal species, in addition to *S. aureus,* can produce yellow colonies; furthermore, not all *S. aureus* are yellow pigmented. Likewise, some species of staphylococci besides *S. aureus* produce hemolysins. The hemolytic zones of *S. aureus* organisms, however, tend to be larger than those of the other staphylococci.

S. epidermidis usually produces pale, translucent, gray-white nonhemolytic colonies; a few may be slightly hemolytic (Plate 5, *F*). *S. saprophyticus* are usually white but can be yellow or orange. They are smooth, slightly convex colonies with entire margins and are usually larger than colonies of *S. epidermidis.* Morphologic descriptions of the other staphylococci can be found in the references.[67,69-71,102]

BIOCHEMICAL IDENTIFICATION
DIFFERENTIATION OF THE GENERA *STAPHYLOCOCCUS* AND *MICROCOCCUS*

Staphylococci and micrococci differ in the base composition of their deoxyribonucleic acid; staphylococci have 30 to 38 mol% G+C in their DNA, and micrococci have 67 to 73 mol%.[70,99] These genera also differ in the chemical composition of their cell walls; staphylococci possess glycine—glycine linkages in the interpeptide bridges of the peptidoglycan, whereas micrococci do not. Although both of these tests are reliable in separating micrococci and staphylococci, they are time consuming and beyond the capability of most clinical laboratories.

Distinguishing characteristics that can easily be determined in the routine clinical laboratory are shown in Table 12-1. Most staphylococci ferment glucose under anaerobic conditions (oxidation-fermentation [OF] test), whereas most micrococci do not. However, some strains of *Micrococcus kristinae* may weakly ferment glucose, and several species of staphylococci, including *S. saprophyticus, S. auricularis, S. hominis, S. xylosus,* and *S. cohnii,* either may fail to grow in the anaerobic portion of OF media or may not produce sufficient quantities of acid to be detected.[45,99] *S. hominis* usually fails to grow or grows only poorly in the anaerobic portions of thioglycolate.[70]

The modified oxidase and benzidine tests detect the presence of cytochrome c.[34] Staphylococci, except *S. sciuri, S. lentus,* and *S. caseolyticus,* do not possess cytochrome c and are negative for both of these tests. The micrococci are positive for both of these tests.

Schleifer and Kloos[103] found the combination of lysozyme and lysostaphin resistance and aerobic production of acid from glycerol in the presence of erythromycin to be a practical scheme for use in the routine laboratory. (These tests are discussed in Appendix A.) Lysozyme is an enzyme that cleaves the glycan strands between *N*-acetyl muramic acid and *N*-acetylglucosamine, both of which are found in the cell walls of staphylococci and micrococci. At certain concentrations of lysozyme most micrococci are susceptible whereas, for reasons not clearly defined, most staphylococci are resistant. Lysostaphin is an enzyme that lyses glycine—glycine bonds. The presence of glycine-containing interpeptide linkages in staphylococci renders them susceptible to lysostaphin; micrococci do not have the glycine—glycine linkages. Finally, most staphylococci are able to produce acid aerobically from glycerol, whereas most micrococci are not. It is important to use both lysozyme-lysostaphin resistance and aerobic production of acid from glycerol in separating staphylococci and micrococci because those organisms that show aberrant reactions in one test show typical reactions in the other. Staphylococci are intrinsically less susceptible to erythromycin than are micrococci. In addition to these tests, Falk and Guering[33] were able to separate staphylococci and micrococci on the basis of their susceptibility to Taxo A bacitracin disks. Staphylococci were resistant to the disks, whereas micrococci were susceptible, producing zones of growth inhibition ranging from 10.5 to 25 mm in diameter.

DIFFERENTIATION AMONG STAPHYLOCOCCAL SPECIES
Distinguishing *Staphylococcus aureus*

The coagulase test is used to distinguish *S. aureus, S. intermedius,* and certain *S. hyicus* strains from the other staphylococcal species.[26,46,65] Coagulase is an enzyme that clots blood plasma. Two types of coagulase tests are used in the laboratory, the slide test and the tube test (see Appendix A).

The slide test is a screening procedure that detects the presence of bound coagulase, or the clumping factor. Bound coagulase is a surface component of the organism that is believed to affect clotting by causing the alpha- and beta-chains of fibrinogen to cross-link.[10] The slide test is performed by making a

TABLE 12-1. Characteristics for Distinguishing Staphylococci from Micrococci

Test	Micrococcus	Staphylococcus
OF-Dextrose	Oxidative or asaccharolytic[a]	Fermentative[b]
Acid (aerobically) from glycerol-erythromycin medium (0.4 μg erythromycin/ml)	−[c]	+/− (rare)
Resistance to:		
Lysozyme (25 μg/ml)	−/+	+
Lysostaphin (200 μg/ml)	+/±	−[d]
Modified oxidase and benzidine tests	+	−[e]

SYMBOLS:	+, Positive reaction
	±, Weak reaction
	−, Negative reaction

Modified from Kloos, W.E.: Clin. Microbiol. Newsletter **4**:75, 1982.
[a] *M. kristinae* may weakly ferment dextrose.
[b] Some strains of *S. auricularis, S. hominis, S. cohnii, S. xylosus,* and *S. saprophyticus* can produce very low amounts of acid from glucose. Indicator may not detect small amounts of acid, and these organisms will appear as *Micrococcus.* In thioglycolate medium, *S. hominis* usually does not produce detectable growth in anaerobic portion within 24 to 48 hours.
[c] *M. kristinae* may produce acid.
[d] *S. sciuri* may be partially resistant.
[e] *S. sciuri, S. lentus,* and *S. caseolyticus* are positive.

heavy suspension of the test organism in a drop of distilled water, adding a drop of plasma, and observing for clumping within 10 seconds. The presence of clumping is a positive test and is indicative of *S. aureus* (Figure 12-1). (It should be noted that some uncommon *S. intermedius* strains are also clumping factor positive; however, this organism is usually isolated from animals and is rarely encountered in the human clinical laboratory.) Although false-positive tests usually do not occur with the slide coagulase test, false-negative results are observed 16.5% of the time.[28] Thus one must confirm all negative slide tests with the more definitive tube test.

The tube test detects the presence of extracellular coagulase. Extracellular coagulase reacts with a component of plasma designated coagulase reacting factor (CRF) to produce coagulase-CRF complex, a substance clinically indistinguishable from thrombin. The coagulase-CRF complex then reacts with fibrinogen to form fibrin.[116] The tube test is performed by inoculating 0.1 ml of either an overnight culture in brain heart infusion broth or an isolated colony into a tube containing 0.5 ml of rabbit plasma. The tube is incubated in a 37° C water bath for 4 hours and observed at 30-minute intervals for clotting. Any degree of clotting is considered a positive test (Figure 12-2). Because some staphylococci produce coagulase slowly, all negative tests should be incubated overnight at room temperature and again observed for clotting. The animal species *S. intermedius* and *S. hyicus* ssp. *hyicus* often require more than 4 hours of incubation for clotting, but these species would most likely be isolated in the veterinary clinical laboratory and not in

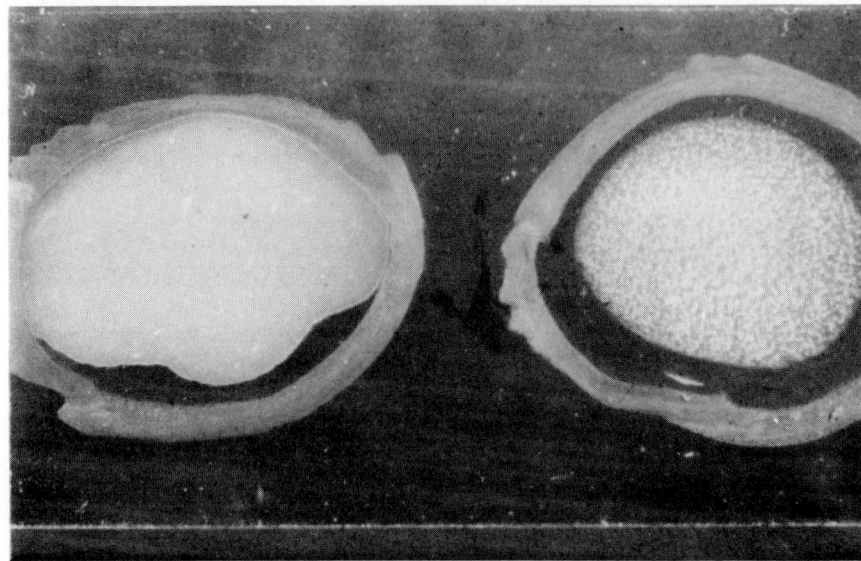

FIGURE 12-1. Positive (*right*) and negative *(left)* slide coagulase test. (Courtesy Dr. Leon J. LeBeau, Department of Biocommunication Arts, Medical Center, University of Illinois at Chicago.)

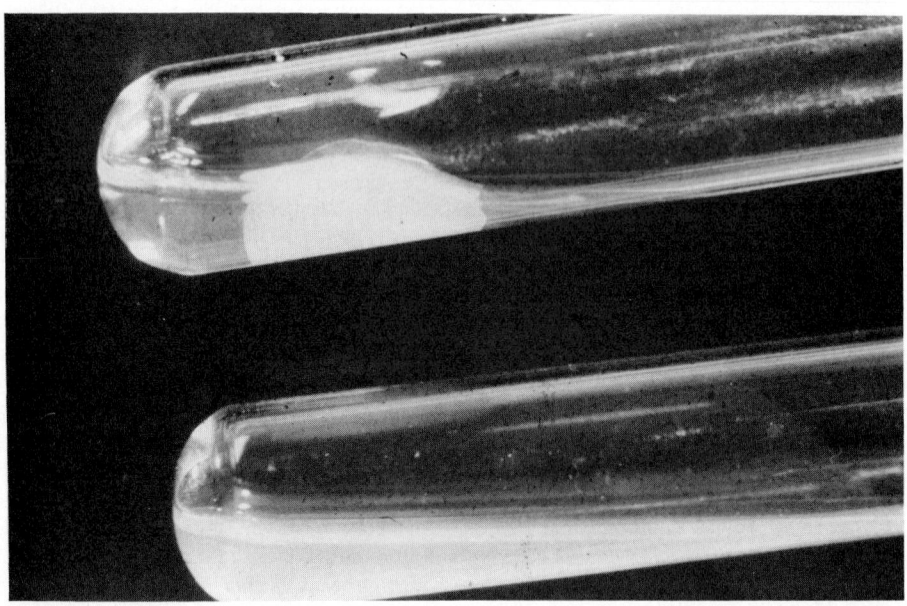

FIGURE 12-2. Positive *(top)* and negative *(bottom)* tube coagulase test. (Courtesy Dr. Leon J. LeBeau, Department of Biocommunication Arts, Medical Center, University of Illinois at Chicago.)

human clinical settings.[65] The tube coagulase test is the most reliable and accurate test for identification of *S. aureus*. It is about 97% predictive of this species in the human clinical laboratory. False-positive reactions can occur when the inoculum contains a mixed culture. *Pseudomonas, Serratia,* and *Enterococcus faecalis* may utilize the citrate in citrated plasma and produce clot formation; hence plasma containing ethylenediamine tetraacetic acid (EDTA) is superior.[12] False-negative reactions can result when *S. aureus* produces so much staphylokinase that it lyses the fibrin clot.

Other tests used to distinguish *S. aureus* are fermentation of mannitol on MSA, DNAse production, and thermonuclease production. These are discussed in Appendix A. Although most *S. aureus* isolates are positive for mannitol fermentation and DNAse production and most of the major human coagulase-negative staphylococci are negative, these two tests are not definitive. Taken as a whole, approximately 21% of human coagulase-negative staphylococci are positive for mannitol fermentation, and 18% of coagulase-negative staphylococci produce DNAse.[115] The thermonuclease test is more definitive than these two tests; 99% of *S. aureus* and less than 2% of coagulase-negative staphylococci are positive. The thermonuclease test has not been used routinely in the clinical laboratory because it is technically more difficult than the coagulase test. A rapid, simpler thermonuclease test, however, has recently been described for identification of *S. aureus* in blood cultures (see Appendix A).

Differentiation among Coagulase-Negative Staphylococci

Definitive identification of coagulase-negative staphylococci (CNS) isolated from humans can be accomplished as described in Tables 12-2 and 12-3. This scheme is based on the original work of Kloos and Schleifer.[70,75] Commercially available systems were recently developed based on the conventional tests in Tables 12-2 and 12-3 and on several other tests. These systems, discussed in Chapter 9, provide the laboratory with an easy, rapid means of definitive identification of CNS. They include API Staph-Ident (Analytab Products, Plainview, N.Y.), API Staph Trac (API Systems S.A., Montalieu-Vercieu, France), Pos Combo panel (Microscan–Baxter Travenol, Sacramento, Calif.), Minitek (BBL Microbiology Systems, Cockeysville, Md.), and the AutoMicrobic system (AMS) (Vitek Systems, Inc., Hazelwood, Mo.) utilizing a Gram Positive Identification Card (GPI).

Until the clinical significance of routine species identification of all CNS can be clearly established, laboratories may choose to restrict complete species identification to isolates from normally sterile sites, such as blood or cerebrospinal fluid, and to routinely distinguish *S. saprophyticus* from other CNS isolated from urine and *S. epidermidis* from other CNS isolated from prosthetic devices, catheters, and shunts.[65] Reports are accumulating that *S. warneri* and *S. haemolyticus* are significant pathogens in native, infectious endocarditis, and they may warrant species identification when isolated from such infections.[17,24] These species are intrinsically less susceptible to methicillin and isoxazolylpenicillins than *S. epidermidis*.[48,93] There may also be occasions when *S. epidermidis* should be identified in urinary tract infections as it can be an opportunistic pathogen in patients with urologic disorders.[86] Susceptibility to novobiocin or nalidixic acid can be used to

presumptively distinguish *S. saprophyticus* from *S. epidermidis*.[54] The former species is resistant to novobiocin and nalidixic acid, whereas the latter is susceptible. A promising 5-hour novobiocin test, which was recently described, may be used for the presumptive identification of *S. saprophyticus* (see Appendix A).[49]

IMMUNOSEROLOGIC AND SEROLOGIC IDENTIFICATION

IMMUNOSEROLOGIC IDENTIFICATION

In 1980 Essers and co-workers[31] described a latex agglutination test for the identification of *Staphylococcus aureus*.[31] The latex particles were coated with human plasma. This reagent contained fibrinogen and IgG and reacted with both the clumping factor and protein A of *S. aureus*. The absence of these two constituents in *S. epidermidis* resulted in a negative reaction with this species. A commercially available modification of this test, the Sero STAT (Scott Laboratories, Inc., Fiskeville, R.I.), can also be used to identify *S. aureus*. The Sero STAT is reportedly as accurate as the tube coagulase test and requires less than 30 seconds to perform.[28] This test is especially useful for the direct identification of *S. aureus* in radiometric blood cultures because it becomes positive before other criteria (that is, the radiometric growth index or the Gram stain of uncentrifuged culture fluid).[29] Other latex agglutination tests include the Staphylatex (Microscan–Baxter Travenol, Sacramento, Calif.) and Accu-Staph (Scarborough Microbiologicals, Inc., Stone Mountain, Ga.).

The Staphyloslide test (BBL Microbiology Systems, Cockeysville, Md.) is a rapid hemagglutination test used for the detection of *S. aureus* on the basis of its clumping factor binding to fibrinogen. Sheep red blood cells sensitized with fibrinogen are mixed with suspect organisms. A positive test is indicated by the clumping of erythrocytes within 15 seconds.

DETECTION OF TEICHOIC ACID ANTIBODIES

Detection of rising or elevated antibodies to teichoic acids can be used to rapidly diagnose *S. aureus* endocarditis[23,120] and to distinguish complicated and uncomplicated *S. aureus* bacteremia.[121] Teichoic acids are major cell wall components of staphylococci and other gram-positive bacteria. Teichoic acids vary in structure depending on the organism. The teichoic acids of *S. aureus* consist of repeating units of ribitol phosphate with *N*-acetyl glucosamine in either alpha- or beta-glycosidic linkage. Antibody detection assays include gel diffusion,[130] counterimmunoelectrophoresis (CIE), radioimmunoassay (RIA),[129,131] and ELISA.[43] Several technical modifications have been suggested to improve the standardization of the gel diffusion and CIE methods and to decrease the variability of results observed among laboratories.[106,129] The introduction of a commercial CIE kit may also reduce the variability reported with these assays.[128]

SEROLOGIC TYPING

In 1937 Cowan divided strains of *S. aureus* into three serologic types, designated Cowan I, II, and III. Since that time numerous serotyping methods have been developed. Although serotyping is of some epidemiologic value, it is rarely used today because of the difficulties in producing specific antisera and the lack of standardization of the method.[37] The systems of *S. aureus* serotyping currently in use include the Cowan-Mer-

TABLE 12-2. Typical Characteristics of Human Coagulase-Negative *Staphylococcus* Spp.

Characteristic	*S. epidermidis*	*S. hominis*	*S. haemolyticus*	*S. warneri*	*S. capitis*	*S. saccharolyticus*	*S. auricularis*	*S. saprophyticus*	*S. cohnii*	*S. xylosus*	*S. simulans*
Colony size[a]	S/M	S/M	M/L	S/M	S	S	VS	M/L	M/L	M/L	L
Pigment	−	+/−	−/+	+/−	−	−	−	+/−	−/+	+/−	−
Anaerobic growth	+	−/±	±/+	+	+/±	+	±/−	+/±	±/+	+/±	+
Aerobic growth	+	+	+	+	+	−	+	+	+	+	+
Nitrate reduction	+/±	+/±	+/−	−/+	+/−	+	±/−	−	−	+/−	+
Alkaline phosphatase	+	−	−	−	−	+/−	−	−	−/±	+/−	±/−
Arginine utilization[b]	+	−/±	+	−/+	+/−	ND	+/−	−	−	−	+
Urease[b]	+	+	−	+	−	ND	−	+	−/±	+	+
Hemolysis	−/±	−/±	+/±	−/±	−/±	−	−	−	−/±	−/±	±/−
Novobiocin resistance	−	−	−	−	−	−	−	+	+	+	−

> **SYMBOLS:** S, Small, 2 to 4 mm
> M, Medium, 5 to 6 mm
> L, Large, >7 mm
> VS, Very small and slow growing, 1 to 2 mm
> −, Negative reactions
> +, Positive reactions
> ±, Weak reactions
> ND, Not determined

Reprinted by permission of the publisher from ''Coagulase-negative staphylococci'' by Wesley E. Kloos, which appeared in Clinical Microbiology Newsletter, Vol. 4, pp. 75-79. Copyright 1982 by Elsevier Science Publishing Co., Inc.
[a]Colony diameter is determined after incubation of P agar at 35° C for 3 days and room temperature for additional 2 days.[65]
[b]Characters determined to be useful, as originally indicated in API Staph Trac and API Staph-Ident Staphylococcal systems, and easily adapted to commercially available media.

cier-Pillet system, which recognizes thermolabile structures on the cell surface, and the Oeding-Haukenes system, which combines the recognition of thermolabile and thermostable surface antigens by using specific antisera for given antigens (that is, factor sera).

Some progress has been made toward the use of serotyping in identifying CNS.[91,118] Only a few different sera have been evaluated for the typing of strains within a species, such as *S. epidermidis*.

EPIDEMIOLOGIC TYPING SYSTEMS
BACTERIOPHAGE TYPING

Bacteriophage typing can be used for epidemiologic investigation of infections resulting from *S. aureus*. The procedure is based on the sensitivity of this organism to bacteriophages, which are viruses capable of infecting and lysing certain bacteria. A set of internationally standardized phages is used in typing. The basic phage typing procedure is performed by first inoculating an agar plate with sufficient bacterial culture to give a lawn of confluent growth.[111,125] A predetermined routine test dilution (RTD) of each phage is then placed at a designated position on the agar plate; a template can be used to mark this placement. The plates are incubated overnight at 30° C, and the degree of lysis or the number of plaques produced by each phage is read semiquantitatively. The phages to which the organisms are strongly susceptible are recorded as the bacteriophage type. The relationships between different isolates of a common outbreak are established on the similarity of these types.

Since phage typing is not of diagnostic or therapeutic importance, it is not recommended as a routine laboratory procedure.[112] Isolates for phage typing should be referred to the state public health laboratories or the Centers for Disease Control.

Although phage typing sets have also been developed for *S. epidermidis*, they offer little practical value at present.

ADDITIONAL TYPING SYSTEMS

Antibiograms can be used epidemiologically, especially when considering strains within a confined area rather than on a larger geographic scale.[65] The emergence of a *Staphylococcus*

TABLE 12-3. Biochemical Activity of Human Coagulase-Negative *Staphylococcus* Spp.: Carbohydrates

Acid Source[a]	*S. epidermidis*	*S. hominis*	*S. haemolyticus*	*S. warneri*	*S. capitis*	*S. saccharolyticus*	*S. auricularis*	*S. saprophyticus*	*S. cohnii*	*S. xylosus*	*S. simulans*
Maltose	+	+	+	+/±	−	−	+/−	+	±/+	+/±	−/±
Trehalose	−	+/−	+	+	−	−	+/±	+/−	+	+	+/−
Mannitol	−	−/+	+/−	+/−	+	−	−	+/−	+/±	+/±	+/±
Xylose	−	−	−	−	−	−	−	−	−	+	−
Cellobiose	−	−	−	−	−	−	−	−	−	−	−
Sucrose	+	+	+	+	+/−	−	−/+	+	−	+	+
Xylitol	−	−	−	−	−	−	−	+/−	−/±	−/±	−
Mannose	+/±	−/+	−	−	+/±	±/+	−/+	−	+/±	+/±	+/−

> **SYMBOLS:** +, Positive reactions
> −, Negative reactions
> ±, Weak reactions

Reprinted by permission of the publisher from "Coagulase-negative staphylococci" by Wesley E. Kloos, which appeared in Clinical Microbiology Newsletter, Vol. 4, pp. 75-79. Copyright 1982 by Elsevier Science Publishing Co., Inc.
[a]Acids produced aerobically. Methods are outlined in simplified scheme of Kloos and Schleifer.[68]

strain with a unique antimicrobial susceptibility pattern can be a valuable signal to the clinical microbiologist and can provide a marker by which similar strains can be detected. Antibiograms in combination with other character analyses, such as plasmid composition, biochemical characters, colony morphologic characters, and phage typing, can identify most strains of staphylococci.[9,20,63,64,88] The accuracy of strain identification is highest when systems incorporate two or more criteria, such as those listed in the previous sections, and when isolates are taken from a single patient or group of patients from a single hospital or facility. Certain unusual strains have some variation with respect to characters used in strain identification. Some of this variation is explained on the basis of a high gene mutation rate, plasmid acquisition or loss, or transposon activity.[63]

CLINICAL SIGNIFICANCE
STAPHYLOCOCCUS AUREUS[109]

S. aureus can cause local infections of the skin, eye, nose and throat, urethra, vagina, and gastrointestinal tract. Local skin infections are by far the most common of these, and in fact are probably the most common of all bacterial infections.

Folliculitis is the most superficial skin infection. This condition follows the infection of a hair follicle and is manifested by minute erythematous nodules around the follicle. The surrounding skin and deeper tissues are not affected. If folliculitis spreads to involve the subcutaneous tissue, the lesion is called a furuncle or boil. Furuncles are characterized by the presence of pus.

More serious invasive staphylococcal conditions rarely occur in healthy individuals but can occur in individuals whose host defenses have been compromised. Predisposing conditions include injury to normal skin (for instance, traumatic wounds, burns, and surgical incisions), prior viral infections (for instance, measles and influenza), leukocyte defects, deficiencies in humoral immunity, presence of foreign bodies (for instance, sutures, pacemakers, and intravenous catheters), alteration of normal flora by use of antimicrobial agents to which *S. aureus* is not susceptible, and presence of miscellaneous illnesses (including diabetes mellitus, alcoholism, coronary artery disease, and various malignant tumors).

The presence of these conditions can lead to serious local or contiguous infections, such as sinusitis, mastitis, and carbuncles (a series of furuncles or large, indurated, and painful lesions with multiple ineffective drainage sites) (Figure 12-3). They may also result in invasion of the bloodstream. From the blood the organisms can spread to numerous body sites. Metastatic infection of the lung can lead to pneumonia, infection of the bone to osteomyelitis and arthritis, infection of the heart to endocarditis and myocarditis, and infection of the central nervous system to brain abscesses or rarely meningitis.

The staphylococcal infections considered up to this point are classified as invasive. *S. aureus* is also responsible for three toxigenic diseases: food poisoning, scalded skin syndrome, and toxic shock syndrome. Toxic shock syndrome is discussed in Chapter 10.

Staphylococcal food poisoning follows the ingestion of preformed enterotoxin.[1] Sufficient enterotoxin to cause disease can be produced in food that has been contaminated with enterotoxin-producing staphylococci by a food handler and then left at 28° C or higher for 2 to 4 hours. Commonly incriminated foods include those containing mayonnaise, custards and cream-filled pastries, cheeses, ham, and processed meats.

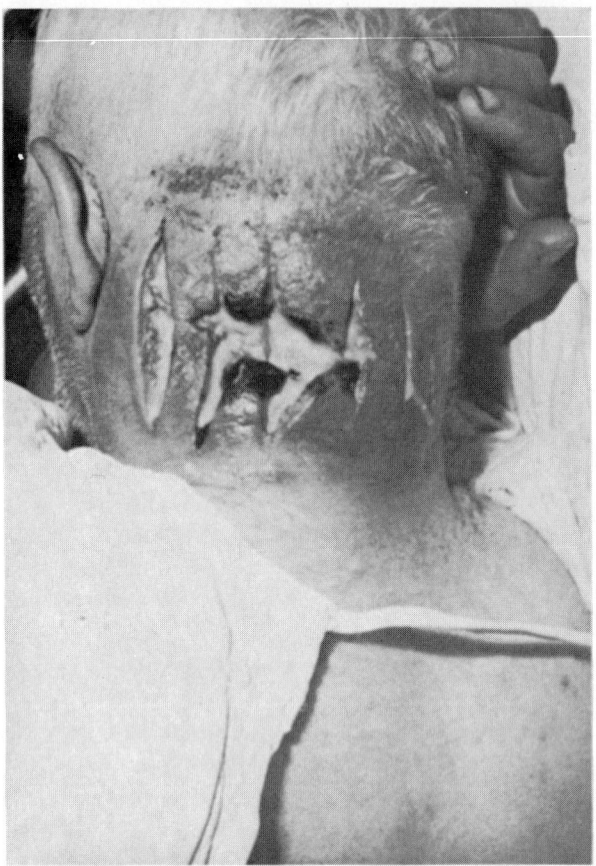

FIGURE 12-3. Carbuncle caused by *Staphylococcus aureus* in diabetic patient admitted to hospital in coma. (From Wehrle, P.F., and Top, F.H.: Communicable and infectious diseases, ed. 9, St. Louis, 1981, The C.V. Mosby Co.)

The characteristic symptoms of staphylococcal food poisoning—nausea, vomiting, abdominal cramps, and frequently watery diarrhea—appear within 2 to 6 hours of consumption of the enterotoxin. The condition is usually self-limited and subsides within 24 hours. The short incubation period and lack of fever distinguish staphylococcal food poisoning from food poisoning resulting from clostridia and salmonellae.

Scalded skin syndrome (SSS) consists of three separate entities, toxic epidermal necrolysis, scarlatiniform erythema, and bullous impetigo, which appear to form a spectrum of disease.[30,85] All three conditions are attributed to the actions of the exfoliatin toxin. Toxic epidermal necrolysis (TEN), also known as generalized exfoliative disease, appears in children under 5 years of age. This condition initially appears as a diffuse generalized erythroderma following conjunctivitis or an upper respiratory tract infection. Shortly thereafter, large flaccid bullae are formed under the epidermis. When the bullae rupture, large sheets of epidermis separate and peel off to reveal the moist, red, "scalded" dermis (Plate 6, *A*). Because staphylococci cannot be recovered from the bullae, it is generally assumed that TEN is caused by exfoliatin that is produced at another site of infection.

Scarlatiniform erythema represents an abortive form of TEN. A generalized scarlatiniform rash resembling the initial erythroderma of TEN is followed by the development of deep cracks and fissures around the eyes and mouth. This leads to a flaky desquamation that ultimately involves the entire skin surface.

Bullous impetigo, a disease of children, is the local form of SSS. This condition is characterized by localized lesions of flaccid bullae that appear on otherwise normal-looking skin. The bullae are filled with staphylococci and polymorphonuclear leukocytes. After the bullae rupture, a thin crust forms over the area.

COAGULASE-NEGATIVE STAPHYLOCOCCI

Most infections resulting from coagulase-negative staphylococci (CNS) are opportunistic in nature. Alteration of the normal integrity of the skin by manipulations, such as implantation of various prostheses and prolonged surgical procedures and trauma, allows these normally commensal organisms to enter the body.[35] CNS are commonly associated with infections of cerebrospinal fluid (CSF) shunts,[38,53] prosthetic heart valves,[51,77,133] prosthetic joints,[55,134] cardiac pacemaker leads and power packs,[81,90] and intravascular catheters.[79,89,107] These organisms are also associated with native infectious endocarditis,[13,39] osteomyelitis,[80] mastitis,[117] continuous ambulatory peritoneal dialysis (CAPD) peritonitis,[42,44] septicemia,[5,92,135] and infections of wounds[87,105] and the urinary tract.[41,57,58,82,87]

The widespread use of vascular and peritoneal access routes and prosthetic devices in modern medicine has resulted in a dramatic increase in the medical importance of *S. epidermidis*. This species is responsible for about 1% to 10% of native heart valve endocarditis and greater than 40% of prosthetic heart valve endocarditis (PVE). During the 1970s, approximately

25% of PVE cases were due to *S. epidermidis*,[25,60] but during the 1980s the rate has increased to between 48% and 80%, depending on the hospital involved.[84,94] The mortality of patients with this infection is high, between 63% and 74%.[84,95]

In experimental endocarditis using a rat model, Baddour and co-workers[11] demonstrated that *S. epidermidis* was considerably more virulent than *S. hominis* in producing endocarditis, colonizing intracardiac catheters, and causing bacteremia. Strains of *S. epidermidis* were significantly more resistant to phagocytic killing in vitro than strains of *S. hominis*. These results affirm the biologic significance of identifying specific CNS in certain infections.

Whereas *S. epidermidis* is by far the major CNS associated with PVE, other CNS (for example, *S. warneri* and *S. haemolyticus*) might account for up to 50% of cases of native heart valve endocarditis.[17]

S. epidermidis is also responsible for 60% to 95% of infections involving CSF shunts and is second only to *S. aureus* as a cause of sepsis after total hip replacement.[21,38,133] CSF shunts and artificial joints, like prosthetic heart valves, are foreign devices regularly infected by CNS. As early as 1969, Holt[52] described the colonization and infection of CSF by *S. epidermidis,* foretelling the potential pathogenicity of this species.

S. epidermidis bacteremias are a growing concern for patients receiving immunosuppressive therapy[135] and in neonatal intensive care units, accounting for 75%, and perhaps as high as 92%, of cases in neonatal intensive care units.[5,36]

S. epidermidis peritonitis as a major complication of CAPD, though usually not severe, can be persistent and remains a therapeutic challenge.[42] This species may account for 30% to 40% of episodes.

As previously mentioned, *S. saprophyticus* is an important pathogen in urinary tract infections, especially in nonhospitalized women aged 16 to 25 years.[41,58,108,123] In fact, it is the second most common cause of urinary tract infection in these patients.[58] *S. epidermidis* also is associated with urinary tract infections.[86,87] Interestingly, infection is not commonly seen in hospitalized women or in men.[123]

Other CNS appear to have less pathogenic potential than the previously mentioned species. *S. haemolyticus,* in addition to causing native endocarditis, is occasionally associated with wound, bone, and joint infections.[83,87,105] *S. hominis* has been associated with wound infections[87,105] and septicemia in patients with cancer.[16] *S. simulans* has been associated with wound infections,[87,105] chronic osteomyelitis and pyarthrosis,[80] and mastitis.[124] *S. xylosus* was considered to be the etiologic agent in a patient with pyelonephritis.[119]

MECHANISMS OF PATHOGENICITY

Proposed mechanisms of pathogenicity of staphylococci include encapsulation, toxin and enzyme production, colonization of specific host sites, and slime production.

ENCAPSULATION

The presence of a capsule in certain strains of *S. aureus* is thought to inhibit phagocytosis through the mechanisms discussed in Chapter 2.

TOXINS

Toxins are produced primarily by *S. aureus*. They include hemolysins, leukocidin, enterotoxin, and exfoliatin.

Hemolysins

There are four distinct hemolysins: alpha, beta, gamma, and delta.[56,136] All of these are capable of lysing red blood cells (RBCs), but they differ in their species specificity (Table 12-4). With the exception of beta-hemolysin, they also lyse the white blood cells of humans and other animals. Their numerous other biologic activities are summarized in Table 12-4.

The mechanism of hemolytic activity is conclusively determined for only the beta-hemolysin. In the presence of magnesium, this toxin hydrolyzes the sphingomyelin of the RBC membrane to phosphorylcholine and *N*-acylsphingosine. The sphingomyelin content of the erythrocyte is correlated with the degree of sensitivity to the toxin. Beta-hemolysin is also known as the hot-cold lysin because its hemolytic activity is increased if incubation at 37° C is followed by incubation at 4° C or at room temperature.

The exact participation of the hemolysins in the production or development of staphylococcal disease is not known. The impressive array of biologic activities, especially in the case of alpha-toxin, certainly suggests a pathogenic role. Alpha-toxin's primary significance may be in producing tissue damage once the focus of infection is established.[7]

Leukocidin

The leukocidin of *S. aureus* is termed the Panton-Valentine leukocidin. This toxin is capable of lysing human and rabbit polymorphonuclear leukocytes and macrophages. Its lytic effects are attributed to an alteration of the sodium-potassium pump, leading to a series of secondary events, including increased permeability to cations, secretion of protein, and accumulation of calcium.[137] The role of leukocidin in staphylococcal pathogenicity remains unknown, although it has been suggested that it inhibits phagocytosis.

Enterotoxins

The enterotoxins and the exfoliatin are pathologically significant in staphylococcal disease. *S. aureus* can produce five distinct enterotoxins, which are designated A through E. Toxins A and D are most commonly associated with food poisoning. However, the mechanisms that permit the effects of enterotoxin have not been resolved.[14] As discussed in Chapter 10, a toxin designated enterotoxin F, pyrogenic exotoxin C, or TSST-1 has been associated with toxic shock syndrome (TSS).[3,15]

Exfoliatin

This toxin, also known as epidermolytic or exfoliative toxin, is responsible for SSS. It cleaves the stratum granulosum layer of the epidermis by splitting the desmosomes that link the cells of this layer. Exfoliatin is produced by *S. aureus* from phage group II.[71] The production of exfoliatin can be both plasmid and chromosomally mediated.[96]

ENZYMES

Among the numerous staphylococcal enzymes are coagulase, lipase, staphylokinase, gelatinase, and phosphatase. With the exception of coagulase, these enzymes are produced in both coagulase-positive and coagulase-negative staphylococci.

Coagulase may contribute to pathogenicity by inhibiting the bactericidal activity of normal serum and by inhibiting phagocytosis through deposition of fibrin on the bacterial cell wall, although this is not known for certain. The lipase enzyme

TABLE 12-4. Hemolysins of *Staphylococcus aureus*[56,136]

Hemolysin	Susceptible Erythrocytes and Leukocytes	Associated Toxicity in Animal and Human Models
Alpha	Rabbit, sheep, and calf erythrocytes susceptible, and rabbit and human leukocytes susceptible	Possesses hemolytic, lethal, and dermonecrotic activities; hemolyzes red blood cells; lyses human macrophages; cytotoxic for large variety of tissue culture cells; degranulates human and rabbit platelets; lethal for mammals and cold-blooded animals; induces circulatory effects and renal cortical necrosis in animals
Beta	Sheep, human, ox erythrocytes susceptible; no susceptible leukocytes	Toxicity controversial with conflicting reports; reported cytotoxic for HeLa cells, human fibroblasts, and human thrombocytes but also reported nontoxic for variety of cultured cells, including HeLa, chick fibroblast, human, bovine, monkey, kidney tissue, and other cells
Delta	Human, rabbit, horse, sheep, rat, and guinea pig erythrocytes susceptible; rabbit, guinea pig, human, and mouse leukocytes susceptible	Cytopathic for large variety of cultured cells; disrupts bacterial protoplasts, lysosomes, and spheroplasts; displays lethal and dermonecrotic effects in certain animals
Gamma	Human, rabbit, horse, sheep, rat, and guinea pig erythrocytes susceptible; rabbit, guinea pig, human, and mouse leukocytes susceptible	Cytopathic for tissue culture cells; causes edema and induration in rabbits and guinea pigs

hydrolyzes lipid. This ability might allow the staphylococci to colonize the sebaceous sites of the skin. The importance of the other proteolytic enzymes appears to be the degradation of host tissue and products, which provides the staphylococci with substrate for growth.[18]

COLONIZATION OF SPECIFIC HOST SITES

S. saprophyticus possesses surface properties that allow it to adhere readily to urogenital cells.[22] This characteristic may play a role in its ability to cause urinary tract infections, although the pathogenic properties of this organism have not yet been adequately assessed.[6] *S. aureus* and *S. epidermidis* demonstrate a selective adherence to nasal epithelial (mucosal) cells.[4] The adherence of *S. aureus* is significantly greater for carriers of this species than for noncarriers.

SLIME PRODUCTION

It has been suggested that the production of slime by staphylococci probably aids in the adherence and accumulation of these organisms on the smooth surfaces of medical devices.[19]

ANTIMICROBIAL SUSCEPTIBILITY

Until the emergence of penicillin-resistant strains, penicillin was considered the drug of choice for *S. aureus* infections. It is now known that approximately 85% of *S. aureus* isolates are resistant to penicillin G. Resistance to penicillin is mediated by the production of the enzyme penicillinase, a beta-lactamase

that inactivates the antibiotic before it has caused irreversible changes in the bacterial cells (see Chapter 8).[97] The ability to produce penicillinase is usually determined by the presence of a plasmid.

Methicillin and other beta-lactamase-resistant penicillins are used to treat the penicillin-resistant *S. aureus*. However, over the past several years increasing numbers of isolates that are resistant to these beta-lactamase-resistant antibiotics have appeared. These isolates are referred to as methicillin-resistant *S. aureus* (MRSA). In 1980, 4.9% of all *S. aureus* isolates from nosocomial infections were methicillin resistant.[127] The MRSA are actually resistant to all beta-lactam antibiotics, including the third-generation cephalosporins. Furthermore, they are usually resistant to streptomycin, tetracycline, and sulfonamides. Methicillin resistance usually is chromosomally mediated.[97] Resistance to methicillin does not depend directly on the action of beta-lactamases but appears to be an intrinsic property of the cell wall. As discussed in Chapter 8, methicillin resistance may be due to altered penicillin-binding proteins.[50,122]

MRSA have been reported in both hospital- and community-acquired infections. Large nosocomial outbreaks have occurred primarily in the large tertiary referral hospitals affiliated with medical schools.[47] It appears that the organisms are introduced into the hospital through transferral of infected patients or on the hands of house staff physicians traveling between hospitals. Community-acquired MRSA infections have occurred primarily among drug addicts.[78,98]

Vancomycin is currently a major drug of choice for MRSA.[113] In fact, in hospitals that have a significant number of MRSA noscomial infections, the initial empirical therapy of serious staphylococcal infections should include vancomycin; therapy should be changed only after susceptibility tests indicate sensitivity to a beta-lactamase-resistant penicillin.[126]

The phenomenom of *S. aureus* tolerance to penicillin and cephalosporins is discussed in Chapter 8.

The major CNS are generally more resistant to antimicrobial agents than is *S. aureus*.[57] Studies of CNS from a variety of sources show that 26% to 74% are resistant to penicillin, and in certain populations up to 67% may be resistant to methicillin.[40,83] Many methicillin-resistant CNS are also resistant to penicillin, sulfamethoxazole, streptomycin, erythromycin, and tetracyclines.[8,132] A recent study of isolates of *S. epidermidis* associated with infective valve endocarditis revealed 79% to be methicillin resistant.[59] Detection of methicillin resistance is discussed in Chapter 8. Karchmer, Archer, and Dismukes[59] suggest that rifampin be used in conjunction with vancomycin to treat prosthetic valve endocarditis caused by methicillin-resistant *S. epidermidis*.

S. epidermidis, *S. hominis*, *S. haemolyticus*, and *S. warneri* are species producing the most multiply-antibiotic-resistant strains, especially in patients receiving prolonged therapy with penicillin, tetracycline, or erythromycin.[63,64] Continued therapy (for instance, in the treatment of acne) results in the accumulation of nearly 100% resistant strains, the majority of which are multiply resistant for penicillin, tetracycline, and erythromycin, in double or triple combinations, even though only one of the antimicrobial agents is administered.

Because of the wide spectrum of resistance to both coagulase-positive and coagulase-negative staphylococci, it is important that proper antimicrobial susceptibility testing be performed on any isolate presumed to be the cause of infection.

REFERENCES

1. Abeyounis, C.J.: *Staphylococcus*. In Milgrom, F., and Flanagan, T.D., editors: Medical microbiology, New York, 1982, Churchill Livingstone.
2. Acar, J.F., Goldstein, F.W., and LaGrange, P.: Human infections caused by thiamine or menadione-requiring *Staphylococcus aureus*, J. Clin. Microbiol. **8**:142, 1978.
3. Altemeier, W.A., et al.: *Staphylococcus aureus* associated with toxic shock syndrome: phage typing and toxin capability testing, Ann. Intern. Med. **96**:978, 1982.
4. Aly, R., Shinefield, H.R., and Maibach, H.I.: *Staphylococcus aureus* adherence to nasal epithelial cells: studies of some parameters. In Maibach, H.I., and Aly, R., editors: Skin microbiology: relevance to clinical infection, New York, 1981, Springer-Verlag.
5. Anday, E.K., and Talbot, G.H.: Coagulase-negative *Staphylococcus* bacteremia—a rising threat in the newborn infant, Ann. Clin. Lab. Sci. **15**:246, 1985.
6. Anderson, J.D., et al.: Urinary tract infections due to *Staphylococcus saprophyticus* biotype 3, Can. Med. Assoc. J. **124**:415, 1981.
7. Arbuthnott, J.P.: Staphylococcal toxins. In Schlessinger, D., editor: Microbiology—1975. Washington, D.C., 1975, American Society for Microbiology.
8. Archer, G.L.: Antimicrobial susceptibilities and selection of resistance among *Staphylococcus epidermidis* isolates recovered from patients with infections of indwelling foreign devices, Antimicrob. Agents Chemother. **14**:353, 1978.
9. Archer, G.L., et al.: Plasmid-pattern analysis for the differentiation of infecting from noninfecting *Staphylococcus epidermidis*, J. Infect. Dis. **149**:913, 1984.
10. Ayers, L.W.: Staphylococci, ASCP teleconferences, Chicago, 1983, American Society of Clinical Pathologists.
11. Baddour, L.M., et al.: Production of experimental endocarditis by coagulase-negative staphylococci: variability in species virulence, J. Infect. Dis. **150**:721, 1984.
12. Bayliss, B.G., and Hall, E.R.: Plasma coagulation by organisms other than *Staphylococcus aureus*, J. Bacteriol. **89**:101, 1965.
13. Bayliss, R., et al.: The microbiology and pathogenesis of infective endocarditis, Br. Heart J. **50**:513, 1983.
14. Bergdoll, M.S.: The enterotoxins. In Cohen, J.O., editor: The staphylococci, New York, 1972, John Wiley & Sons, Inc.
15. Bergdoll, M.S., et al.: An enterotoxin-like protein in *Staphylococcus aureus* strains from patients with toxic shock syndrome, Ann. Intern. Med. **96**:969, 1982.
16. Bowman, R.A., and Buck, M.: *Staphylococcus hominis* septicaemia in patients with cancer, Med. J. Aust. **140**:26, 1984.
17. Caputo, G.M., et al.: Native valve endocarditis due to coagulase-negative staphylococci, Abstracts of the Twenty-fifth Interscience Conference on Antimicrobial Agents and Chemotherapy, No. 898, 1985.
18. Chesbro, W.R., Wamola, I., and Bartley, C.H.: Correlation of virulence with growth rate in *Staphylococcus aureus*, Can. J. Microbiol. **15**:723, 1969.
19. Christensen, G.D., et al.: Adherence of slime-producing strains of *Staphylococcus epidermidis* to smooth surfaces, Infect. Immun. **37**:318, 1982.
20. Christensen, G.D., et al.: Characterization of clinically significant strains of coagulase-negative staphylococci, J. Clin. Microbiol. **18**:258, 1983.
21. Coagulase-negative staphylococci, Lancet **1**:139, 1981.
22. Colleen, S., et al.: Surface properties of *Staphylococcus saprophyticus* and *Staphylococcus epidermidis* as studied by adherence tests and two-polymer, aqueous phase systems, Acta Pathol. Microbiol. Scand. **87B**:321, 1979.
23. Crowder, J.G., and White, A.: Teichoic acid antibodies in staphylococcal and nonstaphylococcal endocarditis, Ann. Intern. Med. **77**:87, 1972.
24. Dan, M., Marien, G.J.R., and Goldsand, G.: Endocarditis caused by *Staphylococcus warneri* on a normal aortic valve following vasectomy, Can. Med. Assoc. J. **131**:211, 1984.
25. Delgado, D.G., and Cobbs, C.G.: Infection of prosthetic valves and intravascular devices. In Mandell, G.L., Douglas, R.G., and Bennett, J.E., editors: Principles and practice of infectious diseases, New York, 1979, John Wiley & Sons, Inc.
26. Devriese, L.A., et al.: *Staphylococcus hyicus* (Sompolinsky 1953) comb. nov. and *Staphylococcus hyicus* subsp. *chromogenes* subsp. nov., Int. J. Syst. Bacteriol. **28**:482, 1978.
27. Devriese, L.A., et al.: *Staphylococcus gallinarum* and *Staphylococcus caprae*, two new species from animals, Int. J. Syst. Bacteriol. **33**:480, 1983.
28. Doern, G.V.: Evaluation of a commercial latex agglutination test for identification of *Staphylococcus aureus*, J. Clin. Microbiol. **15**:416, 1982.
29. Doern, G.V., and Robbie, L.I.: Direct identification of *Staphylococcus aureus* in blood culture fluid with a commercial latex agglutination test, J. Clin. Microbiol. **16**:1048, 1982.
30. Elias, P.M., Fritsch, P., and Epstein, Jr., E.H.: Staphylococcal scalded skin syndrome, Arch. Dermatol. **113**:207, 1977.
31. Essers, L., and Radebold, K.: Rapid and reliable identification of *Staphylococcus aureus* by a latex agglutination test, J. Clin. Microbiol. **12**:641, 1980.
32. Evans, C.A., and Mattern, K.L.: Individual differences in the bacterial flora of the skin of the forehead: *Peptococcus saccharolyticus*, J. Invest. Dermatol. **71**:152, 1978.
33. Falk, D., and Guering, S.J.: Differentiation of *Staphylococcus* and *Micrococcus* spp. with the Taxo A bacitracin disk, J. Clin. Microbiol. **18**:719, 1983.

34. Faller, A., and Schleifer, K.H.: Modified oxidase and benzidine tests for separation of staphylococci from micrococci, J. Clin. Microbiol. **13**:1031, 1981.

35. Fleer, A., and Verhoef, J.: New aspects of staphylococcal infections: emergence of coagulase-negative staphylococci as pathogens, Antonie van Leeuwenhoek **50**:729, 1984.

36. Fleer, A., et al.: Septicemia due to coagulase-negative staphylococci in a neonatal intensive care unit: clinical and bacteriological features and contaminated parenteral fluids as a source of sepsis, Pediatr. Infect. Dis. **2**:426, 1983.

37. Fleurette, J., and Modjadedy, A.: Attempts to combine and simplify two methods for serotyping of *Staphylococcus aureus.* In Jeljaszewicz, J., editor: Staphylococci and staphylococcal diseases, Stuttgart, 1976, Fischer Verlag.

38. Frame, P.T., and McLaurin, R.L.: Treatment of CSF shunt infections with intrashunt plus oral antibiotic therapy, J. Neurosurg. **60**:354, 1984.

39. Garvey, G.J., and Neu, H.C.: Infective endocarditis: an evolving disease; a review of endocarditis at the Columbia-Presbyterian Medical Center, 1968–1973, Medicine **57**:105, 1978.

40. Gemmell, C.G., and Dawson, J.E.: Identification of coagulase-negative staphylococci with the API Staph system, J. Clin. Microbiol. **16**:847, 1982.

41. Gillespie, W.A., et al.: Urinary tract infection in young women with special reference to *Staphylococcus saprophyticus*, J. Clin. Pathol. **31**:348, 1978.

42. Gokal, R., et al.: Peritonitis in continuous ambulatory peritoneal dialysis, Lancet **2**:1388, 1982.

43. Granström, M., et al.: Enzyme-linked immunosorbent assay for antibodies against teichoic acid in patients with staphylococcal infections, J. Clin. Microbiol. **17**:640, 1983.

44. Grefberg, N., Danielson, B.G., and Nilsson, P.: Peritonitis in patients on continuous ambulatory peritoneal dialysis—a changing scene, Scand. J. Infect. Dis. **16**:187, 1984.

45. Gunn, B.A., et al.: Comparison of methods for identifying *Staphylococcus* and *Micrococcus* spp., J. Clin. Microbiol. **14**:195, 1981.

46. Hájek, V.: *Staphylococcus intermedius*, a new species isolated from animals, Int. J. Syst. Bacteriol. **26**:401, 1976.

47. Haley, R.W., et al.: The emergence of methicillin-resistant *Staphylococcus aureus* infections in United States hospitals, Ann. Intern. Med. **97**:297, 1982.

48. Hamilton-Miller, J.M.T., and Iliffe, A.: Antimicrobial resistance in coagulase-negative staphylococci, J. Med. Microbiol. **19**:217, 1985.

49. Harrington, B.J., and Gaydos, J.M.: Five-hour novobiocin test for differentiation of coagulase-negative staphylococci, J. Clin. Microbiol. **19**:279, 1984.

50. Hartman, B., and Tomasz, A.: Altered penicillin-binding proteins in methicillin-resistant strains of *Staphylococcus aureus*, Antimicrob. Agents Chemother. **19**:726, 1981.

51. Hedström, S.A., and Kronvall, G., editors: Symposium on staphylococcal septicaemia and endocarditis, Scand. J. Infect. Dis., Suppl. 41, 1983.

52. Holt, R.J.: The classification of staphylococci from colonized ventriculo-atrial shunts, J. Clin. Pathol. **22**:475, 1969.

53. Holt, R.J.: The colonization of ventriculo-atrial shunts by coagulase-negative staphylococci. In Finland, M., Marget, W., and Bartmann, K., editors: Bacterial infections: changes in their causative agents, trends, and possible basis, Berlin, 1971, Springer-Verlag.

54. Hovelius, B., and Mårdh, P.: On the diagnosis of coagulase-negative staphylococci with emphasis on *Staphylococcus saprophyticus*, Acta Pathol. Microbiol. Scand. **85B**:427, 1977.

55. Inman, R.D., et al.: Clinical and microbial features of prosthetic joint infection, Am. J. Med. **77**:47, 1984.

56. Jeljaszewicz, J.: Toxins (hemolysins). In Cohen, J.O., editor: The staphylococci, New York, 1972, John Wiley & Sons, Inc.

57. John, J.F., Jr., Gramling, P.K., and O'Dell, N.W.: Species identification of coagulase-negative staphylococci from urinary tract isolates, J. Clin. Microbiol. **8**:435, 1978.

58. Jordan, P.A., et al.: Urinary tract infection caused by *Staphylococcus saprophyticus*, J. Infect. Dis. **142**:510, 1980.

59. Karchmer, A.W., Archer, G.L., and Dismukes, W.E.: *Staphylococcus epidermidis* causing prosthetic valve endocarditis: microbiologic and clinical observations as guides to therapy, Ann. Intern. Med. **98**:447, 1983.

60. Karchmer, A.W., and Swartz, M.N.: Infective endocarditis in patients with prosthetic heart valves. In Kaplan, E.L., and Taranta, A.V., editors: Infective endocarditis: an American Heart Association symposium, Monograph 52, Dallas, 1977, American Heart Association.

61. Kloos, W.E.: Natural populations of the genus *Staphyloccus*, Annu. Rev. Microbiol. **34**:559, 1980.

62. Kloos, W.E.: Coagulase-negative staphylococci, Clin. Microbiol. Newsletter **4**:75, 1982.

63. Kloos, W.E.: Community structure of coagulase-negative staphylococci in humans. In Lieve, L., editor: Microbiology—1986, Washington, D.C., 1986, American Society for Microbiology.

64. Kloos, W.E.: Ecology of human skin. In Mårdh, P.A., and Schleifer, K.H., editors: Coagulase-negative staphylococci, Stockholm, 1986, Almquist & Wiksell International.

65. Kloos, W.E., and Jorgensen, J.H.: Staphylococci. In Lennette, E.H., et al, editors: Manual of clinical microbiology, ed. 4, Washington, D.C., 1985, American Society for Microbiology.

66. Kloos, W.E., and Musselwhite, M.S.: Distribution and persistence of *Staphylococcus* and *Micrococcus* and other aerobic bacteria of human skin, Appl. Microbiol. **30**:381, 1975.

67. Kloos, W.E., and Schleifer, K.H.: Isolation and characterization of staphylococci from human skin II—descriptions of four new species: *Staphylococcus warneri, Staphylococcus capitis, Staphylococcus hominis,* and *Staphylococcus simulans*, Int. J. Syst. Bacteriol. **25**:62, 1975.

68. Kloos, W.E., and Schleifer, K.H.: Simplified scheme for routine identification of human *Staphylococcus* species, J. Clin. Microbiol. **1**:82, 1975.

69. Kloos, W.E., and Schleifer, K.H.: *Staphylococcus auricularis* sp. nov.: an inhabitant of the human external ear, Int. J. Syst. Bacteriol. **33**:9, 1983.

70. Kloos, W.E., and Schleifer, K.H.: Genus IV—*Staphylococcus* Rosenbach 1884. In Sneath, P.H.A., Mair, N.S., and Sharpe, M.E., editors (Holt, J.G., editor-in-chief): Bergey's manual of systematic bacteriology, vol. 2, Baltimore, 1986, The Williams & Wilkins Co.

71. Kloos, W.E., Schleifer, K.H., and Noble, W.C.: Estimation of character parameters in coagulase-negative *Staphylococcus* species. In Jeljaszewicz, J., editor: Staphylococci and staphylococcal diseases, Stuttgart, 1976, Fischer Verlag.

72. Kloos, W.E., Schleifer, K.H., and Smith, R.F.: Characterization of *Staphylococcus sciuri* sp. nov. and its subspecies, Int. J. Syst. Bacteriol. **26**:22, 1976.

73. Kloos, W.E., Tornabene, T.G., and Schleifer, K.H.: Isolation and characterization of micrococci from human skin, including two new species: *Micrococcus lylae* and *Micrococcus kristinae*, Int. J. Syst. Bacteriol. **24**:79, 1974.

74. Kloos, W.E., and Wolfshohl, J.F.: Evidence for deoxyribonucleotide sequence divergence between staphylococci living on human and other primate skin, Curr. Microbiol. **3**:167, 1979.

75. Kloos, W.E., and Wolfshohl, J.F.: Identification of *Staphylococcus* species with the API STAPH-IDENT system, J. Clin. Microbiol. **16**:509, 1982.

76. Kloos, W.E., and Wolfshohl, J.F.: Deoxyribonucleotide sequence divergence between *Staphylococcus cohnii* subspecies populations living on primate skin, Curr. Microbiol. **8**:115, 1983.

77. Krayenbühl, H.P., and Rickards, A.F., editors: New aspects of bacterial endocarditis, Eur. Heart J. **5**(suppl. C), 1984.

78. Levine, D.P., et al: Community-acquired methicillin-resistant *Staphylococcus aureus* endocarditis in the Detroit Medical Center, Ann. Intern. Med. **97**:330, 1982.

79. Liekweg, W.G., and Greenfield, L.J.: Vascular prosthetic infections: collected experience and results of treatment, Surgery **81**:335, 1977.

80. Males, B.M., Bartholomew, W.R., and Amsterdam, D.: *Staphylococcus simulans* septicemia in a patient with chronic osteomyelitis and pyarthrosis, J. Clin. Microbiol. **21**:255, 1985.

81. Marrie, T.J., and Costerton, J.W.: Morphology of bacterial attachment to cardiac pacemaker leads and power packs, J. Clin. Microbiol. **19**:911, 1984.

82. Marrie, T.J., et al.: *Staphylococcus saprophyticus* as a cause of urinary tract infections, J. Clin. Microbiol. **16**:427, 1982.

83. Marsik, F.J., and Brake, S.: Species identification and susceptibility to 17 antibiotics of coagulase-negative staphylococci isolated from clinical specimens, J. Clin. Microbiol. **15**:640, 1982.

84. Masur, H., and Johnson, W.D., Jr.: Prosthetic valve endocarditis, J. Thorac. Cardiovasc. Surg. **80**:31, 1980.

85. Melish, M.E., et al.: The staphylococcal epidermolytic toxin. In Jeljaszewicz, J., editor: Staphylococci and staphylococcal diseases, Stuttgart, 1976, Fischer Verlag.

86. Nicolle, L.E., Hoban, S.A., and Harding, G.K.M.: Characterization of coagulase-negative staphylococci from urinary tract specimens, J. Clin. Microbiol. **17**:267, 1983.

87. Nord, C.E., et al.: Characterization of coagulase-negative staphylococcal species from human infections. In Jeljaszewicz, J., editor: Staphylococci and staphylococcal diseases, Stuttgart, 1976, Fischer Verlag.

88. Parisi, J.T.: Coagulase-negative staphylococci and the epidemiological typing of *Staphylococcus epidermidis*, Microbiol. Rev. **49**:126, 1985.

89. Peters, G., Locci, R., and Pulverer, G.: Adherence and growth of coagulase-negative staphylococci on surfaces of intravenous catheters, J. Infect. Dis. **146**:479, 1982.

90. Peters, G., et al.: Investigations on staphylococcal infection of transvenous endocardial pacemaker electrodes, Am. Heart J. **108**:359, 1984.

91. Pillet, J. and Orta, B.: Species and serotypes in coagulase-negative staphylococci. In Jeljaszewicz, J., editor: Staphylococci and staphylococcal infections, Stuttgart, 1981, Fischer Verlag.

92. Ponce DeLeon, S., and Wenzel, R.P.: Hospital-acquired bloodstream infections with *Staphylococcus epidermidis*, Am. J. Med. **77**:639, 1984.

93. Price, S.B., and Flournoy, D.J.: Comparison of antimicrobial susceptibility patterns among coagulase-negative staphylococci, Antimicrob. Agents Chemother. **21**:436, 1982.

94. Richardson, J.F., Marples, R.R., and de Saxe, M.J.: Characters of coagulase-negative staphylococci and micrococci from cases of endocarditis, J. Hosp. Infect. **5**:164, 1984.

95. Richardson, J.V., et al.: Treatment of infective endocarditis: a 10-year comparative analysis, Circulation **58**:589, 1978.

96. Rogolsky, M., Wiley, B.B., and Glasgow, L.A.: Phage group II staphylococcal strains with chromosomal and extrachromosomal genes for exfoliative toxin production, Infect. Immun. **13**:44, 1976.

97. Sabath, L.D.: Mechanisms of resistance to beta-lactam antibiotics in strains of *Staphylococcus aureus*, Ann. Intern. Med. **97**:339, 1982.

98. Saravolatz, L.D., et al.: Methicillin resistant *Staphylococcus aureus*, Ann. Intern. Med. **96**:11, 1982.

99. Schleifer, K.H.: Family I—*Micrococcaceae*. In Sneath, P.H.A., Mair, N.S., and Sharpe, M.E., editors (Holt, J.G., editor-in-chief): Bergey's manual of systematic bacteriology, vol. 2, Baltimore, 1986, The Williams & Wilkins Co.

100. Schleifer, K.H., and Fischer, U.: Description of a new species of the genus *Staphylococcus: Staphylococcus carnosus*, Int. J. Syst. Bacteriol. **32**:153, 1982.

101. Schleifer, K.H., Kilpper-Bälz, R., and Devriese, L.A.: *Staphylococcus arlettae* sp. nov., *S. equorum* sp. nov. and *S. kloosii* sp. nov.: three new coagulase-negative, novobiocin-resistant species from animals, Syst. Appl. Microbiol. **5**:501, 1984.

102. Schleifer, K.H., and Kloos, W.E.: Isolation and characterization of staphylococci from human skin. I. Amended descriptions of *Staphylococcus epidermidis* and *Staphylococcus saprophyticus* and descriptions of three new species: *Staphylococcus cohnii*, *Staphylococcus haemolyticus*, and *Staphylococcus xylosus*, Int. J. Syst. Bacteriol. **25**:50, 1975.

103. Schleifer, K.H., and Kloos, W.E.: Simple test system for the separation of staphylococci from micrococci, J. Clin. Microbiol. **1**:337, 1975.

104. Schleifer, K.H., et al.: Identification of "*Micrococcus candidus*" ATCC 14852 as a strain of *Staphylococcus epidermidis* and of "*Micrococcus caseolyticus*" ATCC 13548 and *Micrococcus varians* ATCC 29750 as members of a new species, *Staphylococcus caseolyticus*, Int. J. Syst. Bacteriol. **32**:15, 1982.

105. Sewell, C.M., et al.: Clinical significance of coagulase-negative staphylococci, J. Clin. Microbiol. **16**:236, 1982.

106. Sheagren, J.N., et al.: Technical aspects of the *Staphylococcus aureus* teichoic acid antibody assay: gel diffusion and counterimmunoelectrophoretic assays, antigen preparation, antigen selection, concentration effects, and cross-reactions with other organisms, J. Clin. Microbiol. **13**:293, 1981.

107. Sheth, N.K., et al.: Colonization of bacteria on polyvinyl chloride and Teflon intravascular catheters in hospitalized patients, J. Clin. Microbiol. **18**:1061, 1983.

108. Shrestha, T.L., and Darrell, J.H.: Urinary infection with coagulase-negative staphylococci in a teaching hospital, J. Clin. Pathol. **32**:299, 1979.

109. Shulman, J.A., and Nahmias, A.J.: Staphylococcal infections: clinical aspects. In Cohen, J.O., editor: The staphylococci, New York, 1972, John Wiley & Sons, Inc.

110. Slifkin, M., et al.: Characterization of CO_2 dependent microcolony variants of *Staphylococcus aureus*, Am. J. Clin. Pathol. **56**:584, 1971.

111. Smith, P.B.: Bacteriophage typing of *Staphylococcus aureus*. In Cohen, J.O., editor: The staphylococci, New York, 1972, John Wiley & Sons, Inc.

112. Smith, P.B.: Staphylococcal infections. In Balows, A., and Hausler, W.J., Jr., editors: Diagnostic procedures for bacterial, mycotic, and parasitic infections, Washington, D.C., 1981, American Public Health Association.

113. Sorrell, T.C., et al.: Vancomycin therapy for methicillin resistant *Staphylococcus aureus*, Ann. Intern. Med. **97**:344, 1982.

114. Spagna, V.A., et al.: Report of a case of bacterial sepsis caused by a naturally occurring variant form of *Staphylococcus aureus*, J. Infect. Dis. **138**:277, 1978.

115. Sperber, W.H.: The identification of staphylococci in clinical and food microbiology laboratories, Crit. Rev. Clin. Lab. Sci. **7**:121, 1976.

116. Tager, M., and Drummond, M.C.: Staphylocoagulase, Ann. N.Y. Acad. Sci. **128**:92, 1965.

117. Thomsen, A.C., Morgensen, S.C., and Jepsen, F.L.: Experimental mastitis in mice induced by coagulase-negative staphylococci isolated from cases of mastitis in nursing women, Acta Obstet. Gynecol. Scand. **64**:163, 1985.

118. Tierno, P.M., and Stotzky, G.: Serological typing of *Staphylococcus epidermidis* biotype 4, J. Infect. Dis. **137**:514, 1978.

119. Tselensis-Kotsowilis, A.D., Koliomichalis, M.P., and Papavassiliou, J.T.: Acute pyelonephritis caused by *Staphylococcus xylosus*, J. Clin. Microbiol. **16**:593, 1982.

120. Tuazon, C.U., and Sheagren, J.N.: Teichoic acid antibodies in the diagnosis of serious infections with *Staphylococcus aureus*, Ann. Intern. Med. **84**:543, 1976.

121. Tuazon, C.U., et al.: *Staphylococcus aureus* bacteremia: relationship between formation of antibodies to teichoic acid and development of metastatic abscesses, J. Infect. Dis. **137:**57, 1978.

122. Ubukata, K., Yamashita, N., and Konno, M.: Occurrence of a β-lactam-inducible penicillin-binding protein in methicillin-resistant staphylococci, Antimicrob. Agents Chemother. **27:**851, 1985.

123. Wallmark, G., Arremark, I., and Telander, B.: *Staphylococcus saprophyticus:* a frequent cause of acute urinary tract infection among female outpatients, J. Infect. Dis. **138:**791, 1978.

124. Watts, J.L., Pankey, J.W., and Nickerson, S.C.: Evaluation of the Staph-Ident and STAPHase systems for identification of staphylococci from bovine intramammary infections, J. Clin. Microbiol. **20:**448, 1984.

125. Wentworth, B.B.: Bacteriophage typing of the staphylococci, Bacteriol. Rev. **27:**253, 1963.

126. Wenzel, R.P.: The emergence of methicillin-resistant *Staphylococcus aureus,* Ann. Intern. Med. **97:**440, 1982.

127. Wenzel, R.P., Donowitz, L., and Miller, G.B.: Methicillin-resistant *Staphylococcus aureus*—United States, MMWR **30:**140, 1981.

128. West, T.E., et al.: Evaluation of a commercial counterimmunoelectrophoresis kit for detection of *Staphylococcus aureus* teichoic acid antibodies, J. Clin. Microbiol. **17:**567, 1983.

129. Wheat, L.J., Kohler, R.B., and White, A.: Solid-phase radioimmunoassay for immunoglobulin G *Staphylococcus aureus* antibody in serious staphylococcal infection, Ann. Intern. Med. **89:**467, 1978.

130. Wheat, L.J., Kohler, R.B., and White, A.: Teichoic acid antibody determination of agar-gel diffusion: effect of using dilute antigen preparations, J. Clin. Microbiol. **10:**138, 1979.

131. Wheat, L.J., et al.: IgM and IgG antibody response to teichoic acid in infections due to *Staphylococcus aureus,* J. Infect. Dis. **147:**1101, 1983.

132. Wilkinson, B.J., Maxwell, S., and Schaus, S.M.: Classification and characteristics of coagulase-negative methicillin-resistant staphylococci, J. Clin. Microbiol. **12:**161, 1980.

133. Wilson, P.D., Jr., et al.: The problem of infection in endoprosthetic surgery of the hip joint, Clin. Orthop. **96:**213, 1973.

134. Wilson, W.R.: Prosthetic valve endocarditis: incidence, anatomic location, cause, morbidity, and mortality. In Duma, R.J., editor: Infections of prosthetic heart valves and vascular grafts, Baltimore, 1977, University Park Press.

135. Winston, D.J., et al.: Coagulase-negative staphylococcal bacteremia in patients receiving immunosuppressive therapy, Arch. Intern. Med. **143:**32, 1983.

136. Wiseman, G.M.: The hemolysins of *Staphylococcus aureus,* Bacteriol. Rev. **39:**317, 1975.

137. Woodin, A.M.: Staphylococcal leucocidin. In Cohen, J.O., editor: The staphylococci, New York, 1972, John Wiley & Sons, Inc.

CHAPTER 13

Streptococci

Barbara J. Howard
Madeline J. Ducate

CLASSIFICATION

Several classification schemes have been used to differentiate among the streptococci. For example, the organisms may be classified according to the hemolytic pattern they exhibit (Table 13-1). This system, as originally proposed by Brown, provides a useful means for preliminary differentiation of streptococci in the clinical laboratory.

In the 1930s Lancefield developed a serologic classification system for differentiating among the streptococci. This system is based on a precipitin reaction between a group-specific antigen (also known as C substance) extracted from the cell wall of the streptococci and specific antisera prepared by immunizing rabbits with heat-killed suspensions of the organisms. The streptococci are divided into serologic groups A to O based on their possession of this specific group antigen. *S. agalactiae* is the only organism that possesses the group B antigen, and thus the names *S. agalactiae* and group B beta-streptococcus are used interchangeably. The names group A beta-streptococcus and *S. pyogenes* are also used interchangeably in the clinical laboratory. It should be noted, however, that although the large majority of organisms with the group A antigen are *S. pyogenes*, a few strains of *S. anginosus* and *S. intermedius* may also possess group A antigen.[35] These latter organisms are not responsible for diseases such as pharyngitis, impetigo, rheumatic fever, or glomerulonephritis, which are associated with *S. pyogenes*.[35] Other groups, such as group C or group D (discussed later), are comprised of several species (Table 13-2). Groups A, B, C, D, F, and G are most commonly associated with human infections. The serologic classification system was originally designed and is primarily used for differentiation of the beta-hemolytic streptococci; however, some hemolytic types of streptococci other than beta may also possess the group C–specific substance and may be grouped but not definitively identified by this method.

Another classification scheme is that of Sherman, who used physiologic characteristics to divide the streptococci into four groups: pyogenic streptococci, lactic streptococci, enterococci, and viridans streptococci. Although Sherman's classification scheme is not used routinely in the clinical laboratory, the terms "enterococci" and "viridans streptococci" are still used to refer to particular groups of organisms. Enterococci are normally found in the human intestine. These organisms, which may be alpha, beta, or nonhemolytic, possess the group D–specific antigen. There are actually two divisions of organisms that possess the group D antigen. In the past, these have been referred to as group D enterococci, including the species *S. faecium*, *S. faecalis*, and *S. durans*, and group D nonenterococci, including the species *S. bovis* and *S. equinus*. *S. equinus* is isolated from horses and is encountered infrequently in the clinical laboratory. Recently it has been proposed that the group D enterococci be removed from the *Streptococcus* genus and given species status, that is, *Enterococcus* spp.[59,82] For the remainder of this chapter these organisms are referred to as enterococci (*Enterococcus* spp.) and the other organisms possessing the group D antigen as group D nonenterococci. These latter organisms are still considered members of the genus *Streptococcus*. In addition to *E. faecalis*, *E. faecium*, and *E. durans*, the following species have also been proposed for inclusion in the genus *Enterococcus*: *E. avium*, *E. casseliflavus*, *E. gallinarum*, and *E. malodoratus*.[25] Of these latter organisms, only *E. avium* has been recovered from humans, specifically from human feces.[25]

The viridans streptococci are the alpha-hemolytic and gamma-hemolytic streptococci found normally in the nasopharyngeal region. Most of these organisms do not have a group antigen and include the numerous species designated in Table 13-1.

It should be noted that the British classification for some of the viridans species differs from that in Tables 13-2 and 13-4 (the classification proposed by the Centers for Disease Control [CDC]).[36] *S. constellatus* and *S. intermedius* are not recognized as viridans streptococci by the British, but rather are designated *Streptococcus milleri*. The CDC and British classification also differ for the species designation of group F beta-hemolytic streptococci, the beta-hemolytic streptococci without group antigens, and the minute colony forms of groups A, C, and G streptococci, which do not grow in normal atmospheres but require increased CO_2. (The beta-hemolytic streptococci without group antigens and the minute colony forms are not considered further in this chapter, since the only organism of these groups to be associated with human disease is the minute colony form of group C.) The British include all of these organisms under the name *S. milleri*, whereas the CDC includes them as subgroups of *S. anginosus*.[34,36]

The interrelationship of the Brown, Lancefield, and Sherman classification systems is summarized in Table 13-2.

Numerous taxonomic changes have recently been proposed for the streptococci. Many of these changes are discussed in *Bergey's Manual of Systematic Bacteriology*[47] but will not be used in this chapter. As previously indicated, the basis of this chapter will be the CDC classification system.

DIRECT ANTIGEN DETECTION

Numerous commercial latex agglutination, coagglutination, or ELISA systems can detect group A streptococci directly

TABLE 13-1. Hemolytic Patterns of the Streptococci

Type of Hemolysis	Description
α or alpha	Greenish or brownish discoloration surrounding colony; indicates partial lysis of red blood cells
β or beta	Clear or colorless zone surrounding colony; indicates complete lysis of red blood cells
γ or gamma (or nonhemolytic)	No lytic activity surrounding red blood cells
α' or alpha prime (or wide-zone hemolysis)	Small zone of alpha-hemolysis surrounded by small zone of beta-hemolysis

from throat swabs. These systems are dependent on the addition of the extracted streptococcal antigen to antibody-coated latex particles, beads, staphylococci, or another solid-phase system.

Some of the commercially available latex agglutination systems use chemical extraction, whereas others employ an enzymatic extraction.

Published studies of some of these latex agglutination kits have demonstrated their high specificity but lower sensitivity as compared with culture.*

The Phadebact Streptococcus coagglutination reagents (Pharmacia Diagnostics, Piscataway, N.J.) may be used with a nitrous acid extraction procedure to identify group A beta-streptococci from throat swabs[31,43,89] and group B beta-strep-

*References 22, 61, 63, 65, 75, 90, and 95.

TABLE 13-2. Classification of Streptococci

Species	Group Antigen (Lancefield Classification)	Sherman Classification	Hemolysis (Brown Classification)	Main Habitat
S. pyogenes	A	Pyogenic	β, γ	Humans
S. agalactiae	B	Pyogenic	β, γ	Cattle; humans
S. equisimilis	C	Pyogenic	β	Many animals; humans
S. zooepidemicus	C	Pyogenic	β	Many animals
S. equi	C	Pyogenic	β	Horses
S. anginosus	F, None (A, C, G)[a]	Pyogenic	β	Humans
E. faecalis	D	Enterococci	α, β, γ	Feces of mammals
E. faecium	D	Enterococci	α, γ	Feces of mammals
E. durans	D	Enterococci	α, β, γ	Feces of mammals
S. avium	D	Enterococci	α, γ	Feces of birds
S. bovis	D	Nonenterococci	γ	Feces of mammals
S. bovis variant	D	Nonenterococci	α, γ	Feces of mammals
S. equinus	D	Nonenterococci	α	Feces of horses
S. mutans	None[b]	Viridans	γ	Humans, other animals
S. uberis	None[b]	Viridans	α	Cattle, soil
S. intermedius	None[b]	Viridans	α, γ	Humans
S. constellatus	None[b]	Viridans	α, γ	Humans
S. sanguis I	None[b]	Viridans	α	Humans
S. sanguis II	None[b]	Viridans	α	Humans
S. salivarius	None[b]	Viridans	γ	Humans
S. mitis	None[b]	Viridans	α	Humans
S. morbillorum	None[b]	Viridans	α	Humans
S. acidominimus	None[b]	Viridans	γ	Cattle

Modified from Facklam, R.R.: Clin. Microbiol. Newsletter 7:91, 1985; and Parker, M.T.: Streptococci and lactobacillus. In Wilson, G., and Miles, A., editors: Topley and Wilson's principles of bacteriology, virology, and immunity, vol. 2, ed. 7, London, 1983, Edward Arnold.
[a]Approximately 75% of S. anginosus have group F antigen, approximately 15% are nongroupable, and approximately 10% possess group C, G, or A antigen (R.R. Facklam, personal communication).
[b]Approximately 75% of viridans streptococci do not have group antigens. Remaining 25% may have any streptococcal group antigen (A-O) with the exception of B and D (R.R. Facklam, personal communication).

tococci from cervical, uterine, and placental swabs.[88] One study also showed the Phadebact system to be useful in detecting groups A, B, C, D, and G streptococci and enterococci (*Enterococcus* spp.) from blood cultures.[102] When blood cultures are tested, however, cross-reactions may be observed between the group C reagent and *Streptococcus pneumoniae;* differentiation of these two organisms is accomplished with bile solubility.[102] The use of the Phadebact system to detect group B streptococci in CSF is discussed in Chapter 8.

The commercially available ELISA test kits are dependent on the principles discussed in Chapter 7. Studies of some of these systems have shown them to be more sensitive and easier to interpret than the latex agglutination assays.[22a,68]

A recent study by Facklam[40a] compared many of the commercially available systems for direct detection of group A streptococci. The high specificity of the systems allows for the immediate treatment of patients with positive test results. However, because of the lower-than-desired sensitivity, negative results must be confirmed with culture.[40a]

The Phadebact Pneumococcus Test (Pharmacia Diagnostics, Inc., Piscataway, N.J.) and the Pneumoslide (BBL Microbiology Systems, Cockeysville, Md.) have also been used for direct detection of pneumococci in clinical specimens. The Phadebact system was more sensitive than counterimmunoelectrophoresis (CIE) in detecting pneumococcal antigen in CSF cultures.[20] The Pneumoslide demonstrated 100% sensitivity and 92% specificity in detecting pneumococci in blood cultures.[19]

GROWTH REQUIREMENTS
MEDIA

Streptococci are fastidious organisms that grow well on infusion media such as trypticase soy, heart infusion, Todd-Hewitt, or proteose peptone supplemented with blood or serum. These media not only provide the necessary nutrients but are also free of fermentable carbohydrates that may influence hemolysis produced by the beta-hemolytic streptococci. For optimal recovery of streptococci the pH of the medium should be 7.3 to 7.4.

Several other factors, such as the type of animal blood, may also affect hemolysis. The enterococci (*Enterococcus* spp.), for example, produce beta-hemolysis on horse, rabbit, or human blood agars but alpha-hemolysis on sheep blood agar, which is recommended for the recovery of the streptococci. Sheep blood agar supports the growth of the commonly encountered clinical isolates, allows easy recognition of beta-hemolysis, and does not support the growth of *Haemophilus haemolyticus,* a beta-hemolytic organism found as normal flora in the human pharynx, which might be confused with beta-hemolytic streptococci.

Different concentrations of blood and the depth of the agar medium also affect the size of the zone of hemolysis. Use of 5% defibrinated sheep blood in agar approximately 4 mm deep appears to be optimal.

Differences in the type of atmospheric environment may also affect the type of hemolysis exhibited by group A beta-hemolytic streptococci. These organisms may produce two types of hemolysins: streptolysin O, which is oxygen labile, and streptolysin S, which is oxygen stable. Most group A beta-hemolytic streptococci produce streptolysin S; however, a few isolates produce only streptolysin O and thus may not be detected if incubated in the presence of oxygen. Anaerobic incubation,

preparation of pour plates, or stabbing the primary isolation plate after inoculation may be used to provide the lowered oxygen tension necessary for detection of these organisms.

The preparation of pour plates involves the inoculation of a loopful of a broth suspension of the specimen into a tube of melted agar containing sheep blood. The mixture is mixed and poured into a sterile Petri dish. After the agar has hardened, the plate is incubated at 35° C in air. The pour plate provides an anaerobic environment for colonies embedded within the agar, so beta-hemolysis is better observed. Although pour plates are an excellent means for observation of beta-hemolysis, they are cumbersome and time consuming and not used routinely in most microbiology laboratories. As an alternative, the inoculating loop may be used to stab the agar in several places after inoculation; this forces some of the organisms beneath the surface, where reduced oxygen tensions allow better observation of hemolysis.

The addition of trimethoprim-sulfamethoxazole (1.25 μg and 23.75 μg, respectively) to sheep blood agar has been recommended to suppress the growth of normal flora and allow better recovery of beta-hemolytic streptococci from throat cultures.[45] Other selective agents, such as gentamicin, crystal violet, colistin, and oxalinic acid, have also been used and are frequently incorporated into the commercially available selective media. Facklam and Carey[36] review the various enrichment, selective, and selective-enrichment techniques available for recovery of streptococci.

Nutritionally Variant Streptococci

Nutritionally variant streptococci (or more specifically, pyridoxal-dependent streptococci) require vitamin B_6 (pyridoxal hydrochloride) for growth. These organisms are most commonly isolated from blood and body fluids, and according to Roberts and co-workers[79] may be responsible for 5% to 6% of all cases of microbial endocarditis. The organisms may be observed in different situations in the laboratory. They may be seen satelliting other bacterial species such as staphylococci, *Escherichia coli, Klebsiella* spp., *Enterobacter* spp., and yeasts. Blood cultures that appear positive by visual or radiometric detection methods and show gram-positive cocci on Gram stain but exhibit no growth on subculture may also harbor these organisms. In fact, these organisms should be considered in cases of culture-negative endocarditis.[18] Good growth of these nutritionally variant streptococci may be achieved by use of a Staph streak (see Chapter 15), by adding pyridoxal HCl (0.001% final concentration) to the growth medium,[26] or by placing sterile disks containing 0.001% pyridoxal HCl (Remel Laboratories, Inc., Kansas City, Mo.)[23] on blood agar plates. In the latter case the organisms exhibit a zone of growth 18 to 20 mm in diameter around the disk.[23]

ENVIRONMENTAL REQUIREMENTS

Streptococci are facultative anaerobes and thus grow both aerobically and anaerobically. Pneumococci require increased CO_2 for best growth and thus should be incubated in a CO_2 incubator or a candle extinction jar. Plates for recovery of the beta-hemolytic streptococci should preferably be incubated under anaerobic conditions with 5% to 10% CO_2 and 85% to 90% N_2.[36] As already discussed, hemolysis of the beta-hemolytic streptococci is more pronounced under reduced oxygen tensions. Non–group A beta-hemolytic streptococci are also isolated significantly more often when incubated in an anaero-

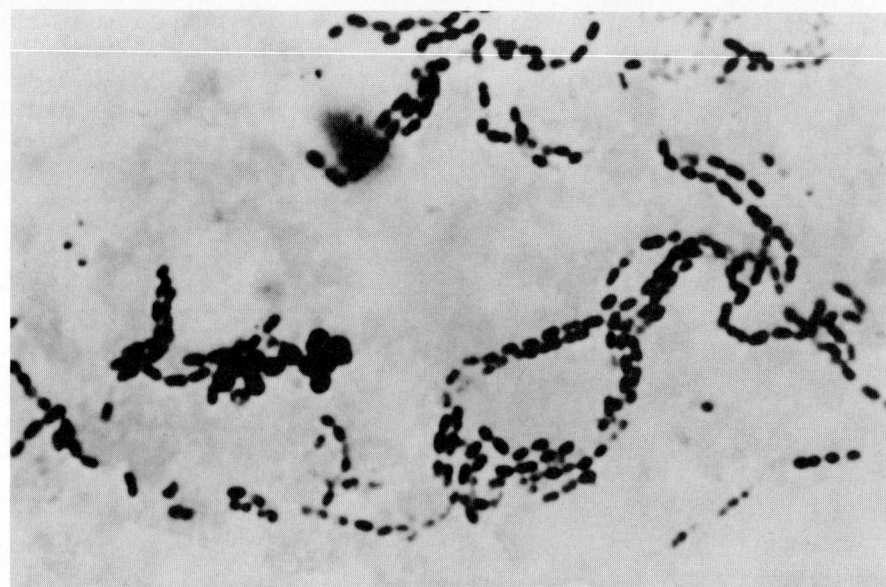

FIGURE 13-1. Gram stain of blood showing streptococci in chains. (Photograph by Dr. Leon J. LeBeau, Department of Biocommunication Arts, Medical Center, University of Illinois at Chicago.)

bic atmosphere.[58] Plates may be incubated in a CO_2 incubator provided that they are stabbed, as mentioned previously.

Some studies have shown comparable recovery or, in one case, enhanced recovery of group A streptococci from throat cultures on plates that have been stabbed and incubated under aerobic conditions—thereby questioning the added expense of anaerobic incubation. Furthermore, because more non–group A streptococci are isolated under anaerobic conditions, some of these studies suggest that these organisms may add confusion when screening for the presence or absence of group A streptococci. Several other studies show a significantly higher isolation rate of group A beta-hemolytic streptococci when throat cultures are incubated under anaerobic conditions.[31,56,84] This increased recovery may be attributed to several reasons: (1) the anaerobic environment prevents the inactivation of streptolysin O; (2) anaerobic conditions prevent the normal flora from forming peroxides that may inhibit the growth of group A beta-hemolytic streptococci; and (3) an anaerobic environment inhibits the growth of the aerobic normal flora that otherwise could overgrow or inhibit the group A beta-hemolytic streptococci.[84] In summary, anaerobic incubation is recommended.

All cultures should be incubated at 35° to 37° C.

CULTURAL CHARACTERISTICS
STAINING REACTIONS

Streptococci generally appear as gram-positive cocci in chains or pairs because of cell division in only one plane and failure of the cocci to separate after division (Figure 13-1). Although streptococci are gram positive, they may appear gram negative with age; therefore Gram stains should be performed on cultures that are less than 24 hours old. (Organisms may also appear gram negative when being phagocytized by PMNs.) Direct Gram stains have been found to be highly reliable in differentiating staphylococci from streptococci in blood cul-

tures. A preponderance of chains, pairs, or both presumptively identifies the organisms as streptococci.[2]

S. pneumoniae is unique since it typically appears as a gram-positive, encapsulated, lancet-shaped coccus occurring singly, in pairs, or in short chains (Plate 6, *B*). It tends to form chains when grown in relatively unfavorable media, particularly in low concentrations of magnesium, or when grown in the presence of type-specific antibody.[28]

COLONIAL MORPHOLOGY

As previously mentioned, streptococci may produce four different types of hemolysis (Table 13-1). The type of hemolysis exhibited is an important aid in their presumptive identification. All four types of hemolysis are best observed in subsurface colonies. Reasonable accuracy in the interpretation of hemolytic reactions can be achieved by examining subsurface or surface colonies with a hand lens or with the naked eye, but the best accuracy is achieved by microscopic examination of colonies growing within the agar or microscopic examination of the area surrounding the stab.

The colonial morphology of the streptococci is variable. Group A beta-hemolytic streptococci tend to be small (0.5 to 1 mm) and transparent with a large zone of hemolysis in relation to the size of the colony (Plate 6, *C*). Group B beta-hemolytic streptococci, on the other hand, are larger, more translucent, grayer, flatter, and creamier in appearance. Furthermore, the zone of hemolysis of group B streptococci is small compared with the colony size—so much so that it is often helpful to scrape the colony aside with a sterile loop to observe the hemolytic effect. Enterococci (*Enterococcus* spp.) are usually large, gray, shiny, and translucent, whereas the viridans streptococci are small, raised, opaque, and convex.

Although colonies of pneumococci are initially dome shaped, they become umbilicated (depressed center with raised margins) with age because of the actions of autolytic enzymes (Plate 6, *D*). Certain strains of pneumococci (for example, types 3 and 37) produce very large capsules and appear much larger and more watery than other strains of pneumococci (Plate 6, *E*). Colonies of *S. pneumoniae* tend to be surrounded by an approximately 2 mm zone of alpha-hemolysis. This hemolysis is produced by a streptolysin O–like lysin, called pneumolysin, which is elaborated under either aerobic or anaerobic conditions. It is active against human, sheep, rabbit, and horse erythrocytes and is inactivated by oxidation. The flatter, concave topography and greenish brown hemolysis of *S. pneumoniae* help distinguish this organism from the other alpha-hemolytic streptococci, which are more raised and convex and surrounded by a more greenish hemolysis.

BIOCHEMICAL IDENTIFICATION
DIFFERENTIATION OF THE GENUS *STREPTOCOCCUS* FROM OTHER GENERA

Staphylococci and micrococci may be confused morphologically with streptococci. This occurs more frequently with young colonies growing on primary isolation media. As discussed in Appendix A, these genera may be distinguished with the catalase test. *Staphylococcus* and *Micrococcus* spp. are catalase positive, and *Streptococcus* spp. are catalase negative. Unfortunately, during testing with hydrogen peroxide, occasional catalase-positive *Streptococcus* or *Aerococcus* spp. are encountered, as are catalase-negative *Micrococcus* spp. Differentiation of these organisms requires the use of the benzidine test to detect the presence or absence of cytochromes.[36] Although benzidine is a potential carcinogen, commercial benzidine disks, such as MicroDent (Remel, Lenexa, Kan.), are available.

Neisseria spp. can also occasionally be confused with the streptococci, especially in aged cultures, from which the streptococci often stain gram negative. Members of the genus *Streptococcus* are cytochrome oxidase negative, whereas the genus *Neisseria* is oxidase positive.

The colonial morphology of *Listeria monocytogenes* is identical to that of the beta-hemolytic streptococci. Furthermore, both of these organisms hydrolyze esculin. *Listeria* spp., however, are gram-positive bacilli and produce catalase.

DIFFERENTIATION WITHIN THE GENUS *STREPTOCOCCUS*

Once an isolate has been determined to be a member of the genus *Streptococcus*, several factors should be considered before proceeding with identification. These include source of specimen, differential diagnosis if available, and morphologic and hemolytic patterns. As in all of clinical microbiology, a knowledge of which organisms are normal flora and which are pathogens in various specimen types is essential before proceeding with identification. For example, an alpha-hemolytic organism in a respiratory culture may be a viridans streptococcus or pneumococcus but probably not *Enterococcus* spp.; alpha-hemolytic organisms in stools are most likely *Enterococcus* spp. and not viridans streptococci or pneumococci. Furthermore, among the beta-hemolytic streptococci, group A accounts for most of the isolates in the upper respiratory tract and group B in the genitourinary tract.[74] Groups C, F, and G may be seen in cases of arthritis, skin infections, and bacteremia.

A knowledge of the differential diagnosis is also helpful, since certain streptococci are most commonly associated with specific clinical conditions. For example, whereas group B streptococci might be suspected from the blood culture of a neonate with meningitis, group A streptococci are generally suspected in the throat specimen of a patient with pharyngitis. The association between groups of streptococci and clinical presentation is discussed more thoroughly later in this chapter.

As previously mentioned, observation of hemolysis is a key feature in differentiating among the streptococci. Once the hemolytic pattern is established, the following approach to identification is recommended.[36] Beta-hemolytic streptococci are most accurately identified by the serologic and immunoserologic procedures discussed later in this chapter. Thus if a strain is beta-hemolytic, it is tested for serologic reaction with groups A, B, C, D, F, and G antisera. If the strain is not beta-hemolytic, it should be tested with groups B and D antisera. This enables detection of the strains of group B streptococci that are nonhemolytic and the alpha-hemolytic or nonhemolytic group D organisms. Streptococci that are neither beta-hemolytic nor members of groups B or D are identified through physiologic tests. These latter organisms must be identified with physiologic tests, since they do not possess group antigens.

Although this approach to identification is the most reliable, some laboratories may not have the economic resources for routine serologic or immunoserologic testing and may depend entirely on physiologic tests. These tests are not as definitive as serologic tests, but they do offer strong presumptive identification.[38] The physiologic tests used for presumptive identification are indicated in Table 13-3. The key physiologic tests for distinguishing clinical isolates are considered next.

DIFFERENTIATION OF GROUP A STREPTOCOCCI

Group A streptococci can be presumptively identified by determination of susceptibility to low levels of bacitracin and trimethoprim-sulfamethoxazole (Figure 13-2 and Table 13-3) and production of the enzyme pyroglutamyl aminopeptidase.

As discussed in Appendix A, to perform the bacitracin susceptibility test, a pure culture of the beta-hemolytic streptococcus is streaked onto a sheep blood agar plate. A disk containing 0.04 unit of bacitracin is placed in the center of the streaked area, and the plate is incubated overnight at 35° to 37° C. Susceptibility to bacitracin, as indicated by any zone of inhibition around the disk, is presumptive identification of group A streptococci (Figure 13-2). When performing this test, it is essential that only beta-hemolytic streptococci be tested, since many alpha-hemolytic streptococci are also susceptible to bacitracin. Although this test is quite sensitive, it is less specific. Groups B, C, and G streptococci may also be inhibited by bacitracin and thus misidentified as group A streptococci.[38,74] The accuracy of this test may be improved by using susceptibility to an SXT disk (1.25 mg of trimethoprim and 23.75 mg of sulfamethoxazole) in combination with bacitracin susceptibility, or by placing the A disk on a plate containing SXT. Organisms that are susceptible to bacitracin and resistant to SXT are presumptively identified as group A streptococci, and those resistant to both bacitracin and SXT are presumptively identified as group B streptococci. Other susceptibility patterns are discussed in Appendix A.

A test for the production of the enzyme pyroglutamyl ami-

TABLE 13-3. Presumptive Identification of Streptococci and Enterococci

Category	Hemolysis	Susceptibility to		Hydrolysis of		CAMP	Bile Esculin	Growth in 6.5% NaCl	Optochin and Bile[a]
		Bacitracin	SXT	Hippurate	PYR				
Group A	Beta	+	−	−	+	−	−	−	−
Group B	Beta[b]	−[b]	−	+	−	+	−	+[b]	−
Beta-hemolytic streptococci (not group A, B, or D)	Beta	−[b]	+	−	−	−	−	−	−
Group D, enterococcus	Alpha, beta, none	−	−	−[b]	+	−	+	+	−
Group D, nonenterococcus	Alpha, none	−	+[b]	−	−	−	+	−	−
Viridans group	Alpha, none	−[b]	+	−[b]	−	−	−[b]	−	−
Pneumococcus	Alpha	±	?	−	−	−	−	−	+

SYMBOLS: SXT, Trimethoprim-sulfamethoxazole
PYR, L-Pyrrolidonyl-β-naphthylamide
+, Positive reaction or susceptible
−, Negative reaction or resistant

From Facklam, R.R., and Carey, R.B.: Streptococci and aerococci. In Lennette, E.H., et al., editors: Manual of clinical microbiology, ed. 4, Washington, D.C., 1985, American Society for Microbiology.
[a] Optochin susceptibility and bile solubility.
[b] Exceptions occasionally occur.

nopeptidase may be used instead of the bacitracin test for presumptive identification of group A streptococci. This test, known as the PYR test, is as sensitive as the bacitracin test but more specific.[40] The PYR test uses the substrate L-pyrrolidonyl-beta-napththylamide (PYR). The test organism is inoculated onto PYR agar, and the plate is incubated overnight at 35° C. The organisms hydrolyze the substrate and produce a red color when the PYR reagent (N, N-dimethylaminocinnamaldehyde) is added to the surface growth. Either a yellow color or no color change is a negative reaction. The test may also be performed by inoculating PYR broth and adding 1 drop of PYR reagent after incubating the broth for 4 to 5 hours. Agar media containing the PYR substrate are available commercially from Remel Laboratories (Lenexa, Kan.), and Carr-Scarborough (Stone Mountain, Ga.). Reagent-impregnated filter paper systems are also commercially available (Strep-A-Chek, E-Y Laboratories, San Mateo, Calif.; Identicult-AE, Scott Laboratories, Fiskeville, R.I.); these systems provide results within 30 minutes. Group A beta-streptococci and enterococci (Enterococcus spp.) are positive for the PYR test; group B streptococci are negative. The use of this test for identification of enterococci (Enterococcus spp.) is discussed later.

The Strep-A-Fluor (Bio Spec, Inc., Dublin, Calif.) has also been used for rapid presumptive identification of group A streptococci.[99] This filter paper strip is impregnated with a substrate similar to PYR. An inoculum of the test organism is placed on the filter paper strip. Buffer is then added to the inoculated portion before the strip is placed in a plastic envelope and incubated for 15 minutes. The strip is examined under ultraviolet light, and any yellowish green fluorescence is a positive reaction for enzymatic hydrolysis of the synthetic substrate. Using this test, Wasilauskas and Hampton[99] correctly categorized 305 beta-hemolytic streptococci as group A or non–group A.

DIFFERENTIATION OF GROUP B STREPTOCOCCI

Determination of the hydrolysis of hippurate or the CAMP test is more specific for presumptive identification of group B streptococci. The hippurate hydrolysis test is discussed in Appendix A. The name CAMP is taken from the initials of the last names of the original investigators of this test: Christie, Atkins, and Munch-Peterson. The CAMP factor produced by group B streptococci is a diffusible, heat-stable, extracellular protein that enhances the hemolysis of sheep red blood cells by the beta-hemolysin of Staphylococcus aureus. In this test a beta-hemolysin-producing S. aureus is streaked down the center of a sheep blood agar plate, and the test organism is streaked perpendicular to but not touching the staphylococcal streak. After 18 to 24 hours of incubation group B streptococci are presumptively identified by the arrowhead type of hemolysis (Plate 6, F) produced by the synergistic actions of the staphylococcal beta-hemolysin and the CAMP factor. Details for performing this test are discussed in Appendix A. The test may also be performed by using a paper disk containing partially purified beta-hemolysin of S. aureus. The disk is placed beside the streak of the streptococcal test isolate.[39]

GROUP D NONENTEROCOCCI AND ENTEROCOCCI (ENTEROCOCCUS SPP.)

In past years most clinical laboratories have differentiated the group D nonenterococci from Enterococcus spp. (throughout this discussion, enterococci) because of their differences in antimicrobial susceptibility. Penicillin is usually adequate for

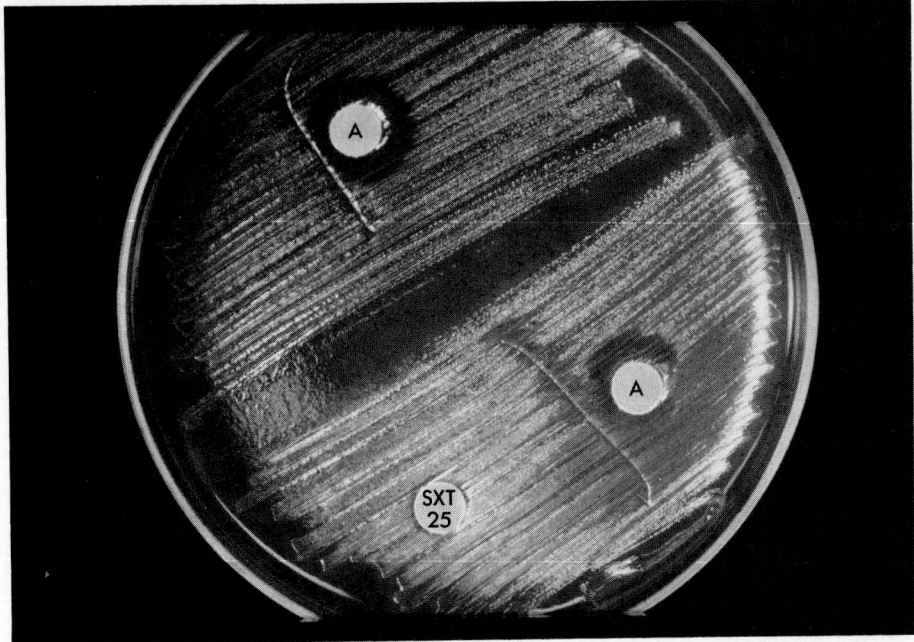

FIGURE 13-2. Group A beta-streptococcus is susceptible to bacitracin and resistant to trimo-theprim-sulfamethoxazole. (Photograph by Dr. Leon J. LeBeau, Department of Biocommuni-cation Arts, Medical Center, University of Illinois at Chicago.)

therapy of infections caused by group D nonenterococci, whereas serious infections caused by enterococci often require the synergistic actions of a penicillin and an aminoglycoside. It should be noted, however, that *E. faecium* has been found to be more resistant to the synergistic effect of penicillin and most aminoglycosides than *E. faecalis*.[67]

These organisms can be presumptively identified with the bile esculin test, growth in 6.5% NaCl, and the PYR test, as already mentioned. Both the enterococci and the group D non-enterococci are bile esculin positive. These two groups may be differentiated with 6.5% NaCl or the PYR test. Enterococci are positive for both of these characteristics, but group D nonente-rococci are negative for both. The PYR test is a much more rapid test than is NaCl and may be used in conjunction with the commercially available serogrouping procedures, such as the Phadebact coagglutination test, for more definitive identifica-tion of these organisms.[15] Organisms that are serogroup D with the coagglutination reagent and are PYR positive are enterococ-ci; those that are serogroup D but PYR negative are group D nonenterococci.[15]

If serologic testing is not used, isolates of *S. bovis* may be misidentified as viridans streptococci, since some isolates of the latter group of organisms are also bile esculin positive, 6.5% NaCl negative, and PYR negative. Ruoff and co-work-ers[80] report that although similarities between *S. bovis* and *S. salivarius*, *S. bovis* and *S. mutans*, and *S. bovis* variant and *S. intermedius* have been noted, their experience indicates that among routine clinical isolates, *S. bovis* is most often confused with *S. salivarius* when a small number of tests are used for presumptive identification. Even when serologic typing is used for definitive identification, *S. salivarius* may type as a group D streptococcus because of the presence of cross-reacting anti-gens. According to these investigators it is important to distin-guish *S. bovis* and *S. salivarius* because *S. bovis* is an agent of

endocarditis and its presence in the bloodstream can be related to underlying gastrointestinal disease (described later). The fol-lowing physiologic tests are recommended for differentiation: fermentation of mannitol, lactose, raffinose, and inulin, hydro-lysis of starch and urea, and the production of polysaccharide from sucrose.[80]

Aerococci may be confused with enterococci if serologic typing is not performed and only a few physiologic tests are used. Aerococci are alpha hemolytic, grow in 6.5% NaCl, and are variable with regard to bile esculin hydrolysis. The Gram stain may help distinguish these two groups of organisms; the aerococci appear as gram-positive cocci in tetrads.[69] Identifica-tion of aerococci requires the use of serologic identification to demonstrate their lack of the group D antigen.[36] Other physio-logic reactions are seen in Table 13-4.

Laboratories that perform serologic identification may fur-ther differentiate among group D organisms with the physio-logic tests in Table 13-4. *E. faecalis*, the most commonly iso-lated *Enterococcus* sp., hydrolyzes arginine and pyruvate, whereas *E. faecium* hydrolyzes arginine but not pyruvate. *S. bovis* and *S. equinus* hydrolyze neither arginine nor pyruvate and are differentiated by hydrolysis of starch and production of acid from mannitol and lactose.

DIFFERENTIATION OF VIRIDANS STREPTOCOCCI AND PNEUMOCOCCI

The viridans streptococci are alpha hemolytic and thus may be confused with the group D nonenterococci, *Enterococcus* spp., and pneumococci. Differentiation from the first two groups of organisms has already been discussed. Both the vir-idans streptococci and the pneumococci are negative with regard to growth in 6.5% NaCl and are usually negative for hydrolysis of bile esculin and hippurate. Susceptibility to opto-chin (ethylhydrocupreine hydrochloride) and bile solubility

TABLE 13-4. Differentiation of Group D Streptococci, *Enterococcus* Spp., Viridans Streptococci, and Aerococci Found in Human Infections

Test	*E. faecalis*	*E. faecium*	*E. avium*	*E. durans*	Aerococci	*S. bovis*	*S. mutans*	*S. uberis*	*S. intermedius*	*S. bovis* (var.)	*S. constellatus*	*S. equinus*	*S. sanguis* I	*S. salivarius*	*S. mitis*	*S. sanguis* II	*S. morbillorum*	*S. acidominimus*
HEMOLYSIS																		
Alpha	+	+	+	+	+	−a	−a	+	−a	−a	+	+	+	−a	+	+	−a	+
Beta	+	−	−	+	−	−	+	−	−	−	−	−	−	−	−	−	−	−
None	+	+	+	+	−a	+	+	+	+	+	−a	−	−a	+	−a	−a	+	−a
PHYSIOLOGIC																		
Bile esculin	+	+	+	+	v	+	−a	−	−a	+	−a	+	−a	−a	−	−	−	−
Growth in 6.5% NaCl	+	+	+	+	+	−	−	−a										
Growth at 10° C	+	+	−	−														
Pyruvate	+	−	+	−	−	−	−	−	−	−	−	−	−a					
Arginine	+a	+	−	+			−a		+a		+a		+			−a		
Esculin	+	+	+	+	v	+	+a	+	+	+	+a	+	+a	+a	−	−	−	−
Starch	−	−	−	−	−	+	−	−	−a	−a	−	+a	−a	−	−	−a		
Hippurate	v	v	−	v	+a	−	−	+a	−	−	−	−	−	−	−	−	−	+a
Sucrose	+a	+	+	−a	+	+	+	+	+	+	+	+	+	+	+	+	+	+
Lactose	+a	+	+	+	+a	+	+	+	+	+	−	+	+a	+	+	−		
Mannitol	+	+	+	−	v	+	+	+	−	−	−	−	−	−	−	−		
Sorbitol	+a	−	+	−	−	−	+	+	−	−	−		−a	−				
Arabinose	−a	+a	+	−	−	−	−a	−	−	−	−a	−						
Sorbose	−	−	+															
Inulin	−	−a	+a	−	−a	+a	+a	+a	−	−	−	+	+	−	−	−		
Raffinose	−a	+a	+	−a	v	+a	+a	+a	v	v	−a	−a	−a	+a	−	+	−	
Glucan	N	N	N	N	N	L	D	N	Na	Na	N	N	Da	La	N	Da	N	N

SYMBOLS:	+, Positive reactions	N, No glucans
	−, Negative reactions	L, Levans
	v, Variable reactions	D, Dextran

Modified from Facklam, R.R., and Carey, R.B.: Streptococci and aerococci. In Lennette, E.H., et al., editors: Manual of clinical microbiology, ed. 4, Washington, D.C., 1985, American Society for Microbiology.
aOccasional exceptions occur.

(Table 13-3) are most commonly used to differentiate the pneumococci, which are usually positive for both of these characteristics. (These procedures are described in Appendix A.) Fermentation of inulin has also been used to identify pneumococci. These three tests do afford presumptive identification, but they are not absolute; it is preferable to use at least two of these tests

simultaneously. Typing should be performed on isolates from sterile sources.

Most viridans streptococci do not possess a group antigen and thus cannot be identified by serologic tests. Definitive identification of these organisms requires the use of extensive physiologic tests (Table 13-4).[32] Although routine differentiation of these organisms is unnecessary, speciation should be performed on isolates from body sites that are normally sterile.

RAPID IDENTIFICATION SYSTEMS

The rapid systems for identification of streptococci are discussed in Chapter 9.

SEROLOGIC AND IMMUNOSEROLOGIC IDENTIFICATION

SEROLOGIC TYPING

Determination of Serogroups

As previously discussed, the Lancefield classification is based on a precipitin reaction between the group-specific antigen extracted from the cell wall and specific antisera. Most of these group antigens are carbohydrate in nature, although the antigens of groups D and N organisms and the pneumococci are teichoic acids. Groups D and N possess glycerol teichoic acid, and the pneumococci possess a choline-containing teichoic acid. The carbohydrate group antigens are attached to the peptidoglycan, and the teichoic acid antigens are found in largest amounts beneath the cell wall.[72] The intracellular location of the teichoic acids has made serologic identification of organisms with this type of group-specific antigen more difficult. As discussed later, routine serologic typing of the pneumococcus depends on the detection of type-specific antigens in the capsule, and not the teichoic acid group-specific antigens.

The group-specific antigen of groups A, B, C, F, and G is carbohydrate in nature. The antigenicity of the group-specific C substance of these organisms depends primarily on the nature of the terminal carbohydrate residue. Cross-reactions with organisms (other than streptococci) that possess the same terminal carbohydrate in their cell walls may be seen. For example, *Listeria* spp. possess an antigen similar to that of group B beta-hemolytic streptococci. Cross-reactions may also occur between groups B and G streptococci and are caused by similar determinant groups.[51]

To perform the Lancefield precipitin test, the group-specific C substance must first be extracted from the cell wall. The original method of Lancefield required use of hot hydrochloric acid for extraction. Alternative extraction procedures, such as hot formamide, nitrous acid autoclave, and enzyme techniques, are described by Facklam.[33]

After extraction the antigen (extract) can be layered over the antisera in a capillary tube, as originally described by Lancefield, or the antisera can be layered over the antigen through use of the CDC capillary ring precipitin test. The latter method works best with a serum of low potency, which is the case with most lots of CDC and commercial antisera.[33]

Determination of Serotypes

Precipitation and agglutination procedures may be used to further differentiate the streptococcal groups into types, based on the presence of type-specific antigens (proteins and carbohydrates) within the group.[72] Group A streptococci may possess type-specific M antigens, T antigens, and R antigens, all of which are protein in nature. There are a total of 80 different M antigens, but with few exceptions each group A streptococcus has only one distinct M antigen. Although M-typing has proven quite useful for epidemiologic studies, many organisms cannot be typed with this system. Over 90% of strains can be T-typed,

but T-typing does not differentiate strains as clearly as M-typing does. There are a total of 26 different T antigens; however, several strains possess more than one antigen and exhibit the same agglutination pattern. Group A streptococci may possess one of two R antigens.

Group B streptococci may also be divided into six serotypes according to type-specific carbohydrate antigens within the group.[49]

Quellung Test

Based on the differences in the type-specific specific soluble substance (SSS) in their capsules, 84 different pneumococcal types are recognized. The Neufeld quellung reaction based on detection of this SSS may be used for the identification of pneumococci. Also known as the capsular "swelling" reaction, this test is performed by adding pneumococcal capsular antiserum directly to a specimen or culture suspected of containing pneumococci. The combination of the capsule and its specific antiserum results in the formation of a clearly defined capsular halo around the pneumococcal organism (Plate 7, *A*). The capsule is best observed microscopically under oblique illumination. Most microbiologists support the theory that the formation of a clearly demarcated capsule is the result of a refractive index change of the precipitate formed in the antigen-antibody reaction. This reaction can be made more visible by adding 1% methylene blue to the slide preparation.

Omniserum, containing antibodies to all pneumococcal types, and monotypic sera are available from the Statens Seruminstitut, Copenhagen. In the United States, commercial antisera to the first 33 capsular types of pneumococci are available (Difco Laboratories, Detroit).

IMMUNOSEROLOGIC IDENTIFICATION

Commercially prepared latex and coagglutination reagents may be used for rapid identification of groups A, B, C, D, F, and G beta-hemolytic streptococci, *Enterococcus* spp., and pneumococci directly from primary isolation plates. The principles of latex agglutination and coagglutination are discussed in Chapter 8.

The Phadebact Streptococcus Test Kit (Pharmacia Diagnostics, Inc., Piscataway, N.J.) is a commercially available coagglutination system used to identify isolates of groups A, B, C, D, F, and G beta-hemolytic streptococci and enterococci (*Enterococcus* spp.). This kit may be used on isolated colonies or on mixed-growth cultures.

The SeroSTAT (Scott Laboratories, Inc., Fiskeville, R.I.) and Streptex (Wellcome Research Laboratories, Beckenham, U.K.) are commercial latex agglutination systems. SeroSTAT contains reagents to detect groups A, B, C, and G streptococci, whereas Streptex detects groups A, B, C, D, F, and G streptococci and enterococci (*Enterococcus* spp.). The Streptex, like the Phadebact, can be used on isolated colonies or mixed cultures, but the SeroSTAT can be used on isolated colonies only. Unlike the SeroSTAT and Phadebact, the Streptex requires extraction of the antigen before testing.

In general, all of these slide methods are both rapid and accurate for the identification of streptococci,[21,91] and the selection of one over another is a matter of personal preference.[36] These systems do appear to be less effective in the identification of group D streptococci and enterococci (*Enterococcus* spp.).[14,24,94] Tests for bile esculin hydrolysis and

TABLE 13-5. Features of Streptococcal Infections of the Skin and Upper Respiratory Tract

Feature	Infections of the Upper Respiratory Tract	Infections of the Skin
EPIDEMIOLOGY		
Seasonal occurrence	Winter and spring	Late summer and early fall
Common-source epidemics	May occur	Not described
Geographic distribution	More common in temperate or cold climates	Common in hot or tropical climates
Age	School-age children	Preschool-age children
Sex	Equal	Equal
Transmission	Direct spread from human reservoirs, particularly nasal carriers	Unknown; insects may be mechanical vectors
Carrier state	Common in pharynx of many populations	Unusual on skin except in certain situations
LABORATORY		
Serologic types of group A streptococci	Many different types	Few types predominate
Antistreptolysin O response	Common	Uncommon

Modified from Wannamaker, L.W. Reprinted by permission of the New England Journal of Medicine **282**:23, 1970.

growth in 6.5% NaCl or PYR should be performed on all suspected isolates of group D nonenterococci and group D enterococci (*Enterococcus* spp.) from tissue and body fluids; testing of oropharyngeal isolates is not necessary.[36]

As discussed in Chapter 7, immunofluorescent staining with fluorescein isothiocyanate–tagged antibody to group A streptococcal antigen may also be used to identify these organisms. Nonspecific staining of *S. aureus* or streptococcal groups can be prevented by adding unlabeled streptococcal group C antiserum or unlabeled nonimmune serum to the conjugate.[36]

The Phadebact Pneumococcus Test (Pharmacia Diagnostics, Inc., Piscataway, N.J.) is used to identify isolates of *S. pneumoniae*. The test, which uses antibody directed against the capsular antigen of the pneumococcus, is reportedly sensitive and specific.[20] As discussed in Chapter 8, this coagglutination test may also be used for direct detection of pneumococcus in cerebrospinal fluid (and pleural fluid), although cross-reactions with *Haemophilus influenzae* have been reported.

The Pneumoslide, a commercially available latex agglutination test (BBL Microbiology Systems, Cockeysville, Md.), is also a rapid and accurate system for identifying isolates of *S. pneumoniae*. When using this test, care must be taken to distinguish between true agglutination and clumping of the latex particles.[92]

CLINICAL SIGNIFICANCE
STREPTOCOCCUS PYOGENES[13,98]

S. pyogenes may be responsible for infections of the upper respiratory tract and for skin infections. The most frequent upper respiratory tract infection is pharyngitis, and the most frequent skin infection is impetigo. Nonsuppurative sequelae—such as otitis media, mastoiditis, peritonsillar abscess, and peritonsillar cellulitis—may follow streptococcal pharyngitis. The suppurative sequelae, acute rheumatic fever and glomerulonephritis, may also occur as a result of previous streptococcal infections. Glomerulonephritis may occur as a sequela of pharyngitis or skin infections, and acute rheumatic fever may occur as a sequela of pharyngitis. Streptococcal infections of the skin and upper respiratory tract differ in several clinical and epidemiologic aspects (Table 13-5).

Pharyngitis[60]

S. pyogenes is one of numerous agents responsible for pharyngitis. Other causes include *Neisseria gonorrhoeae*, *Corynebacterium diphtheriae*, *H. influenzae*, *Chlamydia* spp., *Mycoplasma pneumoniae*, Epstein-Barr virus, cytomegalovirus, rhinovirus, influenza, and several others. Recognition and treatment of pharyngitis caused by *S. pyogenes* is of primary concern because of the risk of developing rheumatic fever and poststreptococcal glomerulonephritis.

Streptococcal pharyngitis occurs most frequently in school-age children in the winter or spring. The infection is spread from person to person via droplets from respiratory secretions. Foodborne and waterborne transmission has also been reported. Clinical manifestations vary, and some patients may be asymptomatic, but in general the most common symptoms are abrupt onset of sore throat, malaise, headache, and fever greater than 101° F. The pharynx is usually erythematous, and a grayish white exudate is present on the enlarged tonsils. Enlarged tender lymph nodes at the angles of the mandibles are a suggestive finding.

Although group A is the most frequent cause of streptococcal pharyngitis, groups B, C, and G streptococci have rarely been implicated.

Scarlet Fever

Scarlet fever results from infection with a group A streptococcus that has been lysogenized with a temperate bacteriophage specifying the production of an erythrogenic toxin. The symptoms of scarlet fever are like those of pharyngitis except for the presence of the characteristic skin rash, which usually appears on the second day of illness. Usually erythematous and punctate in nature, the rash first appears on the upper chest and then spreads to the remainder of the trunk, neck, and extremities. The palms, soles, and face are not affected. The rash fades over the period of a week and is followed by extensive desquamation of the skin for several weeks.

The tongue of patients with scarlet fever is also affected by the generalized inflammation that occurs on the skin. During the first few days of illness red papillae are observed on a yellowish white coated tongue, the so-called strawberry tongue. The tongue also peels and then becomes beefy red, moist, and glistening; this is referred to as the raspberry tongue. An enanthem, a rash characterized by small, bright-red hemorrhagic spots, may also be seen on the soft palate.

Suppurative Sequelae of Upper Respiratory Tract Infections

Complications of upper respiratory tract infection result from the spread of the organism to adjacent tissues and may include peritonsillar cellulitis, peritonsillar abscess, retropharyngeal abscess, otitis media, sinusitis, and in some cases meningitis. These complications occur more often following scarlet fever than after pharyngitis but are rare in either case with early and adequate antimicrobial therapy.

Infections of the Skin

Infections of the skin may range from impetigo, a superficial infection characterized by crusted lesions (Figure 13-3), to myositis, a life-threatening infection of the muscles. The latter condition is quite rare, and only a few cases have been reported in the United States.

Unlike pharyngitis, impetigo occurs most frequently in late summer or early fall, in tropical or subtropical climates (Table 13-6). It may also appear in northern climates in certain epidemiologic settings, such as the American Indian reservations of Minnesota. The infection is associated with low levels of hygiene.

The strains of *S. pyogenes* that are responsible for impetigo belong to different M serotypes than those responsible for pharyngitis. Many of the impetigo-associated strains, however, are untypable in regard to the M antigen, or they belong to several different M serotypes and have not been well characterized. These strains first colonize the skin, which they later invade through abrasions, minor trauma, or insect bites. Patients develop pustular lesions that break down to form thick crusts. Lesions may appear in all exposed areas of the body but are most frequently observed on the lower extremities. Impetigo is treated with penicillin, but adequate therapy does not ensure protection against the subsequent development of glomerulonephritis.

Erysipelas is a diffuse erythematous skin infection that most often remains confined to the face. It usually follows streptococcal pharyngitis, although the mode of spread to the skin is not known.

Cellulitis involves the subcutaneous tissue and may be

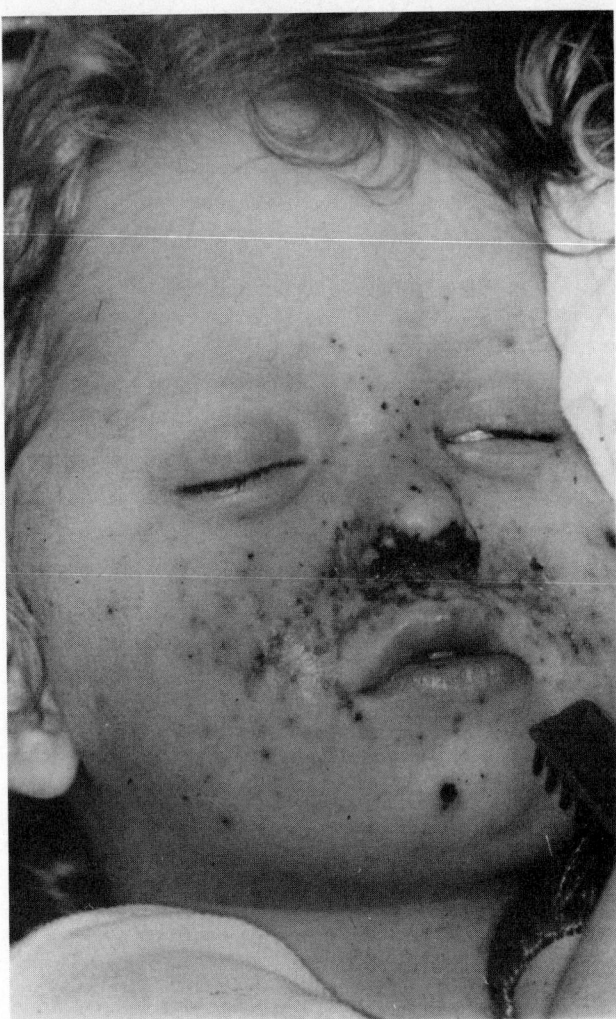

FIGURE 13-3. Impetigo caused by *Streptococcus pyogenes*. (Photograph by Dr. Leon J. LeBeau, Department of Biocommunication Arts, Medical Center, University of Illinois at Chicago.)

accompanied by lymphangitis and abscess formation. Patients with this condition have chills, fever, and marked toxicity. Cellulitis is associated with infection of burns or wounds.

Streptococcal myositis, a rare condition, results in extensive muscle necrosis and overwhelming sepsis.[1] The pathogenesis of this usually fatal infection is unknown. Most patients do not have a local injury, and in those who do the injury is minor; however, blunt trauma to muscles may be involved.[1] Perhaps undefined mechanisms permit these organisms to invade injured muscles following bacteremia.

Rheumatic Fever[12]

Rheumatic fever (RF) is characterized by inflammatory lesions that may involve the heart, joints, subcutaneous tissues, and central nervous system. The classic form of the disease is acute, febrile, and largely self-limited; nevertheless, involvement of the heart may lead to death in the acute stage of the disease or to rheumatic heart disease, a condition characterized by chronic progressive damage to the heart, eventual heart failure, and even death several years after the acute attack. The disease occurs primarily in children 6 to 15 years of age. Rheumatic fever is rampant in the Middle East, the Indian subcontinent, and selected areas of Africa and South America. Furthermore, a resurgence of acute rheumatic fever has recently been reported in the intermountain area of the United States.[94a]

The major manifestations of RF include polyarthritis, carditis, chorea, and erythema marginatum. Polyarthritis occurs in approximately 75% of patients, and carditis in 40% to 50%. Carditis involves all layers of the heart. The characteristic inflammatory lesions of the heart, the Aschoff bodies, arise from injured striated and smooth muscle cells and contain cells with "owl's eyes" or "caterpillar nuclei."[10]

For unknown reasons, RF appears to be a sequela of group A streptococcal pharyngitis but not skin infection. Furthermore, certain strains of *S. pyogenes* appear to be more frequently associated with RF. These strains have large amounts of M protein, possess large hyaluronic acid capsules, and do not produce serum opacity factor.[85] The mechanism by which these strains are able to initiate RF is still undefined, although most lines of evidence suggest that an autoimmune phenomenon is involved. Because of the presence of cross-reactive antigens between streptococci and human tissues, especially the myocardium, it has been suggested that patients produce antistreptococcal antibodies that react with their own hearts. Although this theory is far from being conclusively proved, two recent lines of evidence lend support to its plausibility. First, it has been shown that the group A streptococci contain antigens that cross-react with myosin of the heart.[55] Second, antibodies present in the serum of patients with RF have been shown to react strongly with cardiac myosin; these antibodies can also be absorbed with M proteins from certain serotypes of group A streptococci. Dale and Beachey,[27] the investigators of the latter study, are quick to point out that the cross-reactions between the antibodies and cardiac myosin do not imply a pathologic process. Because patients with RF frequently have exaggerated immune responses, the presence of these antibodies may simply reflect the immune status of the patient and not an abnormal immunologic response to myosin. Further studies should better define the role of these antibodies. Numerous other factors, discussed by Senitzer and Freimer,[85] may play a role in the pathogenesis of RF.

Poststreptococcal Acute Glomerulonephritis[12]

Poststreptococcal acute glomerulonephritis (AGN) is an acute inflammatory disease of the renal glomerulus that may follow group A streptococcal pharyngitis or cutaneous infection. AGN is associated with specific "nephritogenic" serotypes of group A streptococci, and these serotypes differ in pharyngitis and pyoderma-associated AGN. Serotypes 1, 3, 4, 12, and 25 are involved in pharyngitis-associated AGN, whereas serotypes 2, 49, 55, 57, 59, 60, and 61 predominate in pyoderma-associated AGN. In general, the epidemiologic characteristics of AGN vary according to the nature of the antecedent group A streptococcal infection (Table 13-6).

Although the association between group A streptococcal infections and AGN is well established, the precise mechanism by which the initial infection leads to AGN is not known. Most of the available evidence supports the theory that AGN is an immune complex disease resulting from the disposition of preformed complexes of streptococcal antigen and antibody in the kidney.[64] The precise nature of the involved streptococcal antigen is unknown.

The major clinical manifestations of AGN include edema, hypertension, headache, malaise, and circulatory congestion. The urine appears dark or smoky, and hematuria and proteinemia are usually present. The serum levels of total hemolytic complement and C3 complement are reduced. Pathologically the glomeruli of the kidneys appear enlarged and hypercellular as a result of the proliferation of endothelial and mesangial cells. This increased cellularity leads to encroachment of the capillary lumens and the resultant narrowing of these structures. Electron microscopic studies reveal nodular humps on the epithelial side of the basement membrane; these structures are thought to be the deposited immune complexes.

Therapy of AGN is predominantly supportive. Patients are also given pencillin unless they are allergic to it, in which case they receive erythromycin.

GROUP B STREPTOCOCCI[3,42]

The most serious form of group B streptococcal (GBS) disease is neonatal sepsis. This condition is classified as early- or late-onset disease on the basis of several features including the time of onset; early-onset disease occurs at birth or within 7 days of birth, and late-onset disease occurs from 7 days up to 8 to 12 weeks after birth. Early-onset disease is the more common form and has the greater mortality (up to 75%).

Babies who develop early-onset disease become infected in utero or at birth. The degree of colonization of the vagina and cervix of the mother is directly related to the development and severity of disease of the baby. Several risk factors, such as prematurity, prolonged rupture of membranes, and other obstetric complications, are associated with early-onset disease. The most important risk factor, prematurity, is responsible for the diminished immunocompetence of the neonate (described later) and the resulting inability to handle the large numbers of organisms that are introduced by the presence of other obstetric problems. Early-onset disease is associated with group B streptococci of serotypes I, II, and III.

The portal of entry for early-onset disease is probably the upper respiratory tract. Infected neonates usually display some type of respiratory disease plus bacteremia. Bacteremia with or without meningitis may also be seen in the absence of respiratory disease.

The cause of late-onset disease is unknown, but potential sources of infection include the hands or other contacts of colonized mothers or infant-to-infant cross-colonization by the hands of hospital personnel.[6] These infants acquire the organism at mucosal surfaces and display either meningitis or osteomyelitis, both with and without bacteremia. Although the mortality (14% to 18%) is lower than that of early-onset disease, the morbidity secondary to meningitis may be as high as 50%. Type III group B streptococcus is associated with 90% of the cases of late-onset disease.

Adults with diabetes or other underlying conditions, such as genitourinary disorders, are also susceptible to infection by group B streptococci. Disease may be manifest as pyelonephritis, pneumonitis, endometritis, meningitis, and arthritis.[9,73]

GROUP C STREPTOCOCCI[93]

Streptococcus equisimilis is the species of group C streptococci most often associated with human disease, although disease caused by this group of organisms is uncommon. This organism has been associated with pharyngitis, tonsillitis, pneumonia, puerperal sepsis, endocarditis, bacteremia, osteomyelitis, brain abscess, and postoperative wound infection. Approximately 3% of individuals may be asymptomatic pharyngeal carriers of group C streptococci.

The other species of streptococci (*S. zooepidemicus, S. equi,* and *S. dysgalactiae*) are responsible for a wide range of diseases in animals but are rare human pathogens.

GROUP F STREPTOCOCCI[57,69,87]

Group F streptococci* have a marked proclivity for abscess formation in patients with underlying disease or antecedent trauma. These organisms rarely cause disease in otherwise healthy individuals in the absence of trauma. Abscess formation most commonly involves the cutaneous system; the next most common sites (in descending order) are the cervicofacial, dental, and intra-abdominal regions.[57] Group F streptococci have also been associated with empyema, osteomyelitis, meningitis, and bacteremia.

GROUP D STREPTOCOCCI (NONENTEROCOCCI) AND ENTEROCOCCI (*ENTEROCOCCUS* SPP.)

The group D streptococci (nonenterococci) and *Enterococcus* species are significant etiologic agents of urinary tract infections, biliary tract infections, wound infections, intra-abdominal abscesses, endocarditis, and bacteremia.[68] These organisms have also been associated with neonatal septicemia.[8,48]

S. bovis has been associated with neoplasms of the gastrointestinal tract, especially carcinoma of the colon.[54] In fact, it has been suggested that correct identification of *S. bovis* from blood cultures may provide the first clue to the presence of previously unrecognized gastrointestinal disease.[70] It is recommended that patients with *S. bovis* bacteremia undergo a thorough gastrointestinal tract evaluation.[54,67]

GROUP G STREPTOCOCCI[4,100]

Group G streptococci may be carried asymptomatically in the pharynx, gastrointestinal tract, or vagina and on the skin. These organisms are rarely associated with bacteremia, in which case the skin appears to be the most common portal of entry. Predisposing factors for skin entry include the presence of underlying conditions such as alcohol and intravenous drug abuse, diabetes mellitus, and malignancy, which predispose to skin breakdown, subsequent disruption of the skin by surgery or other invasive techniques, and lymphatic obstruction. One study showed the large majority of patients with group G bacteremia to have underlying neurologic malignancies or solid tumors. Other serious infections associated with group G streptococci have included puerperal and neonatal septicemia, joint disease, otitis media, pharyngitis, pneumonia, empyema, meningitis, peritonitis, and cellulitis of the skin. Group G streptococci have also been reported in two outbreaks of pharyngitis caused by contaminated food.[69]

---

*The large majority of organisms reported in these studies as group F streptococci correspond to *S. anginosus* (that is, beta-hemolytic group F organisms).[35]

VIRIDANS STREPTOCOCCI

The viridans streptococci are found as normal flora in the respiratory tract, gastrointestinal tract, and genital tract. These organisms are the most common cause of subacute bacterial endocarditis (SBE). Minor trauma such as cuts or dental manipulations may allow this organism to invade the bloodstream from the pharyngeal region and subsequently infect damaged or undamaged heart valves to cause SBE in susceptible patients. *S. sanguis* I and II, *S. mutans,* and *S. intermedius* are the species implicated most frequently in SBE.[69] It is difficult to assess the rate of the viridans streptococci in infections of the alimentary and genital tracts, since these organisms are often found in mixed culture; however, *S. intermedius* appears to be the species most commonly associated with suppurative infections such as abscesses, cholangitis, empyema, and cellulitis.

S. mutans plays a significant role in tooth decay. As food particles break down in the mouth, the tooth becomes covered with a pellicle of salivary glycoproteins. This action changes the charge at the surface of the tooth and promotes the formation of plaque. Although the first organism to bind to this site is *S. sanguis,* as the plaque matures it is *S. mutans* that produces caries and tooth decay by synthesizing a dextranlike polymer of glucose from the sucrose present.[28]

In the past few years an association between viridans streptococci and neonatal sepsis and meningitis has been observed.[17] A study by Haffar, Fuselier, and Baker[46] showed *S. mitis* to be the single most frequent species of viridans streptococci isolated from neonatal blood cultures. Still, it is interesting that this species was rare in maternal cultures, where *S. sanguis* II and *S. intermedius* predominated. This pronounced discrepancy led the investigators to suggest that *S. mitis* might have increased virulence in neonates. A definitive conclusion awaits further study.

STREPTOCOCCUS PNEUMONIAE

S. pneumoniae is the leading cause of community-acquired bacterial pneumonia, with approximately a half million cases a year being reported in the United States.[36] In infants and children, pneumococci are the most common bacterial cause of pneumonia, otitis media, and bacteremia[53] and a less common cause of meningitis. The types usually associated with bacteremia and meningitis in infants and children are types 6, 14, 18, 19, and 23; type 14 is the most common type associated with invasive disease. Types 3 and 19 are the most common types associated with otitis media.[53] With age the percentage of pneumococcal infections with these types declines, but they still remain among the 14 most important types causing infection in adults.[78] Other common types in adults include 1, 4, 6, 8, and 12.[5]

Pneumococci are carried in the respiratory tract of a significant number of healthy individuals. Transmission of the organism from carrier to susceptible host is directly proportional to the frequency and intimacy of their contact.[77] Individuals with defects of phagocyte function, defects of the humoral system (that is, antibody and complement), and miscellaneous defects in nonimmunologic systems (for instance, skull fracture, ethanol intoxication, and obstruction of the eustachian tube) are predisposed to infection.[52] The most important host defense against this organism is efficient phagocytosis.[52]

It is often difficult to determine the significance of pneumococci present in sputum specimens. Because of the high carriage rate, its presence does not necessarily imply infection. However, if one of the highly pathogenic pneumococcal types is isolated from a rusty-colored sputum that also contains a large number of polymorphonuclear leukocytes, it is usually indicative of a pneumococcal pneumonic process.[36] Additionally, pneumococci isolated from body fluids, blood cultures, or specimens collected via transtracheal or lung puncture from the lower respiratory tract are usually significant.

MECHANISMS OF PATHOGENICITY
STREPTOCOCCUS PYOGENES

Numerous cell-associated and extracellular products may play a role in the virulence of group A beta-hemolytic streptococci.

Extracellular Products
Hemolysins[97]

As previously mentioned, S. pyogenes produces two hemolysins, streptolysin S and streptolysin O.

Streptolysin S. This hemolysin is produced by groups A, C, and G streptococci and is largely responsible for the hemolytic activity observed on blood agar plates. Streptolysin S appears to lyse erythrocytes by an osmotic process after binding to phospholipids in the red blood cell membrane. Streptolysin S can also lyse a wide variety of other eukaryotic cells as well as protoplasts and L forms of bacteria. Other biologic activities include suppression of T lymphocytes and leukotoxicity. The role that this toxin plays in disease is unknown.

Streptolysin O. This hemolysin also lyses a wide variety of mammalian cells but does not affect protoplasts or L forms. Recent studies of the mechanism of lysis of streptolysin O indicate that it first binds to cholesterol in the membrane and then self-associates to form rod-shaped structures that embed within the cell membrane.[11] This embedment generates membrane-penetrating channels, which create large membrane defects and subsequent lysis.

Other biologic activities of streptolysin O include suppression of chemotaxis and motility of neutrophils, inhibition of phagocytosis by macrophages, and cardiotoxicity. Recognition of the latter activity has led to the suggestion that streptolysin O may participate in the cardiac damage of rheumatic fever, perhaps by mediating some type of initial damage, which is followed by the immunologic damage already discussed.

It is interesting to note that cholesterol is a binding site for streptolysin O as well as an inhibitor of streptolysin O. Some investigators have suggested that the inhibitory effects of cholesterol may explain why rheumatic fever follows streptococcal pharyngitis but not skin infections; perhaps the cholesterol in the epidermis inhibits the toxic effects of streptolysin O. Furthermore, patients with throat infections show a strong antibody response to streptolysin O—the basis of the antistreptolysin O titer, which is used diagnostically to prove recent streptococcal infection or to support the diagnosis of acute rheumatic fever and glomerulonephritis. Patients with skin infections, however, show little or no antibody response, again perhaps because of the inhibitory effects of cholesterol in the epidermal tissue.

Erythrogenic toxins

Group A streptococci may produce one or more of three erythrogenic toxins, designated A, B, and C. Erythrogenic tox-

ins are also known as pyogenic exotoxins. These toxins are responsible for a wide range of biologic effects, including pyrogenicity, alteration of the blood-brain barrier, cardiotoxicity, depression of the clearance of the reticuloendothelial system, T-cell mitogenicity, alteration of antibody response to sheep erythrocytes, and the ability to enhance host susceptibility to endotoxin, leading to endotoxin shock.[101] For years it was thought that the erythrogenic toxin was directly responsible for the rash of scarlet fever, but it now appears that the rash is caused by a delayed hypersensitivity reaction to streptococcal antigens that is enhanced by erythrogenic toxin.[83] The primary toxicity of erythrogenic toxin also contributes to the symptoms of scarlet fever. The production of erythrogenic toxin is coded for by a gene carried on a bacteriophage.[59]

Other enzymes

S. pyogenes produces two types of streptokinase enzymes, which activate a substance in plasma to convert plasminogen to plasmin, which in turn lyses fibrin. It has been suggested that these streptokinases may serve as spreading factors for the streptococci by lysing blood clots. Hyaluronidase may also serve as a spreading factor by lysing hyaluronic acid in the basement membrane of tissues. Other spreading factors may include the four deoxyribonucleases, which are designated A, B, C, and D. Although these enzymes do not penetrate mammalian cell membranes, they may degrade the accumulated inflammatory exudate DNA that results from leukocyte disintegration.[28]

The numerous other enzymes include proteinase, nicotinamide adenine dinucleotidase (NADase), esterases, amylase, and neuraminidase—but their role in the pathogenesis of streptococcal infections is unknown. Streptokinase, hyaluronidase, DNAse B, and NADase are all immunogenic, and the demonstration of antibodies to these substances may be used to diagnose infection.

Cell-Associated Factors
M protein

Early studies by Lancefield showed the M protein, a fibrous protein in the cell surface, to be the major virulence determinant for group A streptococci. Strains that lack M protein are avirulent.

The M protein protects the streptococci from opsonization by complement and subsequent phagocytosis by polymorphonuclear neutrophils. This antiphagocytic ability appears to be related to the binding of M protein to fibrinogen.[103]

As previously discussed there are over 70 different types of M protein. Immunity to streptococcal infection depends on the development of antibody to M protein. This immunity is long lasting and type specific, although in rare instances cross-protection by antibody to one type has been demonstrated against organisms of another type.[13]

Lipoteichoic acid

As discussed in Chapter 2, lipoteichoic acid is the adhesive that allows the attachment of S. pyogenes to human epithelial cells (see Figure 2-3).

Peptidoglycan-polysaccharide complexes

The cell walls of streptococci consist of peptidoglycan covalently bound to group-specific polysaccharide.[44] These cell wall components are relatively resistant to digestion and persist

TABLE 13-6. Activity of GBS Enzymes, Toxins, and Other Products and Their Associations with Virulence

Product	Activity	Association with Virulence
EXTRACELLULAR		
CAMP factor	Participates with staphylococcal sphingomyelinase C to cause red blood cell lysis	None
Deoxyribonuclease	Degrades DNA	None
Hyaluronidase	Degrades hyaluronic acid	None
Neuraminidase	Cleavage of sialic acid from bovine submaxillary mucin	May be involved in hyaline membrane disease
Protease	Proteolysis	May be involved in hyaline membrane disease
"Toxin"	Causes pulmonary hypertension and increased pulmonary vascular permeability in sheep	Possible: data from sheep
INTRACELLULAR		
Hippuricase	Hydrolysis of hippuric acid	None
CELL ASSOCIATED		
Hemolysin	Lysis of erythrocytes	Not directly; may be toxic to cells
Lipoteichoic acid	May mediate attachment of GBS to cells	May mediate attachment to cells
Type-specific III antigen	Determines serotype specificity	May activate complement, suppress recruitment of polymorphonuclear leukocytes, or inhibit maturation of macrophages
Sialic acid	Part of cell wall	May enhance invasiveness or act as antiphagocytic factor

Modified from Ferrieri, P.: Antibiot. Chemother. **35**:57, 1985.

for long periods of time within macrophages in inflammatory sites of experimental animal models. These macrophages secrete large amounts of lysosomal enzymes, which are capable of destroying connective tissue. It has been suggested that these undegraded cell wall components may be involved in rheumatic fever.

STREPTOCOCCUS AGALACTIAE

The numerous enzymes, toxins, and other products of group B streptococci and their activities are summarized in Table 13-6. With few exceptions there is little evidence linking any of these substances to virulence. Ayoub and Swingle[6] have proposed that neuraminidase and protease may be involved in the formation of hyaline membrane disease associated with neonatal infection caused by group B streptococci. The type III–specific antigen has been suggested as a virulence factor in neonatal sepsis because its frequency in late-onset disease is out of proportion to its occurrence in colonized patients. This type-specific antigen may contribute to virulence by activating complement, by suppressing the recruitment of polymorphonuclear leukocytes (PMNs), or by inhibiting the maturation of macrophages.[30] Increased levels of sialic acid have also been associated with increased virulence.[86] This substance may directly enhance the invasiveness of the organism, or it may act as a antiphagocytic factor.[86] Evidence suggests that lipoteichoic acid may mediate attachment of group B streptococci to epithelial cells. In neonates this attachment depends on the availability of specific receptor sites that are rich in glycoprotein. The presence of such receptor sites on fetal cell surfaces but not adult cell surfaces may help explain the increased susceptibility of newborn infants to group B streptococcal infections.[71]

Group B beta-hemolytic streptococci produce serious mortality and morbidity in patients with deficient host-defense mechanisms.[62] Individuals with impaired polymorphonuclear function, low complement levels, and lack of type-specific antibody to the infecting group B streptococcal strain appear to be at greater risk for disease.[62] The PMNs of premature infants, for example, show decreased bactericidal activity when exposed to large numbers of organisms. Adults with malfunctions of PMNs are also predisposed to infection. Premature infants have low levels of complement; these low levels decrease the phagocytic effectiveness of PMNs and other phagocytes by depriving them of C3b and C5b opsonins. The lack of type-specific antibody also results in diminished phagocytic ability of PMNs.

OTHER BETA-HEMOLYTIC STREPTOCOCCI

Of the group C streptococci, *S. equisimilis* produces streptolysin O and streptokinase, whereas *S. zooepidemicus* and *S. equi* produce a soluble hemolysin that is unrelated to streptolysin O and S. The streptokinase of group C streptococci is available commercially for the treatment of thromboembolic disease. The hyaluronic acid in the capsule of group C streptococci may impede phagocytosis.[93]

Group F streptococci produce a soluble hemolysin, but their role in pathogenicity, if any, is unknown. Group G streptococci produce streptolysin O, streptokinase, NADase, DNAse, and erythrogenic toxins. An M antigen substance has been reported in the cell wall of one strain of group G streptococci. The in vivo significance of any of these factors has not been determined.

STREPTOCOCCUS PNEUMONIAE

The most important virulence factor of *S. pneumoniae* is the capsule that is responsible for inhibiting phagocytosis. As previously mentioned, efficient opsonization and phagocytosis are necessary for protection against this organism. The inflammatory tissue injury in pneumococcal disease also probably results from the interactions of antibody, complement, and phagocytic cells in this process.[52]

Although the capsule is undoubtedly a virulence factor, it alone can probably not account for the lethality of pneumococcal pneumonia in some hosts. Morbidity may occur after antimicrobial therapy has been initiated, when the organism can no longer be isolated from the blood or tissue, and when the degree of pneumonitis appears to be insufficient to cause death by anoxia.[51] Such consequences have led to the speculation that a toxin such as hemolysin, leukocidin, or neuraminidase may contribute to the virulence of *S. pneumoniae,* but supporting evidence for such a toxin has not been found.[52]

ANTIMICROBIAL SUSCEPTIBILITY

Because streptococci of groups A, B, C, and G are uniformly susceptible to penicillin, antimicrobial susceptibility testing is not routinely performed on these organisms. Such testing may be necessary for serious infections like bacterial endocarditis, in cases of penicillin allergy, or for infections not responding to therapy.

As stated earlier, serious infections caused by *Enterococcus* spp. are treated with penicillin or ampicillin plus an aminoglycoside. These organisms require the synergistic effects of both antimicrobial agents (see Chapter 8 for discussion of synergy screens), since they are resistant to penicillin alone as well as to other beta-lactam antibiotics. The mechanism of this resistance may be attributed in part to the affinity of the enterococcal penicillin-binding proteins for beta-lactams.[66] Because the third-generation cephalosporins are active against a wide range of organisms but are inactive against enterococci, it has been suggested that there is a significant potential for enterococcal superinfection in patients being treated with these antimicrobial agents. The risk of superinfection appears to vary depending on the specific agent. There are several reports of superinfection with moxolactam, for example, but superinfections in patients being treated with cefotaxime are very rare.[66]

S. bovis is generally susceptible to penicillin alone, although resistant strains have been observed.[81] Antimicrobial susceptibility testing should be performed on all isolates of group D streptococci (nonenterococci) and *Enterococcus* spp. from cases of endocarditis.[81]

Most viridans streptococci are susceptible to penicillin, and the large majority of cases of endocarditis caused by these organisms are treated with penicillin alone or with penicillin and an aminoglycoside.[16] Approximately 17% of viridans streptococci, especially *S. sanguis* II and *S. mitis,* are resistant to penicillin.[79] Thus antimicrobial susceptibility testing should be performed on all strains of viridans streptococci recovered from patients with endocarditis or other serious disease states.[16,36]

Strains of viridans streptococci that are multiply resistant to penicillin, oxacillin, the cephalosporins (all generations), piperacillin, azlocillin, and mezlocillin have been reported in South Africa.[41] These multiply resistant strains were more sensitive to vancomycin. Alterations in penicillin-binding proteins appear to be responsible for the resistance of these isolates.[41]

Penicillin is the drug of choice for pneumococcal infection. Over the last 10 years, however, penicillin-resistant as well as multiply resistant strains of *S. pneumoniae* have appeared. Only a few serotypes (4, 6, 9, 14, 19, and 23) are commonly responsible for isolated resistance.[50] Although the mechanism of resistance is unknown, it is possible that it may be due to an R factor capable of conferring multiple resistance. Because of these cases of antimicrobial resistance, it is recommended that routine susceptibility testing be performed on all significant pneumococcal isolates. Performance of susceptibility testing for *S. pneumoniae* was discussed in Chapter 8.

VACCINES

A pneumococcal capsular polysaccharide vaccine has been developed, which incorporates the polysaccharide antigen of the 23 serotypes of pneumococci that are responsible for 87% of pneumococcal disease in the United States. This second-generation vaccine replaces the 14-valent polysaccharide vaccine licensed in 1977.[76,78] Vaccination is primarily recommended for older patients and debilitated patients, including those with sickle cell disease, splenectomized patients, and children aged 2 and older with chronic illnesses specifically associated with increased risk for pneumococcal disease or its complications. It is not suggested for use in children under 2, since it is poorly antigenic in this age group; nor is it recommended for children with recurrent upper respiratory diseases, such as otitis media and sinusitis. In addition, revaccination is not advised.[76]

The development of group B streptococcal vaccines is the focus of ongoing research.[7] Most work has centered on the use of the type III polysaccharide as an immunogen.

REFERENCES

1. Adams, E.M., et al.: Streptococcal myositis, Arch. Intern. Med. **145:**1020, 1985.
2. Agger, W.A., and Maki, D.G.: Efficacy of direct Gram stain in differentiating staphylococci from streptococci in blood cultures positive for gram-positive cocci, J. Clin. Microbiol. **7:**111, 1978.
3. Anthony, B.F.: Epidemiology of GBS in man, Antibiot. Chemother. **35:**10, 1985.
4. Auckenthaler, R., Hermans, P.E., and Washington, J.A., II: Group G streptococcal bacteremia: clinical study and review of the literature, Rev. Infect. Dis. **5:**196, 1983.
5. Austrian, R.: Some observations on the pneumococcus and on the current status of pneumococcal disease and its prevention, Rev. Infect. Dis. **3**(suppl.):S1, 1981.
6. Ayoub, E.M., and Swingle, H.: Pathogenic mechanisms in neonatal GBS infection, Antibiot. Chemother. **35:**128, 1985.
7. Baker, C.J., and Kasper, D.L.: Group B streptococcal vaccines, Rev. Infect. Dis. **7:**458, 1985.
8. Bavikatte, K., et al.: Group D streptococcal septicemia in the neonate, Am. J. Dis. Child. **133:**493, 1979.

9. Bayer, A.S., et al.: Serious infections in adults caused by group B streptococci: clinical and serotypic characterization, Am. J. Med. **61:**498, 1976.

10. Becker, C.G., and Murphy, G.E.: On the pathology of rheumatic heart disease. In Read, S.E., and Zabriskie, J.B., editors: Streptococcal diseases and the immune response, 1980, New York, Academic Press, Inc.

11. Bhakdi, S., et al.: Isolation and identification of two hemolytic forms of streptolysin-O, Infect. Immun. **46:**394, 1984.

12. Bisno, A.L.: Nonsuppurative poststreptococcal sequelae: rheumatic fever and glomerulonephritis. In Mandell, G.L., Douglas, R.G., Jr., and Bennett, J.E., editors: Principles and practice of infectious diseases, ed. 2, New York, 1985, John Wiley & Sons, Inc.

13. Bisno, A.L.: *Streptococcus pyogenes.* In Mandell, G.L., Douglas, R.G., Jr., and Bennett, J.E., editors: Principles and practice of infectious diseases, ed. 2, New York, 1985, John Wiley & Sons, Inc.

14. Bixler-Forell, E., Martin, W.J., and Moody, M.D.: Clinical evaluation of the improved Streptex method for grouping streptococci, Diagn. Microbiol. Infect. Dis. **2:**113, 1984.

15. Bosley, G.S., Facklam, R.R., and Grossman, D.: Rapid identification of enterococci, J. Clin. Microbiol. **18:**1275, 1983.

16. Bourgault, A.-M., Wilson, W.R., and Washington, J.A., II: Antimicrobial susceptibilities of species of viridans streptococci, J. Infect. Dis. **140:**316, 1979.

17. Broughton, R.A., Krafka, R., and Baker, C.J.: Non-group D alpha-hemolytic streptococci, J. Pediatr. **99:**450, 1981.

18. Brown, S., and Fuchs, P.C.: Thiol-dependent streptococci (nutritionally variant streptococci), ASCP Check Sample, Microbiology No. MB80-4 (MD-107), p. 1, 1980.

19. Browne, K., Miegel, J., and Stottmeier, K.D.: Detection of pneumococci in blood cultures by latex agglutination, J. Clin. Microbiol. **19:**649, 1984.

20. Burdash, N.M., and West, M.E.: Identification of *Streptococcus pneumoniae* by the Phadebact coagglutination test, J. Clin. Microbiol. **15:**391, 1982.

21. Burdash, N.M., et al.: Group identification of streptococci: evaluation of three rapid agglutination methods, Am. J. Clin. Pathol. **76:**819, 1981.

22. Campos, J.M., and Charilaou, C.C.: Evaluation of Detect-A-Strep and the Culturette Ten-Minute Strep ID kits for detection of group A streptococcal antigen in oropharyngeal swabs from children. J. Clin. Microbiol. **22:**145, 1985.

22a. Campos, J.M., and Mohla, C.: Comparison of the Quidel Ten Minute Group A Strep Test and the Culturette Brand Ten Minute Group A Strep ID for detection of group A streptococci in throat swabs, Abstracts of the Annual Meeting of the American Society for Microbiology, Abstract C-75, Atlanta, 1987.

23. Carey, R.B.: Handling the nutritionally deficient streptococci in the diagnostic laboratory, Clin. Microbiol. Newsletter **6**(18):131, 1984.

24. Chang, G.T., and Ellner, P.D.: Evaluation of slide agglutination methods for identifying group D streptococci, J. Clin. Microbiol. **17:**804, 1983.

25. Collins, M.D., et al.: *Enterococcus avium* nom. rev., comb. nov.; *E. casseliflavus* nom. rev., comb. nov.: *E. durans* nom. rev., comb. nov.: *E. gallinarum* comb. nov.: and *E. malodoratus* so, nov., Int. J. Syst. Bacteriol. **34:**220, 1984.

26. Cooksey, R.C., Thompson, F.S., and Facklam, R.R.: Physiological characterization of nutritionally variant streptococci, J. Clin. Microbiol. **10:**326, 1979.

27. Dale, J.B., and Beachey, E.H.: Epitopes of streptococcal M proteins shared with cardiac myosin, J. Exp. Med. **162:**583, 1985.

28. Davis, B.D., et al.: Microbiology, ed. 3, Hagerstown, Md., 1980, Harper & Row.

29. Deibel, R.H., and Seeley, H.W., Jr.: Family II: *Streptococcaceae.* In Buchanan, R.E., and Gibbons, N.E., editors: Bergey's manual of determinative bacteriology, ed. 8, Baltimore, 1974, Williams & Wilkins Co.

30. Durham, D.L., et al.: Correlation between the production of extracellular strains and virulence in a mouse model, Infect. Immun. **34:**448, 1981.

31. Dykstra, M.A., McLaughlin, J.C., and Bartlett, R.C.: Comparison of media and techniques for detection of group A streptococci in throat swab specimens, J. Clin. Microbiol. **9:**236, 1979.

32. Facklam, R.R.: Physiological differentiation of viridans streptococci, J. Clin. Microbiol. **5:**184, 1977.

33. Facklam, R.R.: Isolation and identification of streptococci. Part 1. Collection, transportation, and determination of hemolysis, Atlanta, 1978, Center for Disease Control, Department of Health and Human Services.

34. Facklam, R.R.: The major differences in the American and British *Streptococcus* taxonomy schemes with special reference to *Streptococcus milleri*, Eur. J. Clin. Microbiol. **3:**91, 1984.

35. Facklam, R.R.: Serologic identification of streptococci: how useful is serologic grouping? Clin. Microbiol. Newsletter **7:**91, 1985.

36. Facklam, R.R., and Carey, R.B.: Streptococci and aerococci. In Lennette, E.H., et al., editors: Manual of clinical microbiology, ed. 4, Washington, D.C., 1985, American Society for Microbiology.

37. Facklam, R.R., and Smith, P.B.: The gram positive cocci, Hum. Pathol. **7:**187, 1976.

38. Facklam, R.R., et al.: Presumptive identification of group A, B, and D streptococci, Appl. Microbiol. **27:**107, 1974.

39. Facklam, R.R., et al.: Presumptive identification of group A, B, and D streptococci on agar plate media, J. Clin. Microbiol. **9:**665, 1979.

40. Facklam, R.R., et al.: Presumptive identification of streptococci with a new test system, J. Clin. Microbiol. **15:**987, 1982.

40a. Facklam, R.R.: Specificity study of kits for detection of group A streptococci directly from throat swabs, J. Clin. Microbiol. **25:**504, 1987.

41. Farber, B.F., et al.: Multiply resistant viridans streptococci: susceptibility to beta-lactam antibiotics and comparison of penicillin-binding protein patterns, Antimicrob. Agents Chemother. **24:**702, 1983.

42. Ferrieri, P.: GBS infections in the newborn infant: diagnosis and treatment, Antibiot. Chemother. **35:**211, 1985.

43. Gerber, M.A.: Micronitrous acid extraction-coagglutination test for rapid diagnosis of streptococcal pharyngitis, J. Clin. Microbiol. **17:**170, 1983.

44. Ginsberg, I.: *Streptococcus.* In Braude, A.I., Davis, C.E., and Fierer, J., editors: Infectious diseases and medical microbiology, ed. 2, Philadelphia, 1986, W.B. Saunders Co.

45. Gunn, B.A., et al.: Selective and enhanced recovery of group A and B streptococci from throat cultures with sheep blood agar containing sulfamethoxazole and trimethoprim, J. Clin. Microbiol. **5:**650, 1977.

46. Haffar, A.A.M., Fuselier, P.A., and Baker, C.J.: Species distribution of non–group D alpha-hemolytic streptococci in maternal genital and neonatal blood cultures, J. Clin. Microbiol. **18:**101, 1983.

47. Hardie, J.M.: Genus *Streptococcus* Rosenbach 1884, 22[AL]. In Sneath, P.H.A., Mair, N.S., and Sharpe, M.E., editors (Holt, J.G., editor-in-chief): Bergey's manual of systematic bacteriology, vol. 2, Baltimore, 1986, The Williams & Wilkins Co.

48. Headings, D.L., et al.: Fulminant neonatal septicemia caused by *Streptococcus bovis*, J. Pediatr. **92:**282, 1978.

49. Henrichsen, J., et al.: Nomenclature of antigens of group B streptococci, Int. J. Syst. Bacteriol. **34:**500, 1984.

50. Jacobs, M.R., and Koornhof, H.F.: Multiple antibiotic resistance: now the pneumococcus, J. Antimicrob. Chemother. **4:**481, 1978.

51. Jelinkova, J.: Group B streptococci in the human population, Curr. Top. Microbiol. Immunol. **76:**127, 1977.

52. Johnston, R.B., Jr.: The host response to invasion by *Streptococcus pneumoniae:* protection and the pathogenesis of tissue damage, Rev. Infect. Dis. **3:**282, 1981.

53. Klein, J.O.: The epidemiology of pneumococcal disease in infants and children, Rev. Infect. Dis. **3:**246, 1981.

54. Klein, R.S., et al.: *Streptococcus bovis* septicemia and carcinoma of the colon, Ann. Intern. Med. **91:**560, 1979.

55. Krisher, K., and Cunningham, M.W.: Myosin: a link between streptococci and heart, Science **227:**413, 1985.

56. Lauer, B.A., Reller, L.B., and Mirrett, S.: Effect of atmosphere and duration of incubation on primary isolation of group A streptococci from throat cultures, J. Clin. Microbiol. **17:**338, 1983.

57. Libertin, C.R., Hermans, P.E., and Washington, J.A., II: Beta-hemolytic group F streptococcal bacteremia: a study and review of the literature, Rev. Infect. Dis. **7:**498, 1985.

58. Libertin, C.R., Wold, A.D., and Washington, J.A., II: Effects of trimethoprim-sulfamethoxazole and incubation atmosphere on isolation of group A streptococci, J. Clin. Microbiol. **18:**680, 1983.

59. Ludwig, W., et al.: The phylogenetic position of *Streptococcus* and *Enterococcus,* J. Gen. Microbiol. **131:**543, 1985.

60. Mandel, J.H.: Pharyngeal infections: causes, findings, and management, Postgrad. Med. **77:**187, 1985.

61. McCusker, J.J., et al.: Comparison of Directigen Group A Strep Test with a traditional culture technique for detection of group A beta-hemolytic streptococci, Clin. Microbiol. **20:**824, 1984.

62. Meier, F.A., and Hill, H.R.: Host defense deficits in group B streptococcal disease, Clin. Microbiol. Newsl. **7:**97, 1985.

63. Miceika, B.G., Vitous, A.S., and Thompson, K.D.: Detection of group A streptococcal antigen directly from throat swabs with a ten-minute latex agglutination test, J. Clin. Microbiol. **21:**467, 1985.

64. Michael, A.F., and Kim, Y.: Pathogenesis of acute poststreptococcal glomerulonephritis. In Read, S.E., and Zabriskie, J.B., editors: Streptococcal diseases and the immune response, New York, 1980, Academic Press, Inc.

65. Miller, J.M., et al.: Evaluation of the Directigen Group A strep test kit, J. Clin. Microbiol. **20:**846, 1984.

66. Moellering, R.C., Jr., and Eliopoulos, G.M.: Activity of cefotaxime against enterococci, Diagn. Microbiol. Infect. Dis. **2:**85S, 1984.

67. Moellering, R.C., Jr., Korzeniowski, O.M., and Wennersten, C.B.: Species-specific resistant antimicrobial synergism in *Streptococcus faecium* and *Streptococcus faecalis,* J. Infect. Dis. **140:**203, 1979.

68. Moellering, R.C., Jr., Watson, B.K., and Kunz, L.J.: Endocarditis due to group D streptococci, Am. J. Med. **57:**239, 1974.

68a. Mohla, C., and Campos, J.M.: Evaluation of the Tandem ICON Strep A Assay for detection of group A streptococcal antigen in throat swabs, Abstracts of Third European Congress of Clinical Microbiology Interdisciplinary Meeting, May 1987, The Hague, Netherlands.

69. Morello, J.A., and Randall, E.L.: Identification of aerobic gram-positive and gram-negative cocci, Washington, D.C., 1981, American Society for Microbiology.

70. Murray, H.W., and Roberts, R.B.: *Streptococcus bovis* bacteremia and underlying gastrointestinal disease, Arch. Intern. Med. **138:**1097, 1978.

71. Nealon, T.J., and Mattingly, S.J.: Kinetic and chemical analyses of the biologic significance of lipoteichoic acids in mediating adherence of serotype III group B streptococci, Infect. Immun. **50:**107, 1985.

72. Parker, M.T.: Streptococci and lactobacillus. In Wilson, G., and Miles, A., editors: Topley and Wilson's principles of bacteriology, virology, and immunity, vol. 2, ed. 7, London, 1983, Edward Arnold.

73. Pischel, K.D., Weisman, M.H., and Cone, R.O.: Unique features of group B streptococcal arthritis in adults, Arch. Intern. Med. **145:**97, 1985.

74. Pollock, H.M., and Dahlgren, B.J.: Distribution of streptococcal groups in clinical specimens with evaluation of bacitracin screening, Appl. Microbiol. **27:**141, 1974.

75. Radetsky, M., Comparative evaluation of kits for rapid diagnosis of group A streptococcal disease, Pediatr. Infect. Dis. **4:**274, 1985.

76. Recommendations of the Immunization Practices Advisory Committee (ACIP), Update: pneumococcal polysaccharide vaccine usage—United States, MMWR **33:**273, 1984.

77. Riley, I.D., and Douglas, R.M.: An epidemiologic approach to pneumococcal disease, Rev. Infect. Dis. **3:**233, 1981.

78. Robbins, J.B., et al.: Considerations for formulating the second-generation pneumococcal capsular polysaccharide vaccine with emphasis on the cross-reactive types within groups, J. Infect. Dis. **148:**1136, 1983.

79. Roberts, R.B., et al.: Viridans streptococcal endocarditis: the role of various species, including pyridoxal-dependent streptococci, Rev. Infect. Dis. **1:**955, 1979.

80. Ruoff, K.L., et al.: Identification of *Streptococcus bovis* and *Streptococcus salivarius* in clinical laboratories, J. Clin. Microbiol. **20:**223, 1984.

81. Savitch, C.B., Barry, A.L., and Hoeprich, P.D.: Infective endocarditis caused by *Streptococcus bovis* resistant to the lethal effect of penicillin G, Arch. Intern. Med. **138:**931, 1978.

82. Schleifer, K.H., and Kilpper-Balz, R.: Transfer of *Streptococcus faecalis* and *Streptococcus faecium* to the genus *Enterococcus* nom. rev. as *Enterococcus faecalis* comb. nov. and *Enterococcus faecium* comb. nov., Int. J. Syst. Bacteriol. **34:**31, 1984.

83. Schlievert, P.M., Bettin, K.M., and Watson, D.W.: Reinterpretation of the Dick test: rate of group A streptococcal pyrogenic exotoxin, Infect. Immun. **26:**467, 1979.

84. Schwartz, R.H., Gerber, M.A., and McCoy, P.: Effect of atmosphere of incubation on the isolation of group A streptococci from throat cultures, J. Lab. Clin. Med. **106:**88, 1985.

85. Senitzer, D., and Freimer, E.H.: Autoimmune mechanisms in the pathogenesis of rheumatic fever, Rev. Infect. Dis. **6:**832, 1984.

86. Shigeoka, A.O., et al.: Assessment of the virulence factors of group B streptococci: correlation with sialic acid content, J. Infect. Dis. **147:**857, 1983.

87. Shlaes, D.M., et al.: Infections due to Lancefield group F and related streptococci *(S. milleri, S. anginosus),* Medicine **60:**197, 1981.

88. Slifkin, M., Freedel, D., and Gil, G.M.: Direct serogrouping of group B streptococci from urogenital and gastric swabs with nitrous acid extraction and the Phadebact Streptococcus Test, Am. J. Clin. Pathol. **78:**850, 1982.

89. Slifkin, M., and Gil, G.M.: Serogrouping of beta-hemolytic streptococci from throat swabs with nitrous acid extraction and the Phadebact Streptococcus Test, J. Clin. Microbiol. **15:**187, 1982.

90. Slifkin, M., and Gil, G.M.: Evaluation of the Culturette Brand Ten-Minute Group A Strep ID technique, J. Clin. Microbiol. **20:**12, 1984.

91. Slifkin, M., and Pouchet-Melvin, G.R.: Evaluation of three commercially available test products for serogrouping beta-hemolytic streptococci, J. Clin. Microbiol. **11:**249, 1980.

92. Smith, S.K., and Washington, J.A., II: Evaluation of the Pneumo-slide latex agglutination test for identification of *Streptococcus pneumoniae,* J. Clin. Microbiol. **20:**592, 1984.

93. Stamm, A.M., and Cobbs, C.G.: Group C streptococcal pneumonia: report of a fatal case and review of the literature, Rev. Infect. Dis. **2:**889, 1980.

94. Vanzo, S.J., and Washington, J.A., II: Evaluation of a rapid latex agglutination test for identification of group D streptococci, J. Clin. Microbiol. **20:**575, 1984.

94a. Veasy, L.G., et al.: Resurgence of acute rheumatic fever in the inter-mountain area of the United States, N. Engl. J. Med. **316:**421, 1987.

95. Venezia, R.A., et al.: Evaluation of a rapid method for the detection of streptococcal group A antigen directly from throat swabs, J. Clin. Microbiol. **21:**395, 1985.

96. Wannamaker, L.W.: Differences between streptococcal infections of the throat and of the skin, N. Engl. J. Med. **282:**23, 1970.

97. Wannamaker, L.W.: Streptococcal toxins, Rev. Infect. Dis. **5**(suppl.4):S723, 1983.

98. Wannamaker, L.W., Rammelkamp, C.H., and Top, F.H., Sr.: Streptococcal infections. In Wehrle, P.F., and Top, F.H., Sr., editors: Communicable and infectious diseases, ed. 9, St. Louis, 1986, The C.V. Mosby Co.

99. Wasilauskas, B.L., and Hampton, K.D.: Evaluation of the Strep-A-Fluor identification method for group A streptococci, J. Clin. Microbiol. **20:**1205, 1984.

100. Watsky, K.L., Kollisch, N., and Densen, P.: Group G streptococcal bacteremia: the clinical experience at Boston University Medical Center and a critical review of the literature, Arch. Intern. Med. **145:**58, 1985.

101. Weeks, C.R., and Ferretti, J.J.: The gene for type A streptococcal exotoxin (erythrogenic toxin) is located in bacteriophage T 12, Infect. Immun. **46:**531, 1984.

102. Wetkowski, M.A., Peterson, E.M., and de la Maza, L.M.: Direct testing of blood cultures for detection of streptococcal antigens, J. Clin. Microbiol. **16:**86, 1982.

103. Whitnack, E., and Beachey, E.H.: Biochemical and biological properties of the binding of human fibrinogen to M protein in group A streptococci, J. Bacteriol. **164:**350, 1985.

CHAPTER 14

Neisseria

Barbara J. Howard

The organisms in the genus *Neisseria* consist of aerobic gram-negative cocci that inhabit the mucous membranes of humans and other animals. Some species are found as normal flora in the nasopharynx and oropharynx and are usually considered nonpathogenic. The two pathogenic species, *N. gonorrhoeae* and *N. meningitidis,* however, may cause such diseases as gonorrhea and meningitis. Although *N. meningitidis* may be found as normal nasopharyngeal flora in 10% to 15% of the population, under appropriate conditions it may spread to individuals who do not have sufficient antibody protection and result in meningococcemia or meningitis. *N. meningitidis* is isolated from the cerebrospinal fluid, blood, and nasopharynx and is occasionally isolated from the genitourinary tract. The clinical specimens from which *N. gonorrhoeae* may be isolated include urethral exudates, cervical, rectal, and pharyngeal specimens, and occasionally the cerebrospinal fluid, joints, and skin. Since both of these organisms may exist in the same habitat, it is critical that specific identification methods be used to distinguish them.

CLASSIFICATION

Bergey's Manual of Systematic Bacteriology includes the genus *Neisseria* as one of the four genera in family VIII—*Neisseriaceae*—in Section 4, "Gram-Negative Aerobic Rods and Cocci."[104] The other genera in the family *Neisseriaceae* are *Moraxella, Acinetobacter,* and *Kingella* (see Chapter 17). Based on genetic studies, the genus *Branhamella* has been reclassified as a subgenus of *Moraxella.*[9] *B. catarrhalis* is now designated *Moraxella (Branhamella) catarrhalis* in *Bergey's Manual of Systematic Bacteriology* but because of common accepted usage is referred to as *B. catarrhalis* in this chapter.

There are 11 species in the genus *Neisseria: N. gonorrhoeae, N. meningitidis, N. lactamica, N. sicca, N. subflava, N. flavescens, N. mucosa, N. cinerea, N. denitrificans, N. elongata,* and *N. canis. N. subflava* includes the organisms previously designated as *N. subflava, N. perflava,* and *N. flava.* They are now considered collectively as one species because of their close genetic, morphologic, and biochemical relationship. *N. subflava,* as well as *N. lactamica, N. sicca, N. mucosa,* and *N. cinerea,* is found in the nasopharynx of humans. *N. elongata* is isolated from the pharynx of healthy individuals and from individuals with pharyngitis.[104] Unlike the other coccal-shaped *Neisseria* spp., *N. elongata* is a short, slender rod. *N. denitrificans* is isolated from the upper respiratory tract of guinea pigs. *N. canis* is isolated from the upper respiratory tract of cats but has also been recovered from a human cat-bite wound.[44]

The taxonomic status of three other species of previously designated *Neisseria—N. caviae, N. ovis,* and *N. cuniculi*—is uncertain. These species are classified in the current edition of *Bergey's Manual of Systematic Bacteriology* both as *species incertae sedis* of *Neisseria* and as members of the *Branhamella* subgenus of *Moraxella.* Additional studies should resolve the controversial status of these organisms.

SPECIMEN COLLECTION AND PROCESSING[53,72,73]

Successful isolation of the pathogenic species of *Neisseria* organisms depends on careful collection and processing techniques. Specimens must be processed immediately because of the sensitivity of these organisms to drying and temperature extremes. As mentioned in Chapter 11, meningococci are quite sensitive to cold, and specimens suspected of containing this organism should never be refrigerated. Because gonococci are also susceptible to the effects of antiseptics, disinfectants should not be used for preparing the patient or for lubricating the collection equipment.

NEISSERIA GONORRHOEAE

Use of the direct smear or culture of various body sites (or both) for the diagnosis of gonorrhea depends on the sex, sexual practices, and clinical condition of the patient.

When used by properly trained personnel, the direct Gram stain is approximately 95% sensitive and 100% specific for the diagnosis of gonococcal urethritis in symptomatic men (Plate 7, C).[48] Culture of the urethra of these patients may be necessary only if the direct smear is equivocal or negative. The direct smear, however, is not sensitive enough to detect infection in asymptomatic men and a culture must be done. Urethral specimens may be collected from men by inserting a calcium alginate swab or a burr-free platinum inoculating loop into the urethral orifice.

When gonorrhea is suspected in homosexual men, pharyngeal, rectal, and urethral specimens should be cultured. Rectal swabs may be collected by inserting sterile cotton-tipped swabs approximately 1 inch into the anal canal and moving the swab from side to side for 10 to 30 seconds to allow sufficient sampling of the crypts. Direct smears of rectal swabs are not recommended, but smears of rectal mucosa obtained through an anoscope may be useful.[73] Pharyngeal cultures are collected as discussed in Chapter 11. Smears of the oropharynx are not helpful because of the presence of normal *Neisseria* spp.

The sensitivity of endocervical smears in detecting gonorrhea in symptomatic women is only 60%.[53] Thus cervical and rectal cultures should be performed to diagnose infection in these patients as well as in asymptomatic women known to be contacts of infected men. In some instances, especially after antimicrobial therapy, rectal culture findings may be positive when endocervical culture findings are negative. Endocervical specimens are collected with a speculum.

Blood cultures should be drawn in suspected disseminated gonococcal infection in both men and women. Endocervical and rectal cultures should also be obtained from women and urethral cultures from men. Other specimens should be collected depending on the sexual practices of the patient. Biopsies of skin lesions or aspirates of joint fluid may be performed if these sites are thought to be infected. Direct smears should be performed on endocervical and urethral specimens, skin lesions, and joint fluid.

Pharyngeal cultures should be collected whenever pharyngitis is present or there is a history of orogenital contact. Swabs of conjunctival exudates may be collected from infants with conjunctivitis.

To confirm that antimicrobial therapy has been effective, cultures should be collected from the initially infected site 1 week after completion of treatment. Both rectal and endocervical specimens should be collected from women for the reason cited previously.

Ideally, specimens should be plated directly onto culture media and incubated immediately. This is frequently not possible, however, and a transport or holding medium must be used to maintain the viability of the organisms. In hospitals with microbiology laboratories, a holding medium such as Stuart or Amies is usually sufficient. As mentioned in Chapter 11, these nonnutritive media maintain pH, prevent drying, and preserve the organisms in the ratio collected. Because the efficacy of these media depends on good reducing conditions, the tubes should be airtight and almost filled with media, and exposure to the air during insertion of the swab should be absolutely minimal.[53] These media are recommended for transport of swabs from hospital wards or clinics to the laboratory if primary plating cannot be performed within 5 minutes of collection.[53] On receipt, the swabs are removed and inoculated directly onto culture media. If cotton swabs are used, the holding medium must contain charcoal to inhibit toxic lipids present in the cotton. The holding medium should not be used for transport beyond 6 hours.[53]

Physicians' offices or small hospitals or clinics that do not have microbiology laboratories need to use transport systems that will ensure the viability of the Neisseria organisms for longer periods of time. Such systems (Transgrow and Jembec) provide essential nutrients and CO_2 requirements. The Transgrow system is a flat bottle coated with modified Thayer-Martin agar along the inner flat surface and bottled under a partial CO_2 atmosphere. When the Transgrow system was first introduced, it definitely helped resolve the viability problems associated with prolonged transit periods. However, these bottles are rarely used today because of several problems, including variability in their CO_2 content, mechanical difficulties in manipulating the bottle, and the tendency for moisture to collect on the inner surface of the bottle, promoting the spread of contaminants.

The Jembec, an acronym for John E. Martin Biological Environmental Chamber, has gained wider use in laboratories. This system consists of a flat plastic dish containing a culture medium and a well for a CO_2-generating tablet.[63] The tablet, composed of sodium bicarbonate and citric acid, is activated by the moisture in the medium. After inoculation of the medium, the tablet is placed in the well and the entire dish is inserted into a zip-lock plastic pouch and incubated for 18 to 24 hours before shipment to the laboratory. After receiving the specimen in the laboratory, the microbiologist should examine the plate for the typical N. gonorrhoeae colonies. If no growth is observed, the plates should be removed from the pouch and reincubated in a CO_2 incubator or in a candle extinction jar. The media are placed in the candle jar, and a white unscented candle affixed to a Petri dish is placed on top of the media and lighted. Placing a tight-fitting lid on the jar causes the flame to be extinguished, which establishes an atmosphere of 3% to 5% CO_2. Only white unscented wax candles should be used, since certain colored candles emit toxic substances.[73] Candle jars, although clumsy, can also be used to transport cultures to the laboratory.

A variety of other commercial systems are available for transport (and frequently presumptive identification) of N. gonorrhoeae. The Bio-Bag (Marion Scientific, Kansas City, Mo.) discussed in Chapter 11 may be used for transport. The Gono-Pak (BBL Microbiology Systems, Cockeysville, Md.) is a modification of the Jembec system and uses a 60 or 100 mm Petri dish and a CO_2-generating tablet in a larger zip-lock pouch. Other systems are discussed by Lewis.[62]

NEISSERIA MENINGITIDIS

N. meningitidis may be recovered from the blood and cerebrospinal fluid. Nasopharyngeal cultures are used to detect carriers of N. meningitidis. Specific processing techniques for the isolation of meningococci from these sources are discussed in Chapter 11.

The ability to isolate the meningococcus from petechial lesions varies widely.[2] In an early study by Hoyne and Brown[47] meningococci were found in smears from petechiae of 69.8% of the patients examined.

GROWTH REQUIREMENTS
MEDIA

B. catarrhalis and the Neisseria spp. other than N. meningitidis and N. gonorrhoeae grow on nutrient agar devoid of blood. N. meningitidis and N. gonorrhoeae, however, are fastidious and require serum or blood in addition to other accessory growth factors. N. gonorrhoeae is more fastidious than N. meningitidis and requires chocolate agar for growth, whereas N. meningitidis grows on regular blood agar.

A selective medium should be used for isolating the pathogenic Neisseria from sites that may be contaminated with other bacterial flora. With the exception of nasopharyngeal specimens, specimens submitted for recovery of N. meningitidis are not likely to be contaminated and thus do not necessitate the use of selective media. These specimens may be inoculated onto blood agar and chocolate agar. Nasopharyngeal swabs should be plated on blood agar and a selective medium.

Urogenital, urethral, cervical, and most other specimens from which N. gonorrhoeae is recovered are heavily contaminated with normal flora and mandate the use of a selective medium. The observation that certain bacteria such as Citrobacter diversus, Enterobacter cloacae, Serratia marcescens, Pseudomonas, and Candida are strong inhibitors of N. gonorrhoeae growth[61] confirms the importance of using a selective medium.

Selective media include modified Thayer-Martin (MTM) agar, New York City (NYC) agar, and Martin-Lewis (ML)

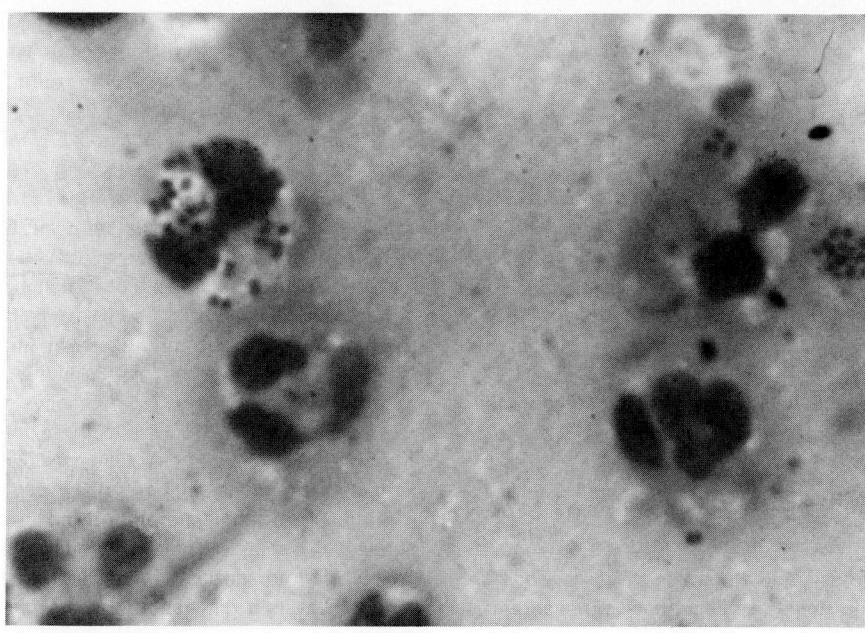

FIGURE 14-1. Typical gram-negative, kidney bean–shaped diplococci of *N. gonorrhoeae.* (Photograph by Dr. Leon J. LeBeau, Department of Biocommunication Arts, Medical Center, University of Illinois at Chicago.)

agar. The antimicrobial agents in these media, which are discussed in Appendix A, account for their selectivity for the pathogenic *Neisseria.* MTM agar contains the antimicrobial agents vancomycin, colistin, nystatin, and trimethoprim lactate. NYC medium contains vancomycin, colistin, amphotericin B, and trimethoprim lactate, and ML medium contains vancomycin, colistin, anisomycin, and trimethoprim lactate. These media are discussed in Appendix A. A modified NYC medium that does not contain hemoglobin will also support the growth of *N. gonorrhoeae,* as well as *Mycoplasma pneumoniae* and urogenital mycoplasmas.[37]

Some strains of *N. gonorrhoeae* are susceptible to vancomycin in selective media and may not be recovered.[11,23,71,83,108] For this reason it has been suggested that chocolate agar (which does not contain vancomycin and thus is noninhibitory) should be used along with a selective medium to isolate gonococci.[40,83] Although use of both media provides optimal recovery, the added expense of chocolate agar may outweigh the benefits for those laboratories in areas of the United States where vancomycin-sensitive strains are rarely recovered.[8] An alternative solution is to use a nonselective medium for patients who are suspected of having gonorrhea but whose initial cultures are negative.[71] For laboratories that use a selective medium only, inoculation of the same plate of selective medium with two separate swabs increases the yield of *N. gonorrhoeae.*[8,51]

Because of the sensitivity of the *Neisseria* organisms to low temperatures, it has become common practice in microbiology laboratories to bring refrigerated culture media to room temperature before inoculation. Two studies, however, have shown no major differences in the isolation rates of *N. gonorrhoeae* on cold or warm media.[21,82] Colonies do tend to be larger and more numerous on room temperature plates after 24 hours, but growth is essentially the same on both room temperature and

refrigerated plates after 48 hours.[82] Occasionally, isolated cold-intolerant strains may not yield colonies if the inoculum is too small.[20]

ENVIRONMENTAL REQUIREMENTS

Members of the genus *Neisseria* and *B. catarrhalis* are aerobic organisms, and little or no growth occurs under anaerobic conditions. *N. gonorrhoeae* and *N. meningitidis* require increased CO_2 (3% to 7%) for growth. Although the exact mechanism of this increased CO_2 requirement is unknown, it has been linked to the initiation of growth and correlated with various phases of the growth cycle. It is required during the lag phase, not required during the exponential phase, but required again later as the colonies age.[79] The additional CO_2 may be supplied by incubation in a CO_2 incubator, a candle jar, or any of the commercial systems previously discussed.

Cultures for isolation of *Neisseria* strains should be incubated at 35° C. Although some strains of *N. gonorrhoeae* grow moderately well after 24 hours, others require 48 or 72 hours before being discarded as negative. Other species of *Neisseria* and *B. catarrhalis* grow moderately well in 18 to 24 hours.

CULTURAL CHARACTERISTICS
STAINING REACTIONS

Members of the genus *Neisseria* (except for *N. elongata*) and *B. catarrhalis* (Plate 7, *B*) typically appear as gram-negative diplococci with adjacent sides flattened. *N. elongata* appear as rods. *Neisseria* and *Branhamella* spp. may occur singly or in masses and tend to form tetrads.

The morphology of *N. gonorrhoeae* in direct smears of urethral or endocervical exudates has classically been described as intracellular, gram-negative, kidney bean–shaped diplococci (Figure 14-1; Plate 7, *C*). Although usually located within the

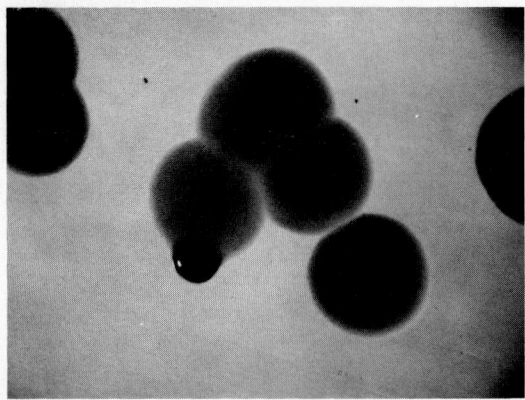

FIGURE 14-2. Colonial types of *N. gonorrhoeae*. Note that types 1 and 2 appear glistening. (From Finegold, S.M., and Baron, E.J.: Bailey and Scott's diagnostic microbiology, ed. 7, St. Louis, 1986, The C.V. Mosby Co.)

polymorphonuclear leukocytes, organisms may also appear extracellularly. In highly contaminated specimens such as endocervical specimens, gram-negative organisms other than gonococci may also be seen within leukocytes, and thus it cannot be assumed that all such forms are *N. gonorrhoeae*.[53] When examining a direct smear for gonococci the microbiologist should note the morphology and staining characteristics of the organism, its location (that is, intracellular versus extracellular), and the presence and quantity of polymorphonuclear leukocytes and epithelial cells. A semiquantitative reporting system such as that described by Kellogg[53] should be used to note the numbers of organisms and cells.

N. meningitidis resembles *N. gonorrhoeae* in direct smears and like *N. gonorrhoeae* may appear intracellularly or extracellularly. Meningococci also tend to be resistant to decolorization in direct smears of cerebrospinal fluid (CSF). Gram stains of isolates of both organisms may reveal oval or spherical cocci without the typical diplococcal arrangement.

COLONIAL MORPHOLOGY

Five colonial types of *N. gonorrhoeae* have been described.[49,56] The microbiologist can most easily discern these with a stereoscopic microscope using the procedures outlined by Jephcott and Reyn[49] or Juni and Heym.[52]

Freshly isolated strains of *N. gonorrhoeae* consist of types 1 and 2. Type 1 is a small, raised, slightly viscid dewdrop colony whereas type 2 is small, raised, and friable. Types 1 and 2 reflect incident light and appear glistening (Figure 14-2). Types 1 and 2 may be maintained in the laboratory by selective transfer.[56] During nonselective transfer, however, types 1 and 2 revert to types 3 to 5, which are larger and slightly convex and do not reflect incident light (Plate 7, *D*). Types 1 and 2 possess pili and are virulent, whereas types 3 to 5 are negative for both of these characteristics.[53] Based on the presence or absence of pili, T_1 and T_2 colonies are now designated P^+ or P^{++}, and T_3, T_4, and T_5 colonies as P^-.

Colonies of *N. meningitidis* appear round, approximately 1 mm in diameter, smooth, glistening, bluish gray, translucent, and butyrous after incubation at 35° C for 24 hours (Plate 7, *E*). Colonies tend to become rubbery with age.

Colonies of *N. lactamica* are convex, smooth, glossy, buty-

rous, and semitranslucent to semiopaque. They may possess a yellowish pigment. Colonies of the other nonpathogenic species of *Neisseria* range from the dry, wrinkled forms of *N. sicca* to the smooth, opaque forms of *N. flavescens* and *N. subflava;* the latter two organisms may produce a yellow pigment. Colonies of the nonpathogenic *Neisseria* spp. tend to be adherent as demonstrated by the ease with which colonies may be pushed across the agar surface or picked up in their entirety with an inoculating loop.

After 24 hours of incubation, colonies of *B. catarrhalis* appear convex, whitish gray, nonhemolytic, opaque, and friable, frequently with a crenated edge. They do not adhere to the agar.

BIOCHEMICAL IDENTIFICATION
PATHOGENIC *NEISSERIA*

After cultures suspected of containing *N. gonorrhoeae* or *N. meningitidis* have incubated for 18 to 24 hours at 35° C in increased CO_2, they should be observed for colonies demonstrating the morphologic characteristics cited previously. An oxidase test (Appendix A) and a Gram stain should be performed on suspect isolates. Kovac's method or commercially available oxidase strips (PathoTec CO, General Diagnostics, Morris Plains, N.J.) are recommended for the oxidase test. With Kovac's method, the colony is touched with a platinum loop (nichrome may give false-positive results) and transferred to a piece of paper containing tetramethyl-*p*-phenylenediamine. If the enzyme cytochrome oxidase is present, it will oxidize the colorless reagent to form a dark blue or black compound within 10 seconds. Oxidase-positive gram-negative diplococci isolated on MTM media from genitourinary specimens may be presumptively identified as *N. gonorrhoeae*. Likewise, oxidase-positive, gram-negative diplococci isolated in pure culture on selective media from CSF are suspicious isolates of *N. meningitidis*. However, because these two organisms may be isolated from the same sites and because other *Neisseria* spp. such as *N. lactamica* or *N. cinerea* may also grow on selective media and resemble the pathogenic *Neisseria* morphologically, definitive identification is mandatory.

Carbohydrate utilization tests have historically been used to differentiate among the *Neisseria* spp. (These tests are sometimes referred to in the literature as fermentation tests. However, use of the term ''fermentation'' is incorrect because most *Neisseria* spp. use carbohydrates oxidatively.[75]) Cystine-tryptic agar (CTA medium; Appendix A) is the most commonly used basal medium for carbohydrate utilization studies. Various carbohydrates (glucose, maltose, sucrose, lactose, or fructose) in impregnated disks or in 1% concentration are added to the CTA basal media. These media are then inoculated with a subculture from the primary isolation plate in one of two ways. A drop of a dense suspension of the organism in 0.5 ml saline may be stabbed into the upper third of the medium using a cotton-plugged capillary pipette. Alternatively, a full 3 mm loopful of growth from the subculture plate may be deposited a few millimeters below the surface of the medium. The latter method provides more rapid and reliable results.[73] With either method the failure to use pure cultures of the test isolate results in misidentification.[40]

The CTA media are incubated at 35° C in a non-CO_2 incubator and observed periodically for 24 hours (or longer). Acid production is indicated by a color change of the phenol red indicator from red to yellow in the upper portion of the tube. *N. gonorrhoeae* utilizes glucose only, whereas *N. meningitidis* uses both glucose and maltose.

Several problems have been reported with the CTA media, especially in the identification of gonococci. First, certain fastidious strains of *N. gonorrhoeae* may grow poorly in CTA media, delaying results for 3 or more days[81] and requiring a large amount of inoculum.[58] This prolonged incubation may result in nonspecific reaction patterns.[110] For example, alkaline products produced from peptone utilization may neutralize the small amounts of acid produced.[58] Finally, certain strains of gonococci may give negative glucose reactions with this method, and occasional strains of meningococci may show negative maltose reactions.[53]

To circumvent these problems, new test media and test methods have been proposed. A modified Hugh and Liefson oxidation-fermentation medium has been suggested as an alternative test medium.[58] Having an increased concentration of carbohydrate relative to peptone, a lowered concentration of phenol red, and an initial pH of 7.2, this medium provides more distinct and consistent reactions, even with problem *Neisseria* spp., when compared with conventional CTA medium.[58]

Because many of the problems with CTA media are associated with the dependency of these media on growth of *Neisseria* spp., Kellogg and Turner[54] subsequently developed a non-growth-dependent test. This so-called rapid fermentation test (RFT), which was later modified by Brown,[12] uses a heavy inoculum of organisms in a small volume of carbohydrate-containing buffered salts solution (see Appendix A for procedure). (''Reagent-grade'' carbohydrates [Sigma, St. Louis, Mo.; Fisher Scientific, Silver Spring, Md.; Mallinkrodt, St. Louis, Mo.] should be used with this method as well as with the CTA procedure.) Although the problems encountered with the CTA method were resolved by the RFT, which yields results in 4 hours, both methods use an inoculum from a subculture of the primary isolation plate, thus increasing the total identification time.

In 1978 Damato reported on the identification of the pathogenic *Neisseria* spp. using enzymatic profiles obtained with chromogenic substrates.[24] *Neisseria* spp. produce certain key enzymes including glycosidases, aminopeptidases, esterases, and acid phosphatases that liberate chromogens (colored products) from selected substrates. This method is advantageous because it can be performed using a single colony from the primary isolation plate and results can be obtained within 4 hours. Furthermore, the test is not dependent on growth of the *Neisseria* organisms nor the use of pure carbohydrates.

Many commercially available rapid systems also use enzyme hydrolysis of chromogenic substrates. The Gonochek II system (E-Y Laboratories, San Mateo, Calif.), for example, uses mixed chromogenic substrates in a single test tube for the identification of *N. gonorrhoeae, N. meningitidis, N. lactamica,* and *B. catarrhalis* within 30 minutes. The RapID NH system (Innovative Diagnostics Systems, Atlanta, Ga.) uses conventional biochemical and single substrate chromogenic tests to identify *N. gonorrhoeae, N. meningitidis,* a variety of other *Neisseria* spp., *B. catarrhalis, Kingella* spp., and *Moraxella* spp. and related M groups. The RapID NH system also identifies *Haemophilus* spp. These systems are discussed in Chapter 9. The Quad-Ferm + (Analytab Products, Plainview, N.Y.) has recently been marketed for identification of *Neisseria.* This system determines utilization of glucose, maltose, sucrose, and lactose, as well as beta-lactamase production.

The Minitek (BBL Microbiology Systems, Cockeysville, Md.) may also be used for rapid identification of members of the genus *Neisseria.*

The Minitek uses carbohydrate-impregnated paper disks to distinguish among *Neisseria* strains (see Chapter 9 for a discussion of the equipment). Most isolates can be identified within 4 hours of inoculation.[74]

DIFFERENTIATION OF *BRANHAMELLA CATARRHALIS* AND OTHER *NEISSERIA* SPP.

B. catarrhalis and the commensal *Neisseria* spp. are not routinely identified in the clinical laboratory, but it is frequently necessary to differentiate these organisms from the pathogenic *Neisseria* spp., since they may be isolated from the same sites. Furthermore, the association of *B. catarrhalis* with disease in immunocompromised patients or in pediatric patients (see below) may necessitate the identification of this organism in these individuals.

B. catarrhalis can be distinguished from the pathogenic *Neisseria* organisms on the basis of its growth on blood agar at 22° C, growth on simple nutrient agar (for example, trypticase soy agar or Mueller-Hinton agar) at 35° C, reduction of nitrate and nitrite, inability to ferment carbohydrates, and production of DNAse.[73] The last characteristic also distinguishes *B. catarrhalis* from the commensal *Neisseria* spp. The inability of *B. catarrhalis* to grow on MTM agar has previously been reported as a distinguishing feature but should not be used because it is frequently unreliable.[27]

Carbohydrate fermentation, reduction of nitrate and nitrite, and production of an iodine-reacting polysaccharide from sucrose may aid in differentiating the commensal *Neisseria* spp. from each other and from the pathogenic species.[44,58,73] Note in Table 14-1 that *N. lactamica* is the only *Neisseria* sp. that produces acid from lactose. The enzyme responsible for lactose fermentation, beta-galactosidase, can be readily detected with an *o*-nitrophenyl-β-galactosidase (ONPG; Appendix A) test.

Among the saccharolytic commensal *Neisseria* spp., *N. sicca, N. mucosa,* and sometimes *N. subflava* produce an iodine-reacting polysaccharide from sucrose but not from other carbohydrates.[43] Polysaccharide synthesis is determined on 48-hour cultures grown at 37° C on brain heart infusion agar containing 5% sucrose. Lugol iodine (1:4 dilution) is added to the culture; a blue color develops around positive colonies.[44] *N. mucosa* may then be separated from the other polysaccharide-producing species by its reduction of nitrate. The nitrate (or nitrite) reduction test is performed by inoculating the organism into Mueller-Hinton or heart infusion broth containing 0.1% KNO_3 or KNO_2. (Growth of fastidious strains may be improved by the addition of serum.) The cultures are incubated for up to 5 days and tested occasionally by adding sulfanilic acid and alpha-naphthylamine, and, when appropriate, zinc dust to an aliquot of the broth solution.

N. cinerea resembles *N. gonorrhoeae* morphologically and may be misidentified as the gonococcus when acid production from glucose is weak.[59] Misidentification has also occurred using commercial systems.[10,28] Differentiation of *N. cinerea* is accomplished by demonstrating its susceptibility to colistin (10 μg) and its growth on simple nutrient media.[59] If findings are

TABLE 14-1. Characteristics of *Neisseria* Spp. and *Branhamella catarrhalis*

Species	Colony Morphology	MTM, ML, or NYC Medium	Growth on Chocolate or Blood Agar at 22°C	Nutrient Agar at 35°C	Acid Production from Glucose	Maltose	Lactose	Sucrose	Fructose	Reduction of NO$_3$	NO$_2$	Polysaccharide Synthesis	DNAse
N. gonorrhoeae	Gray to white, smooth, five colony types on subculture from primary	+	0	0	+	0	0	0	0	0	0	0	0
N. meningitidis	Nonpigmented or gray to white, some yellowish, smooth, transparent, encapsulated strains mucoid	+	0	0	+	+	0	0	0	0	V	0	0
N. lactamica	Nonpigmented or yellowish, smooth, transparent	+	V	+	+	+	+	0	0	0	+	0	0
N. sicca	Nonpigmented, wrinkled, coarse and dry, adherent	0	V	+	+	+	0	+	+	0	+	+	0
N. subflava	Greenish yellow, smooth, often adherent	0	V	V	+	+	0	V	V	0	+	V	0
N. mucosa	Sometimes yellowish, mucoid appearance due to capsule production	0	+	+	+	+	0	+	+	+	+	+	0
N. flavescens	Yellow, opaque, smooth	0	+	+	0	0	0	0	0	0	+	+	0
N. cinerea	Grayish white, slightly granular	V	V	+	0	0	0	0	0	0	+	0	0
N. elongata[a]	Grayish white, slight yellowish tinge, flat, glistening, dry, claylike consistency	0	+	+	0	0	0	0	0	0	+	0	0
B. catarrhalis	Nonpigmented or gray, opaque, smooth	0	+	+	0	0	0	0	0	+	+	0	+

SYMBOLS: +, Strains typically positive, but genetic mutants that lack the requisite enzyme activity are occasionally encountered
0, Most strains negative
V, Variable characteristic

From Morello, J.A., Janda, W.M., and Bohnhoff, M.: *Neisseria* and *Branhamella*. In Lennette, E.H., et al., editors.: Manual of clinical microbiology, ed. 4, Washington, D.C., 1985, American Society for Microbiology.
[a]Weakly positive or negative catalase test, in contrast to other *Neisseria* spp.

positive, the gonococcal coagglutination test may also distinguish *N. cinerea* from *N. gonorrhoeae*, since no cross-reactions between these two organisms have been reported.[61]

SEROLOGIC AND IMMUNOSEROLOGIC IDENTIFICATION

IMMUNOSEROLOGIC DETECTION AND IDENTIFICATION

Neisseria gonorrhoeae

Commercial coagglutination methods are available for identification of the gonococcus. Both the Phadebact Monoclonal GC OMNI test (Pharmacia Diagnostics, Piscataway, N.J.) and the GonoGen test (Micro-Media Systems, Potomac, Md.) use mouse monoclonal antibody to the major outer membrane protein (protein I) of *N. gonorrhoeae*. With both systems, isolates may be tested directly from the primary culture plate. The Phadebact Monoclonal GC OMNI test has only recently been marketed and replaces the previous Phadebact polyvalent test. A recent report shows the Phadebact monoclonal test to be highly sensitive and specific.[1]

A fluorescent monoclonal antibody test for culture confirmation of *N. gonorrhoeae* has recently been marketed (Micro-Trak *Neisseria gonorrhoeae* Culture Confirmation Test, Syva, Palo Alto, Calif.). Studies show this test to be sensitive and specific.[30a,61a]

Gonozyme is a commercially available (Abbott Laboratories, Chicago, Ill.) solid-phase immunoassay recently developed for the direct detection of gonococci in genital specimens. Swabs used to collect the specimens are mixed vigorously in the commercial specimen dilution buffer, and 0.2 ml of this sample solution is added to a well in a test tray. A specially treated bead that absorbs gonococcal antigen from the specimen is then placed in each well. After incubation and washing, rabbit antibody to *N. gonorrhoeae* is added. This mixture is also incubated and washed before antirabbit immunoglobulin goat serum conjugated to horseradish peroxidase is added. Following another incubation and washing, the beads are transferred to polystyrene tubes and *O*-phenylenediamine-2 HC1 substrate is added. If the specimen is positive, a visible color change occurs. The intensity of the color reaction is determined spectrophotometrically in a Quantum spectrophotometer (Abbott Laboratories) and is proportional to the quantity of gonococcal antigen that is present.

Studies by Stamm and others[96] and Schachter and others[88] have shown the Gonozyme test to be equal to the Gram stain in sensitivity and specificity for diagnosis of urethral gonorrhea in symptomatic men, but less sensitive and specific than culture for detection of cervical infection in women. Differences in sampling technique, however, may influence the sensitivity of the test in the diagnosis of cervical gonorrhea.[38,88] A recent study[38] comparing the Gonozyme test to culture showed the Gonozyme test to be 100% sensitive for detection of cervical gonorrhea when the swab containing the specimen was first used to prepare a suspension and the suspension was then used to inoculate both the culture plates and the EIA specimen buffer. Lower sensitivities have been reported when the swab is used to inoculate duplicate cultures before inoculation of the EIA tube.[88] One major drawback of the Gonozyme test is the fact that the swab is inoculated directly into the specimen buffer; therefore no organisms are available for detecting penicillinase production unless a culture is also performed. Furthermore, the system should not be used with pharyngeal or rectal specimens because of the presence of cross-reacting antigens.[38] Additional studies are needed to better define the role of the Gonozyme test in the clinical laboratory.

Neisseria meningitidis

The use of counterimmunoelectrophoresis (CIE), coagglutination (CoA), and latex agglutination (LA) for the rapid direct detection of meningococci in cerebrospinal fluid is discussed in Chapter 9. Although studies have shown the commercial LA and CoA tests to be more sensitive than CIE and useful for rapid diagnosis, these tests should be performed along with Gram stain and culture.[73]

SEROLOGIC TYPING

Neisseria gonorrhoeae

Although not used routinely in a clinical laboratory, the serologic classification of *N. gonorrhoeae* has been important in epidemiologic studies of this organism and in the continued efforts to develop effective vaccines.[45] ELISA, coagglutination, and microimmunofluorescence techniques have been used to type the gonococci. A coagglutination procedure has been used to define three serogroups, WI, WII, and WIII.[86] Serogroup specificity is determined by possession of different antigenic variants of outer membrane protein I (see below); these variants are designated PrIA and PrIB.[87] Serogroup WI strains possess PrIA and serogroups WII and WIII strains possess PrIB.[87] Several studies cited in Bydgeman[14] have shown different serogroups to be correlated with the geographic distribution and antimicrobial susceptibility of *N. gonorrhoeae* and with clinical manifestations of gonorrhea (for example, organisms of serogroup WI are more frequently associated with disseminated gonococcal infection). The availability of commercial coagglutination reagents (Pharmacia Diagnostics, Piscataway, N.J.; Micro-Media, Potomac, Md.) makes serogrouping a much easier and more practical method for typing gonococci.

Using monoclonal antibodies, Knapp and associates[60] have further divided the WI serogroup into 18 serotypes and the WII and WIII serogroups into 28 serotypes. Use of this serotyping system in combination with auxotyping may provide a highly specific means for analyzing the patterns of transmission of gonorrhea.

Neisseria meningitidis

Based on the immunologic specificity of their capsular polysaccharides, the meningococci have been divided into the following established serogroups—A, B, C, D, X, Y, 29E, and W-135. The serogroups H, I, K,[92] and L[3] have also been proposed. Agglutination is the most reliable procedure for routine serogrouping of the meningococci.[103] Commercial antisera are available from Difco Laboratories and Burroughs Wellcome.

To perform the agglutination test,[103] the microbiologist prepares a milky suspension of a young culture of meningococci from a non-carbohydrate-containing medium in 0.5 ml of phosphate-buffered saline (pH 7.2). Clumps in the suspension are allowed to settle for 1 minute and 1 drop is then removed with a Pasteur pipette and placed on a glass slide or in the well of a plastic tray. One drop of antiserum is added, and the mixture is rotated gently up to 4 minutes; higher-titer specific antisera will usually agglutinate in 1 to 2 minutes. All reactions are observed using indirect lighting. If the isolate is ungroupable, the test should be repeated with phosphate-buffered saline of pH 6.8.

Differences in the antigenic composition of outer membrane proteins allow serotyping of the meningococci.[33] Numerous methods, including bactericidal inhibition,[34] immunodiffusion, agglutination, coagglutination, ELISA, and radioimmunoassay, have been used in serotyping. Many serotypes are shared among serogroups and are independent of serogroup.[33]

Using an immunodiffusion procedure, Frasch[32] has identified over 20 serotypes of meningococcal serogroups B and C. The use of serotyping in epidemiologic studies[34] has shown that serotype 2, present in both serogroups B and C, is strongly associated with sporadic and epidemic meningococcal disease.[32] This finding has provided the basis for the development of promising vaccines.

OTHER IDENTIFICATION METHODS

Auxotyping distinguishes *N. gonorrhoeae* on the basis of nutritional requirements.[15] Certain strains of *N. gonorrhoeae*, for example, require certain amino acids such as arginine or uracil for growth, whereas other strains do not. By using a set of chemically defined media, each medium differing from another by the omission of one of these amino acids or other vitamins or selected components, the microbiologist can determine the nutritional profile of an isolate; this profile is called an auxotype. Of particular interest is the multiple requirement for arginine, hypoxanthine, and uracil, among gonococcal strains associated with disseminated gonococcal infection.[57]

It has been observed that the interaction of microbial surfaces with lectins and lectinlike substances can be helpful in the identification of primary isolates.[78] Wheat germ agglutinin (WGA) agglutinates *N. gonorrhoeae* isolates and other *Neisseria* spp., including meningococci.[89] When WGA is used in combination with soybean lectin agglutinins (SBA) and various chromogenic substrates, an accurate means of identifying gonococci within 30 minutes is possible.[29]

Yajko, Chu, and Hadley[109] used a group of five tests (WGA, SBA, ONPG, gamma-glutamyl-beta-naphthylamide, and prolyl-beta-naphthylamide) as a rapid (30 minutes) method for the identification of gonococci.

Restriction endonucleases (bacterial enzymes that cleave DNA at specific sites) have been used to identify bacteria based on their genotype rather than phenotype.[5,102] The bacterial fragments resulting from cleavage by these enzymes may be separated electrophoretically in gel to form unique "fingerprints" of individual isolates. To date, this approach has been used only experimentally for differentiation among the *Neisseria* spp., but it may prove to be a useful epidemiologic technique.

CLINICAL SIGNIFICANCE
NEISSERIA GONORRHOEAE[45]

The clinical spectrum of gonorrhea is broad and includes asymptomatic infections, symptomatic uncomplicated infections, and complicated infections. Uncomplicated infections are defined as those that remain localized to the site of primary inoculation, do not cause disabling symptoms, and with proper treatment rarely cause sequelae.[41] The vast majority (80% to 90%) of the cases of gonorrhea in developed countries are uncomplicated.[41]

Gonorrhea has been the most frequently reported communicable disease in the United States since 1965.[18] From 1975 to 1980, approximately 1 million cases were reported each year; it is estimated that an additional 1 million cases were diagnosed each year but were not reported.[4]

Uncomplicated Infection[41]

Gonorrhea is an acute pyogenic infection of the columnar and transitional epithelium of various mucosal surfaces. The endocervix is the primary site of infection in women, and the urethra the primary site in men. The pharynx and anorectal region of both sexes may be infected. The risk of transmission of urethral gonorrhea from an infected woman to a man is approximately 20% following a single episode of intercourse; the risk increases to 60% to 80% following four exposures.[46] The risk of transmission of urogenital gonorrhea from infected men to women has not been determined in relation to number of exposures. The rates of transmission of pharyngeal and anorectal gonorrhea are not known.

Gonorrhea in men usually appears as acute urethritis with yellow purulent discharge and dysuria following an incubation period of 1 to 14 days. If untreated, ascending spread of the organism may result in prostatitis and epididymitis. With proper antimicrobial therapy, however, these complications are rare.

Precise delineation of the symptoms of uncomplicated gonorrhea in women has been confounded by the frequent coexistence of other organisms such as *Chlamydia trachomatis* and *Trichomonas vaginalis*. Nonetheless, the most frequent symptoms appear to be increased vaginal discharge, burning or frequency of urination, and menstrual abnormalities. Fever and pain may also be present. Depending on the patient population studied, the percentage of women who appear symptomatic has ranged from less than 25% to more than 80%; the true percentage probably lies somewhere within this range.[41]

Infected mothers may transmit the gonococcus to their babies at birth. The conjunctiva is a major site of infection in the newborn, resulting in gonococcal ophthalmia neonatorum. Fortunately, the instillation of silver nitrate or erythromycin drops into the eyes of infants at birth and the routine screening for gonorrhea in pregnant women have greatly reduced the frequency of this disease.

Anorectal gonorrhea has been reported in approximately 35% to 50% of women and homosexual men with gonorrhea and is the only infected site in about 5% of women and 40% of homosexual men. Rectal intercourse is the source of anorectal infection in homosexual men. Anorectal infection occurs rarely in heterosexual men. Most anorectal infections in women occur in the absence of rectal intercourse and are thought to be caused by perineal contamination with the mucopurulent exudate.

Pharyngeal infection is transmitted by orogenital sexual contact. Most pharyngeal infections are asymptomatic.

Complicated Infections[30,64,65,70]

Complications of gonorrhea occur much more frequently in women than in men. In women the spread of organisms from the cervix into the fallopian tubes results in endometritis, salpingitis, and peritonitis, which are collectively called pelvic inflammatory disease (PID) or ESP (endometritis, salpingitis, peritonitis). PID probably occurs in 10% to 20% of women with gonorrhea, although a study by Platt and others[80] suggests that 47% of recently infected women may display nonspecific symptoms suggestive of PID. The signs of PID include lower abdominal pain, abnormal vaginal discharge, purulent cervical exudate, and uterine and adnexal tenderness. These manifestations begin during or shortly after the start of menstruation. PID may result in ectopic pregnancies and infertility.

Spread of *N. gonorrhoeae* from the genitourinary tract, rectum, or pharynx to the bloodstream may result in disseminated gonococcal infection (DGI) in both men and women. Approximately 1% of patients with gonorrhea develop DGI. The most common clinical manifestations of DGI are a maculopapular rash, tenosynovitis, and arthritis. Endocarditis and meningitis are unusual but potentially life-threatening complications.

The risk of primary gonococcal infection progressing to DGI depends on attributes of the organism and of the host. Gonococcal strains associated with this condition are usually of the Arg^- Hyx^- Ura^- auxotype and are typically penicillin sensitive. Patients with deficiencies of complement components C_5, C_6, C_7, and C_8 are especially susceptible to gonococcal dissemination.

NEISSERIA MENINGITIDIS

Asymptomatic nasopharyngeal carriers of *N. meningitidis* appear to be the primary source for the spread of meningococcal disease. The organisms are transmitted via aerosols and colonize the nasopharynx of the new host. Acquisition of the organism from a patient is rare except among close contacts, that is, individuals who sleep and eat with the infected individual.[77] The risk that these individuals will contract the disease is at least several hundred times higher than the risk in the general population.[69,77] The incidence of disease is also high among military recruits where overcrowding and fatigue are thought to predispose individuals to infection.

Colonization of the nasopharynx usually results in subclinical infection but may produce a mild upper respiratory tract infection similar to the common cold. Current evidence suggests that the meningococcus can invade the bloodstream and establish systemic infection only in individuals who lack antibactericidal antibody or in patients deficient in certain complement components.[25] The highest attack rate is in children under 1 year of age.[90] This correlates with the fact that children between 6 months and 24 months of age have the lowest level of antibody.[35] Protective antibodies may be produced in response to oropharyngeal infection with both capsulated and nonencapsulated meningococci or may result from exposure to cross-reactive antigens from bacteria such as *Escherichia coli*.[25]

Invasion of the bloodstream of susceptible individuals may result in septicemia (meningococcemia) or meningitis. Although symptoms vary, patients with meningococcemia usually have fever, shaking, chills, muscle pains, and a petechial rash that is especially prominent on the lower extremities, trunk, and wrists. Meningococcemia may take a chronic, moderate, or fulminant course. In the fulminant form, known as Waterhouse-Friderichsen syndrome, disseminated intravascular coagulation (DIC) develops with subsequent hemorrhaging into the skin, the adrenal glands, and other internal organs. The petechiae on the skin coalesce to form large ecchymotic lesions. The condition progresses rapidly, and without appropriate therapy the patient may die within a few hours.

Chronic meningococcemia is a rare form of meningococcal disease that is characterized by recurrent episodes of fever, arthritis, and a maculopapular or petechial rash. The condition may last for weeks or months.

Patients with meningitis usually display the fever, headache, and classic signs of meningeal irritation (stiffness of the back and neck, Brudzinski's sign, Kernig's sign) typical of all pyogenic meningitides.[106] The presence of a petechial rash suggests meningococcal meningitis.

Unlike other types of bacterial meningitis, meningococcal meningitis may occur in epidemics. Before 1945, epidemics occurred every 8 to 12 years in the United States, but since that time, meningococcal meningitis has occurred primarily as sporadic disease or rarely as small localized clusters of disease.[7] Epidemics of meningitis do continue to occur in other parts of the world.[77] Most epidemics have been associated with group A *N. meningitidis,* but epidemics resulting from groups B and C have occurred occasionally.

N. meningitidis was responsible for 19.6% of the cases of bacterial meningitis in the United States from 1978 to 1981. (*H. influenzae* was responsible for 48.3% and *Streptococcus pneumoniae* for 13.3%.)[90] Serogroup B was the most common *N. meningitidis* serogroup (51.1%), followed by group C (22.3%), group Y (5.8%), and group Z (4.7%).[90] Group Y is also associated with pneumonia, a rare manifestation of meningococcal infection.

OTHER NEISSERIA SPP.[31,50]

The nongonococcal, nonmeningococcal *Neisseria* spp. have occasionally been associated with life-threatening conditions. *N. lactamica* and *N. flavescens* have been reported as the etiologic agents of meningitis and septicemia. *N. mucosa* has been associated with endocarditis and meningitis. *N. sicca* has been reported as a cause of endocarditis and *N. subflava* as a cause of meningitis, endocarditis, and septicemia.

The prevalence or significance of *N. cinerea* is uncertain because of its past misidentification as *B. catarrhalis*, *N. flavescens*, and *N. gonorrhoeae*.[59] Reevaluation of previously reported studies indicates that *N. cinerea* was probably isolated from the genitourinary tract of one patient and from the cerebrospinal fluid of another patient with meningitis.[59] One case of nosocomial pneumonia[10] and one case of proctitis[28] have also been associated with this organism.

BRANHAMELLA CATARRHALIS[21,26]

In the past few years, *B. catarrhalis* has been recognized as a significant cause of otitis media and maxillary sinusitis in children. It is also being increasingly recognized as a cause of pneumonia and bronchitis in immunosuppressed patients, the elderly, and individuals with compromised pulmonary function. *B. catarrhalis* is an infrequent but significant cause of meningitis, endocarditis, and septicemia.

MECHANISMS OF PATHOGENICITY
NEISSERIA GONORRHOEAE
Structural Components

Several structural components of the gonococcus appear to play a role in the pathogenicity of this organism.[45,101] Pili appear to be important in the attachment of the gonococci to

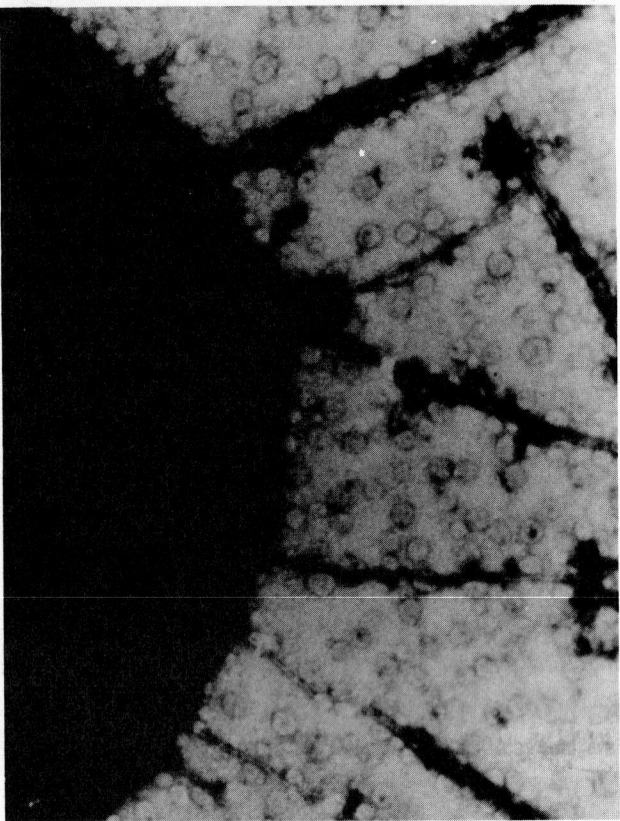

FIGURE 14-3. Pili of *N. gonorrhoeae*. (From Tramont, E.C., and Boslego, J.W.: Pilus vaccines, Vaccine **3**:3, 1985. By permission of the publishers, Butterworth & Co. [Publishers] Ltd.)

human epithelial cells (Figure 14-3). Experimental models of gonococcal infection of human fallopian tube mucosa in organ culture have shown that piliated gonococci attach to and damage the mucosa much more rapidly than nonpiliated gonococci.[66] The mucosal damage, which is manifested by loss of ciliary activity and sloughing of ciliated cells, has been attributed to both the presence of peptidoglycan[68] and the endotoxic properties of the lipopolysaccharide. In addition to these local cytotoxic effects, the lipopolysaccharide may contribute to the fever and systemic toxicity of complicated gonococcal infections.

After attachment and concomitant with mucosal damage, the gonococci are phagocytized (endocytosis) by the epithelial cells of the mucosa and transported in vacuoles to the base of the cells where they are released into subepithelial tissues. How the gonococci are able to evade the mucosal barrier of the host and enter the cell is not known, but interesting studies by Blake and Gotschlich[6] suggest that the presence of protein I may play a role. Protein I is one of several types of proteins that comprise the gonococcal outer membrane along with phospholipids and lipopolysaccharide. Protein I and other groups of proteins designated II and III have been found in the largest amounts. Protein I is the major outer membrane protein; it functions as a porin, allowing small molecules to diffuse through the mem-

brane. The studies of Blake and Gotschlich have shown that protein I is able to leave the membrane of the gonococcus and insert into the membrane of host cells, leading to the speculation that it may initiate the process of endocytosis.

Protein II has also been associated with the virulence of gonococci. Antigen variation of this protein and pili occurs commonly during natural infection.[42] This antigenic variation or antigenic shift might explain the ability of gonococci to colonize anatomically distinct sites, such as the urethra, cervix, and rectum, and persist in these sites despite the host's immune response.[42] Although antibodies would be produced to the specific protein II variant of the invading gonococcus, the high rate of transition of protein II would render these antibodies inactive against subsequent protein II variants. Variations in protein II have also been associated with other characteristics of the gonococci, including attachment to human polymorphonuclear leukocytes and epithelial cells, as well as resistance to antimicrobial agents and serum killing.

After invasion of the subepithelial tissues, the gonococci elicit an inflammatory response that is responsible for the typical symptoms of gonorrhea. The gonococci that cause DGI are able to evade host defenses and invade the bloodstream. These invasive isolates share certain characteristics; they possess certain types of protein I in their outer membrane, they are resistant to the bactericidal activity of normal human serum, and, as mentioned previously, they require arginine, hypoxanthine, and uracil for growth. They also produce transparent colonies and show marked susceptibility to penicillin. The mechanisms by which these isolates are able to resist the bactericidal activity of serum while other isolates are readily killed are unknown, but they have been attributed to possession of certain types of protein I and differences in structure of the polysaccharide.[91] These serum-resistant strains associated with DGI are also resistant to phagocytosis and are able to multiply unchecked in the presence of polymorphonuclear leukocytes.[85] In the appropriate clinical setting, such as menstruation, dissemination may then ensue.[85]

Other Mechanisms

As discussed in Chapter 2, several organisms including *N. gonorrhoeae* produce an IgA1 protease. Another virulence factor of *N. gonorrhoeae* might be its ability to acquire iron from the host (see Chapter 2), but the mechanism by which this is accomplished is unknown. Although evidence is conflicting, recent in vitro studies have shown that *N. gonorrhoeae* does not produce siderophores but does produce certain outer membrane proteins under conditions of iron limitation.[107]

NEISSERIA MENINGITIDIS[25,67]

The ability of the meningococcus to produce invasive disease depends on the lack of protective antibodies in the host and the presence of virulence factors of the organism. This latter tenet is substantiated by the observation that only certain serotypes are isolated from diseased patients during epidemics.

The meningococcus and the gonococcus are similar in structure, and many of the structural components involved in the pathogenicity of the gonococcus may also be virulence factors for the meningococcus. Attachment to and invasion of nasopharyngeal mucosa by meningococci closely parallel the invasion of the fallopian tube mucosa by gonococci.[97] Piliated meningococci attach to the microvilli of nonciliated nasopharyngeal mucosal cells in high numbers.[98] This attachment appears to depend on the presence of specific receptors, since the piliated meningococci attach to cells from other areas of the body in relatively low numbers.[98] Attachment results in a restructuring of the microvilli and subsequent engulfment of the organism.[99] Meningococci appear to penetrate the subepithelial tissues, although the mechanism by which this is accomplished is not known.[99]

Outer membrane proteins and endotoxin may also play a role in the pathogenesis of the meningococcus. Studies by Stephens and McGee[99] have shown that meningococci involved in invasive disease produce transparent colonies and certain large amounts of protein II, whereas nasopharyngeal isolates of asymptomatic carriers usually produce opaque colonies and lack protein II, suggesting that protein II may be required for invasive disease. Although unproven, some studies have suggested that endotoxin may be directly or indirectly responsible for the development of DIC and the subsequent manifestations of fulminant meningococcemia.

Among the other factors that may play a role in the pathogenesis of *N. meningitidis* are the presence of IgA1 protease and the ability to acquire iron from human transferrin.

ANTIMICROBIAL SUSCEPTIBILITY
NEISSERIA GONORRHOEAE[45]

Penicillin was first used for the treatment of gonorrhea in the early 1940s. Although this antibiotic may still be used for susceptible strains of *N. gonorrhoeae*, the emergence of resistant strains has mandated the development of alternative regimens.

Penicillin resistance of *N. gonorrhoeae* may be plasmid mediated or chromosomally mediated. Possession of certain plasmids codes for the production of penicillinase, a TEM beta-lactamase (see Chapter 8). Studies suggest that the gonococcus may have acquired these plasmids from *Haemophilus* spp.[13,94] Penicillinase-producing *N. gonorrhoeae* (PPNG) were first seen in the United States in early 1976 and appear to have been introduced from the Philippines.

Low-level, chromosomally mediated penicillin resistance has been reported in isolates of *N. gonorrhoeae* for several years; these isolates were successfully treated with increased doses of penicillin. Recently, however, isolates with high levels (2 µg/ml or greater) of chromosomally mediated penicillin resistance have emerged. These isolates were first reported in the United States in 1983 in North Carolina[16] and since that time have been reported with increasing frequency from 23 additional states.[17,84] Chromosomal resistance may involve alteration of the permeability of the outer membrane or decreased affinity of penicillin-binding proteins for the beta-lactam antibiotics.[95]

All *N. gonorrhoeae* isolates should be tested for production of beta-lactamase. The acidometric, iodometric, or chromogenic methods discussed in Appendix A may be used. It is important to perform beta-lactamase tests on organisms recovered on primary isolation because the plasmid is unstable and may be lost during subculturing.[76] In an effort to improve surveillance of chromosomally mediated resistant *Neisseria gonorrhoeae* (CMRNG) and monitor gonococcal antibiotic resistance, the Centers for Disease Control (CDC) urges that screening for CMRNG be performed in addition to beta-lactamase testing.[17,84] CMRNG isolates are defined as those that do not

produce beta-lactamase and either grow on media containing 1.5 to 1.6 mg/ml of penicillin or exhibit a zone of growth inhibition of less than 26 mm around a 10-unit penicillin disk.[84] The disk diffusion susceptibility test may be performed using agar plates containing GC agar base supplemented with 1% IsoVitaleX.[73] The inoculum, adjusted to the turbidity of a McFarland 0.5 standard, may be prepared in trypticase soy, brain heart infusion, or Mueller-Hinton broth. All CMRNG isolates should be submitted to a reference laboratory for confirmation by the agar dilution technique.

The CDC proposed guidelines for the treatment of gonorrhea and other sexually transmitted diseases in 1985.[19] Uncomplicated urethral, endocervical, or rectal gonorrhea is treated with a single-dose regimen of amoxicillin plus probenecid, ampicillin plus probenecid, aqueous procaine penicillin G plus probenecid, or ceftriaxone. All of these regimens are followed by tetracycline or doxycycline for 7 days, which is needed for possible coexisting chlamydial infection. Such infections have been shown to be present in up to 45% of gonorrhea cases when adequate chlamydial cultures are performed.[19] Erythromycin may be used in patients when tetracyclines are contraindicated or not tolerated.

Patients with infection resulting from penicillinase-producing *N. gonorrhoeae* (PPNG) or who are likely to have acquired gonorrhea in areas of high prevalence of these organisms should receive spectinomycin or ceftriaxone followed by a 7-day regimen of tetracycline, doxycycline, or erythromycin. Treatment of disseminated gonococcal infection and other considerations for treatment of gonorrhea are discussed in the CDC guidelines.[19]

Studies are ongoing to determine new antimicrobial agents for treatment of gonorrhea. There is special interest in finding a single antimicrobial agent that is effective against both *N. gonorrhoeae* and *C. trachomatis*. Recent studies suggest that spectinomycin derivatives[76] and quinolones such as norfloxacin[22,76] may be effective against penicillin-resistant *N. gonorrhoeae*.

NEISSERIA MENINGITIDIS

Routine susceptibility testing of meningococci is not necessary because these organisms are susceptible to penicillin. Chloramphenicol is used to treat meningococcal disease in patients allergic to penicillin.

Rifampin is used for chemoprophylaxis of close contacts of patients with meningococcal disease, especially members of the same household.[93] Immunoprophylaxis should also be considered for close contacts of individuals known to have meningococcal disease caused by groups A, C, Y, or W135.[93]

VACCINES
NEISSERIA GONORRHOEAE[36]

Ongoing efforts to develop a vaccine for gonorrhea have centered on the use of pili or protein I as the immunogen. Pilus antigens are attractive vaccine candidates because development of antibodies to this portion of the gonococcus might block the initial attachment of the organism to epithelial cells. The problem with pili is their antigenic diversity. Two approaches are being used to develop a pilus-based vaccine that would circumvent the diversity problem. The first approach is to determine the extent of variability among the pili in vivo and then to develop a polyvalent vaccine that would contain a sufficient number of different pilus types to provide protection. The second approach is to determine the specific part of the pilus that is responsible for adhesion and then determine if this portion of the pilus molecule is universal among pili.

Protein I is also an attractive vaccine candidate. Antibodies to this protein are bactericidal, and it does not demonstrate as much antigenic diversity as pili. Studies with partially purified protein I have shown it to be a good immunogen, but protection studies have not been carried out.

NEISSERIA MENINGITIDIS[33]

Vaccines to the polysaccharide capsular antigens of *N. meningitidis* groups A, C, Y, and W135 have been developed and are available as monovalent A or C vaccines, bivalent A and C vaccines, and tetravalent A, C, Y, and W135 vaccines. The vaccines are effective in inducing the production of antibody in adults and have been used successfully to eliminate epidemics of meningitis among military recruits. The vaccines are less effective in young children, the population at greatest risk for meningococcal disease. Group C polysaccharide is not an effective immunogen in children below 18 months of age. Group A polysaccharide vaccine may be effective in children 3 months of age provided booster injections are given.

Currently no vaccine is available for group B meningococci. Earlier studies showed the group B polysaccharide to be poorly immunogenic in humans. Recent studies indicate that a vaccine composed of the outer membrane protein of serotype 2b organisms covalently linked to the group B polysaccharide may be an effective immunogen.[105] As mentioned previously, serotype 2 organisms are found in meningococcal groups B and C and are responsible for 60% to 80% of meningococcal disease caused by these groups. The serotype 2b protein–group B polysaccharide may also provide protection against group C serotype 2 disease in young children.[105] Clinical trials to determine the effectiveness of this vaccine are under way.

REFERENCES

1. Amuso, P., Hester, J., and Frankel, J.: Comparison of coagglutination tests for the identification of *Neisseria gonorrhoeae* (abstract), Abstracts of the Annual Meeting of the American Society for Microbiology, Washington, D.C., 1986.
2. Apicella, M.A.: *Neisseria meningitidis.* In Mandell, G.L., Douglas, R.G., Jr., and Bennett, J.E., editors: Principles and practice of infectious diseases, ed. 2, New York, 1985, John Wiley & Sons, Inc.
3. Ashton, F.E., et al.: A new serogroup (L) of *Neisseria meningitidis,* J. Clin. Microbiol. **17:**722, 1983.
4. Barnes, R.C., and Holmes, K.K.: Epidemiology of gonorrhea: current perspectives, Epidemiol. Rev. **6:**1, 1984.
5. Bjorvatn, B., et al.: Applications of restriction endonuclease fingerprinting of chromosomal DNA of *Neisseria meningitidis,* J. Clin. Microbiol. **19:**763, 1984.
6. Blake, M.S., and Gotschlich, E.C.: Gonococcal membrane proteins: speculation on their role in pathogenesis, Prog. Allergy **33:**298, 1983.
7. Bolan, G., and Barza, M.: Acute bacterial meningitis in children and adults: a perspective, Med. Clin. North Am. **69:**231, 1985.
8. Bonin, P., Tanino, T.T., and Handsfield, H.H.: Isolation of *Neisseria gonorrhoeae* on selective and nonselective media in a sexually transmitted disease clinic, J. Clin. Microbiol. **19:**218, 1984.
9. Bøvre, K.: Genus II. *Moraxella.* Subgenus *Branhamella.* In Krieg, N.R., editor (Holt, J.G., editor-in-chief): Bergey's manual of systematic bacteriology, vol. 1, Baltimore, 1985, Williams & Wilkins Co.
10. Boyce, J.M., et al.: Nosocomial pneumonia caused by a glucose-metabolizing strain of *Neisseria cinerea,* J. Clin. Microbiol. **21:**1, 1985.
11. Brorson, J., et al.: Vancomycin-sensitive strains of *Neisseria gonorrhoeae:* a problem for the diagnostic laboratory, Br. J. Vener. Dis. **49:**452, 1973.
12. Brown, W.J.: Modification of the rapid fermentation test for *Neisseria gonorrhoeae,* Appl. Microbiol. **27:**1027, 1974.
13. Brunton, J.L., et al.: Evolution of antibiotic resistance plasmids in *Neisseria gonorrhoeae* and *Haemophilus* species, Clin. Invest. Med. **6:**221, 1983.
14. Bygdeman, S., editor: Serological classification of *Neisseria gonorrhoeae:* relation to antibiotic susceptibility and auxotypes: epidemiological applications, Stockholm, 1981, Karolinska Institute at Södersjukhuset.
15. Catlin, B.W.: Nutritional profiles of *Neisseria gonorrhoeae, Neisseria meningitidis,* and *Neisseria lactamica* in chemically defined media and the use of growth requirements for gonococcal typing, J. Infect. Dis. **128:**178, 1973.
16. Centers for Disease Control: Penicillin-resistant gonorrhea—North Carolina, MMWR **32:**273, 1983.
17. Centers for Disease Control: Chromosomally mediated resistant *Neisseria gonorrhoeae*—United States, MMWR **33:**408, 1984.
18. Centers for Disease Control: Gonorrhea: sexually transmitted disease (STD) fact sheet no. 35. Atlanta, Georgia, HHS, CDC pub. 81-8195, 1982. As cited in Barnes, R.C., and Holmes, K.K.: Epidemiol. Rev. **6:**1, 1984.
19. Centers for Disease Control: 1985 STD treatment guidelines, MMWR **34:**755, 1985.
20. Chapel, T., et al.: Effect of medium temperature on recovery of gonococci, Am. J. Clin. Pathol. **72:**84, 1979.
21. Chapman, A.J., Jr., et al.: Development of bactericidal antibody during *Branhamella catarrhalis* infection, J. Infect. Dis. **151:**878, 1985.
22. Crider, S.R., et al.: Treatment of penicillin-resistant *Neisseria gonorrhoeae* with oral norfloxacin, N. Engl. J. Med. **311:**137, 1984.
23. Cross, R.C., et al.: VCN-inhibited strains of *Neisseria gonorrhoeae,* HSMHA Health Rep. **86:**990, 1971.
24. D'Amato, R.F., et al.: Rapid identification of *Neisseria gonorrhoeae* and *Neisseria meningitidis* by using enzymatic profiles, J. Clin. Microbiol. **7:**77, 1978.
25. De Voe, I.W.: The meningococcus and mechanisms of pathogenicity, Microbiol. Rev. **46:**162, 1982.
26. Doern, G.V., Miller, M.J., and Winn, R.E.: *Branhamella (Neisseria) catarrhalis* systemic disease in humans: case reports and review of the literature, Arch. Intern. Med. **141:**1690, 1981.
27. Doern, G.V., and Morse, J.A.: *Branhamella (Neisseria) catarrhalis:* criteria for laboratory identification, J. Clin. Microbiol. **11:**193, 1980.
28. Dossett, J.H., et al.: Proctitis associated with *Neisseria cinerea* misidentified as *Neisseria gonorrhoeae* in a child, J. Clin. Microbiol. **21:**575, 1985.
29. Doyle, R.J., et al.: Diagnostic value of interactions between members of the family *Neisseriaceae* and lectins, J. Clin. Microbiol. **19:**383, 1984.
30. Eisenstein, B.I., and Masi, A.T.: Disseminated gonococcal infection (DGI) and gonococcal arthritis (GCA) I. Bacteriology, epidemiology, host factors, pathogen factors, and pathology, Semin. Arthritis Rheum. **10:**155, 1981.
30a. Elliman, D.L., et al.: Evaluation of a fluorescent monoclonal antibody reagent for identification of *Neisseria gonorrhoeae,* Abstract C-273, Abstracts of the Annual Meeting of the American Society for Microbiology, March 1-7, 1987.
31. Feder, H.M., Jr., and Garibaldi, R.A.: The significance of nongonococcal, nonmeningococcal *Neisseria* isolates from blood cultures, Rev. Infect. Dis. **6:**181, 1984.

32. Frasch, C.E.: Noncapsular surface antigens of *Neisseria meningitidis*. In Weinstein, L., and Fields, B.N., editors: Seminars in infectious disease, vol. 2, New York, 1979, Stratton Intercontinental Medical Book Corporation.

33. Frasch, C.E.: Immunization against *Neisseria meningitidis*. In Easmon, C.S.F., and Jeljaszewicz, J., editors: Medical microbiology, vol. 2, New York, 1983, Academic Press, Inc.

34. Frasch, C.E., and Chapman, S.S.: Classification of *N. meningitidis* group B into distinct serotypes. III. Application of a new bactericidal-inhibition technique to distribution of serotypes among cases and carriers, J. Infect. Dis. **127:**149, 1973.

35. Goldschneider, I., Gotschlich, E.C., and Artenstein, M.S.: Human immunity to the meningococcus. I. The role of humoral antibodies, J. Exp. Med. **129:**1307, 1969.

36. Gotschlich, E.C.: Development of a gonorrhoea vaccine: prospects, strategies, and tactics, Bull. W.H.O. **62:**671, 1984.

37. Granato, P.A., Paepke, J.L., and Weiner, L.B.: Comparison of modified New York City medium with Martin-Lewis medium for recovery of *Neisseria gonorrhoeae* from clinical specimens, J. Clin. Microbiol. **12:**748, 1980.

38. Granato, P.A., and Roefaro, M.: Comparative evaluation of enzyme immunoassay and culture for the laboratory diagnosis of gonorrhea, Am. J. Clin. Pathol. **83:**613, 1985.

39. Granato, P.A., Schneible-Smith, C., and Weiner, L.B.: Primary isolation of *Neiserria gonorrhoeae* on hemoglobin-free New York City medium, J. Clin. Microbiol. **14:**206, 1981.

40. Griffin, C.W., III, Mehaffey, M.A., and Cook, E.C.: Five years of experience with a national external quality control program for the culture and identification of *Neisseria gonorrhoeae*, J. Clin. Microbiol. **18:**1150, 1983.

41. Handsfield, H.H.: Gonorrhea and uncomplicated gonococcal infection. In Holmes, K.K., Märdh, P.A., and Sparling, P.F., editors: Sexually transmitted diseases, New York, 1984, McGraw-Hill Book Co.

42. Heckels, J.E.: Molecular studies on the pathogenesis of gonorrhoea, J. Med. Microbiol. **18:**293, 1984.

43. Hehre, E.J., and Hamilton, D.M.: The conversion of sucrose to a polysaccharide of the starch-glycogen class by *Neisseria* from the pharynx, J. Bacteriol. **55:**197, 1948.

44. Hoke, C., and Vedros, N.A.: Characterization of atypical aerobic gram-negative cocci isolated from humans, J. Clin. Microbiol. **15:**906, 1982.

45. Hook, E.W., and Holmes, K.K.: Gonococcal infections, Ann. Intern. Med. **102:**229, 1985.

46. Hooper, R.R., et al.: Cohort study of venereal disease. I. The risk of gonorrhea transmission from infected women to men, Am. J. Epidemiol. **108:**136, 1978.

47. Hoyne, A.L., and Brown, R.H.: 727 meningococcic cases: an analysis, Ann. Intern. Med. **28:**248, 1948.

48. Jacobs, N.F., Jr., and Kraus, S.J.: Gonococcal and nongonococcal urethritis in men: clinical and laboratory differentiation, Ann. Intern. Med. **82:**7, 1975.

49. Jephcott, A.E., and Reyn, A.: *Neisseria gonorrhoeae:* colony variation I, Acta Pathol. Microbiol. Scand. **79B:**609, 1971.

50. Johnson, A.P.: The pathogenic potential of commensal species of *Neisseria*, J. Clin. Pathol. **36:**213, 1983.

51. Judson, F.N., and Werness, B.A.: Combining cervical and anal-canal specimens for gonorrhea on a single culture plate, J. Clin. Microbiol. **12:**216, 1980.

52. Juni, E., and Heym, G.A.: Simple method for distinguishing gonococcal colony types, J. Clin. Microbiol. **6:**511, 1977.

53. Kellogg, D.S., Jr., Holmes, K.K., and Hill, G.A.: Laboratory diagnosis of gonorrhea, Cumitech 4, American Society for Microbiology, Washington, D.C., 1976.

54. Kellogg, D.S., Jr., and Turner, E.M.: Rapid fermentation confirmation of *Neisseria gonorrhoeae*, Appl. Microbiol. **25:**550, 1973.

55. Kellogg, D.S., et al.: *Neisseria gonorrhoeae*. II. Colonial variation and pathogenicity during 35 months in vitro, J. Bacteriol. **96:**596, 1968.

56. Kellogg, D.S., Jr., et al.: *Neisseria gonorrhoeae*. I. Virulence genetically linked to clonal variation, J. Bacteriol. **85:**1274, 1963.

57. Knapp, J.S., and Holmes, K.K.: Disseminated gonococcal infections caused by *Neisseria gonorrhoeae* with unique nutritional requirements, J. Infect. Dis. **132:**204, 1975.

58. Knapp, J.S., and Holmes, K.K.: Modified oxidation-fermentation medium for detection of acid production from carbohydrates by *Neisseria* spp. and *Branhamella catarrhalis*, J. Clin. Microbiol. **18:**56, 1983.

59. Knapp, J.S., et al.: Characterization of *Neisseria cinerea*, a nonpathogenic species isolated on Martin-Lewis medium selective for pathogenic *Neisseria* spp., J. Clin. Microbiol. **19:**63, 1984.

60. Knapp, J.S., et al.: Serological classification of *Neisseria gonorrhoeae* with use of monoconal antibodies to gonococcal outer membrane protein I, J. Infect. Dis. **150:**44, 1984.

61. Kraus, S.J., et al.: Interference of *Neisseria gonorrhoeae* growth by other bacterial species, J. Clin. Microbiol. **4:**288, 1976.

61a. Laughon, B.E., et al.: Fluorescent monoclonal antibody for confirmation of *Neisseria gonorrhoeae* cultures, Abstract C-272, Abstracts of the Annual Meeting of the American Society for Microbiology, Atlanta, Ga., March 1-7, 1987.

62. Lewis, J.S.: New test systems for the identification of *Neisseria gonorrhoeae*. In Facklam, R., Lowell, G., and Lind, I., editors: Recent developments in laboratory identification techniques, Amsterdam, 1980, Excerpta Medica.

63. Martin, J.E., Jr., and Jackson, R.L.: A biological environmental chamber for the culture of *Neisseria gonorrhoeae*, J. Am. Ven. Dis. Assoc. **2:**28, 1975.

64. Masi, A.T., and Eisenstein, B.I.: Disseminated gonococcal infection (DGI) and gonococcal arthritis (GCA). II. Clinical manifestations, diagnosis, complications, treatment, and prevention, Semin. Arthritis Rheum. **10:**173, 1981.

65. McGee, Z.A.: Gonococcal pelvic inflammatory disease. In Holmes, K.K., et al., editors: Sexually transmitted diseases, New York, 1984, McGraw-Hill Book Co.

66. McGee, Z.A., Johnson, A.P., and Taylor-Robinson, D.: Pathogenic mechanisms of *Neisseria gonorrhoeae:* observations on damage to human fallopian tubes in organ culture by gonococci of colony type 1 or type 4, J. Infect. Dis. **143:**413, 1981.

67. McGee, Z.A., and Stephens, D.S.: Common pathways of invasion of mucosal barriers by *Neisseria gonorrhoeae* and *Neisseria meningitidis*, Surv. Synth. Path. Res. **3:**1, 1984.

68. Melly, M.A., McGee, Z.A., and Rosenthal, R.S.: Ability of monomeric peptidoglycan fragments from *Neisseria gonorrhoeae* to damage human fallopian tube mucosa, J. Infect. Dis. **149:**378, 1984.

69. Meningococcal Disease Surveillance Group: Meningococcal diseases: secondary attack rate and chemoprophylaxis in the United States, 1974, JAMA **235:**261, 1976.

70. Mills, J., and Brooks, G.F.: Disseminated gonococcal infection. In Holmes, K.K., et al., editors: Sexually transmitted diseases, New York, 1984, McGraw-Hill Book Co.

71. Mirrett, S., Reller, L.B., and Knapp, J.S.: *Neisseria gonorrhoeae* strains inhibited by vancomycin in selective media and correlation with auxotype, J. Clin. Microbiol. **14:**94, 1981.

72. Morello, J.A.: *Neisseria gonorrhoeae:* methods for laboratory identification, Am. J. Med. Tech. **48:**233, 1982.

73. Morello, J.A., Janda, W.M., and Bohnhoff, M.: *Neisseria* and *Branhamella*. In Lennette, E.H., et al., editors: Manual of clinical microbiology, ed. 4, Washington, D.C., 1985, American Society for Microbiology.

74. Morse, S.A., and Bartenstein, L.: Adaptation of the Minitek system for the rapid identification of *Neisseria gonorrhoeae*, J. Clin. Microbiol. **3:**8, 1976.

75. Morse, S.A., Stein, S., and Hines, J.: Glucose metabolism in *Neisseria gonorrhoeae*, J. Bacteriol. **120:**702, 1974.

76. Peeters, M., Van Dyck, E., and Piot, P.: In vitro activities of the spectinomycin analog U–63366 and four quinolone derivatives against *Neisseria gonorrhoeae*, Antimicrob. Agents Chemother. **26:**608, 1984.

77. Peltola, H.: Meningococcal disease: still with us, Rev. Infect. Dis. **5:**71, 1983.

78. Pistole, T.G.: Interaction of bacteria and fungi with lectins and lectin-like substances, Ann. Rev. Microbiol. **35:**85, 1981.

79. Platt, D.J.: Carbon dioxide requirement of *Neisseria gonorrhoeae* growing on a solid medium, J. Clin. Microbiol. **4:**129, 1976.

80. Platt, R., Rice, P.A., and McCormack, W.M.: Risk of acquiring gonorrhea and prevalence of abnormal adnexal findings among women recently exposed to gonorrhea, JAMA **250:**3205, 1983.

81. Pollock, H.M.: Evaluation of methods for the rapid identification of *Neisseria gonorrhoeae* in a routine clinical laboratory, J. Clin. Microbiol. **4:**19, 1976.

82. Ratner, H.B., et al.: Comparison of the effect of refrigerated versus room temperature media on the isolation of *Neisseria gonorrhoeae* from genital specimens, J. Clin. Microbiol. **21:**127, 1985.

83. Reyn, A., and Bentzon, M.W.: Comparison of a selective and a non-selective medium in the diagnosis of gonorrhoea to ascertain the sensitivity of *Neisseria gonorrhoeae* to vancomycin, Br. J. Vener. Dis. **48:**363, 1972.

84. Rice, R.J., et al.: Changing trends in gonococcal antibiotic resistance in the United States, 1983–84, CDC Surveillance Summaries **33:**11SS, 1985.

85. Ross, S.R., and Densen, P.: Opsonophagocytosis of *Neisseria gonorrhoeae:* interaction of local and disseminated isolates with complement and neutrophils, J. Infect. Dis. **151:**33, 1985.

86. Sandström, E., and Danielsson, D.: Serology of *Neisseria gonorrhoeae* classification by coagglutination, Acta Path. Microbiol. Scand. [B] **88:**27, 1980.

87. Sandström, E.G., Chen, K.C.S., and Buchanan, T.M.: Serology of *Neisseria gonorrhoeae:* coagglutination serogroups WI and WII/III correspond to different outer membrane protein I molecules, Infect. Immun. **38:**462, 1982.

88. Schachter, J., et al.: Enzyme immunoassay for diagnosis of gonorrhea, J. Clin. Microbiol. **19:**57, 1984.

89. Schaefer, R.L., Keller, K.F., and Doyle, R.J.: Lectins in diagnostic microbiology: use of wheat germ agglutinin for the laboratory identification of *Neisseria gonorrhoeae*, J. Clin. Microbiol. **10:**669, 1979.

90. Schlech, W.F., et al.: Bacterial meningitis in the United States 1978–81: the national bacterial meningitis surveillance study, JAMA **253:**1749, 1985.

91. Shafer, W.M., et al.: Serum sensitivity of *Neisseria gonorrhoeae:* the role of lipopolysaccharide, J. Infect. Dis. **149:**175, 1984.

92. Shao-qing, D., Ren-bang, Y., and Huan-chun, Z.: Three new serogroups of *Neisseria meningitidis*, J. Biol. Stand. **9:**307, 1981.

93. Shapiro, E.D.: Prophylaxis for bacterial meningitis, Med. Clin. North Am. **69:**269, 1985.

94. Sparling, P.F., et al.: Antibiotic resistance in the gonococcus: diverse mechanisms of coping with a hostile environment. In Brooks, G.F., Gotschlich, E.C., and Holmes, K.K., editors: Immunobiology of *Neisseria gonorrhoeae*, Washington, D.C., 1978, American Society for Microbiology.

95. Spratt, B.G.: Penicillin-binding proteins and the future of B-lactam antibiotics, J. Gen. Microbiol. **129:**1247, 1983.

96. Stamm, W.E., et al.: Antigen detection for the diagnosis of gonorrhea, J. Clin. Microbiol. **19:**399, 1984.

97. Stephens, D.S., Hoffman, L.H., and McGee, Z.A.: Interaction of *Neisseria meningitidis* with human nasopharyngeal mucosa: attachment and entry into columnar epithelial cells, J. Infect. Dis. **148:**369, 1983.

98. Stephens, D.S., and McGee, Z.A.: Attachment of *Neisseria meningitidis* to human mucosal surfaces: influence of pili and type of receptor cells, J. Infect. Dis. **143:**525, 1981.

99. Stephens, D.S., and McGee, Z.A.: Association of virulence of *Neisseria meningitidis* with transparent colony type and low-molecular weight outer membrane proteins, J. Infect. Dis. **147:**282, 1983.

100. Strauss, R.R., Holderbach, J., and Friedman, H.: Comparison of a radiometric procedure with conventional methods for identification of *Neisseria*, J. Clin. Microbiol. **7:**419, 1978.

101. Swanson, J., and Mayer, L.W.: Biology of *Neisseria gonorrhoeae*. In Holmes, K.K., Mardh, P.-A, and Sparling, P.F., editors: Sexually transmitted diseases, New York, 1984, McGraw-Hill Book Co.

102. Torres, A.R., et al.: Differentiation of *Neisseria gonorrhoeae* from other *Neisseria* species by use of the restriction endonuclease Hae III, J. Clin. Microbiol. **20:**687, 1984.

103. Vedros, N.A.: Serology of the meningococcus. In Bergan, T., and Norris, J.R., editors: Methods in microbiology, vol. 10, New York, 1978, Academic Press, Inc.

104. Vedros, N.A.: Genus I. Neisseria. In Krieg, N.R., editor (Holt, J.G., editor-in-chief): Bergey's manual of systematic bacteriology, vol. 1, Baltimore, 1985, Williams & Wilkins.

105. Wang, L.Y., and Frasch, C.E.: Development of a *Neisseria meningitidis* group B serotype 2b protein vaccine and evaluation in a mouse model, Infect. Immun. **46:**408, 1984.

106. Weinstein, L.: Bacterial meningitis: specific etiologic diagnosis on the basis of distinctive epidemiologic, pathogenetic, and clinical features, Med. Clin. North Am. **69:**219, 1985.

107. West, S.E.H., and Sparling, P.F.: Response of *Neisseria gonorrhoeae* to iron limitation: alterations in expression of membrane proteins without apparent siderophore production, Infect. Immun. **47:**388, 1985.

108. Windall, J.J., Hall, M.M., and Washington, J.A., II: Inhibitory effects of vacomycin on *Neisseria gonorrhoeae* in Thayer-Martin medium, J. Infect. Dis. **142:**775, 1980.

109. Yajko, D.M., Chu, A., and Hadley, W.K,: Rapid confirmatory identification of *Neisseria gonorrhoeae* with lectins and chromogenic substrates, J. Clin. Microbiol. **19:**380, 1984.

110. Yong, D.C.J., and Prytula, A.: Rapid micro-carbohydrate test for confirmation of *Neisseria gonorrhoeae*, J. Clin. Microbiol. **8:**643,1978.

CHAPTER 15

Haemophilus

Barbara J. Howard

Members of the genus *Haemophilus* are small, pleomorphic, nonsporeforming, gram-negative coccobacilli. These strict parasites form part of the indigenous flora of the mucous membranes of the human upper respiratory tract and mouth. Most members of the genus are nonpathogenic or opportunistic; however, some species, such as *H. influenzae*, *H. aegyptius*, and *H. ducreyi*, are pathogens. *H. influenzae* type b (Hib) is responsible for several serious invasive diseases of childhood and is the single most important cause of meningitis in children in the United States.

The word "haemophilus" means "blood loving" and refers to the growth requirement of these organisms for one or both of two factors present in blood—X and V factors. The X factor is protoporphyrin IX or hemin.* The heat-stable X factor is necessary for synthesizing iron-containing respiratory enzymes, cytochrome, cytochrome oxidase, catalase, and peroxidase. The V factor nicotinamide adenine dinucleotide (NAD) is a coenzyme involved in oxidation-reduction reactions. This factor is heat labile.

CLASSIFICATION

Bergey's Manual of Systematic Bacteriology[37] includes the genus *Haemophilus* in the section entitled "Facultatively Anaerobic Gram-Negative Rods." The genus *Haemophilus* is one of the three genera in the family *Pasteurellaceae*. An organism is currently assigned to the genus *Haemophilus* on the basis of its requirements for the X or V factors (or both) previously discussed.

There are 16 species of *Haemophilus* and three species of uncertain status in *Bergey's Manual of Systematic Bacteriology*. Ten of the species are associated with humans. These include *H. influenzae*, *H. aegyptius*, *H. ducreyi*, *H. parainfluenzae*, *H. parahaemolyticus*, *H. paraphrohaemolyticus*, *H. aphrophilus*, *H. segnis*, *H. haemolyticus*, and *H. paraphrophilus*.

The natural habitat of nonencapsulated *H. influenzae* is the nasopharynx. These organisms are found in 75% of healthy children and in a somewhat lower percentage of healthy adults.[37] *H. haemolyticus* is also found in the nasopharynx of a minority of the healthy human population.

The indigenous flora of the human oral cavity comprises *H. parainfluenzae*, *H. parahaemolyticus*, *H. paraphrophilus*, *H. aphrophilus*, and *H. segnis*. These organisms account for approximately 10% of the normal flora. *H. aphrophilus* and *H.*

segnis are especially prevalent in dental plaque. *H. paraphrohaemolyticus* has been isolated from ulcers of the mouth, human sore throats, sputa, and the urethral discharge of adult men; however, its pathogenic significance is unknown.[37] *H. ducreyi* has never been isolated from healthy individuals. It is the etiologic agent of the venereal disease chancroid, or soft chancre.

The taxonomic status of *H. aegyptius* has been questioned for several years. Because this organism is both genetically and phenotypically similar to *H. influenzae* and, like certain biotypes of *H. influenzae*, has been associated with infectious conjunctivitis, it was proposed in 1976 that *H. aegyptius* be reclassified as a biotype of *H. influenzae*.[35] More recently, however, Kilian has stated that *H. aegyptius* should be maintained as a separate species because it is associated with a more acute and contagious form of conjunctivitis than that associated with *H. influenzae*. Like *H. ducreyi*, *H. aegyptius* has never been isolated from healthy individuals.

SPECIMEN COLLECTION AND PROCESSING

Depending on the associated disease, *H. influenzae* may be recovered from the upper and lower respiratory tract, ear, conjunctival scrapings, cerebrospinal fluid (CSF), blood, and other body fluids, including synovial and pleural. *H. parainfluenzae*, *H. aphrophilus*, and *H. paraphrophilus* may occasionally be associated with endocarditis and recovered from blood. *H. aegyptius* is recovered from conjunctival scrapings.

Swabs used in the collection of specimens should be premoistened in broth and transported to the laboratory in transport media. Specimens should be left at room temperature but processed as soon as possible because the *Haemophilus* organisms are susceptible to drying and chilling.

The isolation of *H. ducreyi* from genital ulcers or from the pus of buboes necessitates the use of special collection and processing procedures.[12] The base of the genital ulcer is sampled with a saline-moistened cotton swab, which is immediately streaked across the surface of the isolation medium. Alternatively, the ulcer is irrigated with 0.5 ml of nonbacteriostatic saline and then aspirated with a smooth-tipped Pasteur pipette. The aspirated material is mixed by Vortex agitation for 30 seconds and then used as the inoculum. Although direct Gram stains of the lesion exudate may reveal gram-negative coccobacillary organisms in tangled chains or in parallel arrays (the so-called schools of fish arrangement), these stains are not recommended because of their low sensitivity and specificity.[2,12] *H. ducreyi* frequently does not reveal this characteristic morphology; furthermore, other organisms, such as *Bacteroides*, can give a similar appearance. Culture is the only definitive method for the identification of this organism.[12]

---

*In organisms that possess the ferrochetalase enzyme (for example, *H. influenzae*) the X factor is protoporphyrin IX. For organisms that do not possess this enzyme (for example, *H. aegyptius*) the X factor is hemin (Figure 15-1).

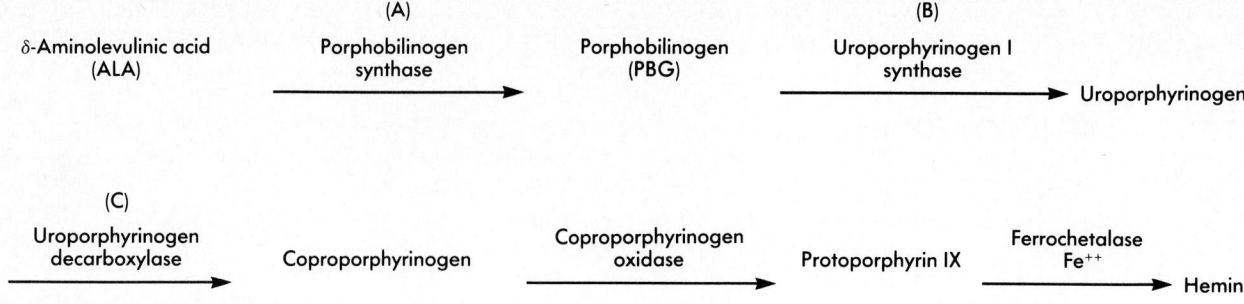

FIGURE 15-1. Biosynthesis of hemin. (From Kilian, M.: Acta Pathol. Microbiol. Scand. **82B:**835, 1974.)

DIRECT EXAMINATION

As discussed later in the chapter, diseases caused by *H. influenzae* can be quite severe. Meningitis, for example, can lead to brain damage, mental retardation, or death. Therefore a presumptive diagnosis must be made rapidly so antimicrobial therapy can be initiated. Rapid diagnostic procedures include examination of a Gram-stained smear of the clinical material, the quellung reaction, and detection of soluble Hib capsular polysaccharide in body fluids.

Gram staining may be performed on uncentrifuged clinical specimens or on the centrifuged sediment. The slide should be examined for the typical short, slender, gram-negative rods of *H. influenzae* (Plate 7, *F*). Slides must be examined carefully because the organisms frequently stain lightly and may not be observed or may be mistaken for debris.

Detection of the soluble capsular polysaccharide of Hib can be accomplished with several procedures, including coagglutination (CoA), latex agglutination (LA), counterimmunoelectrophoresis (CIE), and enzyme-linked immunosorbent assay (ELISA). Coagglutination (Phadebact, Pharmacia Diagnostics, Piscataway, N.J.) and latex agglutination (Bactogen, Wampole, Cranberry, N.J.; Directogen, BBL Microbiology Systems, Cockeysville, Md.; Wellcogen, Wellcome Diagnostics, Research Triangle Park, N.C.) kits are commercially available. These procedures are discussed in Chapter 7. Immunologic procedures are somewhat more sensitive than the Gram stain, and they permit antigen detection in patients who have received prior antimicrobial therapy. They may also offer prognostic information. Several studies have reported that the concentration of Hib capsular polysaccharide in cerebrospinal fluid is correlated with the severity and prognosis of infection (see Chapter 7).

As discussed in Chapter 7, several studies have shown CoA and LA to be more sensitive than CIE in detecting Hib capsular polysaccharide in body fluids. False-positive reactions have been reported, however, especially in serum and urine.

GROWTH REQUIREMENTS
MEDIA

Haemophilus organisms do not grow well on conventional sheep blood agar unless certain modifications are made. The poor growth is attributed to two factors. First, little V factor is available for growth. Although the X factor diffuses from the red cells into the medium, the V factor remains largely imprisoned within the cells. Second, sheep blood possesses NADase,

an enzyme that inactivates V factor. To overcome the inhibitory effects of the NADase and use sheep blood agar for primary isolation, a large exogenous source of V factor must be added to the medium. This is accomplished with a feeder organism, such as *Staphylococcus aureus; S. aureus* produces large amounts of V factor during growth and excretes the excess factor into the medium. With an inoculating wire, *S. aureus* is cross-streaked on a sheep blood agar plate that has been inoculated with the specimen suspected of containing *Haemophilus* organisms. After appropriate incubation, *Haemophilus* organisms appear as small, dewdroplike colonies growing in close proximity to or "satelliting" the *S. aureus* (Plate 8, *A*). The test procedure is called the staphylococcus streak or staph streak. The staph streak may be used for primary isolation of the *Haemophilus* organisms (although chocolate agar is preferred), especially in specimens that are not heavily contaminated with other organisms. It should be noted that other organisms, such as *Neisseria* and *Pseudomonas,* also produce excess V factor. *Haemophilus* spp. may frequently be observed satelliting these organisms in mixed culture.

Although rabbit blood and horse blood do not possess NADase and may support the growth of *Haemophilus* spp., these organisms grow best on media in which the red blood cells have been lysed, resulting in the release of large amounts of V factor. Chocolate agar and Levinthal agar are especially useful. Chocolate agar is prepared by adding red blood cells to the basal agar medium (see Appendix A) and heating the mixture at about 80° C for 15 minutes. Heating lyses the cells, resulting in the brown or chocolate color, and also destroys any NADase that may be present.

Levinthal medium contains horse red blood cells that have been lysed by gentle heating and then filtered through filter paper or glass wool. The medium is colorless, transparent, and especially useful for differentiating encapsulated and nonencapsulated strains of *H. influenzae.* When observed with oblique light, encapsulated strains appear iridescent, whereas nonencapsulated strains appear transparent, bluish, and noniridescent.

Fildes enrichment medium (Difco, Detroit), a peptic digest of sheep blood, may be added to trypticase soy agar or brain heart infusion agar to improve the recovery of *Haemophilus* organisms. The peptic digestion procedure destroys the NADase and liberates V factor from the red blood cells.

The isolation of *H. influenzae* from upper and lower respiratory specimens is difficult because of the overgrowth of normal flora. (The lower respiratory tract does not have a normal flora, but specimens are contaminated as they pass through the upper respiratory tract.) A selective medium may be used in conjunction with a nonselective medium when this organism is suspected as a cause of serious respiratory disease.[8] Selective media include bacitracin-supplemented chocolate agar and chocolate agar plus vancomycin, bacitracin, and clindamycin.[5] The latter medium appears to be especially effective.

A variety of selective agar media have been developed for isolation of *H. ducreyi.* Successful recovery rates have been reported with gonococcal agar base with bovine hemoglobin, IsoVitaleX, and vancomycin,[20] heart infusion agar base with 5% defibrinated rabbit blood and vancomycin,[59] and Mueller-Hinton agar base with chocolatized horse blood, IsoVitaleX, and vancomycin.[5] The addition of fetal bovine serum to selective media frequently improves the isolation rate.[48,59] Hannah and Greenwood[21] have also reported successful recovery of *H. ducreyi* on nonselective chocolate agar. Maximal recovery of *H. ducreyi* is accomplished using more than one medium.[21,48]

ENVIRONMENTAL REQUIREMENTS

Most *Haemophilus* spp. prefer a moist atmosphere of 5% to 10% CO_2. *H. aphrophilus, H. paraphrophilus,* and *H. paraphrohaemolyticus* require increased CO_2 for surface growth. *H. ducreyi* grows well in a candle jar containing a water-saturated gauze pad.[21]

Optimal growth of all *Haemophilus* spp. except *H. ducreyi* occurs at 35° to 37° C. Cultures suspected of containing *H. ducreyi* should be incubated at 33° to 35° C. Cultures for *H. ducreyi* should be incubated for 4 days before being discarded as negative, and cultures for *H. aegyptius* for 2 to 3 days. Other species grow well in 18 to 24 hours.

CULTURAL CHARACTERISTICS
STAINING REACTIONS

The Gram stain of *Haemophilus* isolates reveals gram-negative organisms ranging from coccobacilli to filamentous forms (Plate 8, *B*). Specific reactions are summarized in Table 15-1.

COLONIAL MORPHOLOGY

Descriptions of colonial morphologies are also included in Table 15-1. Calf blood is the most useful medium for detection of hemolysis, followed in decreasing order of suitability by sheep, human, rabbit, poultry, and horse blood.[34] As noted in Table 15-1, many strains of *H. influenzae* emit a distinct "mousy" odor. Indole-producing strains, however, do not have this odor but a dominant, pungent smell of indole. The morphology of *H. influenzae* on chocolate agar can be seen in Plate 8, *C.*

IDENTIFICATION

Most laboratories speciate the genus *Haemophilus* on the basis of hemolysis and X and V factor requirements (Table 15-2). Kilian recommends the use of biochemical tests for species identification and for differentiation of biotypes (Tables 15-2 and 15-3).

DETERMINATION OF X AND V FACTOR REQUIREMENTS
X and V Factor Strips and Disks

Commercially prepared X and V factor–impregnated strips and disks can be used for determination of growth factor

requirements. The test suspension is prepared by inoculating one well-isolated, 24-hour-old colony into 5 ml of trypticase soy broth. Preparation of the suspension is necessary to help dilute any X factor that may be carried over from the primary isolation medium. The suspension is then swabbed onto a trypticase soy agar plate or a brain heart infusion agar plate. (Doern and Chopin[10] recommend the use of trypticase soy agar.*) With aseptic technique, commercial strips (BBL) or disks (Difco) (containing X factor alone, V factor alone, and X and V factors combined) are placed approximately 20 mm apart on the surface of the inoculated medium. After overnight incubation at 35° C in 3% to 10% CO_2, the plates are observed for growth. *Haemophilus* strains such as *H. influenzae* that require both X and V factors grow only around the XV strip. *H. parainfluenzae* and other V factor–requiring species satellite the V and XV factor strips.

Provided the test medium is nutritionally adequate for certain fastidious *H. parainfluenzae* strains, the use of commercially prepared strips or disks is satisfactory for determination of the V factor requirement.[13] There are problems, however, with detection of the X factor requirement. Because probably no single medium is completely devoid of hemin and can otherwise satisfy the growth requirements of the *Haemophilus* strains, avoiding the carryover of X factor with the inoculum is difficult. Thus even when a broth suspension of the test organism is prepared, as many as 18% of the *Haemophilus* strains may be misidentified.[36] For this reason the porphyrin test is considered more reliable in determining the requirements for X factor.

Porphyrin Test[33]

The normal biosynthesis of hemin is seen in Figure 15-1. Strains of *Haemophilus* that require X factor lack the enzymes (designated A, B, and C) necessary to synthesize hemin from delta-aminolevulinic acid (ALA). However, strains that do not require X factor (X-independent strains) do possess these enzymes and are able to convert ALA to porphobilinogen, porphyrin, and, finally, hemin. Furthermore, X-independent strains excrete these porphobilinogens and porphyrins into the medium. The porphyrin test that is described in Appendix A detects these excreted substances.

H. influenzae is negative for the porphyrin test; that is, it does not produce porphyrins and thus requires X factor. *H. aphrophilus* is interesting because it possesses all of the enzymes of the hemin biosynthetic pathway and accordingly gives a positive though weak reaction in the porphyrin test. However, this organism, unlike other X-independent organisms, needs hemin-containing media for primary isolation. The reason for this discrepancy is unknown.[37] Differentiation of *H. aphrophilus* from several similar organisms appears in Table 25-4.

BIOCHEMICAL IDENTIFICATION
Fermentation of Carbohydrates

Fermentation of glucose, sucrose, and lactose is important for species identification.[36] These tests are performed in phenol red broth base (Difco), containing 1% of the respective carbohydrate and supplemented with X and V factors (10 mg of each per liter) after autoclaving.[35]

---

*Special media are required for *H. ducreyi.*[59]

TABLE 15-1. Morphologic Characteristics of *Haemophilus*[37]

Organism	Microscopic Morphology	Colonial Morphology[a]
H. influenzae	Coccobacilli or small, regular rods, 0.3 to 0.5 × 0.3 to 0.5 μm	Small (0.5 to 1 mm), smooth, translucent, grayish, convex with entire edge and a "mousy" odor; encapsulated strains larger (1 to 3 mm) and more mucoid, with tendency to coalesce
H. aegyptius	Long slender rods, 0.2 to 0.3 × 2 to 3 μm	After 48 hr appear small (0.5 mm), smooth, low, convex, grayish, and translucent
H. haemolyticus	Small coccobacilli or short rods with occasional filamentous forms	Resemble *H. influenzae* but are beta-hemolytic on blood agar
H. ducreyi	Slender rods in pairs or chains, 0.5 × 1.5 to 2.0 μm; "schools of fish" arrangement may be observed	After 48 to 72 hr on selective media, most appear small (~0.5 mm in diameter), flat, smooth, yellow-gray, and translucent to opaque; colonies may be pushed intact across agar surface
H. parainfluenzae	Small pleomorphic rods usually with long filamentous forms	Resemble *H. influenzae* except for their slightly larger size (up to 3 mm in diameter)
H. parahaemolyticus	Small pleomorphic rods usually with long filamentous forms	Similar to *H. parainfluenzae* but is beta-hemolytic on blood agar
H. paraphrohaemolyticus	Short- to medium-length rods, 0.75 to 2.5 μm and 0.4 to 0.5 μm in width with occasional short filaments when incubated in 10% CO_2; without extra CO_2 short to long coarse rods with twisted filaments	Resembles *H. aphrophilus* but is beta-hemolytic on blood agar
H. aphrophilus	Short regular rods, 0.45 to 0.55 × 1.5 to 1.7 μm; occasional filamentous forms	Highly convex, opaque, granular, yellowish, ranging in diameter from 1 to 1.5 mm; growth in broth is granular with heavy sediment on bottom of tube, and colonies adhere to walls of tube
H. paraphrophilus	Short regular rods with occasional filamentous forms	Identical to *H. aphrophilus*
H. segnis	Pleomorphic rods; irregular filamentous forms predominate	After 48 hr convex, grayish white, smooth or granular, and 0.5 mm in diameter

[a]On chocolate agar after 24 hours' incubation unless otherwise indicated.

Fermentation of xylose is important in distinguishing *H. aegyptius* from *H. influenzae*. (*H. aegyptius* has the same key biochemical reactions as *H. influenzae* biotype III [Table 15-2]). Other features useful in differentiating *H. aegyptius* include poorer growth on most media, lack of indole production, hemagglutinating activity, distinct bacillary morphology, and susceptibility to troleandomycin.[37] However, none of these features unequivocally differentiate these two species.[36]

Indole, Urease, and Ornithine Decarboxylase

The indole, urease, and ornithine decarboxylase tests can be used to subdivide *H. influenzae* into seven biotypes and *H. parainfluenzae* into four biotypes (Table 15-3). Biotyping procedures can be performed with the conventional tests recommended by Kilian[35] or with the Micro-ID (Organon Teknika, Durham, N.C.), Minitek (BBL Microbiology Systems, Inc.,

Cockeysville, Md.), API 20E (Analytab Products, Plainview, N.Y.), PathoTec strips (Organon Teknika), and rapid spot biochemical tests.[29]

Biotyping is important from an epidemiologic standpoint because it has been shown that certain biotypes of *H. influenzae* are associated with the source of isolation, antimicrobial susceptibility, and invasive disease. *H. influenzae* biotype I is recovered primarily from blood and CSF and is associated with invasive diseases, such as epiglottitis and meningitis.[35,38,39,49] Biotype I is also frequently isolated from children with cystic fibrosis and from children with acute otitis media.[39] *H. influenzae* biotypes II and III are recovered from eye and sputum cultures.[49] Biotypes II and III are also the biotypes most frequently recovered from upper respiratory tracts.[39] Although there are conflicting data,[39] many studies have reported that ampicillin resistance is more frequent among biotype I.[1,17]

TABLE 15-2. Principal Differential Characteristics of *Haemophilus* Spp.

Species	Factor Requirement X[a]	Factor Requirement V	Hemolysis	Fermentation of Glucose	Fermentation of Sucrose	Fermentation of Lactose	Presence of Catalase	CO_2 Enhances Growth
H. influenzae (*H. aegyptius*)[b]	+	+	−	+	−	−	+	−
H. haemolyticus	+	+	+	+	−	−	+	−
H. ducreyi	+	−	−[c]	−[d]	−	−	−	−
H. parainfluenzae [b]	−	+	−	+	+	−	D	−
H. parahaemolyticus[b,e]	−	+	+	+	+	−	D	D
H. segnis[b]	−	+	−	W	W	−	D	−
H. paraphrophilus[b]	−	+	−	+	+	+	−	+
H. aphrophilus	−	−	−	+	+	+	−	+

> **SYMBOLS:** +, 90% or more of strains positive   D, 11%–89% of strains positive
> −, 10% or less of strains positive   W, Weak fermentation reaction

From Kilian, M.: *Haemophilus*. In Lennette, E.H., et al., editors: Manual of clinical micriobiology, ed. 4, Washington, D.C., 1985, American Society for Microbiology.
[a] As determined by porphyrin test.
[b] For further discussion see Table 15-3.
[c] Some strains may show delayed, weak beta-hemolysis.[37]
[d] Clinical isolates usually appear to be asaccharolytic. However, under favorable growth conditions some strains show a late positive reaction for glucose fermentation.[37]
[e] *H. parahaemolyticus* and *H. paraphrohaemolyticus* differ only in their requirement for CO_2.[37,71] *H. paraphrohaemolyticus* requires CO_2, whereas *H. parahaemolyticus* does not.

TABLE 15-3. Differentiation of biotypes of *H. influenzae, H. parainfluenzae, H. aegyptius, H. parahaemolyticus,* and *H. segnis*

Species and Biotype	Indole Production	Urease Activity	Ornithine Decarboxylase Activity
H. influenzae			
Biotype I	+	+	+
Biotype II	+	+	−
Biotype III	−	+	−
Biotype IV	−	+	+
Biotype V	+	−	+
Biotype VI[a]	−	−	+
Biotype VII[b]	+	−	−
H. aegyptius[c]	−	+	−
H. parainfluenzae			
Biotype I	−	−	+
Biotype II	−	+	+
Biotype III	−	+	−
Biotype IV	+	+	+
H. parahaemolyticus	−	+	D
H. segnis	−	−	−

> **SYMBOLS:** +, Positive reaction
> −, Negative reaction
> D, Difference encountered

From Kilian, M.: *Haemophilus*. In Lennette, E.H., et al., editors: Manual of clinical microbiology, ed. 4, Washington, D.C., 1985, American Society for Microbiology.
[a] Biotype VI is characterized according to Oberhofer and Back.[49]
[b] Biotype VII is characterized as proposed by Gratten.[19]
[c] For tests differentiating *H. aegyptius* and *H. influenzae* biotype III, see the text.

ADDITIONAL CHARACTERISTICS FOR IDENTIFICATION OF *HAEMOPHILUS DUCRYEI*

Characteristics that may be especially useful in the identification of *H. ducreyi* include its slow growth, requirement for hemin, and positive reactions for oxidase, nitrate reduction, and alkaline phosphatase. As with all *Haemophilus* organisms, the requirement for hemin is best demonstrated with the porphyrin test. When performing the oxidase test, tetramethyl-*p*-phenylenediamine reagent must be used, since false-negative reactions are observed with the dimethyl-*p*-phenylenediamine reagent.[47] Alkaline phosphatase activity can be determined according to the method of Kilian[35] or with the RapID NH system (Innovative Diagnostic Systems, Inc., Atlanta, Ga.).[21] The nitrate reduction test should be performed in nitrate broth supplemented with 10% fetal bovine serum[59] or 20% rabbit serum.[49]

RAPID IDENTIFICATION

The RapID NH system has been used for rapid identification of *Haemophilus* spp., including *H. ducreyi*.[21] This system is discussed in Chapter 9.

IMMUNOSEROLOGIC AND SEROLOGIC IDENTIFICATION

IMMUNOSEROLOGIC DETECTION

The direct detection of Hib in body fluids using immunoserologic methods is discussed previously in this chapter and in Chapter 7.

SEROLOGIC TYPING

Based on differences in their capsular polysaccharide material, encapsulated *H. influenzae* can be divided into six serologic types, designated A through F. Unencapsulated organisms are designated nontypeable. Serologic typing is important in distinguishing the more virulent type b organisms.

Isolates can be typed with the conventional slide-agglutination method, quellung reaction, CIE, LA, antiserum-agar method, immunofluorescence, and coagglutination. Ingram evaluated the first five of these methods in the serotyping of nasopharyngeal isolates of *H. influenzae*.[26] Nasopharyngeal isolates produce only a moderate amount of capsular polysaccharide. All five methods showed essentially comparable results, with CIE and LA being slightly more sensitive. However, the cross-reactions observed with LA and the expense of both CIE and the antiserum-agar method made these less practical than the slide-agglutination method.

Other studies have reported problems with the slide agglutination method.[57,65] The most common problem is the misidentification of nontypeable isolates as type b.[23] After comparing slide agglutination, coagglutination (Phadebact, Pharmacia Diagnostics), LA, and CIE, Himmelreich, Barenkamp, and Storch[23] recommend the use of slide agglutination or coagglutination because of their simplicity, accuracy, and rapidity. These authors stress, however, that the slide agglutination procedure does contain potential pitfalls and that certain safeguards should be taken. For example, a saline control must be used to detect autoagglutination, and positive reactions should be reported only with those isolates that show strong agglutination and clearing of the background. Furthermore, reactions for both the antiserum and the saline control should be read after 30 to 60 seconds.

To perform the serum agglutination procedure, a suspension of the isolate is prepared in normal saline containing formalin (0.5% vol/vol).[36] This suspension must be prepared from a young (6- to 18-hour) agar culture. A drop of this suspension is added to a drop of antiserum on a slide and observed for agglutination within 1 minute. Interpretation and other precautions are as given previously.

It should be noted that serotyping and biotyping methods are not sufficient for differentiation of *H. influenzae* strains in detailed epidemiologic investigations.[41] Analysis of outer-membrane proteins can be used in those situations.

CLINICAL SIGNIFICANCE
HAEMOPHILUS INFLUENZAE
Diseases of Children

The nasopharynx is usually the initial focus of infection for *H. influenzae* type b (Hib). The organisms may then invade local tissues, causing epiglottitis and pneumonia, or they may enter the bloodstream and localize at distant sites to produce meningitis, septic arthritis, and osteomyelitis. Hib causes about 20,000* invasive infections annually.

Meningitis

The large majority of cases of Hib meningitis occur in children between the ages of 2 months and 3 years; 95% of cases occur before 5 years.[54] Cases are rarely seen in school-age children or in adults. This age-related incidence is thought to be due to the minimal levels of antibodies in children between the ages of 2 months and 3 years. Before the age of 2 months, neonates are protected by maternal antibodies, and active immunity begins to develop in older children. Other factors, such as genetic constitution, may also play a role in susceptibility to disease.[69]

Meningitis appears to be a contagious disease in age-susceptible household contacts.[68] The secondary attack rate among siblings or other close contacts (for instance, day-care center contacts) is several hundred times greater than the attack rate in the general population.[68]

Epiglottitis

Epiglottitis is usually associated with Hib, but some cases are caused by beta-hemolytic streptococci, pneumococci, staphylococci, and, occasionally, other organisms.[54] This dramatic, potentially lethal illness occurs in children between 2 and 4 years of age (peak occurrence); most patients are boys.

The initial symptoms of epiglottitis include a sore throat, barking cough, and fever. These progress rapidly to severe respiratory distress, dyspnea, and prostration. The physical examination reveals the characteristic shiny, cherry-red epiglottis that is enlarged five to 10 times the normal size. This enlarged epiglottis results in the blocking of the air passage. Establishment of the airway by nasotracheal intubation or tracheostomy frequently is necessary to save the patient's life.

Pneumonia[54]

The true incidence of *H. influenzae* pneumonia in infants and children is unknown because of the difficulties in making a precise bacteriologic diagnosis. Sputum is often unobtainable

---

*With use of the vaccine this number is expected to decrease by 25%.[9]

in children less than 4 years of age. Furthermore, the presence of this organism in sputum is not necessarily abnormal or relevant to the etiology of pneumonia. Pneumonia is frequently associated with other conditions, such as otitis media, meningitis, and bacteremia.

Other diseases[30]

Hib may be associated with a variety of other diseases in children. It is the most common organism responsible for septic arthritis in children of 2 years or less. The arthritis may be associated with other infections such as meningitis. Hib is responsible for 5% to 14% of the cases of cellulitis in young children; over 85% of children with Hib cellulitis are 2 years of age or less. Cellulitis is frequently preceded by a nonspecific upper respiratory infection and appears most commonly on the cheek and periorbital region. Hib is also responsible for up to 15% of the cases of pericarditis in children; most children are 2 to 4 years of age. Hib is a relatively uncommon cause of osteomyelitis in children.

In children nonencapsulated *H. influenzae* is responsible for otitis media that is unaccompanied by meningitis or septicemia. Whether these organisms, which are also present as normal flora in the upper respiratory tract, are primary or secondary invaders is not clear.

Diseases of Adults

The nonencapsulated isolates of *H. influenzae* that commonly colonize the nasopharyngeal region are associated with acute sinusitis and bronchitis in adults. In these conditions the organisms act as secondary invaders when the host defenses have been compromised by previous viral infections, allergic reactions, mechanical obstructions, and other dysfunctions.[43,64]

H. influenzae has also been associated with invasive disease in adults, although far less frequently than in children. Many early studies reported Hib to be responsible for adult invasive disease; other studies either assumed the serotype to be b without confirmatory testing or did not perform serotyping at all. Recent studies show nontypeable organisms to be a major cause of invasive disease in adults.*

Most cases of invasive disease in adults are associated with underlying conditions. Meningitis, for example, is commonly seen in patients with head trauma or in patients with antecedent or concurrent infections of sinusitis, otitis media, and pneumonia, as well as in patients with alcoholism, diabetes, splenectomies, or hypogammaglobulinemia.[24,60,65] Thus unlike the situation with children, in whom meningitis is commonly a bacteremic primary infection, meningitis in adults frequently results from a contiguous spread from a local infection.[60] Similarly, pneumonia is associated with chronic obstructive pulmonary disease, chronic alcoholism, diabetes, carcinoma, bronchiectasis, and preceding upper respiratory tract infection.[3,24,45]

H. influenzae may rarely cause a variety of other conditions in adults, including pericarditis, septic arthritis, endocarditis, obstetric and gynecologic infections, urinary and biliary tract infections, and cellulitis.[24] Nontypeable *H. influenzae* associated with maternal bacteremia can lead to serious disease in neonates.[66]

---

*References 3, 27, 44, 45, 60, and 65.

HAEMOPHILUS AEGYPTIUS

This organism is responsible for acute and contagious conjunctivitis, primarily in hot climates. Unlike *H. influenzae*, *H. aegyptius* can colonize eyes without the presence of predisposing conditions.

HAEMOPHILUS DUCREYI[22,46,55]

Chancroid, an *H. ducreyi* infection, is commonly seen in hot tropical climates, such as Southeast Asia, Africa, and the West Indies. Although it is uncommon in the United States, a recent outbreak occurred in California.[6,7] The disease occurs most frequently among men, especially uncircumcised men, and in some environments prostitutes appear to be the most important reservoir of disease.

The characteristic lesion of this disease appears, after an incubation period of 4 to 7 days, as a small, tender papule surrounded by a zone of erythema. The papule rapidly becomes pustular, eroded, and ulcerated. The ulcer is sharply demarcated and nonindurated and has an irregular edge. The base of the ulcer may be covered with a gray or yellow purulent exudate. Autoinoculation may result in the development of multiple ulcers in approximately one half of patients of both sexes. Most of the lesions in men are on the frenulum, in the sulcus, or on the external or internal surface of the prepuce. Most lesions in women are at the entrance to the vagina.

Inguinal lymphadenopathy may develop approximately 1 week after the appearance of the ulcer. These enlarged lymph nodes can progress to form suppurative buboes. Systemic infection does not occur.

HAEMOPHILUS PARAINFLUENZAE

Endocarditis is the most common reported infection with *H. parainfluenzae*.[16,28,63] Several cases of meningitis in children have been attributed to *H. parainfluenzae*.[14] Kilian[38] suggests, however, that some of the reports are due to misidentification of the organism. Other infections caused by *H. parainfluenzae* are rare.[51]

HAEMOPHILUS APHROPHILUS[4]

The majority of diseases associated with *H. aphrophilus* are endocarditis and brain abscesses, but sinusitis, meningitis, pneumonia, bacteremia, and empyema have also been reported. Infections almost always occur in patients with underlying disorders. Most cases of endocarditis are associated with cardiac disease or dental disease. The majority of patients with brain abscesses have congenital heart disease and infection or involvement of the oropharynx. There is an association between the isolation of *H. aphrophilus* and malignancy, cancer chemotherapy, or both.

HAEMOPHILUS PARAPHROPHILUS

H. paraphrophilus has also been associated with endocarditis.[16]

MECHANISMS OF PATHOGENICITY

The type b capsular polysaccharide, a polymer of ribosyl ribose phosphate, is the major virulence determinant of Hib.[43] The way in which elaboration of this polysaccharide promotes invasive infection is not known for certain. Sutton and co-workers[62] propose that the polysaccharide allows the organisms to resist the bactericidal activity of serum complement; this complement resistance permits longer survival and eventual multiplication of Hib in the blood. The fact that the type b capsular material is poorly immunogenic in young children, as demonstrated in human vaccination trials, may also play a role in the pathogenicity of the organism.

Other structural components such as lipopolysaccharide, outer-membrane proteins, and pilus proteins may contribute to the pathogenicity of Hib,[42] as may differences in biotype.[18,39]

Virulent strains of *H. ducreyi* are resistant to the bactericidal action of normal serum and to phagocytosis.[50]

ANTIMICROBIAL SUSCEPTIBILITY

Most *Haemophilus* strains are susceptible to penicillin and its derivatives and to chloramphenicol, sulfonamides, and tetracyclines. Until the early 1970s, virtually all strains of *H. influenzae* were susceptible to ampicillin, and antimicrobial susceptibility testing was unnecessary. Currently, approximately 20% of *H. influenzae* isolates are resistant to ampicillin.[41] This resistance is primarily conveyed by a plasmid-mediated beta-lactamase. Chromosomally mediated ampicillin resistance has also been reported; these strains possess altered penicillin-binding proteins.[40,58]

As discussed in Chapter 8, beta-lactamase testing and antimicrobial susceptibility testing are currently indicated for all clinically significant isolates of *H. influenzae*.[41] Beta-lactamase testing can be accomplished with the iodometric, acidometric, and chromogenic cephalosporin tests (see Appendix A). When performing these tests, microbiologists should be aware that beta-lactamase-positive and beta-lactamase-negative strains may be isolated from the same patient.[61] Plates of *H. influenzae* isolates should be examined carefully for colonies that show different morphologic characteristics; these colonies should be tested separately for beta-lactamase.

Because of the possibility of chromosomally mediated ampicillin resistance in the absence of a beta-lactamase, antimicrobial susceptibility tests should be performed on all beta-lactamase strains, according to the methods discussed in Chapter 8. The performance of agar or broth dilution methods is also discussed in Chapter 8.

Chloramphenicol is used to treat serious disease because of the existence of ampicillin-resistant *H. influenzae*. In 1986 the American Academy of Pediatrics recommended that initial therapy for *H. influenzae* meningitis include chloramphenicol and ampicillin, followed by a change to the appropriate drug when susceptibility data are available. Unfortunately, although rare, isolates resistant to chloramphenicol[67] and to both chloramphenicol and ampicillin[32] have been reported. (Resistance to other antimicrobial agents has also been reported.[70]) Chloramphenicol resistance is most frequently associated with the enzyme chloramphenicol acetyltransferase[70] and can be detected with commercially available filter paper disks (C.A.T., Remel Laboratories, Lenexa, Kan.). The development of resistance to chloramphenicol (as well as ampicillin) and the toxicity of chloramphenicol have prompted the search for alternative antimicrobics.[15] Several studies show the newer cephalosporins to be effective.[15,31,70]

The Centers for Disease Control recommends that chancroid be treated with erythromycin or, alternatively, with sulfamethoxazole and trimethoprim.[7] Antimicrobial susceptibility testing is necessary only for isolates from patients who do not respond to this treatment.[12]

PREVENTION

Even with appropriate antimicrobial therapy, Hib meningitis can cause serious sequelae, such as mental retardation and hearing loss.[56] The high morbidity and mortality of this disease have prompted much research in the development of a vaccine, and in fact a polysaccharide vaccine against *H. influenzae* type b has recently been licensed in the United States. This vaccine is recommended for all children at 24 months of age. However, it is not effective in children less than 18 months of age, and its precise efficacy in children of 18 to 23 months is unknown.[52] Ongoing research is aimed at developing a vaccine that could be used in infants, the population at greatest risk for this disease. Hib polysaccharide-protein conjugate vaccines may prove to be effective in this age group.[18,29a,52]

REFERENCES

1. Albritton, W.L., et al.: Biochemical characteristics of *Haemophilus influenzae* in relationship to source of isolation and antibiotic resistance, J. Clin. Microbiol. **7:**519, 1978.
2. Albritton, W.L., et al.: *Haemophilus ducreyi* and *Calymmatobacterium granulomatis*. In Lennette, E.H., et al, editors: Manual of clinical microbiology, ed. 4, Washington, D.C., 1985, American Society for Microbiology.
3. Berk, S.L., et al.: Nontypeable *Haemophilus influenzae* in the elderly, Arch. Intern. Med. **142:**537, 1982.
4. Bieger, R.C., Brewer, N.S., and Washington, J.A., II: *Haemophilus aphrophilus:* a microbiologic and clinical review and report of 42 cases, Medicine **57:**345, 1978.
5. Bilgeri, Y.R., et al.: Antimicrobial susceptibility of 103 strains of *Haemophilus ducreyi* isolated in Johannesburg, Antimicrob. Agents Chemother. **22:**686, 1982.
6. Blackmore, C.A., et al.: An outbreak of chancroid in Orange County, California: descriptive epidemiology and disease-control measures, J. Infect. Dis. **151:**840, 1985.
7. Centers for Disease Control: Chancroid—California, MMWR **31:**173, 1982.
8. Chapin, K.C., and Doern, G.V.: Selective media for recovery of *Haemophilus influenzae* from specimens contaminated with upper respiratory tract microbial flora, J. Clin. Microbiol. **17:**1163, 1983.
9. Daum, R.S., and Granoff, D.M.: A vaccine against *Haemophilus influenzae* type b, Pediatr. Infect. Dis. **4:**355, 1985.
10. Doern, G.V., and Chapin, K.C.: Laboratory identification of *Haemophilus influenzae:* effects of basal media on the results of the satellitism test and evaluation of the RapID NH system, J. Clin. Microbiol. **20:**599, 1984.
11. Edberg, S.C., Melton, E., and Singer, J.M.: Rapid biochemical characterization of *Haemophilus* species by using the Micro-ID, J. Clin. Microbiol. **11:**22, 1980.
12. Eschenbach, D., Pollock, H.M., and Schacter, J.: Laboratory diagnosis of female genital tract infections. In Rubin, S.J., editor: Laboratory diagnosis of female genital tract infections, Cumitech 17, Washington, D.C., 1983, American Society for Microbiology.
13. Evans, N.M., and Smith, D.D.: The effect of the medium and source of growth factors on the satellitism for *Haemophilus* species, J. Med. Microbiol. **5:**509, 1972.
14. Frazier, J.P., Cleary, T.G., and Pickering, L.K.: Meningitis due to *Haemophilus parainfluenzae:* report of three cases and review of the literature, Pediatr. Infect. Dis. **1:**117, 1982.
15. Freedman, J.M., et al.: Moxalactam for the treatment of bacterial meningitis in children, J. Infect. Dis. **148:**886, 1983.
16. Geraci, J.E., et al.: *Haemophilus* endocarditis, Mayo Clin. Proc. **52:**209, 1977.
16a. Gerber, M.A.: Critical appraisal of the clinical relevance of rapid diagnosis in pediatrics, Diagn. Microbiol. Infect. Dis. **3:**39S, 1985.

17. Granato, P.A., Jurek, E.A., and Weiner, L.B.: Biotypes of *Haemophilus influenzae:* relationship to clinical source of isolation, serotype, and antibiotic susceptibility, Am. J. Clin. Pathol. **79:**73, 1983.

18. Granoff, D.M., and Cates, K.L.: *Haemophilus influenzae* type b polysaccharide vaccines, J. Pediatr. **107:**330, 1985.

19. Gratten, M.: *Haemophilus influenzae* biotype VII, J. Clin. Microbiol. **18:**1015, 1983.

20. Hammond, G.W. et al.: Comparison of specimen collection and laboratory techniques for isolation of *Haemophilus ducreyi,* J. Clin. Microbiol. **7:**39, 1978.

21. Hannah, P., and Greenwood, J.R.: Isolation and rapid identification of *Haemophilus ducreyi,* J. Clin. Microbiol. **16:**861, 1982.

22. Hart, G.: Chancroid, donovanosis, and lymphogranuloma venereum, Dermatol. Clin. **1:**75, 1983.

23. Himmelreich, C.A., Barenkamp, S.J., and Storch, G.A.: Comparison of methods for serotyping isolates of *Haemophilus influenzae,* J. Clin. Microbiol. **21:**158, 1985.

24. Hirschmann, J.V., and Everett, E.D.: *Haemophilus influenzae* infections in adults: report of nine cases and a review of the literature, Medicine **58:**80, 1979.

25. Holmes, R.L., DeFranco, L.M., and Otto, M.: Novel method of biotyping *Haemophilus influenzae* that uses API 20E, J. Clin. Microbiol. **15:**1150, 1982.

26. Ingram, D.L., et al.: Methods for serotyping nasopharyngeal isolates of *Haemophilus influenzae:* slide agglutination, quellung reaction, countercurrent immunoelectrophoresis, latex agglutination, and antiserum agar, J. Clin. Microbiol. **9:**570, 1979.

27. Ispahani, P., and Youngs, E.R.: Non-capsulate *Haemophilus influenzae:* a neglected pathogen in adults, Br. Med. J. **290:**1870, 1985.

28. Jemsek, J.G., et al.: *Haemophilus parainfluenzae* endocarditis: two cases and review of the literature in the past decade, Am. J. Med. **66:**51, 1979.

29. Juni, B.A., Rysavy, J.M., and Blazevic, D.J.: Rapid biotyping of *Haemophilus influenzae* and *Haemophilus parainfluenzae* with PathoTec strips and spot biochemical tests, J. Clin. Microbiol. **15:**976, 1982.

29a. Käyhty, H., et al.: Immunogenicity in infants of a vaccine composed of *Haemophilus influenzae* type b capsular polysaccharide mixed with DPT or conjugated to diphtheria toxoid, J. Infect. Dis. **155:**100, 1987.

30. Kaplan, S.L., and Feigin, R.D.: Infections due to *Haemophilus influenzae.* In Behrman, R.E. and Vaughn, V.C., III, editors: Textbook of pediatrics, ed. 12, Philadelphia, 1983, W.B. Saunders Co.

31. Kaplan, S.L., et al.: Moxalactam treatment of serious infections primarily due to *Haemophilus influenzae* type b in children, Pediatrics **71:**187, 1983.

32. Kenny, J.F., Isburg, C.D., and Michaels, R.H.: Meningitis due to *Haemophilus influenzae* type b resistant to both ampicillin and chloramphenicol, Pediatrics **66:**14, 1980.

33. Kilian, M.: A rapid method for the differentiation of *Haemophilus* strains—the porphyrin test, Acta Pathol. Microbiol. Scand. **82B:**835, 1974.

34. Kilian, M.: The haemolytic activity of *Haemophilus* species, Acta Pathol. Microbiol. Immunol. Scand. **84B:**339, 1976.

35. Kilian, M.: A taxonomic study of the genus *Haemophilus* with the proposal of a new species, J. Gen. Microbiol. **93:**9, 1976.

36. Kilian, M.: *Haemophilus.* In Lennette, E.H., et al., editors: Manual of clinical microbiology, ed. 4. Washington, D.C., 1985, American Society for Microbiology.

37. Kilian, M., and Biberstein, E.L.: Genus II—*Haemophilus.* In Krieg, N.R., editor (Holt, J.G., editor-in-chief): Bergey's manual of systematic bacteriology, Baltimore, 1984, Williams & Wilkins Co.

38. Kilian, M., Sorensen, I., and Frederiksen, W.: Biochemical characteristics of 130 recent isolates from *Haemophilus influenzae* meningitis, J. Clin. Microbiol. **9:**409, 1979.

39. Long, S.S., Teter, M.J., and Gilligan, P.H.: Biotype of *Haemophilus influenzae:* correlation with virulence and ampicillin resistance, J. Infect. Dis. **147:**800, 1983.

40. Mendelman, P.M., et al.: Characterization of non-β-lactamase-mediated ampicillin resistance in *Haemophilus influenzae,* Antimicrob. Agents Chemother. **26:**235, 1984.

41. McCarthy, L.R.: Advances in the understanding of *Haemophilus* spp., Clin. Microbiol. Newsletter **5:**27, 1983.

42. Moxon, E.R.: The molecular basis of *Haemophilus influenzae* virulence, J. R. Coll. Phys. Lond. **19:**174, 1985.

43. Moxon, E.R., and Vaughn, K.A.: The type b capsular polysaccharide as a virulence determinant of *Haemophilus influenzae:* studies using clinical isolates and laboratory transformants, J. Infect. Dis. **143:**517, 1981.

44. Musher, D.M., and Wallace, R.J.: Nontypeable *Haemophilus influenzae* definitely pathogenic for adults, Arch. Intern. Med. **142:**448, 1982.

45. Musher, D.M., et al.: Pneumonia and acute febrile tracheobronchitis due to *Haemophilus influenzae,* Ann. Intern. Med. **99:**444, 1983.

46. Noble, R.C.: Chancroid. In Sexually transmitted diseases, ed. 3, New York, 1985, Medical Examination Publishing Co.

47. Nobre, G.N.: Identification of *Haemophilus ducreyi* in the clinical laboratory, J. Med. Microbiol. **15:**243, 1982.

48. Nsanze, H., et al.: Comparison of media for the primary isolation of *Haemophilus ducreyi,* Sex. Transm. Dis. **11:**6, 1984.

49. Oberhoefer, T.R., and Back, A.E.: Biotypes of *Haemophilus* encountered in clinical laboratories, J. Clin. Microbiol. **10:**168, 1979.

50. Odumeru, J.A., Wiseman, G.M., and Ronald, A.R.: Virulence factors of *Haemophilus ducreyi,* Infect. Immun. **43:**607, 1984.

51. Oill, P.A., Chow, A.W., and Guze, L.B.: Adult bacteremic *Haemophilus parainfluenzae* infections: seven reports of cases and a review of the literature, Arch. Intern. Med. **139:**985, 1979.

52. Recommendations of the Immunization Practices Advisory Committee (ACIP)—polysaccharide vaccine for prevention of *Haemophilus influenzae* type b disease, MMWR **34:**201, 1985.

53. Retter, M.E., and Bannatyne, R.M.: A comparison of conventional and Minitek systems for biotyping *Haemophilus influenzae,* Am. J. Clin. Pathol. **75:**827, 1981.

54. Riley, H.D., Jr.: *Haemophilus influenzae* infections, Part II, Crit. Rev. Clin. Lab. Sci. **15:**277, 1981.

55. Ronald, A.R., and Albritton, W.L.: Chancroid and *Haemophilus ducreyi.* In Holmes, K.K., et al., editors: Sexually transmitted diseases, New York, 1984, McGraw-Hill Book Co.

56. Sell, S.H.W., et al.: Long-term sequelae of *Haemophilus influenzae* meningitis, Pediatrics **49:**206, 1972.

57. Shively, R.G., et al.: Typing of *Haemophilus influenzae* by coagglutination and conventional slide agglutination, J. Clin. Microbiol. **14:**706, 1981.

58. Smith, A.: Antibiotic resistance. In Session 208 *Haemophilus influenzae,* Annual Meeting, American Society for Microbiology, New Orleans, March 10, 1983.

59. Sottnek, F.O., et al.: Isolation and identification of *Haemophilus ducreyi* in a clinical study, J. Clin. Microbiol. **12:**170, 1980.

60. Spagnuolo, P.J., et al.: *Haemophilus influenzae* meningitis—the spectrum of disease in adults, Medicine **61:**74, 1982.

61. Stewardson-Krieger, P., and Naidu, S.: Simultaneous recovery of β-lactamase-negative and β-lactamase-positive *Haemophilus influenzae* type b from cerebrospinal fluid of a neonate, Pediatrics **68:**253, 1981.

62. Sutton, A., et al.: Differential complement resistance mediates virulence of *Haemophilus influenzae* type b, Infect. Immun. **35:**95, 1982.

63. Trollfors, B., et al.: Invasive infections caused by *Haemophilus* species other than *Haemophilus influenzae,* Infection **13:**12, 1985.

64. Turk, D.C.: Clinical importance of *Haemophilus influenzae*—1981. In Sell, S.H., and Wright, P.F., editors: *Haemophilus influenzae:* epidemiology, immunology, and prevention of disease, New York, 1981, Elsevier Biomedical.

65. Wallace, R.J., et al.: *Haemophilus influenzae* infections in adults: characterization of strains by serotypes, biotypes, and β-lactamase production, J. Infect. Dis. **144:**101, 1981.

66. Wallace, R.J., et al.: Nontypeable *Haemophilus influenzae* (biotype 4) as a neonatal, maternal, and genital pathogen, Rev. Infect. Dis. **5:**123, 1983.

67. Ward, J.I., et al.: Prevalence of ampicillin- and chloramphenicol-resistant strains of *Haemophilus influenzae* causing meningitis and bacteremia: national survey of hospital laboratories, J. Infect. Dis. **138:**421, 1978.

68. Ward, J.I., et al.: *Haemophilus influenzae* meningitis—a national study of secondary spread in household contacts, N. Engl. J. Med. **301:**122, 1979.

69. Whisnant, J.K., et al.: Host factors and antibody response in *Haemophilus influenzae* type b meningitis and epiglottitis, J. Infect. Dis. **133:**448, 1976.

70. Williams, J.D., and Moosdeen, F.: Antibiotic resistance in *Haemophilus influenzae:* epidemiology, mechanisms, and therapeutic possibilities, Rev. Infect. Dis. **8:**S555, 1986.

71. Zinnemann, K., et al.: A haemolytic V-dependent CO_2-preferring *Haemophilus* species *Haemophilus paraphrohaemolyticus* nov. spec., J. Med. Microbiol. **4:**139, 1971.

CHAPTER 16

Enterobacteriaceae

J. J. Farmer III
Barbara J. Howard
Alice S. Weissfeld

The family *Enterobacteriaceae* is comprised of a large group of gram-negative, nonsporeforming bacilli that are oxidase negative, ferment glucose with the production of acid and gas, reduce nitrate to nitrite (with the exception of certain biogroups of *Enterobacter agglomerans* and members of the genus *Erwinia*), and are peritrichously flagellated if motile. Many genera in this family (such as *Escherichia*, *Enterobacter*, and *Klebsiella*) are normal inhabitants of the intestinal tract of humans and other animals. Other genera, such as *Salmonella*, *Shigella*, and *Yersinia*, are important enteric pathogens that are responsible for a variety of diseases, including dysentery, gastroenteritis, and enteric fever.

CLASSIFICATION

Over the last dozen years, there has been a considerable change in the family *Enterobacteriaceae*.* This can best be seen by comparing the classification of the family given in the third edition of Edwards and Ewing's *Identification of Enterobacteriaceae*[39] and the eighth edition of *Bergey's Manual of Determinative Bacteriology*[27] (see box on p. 290) with the following classification, which is an update of that given in the 1984 edition of *Bergey's Manual of Systematic Bacteriology*:

Genus *Buttiauxella*
  Buttiauxella agrestis
Genus *Cedecea*†
  Cedecea davisae†
  Cedecea lapagei†
  Cedecea neteri† (*Cedecea* species 4)‡
  "*Cedecea* species 3"†
  "*Cedecea* species 5"†
Genus *Citrobacter*†
  Citrobacter freundii†
  Citrobacter amalonaticus† (*Levinea amalonatica*, *Citrobacter freundii* indole⁺, H₂S⁺)
    Citrobacter amalonaticus biogroup 1†
  Citrobacter diversus† (*Citrobacter koseri*, *Levinea malonatica*)
Genus *Edwardsiella*†
  Edwardsiella tarda† (*Edwardsiella anguillimortifera*)
    Edwardsiella tarda biogroup 1†
  Edwardsiella hoshinae
  Edwardsiella ictaluri
Genus *Enterobacter*†
  Enterobacter cloacae†
  Enterobacter aerogenes† (*Klebsiella mobilis*)
  Enterobacter agglomerans† (*Erwinia herbicola*, *Erwinia* sp.)
  Enterobacter amnigenus†

Enterobacter amnigenus biogroup 1†
Enterobacter amnigenus biogroup 2
Enterobacter gergoviae†
Enterobacter intermedium
Enterobacter sakazakii†
Enterobacter taylorae† (Enteric Group 19)
Genus *Erwinia*
  The "true *Erwinia* species"
    Erwinia amylovora—type species for the genus§
    Erwinia herbicola = *Enterobacter agglomerans*
Genus *Escherichia* (including *Shigella*)†
  Escherichia coli†
  Shigella dysenteriae†
  Shigella flexneri† ‖
  Shigella boydii†
  Shigella sonnei†
  Escherichia blattae
  Escherichia fergusonii† (Enteric Group 10)
  Escherichia hermannii† (Enteric Group 11)
  Escherichia vulneris†
Genus *Ewingella*†
  Ewingella americana†
Genus *Hafnia*†
  Hafnia alvei† (*Enterobacter hafinae*)
    Hafnia alvei biogroup 1 (*Obesumbacterium proteus* biogroup 1)

Dr. Farmer is Chief of the Enteric Identification Laboratories of the Enteric Bacteriology Section, Center for Infectious Diseases, Centers for Disease Control, Atlanta, Ga. The contribution to this chapter was written by Dr. Farmer in his private capacity. No official support or endorsement by the Public Health Service or the Department of Health and Human Services is intended or should be inferred. Some of the material in the text and tables is from, or adapted from, public domain government publications. These are considered to be noncopyrightable works of the U.S. government.[56,59,60]
*References 17-20, 23, 27, 34, 35, 43, 47, 53, 54, 56, 60, 66-68, 76, 77, 115-117, 132, 157, 162, 171, and 175.
†Genera and species that have been reported to occur in clinical specimens.
‡Synonyms are given in parentheses.
§Other named species have been included in the genus *Erwinia*. Their inclusion makes it a very heterogeneous genus but one that seems to be of value to plant pathologists and to others who work with isolates from plants. Many of the named *Erwinia* spp. can be classified in the other genera of *Enterobacteriaceae*.
‖All five species are closely related.

Earlier Classifications of the Family *Enterobacteriaceae*

EDWARDS AND EWING

Tribe I: *Escherichieae*
    Genus I: *Escherichia*
        Species: *E. coli*
    Genus II: *Shigella*
        Species: *S. dysenteriae*
                 S. flexneri
                 S. boydii
                 S. sonnei
Tribe II: *Edwardsielleae*
    Genus I: *Edwardsiella*
        Species: *E. tarda*
Tribe III: *Salmonelleae*
    Genus I: *Salmonella*
        Species: *S. cholerae-suis*
                 S. typhi
                 S. enteritidis
    Genus II: *Arizona*
        Species: *A. hinshawii*
    Genus III: *Citrobacter*
        Species: *C. freundii*
Tribe IV: *Klebsielleae*
    Genus I: *Klebsiella*
        Species: *K. pneumoniae*
                 K. ozaenae
                 K. rhinoscleromatis
    Genus II: *Enterobacter*
        Species: *E. cloacae*
                 E. aerogenes
                 E. hafnia
                 E. liquefaciens
    Genus III: *Pectobacterium*
        Species: *P. carotovorum*
    Genus IV: *Serratia*
        Species: *S. marcescens*
Tribe V: *Proteeae*
    Genus I: *Proteus*
        Species: *P. vulgaris*
                 P. mirabilis
                 P. morganii
                 P. rettgeri
    Genus II: *Providencia*
        Species: *P. stuartii*
                 P. alcalifaciens

BERGEY'S MANUAL (ED. 8)

Genus I: *Escherichia*
    Species: *E. coli*
Genus II: *Edwardsiella*
    Species: *E. tarda*
Genus III: *Citrobacter*
    Species: *C. freundii*
             C. intermedius
Genus IV: *Salmonella*
    Subgenus I
        Species: *S. cholerae-suis*
             S. hirschfeldii (S. paratyphi-C)
             S. typhi
             S. paratyphi-A
             S. schottmuelleri (S. paratyphi-B)
             S. typhimurium
             S. enteritidis
             S. gallanarum
    Subgenus II
        Species: *S. salamae*
    Subgenus III
        Species: *S. arizonae*
    Subgenus IV
        Species: *S. houtenae*
Genus V: *Shigella*
    Species: *S. dysenteriae*
             S. flexneri
             S. boydii
             S. sonnei
Genus VI: *Klebsiella*
    Species: *K. pneumoniae*
             K. ozaenae
             K. rhinoscleromatis
Genus VII: *Enterobacter*
    Species: *E. cloacae*
             E. aerogenes
Genus: VIII: *Hafnia*
    Species: *H. alvei*
Genus IX: *Serratia*
    Species: *S. marcescens*
Genus X: *Proteus*
    Species: *P. vulgaris*
             P. mirabilis
             P. morganii
             P. rettgeri
             P. inconstans
Genus XI: *Yersinia*
    Species: *Y. pestis*
             Y. pseudotuberculosis
             Y. enterocolitica
Genus XII: *Erwinia*
    Amylovora Group
        Species: *E. amylovora*
             E. salicis
             E. tracheiphila
             E. nigrifluens
             E. guercina
             E. rubrifaciens
    Herbicola Group
        Species: *E. herbicola*
             E. stewartii
             E. uredovora
    Carotovora Group
        Species: *E. carotovora*
             E. chrysanthemi
             E. cypripedii
             E. rhapontici

Genus *Klebsiella**
  *Klebsiella pneumoniae**
  *Klebsiella ozaenae**   ⎫
  *Klebsiella rhinoscleromatis** ⎬ †
                  ⎭
  *Klebsiella oxytoca** (*Klebsiella pneumoniae* indole positive)
  *Klebsiella planticola**
  Klebsiella terrigena (*Klebsiella trevisanii*)
  Klebsiella Group 47—indole and ornithine positive*
Genus *Kluyvera**
  *Kluyvera ascorbata**
  *Kluyvera cryocrescens**
Genus *Moellerella**
  *Moellerella wisconsensis**
Genus *Morganella**
  *Morganella morganii** (*Proteus morganii*)
Genus *Obesumbacterium*
  Obesumbacterium proteus biogroup 2 (*Hafnia proteae*)
Genus *Proteus**
  *Proteus mirabilis**
  Proteus myxofaciens
  *Proteus penneri** (*Proteus vulgaris* indole negative)
  *Proteus vulgaris**
Genus *Providencia**
  *Providencia alcalifaciens** (*Proteus inconstans* biogroup A)
  *Providencia rettgeri** (*Proteus rettgeri*)
  *Providencia rustigianii** (*Providencia alcalifaciens* biogroup 3)
  *Providencia stuartii** (*Proteus inconstans* biogroup B)
Genus *Rahnella**
  *Rahnella aquatilis**
Genus *Salmonella**
  Subgroup 1* (Subgenus I)—over 1200 named serotypes, such as:
    Salmonella typhimurium‡
    Salmonella newport‡
    Salmonella anatum‡
    Salmonella infantis‡
    Salmonella enteritidis‡
    Salmonella heidelberg‡
    Salmonella saint-paul‡
    Salmonella typhi§
    Salmonella paratyphi A§
    Salmonella choleraesuis§
    Salmonella sendai§
    Salmonella abortusovis§
    Salmonella typhisuis§
    Salmonella gallanarum§
    Salmonella pullorum§
  Subgroup 2*(Subgenus II)
  Subgroup 3a* (Arizona group; Subgenus III with monophasic flagella antigens)
  Subgroup 3b* (Arizona group; Subgenus III with diphasic flagella antigens)
  Subgroup 4* (Subgenus IV)
  Subgroup 5* (Subgenus V)
Genus *Serratia**
  *Serratia marcescens**
  *Serratia ficaria**
  Serratia liquefaciens Group*‖

*Serratia odorifera**
*Serratia plymuthica**
*Serratia rubidaea** (*Seratia marinorubra*)
*Serratia fonticola**—a candidate for removal from genus
Genus *Shigella**¶
  *Shigella dysenteriae** (*Shigella* serogroup A)
  *Shigella flexneri** (*Shigella* serogroup B)
  *Shigella boydii** (*Shigella* serogroup C)
  *Shigella sonnei** (*Shigella* serogroup D)
Genus *Tatumella** (Group EF-9)
  *Tatumella ptyseos**
Genus *Yersinia**
  *Yersinia pestis**   ⎫
  *Yersinia pseudotuberculosis** ⎬**
  *Yersinia enterocolitica**   ⎭
  *Yersinia frederiksenii**
  *Yersinia intermedia**
  *Yersinia kristensenii**
  Yersinia ruckeri—a candidate for removal from genus
Genus *Xenorhabdus*
  Xenorhabdus luminescens
  Xenorhabdus nematophilus
Unclassified organisms which have been given a vernacular name
  Enteric Group 17* (now *Enterobacter asburiae*)††
  Enteric Group 41* (now *Leclercia*)††[162a]
  Enteric Group 45* (now *Koserella*)††[90a]
  Enteric Group 57* (now *Leminorella*)††[90b]
  Enteric Group 58*
  Enteric Group 59*
  Enteric Group 60*
  Enteric Group 63
  Enteric Group 64
  Enteric Group 68*
  Enteric Group 69
  The genera that are new to the family *Enterobacteriaceae,* as described by Edwards and Ewing in 1972, include the following:
  Buttiauxella[62]
  Cedecea[3,58,82,120]

---

*Genera and species that have been reported to occur in clinical specimens.
†All three species are closely related.
‡Examples of serotypes that are biochemically typical and usually cause uncomplicated gastroenteritis.
§Serotypes that are biochemically atypical and often cause extraintestinal diseases in humans or animals.
‖Grimont and co-workers have proposed a more complex classification for the *Serratia liquefaciens* Group in which three species (one with two subspecies) are recognized: *Serratia liquefaciens, Serratia grimesii, Serratia proteamaculans* ssp. *proteamaculans,* and *Serratia proteamaculans* ssp. *quinovora.*
¶See also the genus *Escherichia.*
**These two species are closely related.
††These enteric groups have been assigned the indicated names since this chapter was written.

Erwinia[70,123,146,160,161,173]
Ewingella[83]
Hafnia[84]
Kluyvera[1,2,15,51,57,147]
Moellerella[90]
Morganella[20,87]
Obesumbacterium[29,139,152-155]
Rahnella[101]
Tatumella[94]
Yersinia[7-9,12,14,21,24,50,143,165,166]
Xenorhabdus[133-136,164]

The species that are new to previously described genera include the following:

Citrobacter amalonaticus[53,176]
Citrobacter diversus[46,176]
Edwardsiella hoshinae[81]
Edwardsiella ictaluri[85]
Enterobacter agglomerans[48]
Enterobacter amnigenus[102]
Enterobacter gergoviae[22,141]
Enterobacter intermedium[100]
Enterobacter sakazakii[55]
Enterobacter taylorae[61]
Escherichia adecarboxulata[114]
Escherichia blattae[28]
Escherichia fergusonii[61]
Escherichia hermannii[25]
Escherichia vulneris[26]
Klebsiella oxytoca[104]
Klebsiella planticola[4,63,174]
Klebsiella terrigena[103]
Proteus myxofaciens[33]
Proteus penneri[88]
Providencia rustigianii[89]
Serratia ficaria[71,78]
Serratia fonticola[69]
Serratia liquefaciens[49,79]
Serratia odorifera[80]
Serratia plymuthica[80]
Serratia rubidaea[49,159]

Synonyms for some of these new organisms are given in parentheses in the list beginning on p. 289. When names change, it is a good idea to list both the new designation and the previous designation for a period of time so physicians and allied health professionals have a chance to familiarize themselves with the new nomenclature.

Other changes include the addition of a number of biogroups or subdivisions of existing species that have been defined for more precise identification.[60] There are also a number of biochemically defined ''enteric groups'' that have not yet been given scientific names. The genera *Escherichia* and *Shigella* can be considered together because recent data from DNA-relatedness studies suggest that they are closely related.[125] *Pectobacterium* is no longer used as a subdivision within *Erwinia*. *Arizona* is no longer a separate genus; it is now included as subgroups 3a and 3b of the genus *Salmonella*.[116,117] The genus *Salmonella* currently can be further subdivided into six major subgroups and into over 2000 serotypes. However, for convenience, the named serotypes can be artificially treated as species; for instance, *Salmonella* serotype *typhimurium* is called *Salmonella typhimurium*. (This is discussed more thoroughly on p. 306.)

The new classification scheme is based on a polyphasic approach to taxonomy[23] that utilizes DNA-DNA hybridization, computer analysis, and phenotypic testing (biochemical reactions, antimicrobial susceptibility patterns, and other tests) to show that a group of strains belongs to a new genus, species, or biogroup (see Chapter 1). Simple tests are then found to differentiate the new organism from existing species in the family; these tests are used by clinical microbiologists to identify an unknown isolate.

Although the current scheme is more complex, most of the new genera, species, biogroups, and enteric groups are rarely found in human specimens. A typical hospital microbiology laboratory isolates many hundreds, perhaps thousands, of strains of *Escherichia coli*, *Klebsiella pneumoniae*, and *Proteus mirabilis*, but only a handful of isolates of many of these new organisms. This fact must always be kept in mind when one is trying to identify a clinical isolate. For example, a strain from urine is about 100,000 times more likely to be *E. coli* than a *Kluyvera* sp.

SPECIMEN COLLECTION AND PROCESSING

Clinical specimens often contain *Enterobacteriaceae* in combination with many other bacterial species. Thus specimens should be transported to the laboratory rapidly or placed in transport media (such as Cary-Blair medium, Amies medium, or Stuart medium) so the *Enterobacteriaceae* do not outgrow the more fastidious pathogens. Cary-Blair transport medium is preferred for transporting and maintaining tissues infected with *Yersinia pestis*.[140] Cary-Blair medium is also useful for transporting stool for isolation of the genera *Salmonella*, *Shigella*, or *Yersinia*.

GROWTH REQUIREMENTS
MEDIA

In general, *Enterobacteriaceae* grow well on a variety of laboratory plating media, including numerous differential and selective media that were initially developed for the isolation of the enteric pathogens from stool. These media are selective by virtue of the incorporation of dyes (for instance, brilliant green or crystal violet) and bile salts (for instance, sodium deoxycholate) that inhibit both gram-positive bacteria and some nonpathogenic species of *Enterobacteriaceae* present in stool. Depending on the concentration of inhibitory agents, the media are defined as possessing (1) low selectivity, for instance, MacConkey (MAC) agar or eosin–methylene blue (EMB) agar, (2) moderate selectivity, for instance, Salmonella-Shigella (SS) agar, deoxycholate citrate (DC) agar, Hektoen enteric (HE) agar, or xylose lysine deoxycholate (XLD) agar, or (3) high selectivity, for instance, brilliant green (BG) agar or bismuth sulfite (BS) agar. (All of these media are discussed in Appendix A.) Most of these selective media are also differential media; that is, the majority of them differentiate among organisms on the basis of whether the organisms ferment lactose. pH indicators (for example, neutral red) are incorporated into the media to detect acid produced by the bacteria as they ferment lactose. Enrichment broths (for example, gram-negative [GN] broth, selenite F [SF] broth, or tetrathionate broth with brilliant green) have also been developed to promote the growth of *Salmonella* or *Shigella* spp. while inhibiting the growth of normal intestinal flora. Following incubation at 35° C for specified intervals, these broths are subcultured to the same media used for primary isolation (see Appendix A).

Isolation of *Enterobacteriaceae* from extraintestinal sources is relatively simple. Specimens of any type may be submitted, including urine, sputum, pus, blood, and body fluids. Most commercial blood culture media are acceptable for isolation of organisms from blood. Other specimens are usually plated on a noninhibitory medium, such as blood agar, and on a differential medium with low selectivity, such as MacConkey or EMB agar.

Isolation of the genera *Salmonella, Shigella,* or *Yersinia* from intestinal sources is somewhat more complicated. An occasional strain of *Shigella* may not grow on MacConkey, SS, or DC agar, and some strains of *Salmonella* do not grow on BG agar. Therefore a variety of media are included to ensure maximal recovery of these organisms. In general, specimens from intestinal sources are plated onto one medium of low selectivity, one of moderate selectivity, and one of high selectivity. BS agar is not widely used in clinical laboratories for a number of reasons, including its very short shelf life (48 to 72 hours). However its use is sometimes more advantageous than BG agar because it allows detection of rare strains of *Salmonella* that ferment lactose. An enrichment broth is also included in the primary setup for isolation of the genera *Salmonella* and *Shigella.*

Yersinia enterocolitica is often overgrown by other intestinal flora on MacConkey and other enteric agars. Therefore a selective medium, such as cefsulodin-irgasan-novobiocin (CIN) agar, can be used to isolate this organism from stool.[145] The low yield of *Y. enterocolitica* in most studies, however, has limited the use of a specific plate for this organism. Nonetheless, a selective medium may be necessary in areas such as Canada and the northeastern United States where the incidence of *Y. enterocolitica* infection is high. Cold enrichment techniques or alkaline treatment have also been used successfully to recover these organisms from intestinal sources, but these are seldom used routinely in the clinical laboratory.[172] A more complete discussion of the collection and processing of gastrointestinal specimens is included in Chapter 11.

Microbiologists must be cautious in handling isolates of *Salmonella typhi*. Numerous laboratory-acquired infections, some fatal, have occurred because of failure to adhere to recognized standards of safety.

Special care must also be taken with specimens from patients with suspected *Yersinia pestis* infection (bubonic or pneumonic plague). Such infections have been recently reported in the western United States, especially California and New Mexico. All work with this organism must be performed in a biologic safety cabinet by personnel wearing masks and gloves.

ENVIRONMENTAL REQUIREMENTS

Members of the family *Enterobacteriaceae* grow in both the presence and absence of oxygen and thus are facultative anaerobes. Most of the *Enterobacteriaceae* form 1 to 3 mm diameter colonies within 18 to 24 hours on standard laboratory media.

Although the optimum temperature for the isolation of *Enterobacteriaceae* is 35° to 37° C, individual species show a wide temperature tolerance, with some species growing at temperatures as low as 1° to 5° C (*Serratia* and *Yersinia*), and others growing at temperatures as high as 45° to 50° C (*Escherichia coli*). Some organisms, such as *Yersinia enterocolitica* and *Hafnia alvei,* have different biochemical reactions at different temperatures.

CULTURAL CHARACTERISTICS
STAINING REACTIONS

The members of the family *Enterobacteriaceae* cannot be identified on the basis of their Gram stain morphology. Most are gram-negative, rod-shaped bacteria with straight sides and rounded ends, ranging in size from 0.5 to 2 µm wide and 2 to 4 µm long (Figure 16-1). Some strains appear coccobacillary. In addition, some young cultures of swarming *Proteus* appear as long, curved filaments, reaching 10 to 30 µm in length. *Klebsiella* strains may appear shorter or thicker than other members of the family; encapsulated strains may be observed (Plate 8, *D*).

Yersinia pestis can be stained with a polychromatic stain, such as the Wayson stain. The organisms are characteristically light blue to reddish with dark blue polar bodies; they appear swollen, barrel shaped, or like closed safety pins.

COLONIAL MORPHOLOGY

Most members of the *Enterobacteriaceae* family produce similar growth on blood agar. Colonies are relatively large and dull gray. Colonies of some species are watery or mucoid. Members of the genus *Klebsiella,* for example, produce large, mucoid colonies that frequently form a string when touched with an inoculating needle (Figure 16-2). Hemolysis on blood agar is usually variable and not distinctive, although *Escherichia coli* is often distinctly hemolytic on primary isolation from significant infection.

Proteus mirabilis, Proteus penneri, and *Proteus vulgaris* tend to swarm on blood and other moist agar, producing a thin film of confluent surface growth (Plate 8, *E*). Swarming may be inhibited on MacConkey and EMB plates by increasing concentration of the agar in the medium from 1.5% to 5%.

Yersinia pestis grows from pinpoint colonies (0.1 to 0.5 mm) at 24 hours to 1 to 1.5 mm colonies by 48 hours. Colonies usually exhibit a characteristically rough, hammered copper or cauliflower appearance within 48 hours. *Yersinia enterocolitica* produces bright burgundy, "bull's-eye" colonies on CIN medium.

Most *Enterobacteriaceae* produce turbid growth in common broth media (such as thioglycolate and brain heart infusion) within 24 hours. One exception is *Yersinia pestis,* which exhibits a stalactite pattern of growth with floccules that adhere to one side of the tube.

Table 16-1 describes the colonial appearance of the most commonly isolated clinical genera on a variety of enteric media.

BIOCHEMICAL IDENTIFICATION

There are many different approaches to the identification of the family *Enterobacteriaceae*. Until the 1970s almost all clinical and public health microbiology laboratories performed conventional biochemical tests in tubes.[39,45,52] This often involved inoculating 25 to 50 separate media. Today, more and more laboratories are using miniaturized or automated commer-

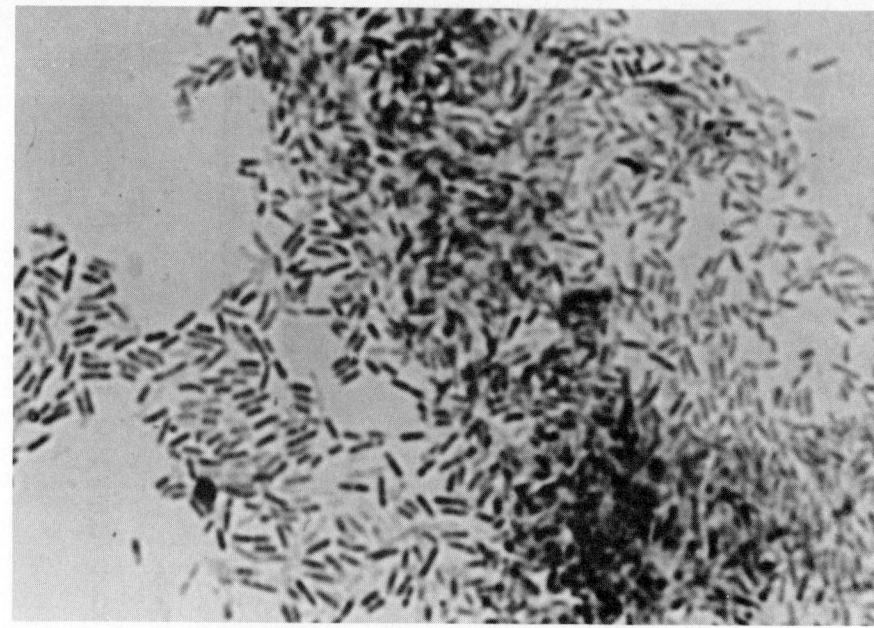

FIGURE 16-1. *Enterobacteriaceae* typically appear as gram-negative, rod-shaped bacteria with straight sides and rounded ends. (Photograph by Dr. Leon J. LeBeau, Department of Biocommunication Arts, Medical Center, University of Illinois at Chicago.)

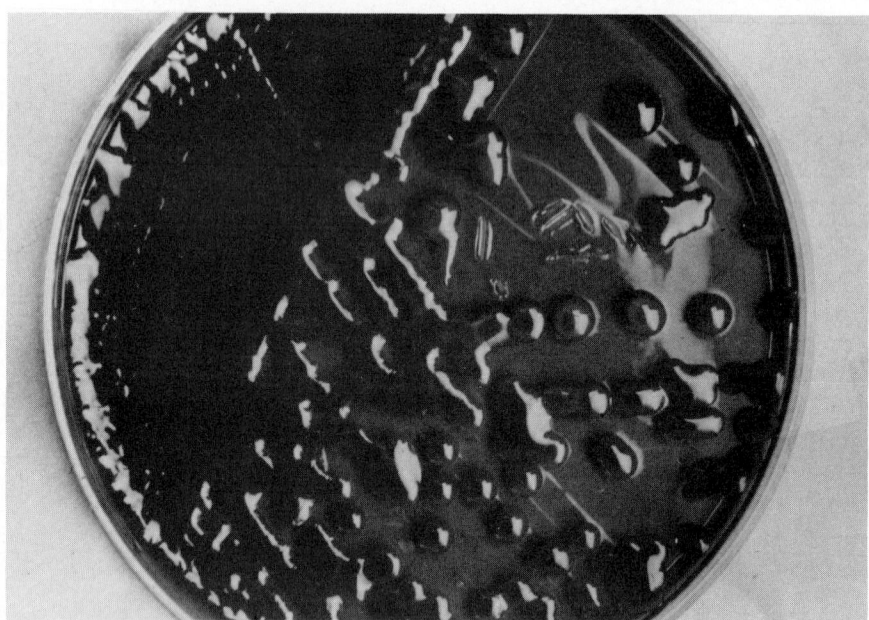

FIGURE 16-2. Mucoid colonies of *Klebsiella pneumoniae* on eosin–methylene blue (EMB) agar.

TABLE 16-1. Appearance of Commonly Isolated *Enterobacteriaceae* on Various Enteric Media

	MacConkey (MAC) Agar	Eosin–Methylene Blue (EMB) Agar	Hektoen Enteric (HE) Agar	Xylose–Lysine Deoxycholate (XLD) Agar	Salmonella-Shigella (SS) Agar	Deoxycholate Citrate (DC) Agar	Bismuth Sulfite (BS) Agar	Brilliant Green (BG) Agar
Escherichia coli Lac+	Flat; red or dark pink; surrounded by zone of precipitated bile	Red black with metallic sheen[a] (Plate 9, A)	Yellow-orange	Yellow	Pink	Deep red-pink	Usually do not grow	Usually do not grow
Lac−	Colorless	Colorless	Yellow-orange or green	Yellow	Colorless	Colorless	Usually do not grow	Usually do not grow
Klebsiella	Pink; mucoid	Purple	Yellow-orange	Yellow	Pink	Pink	Usually do not grow	Usually do not grow
Enterobacter	Pink; not usually as mucoid as *Klebsiella*	Purple	Yellow-orange	Yellow	Pink	Pink	Usually do not grow	Usually do not grow
Citrobacter, Serratia, Hafnia, Providencia	May appear colorless after 24 hr or slightly pink in 24 to 48 hr	Lavender or colorless	Colorless	Red, yellow, or colorless with or without black centers	Colorless	Colorless	Usually do not grow	Usually do not grow
Proteus, Morganella, Edwardsiella	Colorless[b]	Colorless	Colorless	Red, yellow, or colorless with or without black centers	Colorless	Colorless	Usually do not grow	Usually do not grow
Salmonella	Colorless	Colorless	Green or blue-green	Pink to red with black center	Colorless with black center	Colorless	Green-black	Pink-white opaque; surrounded by brilliant red medium
Shigella	Colorless	Colorless	Green or blue-green	Colorless	Colorless	Colorless	Usually do not grow	Usually do not grow
Yersinia	Colorless to peach	Colorless or purple[c]	Salmon	Yellow	Colorless	Colorless	Usually do not grow	Usually do not grow

[a]Not all strains produce a metallic sheen; on the other hand, other species of enteric bacilli (for instance, *Yersinia enterocolitica*) may produce a sheen.

[b]*Proteus mirabilis, Proteus vulgaris,* and *Proteus penneri* may swarm.

[c]*Yersinia enterocolitica,* a non-lactose-fermenter that ferments sucrose, produces colorless colonies on Levine EMB agar and purple colonies on the modified Holt-Harris Teague formula, which contains sucrose.

cial identification systems to identify members of the family. The use of these test kits and automated instruments is described in Chapter 8. Conventional methodology is considered in this chapter. More specialized methods (that is, computer analysis, DNA-DNA hybridization, and chemical analysis) are seldom used in clinical laboratories but can be useful in reference and research laboratories.[6,20,36,112]

The question "How many tests are needed for correct identification of the family *Enterobacteriaceae?*" is sometimes asked. There is no single answer to this question. Before it can be answered, another question must be asked and answered—"What is the acceptable percentage of incorrect identifications?" Because reference centers must strive for 100% accuracy in identification, 25 to 50 biochemical and other tests, such as serologic typing and computer analysis, may be done on each culture sent for identification. Reference laboratories are not required to obtain results as rapidly as are primary hospital microbiology laboratories and can work for 100% accuracy with essentially no time or cost constraints. Obviously a busy hospital microbiology laboratory cannot afford to spend that much time and effort on identification. Thus most clinical laboratories that use conventional biochemical tests have developed their own flowcharts or abbreviated differentiation charts for identification.[91] These charts are usually based on an analysis of key tests for identification of each genus. Since a few species of the family *Enterobacteriaceae* represent 95% to 98% of all those found, such shortcuts yield acceptable results most of the time. Misidentifications sometimes occur, however, because of the biochemical similarity of some species.

Table 16-2 lists the test results that are useful for differentiating the genera of *Enterobacteriaceae.* (These values are weighted to reflect data for those species in the genus that are most common in clinical specimens.) Before reviewing key reactions for each genus, several salient points should be noted.

First, the oxidase and nitrate reduction tests are critical. Strains of *Enterobacteriaceae* may be separated from the genus *Pseudomonas,* as well as from certain other miscellaneous gram-negative rods, on the basis of a negative result with the cytochrome oxidase test. Similarly, most genera (except certain biogroups of *Enterobacter agglomerans* and members of the genus *Erwinia*) reduce nitrate to nitrite.

Second, experienced microbiologists can presumptively identify many organisms by simply observing the colonial growth (lactose versus non-lactose-fermenter) on MacConkey or EMB agar.

Third, three media, triple sugar iron (TSI) agar, lysine iron agar (LIA), and urea agar, are extremely helpful in screening stool cultures for potential pathogens. (Table 16-3 lists the reactions observed in TSI and LIA for various genera and species of *Enterobacteriaceae.*) Urea is included to screen out rapid urease-positive organisms, such as *Proteus* and *Providencia* (Plate 9, *D*). The TSI, LIA, and urea slants are inoculated by touching the inoculating needle to the center of a well-isolated colony and (1) stabbing the butt of the TSI and streaking the slant as the needle is removed, (2) stabbing the butt of the LIA twice, and (3) stabbing the butt of the urea agar once and streaking the slant as the needle is removed. The needle should not be flamed between inoculating different tubes nor returned to the original colony to pick up additional inoculum. Kligler iron agar (KIA) can be substituted for TSI. A complete descrip-

tion of the purpose, mechanism, and interpretation of these media and other biochemical tests for identification of *Enterobacteriaceae* is presented in Appendix A.

Another point to note concerns IMViC reactions. These reactions are now seldom used in clinical microbiology laboratories because of the introduction of rapid systems; however, they are still used in food and dairy microbiology and may be of use to clinical laboratories that still rely on standard biochemicals. The acronym IMViC refers to a combination of four tests—*I*ndole, *M*ethyl red, *V*oges-Proskauer, and *C*itrate (the "i" is inserted for euphony)—that are useful in distinguishing certain members of the family *Enterobacteriaceae,* especially the lactose-fermenting normal intestinal flora.* For example, a lactose fermenter that produces a flat, red colony on MacConkey agar, is surrounded by a red zone of precipitated bile salts, and is indole positive, methyl red positive, Voges-Proskauer negative, and citrate negative is, most probably, *Escherichia coli.* Similarly, a lactose-positive mucoid colony that is indole negative, methyl red negative, Voges-Proskauer positive, and citrate positive is, most probably, *Klebsiella pneumoniae.*

Finally, it should be noted that the appearance of an atypical character in a culture that is otherwise typical (for instance, H_2S-producing variants of *Escherichia coli*[113]) may be explained by the acquisition of a plasmid for the phenotypic trait. Therefore the overall biochemical profile should be considered when identifying an unknown isolate.

BIOCHEMICAL CHARACTERISTICS

Table 16-4 lists the named genera, species, and biogroups of *Enterobacteriaceae* and their reactions in the biochemical tests most often used for identification. Each number in the table represents the percentage of organisms positive for a given test after 48 hours of incubation. No delayed reactions were considered, and it should be noted that the vast majority of the organisms had positive reactions after 24 hours. All incubations were at $36° \pm 1°$ C, except for *Xenorhabdus* organisms, which do not grow well at $36°$ C and were incubated at $25°$ C.

Cedecea

Cedecea spp. resemble *Serratia* spp. but differ from them in being DNAse negative and gelatinase negative. Differentiation of species within the genus is shown in Table 16-5.

Citrobacter

Members of the genus *Citrobacter* are motile rods that are both rapid and late lactose fermenters. They are often confused with strains of the genus *Salmonella* because their biochemical reactions in TSI, LIA, and urea are similar on initial screening. Many serologic cross-reactions also occur between these genera. Unlike the *Salmonella,* however, *Citrobacter* spp. are lysine decarboxylase negative. As shown in Table 16-6, the three species within the genus may be distinguished on the basis of their reactions in a small number of media.

Edwardsiella

The *Edwardsiella* spp. resemble both *Citrobacter* and *Salmonella* in being H_2S positive. They can be separated from these other genera, however, on the basis of their inability to grow on Simmons' citrate agar and their inability to ferment

---

*These organisms were previously referred to as coliforms.

Text continued on p. 302.

TABLE 16-2. Reaction of the Genera of *Enterobacteriaceae* in Tests Commonly Used for Identification[a]

Genus	IMViC Reactions				Decarboxylases			Miscellaneous Tests					Hydrolytic Enzymes			Fermentation Reactions														
	IND	MR	VP	CIT	LYS	ARG	ORN	H₂S	URE	PHE	MOT	GAS	DNA	GEL	LIP	LAC	SUC	MNT	DUL	SAL	ADO	INO	SRT	ARN	RAFF	RHAM	MALT	XYL	TRE
CORE GENERA																													
Escherichia	+	+	−	−	+	v	v	−	−	−	+	+	−	−	−	+	v	+	v	v	−	−	+	+	v	(+)	+	+	+
Shigella	(−)	+	−	−	−	(−)	v	−	−	−	−	−	−	−	−	−	v	+	v	−	−	−	(−)	(+)	v	v	v	−	(+)
Citrobacter	v	+	−	+	−	v	v	+	(+)	−	+	+	−	−	−	v	v	+	v	v	v	−	+	+	v	+	+	+	+
Salmonella	−	+	−	+	+	(+)	+	+	−	−	+	+	−	−	−	−	−	+	+	−	−	v	+	+	−	+	+	+	+
KES GROUP																													
Klebsiella	(−)	(−)	+	+	+	−	−	−	+	−	−	+	−	−	−	+	+	+	v	+	+	+	+	+	+	+	+	+	+
Enterobacter	−	−	+	+	v	(+)	+	−	v	−	+	+	−	−	−	+	+	+	(−)	(+)	v	v	+	+	+	+	+	+	+
Serratia	−	(−)	+	+	+	−	+	−	(−)	−	+	v	+	+	+	−	+	+	−	+	v	(+)	+	−	−	−	+	−	+
PROTEUS GROUP																													
Proteus	v	+	(−)	v	−	−	v	+	+	+	+	+	v	+	(+)	−	v	−	−	v	−	−	−	−	−	−	v	+	v
Providencia	+	+	−	+	−	−	−	−	v	+	+	v	−	−	−	−	v	v	−	v	v	v	+	−	v	v	−	−	v
Morganella	+	+	−	−	−	−	+	−	+	+	+	(+)	−	−	−	−	−	−	−	−	−	−	−	+	−	−	−	−	(−)
MISCELLANEOUS GENERA																													
Yersinia	v	+	−	−	−	−	v	−	(+)	−	−	−	v	−	v	−	+	+	−	v	−	v	+	+	−	−	(+)	(+)	+
Hafnia	−	v	(+)	−	+	−	+	−	−	−	+	+	−	−	−	−	−	+	−	(−)	−	−	−	+	+	+	+	+	+
RARELY ISOLATED GENERA																													
Kluyvera	(+)	+	−	+	+	v	+	−	−	−	+	(+)	−	−	−	+	+	+	(−)	+	−	−	+	+	+	+	+	+	+
Cedecea	−	+	v	+	−	v	v	−	−	−	+	+	−	−	+	(−)	(+)	+	−	−	−	−	v	+	−	+	(−)	(+)	+
Edwardsiella	+	+	−	−	+	v	+	+	−	−	+	+	−	−	−	−	−	−	v	−	−	−	−	−	−	−	+	−	+
Ewingella	−	(+)	+	+	−	−	−	−	−	−	v	+	−	−	−	v	v	+	−	−	−	−	+	+	−	−	+	(−)	+
Rahnella	−	(+)	+	+	−	−	−	−	−	−	−	+	−	−	−	+	+	+	(+)	+	+	−	+	+	(−)	+	+	+	+
Tatumella	−	+	−	−	−	−	−	−	−	+	+	−	−	−	−	−	+	+	v	v	−	−	−	−	−	−	+	+	−
"NONCLINICAL" GENERA																													
Butiauxella	−	+	−	−	+	−	+	−	−	−	+	+	−	−	−	+	−	+	−	+	−	−	+	+	+	+	(+)	+	+
Obesumbacterium	−	(−)	−	−	+	−	+	−	−	−	−	−	−	−	−	−	−	−	−	−	−	−	−	−	−	(−)	v	(−)	(+)
Xenorhabdus	v	−	−	v	−	−	−	−	(−)	−	+	−	−	v	−	−	−	−	−	v	−	−	−	−	−	−	(−)	−	−

SYMBOLS:
+, Vast majority (perhaps ≥ 90%) positive
(+), Most strains (75%-85%) positive
v, Variable (26%-74%) positive
(−), Most strains negative (11%-25% positive)
−, Vast majority negative (≤10% positive)

IND, Indole	H₂S, Hydrogen sulfide production on TSI	LIP, Lipase (corn oil)	INO, myo-Inositol
MR, Methyl red	URE, Urea hydrolysis	LAC, Lactose	SRT, D-Sorbitol
VP, Voges-Proskauer	PHE, Phenylalanine	SUC, Sucrose	ARN, L-Arabinose
CIT, Simmons' citrate	MOT, Motility	MNT, D-Mannitol	RAFF, Raffinose
LYS, Lysine	GAS, Gas from D-glucose	DUL, Dulcitol	RHAM, L-Rhamnose
ARG, Arginine	DNA, DNAse (25° C)	SAL, Salicin	MALT, Maltose
ORN, Ornithine	GEL, Gelatin (22° C)	ADO, Adonitol	XYL, D-Xylose
			TRE, Trehalose

[a]See text for explanation of how data for each genus are weighted for species that are most commonly encountered in clinical specimens.

TABLE 16-3. Typical Reaction Patterns of *Enterobacteriaceae* on Triple Sugar Iron Agar and Lysine Iron Agar

LYSINE IRON AGAR	Triple Sugar Iron Agar (Plate 9, E)					
	K/Ⓐ H₂S+	K/Ⓐ	K/A	A/Ⓐ H₂S+	A/Ⓐ	A/A
R/A	Proteus vulgaris, Proteus mirabilis	Morganella morganii, Providencia spp.	M. morganii (rare), Providencia spp.	P. vulgaris, P. mirabilis (rare), Proteus penneri	P. penneri	Providencia spp., P. penneri
K/K or K/NC H₂S+	Salmonella typhi, Salmonella spp.	Salmonella spp., Edwardsiella spp.	Salmonella spp. (rare)	Salmonella spp. (rare)	S. typhi	
K/K or K/NC	Salmonella spp. (rare)	Escherichia coli, Hafnia alvei, Klebsiella spp. (rare), Serratia spp. (rare), Enterobacter gergoviae	S. typhi, Serratia spp. (rare), Klebsiella spp. (rare), E. coli		Klebsiella spp., E. coli, Serratia spp., Enterobacter aerogenes, E. gergoviae	Serratia spp.
K/A H₂S+	Citrobacter freundii	Salmonella paratyphi A		C. freundii		
K/A		Escherichia agglomerans (occ), Enterobacter cloacae, Enterobacter taylorae, E. coli (occ), M. morganii, S. paratyphi A, Shigella flexneri, Citrobacter diversus, Citrobacter amalonaticus	E. coli, Shigella spp., M. morganii, E. agglomerans, Yersinia spp., Serratia spp. (rare)			E. coli, Enterobacter spp., Citrobacter spp., Yersinia spp., E. agglomerans, Serratia spp.

SYMBOLS: R, Red, oxidative deamination of lysine /A, Acid butt
K, Alkaline slant Ⓐ, Acid + gas in butt
A, Acid slant /NC, No change in butt
/K, Alkaline butt H₂S+, Hydrogen sulfide production

Modified from Hall, C.T.: Bacteriology 1; January 1973 summary analysis—proficiency survey, Atlanta, 1973, Centers for Disease Control.

TABLE 16-4. Biochemical Reactions of the Named Species, Biogroups, and Enteric Groups of the Family *Enterobacteriaceae*

	Voges-Proskauer	Urea Hydrolysis	Sucrose Fermentation	D-Sorbitol Fermentation	Salicin Fermentation	Phenylalanine Deaminase	Ornithine Decarboxylase	myo-Inositol Fermentation	Motility (36° C)	Methyl Red	D-Mannitol Fermentation	Malonate Utilization	Lysine Decarboxylase	Lactose Fermentation	KCN (Growth in)	Indole Production	Hydrogen Sulfide (TSI)	D-Glucose—Gas	D-Glucose—Acid	Gelatin Hydrolysis (22° C)	Dulcitol Fermentation	Citrate (Simmons')	Arginine Dihydrolase	L-Arabinose Fermentation	Adonitol Fermentation
Buttiauxella																									
B. agrestis	0	0	0	0	100	0	100	0	100	100	100	60	0	100	80	0	0	100	100	0	0	100	0	100	0[a]
Cedecea																									
C. davisae[b]	50	0	100	0	99	0	95	0	95	100	100	91	0	19	86	0	0	70	100	0	0	95	50	0	0
C. lapagei[b]	80	0	0	0	100	0	0	0	80	100	100	99	0	60	100	0	0	100	100	0	0	99	80	0	0
C. neteri[b]	50	0	100	100	100	0	0	0	100	40	100	100	0	35	65	0	0	100	100	0	0	100	100	0	0
C. species 3[b]	50	0	50	0	100	0	0	0	100	100	100	0	0	0	100	0	0	100	100	0	0	100	100	0	0
C. species 5[b]	50	0	100	100	100	0	50	0	100	100	100	0	0	0	100	0	0	100	100	0	0	100	50	0	0
Citrobacter																									
C. freundii[b]	0	70	30	98	5	0	20	3	95	100	99	15	0	50	96	5	80	95	100	0	55	95	65	100	0
C. diversus[b]	0	75	45	99	20	0	99	0	95	100	100	90	0	35	0	99	0	98	100	0	50	99	65	100	98
C. amalonaticus[b]	0	80	15	100	40	0	95	0	98	100	100	0	0	50	95	100	0	97	100	0	0	85	85	100	0
C. amalonaticus biogroup 1[b]	0	45	100	100	0	0	100	0	99	100	100	0	0	19	96	100	0	93	100	0	4	1	85	100	0
Edwardsiella																									
E. tarda[b]	0	0	0	0	0	0	100	0	98	100	0	0	100	0	0	99	100	100	100	0	0	1	0	9	0
E. tarda biogroup 1[b]	0	0	100	0	0	0	100	0	100	100	0	0	100	0	0	100	100	50	100	0	0	0	0	100	0
E. hoshinae	0	0	100	0	50	0	95	0	100	100	100	100	100	0	0	13	0	35	100	0	0	0	0	13	0
E. ictaluri	0	0	0	0	0	0	65	0	0	0	0	0	100	0	0	0	0	50	100	0	0	0	0	0	0
Enterobacter																									
E. aerogenes[b]	98	2	100	100	100	0	98	95	97	5	100	95	98	95	98	0	0	100	100	0	5	95	0	100	98
E. cloacae[b]	100	65	97	95	75	0	96	15	95	5	100	75	0	93	98	0	0	100	100	0	15	100	97	100	25
E. agglomerans[b]	70	20	75	30	65	20	0	15	85	50	100	65	0	40	35	20	0	20	100	2	15	50	0	95	7
E. gergoviae[b]	100	93	98	0	99	0	100	0	90	5	99	96	90	55	0	0	0	98	100	0	0	99	0	99	0
E. sakazakii[b]	100	1	100	0	99	50	91	75	96	5	100	18	0	99	99	11	0	98	100	0	5	99	99	100	0
E. taylorae[b]	100	1	0	1	92	0	99	0	99	5	100	100	0	10	98	0	0	100	100	0	0	100	94	100	0
E. amnigenus biogroup 1[b]	100	1	100	9	91	0	55	0	92	7	100	91	0	70	100	0	0	100	100	0	0	70	9	100	0
E. amnigenus biogroup 2	100	0	0	100	100	0	100	0	100	65	100	100	0	35	100	0	0	100	100	0	0	100	35	100	0
E. intermedium	100	0	65	100	100	0	89	0	89	100	100	100	0	100	65	0	0	100	100	0	100	65	0	100	0
Escherichia-Shigella																									
E. coli[b]	0	1	50	94	40	0	65	1	95	99	98	0	90	95	3	98	1	95	100	0	60	1	17	99	5
E. coli—inactive[b]	0	1	15	75	10	0	20	1	5	95	93	0	40	25	1	80	1	5	100	0	40	1	3	85	3
Shigella—serogroups A, B, and C[b]	0	0	0	30	0	0	1	0	0	100	93	0	0	0	0	50	0	2	100	0	2	0	5	60	0
S. sonnei[b]	0	0	1	2	0	0	98	0	0	100	99	0	0	2	0	0	0	0	100	0	0	0	2	95	0
E. fergusonii[b]	0	0	0	0	65	0	100	0	98	100	98	35	95	45	0	98	0	95	100	0	60	17	5	98	98
E. hermannii[b]	0	0	45	0	40	0	100	0	93	100	100	0	6	45	94	99	0	97	100	0	19	1	0	100	0
E. vulneris[b]	0	0	8	1	30	0	0	0	99	100	100	85	85	15	15	0	0	97	100	0	0	0	30	100	0
E. blattae	0	0	0	0	0	0	100	0	100	100	100	100	100	0	100	0	0	100	100	0	0	50	0	100	0

Continued.

TABLE 16-4. Biochemical Reactions of the Named Species, Biogroups, and Enteric Groups of the Family *Enterobacteriaceae*—cont'd

	Adonitol Fermentation	L-Arabinose Fermentation	Arginine Dihydrolase	Citrate (Simmons')	Dulcitol Fermentation	Gelatin Hydrolysis (22°C)	D-Glucose—Acid	D-Glucose—Gas	Hydrogen Sulfide (TSI)	Indole Production	KCN (Growth in)	Lactose Fermentation	Lysine Decarboxylase	Malonate Utilization	D-Mannitol Fermentation	Methyl Red	Motility (36°C)	myo-Inositol Fermentation	Ornithine Decarboxylase	Phenylalanine Deaminase	Salicin Fermentation	D-Sorbitol Fermentation	Sucrose Fermentation	Urea Hydrolysis	Voges-Proskauer
Ewingella																									
E. americana[b]	0	0	0	95	0	0	100	0	0	0	5	70	0	0	100	84	60	0	0	0	80	0	0	0	95
Hafnia																									
H. alvei[b]	0	95	6	10	0	0	100	98	0	0	95	5	100	50	99	40	85	0	98	0	13	0	10	4	85
H. alvei biogroup 1	0	0	0	0	0	0	100		0	0	100	0	100	45	55	85	0	0	45	0	55	0	0	0	70
Klebsiella																									
K. pneumoniae[b]	90	99	0	98	30	0	100	97	0	0	98	98	98	93	99	10	0	95	0	0	99	99	99	95	98
K. oxytoca[b]	99	98	6	95	55	0	100	97	0	99	97	100	99	98	99	20	0	98	0	1	100	99	100	90	95
K. Group 47 (indole and ornithine positive)	100	100	0	100	10	0	100	100	0	100	100	100	100	100	100	96	0	95	100	0	100	100	100	100	70
K. planticola[b]	100	100	0	100	15	0	100	100	0	20	100	100	100	100	100	100	0	100	0	0	100	92	100	98	98
K. ozaenae[b]	97	98	6	30	2	0	100	50	0	0	88	30	40	3	100	98	0	55	3	0	97	65	20	10	0
K. rhinoscleromatis[b]	100	100	0	0	0	0	100	0	0	0	80	0	0	95	100	100	0	95	0	0	98	100	75	0	0
K. terrigena	100	100	0	40	20	0	100	80	0	0	100	100	100	100	100	60	0	80	20	0	100	100	100		100
Kluyvera																									
K. ascorbata[b]	0	100	0	96	25	0	100	93	0	92	92	98	97	96	100	100	98	0	100	0	100	40	98	0	0
K. cryocrescens[b]	0	100	0	80	0	0	100	95	0	90	86	95	23	86	95	100	90	0	100	0	100	45	81	0	0
Moellerella																									
M. wisconsensis	100	0	0	80	0	0	100	0	0	0	70	100	0	0	60	100	0	0	0	0	0	0	100	0	0
Morganella																									
M. morganii[b]	0	0	0	0	0	0	100	90	5	98	98	1	0	1	0	97	95	0	98	95	0	0	0	98	0
M. morganii biogroup 1[b]	0	0	0	0	0	0	100	91	41	100	91	0	100	5	0	95	0	0	95	100	0	0	0	100	0
Obesumbacterium																									
O. proteus biogroup 2	0	0	0	0	0	0	100	0	0	0	0	0	100	0	0	15	0	0	100	0	0	0	0	0	0
Proteus																									
P. mirabilis[b]	0	0	0	65	0	90	100	96	98	2	98	2	0	2	0	97	95	0	99	98	0	0	15	98	50
P. vulgaris[b]	0	0	0	15	0	91	100	85	95	98	99	2	0	0	0	95	95	0	0	99	50	0	97	95	0
P. penneri[b]	0	0	0	0	0	50	100	45	30	0	99	1	0	1	0	100	85	0	0	99	0	0	100	100	0
P. myxofaciens	0	0	0	50	0	100	100	100	0	0	100	0	0	0	0	100	100	0	0	100	0	0	100	100	100
Providencia																									
P. rettgeri[b]	100	0	0	95	0	0	100	10	0	99	97	5	0	0	100	93	94	90	0	98	50	1	15	98	0
P. stuartii[b]	5	1	0	93	0	0	100	0	0	98	100	2	0	0	10	100	85	95	0	95	2	1	50	30	0
P. alcalifaciens[b]	98	1	0	98	0	0	100	85	0	99	100	0	0	0	2	99	96	1	1	98	1	1	15	0	0
P. rustigianii[b]	0	0	0	15	0	0	100	35	0	98	100	0	0	0	0	65	30	0	0	100	0	0	35	0	0
Rahnella																									
R. aquatilis[b]	0	100	0	94	88	0	100	98	0	0	0	100	0	100	100	88	6	0	0	0	100	94	100	0	100

Salmonella

Organism																																									
Subgroup 1 serotypes[b]—most
S. typhi[b]
S. choleraesuis[b]
S. paratyphi A[b]
S. gallinarum[b]
S. pullorum[b]
Subgroup 2 strains[b]
Subgroup 3a strains[b] (Arizona)
Subgroup 3b strains[b] (Arizona)
Subgroup 4 strains[b]
Subgroup 5 strains[b]

Serratia

S. marcescens[b]
S. marcescens biogroup 1[b]
S. liquefaciens group[b]
S. rubidaea[b]
S. odorifera biogroup 1[b]
S. odorifera biogroup 2[b]
S. plymuthica[b]
S. ficaria[b]

Serratia fonticola[b]

Tatumella

T. ptyseos[b]

Yersinia

Y. enterocolitica[b]
Y. frederiksenii[b]
Y. intermedia[b]
Y. kristensenii[b]
Y. pestis[b]
Y. pseudotuberculosis[b]

Yersinia ruckeri

Xenorhabdus

X. luminescens (25° C)
X. nematophilus (25° C)

Enteric Group 17[b]
Enteric Group 41[b]
Enteric Group 45[b]
Enteric Group 57[b]
Enteric Group 58[b]
Enteric Group 59[b]
Enteric Group 60[b]
Enteric Group 63
Enteric Group 64
Enteric Group 68[b]
Enteric Group 69

From Farmer, J.J., III, et al.: J. Clin. Microbiol. **21:**46, 1985.

[a]Each number gives the percentage of positive reactions after 2 days of incubation at 36° C (except *Xenorhabdus* organisms, which were incubated at 25° C). The vast majority of these positive reactions occur within 24 hours. Reactions that become positive after 2 days are not considered in the table.

[b]Organism is known to occur in clinical specimens.

TABLE 16-5. Differentiation within the Genus *Cedecea*[a]

Test	*C. davisae*	*C. lapagei*	*C. neteri*	*Cedecea* Species 3	*Cedecea* Species 5
Ornithine decarboxylase	+	−	−	−	v
Fermentation of:					
Sucrose	+	−	+	v	+
D-Sorbitol	−	−	+	−	+
Raffinose	−	−	−	+	+
D-Xylose	+	−	+	+	+
Melibiose	−	−	−	+	+
Malonate utilization	+	+	+	−	−

> **SYMBOLS:** +, 90%-100% positive
> −, ≤ 10% positive
> v, 25.1%-74.9% positive

From Farmer, J.J., III, et al.: J. Clin. Microbiol. **21**:46, 1985.
[a]All data for reaction within 2 days unless otherwise specified.

mannitol, sorbitol, arabinose, rhamnose, xylose, or trehalose. The three species of *Edwardsiella* include *E. tarda*, *E. hoshinae*, and *E. ictaluri*. Only *E. tarda* is found in clinical specimens. *E. tarda* is differentiated from the other *Edwardsiella* spp. on the basis of its positive results in tests for indole production, H_2S production, and motility, and its negative results in tests for malonate utilization and fermentation of D-mannitol, sucrose, trehalose, and L-arabinose.

Enterobacter

The ornithine decarboxylase test is extremely useful in separating the genus *Klebsiella* (which gives a negative result) from the genus *Enterobacter* (most of which give a positive result). In addition, the genus *Enterobacter* is usually motile, whereas the genus *Klebsiella* is nonmotile. *E. agglomerans* is quite variable biochemically and thus may present an identification problem. It is best to consider several reactions simultaneously in attempting to identify this organism. For example, *E. agglomerans* is one of the few members of the *Enterobacteriaceae* family isolated from human clinical specimens that is ornithine decarboxylase, arginine dihydrolase, and lysine decarboxylase negative. Differentiation of the genus *Enterobacter* is shown in Table 16-7.

Escherichia-Shigella

Table 16-8 lists key tests that are useful for differentiation within the genera *Escherichia-Shigella*. These organisms are closely related, and sometimes *Escherichia coli* strains are serologically identified as *Shigella*. In fact, many of the nonmotile, anaerogenic strains of *E. coli* that belong to the old Alkalescens-Dispar group were once classified as *Shigella alkalescens* and *Shigella dispar*.

E. coli can be differentiated from *Shigella* on the basis of the following criteria: (1) *Shigella* isolates are always nonmotile and lysine decarboxylase negative; (2) with the exception of the

TABLE 16-6. Differentiation within the Genus *Citrobacter*[a]

Characteristic	*C. amalonaticus*	*C. freundii*	*C. diversus*
BIOCHEMICAL TESTS			
Indole production	+	−	+
H_2S production (TSI)	−	+	−
Malonate utilization	−	−	+
Growth in KCN	+	+	−
Tyrosine clearing[b]	−	−	+
Adonitol fermentation	−	−	+
ANTIBIOGRAM—ZONE SIZES			
Cephalothin (30 μg)[c]	18 (2.0)[d]	10.9 (2.9)	23.5 (1.2)
Ampicillin (10 μg)	8.7 (2.4)	14.3 (3.1)	7.1 (1.2)
Carbenicillin (100 μg)	16.5 (2.4)	24.1 (0.9)	12.6 (1.6)

> **SYMBOLS:** +, 90%-100% positive
> −, ≤ 10% positive

Modified from Farmer, J.J., III, et al.: J. Clin. Microbiol. **21**:46, 1985.
[a]All data for reaction within 2 days unless otherwise specified.
[b]More useful in reference laboratories than in clinical laboratories.
[c]Number in parentheses is the strength of antimicrobial agent.
[d]First number is mean; number in parentheses is standard deviation of zones of inhibition.

Manchester and Newcastle bioserotypes of *Shigella flexneri* 6, strains of *Shigella* do not produce gas during carbohydrate fermentation; and (3) cultures that ferment mucate or utilize acetate are much more likely to be *E. coli* than *Shigella*. Table 16-9 lists several biochemical tests useful in differentiating strains of *E. coli* and *Shigella*.

Ewingella

E. americana is the only member of the genus *Ewingella*. This organism is negative for deoxyribonuclease, lysine decarboxylase, ornithine decarboxylase, arginine dihydrolase, and lipase, and does not ferment L-arabinose, melibiose, raffinose, D-sorbitol, or sucrose. *E. americana* is Voges-Proskauer positive and like all members of the family *Enterobacteriaceae* produces acid from glucose.

Hafnia

H. alvei is the only species in the genus *Hafnia*. It may be separated from the genus *Enterobacter*, of which it was once a member, on the basis of negative reactions for citrate utilization and fermentation of lactose, sucrose, sorbitol, and raffinose.

Klebsiella

Strains of the genus *Klebsiella* are nonmotile, encapsulated short rods. *K. ozaenae* and *K. rhinoscleromatis* are probably host-adapted strains of *K. pneumoniae*, although they are treated as distinct subspecies of *K. pneumoniae* in *Bergey's Manual of Systematic Bacteriology*. Separation of the species of the *Klebsiella* is shown in Table 16-10.

TABLE 16-7. Differentiation within the Genus *Enterobacter*[a]

Test	*E. aerogenes*	*E. agglomerans*	*E. amnigenus* Biogroup 1	*E. amnigenus* Biogroup 2	*E. cloacae*	*E. gergoviae*	*E. intermedium*	*E. sakazakii*	*E. taylorae*
Lysine decarboxylase	+	−	−	−	−	+	−	−	−
Arginine dihydrolase	−	−	−	v	+	−	−	+	+
Ornithine decarboxylase	+	−	v	+	+	+	(+)	+	+
Growth in KCN	+	v	+	+	+	−	v	+	+
Fermentation of:									
Sucrose	+	(+)	+	−	+	+	v	+	v
Dulcitol	−	(−)	−	−	(−)	−	+	−	−
Adonitol	+	−	−	−	(−)	−	−	−	−
D-Sorbitol	+	v	−	+	+	−	+	−	−
Raffinose	+	v	+	−	+	+	+	+	−
Alpha-methyl-D-glucoside	+	−	v	+	(+)	−	+	+	v
D-Arabitol	+	v	−	−	(−)	+	−	−	−
Yellow pigment	−	(+)	−	−	−	−	−	+	−
Present in human clinical specimens	+	+	−	−	+	+	−	+	+

> **SYMBOLS:**   +, 90%-100% positive
>   (+), 75%-89.9% positive
>   v, 25.1%-74.9% positive
>   (−), 10.1%-25% positive
>   −, ≤ 10% positive

From Farmer, J.J., III, et al.: J. Clin. Microbiol. **21:**46, 1985.
[a]All data for reaction within 2 days unless otherwise specified.

TABLE 16-8. Differentiation within the Genera *Escherichia-Shigella*[a]

Test	*Shigella* Serogroups A, B, and C	*S. sonnei*	*E. coli* ("Inactive")	*E. coli* ("Normal")	*E. blattae*	*E. fergusonii*	*E. hermannii*	*E. vulneris*
Indole production	v	−	(+)	+	−	+	+	−
Lysine decarboxylase	−	−	v	+	+	+	−	(+)
Ornithine decarboxylase	−	+	−	v	+	+	+	−
Motility	−	−	−	+	−	+	+	+
Gas produced during fermentation	−	−	−	+	+	+	+	+
Acetate utilization	−	−	v	+	−	+	(+)	v
Mucate fermentation	−	−	v	+	v	−	+	(+)
Lactose fermentation	−	−	(−)	+	−	−	v	(−)
Growth in KCN	−	−	−	−	−	−	+	(−)

Continued.

TABLE 16-8. Differentiation within the Genera *Escherichia-Shigella*[a]—cont'd

Test	Shigella Serogroups A, B, and C	S. sonnei	E. coli ("Inactive")	E. coli ("Normal")	E. blattae	E. fergusonii	E. hermannii	E. vulneris
Yellow pigment	−	−	−	−	−	−	+	v
D-Mannitol fermentation	(+)	+	+	+	−	+	+	+
Adonitol fermentation	−	−	−	−	−	+	−	−
D-Sorbitol fermentation	v	−	(+)	+	−	−	−	−
Cellobiose fermentation	−	−	−	−	−	+	+	+
D-Arabitol fermentation	−	−	−	−	−	+	−	−
Present in human clinical specimens	+	+	+	+	−	+	+	+
Isolated from cockroaches	−	−	−	−	+	−	−	−

> **SYMBOLS:**   +, 90%-100% positive
> (+), 75%-89.9% positive
> v, 25.1%-74.9% positive
> (−), 10.1%-25% positive
> −, ≤ 10% positive

From Farmer, J.J., III, et al.: J. Clin. Microbiol. **21**:46, 1985.
[a]All data for reactions within 2 days unless otherwise specified.

TABLE 16-9. Biochemical Tests Useful in Differentiating Strains of *Escherichia coli* and *Shigella* Spp.

Test	Escherichia coli ("Normal")	Escherichia coli ("Inactive")	Shigella dysenteriae	Shigella flexneri O Groups 1 to 5	Shigella flexneri O Group 6	Shigella boydii	Shigella sonnei
Motility	95[a]	0	0	0	0	0	0
Gas production from glucose	95	0	0	0	18	0	0
Lactose fermentation	95	0	0	0	0	1	2
Indole production	99	90	44	62	0	29	0
Acetate utilization	95	60	0	0	0	0	0
Mucate fermentation	95	25	0	0	0	0	15
Lysine decarboxylase	88	43	0	0	0	0	0
Arginine dihydrolase	17	2	2	0	49	18	1
Ornithine decarboxylase	63	18	0	0	0	3	99
Sucrose fermentation	51	11	0	2	0	0	0.1
Salicin fermentation	37	3	0	0	0	0	0

Modified from Farmer, J.J., III, et al.: J. Clin. Microbiol. **21**:46, 1985.
[a]Numbers represent percentage of strains positive within 2 days' incubation.

TABLE 16-10. Differentiation within the Genus *Klebsiella*[a]

Test	*K. pneumoniae*	*K. oxytoca*	*K. terrigena*	*K. planticola*	*Klebsiella* Group 47 (Indole and Ornithine Positive)
Indole production	−	+	−	(−)	+
Ornithine decarboxylase	−	−	−	−	+
Growth and D-glucose fermentation at:					
5° C	−	−	+	+	+
10° C	−	+	+	+	+
41° C	+	+	−	+	+
44.5° C	+	v	−	−	(−)

> **SYMBOLS:** +, 90%-100% positive
> v, 25.1%-74.9% positive
> (−), 10.1%-25% positive
> −, ≤ 10% positive

From Farmer, J.J., III, et al.: J. Clin. Microbiol. **21**:46, 1985.
[a]All data for reaction within 2 days unless otherwise specified.

TABLE 16-11. Differentiation within the Genus *Kluyvera*[a]

Test	*K. ascorbata*	*K. cryocrescens*
Ascorbate test	+	−
D-Glucose fermentation at 5° C (21 days)	−	+
Zone sizes for cephalothin and carbenicillin	Small	Large

> **SYMBOLS:** +, 90%-100% positive
> −, ≤ 10% positive

From Farmer, J.J., III, et al.: J. Clin. Microbiol. **21**:46, 1985.
[a]All data for reaction within 2 days unless otherwise specified.

Kluyvera

Kluyvera spp. must be differentiated from *Escherichia coli;* unlike *E. coli* they utilize citrate, grow in KCN broth, decarboxylate lysine, and ferment sorbitol and raffinose. The differentiation of the *Kluyvera* spp. is shown in Table 16-11.

Moellerella[90]

Colonies of *M. wisconsensis* resemble *Escherichia coli* on MacConkey and EMB agars. Characteristics that help distinguish this organism from *E. coli* and other *Enterobacteriaceae* include its positive reactions for methyl red, citrate (Sim-

TABLE 16-12. Differentiation of the Three Genera in "*Proteus*" Group[a]

Test	*Proteus*	*Providencia*	*Morganella*
Citrate utilization	v	+	−
H₂S production (TSI)	+	−	−
Ornithine decarboxylase	v	−	+
Gelatin liquefaction	+	−	−
Lipase (corn oil)	+	−	−
D-Mannose fermentation	−	+	+
Swarming on trypticase soy agar or blood agar	+	−	−

> **SYMBOLS:** +, 90%-100% positive
> v, 25.1%-74.9% positive
> −, ≤ 10% positive

From Farmer, J.J., III, et al.: J. Clin. Microbiol. **21**:46, 1985.
[a]All data for reaction within 2 days unless otherwise specified.

mons'), and acid production from lactose and raffinose, and negative reactions for the Voges-Proskauer test and tests for indole, H₂S production, urea hydrolysis, phenylalanine deaminase, lysine and ornithine decarboxylases, arginine dihydrolase, gas production from D-glucose, motility, and acid production from trehalose. All strains of *M. wisconsensis* are resistant (produce no zone of inhibition) to colistin.

Morganella

The genus *Morganella* has a single species, *M. morganii.* The genus is differentiated from the genus *Proteus* in being H₂S negative, gelatin negative, and D-mannose positive. It is distinguished from the genus *Providencia* by its ability to decarboxylate ornithine and its inability to utilize citrate (Table 16-12).

Proteus

The *Proteus* group includes three genera: *Proteus, Providencia,* and *Morganella.* Most of the members of these genera are motile, phenylalanine deaminase positive, and lysine deaminase positive. They may be differentiated as shown in Table 16-12.

Members of the genus *Proteus* are lactose negative and may be mistaken for salmonellae or shigellae on some common enteric agars. This is one reason that TSI (or KIA), LIA, and urea are recommended for screening isolates from stools. *Proteus* spp. are rapidly (4 hours) urea positive. Species identification is important because *P. mirabilis* is susceptible to a broader range of antimicrobial agents than other species found in human clinical specimens. *P. mirabilis* and *P. penneri* are indole negative, whereas *P. vulgaris* is indole positive. *P. penneri* characteristically produces a small zone of inhibition around the chloramphenicol disk (Table 16-13).

TABLE 16-13. Differentiation within the Genus *Proteus*[a]

Test or Property	*P. mirabilis*	*P. myxofaciens*	*P. penneri*	*P. vulgaris* biogroup 2	*P. vulgaris* biogroup 3
Indole production	−	−	−	+	+
Ornithine decarboxylase	+	−	−	−	−
Maltose fermentation	−	+	+	+	+
D-Xylose fermentation	+	−	+	+	+
Salicin fermentation	−	−	−	+	−
Esculin hydrolysis	−	−	−	+	−
Chloramphenicol susceptibility	S	S	R	V	S
Present in human clinical specimens	+	−	+	+	+
Occurs as a pathogen of gypsy moth larvae	−	+	−	−	−

> **SYMBOLS:** +, 90%-100% positive
> −, ≤ 10% positive
> S, Susceptible
> R, Resistant
> V, Variable susceptibility

From Farmer, J.J., III, et al.: J. Clin. Microbiol. **21:**46, 1985.
[a]All data for reaction within 2 days unless otherwise specified.

Providencia

Providencia spp. are lactose and H$_2$S negative and may or may not produce gas in glucose. Thus they often resemble *Shigella* isolates in TSI (or KIA). They may be differentiated from *Shigella* spp. on the basis of positive reactions in tests for motility and citrate utilization. Differentiation of the four species within the genus is shown in Table 16-14.

Salmonella

Until recently, three species of *Salmonella* were recognized in the classification widely used in the United States.[39] These included *S. choleraesuis, S. typhi,* and *S. enteritidis.* The Arizona group was classified in a separate genus as *Arizona hinshawii.* DNA-DNA hybridization studies[116,117] did not support this classification, however. These studies showed that *Salmonella* and *Arizona* should be classified as one genus and that all strains are closely related. According to LeMinor and associates,[116,117] only one species of *Salmonella* is recognized based on genetic studies; this species, *S. choleraesuis,* can further be divided into six formally named subspecies (Table 16-15). Fortunately, to avoid the confusion that would result if the new nomenclature were used, serotype names are being used. For example, an organism identified as the typhoid bacillus would be reported as *S. typhi* or *Salmonella* serotype *typhi* rather than as the extremely awkward *Salmonella choleraesuis* subspecies *choleraesuis* serotype *typhi.*

TABLE 16-14. Differentiation within the Genus *Providencia*[a]

Test	*P. alcalifaciens*	*P. rustigianii*	*P. stuartii*	*P. rettgeri*
Urea hydrolysis	−	−	v	+
myo-Inositol	−	−	+	+
Adonitol	+	−	−	+
D-Arabitol	−	−	−	+
Trehalose	−	−	+	−
D-Galactose	−	+	+	+

> **SYMBOLS:** +, 90%-100% positive
> v, 25.1%-74.9% positive
> −, ≤ 10% positive

From Farmer, J.J., III, et al.: J. Clin. Microbiol. **21:**46, 1985.
[a]All data for reaction within 2 days unless otherwise specified.

The salmonellae are usually motile, and with the exception of *S. pullorum* and *S. gallinarum,* most produce gas in glucose. Isolates that produce an alkaline slant and acid, gas, and H$_2$S in the butt of TSI (or KIA) and are urease negative should be tested with *Salmonella* polyvalent antisera. Kelly[110a] recommends that three important *Salmonella* organisms be identified biochemically and serologically: *S. choleraesuis, S. typhi,* and *S. paratyphi* A. Identification of these organisms is important because of their association with life-threatening conditions. These three organisms can be distinguished by tests for citrate utilization, lysine decarboxylase, ornithine decarboxylase, gas from glucose, and fermentation of arabinose, rhamnose, and trehalose (see Table 6-4).[110a] *S. typhi* should be suspected if a non-lactose-fermenter produces small amounts of H$_2$S in TSI (or KIA) and is anaerogenic and citrate negative. The small amount of H$_2$S produced by *S. typhi* is said to resemble a button or mustache at the point of inoculation of the butt. Other *Salmonella* isolates should be identified to the genus and subgroup level (such as *Salmonella* serogroup C1) and referred to reference laboratories for serotype determination.[110a] Most strains isolated in hospital laboratories belong to *Salmonella* serogroups A to E (subgroup 1) (Table 16-15). Organisms formerly classified as *A. hinshawii* are now included in *Salmonella* as subgroup 3 (Table 16-15).

Serratia

Members of the genus *Serratia* hydrolyze DNA, liquefy gelatin, are lipase positive, and ferment sorbitol. These reactions may be used to differentiate them from many species of the genus *Enterobacter,* which they resemble. A small percentage of strains produce a distinctive red pigment (prodigiosin) at room temperature but not at 35° C (Plate 9, *F*). The ability to ferment arabinose may be used to differentiate *S. marcescens* (negative) from the other species (positive). Differentiation within the genus is shown in Table 16-16.

TABLE 16-15. Differentiation of the Six Subgroups within the Genus *Salmonella* (''*Salmonella-Arizona* Group'')

	Salmonella Subgroup 1	*Salmonella* Subgroup 2	*Salmonella* Subgroup 3a	*Salmonella* Subgroup 3b	*Salmonella* Subgroup 4	*Salmonella* Subgroup 5
CHARACTERISTICS						
DNA-hybridization group of Crosa et al.[34]	1	2	3	4	5	Not studied
Salmonella subgenus names formerly used	I	II	III	III	IV	V
Genus according to Ewing[44]	*Salmonella*	*Salmonella*	*Arizona*	*Arizona*	*Salmonella*	*Salmonella*
Subspecies according to Le Minor et al.[116]	*choleraesuis*	*salamae*	*arizonae*	*diarizonae*	*houtenae*	*bongori*
Usually monophasic or diphasic flagella	Di	Di	Mono	Di	Mono	Mono
Usually isolated from humans and other warm-blooded animals	Yes	No	No	No	No	No
Usually isolated from cold-blooded animals and the environment	No	Yes	Yes	Yes	Yes	Yes
Pathogenic for humans	Highly	Yes	Yes	Yes	Yes	Possibly
TESTS						
Dulcitol fermentation	96[a]	90	0	1	0	100
Lactose fermentation	1	1	15	85	0	0
ONPG test	2	15	100	100	0	100
Malonate utilization	1	95	95	95	0	0
Growth in KCN medium	1	1	1	1	95	100
Mucate fermentation	90	96	90	30	0	100
Gelatin hydrolysis[b]	−	+	+	+	+	−
D-Galacturonate fermentation[b]	−	+	−	+	+	+
Lysis by 01 bacteriophage[b]	+	+	−	+	−	v

> **SYMBOLS:** Di, Diphasic
> Mono, Monophasic
> +, 90%-100% positive
> v, 25.1%-74.9% positive
> −, ≤ 10% positive

From Farmer, J.J., III, et al.: J. Clin. Microbiol. **21**:46, 1985.
Data from references 34, 44, 59, 116, and 117.
[a]Numbers give percentage positive for tests after 2 days' incubation at 36° C. Most positive results occur within 24 hours; reactions positive after 2 days are not considered.
[b]Based on data of LeMinor et al.[116,117] Test for gelatin hydrolysis is rapid ''film'' method at 36° C (almost all strains are negative by tube method at 22° C within 2 days).

Tatumella

T. ptyseos is the only species in the genus *Tatumella*. It is biochemically inactive compared with other members of the family *Enterobacteriaceae* and grows poorly on most commonly used media. Furthermore, it is the only member of the family that is motile by means of a polar-lateral flagellum.

Yersinia

With a few exceptions the yersiniae are nonmotile at 37° C. *Y. enterocolitica* and *Y. pseudotuberculosis* may be motile at temperatures below 30° C. *Y. enterocolitica* or *Y. pseudotuberculosis* may be suspected if a TSI slant appears orange-yellow after 24 hours' incubation at 35° C. The biochemical reactions

TABLE 16-16. Differentiation within the Genus *Serratia*[a]

Test	*S. ficaria*	*S. liquefaciens* Group	*S. marcescens*	*S. odorifera*	*S. plymuthica*	*S. rubidaea*	*S. fonticola*
DNAse (25° C)	+	(+)	+	+	+	+	−
Lipase (corn oil)	(+)	(+)	+	v	v	+	−
Gelatinase (22° C)	+	+	+	+	v	(+)	−
Lysine decarboxylase	−	+	+	+	−	v	+
Ornithine decarboxylase	−	+	+	v	−	−	+
Fermentation of:							
L-Arabinose	+	+	−	+	+	+	+
D-Arabitol	+	−	−	−	−	(+)	+
D-Sorbitol	+	+	+	+	v	−	+
Adonitol	−	−	v	v	−	+	+
Dulcitol	−	−	−	−	−	−	+
Odor of *Serratia odorifera*	+	−	−	+	−	(−)	−
Red, pink, or orange pigment	−	−	v	−	v	v	−

SYMBOLS: +, 90%-100% positive
(+), 75%-89.9% positive
v, 25.1%-74.9% positive
(−), 10.1%-25% positive
−, ≤ 10% positive

From Farmer, J.J., III, et al.: J. Clin. Microbiol. **21**:46, 1985.
[a]All data for reaction within 2 days unless otherwise specified.

used to speciate *Y. enterocolitica, Y. kristensenii, Y. intermedia,* and *Y. frederiksenii* are listed in Table 16-17. The differentiation of *Y. enterocolitica* and *Y. pseudotuberculosis* is shown in Table 16-18.

The biochemical reactions used to differentiate *Y. pestis* and *Y. pseudotuberculosis* are shown in Table 16-19; however, these reactions are not the primary means of identification of *Y. pestis.* Identification of this organism usually depends on the macroscopic and microscopic appearance of cultures both on agar and in broth, the sensitivity to a specific bacteriophage, the production of an envelope antigen (F1), and pathogenicity for rats or guinea pigs. These tests are performed in a reference laboratory.

Buttiauxella, Erwinia, Obesumbacterium, Rahnella, Xenorhabdus

The genera *Buttiauxella, Erwinia, Obesumbacterium, Rahnella,* and *Xenorhabdus* are not considered here, since they are rarely or never found in clinical specimens.

SEROLOGIC AND IMMUNOSEROLOGIC IDENTIFICATION

Enterobacteriaceae are usually simple to isolate, so the technique of looking for serum antibodies is seldom used. Two

exceptions are in the diagnosis of typhoid fever, in which agglutinating antibodies are often measured (the Widal test), and in the diagnosis of plague. Serologic typing plays an important role in identifying members of the genera *Salmonella* and *Shigella* and is an important tool for dividing various species of *Enterobacteriaceae* into serogroups during epidemiologic investigations.

Genera in the family *Enterobacteriaceae* possess a variety of antigens that may be categorized into three general groups: O antigens (from the German *Ohne Hauch,* nonspreading), H antigens (from the German *Hauch,* spreading), and K antigens (from the German *Kapsel,* capsule). The O, or heat-stable lipopolysaccharide somatic, antigens are located primarily in the cell wall. Typing with O antisera determines group identification. The specific O antigens are usually designated with Arabic numerals. The H antigens are heat-labile proteins located in the flagella. These antigens are important in further subdividing the O serogroups into serotypes in motile genera of *Enterobacteriaceae* (such as *Salmonella*). The K antigen is present in the envelope (or capsule) surrounding the bacterial cell wall and is often heat labile. The K antigens often mask the O antigens, causing living cells to be inagglutinable in O antisera. When this happens, a suspension of the organism should be boiled for 15 to 30 minutes to destroy the K antigens and unmask the O

TABLE 16-17. Differentiation of the Four Species Formerly Included in *Yersinia enterocolitica*[a]

Test	*Y. enterocolitica*	*Y. kristensenii*	*Y. intermedia*	*Y. frederiksenii*
Sucrose fermentation	+	−	+	+
L-Rhamnose fermentation	−	−	+	+
Raffinose fermentation	−	−	+	−
Melibiose fermentation	−	−	+	−

SYMBOLS: +, Vast majority positive
−, Vast majority negative

From Farmer, J.J., III, et al.: J. Clin. Microbiol. **21**:46, 1985.
[a]These characteristic fermentation patterns occur rapidly at 25° C but are sometimes delayed 3 to 7 days at 36° C.

antigens. K antigens are important in typing isolates of the genus *Klebsiella*.

In hospital microbiology laboratories serologic identification of the family *Enterobacteriaceae* is usually limited to preliminary grouping of the genera *Salmonella* and *Shigella*. Ideally, typing should be performed from a non-sugar-containing medium. Sugar-containing media such as MacConkey or TSI can be used with appropriate controls but sometimes cause an isolate to become rough, or autoagglutinable. The serologic procedure usually employed for grouping *Salmonella* and *Shigella* is the slide agglutination test. The agglutination test is performed as follows:

1. A single drop of properly diluted antiserum is added to a glass slide.
2. A loopful of growth (preferably from a sugar-free medium) is suspended in a few drops of phenolized saline (or mercuric iodide saline) in a glass tube; the suspension should be prepared to the density of skim milk. (Phenolized saline will kill the organism.)
3. A single drop of the bacterial suspension is added to the drop of antiserum on the slide.
4. The slide is tilted back and forth several times for up to 1 minute.
5. A positive result is indicated by rapid, complete agglutination of the bacterial cells.
6. If suspected *Salmonella* or *Shigella* organisms fail to agglutinate in the polyvalent antiserum, a suspension should be heated in a beaker of boiling water for 15 to 30 minutes, cooled, and retested. As mentioned previously, the initial inagglutinability may be due to the presence of an envelope antigen that is destroyed by heating.

SALMONELLA

The extensive scheme used for serologic classification of the genus *Salmonella* was developed by Kauffman and White.[39] At a minimum, all clinical laboratories should be able to detect the Vi capsular antigen of *S. typhi* and the common O antigen groups of *Salmonella*—specifically A, B, C, C_2, D, and E.

TABLE 16-18. Differentiation of *Yersinia enterocolitica* and *Yersinia pseudotuberculosis*

Test	*Y. enterocolitica*	*Y. pseudotuberculosis*
Fermentation of:		
Sucrose	+	−
D-Sorbitol	+	−
Ornithine decarboxylase	+	−

SYMBOLS: +, Vast majority (perhaps ≥ 90%) positive
−, Vast majority (perhaps ≥ 90%) negative

TABLE 16-19. Differentiation of *Yersinia pestis* and *Yersinia pseudotuberculosis*

Test	*Y. pestis*	*Y. pseudotuberculosis*
Urea hydrolysis	−	+
Motility, 20° to 25° C	−	+
Melibiose fermentation	−	+
L-Rhamnose fermentation	−	+
Phage[a] susceptibility		
20° C	+	−
36° C	+	−
Reaction with *Y. pestis* fraction 1 antiserum	+	−
Pathogenic for:		
Guinea pigs	+	+
White rats	+	−

SYMBOLS: +, Vast majority (perhaps ≥ 90%) positive
−, Vast majority (perhaps ≥ 90%) negative

Modified from Quan, T.J.: *Yersinia pestis*. In Starr, M.P., et al., editors: The prokaryotes: a handbook on habitats, isolation, and identification of bacteria, New York, 1981, Springer-Verlag.

Ninety-five percent of the *Salmonella* serotypes isolated from humans belong to these few serogroups. Complete serologic typing of salmonellae is then done by reference laboratories. Both salmonellosis and shigellosis are reportable diseases; laboratories must furnish public health institutions with the names and addresses of individuals from whom these organisms are recovered. Furthermore, clinical laboratories usually forward the bacterial isolate to a reference laboratory for further studies. In the case of strains of *Salmonella*, this often involves identifying the specific H antigen(s). This is no easy task because the majority of salmonellae are diphasic; that is, they possess two antigenic forms of H antigens. Phase-reversal procedures may be necessary to reveal both phases. This can be accomplished by inoculating the organisms into a small Petri dish with semisolid agar containing specific antisera against the antigen(s) of the first phase. The first phase is arrested at the site of inoculation, whereas the other phase expresses itself and may then be identified. When fully identified, each of the *Salmonella* strains may be described by an antigenic formula that is composed of three parts: the somatic O antigens, the H antigen(s) of phase 1, and the H antigen(s) of phase 2. These three parts of the formula are separated by colons; components within each part are separated by commas.[39] For example, the antigenic formula 1,4,5,12:i:1,2 means that the strain has O antigen components 1, 4, 5, and 12; flagella phase 1 antigen i; and flagella phase 2 antigens 1 and 2. An organism with this antigenic formula is reported as *S. typhimurium*.

Organisms suspected to be *S. typhi* should be first tested in the unheated (living) state in group D antiserum and in Vi antiserum. Then, after boiling for 15 minutes, the suspension should be cooled and retested. The following reaction pattern is typical of *S. typhi:*

Suspension	*Salmonella* polyvalent	*Salmonella* O group D	Vi
Living	4+	−	4+
Heated	4+	4+	−

The Vi antigen is the capsular antigen of *S. typhi*. This antigen masks the O antigens and thus is responsible for the initial inagglutinability in the *Salmonella* O group D antiserum. The living suspension agglutinates in the *Salmonella* polyvalent antiserum, however, because this antiserum also contains agglutinins to the Vi antigen.

SHIGELLA

The genus *Shigella* is divided into four species or subgroups based on biochemical and antigenic characteristics. The four subgroups are *S. dysenteriae* (subgroup A), *S. flexneri* (subgroup B), *S. boydii* (subgroup C), and *S. sonnei* (subgroup D). These subgroups may be further divided into subtypes or serotypes on the basis of type-specific O antigens. Since *Shigella* strains are nonmotile, they do not possess H or flagellar antigens. Some species, however, do possess a K antigen. If a suspected *Shigella* isolate fails to agglutinate in one of the four polyvalent antisera, the suspension should be boiled for 15 to 30 minutes and retested. If the reaction continues to be negative, the organism should be tested with the *Salmonella* Vi and polyvalent grouping sera. The isolate may be a strain of *S. typhi* that fails to produce H_2S.

EPIDEMIOLOGIC TYPING SYSTEMS

Knowing the relationship of a group of strains that belong to the same species is often desirable. This is important, for example, in any epidemiologic investigation of a cluster of nosocomial (hospital-acquired) infections. The following marker systems have been used to differentiate strains of the family *Enterobacteriaceae:*

1. Simple techniques
   a. Biotyping
   b. Antibiogram
   c. Serotyping with commercial sera
   d. Resistogram
   e. Dienes reaction for *Proteus*
   f. Colony incompatibility
2. Reference techniques
   a. Complete antigenic analysis (serologic typing)
   b. Bacteriophage susceptibility
   c. Bacteriocin susceptibility
   d. Bacteriocin production
   e. Plasmid profile analysis
   f. Genome sequence determination

The simple techniques do not require specialized equipment, instruments, or strains, whereas reference techniques do. The simple techniques are most applicable in a hospital microbiology laboratory, whereas the reference techniques are performed in a research laboratory or in state, regional, or national reference centers.

BIOTYPING

Biotyping is the characterization of strains by biochemical and physiologic characteristics.[16,52] In biotyping one tries to find a unique biochemical characteristic or biochemical profile of the test organism. This may be accomplished by finding a biochemical marker that rarely varies within the species. For example, *Escherichia coli* is rarely citrate positive. Thus the observation of several citrate-positive strains immediately suggests the possibility of an outbreak. Biotyping may also be accomplished by comparing several reactions that usually vary within a species, for example, reactions that are 15% to 85% positive. This profile or "fingerprint" provides the basis for comparing strains. The profile numbers generated by many of the commercial kits used for identification of the *Enterobacteriaceae* represent biotypes but are often poorly reproducible and should be used with caution in epidemiologic investigations.

ANTIBIOGRAM

An antibiogram is the pattern of susceptibility of an organism to antimicrobial agents. Antibiograms are useful epidemiologic tools if the strains show unusual susceptibility patterns but are of little use if the susceptibility patterns are typical of most strains.

SEROTYPING

Biotyping and analysis of antibiograms are easy to perform. Although these techniques can distinguish unusual isolates, serotyping is much more sensitive in differentiating among closely related strains. Serotyping is normally considered a reference technique but can become a simple technique if commercial antisera are available.

RESISTOGRAM

The resistogram technique is similar to the antibiogram except that organic and inorganic chemicals are used instead of antimicrobial agents to inhibit the test strains. Using these chemicals has the advantage that the susceptibility patterns are less likely to change because there is little or no selective pressure in the hospital. This is in contrast to the intense selective pressure for antimicrobial agents.

DIENES REACTION FOR *PROTEUS*

The Dienes test may be used to type swarming *Proteus* organisms.[158] If the same strain of a swarming *Proteus* is inoculated at two different ends of a blood agar plate, swarms of cells soon migrate from the original point of inoculation. Eventually the two swarms meet and merge completely. This is considered a negative Dienes reaction, indicating that the two isolates are probably the same strain. However, if two different strains of swarming *Proteus* are similarly inoculated, they eventually come close together but a zone remains between them where there is no growth. This is a positive Dienes reaction, indicating that the isolates are different strains.

COLONY INCOMPATIBILITY

Colony incompatibility[10] is probably similar in mechanism to the Dienes reaction. Only motile species of *Enterobacteriaceae* can be compared. Two isolates are inoculated at different ends of a Petri dish and allowed to migrate together. The difference between this and the Dienes reaction is that colony incompatibility is tested in a semisolid medium. If the two isolates are different strains, they do not come completely together and a zone of inhibition, varying from a few millimeters to more than 10 mm,[10] remains between them. The definition of positive and negative findings is similar to the Dienes reaction, as is the interpretation for use in epidemiologic analysis.

COMPLETE ANTIGENIC ANALYSIS (SEROLOGIC TYPING)

Complete antigenic analysis is listed as a reference technique because it may require a large number of antisera, most of which are not available commercially. This method is the preferred typing technique because the antisera are stable and because the results are reproducible and usually correlate well with epidemiologic findings. Organisms are first tested with O (somatic) antigens and then if necessary with antisera to H (flagellar) or K (capsular) antigens, or with antisera to fimbriae or other cell structures.

BACTERIOPHAGE SUSCEPTIBILITY

As explained in Chapter 12, bacteriophage susceptibility determines the susceptibility of a group of isolates to a group of standard bacteriophages. When the phages are carefully selected, different lysis patterns occur if the isolates are different strains. This technique is not as reproducible as serologic typing and usually does not correlate as well with epidemiologic findings.

BACTERIOCIN SUSCEPTIBILITY

Bacteriocin susceptibility[5] is almost identical to bacteriophage susceptibility except that a set of standard bacteriocins is used. Bacteriocins, which are produced by gram-negative enteric bacteria, are antibiotic-like substances that may have a lethal effect on other bacteria from the same habitat. Different isolates usually have different bacteriocin susceptibility patterns. This technique has all the drawbacks mentioned for bacteriophage susceptibility studies.

BACTERIOCIN PRODUCTION

In bacteriocin production the patterns of a group of isolates are tested against a set of standard indicator strains. The indicator strains are chosen on the basis of their ability to differentiate a large collection of strains of the species. Reproducibility of bacteriocin production patterns can be a problem, but the correlation with epidemiologic findings is usually better than with bacteriophage and bacteriocin susceptibility and often approaches that of serologic typing.

PLASMID PROFILE ANALYSIS

Plasmid profile analysis is a relatively new typing method. In this technique bacterial strains are lysed and their plasmids are extracted in a standardized way. The plasmids are then separated by agarose gel electrophoresis. The size of the plasmids is calculated by comparison with molecular weight standards. The use of plasmid profile analysis is illustrated in the following example:

	Plasmids present (weight in megadaltons)						
Isolate 1	2.8	3.2	4.5	—	60	—	86
Isolate 2	2.8	3.2	4.5	—	60	—	86
Isolate 3	—	—	—	40	—	78	—

In this case plasmid profile analysis has shown the similarity of isolates 1 and 2 and their difference from isolate 3.

GENOME SEQUENCING

Genome sequencing is a technique that has become more available as improvements have been made in the technology. In this method the exact nucleotide sequence is determined for specific pieces of DNA. These sequences can then be compared for different isolates to see whether they are identical or different. DNA sequencing is an extremely accurate measurement of how similar or different isolates are; the only disadvantage is the great amount of work required to make just a few comparisons.

• • •

Table 16-20 is an example of the use of typing methods to study the relationship of several strains of *Klebsiella pneumoniae*. Strains 6, 7, 8, and 9 are all resistant to antimicrobial agents and are the same serologic type. They are most likely the same strain in an evolutionary or epidemiologic sense. Isolate 9 differs from isolates 6 to 8 in its API 20E profile, but this is a difference of only one test out of 21. This is probably not a significant difference, and the test should be repeated for each strain using both the API system and a standard tube test to see whether the difference is reproducible. Antimicrobial-resistant strains of the same serotype are usually acquired in the hospital and are not part of the person's normal flora. In contrast to isolates 6 to 9, isolates 1 to 5 are all generally sensitive to antimicrobial agents and belong to five different serotypes. These five isolates are more likely to have been acquired from the patient's own flora. Thus typing methods, in conjunction with antimicrobial susceptibility patterns, are useful in analyzing many different situations in hospitals.

ASSOCIATED DISEASES
DISTRIBUTION OF *ENTEROBACTERIACEAE* IN CLINICAL SPECIMENS

Members of the family *Enterobacteriaceae* represent important causes of both community and nosocomial infections. At one time or another, most of the species of *Enterobacteriaceae* have been incriminated in human disease. However, the relative frequency of isolation of each of these organisms in the hospital laboratory varies considerably. *Escherichia coli*, for example, is a common organism whereas *Enterobacter sakazakii* is a rare one; even a large laboratory serving a 1000-bed hospital sees only one or two isolates of *E. sakazakii* each year in contrast to thousands of isolates of *E. coli*. Likewise, *Proteus mirabilis* and *Klebsiella pneumoniae* are extremely common, with many isolates each week, although not nearly as common as *E. coli*. *Enterobacter cloacae, Citrobacter freun-*

TABLE 16-20. Use of Typing Methods to Study Relationship of *Klebsiella pneumoniae* Strains

Strain	Patient Number	Hospital Location	Specimen	API Biochemical Profile	Resistance	Capsule Type (K Antigen)
Endemic strains	1	2 East	Urine	5 215 773	AM, CB	16
	2	6 East	Urine	5 215 773	AM, CB	32
	3	6 East	Urine	5 214 773	AM, CB, TE	2
	4	6 West	Wound	5 205 773	AM, CB	30
	5	Emer.	Stool	5 215 773	AM, CB	7
Hospital-acquired strains	6	ICU	Urine	5 215 773	AM, CB, TE, C, NA, S, K, GM, NN, AN	2
	7	ICU	Urine	5 215 773	AM, CB, TE, C, NA, S, K, GM, NN, AN	2
	8	ICU	Wound	5 215 773	AM, CB, TE, C, NA, S, K, GM, NN, AN	2
	9	2 East	Blood	5 214 773	AM, CB, TE, C, NA, S, K, GM, NN, AN	2

SYMBOLS: Emer., Emergency room   NA, Nalidixic acid
ICU, Intensive care unit   S, Streptomycin
AM, Ampicillin   K, Kanamycin
CB, Carbenicillin   GM, Gentamicin
TE, Tetracycline   NN, Tobramycin
C, Chloramphenicol   AN, Amikacin

dii, and *Serratia marcescens* are quite common but less so than the species named previously.

The expected number of isolates of each species of *Enterobacteriaceae* follows a general pattern in most hospitals; the exact distribution of the different species varies depending on a number of factors, including hospital size, patient population served, and the extent of the laboratory's testing to identify strains. Table 16-21 gives the relative frequency of the different species in clinical specimens. This estimate is based on many reports in the literature (summarized in reference 60). The numbers in the table represent the relative frequency of the organisms' occurrence in clinical specimens. Because it is an estimate, it should be taken only as a guide. These values will need to be updated as more clinical microbiology laboratories report their experiences with the new species. The high numbers signify the common organisms, and the low numbers the rare organisms. The definitions below are used:

Relative frequency 10—most common by far (one organism: *Escherichia coli*). *E. coli* is by far the most common species of *Enterobacteriaceae* isolated in clinical laboratories and is usually far ahead of *Klebsiella pneumoniae, Proteus mirabilis,* and the other species that follow.

Relative frequency 8—extremely common (two organisms: *Klebsiella pneumoniae* and *Proteus mirabilis*). These two species follow *E. coli* in frequency.

Relative frequency 7—common (examples: *Enterobacter cloacae* and *Serratia marcescens*). Organisms in this category are common in clinical specimens.

Relative frequency 6—often isolated (examples: *Citrobacter diversus* and *Enterobacter agglomerans*). Organisms in this category are well known to clinical microbiologists and are often isolated and identified.

Relative frequency 5—occasional (examples: *Serratia liquefaciens* and *Providencia alcalifaciens*). Organisms in this

category are still well known to most clinical microbiologists but may give rise to the comment, ''We have not seen one of these in quite a while.''

Relative frequency 4—rare (examples: *Edwardsiella tarda* and *Serratia rubidaea*). Organisms in this category are seen a few times each year at most.

Relative frequency 3—very rare (examples: *Enterobacter sakazakii* and *Yersinia fredericksenii*). Organisms in this category are not isolated in many laboratories over the course of a year. Most of these have been described relatively recently and when reported may give rise to comments such as, ''What in the world is that?'' The names are more familiar to microbiologists than to physicians.

Relative frequency 2—extremely rare (examples: *Cedecea davisae, Tatumella ptyseos,* and Enteric Group 17). Most organisms in this category have been described only recently. They are so rare that often case reports are written when the organism is isolated from a patient with significant disease. Most laboratories do not see one isolate in a year's time.

Relative frequency 1—only a few clinical isolates known (examples: *Serratia ficaria, Cedecea lapagei, Edwardsiella ictaluri,* and Enteric Group 53). Organisms in the category can occur in clinical specimens, but even their occurrence is so unusual that a case report is often written.[71,120]

Relative frequency 0—not known to occur in clinical specimens (examples: *Proteus myxofaciens* and *Xenorhabdus*). Organisms in this category often have a specialized ecologic niche (water, soil, plants, insects, invertebrates) and perhaps for that reason do not occur in clinical specimens. A case report would probably be written if one occurred in a clinical specimen.

TABLE 16-21. Sources of the New Genera, Species, Biogroups, and Enteric Groups of *Enterobacteriaceae*

Genus and Species	Relative Frequency	Clinical Significance		Human Sources							Other Sources				
		Diarrhea	Other	Spinal Fluid	Blood	Urine	Wounds	Respiratory Tract	Stool	Other	Animals	Water	Soil	Environment	Food
Buttiauxella															
B. agrestis	0	−	−	−	−	−	−	−	−	−	−	+	−	−	−
Cedecea															
C. davisea	2	−	(−)	−	−	+	+	+	+	+	−	−	−	−	−
C. lapagei	1	−	(−)	−	−	+	−	+	+	−	−	−	−	−	−
C. neteri	1	−	+	+	+	+	+	+	−	−	−	−	−	−	−
C. species 3	1	−	(−)	+	+	+	+	+	−	−	−	−	−	−	−
C. species 5	1	−	(−)	−	−	−	+	−	−	−	−	−	−	−	−
Citrobacter															
C. amalonaticus	5	−	+	−	+	+	+	+	+	+	+	+	−	−	−
C. amalonaticus biogroup 1	4	−	+	−	+	+	+	−	+	+	−	−	−	−	−
C. diversus	6	−	++	+	+	+	+	+	+	+	−	+	+	−	+
C. freundii	7	(+)	++	−	+	+	+	+	+	+	+	+	+	−	+
Edwardsiella															
E. hoshinae	1	−	−	−	−	−	−	−	−	−	+	+	−	−	−
E. ictaluri	0	−	−	−	−	−	−	−	−	−	+	−	−	−	+
E. tarda	4	(+)	+	−	+	+	+	+	+	+	+	+	+	−	−
E. tarda biogroup 1	0	−	−	−	−	−	−	−	−	+	+	−	−	−	−
Enterobacter															
E. aerogenes	7	−	++	+	+	+	+	+	+	+	+	+	−	+	−
E. agglomerans	6	−	+	+	+	+	+	+	+	+	+	+	−	+	+
E. amnigenus biogroup 1	1	−	−	−	−	+	−	−	+	−	−	+	−	−	−
E. amnigenus biogroup 2	0	−	+++	+	+	+	+	+	+	+	+	+	−	+	+
E. cloacae	7	−	+	+	+	+	+	+	+	+	+	+	−	+	+
E. gergoviae	3	−	+	−	−	+	−	+	+	+	−	−	−	−	−
E. intermedium	0	−	−	−	−	−	−	−	−	−	−	+	−	−	+
E. sakazakii	3	−	(−)	+	+	+	+	+	+	+	+	+	−	+	+
E. taylorae	2	−	(−)	+	−	+	−	−	−	+	−	−	−	+	−
Escherichia															
E. blattae	0	−	(−)	−	+	+	+	+	+	+	+	−	−	−	−
E. fergusonii	2	−	(−)	+	+	+	+	+	+	+	+	−	−	−	+
E. hermanii	2	−	(−)	+	+	+	+	+	+	+	−	+	+	+	+
E. vulneris	2	−	−	−	+	+	+	+	−	−	+	−	−	+	−
Ewingella															
E. americana	1	−	+	−	+	+	+	+	+	+	−	−	−	−	+

Continued.

TABLE 16-21. Sources of the New Genera, Species, Biogroups, and Enteric Groups of *Enterobacteriaceae*—cont'd

Genus and Species	Relative Frequency	Clinical Significance		Human Sources							Other Sources				
		Diarrhea	Other	Spinal Fluid	Blood	Urine	Wounds	Respiratory Tract	Stool	Other	Animals	Water	Soil	Environment	Food
Hafnia															
H. alvei	6	(+)	+	+	+	+	+	+	−	+	−	−	−	−	−
H. alvei biogroup 1	0	−	−	−	−	−	−	−	−	+	−	−	−	−	−
Klebsiella															
K. oxytoca	7	(+)	+++	−	+	+	+	+	+	+	+	+	−	+	+
K. planticola	4	−	(−)	−	−	+	−	−	+	+	+	+	−	+	+
K. terrigena	0	−	−	−	−	−	−	−	−	−	−	+	−	−	−
K. group 47 ind⁺ orn⁺	2	−	(+)	−	+	+	−	+	−	+	−	−	−	−	−
Kluyvera															
K. ascorbata	4	(−)	(+)	−	+	+	+	+	+	+	+	+	−	−	+
K. cryocrescens	2	−	(−)	−	+	+	−	+	−	+	−	−	+	+	+
Moellerella															
M. wisconsensis	1	(−)	(−)	−	−	−	−	−	−	+	−	−	−	−	−
Morganella															
M. morganii biogroup 1	4	−	(+)	−	−	+	+	+	+	+	−	−	−	−	−
Obesumbacterium															
O. proteus biogroup 2	0	−	−	−	−	−	−	−	−	−	−	−	−	−	−
Proteus															
P. myxofaciens	0	−	−	−	−	−	−	−	−	−	+	−	−	−	−
P. penneri	3	−	+	−	+	+	+	+	+	+	−	−	−	−	−
Providencia															
P. rustigianii	3	−	(−)	−	−	−	−	−	+	−	−	−	−	−	−
Rahnella															
R. aquatilis	1	−	(−)	−	−	−	+	−	−	−	−	+	−	−	−
Serratia															
S. ficaria	1	−	(−)	−	−	−	+	+	−	+	+	−	−	−	+
S. fonticola	0	−	(−)	−	−	−	+	+	−	+	−	+	−	+	−
S. liquefaciens group	5	−	(−)+	−	−	−	+	+	+	+	−	−	+	−	−
S. marcescens biogroup 1	5	−	(−)	−	−	+	+	+	+	+	−	−	−	−	−
S. odorifera biogroup 1	2	−	(−)	+	+	+	+	+	+	+	−	+	+	+	+
S. odorifera biogroup 2	3	−	(−)	−	+	+	−	+	+	+	−	−	−	−	−
S. plymuthica	2	−	(−)	−	−	+	+	+	+	+	+	+	−	+	−
S. rubidaea	4	−	(−)	−	+	+	+	+	+	+	+	+	−	−	−
Tatumella															
T. ptyseos	2	−	(+)	−	+	+	−	+	+	+	−	−	−	−	−

Yersinia

	Relative Frequency	Clinical Significance—Diarrhea
Y. enterocolitica	6	++
Y. frederiksenii	3	(+)
Y. intermedia	3	(+)
Y. kristensenii	3	(+)
Y. ruckeri	1	−

Xenorhabdus

X. luminescens	0	−
X. nematophilus	0	−
Enteric Group 17	2	(+)
Enteric Group 41	1	−
Enteric Group 46	1	−
Enteric Group 53	1	(−)
Enteric Group 57	1	(−)
Enteric Group 58	1	(−)
Enteric Group 59	1	(−)
Enteric Group 60	1	(−)
Enteric Group 61	1	(−)
Enteric Group 63	0	
Enteric Group 64	0	
Enteric Group 68	1	(−)
Enteric Group 69	0	

SYMBOLS:

For "Relative Frequency" (See text for more details):
10, Most common by far
8, Extremely common
7, Common
6, Occasional
5, Uncommon
4, Rare
3, Very rare
2, Extremely rare
1, Only a few clinical isolates known
0, Not known to occur in clinical specimens

For "Clinical Significance—Diarrhea":
+++, Intrinsic cause
++, Documented cause but not all strains are able
(+), mentioned as a possible cause but there is not universal agreement
(−), Unlikely cause but mentioned in literature
−, Not a cause

For "Clinical Significance—Other":
+++ and ++, Clinically significant
+, Reported to be clinically significant at least at some sites; may not be significant at other sites
(+), Clinical significance at least suggested in the literature, but more data are needed
(−), No data at present to suggest significance, but significance can not be totally excluded because of occurrence in clinical specimens
−, Not significant

For "Sources":
+, Organism has been found at that source
−, It has not been reported

Modified from Farmer, J.J., III, et al.: J. Clin. Microbiol. **21**:46, 1985.

CLINICAL SIGNIFICANCE OF *ENTEROBACTERIACEAE*

Table 16-21 also rates the species of *Enterobacteriaceae* as to their clinical significance in intestinal (diarrheal) or extraintestinal infections. The *Enterobacteriaceae* spp. that cause infections of the intestinal tract are rated according to the following definitions:

Clinical significance +++. Intrinsic cause (examples: *Shigella dysenteriae* and *Salmonella typhimurium*). Organisms in this category are well-known causes of diarrhea, and most (if not all strains) can cause diarrhea. The organisms are always mentioned in textbooks as causes of diarrhea.

Clinical significance ++. Documented cause of diarrhea, but not all strains are capable (examples: *Escherichia coli* and *Yersinia enterocolitica*). Organisms in this category have been well documented as a cause of diarrhea and are usually mentioned in textbooks. However, the ability to cause diarrhea is not present in all strains of the species. For example, most "normal" gut strains of *Escherichia coli* do not. A number of mechanisms of pathogenicity (enterotoxins, cytotoxins, invasiveness, colonization factors) have usually been associated with strains that have the ability to cause diarrhea.

Clinical significance + or (+). Implicated cause, but there is not universal agreement (examples: *Edwardsiella tarda,* *Hafnia alvei,* and *Klebsiella oxytoca*). Organisms in this category are seldom mentioned in textbook discussions of bacteria causing diarrhea; however some reports in the literature incriminate them as causes. Thus there is disagreement as to whether they can cause diarrhea.

Clinical significance (−). Unlikely cause, but mentioned in literature (example: *Kluyvera*). Organisms in this category have been mentioned in relationship to diarrhea,[51] but there is no strong evidence that they actually cause diarrhea.

Clinical significance −. No association with diarrhea. These organisms have not been associated with diarrhea. They may or may not be found in feces (Table 16-21).

CLINICAL SYNDROMES

Some members of the family *Enterobacteriaceae* such as the genera *Shigella* and *Salmonella* are primary pathogens capable of causing disease in healthy hosts. Others, including the genera *Klebsiella, Enterobacter,* and *Serratia,* are opportunistic pathogens and usually cause disease in immunocompromised hosts. As discussed in Chapter 4, the latter organisms have become primary causes of nosocomial infections over the past few years. Because of the selective pressure of antimicrobial agents these nosocomial pathogens are frequently resistant to multiple drugs and thus are of major concern in hospitals.

Specific clinical syndromes of species of the *Enterobacteriaceae* are considered in the following sections.

Cedecea

Most isolates of the genus *Cedecea* are from the respiratory tract. The clinical relevance of these organisms is unknown. *C. neteri* has been associated with a case of bacteremia.[56]

Citrobacter[93]

Citrobacter spp. are opportunists that may be responsible for community-acquired and nosocomial infections. Most *Citrobacter* infections involve the urinary or respiratory tract. *C. freundii* has also been associated with septicemia related to bacterial contamination of intravenous fluids and urinary tract, respiratory tract, wound, and cutaneous infections. *C. diversus* has been associated with brain abscesses and meningitis in neonates.[75] *C. amalonaticus* has been isolated from a number of specimen types and has been reported as a cause of urinary tract infections.

Edwardsiella

E. tarda is the only species of *Edwardsiella* implicated in human disease. This organism may be isolated from the environment and from a large variety of cold- and warm-blooded animals. The primary reservoirs are reptiles, and freshwater fish including aquarium fish may serve as a source of human infection.[167]

E. tarda appears to be a cause of gastrointestinal disease, primarily in tropical and subtropical countries. Extraintestinal infections have been reported infrequently.[32] These include septic shock, hepatic abscesses, cholangitis, meningitis, cellulitis, and wound infections.

Enterobacter[107]

Members of the genus *Enterobacter* are opportunistic pathogens. *E. cloacae* and *E. aerogenes* are the most frequently isolated species. These organisms may account for 4% to 12% of all cases of gram-negative bacteremia, most of which is hospital acquired. Most studies of bacteremia have not differentiated among the *Enterobacter* spp. so it is difficult to determine species-specific rates; those studies in which speciation has been performed show *E. cloacae* to be the predominant isolate. *E. cloacae* is frequently the cause of bacteremia and wound infections among patients in burn units.

E. cloacae tends to contaminate intravenous fluids and hospital equipment. In fact, the genera *Klebsiella, Enterobacter,* and *Serratia* are the primary cause of sepsis resulting from contaminated intravenous fluids. These organisms are able to multiply in glucose-containing intravenous fluid, whereas most other organisms either die or are unable to multiply.[119] Thus bacteremia from *Enterobacter, Klebsiella,* or *Serratia* spp. should prompt an epidemiologic investigation of exposure to contaminated materials, especially those introduced into the bloodstream.

E. aerogenes and *E. cloacae* have been associated with a variety of other infections, the most serious being endocarditis, ventriculitis, and gram-negative meningitis. These organisms may also be responsible for urinary and lower respiratory tract infections. They are unusual causes of gram-negative septic arthritis and osteomyelitis.

E. sakazakii is a rare cause of neonatal meningitis and sepsis.[127] The route of transmission of the organism in most cases of neonatal meningitis is unknown; the organism may be acquired from passage through the birth canal or from exogenous hospital sources. In adults *E. sakazakii* has also been isolated from sputum, feces, and wounds, but it is probably a colonizer or transient organism and not clinically significant in these specimens.

E. gergoviae has been isolated from a variety of specimens including sputum, wounds, and urine. It has been implicated as the cause of an outbreak of urinary tract disease.[22] Four clinical isolates of *E. amnigenus* have been reported, but their role in infection is unknown. *E. taylorae* has been isolated from the blood and cerebrospinal fluid, but its clinical significance is unknown.[61] *E. intermedium* has not been associated with clinical infection.

Erwinia

The *Erwinia* organisms are plant pathogens and not involved in human infection. Reports in the literature that cite the association of the *Erwinia herbicola* group with human infections are referring to the organism also known as *Enterobacter agglomerans*.

Escherichia-Shigella

Three species of *Escherichia* are isolated from human infections. *E. hermannii* and *E. vulneris* are sometimes isolated from wound infections. *E. coli* is associated with a number of syndromes including diarrhea, gastroenteritis, cystitis, pyelitis, pyelonephritis, appendicitis, peritonitis, gallbladder infections, septicemia, neonatal meningitis, pneumonia, and endocarditis.

E. coli causes approximately 90% of all acute urinary tract infections in nonhospitalized patients without urologic abnormalities. The *E. coli* strains responsible for these infections are those comprising the normal intestinal flora. *E. coli* is also responsible for approximately 30% of nosocomial urinary tract infections.

Several distinct types of *E. coli* are involved in gastroenteritis. These types are differentiated on the basis of the mechanism by which they cause disease. Enterotoxigenic *E. coli* (ETEC) produces enterotoxins. Enteroinvasive *E. coli* (EIEC) invades the intestinal epithelium. Enteropathogenic *E. coli* (EPEC) is noninvasive and does not produce toxins; the mechanism of pathogenicity is unknown. An unusual serotype of *E. coli*, O157:H7, not belonging to any of the other three types, has also been associated with hemorrhagic colitis and hemolytic uremic syndrome.[142]

ETEC is a common cause of travelers' diarrhea, accounting for 40% to 70% of all cases in some geographic areas.[74] It is also a common cause of diarrhea in children in developing countries and may produce a cholera-like illness in adults in these countries. The latter condition is the most severe form of ETEC gastroenteritis and is clinically similar to cholera. The other forms of ETEC gastroenteritis are much milder and are characterized by diarrhea, vomiting, chills, headache, and fever following an incubation period of 1 to 2 days. The illness may last 5 to 10 days. ETEC gastroenteritis is usually transmitted through contaminated food and water.

Gastroenteritis caused by EIEC is clinically similar to shigellosis. Fever, tenesmus, abdominal cramping, and bloody diarrhea with pus occur after an incubation period of 12 to 24 hours. Cases occur primarily in Eastern Europe and rarely in Southeast Asia and North America. Outbreaks in the United States have been linked with the consumption of contaminated food.

EPEC has historically been associated with outbreaks of hospital-acquired infantile diarrhea. This disease, characterized by diarrhea without blood or mucus, and by infrequent vomiting and fever, may progress to dehydration, shock, and death. Recent studies have shown that enteropathogenic strains of *E. coli* continue to be isolated in many parts of the world, especially in developing countries.[38]

Strains of *E. coli* O157:H7 appear to be responsible for hemorrhagic colitis. This illness is characterized by severe abdominal pain, initially watery diarrhea followed by grossly bloody diarrhea, and little or no fever. Outbreaks of hemorrhagic colitis occurred in Oregon and Michigan in 1982.[142] They were associated with the consumption of undercooked hamburger from a fast-food chain.

Shigellosis or bacillary dysentery is caused by all four species of *Shigella*. Following an incubation period of 1 to 7 days, shigellosis typically begins with fever, cramping, abdominal pain, and diarrhea. The diarrhea is initially watery and may last 1 to 3 days. This phase of shigellosis may be followed by a second phase characterized by frequent, scant stools containing blood, mucus, and pus. Microscopic examination of these stools stained with methylene blue usually reveals numerous sheets of polymorphonuclear leukocytes. The second phase of shigellosis, most often referred to as dysentery, is also characterized by tenesmus, fever, and severe abdominal cramps. Convulsions may occur in children.

The severity of shigellosis varies depending on the species. Although all species may cause mild diarrhea or fulminant dysentery, infections resulting from *S. sonnei* tend to be much milder than those from *S. flexneri* and *S. dysenteriae*. *Shigella* bacteremia is rare in immunocompetent hosts.

In the United States shigellosis is usually restricted to populations characterized by poverty, crowded living conditions, inadequate water supplies, poor sanitation, or poor personal hygiene. Outbreaks also occur in nurseries and day-care centers. *S. sonnei* accounts for approximately 70% of the *Shigella* isolates reported in the United States.[11] The highest reported rates of shigellosis are in the Western states and among children between the ages of 1 and 5 years.[11]

As few as 10 to 200 *Shigella* organisms may cause shigellosis. This infectious dose is 100 to 100,000 times smaller than that of many other enteric pathogens and is responsible for the transmission of *Shigella* organisms from person to person via the fecal-oral route. Contaminated food and water may serve as a vehicle of transmission, especially in developing countries. Shigellae can also be transmitted venereally among homosexual men.[37,124]

Ewingella

Only a few clinical isolates of *Ewingella americana* have been reported. Sputum is the most common source, but recently two nosocomial outbreaks of bacteremia occurred.

Hafnia

Hafnia alvei has been recovered from a variety of clinical specimens but is rarely if ever pathogenic.

Klebsiella[105,126]

Approximately 95% of *Klebsiella* isolates are *K. pneumoniae*. *K. oxytoca* makes up the majority of the remaining 5%. These organisms may be responsible for pneumonia, lung abscess, septicemia, meningitis, infections of the intestinal tract and biliary tree, soft tissue infections, and urinary tract infections; most infections are extraintestinal.

Many *Klebsiella* infections (with the exception of primary lobar pneumonia and urinary tract infections) are hospital acquired. Epidemics have occurred primarily in newborns and among patients in urologic wards and intensive care units. Over

50% of the nosocomial outbreaks reported from 1965 to 1982 were in neonatal intensive care units.[105] Colonization of the bowel or other body sites serves as the primary reservoir of infection, and the hands of hospital personnel are the major transmitters of the organism. Other means of transmission include contaminated medications, hand cream, intravenous solutions, and respiratory equipment.

K. ozaenae is a rare clinical isolate. This organism is responsible for atrophy of the nasal mucosa. *K. rhinoscleromatis* is a rare isolate in the United States but is more common in Central and South America and North Africa. It causes a granulomatous disease affecting the nose, nasal mucosa, paranasal sinuses, larynx, pharynx, trachea, bronchi, and rarely the middle ear. *K. planticola* (from plants) is a rare clinical isolate. *K. terrigena* (from soil) has not been recovered from clinical specimens.

Kluyvera

Strains of *Kluyvera* have been isolated from a variety of human clinical specimens, but their role in disease is unknown.

Moellerella[90]

Eight of nine *Moellerella wisconsensis* strains have been isolated from stool samples, but there is no evidence that it causes diarrhea.

Morganella

Morganella morganii produces infections mainly in hospitalized patients. The primary sites of infection are the urinary tract and postoperative wounds. These infections occur in older patients with serious underlying disease and particularly in surgical patients who have had prior antimicrobial therapy.[122] The genus *Morganella* has been regarded as a relatively unimportant human pathogen in the past. However, its recent association with bacteremia[122] and septicemia suggests that it may become an important cause of nosocomial infection in the future.[173]

Proteus

P. mirabilis is by far the most frequently isolated species of *Proteus*. This organism is most commonly associated with urinary tract infections and wound infections but may also be responsible for pneumonia and septicemia. *P. mirabilis* causes approximately 10% of community-acquired urinary tract infections, many of which are observed in male children. Nosocomial urinary tract infections usually occur in patients with obstructive lesions of the urinary tract or in association with instrumentation or prolonged catheterization. As with *Klebsiella pneumoniae*, intestinal colonization of patients appears to be a major reservoir of these infections.[30]

P. vulgaris may be responsible for the same clinical syndromes observed with *P. mirabilis*, but urinary tract infections associated with this organism are almost always nosocomial in origin. Although the clinical significance of *P. penneri* is unknown, this organism was recently associated with a urinary tract infection.[111]

Providencia

Providencia stuartii and *Providencia rettgeri* are the most common isolates and are associated with nosocomial infections of the urinary tract or skin. Urinary tract infections are almost invariably associated with underlying urologic disorders and catheterization. Elderly patients are especially susceptible. The major reservoir in outbreaks of urinary tract infection caused by *P. rettgeri* appears to be the genitourinary tract of catheterized patients.[144] Fecal colonization may be an important nosocomial reservoir for *P. stuartii*.[86] *P. stuartii* is a significant cause of burn infections.

Salmonella
Nontyphoid *Salmonella*[96]

Nontyphoid salmonellae *(Salmonella* other than *S. typhi)* are primarily pathogens of humans and animals. In fact these organisms have been isolated from almost every animal source known, including poultry (chicken, ducks, turkeys), pets (turtles, cats, dogs, mice, guinea pigs, hamsters), cows, pigs, sheep, seals, donkeys, lizards, snakes, and birds (doves, pigeons, parrots, starlings, sparrows, cowbirds). Spread of infection among animals may occur by direct transmission or by ingestion of contaminated animal feed.

Human infection is primarily acquired by ingestion of contaminated poultry or meat (beef or pork). Water that has been contaminated by feces or urine from humans or animals may also serve as a vehicle of transmission. Other cases of human salmonellosis have been traced to contact with infected dogs, cats, turtles, chicks, and ducks.

Current food processing methods may augment the spread of *Salmonella* among domestic animals used as human food resources. For example, if tools used in a slaughterhouse are contaminated by one infected animal, their subsequent use in a slaughter run may contaminate the carcasses of numerous animals. As a result 1% to more than 50% of raw meat purchased in retail markets may be contaminated with salmonellae.

One must be careful when preparing foods that are likely to be contaminated with salmonellae. Cooking destroys these organisms, but failure to reach sufficiently high temperatures in the innermost areas of a large piece of meat will result in continued contamination. Precautions must also be taken to avoid recontaminating cooked food with cooking utensils previously exposed to the raw infected meat.

A few of the *Salmonella* serotypes other than *S. typhi* produce bacteremia. This may lead to the localization of the organism in numerous body sites, especially those that are the site of preexisting disease. Bronchopneumonia, empyema, endocarditis, osteomyelitis, pyelonephritis, arthritis, and meningitis are relatively common.

S. paratyphi A, *S. paratyphi* B, and *S. choleraesuis* can cause enteric fever, which is similar to but milder than typhoid fever.

Salmonella typhi[97]

Humans are the only reservoir of *S. typhi*. Typhoid fever is acquired by ingestion of food or water that has been directly or indirectly contaminated by the excreta (primarily feces) of infected individuals including carriers. The incidence of typhoid fever is high in countries with substandard sanitation measures. Between 1977 and 1979 international travel led to 63% of the cases of typhoid fever reported in the United States.[163]

The incubation period of typhoid fever is typically 8 to 14 days. Onset is usually insidious; the most marked symptoms are fever, headache, myalgia, and gastrointestinal problems. A dry cough and bronchitis may also be present. The patient appears acutely ill during the second and third weeks. A high fever is present, and prostration and delirium are common. Rhonchi and scattered moist rales (abnormal sounds produced by passage of air through bronchi that contain secretion or exudate), splenomegaly, and rose spots may occur. Rose spots, 2 to 4 mm erythematous maculopapular lesions that blanch on pressure, appear on the abdomen in crops of 10 to 20 but disappear in hours to days. If no complications occur, the fever begins to decline and the patient begins to improve toward the end of the third week. Recovery continues through the fourth week.

The site of isolation of *S. typhi* depends on the stage of illness. In the absence of antimicrobial therapy, organisms may be recovered from the blood of 90% of patients during the first week of disease. Up to 50% of patients may have positive blood cultures as late as the third week, but the incidence of positive cultures rapidly decreases after this time. Stool culture findings are positive in only 10% of patients during the first week of disease, but the frequency of positive stool cultures increases to 85% during the third to fifth weeks. Urine cultures may be positive in 25% of patients during the third to fourth week of illness.

Prior administration of antimicrobial agents decreases the recovery rate of *S. typhi* from the blood, urine, and stool.[72] The bone marrow and rose spots may be better sources for isolation of the organism after antimicrobial therapy.[72]

The Widal test has been used for serologic diagnosis of typhoid fever. This test detects antibody rises to the O and H antigens of *S. typhi;* antibody titers to the O antigen are generally considered more specific than those to the H antigen. Antibodies to O antigens appear during the first week of illness and peak during the third week of illness. A fourfold or greater increase in titer between the acute phase and convalescent phase sera may be significant. However, results must be interpreted cautiously for several reasons. First, other serologically related *Salmonella* spp. may cause the antibody rise. Second, low titers of antibody may be present because of previous immunizations. Finally, antibodies may not be present because of previous antimicrobial therapy.

Chloramphenicol is still probably the drug of choice for typhoid fever and reduces the frequency of complications, notably intestinal hemorrhage and perforation. Vaccines are also available for individuals residing or traveling in highly endemic areas or for exposed laboratory workers.

Serratia[177]

The majority of human isolates of *Serratia* are *S. marcescens*. This organism has been associated with urinary and respiratory tract infections, septicemia, and endocarditis. Almost all infections are hospital acquired. Endocarditis may be community acquired among drug addicts.

Nosocomial infections usually occur in patients subjected to instrumentation, especially urinary catheters and tracheostomy tubes, in debilitated patients, and in patients receiving antimicrobial therapy. The genitourinary tracts of catheterized patients are the primary reservoir of outbreaks of urinary tract infections, and the hands of hospital personnel are the primary mode of transmission. Contaminated solutions or medical equipment have also been responsible for outbreaks of noso-

comial infections. Incriminated sources have included disinfectants, water from ultrasonic nebulizers and the nebulizers themselves, intravenous solutions, hand lotions, mechanical respirators, polyethylene intravenous catheters, and fiberoptic bronchoscopes.

Yersinia enterocolitica[12,168]

Y. enterocolitica may cause a wide spectrum of infections depending on the age and physical state of the host. Enterocolitis is the most frequently encountered infection and occurs primarily in infants and young children. It is characterized by diarrhea lasting from 2 to several weeks. Abdominal pain, frequently in the right lower quadrant, is usually present, and fever may occur.

Acute mesenteric lymphadenitis and terminal ileitis are observed among older children and younger adults. The presentation of these conditions is clinically indistinguishable from acute appendicitis. Patients often undergo appendectomies that reveal a normal appendix but an inflamed, thickened, hyperemic terminal ileum and enlarged mesenteric lymph nodes.

Sequelae of *Yersinia* infection observed in adults include erythema nodosum, septic arthritis, and septicemia. Septicemia is most often reported in aged or debilitated patients. Other manifestations reported in adults include meningitis, panophthalmitis, cellulitis, hemolytic anemia, Reiter's syndrome, and intra-abdominal and lung abscesses.

Y. enterocolitica has an interesting geographic distribution. Serotypes 0:3 and 0:9 are the most common in Europe and Canada but are relatively rare in the United States, where serotypes 0:5 and 0:8 are common. Furthermore, as previously stated, infections tend to be more common in the North than in the South.

Animals serve as a significant reservoir of *Y. enterocolitica*. Evidence suggests that swine may be important in the epidemiology of *Y. enterocolitica* infections in Belgium. Isolates of the same serotype (0:9) have been recovered from pigs and from humans suffering from yersiniosis following consumption of pork or direct contact with pigs.

Consumption of contaminated food and milk products has been associated with outbreaks of yersiniosis in the United States. Person-to-person transmission has been strongly suggested in certain family and hospital outbreaks. In most sporadic cases of yersiniosis, however, the source of infection and mode of transmission remain obscure.

MECHANISMS OF PATHOGENICITY
ESCHERICHIA-SHIGELLA
Escherichia

As discussed previously, *Escherichia coli* may cause diarrheal disease by several mechanisms. ETEC strains may produce one or both of two enterotoxins, LT and ST. ST is a heat-labile toxin, and ST is heat stable. Production of these toxins is plasmid mediated.

LT is similar to cholera toxin (see Chapter 18) in structure, antigenicity, and mode of action. Both LT and cholera toxins cause diarrhea by binding to specific Gm_1 gangliosides on the epithelial cells of the small intestine and stimulating the production of the enzyme adenyl cyclase. Adenyl cyclase then causes increased production of cyclic adenosine monophosphate (cyclic AMP), which stimulates fluid transport into the lumen of the bowel, resulting in diarrhea.

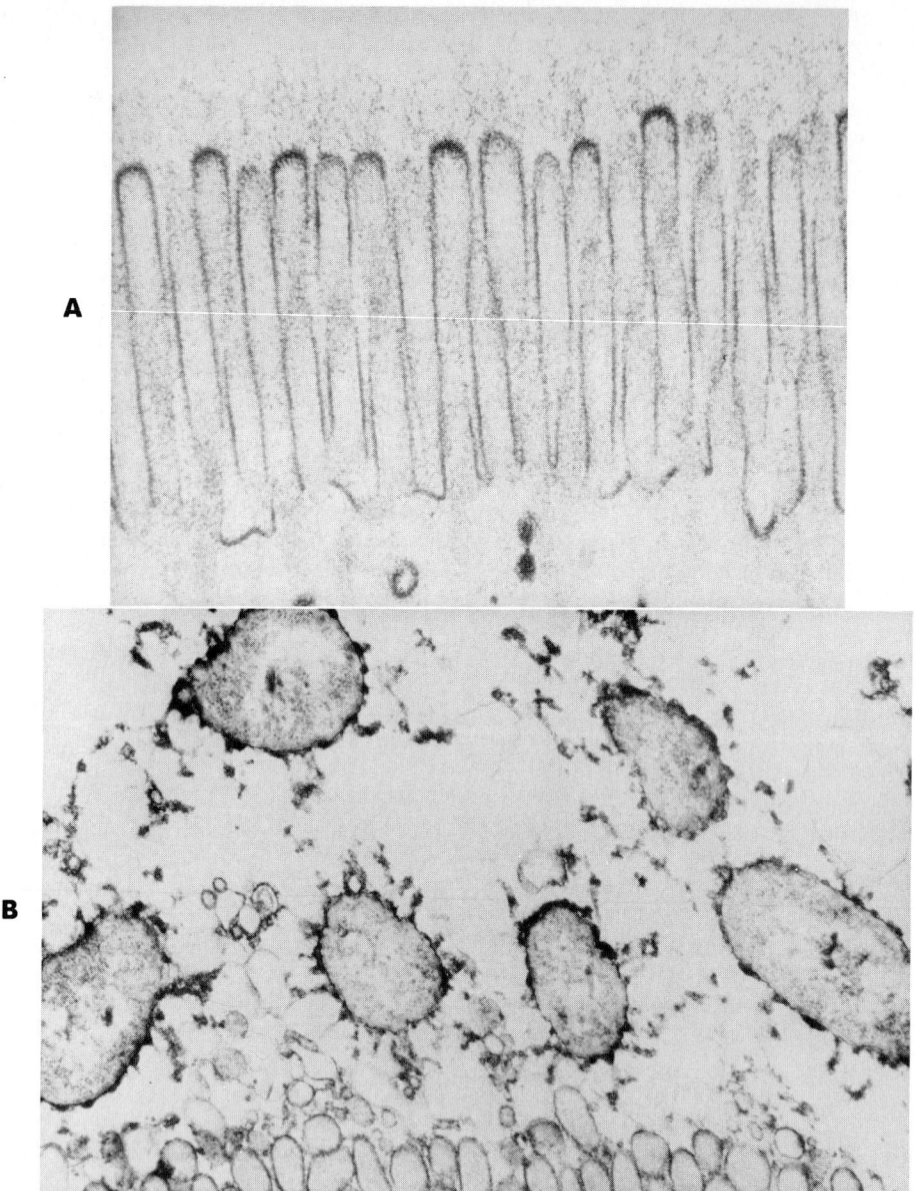

FIGURE 16-3. A, Transmission electron micrograph of intestinal epithelium stained with ruthenium red. Note electron-dense fibrous glycocalyx extending above the tips of microvilli. (×40,000.) **B,** Electron micrograph of ileal mucosa from calf infected with enterotoxigenic strain of *Escherichia coli* (ETEC). Tissue was treated with anti-K99 monoclonal antibody before staining with ruthenium red. Note thickened K99 fimbriae *(arrows)* that appear as fine, electron-dense projections from bacterial surface. Extracellular polysaccharide capsule became dehydrated during fixation and collapsed to form amorphous accretions on bacterial surface and fimbriae. (×20,000.)

The mechanism of action of ST differs from that of LT. This toxin also binds to specific receptors on the cell surface of intestinal cells,[65] but it activates the enzyme guanylate cyclase. Guanylate cyclase leads to increased production of cyclic guanosine monophosphate (cyclic GMP), the mediator responsible for diarrhea.

To cause diarrhea, ETEC must also adhere to the small intestine. This adherence appears to be mediated by fimbriae (or pili), which are hairlike projections extending from the cell surface. (Many gram-negative bacteria adhere by means of fimbriae.) There are several fimbrial antigens involved in the adherence of ETEC. The K88 antigen (and others) is responsible for adherence in pigs and calves (Figure 16-3, *B*). The fimbriae that mediate colonization of the human small intestine have been designated colonization factors. Earlier studies showed two major colonization factors, CF 1 and CF II,[41] but

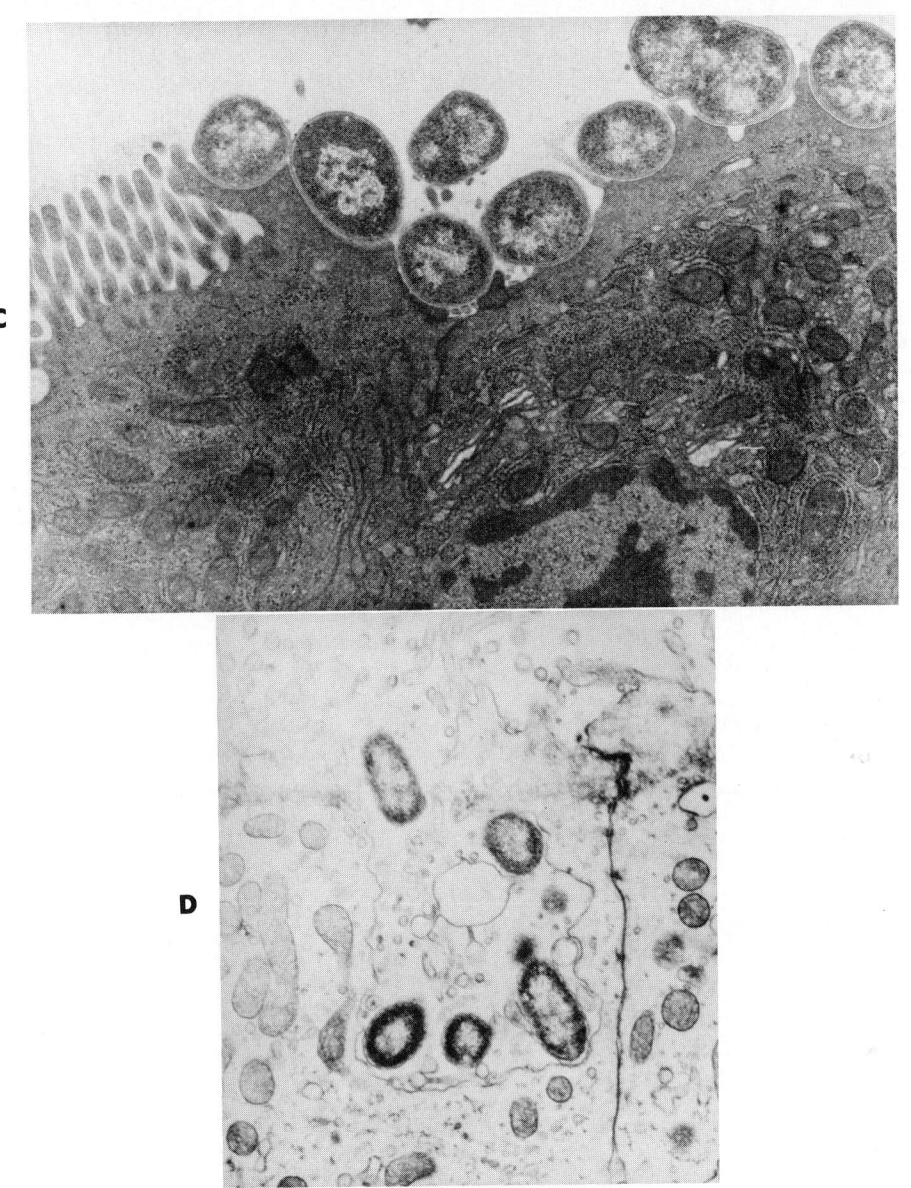

FIGURE 16-3, cont'd. C, Electron micrograph of enteropathogenic *E. coli* (EPEC) adhering to jejunal epithelium of infected infant. At areas of bacterial contact, microvilli are obliterated and adherent organisms are found in cuplike depressions of simplified plasma membrane. (×18,000.) **D,** Electron micrograph of *Salmonella typhimurium* invading ileal epithelium of guinea pig. Microvilli, terminal web, and apical cytoplasm are replaced by cavity lined with bleblike projections *(A),* some of which contain small vesicles *(B, C).* Intercellular junctional complex is displaced laterally *(arrows)* while bacteria are being internalized. (×18,000.) (**A** courtesy J. Trier. **D** courtesy A. Takeuchi. Both from Formal, S.B., Hale, T.L., and Boedeker, E.C.: Phil. Trans. R. Soc. Lond. [B] **303:**65, 1983. **B** courtesy J.W. Costerton. **C** courtesy R. Giannella.)

more recent studies reported several possible additional colonization factors.[95] Production of colonization factors is plasmid mediated. In fact, several studies have shown that a single plasmid carries genes for both enterotoxin and colonization factor production.

Enterotoxin production usually occurs in a limited number of O groups, the most common being O6, O8, O15, O25, O63, O78, O148, and O159. Certain of these serotypes are usually correlated with a particular pattern of enterotoxin production; that is, some strains produce LT and ST, some only ST, and others only LT.[148] Colonization factors also appear to be associated with selected serotypes; CFA I is produced by certain strains, and CFA II is produced by others.[41]

Colonies of ETEC are usually indistinguishable from those of normal intestinal *Escherichia coli* and must be identified on the basis of toxin production. Classical tests for enterotoxin production are impractical for the routine clinical laboratory and have been performed in research laboratories. An infant mouse assay has been used to detect ST. Rabbit ileal loop tests and detection of morphologic changes in either of two tissue culture systems, Chinese hamster ovary or mouse Y_1 adrenal cells, have been used to detect LT. Three simple and rapid immunologic methods, ELISA, gel immunodiffusion, and staphylococcal coagglutination, were recently developed for assay of LT.[149] These may be suitable for use in clinical laboratories.

EIEC, like *Shigella*, causes disease by penetrating and multiplying in the epithelial cells of the intestinal mucosa (Figure 16-3, *D*). The ability to invade the epithelial cells is associated with the presence of a plasmid.[64]

EIEC is associated with the following O groups: 28, 112, 115, 124, 136, 143, 144, 147, and 152. It is biochemically and serologically similar to *Shigella* organisms (lysine decarboxylase negative and nonmotile). Techniques used to identify EIEC include the penetration of HeLa cell monolayers and the Sereny test. In the latter test the organisms are inoculated into a guinea pig's eye. *E. coli* that are enteroinvasive are able to invade the eye, causing keratoconjunctivitis. This is a positive Sereny test. The test may be used to detect other enteroinvasive organisms as well as EIEC.

The pathogenesis of *E. coli* O157:H7 may be associated with production of a cytotoxin,[108,130] which is assayed in the Vero cell culture line. This toxin resembles that of *S. dysenteriae* type 1 (Shiga toxin) in that the cytotoxicity can be neutralized by antisera to Shiga toxin. The cytotoxin has been named Shiga-like toxin.[129,130]

EPEC belongs to a limited number of serotypes (O antigen plus H antigen). Its pathogenic mechanism is largely unknown, but the subject is being investigated intensely. Production of the Shiga-like toxin has been associated with some strains.[129] Plasmid-mediated adhesiveness has also been reported.[128] Unlike the enterotoxigenic *E. coli*, the EPEC disrupt the epithelial cell microvilli with close bacterial attachment (Figure 16-3, *C*).[63a] However, they do not invade the epithelial cells as do EIEC.

In the last few years there has been confusion as to the importance of the identification of EPEC in the clinical laboratory. This confusion largely stems from historical events. From 1945 to 1950 several studies implicated strains of *E. coli* in nursery outbreaks of diarrhea. Kaufman and Dupont[110] then showed that almost all of the strains that were causing nursery outbreaks belonged to only six serotypes: O55:H2, O55:H6, O55:nonmotile, O111:H2, O111:H12, and O111:nonmotile. When commercial antisera became available, these strains were sought in the feces of infants with diarrhea. They were soon shown to be important etiologic agents of infant diarrhea in most parts of the world. Other strains of *E. coli* were then implicated as causes of infantile diarrhea, and they were added to the list of enteropathogenic serotypes. Commercial antisera became available to search for strains with these O groups: serum "polyvalent A": O26, O55, O111, and O127; and serum "polyvalent B": O86, O119, O124, O125, O126, and 128.

It was at this time that the confusion began. The documented enteropathogenic strains of *E. coli* were originally defined in terms of both O and H antigens, but no commercial antisera were available to determine the H antigens. Thus clinical laboratories could do only half of the required serologic analysis. Another problem was that many strains of *E. coli* found in the feces of normal infants and adults cross-reacted with the commercial screening sera. Further serologic typing is necessary to eliminate these false-positive results. These two factors have resulted in many strains being incorrectly reported as "enteropathogenic *E. coli*." The "true" enteropathogenic *E. coli* strains have greatly declined since the mid-1950s, so those false-positive reports have become more and more of a problem. Serotyping continued in many laboratories until the early to mid-1970s but was then dropped by most clinical and public health laboratories. No laboratory method for identifying EPEC can be recommended at present, but in the future, antisera may become available to identify these organisms, based either on the O or H antigens or on colonization factor antigens.

The *E. coli* serotypes of the normal flora of the human intestine differ from the serotypes of ETEC, EIEC, and EPEC discussed above. *E. coli* of the normal intestinal flora are not usually responsible for intestinal infections, but certain serotypes may cause extraintestinal infections such as bacteremia, neonatal meningitis, and urinary tract infections. The ability of these opportunistic organisms to cause disease depends on the presence of predisposing host factors and the possession of a complex system of mechanisms of pathogenicity. Among these mechanisms are hemolysin production, possession of certain capsular (K) antigens and O antigens, and the presence of fimbriae that are responsible for adherence.[42] Of particular interest is the K1 capsular antigen. This antigen is a polysaccharide composed of sialic acid; it is identical or very similar to the capsular polysaccharide of group B *Neisseria meningitidis*. Studies have shown that more than 80% of the serotypes of *E. coli* isolated from cases of neonatal meningitis possess the K1 capsular antigen.[73]

Shigella[64]

The pathogenesis of *Shigella* (and *Salmonella*) organisms is associated with their ability to penetrate the intestinal mucosa and invade the epithelial cells. On contact with the epithelial cells, these organisms cause a degeneration of the brush border of the cells and are then engulfed by an invagination of the cell membrane. This results in the formation of vacuoles around the organisms. *Shigella*, but not *Salmonella*, organisms are able to digest these vacuoles and then spread laterally to adjacent epithelial cells. Invasion by itself, however, is insufficient to cause overt disease. Virulent *Shigella* strains must also be able to multiply in the epithelial cells, since studies show that organisms that can penetrate but cannot multiply cause an inflammatory reaction but no overt disease.

After penetration and multiplication, a complex series of events results in ulceration of the mucosa. The Shiga toxin produced by *S. dysenteriae* may play a role in this ulceration; this toxin is cytotoxic, enterotoxic, and neurotoxic.[40] The Shiga toxin may also be responsible for the watery diarrhea that precedes the dysenteric phase of shigellosis. *S. flexneri* and *S. sonnei* elaborate the toxin but in much smaller amounts.

KLEBSIELLA[92]

Three factors appear to contribute to the virulence of *Klebsiella pneumoniae*. The first is the presence of cell wall receptors that enable the organism to attach to host cells and also protect the organism from phagocytosis and intracellular killing by polymorphonuclear leukocytes. The second factor is the large polysaccharide capsule, which protects the bacterial cell from phagocytosis and directly suppresses the immune response. Finally, the production of endotoxin may contribute directly or indirectly to pathogenicity.

PROTEUS

The enzyme urease is thought to play a major role in the pathogenicity of urinary tract infections caused by the genera *Proteus* (and *Morganella*).[31] Urease hydrolyzes urea to ammonia and CO_2. Ammonia may damage the epithelium of the urinary tract. Furthermore, ammonia increases the alkalinity of the urine and potentiates the deposition of calcium and magnesium phosphates and of ammonium magnesium phosphate. These deposits become calcified and form stones. Members of the genus *Proteus* may survive within the matrix of the stones and resist the effects of antimicrobial therapy. These organisms may cause recurrent bacteriuris following the discontinuation of therapy.

Although all species of *Proteus* (and *Morganella morganii*) produce urease, the marked prevalence of urinary tract infections caused by *P. mirabilis* may be related to two factors: the rapid generation time of *P. mirabilis* and its rapid liberation of ammonia and rapid production of alkaline conditions.[150] Other virulence factors of *P. mirabilis* may include invasiveness,[131] possession of pili, and production of proticine (a bacteriocin).[151]

SALMONELLA
Nontyphoid *Salmonella*

The mechanisms of pathogenicity of the nontyphoidal salmonellae have not been well defined nor generally accepted. As stated previously, species of *Salmonella* (including *typhi*) are able to penetrate the intestinal mucosa and invade the intestinal epithelial cells. Studies with *S. typhimurium* suggest that this ability may be plasmid mediated.[109] Figure 16-3, *D*, shows the changes that occur in the epithelium after invasion. For unknown reasons, invasion by *S. typhi* elicits a mononuclear response with subsequent bloodstream invasion, whereas nontyphoidal salmonellae stimulate a polymorphonuclear leukocyte response with infection usually confined to the mucosa.

Development of diarrhea caused by nontyphoid salmonellae is related to the stimulation of the adenyl cyclase system although the precise mechanism is unresolved. The adenyl cyclase enzyme may be stimulated by enterotoxins that are produced by the organisms or by prostaglandins that are released from the polymorphonuclear leukocytes that are present in the inflammatory response.[106]

Salmonella typhi[97,99]

The pathogenesis of *S. typhi* is associated with the ability of the organism to multiply within mononuclear phagocytes. After consumption the organisms penetrate the intestinal mucosa with minimal epithelial damage. They are transported through the cells in vacuoles, pass via the lymphatics to the intestinal lymph nodes, and are carried to the bloodstream. They are disseminated to the liver and spleen where they are phagocytized by mononuclear cells. The organisms are able to persist and multiply within these cells for several days. Organisms subsequently invade the bloodstream, producing a continuous bacteremia. This marks the end of the incubation period and the beginning of the symptomatic phase of typhoid fever. Bacteremia results in the spread of large numbers of organisms to all organs of the body, including the gallbladder and small intestine. Invasion of the intestine lymph follicles leads to hyperplasia, necrosis, and in severe cases, hemorrhage and perforation of the bowel.

Experimental typhoid in mice has demonstrated the importance of cellular immune mechanisms in the control of typhoid fever. The lymphokines of sensitized T lymphocytes stimulate increased intracellular bactericidal activity of the macrophages containing *S. typhi*.

Additional pathogenic mechanisms of *S. typhi* include the Vi antigen, which may inhibit phagocytosis and serum bactericidal activity. The sustained pyrexia of typhoid fever may be due to the local effects of endotoxin, which stimulates the synthesis and release of endogenous pyrogen from leukocytes within local inflammatory cell populations.[98]

SERRATIA

The virulence of *Serratia marcescens* has been associated with the ability of this organism to resist the bacterial and opsonic activity of serum[156] and the possession of a protease.[118] The latter enzyme may be involved in the pathogenesis of pneumonia.[118]

YERSINIA

Some strains of *Y. enterocolitica* (and the other *Yersinia* spp.) possess virulence plasmids that encode the production of certain outer membrane proteins, including the V (virulence) antigen.[138] These plasmid-associated proteins appear to be involved in pathogenesis. The outer membrane proteins of *Y. enterocolitica* are only produced at 37° C under the calcium limitation. The concentration of calcium is very low in eukaryotic cells; thus it is possible that *Y. enterocolitica* is induced to synthesize these proteins during its intracellular existence.[137] The exact pathogenic role of these proteins is unknown, but evidence suggests that they afford the bacteria altered surface properties that allow them to resist the bactericidal activity of normal human serum and perhaps phagocytosis by phagocytic cells.[121,138]

Invasiveness also appears to play a role in the pathogenesis of *Y. enterocolitica*, but the specific invasive properties have not been defined. Martinez[121] offers the following hypothetical scenario of host invasion by *Y. enterocolitica*. The organisms are ingested in contaminated food or water. They travel to the base of the small intestine where they contact the columnar epithelial cells lining the lumen of the ileum. The organisms are subsequently transported to the lamina propria where they generate an inflammatory response and encounter local macrophages. The outer membrane proteins may provide protection from these host defenses, allowing the organisms to survive and cause infection.

ANTIMICROBIAL SUSCEPTIBILITY

The antimicrobial agents used to treat diseases caused by the *Enterobacteriaceae* are discussed in Chapter 8. Antimicrobial resistance in *Enterobacteriaceae* is either common or rare, depending on the sample being considered. Those who work with strains isolated from the environment such as unpolluted water are much less likely to encounter resistant strains than those who work in hospitals.

TABLE 16-22. Intrinsic Antimicrobial Resistance in *Enterobacteriaceae*

Organism	Antimicrobial Agent
COMMON SPECIES	
Citrobacter amalonaticus	Ampicillin
Citrobacter freundii	Cephalothin
Citrobacter diversus	Ampicillin, carbenicillin
Edwardsiella tarda	Colistin
Enterobacter cloacae[a]	Cephalothin
Enterobacter aerogenes[a]	Cephalothin
Many other *Enterobacter*	Cephalothin
Hafnia alvei	Cephalothin
Klebsiella	Ampicillin, carbenicillin
Proteus mirabilis	Polymyxins, tetracycline, nitrofurantoin
Proteus vulgaris	Polymyxins, ampicillin, cephalothin, nitrofurantoin
Morganella morganii	Polymyxins, ampicillin, cephalothin
Providencia rettgeri	Polymyxins, cephalothin, nitrofurantoin, tetracycline
Other *Providencia*	Polymyxins, nitrofurantoin[b]
Serratia marcescens	Polymyxins, cephalothin[c]
LESS COMMON GENERA AND SPECIES	
Buttiauxella	Cephalothin
Cedecea	Polymyxins, ampicillin, cephalothin
Escherichia hermannii	Ampicillin, carbenicillin
Ewingella americana	Cephalothin
Kluyvera ascorbata	Ampicillin, cephalothin
Kluyvera cryscrescens	Ampicillin
Serratia fonticola	Ampicillin, carbenicillin, cephalothin
Other *Serratia*	Polymyxins,[d] cephalothin

Data from references 56 and 169 and from original papers describing new genera and species.
[a]Most strains are also resistant to ampicillin.
[b]Most strains of *Providencia stuartii* are also resistant to cephalothin and tetracycline.
[c]*Serratia marcescens* can also have intrinsic resistance to ampicillin, carbenicillin, streptomycin, and tetracycline.
[d]Resistance to polymyxins is common, but many strains have zones of 12 mm or more.

Intrinsic resistance is discussed in Chapter 8. The well-documented intrinsic resistances in *Enterobacteriaceae* are included in Table 16-22.

As also discussed in Chapter 8, nonintrinsic plasmid-mediated resistance is quite common among the *Enterobacteriaceae*. Use of antimicrobial agents exerts a strong selection for these resistant strains, which are often isolated from hospital outbreaks (see Chapter 4). Resistant strains of *Klebsiella pneumoniae, Serratia marcescens, Providencia rettgeri,* and *Providencia stuartii* are common in many hospitals. Other common species that are sometimes resistant include *Escherichia coli, Citrobacter freundii, Citrobacter diversus, Proteus mirabilis,* and the genera *Salmonella* and *Shigella*. Antimicrobial resistance is rare in most of the other species. Use of antimicrobial agents in animal husbandry is thought to be the main contributing factor for antimicrobial resistance in *Salmonella* spp., and resistance in *S. typhimurium* has become more common in recent years.

REFERENCES

1. Asai, T., Iizuka, H., and Komagata, K.: The flagellation of genus *Kluyvera,* J. Gen. Appl. Microbiol. **8:**187, 1962.
2. Asai, T., Okumura, S., and Tsunoda, T.: On a new genus, *Kluyvera,* Proc. Jpn. Acad. **32:**488, 1956.
3. Bae, B.H.C., Sureka, S.B., and Ajamy, J.A.: Enteric Group 15 (*Enterobacteriaceae*) associated with pneumonia, J. Clin. Microbiol. **14:**596, 1981.
4. Bagley, S.T., Seidler, R.J., and Brenner, D.J.: *Klebsiella planticola* sp. nov.: a new species of *Enterobacteriaceae* found primarily in nonclinical environments, Curr. Microbiol. **6:**105, 1981.
5. Bauernfeind, A., Petermuller, C., and Schneider, R.: Bacteriocins as tools in analysis of nosocomial *Klebsiella pneumoniae* infections, J. Clin. Microbiol. **14:**15, 1981.
6. Baumann, L., Bang, S.S., and Baumann, P.: Study of relationship among species of *Vibrio, Photobacterium,* and terrestrial enterobacteria by an immunological comparison of glutamine synthetase and superoxide dismutase, Curr. Microbiol. **4:**133, 1980.
7. Bercovier, H., et al.: Characterization of *Yersinia enterocolitica sensu stricto,* Curr. Microbiol. **4:**201, 1980.
8. Bercovier, H., et al.: Intra- and interspecies relatedness of *Yersinia pestis* by DNA hybridization and its relationship to *Yersinia pseudotuberculosis,* Curr. Microbiol. **4:**225, 1980.
9. Bercovier, H., et al.: *Yersinia kristensenii:* a new species of *Enterobacteriaceae* composed of sucrose-negative strains (formerly called *Yersinia enterocolitica* or *Yersinia enterocolitica*-like), Curr. Microbiol. **4:**219, 1980.
10. Bettelheim, K.A.: Colony incompatibility among New Zealand isolates of *Salmonella typhimurium,* J. Gen. Microbiol. **107:**249, 1978.
11. Blaser, M.J., Pollard, R.A., and Feldman, R.A.: *Shigella* infections in the United States: 1974-1980, J. Infect. Dis. **147:**771, 1983.
12. Bottone, E.J.: *Yersinia enterocolitica:* a panoramic view of a charismatic microorganism, CRC Crit. Rev. Microbiol. **5:**211, 1977.
13. Bottone, E.J.: Atypical *Yersinia enterocolitica:* clinical and epidemiological parameters, J. Clin. Microbiol. **7:**562, 1978.
14. Bottone, E.J., editor: *Yersinia enterocolitica,* Boca Raton, Fla., 1981, CRC Press, Inc.
15. Braunstein, H., et al.: A biotype of *Enterobacteriaceae* intermediate between *Citrobacter* and *Enterobacter,* Am. J. Clin. Pathol. **73:**114, 1980.
16. Brenner, D.J.: Biotyping of *Enterobacteriaceae* in the clinical laboratory. In Balows, A., and Isenberg, H.D., editors: Biotyping in the clinical microbiology laboratory, Springfield, Ill., 1978, Charles C Thomas, Publisher.

17. Brenner, D.J.: The genus *Enterobacter*. In Starr, M.P., et al., editors: The prokaryotes: a handbook on habitats, isolation, and identification of bacteria, vol. 2, New York, 1981, Springer-Verlag.

18. Brenner, D.J.: Introduction to the family *Enterobacteriaceae*. In Starr, M.P., et al., editors: The prokaryotes: a handbook on habitats, isolation, and identification of bacteria, vol. 2, New York, 1981, Springer-Verlag.

19. Brenner, D.J., Steigerwalt, A.G., and Fanning, G.R.: Differentiation of *Enterobacter aerogenes* from klebsiellae by deoxyribonucleic acid reassociation, Int. J. Syst. Bacteriol. **22:**193, 1972.

20. Brenner, D.J., et al.: Deoxyribonucleic acid relatedness of *Proteus* and *Providencia* species, Int. J. Syst. Bacteriol. **28:**269, 1978.

21. Brenner, D.J., et al.: Deoxyribonucleic acid relatedness in *Yersinia enterocolitica* and *Yersinia enterocolitica*-like organisms, Curr. Microbiol. **4:**195, 1980.

22. Brenner, D.J., et al.: *Enterobacter gergoviae* sp. nov.: a new species of *Enterobacteriaceae* found in clinical specimens and the environment, Int. J. Syst. Bacteriol. **30:**1, 1980.

23. Brenner, D.J., et al.: Taxonomic and nomenclatural changes in *Enterobacteriaceae*, Atlanta, 1980, Centers for Disease Control.

24. Brenner, D.J., et al.: *Yersinia intermedia:* a new species of *Enterobacteriaceae* composed of rhamnose-positive, melibiose-positive, raffinose-positive strains (formerly called atypical *Yersinia enterocolitica* or *Yersinia enterocolitica*-like), Curr. Microbiol. **4:**207, 1980.

25. Brenner, D.J., et al.: Atypical biogroups of *Escherichia coli* found in clinical specimens and descriptions of *Escherichia hermannii* sp. nov., J. Clin. Microbiol. **15:**703, 1982.

26. Brenner, D.J., et al.: *Escherichia vulneris:* a new species of *Enterobacteriaceae* associated with human wounds, J. Clin. Microbiol. **15:**1133, 1982.

27. Buchanan, R.E., and Gibbons, N.E., editors: Bergey's manual of determinative bacteriology, ed. 8, Baltimore, 1974, Williams & Wilkins Co.

28. Burgess, N.R.H., McDermott, S.N., and Whiting, J.: Aerobic bacteria occurring in the hind-gut of the cockroach, *Blatta orientalis,* J. Hyg. (Lond.) **71:**1, 1973.

29. Case, A.C.: Conditions controlling *Flavobacterium proteus* in brewery fermentation, J. Inst. Brew. **71:**250, 1965.

30. Chow, A.W., et al.: A nosocomial outbreak of infections due to multiply resistant *Proteus mirabilis:* role of intestinal colonization as a major reservoir, J. Infect. Dis. **139:**621, 1979.

31. Chute, R., and Suby, H.I.: Prevalence and importance of urea-splitting bacterial infections of the urinary tract in the formation of calculi, J. Urol. **44:**590, 1940.

32. Clarridge, J..E., et al.: Extraintestinal human infection caused by *Edwardsiella tarda,* J. Clin. Microbiol. **11:**511, 1980.

33. Cosenza, B.J., and Podgwaite, J.D.: A new species of *Proteus* isolated from larvae of the gypsy moth *Porthetria dispar* (L.), Antonie van Leeuwenhoek, J. Microbiol. Serol. **32:**187, 1966.

34. Crosa, J.H., et al.: Molecular relationships among the salmonellae, J. Bacteriol. **115:**307, 1973.

35. Crosa, J.H., et al.: Polynucleotide sequence divergence in the genus *Citrobacter,* J. Gen. Microbiol. **83:**271, 1974.

36. Darland, G.: Discriminant analysis of antibiotic susceptibility as a means of bacterial identification, J. Clin. Microbiol. **2:**391, 1975.

37. Dritz, S.K., et al.: Patterns of sexually transmitted enteric diseases in a city, Lancet **2:**3, 1977.

38. Edelman, R., and Levine, M.M.: Summary of a workshop on enteropathogenic *Escherichia coli,* J. Infect. Dis. **147:**1108, 1983.

39. Edwards, P.R., and Ewing, W.H.: Identification of *Enterobacteriaceae,* ed. 3, Minneapolis, 1972, Burgess Publishing Co.

40. Eiklid, K., and Olsnes, S.: Animal toxicity of *Shigella dysenteriae* cytotoxin: evidence that the neurotoxic, enterotoxic, and cytotoxic activities are due to one toxin, J. Immunol. **130:**380, 1983.

41. Evans, D.J., Jr., and Evans, D.G.: Classification of pathogenic *Escherichia coli* according to serotype and the production of virulence factors with special reference to colonization-factor antigens, Rev. Infect. Dis. (suppl. 5): S692, 1983.

42. Evans, D.J., Jr., et al.: Hemolysin and K antigens in relation to serotype and hemagglutination types of *Escherichia coli* isolated from extraintestinal infections, J. Clin. Microbiol. **13:**171, 1981.

43. Ewing, W.H.: The tribe *Proteeae:* its nomenclature and taxonomy, Int. Bull. Bacteriol. Nomencl. Taxon. **12:**92, 1962.

44. Ewing, W.H.: The nomenclature of *Salmonella,* its usage and definitions for the three species, Can. J. Microbiol. **18:**1629, 1972.

45. Ewing, W.H.: Differentiation of *Enterobacteriaceae* by biochemical reactions, Atlanta, 1973, Centers for Disease Control.

46. Ewing, W.H., and Davis, B.R.: Biochemical characterization of *Citrobacter diversus* (Burkey) Werkman and Gillen and designation of the neotype strain, Int. J. Syst. Bacteriol. **22:**12, 1972.

47. Ewing, W.H., Davis, B.R., and Sikes, S.V.: Biochemical characterization of *Providencia,* Pub. Health Lab. **30:**25, 1972.

48. Ewing, W.H., and Fife, M.A.: *Enterobacter agglomerans* (Beijerinck) comb. nov. (the *herbicola-lathyri* bacteria), Int. J. Syst. Bacteriol. **22:**4, 1972.

49. Ewing, W.H., et al.: Biochemical characterization of *Serratia liquefaciens* (Grimes and Hennerty) Bascomb et. al. (Formerly *Enterobacter liquefaciens*) and *Serratia rubidaea* (Stapp) comb. nov. and designation of type and neotype strains, Int. J. Syst. Bacteriol. **23:**217, 1973.

50. Ewing, W.H., et al.: *Yersinia ruckerii* sp. nov., the redmouth (RM) bacterium, Int. J. Syst. Bacteriol. **28:**37, 1978.

51. Fainstein, V., et al.: Colonization by or diarrhea due to *Kluyvera* species, J. Infect. Dis. **145:**127, 1982.

52. Farmer, J.J., III: Standardization and automation in biotyping. In Balows, A., and Isenberg, H., editors: Biotyping in the clinical microbiology laboratory, Springfield, 1978, Charles C Thomas, Publisher.

53. Farmer, J.J., III: The genus *Citrobacter*. In Starr, M.P., et al., editors: The prokaryotes: a handbook on habitats, isolation, and identification of bacteria, vol. 2, New York, 1981, Springer-Verlag.

54. Farmer, J.J., III: The genus *Edwardsiella*. In Starr, M.P., et al., editors: The prokaryotes: a handbook on habitats, isolation, and identification of bacteria, vol. 2, New York, 1981, Springer-Verlag.

55. Farmer, J.J., III, et al.: *Enterobacter sakazakii:* a new species of *Enterobacteriaceae* isolated from clinical specimens, Int. J. Syst. Bacteriol. **30:**569, 1980.

56. Farmer, J.J. III, et al.: *Enterobacteriaceae*. In Balows, A., and Hausler, W.J. Jr., editors: Diagnostic procedures for bacterial, mycotic and parasitic infections, ed. 6, Washington, D.C., 1981, American Public Health Association.

57. Farmer, J.J., III, et al.: *Kluyvera:* a new (redefined) genus in the family *Enterobacteriaceae*—identification of *Kluyvera ascorbata* sp. nov. and *Kluyvera cryocrescens* sp. nov. in clinical specimens, J. Clin. Microbiol. **13:**919, 1981.

58. Farmer, J.J., III, et al.: Bacteremia due to *Cedecea neteri* sp. nov., J. Clin. Microbiol. **16:**775, 1982.

59. Farmer, J.J., III, et al.: The *Salmonella-Arizona* group of *Enterobacteriaceae:* nomenclature, classification, and reporting, Clin. Microbiol. Newsletter 6:63, 1984.

60. Farmer, J.J., III, et al.: Biochemical identification of new species and biogroups of *Enterobacteriaceae* isolated from clinical specimens, J. Clin. Microbiol. **21:**46, 1985.

61. Farmer, J.J., III, et al.: *Escherichia fergusonii* and *Enterobacter taylorae:* two new species of *Enterobacteriaceae* isolated from clinical specimens, J. Clin. Microbiol. **21:**77, 1985.

62. Ferragut, C., et al.: *Buttiauxella,* a new genus of the family *Enterobacteriaceae,* Zentralbl. Bakteriol. **C2:**33, 1981.

63. Ferragut, C., et al.: *Klebsiella trevisanii:* a new species from water and soil, Int. J. Syst. Bacteriol. **33:**133, 1983.

63a. Formal, S.B., Hale, T.L., and Boedeker, E.C.: Interactions of enteric pathogens and the intestinal mucosa, Phil. Trans. R. Soc. Lond. [B] **303:**65, 1983.

64. Formal, S.B., Hale, T.L., and Sansonetti, P.J.: Invasive enteric pathogens, Rev. Infect. Dis. **4**(suppl. 5):S702, 1983.

65. Frantz, J.C., Jaso-Friedman, L., and Robertson, D.C.: Binding of *Escherichia coli* heat-stable enterotoxin to rat intestinal cells and brush border membranes, Infect. Immun. **43**:622, 1984.

66. Gavini, F., Lefebre, B., and Leclerc, H.: Positions taxonomiques d'entérobactéries H₂S par rapport au genre *Citrobacter,* Ann. Microbiol. (Paris) **127A**:275, 1976.

67. Gavini, F., et al.: Étude taxonomique d'entérobactéries appartenant ou apparentées au genre *Enterobacter,* Ann. Microbiol. (Paris) **127B**:317, 1976.

68. Gavini, F., et al.: Étude taxonomique d'entérobactéries appartenant ou apparentees au genre *Klebsiella,* Ann. Microbiol. (Paris) **128B**:45, 1977.

69. Gavini, F., et al.: *Serratia fonticola,* a new species from water, Int. J. Syst. Bacteriol. **29**:92, 1979.

70. Gilardi, G.L., Bottone, E., and Birnabaum, M.: Unusual fermentative, gram-negative bacilli isolated from clinical specimens. I. Characterization of *Erwinia* strains of the "lathyri-herbicola group," Appl. Microbiol. **20**:151, 1970.

71. Gill, V.J., et al.: *Serratia ficaria* isolated from a human clinical specimen, J. Clin. Microbiol. **14**:234, 1981.

72. Gilman, R.H., et al.: Relative efficacy of blood, urine, rectal swab, bone-marrow, and rose-spot cultures for recovery of *Salmonella typhi* in typhoid fever, Lancet **1**:1211, 1975.

73. Glode, M.P.: Neonatal meningitis due to *Escherichia coli* Kl, J. Infect. Dis. **136**(suppl.):S93, 1977.

74. Gorbach, S.L.: Travelers diarrhea, N. Engl. J. Med. **307**:881, 1982.

75. Graham, D.R., et al.: Epidemic nosocomial meningitis due to *Citrobacter diversus* in neonates, J. Infect. Dis. **144**:203, 1981.

76. Grimont, P.A.D., and Grimont, F.: The genus *Serratia,* Annu. Rev. Microbiol. **32**:221, 1978.

77. Grimont, P.A.D., and Grimont F.: The genus *Serratia.* In Starr, M.P., et al., editors: The prokaryotes: a handbook on habitats, isolation and identification of bacteria, New York, 1981, Springer-Verlag.

78. Grimont, P.A.D., Grimont, F., and Starr, M.P.: *Serratia ficaria* sp. nov., a bacterial species associated with smyrna figs and the fig wasp *Blastophaga psenes,* Curr. Microbiol. **2**:277, 1979.

79. Grimont, P.A.D., Irino, K., and Grimont, F.: The *Serratia liquefaciens–S. proteamaculans–S. grimesii* complex: DNA relatedness, Curr. Microbiol. **7**:63, 1982.

80. Grimont, P.A.D., et al.: Deoxyribonucleic acid relatedness between *Serratia plymuthica* and other *Serratia* species with a description of *Serratia odorifera* sp. nov. (type strain: ICPB 3995), Int. J. Syst. Bacteriol. **28**:453, 1978.

81. Grimont, P.A.D., et al.: *Edwardsiella hoshinae,* a new species of *Enterobacteriaceae,* Curr. Microbiol. **4**:347, 1980.

82. Grimont, P.A.D., et al.: *Cedecea davisae* gen. nov., sp. nov. and *Cedecea lapagei* sp. nov.: new *Enterobacteriaceae* from clinical specimens, Int. J. Syst. Bacteriol. **31**:317, 1981.

83. Grimont, P.A.D., et al.: *Ewingella americana* gen. nov., sp. nov., a new *Enterobacteriaceae* isolated from clinical specimens, Ann. Microbiol. (Paris) **134A**:39, 1983.

84. Guinée, P.A.M., and Valkenburg, J.J.: Diagnostic value of a *Hafnia*-specific bacteriophage, J. Bacteriol. **96**:564, 1968.

85. Hawke, J.P., et al.: *Edwardsiella ictaluri* sp. nov.: the causative agent of enteric septicemia of catfish, Int. J. Syst. Bacteriol. **31**:396, 1981.

86. Hawkey, P.M., et al.: Prospective survey of fecal, urinary tract, and environmental colonization by *Providencia stuartii* in two geriatric wards, J. Clin. Microbiol. **16**:422, 1982.

87. Hickman, F.W., et al.: Unusual groups of *Morganella ("Proteus") morganii* isolated from clinical specimens: lysine-positive and ornithine-negative biogroups, J. Clin. Microbiol. **12**:88, 1980.

88. Hickman, F.W., et al.: Identification of *Proteus penneri* sp. nov., formerly known as *P. vulgaris* indole negative or as *Proteus vulgaris* biogroup 1, J. Clin. Microbiol. **15**:1097, 1982.

89. Hickman-Brenner, F.W., et al.: *Providencia rustigianii:* a new species in the family *Enterobacteriaceae* formerly known as *Providencia alcalifaciens* biogroup 3, J. Clin. Microbiol. **17**:1057, 1983.

90. Hickman-Brenner, F.W., et al.: *Moellerella wisconsensis,* a new genus and species of *Enterobacteriaceae* found in human stool specimens, J. Clin. Microbiol. **19**:460, 1984.

90a. Hickman-Brenner, F.W., et al.: *Koserella trabulsii,* a new genus and species of *Enterobacteriaceae* formerly known as Enteric Group 45, J. Clin. Microbiol. 21:39, 1985.

90b. Hickman-Brenner, F.W., et al.: *Leminorella,* a new genus of *Enterobacteriaceae:* identification of *Leminorella grimontii* sp. nov. and *Leminorella richardii* sp. nov. found in clinical specimens, J. Clin. Microbiol. 21:234, 1985.

91. Hicks, M.J., and Ryan, K.J.: Simplified scheme for identification of prompt lactose-fermenting members of the *Enterobacteriaceae,* J. Clin. Microbiol. **4**:511, 1976.

92. Highsmith, A.K., and Jarvis, W.R.: *Klebsiella pneumoniae:* selected virulence factors that contribute to pathogenicity, Infect. Control **6**:75, 1985.

93. Hodges, G.R., Degener, C.E., and Barnes, W.G.: Clinical significance of *Citrobacter* isolates, Am. J. Clin. Pathol. **70**:37, 1978.

94. Hollis, D.G., et al.: *Tatumella ptyseos* gen. nov., sp. nov., a member of the family *Enterobacteriaceae* found in clinical specimens, J. Clin. Microbiol. **14**:79, 1981.

95. Honda, T., Arita, M., and Miwatani, T.: Characterization of new hydrophobic pili of human enterotoxigenic *Escherichia coli:* a possible new colonization factor, Infect. Immun. **43**:959, 1984.

96. Hornick, R.B.: Nontyphoidal salmonellosis. In Hoeprich, P.D., editor: Infectious diseases, ed. 3, Philadelphia, 1983, Harper & Row, Publishers.

97. Hornick, R.B.: Typhoid fever. In Hoeprich, P.D., editor: Infectious diseases, ed. 3, Philadelphia, 1983, Harper & Row, Publishers.

98. Hornick, R.B., and Greisman, S.: On the pathogenesis of typhoid fever, Arch. Intern. Med. **138**:357, 1978.

99. Hornick, R.B., et al.: Typhoid fever: pathogenesis and immunologic control, N. Engl. J. Med. **283**:686, 1970.

100. Izard, D., Gavini, F., and Leclerc, H.: Polynucleotide sequence relatedness and genome size among *Enterobacter intermedium* sp. nov. and the species *Enterobacter cloacae* and *Klebsiella pneumoniae,* Zentralbl. Bakteriol. **C1**:51, 1980.

101. Izard, D., et al.: *Rahnella aquatilis,* nouveau membre de la famille des *Enterobacteriaceae,* Ann. Microbiol. (Paris) **130A**:163, 1979.

102. Izard, D., et al.: Deoxyribonucleic acid relatedness between *Enterobacter cloacae* and *Enterobacter amnigenus* sp. nov., Int. J. Syst. Bacteriol. **31**:35, 1981.

103. Izard, D., et al.:, *Klebsiella terrigena,* a new species from soil and water, Int. J. Syst. Bacteriol. **31**:116, 1981.

104. Jain, K., Radsak, K., and Mannheim, W.: Differentiation of the Oxytocum group from *Klebsiella* by deoxyribonucleic acid-deoxyribonucleic acid hybridization, Int. J. Syst. Bacteriol. **24**:402, 1974.

105. Jarvis, W.R., et al.: The epidemiology of nosocomial infections caused by *Klebsiella pneumoniae,* Infect. Control **6**:68, 1985.

106. Jiwa, S.F.H.: Probing for enterotoxigenicity among the *Salmonella:* an evaluation of biological assays, J. Clin. Microbiol. **14**:463, 1981.

107. John, J.F., Jr., Sharbaugh, R.J., and Bannister, E.R.: *Enterobacter cloacae:* bacteremia, epidemiology and antibiotic resistance, Rev. Infect. Dis. **4**:13, 1982.

108. Johnson, W.M., Lior, H., and Bezanson, G.S.: Cytotoxic *Escherichia coli* 0157:H7 associated with haemorrhagic colitis in Canada, Lancet **1**:76, 1983.

109. Jones, G.W., et al.: Association of adhesive, invasive, and virulent phenotypes of *Salmonella typhimurium* with autonomous 60-megadalton plasmids, Infect. Immun. **38**:476, 1982.

110. Kauffmann, F., and DuPont, A.: *Escherichia* strains from infantile gastro-enteritis, Acta Pathol. Microbiol. Scand. **27**:552, 1950.

110a. Kelly, M.T., Brenner, D.J., and Farmer, J.J., III: *Enterobacteriaceae*. In Lennette, E.H., et al., editors: Manual of clinical microbiology, ed. 4, Washington, D.C., 1985, American Society for Microbiology.

111. Krajden, S., et al.: *Proteus penneri* and urinary calculi formation, J. Clin. Microbiol. **19**:541, 1984.

112. Lapage, S.P., et al.: Identification of bacteria by computer: general aspects and perspectives, J. Gen. Microbiol. **77**:273, 1973.

113. Lautrop, H., Ørskov, I., and Gaarslev, K.: Hydrogen-sulfide producing variants of *Escherichia coli*, Acta Pathol. Microbiol. Immunol. Scand. **79**:641, 1971.

114. Leclerc, H.: Étude biochimique d *Enterbacteriaceae* pigmentées, Ann. Inst. Pasteur (Paris) **102**:726, 1962.

115. Leclerc, H., and Buttiaux, R.: Les *Citrobacter*, Ann. Inst. Pasteur (Lille) **16**:67, 1965.

116. LeMinor, L., Véron, M., and Popoff, M.: Proposition pour une nomenclature des *Salmonella*, Ann. Microbiol. (Paris) **133B**:245, 1982.

117. LeMinor, L., Véron, M., and Popoff, M.: Taxonomie des *Salmonella*, Ann. Microbiol. (Paris) **133B**:223, 1982.

118. Lyerly, D.M., and Kreger, A.S.: Importance of *Serratia* protease in the pathogenesis of experimental *Serratia marcescens* pneumonia, Infect. Immun. **40**:113, 1983.

119. Maki, D.G., and Martin, W.T.: Nationwide epidemic of septicemia caused by contaminated infusion products. IV. Growth of microbial pathogens in fluids for intravenous infusion, J. Infect. Dis. **131**:267, 1975.

120. Mangum, M.E., and Radisch, D.: *Cedecea* species: unusual clinical isolate, Clin. Microbiol. Newsletter **4**:117, 1982.

121. Martinez, R.J.: Plasmid-mediated and temperature-regulated surface properties of *Yersinia enterocolitica*, Infect. Immun. **41**:921, 1983.

122. McDermott, C., and Mylotte, J.M.: *Morganella morganii*: epidemiology of bacteremic disease, Infect. Control **5**:131, 1984.

123. Meyers, B.R., et al.: Infections caused by microorganisms of the genus *Erwinia*, Ann. Intern. Med. **79**:9, 1972.

124. Mildvan, D., Gelb, A.M., and William, D.: Venereal transmission of enteric pathogens in male homosexuals: two case reports, JAMA **238**:1387, 1977.

125. Miller, J.M.: New genera and species of *Enterobacteriaceae*, Clin. Microbiol. Newsletter **5**:149, 1983.

126. Montgomerie, J.: Epidemiology of *Klebsiella* and hospital-associated infections, Rev. Infect. Dis. **1**:736, 1979.

127. Muytjens, H.L., et al.: Analysis of eight cases of neonatal meningitis and sepsis due to *Enterobacter sakazakii*, J. Clin. Microbiol. **18**:115, 1983.

128. Nataro, J.: Enteroadherence of EPEC. In Session 187: New concepts in the pathogenesis of *Escherichia coli* diarrhea, Annual Meeting, American Society for Microbiology, St. Louis, 1984.

129. O'Brien, A.D., et al.: Production of *Shigella dysenteriae* type 1-like cytotoxin by *Escherichia coli*, J. Infect. Dis. **146**:763, 1982.

130. O'Brien, A.D., et al.: *Escherichia coli* 0157:H7 strains associated with haemorrhagic colitis in the United States produce a *Shigella dysenteriae* 1 (Shiga) like cytotoxin, Lancet **1**:702, 1983.

131. Peerbooms, P.G.H., et al.: Vero cells invasiveness of *Proteus mirabilis*, Infect. Immun. **43**:1068, 1984.

132. Penner, J.L.: The tribe *Proteeae*. In Starr, M.P., et al., editors: The prokaryotes: a handbook on habitats, isolation, and identification of bacteria, New York, 1981, Springer-Verlag.

133. Poinar, G.O., Jr., and Thomas, G.M.: A new bacterium, *Achromo-*

bacter nematophilus sp. nov. *(Achromobacteriaceae: Eubacteriales)* associated with a nematode, Int. Bull. Bacteriol. Nomen. Taxon. **15**:249, 1965.

134. Poinar, G.O., Jr., and Thomas, G.M.: The nature of *Achromobacter nematophilus* as an insect pathogen, J. Invertebr. Pathol. **9**:510, 1967.

135. Poinar, G.O., Jr., Thomas, G.M., and Hess, R.: Characteristics of the specific bacterium associated with *Heterorhabditis bacteriophora (Heterorhabditidae: Rhabditida)*, Nematologica **23**:97, 1977.

136. Poinar, G.O., Jr.: Further characterization of *Achromobacter nematophilus* from American and Soviet populations of the nematode *Neoaplectana carpocapsae*, Weiser. Int. J. Syst. Bacteriol. **21**:78, 1971.

137. Portnoy, D.A., Moseley, S.L., and Falkow, S.: Characterization of plasmids and plasmid-associated determinants of *Yersinia enterocolitica* pathogenesis, Infect. Immun. **31**:775, 1981.

138. Portnoy, D.A., et al.: Characterization of common virulence plasmids in *Yersinia* species and their role in the expression of outer membrane proteins, Infect. Immun. **43**:108, 1984.

139. Priest, F.G., et al.: The taxonomic position of *Obesumbacterium proteus*, a common brewery contaminant, J. Gen. Microbiol. **75**:295, 1973.

140. Quan, T.J.: *Yersinia pestis*. In Starr, M.P., et al., editors; The prokaryotes: a handbook on habitats, isolation, and identification of bacteria, New York, 1981, Springer-Verlag.

141. Richard, C., et al.: Étude de souches de *Enterobacter* appartenant a un groupe particulier proche de *E. aerogenes*, Ann. Microbiol. (Paris) **127A**:545, 1976.

142. Riley, L.W., et al.: Hemorrhagic colitis associated with a rare *Escherichia coli* serotype, N. Engl. J. Med. **308**:681, 1983.

143. Ross, A.J., Rucker, R.R., and Ewing, W.H.: Description of a bacterium associated with redmouth disease of rainbow trout *(Salmo gairdneri)*, Can. J. Microbiol. **12**:763, 1966.

144. Schaberg, D.R., Weinstein, R.A., and Stamm, W.E.: Epidemics of nosocomial urinary tract infection caused by multiply resistant gram-negative bacilli: epidemiology and control, J. Infect. Dis. **133**:363, 1976.

145. Schiemann, D.A.: Synthesis of a selective agar medium for *Yersinia enterocolitica*, Can. J. Microbiol. **25**:1298, 1979.

146. Schneierson, S.S., and Bottone, E.J.: *Erwinia* infections in man, CRC Crit. Rev. Clin. Lab. Sci., **4**:341, 1973.

147. Schwach, T.: Case report, Clin. Microbiol. Newsletter **1**(16):4, 1979.

148. Scotland, S.M., Day, N.P., and Rowe, B.: Acquisition and maintenance of enerotoxin plasmids in wild-type strains of *Escherichia coli*, J. Gen. Microbiol. **129**:3111, 1983.

149. Sen, D., Saha, M.R., and Sudhir, C.P.: Evaluation of three simple and rapid immunological tests for detection of heat-labile enterotoxin of enterotoxigenic *Escherichia coli*, J. Clin. Microbiol. **19**:194, 1984.

150. Senior, B.W.: *Proteus morgani* is less frequently associated with urinary tract infections than *Proteus mirabilis*—an explanation, J. Clin. Microbiol. **16**:317, 1983.

151. Senior, B.W.: The purification, structure, and synthesis of proticine 3, J. Med. Microbiol. **16**:323, 1983.

152. Shimwell, J.L.: A study of the common rod bacteria of brewers' yeast, J. Inst. Brew. **42**:119, 1936.

153. Shimwell, J.L.: *Obesumbacterium* gen. nov., Brewers' J. **99**:759, 1963.

154. Shimwell, J.L.: *Obesumbacterium*, a new genus for the inclusion of "*Flavobacterium proteus*," J. Inst. Brew. **70**:247, 1964.

155. Shimwell, J.L., and Grimes, M.: The distinguishing characteristics of *Flavobacterium proteus* (sp. nov.): the common rod bacterium of brewers' yeast, J. Inst. Brew. **42**:348, 1936.

156. Simberkoff, M.S., Ricupero, I., and Rahal, J.J., Jr.: Host resistance to *Serratia marcescens* infection: serum bactericidal activity

and phagocytosis by normal blood leucocytes, J. Lab. Clin. Med. **87**:206, 1976.

157. Skerman, V.B.D., McGowan, V., and Sneath, P.H.A.: Approved lists of bacterial names, Int. J. Syst. Bacteriol. **30**:225, 1980.

158. Skirrow, M.B.: The Dienes (mutual inhibition) test in the investigation of *Proteus* infections, J. Med. Microbiol. **2**:471, 1969.

159. Stapp, C.: *Bacterium rubidaeum* nov. sp., Zentralbl. Bakteriol. Abt. II **102**:251, 1940.

160. Starr, M.P.: The genus *Erwinia*. In Starr, M.P., et al., editors: The prokaryotes: a handbook on habitats, isolation, and identification of bacteria, New York, 1981, Springer-Verlag.

161. Starr, M.P., and Chatterjee, A.K.: The genus *Erwinia*: enterobacteria pathogenic to plants and animals, Annu. Rev. Microbiol. **26**:389, 1972.

162. Steigerwalt, A.G., et al.: DNA relatedness among species of *Enterobacter* and *Serratia*, Can. J. Microbiol. **22**:121, 1976.

162a. Tamura, K., et al.: *Leclercia adecarboxylata* gen. nov., formerly known as *Escherichia adecarboxylata*, Curr. Microbiol. **13**:179, 1986.

163. Taylor, D.N., Pollard, R.A., and Blake, P.A.: Typhoid in the United States and the risk to the international traveler, J. Infect. Dis. **148**:599, 1983.

164. Thomas, G.M., and Poinar, G.O., Jr.: *Xenorhabdus* gen. nov., a genus of entomopathogenic nematophilic bacteria of the family *Enterobacteriaceae*, Int. J. Syst. Bacteriol. **29**:352, 1979.

165. Ursing, J., Steigerwalt, A.G., and Brenner, D.J.: Lack of genetic relatedness between *Yersinia philomiragia* (the ''Philomiragia'' bacterium) and *Yersinia* species, Curr. Microbiol. **4**:231, 1980.

166. Ursing, J., et al.: *Yersinia frederiksenii:* a new species of *Enterobacteriaceae* composed of rhamnose-positive strains (formerly called atypical *Yersinia enterocolitica* or *Yersinia enterocolitica*-like), Curr. Microbiol. **4**:213, 1980.

167. Vandepitte, J., Lemmens, P., and DeSwert, L.: Human edwardsiellosis traced to ornamental fish, J. Clin. Microbiol. **17**:165, 1983.

168. Vantrappen, G., Geboes, K., and Ponette, E.: *Yersinia* enteritis, Med. Clin. North Am. **66**:639, 1982.

169. von Graevenitz, A.: Recognition and differential diagnosis of *Erwinia herbicola* strains isolated in the hospital, Pathol. Microbiol. **37**:84, 1971.

170. von Graevenitz, A.: Are microbial identification and sensitivity testing necessary for effective chemotherapy? In Borchi, A., Bartola, J.T., and Prior, J.E., editors: The clinical laboratory as an aid in chemotherapy of infectious diseases, Baltimore, 1977, University Park Press.

171. von Graevenitz, A., and Rubin, S.J., editors: The genus *Serratia*, Boca Raton, Fla., 1980, CRC Press, Inc.

172. Weissfeld, A.S.: *Yersinia enterocolitica*, Clin. Microbiol. Newsletter **3**:91, 1981.

173. Williams, E.W., et al.: Serious nosocomial infection caused by *Morganella morganii* and *Proteus mirabilis* in a cardiac surgery unit, J. Clin. Microbiol. **18**:5, 1983.

174. Woodward, B.W., Carter, M., and Seidler, R.J.: Most nonclinical *Klebsiella* strains are not *K. pneumoniae sensu stricto*, Curr. Microbiol. **2**:181, 1979.

175. World Health Organization Centre for Reference and Research on *Salmonella*: Antigenic formulae of the *Salmonella*, Paris, 1980, WHO International *Salmonella* Center, Institut Pasteur.

176. Young, V.M., et al.: *Levinea*, a new genus of the family *Enterobacteriaceae*, Int. J. Syst. Bacteriol. **21**:58, 1971.

177. Yu, V.L.: *Serratia marcescens:* historical perspective and clinical review, N. Engl. J. Med. **300**:887, 1979.

CHAPTER 17

Nonfermentative Gram-Negative Bacteria

Thomas R. Oberhofer
Barbara J. Howard

Nonfermentative gram-negative bacteria (NFB) are ubiquitous organisms that can be recovered from most natural sources, exploiting wet environments (such as respiratory therapy equipment, sinks, faucet aerators, and water baths) and contaminating sterile solutions, medications, and other fluids for consumer use. NFB respond poorly to chemical controls, often thriving in their presence.

As pathogens the NFB are opportunistic and are often recovered from patients with serious underlying disease, from those who have had prior antimicrobial therapy, from those receiving concurrent treatment with immunosuppressive agents, and from those undergoing extensive intubation or instrumentation. The possibility of contaminating wounds and instruments with soil is ever present. Reports are increasing, however, that point to the NFB as primary causes of infections rather than as incidental organisms. Hospital-acquired infections are common.

CLASSIFICATION

The NFB are classified for diagnostic purposes according to their physiologic similarities and their relatedness based on DNA homology and DNA base composition studies. The systems of classification currently in use have been developed from work of the late Elizabeth O. King at the Centers for Disease Control (CDC) in Atlanta and from *Bergey's Manual of Determinative Bacteriology* and *Bergey's Manual of Systematic Bacteriology*.[34] Many of the organisms that are of clinical significance and discussed in this chapter, however, are not included in the recent edition of *Bergey's Manual of Systematic Bacteriology* because they do not possess characteristics in accord with the generic description or because they have not been clearly defined taxonomically. These latter organisms are referred to with letter and number designations (for example, CDC Ve-1) and are called "alphanumerics." Furthermore, some organisms are recognized in the clinical literature and in this chapter but are no longer considered valid species in *Bergey's Manual of Systematic Bacteriology*. The first is *Alcaligenes odorans*, which is currently considered part of *Alcaligenes faecalis* in *Bergey's Manual of Systematic Bacteriology*, although *A. odorans* has distinct morphologic and biochemical features. *Achromobacter xylosoxidans* is classified as *Alcaligenes denitrificans* ssp. *xylosoxydans* (note the difference in spelling), even though *Achromobacter xylosoxidans* oxidizes carbohydrates but *Alcaligenes* does not. In fact, the genus *Achromobacter* is no longer recognized in *Bergey's Manual*. Yabuuchi and Yano[85] have proposed that the genus name *Achromobacter* be revived. The genus name is still recognized by the CDC[80] and is included in this chapter because of its common accepted usage among clinical microbiologists. Another example is *Alcaligenes denitrificans*, which is currently classified as *Alcaligenes denitrificans* subspecies *denitrificans*. *Pseudomonas putrefaciens* has been reclassified as *Alteromonas putrefaciens* in *Bergey's Manual of Systematic Bacteriology* but is listed under *species incertae sedis*. This means that its taxonomic classification is uncertain and that more extensive classification is necessary before it can be formally assigned to the genus *Alteromonas*.

In this chapter all of these organisms are referred to by their former names and not the reclassified names used in *Bergey's Manual of Systematic Bacteriology*.

Other taxonomic changes that have been proposed since the publication of *Bergey's Manual of Systematic Bacteriology* include the transfer of *Flavobacterium multivorum* to the genus *Sphingobacterium* as *Sphingobacterium multivorum*[84] and the transfer of *Pseudomonas maltophilia* to the genus *Xanthomonas* as *Xanthomonas maltophilia*.[77]

The organisms included in this chapter are classified according to genus in Table 17-1. Synonyms are included to point out the variety of names under which these organisms may be found in the older literature. The organisms designated by alphanumerics in Table 17-1 are not species but are closely related to other members of the genus in their morphologic, physiologic, and biochemical characteristics. Note that *Bordetella bronchiseptica* is included in Table 17-1. This organism is discussed more thoroughly in Chapter 22 but is also included here because of its similarity to members of the genus *Alcaligenes*. In fact, *B. bronchiseptica* was previously classified as *Alcaligenes bronchiseptica*.

The nonfermentative gram-negative bacteria by definition do not ferment glucose. The genera that meet this definition include *Pseudomonas, Acinetobacter, Alcaligenes, Achromobacter, Moraxella, Eikenella,* and the alphanumerics. The flavobacteria oxidize glucose, but in some instances the reaction is so intense that the slant on triple sugar iron (TSI) agar is acidified and appears as a weak fermentation reaction. The genus *Kingella* and EF-4, however, are true fermenters, although reactions may be delayed and subtle. They are discussed in this chapter because they are somewhat fastidious and their carbohyrate reactions may be mistaken for those of nonfermentative bacteria.

GROWTH REQUIREMENTS
MEDIA

The isolation methods that are used for recovery of the *Enterobacteriaceae* also recover the NFB from body fluids, wounds, urine, stool, environmental sources, and other specimens. Most NFB are considered nonfastidious because they

TABLE 17-1. Nomenclature of Nonfermentative Bacteria

Genus	Current Name	Synonyms
Pseudomonas		
Glucose oxidizer	*P. aeruginosa*	*Bacillus pyocyaneous*
	P. putida	*P. ovalis*
	P. fluorescens	*P. aureofaciens, P. chlororaphis*
	P. pseudomallei	*Loefferella/Malleomyces pseudomallei*
	P. cepacia	*P. multivorans, P. kingii,* EO-1
	P. stutzeri	*P. stanieri,* CDC Vb-1
	P. mendocina	CDC Vb-2
	P. stutzeri–like	CDC Vb-3
	P. maltophilia[a]	*P. melanogena, Alcaligenes bookeri,* CDC 1
	P. paucimobilis	CDC IIk-1, *Xanthomonas, P. campestris*
	CDC Ve-1 and Ve-2	
	P. pickettii	CDC Va-1, CDC Va-2, CDC IVd, *P. thomasii*
Glucose nonoxidizer	*P. alcaligenes*	*Bacterium alcaligenes, P. alcaligenes* A
	P. pseudoalcaligenes	*P. alcaligenes* B
	P. diminuta	CDC 1a
	P. vesicularis	
	P. acidovorans	*Comamonas terrigena, P. indoloxidans*
	P. testosteroni	*Comamonas terrigena*
	P. putrefaciens[b]	*P. rubescens,* CDC 1b-1, 1b-2
Achromobacter[c]	*A. xylosoxidans*[d]	CDC IIIa, CDC IIIb
	CDC Vd-1[e]	
	CDC Vd-2[e]	
Alcaligenes/Bordetella	*A. faecalis*	CDC VI
	A. denitrificans[f]	CDC Vc
	A. odorans[g]	*Pseudomonas odorans*
	B. bronchiseptica	*B. bronchicanis,* CDC IVa
	CDC IVc	
	CDC IVe	
Acinetobacter	*A. calcoaceticus* var. *anitratus*	*Achromobacter anitratus, Herellea vaginicola, Bacterium anitratum*

grow on simple media such as trypticase soy broth or nutrient agar or on unsupplemented blood agar. *P. maltophilia* requires methionine for growth, and *P. diminuta* requires cystine and biotin, but these factors are present in most laboratory media in sufficient quantities to support growth. The genera *Moraxella, Eikenella,* and *Kingella* are more nutritionally demanding than the other NFB but less demanding than such genera as *Haemophilus* or *Neisseria*. Blood agar should be used for primary isolation of these organisms. *M. lacunata* and *Kingella* strains do not grow in oxidative-fermentative (OF) carbohydrates, TSI agar, or other peptone-based carbohydrate media without the addition of serum.

With the exception of the genera *Kingella, Eikenella, Moraxella,* and certain *Flavobacterium* strains, NFB grow on MacConkey agar. The ability to grow on MacConkey agar is a criterion used in the identification and characterization of NFB.

ENVIRONMENTAL REQUIREMENTS

The NFB are obligate aerobes and use molecular oxygen as the hydrogen acceptor. NFB do not grow well, if at all, under anaerobic conditions except for strains that can respire and grow in the presence of nitrate or arginine as an electron acceptor. To permit access to oxygen during the growth phase, the tops of all biochemical tubes must be kept loosened during incubation.

A constant temperature of 35° C is customarily used to incubate tests for the *Enterobacteriaceae* and has arbitrarily been selected for the NFB as well. Most data bases and identification charts are an accumulation of results obtained at a 35° C incubation. However, some NFB grow poorly or not at all at this high temperature and must be incubated at room temperature (22° to 25° C), whereas others have an optimal temperature closer to 30° C. Indications for room-temperature incubation are poor growth at 35° C or biochemical characteristics that

TABLE 17-1. Nomenclature of Nonfermentative Bacteria—cont'd

Genus	Current Name	Synonyms
Acinetobacter	var. *haemolyticus*	
	var. *lwoffi*	*Mima polymorpha, Moraxella lwoffi*
	var. *alcaligenes*	
Flavobacterium	*F. meningosepticum*	CDC IIa
	F. odoratum	CDC M4-f
	F. breve	
	F. multivorum[h]	CDC IIk-2
	F. indologenes	*Flavobacterium* IIb
	Flavobacterium sp. group IIf	
Moraxella	*M. osloensis*	*Moraxella duplex, Mima polymorpha* var. *oxidans*
	M. nonliquefaciens	*Moraxella duplex* var. *nonliquefaciens*
	M. lacunata	
	M. atlantae	CDC M-3
	M. urethralis	CDC M-4
	M. phenylpyruvica	
	M-5	
	M-6	
Others	*Eikenella corrodens*	HB-1
	Kingella denitrificans	TM-1
	Kingella kingae	*Moraxella kingii, Moraxella kingae*
	Kingella indologenes	
	CDC EF-4	

[a]Proposed name, *Xanthomonas maltophilia*.

[b]*P. putrefaciens* is classified as *Alteromonas putrefaciens* in *Bergey's Manual of Systematic Bacteriology*.

[c]The genus *Achromobacter* is not included in *Bergey's Manual of Systematic Bacteriology*.

[d]Classified as *Alcaligenes denitrificans* ssp. *xylosoxydans* in *Bergey's Manual of Systematic Bacteriology*.

[e]According to *Bergey's Manual of Systematic Bacteriology* the taxonomic position of these organisms remains unknown.

[f]Classified as *Alcaligenes denitrificans* ssp. *denitrificans* in *Bergey's Manual of Systematic Bacteriology*.

[g]Not listed as separate species in *Bergey's Manual of Systematic Bacteriology*; included as part of *A. faecalis*.

[h]Proposed name, *Sphingobacterium multivorum*.

point to a species identification but that are incomplete at 35° C (for example, fluorescein production). The most notable organisms that thrive at the lower temperatures are the *Pseudomonas fluorescens–P. putida* group.

The NFB grow slowly, in contrast to the *Enterobacteriaceae*. NFB require at least 24 hours and, at times, 48 to 72 hours of incubation before they can be identified.

CULTURAL CHARACTERISTICS
STAINING REACTIONS

A Gram stain is performed from the blood or MacConkey agar plates to obtain not only the Gram reaction but the cellular morphology (rod, coccobacillus, coccus) and size of the cell (a long rod is 1.2 to 2.5 μm, a short rod is 0.5 to 1 μm). All of the NFB are gram negative. Members of the genus *Pseudomonas* generally appear as long, thin rods (Plate 10, *A*). *A. xylosoxidans* is a long rod with a beaded or barred stain. Members of the

genus *Acinetobacter* are coccoid, coccobacillary (Plate 10, *B*), or even filamentous, and members of the *Moraxella* may be short, fat rods (coccobacilli) or short, thin rods. The coccobacilli of the genera *Moraxella* and *Acinetobacter* may occur in pairs and thus be confused with *Neisseria* spp. in cervical and urethral smears. *Kingella* organisms are short rods that occur in pairs and sometimes short chains; these organisms may resist decolorization. *Eikenella* organisms characteristically appear as coccobacilli in direct smears but as uniformly thin rods with rounded ends in smears prepared from growth on solid media.

COLONIAL MORPHOLOGY

Primary isolation media are often overlooked as a source of immediate and valuable information to aid in the identification of NFB. Blood agar is used to examine colonial morphology, colony size, hemolytic activity, and pigmentation. Colonies

TABLE 17-2. Colonial Morphology of the Nonfermentative Bacteria

Organism	Description
Pseudomonas aeruginosa	Several colonial forms (Plate 10, *C* to *E*); usually large (2 mm in diameter), irregularly round, effuse colonies with matte surface and floccular internal structure; colonies have ground-glass appearance with raised butyrous centers and usually produce metallic sheen on blood agar and distinct grapelike odor; mucoid forms commonly seen in patients with cystic fibrosis
Pseudomonas fluorescens	Tiny colonies (less than 1 mm); increase in size after extended incubation
Pseudomonas cepacia	May appear as sulfur-yellow colonies or as colorless colonies
Pseudomonas diminuta	Colonies brown
Pseudomonas putida	Circular, smooth, raised, amorphous with entire edge
Pseudomonas stutzeri	Usually buff colored to yellow, wrinkled, and coherent, although smooth stains not uncommon (Plate 10, *F*)
Pseudomonas (Xanthomonas) maltophilia	Young colonies lavender colored but become gray-green with age (yellow colonies seen on peptone medium); colonies produce odor of ammonia (Plate 11, *A*)
Pseudomonas putrefaciens	Colonies slightly mucoid and initially tan in color; color becomes reddish brown or pink after 48 hr
Pseudomonas pseudomallei	Young colonies white but become buff to brown after few days; colonies may produce earthy smell
CDC Ve	Form wrinkled yellow colonies after 48 hr of incubation (Plate 11, *B*); wrinkles may be lost after numerous subcultures
Achromobacter xylosoxidans	Small, convex, circular, smooth, glistening, and butyrous with an entire margin; may or may not exhibit indeterminate lysis of blood cells
Alcaligenes faecalis	Nonpigmented, glistening, convex, almost clear colonies surrounded by greenish brown discoloration
Alcaligenes odorans	Feather-edged colonies usually surrounded by zone of green discoloration; produce highly characteristic fruity odor

can be described as large (2 mm or greater) or small (less than 1 mm). *Moraxella* spp. and *P. fluorescens* (at 35° C) form tiny colonies (less than 1 mm) after overnight incubation and increase in size only after extended incubation. Although most organisms form smooth colonies with entire edges, *P. pseudomallei*, *P. stutzeri*, and CDC Ve form wrinkled colonies, especially after 48 hours of incubation. Beta-hemolysis is restricted to *P. aeruginosa*, *A. haemolyticus*, *A. alcaligenes*, *K. kingae*, and *P. fluorescens* (only at 25° C). Detailed colonial descriptions are included in Table 17-2. Plates 10, *C* to *F*, and 11, *A* to *E*, depict the colonial morphologies of these organisms.

BIOCHEMICAL IDENTIFICATION
CLUES TO PRESENCE OF NONFERMENTATIVE ORGANISMS

Observation of the primary MacConkey agar plate and performance of a spot oxidase test aid the microbiologist in distinguishing potential nonfermenters from members of the family *Enterobacteriaceae*. As previously mentioned, the presence of a nonfermentative organism should be considered if a gram-negative rod grows on blood agar but fails to grow on MacConkey agar. All nonfermenters that do grow on MacConkey are lactose negative, in contrast to *Enterobacteriaceae*, which may be positive or negative. Furthermore, all *Enterobacteriaceae* are oxidase negative, whereas the nonfermenters may be positive or negative.

Two additional tests, motility and determination of whether organisms utilize glucose fermentatively, oxidatively, or not at all, are also useful in distinguishing nonfermenters and, in conjunction with growth on MacConkey agar and oxidase, may offer clues as to the genus of the isolate (Table 17-3). The motility slide test (Appendix A) may be performed with growth from the blood agar plate. Motile organisms may be further differentiated on the basis of the number and arrangement of their flagella through use of a flagella stain. As discussed in Chapter 6, the basic principle of all flagella stains is to precipitate a colored compound on an otherwise invisible flagellum to

TABLE 17-2. Colonial Morphology of the Nonfermentative Bacteria—cont'd

Organism	Description
Acinetobacter	Raised, creamy, circular, smooth, opaque, grayish white (Plate 11, *C*); resembles *Enterobacteriaceae*; *A. alcaligenes* and *A. haemolyticus* beta-hemolytic
Flavobacterium meningosepticum	Circular with entire edge, convex, smooth or slightly mottled, glistening, butyrous, and pale yellow (cream) in color
Flavobacterium breve	Same as for *F. meningosepticum,* except yellow-orange in color
Flavobacterium (Sphingobacterium) multivorum	Small, circular, convex, smooth, opaque with pale yellow pigment; pigmentation develops after overnight incubation at room temperature
Flavobacterium indologenes	Same as for *F. breve*
Flavobacterium sp. group IIf	Small colonies at 24 hours but increasing in size and developing a distinctive, tan, mucoid appearance with continued incubation
Moraxella	Form tiny (less than 1 mm), translucent to semiopaque colonies after overnight incubation; *M. osloensis* and *M. nonliquefaciens* may form slightly larger colonies; *M. lacunata, M. nonliquefaciens,* and *M. atlantae* may show pitting; pitting colonies of *M. atlantae* and *M. nonliquefaciens* may also show surface spreading; all colonies are white except for *M. atlantae* and *M. phenylpyruvica,* which may appear slightly pink
Eikenella corrodens[6]	Forms characteristic grayish, dry, flat, radially spreading colony with irregular periphery and moist central core; when colonies are examined with stereoscopic microscope, three distinct zones of growth may be noted: (1) innermost clear, moist center, apparently devoid of growth, (2) highly refractile, speckled, pearl-like zone resembling mercury droplets, and (3) outer refractile spreading perimeter; when colonies are scraped from agar surface, pitting or corroding may be observed
Kingella	May appear as smooth, entire, convex colonies or as colonies that pit the agar and have thin, spreading zone of growth around outer edge

render it visible by ordinary light microscopy. Types of flagellar arrangement are described in Table 17-4.

Unlike the *Enterobacteriaceae,* the NFB do not utilize glucose fermentatively. Thus on TSI agar they produce no change in the butt; the slant also remains unchanged or may become alkaline as a result of protein metabolism. Although they do not ferment glucose, NFB may utilize glucose oxidatively.

Fermentation and oxidation both depend on a series of oxidation-reduction reactions that provide bacteria with energy in the form of adenosine triphosphate (ATP). However, in fermentation the final electron acceptor is an organic compound, and in oxidation the final electron acceptor is usually oxygen. The practical distinction between oxidation and fermentation of carbohydrates depends on the role played by atmospheric oxygen.[30] Fermentation is an anaerobic process, and most fermentative organisms are facultative anaerobes. Oxidation, on the other hand, is an aerobic process, and most oxidative organisms are obligate aerobes.

Fermentative organisms degrade glucose primarily by the Embden-Meyerhof (EM) pathway. Glucose is first phosphorylated and later split into two molecules of glyceraldehyde phosphate, which undergo further changes to produce pyruvic acid. Depending on the species, pyruvic acid is further oxidized to a variety of products, including acetic acid, succinic acid, formic acid, lactic acid, and acetoin.

Oxidative organisms depend on the Entner-Doudoroff pathway or hexose monophosphate shunt for glucose catabolism. Pyruvic acid is produced by both of these pathways. The pyruvic acid is oxidized to acetyl coenzyme A (acetyl CoA) and enters the tricarboxylic acid cycle (Krebs cycle), where it is oxidized completely to CO_2 and H_2O.

Fermentation of glucose results in the production of large amounts of acid, whereas oxidation produces little acid. Although TSI agar (and other fermentative media) can detect fermentation or nonfermentation of glucose, they cannot detect oxidation of glucose. These media contain a large ratio of pep-

TABLE 17-3. Characteristics of Genera of Nonfermentative Bacteria

Genus	Oxidase	Growth on MacConkey Agar	Motility	Utilization of Glucose
Pseudomonas	+[a]	Good	Motile by means of polar flagella	Oxidative
Achromobacter	+	Good	Motile by means of peritrichous flagella	Oxidative
Alcaligenes	+	Good	Motile by means of peritrichous flagella	Inactive
Acinetobacter	−	Good, except for few strains of var. *lwoffi*	Nonmotile	Oxidative or inactive
Flavobacterium	+	Variable according to species (see Table 17-9)	Nonmotile	Oxidative
Moraxella	+	Variable according to species (see Table 17-12)	Nonmotile	Inactive
Eikenella	+	Negative	Nonmotile	Inactive
Kingella	+	Variable according to species (see Table 17-13)	Nonmotile	Delayed fermentative

SYMBOLS: +, Positive
−, Negative

[a]*P. maltophilia* is usually oxidase negative. *P. cepacia* may be negative.

TABLE 17-4. Types of Flagellation

Type	Definition
Polar	Monotrichous—a single flagellum at one or both poles
	Multitrichous—two or more flagella at one or both poles
Subpolar	Monotrichous—a single flagellum located near but not at the pole
	Multitrichous—several flagella near the pole
Peritrichous	Flagella seemingly haphazardly arranged either singly or multiply

From Liefson, E.: Atlas of bacterial flagellation, New York, 1960, Academic Press, Inc.

tone to carbohydrate, and the small amounts of acid produced from oxidation are neutralized by the alkaline products produced from the large amounts of peptone. Hugh and Liefson oxidative-fermentative (OF) media should be used to detect oxidative activity (Appendix A). OF medium contains less peptone, resulting in an increased carbohydrate-to-peptone ratio. Thus it is able to detect small amounts of acid. OF medium also contains agar to prevent convection currents and diffusion of the acid in the medium, thereby retaining the acid at the surface for a more effective test reaction.

GENERAL CONSIDERATIONS

The identification of NFB is based on three considerations.

1. The methods used for identification must be specified. Several schemes have been proposed for identification of the NFB: those of Weaver and co-workers[80] and Tatum, Ewing and Weaver from the CDC,[78] Gilardi,[18,20] Oberhofer and co-workers,[48,50] and Pickett and Pederson,[56,57] wherein the approaches to the problems of identification and the criteria used for identification differ to some extent. Personal preferences and resources may determine the selection of one scheme over another, but once a scheme is selected, it must be strictly followed. Under no circumstances should the microbiologist use the results of one scheme and the methods of another.

2. The frequency of isolation of an organism must be examined to select the tests that will best assist in identification. Most conventional definitive identification schemes require numerous biochemical tests and are prohibitively expensive for the smaller clinical laboratory. These laboratories may elect to use the screening method discussed later, a commercial rapid identification system, or a smaller battery of tests selected from the extensive identification schemes. If the last approach is used, the microbiologist must select the tests that identify the isolates most commonly encountered in the clinical laboratory.

Pseudomonas aeruginosa, for example, is by far the most frequently isolated nonfermenter. Most, but not all, isolates of *P. aeruginosa* produce pyocyanin, a water-soluble, chloroform-soluble blue phenazine pigment. Furthermore, *P. aeruginosa* is the only organism in the clinical laboratory to produce this pigment. Most pyocyanin-positive strains of *P. aeruginosa* produce the pigment on ordinary isolation media such as blood or MacConkey agar and are easily identified. Some strains, however, must be induced to produce the pigment with the special pyocyanin media mentioned on p. 337. In any event, whenever a pyocyanin-producing organism is isolated, it can be reported as *P. aeruginosa* without further identification.

Of the other nonfermentative organisms, the nonpigmented *P. aeruginosa, P. putida, P. fluorescens, P. maltophilia, Acinetobacter anitratus,* and *A. lwoffi* make up 55% of the total (Table 17-5). (The values may vary between institutions, and *P. cepacia* may account for a significant number of isolates in institutions that have an in-house strain.) Therefore, based on expected frequency of isolation, a routine battery of tests does not include the indole test (for flavobacteria) or the catalase test (for moraxellae). Both of these tests are indicated only in an examination of an oxidase-positive, nonmotile, MacConkey-negative organism.

3. The degree of accuracy desired for identification is important. This consideration goes hand in hand with the previous consideration because the degree of accuracy determines the extent of identification. Although clear speciation or biotyping is desirable, not all organisms need such identification to be clinically relevant. Some NFB, for example, may be grouped, the most notable examples being the *P. fluorescens–putida* group and *Moraxella* spp. If differentiation of *P. fluorescens* from *P. putida* is needed, a test for gelatin liquefaction may be used (Figure 17-1). Otherwise, isolates that produce fluorescein but fail to grow at 42° C or to alkalinize acetamide may be reported as *P. fluorescens–putida* group without further differentiation. Similarly, *Moraxella* spp. may be reported when a nonpitting, oxidase-positive isolate that fails to grow on MacConkey agar is also negative in tests for motility, glucose oxidation, and indole production.

SCREENING METHODS

A two-tube screening system in combination with a quadrant plate may be used for presumptive identification of the most common NFB and those that grow on MacConkey agar. MacConkey-negative organisms must be identified by more definitive means. After the oxidase test is performed, fluorescein-denitrification lactose (FDL) and motility-glucose medium (MGM) (see Appendix A) are inoculated with growth taken directly from the primary isolation medium. A quadrant plate containing acetamide, agar gelatin, bile esculin, and DNA agars is spot-inoculated in each test area. A susceptibility test is performed, and a TSI slant is inoculated to ensure that the organism tested is a nonfermenter. All tests are incubated overnight at 35° C, and all negative tests are reincubated for an additional 24 hours at room temperature. Figure 17-1 presents the results of the screening method and accounts for the most common isolates. The screening method cannot identify all organisms to the species level.

DEFINITIVE IDENTIFICATION

The definitive identification scheme presented in this chapter is depicted in Tables 17-6 through 17-13. The remainder of this

TABLE 17-5. Frequency of Isolation of 1781 Nonfermentative Bacteria[a] (1975 to 1983)

Organism	Isolation (%)
Acinetobacter anitratus	14.9
Pseudomonas maltophilia	10.5
Pseudomonas aeruginosa (apyocyanogenic)	9.7
Pseudomonas putida	8.4
Acinetobacter lwoffi	7.7
Pseudomonas fluorescens	3.7
P. aeruginosa (delayed pyocyanin)	2.9
Flavobacterium indologenes	2.7
Achromobacter xylosoxidans	2.6
P. aeruginosa (pyomelanine), *P. aeruginosa* (mucoid), *Pseudomonas stutzeri, Pseudomonas pseudoalcaligenes, Flavobacterium* sp. group IIf	1.5 to 1.9
P. stutzeri–like, *Alcaligenes haemolyticus, Pseudomonas paucimobilis,* CDC Ve-2, *Pseudomonas acidovorans, Pseudomonas testosteroni, Alcaligenes odorans, Moraxella osloensis, Eikenella corrodens*	1.0 to 1.4
UFP, *Pseudomonas pickettii,* CDC Vd-1, *Pseudomonas cepacia, Flavobacterium meningosepticum, Pseudomonas diminuta, Flavobacterium multivorum, Pseudomonas alcaligenes, Alcaligenes faecalis,* CDC IVc, *Moraxella nonliquefaciens,* M-5, *Kingella denitrificans,* EF-4	0.5 to 0.9
Pseudomonas mendocina, Pseudomonas vesicularis, CDC Vd-2, *Flavobacterium breve, P. aeruginosa* (nonglucolytic), CDC Ve-1, *Pseudomonas putrefaciens, Pseudomonas denitrificans, Alcaligenes denitrificans, Acinetobacter alcaligenes, Bordetella bronchiseptica, Flavobacterium odoratum, Moraxella atlantae, Moraxella urethralis, Moraxella phenylpyruvica*	0.5

[a] See identification tables for number of isolates.

section discusses the media and methodology of this scheme. More detailed information regarding the preparation, principle, and interpretation of the media is included in Appendix A.

Media
Triple sugar iron agar[50]

The value of TSI for determination of fermentative ability has been discussed. Again, because glucose is not fermented by NFB, the butt of the agar remains unchanged, and the slant remains unchanged or becomes alkaline as a result of protein metabolism (Plate 9, *E*). *P. pseudomallei* and occasional strains of *F. indologenes* and *P. paucimobilis* oxidize the sugars in the slant, giving a delayed, weak acid change. The CDC EF-4, technically a glucose-fermenting organism, gives a "no change" butt in 24 hours but an acid butt at 48 hours.

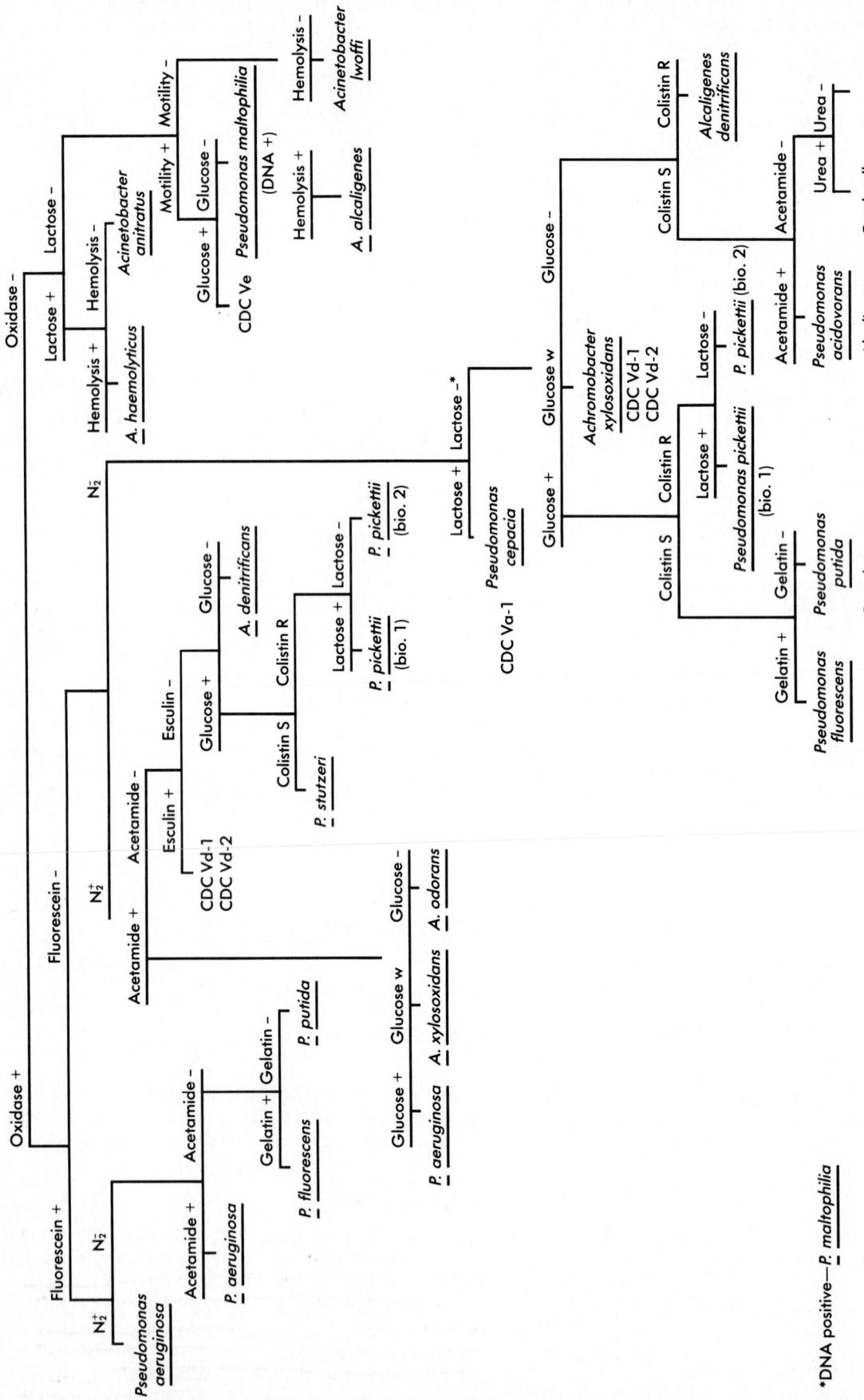

FIGURE 17-1. Diagrammatic scheme using selected tests to identify nonfermentative bacteria.

*DNA positive—*P. maltophilia*

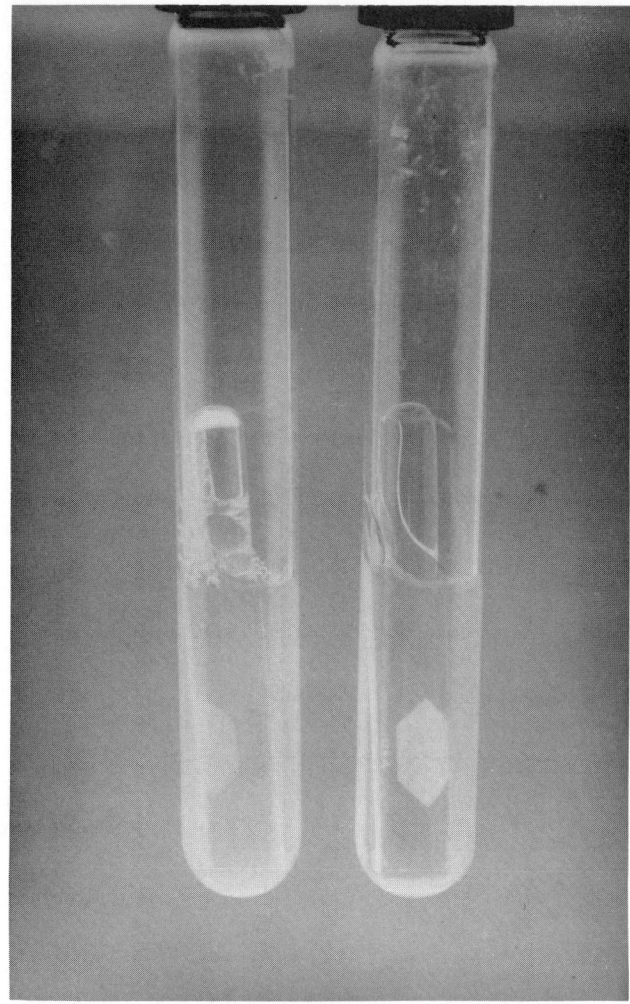

FIGURE 17-2. Test for nitrogen gas production. Test on left is positive for gas production. Note gas bubbles, as well as space in inverted tube.

Motility test[50,78]

Common to the identification of all gram-negative bacteria is the test for bacterial motility. MGM is preferred over the semi-solid motility medium used for the *Enterobacteriaceae* not only because it is a combination medium, but also because it contains less agar (0.3%) to impede the movement of the cells (Plate 11, *F*). The NFB are not as vigorous in their motility as the *Enterobacteriaceae* and this medium presents less resistance to their motile action. Organisms that are nonmotile in MGM should be examined with the slide technique.

Oxidase test[33,50,70]

Many of the NFB produce indophenol (cytochrome) oxidase during the later phases of respiration. The Kovacs spot test, which uses 1% tetramethyl-*p*-phenylenediamine dihydrochloride, is preferred for identification of the NFB. Neither the use of the dimethyl compound in the spot test nor the flooding of a plate or slant with the reagent is as sensitive or rapid a test. Commercial oxidase reagents containing ascorbic acid for stability also are available. When performing the test, the follow-

ing safeguards must be taken: (1) the growth used should be from a 24-hour culture, since the oxidase-negative *P. maltophilia* can give a weak but definite positive reaction at 48 hours; (2) the test should not be read after 10 seconds, since false-positive reactions may occur; (3) growth should not be taken from a MacConkey agar plate, since the dyes may impart a blue color; (4) a TSI slant as a source of growth should be avoided since oxidase-positive, fermentative organisms (such as *Pasteurella* and *Aeromonas* spp.) may give a false-negative reaction owing to interference by acids in the slant; (5) a platinum—not Nichrome—loop should be used, since the Nichrome can contribute to a false-positive test; and (6) any discolored reagent should be discarded.

Oxidative-fermentative medium[50,80]

The importance of OF medium in determining oxidative ability has been discussed. The OF medium, containing casitone as enrichment and phenol red as indicator, is also used to detect motility (see the section on MGM). A single tube containing glucose can be used as a screening medium or as a battery (in combination with lactose, sucrose, maltose, mannitol, xylose, and fructose).

Fluorescein medium[32,50]

Only four species of pseudomonads produce fluorescein: *P. aeruginosa, P. putida, P. fluorescens,* and UFP (unidentified fluorescent pseudomonads). Fluorescein is a combination of fluorescent, water-soluble, yellow-green pigments that can be detected on Pseudomonas agar F (Difco Laboratories, Detroit) or FLO agar (BBL Microbiology Systems, Cockeysville, Md.). The pigments are released into the media and usually produce a visible yellow or yellow-green color (Plate 12, *A*). Tubes negative for fluorescein to the unaided eye are examined under an ultraviolet light (366 nm) or Wood's lamp and observed for a definitive fluorescence. *P. cepacia* can produce a nonfluorescing, sulfur-yellow pigment that mimics a positive test on Pseudomonas agar F medium. Also, a dried medium should not be used because the absence of moisture tends to quench fluorescein production.

Pyocyanin medium[32,50]

Pyocyanin is a water-soluble, chloroform-soluble, blue phenazine pigment that, when produced in combination with pyoverdin (fluorescein), pyorubin (red), or pyomelanin (brown), displays a mosaic of colors. The strains of *P. aeruginosa* that do not readily produce pyocyanin on ordinary isolation media must be induced to do so by use of a specially formulated medium such as Pseudomonas agar P (Difco) or TECH agar (BBL). In both of these media pyocyanin appears as light green, green, dark green, blue-green, or dark blue in various degrees of intensity (Plate 12, *B*).

Denitrification[43,50]

Some NFB reduce nitrate to nitrite, and some reduce nitrite further to nitrogen gas. The latter step is called denitrification. Denitrification is useful in differentiating *P. aeruginosa, P. stutzeri, A. xylosoxidans,* and *A. denitrificans* from biochemically similar organisms. Nitrite production is determined by adding specific reagents to the test medium, whereas nitrogen gas is detected visually by bubble formation or entrapment of the gas in a Durham tube (Figure 17-2).

Fluorescein-denitrification-lactose medium[55,65]

FDL medium is a combination medium designed to detect fluorescein production, nitrogen gas production, and lactose oxidation (Plate 12, *C*). It is especially useful in screening oxidase-positive organisms to identify nonpigmented *P. aeruginosa* and *P. cepacia* rapidly.

Decarboxylase medium[42,50,51]

Decarboxylation of lysine and ornithine to cadaverine and putrescine, respectively, and dihydrolation of arginine to putrescine and ammonia result in binding of the hydrogen ions by these products. This raises the pH of the medium, changing the color indicator to the alkaline range. The Moeller medium is suitable for use with the *Enterobacteriaceae,* but when used with the NFB, reactions are delayed until sufficient alkaline products are formed to contrast with the initial color of the medium. The rapid medium (Plate 12, *D,* and discussed in Appendix A) is preferred over the Moeller medium because more rapid and uniform results are obtained. The rapid method utilizes a lower initial pH, allowing changes to occur and to be visualized more rapidly.

Urea agar[9,50]

Christensen urea agar is valuable in detecting urease production by *Bordetella bronchiseptica* and a *Bordetella*-like organism (CDC IVc). Both produce a strong and rapid change in the slant and in the butt (Plate 12, *E*). Urease production by the NFB is scored as positive only when the slant turns a definite pink; pinkness in the agar is nonspecific alkalinization and is a negative result.

Gelatin liquefaction[3,50,78]

Many NFB produce an enzyme that degrades gelatins prepared from different animal and plant sources. Gelatin liquefaction is particularly useful in differentiating *P. fluorescens* from *P. putida* and for characterizing the flavobacteria. Nutrient gelatin (Figure 17-3) is customarily used for microbiologic and taxonomic studies, although it is a growth test and requires at least overnight incubation. The agar gelatin test is also an overnight test. The film strip method is a rapid method that detects preformed enzymes in 4 hours (Plate 12, *F*) and is better suited for routine use.

Litmus milk peptonization[50]

Litmus milk is a multipurpose medium that detects several reactions (see Milk Medium, Appendix A); however, the only reaction that is observed with NFB is peptonization, or the digestion of casein to produce a clearing at the surface of the milk (Plate 13, *A*). This is often accompanied by a change in the phenolphthalein indicator from blue to lavender as a result of alkalinization. Similar to gelatin liquefaction, peptonization is useful to differentiate *P. fluorescens* from *P. putida* and to characterize the flavobacteria. Some strains of *Acinetobacter* actively oxidize the milk lactose, changing the color indicator to white or pink.

Cetrimide tolerance[50,80]

The fluorescent pseudomonads and *A. xylosoxidans* and *P. cepacia* grow uniformly in the presence of cetrimide (hexadecyltrimethyl ammonium bromide) at a concentration of 0.09% in trypticase soy or brain heart infusion agars. Some formulations

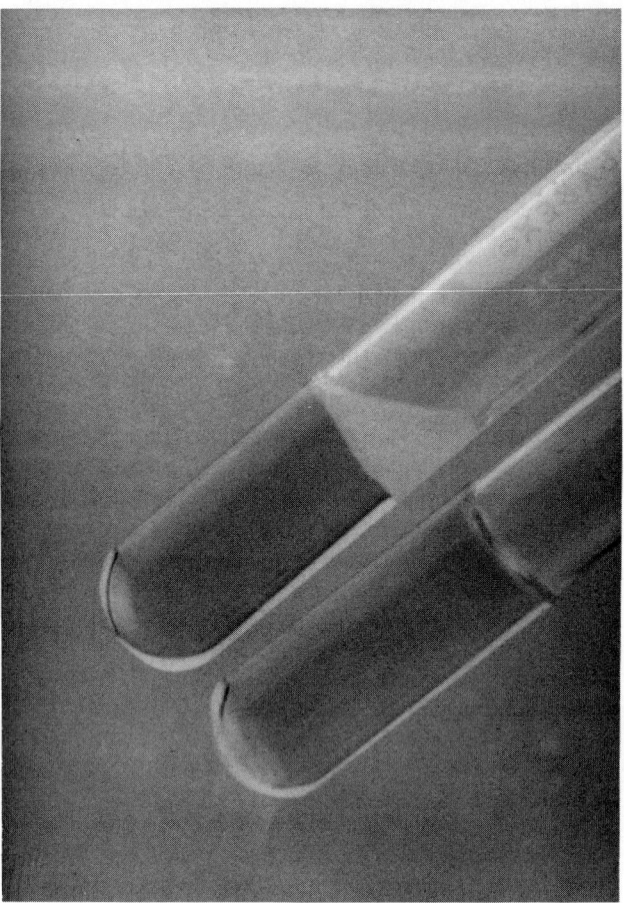

FIGURE 17-3. Test for gelatin liquefaction using nutrient gelatin. Test at top is positive.

of cetrimide agar have a concentration of 0.03%, giving a wider range of growth with less discrimination. In all instances cetrimide must be pretested because of a lot-to-lot variation in potency.

Esculin hydrolysis[50]

Most NFB grow on bile-esculin agar (BEA), and some hydrolyze esculin to esculetin, which combines with ferric ions present in the medium to form a brown-black color (Plate 13, *B*). This latter reaction is a positive reaction for esculin hydrolysis. Of the esculin-positive NFB, *P. paucimobilis* and *P. vesicularis* do not grow on BEA but do blacken the slant to a slight degree owing to preformed enzymes, whereas *P. cepacia, P. maltophilia,* and the flavobacteria do grow and blacken the medium. Esculin agar and esculin disks may be used for testing. Caution must be taken not to confuse pyocyanin produced by *P. aeruginosa* on BEA with esculin hydrolysis.

Gluconate oxidation[18,43,50]

Oxidation of potassium gluconate serves to distinguish the fluorescent pseudomonads from other NFB, although *A. xylosoxidans, P. cepacia,* and CDC Ve-2 may also be positive. Gluconate is oxidized to a reducing compound (2-ketogluconate), which in turn reduces copper sulfate to produce a color reaction (Plate 13, *C*).

Deoxyribonuclease (DNAse) test[18,50]

Deoxyribonucleic acid (DNA) test agar containing methyl green is used to detect DNAse production by *P. maltophilia, F. meningosepticum, P. putrefaciens,* and *P. diminuta* (Plate 13, *D*). DNAse hydrolyzes DNA into smaller nonprecipitable fragments. In the conventional test, hydrochloric acid is used to precipitate unhydrolyzed DNA, leaving a clear zone of hydrolyzed DNA surrounding the growth. When methyl green is added to the medium, unhydrolyzed DNA (acid) appears green, whereas the hydrolyzed DNA (neutral pH) is colorless. Although the reactions in the methyl green medium are less intense than on the conventional medium, the methyl green medium may be reincubated, since it is not obliterated by flooding with acid. DNA test agar with toluidine blue may also be used.

Starch hydrolysis[35,50]

The test for starch hydrolysis is useful to differentiate *P. stutzeri* from the biochemically similar achromobacteria (Plate 13, *E*). Starch binds to iodine to form a purple color. *P. stutzeri* and *Flavobacterium indologenes* produce amylase, hydrolyzing the starch into soluble end products, which are no longer available to bind iodine.

Lecithinase test[48,50]

The ability to produce lecithinase distinguishes *P. fluorescens, P. pseudomallei, Acinetobacter calcoaceticus* var. *haemolyticus,* and *A. calcoaceticus* var. *alcaligenes* from biochemically similar organisms. Lecithinase acts on the lipoprotein component of egg yolk in egg yolk agar (Appendix A) to produce an opaque zone of precipitation (Plate 13, *F*). Lipase activity, which should not be confused with lecithinase activity, is seen as an iridescent ''pearly layer'' at the edge of the growth. Lipase production is neither a consistent nor a reliable characteristic for the NFB and is ignored. A slight clearing around the spot inoculum is a result of proteolysis and should also be ignored.

Beta-D-galactosidase[50]

Although the NFB do not ferment lactose, some strains produce a beta-D-galactosidase. The test is particularly useful to identify some of the yellow-pigmented pseudomonads and flavobacteria. Beta-D-galactosidase hydrolyzes *o*-nitrophenyl-beta-D-galactopyranoside (ONPG) to form the yellow compound *o*-nitrophenyl (see ONPG test in Appendix A).

Acetamide utilization[46,49,50]

Deamidation of acetamide results in an alkalinization of the medium and a pronounced change to a blue color (Plate 14, *A*). This test is useful in differentiating nonpigmented *P. aeruginosa, A. xylosoxidans, P. acidovorans,* and *A. odorans* from biochemically similar organisms. Alkalinization of other amides and organic salts—including allantoin, citrate, and tartrate—may also aid in differentiating among the NFB.

Growth at 42° C[46,49,50]

Growth at 42° C has been used to differentiate *P. aeruginosa* from *P. fluorescens* and *P. putida,* as well as to distinguish *P. stutzeri, A. xylosoxidans,* and *P. pseudoalcaligenes* from related organisms. Because the alkalinization of acetamide is closely correlated to growth at 42° C, either of these two tests may be

used to identify *P. aeruginosa* (see temperature tolerance test in Appendix A).

KOH distinction test[48]

The principle of the potassium hydroxide (KOH) test is discussed in Chapter 6. The test may be used to distinguish gram-negative variants of *Bacillus* spp. that closely resemble the NFB in morphology, growth characteristics, oxidase reaction, and motility. Gram-positive bacteria are unaffected by dilute concentrations of alkali. Gram-negative bacteria, however, are disrupted, become viscous, and string out when touched with a wire or loop (Figure 17-4.)

Indole test[50,78]

Among the NFB only the flavobacteria and *K. indologenes* produce indole. Often the amount of indole produced is quite small and cannot be demonstrated with Kovacs reagent, necessitating the use of the xylene extraction technique (Plate 14, *B*). Xylene extracts the indole from the broth and concentrates it in a layer between the broth and the xylene. The Ehrlich reagent reacts with the indole in the extract to produce a red color. The peptone water customarily used as the substrate with the *Enterobacteriaceae* is not satisfactory for testing the NFB; casitone broth or trypticase soy broth should be used. It should be noted that the indole test is performed only with oxidase-positive, nonmotile NFB.

Phenylalanine deaminase[8,50]

The test for phenylalanine deaminase is used to distinguish the *stutzeri* group* and members of the genus *Achromobacter* from biochemically similar organisms. Phenylalanine is oxidatively deaminated to phenylpyruvic acid, which reacts with ferric chloride to form a green color.

Catalase test[80]

The catalase test may be used to identify the *Moraxella* group (nonmotile, MacConkey negative). These organisms produce catalase, which degrades hydrogen peroxide to water and oxygen.

Flagella stain[18,50,78,82]

The importance of the flagella stain has been discussed. Details of the procedure are in Chapter 6.

Colistin susceptibility[18,50]

Susceptibility of NFB to antimicrobial agents is useful in their differentiation. Susceptibility to colistin (or polymyxin) clearly separates various groups of NFB. Except for *P. maltophilia* and CDC Ve, the yellow-pigmented NFB are uniformly resistant to colistin (with a zone size of less than 9 mm). Of the pseudomonads, *P. pseudomallei, P. pickettii,* and *P. vesicularis* are resistant to colistin, as is *A. denitrificans.* Colistin can be included in a battery of antimicrobial agents for routine testing or tested separately with a small blood agar plate.

Inoculation and Incubation of Media

The standard inoculum when using a battery of tests for definitive identification is 1 drop of a 4- to 6-hour trypticase soy

---

*The *stutzeri* group includes *P. stutzeri, P. mendocina,* and CDC Vb3. CDC Vb3 includes the arginine-positive *P. stutzeri.*

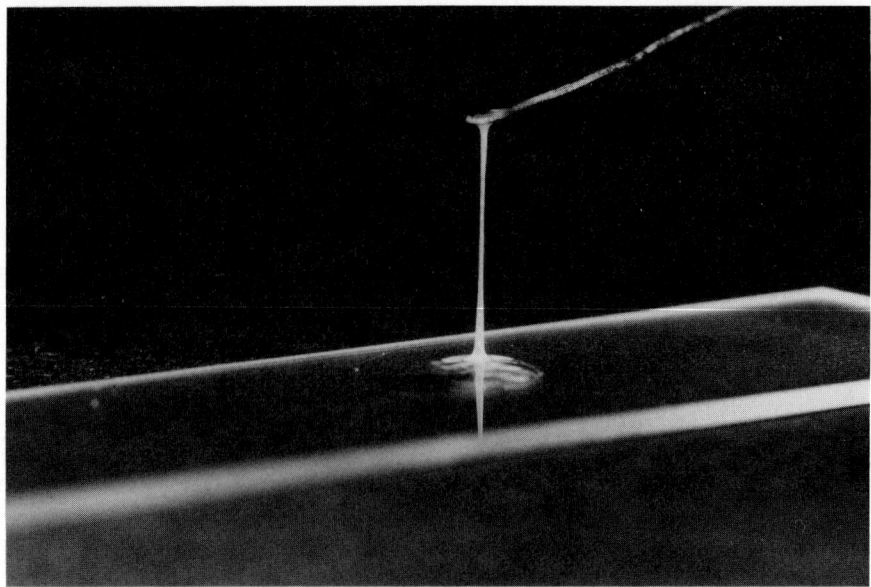

FIGURE 17-4. Test for potassium hydroxide (KOH) solubility. In positive test the organism becomes viscous and "strings" with pull of a loop.

or brain heart infusion broth culture. The inoculum for rapid tests or for individual tests can be prepared in one of two ways. Either a portion of growth is taken from a solid medium to inoculate each tube, or a dense suspension of the organism is prepared in saline and 1 drop added to each tube. The tubed media are incubated with the tops loose, since most biochemical reactions are oxidative. After overnight incubation the tubes are checked and the caps are loosened if necessary. Negative tests are reincubated for at least an additional 24 hours, and longer if possible.

Identification Schema

A few simple tests, including utilization of glucose and oxidase, motility, and pigment production, help to separate NFB into the groups depicted in Tables 17-6 through 17-13. Differentiation of the organisms within each of these groups is considered in the following sections.

Fluorescent pseudomonads (Table 17-6)

The fluorescent pseudomonads are polar flagellated organisms of aquatic origin. Although *P. aeruginosa* grows well at temperatures of 35° C and above, *P. fluorescens* and *P. putida* have an optimal temperature of 30° C or less. The latter organisms show a wide range of growth characteristics, with some strains growing well at 35° C and others not growing at all. This may account for a lower recovery rate on primary isolation media when incubated at 35° C. Furthermore, as previously mentioned, identification tests may have to be incubated at room temperature before characteristic reactions take place.

Although there is little difference between pigmented strains and nonpigmented (apyocyanogenic) strains of *P. aeruginosa* in the extent or rate of biochemical activity, mucoid strains are usually slow reacting, in contrast to nonmucoid strains. As already noted, strains of *P. aeruginosa* that produce pyocyanin can be identified on this criterion. Other strains, including those producing the brown pigment pyomelanin or those that are delayed pyocyanin producers, can be differentiated as in

Table 17-6. The strains of *P. aeruginosa* designated nonglucolytic in Table 17-6 do not oxidize glucose or do so only after a long incubation. These strains also do not oxidize gluconate and are not proteolytic by conventional means, such as gelatin, litmus milk, and lecithinase.

P. aeruginosa is distinguished from *P. fluorescens* and *P. putida* by growth at 42° C, flagellar arrangement, acetamide alkalinization, and the occasional production of a characteristic grapelike odor. *P. fluorescens* is distinguished from *P. putida* by producing gelatinase and lecithinase and by peptonizing litmus milk.

The unidentified fluorescent pseudomonads (UFPs)[47] have characteristics resembling both *P. aeruginosa* (growth at 42° C, hemolytic, mucoid, and monotrichous) and *P. fluorescens* (negative for pyocyanin, nitrogen gas, and acetamide utilization, but very susceptible to kanamycin). They uniformly fail to oxidize gluconate.

Nonfluorescent, oxidative pseudomonads (Table 17-7)

The nonfluorescent, oxidative pseudomonads do not produce fluorescein or pyocyanin and do not oxidize gluconate or hemolyze sheep red cells, but usually produce nitrogen gas. *P. pseudomallei*, an organism believed not to be indigenous to the United States, is genetically related to *P. cepacia*. It is multitrichous and actively proteolytic; it avidly attacks carbohydrates and arginine but does not grow on Salmonella-Shigella (SS) agar and is resistant to colistin. *P. stutzeri* and *P. stutzeri*-like (CDC Vb-3) organisms have monotrichous flagella, produce nitrite and gas, hydrolyze starch, and grow on SS agar, but they are not proteolytic and do not oxidize lactose. *P. stutzeri* is arginine negative by the Moeller method and usually arginine positive by the rapid method. Tests for lactose, starch hydrolysis, growth on SS agar, and susceptibility to colistin separate the *stutzeri* group from *P. pseudomallei*. *P. mendocina* is arginine positive but fails to hydrolyze starch or to oxidize maltose and mannitol. *P. mendocina* does not form wrinkled colonies.

TABLE 17-6. Biochemical and Morphologic Characteristics of Fluorescent *Pseudomonas* Spp.

Test or Substrate[a]	P. aeruginosa (31)[b] (Pyomelanine)	P. aeruginosa (52) (Delayed Pyocyanin)	P. aeruginosa (173) (Nonpigmented)	P. aeruginosa (28) (Mucoid)	P. aeruginosa (7) (Nonglucolytic)	UFP-1 (7)	UFP-2 (7)	P. fluorescens (66)	P. putida (150)
Motility									
Slide[c]	100[d]	100	90	89	29	100	100	82	97
Tube[c]	100	88	90	75	57	100	100	77	89
Flagella	1	1	1	1	1	1	1	>2	>2
Oxidase	100	100	100	100	100	100	100	100	100
Pyocyanin (35° C)[c]	84	92	60	82	100	0	0	0	0
Fluorescein (25° C)[c]	90	88	78	57	14	86	71	85	83
Gluconate oxidation	97	98	90	93	0	0	0	85	73
Urease	84	88	90	68	29	71	100	17	33
Arginine dihydrolase	100	100	99	100	86	100	100	77	95
Nitrite production	23	35	30	29	100	14	29	9	5
Denitrification (N$_2$)[c]	97	100	97	93	100	0	14	0	0
Gelatinase[c]	90	77	69	75	0	100	0	97	0
Litmus milk peptonized[c]	90	100	93	89	0	100	0	80	0
Deoxyribonuclease	0	6	9	14	0	0	0	0	0
Lecithinase	3	18	26	36	0	0	0	45	0
Starch hydrolysis	0	0	0	0	0	0	71	0	0
Growth on cetrimide[c]	97	100	99	100	100	100	86	85	84
Growth at 42° C[c]	97	100	100	100	100	100	60	0	5
Growth on SS agar	94	100	97	93	100	100	100	86	95
Growth on MacConkey agar	100	100	100	100	100	100	100	100	100
Hemolysis	84	85	80	61	57	100	0	6	0
Pigment	100	100	0	11	0	86	29	12	10
Mucoid colonies	0	2	0	100	100	67	0	9	0
Oxidative-fermentative									
Glucose[c]	100	100	100	100	14[e]	100	100	100	100
Lactose[c]	0	0	0	0	0	0	86	8	3
Sucrose	0	0	0	0	0	0	0	27	0
Maltose	0	0	0	0	0	0	100	11	1
Mannitol	90	83	87	82	0	0	0	56	20
Xylose[c]	87	96	90	96	0	0	43	92	98
Fructose	93	83	86	93	14[e]	100	100	91	89
Amides/salts									
Acetamide[c]	100	100	99	100	57[e]	0	0	2	2
Allantoin	45	81	77	82	0	0	0	5	2
Citrate	100	100	100	100	57	100	100	100	100
Tartrate	0	0	0	0	0	0	0	8	26
Colistin susceptible	99	100	100	100	100	100	100	100	100

[a]All strains were negative in tests for phenylalanine deaminase, lysine and ornithine decarboxylase, esculin hydrolysis, and beta-D-galactosidase.
[b]Figures in parentheses indicate number of strains tested.
[c]Key characteristics.
[d]Results expressed as percent positive after 7 days' incubation.
[e]Weak reaction.

Miscellaneous pseudomonads and achromobacteria
(Table 17-8)

P. pseudoalcaligenes organisms are long rods with polar, monotrichous flagella. They grow on SS and cetrimide agars but are variable in phenylalanine and arginine activity. Oxidation of glucose is delayed, although activity against fructose is prompt. *P. pseudoalcaligenes* is nutritionally and biochemically similar to the inert *P. alcaligenes*.

P. pickettii is a heterogeneous species comprised of up to seven biovars.[21] *P. pickettii* biovar 1 includes organisms formerly designated CDC Va-1 and differs from *P. pickettii* biovar 2 (formerly CDC Va-2) in its production of acid from lactose

TABLE 17-7. Biochemical and Morphologic Characteristics of Nonfluorescent, Oxidative *Pseudomonas* Spp.

Test or Substrate[a]	*P. pseudomallei* (6)[b]	*P. stutzeri* (28)	*P. mendocina* (5)	*P. stutzeri*-like (20)
Motility				
Slide[c]	100[d]	100	100	95
Tube[c]	100	100	100	85
Flagella[c]	>2	1	1	1
Oxidase	100	100	100	100
Urease	67	64	100	40
Phenylalanine deaminase[c]	0	89	80	70
Arginine dihydrolase				
Moeller broth[b]	100	0	100	100
Rapid broth	100	68	100	100
Nitrite production[c]	100	55	60	65
Denitrification (N$_2$)[c]	100	79	100	60
Gelatinase[c]	100	0	0	0
Litmus milk peptonized[c]	100	5	0	5
Lecithinase	100	0	0	10
Starch hydrolysis[c]	0	75	0	85
Esculin hydrolysis	17	0	0	0
Growth on cetrimide[c]	67	28	80	50
Growth at 42° C[c]	NT[e]	90	100	100
Growth on SS agar[c]	0	86	100	85

TABLE 17-7. Biochemical and Morphologic Characteristics of Nonfluorescent, Oxidative *Pseudomonas* Spp.—cont'd

Test or Substrate[a]	*P. pseudomallei* (6)[b]	*P. stutzeri* (28)	*P. mendocina* (5)	*P. stutzeri*-like (20)
Growth on MacConkey agar	100	100	100	100
Wrinkled colonies	50	59	0	75
Pigment (buff, slightly yellow)	33	59	80	35
Beta-D-galactosidase (ONPG)	0	0	0	0
Oxidative-fermentative				
Glucose	100	100	100	100
Lactose[c]	100	0	0	0
Sucrose	50	0	0	0
Maltose[c]	100	76	0	95
Mannitol	100	69	0	55
Xylose[c]	83	90	80	80
Fructose	100	83	100	90
Amides/salts				
Acetamide	33	17	0	10
Allantoin[c]	0	0	0	0
Citrate	100	90	100	100
Tartrate[c]	0	3	0	15
Colistin susceptible[c]	0	100	100	100

[a]All strains tested were negative in tests for pyocyanin, fluorescein, gluconate oxidation, lysine and ornithine decarboxylase, deoxyribonuclease, and hemolysis on blood agar.
[b]Figures in parentheses indicate number of strains tested.
[c]Key characteristics.
[d]Results expressed as percent positive after 7 days' incubation.
[e]Not tested.

and maltose. *P. pickettii* is distinguished by its inability to grow on SS agar. Other characteristics are noted in Table 17-8. These organisms may require 2 days or more of incubation to effect changes in biochemical tests. There is a tendency for cultures of *P. pickettii* biovar 1 to die after 4 to 7 days, and the organisms should be preserved by freezing in skim milk or by other suitable means of storage.

The achromobacteria are motile, peritrichous organisms that grow well on artificial media. *A. xylosoxidans* is distinguished by its reduction of nitrate to nitrite and gas, growth on cetrimide and SS agars, growth at 42° C, and alkalinization of acetamide. It consistently oxidizes xylose but varies in the oxidation of glucose and fructose. Most achromobacteria are denitrifiers. CDC Vd-1 and Vd-2 organisms are characterized by rapid urea hydrolysis, phenylalanine deamination, esculin hydrolysis, alkalinization of allantoin, and failure to grow at 42° C. Whereas *A. xylosoxidans* is characteristically resistant to the aminoglycosides, the unnamed achromobacteria are susceptible.

Yellow-pigmented oxidative bacteria (Table 17-9)

P. (Xanthomonas) maltophilia, *P. cepacia*, and *Eikenella corrodens* are the only species of NFB that produce detectable lysine decarboxylase. *P. maltophilia* and *P. cepacia* are multitrichous and proteolytic and generally fail to grow on SS agar. *E. corrodens* does not grow on either MacConkey or SS agar.

As noted in Table 17-2, on blood and MacConkey agars young colonies of *P. maltophilia* are lavender colored but become gray-green with age. Yellow colonies are produced on peptone media. Colonies of *P. maltophilia* emit an odor of ammonia. *P. cepacia* produces two colonial forms—a sulfur-yellow colony and a colorless colony. The colorless organism may produce an orange-yellow pigment on TSI agar. *P. cepacia* and *P. maltophilia* differ biochemically in that the former is oxidase positive, oxidizes gluconate, decarboxylates ornithine, produces lecithinase, and avidly oxidizes carbohydrates. *P. maltophilia* produces extracellular deoxyribonuclease and is a weak oxidizer of carbohydrates, except for maltose.

P. vesicularis resembles *P. diminuta* (Table 17-9) but differs in its oxidation of glucose and maltose and its production of a yellow-orange pigment. *P. paucimobilis* is a bright yellow, weakly motile, short rod with polar monotrichous flagella (Plate 11, *E*). The oxidase reaction of *P. paucimobilis* can be slow, very weak, or negative. It fails to split urea or to grow on

TABLE 17-8. Biochemical and Morphologic Characteristics of Miscellaneous Oxidative *Pseudomonas* and *Achromobacter* Spp.

Test or Substrate[a]	*P. pseudoalcaligenes* (27)[b]	*P. picketti* bio. 1 (14)	*P. picketti* bio. 2 (11)	*A. xylosoxidans*—1 (41)	*A. xylosoxidans*—2 (5)	CDC Vd-1 (12)	CDC Vd-2 (3)
Motility							
Slide[c]	96[d]	64	70	100	100	92	100
Tube[c]	78	43	20	95	100	83	100
Flagella[c]	1	1	1	Peri[e]	Peri[e]	Peri[e]	Peri[e]
Oxidase	100	100	100	100	100	100	100
Gluconate oxidation	0	0	0	29	20	0	0
Urease[c]	7	100	100	0	0	100	100
Phenylalanine deaminase	22	7	10	0	0	75	100
Arginine dihydrolase[c]	74	0	0	0	0	42	0
Nitrite production[c]	100	71	100	44	100	42	100
Denitrification (N_2)[c]	0	57	10	93	20	67	67
Gelatinase	0	43	30	0	0	0	0
Litmus milk peptonized	0	0	0	0	0	0	33
Starch hydrolysis	0	43	50[f]	0	0	0	0
Esculin hydrolysis[c]	0	0	0	0	0	73	100
Growth at 42° C[c]	82	44	100	98	80	0	0
Growth on SS agar[c]	67	0	0	100	100	83	100
Growth on MacConkey agar	100	100	100	100	100	100	100
Mucoid colonies	0	0	0	0	60	75	100
Pigment (tan)	0	38	10	37	20	0	0
Beta-D-galactosidase (ONPG)	0	21	0	0	0	0	0
Oxidative-fermentative							
Glucose[c]	30	100	100	68[f]	80[f]	67	100
Lactose	0	86	0	0	0	0	0
Sucrose	0	0	0	0	0	0	100
Maltose	0	79	0	0	0	0	67
Mannitol[c]	15	21	0	0	0	17	100
Xylose	4	100	100	100	100	100	100
Fructose	96	64	100	12[f]	40[f]	92	100
Amides/salts							
Acetamide[c]	0	0	0	95	20	0	0
Allantoin	0	86	100	27	20	100	100
Citrate	37	100	100	100	100	67	100
Tartrate[c]	0	15	100	2	0	8	0
Colistin susceptible	100	0	0	85	33	82	67

[a]All strains were negative in tests for pyocyanin, fluorescein, lysine and ornithine decarboxylase, DNAse, lecithinase, and hemolysis on blood agar.
[b]Figures in parentheses indicate number of strains tested.
[c]Key characteristics.
[d]Results expressed as percent positive after 7 days' incubation.
[e]Peritrichous.
[f]Weak reaction.

TABLE 17-9. Biochemical and Morphologic Characteristics of Yellow-Pigmented, Oxidative Species

Test or Substrate[a]	Pseudomonas maltophilia (187)[b]	Pseudomonas cepacia (16)	Pseudomonas vesicularis (7)	Flavobacterium meningosepticum (10)	Flavobacterium indologenes (48)	Flavobacterium breve (2)	Pseudomonas paucimobilis (24)	Flavobacterium multivorum (11)	CDC Ve-1 (7)	CDC Ve-2 (25)
Motility										
Slide[c]	99[d]	88	14	0	0	0	25	0	100	80
Tube[c]	92	75	29	0	0	0	8	0	86	72
Flagella	>2	>2	1	0	0	0	1	0	>2	1
Oxidase[c]	17	88	100	100	100	100	71	100	0	0
Gluconate oxidation	0	69	0	0	0	0	0	0	0	36
Indole production[c]	0	0	0	100	72	100	0	0	0	0
Urease	26	94	0	0	10	0	0	100	86	60
Phenylalanine deaminase	13	0	14	0	17[e]	0	17	18	0	48
Lysine decarboxylase[c]	99	100	0	0	0	0	0	0	0	0
Arginine dihydrolase	0	0	0	0	0	0	0	0	57	0
Ornithine decarboxylase	0	50	0	0	0	0	0	0	0	0
Nitrite production[c]	31	50	14	10	25	0	0	11	14	4
Gelatinase[c]	100	88	14	90	100	100	4	0	71	12
Litmus milk peptonized	98	94	14	100	96	0	4	0	29	24
Deoxyribonuclease[c]	93	0	14	100	34	100	4	9	0	0
Lecithinase	0	73	0	0	0	0	0	0	0	0
Starch hydrolysis[c]	0	0	0	80	68	50	4	18[e]	14	32[e]
Esculin hydrolysis[c]	98	75	100	100	92	50	100	100	86	0
Growth on cetrimide	21	81	0	0	0	0	0	0	43	36
Growth at 42° C	60	78	0	67	31	50	40	13	100	13

MacConkey agar but oxidizes carbohydrates except for mannitol. The latter feature may distinguish this organism from the CDC Ve group. Other characteristics of the CDC Ve group include their positive reaction for motility, negative reaction for oxidase, and a tendency to form wrinkled colonies after 48 hours of incubation. All members of the group grow well on MacConkey agar and produce yellow colonies on this medium as well as on blood agar. CDC Ve-1 is multitrichous and is usually positive for arginine dihydrolase and esculin hydrolysis. It varies with regard to beta-galactosidase. CDC Ve-2 is monotrichous and negative for arginine dihydrolase, esculin hydrolysis, and beta-galactosidase. CDC Ve-2 is usually active against tartrate and may oxidize gluconate and deaminate phenylalanine. Members of the Ve group and *P. maltophilia* are susceptible to colistin, whereas *P. cepacia*, *P. paucimobilis*, and the flavobacteria are resistant.

The flavobacteria are nonmotile organisms that fail to grow on SS agar and grow poorly on MacConkey agar. As previously mentioned, except for *K. indologenes*, the flavobacteria are the only NFB that produce indole. On blood agar, *F. meningosepticum* is pale yellow (cream) in color, whereas *F. breve* and *F. indologenes* are yellow-orange. *F. meningosepticum* and *F. indologenes* are biochemically similar, although *F. meningosepticum* is more active in tests for deoxyribonuclease, beta-galactosidase, and mannitol oxidation, and *F. indologenes* usually produces a fruity odor. *F. (Sphingobacterium) multivorum* grows on MacConkey agar, is indole negative and urease positive, and oxidizes all carbohydrates except mannitol. Pigmentation of this organism develops after overnight incubation at room temperature.

Oxidase-negative, nonmotile bacteria (Table 17-10)

There is one species of *Acinetobacter: A. calcoaceticus*. This species includes the four varieties *anitratus, lwoffi, haemolyticus,* and *alcaligenes*. All members of the genus are oxidase-negative, nonmotile organisms that grow well on MacConkey agar and mimic the *Enterobacteriaceae* on blood agar. The cellular morphology varies considerably with most cultures

TABLE 17-9. Biochemical and Morphologic Characteristics of Yellow-Pigmented, Oxidative Species–cont'd

Test or Substrate[a]	Pseudomonas maltophilia (187)[b]	Pseudomonas cepacia (16)	Pseudomonas vesicularis (7)	Flavobacterium meningosepticum (10)	Flavobacterium indologenes (48)	Flavobacterium breve (2)	Pseudomonas paucimobilis (24)	Flavobacterium multivorum (11)	CDC Ve-1 (7)	CDC Ve-2 (25)
Growth on SS agar[c]	29[e]	0	0	0	0	0	0	0	14	16[e]
Growth on MacConkey agar[c]	100	94	29	30[e]	8[e]	100	0	18	100	100
Hemolysis	5	13	0	0	15	0	0	0	0	0
Wrinkled colonies[c]	0	0	0	0	0	0	0	0	60	88
Pigment (yellow)[c]	44	56	57	30	100	100	100	64	100	100
Beta-D-galactosidase (ONPG)[c]	64	100	43	100	36	0	79	91	29	0
Oxidative-fermentative										
Glucose[c]	52[e]	100	100	100	100	100	100	100	100	100
Lactose	7[e]	100	0	40	4	0	83	100	0	0
Sucrose	5[e]	88	0	0	29	0	96	100	14	24
Maltose[c]	99	94	86	90	100	100	100	100	86	100
Mannitol	0	88	0	90	8	0	0	0	57	96
Xylose[c]	8[e]	94	43	0	40	0	100	100	100	100
Fructose	66[e]	94	0	100	89	0	90	100	100	95
Amides/salts										
Acetamide	5	75	0	10	0	0	0	0	0	10
Allantoin	0	6	0	10	41	0	0	75	0	0
Citrate	96	100	0	40	65	0	4	0	100	100
Tartrate	5	100	0	0	0	0	11	0	0	71
Colistin susceptible[c]	85	6	17	0	0	0	14	0	100	100

[a]All strains were negative in tests for pyocyanin, fluorescein, and denitrification.
[b]Figures in parentheses indicate number of strains tested.
[c]Key characteristics.
[d]Results expressed as percent positive after 7 days' incubation.
[e]Weak reaction.

showing coccobacilli and diplococci, although diplobacilli, short rods, and even filaments are often present. *A. calcoaceticus* var. *anitratus* (Plate 11, *C*) and *A. calcoaceticus* var. *lwoffi* are nonhemolytic, whereas the other varieties are hemolytic. *A. calcoaceticus* var. *anitratus* and *A. calcoaceticus* var. *haemolyticus* oxidize glucose, lactose, and xylose, whereas *A calcoaceticus* var. *lwoffi* and *A. calcoaceticus* var. *alcaligenes* do not. *A. calcoaceticus* var. *haemolyticus* and *A. calcoaceticus* var. *alcaligenes* differ from the nonhemolytic varieties in proteolytic activity (gelatinase, caseinase, lecithinase) and growth on SS agar. *A. calcoaceticus* var. *lwoffi* is generally susceptible to ampicillin and chloramphenicol, whereas *A. calcoaceticus* var. *anitratus* is not.

Motile, nonoxidative bacteria (Table 17-11)

The nonoxidative pseudomonads have polar flagella, and the genus *Alcaligenes* has peritrichous flagella.

Pseudomonas. *P. acidovorans* and *P. testosteroni* are multitrichous, often exhibiting tufts of flagella at both poles.

Although *P. acidovorans* is technically an oxidizer because acid is produced from mannitol and fructose, activity is usually weak and late, and oxidation of glucose may be weak, equivocal, or negative. *P. acidovorans* is differentiated from *P. testosteroni* on the basis of its inability to grow at 42° C and its rapid alkalinization of acetamide, allantoin, and tartrate.

P. alcaligenes is monotrichous, with an ability to grow on cetrimide, reduce nitrate, and occasionally hydrolyze arginine. *P. putrefaciens* is proteolytic and has an unpleasant odor. It is the only pseudomonad other than *P. cepacia* to decarboxylate ornithine and is the only one to produce hydrogen sulfide in the stabbed portion of a TSI slant. *P. diminuta* usually fails to grow on amide media because of complex growth factor requirements and is variable in tests for gelatin liquefaction and DNAse production. The single polar flagellum of short wavelength is distinctive and has a corkscrew appearance. Colonies on solid medium produce a brown color.

Alcaligenes. These peritrichous NFB are short rods, almost coccobacillary, with flagellar arrangements varying from

TABLE 17-10. Biochemical Characteristics of Oxidase-Negative, Nonmotile *Acinetobacter* Spp.

Test or Substrate[a]	*A. anitratus*[b] (265)[c]	*A. haemolyticus* (25)	*A. lwoffi* (137)	*A. alcaligenes* (7)
Motility[d]	0[e]	0	0	0
Oxidase[d]	0	0	0	0
Urease	53	4	11	0
Phenylalanine deaminase	0	0	15	29
Nitrite production	0	0	6	0
Gelatinase[d]	1	64	1	57
Litmus milk peptonized[d]	5	88	3	86
Lecithinase	3[f]	56	9	100
Growth at 42° C	99	54	59	42
Growth on SS agar[d]	5	52	7	43
Growth on MacConkey agar	100	100	94	100
Hemolysis[d]	0	100	0	100
Oxidative-fermentative				
Glucose[d]	100	100	0	0
Lactose	95	88	0	0

TABLE 17-10. Biochemical Characteristics of Oxidase-Negative, Nonmotile *Acinetobacter* Spp.—cont'd

Test or Substrate[a]	*A. anitratus*[b] (265)[c]	*A. haemolyticus* (25)	*A. lwoffi* (137)	*A. alcaligenes* (7)
Sucrose	0	0	0	0
Maltose	13[f]	16[f]	0	0
Mannitol	0	0	0	0
Xylose[d]	100	100	0	0
Fructose	0	0	0	0
Amides/salts				
Acetamide	2	0	12[f]	0
Allantoin	3	4	1	0
Citrate	98	88	47	100
Malonate	83	48	30	71
Tartrate	49	16	3	0
Colistin susceptible	100	100	100	100

[a]All strains tested were negative for pyocyanin, fluorescein, gluconate oxidation, lysine and ornithine decarboxylase, arginine dihydrolase, denitrification, DNAse, starch hydrolysis, esculin hydrolysis, cetrimide tolerance, pigment, and beta-D-galactosidase.
[b]All organisms are biotypes of *A. calcoaceticus*.
[c]Figures in parentheses indicate number of strains tested.
[d]Key characteristics.
[e]Results expressed as percent positive after 7 days' incubation.
[f]Weak reaction.

degenerate to conspicuous. All species grow well on MacConkey agar. About half of the *A. faecalis* strains are able to reduce nitrate to nitrite. Gas is not produced. *A. denitrificans* reduces nitrate to nitrite and gas. *A. odorans* cannot reduce nitrate but can reduce nitrite to gas. Other differences among these species are the ability of *A. odorans* to grow at 42° C and on cetrimide agar and to alkalinize acetamide. *A. denitrificans* lacks these attributes but alkalinizes allantoin. A few strains of *A. faecalis* may alkalinize acetamide and tartrate. *A. odorans* has a highly characteristic fruity odor on solid medium and usually produces feather-edged colonies surrounded by a zone of green discoloration on blood agar. *Bordetella bronchiseptica* may be differentiated from *Alcaligenes* strains on the basis of urease activity. Strains of the rapid urea-splitting *B. bronchiseptica* and CDC IVc-2 are biochemically similar, except that the former reduces nitrate to nitrite and grows on SS agar and the latter fails to do so. Similar to the achromobacteria, CDC IVc-2 actively alkalinizes allantoin and tartrate.

Oxidase-positive, nonmotile, nonoxidative bacteria
(Table 17-12)

Flavobacterium sp. group IIf is an indole-positive organism that grows well on Martin-Lewis medium and is isolated almost exclusively from cervical cultures. It forms small colonies at 24 hours but increases in size and takes on a distinctive tan, mucoid appearance with continued incubation. *F. odoratum* is yellow and produces a strong, sweet odor similar to that of *F. indologenes*. *Flavobacterium* sp. group IIf is positive for indole and negative for urease, whereas *F. odoratum* is negative for indole and positive for urease.

The moraxellae are relatively inert biochemically but are susceptible to penicillin. Penicillin susceptibility can be determined by streaking a blood agar plate with growth from an 18- to 36-hour culture. A 10-unit penicillin disk is added to the plate before incubation. A zone of inhibition is considered a positive test. *M. phenlpyruvica* grows well on MacConkey agar and produces phenylalanine deaminase and urease, which distinguish it from the other *Moraxella* spp. Most strains of *M. urethralis* grow well on MacConkey agar. This organism alkalinizes citrate and may produce phenylalanine deaminase and lecithinase. *M. osloensis* grows well on blood and TSI agars, but the other species of *Moraxella* do not. This organism may also grow on MacConkey agar. *M. lacunata* is gelatinase positive and liquefies inspissated bovine serum in Loeffler serum slants, a characterisitic infrequently employed in the clinical laboratory. *M. nonliquefaciens* is inert except for its reduction

TABLE 17-11. Biochemical and Morphologic Characteristics of Motile, Nonoxidative Bacteria

Test or Substrate[a]	Pseudomonas acidovorans (24)[b]	Pseudomonas testosteroni (13)	Pseudomonas alcaligenes (14)	Pseudomonas diminuta (13)	Pseudomonas putrefaciens (4)	Pseudomonas aeruginosa (7) (Nonglucolytic)	Pseudomonas denitrificans (2)	Alcaligenes faecalis (12)	Alcaligenes denitrificans (8)	Alcaligenes odorans (21)	Bordetella bronchiseptica (6)	CDC IVc (15)
Motility												
Slide[c]	100[d]	100	100	100	100	29	100	100	100	100	100	87
Tube[c]	67	89	100	92	100	57	100	67	100	95	100	67
Flagella[c]	>2	>2	1	1	1	1	1	Peri[e]	Peri[e]	Peri[e]	Peri[e]	Peri[e]
Oxidase	100	100	100	100	100	100	100	100	100	100	100	100
Fluorescein	0	0	0	0	0	14	0	0	0	0	0	0
Urease[c]	0	11	7	15	80	29	0	0	0	0	100	100
Phenylalanine deaminase	0	6	14	23	0	0	100	17	0	0	0	0
Arginine dihydrolase	0	0	21	0	0	86	100	0	0	0	0	0
Ornithine decarboxylase[c]	0	0	0	0	100	0	0	0	0	0	0	0
Nitrite production[c]	100	83	100	0	100	100	50	50	38	0	100	0
Denitrification (N_2)[c]	0	0	0	0	0	100	100	0	88	0[f]	0	0
Gelatinase	13	6	0	69	100	0	0	0	0	0	0	0
Litmus milk peptonized	8	0	0	0	100	0	0	0	38	0	0	0
Deoxyribonuclease	0	0	0	15	100	0	0	0	0	0	0	0
Growth on cetrimide[c]	13	0	57	0	0	100	50	25	0	52	0	0
Growth at 42° C[c]	0	63	88	11	100	100	100	67	0	85	50	90
Growth on SS agar[c]	63	11	50	0	60	100	100	75	0	57	100	0
Growth on MacConkey agar	100	94	100	92	100	100	100	100	100	100	100	100
Pigment (tan, yellow)	0	0	7	69	80	0	100	0	13	19	0	0
Hydrogen sulfide[c]	0	0	0	0	100	0	0	0	0	0	0	0
Hemolysis	0	0	0	0	0	57	100	0	0	0	0	0
Amides/salts												
Acetamide[c]	100	0	0	0	0	100	0	25	0	100	0	0
Alantoin	96	33	0	0	0	80	0	8	88	0	33	100
Tartrate	100	12	0	0	0	0	0	17	0	14	0	91
Colistin susceptible[c]	13	100	100	18	60	100	100	100	0	100	100	92

[a]All strains were negative for pyocyanin, gluconate oxidation, lysine decarboxylase, indole, lecithinase, starch hydrolysis, esculin hydrolysis, oxidation of carbohydrates, and beta-D-galactosidase.

[b]Figures in parentheses indicate number of strains tested.

[c]Key characteristics.

[d]Results expressed as percent positive after 7 days' incubation.

[e]Peritrichous.

[f]Gas negative in nitrate broth; 100% positive in Sellers agar.

TABLE 17-12. Biochemical and Morphologic Characteristics of Oxidase-Positive, Nonmotile, Nonoxidative Bacteria

Test or Substrate[a]	Flavobacterium Sp. Group IIf (29)[b]	Flavobacterium odoratum (7)	Moraxella osloensis (26)	Moraxella nonliquefaciens (16)	Moraxella atlantae (5)	Moraxella urethralis (5)	Moraxella phenylpyruvica (2)	M-5 (16)[c]
Motility[d]	0[e]	0	0	0	0	0	0	0
Oxidase[d]	100	100	100	100	100	100	100	100
Indole[d]	97	0	0	0	0	0	0	0
Urease[d]	0	100	0	0	0	0	100	0
Phenylalanine deaminase	76	14	0	0	0	20	100	0
Nitrite production	0	0	15	100	0	0	100	19
Gelatinase[d]	93	100	0	0	0	20	0	0
Litmus milk peptonized	59	100	0	0	0	0	0	0
Deoxyribonuclease	72	29	4	0	20	0	0	14
Lecithinase	0	0	0	0	0	60	0	0
Growth on MacConkey agar[d]	3	43	27	0	0	80	100	0
Growth on blood abundant[d]	100	100	100	0	0	0	0	100
Pigment[d]	100	100	0	0	0	0	0	93
Mucoid	100	0	0	0	0	0	0	0
Amides/salts								
Acetamide	0	0	0	0	0	0	0	0
Allantoin	0	14	0	0	0	0	0	0
Citrate	0	0	0	0	0	100	0	0
Tartrate	0	0	0	0	0	20	0	0

[a]All strains were negative in tests for pyocyanin, fluorescein, gluconate oxidation, lysine and ornithine decarboxylase, arginine dihydrolase, cetrimide tolerance, starch hydrolysis, esculin hydrolysis, oxidation of carbohydrates, denitrification, beta-D-galactosidase, and growth on SS agar.
[b]Figures in parentheses indicate number of strains tested.
[c]M-6 and *Moraxella lacunata* are not included here because they are rarely seen in the clinical laboratory. See text for differentiating features.
[d]Key characteristics.
[e]Results expressed as percent positive after 7 days' incubation.

of nitrate to nitrite. *M. atlantae* is relatively inert, except for a few strains that are DNAse positive. It is negative for nitrite production, alkalinization of citrate, phenylalanine deaminase, and urease.

M-5 and M-6, yellow-pigmented *Moraxella*-like organisms, are recovered from mouths of dogs and cats and have been associated with bites and scratches from these animals. M-6 reduces nitrate to nitrite and is catalase negative. M-5 is catalase positive and usually does not produce nitrite.

Fastidious, nonoxidative bacteria (Table 17-13)

Members of the genus *Kingella* differ from the moraxellae in that they are usually catalase negative and ferment glucose. *Kingella denitrificans* and *Eikenella corrodens* require blood or blood products to grow and often exhibit pitting on blood agar. CO_2 enhances their growth, although both can grow in its absence. *K. kingae* and *K. indologens* do not require blood for growth, but they both can pit the agar, especially when freshly

isolated. *K. denitrificans* is a denitrifier that grows well on Martin-Lewis medium and is frequently recovered during surveys for *Neisseria* spp.

E. corrodens does not grow on Martin-Lewis medium. This organism frequently produces a characteristic odor of bleach. Nitrites are produced and lysine and ornithine are decarboxylated when a heavy inoculum is used.

EF-4 is a fermentative organism (in TSI agar) in 48 but not in 24 hours, and it frequently oxidizes glucose in OF medium. It usually produces nitrogen gas and is positive for arginine dihydrolase. *K. kingae* and *K. indologenes* both ferment glucose but differ from EF-4 in that *K. kingae* is beta-hemolytic and *K. indologenes* produces indole.

RAPID IDENTIFICATION SYSTEMS (see Chapter 9)

The introduction of commercial microtest systems has provided the clinical microbiology laboratory with simple, rapid, and relatively inexpensive means to facilitate the identification

TABLE 17-13. Biochemical and Morphologic Characteristics of Fastidious, Nonoxidative, Gram-Negative Bacteria

Test or Substrate[a]	*Kingella denitrificans* (15)[b]	*Kingella kingae* (3)	*Kingella indologenes* (2)	*Eikenella corrodens* (18)	EF-4 (10)
Motility[c]	0[d]	0	0	0	0
Oxidase[c]	100	100	100	94	100
Indole[c]	0	0	100	0	0
Urease	0	0	0	0	0
Phenylalanine	0	0	0	0	20
Nitrite production[c]	80	0	0	100	100
Denitrification[c]	100	0	0	0	60
Lysine decarboxylase	0	0	0	50	0
Arginine dihydrolase	0	0	0	0	50
Ornithine decarboxylase[c]	0	0	0	94	0
Gelatinase	0	0	0	0	10
Litmus milk peptonized[c]	0	100	100	0	0
Growth on TSI agar[c]	Poor	100	100	Poor	100
Growth on MacConkey agar	0	0	0	0	0
Growth on Martin-Lewis agar	93	0	0	0	0

TABLE 17-13. Biochemical and Morphologic Characteristics of Fastidious, Nonoxidative, Gram-Negative Bacteria—cont'd

Test or Substrate[a]	*Kingella denitrificans* (15)[b]	*Kingella kingae* (3)	*Kingella indologenes* (2)	*Eikenella corrodens* (18)	EF-4 (10)
Growth at 42° C	NT[e]	0	0	NT[e]	100
Hemolysis[c]	0	100	0	0	0
Pitting					
Blood agar	38	67	50	78	0
Chocolate agar	46	67	50	61	0
TSA plate					
Growth[c]	0	100	100	0	100
X factor[c]	0	0	0	94	0
CO_2 enhanced[c]	100	0	0	100	0
Odor (bleach)	0	0	0	78	0
Glucose-fermentation[c]	13	100	100	0	100

[a]All strains were negative in tests for pyocyanin, fluorescein, gluconate, cetrimide, starch hydrolysis, esculin hydrolysis, H_2S, alkalinization of amides and salts, beta-D-galactosidase, lecithinase, and deoxyribonuclease.
[b]Figures in parentheses indicate number of strains tested.
[c]Key characteristics.
[d]Results expressed as percent positive after 7 days' incubation.
[e]Not tested.

of NFB. These rapid systems include computer-generated interpretation manuals for convenience and standardization.

OTHER IDENTIFICATION PROCEDURES[7]
EPIDEMIOLOGIC TYPING

Typing of *P. aeruginosa* is extremely important in tracing the source of outbreaks caused by this organism. Typing enables the microbiologist to trace its travels between patients, hospital personnel, and the environment. It is important to know whether strains are nosocomially acquired and of exogenous or endogenous origin. Typing can save lives by revealing the sources of contamination leading to life-threatening situations.[86]

Many of the methods used for epidemiologic investigations of the *Enterobacteriaceae* are also used for *P. aeruginosa*. These include biotyping, antibiograms, serotyping, bacteriocin (pyocin) production, bacteriocin susceptibility, and bacteriophage typing.

Although biotyping and antibiograms are easy to perform, they are the least sensitive of the typing methods. They are able to distinguish unusual isolates but unable to differentiate more closely related strains. Serologic typing provides more reliable evidence for relatedness among strains. Until recently serologic

typing was not widely used for *Pseudomonas* isolates because of the lack of a standard set of antigenic strains and of commercially available antisera. The Subcommittee on *Pseudomonadaceae* and Related Organisms of the International Committee on Systematic Bacteriology has proposed an International Antigenic Typing Scheme (IATS). This scheme uses a total of 17 antigenic strains. Antisera to these 17 antigens are available from Difco (Detroit). Although Brokopp and Farmer[7] find serotyping to be the best and most practical typing procedure, it has limitations. Most important is its inability to differentiate among isolates that belong to the more common serogroups, especially O antigen 6. Bacteriocin typing or bacteriophage typing may be used for this purpose. Both of these procedures are usually performed in a reference laboratory.

Pyocins are the bacteriocins produced by *P. aeruginosa*. Pyocins are different from pyocyanin, the green-blue pigment produced by this organism. As with the *Enterobacteriaceae*, bacteriocin (pyocin) typing can be completed by a bacteriocin production procedure or by a bacteriocin susceptibility procedure. The former is most often used for *P. aeruginosa*. Pyocin typing is the most sensitive method for the study of nosocomial infections, especially when variation among strains is minimal. This is often the case in outbreaks caused by *P. aeruginosa*.

Although bacteriophage typing can be useful, it should not be used as the only typing method, since biologic and procedural variations often affect the lytic reactions.

The use of more than one typing method bolsters the confidence level of type designation of a strain.[86] Brokopp and Farmer[7] recommend the combined use of the antibiogram and serotyping as the most practical procedure. For situations in which serotyping cannot differentiate isolates with the same O antigen, the test organism should be sent to a reference laboratory for further characterization by pyocin or bacteriophage typing.

CLINICAL SIGNIFICANCE
PSEUDOMONADS

P. mallei and *P. pseudomallei* are serious obligate pathogens but are rarely isolated in the United States. The other pseudomonads, if pathogenic, are opportunistic pathogens. Their ability to grow in water with minimal nutrients enables them to thrive in the hospital environment.

The frequency of isolation of the pseudomonads varies according to species, as the following shows*:

Frequency	Organisms
Predominant	*P. aeruginosa*
Infrequent	*P. cepacia, P. fluorescens, P. maltophilia, P. putida, P. stutzeri*
Rare	*P. acidovorans, P. alcaligenes, P. pseudoalcaligenes, P. putrefaciens*
Very rare	*P. diminuta, P. mendocina, P. pickettii, P. testosteroni, P. thomasii, P. vesicularis,* Va-1, *P. denitrificans*
Very rare in United States but frequent in other geographic areas	*P. mallei, P. pseudomallei*

It is often difficult to evaluate the clinical significance of these isolates because they are usually recovered in combination with other bacteria. Furthermore, as with all nonfermenters, colonization occurs much more frequently than infection does. Nonetheless, the potential pathogenicity of many of these organisms under certain conditions should not be ignored.[17]

Pseudomonas aeruginosa[4,45]

P. aeruginosa has become a major cause of nosocomial infections over the past 30 to 40 years, currently accounting for approximately 10% of these infections.[62] This increased incidence has been largely attributed to the widespread use of antibiotics; the resistance of *P. aeruginosa* to most antimicrobial agents has allowed this organism to flourish while more susceptible organisms have been suppressed.

Hospitalized patients may become infected with *P. aeruginosa* from exogenous or endogenous sources. There are a multitude of potential reservoirs of *P. aeruginosa* in the hospital environment. In fact, serious infections have been traced to

---

*Modified from Bergan, T.: Human and animal pathogenic members of the genus *Pseudomonas*. In Starr, M.P., et al., editors: The prokaryotes: a handbook on habitats, isolation, and identification of bacteria, vol. 1, New York, 1981, Springer-Verlag.

infusion fluids, ophthalmologic solutions, soaps, hand creams, aqueous disinfectant quaternary ammonium solutions, and hydrotherapy tanks.[45] Person-to-person transfer may be a more important means of transmission.[19,38] The hands of hospital personnel may transmit organisms from patient to patient or from inanimate reservoir to patient.

Patients may become endogenously infected with organisms from their own respiratory or gastrointestinal (GI) tracts.[19] Only 5% to 10% of healthy individuals carry *P. aeruginosa* in their GI tracts; however, this percentage rapidly increases among hospitalized patients, largely because of the selective pressure of antibiotics.

P. aeruginosa infection rarely occurs in individuals with normal defenses but occurs frequently in patients who are granulocytopenic or immunosuppressed. Other predisposing conditions include the presence of extensive burns, immunologic immaturity, prior or concomitant antibiotic therapy, intravenous drug abuse, the presence of an indwelling foreign device (for instance, a vascular or urinary catheter), and cystic fibrosis. These conditions may lead to the following infections.

Burn wound infections[58]

Patients with extensive burns may become colonized with organisms from other patients or with organisms from their own GI tract. Burn injuries not only destroy the mechanical barrier of the skin but also adversely affect all other aspects of the immune system. Once the opportunistic *P. aeruginosa* has colonized the burn wound, it may multiply in the avascular eschar and spread to subeschar space. When the bacterial density exceeds 10^5 organisms/g of tissue, the organisms may pass through the subeschar space into viable tissue. Hematogenous dissemination and burn wound septicemia may occur.

Septicemia

Pseudomonas septicemia may occur in infants and immunocompromised patients, as well as in burn patients. Although not always present, ecthyma gangrenosum may be a clue to *Pseudomonas* septicemia. This skin lesion appears as a round, indurated, purple, blanched area about 1 cm in diameter with an ulcerated center and a surrounding zone of erythema. Lesions are most commonly seen on the buttocks, extremities, and perineum.

Respiratory disease

Hospital-acquired pneumonia occurs in patients with hematologic malignancies, diabetes, or chronic lung or heart disease, or in those who have undergone surgery or tracheostomy.

P. aeruginosa is also associated with the chronic pulmonary disease of patients with cystic fibrosis (CF). CF is a hereditary disorder characterized by a dysfunction of the exocrine glands. These glands secrete abnormal viscid mucus, which obstructs secretory ducts and organ passages, especially the bronchi, intestine, and pancreatic and biliary ducts. Chronic pulmonary disease is the primary cause of morbidity and mortality in these patients.

The pathogenesis of the pulmonary disease in CF is unresolved, although bacterial infection plays a large role and is responsible for the irreversible lung damage that occurs.[13] The abnormal, thick secretions in the lung may lead to impaired ciliary function, obstruction, and infection. Chronic infection may lead to bronchitis, bronchiectasis, fibrosis, and eventually respiratory failure and cor pulmonale.[37]

P. aeruginosa is isolated from the sputum of over 50% of patients with CF.[37] The isolates are quite mucoid. The propensity for *Pseudomonas* colonization is not understood, although the widespread use of antibiotics in these patients may play a role.[37] The inability of CF sera to opsonize *Pseudomonas* organisms and promote phagocytosis by alveolar macrophages may also contribute to colonization.

Other infections

P. aeruginosa causes approximately 70% of the cases of otitis externa. This is frequently observed among swimmers ("swimmer's ear") and is one of the few *Pseudomonas* infections that occurs in healthy individuals. Folliculitis, a dermatologic infection characterized by a syndrome of rash, malaise, otitis externa, and mastitis, may also occur in healthy hosts. This condition results from bathing in contaminated water and has been associated with the use of whirlpools, swimming pools,[26] and in one case a waterslide.[53] There have also been rare cases of community-acquired *Pseudomonas* pneumonia in individuals having no underlying disease.[15]

The most serious type of ear infection caused by *P. aeruginosa* is malignant otitis externa. Most frequently seen in diabetic patients, this condition begins as ordinary otitis externa but fails to respond to therapy. The condition may spread to involve the temporal bone and to cause osteomyelitis of the base of the skull and paralysis of certain cranial nerves.

P. aeruginosa may be responsible for the formation of corneal ulcers. This follows eye trauma involving a foreign body. If not treated properly or sometimes despite treatment, the ulcer may progress to panophthalmitis (an inflammation involving all the tissue of the eyeball) and blindness.

Meningitis is uncommon but may occur as the result of infection at a contiguous focus (such as otitis media) or as the result of direct inoculation of the organism into the nervous system during lumbar puncture or neurologic procedures. This disease is mostly seen in neonates or in patients with cancer.

Urinary tract infections usually occur in patients who have been treated with antibiotics or who have undergone genitourinary manipulations (for instance, insertion of a catheter). Endocarditis and osteomyelitis are most commonly seen in intravenous drug addicts. Why this population is predisposed to *Pseudomonas* infection is unknown, but it is probably related to the use of contaminated intravenous devices.

Pseudomonas maltophilia[87]

P. maltophilia is the second most frequently isolated pseudomonad. It is thought to be a common commensal or contaminant of clinical specimens and part of the transient flora of hospitalized patients.[21] This occasional opportunistic pathogen has been associated with a wide spectrum of disease, including pneumonia, endocarditis, cholangitis, meningitis, and urinary tract infections. With few exceptions these infections are nosocomial in origin and occur in compromised hosts. Endocarditis occurs in association with intravenous administration of drugs or as a complication of open-heart surgery, usually the insertion of a prosthetic valve. Meningitis is exceedingly rare, and infection of the urinary tract is uncommon. The latter infection is associated with instrumentation or manipulation of the urinary tract.

Pseudomonas cepacia[40,60]

P. cepacia organisms have been associated with nosocomial outbreaks of pneumonia, septicemia, urinary tract infections, and wound infections. Outbreaks are almost invariably related to the use of contaminated disinfectants used for antisepsis of the skin or for disinfecting devices later inserted into the patient, contaminated anaesthetics applied to wounds or other body sites, and contaminated parenteral solutions. Epidemic bloodstream infections have been traced to normal saline, human serum albumin, contaminated injectable anesthetics, aqueous chlorhexidine solution, and others. Epidemic infections or colonization of the respiratory tract, the urinary tract, and wounds have been traced to aqueous chlorhexidine, aqueous benzalkonium chloride, water, and topical tetracaine and cocaine solutions. Commercially prepared catheter kits have also been the source of urinary tract infections. Pseudobacteremias may occur when contaminated skin disinfectants are used.

Community-acquired infections are rare except in two instances. *P. cepacia* endocarditis is associated with intravenous drug abusers, and dermatitis has been observed among military troups training in swampy areas.

A recent development is the association of *P. cepacia* with respiratory infections in patients with cystic fibrosis.[31,41] These isolates have been shown to produce protease and lipase enzymes. Studies are under way to determine the role of these factors in disease.

Pseudomonas fluorescens and Pseudomonas putida[18]

P. fluorescens and *P. putida* represent part of the normal oropharyngeal flora, and most isolates are from respiratory tract specimens. Less common sources include wounds, pleural fluid, cerebrospinal fluid, urine, feces, skin lesions, and blood. These species have also been isolated from many sources in the hospital environment, including water sources, sinks, floors, contaminated blood and blood products stored in the refrigerator, benzalkonium chloride solution, and fluid from an ultrasonic nebulizer.

P. fluorescens and *P. putida* are usually environmental contaminants and only rarely opportunistic pathogens. The growth and release of endotoxins of these organisms into contaminated blood and blood products have resulted in cases of posttransfusion septicemia. Other associated infections include septic arthritis, abscesses, urinary tract infections, and wound infections.

Pseudomonas stutzeri

P. stutzeri has been isolated from urine, blood, wounds, cerebrospinal fluid, sputum, and middle ear discharge. It has been considered the cause of otitis media, a tibia wound infection, septic arthritis, urinary tract infections, and bacteremia.[23]

Pseudomonas pseudomallei[29]

P. pseudomallei causes melioidosis, a glanderslike or "melioid" disease of humans. This disease is primarily seen in Southeast Asia and less frequently in Central and South America, the West Indies, Madagascar, Australia, and Guam. Melioidosis has also been observed in the United States among military personnel who returned from Southeast Asia, especially Vietnam.[66] Melioidosis presents a wide spectrum of disease

TABLE 17-14. Clinical Significance of the Rare Pseudomonads

Organism	Specimens	Associated Conditions
P. acidovorans	Blood, abscess, urine, wound, urinary tract	One case of septicemia
P. alcaligenes	Blood, urine, respiratory tract	Empyema, endocarditis, neonatal septicemia
P. denitrificans	Blood, spinal fluid, wound	One case of bacteremia and meningitis[14]
P. mendocina	Urine	None
P. paucimobilis	Wound, blood, spinal fluid	Infected leg ulcer following trauma, a case of septicemia, a case of meningitis, a case of bacteremia following surgery for occlusive vascular disease of lower extremities[69]
P. pickettii	Blood, urine, wound, spinal fluid, abscess	Bacteremia, meningitis, outbreak of hospital-acquired colonization of the respiratory tract[59]
P. putrefaciens	Blood, urine, feces, sputum, wound secretion, abscess, ulcer, throat swab	Otitis media, a tibia wound infection, septicemia, purulent skin ulcerations of diabetic and debilitated patients
P. pseudoalcaligenes	Blood, urine, respiratory tract, spinal fluid	Postoperative knee infection, pneumonitis, septicemia, meningitis
P. stutzeri–like	Sputum, wound, ear	Unknown
P. testosteroni	Blood, abscess, urine, wound, urinary tract	One case of septicemia
P. vesicularis	Cervical	None
UFP-1[47]	Ear	Severe ear infections
UFP-2[47]	Sputum, stool	None

Data from references 18 and 21.

ranging from inapparent infection to acute pulmonary infection to overwhelming septicemia. In this last case the widespread dissemination of the organism is responsible for the multiple abscesses observed in nearly every organ of the body.

P. pseudomallei appears to be a normal inhabitant of soil and water in the regions just cited. Persons acquire the organism through wounds or abrasions that have been contaminated with soil, by inhalation of dust, or by ingestion.

Pseudomonas mallei[11,29]

P. mallei causes glanders, an equine infection that was prevalent when horses were the mainstay of civil and military transport but which has been largely eliminated today except in areas of Asia, Africa, and the Middle East. Sporadic cases are extremely rare in the Western world.

Glanders may appear in three forms in horses as well as in humans: an acute fatal septicemia, a chronic pulmonary form, and a form characterized by multiple abscesses in the skin, subcutaneous tissue, and lymphatics. This last form is known as farcy. Persons acquire the disease by contact with infected nasal secretions of equines. The organism usually enters the body through an abrasion or scratch, although primary nasal infection may occur. Laboratory-acquired infections may also occur, presumably as the result of aerosol transmission.

Other Pseudomonads

The sources of isolation and clinical significance of the other pseudomonads are summarized in Table 17-14.

ACINETOBACTER[22,61]

Members of the genus Acinetobacter are found universally in soil and water. They are also found as indigenous skin flora on approximately 25% of individuals and less frequently as normal flora of the pharyngeal region and genitourinary tract.

Acinetobacter is a common colonizer but an uncommon nosocomial opportunist. It has been associated with pneumonia, tracheobronchitis, urinary tract infections, surgical and burn wound infections,[25] skin infections, and septicemia. Most infections are associated with A. calcoaceticus var. anitratus.

Virtually all hospital-acquired infections occur in patients with one or more of the following predisposing conditions: prior antimicrobial therapy; surgery; residence in intensive care unit; instrumentation and manipulation including endotracheal intubation, urinary bladder catheterization, and arterial and venous cannulation; and severe underlying disease, either systemic (for instance, chronic obstructive pulmonary disease, malignancy) or localized to the infected area. Nosocomial infections have been traced to contaminated hospital equipment and instrumentation (including respiratory therapy equipment, dialysis baths, and tracheostomy equipment) and to the hands of hospital personnel. For unknown reasons there is a definite increase in the incidence of nosocomial infections caused by A. calcoaceticus var. anitratus during July through September.

Acinetobacter may also be responsible for community-acquired pneumonia; this occurs in older persons with chronic disease, especially alcoholism.[64] Community-acquired pneumonia has also been reported in foundry workers who were exposed to unacceptably high levels of free silica, metallic dusts, and total particulates.[10]

ALCALIGENES AND ACHROMOBACTER

A. faecalis is the most frequently isolated species of Alcaligenes. This organism has been recovered from blood, sputum, and urine specimens. It has been associated with nosocomially acquired septicemia and pyrexic reactions without septicemia. These cases were attributed to the contamination of hemodialysis fluid and intravenous solutions.

A. denitrificans has been isolated from blood, spinal fluid, urine, and ear discharges. A. odorans is recovered primarily from urine but is also seen in wounds, sputum, feces, and ear discharges.

Achromobacter xylosoxidans has been isolated from a wide variety of clinical material, including blood, sputum, wounds, urine, spinal fluid, and ears. This opportunistic pathogen has been associated with rare cases of meningitis, cervical lymphadenopathy,[28] pneumonia,[81] and ventriculitis following neurosurgical operations.[67] Contaminated chlorhexidine solution used to wash the surgeon's hands and to prepare the patient's skin for surgery was thought to be the source of those cases of ventriculitis.

MORAXELLA[27,63]

Members of the genus Moraxella are generally harmless parasites of the mucous membranes of humans and other warm-blooded animals. These organisms are rarely found in the inanimate environment.

Moraxella infections may be seen in noncompromised hosts outside of the hospital. Most Moraxella infections involve the eyes.

M. lacunata organisms appeared to have been a significant cause of human conjunctivitis and keratitis before 1920 but are currently isolated from these infections only rarely. One hospital study showed it to be responsible for 4% of all corneal ulcers* from 1970 to 1979.[1] A more recent report attributes less than 2% of corneal ulcers to this organism.[71] Almost all cases occur in the malnourished alcoholic population. Although infrequent, these infections are serious and respond poorly to antimicrobial therapy.[71]

M. nonliquefaciens is found as a harmless commensal of the respiratory tract. This organism is an extremely rare cause of meningitis, endocarditis,[72] bronchitis, and infections of the eye.

M. osloensis is part of the flora indigenous to the genitourinary tract, probably the skin, and less commonly the upper respiratory tract.[52] This organism is a rare cause of disease. It has been cultured from cases of septic arthritis, meningitis, urethritis, a necrotic mouth lesion, bacteremia, osteomyelitis,[73] and endocarditis.[72]

The natural habitat of M. phenylpyruvica is unknown. This organism has been recovered from blood, pus, the genitourinary tract, and cerebrospinal fluid. It is an opportunistic pathogen that is etiologically significant in the spinal fluid and potentially significant in the urinary tract.[52]

M. atlantae strains have been isolated from blood and cerebrospinal fluid. The pathogenicity of these organisms is

unknown. M. urethralis has been recovered from human genitourinary tract infections. As previously mentioned, M-5 and M-6, the unnamed organisms that resemble Moraxella, have been isolated from animal bites. M-6 has been associated with one case of endocarditis in a patient with mitral valve prolapse.[68]

FLAVOBACTERIUM[79]

The flavobacteria are rarely isolated from clinical specimens. With the exception of F. meningosepticum, the pathogenicity of these organisms is low grade or questionable.

F. meningosepticum is a cause of neonatal meningitis. There have been 100 cases of neonatal meningitis published since the first description of this disease in 1944. The overall case-fatality rate in these reports was 55%, and hydrocephalus developed in most of the survivors. Whether the organisms have an environmental or a maternal origin is unknown, although evidence points to the former. In either case the probable portal of entry is the pharynx. Only six cases of adult meningitis have been reported in the literature, and all of these patients had underlying diseases predisposing to gram-negative meningitis.

F. meningosepticum has been responsible for rare cases of pneumonia in adults and children. Colonization of the respiratory tract of compromised hosts may occur under epidemic situations.

Flavobacterium sp. group IIf and F. odoratum are most commonly recovered from the urogenital tract but are rarely clinically significant. Two wound isolates of F. odoratum have been considered significant; one was from an amputation site on a foot and the other from a gangrenous foot. F. indologenes has been associated with exceedingly rare cases of meningitis and septicemia, and F. multivorum with one case of peritonitis.

KINGELLA[5]

K. kingae is not commonly encountered in clinical specimens. The majority of isolates are from the blood or from bone- or joint-associated sites. Less common sources include the throat, pustules, wounds, and urine. The organism is an occasional normal inhabitant of the upper respiratory tract.

K. kingae is an opportunistic organism with pathogenic potential. It has been associated with cases of endocarditis, arthritis,[12] osteomyelitis,[12] diskitis, and septicemia.[16] Infections have been reported more frequently in children, both normal and immunosuppressed, than in adults. It is not known whether this prevalence represents a true predominance in the pediatric population or a pediatric reporting bias.

K. indologenes has been isolated from ocular lesions.[74] K. denitrificans has been responsible for two cases of endocarditis.[24,76]

EIKENELLA[39,75]

E. corrodens is part of the normal flora of human mucous membranes, especially the oronasopharynx and digestive tract. Disruption of these surfaces by trauma (for instance, dental manipulation) or surgery predisposes to infection. The organism may spread to contiguous areas or enter the bloodstream and be distributed to other parts of the body. E. corrodens is usually isolated in mixed culture, frequently with streptococci from human bite wounds. However, it has also been isolated in pure culture from patients with meningitis, endocarditis, subdural empyema, soft tissue abscesses, and various infections of

---

*Severe keratitis may lead to ulceration of the cornea.

the head and neck. Many of these patients have been immunocompromised.

EF-4

These organisms have been recovered from wounds, primarily dog bites and, less commonly, cat bites.

MECHANISMS OF PATHOGENICITY OF *PSEUDOMONAS AERUGINOSA*[4,36,54]

P. aeruginosa produces a number of virulence factors, including extracellular enzymes, toxins, and cell surface components (Table 17-15). The exact contribution of each of these structures or products to the pathogenicity of *P. aeruginosa* remains unclear; it probably varies according to the host's underlying disease and the anatomic location of the infection.[83]

PROTEOLYTIC ENZYMES

P. aeruginosa produces several proteolytic enzymes or proteases. The two major ones are elastase, an enzyme with activity against elastin, and a nonelastolytic alkaline proteinase, referred to as protease. The proteolytic enzymes are thought to be responsible for the hemorrhagic lesions that are frequently seen in the skin or internal organs. Furthermore, they are probably responsible for the destruction of the cornea when *P. aeruginosa* invades the eye. The elastase has also been associated with the lung damage of pneumonia[2] and, as mentioned in Chapter 2, with the inactivation of several complement components.

EXOTOXIN A[2]

Exotoxin A is the most toxic product produced by *P. aeruginosa*. It is cytotoxic for cultured eukaryotic cells and lethal for various mammalian species. The mechanism of exotoxin A is like that of diphtheria toxin; it interferes with protein synthesis by inhibiting the action of elongation factor 2 (see Chapter 21).

The extreme toxicity of exotoxin A, its production by most clinical isolates in vivo and in vitro, and the decreased virulence of non–toxin A–producing mutants all suggest a potential role for the exotoxin in the pathogenesis of *P. aeruginosa* infections. The precise role, however, is unknown.

PHOSPHOLIPASE AND GLYCOLIPIDS

These enzymes may play a significant role in *Pseudomonas* pneumonia. Phospholipase liberates phosphorylcholine from lecithin. Lecithin is the major component of the pulmonary surfactant, the substance that reduces the surface tension of the lung and prevents atelectasis (pulmonary collapse). Thus the production of phospholipase may result in destruction of the surfactant and consequent atelectasis. The glycolipids appear to enhance the activity of the phospholipase by acting as detergents and solubilizing the phospholipids.

CELL SURFACE COMPONENTS

Several cellular factors may contribute to the pathogenicity of *P. aeruginosa*. The pili may mediate attachment to epithelial cells and thus affect colonization.

The slime polysaccharide that forms the outermost part of the cell is composed of polysaccharide, nucleic acids, hyaluronic acid, lipid, and protein. This material can produce many

TABLE 17-15. Virulence Factors of *Pseudomonas aeruginosa*

Virulence Factors	Biologic Effects
EXTRACELLULAR PRODUCTS	
Proteases	Tissue invasion, cellular damage, decreased complement-mediated defense mechanisms
Exotoxin A	Cellular damage, toxicity for macrophages
Phospholipase	Destruction of pulmonary surfactant
CELL SURFACE COMPONENTS	
Pili	Adherence to epithelial cells (colonization)
Slime polysaccharide	Toxicity for neutrophils, endotoxin-like properties
Mucoid polysaccharide	Antiphagocytic effects, decreased pulmonary clearance
Lipopolysaccharide	Antiphagocytic, endotoxic

Modified from Peterson, P.K.: Host defense against *Pseudomonas aeruginosa*. In Sabath, L.D., editor: *Pseudomonas aeruginosa:* the organism, diseases it causes, and their treatment, Bern, Switzerland, 1980, Hans Huber Publications.

toxic effects, including leukopenia and death. The toxicity may reflect the presence of exotoxin.

The mucoid polysaccharide enables the organism to resist phagocytosis; this may be related to the inhibition of complement-mediated opsonization.

The lipopolysaccharide (LPS) of *P. aeruginosa* is much less potent than the endotoxin of other gram-negative bacilli. The endotoxic properties of the LPS reside in the lipid A portion. The O antigen portion of the LPS may inhibit phagocytosis.

ANTIMICROBIAL SUSCEPTIBILITY

Antimicrobial susceptibility results obtained using the standardized disk diffusion technique must be interpreted cautiously for several reasons when testing the NFB. First, the NCCLS standards for disk susceptibility tests (see Chapter 8) apply only to *P. aeruginosa;* none of the NFB zone sizes other than for *P. aeruginosa* have been adequately correlated with minimum inhibitory concentration (MIC) values. Second, Mueller-Hinton agar may not be the best medium for testing *all* NFB because of different nutritional requirements. Third, the NCCLS standards were designed for rapid growers, and the NFB grow at different rates. The balance between the rate of growth of the NFB and the diffusion of antimicrobial agents in the agar may not be realistic. Furthermore, the correct temperature for incubation of susceptibility tests of the NFB has not been determined. Temperature substantially affects the rate of growth of each species and can have profound effects on susceptibility results. Finally, there is insufficient data to correlate the results of the disk diffusion and MIC tests with clinical relevance. The NFB are viewed as being similar to the *Enterobacteriaceae* in their in vivo response to antimicrobial agents,

TABLE 17-16. Susceptibility of Nonfermentative Bacteria to Penicillin and Cephalosporin Group

Organism (Number of Isolates Tested)[a]	Ampicillin	Carbenicillin	Mezlocillin	Piperacillin	Cephalothin	Cefoxitin	Cefotaxime	Cefoperazone	Moxalactam
Pseudomonas aeruginosa (101)	0[b]	81	85	96	0	0	75	96	83
UFP-1 (7)	0	57	100	100	0	0	100	100	100
UFP-2 (6)	0	17	—	—	0	0	100	—	—
Pseudomonas putida (130)	0	1	81	94	0	0	56	80	21
Pseudomonas fluorescens (50)	0	0	83	100	0	3	33	95	14
Pseudomonas pseudomallei (6)	84	84	—	—	0	—	—	—	—
Pseudomonas stutzeri group (45)	90	98	93	100	2	86	86	100	93
Pseudomonas mendocina (4)	0	100	100	100	0	0	100	100	100
Pseudomonas pickettii bio. 1 (8)	44	55	100	100	100	100	100	100	90
Pseudomonas pickettii bio. 2 (5)	40	100	100	100	100	100	100	100	100
Pseudomonas vesicularis (6)	83	100	100	100	83	83	83	75	50
Pseudomonas pseudoalcaligenes (23)	56	100	100	100	0	20	100	100	100
Achromobacter xylosoxidans (39)	65	100	100	100	4	0	0	100	100
CDC Vd-1 (9)	9	18	0	0	9	20	20	100	60
CDC Vd-2 (3)	0	33	0	33	33	33	33	100	67
Pseudomonas maltophilia (160)	8	39	73	80	2	0	24	100	100
Pseudomonas cepacia (14)	0	6	100	100	0	0	93	—	62
Flavobacterium meningosepticum (9)	0	0	67	33	0	50	33	100	100
Flavobacterium indologenes (41)	8	32	100	100	8	91	35	100	17
Flavobacterium multivorum (7)	14	100	50	86	22	0	100	86	71
Pseudomonas paucimobilis (18)	81	95	10	11	24	100	100	0	0
CDC Ve (25)	96	96	100	100	11	25	100	100	100
Acinetobacter anitratus (221)	17	98	100	96	1	14	100	45	22
Acinetobacter lwoffi (113)	69	99	84	100	16	55	73	73	63
Pseudomonas acidovorans (22)	0	52	100	100	0	100	100	100	100
Pseudomonas testosteroni (14)	59	100	100	100	76	100	100	100	75
Pseudomonas alcaligenes (8)	45	100	100	100	36	100	100	100	100
Pseudomonas diminuta (10)	9	100	100	100	64	—	100	100	33
Pseudomonas putrefaciens (5)	80	100	100	100	0	100	100	100	100
Pseudomonas denitrificans (2)	0	100	—	—	0	0	—	—	—
Alcaligenes faecalis (11)	67	83	100	100	58	33	50	100	100
Alcaligenes odorans (19)	84	100	100	100	100	80	100	100	100
Alcaligenes denitrificans (5)	100	100	100	100	0	50	100	100	100
Bordetella bronchiseptica (6)	34	100	100	100	100	0	0	100	100
CDC IVc (11)	25	92	100	100	83	83	100	100	100
Flavobacterium sp. group IIf	100	100	—	—	100	100	100	—	—
Flavobacterium odoratum (7)	71	86	100	100	0	100	33	0	33
Moraxella spp. (44)	100	100	—	—	100	100	100	—	—
Kingella denitrificans (11)	100	100	—	—	100	100	—	—	—
Eikenella corrodens (14)	100	100	—	—	100	100	—	—	—
EF-4 (7)	100	100	100	100	55	100	100	100	100

[a]Not all organisms were tested with all agents.
[b]Results are expressed as percent susceptible.

but there is no supporting evidence for this.

Nevertheless, antibiograms are readily available and can offer supplemental information for identification of the NFB. Antibiograms of the NFB are shown in Tables 17-16 and 17-17, with the intermediate category of susceptibility included as susceptible.

The fluorescent pseudomonads are susceptible to the newer penicillins and cephalosporins (piperacillin and cefoperazone, respectively) as well as to the aminoglycosides. There is an inverse relationship in susceptibility to carbenicillin and kanamycin among the fluorescent organisms. Whereas *P. aerugino-*

TABLE 17-17. Susceptibility of Nonfermentative Bacteria to Aminoglycosides and Miscellaneous Antimicrobial Agents

Organism (Number of Isolates Tested)[a]	Kanamycin	Gentamicin	Tobramycin	Amikacin	Netilmicin	Chloramphenicol	Tetracycline	Nitrofurantoin	Trimethoprim-Sulfamethoxazole
Pseudomonas aeruginosa (101)	18[b]	91	100	77	100	7	7	0	2
UFP-1 (7)	100	100	100	100	100	0	86	0	—
UFP-2 (6)	100	100	100	100	—	0	50	0	0
Pseudomonas putida (130)	93	91	95	97	92	9	44	0	3
Pseudomonas fluorescens (150)	96	100	100	100	86	29	81	0	33
Pseudomonas pseudomallei (6)	100	0	—	—	—	100	100	0	—
Pseudomonas stutzeri (45)	100	100	100	100	100	67	100	0	100
Pseudomonas mendocina (4)	100	100	100	100	100	20	100	0	100
Pseudomonas pickettii bio. 1 (8)	89	78	78	78	75	89	100	0	100
Pseudomonas pickettii bio. 2 (5)	60	0	0	0	0	100	100	0	100
Pseudomonas vesicularis (6)	83	83	83	83	100	100	100	33	100
Pseudomonas pseudoalcaligenes (23)	92	100	100	100	100	68	100	0	100
Achromobacter xylosoxidans (39)	0	0	0	0	0	54	0	0	78
CDC Vd-1 (9)	18	91	100	100	100	18	100	20	100
CDC Vd-2 (3)	0	67	100	100	67	0	100	0	67
Pseudomonas maltophilia (160)	27	44	54	26	64	93	9	0	62
Pseudomonas cepacia (14)	56	31	13	0	0	100	0	0	0
Flavobacterium meningosepticum (9)	0	20	0	0	33	50	20	0	81
Flavobacterium indologenes (41)	20	52	0	37	17	44	24	33	100
Flavobacterium multivorum (7)	0	22	0	25	43	100	100	50	100
Pseudomonas paucimobilis (18)	71	95	86	86	100	95	100	25	100
CDC Ve (25)	100	100	100	100	100	93	100	17	89
Acinetobacter anitratus (221)	97	99	97	96	86	9	77	0	90
Acinetobacter lwoffi (113)	96	99	96	96	100	67	79	25	100
Pseudomonas acidovorans (22)	43	0	22	44	0	100	100	95	100
Pseudomonas testosteroni (14)	100	88	100	100	75	100	100	75	100
Pseudomonas alcaligenes (8)	100	91	100	100	100	73	100	36	100
Pseudomonas diminuta (10)	91	91	100	100	100	100	100	0	—
Pseudomonas putrefaciens (5)	100	100	100	100	100	100	100	100	100
Pseudomonas denitrificans (2)	100	100	100	100	—	0	100	—	—
Alcaligenes faecalis (11)	92	67	100	100	80	75	75	9	100
Alcaligenes odorans (19)	27	95	88	88	91	79	89	87	50
Alcaligenes denitrificans (5)	0	0	0	0	0	0	100	0	100
Bordetella bronchiseptica (6)	100	100	100	50	100	100	100	0	100
CDC IVc (11)	25	42	14	17	0	50	92	9	100
Flavobacterium sp. group IIf (19)	4	92	0	30	—	100	85	40	50
Flavobacterium odoratum (7)	0	0	0	0	0	29	29	0	—
Moraxella spp. (44)	100	100	100	100	—	100	100	—	—
Kingella denitrificans (11)	100	100	100	100	—	100	100	—	—
Eikenella corrodens (14)	100	100	100	100	—	100	100	—	—
EF-4 (7)	100	100	100	78	100	100	100	100	100

[a]Not all organisms were tested with all agents.
[b]Results are expressed as percent susceptible.

sa is usually susceptible to carbenicillin and resistant to kanamycin, the reverse is seen for *P. putida* and *P. fluorescens*. The unidentified fluorescent pseudomonads are similar to *P. putida* and *P. fluorescens* in being susceptible to kanamycin and tetracycline and similar to *P. aeruginosa* in partial susceptibility to carbenicillin.

The *stutzeri* group, in contrast to *P. pseudomallei*, is sensi-

tive to a wide range of agents, especially the aminoglycosides. The response to ampicillin is also marked. *P. pickettii* biovars 1 and 2 are similar in their susceptibility to antimicrobial agents, with the exception of the aminoglycosides. A striking difference in susceptibility is seen with the various species of achromobacteria. Whereas *A. xylosoxidans* is susceptible to the penicillins, newer cephalosporins, and chloramphenicol and resistant to all of the aminoglycosides and tetracycline, the exact opposite holds for groups Vd-1 and Vd-2.

For the most part the yellow-pigmented organisms are resistant to antimicrobial agents, especially the aminoglycosides. However, the newer penicillins (mezlocillin and piperacillin) and cephalosporins (cefoperazone and moxalactam) have activity against this group. Most strains are susceptible to chloramphenicol and trimethoprim-sulfamethoxazole; the exception is *P. cepacia,* which is resistant to trimethoprim-sulfamethoxazole. *P. paucimobilis* and CDC Ve are susceptible to a wide range of agents, especially ampicillin and carbenicillin. Responses to cefoperazone and moxalactam, however, are markedly different; *P. paucimobilis* is resistant to these agents.

The susceptibility patterns of *P. acidovorans* and *P. testosteroni* are noticeably different; the latter organism is more susceptible to ampicillin, cephalothin, and the aminoglycosides. *P. alcaligenes* and the closely related *P. pseudoalcaligenes* are similar in susceptibility, except against ampicillin. The nonoxidative pseudomonads (except for *P. diminuta*) are usually susceptible to nitrofurantoin, whereas the *Alcaligenes* spp. (except for *A. odorans*) are not.

A. faecalis and *A. odorans* are susceptible to a wide range of antimicrobial agents, unlike *A. denitrificans,* which is resistant to the aminoglycosides, cephalothin, and chloramphenicol. *B. bronchiseptica* is resistant to cefoxitin and cephotaxime but susceptible to the aminoglycosides, whereas CDC IVc is just the opposite.

The moraxellae are usually susceptible to a wide range of antimicrobial agents, with a unique feature of being susceptible to penicillin.

REFERENCES

1. Ashell, P. and Stenson, S.: Ulcerative keratitis: survey of 30 years' laboratory experience, Arch. Ophthalmol. **100:**77, 1982.
2. Blackwood, L.L., et al.: Evaluation of *Pseudomonas aeruginosa* exotoxin A and elastase as virulence factors in acute lung infection, Infect. Immun. **39:**198, 1983.
3. Blazevic, D.J., Koepcke, M.H., and Matsen, J.M.: Incidence and identification of *Pseudomonas fluorescens* and *Pseudomonas putida* in the clinical laboratory, Appl. Microbiol. **25:**107, 1973.
4. Bodey, G.P., et al.: Infection caused by *Pseudomonas aeruginosa,* Rev. Infect. Dis. **5:**279, 1983.
5. Bosworth, D.E.: *Kingella (Moraxella) kingae* infections in children, Am. J. Dis. Child. **137:**650, 1983.
6. Bottone, E.J., Kittick, J., and Schneierson, S.S.: Isolation of bacillus HB-1 from human clinical sources, Am. J. Clin. Pathol. **59:**560, 1973.
7. Brokopp, C.D., and Farmer, J.J., III: Typing methods for *Pseudomonas aeruginosa.* In Doggett, R.G., editor: *Pseudomonas aeruginosa:* clinical manifestations of infection and current therapy, New York, 1979, Academic Press, Inc.
8. Chester, B., and Cooper, L.H.: *Achromobacter* species (CDC group Vd): morphologic and biochemical characterization, J. Clin. Microbiol. **9:**425, 1979.
9. Christensen, W.B.: Urea decomposition as a means of differentiating *Proteus* and paracolon cultures from each other and from *Salmonella* and *Shigella* types, J. Bacteriol. **52:**461, 1946.
10. Cordes, L.G., et al.: A cluster of *Acinetobacter* pneumonia in foundry workers, Ann. Intern. Med. **95:**688, 1981.
11. Davis, C.E.: Glanders (farcy). In Braude, A., editor: Medical microbiology and infectious diseases, Philadelphia, 1981, W.B. Saunders Co.
12. Davis, J.M., and Peel, M.M.: Osteomyelitis and septic arthritis caused by *Kingella kingae,* J. Clin. Pathol. **35:**219, 1982.
13. Fick, R.B., Jr.: *Pseudomonas* in cystic fibrosis: sylph or sycophant? Clin. Chest Med. **2:**91, 1981.
14. Fischer, R.A., Doern, G.V., and Cheeseman, S.H.: *Pseudomonas dentrificans* meningitis, J. Clin. Microbiol. **13:**1004, 1981.
15. Fishman, H., et al.: Primary *Pseudomonas* pneumonia in a previously healthy man, South. Med. J. **76:**260, 1983.
16. Förstl, H., et al.: Septicemia caused by *Kingella kingae,* Eur. J. Clin. Microbiol. **3:**267, 1984.
17. Gilardi, G.L.: Infrequently encountered *Pseudomonas* species causing infection in humans, Ann. Intern. Med. **77:**211, 1972.
18. Gilardi, G.L.: *Pseudomonas* species in clinical microbiology, Mt. Sinai J. Med. **43:**710, 1976.
19. Gilardi, G.L.: Medical microbiology. In Sabath, L.D., editor: *Pseudomonas aeruginosa:* the organism, diseases it causes, and their treatment, Bern, Switzerland, 1980, Hans Huber Publishers.
20. Gilardi, G.L., editor: Nonfermentative gram-negative rods: laboratory identification and clinical aspects, New York, 1985, Marcel Decker, Inc.
21. Gilardi, G.L.: *Pseudomonas.* In Lennette, E.H., et al., editors: Manual of clinical microbiology, ed. 4, Washington, D.C., 1985, American Society for Microbiology.
22. Glew, R.H., Moellering, R.C., and Kunz, L.J.: Infections with *Acinetobacter calcoaceticus (Herellea vaginicola):* clinical and laboratory studies, Medicine **56:**79, 1977.
23. Goetz, A., et al.: *Pseudomonas stutzeri* bacteremia associated with hemodialysis, Arch. Intern. Med. **143:**1909, 1983.
24. Goldman, I.S., et al.: Infective endocarditis due to *Kingella denitrificans,* Ann. Intern. Med. **93:**152, 1980.
25. Green, A.R., and Milling, M.A.P.: Infection with *Acinetobacter* in a burns unit, Burns Incl. Therm. Inj. **9:**292, 1983.
26. Gustafson, T.L., et al.: *Pseudomonas folliculitis:* an outbreak and review, Rev. Infect. Dis. **5:**1, 1983.
27. Henriksen, S.D.: *Moraxella, Acinetobacter,* and the *Mimeae,* Bacteriol. Rev. **37:**522, 1973.
28. Holmes, B., Snell, J.J.S., and Lapage, S.P.: Strains of *Achromobacter xylosoxidans* from clinical material, J. Clin. Pathol. **30:**595, 1977.
29. Howe, C., Sampath, A., and Spotnitz, M.: The *Pseudomallei* group: a review, J. Infect. Dis. **124:**598, 1971.
30. Hugh, R., and Leifson, E.: The taxonomic significance of fermentative versus oxidative metabolism of carbohydrates by various gram-negative bacteria, J. Bacteriol. **66:**24, 1953.
31. Isles, A., et al.: *Pseudomonas cepacia* infection in cystic fibrosis: an emerging problem, J. Pediatr. **104:**206, 1984.
32. King, E.O., Ward, M.K., and Raney, D.E.: Two simple media for the demonstration of pycocyanin and fluorescin, J. Lab. Clin. Med. **44:**301, 1954.
33. Kovacs, N.: Identification of *Pseudomonas pyocyanea* by the oxidase reaction, Nature **178:**703, 1956.
34. Krieg, N.R., editor (Holt, J.G., editor-in-chief): Bergey's manual of systematic bacteriology, vol. 1, Baltimore, 1984, Williams & Wilkins Co.
35. Lee, W.: Use of Mueller-Hinton agar as amylase-testing medium, J. Clin. Microbiol. **4:**312, 1976.
36. Liu, P.V.: Extracellular toxins of *Pseudomonas aeruginosa,* J. Infect. Dis. **130**(suppl.):94, 1974.
37. Lloyd-Still, J.D., editor: Textbook of cystic fibrosis, Littleton, Mass., 1983, John Wright Publishing, Inc.
38. Lowbury, E.J.L., et al.: Sources of infection with *Pseudomonas aeruginosa* in patients with tracheostomy, J. Med. Microbiol. **3:**39, 1970.
39. Maia, A., et al.: Isolation of *Eikenella corrodens* from human infections: report of six cases, J. Infect. **2:**347, 1980.
40. Martone, W.J., et al.: *Pseudomonas cepacia:* implications and control of epidemic nosocomial colonization, Rev. Infect. Dis. **3:**708, 1981.

41. McKevitt, A.I., and Woods, D.E.: Characterization of *Pseudomonas cepacia* isolates from patients with cystic fibrosis, J. Clin. Microbiol. **19:**291, 1984.

42. Moeller, V.: Simplified tests for some amino acid decarboxylases and for the arginine dihydrolase system, Acta Pathol. Microbiol. Scand. **36:**153, 1955.

43. Moore, H.B., and Pickett, M.J.: The *Pseudomonas-Achromobacter* group, Can. J. Microbiol. **6:**35, 1960.

44. Neu, H.C.: Clinical role of *Pseudomonas aeruginosa*. In Gilardi, G.L., editor: Glucose nonfermenting gram-negative bacteria in clinical microbiology, Boca Raton, Fla., 1978, CRC Press, Inc.

45. Neu, H.C.: The role of *Pseudomonas aeruginosa* in infections, J. Antimicrob. Chemother. **2**(suppl. B):1, 1983.

46. Oberhofer, T.R.: Growth of nonfermentative bacteria at 42° C, J. Clin. Microbiol. **10:**800, 1979.

47. Oberhofer, T.R.: Characteristics of human isolates of unidentified fluorescent pseudomonads capable of growth at 42° C, J. Clin. Microbiol. **14:**492, 1981.

48. Oberhofer, T.R.: Manual of nonfermentative gram-negative bacteria, New York, 1985, John Wiley & Sons, Inc.

49. Oberhofer, T.R., and Rowen, J.W.: Acetamide agar for differentiation of nonfermentative bacteria, Appl. Microbiol. **28:**720, 1974.

50. Oberhofer, T.R., Rowen, J.W., and Cunningham, G.F.: Characterization and identification of gram-negative, nonfermentative bacteria, J. Clin. Microbiol. **5:**208, 1977.

51. Oberhofer, T.R., et al.: Evaluation of the rapid decarboxylase and dihydrolase tests for the differentiation of nonfermentative bacteria, J. Clin. Microbiol. **3:**137, 1976.

52. Pedersen, M.M., Marso, E., and Pickett, M.J.: Nonfermentative bacilli associated with man. III. Pathogenicity and antibiotic susceptibility, Am. J. Clin. Pathol. **54:**178, 1970.

53. Perrotta, D.M., et al.: An outbreak of *Pseudomonas* folliculitis associated with a waterslide—Utah, JAMA **250:**1259, 1983.

54. Peterson, P.K.: Host defense against *Pseudomonas aeruginosa*. In Sabath, L.D., editor: *Pseudomonas aeruginosa*: the organism, diseases it causes, and their treatment, Bern, Switzerland, 1980, Hans Huber Publishers.

55. Pickett, M.J., and Pedersen, M.M.: Screening procedure for partial identification of nonfermentative bacilli associated with man, Appl. Microbiol. **36:**1631, 1968.

56. Pickett, M.J., and Pedersen, M.M.: Characterization of saccharolytic nonfermentative bacteria associated with man, Can. J. Microbiol. **16:**351, 1970.

57. Pickett, M.J., and Pedersen, M.M.: Salient features of non-saccharolytic and weakly saccharolytic rods, Can. J. Microbiol. **16:**401, 1970.

58. Pruitt, B.A.: Infections of burns and other wounds caused by *Pseudomonas aeruginosa*. In Sabath, L.D., editor: *Pseudomonas aeruginosa*: the organism, diseases it causes, and their treatment, Bern, Switzerland, 1980, Hans Huber Publishers.

59. *Pseudomonas pickettii* colonization associated with a contaminated respiratory therapy solution—Illinois, MMWR **32:**495, 1983.

60. Randall, C.: The problem of *Pseudomonas cepacia* in a hospital, Can. J. Pub. Health **71:**119, 1980.

61. Retailliau, H.F., et al.: *Acinetobacter calcoaceticus*: a nosocomial pathogen with an unusual seasonal pattern, J. Infect. Dis. **139:**371, 1979.

62. Rhame, F.S.: The ecology and epidemiology of *Pseudomonas aeruginosa*. In Sabath, L.D., editor: *Pseudomonas aeruginosa*: the organism, diseases it causes, and their treatment, Bern, Switzerland, 1980, Hans Huber Publishers.

63. Rosenthal, S.L.: Clinical role of *Acinetobacter* and *Moraxella*. In Gilardi, G.L., editor: Glucose nonfermenting gram-negative bacteria in clinical microbiology, Boca Raton, Fla., 1978, CRC Press, Inc.

64. Rudin, M.L., Michael, J.R., and Huxley, E.J.: Community-acquired *Acinetobacter* pneumonia, Am. J. Med. **67:**39, 1979.

65. Sellers, W.: Medium for differentiating the gram-negative, nonfermenting bacilli of medical interest, J. Bacteriol. **87:**46, 1964.

66. Shaefer, C.F., Trincher, R.C., and Rissing, J.P.: Melioidosis: recrudescence with a strain resistant to multiple antimicrobials, Am. Rev. Respir. Dis. **128**(suppl.):173, 1983.

67. Shigeta, S., et al.: Cerebral ventriculitis associated with *Achromobacter xylosoxidans*, J. Clin. Pathol. **31:**156, 1978.

68. Simor, A.E., and Salit, I.E.: Endocarditis caused by M6, J. Clin. Microbiol. **17:**931, 1983.

69. Southern, P.M., Jr., and Kutscher, A.E.: *Pseudomonas paucimobilis* bacteremia, J. Clin. Microbiol. **13:**1070, 1981.

70. Steel, K.J.: The oxidase reaction as a taxonomic tool, J. Gen. Microbiol. **25:**297, 1961.

71. Stern, G.A.: *Moraxella* corneal ulcers: poor response to medical treatment, Ann. Ophthalmol. **14:**295, 1982.

72. Stryker, T.D., Stone, W.J., and Savage, A.M.: Renal failure secondary to *Moraxella osloensis* endocarditis, Johns Hopkins Med. J. **150:**217, 1982.

73. Sugarman, B., and Clarridge, J.: Osteomyelitis caused by *Moraxella osloensis*, J. Clin. Microbiol. **15:**1148, 1982.

74. Sutton, R.G.A., et al.: Isolation of a new *Moraxella* from a corneal abscess, J. Med. Microbiol. **5:**148, 1972.

75. Suwanagool, S., et al.: Pathogenicity of *Eikenella corrodens* in humans, Arch. Intern. Med. **143:**2265, 1983.

76. Swann, R.A., and Holmes, B.: Infective endocarditis caused by *Kingella denitrificans*, J. Clin. Pathol. **37:**1384, 1984.

77. Swings, J., et al.: Transfer of *Pseudomonas maltophilia* (Hugh 1981) to the genus *Xanthomonas*, *Xanthomonas maltophilia* (Hugh 1981) comb. nov., Int. J. Syst. Bacteriol. **33:**409, 1983.

78. Tatum, H.W., Ewing, W.H., and Weaver, R.E.: Miscellaneous gram-negative bacteria. In Lennette, E.H., Spaulding, E.H., and Truant, J.P., editors: Manual of clinical microbiology, ed. 2, Washington, D.C., 1974, American Society for Microbiology.

79. von Graevenitz, A.: Clinical significance and antimicrobial susceptibility of *Flavobacteria*. In Reichenbach, H., and Weeks, O.B., editors: The *Flavobacterium-cytophaga* group, Verlag Cheme, 1981, Gesellschaft fur Biotechnologische Forschung.

80. Weaver, R.E., et al.: The identification of unusual pathogenic gram-negative bacteria, Atlanta, 1983, Centers for Disease Control.

81. Welk, S.W.: *Achromobacter* pneumonia, West. J. Med. **136:**349, 1982.

82. West, M., Burdash, N.M., and Freimuth, F.: Simplified silver-plating stain for flagella, J. Clin. Microbiol. **6:**414, 1977.

83. Woods, D.E., and Iglewski, B.H.: Toxins of *Pseudomonas aeruginosa*: new perspectives, Rev. Infect. Dis. **5**(suppl. 4):S715, 1983.

84. Yabuuchi, E., et al.: *Sphingobacterium* gen. nov., *Sphingobacterium spiritivorum* comb. nov., *Sphingobacterium mizutae* sp. nov., and *Flavobacterium indologenes* sp. nov.: glucose-nonfermenting gram-negative rods in CDC groups IIK-2 and IIb, Int. J. Syst. Bacteriol. **33:**580, 1983.

85. Yabuuchi, E., and Yano, I.: *Achromobacter* gen. nov. and *Achromobacter xylosoxidans* (ex Yabuuchi and Ohyama 1971) nom. rev., Int. J. Syst. Bacteriol. **31:**477, 1981.

86. Zierdt, C.H.: Systems for typing *Pseudomonas aeruginosa*. In Gilardi, G.L., editor: Glucose nonfermenting gram-negative bacteria in clinical microbiology, West Palm Beach, Fla., 1978, CRC Press.

87. Zuravleff, J.J., and Yu, V.L.: Infections caused by *Pseudomonas maltophilia* with emphasis on bacteremia: case reports and a review of the literature, Rev. Infect. Dis. **4:**1236, 1982.

CHAPTER 18

Vibrio

Edward J. Bottone
J. Michael Janda

The genus *Vibrio* contains a large group of organisms that are found in surface and marine waters. The greater utilization of aquatic environments for leisure time and scientific activities has heightened exposure to marine bacteria, and as a result more individuals are seeking medical attention for infections caused by *Vibrio* spp.

CLASSIFICATION

The genus *Vibrio* is one of four genera in the family *Vibrionaceae*. This family is classified in *Bergey's Manual of Systematic Bacteriology*[1] as family II in section 5, "Facultatively Gram-Negative Rods." *Aeromonas, Plesiomonas*, and *Photobacterium* are the other genera in the family *Vibrionaceae*. *Photobacterium* has not been implicated in human pathology and is not considered in this book. *Aeromonas* and *Plesiomonas* are discussed in Chapter 19.

The requisite features for inclusion in the genus *Vibrio* are as follows[1]:

1. Gram-negative, straight or curved rods, spheroplasts
2. Flagella: polar, sheathed after growth in liquid media
3. Fermentative—anaerogenic, rare aerogenic
4. Butylene glycol production (variable)
5. Indole-positive members
6. Urease negative (except that *V. damsela* and rare strains of *V. parahaemolyticus* are urease positive)
7. Oxidase positive (except that *V. metschnikovii* is oxidase negative)
8. 0/129 sensitivity (2,4,diamino-6,7-diisopropylpteridine phosphate)
9. Found in fresh and salt water
10. Halotolerant (most species)
11. Nitrate reduction

For several years, various investigators in Europe, the United States, and Bangladesh have been studying a number of *Vibrio*-like organisms isolated from patients with diarrhea, soft tissue, or bacteremic infections. Since these *Vibrio*-like isolates had not been assigned species status, they were given various appellations as group F vibrios[9] or group EF6,[14] group EF5,[29] group EF13,[11] and "lactose-positive marine vibrios."[31] Subsequent DNA/DNA hybridization studies and biochemical (phenotypic) characterization have led to the following proposed species: *V. fluvialis* (EF6),[26] *V. damsela* (EF5),[29] *V. hollisae* (EF13),[11] and *V. (Beneckea) vulnificus*[7] for the lactose-positive species. The genus *Beneckea*, which formerly included a number of *Vibrio*-like species, has been abolished with assignment of its constituent species to the genus *Vibrio*.[2] *V. metschnikovii*, a recently redefined,[25] oxidase-negative organism, has also been implicated in human bacteremic disease,[15] while *V. mim-*

icus (formerly thought to be an "atypical *V. cholerae*") has received species status distinct from the cholera bacillus.[5] *V. mimicus* differs from true *V. cholerae* because it is sucrose and Voges-Proskauer negative. As a result of these studies, the genus *Vibrio* now contains at least 25 species, 11 of which have been implicated in human disease. The *Vibrio* spp. follow:

1. Species associated with human disease
   a. *V. alginolyticus*
   b. *V. cholerae*
   c. *V. cincinnatiensis*
   d. *V. damsela*
   e. *V. fluvialis*
   f. *V. furnissii*
   g. *V. hollisae*
   h. *V. metschnikovii*
   i. *V. mimicus*
   j. *V. parahaemolyticus*
   k. *V. vulnificus*
2. Species not associated with human disease
   a. *V. anguillarum*
   b. *V. campbellii*
   c. *V. costicola*
   d. *V. fischeri*
   e. *V. gazogenes*
   f. *V. harveyi*
   g. *V. logei*
   h. *V. marinus*
   i. *V. natriegens*
   j. *V. nereis*
   k. *V. nigripulchritudo*
   l. *V. pelagius*
   m. *V. proteolyticus*
   n. *V. splendidus*

SPECIMEN COLLECTION AND PROCESSING

Formed or liquid (rice water) stool or swab specimens should be transported in Cary-Blair medium; buffered glycerol saline is unsuitable. Rectal swabs should be submitted only during the acute phase of diarrheal illness. In the absence of suitable transport media, strips of blotting paper may be soaked in rice water stool and submitted to the laboratory in zip-lock specimen bags.

GROWTH REQUIREMENTS
MEDIA

Vibrios are not fastidious in their growth factor requirements. Colonies develop quite readily on a variety of routinely used bacteriologic media. The introduction of thiosulfate-

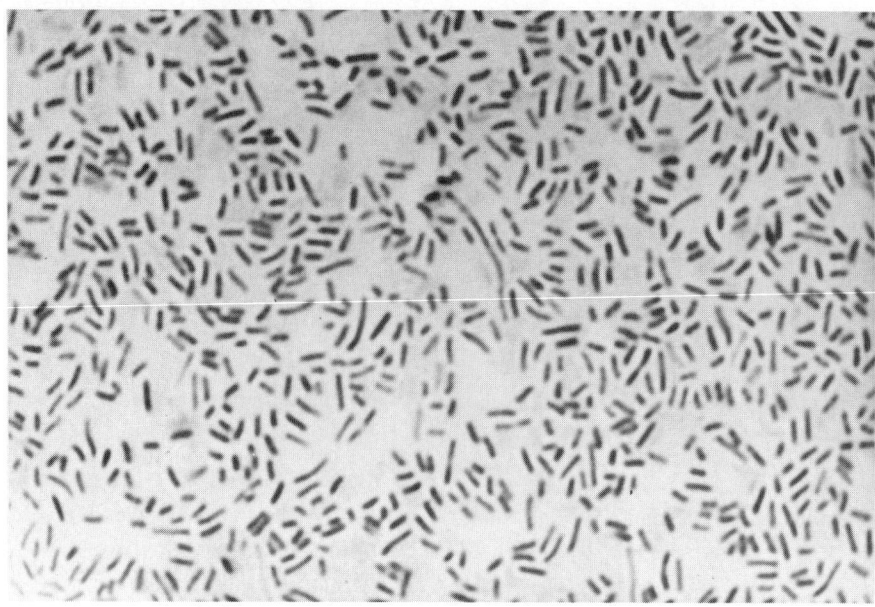

FIGURE 18-1. Typical slightly curved rods of *Vibrio* spp.

citrate–bile salts–sucrose (TCBS) agar[21] has greatly facilitated the recovery of *Vibrio* spp. from highly contaminated specimens such as feces. However, not all species grow on TCBS. Indeed, *V. hollisae* and some strains of *V. metschnikovii* may fail to initiate growth on this selective medium.[25,26,29] Inoculation of an enrichment broth (such as alkaline peptone water) is also recommended for recovery of *Vibrio* spp. Enrichment should be routine for possible *V. cholerae* carriers, contacts of cholera patients, and patients receiving antimicrobial therapy. In these instances bulk stool specimens should be submitted to enhance recovery.[32]

ENVIRONMENTAL REQUIREMENTS

The vibrios are facultative anaerobes. All cultures should be incubated at 35° C in air or a CO_2 incubator. Most species form 1 to 2 mm colonies within 24 hours.

CULTURAL CHARACTERISTICS
MICROSCOPIC MORPHOLOGY

Vibrios may be characterized as gram-negative, straight or slightly curved rods (Figure 18-1) with a tendency to produce spheroplasts, especially after prolonged incubation. The flagella, which impart a rapid, darting motility, are usually polar and are sheathed after growth in liquid medium. Some strains may have lateral flagella.[1] Spores and capsules have not been observed.

COLONIAL MORPHOLOGY

The appearance of colonies on TCBS agar depends on whether the organism can ferment sucrose. Species fermenting sucrose, for example, *V. cholerae* and *V. alginolyticus*, form yellow colonies in contrast to the green colonies of species, such as *V. mimicus* and *V. parahaemolyticus*, that do not ferment sucrose (Plate 14, *C*). On 5% sheep blood and chocolate agars, most *Vibrio* spp. produce colonies that are iridescent with a greenish hue. *V. fluvialis* is beta-hemolytic on sheep

blood agar (Figure 18-2). On human, but not sheep blood, agar *V. parahaemolyticus* isolates from patients with diarrhea produce hemolytic colonies, a characteristic termed the Kanagawa phenomenon.[19]

BIOCHEMICAL IDENTIFICATION

Metabolically, vibrios resemble the *Enterobacteriaceae* in their fermentative metabolism (usually anaerogenic) and *Pseudomonadaceae*, since most species are oxidase positive and use molecular oxygen as an electron acceptor. *V. metschnikovii* and *V. gazogenes* are oxidase negative.

Once a suspect organism has been isolated, characterization as a *Vibrio* spp. may be rapidly achieved by evaluation of characteristics such as oxidase reaction, oxidative-fermentative (OF) test, ''stringing'' after emulsification of colonies in 0.5% sodium deoxycholate (Figure 18-3),[38] and susceptibility to the vibriostatic agent 2,4,diamino-6,7-diisopropylpteridine phosphate (0/129).[27] Regarding 0/129 sensitivity, *Vibrio* spp. may show variability based on the concentration of 0/129 used (Table 18-1).[25] Disks containing between 10 and 150 µg/ml should be used to discern vibrios, since *Aeromonas* spp. are inhibited by concentrations greater than or equal to 320 µg/ml. Since vibrios are rather heterogeneous, variability in any of these tests may be observed (Table 18-1).

Vibrio spp. display a range of halotolerance. The presence of NaC1 stimulates growth, but the concentration of NaC1 required for stimulation varies among the species (Table 18-1). Thus species may be regarded as nonhalophilic (for example, *V. cholerae*) and halophilic (such as *V. parahaemolyticus* and *V. alginolyticus*). Most conventional media used for identification must be supplemented with 3% NaC1 for the halophilic species to grow.

Vibrio spp. are highly active in producing a number of extracellular hydrolases (such as amylase, chitinase, deoxyribonuclease, gelatinase, mucinase, and lipase). They are also capable of utilizing a wide range of organic substrates, including amino

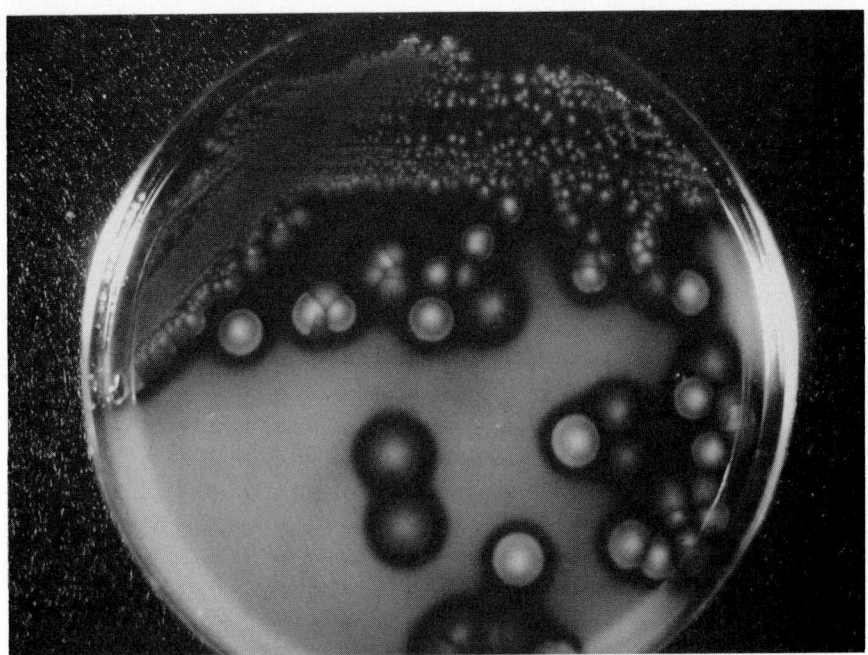

FIGURE 18-2. *Vibrio fluvialis* on sheep blood agar.

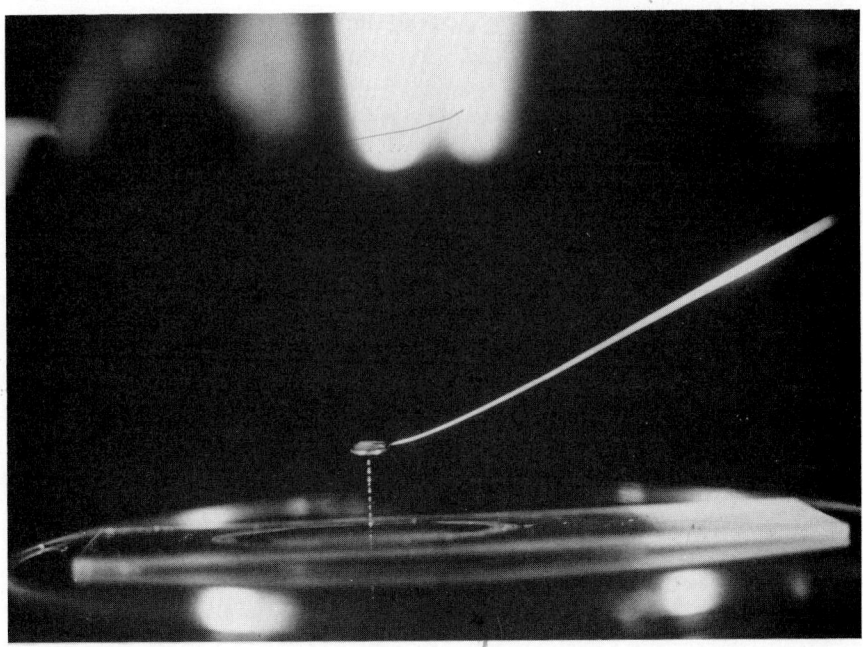

FIGURE 18-3. Stringing of *Vibrio* spp. after emulsification of colonies in 0.5% sodium deoxycholate.

TABLE 18-1. Differential Biochemical Characteristics of *Vibrio* Spp.

Test	*V. cholerae*	*V. parahaemolyticus*	*V. hollisae*	*V. alginolyticus*	*V. vulnificus*	*V. damsela*	*V. fluvialis*	*V. metschnikovii*	*V. cincinnatiensis*
Oxidase	+	+	+	+	+	+	+	−	+
Indole	+	+	+	+	+	−	−	v	−
Voges-Proskauer	v[a]	−	−	+	−	+	−	+	+
Lactose	+(D)	−	−	−	+	−	−	v	
Sucrose	+[a]	−	−	+	−	−	+(gas)[b]	+	+
Growth in									
0% NaCl	+	−	−	−	−	−	−	−	−
1% NaCl	+	+	−	+	+	+	+	+	+
6% NaCl	v	+	v	+	+	+	+	+	+
7% NaCl	−	+	v	+	−	−	+	+	−
10% NaCl	−	−	−	+	−	−	v	−	−
Inhibition by 0/129									
10 µg	S	R	S	R	S	S	R	S	R
150 µg	S	S	S	S	S	S	S	S	S

SYMBOLS:	+(D), Positive delayed	−, Negative
	v, Variable	S, Susceptible
	+, Positive	R, Resistant

[a]*V. mimicus* negative.

[b]*V. furnissii.*

acids, as sources of carbon and nitrogen for synthetic activities. *Vibrio* spp. may be distinguished and identified by the characteristics listed in Table 18-1. The tests listed in Table 18-2 provide a means for rapid selection of a given species while awaiting results of more extensive testing.

SEROLOGIC IDENTIFICATION

V. cholerae may be divided into six serogroups. Only toxigenic strains of serogroup 01 are involved in epidemic infections. Serogroup 01 is comprised of two or three antigenic factors (A, B, and C) that determine the serotype (Table 18-3). *V. cholerae* that do not fall into serogroup 01 are referred to collectively as non-01 *V. cholerae* strains.

Isolates identified as *V. cholerae* should be tested by slide agglutination with polyvalent 01 antiserum. Cultures agglutinating in polyvalent antiserum should be further tested with absorbed, monospecific Ogawa and Inaba antisera to determine the serotype. Reaction in both antisera is usually interpreted as the Hikojima serotype. This serotype is rare and should be confirmed by a state or federal reference laboratory. In fact, although antisera are available commercially, all serologic typing of *V. cholerae* is usually performed by state or federal reference laboratories, since most hospital laboratories do not maintain stocks of these antisera.

An immunoserologic diagnosis of cholera may be made by examining acute and convalescent sera in agglutination, vibriocidal, or antitoxin tests.[8]

OTHER IDENTIFICATION PROCEDURES

Epidemic *V. cholerae* 01 isolates may be differentiated into classical and El Tor biotypes in epidemiologic studies. El Tor biotypes differ from classical biotypes in that they produce a soluble hemolysin, are Voges-Proskauer positive, and are resistant to polymyxin B. These two groups also differ in their phage susceptibility. The El Tor biotypes are so named because they were originally recognized among Mecca pilgrims at the quarantine camp of El Tor on the Sinai Peninsula. Both classical and El Tor biotypes of *V. cholerae* possess the antigenic determinants discussed previously and thus can be divided into the serotypes in Table 18-3.

CLINICAL SIGNIFICANCE
VIBRIO CHOLERAE 01

V. cholerae 01 is the etiologic agent of cholera. The clinical severity of this disease varies greatly. Asymptomatic or mild disease occurs most commonly. In its most severe form the disease is characterized by massive loss of fluid and electrolytes and the production of voluminous amounts of liquid feces (rice water stools). Hypovolemic shock and metabolic acidosis develop, and the cardiovascular system collapses; if untreated, patients may die within a few hours.

Contaminated food and water are responsible for outbreaks of cholera. Person-to-person transmission is rare. Improperly preserved or handled foods that have been refrigerated or fro-

TABLE 18-2. Separation of Clinically Significant *Vibrio* Spp. on Basis of Minimal Criteria

Test	Species Selected
String test negative	*V. damsela, V. parahaemolyticus*
Oxidase negative	*V. metschnikovii*
Nitrate reduction negative	*V. metschnikovii*
Halotolerance 0% 10%	*V. cholerae, V. mimicus* *V. alginolyticus, V. fluvialis* (variable)
Aerogenic fermentation	*V. furnissii, V. damsela*
Sucrose negative	*V. mimicus, V. parahaemolyticus, V. hollisae, V. vulnificus* (most), *V. damsela*
Lactose fermentation	*V. vulnificus, V. fluvialis* (4%), *V. metschnikovii* (59%)[a]
Indole negative	*V. damsela, V. metschnikovii, V. cincinnatiensis*
Urease positive	*V. damsela, V. parahaemolyticus* (rare)
Beta-hemolysis—sheep blood	*V. fluvialis*
TCBS: no growth	*V. hollisae, V. metschnikovii* (variable)
0/129 resistance (10 μg)	*V. fluvialis, V. alginolyticus, V. parahaemolyticus*

[a]Numbers in parentheses are percent positive.

zen are particularly prone to harbor *V. cholerae.* Examples include unpreserved meat, fish and seafood, milk, and ice cream.

Cholera is an internationally reportable disease. It has been responsible for a number of life-threatening pandemics in areas with poor sanitation, especially southern Asia and Africa. The cholera outbreak in Louisiana in 1978[3] was the first in the United States in almost a century; one unexplained case also occurred in Port LaVaca, Texas, in 1973.[42]

OTHER *VIBRIO* ORGANISMS

A remarkable overlapping of clinical syndromes is associated with *V. cholerae* 01 and the other pathogenic *Vibrio* spp. (Table 18-4). Each of these organisms seems capable of eliciting one to three manifestations of infection: gastroenteritis, soft tissue infections, and systemic infections including bacteremia.[13] Ingestion of human pathogenic *Vibrio* organisms, usually in contaminated shellfish, may lead to a diarrheal illness ranging in clinical presentation from mild watery diarrhea to frank dysentery-like syndromes. In the case of *V. vulnificus,* fulminating bacteremia with metastatic, hemorrhagic ecthyma gangrenosum lesions (myonecrosis) of the extremities may occur in a susceptible host.[6,20,30] When *V. parahaemolyticus* and *V. alginolyticus* are introduced traumatically as a result of injury at seashores or in other aquatic environments, severe and extensive cellulitis may result.[10,33] In compromised patients septicemia is not an uncommon presentation following infec-

TABLE 18-3. Serotypes of *Vibrio cholerae* Serogroup 01

Serotype	Antigenic Determinants
Inaba	A, C
Ogawa	A, B
Hikojima	A, B, C

TABLE 18-4. Primary Clinical Infections Associated with Members of the Family *Vibrionaceae*

Species	Infections
V. cholerae 01	Cholera, gastroenteritis, wound infections, bacteremia
V. cholerae non-01	Gastroenteritis
V. mimicus	Gastroenteritis
V. parahaemolyticus	Gastroenteritis, wound infections
V. alginolyticus	Ear infections, conjunctivitis, wound infections, bacteremia
V. vulnificus	Septicemia, fasciitis, myonecrosis, gastroenteritis[17a]
V. metschnikovii	Bacteremia, peritonitis, gastroenteritis (?)
V. fluvialis	Gastroenteritis
V. furnissii	Gastroenteritis[36]
V. hollisae	Gastroenteritis
V. damsela	Wound infections
V. cincinnatiensis	Meningitis

tion with *Vibrio* organisms.[15a,16,36,40] Unusual manifestations of *Vibrio* infections include panophthalmitis caused by *V. parahaemolyticus,* resulting from contamination of an eye injury with pond water,[40] the incrimination of nontoxigenic serogroup 01 *V. cholerae* in wound infections,[17] and meningitis caused by *V. cincinnatiensis.*[3a]

MECHANISMS OF PATHOGENICITY

It should be evident from the associated disease spectrum that *Vibrio* spp. are multifaceted in their human pathogenic potential, running the gamut of pathogenic mechanisms from the purely enterotoxigenic *V. cholerae* 01 to the highly invasive *V. vulnificus.*

The epidemic *V. cholerae* 01 colonize the small intestine, multiply, and elaborate a protein enterotoxin called choleragen. Choleragen binds to ganglioside GM_1 in the plasma membrane and through a complex mechanism stimulates the production of adenylate cyclase. This enzyme converts adenosine triphosphate (ATP) into cyclic adenosine 3'5'-monophosphate (cAMP). The accumulation of cAMP stimulates the secretion of electrolytes osmotically with water from the extracellular space to the intestinal lumen.[35] The large volumes of secretion overpower the absorptive capacity of the gastrointestinal tract, resulting in the voluminous outpouring of liquid feces.

Non-01 *V. cholerae* and other *Vibrio* spp. may produce diarrheal illness or extraintestinal infection by a variety of mechanisms (Table 18-5).

Examination for the presence of potential virulence factors involved in the pathogenicity of vibrios other than *V. cholerae*

is an area of increasing scientific interest. Excluding the association of the Kanagawa reaction (hemolysin) with diarrhea-producing strains of *V. parahaemolyticus*,[34] a number of new virulence-associated factors have been described for other *Vibrio* spp. Operative in the bowel are cytolysins (*V. fluvialis, V. vulnificus, V. damsela*)[22,24,28] and enterotoxins (*V. fluvialis, V. mimicus*).[28,41] Recently a cholera-like enterotoxin was isolated from two strains of *V. mimicus*. In biochemical and immunologic studies this enterotoxin appears identical to that produced by *V. cholerae*.[39] Factors thought to enhance invasiveness include proteases (*V. fluvialis, V. vulnificus*),[28,37] undefined cell-killing factors (*V. fluvialis*),[28] and resistance to the bactericidal activity of normal human sera (*V. vulnificus, V. parahaemolyticus*)[4,41] and to phagocytosis (*V. vulnificus*).[23] The precise role these factors play in human infections remains to be clarified. A number of these factors may correlate with specific disease-associated syndromes, such as localized gastroenteritis or the ability to invade the intestinal mucosa and produce fulminating septicemia accompanied by cutaneous manifestations (ecthyma gangrenosum).

ANTIMICROBIAL SUSCEPTIBILITY

Antimicrobial susceptibility patterns are not characteristic for any particular member of the *Vibrio* genus. While certain species have been reported to be susceptible to ampicillin, carbenicillin, and penicillin,[11,24] enough variability exists among the species to warrant individual testing. Table 18-6 lists the overall susceptibility patterns reported for the more commonly used antimicrobial agents against *Vibrio*.*

*References 5, 11, 12, 18, 26, and 33.

TABLE 18-5. Mechanisms of Pathogenicity Associated with *Vibrio* Spp.

Species	Mechanisms
V. cholerae	Adherence, enterotoxin, motility, mucinase, protease
V. mimicus	Enterotoxin
V. parahaemolyticus	Adherence, hemolysin
V. vulnificus	Cytolysins, proteases, serum resistance, inhibition of phagocytosis
V. fluvialis	Cytolysins, enterotoxin, proteases
V. damsela	Cytolysin

TABLE 18-6. Antimicrobial Susceptibility of *Vibrio* Spp.

Antimicrobial Agent	*V. cholerae*	*V. mimicus*	*V. vulnificus*	*V. parahaemolyticus*	*V. alginolyticus*	*V. damsela*	*V. hollisae*
Tetracycline	100[a]	100	100	100	100	80	90
Colistin	16	96	0	29	—[b]	—[b]	—[b]
Nalidixic acid	99	96	100	100	100	—[b]	—[b]
Sulfadiazine	31	13	100	100	100	0	60
Gentamicin	100	100	100	100	100	100	100
Chloramphenicol	99	100	100	100	100	100	100
Penicillin	92	87	100	4	0	0	100
Ampicillin	100	100	100	4	0	0	100
Carbenicillin	100	100	100	4	0	—[b]	—[b]
Cephalothin	99	100	100	100	100	80	100

Data from references 5, 11, 12, 18, 26, and 33.
[a]Numbers throughout indicate percent susceptible.
[b]Not determined.

Antimicrobial susceptibility testing may be performed with the Bauer-Kirby method, since halophilic vibrios grow on Mueller-Hinton agar without added salt.[12] Minimal inhibitory concentrations (MICs) to gentamicin cannot be determined because the increased NaCl required for growth decreases gentamicin activity.[18]

REFERENCES

1. Baumann, P., and Schubert, R.H.W.: Family II. *Vibrionaceae* Veron 1965, 5245[AL]. In Krieg, N.R., editor (Holt, J.G., editor-in-chief): Bergey's manual of systematic bacteriology, Baltimore, 1984, The Williams & Wilkins Co.

2. Baumann, P., et al.: Reevaluation of the taxonomy of *Vibrio, Beneckea,* and *Photobacterium:* abolition of the genus *Beneckea,* Curr. Microbiol. **4**:127, 1980.

3. Blake, P.A., et al.: Cholera: a possible endemic focus in the United States, N. Engl. J. Med. **302**:305, 1980.

3a. Bode, R.B., et al.: A new *Vibrio* species, *Vibrio cincinnatiensis,* causing meningitis: successful treatment in an adult, Ann. Intern. Med. **104**:55, 1986.

3b. Brenner, D.J., et al.: *Vibrio furnissii* (formerly aerogenic biogroup of *Vibrio fluvialis*), a new species isolated from human feces and the environment, J. Clin. Microbiol. **18**:816, 1983.

4. Carruthers, M.M., and Kabat, W.J.: *Vibrio vulnificus* (lactose-positive *Vibrio*) and *Vibrio parahaemolyticus* differ in their susceptibilities to human serum, Infect. Immun. **32**:964, 1981.

5. Davis, B.R., et al.: Characterization of biochemically atypical *Vibrio cholerae* strains and designation of a new pathogenic species, *Vibrio mimicus,* J. Clin. Microbiol. **14**:631, 1981.

6. Ellington, E.P., Wood, J.G., and Hill, E.O.: Disease caused by a marine vibrio—*Vibrio vulnificus,* N. Engl. J. Med. **307**:1642, 1982.

7. Farmer, J.J., III: *Vibrio* (''*Beneckea''*) *vulnificus,* the bacterium associated with sepsis, septicemia, and the sea, Lancet **2**:903, 1979.

8. Feely, J.C., and DeWitt, W.E.: Immune response to *Vibrio cholerae.* In Rose, N.R., and Friedman, H., editors: Manual of clinical immunology, Washington, D.C., 1976, American Society for Microbiology.

9. Furniss, A.L., Lee, J.V., and Donovan, T.J.: Group F, a new vibrio? Lancet **2**:565, 1977.

10. Ghost, H.K., and Bowen, T.E.: Halophilic vibrios from human tissue infections on the Pacific coast of Australia, Pathology **12**:397, 1980.

11. Hickman, F.W., et al.: Identification of *Vibrio hollisae* sp. nov. from patients with diarrhea, J. Clin. Microbiol. **15**:395, 1982.

12. Hollis, D.G., et al.: Halophilic *Vibrio* species isolated from blood cultures, J. Clin. Microbiol. **3**:425, 1976.

13. Hughes, J.M., et al.: Non-cholera vibrio infections in the United States: clinical, epidemiology, and laboratory features, Ann. Intern. Med. **88**:602, 1978.

14. Huq, M.I., et al: Isolation of *Vibrio*-like group EF6 from patients with diarrhea, J. Clin. Microbiol. **11**:621, 1980.

15. Jean-Lacques, W., et al.: *Vibrio metschnikovii* bacteremia in a patient with cholecystitis, J. Clin. Microbiol. **14**:711, 1981.

15a. Janda, J.M., et al.: *Vibrio alginolyticus* bacteremia in an immunocompromised patient, Clin. Microbiol. Newsletter **8**:125, 1986.

16. Johnston, J.M., Andes, A., and Glasser, C.: *Vibrio vulnificus:* a gastronomic hazard, JAMA **249**:1756, 1983.

17. Johnston, J.M., et al.: Isolation of nontoxigenic *Vibrio cholerae* 01 from human wound infections, J. Clin. Microbiol. **17**:918, 1983.

17a. Johnson, J.M., Becker, S.F., and McFarland, L.M.: Gastroenteritis in patients with stool isolates of *Vibrio vulnificus,* Am. J. Med. **80**:336, 1986.

18. Joseph, S.W., DeBell, R.N., and Brown, W.P.: In vitro response to chloramphenicol, tetracycline, ampicillin, gentamicin, and beta-lactamase production by halophilic vibrios from human and environmental sources, Antimicrob. Agents Chemother. **13**:244, 1978.

19. Kato, T., et al.: Grouping of *Vibrio parahaemolyticus* (biotype 1) by hemolytic reaction, Shokuhin Eisei Kenkyu **15**:83, 1965.

20. Kelly, M.T., and McCormick, W.F.: Acute bacterial myositis caused by *Vibrio vulnificus,* JAMA **246**:72, 1981.

21. Kobayashi, T., et al: A new selective isolation medium for the vibrio group (modified Nakanishi medium–TCBS agar), Jpn. J. Bacteriol. **18**:387, 1973.

22. Kreger, A.S.: Cytolytic activity and virulence of *Vibrio damsela,* Infect. Immun. **44**:326, 1984.

23. Kreger, A.S., DeChatelet, L., and Shirley, P.: Interaction of *Vibrio vulnificus* with human polymorphonuclear leukocytes: association of virulence with resistance to phagocytosis, J. Infect. Dis. **144**:244, 1981.

24. Kreger, A.S. and Lockwood, D.: Detection of extracellular toxin(s) produced by *Vibrio vulnificus,* Infect. Immun. **33**:583, 1981.

25. Lee, J.V., Donovan, T.J., and Furniss, A.L.: Characterization, taxonomy and emended description of *Vibrio metschnikovii,* Int. J. Syst. Bacteriol. **28**:99, 1978.

26. Lee, J.V., et al.: Taxonomy and description of *Vibrio fluvialis* sp. nov. (synonym group F *Vibrios,* group EF6), J. Appl. Bacteriol. **50**:73, 1981.

27. Lee, J.V., et al: The taxonomic significance of the MIC of the vibriostatic compound 0/129 and other agents against the *Vibrionaceae* (abstract), J. Appl. Bacteriol. **45**:VIII, 1978.

28. Lockwood, D.I., Kreger, A.S., and Richardson, S.H.: Detection of toxins produced by *Vibrio fluvialis,* Infect. Immun. **35**:702, 1982.

29. Love, M., et al.: *Vibrio damsela,* a marine bacterium, causes skin ulcers on the damselfish *Chromis punctipinnis,* Science **214**:1139, 1981.

30. McManus, R.: Highly invasive new bacterium isolated from U.S. east coast waters, JAMA **251**:323, 1984.

31. Reichelt, J.L., Baumann, P., and Baumann, L.: Study of genetic relationships among marine species of the genera *Beneckea* and *Photobacterium* by means of in vitro DNA/DNA hybridization, Arch. Microbiol. **110**:101, 1976.

32. Rennels, M.B., et al.: Selective vs. nonselective media and direct plating vs. enrichment technique in isolation of *Vibrio cholerae*: recommendations for clinical laboratories, J. Infect. Dis. **142**:328, 1980.

33. Rubin, S.J., and Tilton, R.C.: Isolation of *Vibrio alginolyticus* from wound infections, J. Clin. Microbiol. **2**:556, 1975.

34. Sakazaki, R., et al.: Studies on the enteropathogenic facultatively halophilic bacteria, *Vibrio parahaemolyticus.* III. Enteropathogenicity, Jpn. J. Med. Sci. Biol. **21**:325, 1968.

35. Sherwood, L.M., and Davis, E.E.: Intestinal secretion: effect of cyclic AMP and its role in cholera, N. Engl. J. Med. **284**:1137, 1971.

36. Siegel, M.I., and Rogers, A.I.: Fatal non-01 *Vibrio cholerae* septicemia in chronic lymphocytic leukemia, Gastroenterology **83**:1130, 1982.

37. Smith, G.C., and Merkel, J.R.: Collagenolytic activity of *Vibrio vulnificus:* potential contribution to its invasiveness, Infect. Immun. **35**:1155, 1982.

38. Smith, H.L.: A presumptive test for vibrios: the ''string'' test, Bull. WHO **42**:817, 1970.

39. Spira, W.M., and Fedorka-Cray, P.J.: Production of cholera toxin-like toxin by *Vibrio mimicus* and non-01 *Vibrio cholerae:* batch culture conditions for optimum yields and isolation of hypertoxigenic lincomycin-resistant mutants, Infect. Immun. **42**:501, 1983.

40. Tacket, C.O., et al.: Panophthalmitis caused by *Vibrio parahaemolyticus,* J. Clin. Microbiol. **16**:195, 1982.

41. Tamplin, M.L., et al.: Differential complement activation and susceptibility to human serum bactericidal action by *Vibrio* species, Infect. Immun. **42**:1187, 1983.

42. Weissman, J.B., et al.: A case of cholera in Texas, Am. J. Epidemiol. **100**:487, 1974.

CHAPTER 19

Aeromonas and *Plesiomonas*

Alexander von Graevenitz

The genera *Aeromonas* and *Plesiomonas* are still classified in the family *Vibrionaceae* by virtue of their flagellation, facultative anaerobiosis, oxidase reaction, and guanine-cytosine ratio of the DNA (57 to 63 mol%). Both species are aquatic, but not marine, in origin. Although there are variations between the species, most strains grow at between 10° and 38° C and at pH values of 5.5 to 8.0. Infections occur chiefly in cold-blooded animals but occasionally in humans and other warm-blooded animals.

CLASSIFICATION

Bergey's Manual of Systematic Bacteriology[17] recognizes four species in the genus *Aeromonas: A. hydrophila, A. caviae, A. sobria,* and *A. salmonicida. A. salmonicida* (with three subspecies) does not grow at 37° C, has not been reported from humans, and is therefore disregarded here. The genus *Plesiomonas* has one species, *P. shigelloides.*[22]

GROWTH REQUIREMENTS
TRANSPORT MEDIA

Aeromonas and *Plesiomonas* survive in glycerol-buffered phosphate medium for only 5 days.[15] Cary-Blair medium seems to be more useful (own observations).

CULTURE MEDIA

Aeromonas and *Plesiomonas* are able to initiate growth on a variety of nonselective (blood) and very often on selective (for example, MacConkey and Salmonella-Shigella) agars. In contrast to *Vibrio* spp., growth of *Aeromonas* and *Plesiomonas* on thiosulfate–citrate–bile salts–sucrose (TCBS) medium occurs irregularly.[28]

Selective techniques are often necessary for isolation of *Aeromonas* or *Plesiomonas* from mixed cultures, particularly stool. The most sensitive and specific agars for *Aeromonas*[28] are dextrin-fuchsin-sulfite agar[20] (Aeromonas Differential Agar, E. Merck, Darmstadt, Germany), inositol–brilliant green–bile salts agar[22] (Plesiomonas Agar, E. Merck), pril-xylose-ampicillin agar,[19] and xylose-deoxycholate-citrate agar.[23] Recently, certain preparations of cefsulodin-irgasan-novobiocin (CIN) agar has been found suitable for the isolation of *Aeromonas* spp.[1]; thus *Yersinia* spp. and *Aeromonas* spp. can be isolated at 25° to 29° C on one and the same medium. As an enrichment broth, alkaline peptone water or trypticase soy broth with ampicillin[28] is optimal.

Optimal selective media for *P. shigelloides* are inositol–brilliant green–bile salts agar and alkaline peptone water.[28]

In light of recent data,[4,8,16] routine isolation of aeromonads from stool seems justified.

CULTURAL CHARACTERISTICS

Aeromonas and *Plesiomonas* are facultative anaerobes that grow well at 35° C and produce 1 to 3 mm colonies on a variety of media within 24 hours.

MICROSCOPIC MORPHOLOGY

Members of the genus *Aeromonas* are asporogenous, gram-negative rods, 1 to 4.4 μm long and 0.4 to 1 μm wide. Except for *A. salmonicida,* which is nonmotile, the aeromonads possess polar, usually monotrichous flagella with a wavelength of 1.7 μm.[17]

P. shigelloides is an asporogenous, gram-negative rod measuring 2 to 3 μm by 0.8 to 1 μm. It possesses polar, generally lophotrichous flagella with a wavelength of 3.5 to 4 μm.[21]

COLONIAL MORPHOLOGY

Most strains of *A. hydrophila* and *A. sobria* show a large zone of beta-hemolysis on blood agar; however, nonhemolytic strains do occur (see Table 19-2). The majority of strains are non–lactose fermenters on enteric agars; a smaller number produce lactose-fermenting colonies.[28] On CIN medium, colonies are mannitol positive.

P. shigelloides is not beta-hemolytic on blood agar and generally does not ferment lactose on enteric agars.[18]

BIOCHEMICAL IDENTIFICATION

Aeromonas spp. can be separated from the *Enterobacteriaceae* by means of the oxidase reaction, which has to be done from blood agar, since the reaction may be negative if the medium contains a fermentable sugar.[9] If colonies must be taken from enteric agars, a buffered reagent or a centrifugate of a broth subculture has to be used.[9]

Separation of *Aeromonas* spp. from *Vibrio* spp. is best done with 0/129 disks and growth in 6% NaCl broth (the latter reaction is positive only for halophilic vibrios). The 0/129 test can be performed by using 150 μg disks (Oxoid) whereby any zone indicates sensitivity[7] or by using 500 μg disks (Institut Pasteur) whereby zones of 15 mm or greater indicate sensitivity.[18] *P. shigelloides* is susceptible to 0/129. Separation of this organism from *Vibrio* may be accomplished by growth in 6% NaCl broth and a test for deoxyribonuclease. *P. shigelloides* is negative for both of these characteristics. *V. hollisae* and some strains of *V. mimicus, V. damsela,* and *V. metschnikovii* are also negative for deoxyribonuclease; however, they usually grow in 6% NaCl (NaCl-negative strains of *V. mimicus* are arginine negative).

Most strains of *Aeromonas* produce acid butts and slants with no H_2S on triple sugar iron (TSI) agar or Kligler iron agar

TABLE 19-1. Differentiation of *Aeromonas* and *Plesiomonas* in the Routine Laboratory

Test	*Aeromonas* (Motile Species)	*Plesiomonas*
DNAse	+ (99)	− (0)
Amylase	+(100)	− (0)
Ornithine decarboxylase	− (0)	+(100)
Gelatin liquefaction (22° C)	+ (99)	− (0)
Acid from mannitol	+ (99)	− (0)

SYMBOLS: +, Positive reaction
−, Negative reaction
( ), Percents of strains positive within 48 hours

TABLE 19-2. Biochemical Characteristics of *Aeromonas* and *Plesiomonas shigelloides*

Test	*A. hydrophila*	*A. caviae*	*A. sobria*	*P. shigelloides*
Oxidase	+	+	+	+
Catalase	+	+	+	+
Indole[a]	+	+	+	+
Motility	+	+	+	+
Nitrate to nitrite	+	+	+	+
Nitrate to gas	−	−	−	−
o-Nitrophenyl-β-D galactopyranoside (ONPG)	+	+	+	V
Hemolysis (sheep RBC)	+	−	+	−
Growth on MacConkey agar	+	+	+	+
Growth on Salmonella-Shigella (SS) agar	+	+	+	+
Deoxyribonuclease[a]	+	+	+	−
Amylase	+	+	+	−
Elastase	+	−	−	−
Caseinase	+	+	+	−
Gelatinase	+	+	+	−
Lipase (corn oil)	+	+	+	−
Gas from glucose	+	−	+	−
Acid from: Adonitol	−	−	−	−

TABLE 19-2. Biochemical Characteristics of *Aeromonas* and *Plesiomonas shigelloides*—cont'd

Test	*A. hydrophila*	*A. caviae*	*A. sobria*	*P. shigelloides*
Arabinose	+	+	−	−
Dulcitol	−	−	−	−
Glucose	+	+	+	+
Inositol	−	−	−	+
Lactose	V	V	V	V
Maltose	+	+	+	+
Mannitol	+	+	+	−
Raffinose	−	−	−	−
Rhamnose	−	−	−	−
Salicin	+	+	−	V
Sorbitol	−	−	−	−
Sucrose	+	+	+	−
Trehalose	+	+	+	+
Xylose	−	−	−	−
Voges-Proskauer	+	−	+	−
Simmons' citrate	V	V	V	−
Lysine decarboxylase[b]	+	−	+	+
Ornithine decarboxylase	−	−	−	+
Arginine dihydrolase[a]	+	+	+	+
Growth in potassium cyanide	+	+	V	−
Phenylalanine deaminase	V,W	V,W	V,W	V
Urease	−	−	−	−
H$_2$S (triple sugar iron or Kligler iron agar)	−	−	−	−
Malonate	−	−	−	−
Growth in 6.5% NaCl broth	−	−	−	−
Gluconate oxidation	+	−	+	−
Esculin hydrolysis	+	+	−	−

SYMBOLS: +, ≥ 85% of strains positive
−, ≥ 85% of strains negative
V, Variable
W, Weak

Data from references 10, 17, 18, 21, and 26.
[a]Reactions may be delayed 48 hours or more.
[b]Reactions vary with method used (own observations: Current Microbiology, in print).

(KIA); a few strains show alkaline slants or gas or both. The yellow butt helps to distinguish the organism from the nonfermentative gram-negative rods.

P. shigelloides produces acid butts and acid or alkaline slants with no H_2S on TSI agar. A few strains share a common O antigen with *Shigella sonnei* phase 1 but may be distinguished from *Shigella* on the basis of positive oxidase test findings.

Table 19-1 lists key tests for the differentiation of *Aeromonas* and *Plesiomonas*. Complete biochemical profiles of each genus are shown in Table 19-2.

SEROLOGIC IDENTIFICATION

Serologic testing of *Aeromonas* has not progressed to the point of practical applicability.[11] Serotyping of *P. shigelloides* has been successful with only part of the strains.[2]

CLINICAL SIGNIFICANCE
AEROMONAS

Cold-blooded animals (amphibians, reptiles, fish) may be infected by aeromonads or may be carriers. Human infections usually originate from water sources (including foodstuffs and muddy areas) or from the intestinal flora. Earlier investigations in the United States found intestinal carrier rates between 0.2% and 3.2%,[30] but a recent study from Thailand found up to one quarter of a population in one area to be carriers.[16]

Human infections are of several types:

1. Wound infections, cellulitis, or even myonecrosis with gas formation following contact with contaminated water or soil.[3,29,31] These are mostly outpatient infections.
2. Septicemia, mostly associated with acute leukemia, bone marrow aplasia, or liver disease (cirrhosis, cholangitis).[3,29,31] The source is usually the intestine. Septicemia in noncompromised hosts is rare.[3]
3. Other nonintestinal infections (postoperative wound infections, urinary infections, peritonitis, pneumonia, meningitis, otitis media, conjunctivitis, endocarditis). These are rare and may have their origin in either source mentioned previously.[3,29,31]
4. Diarrheal disease. This most numerous infection associated with *Aeromonas* is ubiquitous, affects any age group (more often children than adults), and occurs more frequently during the warm seasons.* It may be watery or bloody and is sometimes choleriform. It probably accounts for many cases of traveler's diarrhea[4] and as such is self-limited.

PLESIOMONAS

P. shigelloides occurs in both cold- and warm-blooded animals.[2] Few extraintestinal strains have been isolated from humans[14]; most strains come from diarrheic stools of patients residing in subtropical or tropical areas, Japan, Australia, and only occasionally Europe or the United States.[18,25,27,29] Carriers are rare but have recently been found with higher frequency in Thai populations.[16] Diarrhea resulting from *P. shigelloides* resembles that caused by *Aeromonas*.[8]

MECHANISMS OF PATHOGENICITY

Aeromonads have been shown to produce a heat-labile enterotoxin, as well as cytotoxins.[12,13] An association has been

demonstrated between positive ileal loop and infant mouse tests and certain biochemical traits (positive findings for lysine decarboxylase, Voges-Proskauer, gluconate oxidation, hemolysis, and gas formation from glucose tests).[10,26] The clinical relevance of these factors is still under debate.

Enterotoxin production by *P. shigelloides* has not been proved unequivocally.[16]

ANTIMICROBIAL SUSCEPTIBILITY

A. hydrophila is usually sensitive to second- and third-generation cephalosporins, aminoglycosides, nitrofurantoin, nalidixic acid, trimethoprim-sulfamethoxazole, and chloramphenicol. Some strains are resistant to tetracycline, and most are resistant to penicillin, carbenicillin, ampicillin, and cephalothin.[5,6]

P. shigelloides is sensitive to the same drugs to which *A. hydrophila* is sensitive except that more strains are susceptible to ampicillin, carbenicillin, and cephalothin.[14,18,29]

REFERENCES

1. Altorfer, R., et al.: Growth of *Aeromonas* spp. on cefsulodin-irgasan-novobiocin agar selective for *Yersinia enterocolitica*, J. Clin. Microbiol. **22**:478, 1985.
2. Arai, T., et al.: A survey of *Plesiomonas shigelloides* from aquatic environments, domestic animals, pets and humans, J. Hyg. (Camb.) **84**:203, 1980.
3. Davis, W.A., Kane, J.G., and Garagusi, V.F.: Human *Aeromonas* infections: a review of the literature and a case report of endocarditis, Medicine (Baltimore) **57**:267, 1978.
4. Echeverria, P., et al.: Travelers' diarrhea among American Peace Corps volunteers in rural Thailand, J. Infect. Dis. **143**:767, 1981.
5. Fainstein, V., Weaver, S., and Bodey, G.P.: In vitro susceptibilities of *Aeromonas hydrophila* against new antibiotics, Antimicrob. Agents Chemother. **22**:513, 1982.
6. Fass, R.J., and Barnishan, J.: In vitro susceptibilities of *Aeromonas hydrophila* to 32 antimicrobial agents, Antimicrob. Agents Chemother. **19**:357, 1981.
7. Furniss, A.L., Lee, J.V., and Donovan, T.J.: The vibrios, Pub. Health Lab. Monogr. Ser. 11, London, 1978, Her Majesty's Stationery Office.
8. Holmberg, S.D., and Farmer, J.J., III: *Aeromonas hydrophila* and *Plesiomonas shigelloides* as causes of intestinal infections, Rev. Infect. Dis. **6**:633, 1984.
9. Hunt, L.K., Overman, T.L., and Otero, R.B.: Rapid oxidase method for testing oxidase-variable *Aeromonas hydrophila* strains, J. Clin. Microbiol. **13**:1117, 1981.
10. Janda, J.M., Reitano, M., and Bottone, E.J.: Biotyping of *Aeromonas* isolates as a correlate to delineating a species-associated disease spectrum, J. Clin. Microbiol. **19**:44, 1984.
11. Leblanc, D., et al.: Serogrouping of motile *Aeromonas* species isolated from healthy and moribund fish, Appl. Microbiol. **42**:56, 60, 1981.
12. Ljungh, A., Popoff, M., and Wadström, T.: *Aeromonas hydrophila* in acute diarrheal disease: detection of enterotoxin and biotyping of strains, J. Clin. Microbiol. **6**:96, 1977.
13. Ljungh, A., and Wadström, T.: *Aeromonas* toxins, Pharmacol. Ther. **15**:339, 1982.
14. McNeeley, D., et al.: *Plesiomonas*: biology of the organism and diseases in children, Pediatr. Infect. Dis. **3**:176, 1984.
15. Morgan, D.R., et al.: Isolation of enteric pathogens from patients with traveler's diarrhea using fecal transport media, FEMS Microbiol. Lett. **23**:59, 1984.
16. Pitarangsi, C., et al.: Enteropathogenicity of *Aeromonas hydrophila* and *Plesiomonas shigelloides:* prevalence among individuals with and without diarrhea in Thailand, Infect. Immun. **35**:666, 1982.

---

*References 3, 8, 10, 12, 24, and 29.

17. Popoff, M.: Genus III: *Aeromonas* Kluyver and van Niel 1936, 398. In Krieg, N.R., editor (Holt, J.G., editor-in-chief): Bergey's manual of systematic bacteriology, vol. 1, Baltimore, 1984, The Williams & Wilkins Co.

18. Richard, C., Lhuillier, M., and Laurent, B.: *Plesiomonas shigelloides:* une Vibrionacée enteropathogène exotique, Bull. Inst. Pasteur Paris **76:**187, 1978.

19. Rogol, M., et al.: Pril-xylose-ampicillin agar, a new selective medium for the isolation of *Aeromonas hydrophila,* J. Med. Microbiol. **12:**229, 1979.

20. Schubert, R.H.W.: Die Pathogenität der Aeromonaden für Mensch und Tier, Arch. Hyg. **150:**709, 1967.

21. Schubert, R.H.W.: Ueber den Nachweis von *Plesiomonas shigelloides* Habs und Schubert, 1962, und ein Elektivmedium, den Inositol-Brillantgrün-Gallesalz-Agar, E. Rodenwaldt-Arch. **4:**97, 1977.

22. Schubert, R.H.W.: Genus IV: *Plesiomonas* Habs and Schubert 1962, 324. In Krieg, N.R., editor (Holt, J.G., editor-in-chief): Bergey's manual of systematic bacteriology, vol. 1, Baltimore, 1984, The Williams & Wilkins Co.

23. Shread, P., Donovan, T.J., and Lee, J.V.: A survey of the incidence of *Aeromonas* in human faeces, Soc. Gen. Microbiol. Q. **8:**184, 1981.

24. Simon, G., and von Graevenitz, A.: Intestinal and water-borne infections due to *Aeromonas hydrophila,* Public Health Lab. **27:**159, 1969.

25. Tsukamoto, T., et al.: Two epidemics of diarrhoeal disease possibly caused by *Plesiomonas shigelloides,* J. Hyg. **80:**275, 1978.

26. Turnbull, P.C.B., et al.: Enterotoxin production in relation to taxonomic grouping and source of isolation of *Aeromonas* species, J. Clin. Microbiol. **19:**175, 1984.

27. Vandepitte, J., Makulu, A., and Gatti, F.: *Plesiomonas shigelloides:* survey and possible association with diarrhea in Zaire, Ann. Soc. Belg. Med. Trop. **54:**503, 1974.

28. von Graevenitz, A., and Bucher, C.: Evaluation of differential and selective media for isolation of *Aeromonas* and *Plesiomonas* spp. from human feces, J. Clin. Microbiol. **17:**16, 1983.

29. von Graevenitz, A., and Mensch, A.H.: The genus *Aeromonas* in human bacteriology: report of 30 cases and review of the literature, N. Engl. J. Med. **278:**245, 1968.

30. von Graevenitz, A., and Zinterhofer, L.: The detection of *Aeromonas hydrophila* in stool specimens, Health Lab. Sci. **7:**124, 1970.

31. Washington, J.A.: *Aeromonas hydrophila* in clinical bacteriologic specimens, Ann. Intern. Med. **76:**611, 1972.

CHAPTER 20

Anaerobic Bacteria

Barbara J. Howard
Madeline J. Ducate

Anaerobic bacteria have been defined as organisms that fail to grow in the presence of air or molecular oxygen. Actually, there is a wide variety in oxygen sensitivity among bacteria in this group and more specific terms have been suggested to allow their differentiation.

Loesche[70] divided anaerobes into two groups: strict anaerobes are incapable of agar surface growth at Po_2 levels greater than 0.5%, and moderate anaerobes are capable of growth in the presence of oxygen levels as high as 2% to 8%. Neblett and Brown[97] have described three groups of anaerobes: aerotolerant, obligate, and strict.

Although aerotolerant anaerobes grow better in the absence of oxygen than in its presence, they are able to produce colonies on freshly prepared, nutritionally adequate media when heavily inoculated. They can be isolated with relatively unsophisticated anaerobic techniques. *Clostridium tertium* is such an aerotolerant anaerobe.

Obligate anaerobes usually do not grow (even on freshly prepared media and from heavy inocula) when exposed to molecular oxygen in greater than a minute amount. Depending on conditions these organisms may survive from minutes to hours in clinical specimens. Obligate anaerobes may require prereduced media and stringent oxygen-excluding techniques for isolation. Most of the commonly encountered clinical isolates discussed in this chapter are obligate anaerobes.

Strict anaerobes such as the family *Treponemataeae* are extremely oxygen sensitive and demand chemically reduced media and exacting oxygen-excluding techniques. When exposed to ambient conditions, they die readily.

It should be noted that no definitive limits divide these three groups and that variations exist within each group.

Numerous hypotheses have been offered over the past few years to explain the oxygen sensitivity of anaerobes.[86-88] The two hypotheses explained in the following paragraphs have been the most widely accepted.

Hypothesis 1. The toxic agent for anaerobic bacteria is not molecular oxygen per se but rather products of the interaction of oxygen with cellular components or components of the culture media.

Interaction of oxygen with bacteria or components of the culture media may result in the production of several toxic products including hydrogen peroxide, superoxide anion, singlet oxygen, and the hydroxyl radical. These toxic products are invariably formed by the interaction of oxygen with various cellular constituents such as reduced flavoproteins and iron sulfur proteins, as well as by the interaction of oxygen with several common media constituents including agar, yeast extract, reducing agents, and certain metals such as manganese.[127] Bacteria produce certain key enzymes that allow protection from these toxic substances. The enzyme catalase, for example, degrades hydrogen peroxide, and the enzyme superoxide dismutase (SOD) degrades the superoxide anion.

Several studies have suggested that anaerobes, unlike aerobes, cannot grow in the presence of oxygen because they do not produce these protective enzymes. The early studies of McLeod and Gordon,[79] for example, suggested that oxygen toxicity in anaerobes was due to hydrogen peroxide accumulation because of the lack of the enzyme catalase. This theory was later disproved, however, when several anaerobes were found that produced catalase but still could not grow in the presence of oxygen, and conversely, when organisms such as streptococci that were capable of aerobic growth were determined to be catalase negative.

Subsequently, McCord, Keele, and Fridovich[78] studied the levels of catalase and SOD in selected aerobic organisms, strict anaerobic organisms, and aerotolerant anaerobic organisms. The aerobic organisms had both catalase and SOD. Strict anaerobes were SOD negative and usually catalase negative. Aerotolerant anaerobes initially seemed paradoxic in that they produced hydrogen peroxide but did not produce catalase; they also produced 30% of the level of SOD as did anaerobic strains. These aerotolerant organisms were able to survive without catalase production because of their low rate of production of hydrogen peroxide and the utilization of other catalysts in the medium (or other organisms in a mixed culture) to degrade the small amount of hydrogen peroxide. McCord and associates concluded that dismutation of superoxide radicals by SOD was the single most important enzymatic activity for allowing organisms to survive in the presence of molecular oxygen. Organisms without the SOD enzyme could survive in oxygen only if they did not produce large quantities of the superoxide radical.

Tally and co-workers[137] confirmed that aerotolerant organisms possessed SOD, whereas the extremely oxygen-sensitive isolates had low or undetectable SOD levels; however, this correlation was not universal. Thus, although there is a correlation between SOD activity and oxygen tolerance, SOD is not the sole basis for an organism's ability or inability to withstand oxygen exposure.[110] Nevertheless, the toxic derivatives of oxygen do appear to play a role in the oxygen sensitivity of anaerobic organisms.

Hypothesis 2. Normal growth and metabolism of anaerobic bacteria are possible only within certain oxidation-reduction (redox) potential limits, and because oxygen is the cause of high oxidation-reduction potentials, its presence is incompatible with the attainment and maintenance of the necessary low potentials.

Bacteria require certain redox potential levels for growth and function of their metabolic systems. (When the redox potential is determined with a hydrogen electrode as the reference electrode, it is expressed as E_h.) Anaerobic bacteria generally require reduced conditions, although some must have more reduced conditions than others. These low potentials are vital in keeping the reversible components of various enzymes in their active reduced form rather than their inactive oxidizable form.

Anaerobic bacteria differ in the redox potential at which they can initiate growth. Some anaerobic bacteria, by their normal reducing metabolism, can establish sufficient reduced conditions, provided that oxygen exposure of the media is minimal, a sufficient inoculum is used, and anaerobic incubation methods are used. However, other anaerobic bacteria require very reduced conditions that can be established only with strict oxygen-excluding techniques and the addition of reducing agents. Thus, according to hypothesis 2, oxygen is toxic because its presence precludes the establishment of these reduced conditions.

As previously indicated, these are two of several hypotheses that have been offered to explain the oxygen sensitivity of anaerobic bacteria. Morris,[86] however, suggests that probably no one unitary hypothesis can account for the oxygen sensitivity of all anaerobic strains in all media. Rather, a comprehensive explanation that includes elements from these two theories, as well as from the other, less accepted theories, probably best describes the complex interaction between these organisms and oxygen. According to Morris,[86] oxygen toxicity probably occurs in two phases. During the first phase, incoming oxygen may initially be reduced but only at the expense of considerable reducing power. Reversible metabolic dysfunctions might develop at this stage because of the elevation of the intracellular oxidation-reduction potential in oxygen's presence. Since the initial reduction of molecular oxygen would exert few additional effects on the organism, a return to anaerobic conditions within a short time might reverse these metabolic dysfunctions. However, if oxygen exposure is continued, the reducing power of the organism would be overwhelmed, growth would be halted, and phase two of oxygen toxicity would ensue. The resulting free ingress of oxygen into the cell would probably mark the initiation of the bactericidal phase and would result in irreversible structural damage from direct interaction with oxygen-labile cell components (such as sulfhydryl groups) and generation of toxic by-products (such as superoxide anion, hydrogen peroxide, and numerous oxygen-derived free radicals).

CLASSIFICATION

The classification used in this chapter reflects that in *Bergey's Manual of Systematic Bacteriology*. Some of the numerous nomenclature changes that have occurred over the past few years are shown in Table 20-1. The clinically significant anaerobic bacteria are indicated in the box on pp. 373 and 374.*

SPECIMEN COLLECTION AND PROCESSING

Numerous studies stress the importance of proper collection and transport of specimens containing suspected anaerobic pathogens.[50,81,132] If these procedures are not used, contami-

---

*References 15, 19, 52-54, 83, 84, and 116-118.

nation by normal flora, overgrowth of facultative organisms, or death of certain anaerobic organisms when exposed to air may result in changes in the sample microbial population and thus provide erroneous and misleading results.[81]

Four cardinal principles should be strictly adhered to in the cultivation of anaerobic bacteria[23]:

1. Proper collection and transport of the specimen
2. Culture of the specimen as soon as possible after collection
3. Use of appropriate media that are either freshly prepared or properly reduced
4. Incubation under appropriate anaerobic conditions

Proper collection is mandatory because anaerobes are present in large numbers as indigenous flora on the mucosal surfaces of numerous body sites (Table 20-2) and even minimal contamination of the specimen with these indigenous anaerobic organisms can lead to erroneous and misleading culture results.[132] Accordingly, only specimens that are free of these organisms should be cultured for anaerobic pathogens. The following specimens are likely to be contaminated and are thus generally unacceptable for anaerobic culture:

1. Oral
   a. Throat
   b. Nasopharyngeal
   c. Gingival
   d. Expectorated sputum (except in cases of suspected actinomycosis)
   e. Sputum obtained by nasotracheal or orotracheal suction and bronchial washings
2. Intestinal
   a. Gastric and small bowel contents (except in blind loop and similar syndromes)
   b. Large bowel contents
   c. Ileostomy and colostomy effluents
   d. Feces (except in suspected *C. difficile* gastrointestinal illness)
   e. Rectal swabs
3. Genitourinary
   a. Voided and catheterized urine
   b. Vaginal and cervical swabs
4. Superficial
   a. Swabs of open skin lesions

On the other hand, the following clinical specimens are acceptable for anaerobic culture[21]:

1. Central nervous system
   a. Cerebrospinal fluid
   b. Abscess material
   c. Tissue biopsy specimen
2. Oral cavity, ears, nose, and throat
   a. Material aspirated from abscesses
   b. Tissue biopsy specimen
3. Pulmonary
   a. Transtracheal aspirate
   b. Direct lung aspirate
   c. Pleural fluid
   d. Tissue biopsy specimen
   e. "Sulfur granules" from draining fistula
4. Intra-abdominal
   a. Ascitic fluid
   b. Aspirate of loculated abscess
   c. Tissue biopsy specimen

TABLE 20-1. Recent Nomenclature Changes of Anaerobic Bacteria[a]

Current Name	Former Name
Bacteroides	
B. asaccharolyticus	B. melaninogenicus ssp. asaccharolyticus
B. bivius	New species
B. buccae	New species
B. buccalis	New species, formerly included in B. oralis
B. corporis	B. melaninogenicus ssp. intermedius (in part)
B. denticola	B. melaninogenicus ssp. melaninogenicus (in part)
B. disiens	New species
B. distasonis	B. fragilis ssp. distasonis
B. eggerthii	New species
B. fragilis	B. fragilis ssp. fragilis
B. gingivalis	B. melaninogenicus ssp. asaccharolyticus (oral strains)
B. intermedius	B. melaninogenicus ssp. intermedius (in part)
B. loescheii	B. melaninogenicus ssp. melaninogenicus (in part)
B. melaninogenicus	B. melaninogenicus ssp. melaninogenicus (in part)
B. oris	New species
B. ovatus	B. fragilis ssp. ovatus
B. splanchnicus	New species
B. thetaiotaomicron	B. fragilis ssp. thetaiotaomicron
B. uniformis	New species; previously identified as B. thetaiotaomicron
B. ureolyticus	Anaerobic strains included in B. corrodens
B. veroralis	B. oralis (in part)
B. vulgatus	B. fragilis ssp. vulgatus
Clostridium	
C. baratii	Includes C. perenne and C. paraperfringens
C. clostridioforme	Bacteroides clostridiiformis ssp. clostridiiformis and ssp. girans
C. hastiforme	Previously misidentified as C. subterminale
Peptostreptococcus-Peptococcus	
Peptostreptococcus asaccharolyticus	Peptococcus asaccharolyticus
Peptostreptococcus indolicus	Peptococcus indolicus
Peptostreptococcus magnus	Peptococcus magnus
Peptostreptococcus prevotii	Peptococcus prevotii
Peptostreptococcus tetradius	Gaffkya anaerobia
Veillonella	
V. parvula	Includes V. alcalescens
V. atypica	V. parvula ssp. atypica
V. dispar	V. alcalescens ssp. dispar

Modified from Holdeman, L.V., Cato, E.P., and Moore, W.E.C.: Rev. Infect. Dis. **6**(suppl. 1):S3, 1984.
[a]References for these nomenclature changes are cited throughout this chapter and in Holdeman.[51]

Anaerobic gram-negative straight, curved, and helical rods
Family I.   *Bacteroidaceae*
   Genus I.   *Bacteroides*
      B. asaccharolyticus
      B. bivius
      B. buccae
      B. capillosus
      B. corporis
      B. disiens
      B. distasonis
      B. eggerthii
      B. fragilis
      B. gingivalis
      B. intermedius
      B. melaninogenicus

Anaerobic gram-negative straight, curved, and helical rods—cont'd
Family I.   *Bacteroidaceae*
   Genus I.   B. oralis
      B. oris
      B. ovatus
      B. praecutus (now *Tissierella praeacuta*[18])
      B. putredinis
      B. splanchnicus
      B. thetaiotaomicron
      B. uniformis
      B. ureolyticus
      B. veroralis
      B. vulgatus
      B. zoogleoformans

Continued.

Anaerobic gram-negative straight, curved, and helical
rods—cont'd
  Family I.   *Bacteroidaceae*
    Genus II.   *Fusobacterium*
                F. gonidiaformans
                F. mortiferum
                F. naviforme
                F. necrogenes
                F. necrophorum
                F. nucleatum
                F. perfoetens
                F. prausnitizii
                F. russii
                F. varium
    Genus III.   *Leptotrichia*
    Genus IV.   *Butyrivibrio*
    Genus V.   *Succinimonas*
    Genus VII.   *Anaerobiospirillum*
    Genus VIII.   *Wolinella*
    Genus IX.   *Selenomonas*
    Genus X.   *Anaerovibrio*
    Genus XI.   *Pectinatus*
    Genus XII.   *Acetivibrio*
    Genus XIII.   *Lachnospira*
Anaerobic gram-negative cocci
  Family I.   *Veillonellaceae*
    Genus I.   *Veillonella*
                V. atypica
                V. dispar
                V. parvula
    Genus II.   *Acidaminococcus*
                A. fermentans
    Genus III.   *Megasphaera*
                M. elsdenii
Anaerobic gram-positive cocci
  Genus   *Peptococcus*
                P. niger
  Genus   *Peptostreptococcus*
                P. anaerobius
                P. asaccharolyticus
                P. indolicus
                P. magnus
                P. micros
                P. productus
                P. prevotii
                P. tetradius
Endospore-forming gram-positive rods and cocci
  Genus   *Clostridium*
                C. baratii
                C. bifermentans
                C. botulinum
                C. butyricum
                C. cadaveris

Endospore-forming gram-positive rods and cocci—cont'd
  Genus   *C. chauvoei*
                C. clostridioforme
                C. difficile
                C. hastiforme
                C. histolyticum
                C. innocuum
                C. limosum
                C. novyi
                C. paraputrificum
                C. perfringens
                C. ramosum
                C. septicum
                C. sordellii
                C. sphenoides
                C. sporogenes
                C. subterminale
                C. tertium
                C. tetani
Regular, nonsporing, gram-positive rods
  Genus   *Lactobacillus*
                L. acidophilus
                L. casei
                L. catenaforme[a]
                L. gasseri
                L. plantarum
                L. salivarius
Irregular, nonsporing, gram-positive rods
  Genus   *Arachnia*
                A. propionica
  Genus   *Propionibacterium*
                P. acnes
                P. granulosum
  Genus   *Eubacterium*[b]
                E. aerofaciens
                E. alactolyticum
                E. brachy
                E. combesii
                E. contortum
                E. lentum
                E. limosum
                E. moniliforme
                E. nodatum
                E. tenue
                E. timidum
  Genus   *Actinomyces*
                A. israelii
                A. meyeri
                A. naeslundii
                A. odontolyticus
                A. viscosus
  Genus   *Bifidobacterium*
                B. dentium (eriksonii)

[a]This species is listed in *Bergey's Manual of Systematic Bacteriology* in the addendum to the genus *Lactobacillus* and not as a species in the genus. At the current time its taxonomic position is undetermined, but it is treated as a species of *Lactobacillus* in this chapter.
[b]Several of these species have been isolated from various human infections, although their precise role in these infections is unknown.

TABLE 20-2. Incidence of Various Anaerobes as Normal Flora in Humans

Body Site	Clostridium	Nonsporeforming Bacilli							Cocci	
		Gram-Positive					Gram-Negative			
		Actinomyces	Bifidobacterium	Eubacterium	Lactobacillus[a]	Propionibacterium	Bacteroides	Fusobacterium	Gram-positive	Gram-negative
Skin	0	0	0	±	0	2	0	0	1	0
Upper respiratory tract[b]	0	1	0	±	0	1	1	1	1	1
Mouth	±	1	1	1	1	±	2	2	2	2
Intestine	2	±	2	2	1-2	±	2	±	2	±
External genitalia	0	0	0	U	0	U	1	1	1	0
Urethra	±	0	0	U	±	0	1	1	±	U
Vagina	±	0	±	±	2	1	1	±	2	1

> **SYMBOLS:** U, Unknown 1, Usually present
> 0, Not found or rare 2, Usually present in large numbers
> ±, Irregular

Reprinted from Sutter, V.L., et al.: Wadsworth anaerobic bacteriology manual, 4th edition, Copyright 1985, Star Publishing Company, Belmont, Calif.

[a]Includes anaerobic, microaerophilic, and facultative strains.
[b]Includes nasal passages, nasopharynx, oropharynx, and tonsils.

5. Genitourinary
   a. Suprapubic urine aspirate
   b. Aspirate from loculated abscess
   c. Tissue biopsy specimen from normally sterile site
   d. Culdoscopy specimen
   e. Endometrial specimens obtained through catheter
6. Other
   a. Blood
   b. Bone marrow
   c. Bile
   d. Aspirated joint fluid
   e. Tissue biopsy specimen from any normally sterile site

Generally all abscess material, necrotic tissue, and aspirated fluids from infections of normally sterile sites should be cultured anaerobically.

The use of precise collection techniques to obtain specimens for anaerobic culture cannot be overemphasized. Material for anaerobic culture is best obtained using a needle and syringe from which all air has been expelled. The specimen may then be transported to the laboratory in the syringe and should be processed within 30 minutes. Swabs are generally not recommended for anaerobic culture because they are more easily contaminated during collection, become desiccated easily, and retain organisms within their fibers.[17] If swabs must be used, they should be transported to the laboratory in one of the anaer-

obic transport systems discussed in Chapter 11. Gassed-out, rubber-stoppered tubes or vials are the method of choice for transportation of fluid specimens. If specimens in these systems cannot be processed within 2 to 3 hours, they should be stored at room temperature. Gassed-out, oxygen-free, rubber-stoppered tubes or Bio-Bags (Marion Scientific, Kansas City, Mo.) are suitable for transporting tissue.

Although oxygen intolerance among the anaerobic organisms is variable, and some studies have demonstrated the survival of anaerobic organisms in clinical specimens despite delayed processing,[7] the immediate processing of specimens enhances the recovery of organisms.

DIRECT EXAMINATION

Clues to anaerobic infection and even to the species present may be obtained by macroscopic and microscopic direct examination of the specimen.

MACROSCOPIC EXAMINATION

Specimens that have a foul odor caused by production of metabolic products or that possess large amounts of gas strongly suggest the presence of anaerobic infections. Members of the genera *Peptostreptococcus, Bacteroides,* and *Clostridium* may produce gas during anaerobic sepsis. *Bacteroides* and *Peptostreptococcus* spp. are often associated with a putrid odor.

Exudates with black discoloration that fluoresce red under

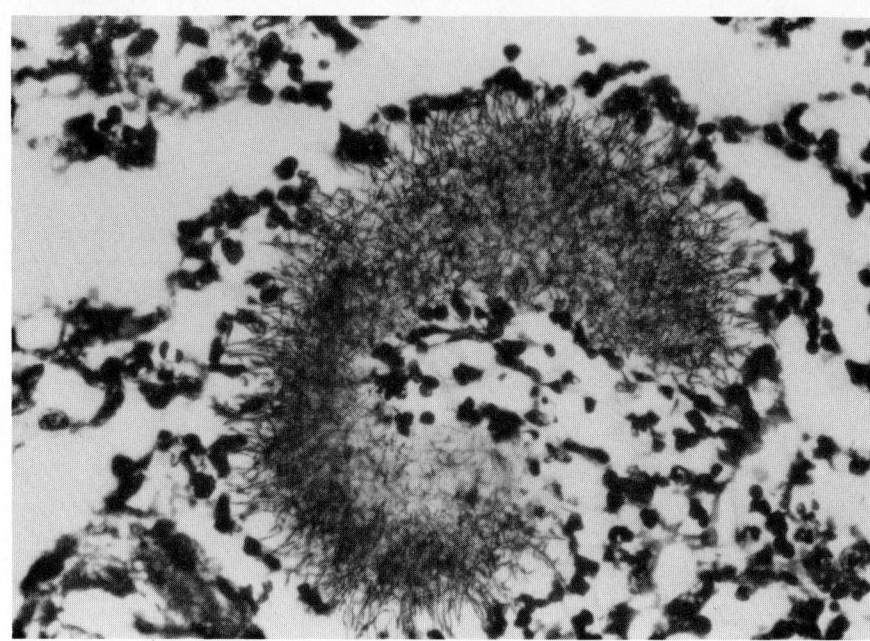

FIGURE 20-1. Brown and Brenn stain of *Actinomyces israelii* in tissue.

long-wave (366 nm) ultraviolet light constitute strong presumptive evidence of the presence of the pigmented *Bacteroides* group (see p. 393). The presence of sulfur granules (white or yellowish firm grains up to 5 mm in diameter) suggests actinomycosis, a disease usually associated with the genus *Actinomyces*. These granules may be detected macroscopically (or with a dissecting microscope or a light microscope at ×100) in sputum, suppurative exudates, or gauze dressings that have been in contact with the draining sinuses associated with actinomycosis. The granule should be placed in a drop of water or potassium hydroxide (KOH) on a glass slide, pressed gently with a coverslip, and examined under high power or oil immersion for the presence of a dense mass of entangled filaments that may end in hyaline, club-shaped structures (Figure 20-1). These filaments are composed of colonies of the organisms embedded in a calcium phosphate matrix that is formed by the host in response to tissue invasion. If the granules are crushed, smeared, and Gram stained, the characteristic gram-positive filaments can be observed (Plate 14, *D*). Smears of the crushed granules should also be stained with the Ziehl-Neelsen or Kinyoun acid-fast stain to differentiate the morphologically similar, partially acid-fast *Nocardia asteroides*. Finally, the granules should be washed several times with sterile saline, drained, and crushed with a loop or sterile glass rod to prepare a suspension that is used as an inoculum.

MICROSCOPIC EXAMINATION

The direct microscopic examination is of utmost importance because it may furnish early presumptive evidence of the presence of anaerobes and may assist the physician in prescribing appropriate therapy. The direct smear is especially valuable in diagnosis of the clostridial infections, ranging from severe gas gangrene myonecrosis to the serious but considerably less severe and more treatable cellulitis. The presence of serosan-

guineous fluid, often accompanied by gas in the tissues, and a direct smear revealing typical gram-positive, rod-shaped clostridia with few if any leukocytes is characteristic of myonecrosis. On the other hand, the purulent exudate of cellulitis may reveal clostridia in the presence of numerous leukocytes.

Direct microscopic examination can also serve as a guide to the selection of media and as a check on the adequacy of the isolation technique employed. The Kopeloff modified Gram stain (see Appendix A) is recommended for staining anaerobes.[50]

Several species commonly appear in characteristic morphologic forms on direct smear. *Bacteroides* organisms appear as pleomorphic, pale, gram-negative bacilli showing irregular and often bipolar staining. Pale, long, slender, spindle-shaped, gram-negative bacilli with sharply pointed ends, often appearing in pairs or end to end, suggest *Fusobacterium nucleatum* (Plate 14, *E*). Pale, irregularly staining, extremely pleomorphic, gram-negative bacilli with swollen areas, filaments, and large round bodies suggest *Fusobacterium necrophorum* (Plate 14, *F*) or *Fusobacterium mortiferum*.

The presence or absence of spores, their location (terminal, subterminal, or central), and shape (round or oval) should also be noted on the direct Gram stain. Spores may also be seen with a spore stain such as malachite green, although spore stains are usually unnecessary.

When spirochetes are suspected, the direct microscopic examination should include the observation of a wet mount by darkfield or phase contrast microscopy.

Other identification procedures that may be used directly on the specimen are the direct fluorescent antibody technique, gas-liquid chromatographic analysis, and detection of bacterial antigens by counterimmunoelectrophoresis, radioimmunoassay, and other serologic procedures. These are discussed later in the chapter.

GROWTH REQUIREMENTS

Because of their unique oxygen sensitivity and in some cases their specific nutritional requirements, the isolation of anaerobic bacteria requires the use of special cultural and incubation methods.

MEDIA
Growth Factors

The use of enriched media provides optimal growth of anaerobes.[47] Among the common supplements are yeast extract, blood, hemin, and vitamin K_1. Hemin or vitamin K_1 or both are required for the growth of *B. melaninogenicus* and certain other *Bacteroides* spp. and stimulate the growth of many other organisms.

Although not a routine supplement, sodium bicarbonate may be added to various media such as thioglycolate to provide a source of CO_2. CO_2 greatly improves the growth of most anaerobes and stimulates the formation of spores of clostridia. Most organisms can assimilate CO_2 directly from the atmosphere; however, some cannot and thus need CO_2 to be provided as bicarbonate ions in the medium.[107]

Various amino acids may also be added to culture media to promote the growth of selected organisms. The addition of L-cystine permits the growth of certain thiol-dependent or sulfur-containing, amino acid–requiring bacteria such as *Fusobacterium necrophorum*. L-Cystine is also a required growth factor of *Clostridium novyi* B.

Reducing Agents

Reducing agents may be added to media to absorb oxygen and lower the oxidation-reduction potential. In the laboratory the most commonly used reducing agents are thioglycolic acid or its sodium salt, sodium thioglycolate, and cysteine in concentrations not exceeding 0.05%. Although reducing agents are commonly included in liquid or biochemical fermentation media, their addition to primary plating media is not essential and is influenced by the composition and length of storage of the media, as well as the specific organism being recovered.[92]

For laboratories that use reducing agents, prereduced anaerobically sterilized (PRAS) media and "reducible" media are available. PRAS media are sterilized in a reduced condition and remain reduced until and during inoculation. Preparation of such media is accomplished by (1) driving off the oxygen and partially reducing the ingredients by boiling, (2) cooling while simultaneously bubbling oxygen-free CO_2 through the media to introduce CO_2 and keep out air, (3) further reducing with the reducing agent cysteine hydrochloride, (4) adjusting the pH before dispensing into tubes that are being flushed with oxygen-free nitrogen, and (5) placing the tubes into a special press before autoclaving to keep the rubber stoppers in place. Thus oxygen exposure is minimal throughout preparation and subsequent use. The boiling before addition of reducing agents is important, since reducing agents themselves may become oxidized to form various toxic products. Boiling helps rid the medium of free oxygen and thus eliminates this possibility. The final E_h established in PRAS media is about -150 mV.

Reducible media also contain reducing agents; however, unlike PRAS media they are prepared under ambient conditions and not vigorous oxygen-excluding conditions. Reducing these media before use by placing them in an anaerobic environment overnight is generally recommended. Commercially prepared reducible media (for example, that available from Scott Laboratories, Inc., Fiskeville, R.I.) often contain L-cysteine hydrochloride, dithiothreitol, and palladium chloride. Both L-cysteine hydrochloride and dithiothreitol serve as reducing agents in the medium, whereas the palladium chloride functions as a catalyst, permitting the medium to remain semireduced when culture plates are stored aerobically provided they are placed in an oxygen-free atmosphere containing hydrogen for 24 hours before use. Hydrogen reacts to form H_2O in the presence of the catalyst.

PRAS media are excellent in supporting anaerobic growth, including that of the strict anaerobes, but their expense precludes their use in many clinical laboratories. Both freshly prepared media and commercial reducible media support the growth of the commonly encountered clinical anaerobic bacteria.

PRIMARY ISOLATION

Specimens recommended for anaerobic culture should be inoculated to nonselective anaerobic blood agar plates, anaerobic selective media, liquid enrichment media, and appropriate media for microaerophilic and aerobic organisms. A single agar medium is inadequate for isolation of anaerobes, since the recovery of anaerobic organisms is ordinarily lower with selective media, and overgrowth of facultative organisms occurs in nonselective media.[130] Both nonselective and selective media should be used during primary isolation. All primary plating media should be reduced by placing them in an anaerobic environment overnight unless freshly prepared media are used.[132] A liquid enrichment medium should also be employed as a check for the primary culture plates to recover low numbers of organisms and for the isolation of slow-growing anaerobes.

The choice of specific types of selective media varies with the source and nature of the specimen, as well as the number and appearance of the organisms on the Gram-stained direct smear. Table 20-3 offers a general guide for selection of anaerobic media for various specimen types.

Nonselective Media

Numerous nonselective blood agar media are available for culture of anaerobes. These media differ in their blood agar base and their growth supplements. The most commonly used blood agar bases include Columbia, Brucella, Schaedler, brain heart infusion (BHI), and tryptic soy agar (TSA).* Vitamin K_1 and hemin should be added during media preparation. As previously mentioned, enriched media allow optimal growth of anaerobes. Blood agar media intended solely for aerobic use are insufficient for the cultivation of these organisms.[47]

A study comparing the quantitative growth, rate of growth, and colony size of 47 clinical anaerobe isolates (10 different species) on commercially prepared Brucella, BHI, Columbia, TSA, and Schaedler agars showed similar quantitative bacterial growth on all media.[92] CDC anaerobe blood agar (see blood

---

*For examples of these nonselective media see blood agar, anaerobic Brucella base (Wadsworth), and blood agar, anaerobic, Columbia base in Appendix A.

TABLE 20-3. Guide to Media for Primary Isolation of Anaerobic Bacteria from Various Specimen Types

Source of Specimen	Media[a]
Central nervous system (abscess)	AnBA, Thio
Eye (intraocular)	AnBA, AnPEA, Thio
Pulmonary	AnBA, AnPEA, Thio
Intra-abdominal	AnBA, AnPEA, PV,[b] Thio (BBE)[c]
Genitourinary (endometrium upper tract disease)	AnBA, AnPEA, PV, Thio
Muscle tissue	AnBA, AnPEA, CMG (NEYA)
Bone marrow	AnBA, Thio
Body fluids (other than blood and urine)	AnBA, Thio

> SYMBOLS: AnBA, Anaerobic blood agar
> Thio, Enriched thioglycolate medium
> AnPEA, Anaerobic phenylethyl alcohol agar
> PV, Paromomycin-vancomycin blood agar
> BBE, Bacteroides bile esculin agar
> CMG, Chopped meat–glucose medium
> NEYA, Neomycin–egg yolk agar

Modified from Allen, S.D., Siders, J.A., and Marler, L.M.: Isolation and examination of anaerobic bacteria. In Lennette, E.H., et al., editors: Manual of clinical microbiology, ed. 4, Washington, D.C., 1985, American Society for Microbiology.
[a]These media are used for the recovery of anaerobic organisms. Other routine media that should be used for culture of these specimen types are cited in Table 11-5.
[b]Kanamycin-vancomycin blood agar may be used instead of paromomycin-vancomycin blood agar. The latter is recommended because some facultatively anaerobic, gram-negative bacilli are occasionally resistant to kanamycin but not to paromomycin.[4]
[c]Media in parentheses are optional.

agar, anaerobic [CDC] in Appendix A), although not included in this study, has the advantage that its inclusion of L-cystine enhances the growth of *Clostridium novyi* and thiol-dependent or sulfur-containing, amino acid–requiring bacteria.[128]

Selective Media

Among the numerous selective media are anaerobic phenylethyl alcohol blood agar,* kanamycin-vancomycin blood agar or laked blood agar,* Bacteroides bile esculin agar, paromomycin-vancomycin blood agar and cycloserine–cefoxitin–egg yolk–fructose agar. These media are discussed in Appendix A.

---

*See blood agar, anaerobic with kanamycin-vancomycin (CDC); blood agar, laked, anaerobic with kanamycin-vancomycin (Wadsworth); blood agar, phenylethyl alcohol, anaerobic (CDC); and blood agar, phenylethyl alcohol, anaerobic (Wadsworth) in Appendix A.

Liquid Media

Satisfactory liquid media for primary isolation include thioglycolate without indicator (Appendix A) and chopped meat–glucose (CMG) broth (Appendix A), provided they are supplemented with hemin (5 μg/ml) and vitamin K_1 (0.1 μg/ml). Thioglycolate medium is especially useful for the culture of slow-growing *Actinomyces* and *Arachnia* organisms, whereas CMG agar slant is valuable as a holding medium for anaerobes and for isolating clostridia by spore selection.

If liquid media are not stored anaerobically, they should be boiled for 10 minutes before inoculation to drive off dissolved oxygen. Tubes that are not used on the day of boiling should be discarded.[33] Liquid media should be incubated in an anaerobic system with the caps loosened.

Inoculating Procedures

Specimens for primary isolation should be inoculated according to the following procedures.[4,23]

Fluid specimens

A capillary pipette should be used to inoculate liquid or semisolid media near the bottom of the tube with 1 or 2 drops of the inoculum. When thioglycolate is inoculated, agitation should be avoided, since it might result in aeration of the medium. One drop is placed on each plating medium, and the medium is streaked for isolation with a platinum-iridium loop. Nichrome is not acceptable because it oxidizes the inoculum. A smear for Gram stain should be performed before the pipette is discarded.

Tissue or other solid specimens

A solid specimen should be minced with sterile scissors and sufficient prereduced broth added to emulsify the specimen. The specimen can be broken up by grinding with a mortar and a pestle, using sterile sand as necessary. The specimen can then be treated like the liquid specimen noted previously.

Swabs

If two swabs are received, the agar media and then the liquid media should be inoculated with one swab. The swab should be placed directly into the liquid medium and gently swirled, avoiding agitation. The second swab is used to prepare a smear for Gram stain examination. If only one swab is received, an inoculating suspension can be prepared by gently scrubbing the inoculum off the swab in approximately 2 ml of prereduced broth or 0.5 to 1 ml thioglycolate. The suspension is then used to inoculate the media in the same manner as the previously described liquid specimen.

SPECIAL ISOLATION PROCEDURES

Although not used routinely in the clinical laboratory, under certain circumstances the following special procedures may be helpful for the isolation of clostridia.[23,67,126,128] (Other special procedures are discussed in the text.)

Clostridia

Clostridia usually occur in mixed culture with gram-negative bacteria and nonsporeforming anaerobes. Their selective isolation is accomplished through the use of heat and alcohol treatments that kill vegetative forms of organisms present but allow clostridial spores to survive and subsequently germinate.

The following heat isolation method is recommended[23]:

1. Inoculate the specimen into three tubes of chopped meat–glucose with starch or another chopped meat medium.
2. Maintain all three tubes at 70° C for 10 minutes.
3. Cool one tube quickly, but transfer each of the other two tubes to an 80° C water bath for 10 and 20 minutes, respectively.
4. After designated incubation, cool tubes quickly in cold water.
5. Incubate all three tubes anaerobically at 30° C.
6. After 24 to 48 hours, streak inoculum onto blood agar plates.

Alternatively the original culture may be heat shocked at 80° C for 10 minutes and then inoculated onto blood agar and egg yolk agar or egg yolk agar with neomycin plates. The clostridial spores of some organisms, however, especially those of *C. botulinum* type E, may be as sensitive to heat as are the vegetative cells. Treatment of the specimen with 50% ethanol for 1 hour[67] is effective for the selective isolation of these clostridia. Spores are not sensitive to ethanol.

Clostridium tetani[126,128]

The isolation of *C. tetani* from lesions is difficult and often requires special procedures. When clinical and microscopic evidence suggests the presence of this organism, the specimen should be lightly inoculated onto a freshly poured blood agar plate and incubated anaerobically for 24 hours. The plate is examined for characteristic "swarming" appearing as a thin layer of growth across the agar surface. The cells are transferred from the edge of the swarming area to a tube of broth, and then the broth is streaked onto a plated medium containing 5% agar. Plates with this increased amount of agar (three times the concentration of routine medium) inhibit the swarming of *C. tetani*.

Clostridium perfringens[126]

The ability of *C. perfringens* to grow rapidly at 45° C allows for its selective isolation. When the clinical symptoms and microscopic features suggest the presence of *C. perfringens* but the specimen is contaminated, the specimen should be inoculated into chopped meat–glucose medium and incubated at 45° C. During the first 4 to 6 hours of incubation *C. perfringens* rapidly outgrows all other organisms, but after this time the contaminating flora outgrow *C. perfringens*. Thus, as soon as growth is observed but no longer than 6 hours after primary inoculation, the broth should be subcultured to blood agar and egg yolk agar and incubated overnight at 37° C. The cultures should be observed for characteristic morphology.

ANAEROBIC SYSTEMS

The incubation of anaerobes must be carried out in the absence of air. Three systems are available for anaerobic incubation: the anaerobic jar, the anaerobic glove box, and the roll tube method. These systems can be seen in Figures 20-2 to 20-4. The Bio-Bag chambers mentioned previously are basically individual anaerobic jars or containers.

Anaerobic Jars

Anaerobic conditions were achieved in the early anaerobic jars through the use of a catalyst system (to catalyze the combination of H_2 and O_2 to form water) that was activated by an electric current. The anaerobic jars used today, such as the GasPak jar (BBL, Cockeysville, Md.) or Oxoid jar (Oxoid USA, Columbia, Md.), are much more practical in that they use a "cold" catalyst system that does not require heat and obviates the potential for explosion.

The GasPak jar (Figure 20-2) is a cylindric polycarbonate plastic jar that is flanged at the top so the airtight lid can be clamped firmly into place. A wire mesh basket on the undersurface of the lid contains the room-temperature catalyst—palladium-coated aluminum pellets. (The catalysts should be rejuvenated at 160° C for 2 hours after each use because the accumulation of moisture and H_2S renders them nonfunctional.) Anaerobic conditions may be achieved in the GasPak jar (or other anaerobic jars) by using disposable hydrogen–carbon dioxide generators or an evacuation-replacement technique. The GasPak envelope (BBL) is a disposable envelope that serves as a hydrogen–carbon dioxide generator for the GasPak jar. This envelope contains two tablets, one consisting of citric acid and sodium bicarbonate and the other of sodium borohydride and cobalt chloride. After one corner of the envelope is torn off, the system is activated by adding 10 ml of water with a syringe or pipette. The envelope is then placed in the jar alongside the culture plates, and the lid is clamped securely. Paper towels are added to the jar to absorb moisture. The following reactions are responsible for the establishment of anaerobic conditions:

(a) $C_6H_8O_7 + 3\ NaHCO_3 \rightarrow Na_3\ (C_6H_5O_7) + 3\ H_2O + 3\ CO_2$
(b) $NaBH_4 + 2\ H_2O \rightarrow NaBO_2 + 4\ H_2$

The CO_2 generated in reaction *a* stimulates anaerobic growth. In the presence of the catalyst, the hydrogen produced in reaction *b* reacts with the oxygen in the jar to form water that condenses as a fine mist along the sides of the jar.

A GasPak Plus system is also available through BBL. This system incorporates the palladium catalyst within the disposable H_2 and CO_2 generator envelope. All reactions occurring in the GasPak Plus system are the same as those discussed previously.

A study of the atmospheric conditions established in an anaerobic jar with an activated GasPak envelope showed that the O_2 concentration in the jar was reduced to less than 0.4% in 100 minutes.[120] The E_h of the media reached -100 mV within 60 to 100 minutes, and the CO_2 concentration increased to between 4% and 7% in 60 minutes depending on the number of plates present. The heat on the lid* reached a maximum between 20 and 40 minutes, and the condensate appeared on the sides of the jar within 10 to 15 minutes. Although this study was conducted at 20° to 25° C and not at 37° C, it can be concluded that when a GasPak generator is used an anaerobic environment can be reached in approximately 100 minutes.[120]

Advantages of the GasPak system include its commercial availability, simplicity, and requirement for relatively little space. Its greatest disadvantage is that it must be opened for examination of the cultures, which results in oxygen exposure.

An evacuation-replacement (E-R) procedure[4] may also be used to establish anaerobiosis. With the E-R procedure the

---

*The lid of the jar directly above the catalyst basket becomes warm as a result of the reaction that is occurring.

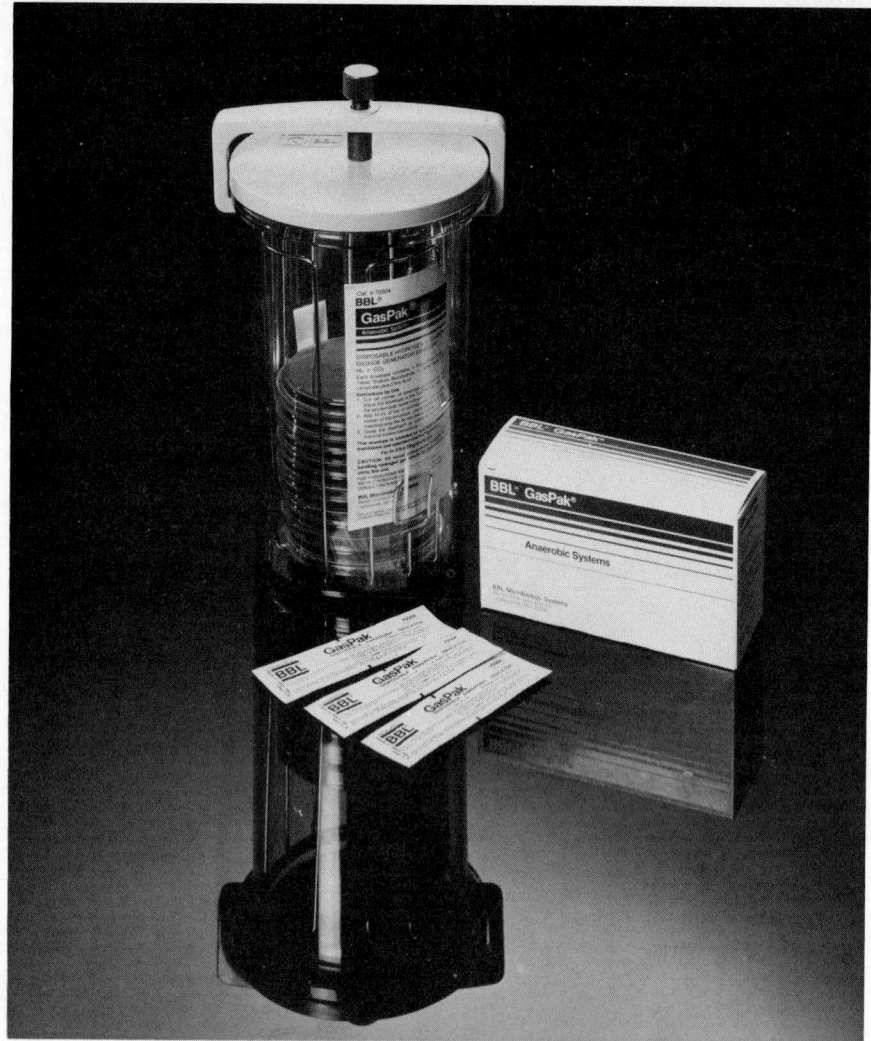

FIGURE 20-2. GasPak anaerobic jar. (Courtesy BBL Microbiology Systems, Division of Becton Dickinson & Co., Cockeysville, Md.)

vented lid on the cold catalyst jar is attached to an outlet tubing that in turn is attached to a vacuum pump. The jar is evacuated until the mercury column stands 50 to 60 cm (20 to 24 inches) and then filled with commercial-grade nitrogen. This procedure is repeated. When the jar is evacuated for the third time, it is refilled with an anaerobe gas mixture (10% H_2, 5% CO_2, 85% N_2) instead of commercial-grade nitrogen. The rubber tubing attached to the vented jar is then clamped, and the jar is disconnected from the vacuum and the gas line and placed in the incubator.

Holding Jars[4]

When anaerobic jars are used for incubation, the use of the holding jar technique is recommended to minimize oxygen exposure of cultures while primary plating, inspection of colonies, or subculturing is performed. Holding jars are simply anaerobic jars with loosely fitted, vented lids attached by rubber tubing to a tank of inexpensive, commercial-grade nitrogen gas.

Generally, three holding jars are used. One jar holds reduced

uninoculated media, the second jar freshly inoculated plates awaiting incubation, and the third jar plates with colonies that need to be subcultured. The uninoculated plating media, which have been previously reduced by placing them in an anaerobic jar or glove box for 6 to 24 hours, are placed in the first jar. After the lid is closed, the jar is flushed continuously with a gentle stream of N_2 or CO_2. The plates requiring subculture can be removed and appropriately subcultured. As soon as each plate is streaked, it is immediately placed in the second holding jar, which is also flushed with N_2 or CO_2. Primary plating may also be completed in a similar manner. After the second holding jar is filled with freshly inoculated plates, the holding jar lid is removed and the plates can be incubated with either the GasPak or E-R jar technique.

As an alternative to nitrogen gas, commercial-grade CO_2 that has been passed through a copper catalyst may be used. The flow rate of gas to the holding jars can be regulated by opening the small needle valve on the gas manifold and adjusting the gas tank regulator to 4 pounds/inch^2 for 1 to 2 minutes to purge the jar of air. The regulator pressure should be reduced to

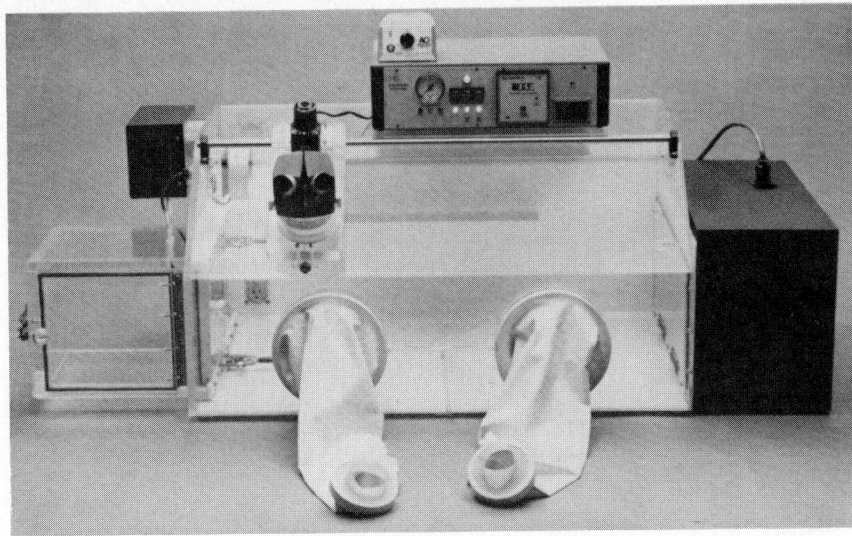

FIGURE 20-3. Anaerobic glove box. (Courtesy Anaerobe Systems, Santa Clara, Calif.)

½ to 1 pound/inch^2 and the flow rate to each jar regulated at 50 to 100 ml/min. If a flow meter is not available, this rate is equivalent to a flow rate of 1 to 2 bubbles per second when the rubber tubing in the jar is placed just beneath the surface of water in a small beaker.

Anaerobic Glove Box[61]

The glove box is a flexible vinyl plastic box or a rigid chamber that functions as a self-contained anaerobic system. This system not only provides the appropriate environment for incubation of cultures but also provides an oxygen-free environment in which the microbiologist can process specimens and perform other isolation and identification procedures. An anaerobic environment is initially achieved in the plastic glove box by inflation with a gas mixture of 5% CO_2, 10% H_2, and 85% N_2. Anaerobiosis is then maintained through the combined action of a palladium catalyst within the box with the 10% H_2 in the atmosphere.

Figure 20-3 illustrates the components of a glove box. Neoprene gloves attached to boxes permit manipulations inside the box by the microbiologist. More recently available glove boxes permit the use of bare hands within the chamber. The airlock system permits the movement of material into and out of the box without disturbance to the anaerobic atmosphere. To pass materials into the box, the operator opens the outer door of the airlock and places the materials inside. After the outer door is closed, the airlock atmosphere is evacuated and replaced with an oxygen-free gas for a total of three times. The inner door of the airlock leading to the chamber is then opened, materials are removed from the airlock into the chamber, and the inner door is reclosed to maintain the anaerobic atmosphere. The inclusion of a separate incubator in the glove box, as depicted in Figure 20-3, is generally preferred over maintaining the entire box at 37° C.

The greatest advantage of the glove box is that it permits examination of a culture without oxygen exposure. Disadvantages, however, include the large space requirement, the initial difficulty in manual dexterity encountered when working with the gloves, and the possibility of leaks.

Roll Tube Method[50]

The roll tube method uses rubber-stoppered tubes of PRAS agar media that have been cooled in a rolling machine to coat the entire inner surface of the tube with a thin layer of agar. To maintain the anaerobic environment in each tube, all inoculations and transfers are completed by removing the stopper and immediately inserting a cannula carrying a stream of oxygen-free CO_2. These manipulations are facilitated through the use of the V.P.I. Anaerobic Culture System (Bellco, Inc., Vineland, N.J.), which consists of (1) a streaker that rotates the PRAS tubes, permitting inoculation of the entire agar surface, (2) a treadle-operated gas cannula carrying the oxygen-free CO_2 gas inserted into the neck of each tube, and (3) a treadle-operated inoculator for rapid inoculation of differential media (Figure 20-4).

The primary advantage of this system is that each tube serves as its own anaerobic environment. The tubes can be placed in an ambient air incubator for incubation and can be examined at any time without oxygen exposure. The primary disadvantage is the necessity of special equipment.

Indicators of Anaerobiosis

Redox dyes are used to estimate the E_h potential of an anaerobic system. These dyes act as electron acceptors or donors and are generally colored in the oxidized form and colorless in the reduced form. Individual redox dyes are reduced or become colorless at different oxidation-reduction potentials.

Methylene blue indicators are available commercially for use in anaerobe jars. These indicators consist of glucose and methylene blue in an alkaline buffer. In the presence of the alkaline buffer the glucose reduces the methylene blue to its colorless form; however, when exposed to oxygen the indicator converts to its colored form.

Indicators such as resazurin or phenosafranin change color at lower oxidation-reduction potentials than methylene blue and can be used in the glove box. Resazurin is added to PRAS media. The ability to isolate extremely oxygen-sensitive organisms such as *Clostridium novyi* B may also be used to monitor anaerobiosis in the glove box.[61] If a culture of this organism is

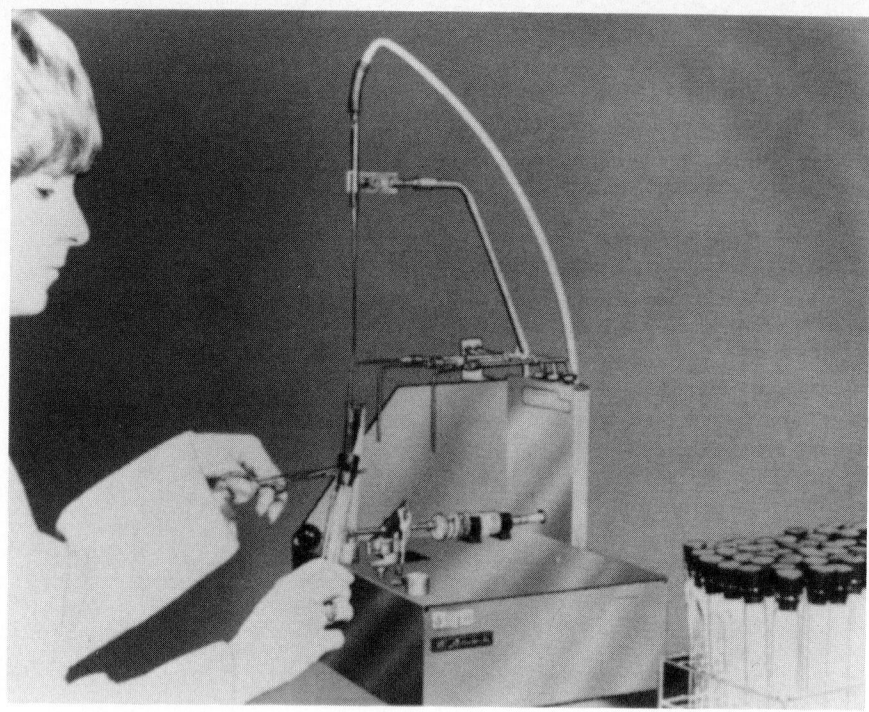

FIGURE 20-4. VPI anaerobic culture system. (Courtesy Bellco, Inc., Vineland, N.J.)

able to grow when maintained in the system, sufficiently anaerobic conditions have been achieved.

Comparison of Systems

Early studies comparing the efficacy of anaerobe jars, the anaerobic glove box, and roll tubes showed all three systems to give comparable results with clinical isolates.[64] Rosenblatt[111] has suggested that the anaerobic jar may be more effective because coincubation of cultures in the closed space of the jar stimulates the growth of certain anaerobes. This stimulation may be due to the production of a volatile gas by organisms such as *Clostridium perfringens*.

CULTURAL CHARACTERISTICS
OBSERVATION OF 24-HOUR PLATES

It is generally recommended that cultures in anaerobic jars be incubated for 48 hours at 35° C before examination. Examination in less than 48 hours may result in potentially bactericidal oxygen exposure that inhibits subsequent growth. In special circumstances when it is necessary to observe 18- to 24-hour plates, duplicate cultures may be inoculated and placed in separate anaerobe jars. (Roll tubes or culture plates incubated in a glove box may be examined at any time during incubation.)

OBSERVATION OF 48-HOUR PLATES AND LIQUID MEDIA

After 48 hours' incubation the colonial morphology of all isolates from the primary cultures should be examined, preferably with the use of a stereoscopic microscope or alternatively with a hand lens. Each colony type should be Gram stained, and the presence or absence of spores noted. The primary plating media should be examined with an ultraviolet light to note

any fluorescence of the colonies. The typical cellular and colonial morphologic characteristics of the most commonly isolated anaerobes are included in Tables 20-4 to 20-10. The colonial morphologies of many of these organisms are seen in Plates 15 to 17.

When Gram stained, some anaerobic gram-positive bacteria tend to decolorize more readily than others. If the Gram stain appears variable, the potassium hyroxide (KOH) test[45] or other methods discussed in Chapter 6 can be used to distinguish between gram-positive and gram-negative bacteria.[45]

Antimicrobial susceptibility tests may also be useful in distinguishing between gram-positive and gram-negative organisms. Susceptibility to a vancomycin disk (5 µg) and resistance to a colistin disk (10 µg) strongly suggest a gram-positive organism, whereas susceptibility to colistin and resistance to vancomycin strongly suggest a gram-negative organism.[132]

Many facultative and obligate anaerobic bacteria are morphologically similar. Thus, to ensure that an isolate is indeed an anaerobe, its relationship to oxygen or aerotolerance must be determined. Each colony type should be subcultured to an anaerobic blood agar purity plate incubated anaerobically, a chocolate agar plate incubated under 5% to 10% CO_2, and an aerobic blood agar plate incubated aerobically. The aerobic and anaerobic blood agar should contain the same base (W.J. Brown, personal communication, 1986). After 24 hours' incubation (or more depending on the amount of time required for primary isolation), each colony type should be classified according to its growth patterns (Table 20-11). The microaerophilic streptococci may give deceiving results when the aerotolerance test is performed.[112] On initial subculture these organisms may grow only anaerobically; however, a second subculture reveals their ability to grow also under CO_2 (capnophilic) (Figure 20-6). *Text continued on p. 391.*

TABLE 20-4. Microscopic Characteristics of the Clostridia

| Species | Gram Stain | | Spores | |
	Appearance and Arrangement	Size (μm)	Shape	Location
C. bifermentans	Gram-positive, straight rods occurring singly, in pairs, or in short chains	0.6-1.9 × 1.6-11	Oval; usually do not swell cells	Central to subterminal
C. botulinum type A and proteolytic strains of types B and F	Gram-positive, straight to slightly curved rods occurring singly or in pairs	0.6-1.4 × 3-20.2	Oval; swell cells	Subterminal
C. botulinum type E and saccharolytic strains of types B and F	Gram-positive straight rods occurring singly or in pairs	0.8-1.6 × 1.7-15.7	Oval; usually swell cells	Eccentric to subterminal
C. botulinum types C, D	Gram-positive straight rods occurring singly or in pairs	0.5-2.4 × 3-22	Oval; swell cells	Subterminal
C. butyricum	Gram-positive straight rods with rounded ends occurring singly, in pairs, or in short chains; occasionally occur as long filaments	0.5-1.7 × 2.4-7.6	Oval; usually do not swell cells	Central to subterminal
C. cadaveris	Gram-positive, straight rods occurring singly or in pairs	0.5-1.3 × 1.4-9.4	Oval; swell cells	Terminal; occasionally subterminal
C. difficile	Gram-positive straight rods; may produce chains of two to six cells aligned end to end	0.5-1.9 × 3-16.9	Oval; swell cells	Subterminal; rarely terminal
C. histolyticum	Gram-positive straight rods occurring singly, in pairs, or in short chains	0.5-0.9 × 1.3-9.2	Oval; may swell cells	Central to subterminal
C. innocuum	Gram-positive straight rods with rounded or tapered ends occurring singly or in pairs	0.4-1.6 × 1.6-9.4	Oval; wider than cells	Terminal to subterminal or free
C. limosum	Gram-positive straight rods occurring singly, in pairs, or in short chains	0.6-1.6 × 1.7-16	Oval; swell cells	Central to subterminal
C. novyi type A	Gram-positive rods occurring singly or in pairs	0.6-1.4 × 1.6-17	Oval; may swell cells	Central or subterminal
C. novyi type B	Similar to type A but larger (Plate 15, *A*)	1.1-2.5 × 3.3-22.5	Oval	Subterminal
C. perfringens	Gram-positive straight rods with blunt ends occurring singly or in pairs (Plate 15, *B*)	0.6-2.4 × 1.3-19	Seldom seen but when present are large and oval and swell cells	Central to subterminal

Continued.

TABLE 20-4. Microscopic Characteristics of the Clostridia—cont'd

| Species | Gram Stain | | Spores | |
	Appearance and Arrangement	Size (μm)	Shape	Location
C. ramosum	Gram-positive or gram-negative straight rods, often in short chains in V arrangements	0.5-0.9 × 2-12.8	Usually round; some oval; swell cells	Terminal (rarely seen and difficult to detect by heat test)
C. septicum	Gram-positive in young cultures but become gram negative with age; stain unevenly; straight or curved rods occurring singly or in pairs	0.6-1.9 × 1.9-35	Oval; swell cells	Subterminal
C. sordellii	Gram-positive straight rods occurring singly or in pairs	0.5-1.7 × 1.6-20.6	Oval; swell cells slightly	Central to subterminal
C. sporogenes	Gram-positive rods occurring singly	0.3-1.4 × 1.3-16	Oval; swell cells	Subterminal; sporulates readily
C. subterminale	Gram-positive straight rods occurring singly or in pairs	0.5-1.9 × 1.6-11	Oval; swell cells	Subterminal; occasionally central
C. tertium	Gram-positive straight rods occurring singly or in pairs	0.5-1.4 × 1.5-10.2	Large, oval; markedly swell cells	Terminal or occasionally subterminal
C. tetani	Gram positive becoming gram negative after 24 hours' incubation; occur singly or in pairs (Plate 15, *C*)	0.5-1.7 × 2.1-18.1	Oval; occasionally round	Terminal or subterminal; "drumstick" or "tennis-racket" appearance

[a]Descriptions are from Cato et al.[14] and are based on PYG broth.

TABLE 20-5. Colonial Characteristics of Some Commonly Encountered Clostridia[a]

Species	Size (mm)	Appearance	Hemolysis
C. bifermentans	0.5-4	Circular with irregular margins; flat or raised; lobate or scalloped; translucent or opaque; gray; smooth; shiny	Usually beta
C. butyricum	1-6	Large circular to irregular; smooth; raised; convex; lobate to slightly scalloped; gray-white; shiny or dull	None
C. difficile	2-5	Circular; matte to glossy; flat to low convex; occasionally rhizoid; opaque; white (Plate 15, *D*); fluoresce under UV light on KVA	None
C. histolyticum	0.5-2	Small circular to irregular; shiny; mosaic or granular surface; flat to low convex; entire to undulate margin; translucent or semiopaque; gray-white (Plate 15, *E*)	Beta

TABLE 20-5. Colonial Characteristics of Some Commonly Encountered Clostridia[a]—cont'd

Species	Size (mm)	Appearance	Hemolysis
C. innocuum	0.5-3	Circular; smooth, shiny; mottled or mosaic internal appearance; raised or convex; entire or slightly scalloped edge; translucent; gray-white or yellowish	Beta
C. limosum	1-4	Circular or irregular; shiny or dull; smooth; raised to convex; entire; translucent; gray; scalloped or undulate edge	Beta
C. novyi	1-5	Circular or irregular; crystalline or mosaic internal structure; flat or raised; translucent or opaque; gray; scalloped, undulate or lobate margins; some strains so thin and transparent that they are impossible to detect unless agar is "sloppy" streaked or surface is streaked immediately after solidification (Plate 15, *F*)	Beta (type B wider than A)
C. perfringens	2-5	Circular; glossy; dome shaped; entire; translucent; gray to grayish yellow; other morphologies including dwarfs, rough colonies with lobate edge, or flat colonies with irregular surface and filamentous margins may occur in same culture (Plate 16, *A*)	Double-zone beta
C. ramosum	0.5-2	Circular to slightly irregular; smooth; mottled or mosaic or granular internal structure; convex or raised; translucent to semiopaque; gray-white to colorless; entire, scalloped, or erose margin	None
C. septicum	1-5	Swarming; circular; glossy; slightly raised; markedly irregular to rhizoid margins; translucent; gray	Beta
C. sordellii	1-4	Circular to irregular; dull or shiny surface; granular or mottled internal structure; flat or raised; translucent to opaque; gray or chalklike; and a scalloped, lobate, or entire margin (Plate 16, *B*)	Variable (beta on rabbit blood)
C. sporogenes	2-6	Raised yellowish gray center and flattened periphery composed of entangled filaments ("Medusa head" colony); opaque; matte surface; coarse rhizoid edge (Plate 16, *C*)	Usually beta
C. subterminale	1-4	Matte surface; low convex or raised; translucent; gray; crystalline, mottled or mosaic internal structure; lobate or scalloped margin	Beta
C. tetani	2-5	Matte surface; may swarm; flat; irregular to rhizoid margin; translucent; gray	Usually narrow beta

[a]Descriptions are from Cato et al.[14] and are based on blood agar.

TABLE 20-6. Microscopic Characteristics of Common Anaerobic Gram-Negative Bacilli[a]

Genus and Species	Appearance and Arrangement	Size (μm)
Bacteroides		
B. disiens	Rods occur in pairs or occasionally in short chains	0.6-0.9 × 2-7
B. distasonis	Straight rods with rounded ends occurring singly or occasionally in pairs	0.6-1 × 1.6-11
B. fragilis	Pale-staining, pleomorphic rods with round ends occurring singly or in pairs; vacuoles often seen (Plate 16, *D*)	0.8-1.3 × 1.6-8
B. melaninogenicus	Coccobacillary rods	0.5-0.8 × 0.9-2.5 (occasionally up to 10)
B. ovatus	Oval cells with rounded ends occurring singly and occasionally in pairs	0.6-0.8 × 1.6-5
B. thetaiotaomicron	Irregularly staining, pleomorphic rods with rounded ends occurring singly or in pairs	0.7-1.1 × 1.3-8
B. vulgatus	Pleomorphic rods with rounded ends occurring singly and occasionally in pairs or short chains; swellings or vacuoles seen	0.5-0.8 × 1.5-8
Fusobacterium		
F. mortiferum	Pale, irregularly staining, highly pleomorphic rods with swollen areas, filaments, and large round bodies	0.8-1 × 1.5-10
F. necrophorum	Pleomorphic rods with round to tapered ends; may be filamentous or contain round bodies (Plate 14, *F*)	0.5-0.7 (to 1.8) × up to 10
F. nucleatum	Pale staining; long, slender, spindle shaped with sharply pointed or tapered ends; in pairs or end to end (Plate 14, *E*)	0.4-0.7 × 3-10
F. varium	Unevenly staining; pleomorphic, coccoid and rod shapes occurring singly or in pairs	0.3-0.7 × 0.7-2

[a]Descriptions are from Holdeman et al.[54] and Moore et al.[83] and are based on appearance in PYG broth.

TABLE 20-7. Colonial Characteristics of Some Commonly Encountered Anaerobic Gram-Negative Bacilli[a]

Genus and Species	Size (mm)	Appearance	Hemolysis
Bacteroides			
B. fragilis	1-3	Circular; entire; low convex; translucent to semiopaque (Plate 16, *E*)	Few strains slightly beta-hemolytic
B. thetaiotaomicron	1-3	Circular; entire; punctiform; convex; semiopaque; soft; shiny whitish	None

TABLE 20-7. Colonial Characteristics of Some Commonly Encountered Anaerobic Gram-Negative Bacilli[a]—cont'd

Genus and Species	Size (mm)	Appearance	Hemolysis
B. distasonis	Pinpoint to 0.5	Circular; entire; convex; smooth; translucent to opaque; gray-white	Some alpha
B. ovatus	0.5-1	Circular; entire; convex; pale buff color; semi-opaque; occasionally mottled in appearance	None
B. vulgatus	1-2	Circular; entire; convex; grayish; semiopaque	None
B. melaninogenicus	0.5-2	Circular; entire; convex; shiny; usually darker in center with gray to light brown edges; darker with continued incubation (Plate 16, *F*); dark pigment best on KVLBA; young colonies fluoresce under UV light (Plate 17, *A*)	None
B. disiens	Pinpoint to 2	Circular; entire; convex; translucent to opaque; smooth; shiny; white; some strains show light orange to pink fluorescence on blood agar	None
Fusobacterium *F. nucleatum*	1-2	Circular to slightly irregular; convex to pulvinate; translucent; often with "flecked" appearance when viewed by transmitted light (Plate 17, *B*)	Usually none
F. varium	Punctiform to 1	Circular; entire; flat to low convex; translucent; usually gray-white center with colorless edge	None
F. necrophorum	1-2	Circular with scalloped or erose edges; convex to umbonate; bumpy or ridged surface; translucent to opaque (Plate 17, *C*)	Alpha or beta (on rabbit)
F. mortiferum	1-2	Circular with entire, diffuse, or slightly scalloped edge; convex or slightly umbonate; translucent; smooth	None

[a]Descriptions are from Holdeman et al.[54] and Moore et al.[83] and are based on blood agar.

TABLE 20-8. Microscopic and Colonial Characteristics of More Commonly Isolated Anaerobic, Gram-Positive, Nonsporeforming Bacilli

Genus and Species	Microscopic Characteristics[a]		Colonial Characteristics[b]	
	Appearance and Arrangement	Size (μm)	Size (mm)[c]	Appearance
Eubacterium				
E. lentum	Diphtheroidal; small pleomorphic rods occurring singly and in pairs and short chains	0.2-0.4 × 0.2-2	0.5-2	Circular; entire to erose; raised to low convex; translucent to semiopaque; dull to shiny; smooth
E. limosum	Often appear with swollen ends and bifurcations; occur singly, in pairs, and in small clumps	0.6-0.9 × 1.6-4.8	Punctiform up to 2 mm in diameter	Circular; entire; convex; translucent to slightly opaque; sometimes mottled when viewed by obliquely transmitted light (Plate 17, *D*)
E. alactolyticum	Diphtheroidal; small rods with or without metachromatic staining and long filaments; "Chinese letter" configuration common	0.3-0.6 × 1.6-7.5	Punctiform to 0.5	Circular; entire; convex to pulvinate; smooth, shiny; translucent to opaque
Lactobacillus				
L. catenaforme	Short to medium rods; usually in chains; long, curved swollen rods and coccoid forms occasionally seen	—	—	Small; rough; nonpigmented; gray-white
Propionibacterium				
P. acnes	Pleomorphic small rods with or without metachromatic granules; club-shaped; "Chinese letter" configurations common	0.3-1.3 × 1-10	Punctiform to 0.5	Circular; entire to pulvinate; translucent to opaque; white to gray; glistening

Data from references 19 and 84.
[a]From PYG broth.
[b]From blood agar.
[c]Maximum size after approximately 4 days of incubation.

TABLE 20-9. Microscopic and Colonial Characteristics of Commonly Encountered *Actinomyces*, *Arachnia*, and *Bifidobacterium* Spp.

Genus and Species	Microscopic Characteristics— Appearance and Arrangement	Colonial Characteristics	
		Microcolony[a]	Macrocolony[b]
Actinomyces			
A. israelii	Groups of intertwining, branching filaments resembling microcolony; club-shaped rods also seen[c]	"Spider colony" (branching filaments radiating from single point) most common; filaments long, slender with branches arising at acute angles; also tiny colonies with one or two branching filaments, or larger with many filaments but no tangled central mass	Rough with or without central depression; circular or irregular with undulate, lobate, or erose edges; "molar tooth" (Figure 20-5), "breadcrumb," or "raspberry-like"; surface texture often granular with ground-glass appearance; elevation from convex to pulvinate to umbonate; opaque; cream or gray-white

TABLE 20-9. Microscopic and Colonial Characteristics of Commonly Encountered *Actinomyces, Arachnia,* and *Bifidobacterium* Spp.—cont'd

Genus and Species	Microscopic Characteristics— Appearance and Arrangement	Colonial Characteristics	
		Microcolony[a]	Macrocolony[b]
A. naeslundii	Variable; groups of intertwining branching filaments; club-shaped rods; thin filaments; rods with bifurcated ends; small rods with or without metachromatic staining[c]	Dense center or mass of diphtheroidal cells or filaments surrounded by long, branched filaments projecting in all directions	Smooth; 1-2 mm; circular; low convex to umbonate; entire edge; may produce rough colonies—simple granular surface to "raspberry-like"
A. odontolyticus	Variable; club-shaped rods; rods with bifurcated ends; thin filaments; small rods with or without metachromatic staining[c]	Smooth to finely granular; entire to irregular edge; slightly raised to convex; soft and white	Circular to irregular; 1-2 mm; entire or irregular edge; low convex to umbonate; smooth to finely granular; white, soft, opaque; deep red color on sheep blood agar
Arachnia *A. propionica*	Diphtheroidal cells; branching filaments; swollen spherical cells also seen	Branching, filamentous resembling *A. israelii;* smooth colonies rare	Variable; rough resembling molar tooth or breadcrumb; also smooth, convex with undulate edges seen
Bifidobacterium *B. eriksonii*	Diphtheroidal; coccoid or thin-pointed shape, or larger, highly irregular curved with branching; terminating in clubs or thick bifurcated ends	Tiny, glistening colonies at 48 hr; under ×100, circular, flat, granular with central core of denser growth and finely serrated to fuzzy edge	Dull white, soft, slightly convex to conical, smooth with entire edge; with age, more heaped in central areas and more spreading at edges; central areas smooth or pebbly; flattened border thin and transparent or denser with irregular grooves and scallops

Data from references 35 and 124.
[a]At 24 hours with magnification.
[b]At 7 to 14 days.
[c]From thioglycolate broth.

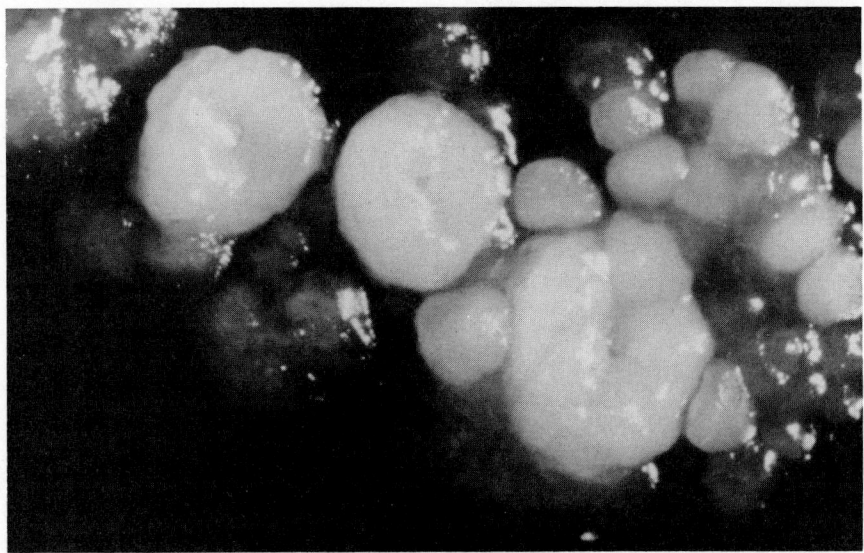

FIGURE 20-5. Typical "molar-tooth" colonies of *Actinomyces israelii.* (Courtesy Jill E. Clarridge.)

TABLE 20-10. Microscopic and Colonial Characteristics of Commonly Encountered Anaerobic Cocci

Genus and Species	Microscopic Characteristics[a]		Colonial Characteristics[b]	
	Appearance and Arrangement	Size (μm)	Size (mm)	Appearance
Peptostreptococcus spp.[c]	Gram-positive, spherical to ovoid cells occurring in pairs and chains	0.5-0.6	0.5-2	Smooth; shiny or dull; low convex with entire edges; gray to white; translucent to opaque (Plate 17, *E*)
Peptococcus niger	Gram-positive, spherical cells occurring singly and in pairs, tetrads, and irregular masses	0.3-1.3	0.5	Tiny, black, convex, shiny, smooth, circular colonies with entire edge; become light gray when exposed to air
Veillonella parvula	Gram-negative diplococci in masses and short chains	0.3-0.5	1-3	Smooth; entire; opaque; grayish white; butyrous (Plate 17, *F*); may show red fluorescence under ultraviolet light (360 nm)
Acidaminococcus fermentans	Gram-negative, oval or kidney-shaped diplococci	0.6-1	0.1-0.2	Round; slightly raised; entire; grayish white to nearly translucent
Megasphaera elsdenii	Gram-negative, spherical cocci in pairs, occasionally chains	2.4-2.6	0.5-2	Circular; entire; slightly raised; glistening to slightly rough surface; adherent to butyrous

Data from references 52 and 53.
[a]From PYG broth.
[b]On blood agar.
[c]All species have similar morphology.

TABLE 20-11. Relative Growth of Various Groups of Bacteria on the Basis of Their Relationships to Oxygen

Group	Examples	Relative Growth on Anaerobe Blood Agar in			
		Ambient Air	Candle Jar or 5% to 10% CO₂-Air Incubator	Mixture of 5% O₂, 10% CO₂, and 85% N₂	Anaerobic System without O₂
AEROBES					
Obligate	*Micrococcus luteus*	++++	++	±	−
	Nocardia asteroides	++++	++	±	−
Microaerophiles	*Campylobacter jejuni*	−	+ or ++	++++	−
ANAEROBES					
Facultative	*Escherichia coli*	++++	++++	++++	+++
	Pseudomonas aeruginosa	++++	+++	++	+ or ±
Aerotolerant	*Clostridium tertium*	+	+ or ++	+++	++++
	Clostridium histolyticum	+	+ or ++	+++	++++
Obligate	*Bacteroides fragilis*	−	−	−	++++
	Peptostreptococcus magnus	−	−	−	++++

SYMBOLS: ++++, Best growth	±, Scant growth
+++ or ++, Degrees of moderate growth	−, No growth
+, Poor growth	

From Allen, S.D., Siders, J.A., and Marler, L.M.: Isolation and examination of anaerobic bacteria. In Lennette, E.H., et al., editors: Manual of clinical microbiology, ed. 4, Washington, D.C., 1985, American Society for Microbiology.

The primary liquid enrichment media should also be Gram stained and examined for growth characteristics. If any morphologic forms that do not appear on the primary culture plates are observed on Gram stain, the liquid enrichment medium should be subcultured to appropriate plating media and then reincubated. Growth characteristics that should be noted in enriched thioglycolate without indicator are rate of growth (rapid, moderate, or slow), appearance (granular or diffuse), gas production, and odor.[4]

After appropriate identification procedures are performed, primary isolation plates should be reincubated for at least 48 hours and ideally for 5 to 7 days and examined periodically for any new colony types. Chopped meat–glucose and thioglycolate media should be held for a minumum of 7 days before being discarded as negative. In cases of suspected actinomycosis, osteomyelitis, endocarditis, or other serious infections, the broth cultures should be held for a minimum of 2 weeks before being discarded as negative[4] (preferably for 4 weeks when actinomycosis is suspected[3]).

OVERVIEW OF IDENTIFICATION PROCEDURES

The questions of how far to go in the identification of anaerobes and what identification method to use do not have clearcut answers.[1] These questions must be addressed based on an assessment of the technical competence of the personnel, resources available, patient population served, and needs of the physician. Definitive identification requires a multiplicity of biochemical tests, serologic tests, gas-liquid chromatographic (GLC) analysis, toxicity and toxin neutralization studies, and possibly animal pathogenicity tests. The three definitive identification schemes in anaerobic bacteriology are the Virginia Polytechnic Institute (VPI) method,[50] the Wadsworth method,[132] and the Centers for Disease Control (CDC) method.[23]

The *VPI Manual* initially classifies an organism to a genus on the basis of the Gram stain, aerotolerance test, and GLC analysis. Numerous biochemical tests are then performed for differentiation of species within the various genera. Analysis of the biochemical test results and chromatographic patterns permits definitive identification. Any laboratory performing GLC will find the manual's depicted chromatograms of each organism an invaluable aid. The VPI method uses PRAS media and the VPI inoculator or roll tube apparatus previously discussed. Fermentation of carbohydrates in PRAS media is determined with a pH meter.

The *Wadsworth Manual* offers both presumptive and definitive identification schemes. In this protocol, when the aerotolerance test is performed, a Brucella blood agar plate for anaerobic incubation is streaked for purity and then five disks are placed on its surface: 1000 μg kanamycin, 10 μg colistin, 5 μg vancomycin, a sodium polyanethol sulfonate (SPS) disk, and a nitrate disk. After appropriate incubation the results of the susceptibility, nitrate, and SPS tests are recorded, and colonial morphology, pigment, hemolysis, fluorescence, and pitting of the agar are noted. A Gram stain, spot indole test, and catalase test are also performed. Based on results of all these test findings and characteristics, isolates may be presumptively classified into groups. GLC analysis and various biochemical media are then recommended to allow definitive speciation within each group. The Wadsworth method uses PRAS carbohydrate fermentation media. These media may be inoculated using the VPI apparatus or, if prepared in Hungate-type tubes (tubes with

a rubber diaphragm stopper), they may be inoculated with a syringe.

After aerotolerance is determined and pure cultures of each anaerobic isolate in thioglycolate and chopped meat broths are obtained, the *CDC Manual* recommends the inoculation of a basic set of differential media: chopped meat, fermentation base, glucose, mannitol, lactose, sucrose, maltose, salicin, thiogel, iron-milk, indole nitrate, H_2S, motility, esculin, peptone-yeast-glucose (PYG) agar, infusion agar slant, and PYG broth (for GLC analysis). Additional biochemical media are added to this basic set for the gram-positive sporeformers, gram-negative rods, and gram-positive nonsporeforming rods. Unlike the VPI and Wadsworth methods, the CDC method uses a thioglycolate-based carbohydrate fermentation medium with a bromthymol blue indicator for determination of carbohydrate fermentation. The formulations for many of the other biochemical and culture media also vary according to the scheme used. The reader should consult the *CDC Laboratory Manual*,[23] *V.P.I. Anaerobe Laboratory Manual*,[50] and *Wadsworth Anaerobic Bacteriology Manual*[132] for details of media preparation and use.

Although definitive identification should be made whenever possible, many clinical laboratories do not have the resources to complete these procedures. Fortunately, presumptive identification methods involve a few key characteristics that are relatively easy to determine. Furthermore, some of these key features may be determined with rapid tests. All laboratories should be capable of presumptive identification of isolates from primary plates and of isolation and maintenance of the organisms in pure culture so that in important cases the isolate can be sent to a reference laboratory for complete identification and susceptibility testing.[132]

BIOCHEMICAL IDENTIFICATION
ANAEROBIC, NONSPOREFORMING, GRAM-NEGATIVE BACILLI

The genera comprising the anaerobic, gram-negative bacilli are listed on pp. 373 and 374. Members of the genus *Bacteroides* are by far the most common isolates among this group of organisms.[74,148]

Bacteroides
Bacteroides fragilis group

B. fragilis, B. distasonis, B. ovatus, B. thetaiotaomicron, B. vulgatus, and *B. uniformis* make up what is known as the *B. fragilis* group. These organisms are distinguished by their ability to grow in the presence of bile as determined by the 20% bile tube test, disk test, or growth on BBE agar. The *B. fragilis* group is also resistant to several antimicrobial agents, and these two characteristics, bile resistance and antimicrobial resistance, form the basis of presumptive identification schemes. Draper and Barry,[24] for example, proposed that bile resistance and kanamycin resistance be used for presumptive identification of these organisms. Paper disks impregnated with oxgall (25 mg) and kanamycin (100 μg) may be placed on the surface of a Brucella blood agar plate that has been inoculated with a thioglycolate broth culture of the test organism adjusted to the turbidity of a McFarland no. 0.5 standard. After incubation for 24 to 48 hours in an anaerobic environment, isolates that are resistant to both kanamycin (zone of inhibition greater than 12 mm) and bile (confluent growth to the edge of the disk) are presump-

TABLE 20-12. Characteristics of Bile-Resistant *Bacteroides* Spp.

Genus and Species	Growth in 20% Bile	Indole Production	Catalase	Esculin Hydrolysis	Fermentation of							Fatty Acids from PYG[a]
					Sucrose	Maltose	Rhamnose	Salicin	Trehalose	Arabinose	Xylan	
B. FRAGILIS GROUP												
B. distasonis	+	−	+⁻	+	+		v	+	+	−⁺		A, p, S, (pa), (ib), (iv), (l)
3452A homology group[b]	+	−	−	+	+		+⁻	+⁻	+	+		
B. fragilis	+	−	+	+	+		−	−	−	−		A, p, S, pa
B. vulgatus	+	−	−⁺	−⁺	+		+	−	−	+		A, p, S
B. ovatus	+	+	−⁺	+	+		+	+	+	+	+	A, p, S, pa, (ib), (iv), (l)
B. thetaiotaomicron	+	+	+⁻	+	+		+	−⁺	+	+	−	A, p, S, pa
B. uniformis	W⁺	+	−⁺	+	+		−⁺	+⁻	−	+		a, p, l, S, (ib), (iv)
OTHER												
B. eggerthii	+	+	−	+	−	+	+⁻	−	−	+		A, p, S, (ib), (iv), (l)
B. splanchnicus	W⁺	+	−	+	−	−	−	−	−	+		A, P, ib, b, iv, S, (l)

SYMBOLS: +, Positive reaction for majority of strains; includes weak as well as strong acid production from carbohydrates in saccharolytic organism
−, Negative reaction
+⁻, Most strains positive; reaction helpful if positive
−⁺, Most strains negative, some weakly positive
W⁺, Most strains weakly positive, some positive
W⁻, Most strains weakly positive, some negative
v, Variable reaction
PRAS carbohydrates: +, pH < 5.5
W, pH 5.5–5.7
−, pH > 5.7

A, Acetic acid
P, Propionic acid
S, Succinic acid
L, Lactic acid
B, Butyric acid
PA, Phenylacetic acid
IB, Isobutyric acid
IV, Isovaleric acid

Reprinted from Sutter, V.L., et al.: Wadsworth anaerobic bacteriology manual, 4th edition, copyright 1985, Star Publishing Company, Belmont, Calif.

[a]Capital letters indicate major metabolic products, and small letters minor metabolic products. Parentheses indicate a variable reaction. Isoacids are primarily from carbohydrate-free media (such as PY) in the case of saccharolytic organisms.
[b]This group has recently been named *Bacteroides caccae*.[60a]

tively identified as members of the *B. fragilis* group. *B. eggerthii* and *B. splanchnicus,* however, are also kanamycin susceptible and bile resistant and thus must be differentiated from the *B. fragilis* group as discussed in the following paragraph.

Weinberg, Smith, and McTighe[142] have suggested the use of bile susceptibility and catalase for presumptive identification of *Bacteroides* organisms. In this scheme anaerobic, gram-negative bacilli are subcultured directly on chocolate agar, a 15 mg bile disk is placed in the area of heaviest inoculum, and the plate is incubated for 24 to 48 hours at 35° C in an anaerobic glove box. The catalase test is performed directly on the chocolate agar plate after exposure to air for 30 minutes. Although several species of the *B. fragilis* group are catalase negative (Table 20-12), most isolates of *B. thetaiotaomicron* and *B. fragilis,* the most commonly isolated species, are positive. Thus organisms that are bile resistant and catalase positive are pre-

sumptively identified as the *B. fragilis* group, whereas those that are bile sensitive and catalase negative are presumptively identified as anaerobic, gram-negative bacilli not of the *B. fragilis* group. Organisms that are neither positive nor negative for both of these characteristics require further work, since *Fusobacterium mortiferum, Fusobacterium varium, B. eggerthii,* and *B. splanchnicus* are all bile resistant and catalase negative. Fermentation of sucrose distinguishes the latter two organisms from the *B. fragilis* group; *B. eggerthii* and *B. splanchnicus* are sucrose negative and the *B. fragilis* group is sucrose positive.

Indole production is determined by the rapid spot test (growth from blood agar is rubbed onto filter paper containing paradimethylaminocinnamaldehyde; blue color is a positive finding) or by the conventional tube test using a tryptophan-rich medium. Fermentation of various carbohydrates further differ-

TABLE 20-13. Characteristics of Pigmented *Bacteroides* Spp.

| Genus and Species | Indole Production | Lipase | Fermentation of | | | Esculin Hydrolysis | Phenylacetic Acid Production | Fatty Acids from PYG[a] |
			Glucose	Lactose	Cellobiose			
B. asaccharolyticus[b]	+	−	−	−	−		−	A, p, ib, B, iv, S
B. gingivalis	+	−	−	−	−		+	a, p, ib, B, IV, s, pa
B. intermedius	+	+	+	−	−			A, iv, S, (p), (ib)
B. corporis	−	−	+	−	−			A, ib, iv, S, (b)
B. melaninogenicus	−	−	+	+	−	−		A, S, (ib), (iv), (l)
B. denticola	−	−	+	+	−	+		A, S, (ib), (iv), (l)
B. loescheii	−	−+	+	+	+	v		a, S, (l)

SYMBOLS:	+, Positive reaction for majority of strains; includes weak as well as strong acid production from carbohydrates in saccharolytic organisms
	−, Negative reaction
	−+, Most strains negative, some weakly positive
	v, Variable reaction
	A or a, Acetic acid ib, Isobutyric acid
	p, Propionic acid IV or iv, Isovaleric acid
	B or b, Butyric acid l, Lactic acid
	S or s, Succinic acid pa, Phenylacetic acid

Reprinted from Sutter, V.L., et al.: Wadsworth anaerobic bacteriology manual, 4th edition, copyright 1985, Star Publishing Company, Belmont, Calif.

[a]Capital letters indicate major metabolic products, and small letters minor metabolic products. Parentheses indicate a variable reaction. Isoacids are primarily from carbohydrate-free media (such as PY) in the case of saccharolytic organisms.

[b]*B. endodontalis*, a newly described pigmented *Bacteroides* sp., is phenotypically indistinguishable from *B. asaccharolyticus*.

entiates among the members of the *B. fragilis* group (Table 20-12). Organisms previously known as the 3452A homology group (Table 20-12) have recently been named *Bacteroides caccae*.[60a] These organisms are phenotypically very similar to *B. distasonis*. The fermentation of arabinose by *B. caccae* but by only a few strains of *B. distasonis* helps to differentiate these organisms.[51]

Pigmented *Bacteroides*

DNA homology studies have identified several new species of pigmented *Bacteroides* that were originally classified as subspecies of *B. melaninogenicus*. Of these species, *B. melaninogenicus*, *B. denticola*, *B. loescheii*, and *B. intermedius* are frequently isolated from the saliva and gingival margins of individuals with periodontitis and are also commonly seen in clinical specimens. *B. gingivalis* is common in the human mouth but is a rare clinical isolate. *B. asaccharolyticus* and *B. corporis* are not isolated from the human mouth but are recovered from clinical specimens.

These organisms produce pigments ranging from buff to tan to black after 2 to 21 days' incubation. The degree and rapidity of pigmentation vary according to the type of blood used; rabbit and human blood are the best supporters of pigmentation.[51] Because of the variability of pigment production, characteristics other than pigmentation should be used for recognition of

these organisms.[51] As discussed previously, presumptive identification of the pigmented *Bacteroides* spp. is indicated by brick-red fluorescence of the clinical specimen or of isolated colonies (Plate 17, *A*). These organisms may also fluoresce pink, orange, or chartreuse. Brick red is the only reliable color for presumptive identification if pigment has not been produced because nonpigmented *Bacteroides* spp. may also fluoresce pink or orange.[132]

Characteristics for differentiation of these organisms are shown in Table 20-13. *B. asaccharolyticus* does not utilize carbohydrates. The oral strains of *B. asaccharolyticus* are now called *B. gingivalis*.[54] *B. gingivalis* differs from other *B. asaccharolyticus* strains in the production of phenylacetic acid[62] and the ability to agglutinate sheep erythrocytes.[125] As noted in Table 20-13, *B. endodontalis* is phenotypically indistinguishable from *B. asaccharolyticus*.

Bile-sensitive, nonpigmented *Bacteroides*

Bile-sensitive, nonpigmented *Bacteroides* strains do not grow well in 20% bile (2% oxgall) and do not form a black pigment. Sutter and co-workers[132] divide this group into three subgroups: saccharolytic and proteolytic species, saccharolytic species, and nonsaccharolytic or weakly saccharolytic species (Table 20-14). The saccharolytic species may be further divided into pentose fermenters and pentose nonfermenters. *B. oris*

TABLE 20-14. Characteristics of Nonpigmented, Bile-Sensitive *Bacteroides* Spp.

Genus and Species	Fermentation of							Esculin Hydrolysis	Beta-Glucosidase	Zoogleal Mass	Indole Production	Gelatin Hydrolysis	Fatty Acids from PYG[a]
	Glucose	Sucrose	Lactose	Arabinose	Xylose	Salicin	Xylan						
SACCHAROLYTIC													
Pentose fermenters													
B. oris	+	+	+	+	+	+		+	−	−	−		A, S, (p), (ib), (iv)
B. buccae	+	+	+	+	+	+		+	+	−	−		A, S, (p), (ib), (b), (iv), (l)
B. zoogleoformans	+	+	+	v	v	v		+		+	+⁻		A, P, S, (iv), (ib)
Pentose nonfermenters													
B. oralis	+	+	+	−	−	+		+			−		A, S, (l)
B. buccalis	+	+	+	−	−	−	−	+			−		a, iv, S
B. veroralis	+	+	+	−	−	−	+	+			−		a, S
SACCHAROLYTIC AND PROTEOLYTIC													
B. bivius	+	−	+	−	−	−		−			−	+	A, iv, S, (ib)
B. disiens	+	−	−	−	−	−		−			−	+	A, S, (p), (ib), (iv)
NONSACCHAROLYTIC OR WEAKLY SACCHAROLYTIC													
B. capillosus	w⁻	−	−	−	−	−		+			−	−	a, s, (p), (l)
B. praeacutus[b]	−	−	−	−	−	−		−			−	+	A, p, ib, B, IV, a, (l)
B. putredinis	−	−	−	−	−	−		−			+	+	a, P, ib, b, IV, S, (l)

> **SYMBOLS:** +, Positive reaction for majority of strains; includes weak as well as strong acid production from carbohydrates in saccharolytic organisms
> −, Negative reaction
> v, Variable reaction
> w⁻, Most strains weakly positive, some negative
> +⁻, Most strains positive, reaction helpful if positive
> A, Acetic acid
> S, Succinic acid
> P, Propionic acid
> l, Lactic acid
> ib, Isobutyric acid
> IV, Isovaleric acid
> B, Butyric acid

Reprinted from Sutter, V.L., et al.: Wadsworth anaerobic bacteriology manual, 4th edition, Copyright 1985, Star Publishing Company, Belmont, Calif.
[a]Capital letters indicate major metabolic products, and small letters minor metabolic products. Parentheses indicate a variable reaction. Isoacids are primarily from carbohydrate-free media (such as PY) in the case of saccharolytic organisms.
[b]Now *Tissierella praeacuta*.[18]

and *B. buccae* are pentose fermenters that are frequently found in clinical specimens and in the sulci and gingival crevices of individuals with periodontitis. These two species are separated by testing with beta-glucosidase. *B. zoogleoformans*, another pentose fermenter, may also be found in the gingival crevices of patients with periodontal disease.[15] The name of this organism is derived from the Greek adjective *zoos*, alive or living, and the Greek noun *glois*, gum or glue; "living glue" describes the viscous, glutinous type of growth exhibited by these organisms in broth cultures.[15]

The three pentose nonfermenters, *B. oralis*, *B. buccalis*, and *B. veroralis*, are part of the flora of the oral cavity but are relatively rare in clinical specimens. They may be differentiated by fermentation of salicin and xylan. Sutter and co-workers[132] stress that these three pentose nonfermenters may be confused with members of the pigmented *Bacteroides* spp., especially *B. loescheii*, *B. melaninogenicus*, and *B. denticola*, if the development of pigment is delayed in the latter group.

B. bivius and *B. disiens* are saccharolytic and proteolytic. The latter characteristic is indicated by their hydrolysis of gelatin within 2 to 3 days. These organisms ferment glucose and, in the case of *B. bivius*, also lactose. They do not ferment sucrose or the pentose carbohydrates as do the saccharolytic species described previously.

B. ureolyticus and *B. gracilis* are asaccharolytic *Bacteroides* spp. that usually "pit" the agar. The previous taxonomy of these organisms is confusing.[60] *Bacteroides corrodens* was the original name given to all organisms, both facultative and anaerobic, that produced "corroding" colonies on agar. Subsequently the facultative strains were designated *Eikenella corrodens* (see Chapter 17) and the name *Bacteroides corrodens* was reserved for the anaerobic strains only. In 1978, *B. corrodens* was renamed *B. ureolyticus*.[58] Subsequent DNA homology studies have helped to redefine *B. ureolyticus* and all the other organisms that "pit" or "corrode" the agar.[138] The new species *B. gracilis* has been proposed for the urease-negative strains of *B. ureolyticus*. The other anaerobic organisms that pit or corrode the agar are members of the genus *Wolinella*. (The facultative organisms that corrode the agar include *E. corrodens* and *Campylobacter concisus*.) In addition to pitting the agar, *B. ureolyticus*, *B. gracilis*, and the genus *Wolinella* grow poorly or not at all in broth culture without the addition of formate and fumarate. These substances act as an electron donor-acceptor pair; the transfer of electrons provides energy for growth of the organisms. (Hydrogen may replace formate as the electron donor.) Differentiation of members of the genus *Wolinella* is discussed in the following paragraph. If susceptibility to kanamycin, colistin, and vancomycin is used for initial screening of the anaerobes as recommended by Sutter and co-workers,[132] *B. ureolyticus* and *B. gracilis* can be distinguished from other *Bacteroides* spp. by their susceptibility to kanamycin and colistin. Concomitant demonstration of pitting and the requirement for formate and fumarate offers strong presumptive identification of these organisms provided they are distinguished from *Wolinella* organisms.

Wolinella

In addition to pitting the agar and requiring formate-fumarate for growth, *Wolinella*, like *B. ureolyticus* and *B. gracilis*, is asaccharolytic and reduces nitrate. Motility is used to distinguish *Wolinella* from *Bacteroides* spp.; *B. ureolyticus* and *B. gracilis* are nonmotile, and members of the genus *Wolinella* are motile. Differentiation of the three species of *Wolinella*—*W. succinogenes*, *W. recta*, and *W. curva*—is discussed in other sources.[138,139]

Fusobacterium

F. nucleatum and *F. necrophorum* are by far the most frequently isolated and most pathogenic members of the genus *Fusobacterium*. A 6-year study at Wadsworth Medical Center[38] demonstrated that *F. gonidiaformans*, *F. naviforme*, *F. russii*, *F. mortiferum*, and *F. varium* were the most commonly isolated "other gram-negative bacilli" (OGNB). The OGNB group included all gram-negative, anaerobic bacilli other than *F. nucleatum*, *F. necrophorum*, and members of the genus *Bacteroides*.

Differentiation among the fusobacteria is shown in Table 20-15. As with the genus *Bacteroides*, growth in 20% bile divides members of the genus *Fusobacterium* into bile-sensitive and bile-resistant species. The three bile-resistant species—*F. mortiferum*, *F. varium*, and *F. necrogenes*—can be differentiated on the basis of indole production, esculin hydrolysis, and lactose fermentation.

Among the bile-sensitive fusobacteria, *F. gonidiaformans* is weakly saccharolytic and produces indole. It is distinguished

from *F. nucleatum* on the basis of cellular morphology and from *F. necrophorum* by its inability to convert lactate to propionate and to produce lipase. *F. naviforme* is inactive except for indole production, which distinguishes it from the totally inactive *F. russii*. All the fusobacteria are glutamic acid decarboxylase negative.

GLC is useful in differentiating among the *Bacteroides* and *Fusobacterium* genera, as well as among some species of fusobacteria. Gram-negative, nonsporeforming rods forming butyric acid as a major product are members of the genus *Fusobacterium*, whereas rods that generally do not produce butyric acid are members of the genus *Bacteroides*. Although some *Bacteroides* spp. do produce butyric acid, it is generated in combination with isobutyric and isovaleric acids, unlike *Fusobacterium* spp., which produce butyric acid and not isobutyric or isovaleric.

Other Anaerobic, Nonsporeforming, Gram-Negative Bacilli[38]

The remaining genera of the anaerobic, nonsporeforming, gram-negative bacilli include *Leptotrichia*, *Succinimonas*, *Selenomonas*, *Butyrivibrio*, *Anaerovibrio*, *Succinivibrio*, *Anaerobiospirillum*, *Pectinatus*, *Acetivibrio*, and *Lachnospira*. Several of these genera have been reported in the literature as anaerobic vibrios on the basis of polar flagella and curved morphology. Although most of these organisms are infrequently isolated from clinical specimens and thus have not been well defined or identified in most clinical laboratories, they are occasionally associated with human infection and their identification aids in appreciation of their pathogenic potential.[38] Differentiation among genera of these organisms is shown in Table 20-16.

Special mention should be made of *Leptotrichia buccalis*, a potentially virulent organism, especially in compromised hosts.[85] This organism presents a characteristic morphology and Gram stain appearance. It is a long, plump, straight or slightly curved, gram-negative bacillus growing end to end in pairs or chains. The joined ends of the cells are flattened, whereas the unjoined ends are tapered. On blood agar after incubation for 24 hours, the colonies are 2 to 3 mm in diameter with a characteristic cerebriform or convoluted appearance. Definitive identification is accomplished with GLC. Unlike the other gram-negative anaerobic bacilli, *L. buccalis* produces lactic acid as the sole metabolic organic acid end product.

ANAEROBIC, SPOREFORMING, GRAM-POSITIVE BACILLI

The clostridia vary with regard to oxygen requirements and Gram stain reaction.[126] *C. tertium* and *C. histolyticum* are aerotolerant and form colonies on freshly prepared blood agar incubated aerobically. *C. novyi* type B and *C. haemolyticum* are strict anaerobes and require stringent oxygen-excluding techniques for isolation. Occasionally the aerotolerant clostridia may be confused with the facultative *Bacillus* spp. Differentiation is accomplished with the catalase test; bacilli are usually catalase positive, whereas clostridia are catalase negative.

Some clostridia may appear gram negative, especially in overnight broth cultures. Furthermore, spores are not always obvious unless spore selection techniques are used. Because clostridia are usually larger than other organisms, their pres-

TABLE 20-15. Identification of *Fusobacterium* Spp.

Genus and Species	Growth in 20% Bile	Indole	Esculin Hydrolysis	Propionate from Lactate	Propionate from Threonine	Fermentation of[a] Glucose	Fermentation of[a] Mannose	Fermentation of[a] Lactose	Fatty Acids from PYG Broth[b]
F. nucleatum	1	+	−	−	+	−, w	−	−	B, a, p, (F), (L), (s)
F. gonidiaformans	NG, 2	+	−	−	+	−	−	−	B, A, p, (l), (f), (s)
F. varium	4, 2	d	−	−	+	w, +	w, +	−	B, L, a, p, (s)
F. necrophorum	NG, 4	+	−	+	+	−, w	−	−	B, p, a, (l), (s)
F. perfoetens	NG	−	−	−	+	w	−	−	B, a, p, (L)
F. naviforme	NG, 2	+	−	−	−	w, −	−	−	B, L, a, (f), (p), (s)
F. russii	NG, 2	+	−	−	−	−	−	−	B, L, a, (f)
F. mortiferum	4, St	−	+	−	+	+, w	w, +	+, w	B, a, p, (s), (f), (l), (v)
F. necrogenes	4, 2	−	+	−	+	w, +	w, +	−	B, a, p, (f), (s), (l)
F. prausnitzii	2, NG	−	+	−	−	w, −	−, w	w, −	B, L, F, (s)

SYMBOLS:
NG, No growth
1, Very poor
2, Poor
3, Moderate
4, Excellent
St, Stimulated (more growth than in PYG control tube)
−, Negative

+, Positive
A, Acetic acid
B, Butyric acid
P, Propionic acid
F, Formic acid
L, Lactic acid
S, Succinic acid
V, Valeric acid

For carbohydrate reactions:
+, pH below 5.5
−, pH 5.7 or above
w, Weak reaction, pH 5.5 to 5.7

Modified from Moore, W.E.C., Holdeman, L.V., and Kelley, R.W.: Genus II. *Fusobacterium*. In Krieg, N.R., editor (Holt, J.G., editor-in-chief): Bergey's manual of systematic bacteriology, vol. 1, Baltimore, 1984, Williams & Wilkins Co.
[a]When two reactions are given, the first is the more common.
[b]Products from 1% peptone–1% yeast extract–1% glucose (PYG) broth cultures. Capital letters indicate an average (from multiple cultures) of >1 mEq of acid/100 ml broth. Lower-case letters indicate <1 mEq/100 ml. Products in parentheses may or may not be detected.

ence should be suspected when large cells are seen in the Gram stain of a clinical specimen.[126]

Definitive identification of the clostridia is shown in Table 20-17. The characteristics in Table 20-18 may be used for presumptive identification; determination of lecithinase and lipase and the Nagler reaction on egg yolk agar are especially useful (see egg yolk agar, Appendix A).

C. perfringens is the most frequently isolated pathogenic species. Its characteristic double zone of hemolysis, an inner zone of complete hemolysis caused by theta toxin and an outer zone of incomplete hemolysis caused by alpha toxin (Plate 16, *A*), typical Gram stain reaction (Plate 15, *B*), stormy fermentation of milk (see milk medium, Appendix A), and production of lecithinase are useful for presumptive identification. Several other species of *Clostridium* are also lecithinase positive (Table 20-18). Among these lecithinase-positive organisms, *C. perfringens*, *C. baratii*, *C. bifermentans*, and *C. sordellii* are also positive in the Nagler test (see Appendix A for description). Differentiation of these four Nagler-positive species may be accomplished on the basis of the characteristic morphology of

C. perfringens and the reactions for indole, motility, lactose, gelatin, and urease (Table 20-18). *C. sordellii* is the only urease-positive clostridial species, but not all *C. sordellii* strains are urease positive.

A reverse CAMP test has been suggested for the presumptive identification of *C. perfringens*.[11,44,46] The test is based on the synergistic hemolysis shown by *Clostridium perfringens* and group B streptococci. To perform the test, a blood agar plate is inoculated with a single streak of the suspected isolate of *C. perfringens*. A group B beta-hemolytic *Streptococcus* is then inoculated at a 90-degree angle in a single streak to within a few millimeters of the *Clostridium*. After anaerobic incubation for 24 to 48 hours, an arrowhead zone of synergistic hemolysis is presumptive identification of *C. perfringens*.

The identification of *C. difficile* is discussed on p. 409.

GRAM-POSITIVE, NONSPOREFORMING BACILLI

The genera *Actinomyces*, *Arachnia*, *Propionibacterium*, *Lactobacillus*, *Bifidobacterium*, and *Eubacterium* are gram-positive, nonsporeforming bacilli. The genera *Actinomyces*,

TABLE 20-16. Differentiation of Anaerobic, Nonsporeforming, Gram-Negative Bacilli

Characteristics	Genus
I. Nonmotile	
A. Produce butyric acid as a major product	*Fusobacterium*
B. Produce only lactic acid	*Leptotrichia*
II. Possess peritrichous flagella; produce a mixture of fermentative products; butyric acid not a major product	*Bacteroides*
III. Motile, not peritrichous	
A. Curved rod; polar flagella; butyric acid as a major product	*Butyrivibrio*
B. Produce succinate and acetate as major product	
1. Short rod/coccobacilli, single polar flagellum	*Succinimonas*
2. helical or spiral shaped	
a. Single polar flagellum	*Succinivibrio*
b. Bipolar tufts of flagella	*Anaerobiospirillum*
C. Produces succinate from fumarate; single polar flagellum; asaccharolytic	*Wolinella*

TABLE 20-16. Differentiation of Anaerobic, Nonsporeforming, Gram-Negative Bacilli—cont'd

Characteristics	Genus
D. Produce proprionate and acetate; curved cells	
1. Tufts of flagella on concave side	*Selenomonas*
2. Curved; lipolytic; single polar flagellum	*Anaerovibrio*
3. Lateral flagella aligned on concave side	*Pectinatus*
E. Produce acetic acid, ethanol, hydrogen, carbon dioxide as major products; straight to curved rods; nonpolar or lateral flagella	*Acetivibrio*
F. Produce ethanol, formate, lactate, acetate, carbon dioxide, hydrogen; straight to slightly curved rods; single lateral/subpolar flagellum	*Lachnospira*

Modified from Holdeman, L.V., Kelley, R.W., and Moore, W.E.C.: Family I *Bacteroidaceae* and genus I. *Bacteroides*. In Krieg, N.R., editor (Holt, J.G., editor-in-chief): Bergey's manual of systematic bacteriology, vol. 1, Baltimore, 1984, Williams & Wilkins Co.

TABLE 20-17. Identification of the Genus *Clostridium*[a]

Species	Gelatin Hydrolyzed	Milk Digested	Glucose Acid	Sucrose Acid	Starch Acid	Lactose Acid	Mannose Acid	Xylose Acid	Mannitol Acid	Indole	Lecithinase	Lipase	Urease	Esculin Hydrolyzed	Growth on Aerobic Plate	Spore Location	Hydrogen Produced	Products[b]
C. baratii	−	−	+	+	d	+w	+	−	−	−	+	−	−	+	−	ST[T]	4	B, A, L, (f), (p), (s)
C. bifermentans	+	+	+	−	−	−	−w	−	−	+	+	−	−	+−	−	ST	4	A, F, (iv), (ic), (p), (ib), (b), (l), (s), (2)
C. botulinum																		
ABF (proteolytic)	+	+	+	−	−	−	−	−	−	−	+	−	+	−	−	ST	4	A, B, iv, b, (ic), (v), (p), (2), (3), (4)
BEF (saccharolytic)	+	−	+	+w	d	−	+w	−	−	−	+	−	−	−	−	ST	4	B, A
CD	+	+−	+	−	−	−	d	−	−	−+	−+	+	−	−	−	ST	4	B, P, A, (v), (l), (s)
G	+	+	−	−	−	−	−	−	−	−	−	−	−	−	−	ST	4	A, b, iv, ib
C. butyricum	−	−	+	+	+	+	+	+	−+	−	−	−	−	+	−	ST	4	B, A, F, (l), (s), (2), (4)
C. cadaveris	+	+−	+	−	−	−	−w	−	−	+	−	−	−	−	−	T	4	B, A, 2, 4, (f), (p), (l), (s)
C. chauvoei	+	−	+	+w	−	+w	+w	−	−	−	−	−	−	+	−	ST	4	A, B, F, (l), (s), (4)
C. clostridioforme	−	−	+	+	−w	+−	+w	+	−	−	−+	−	−	+	−	ST	4	A, (F), (l), (s), (2)

Continued.

TABLE 20-17. Identification of the Genus *Clostridium*—cont'd

Species	Gelatin Hydrolyzed	Milk Digested	Glucose Acid	Sucrose Acid	Starch Acid	Lactose Acid	Mannose Acid	Xylose Acid	Mannitol Acid	Indole	Lecithinase	Lipase	Urease	Esculin Hydrolyzed	Growth on Aerobic Plate	Spore Location	Hydrogen Produced	Products[b]
C. difficile	+	−	+	−	−	−	+−	−w	+−	−	−	−	−	+	−	ST^T	4	B, A, ic, iv, ib, (f), (v), (l), (2), (4)
C. hastiforme	+	−+	−	−	−	−	−	−	−	−	−	−	−	−	−	T	−, 1	A, B, iv, ib, (f), (p), (ic)
C. histolyticum	+	+	−	−	−	−	−	−	−	−	−	−	−	−	−	ST	−, 2	A, (f), (l), (s)
C. innocuum	−	−	+	+	−	−	+	−w	+	−	−	−	−	+	−	T^ST	4	B, L, a, (f), (s)
C. limosum	+	+	−	−	−	−	−	−	−	−	+	−	−	−	−	ST	−1	A, (f), (l), (s)
C. novyi A	+	−	+	−	−	−	−	−	−	−	+	+	−	−	−	ST	4	A, B, P
C. novyi B	+	+	+	−	−	−	+w	−	−	+−	+	−	−	−	−	ST	d	P, B, A
C. paraputrificum	−	−	+	+	+	+	+	−	−	−	−	−	−	+	−	T^ST	4	B, A, L, (s), (f)
C. perfringens	+	+	+	+	d	+	+	−	−	−	+	−	−	d	−	ST	4	A, B, L, (p), (f), (s)
C. ramosum	−	−	+	+	−+	+	+	−w	+−	−	−	−	−	+	−	T	d	F, A, l, (s), (2)
C. septicum	+	+−	+	−	−	−	+	+	−	−	−	−	−	+	−	ST	4	B, A, (F), (p), (l), (2)
C. sordellii	+	+	+	−	−	−	−w	−	+	+	+	−	+	−+	−	ST	4	A, (F), (iC), (p), (ib), (iv), (l)
C. sphenoides	−	−	+	w−	w−	w+	w+	d	w+	+	−	−	−	+	−	ST^T	4	A, F, (l), (s), (2)

Arachnia, and *Bifidobacterium* are most commonly associated with infection. These latter three genera are fermentative actinomycetes found in the natural cavities of humans and other animals. They are morphologically similar, primarily anaerobic or microaerophilic organisms that do not form aerial mycelia or spores. The filaments produced by these organisms frequently segment during growth, yielding pleomorphic, club-shaped or diphtheroidal cells that closely resemble the corynebacteria. The genera *Streptomyces* and *Nocardia,* discussed in Chapter 30, are oxidative aerobic actinomycetes; they are primarily soil inhabitants. All actinomycetes are slow growers; a division cycle of these organisms may take 2 to 3 hours as compared with 20 minutes for *Escherichia coli.*

The gram-positive, nonsporeforming bacilli may present cellular morphologic characteristics similar to those of nonsporulating *Clostridium* spp. or even *Bacteroides* spp. if they decolorize during Gram staining, but lack of spores can be demonstrated by susceptibility to 70° C for 10 minutes. Differentiation from gram-negative organisms may be accomplished with either antimicrobial susceptibility or the KOH test discussed previously.

GLC differentiates among the genera of gram-positive, nonsporeforming bacilli (Table 20-19). Other characteristics that aid in presumptive identification include observation of colonial morphology (smooth versus rough) on anaerobe blood agar, red pigmentation of colonies on blood agar, appearance in enriched thioglycolate broth, cellular morphology in enriched thioglycolate broth, production of catalase and indole, glucose fermentation, and analysis by GLC. GLC analysis is required for reliable presumptive identification of these organisms. Analysis is performed on PYG broth after the broth is checked with a pH meter to ascertain glucose fermentation. The catalase test may be performed by adding 3% H_2O_2 to a medium that does not contain blood. Definitive identification of the gram-positive, nonsporeforming bacilli requires GLC and the use of extensive carbohydrate fermentation and other biochemical tests (Table 20-20). Information regarding definitive identification of these organisms is available in Allen,[3] Dowell and Hawkins,[23] Holdeman, Cato, and Moore,[50] and Sutter and co-workers.[132] Some of the key characteristics for differentiating these organisms are noted in the following paragraphs.

TABLE 20-17. Identification of the Genus *Clostridium*—cont'd

Species	Gelatin Hydrolyzed	Milk Digested	Glucose Acid	Sucrose Acid	Starch Acid	Lactose Acid	Mannose Acid	Xylose Acid	Mannitol Acid	Indole	Lecithinase	Lipase	Urease	Esculin Hydrolyzed	Growth on Aerobic Plate	Spore Location	Hydrogen Produced	Products[b]
C. sporogenes	+	+	+	−	−	−	−	−	−	−	−	+	−+	+	−	ST	4	A, B, iv, ib, 2, (p), (ic), (v), (l), (s), (4)
C. subterminale	+	+−	−	−	−	−	−	−	−	−+	−	−	−	−	−	ST	4	A, B, iV, ib, (f), (p), (ic), (l), (s), (2)
C. tertium	−	−	+	+	+w	+	+	+−	+w	−	−	−	−	+	+	TST	4	A, B, L, (f), (s), (2)
C. tetani	+	+−	−	−	−	−	−	−	−	d	−	−	−	−	−	TST	4	A, B, p, 4, (2), (l), (s)

SYMBOLS: +, 90%-100% of strains positive (pH of sugars below 5.5)
−, 90%-100% of strains negative
w, Weak reaction (pH of sugars 5.5-5.9)
d, 40%-60% of strains positive
Numbers (hydrogen), Negative to abundant on scale of − to 4+

ST, Subterminal	iv, Isovaleric acid
T, Terminal	ib, Isobutyric acid
A, Acetic acid	v, Valeric acid
B, Butyric acid	c, Caproic acid
L, Lactic acid	ic, Isocaproic acid
S, Succinic acid	2, Ethanol
P, Propionic acid	3, Propanol
F, Formic acid	4, Butanol

Table prepared by E.P. Cato, Anaerobe Laboratory, Virginia Polytechnic Institute, Blacksburg, Va.
[a]Where two reactions are listed, the first is the more usual and occurs in 60% to 90% of strains.
[b]Products listed in order of amounts usually detected. Capital letters indicate at least 1 mEq/100 ml of culture; small letters indicate less than 1 mEq/100 ml. Products in parentheses are not detected uniformly.

TABLE 20-18. Characteristics Particularly Useful for Identification of Commonly Encountered *Clostridium* Spp.

Characteristic	Species
Aerotolerant	*C. histolyticum, C. tertium*
Nonmotile	*C. innocuum, C. perfringens, C. ramosum*
Terminal spores	*C. cadaveris, C. innocuum, C. tertium, C. tetani*
Lecithinase positive (on EYA)	*C. bifermentans, C. limosum, C. novyi, C. perfringens, C. sordellii, C. subterminale*
Lipase positive (on EYA)	*C. botulinum, C. novyi* type A, *C. sporogenes*

TABLE 20-18. Characteristics Particularly Useful for Identification of Commonly Encountered *Clostridium* Spp.—cont'd

Characteristic	Species
Asaccharolytic	*C. histolyticum, C. limosum, C. subterminale, C. tetani*
Urease positive	*C. sordellii*
Gelatin negative	*C. butyricum, C. innocuum, C. ramosum, C. tertium*

Modified from Dowell, V.R., and Hawkins, T.M.: Laboratory methods in anaerobic bacteriology—CDC laboratory manual, Atlanta, 1981, Centers for Disease Control, U.S. Department of Health and Human Services, Pub. No. (CDC) 81-8272.

Almost all isolates of the genus *Propionibacterium* are *P. acnes*. This organism is identified presumptively on the basis of positive reactions for indole and catalase. Indole-negative, catalase-positive organisms may be *P. acnes*, *P. granulosum*, or *Actinomyces viscosus*. Differentiation is accomplished with carbohydrate fermentation and esculin hydrolysis.

Eubacterium lentum is biochemically inactive except for its variable nitrate reduction reaction and its occasionally positive catalase reaction. *E. limosum* and *E. alactolyticum*, both saccharolytic, may be differentiated with esculin hydrolysis and selected carbohydrate fermentations. Differentiation of other *Eubacterium* spp. is discussed by Moore and Moore.[84]

The characteristics of *Bifidobacterium eriksonii* are its ability to form distinctly branched forms but generally smooth colonies, a requirement for strict anaerobiosis and stimulation by CO_2, coagulation of milk and hydrolysis of starch, inability to reduce nitrate, and marked fermentation of carbohydrates.[35]

Members of the genus *Lactobacillus* produce large amounts of lactic acid from glucose. *L. catenaforme*, the species isolated most often from clinical specimens, has been recovered from infections of the head, neck, and respiratory tract, but its clinical significance is uncertain.[3,126] Other species less commonly recovered from clinical specimens are described by Kandler.[63]

The isolation and identification of *Actinomyces* spp. may be difficult. As previously mentioned, if granules are observed, they should be washed, crushed, and inoculated to appropriate media such as enriched thioglycolate, anaerobe blood agar, anaerobe PEA, and brain heart infusion agar.[3,123,124] The genus *Actinomyces* requires CO_2, so all media must be incubated in an anaerobic environment containing CO_2. (Schaal and Pulverer[119] recommend the Fortner principle for isolation of these organisms.) *Actinomyces* organisms are difficult to isolate in pure culture, and the presence of contaminating organisms will give confusing results.[123] Biochemical test results also vary with the media and method used.[123] Furthermore, differentiation of *A. israelii*, the most common species of *Actinomyces*, from *Arachnia propionica* can be accomplished with GLC or fluorescent antibody studies. Readers should consult Allen,[3] Holdeman, Cato, and Moore,[50] Slack,[123] and Slack and Gerencser[124] for detailed discussions of the identification of *Actinomyces* isolates.

ANAEROBIC COCCI

The anaerobic, gram-positive cocci are classified within the genera *Peptococcus*, *Peptostreptococcus*, *Streptococcus*, *Ruminococcus*, *Sarcina*, and *Coprococcus*, and the gram-negative cocci within the genera *Veillonella*, *Acidaminococcus*, and *Megasphaera*. Among these organisms *Peptostreptococcus* spp. are more often associated with human disease. In general the anaerobic cocci are slow growers that may require prolonged incubation of their biochemical tests. Biochemical reactions should not be read until sufficient growth can be observed.

Gram-Positive Cocci

The classification of the genera *Peptostreptococcus* and *Peptococcus* has recently been revised. There are currently nine species of *Peptostreptococcus* and one species of *Peptococcus* (see box on p. 374).[26] The anaerobic, gram-positive cocci that metabolize peptones and amino acids and have a G+C content of 28 to 35 mol% have been placed into the genus *Peptostrep-*

TABLE 20-19. Differentiation of Gram-Positive, Nonsporeforming, Anaerobic Bacilli to the Genus Level

Characteristic	Genus
I. Produce propionic acid	
A. Catalase usually produced	*Propionibacterium*
B. Catalase not produced	*Arachnia*
II. Propionic acid and catalase not produced	
A. Ratio of lactic to acetic acid produced greater than 1:1	
1. Lactic acid only major product	*Lactobacillus*
2. Succinic acid is a major product	*Actinomyces*
B. Ratio of lactic to acetic acid produced less than 1:1	
1. Produce butyric acid plus other acids or no major acids	*Eubacterium*
2. Butyric acid not produced	*Bifidobacterium*

From Dowell, V.R., and Hawkins, T.M.: Laboratory methods in anaerobic bacteriology—CDC laboratory manual, Centers for Disease Control, U.S. Department of Health and Human Services, Pub. No. (CDC) 81-8272, 1981.

tococcus. *Peptostreptococcus productus* is the only exception to this rule. *P. niger*, the sole species of the genus *Peptococcus*, has a G+C content of 50 mol%. *Peptostreptococcus saccharolyticus* has been transferred to the genus *Staphylococcus*, and *Peptostreptococcus parvulus* to the genus *Streptococcus*.[13] Several other species formerly recognized as members of the genera *Peptococcus* or *Peptostreptococcus* have also been transferred to the genus *Streptococcus* as *S. morbillorum*, *S. constellatus*, and *S. intermedius*. Streptococci are defined as facultative anaerobes that occur in chains and are fermentative, producing large amounts of lactic acid. Although these reclassified organisms are not facultative anaerobes, they do grow in chains and produce large amounts of lactic acid. Thus they are best considered members of the genus *Streptococcus*.[55,109] The production of lactic acid distinguishes these organisms from members of the genus *Peptostreptococcus*, which produce the fatty acids indicated in Table 20-21. Actually many strains of *S. morbillorum*, *S. constellatus*, and *S. intermedius* grow in 5% to 10% CO_2 after one or more subcultures (Figure 20-6). These capnophilic or microaerophilic strains should be identified as viridans streptococci.[27]

The majority of clinical isolates of anaerobic, gram-positive cocci are species of *Peptostreptococcus*. As currently defined, the major difference between the genera *Peptostreptococcus* and *Peptococcus* is the G+C content of the DNA. Neither arrangement of cells (tetrad, chains, and so on) nor production of catalase is useful in differentiating between these two genera. Differentiation is seldom a problem, however, since the only species in the genus *Peptococcus* is *P. niger* and this organism can be distinguished by its production of black colonies (Table 20-10) and major peaks of butyric and caproic acids (Table 20-21). *P. niger* is a rare clinical isolate.

The sole use of the biochemical tests in Table 20-21 provides

TABLE 20-20. Identification of Gram-Positive, Nonsporeforming Bacilli

Genus and Species	Relationship to Oxygen	Enriched Thioglycolate Medium — Appearance	Cellular Morphology	Red Pigment on Blood Agar	Catalase	Esculin	Indole	Nitrate Reduction	Urease	Fermentation of — Glucose	Mannitol	Lactose	Sucrose	Maltose	Salicin	Glycerol	Xylose	Arabinose	Fatty Acids from PYG Broth[a]
Actinomyces																			
A. israelii	M or OA	Granular or diffuse (Plate 18, A)	Branching filaments or diphtheroidal	−	−	+⁻	−	V	−	+	v	+⁻	+	+	v	−	+⁻	v	A, L, S
A. naeslundii	F	Diffuse	Diphtheroidal or branching	−	−	+⁻	−	+⁻	+	+	−	+⁻	+⁻	+	v	−	+⁻	−⁺	A, L, S
A. odontolyticus	M or OA	Diffuse	Diphtheroidal or branching	+	−	v	−	+	−	+	−	+⁻	+⁻	+⁻	v	v	v	−⁺	A, L, S
A. viscosus	F	Diffuse	Diphtheroidal or branching	−	+	+	−	+⁻	+	+	−	+⁻	+⁻	+	+⁻	+	v	v	A, L, S
A. meyeri	OA, F	Diffuse	Diphtheroidal or branching	−	−	−⁺	−	+	−	+	+	+⁻	+	+	+⁻	+	+	v	A, L, S
Arachnia propionica	M or OA	Granular or diffuse	Branching filaments or diphtheroidal	−	−	−⁺	−	+	−	+	+	+	+	+	−⁺	−⁺	−	−	A, P, (L), (S)
Bifidobacterium dentium (eriksonii)	OA	Diffuse	Thin rods; bifid ends; bulbous ends	−	−	+⁻	−	−	−	+	v	+	+	+	+	−	+	+	A, L
Eubacterium																			
E. lentum	OA	Diffuse	Short, coccoidal rods; diphtheroidal	−	−	−	−	v	−	−	−	−	−	−	−	−	−	−	
E. limosum	OA	Diffuse	Plump rods; bulbous and bifid forms	−	−	+	−	−	−	+	+⁻	−	+⁻	−	+⁻	+	−	−	A, B
E. alactolyticum	OA	Diffuse	Thin rods; V forms; cross-stick arrangement	−	−	−	−	−	−	+	+⁻	−	−	−	−	−	−	−	A, B, C
Propionibacterium																			
P. acnes	OA[b]	Diffuse (granular)	Diphtheroidal	−	+[c]	−	+[c]	+⁻	−	+	v	−	−	−	−	−⁺	−	−	A, P, L, S
P. granulosum	F	Diffuse	Diphtheroidal	−	+	−	−	−	−	+	−	−	+	+	−⁺	+⁻	−	−	A, P, (L), S
Lactobacillus catenaforme	OA	Diffuse (granular)	Short rods in chains or singly	−	−	−	−	−	−	+	−	−	−	−	−	−	−	−	A, L

Symbols:

+, Positive		blank, No data available	P, Propionic acid
−, Negative		A, Acetic acid	S, Succinic acid
+⁻, Most strains positive, occasional strains negative		B, Butyric acid	M, Microaerophilic
−⁺, Most strains negative, occasional strains positive		C, Caproic acid	OA, Obligately anaerobic
v, Variable reaction		L, Lactic acid	F, Facultatively anaerobic

Modified from Allen, S.D.: Gram-positive, nonsporeforming anaerobic bacilli. In Lennette, E.H., et al., editors: Manual of clinical microbiology, ed. 4, Washington, D.C., 1985, American Society for Microbiology.

[a]Acids in parentheses are produced variably or, if produced, are usually present only in trace amounts.
[b]11% to 25% of strains may be facultative.
[c]11% to 25% of strains may be negative.

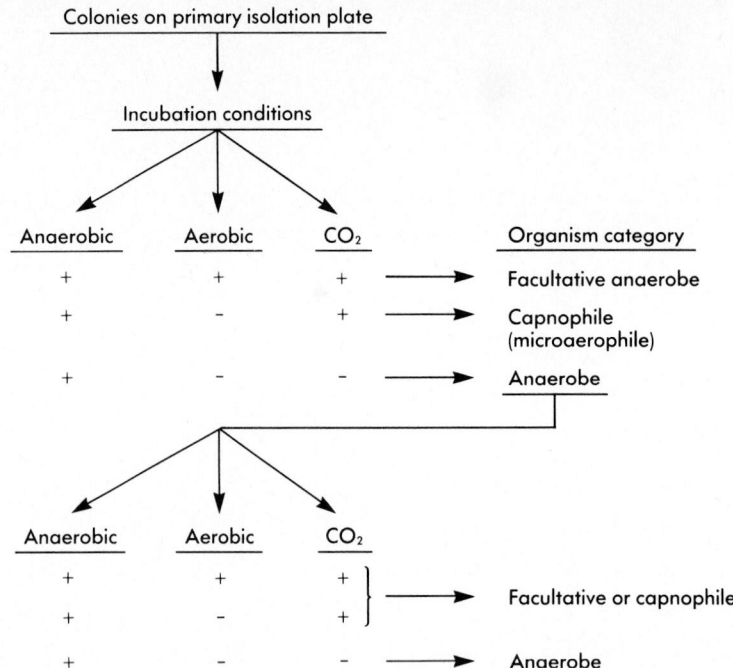

Colonies on primary isolation plate

↓

Incubation conditions

Anaerobic	Aerobic	CO₂	Organism category
+	+	+	Facultative anaerobe
+	-	+	Capnophile (microaerophile)
+	-	-	Anaerobe

Anaerobic	Aerobic	CO₂	
+	+	+	Facultative or capnophile
+	-	+	
+	-	-	Anaerobe

FIGURE 20-6. Subculture scheme to determine aerotolerance of gram-positive cocci. (From Rosenblatt, J.E.: Anaerobic bacteria. In Washington, J.A., editor: Laboratory procedures in clinical microbiology, New York, 1985, Springer-Verlag.)

a presumptive identification of the anaerobic cocci; definitive identification requires the use of GLC. Among the anaerobic gram-positive cocci, the most common clinical isolates are *P. micros, P. magnus, P. prevotii,* and *P. anaerobius. P. magnus* and *P. micros* are relatively inert. Differentiation of these organisms from *P. prevotii* is accomplished with GLC; *P. prevotii* produces butyric acid, whereas *P. magnus* and *P. micros* do not. *P. magnus* is microscopically larger (1 to 2 μm in diameter) than *P. micros* and unlike *P. prevotii* does not produce butyric acid.

Presumptive identification of *P. anaerobius* is provided by determining its sensitivity to sodium polyanethol sulfonate (SPS).[146] The test is performed by streaking the test organism to Schaedler or Brucella blood agar or another medium that does not contain protease peptone, gelatin, or casein,[147] placing a disk containing 20 μl of 5% SPS on the agar surface, and incubating for 48 hours. Gram-positive cocci showing zones of inhibition of 12 mm or greater may be reported as *P. anaerobius.* This test has an overall accuracy of 98%.[146]

P. asaccharolyticus is inert except for indole production. Although rarely encountered, *P. indolicus* has been isolated from the finger of a sheep-herder.[10] *P. indolicus* and *P. asaccharolyticus* are the only indole-positive species among the anaerobic cocci. *P. indolicus* also reduces nitrate, whereas *P. asaccharolyticus* does not.

Gram-Negative Cocci

Members of the gram-negative cocci include *Veillonella parvula, Veillonella atypica, Veillonella dispar,*[77] *Megasphaera elsdenii,* and *Acidaminococcus fermentans. V. parvula* is by far the most frequent isolate among this group of organisms.[97,113]

The use of GLC is essential to differentiate among the three genera of gram-negative cocci. The typical fatty acids produced by these organisms are listed in Table 20-21. Differentiation on the basis of size, although not totally reliable, may also help. *Veillonella* colonies tend to be very small, *Acidaminococcus* of moderate size, and *Megasphaera* very large. *Megasphaera* organisms, although gram negative according to cell wall composition, often appear gram positive. Colonies of *Veillonella,* like those of the pigmented *Bacteroides,* may fluoresce red under ultraviolet light.[16]

COMMERCIALLY AVAILABLE IDENTIFICATION SYSTEMS

The commercial systems that have been used for anaerobe identification include the API 20A, AN-IDENT, Minitek, Rap-ID ANA system, Automicrobic system, and various microdilution systems. These are discussed in Chapter 9.

Commercially available Presumpto plates (Carr-Scarborough, Stone Mountain, Ga.) have been developed by Dowell and Lombard for presumptive identification of anaerobes. These three plates, each divided into quadrants, allow determination of the following characteristics: indole; catalase; H₂S production; lipase; lecithinase; proteolysis; growth in presence of 20% bile; hydrolysis of starch, esculin, casein, and gelatin; DNAse; and fermentation of glucose, mannitol, lactose, and rhamnose. Details concerning the use of this system are given in other texts.[66]

GAS-LIQUID CHROMATOGRAPHY[97]

During cellular metabolism anaerobes produce distinguishing by-products including alcohols, fatty acids, and nonvolatile organic acids. Determination of these products by GLC may be used for presumptive and definitive identification.

TABLE 20-21. Identification of Anaerobic Cocci

Genus and Species	Gram Stain	Catalase	Indole	Nitrate	Esculin	Gelatin	Fermentation of Glucose	Lactose	Maltose	Sucrose	Fatty Acids from PYG Broth[a]
Peptostreptococcus											
P. anaerobius	+	−	−	v	−	−	+	−	−	−	A, IB, B, IV, IC, (P)
P. micros	+	−	−	−	−	−	−	−	−	−	A, (L), (S)
P. productus	+	−	−	−	+	−	+	+	+	+	A, L, S
P. asaccharolyticus	+	−	+	−	−	−	−	−	−	−	A, B, P
P. indolicus	+	−	+	+	−	−	−	−	−	−	A, P, B
P. magnus	+	−	−	−	−	v	w	−	−	−	A, (L), (S)
P. prevotii	+	−	−	±	−	−	−	−	−	−	B, L, (A), (P), (S)
P. tetradius	+	v	−	−	−,w	−	+	−	+	+	A, B, L
Peptococcus niger	+	w	−	−	−	−	−	−	−	−	A, IB, B, IV, C
Veillonella parvula	−	v	−	+	−	−	−	−	−	−	A, P, (S)
Acidaminococcus fermentans	−	−	−	−	−	−	−	−	−	−	A, B, (P), (L)
Megasphaera elsdenii	−	−	−	−	−	−	+	−	+	−	A, IB, B, IV, V, C, L, (F)

Symbols:	+, 90% or more positive	P, Propionic acid	S, Succinic acid
	−, 90% or more negative	B, Butyric acid	V, Valeric acid
	w, Weak	C, Caproic acid	IB, Isobutyric acid
	v, Variable	L, Lactic acid	IV, Isovaleric acid
	A, Acetic acid	F, Formic acid	IC, Isocaproic acid

Data from references 52, 53, and 108.
[a]Acids in parentheses are not produced uniformly.

COMPONENTS

The basic components of a gas chromatograph include the following:

1. *Injector port.* The properly prepared sample is injected into the system through the injector port, which is heated to a critical temperature, allowing volatilization of the sample.
2. *Inert carrier gas.* The carrier gas, commonly helium or nitrogen, transports the solute vapors through the column at a constant flow.
3. *Column.* The column, consisting of a solid support packing coated with a stationary liquid phase, allows separation of the sample.
4. *Oven.* The critical temperature of the oven surrounding the column is responsible for the maintenance of the sample in its volatilized state.
5. *Detector.* The detector measures the concentration of the sample components by generating an electrical signal proportional to the sample concentration. Although there are several types of detectors, the thermal conductivity detector (TCD) and flame ionization detector (FID) are most commonly used in anaerobic bacteriology. With the TCD the rate of heat loss serves as a measure of gas composition because a hot body loses heat at a rate that depends on the composition of the surrounding gas. In contrast, the FID operates on the principle that the electrical conductivity of a gas is directly proportional to the concentration of charged particles within the gas.[80] Although the FIC is much more sensitive than the TCD, the latter is quite adequate for anaerobic bacteriology work. In addition, the TCD is relatively inexpensive, and, unlike the FID, responds to formic acid. The operating parameters for both of these systems are discussed by Sutter and co-workers.[132]

6. *Recorder.* After receipt of signals from the detector, the recorder converts them into mechanical energy that is recorded in graphic form on chart paper.

PRINCIPLE

GLC is actually a type of partitioning whereby the solute (sample) is separated into its components based on its relative solubility in the two phases, the mobile inert gas and the stationary liquid phase. The components of the sample that are least soluble in the stationary phase move rapidly through the column, whereas the components that are most soluble in the stationary phase are retained longer and emerge from the column much later. The retention time of the solute in the stationary phase is a function of its boiling point; a substance with a low boiling point enters the stationary phase and returns to the carrier stream with low retention time, whereas substances with higher boiling points remain longer in the stationary liquid phase. In summary, fractions of a mixture dissolve in the stationary phase from the moving phase based on their similarity to it. These fractions then revolatilize into the moving phase relative to their boiling points.

SAMPLE PREPARATION

Except in cases where FIDs are used, the samples must be prepared before their injection into the chromatograph. The ether extract sample preparation procedure is used to detect the ether-soluble, volatile, short-chain fatty acids including acetic, propionic, isobutyric, butyric, isovaleric, valeric, isocaproic, and caproic. Ether is an effective solvent not only because it removes most of the organic products from the broth cultures, but also because it has a low boiling point and is readily vaporized when injected into the injector port. The procedure is as follows[50]:

1. Inoculate 0.1 ml of a 24- to 48-hour chopped meat–glucose broth (or supplemented thioglycolate broth) culture of the test organism into 7 to 8 ml tubes of prereduced peptone-yeast-glucose (PYG) broth medium.
2. Incubate for 48 hours or until adequate growth is obtained.
3. With a pipette, transfer 1 ml of the PYG culture into a 12 × 75 mm tube. Add 0.2 ml of 50% H_2SO_4, 0.4 g NaCl, and 1 ml ethyl ether.
4. Stopper the tube and mix gently by inverting the tube approximately 20 times.
5. Centrifuge briefly to break the ether-culture emulsion.
6. With a pipette carefully remove the ether layer from the aqueous layer, avoiding contamination of the ether with water. Add anhydrous 4-20 mesh $CaCl_2$ to equal about one-fourth the volume of ether in the tube. Stopper the tube and let stand about 5 minutes. The $CaCl_2$ will remove traces of water from the ether.
7. Inject approximately 14 μl of the ether extract into the chromatograph.
8. Identify volatile acids by comparing elution times of products in the extracts with those of the volatile fatty acid standards on which chromatography was performed on the same day.
9. Examine a tube of uninoculated PYG medium in the same manner, since some lots of peptones and yeast extract may contain significant quantities of these acids.

The nonvolatile acids (pyruvic, lactic, and succinic) must first be methylated before they can be volatilized and analyzed. Either the boron trifluoride–methanol method or the methanol procedure (see below) may be used to prepare methyl derivatives. (Because of the potential hazards associated with the use of ethyl ether and chloroform, Thomann and Hill[140] have recently suggested the use of methyl tert-butyl ether in modified extraction procedures.) The methanol procedure of GLC sample preparation to detect the nonvolatile acids follows[50]:

1. Transfer 1 ml of the PYG broth culture (see procedure for volatile acids) into a 12 × 75 mm tube.
2. Add 2 ml of methanol and 0.4 ml of 50% H_2SO_4. Stopper

the tube and heat at 60° C in a water bath or temperature block for 30 minutes.
3. Add 1 ml of water and 0.5 ml of chloroform. Replace the stopper in the tube and mix by inverting the tube gently about 20 times. If an emulsion forms, centrifuge the tube briefly to break the emulsion.
4. Place the tip of the needle of a syringe in the bottom chloroform layer and fill the syringe with the chloroform extract.
5. After wiping off the outside of the needle with a clean tissue, inject 14 μl of the chloroform extract into the column. (NOTE: After testing of approximately 15 to 20 methylated samples, the column should be reconditioned by injecting 14 μl of methanol.)
6. Identify the nonvolatile methylated acids by comparing the elution times of the components with those of the nonvolatile acid standards on which chromatography was performed on the same day.
7. Test an uninoculated medium by the same method to detect the presence of nonvolatile acids, especially lactic and succinic. If these acids are present, corrections must be made or the medium discarded.

In addition to the volatile and nonvolatile standards, Mayhew and Gorbach[76] suggest that internal standards be used in the gas chromatographic analysis to facilitate identification and quantification of short-chain organic acids and to function as monitors of the analytic techniques. They recommend that 2-methylpentanoic acid be used as a volatile marker and benzoic acid be employed as a nonvolatile marker.

It is important to remember that different gas chromatographic profiles may be observed when different growth media, extraction procedures, or detectors are used. Because of these variations in methods and systems, various anaerobic bacteriology manuals may show different chromatographic profiles for the same organism. Laboratories should make sure that their methods of analysis are consistent with the identification protocol being used.

DIRECT ANALYSIS

Direct GLC on clinical specimens has been suggested for rapid tentative identification of anaerobes. Gorbach and co-workers[43] showed that direct GLC analysis of pus and various body fluids provided a rapid presumptive test for identification of the genera *Bacteroides* and *Fusobacterium*. In their analysis of pus samples, Phillips, Tearle, and Willis[105] found direct GLC analysis to be reliable for presumptive differentiation of aerobic and anaerobic infections. Samples containing pure and mixed cultures of facultative organisms demonstrated only acetic acid, whereas pure and mixed cultures of obligate anaerobes and mixed cultures of anaerobes and facultative organisms yielded multiple volatile fatty acids in addition to acetic acid. Pus specimens that contained acetic acid alone or no volatile fatty acids never yielded obligate anaerobes only. Rapid presumptive identification of anaerobes in blood cultures has also revealed characteristic acid patterns.[130]

SEROLOGIC IDENTIFICATION
BACTEROIDES

A commercial diagnostic fluorescent antibody kit (Fluoretec, General Diagnostics, Morris Plains, N.J.) has been developed for rapid detection of the *B. fragilis* group (BFG) and the *B. melaninogenicus* group (BMG) from colonies or directly from clinical material; Fluoretec F is used for the former and Fluoretec M for the latter. An evaluation of this kit showed it to be a useful adjunct to standard techniques for the rapid presumptive identification of *B. melaninogenicus* and *B. fragilis*.[144]

Other potentially useful serologic methods for rapid detection of *B. fragilis* organisms or infections include immunoperoxidase and radioimmunoassay.

CLOSTRIDIUM

Commercially available fluorescent antibody reagents can be used with confidence for presumptive identification of the clostridia *C. novyi, C. septicum,* and *C. sordellii*.[2]

GRAM-POSITIVE, NONSPOREFORMING BACILLI

The fluorescent antibody technique can be used to detect and identify *Actinomyces* spp. in clinical material or in culture.

ANAEROBIC COCCI

Numerous serologic procedures, including fluorescent antibody methods, agglutination tests, immunodiffusion, immunoelectrophoresis, coagglutination, and counterimmunoelectrophoresis, have been used to differentiate the gram-positive cocci. However, none of these procedures is used in the laboratory for routine identification.

CLINICAL SIGNIFICANCE[29]

Anaerobic bacteria are present as indigenous flora of the skin and all mucous membrane surfaces of the body. Under normal circumstances these organisms are contained by the mucous membranes and natural barriers of the host; however, when these barriers are disrupted by conditions such as trauma and manipulations (for example, oral manipulations, various instrumentation) or the host is compromised by various disorders (such as cancer), the normal anaerobic inhabitants may penetrate neighboring tissues and establish infection. One reason these conditions and numerous associated conditions (such as vascular disease, shock, edema, and presence of foreign bodies) predispose the host to anaerobic infection is that they result in poor blood supply and tissue necrosis that lower the oxidation-reduction potential of the tissue to a level favoring anaerobic growth. Most pathogenic anaerobic clinical isolates are relatively aerotolerant. Possibly this tolerance to oxygen functions as a mechanism of pathogenicity by allowing these organisms to survive until the oxidation-reduction potential is lowered enough for subsequent multiplication.[137]

Anaerobic infections are often polymicrobial in nature, consisting of both aerobes and anaerobes. Studies in experimental animals have shown that these organisms act synergistically to cause many infections; that is, a mixed inoculum of aerobes and anaerobes is able to produce disease that cannot be induced by either group of organisms alone.[101,102,143]

Two hypotheses have been proposed to explain the mechanism of this synergy. The first hypothesis suggests that facultative organisms may enhance the growth and pathogenic potential of anaerobes by providing lowered oxidation potentials or essential growth factors. For example, in mixed dental infections facultative diphtheroids produce vitamin K, which is required by *B. melaninogenicus*.[72] The second hypothesis suggests that anaerobes interfere with the phagocytosis and killing of aerobes that when present alone may not be overtly pathogenic.[57,95] Anaerobes may also inhibit the chemotaxis of leukocytes to aerobes.[96]

Anaerobes may be involved in oral and dental infections; ear, nose, throat, head, and neck infections; skin and soft tissue infections; infections of the lung and pleural space; intra-abdominal infections; female genital tract infections; central nervous system infections; and cardiovascular infections. Thoracic, intra-abdominal, and obstetric-gynecologic infections are most commonly associated with anaerobes; in fact, anaerobes are responsible for 70% to 95% of these infections. Anaerobes are found in pure culture in one half to two thirds of certain thoracic infections and in one third of obstetric-gynecologic infections.

ORAL AND DENTAL INFECTIONS

Anaerobes are able to establish infection in an area, such as the mouth, that is exposed to large amounts of air, because the presence of facultative organisms may lower the oxidation-reduction potential to levels favoring anaerobic growth. The facultative streptococci in human dental plaque create a suitable environment for the establishment of anaerobes, even in sites exposed to air.

When host tissue integrity is compromised, the normal flora of the oral cavity may contribute to the development of a variety of oral and dental infections. These infections may remain local or disseminate widely to produce serious infections of the jaw, face, neck, brain, and meninges.

Examples of oral and dental infections are periodontal disease, dental abscesses, and dental phlegmons (acute suppurative inflammation of tissue). *Fusobacterium nucleatum, Eubacterium nodatum, Peptostreptococcus micros, Eubacterium timidum, Bacteroides gingivalis, B. intermedius, B. oralis,* and *B. buccae* appear to be the anaerobes most frequently isolated from periodontal lesions.[56,84a,84b,98]

EAR, NOSE, THROAT, HEAD, AND NECK INFECTIONS[12]

Although the role of anaerobes in acute otitis media remains undefined, chronic otitis media is commonly caused by anaerobic bacteria. Among the numerous organisms associated with chronic otitis media are *Bacteroides* spp., anaerobic streptococci, *Clostridium perfringens,* and fusobacteria. *Bacteroides fragilis* is commonly found.

There are conflicting data regarding the importance of anaerobes in acute sinusitis, but their role in chronic sinusitis is unquestioned. The genera *Peptostreptococcus, Fusobacterium,* and *Bacteroides* are commonly associated with chronic sinusitis.

Soft tissue infections of the head and neck usually originate in the posterior pharynx or in periodontal tissue. The normal flora surrounding the teeth, especially those organisms in the gingival crevice, are responsible for soft tissue infections of dental origin. Members of the genera *Bacteroides, Fusobacterium,* and *Peptostreptococcus* are frequent isolates.

Actinomyces and *Arachnia* spp. also normally reside in periodontal tissue and after oral trauma may be responsible for actinomycosis, a chronic granulomatous inflammation leading to suppuration, abscess formation, and draining sinuses. The abscesses expand into contiguous tissues and form burrowing, tortuous sinuses to the skin surface where they discharge purulent material. Pus from these abscesses reveals the characteristic sulfur granules. Cervicofacial actinomycosis is most commonly observed, but actinomycosis of the thoracic and abdominal areas may also be seen. Thoracic actinomycosis may result from extension of cervicofacial actinomycosis or from aspiration of *Actinomyces* organisms from the oral cavity.

SKIN AND SOFT TISSUE INFECTIONS

Anaerobic infections may develop in traumatized or devitalized skin and soft tissue such as surgical and traumatic wounds, human and animal bites, and ischemic extremities associated with arteriosclerosis or diabetes mellitus. In a series of studies on bite wounds, anaerobes were found in significant quantities in 39% of animal bite wounds, 50% of human bite wounds, and 56% of clenched fist injuries.[40] (Clenched fist injuries occur when one person strikes another in the mouth with a clenched fist; this usually results in injury to the metacarpophalangeal or interphalangeal joints of the hand.) Bite wounds usually contain several species of anaerobes that are always present in mixed culture with aerobic oral flora. The most common anaerobic isolates are *Bacteroides asaccharolyticus, B. bivius,*[65] *B. disiens,*[65] *B. melaninogenicus, B. oralis, B. ureolyticus, Fusobacterium nucleatum, F. russii, Peptostreptococcus* spp., and *Veillonella* spp. Most animal bite wounds are from dogs, although infections have resulted from bites of cats, a squirrel, and a sheep.[9]

Foot infections in diabetic patients are also polymicrobial in nature. Gram-negative enteric bacilli and group D enterococci are the most frequently observed aerobes, and members of the genera *Bacteroides, Clostridium,* and *Peptostreptococcus* are the most frequently encountered anaerobes.[115]

INFECTIONS OF LUNG AND PLEURAL SPACE

Anaerobes are commonly implicated in pneumonia (acute or chronic), aspiration pneumonia, necrotizing pneumonia, lung abscess, or empyema. Most anaerobic pleuropulmonary infections involve two to nine species of anaerobes in addition to aerobes or facultative organisms.[34] Peptostreptococci, *Bacteroides melaninogenicus,* and *Fusobacterium nucleatum* are the most common isolates.[29,42] *B. gracilis* also appears to be an important, previously unrecognized pathogen in pleuropulmonary infections.[60]

Conditions that predispose to anaerobic pleuropulmonary disease include aspiration usually related to altered consciousness, preceding extrapulmonary anaerobic infection, penetrating chest wounds, and local or systemic underlying conditions such as bronchiectasis, diabetes mellitus, and malignancy.[34] The overall mortality in anaerobic pleuropulmonary disease is 15% with proper antimicrobial therapy.[34]

FEMALE GENITAL TRACT INFECTIONS[29,34,41]

Female genital tract infections include postabortal sepsis, puerperal sepsis, tubo-ovarian infections, pelvic abscess, Bartholin's gland abscess, endometritis, and postoperative infections. Anaerobes appear to be the predominant pathogens in these infections. The most common isolates are *Bacteroides* spp. (including *B. fragilis, B. melaninogenicus, B. bivius,* and *B. disiens*)[65,129] and anaerobic gram-positive cocci. *Clostridium perfringens* causes a rare but serious septic infection.

The following conditions predispose to or are associated with anaerobic infections of the female genital tract: pregnancy, abortion, malignancy, irradiation, obstetric or gynecologic surgery, endocervical or vaginal stenosis, uterine fibroids, intrauterine contraceptive devices, and childbirth associated with premature rupture of membranes, prolonged labor, or postpartum hemorrhage.

INTRA-ABDOMINAL INFECTIONS[25,41]

Intra-abdominal sepsis results from the perforation of the bowel and the subsequent contamination of the normally sterile peritoneal cavity. This may be triggered by trauma, surgery, appendicitis, inflammatory bowel disease, or cancer. Generalized or localized peritonitis is the initial event, followed by abscess formation. Aerobes and anaerobes are present at each stage, but aerobes predominate during the peritonitis stage and anaerobes in the later abscess stage. Experimental studies suggest that anaerobes predispose to abscess formation.[101,102,143] As discussed later in the chapter the capsule of *Bacteroides fragilis* may be a contributing factor. The anaerobes that are consistently associated with intra-abdominal sepsis are *B. fragilis, Clostridium* spp., and anaerobic cocci. *B. gracilis* has been associated with intra-abdominal abscess or peritonitis resulting from underlying biliary tree obstruction or appendiceal perforation.[60]

Pyogenic liver abscesses are usually polymicrobial in nature containing both aerobes and anaerobes. The most commonly isolated anaerobes are gram-positive cocci including microaerophilic streptococci, *B. fragilis* and other *Bacteroides* spp., and *Fusobacterium necrophorum*. Members of the genera *Clostridium* and *Actinomyces* are slightly less common.[114]

URINARY TRACT INFECTIONS

Anaerobes rarely cause significant urinary tract infections (UTIs). Of the numerous types of UTI, ranging from cystitis to pyelonephritis to renal or perirenal abscesses, anaerobes are responsible for approximately 1% to 2%.[34] The most common isolates include anaerobic cocci, *B. fragilis,* other *Bacteroides* spp., and *C. perfringens.*

Because anaerobes are normally present in the urethral mucosa, urethral trauma, especially instrumentation, may introduce organisms from the urethra to the bladder. Other causes of UTI include bacteremia, obstruction, direct extension from adjacent organs such as the uterus or bowel, and introduction during surgery.

CENTRAL NERVOUS SYSTEM INFECTIONS

Anaerobes are a major cause of brain abscess but an uncommon cause of meningitis. Organisms associated with brain abscess and cerebritis include *Bacteroides* and *Fusobacterium* spp. and microaerophilic and anaerobic streptococci.[75]

CARDIOVASCULAR INFECTIONS[34]

Bacteremia and endocarditis may be associated with anaerobes. It is difficult to assess the incidence of anaerobic bacteremia from earlier studies, since it is not clear that optimal techniques were used and that all anaerobes recovered were clinically significant; however, a 2% to 10% incidence has been more recently reported.[34] The nonsporeforming gram-negative rods or *Bacteroidaceae* are the most common isolates, and *Bacteroides fragilis* is the most common species. Clostridia and anaerobic cocci are found less often.

Earlier studies reported the incidence of endocarditis to be 1% to 2%. As with bacteremia, however, this incidence is probably low because of the use of inadequate culture techniques. *B. fragilis*, fusobacteria, clostridia, and peptostreptococci are the most commonly isolated organisms. The primary portals of entry for these agents of endocarditis are the mouth (especially with poor oral hygiene, periodontal disease, and tooth extraction), the gastrointestinal tract, and to a lesser extent the genitourinary tract.

BONE AND JOINT INFECTIONS[94]

Anaerobes have been isolated from cases of osteomyelitis and arthritis, although their specific role in these infections remains undefined. *Actinomyces* spp. are responsible for bone infections that occur in conjunction with cervicofacial actinomycosis. The frequent isolates from anaerobic nonactinomycotic bone infections are *Bacteroides* and *Fusobacterium* spp. and anaerobic or microaerophilic cocci. *Fusobacterium, Bacteroides, Clostridium*, anaerobic cocci, and *Propionibacterium acnes*, have been isolated from anaerobic joint infections.

CLOSTRIDIAL INFECTIONS[49,126]

The clostridial infections are reviewed here in detail to illustrate the pathogenic potential of anaerobes.

Clostridium tetani and Tetanus[126]

C. tetani produces two primary toxins: the highly toxic spasmogenic neurotoxin, or tetanospasmin, and the hemolytic toxin, or tetanolysin. Although the first of these is the only one largely responsible for the characteristic signs of tetanus, there is some evidence that the tetanolysin may also be involved.

The spores of *C. tetani*, found in feces of humans and various animals, are ubiquitous in soil and street dust throughout the world and are able to survive in this environment for years. They enter the body through a wide variety of wounds, which are in turn contaminated with soil or feces. The germination of these spores into vegetative cells and subsequent production of toxin depend on the establishment of a sufficiently low oxidation-reduction potential in the infected tissue. The toxin apparently can travel by two routes to the central nervous system: humorally through the lymph and blood or neurally through the tissue spaces of the peripheral nerves.

Tetanus toxin binds avidly and specifically to the sialic acid–containing gangliosides of the nervous tissue. It then acts primarily by inhibiting the release of the transmitter substance, glycine or gamma-aminobutyric acid, in the inhibitory nerve system of the spinal cord. This system prevents the contraction of a muscle when the muscle with the opposite action contracts.

The incubation period of tetanus varies from 1 to 54 days but is generally 6 to 15 days.[29] Early signs and symptoms include tension or cramps and twitching in muscles around the wound, increased reflexes in the wounded extremity, slight dysphagia, stiffness of the neck and jaw muscles, headache, backache, general irritability, tachycardia, and anxious facial expressions. These are followed by trismus (lockjaw), spasms of the jaw and mouth, and finally spasticity of the neck, trunk, and limbs.[29]

Therapy for tetanus is aimed at neutralizing the circulating toxin by the administration of antitoxin, relieving the muscular spasms, maintaining an open airway, and preventing further toxin synthesis by surgical removal of infected tissue and administration of antimicrobial agents.

Clostridium botulinum and Botulism[126]

Clostridium botulinum is responsible for the paralyzing disease botulism. This species is divided into eight types (A, B, C alpha, C beta, D, E, F, and G) on the basis of the serologic specificity of the toxins that it produces. Not all types produce a single toxin, but the predominant or only toxin from each type is designated by the same capital letter as the *C. botulinum* type.

All *C. botulinum* types are found in the soil or in freshwater or seawater sediments. Types A and B are found in cultivated or noncultivated soil; type A is found most frequently in the western United States and type B in the eastern United States. Types C, D, E, and F are common in damp soil, mud, or sediment.

Types A, B, and E are most frequently associated with human botulism. Type F has been associated with several human outbreaks and type G with several human cases.[131] Types C and D are primarily associated with botulism in birds and nonhuman animals.

Botulinal toxin is the most powerful toxin known. This toxin acts on the neuromuscular junctions of the peripheral nervous system by blocking the release of the transmitter acetylcholine.[122] As a result, no impulse can be passed along to the motor end-plate, muscle contraction is not induced, and paralysis results.

Three clinical forms of botulism may occur: foodborne, infant, and wound. Foodborne botulism follows ingestion of preformed toxin in contaminated food; infant botulism and wound botulism follow production of the toxin in vivo.

Foodborne botulism

In the United States inadequately processed home-canned food is the most frequent source of botulism, although commercially prepared foods have also been incriminated. Outbreaks have been attributed to green beans, mushrooms, peppers, corn, beets, asparagus, spinach, and chard. Type A and type B outbreaks usually involve vegetables or condiments prepared from vegetables, and type E outbreaks usually involve fish or fish products.[22]

For an outbreak of foodborne botulism to occur, several conditions must be met. First, food must be contaminated with *C. botulinum* spores. Second, the food must possess the composition and nutritive properties that allow the spores to germinate and the resulting vegetative forms to grow and produce toxin. Certain environmental conditions such as suitable pH and temperature must also be met. Even in the presence of these conditions, spores are able to survive only because of inadequate heating in canning or inadequate processing. Although sufficient cooking of the food inactivates the toxin, highly suspect food must not be consumed regardless of the amount of heating. Following consumption, toxin is absorbed from the intestinal tract and transported via lymph and blood to the peripheral nervous system.

Nausea, vomiting, and diarrhea may be the first clinical signs of botulism. The classic neurologic symptoms usually appear 18 to 36 hours after consumption of the contaminated food, although they may occur as early as 8 hours or as late as 8 days. The cardinal feature is the symmetric descending paralysis that begins with the ocular muscles (disturbances of vision) and progresses rapidly to the pharyngeal muscles (dysphagia, hoarseness) and the muscles of the neck, trunk, and limbs.

Paralysis of the respiratory muscles usually results in death. Fever is usually absent.

Therapy for foodborne botulism includes administration of type-specific antitoxin or trivalent A,B,E antitoxin when the toxin has not been definitively identified. Pharmacologic and respiratory therapy may also be used. Scrupulous supportive care is essential.

Infant botulism[126]

Infant botulism follows the ingestion of *C. botulinum* spores and the germination of these spores in the infant's colon. Almost all cases occur in infants under 6 months of age.[22] The illness may range from subclinical to sudden infant death. The latter results from production of large amounts of toxin in the bowel and subsequent rapid paralysis of the airway and respiratory muscles. Direct or indirect contamination of food or the immediate environment may be the source of infection, although few specific agents have been identified. Honey has been implicated as a source of infection.

Wound botulism

Wound botulism may occur following *C. botulinum* toxin production in a traumatic wound.[141] The toxin is absorbed from the infected wound and transported via lymph and blood to individual motor nerve terminals. The clinical symptoms are similar to those of foodborne botulism. Differences may include the presence of fever and absence of gastrointestinal symptoms in wound botulism and a slightly longer (4 to 14 days) incubation period for wound botulism than for foodborne botulism.[82] Treatment should include aggressive respiratory support and administration of antimicrobial agents and antitoxin.[141]

Clostridial Wound Infections[73]

Most clostridial wound infections occur as simple contamination of a fresh wound. A Gram stain reveals the presence of typical clostridial organisms, but there is no toxin production and no invasion of the underlying tissue. The wound heals normally with simple therapeutic measures.

Anaerobic cellulitis follows the invasion of necrotic wound tissue by the proteolytic clostridia. It is characterized by gas accumulation, discoloration of the underlying skin, and the presence of a malodorous, brownish, purulent discharge. Although more severe than simple contamination, anaerobic cellulitis is usually contained by prompt debridement and intensive antimicrobial and supportive therapy.

Clostridial myonecrosis or gas gangrene involves the invasion of normal healthy muscle surrounding the wound site. Gas gangrene is associated with severe deep wounds such as those of warfare.[126] Two or three species of clostridia are almost always present. *Clostridium perfringens* is the most common species; others include *C. novyi*, *C. septicum*, *C. bifermentans*, *C. histolyticum*, and *C. sordellii*.

For clostridial myonecrosis to develop, a lowered oxidation-reduction potential must be present in the wound. This may be precipitated by the presence of foreign bodies in the wound, failure of the blood supply to the infected area, the presence of necrotic tissue and hemorrhage in the wound, and the presence and multiplication of other bacteria. The lowered oxidation-reduction potential results in the reduction of pyruvate to lactate, causing a drop in pH in the muscle. As a result of these changes, proteolytic enzymes of the muscles are activated to hydrolyze protein and release amino acids required for further growth of the clostridia.

Clinical features of gas gangrene include marked systemic toxicity, drowsiness, fever, tachycardia, and a tender, painful edematous wound with a sweet- or foul-smelling discharge. Gas is present, but it is not as obvious as in cellulitis. The underlying skin appears gangrenous or erythematous with a coppery hue and bullae. If the condition is untreated, death may occur.

Clostridium difficile–Associated Diseases[5]

Diarrhea is one of the adverse side effects of antimicrobial therapy. The severity of this disorder as manifested by pathologic changes in the colonic mucosa may range from antibiotic-associated diarrhea without colitis to antibiotic-associated colitis and finally to the severe antibiotic-associated pseudomembranous colitis (PMC). PMC is characterized by the presence of raised, adherent, whitish yellow or greenish yellow, colonic plaques ranging from a few millimeters to 10 to 20 mm in diameter. These plaques often coalesce to form a pseudomembrane composed of mucin, fibrin, sloughed epithelial cells, and acute inflammatory cells. Complications of PMC include dehydration and electrolyte imbalance as a result of fluid loss, toxic megacolon, colonic perforation, and, rarely, extraintestinal symptoms such as polyarthritis.

PMC usually occurs in association with antibiotic usage and is almost invariably due to *C. difficile*.[6] *C. difficile* is also responsible for most cases of antibiotic-associated colitis without pseudomembrane formation and up to one third of cases of antibiotic-associated diarrhea without colitis.[78a] The key factor in the pathogenesis of *C. difficile* disease is a disturbance of the normal bowel flora that permits *C. difficile* organisms that are either present in the bowel of a healthy carrier or are acquired from exogenous sources to overgrow the endogenous flora, produce toxin, and induce disease.[28] Antimicrobial agents are the most frequent inciting agents, although other conditions such as disease or surgery of the colon that alter the normal flora may also be responsible.[28,78a] The antimicrobial agents most frequently implicated are ampicillin, clindamycin, and the cephalosporins, but nearly any antimicrobial agent may be responsible.

C. difficile has been found in the feces of approximately 2% to 3% of asymptomatic healthy adults or children over 2 years of age. Between 25% and 60% of healthy children under 1 year of age are colonized by *C. difficile*.[6] As discussed in Chapter 4, evidence suggests that this organism may be an important nosocomial pathogen.[28,39,48,91] It has also been isolated from numerous environmental sources including toilets, bedpans, floors, and the hands and stools of asymptomatic hospital personnel.[90] Spores may remain viable for a long time in the hospital environment; only a few spores are necessary for ingestion and subsequent colonization of the colon.[28] Although not known for certain, evidence suggests that patients acquire *C. difficile* from the environment or from the hands of contaminated hospital personnel.[78a] The recent development of typing schemes for *C. difficile* should provide the means for better defining the epidemiology of this organism in nosocomial infections.[48,91]

The pathogenicity of *C. difficile* is associated with its ability to produce toxin; not all isolates are toxigenic. Two toxins, A and B, have been identified. These toxins can be distinguished based on separation by anion exchange chromatography, antigenic differences, and differences in biologic activity. Toxin B is an extremely potent cytotoxin that is responsible for the cytopathic effect in the cell culture assay discussed below. Toxin A is an enterotoxin but may be cytopathic in very large quantities.[28] Although the precise role of each of these toxins in human disease has not been defined, isolates from human disease have been shown to produce both toxins, and thus the presence of either toxin is currently accepted as evidence for *C. difficile*–induced disease.[69,71]

The laboratory diagnosis of antibiotic-associated diarrhea, colitis, and PMC depends on detection of the toxin or culture of *C. difficile*. Detection of toxin B by a tissue culture cytotoxicity assay (see Appendix A) is the standard and most definitive method. This technique involves preparing cell-free fecal extracts, demonstrating that these extracts produce a cytopathic effect (because of the toxin) in cell culture lines, and showing that this effect is neutralized by *C. sordellii* antitoxin or specific *C. difficile* antitoxin.[93] The neutralization of *C. difficile* toxin by *C. sordellii* antitoxin is attributed to the cross-reactivity between these two organisms. The tissue culture assay (Appendix A) is quite sensitive and specific, although false-positive findings may occur, especially in infants during the first year of life. (Unlike the situation in adults, asymptomatic carriage in infants under 1 year of age is commonly accompanied by the presence of *C. difficile* toxin; thus assay is not recommended in this age group.[6]) A commercial cytotoxicity assay is also available (Bartels Immunodiagnostics, Bellevue, Wash.).[93] Because patients with PMC are quite ill and require treatment as soon as possible, more rapid methods for diagnosis of this disease have been proposed. Counterimmunoelectrophoresis was recommended as an alternative to the tissue culture assay but is no longer widely used because of the high false-positive and false-negative rates, probably caused by the use of crude antitoxin.[59,104] Enzyme-linked immunosorbent assay (ELISA) has shown good sensitivity for detection of toxin A, and studies show it to be comparable to tissue culture assay.[69,104] A latex agglutination (LA) test is also commercially available (Marion Scientific) for detection of *C. difficile*–associated disease. This test detects *C. difficile* antigen and has been recommended as a screening test. Negative results are reported as ''no *C. difficile* present.'' Positive results are followed by a cytotoxin assay.[113b]

Cycloserine–cefoxitin–egg yolk–fructose agar (CCFA) is used for the selective isolation of *C. difficile* (see Appendix A). (It has recently been reported that cycloserine mannitol agar [CMA] and cycloserine mannitol blood agar [CMBA] are superior to CCFA for recovery of *C. difficile*.[8]) However, culture is less specific than toxin assay; cultures may be positive in 2% to 3% of healthy adults or children over 2 years of age, in 10% to 20% of adults who have had recent antimicrobial exposure without gastrointestinal complications, and in hospitalized patients who have had neither recent antimicrobial exposure nor gastrointestinal symptoms. Thus there are problems associated with the interpretation of culture results for *C. difficile*.[36,37,68]

MECHANISMS OF PATHOGENICITY

With few exceptions (such as the botulinal and tetanus toxins of clostridia) the specific mechanisms that are responsible for the infections and diseases of anaerobic bacteria are largely speculative. Toxins, enzymes, encapsulation, and inhibition of phagocytosis and chemotaxis have been suggested as potential virulence determinants.

EXOTOXINS

In general the clostridia are not invasive, and their pathogenicity is attributed to their elaboration of enzymes and toxins. Although exotoxins are produced by several clostridial species, the numerous toxins elaborated by *C. perfringens* have probably been the most thoroughly studied. These toxins are summarized in Table 20-22.

C. perfringens is divided into five types, A to E, on the basis of the major lethal toxins produced (Table 20-23). These toxins are the alpha, beta, epsilon, iota, and delta toxins. Although all types of *C. perfringens* produce the alpha toxin, type A produces more than the others. The lethal, necrotizing alpha-toxin is the lecithinase responsible for the characteristic in vitro egg yolk agar reactions. Since lecithin is also present in vivo in the membranes of numerous different cell types, this toxin has the potential for causing extensive tissue damage. It has been suggested that the lack of leukocytes in the exudate of gas gangrene may be due to the action of the toxin. Other important exotoxins include the potent neurotoxins of *C. botulinum* and *C. tetani*. These are discussed on p. 407.

ENDOTOXIN

The gram-negative anaerobic bacteria, like other gram-negative bacteria such as the *Enterobacteriaceae*, produce lipopolysaccharide. The endotoxic activity of the lipopolysaccharides of *Fusobacterium* and *Veillonella* spp. is similar to that of *Salmonella* and other *Enterobacteriaceae* endotoxins, whereas the endotoxicity of the *Bacteroides* lipopolysaccharide is quite low.[134] These differences in endotoxicity are probably related to differences in chemical composition of the lipid A component,[20] which is responsible for the toxicity of the lipopolysaccharide. The lipopolysaccharide of anaerobes, like that of other gram-negative organisms, is able to activate complement,[100] is chemotactic for polymorphonuclear leukocytes, and has been shown to activate histamine release in animal models.[99] All these factors are important in the induction of the inflammatory response. Because of these characteristics, it is thought that the endotoxin-elaborating anaerobes in human gingival plaque may contribute to the initiation of the inflammatory response and the subsequent tissue destruction of periodontitis.[133]

ENZYMES[9,30]

Anaerobes may produce a variety of enzymes including hyaluronidase, collagenase, fibrinolysin, heparinase, other proteases, elastase, lecithinase, phosphatase, RNAse, DNAse, neuraminidase, glucuronidase, and chondroitin sulfatase. Studies have suggested that some of these enzymes may participate in the development of infection. The collagenase and IgA protease[89] of *Bacteroides melaninogenicus*, for example, may be important in the establishment of periodontal disease, the protease of *Propionibacterium acnes* may contribute to the development of acne vulgaris, and the phosphatase, RNAse, and DNAse of *Bacteroides* species may facilitate invasion of tissue. While it is true that many of these enzymes have the potential to damage host tissue and participate in the pathogenesis of anaerobic infection, their precise role remains undefined.

TABLE 20-22. Toxins of *Clostridium perfringens*

Toxin	Biologic Activity	Role in Disease
Alpha (lecithinase, phospholipase C)	Lethal, necrotizing, hemolytic	Although usually associated with gas gangrene, exact involvement in this disease is unknown; probably interacts with several other toxins in producing disease
Beta	Lethal, necrotizing	Of most concern to veterinary medicine; also thought to be responsible for necrotizing jejunitis in humans
Epsilon	Lethal, necrotizing	Rare or nonexistent as cause of human disease; responsible for acute enterotoxemia in sheep, goats, and cattle
Iota	Lethal, necrotizing	Reportedly does not play role in disease; recent evidence suggests enterotoxicity in rabbits
Delta	Lethal, hemolytic	Very little known about role, if any, in disease
Theta	Lethal, hemolytic	Role in disease unknown
Eta	Lethal	Probably not important in disease
Kappa (collagenase)	Lethal, necrotizing, gelatinase	May play role in gas gangrene by softening muscle tissue
Lambda (protease)	Proteolytic	Role in disease unclear; probably contributes to breakdown of muscle and connective tissue
Mu (hyaluronidase)	Lethal, hemolytic, necrotizing	Role in disease unclear
Nu (deoxyribonuclease)	Leukocidin	May be responsible for destruction of leukocytes often seen in gas gangrene and postabortal uterine infections
Neuraminidase		May contribute to virulence and invasiveness
Enterotoxin		One of most common types of food poisoning in United States; primarily associated with meat, poultry, and gravy-containing dishes

TABLE 20-23. Major Toxins Produced by the Five Different Types of *Clostridium perfringens*

Type	Major Toxins			
	Alpha	Beta	Epsilon	Iota
A	+	−	−	−
B	+	+	+	−
C	+	+	−	−
D	+	−	+	−
E	+	−	−	+

SYMBOLS: +, Present
−, Absent

CAPSULE

The polysaccharide capsule of *Bacteroides fragilis* appears to be an important virulence factor. Studies have shown that this capsule promotes abscess formation[103] and inhibits opsonophagocytic killing.[121] *B. fragilis* is the most common anaerobic organism encountered in clinical specimens and is the most common species of intestinal anaerobe isolated from intra-abdominal infection, bacteremia, pelvic inflammatory disease, wounds and abscesses, and infections associated with appendicitis.[106]

INHIBITION OF PHAGOCYTIC KILLING AND CHEMOTAXIS

As previously mentioned, anaerobes may inhibit chemotaxis and phagocytic killing of aerobes. Studies have shown that *Bacteroides* spp. inhibit killing of *Proteus mirabilis*. Some

TABLE 20-24. In Vitro Susceptibility of Anaerobes to Antimicrobial Agents

Bacteria	Chloramphenicol	Clindamycin	Erythromycin[a]	Metronidazole	Cefoxitin	Ureido- and Carboxypenicillins[b]	Penicillin G[c]	Tetracycline	Vancomycin[a]
Anaerobic cocci	+++	++ to +++	++ to +++	+++[d,e]	+++	+++	+++	+ to ++	+++
Bacteroides fragilis group	+++	++ to +++	+ to ++	+++	++ to +++	++ to +++	+	+ to ++	+
Other *Bacteroides* spp.	+++	+++[d]	++ to +++	+++	+++[d]	+++[d]	++ to +++	++	+
Fusobacterium varium	+++	+ to ++	+	+++	+++[d]	+++[d]	+++[d]	++	
Other *Fusobacterium* spp.	+++	+++	+	+++	+++[f]	+++[f]	++++	+++	+
Clostridium perfringens	+++	+++[f]	+++	+++	+++	+++	+++	++	+++
Other *Clostridium* spp.	+++	++	++ to +++	+++	+ to ++	+++	+++	++	++ to +++
Nonsporeforming GPR	+++	++ to +++	+++	+ to ++	+++	+++	++++	++ to +++	++ to +++

SYMBOLS: +, Poor or inconsistent activity
++, Moderate activity
+++, Good activity
++++, Good activity, good pharmacologic characteristics, low toxicity, drug of choice

Reprinted from Sutter, V.L., et al.: Wadsworth anaerobic bacteriology manual, 4th edition, copyright 1985, Star Publishing Company, Belmont, Calif.
[a]Not approved by Food and Drug Administration for anaerobic infections.
[b]Piperacillin, mezlocillin, azlocillin, carbenicillin, ticarcillin.
[c]Other penicillins and cephalosporins are frequently less active. Ampicillin and amoxicillin are roughly comparable to penicillin G in activity. Addition of beta-lactamase inhibitors such as clavulanic acid and sulbactam remarkably increase activity against beta-lactamase producers such as *B. fragilis* group.
[d]A few strains are resistant.
[e]Microaerophilic streptococci (officially in genus *Streptococcus*) are often resistant to metronidazole.
[f]Rare strains are resistant.

Bacteroides spp. show greater inhibitory effects than others.[95]

ANTIMICROBIAL SUSCEPTIBILITY

Incision and drainage is frequently the best approach to anaerobic infections. In situations where antimicrobial therapy is necessary, clindamycin, metronidazole, chloramphenicol, cefoxitin, several third-generation cephalosporins (such as moxalactam and cefoperazone), and imipenem[145] may be used, although these agents are not interchangeable because of their different spectra of activity and pharmacologic properties.[49a]

Metronidazole and chloramphenicol show consistent activity against the *B. fragilis* group, *Bacteroides* spp. other than the *B. fragilis* group, and *Flavobacterium* spp. (Table 20-24). The ureidopenicillins, carboxypenicillins, and piperazine penicillins, as well as cefoxitin, show moderate to good activity against other *Bacteroides* spp. and *Fusobacterium* (Table 20-24).[31] Chloramphenicol is the drug of choice for cerebritis and brain abscess, and clindamycin, metronidazole, and chloramphenicol may be used for lung abscess.[49a] Although penicillin G was previously considered effective against *B. fragilis* and other *Bacteroides* spp. more recent studies have shown the striking resistance of these organisms to penicillin G.[113a] Penicillin resistance is mediated by the production of beta-lactamase and can be detected with the chromogenic cephalosporin method discussed in Appendix A.

Pencillin G is generally the drug of choice for clostridial infections, although occasional strains may be resistant. Chloramphenicol, carbenicillin, and metronidazole are active against nearly all the clostridia.[2] Orally administered metronidazole and vancomycin may be used to treat *C. difficile* diarrhea and PMC; the former drug is considerably less expensive.

Penicillin G is the drug of choice for anaerobic infections caused by gram-positive cocci and in high concentrations is the drug of choice for actinomycosis.[3] Strains of gram-positive cocci requiring high concentrations of penicillin may be treated with chloramphenicol, carboxypenicillin, or ureidopenicillins. Penicillin G, metronidazole, clindamycin, chloramphenicol, the cephalosporins, and imipenem are effective against gram-negative cocci, although therapy directed against these organisms is rarely indicated.[113]

Antimicrobial susceptibility testing of anaerobic bacteria is discussed in Chapter 8 and by Finegold.[32] Mechanisms of resistance of anaerobic bacteria to antimicrobial agents are reviewed by Tally.[135,136]

REFERENCES

1. Allen, S.D.: Identification of anaerobic bacteria, Clin. Microbiol. Newsletter **1**:3, 1979.
2. Allen, S.D.: *Clostridium.* In Lennette, E.H., et al., editors: Manual of clinical microbiology, ed. 4, Washington, D.C. 1985, American Society for Microbiology.
3. Allen, S.D.: Gram-positive, nonsporeforming anaerobic bacilli. In Lennette, E.H., et al., editors: Manual of clinical microbiology, ed. 4, Washington, D.C., 1985, American Society for Microbiology.
4. Allen, S.D., Siders, J.A., and Marler, L.M.: Isolation and examination of anaerobic bacteria. In Lennette, E.H., et al., editors: Manual of clinical microbiology, ed. 4, Washington, D.C., 1985, American Society for Microbiology.
5. Bartlett, J.G.: Antibiotic-associated colitis, DM **30**:6, 1984.
6. Bartlett, J.G.: *Clostridium difficile:* pseudomembranous colitis and antibiotic-associated diarrhea. In Gorbach, S.L., editor: Infectious diarrhea, Boston, 1986, Blackwood Scientific Publications.
7. Bartlett, J.G., et al.: Anaerobes survive in clinical specimens despite delayed processing, J. Clin. Microbiol. **3**:133, 1976.
8. Bartley, S.L., and Dowell, V.R., Jr.: Comparison of media for the isolation of *Clostridium difficile* from fecal specimens, Abstract C-1, Abstracts of the Annual Meeting of the American Society for Microbiology, March 1-6, 1987, Atlanta.
9. Bjornson, H.S.: Enzymes associated with the survival and virulence of gram negative anaerobes, Rev. Infect. Dis. **6**(suppl. 1):S521, 1984.
10. Bourgault, A.M., and Rosenblatt, J.E.: First isolation of *Peptostreptococcus indolicus* from a human clinical specimen, J. Clin. Microbiol. **9**:549, 1979.
11. Buchanan, A.G.: Clinical laboratory evaluation of a reverse CAMP test for presumptive identification of *Clostridium perfringens,* J. Clin. Microbiol. **16**:761, 1982.
12. Busch, D.F.: Anaerobes in infections of the head and neck and ear, nose, and throat, Rev. Infect. Dis. **6**(suppl. 1):S115, 1984.
13. Cato, E.P.: Transfer of *Peptostreptococcus parvulus* (Weinberg, Nativelle, and Prevot 1937), Smith 1957 to the genus *Streptococcus: Streptococcus parvulus* (Weinberg, Nativelle, and Prevot 1937), comb. nov., nom. rev., emend., Int. J. Syst. Bacteriol. **33**:82, 1983.
14. Cato, E.P., George, W.L., and Finegold, S.M.: Genus *Clostridium.* In Sneath, P.H.A., Mair, N.S., and Sharpe, M.E., editors (Holt, J.G., editor-in-chief): Bergey's manual of systematic bacteriology, vol. 2, Baltimore, 1986, Williams & Wilkins Co.
15. Cato, E.P., et al.: *Bacteroides zoogleoformans* (Weinberg, Nativelle and Prevot 1937) corrig., comb. nov.: emended description, Int. J. Syst. Bacteriol. **32**:271, 1982.
16. Chow, A.W., Patten, V., and Guze, L.B.: Rapid screening of *Veillonella* by ultraviolet fluorescence, J. Clin. Microbiol. **2**:546, 1975.
17. Collee, J.G.: Factors contributing to the loss of anaerobic bacteria in transit from the patient to the laboratory, Infection **8**(suppl. 2):S145, 1980.
18. Collins, M.D., and Shah, H.N.: Reclassification of *Bacteroides praecutus* Tissier (Holdeman and Moore) in a new genus, *Tissierella,* as *Tissierella praecuta* comb. nov., Int. J. Syst. Bacteriol. **36**:461, 1986.
19. Cummins, C.S., and Johnson, J.L.: Genus I. *Propionibacterium* Orla-Jensen 1909, 337.[AL] In Sneath, P.H.A., Mair, N.S, and Sharpe, M.E., editors (Holt, J.G., editor-in-chief): Bergey's manual of systematic bacteriology, vol. 2, Baltimore, 1986, Williams & Wilkins Co.
20. Dahlen, G., and Mattsby-Baltzer, I.: Lipid A in anaerobic bacteria, Infect. Immun. **39**:466, 1983.
21. Dowell, V.R., Jr.: Collection of clinical specimens and primary isolation of anaerobic bacteria. In Balows, A., et al., editors: Anaerobic bacteria: role in disease, Springfield, Ill., 1972, Charles C Thomas, Publishers.
22. Dowell, V.R., Jr.: Botulism and tetanus: selected epidemiologic and microbiologic aspects, Rev. Infect. Dis. **6**(suppl. 1):S202, 1984.
23. Dowell, V.R., and Hawkins, T.M.: Laboratory methods in anaerobic bacteriology—CDC laboratory manual, Centers for Disease Control, U.S. Dept. of Health and Human Services, Pub. No. (CDC) 81-8272, 1981.
24. Draper, D.L., and Barry, A.L.: Rapid identification of *Bacteroides fragilis* with bile and antibiotic discs, J. Clin. Microbiol. **5**:439, 1977.
25. Dunn, D.L., and Simmons, R.L.: The role of anaerobic bacteria in intraabdominal infections, Rev. Infect. Dis. **6**(suppl. 1):S139, 1984.
26. Ezaki, T., et al.: Transfer of *Peptococcus indolicus, Peptococcus asaccharolyticus, Peptococcus prevotii,* and *Peptococcus magnus* to the genus *Peptostreptococcus* and proposal of *Peptostreptococcus tetradius* sp. nov., Int. J. Syst. Bacteriol. **33**:683, 1983.
27. Facklam, R.R.: Physiological differentiation of viridans streptococci, J. Clin. Microbiol. **5**:184, 1977.

28. Fekety, R.: Pathology and pathogenesis of *C. difficile* colitis, presented in session 113 Annual Meeting of the American Society for Microbiology, Washington, D.C., March 23-28, 1986.

29. Finegold, S.M.: Anaerobic bacteria in human disease, New York, 1977, Academic Press, Inc.

30. Finegold, S.M.: Taxonomy, enzymes and clinical relevance of anaerobic bacteria, Rev. Infect. Dis. **1**:248, 1979.

31. Finegold, S.M., and Edelstein, M.A.C.: Gram-negative nonsporeforming anaerobic bacilli. In Lennette, E.H., et al., editors: Manual of clinical microbiology, ed. 4, Washington, D.C., 1985, American Society for Microbiology.

32. Finegold, S.M., and Rolfe, R.D.: Susceptibility testing of anaerobic bacteria, Diagn. Microbiol. Infect. Dis. **1**:33, 1983.

33. Finegold, S.M., Shepherd, W.E., and Spaulding, E.H. (Shepherd, W.E., coordinating editor): Practical anaerobic bacteriology, Cumitech 5, Washington, D.C., 1977, American Society for Microbiology.

34. Finegold, S.M., and Sutter, V.L.: Anaerobic infections, Kalamazoo, Mich., 1982, The Upjohn Co.

35. Georg, L.K., et al.: A new pathogenic anaerobic *Actinomyces* species, J. Infect. Dis. **115**:88, 1965.

36. George, W.L.: Antimicrobial agent–associated colitis and diarrhea: historical background and clinical aspects, Rev. Infect. Dis. **6**(suppl. 1):S208, 1984.

37. George, W.L., Rolfe, R.D., and Finegold, S.M.: *Clostridium difficile* and its cytotoxin in feces in patients with antimicrobial agent–associated diarrhea and miscellaneous conditions, J. Clin. Microbiol. **15**:1049, 1982.

38. George, W.L., et al.: Gram negative anaerobic bacilli: their role in infection and patterns of susceptibility to antimicrobial agents. II. Little-known *Fusobacterium* species and miscellaneous genera, Rev. Infect. Dis. **3**:599, 1981.

39. Gerding, D.N., et al.: *Clostridium difficile*–associated diarrhea and colitis in adults, Arch. Intern. Med. **146**:95, 1986.

40. Goldstein, E.J.C., Citron, D.M., and Finegold, S.M.: Role of anaerobic bacteria in bite-wound infections, Rev. Infect. Dis. **6**(suppl. 1):S177, 1984.

41. Gorbach, S.L., and Bartlett, J.G.: Anaerobic infections (first of three parts), N. Engl. J. Med. **290**:1177, 1974.

42. Gorbach, S.L., and Bartlett, J.G.: Anaerobic infections (second of three parts), N. Engl. J. Med. **290**:1237, 1974.

43. Gorbach, S.L., et al.: Rapid diagnosis of anaerobic infections by direct gas liquid chromatography of clinical specimens, J. Clin. Invest. **57**:478, 1976.

44. Gubash, S.M.: Synergistic haemolysis test for presumptive identification and differentiation of *Clostridium perfringens, C. bifermentans, C. sordellii,* and *C. paraperfringens,* J. Clin. Pathol. **33**:395, 1980.

45. Halebian, S., et al.: Rapid method that aids in distinguishing gram positive from gram negative bacteria, J. Clin. Microbiol. **13**:444, 1981.

46. Hansen, M.V., and Elliott, L.P.: New presumptive identification test for *Clostridium perfringens:* reverse CAMP test, J. Clin. Microbiol. **12**:617, 1980.

47. Hanson, C.W., and Martin, W.J.: Evaluation of enrichment, storage and age of blood agar medium in relation to its ability to support growth of anaerobic bacteria, J. Clin. Microbiol. **4**:394, 1976.

48. Heard, S.R., et al.: The epidemiology of *Clostridium difficile* with use of a typing scheme: nosocomial acquisition and cross-infection among immunocompromised patients, J. Infect. Dis. **153**:159, 1986.

49. Henderson, D.K., et al.: Infectious disease emergencies: the clostridial syndromes, West. J. Med. **129**:101, 1978.

49a. Hermans, P.E.: Lincosamides. In Peterson, P.K., and Verhoef, J., editors: The antimicrobial agents annual 1, New York, 1986, Elsevier Science Publishing Co., Inc.

50. Holdeman, L.V., Cato, E.P., and Moore, W.E.C.: Anaerobe laboratory manual, ed. 4, Blacksburg, Va., 1977, Virginia Polytechnic Institute and State University.

51. Holdeman, L.V., Cato, E.P., and Moore, W.E.C.: Taxonomy of anaerobes: present state of the art, Rev. Infect. Dis. **6**(suppl. 1):S3, 1984.

52. Holdeman, L.V., Johnson, J.L., and Moore, W.E.C.: Genus *Peptococcus* Klyyver and van Neil 1936, 400.[AL] In Sneath, P.H.A., Mair, N.S., and Sharpe, M.E., editors (Holt, J.G., editor-in-chief): Bergey's manual of systematic bacteriology, vol. 2, Baltimore, 1986, Williams & Wilkins Co.

53. Holdeman, L.V., Johnson, J.L., and Moore, W.E.C.: Genus *Peptostreptococcus* Klyyver and van Neil 1936, 401.[AL] In Sneath, P.H.A., Mair, N.S., and Sharpe, M.E., editors (Holt, J.G., editor-in-chief): Bergey's manual of systematic bacteriology, vol. 2, Baltimore, 1986, Williams & Wilkins Co.

54. Holdeman, L.V., Kelley, R.W., and Moore, W.E.C.: Family I. *Bacteroidaceae* and genus I. *Bacteroides*. In Krieg, N.R., editor (Holt, J.G., editor-in-chief): Bergey's manual of systematic bacteriology, vol. 1, Baltimore, 1984, Williams & Wilkins Co.

55. Holdeman, L.V., and Moore, W.E.C.: New genus, *Coprococcus,* twelve new species, and emended descriptions of four previously described species of bacteria from human feces, Int. J. Syst. Bacteriol. **24**:260, 1974.

56. Holdeman, L.V., et al.: *Bacteroides oris* and *Bacteroides buccae,* new species from human periodontitis, and other human infections, Int. J. Syst. Bacteriol. **32**:125, 1982.

57. Ingham, H.R., et al.: Inhibition of phagocytosis in vitro by obligate anaerobes, Lancet **2**:1252, 1977.

58. Jackson, F.L., and Goodman, Y.E.: *Bacteroides ureolyticis,* a new species to accommodate strains previously identified as "Bacteroides corrodens, Anaerobic," Int. J. Syst. Bacteriol. **28**:197, 1978.

59. Jarvis, W., et al.: Comparison of bacterial isolation, cytotoxicity assay, and counterimmunoelectrophoresis for the detection of *Clostridium difficile* and its toxin, J. Infect. Dis. **147**:778, 1983.

60. Johnson, C.C., et al.: *Bacteroides gracilis,* an important anaerobic bacterial pathogen, J. Clin. Microbiol. **22**:799, 1985.

60a. Johnson, J.L., Moore, W.E.C., and Moore, L.V.H.: *Bacteroides caccae* sp. nov. *Bacteroides merdae* sp. nov., and *Bacteroides stercoris* sp. nov. isolated from human feces, Int. J. Syst. Bacteriol. **36**:499, 1986.

61. Jones, G.L., Whaley, D.N., and Dever, S.M.: Use of the flexible anaerobic glove box, Atlanta, 1977, Centers for Disease Control.

62. Kaczmarek, F.S., and Coykendall, A.L.: Production of phenylacetic acid by strains by *Bacteroides asaccharolyticus* and *Bacteroides gingivalis* (sp. nov.), J. Clin. Microbiol. **12**:288, 1980.

63. Kandler, O., and Weiss, N.: Genus *Lactobacillus* Beijerinck 1901, 212.[AL] In Sneath, P.H.A, Mair, N.S., and Sharpe, M.E., editors (Holt, J.G., editor-in-chief): Bergey's manual of systematic bacteriology, vol. 2, Baltimore, 1986, Williams & Wilkins Co.

64. Killgore, G.E., et al.: Comparison of three anaerobic systems for the isolation of anaerobic bacteria from clinical specimens, Am. J. Clin. Pathol. **59**:552, 1973.

65. Kirby, B.D., et al.: Gram negative anaerobic bacilli: their role in infection and patterns of susceptibility to antimicrobial agents. I. Little-known *Bacteroides* species, Rev. Infect. Dis. **2**:914, 1980.

66. Koneman, E.W., et al.: Color atlas and textbook of diagnostic microbiology, ed. 2, Philadelphia, 1983, J.B. Lippincott Co.

67. Koransky, J.R., Allen, S.D., and Dowell, V.R., Jr.: Use of ethanol for selective isolation of sporeforming microorganisms, Appl. Environ. Microbiol. **35**:762, 1978.

68. Lashner, B.A., et al.: *Clostridium difficile* culture-positive toxin-negative diarrhea, Am. J. Gastroenterol. **81**:940, 1986.

69. Laughon, B.E., et al.: Enzyme immunoassays for detection of *Clostridium difficile* toxins A and B in fecal specimens, J. Infect. Dis. **149**:781, 1984.

70. Loesche, W.J.: Oxygen sensitivity of various anaerobic bacteria, Appl. Microbiol. **18**:723, 1969.

71. Lyerley, D.M., and Wilkins, T.D.: Commercial latex test for *Clostridium difficile* toxin A does not detect toxin A, J. Clin. Microbiol. **23**:622, 1986.

72. MacDonald, J.B., Socransky, S.S., and Gibbons, R.J.: Aspects of the pathogenesis of mixed anaerobic infections of mucous membranes, J. Dent. Res. **42**:529, 1962.

73. MacLennan, J.D.: The histotoxic clostridial infections of man, Bacteriol. Rev. **26**:177, 1962.

74. Martin, W.J.: Isolation and identification of anaerobic bacteria in the clinical laboratory—a two year experience, Mayo Clin. Proc. **49**:300, 1974.

75. Mathisen, G.E., et al.: Brain abscess and cerebritis, Rev. Infect. Dis. **6**(suppl. 1):S101, 1984.

76. Mayhew, J.W., and Gorbach, S.L.: Internal standards for gas chromatographic analysis of metabolic end products from anaerobic bacteria, Appl. Environ. Microbiol. **33**:1002, 1977.

77. Mays, T.D., et al.: Taxonomy of the genus *Veillonella* Prévot, Int. J. Syst. Bacteriol. **32**:28, 1982.

78. McCord, J.M., Keele, B.B., Jr., and Fridovich, I.: An enzyme-based theory of obligate anaerobiosis: the physiological function of superoxide dismutase, Proc. Natl. Acad. Sci. USA **68**:1024, 1971.

78a. McFarland, L.V., and Stamm, W.E.: Review of *Clostridium difficile* associated diseases, Am. J. Infect. Control **14**:99, 1986.

79. McLeod, J.W., and Gordon, J.: The problem of intolerance of oxygen by anaerobic bacteria, J. Pathol. Bacteriol. **26**:332, 1923.

80. McNair, H.M.: Instrumentation in gas chromatography. In Heftmann, E., editor: Chromatography, ed. 3, New York, 1975, Van Nostrand Reinhold Co.

81. Mena, E., et al.: Evaluation of port-a-cul transport system for protection of anaerobic bacteria, J. Clin. Microbiol. **8**:28, 1978.

82. Merson, M.H., and Dowell, V.R., Jr.: Epidemiologic, clinical, and laboratory aspects of wound botulism, N. Engl. J. Med. **289**:1005, 1973.

83. Moore, W.E.C., Holdeman, L.V., and Kelley, R.W.: Genus II. *Fusobacterium*. In Krieg, N.R., editor (Holt, J.G., editor-in-chief): Bergey's manual of systematic bacteriology, vol. 1, Baltimore, 1984, Williams & Wilkins Co.

84. Moore, W.E.C., and Moore, L.V.H.: Genus *Eubacterium* Prevot 1938, 294.[AL] In Sneath, P.H.A., Mair, N.S., and Sharpe, M.E., editors (Holt, J.G., editor-in-chief): Bergey's manual of systematic bacteriology, vol. 2, Baltimore, 1986, Williams & Wilkins Co.

84a. Moore, W.E.C., et al.: Bacteriology of moderate (chronic) periodontitis in mature adult humans, Infect. Immun. **42**:510, 1983.

84b. Moore, W.E.C., et al.: Comparative bacteriology of juvenile periodontitis, Infect. Immun. **48**:507, 1985.

85. Morgenstein, A.A., et al.: Serious infection with *Leptotrichia buccalis:* report of a case and review of the literature, Am. J. Med. **69**:782, 1980.

86. Morris, J.G.: The physiology of obligate anaerobiosis, Adv. Microb. Physiol. **12**:169, 1975.

87. Morris, J.G.: Fifth Stenhouse-Williams memorial lecture: oxygen and the obligate anaerobe, J. Appl. Bacteriol. **40**:229, 1976.

88. Morris, J.G., and O'Brien, R.W.: Oxygen and clostridia: a review. In Barker, A.N., Gould, G.W., and Wolf, J., editors: Spore research, New York, 1971, Academic Press, Inc.

89. Mortensen, S.B., and Kilian, M.: Purification and characterization of an immunoglobulin Al protease from *Bacteroides melaninogenicus*, Infect. Immun. **45**:550, 1984.

90. Mulligan, M.E., et al.: Epidemiolgical aspects of *Clostridium difficile*-induced diarrhea and colitis, Am. J. Clin. Nutr. **33**(suppl. 11):2533, 1980.

91. Mulligan, M.E., et al.: Bacterial agglutination and polyacrylamide gel electrophoresis for typing *Clostridium difficile*, J. Infect. Dis. **153**:267, 1986.

92. Murray, P.R.: Growth of clinical isolates of anaerobic bacteria on agar media: effects of media composition, storage conditions, and

93. Nachamkin, I., Lotz-Nolan, L., and Skalina, D.: Evaluation of a commercial cytotoxicity assay for detection of *Clostridium difficile* toxin, J. Clin. Microbiol. **23**:954, 1986.

94. Nakata, M.M., and Lewis, R.P.: Anaerobic bacteria in bone and joint infections, Rev. Infect. Dis. **6**(suppl. 1):S165, 1984.

95. Namavar, F., et al.: Effect of anaerobic bacteria on killing of *Proteus mirabilis* by human polymorphonuclear leukocytes, Infect. Immun. **40**:930, 1983.

96. Namavar, F., et al.: Polymorphonuclear leukocyte chemotaxis by mixed anaerobic and aerobic bacteria, J. Med. Microbiol. **18**:167, 1984.

97. Neblett, T.R., and Brown, W.J.: Fundamentals of anaerobic bacteriology as related to the clinical laboratory, Washington, D.C., 1980, American Society for Microbiology.

98. Newman, M.G.: Anaerobic oral and dental infection, Rev. Infect. Dis. **6**(suppl. 1):S107, 1984.

99. Nygen, H., and Dahlen, G.: Complement-dependent histamine release from rat peritoneal mast cells, induced by lipopolysaccharides from *Bacteroides oralis, Fusobacterium nucleatum* and *Veillonella parvula*, J. Oral Pathol. **10**:87, 1981.

100. Nygen, H., Dahlen, G., and Nilsson, L.: Human complement activation by lipopolysaccharides from *Bacteroides oralis, Fusobacterium nucleatum* and *Veillonella parvula*, Infect. Immun. **26**:391, 1979.

101. Onderdonk, A.B., et al.: Experimental intra-abdominal abscesses in rats: quantitative bacteriology of infected animals, Infect. Immun. **10**:1256, 1974.

102. Onderdonk, A.B., et al.: Microbial synergy in experimental intra-abdominal abscess, Infect. Immun. **13**:22, 1976.

103. Onderdonk, A.B., et al.: The capsular polysaccharide of *Bacteroides fragilis* as a virulence factor: comparison of the pathogenic potential of encapsulated and unencapsulated strains, J. Infect. Dis. **136**:82, 1977.

104. Peterson, L.: Laboratory diagnosis of *C. difficile* colitis. Presented in session 113, Annual Meeting of the American Society for Microbiology, Washington, D.C., March 23-28, 1986.

105. Phillips, K.D., Tearle, P.V., and Willis, A.T.: Rapid diagnosis of anaerobic infections by gas liquid chromatography of clinical material, J. Clin. Pathol. **29**:428, 1976.

106. Polk, B.F., and Kasper, D.L.: *Bacteroides fragilis* subspecies in clinical isolates, Ann. Intern. Med. **86**:569, 1977.

107. Reilly, S.: The carbon dioxide requirements of anaerobic bacteria, J. Med. Microbiol. **13**:573, 1980.

108. Rogosa, M.: Family I. *Veillonellaceae* Rogosa 1971, 232.[AL] In Krieg, N.R., editor (Holt, J.G., editor-in-chief): Bergey's manual of systematic bacteriology, vol. 1, Baltimore, 1984, Williams & Wilkins Co.

109. Rogosa, M.: *Peptococcaceae*, a new family to include in the gram-positive, anaerobic cocci of the genera *Peptococcus, Peptostreptococcus,* and *Ruminococcus*, Int. J. Syst. Bacteriol. **21**:234, 1971.

110. Rolfe, R.D., et al.: Factors related to the oxygen tolerance of anaerobic bacteria, Appl. Environ. Microbiol. **36**:306, 1978.

111. Rosenblatt, J.E.: Reevaluation of current methods for anaerobic incubation, Clin. Microbiol. Newsletter **6**:41, 1982.

112. Rosenblatt, J.E.: Anaerobic bacteria. In Washington, J.A., editor: Laboratory procedures in clinical microbiology, ed. 2, New York, 1985, Springer-Verlag.

113. Rosenblatt, J.E.: Anaerobic cocci. In Lennette, E.H., et al.: editors: Manual of clinical microbiology, ed. 4, Washington, D.C., 1985, American Society for Microbiology.

113a. Rosenblatt, J.E.: Antimicrobial susceptibility testing of anaerobes. In Lorian, V., editor: Antibiotics in laboratory medicine, ed. 2, Baltimore, 1986, The Williams & Wilkins Co.

113b. Ryan, R., et al.: Utility of a rapid latex test for detection of *C. difficile* in fecal specimens, Ann. Clin. Lab. Sci. In press.

reduction under anaerobic conditions, J. Clin. Microbiol. **8**:708, 1978.

114. Sabbaj, J.: Anaerobes in liver abscess, Rev. Infect. Dis. **6**(suppl. 1):S152, 1984.

115. Sapico, F.L., et al.: The infected foot of the diabetic patient: quantitative microbiology and analysis of clinical features, Rev. Infect. Dis. **6**(suppl. 1):S171, 1984.

116. Scardovi, V.: Genus *Bifidobacterium* Orla-Jensen 1924, 472.[AL] In Sneath, P.H.A., Mair, N.S., and Sharpe, M.E., editors (Holt, J.G., editor-in-chief): Bergey's manual of systematic bacteriology, vol. 2, Baltimore, 1986, Williams & Wilkins Co.

117. Schaal, K.P.: Genus *Actinomyces* Harz 1877, 133.[AL] In Sneath, P.H.A., Mair, N.S., and Sharpe, M.E., editors (Holt, J.G., editor-in-chief): Bergey's manual of systematic bacteriology, vol. 2, Baltimore, 1986, Williams & Wilkins Co.

118. Schaal, K.P.: Genus *Arachnia* Pine and Georg 1969, 269.[AL] In Sneath, P.H.A., Mair, N.S., and Sharpe, M.E., editors (Holt, J.G., editor-in-chief: Bergey's manual of systematic bacteriology, vol. 2, Baltimore, 1986, Williams & Wilkins Co.

119. Schaal, K.P., and Pulverer, G.: The genera *Actinomyces, Agromyces, Arachnia, Bacterionema,* and *Rothia.* In Staff, M.P., et al., editors: The prokaryotes: a handbook on habitats, isolation, and identification of bacteria, New York, 1981, Springer-Verlag.

120. Siep, W.F., and Evans, G.L.: Atmospheric analysis and redox potentials of culture media in the Gas Pak system, J. Clin. Microbiol. **11**:226, 233, 1980.

121. Simon, G.L., et al.: Alterations in opsonophagocytic killing by neutrophils of *Bacteroides fragilis* associated with animal and laboratory passage: effect of capsular polysaccharide, J. Infect. Dis. **145**:72, 1982.

122. Simpson, L.L.: The action of botulinal toxin, Rev. Infect. Dis. **1**:656, 1979.

123. Slack, M.A.: Actinomycosis. In Balows, A., and Hausler, W.J., Jr., editors: Bacterial, mycotic, and parasitic infections, ed. 6, Washington, D.C., 1981, American Public Health Association.

124. Slack, J.M., and Gerencser, M.A.: *Actinomyces,* filamentous bacteria: biology and pathogenicity, Minneapolis, 1975, Burgess Publishing Co.

125. Slots, J., and Genco, R.J.: Direct hemagglutination technique for differentiating *Bacteroides asaccharolyticus* oral strains from normal strains, J. Clin. Microbiol. **10**:371, 1979.

126. Smith, L.DS.: The pathogenic anaerobic bacteria, Springfield, Ill., 1984, Charles C Thomas, Publisher.

127. Smith, L.DS.: Anaerobes and oxygen. In Fredette, V., editor: The anaerobic bacteria, Montreal, 1967, The Institute of Microbiology Hygiene of Montreal University.

128. Smith, L.DS., and Dowell, V.R., Jr.: Clostridium. In Lennette, E.H., et al., editors: Manual of clinical microbiology, ed. 3, Washington, D.C., 1980, American Society for Microbiology.

129. Snydman, D.R., et al.: *Bacteroides bivius* and *Bacteroides disiens* in obstetrical patients: clinical findings and antimicrobial susceptibilities, J. Antimicrob. Chemother. **6**:519, 1980.

130. Sondag, J.E., Ali, M., and Murray, P.R.: Rapid presumptive identification of anaerobes in blood cultures by gas liquid chromatography, J. Clin. Microbiol. **11**:274, 1980.

131. Sonnabend, O., et al.: Isolation of *Clostridium botulinum* type G and identification of type G botulinal toxin in humans; a report of five sudden unexpected deaths, J. Infect. Dis. **144**:22, 1981.

132. Sutter, V.L., et al.: Wadsworth anaerobic bacteriology manual, ed. 4, Belmont, Calif., 1985, Star Publishing Co.

133. Sveen, K.: Rabbit polymorphonuclear leukocytes migration in vitro in response to lipopolysaccharides from *Bacteroides, Fusobacterium,* and *Veillonella,* Acta Pathol. Microbiol. Scand. (B) **85**:374, 1977.

134. Sveen, K., Hofstad, T., and Milner, K.C.: Lethality for mice and chick embryos, pyrogenicity in rabbits and ability to gelate lysate from amoebocytes of *Limulus polyphemus* by lipopolysaccharides from *Bacteroides, Fusobacterium* and *Veillonella,* Acta Pathol. Microbiol. Scand. **85**:388, 1977.

135. Tally, F.P., Cuchural, G.J., and Malamy, M.H.: Mechanisms of resistance and resistance transfer in anaerobic bacteria: factors influencing antimicrobial therapy, Rev. Infect. Dis. **6**(suppl. 1):S260, 1984.

136. Tally, F.P., and Malamy, M.H.: Antimicrobial resistance and resistance transfer in anaerobic bacteria: a review, Scand. J. Gastroenterol. **91**:21, 1984.

137. Tally, F.P., et al.: Superoxide dismutase in anaerobic bacteria of clinical significance, Infect. Immun. **16**:20, 1977.

138. Tanner, A.C.R., Listgarten, M.A., and Ebersole, J.L.: *Wolinella curva* sp. nov.: "Vibrio succinogenes" of human origin, Int. J. Syst. Bacteriol. **34**:275, 1984.

139. Tanner, A.C.R., et al.: *Wolinella* gen. nov., *Wolinella succinogenes* (*Vibrio succinogenes* Wolin et al.) comb. nov., and description of *Bacteroides gracilis* sp. nov., *Wolinella recta* sp. nov., *Campylobacter concisus* sp. nov., and *Eikenella corrodens* from humans with periodontal disease, Int. J. Syst. Bacteriol. **31**:432, 1981.

140. Thomann, W.R., and Hill, G.B.: Modified extraction procedure for gas-liquid chromatography applied to the identification of anaerobic bacteria, J. Clin. Microbiol. **23**:392, 1986.

141. Thorne, F.L., and Kropp, R.J.: Wound botulism: a life-threatening complication of hand injuries, Plast. Reconstr. Surg. **71**:548, 1983.

142. Weinberg, L.G., Smith, L.L., and McTighe, A.H.: Rapid identification of the *Bacteroides fragilis* group by bile disk and catalase tests, Lab. Med. **14**:785, 1983.

143. Weinstein, W.M., et al.: Experimental intra-abdominal abscesses in rats: development of an experimental model, Infect. Immun. **10**:1250, 1974.

144. Weissfeld, A.S., and Sonnenwirth, A.C.: Rapid detection and identification of *Bacteroides fragilis* and *Bacteroides melaninogenicus* by immunofluorescence, J. Clin. Microbiol. **13**:798, 1981.

145. Wexler, H.M., and Finegold, S.M.: In vitro activity of imipenem against anaerobic bacteria, Rev. Infect. Dis. **7**:S417, 1985.

146. Wideman, P.A., et al.: Evaluation of the sodium polyanethol sulfonate disk test for the identification of *Peptostreptococcus anaerobius,* J. Clin. Microbiol. **4**:330, 1976.

147. Wilkins, T.D., and West, S.E.H.: Medium-dependent inhibition of *Peptostreptococcus anaerobius* by sodium polyanethol sulfonate in blood culture media, J. Clin. Microbiol. **3**:393, 1976.

148. Zabransky, R.J.: Isolation of anaerobic bacteria from clinical specimens, Mayo Clin. Proc. **45**:256, 1970.

CHAPTER 21

Gram-Positive Bacilli

Bacillus, *Corynebacterium*, *Listeria*, and *Erysipelothrix*

Jill E. Clarridge

The group of aerobic or facultatively anaerobic, gram-positive, rod-shaped bacteria is taxonomically heterogeneous, and its lines of relatedness are not clearly defined at this time. When an organism of such morphology is confronted, the genera that need to be considered include *Listeria, Erysipelothrix, Lactobacillus, Bacillus, Corynebacterium,* occasional strains of *Clostridium, Propionibacterium, Mycobacterium, Actinomyces,* and *Nocardia* and genera related to *Nocardia.* Species of all these genera have been associated with disease. Some genera that are rarely isolated in the clinical laboratory and yet fit the group description are *Arthrobacter, Brevibacterium, Cellomonas, Microbacterium, Oerskovia, Rothia, Kurthia,* and *Rhodococcus.* Of this last group only *Rothia* and some *Brevibacterium* are normal human flora; the others are found in soil, water, and food. *Oerskovia, Rothia, Kurthia,* and *Rhodococcus* have been reported as occasionally associated with disease. Members of the genera *Actinomyces, Clostridium, Propionibacterium,* and *Lactobacillus* usually grow better anaerobically and were considered in Chapter 20; however, initial isolation of some strains may be achieved aerobically, especially with incubation under 3% to 8% CO_2. Some of the Runyon group IV mycobacteria grow on ordinary laboratory media (for example, *Mycobacterium fortuitum* grows on MacConkey agar at 35° C in air) and can appear as gram-positive rods. These organisms are acid fast and are considered in Chapter 26. Members of the genus *Nocardia* are generally branched and also are discussed elsewhere (Chapter 30). Differential tests to identify the genera of the clinically significant gram-positive rods are given in Table 21-1 and Figure 21-1.

CORYNEBACTERIUM

Corynebacterium organisms are gram-positive, catalase-positive, aerobic or facultatively anaerobic, asporogenous rods that are usually nonmotile. The cell wall of some species is weaker at the ends, allowing the organism to assume a club shape and suggesting its name (*coryne* means "club" in Greek). At cell division the daughter cells can remain attached on one side, forming Ls and Vs. The arrangement and cuneiform shape of these cells can suggest Chinese characters. Corynebacteria are found in the environment, on plants, and as part of the normal flora of humans and animals. They are also associated with diseases of humans, animals, and plants. The major pathogen and the type species of the genus is *C. diphtheriae,* the causative agent of diphtheria.

Corynebacteria are common isolates in the clinical laboratory. It is important to realize that although most isolates are commensal, some can be pathogens and these should be identified. Only species that have been isolated from humans or animals associated with humans are discussed here.

CLASSIFICATION

In *Bergey's Manual of Systematic Bacteriology*[26] the genus *Corynebacterium* includes only 16 species, many of which have been isolated from only plants and animals. To be assigned to this genus, an organism must have a cell wall with meso-diaminopimelic acid, arabinose, galactose, and short-chain mycolic acids (22 to 36 carbon atoms). The DNA base composition ranges from 51 to 63 mol% G+C.[2]

Many organisms that are encountered clinically resemble the genus *Corynebacterium* morphologically (that is, pleomorphic gram-positive rods with angular shapes), but their classification is not yet complete and they may not necessarily meet the definition of the genus. These organisms have been designated by the Centers for Disease Control as coryneform groups (Table 21-2). In fact, it is common practice to refer to all bacteria that display this characteristic morphology as coryneform organisms.

Hollis and Weaver[43] and others[19,25] have described approximately 30 species or groups of corynebacteria and other coryneform organisms isolated from humans or animals. The classification from *Bergey's Manual of Systematic Bacteriology,*[19] with the addition of some of the coryneform groups defined by the CDC, is used in this chapter. A condensed form of their data is shown in Table 21-2.

The classification of coryneform bacteria on the basis of DNA homology and chemotaxonomic characteristic is ongoing.[23,36,90]

CORYNEBACTERIUM DIPHTHERIAE
Specimen Collection and Handling

For cases of suspected diphtheria, material for culture is taken by swab from the inflamed areas of the membranes that are formed in the throat and nasopharynx. Similar specimens from the nasopharynx and throat of suspected carriers are also cultured. Material from wounds should be removed by swab or aspiration, with care taken to avoid normal skin flora. Gram stains are made of the original material.

Growth Requirements
Media

The swabs or exudate should be plated to a Loeffler agar slant, blood agar plate, and a medium containing tellurite, such as cystine-tellurite agar or Tinsdale medium (Appendix A). Cystine-tellurite agar is preferred over Tinsdale medium for primary isolation because of the short shelf life of the latter. However, Tinsdale medium may be useful in differentiating among the corynebacteria (see the section on identification). The blood agar and cystine-tellurite agar are streaked for isolation.

TABLE 21-1. Abbreviated Scheme for Identification of Gram-Positive Bacilli

Genus or Species	Microscopic Morphology[a]	Catalase	Grows Better Anaerobically	Motility	Esculin	H₂S (TSI)	TSI Acid Slant/Butt[b]	Nitrate Reduction	Urease	Hemolysis	Comments
Bacillus	Medium-large regular rods, spores	+	-	v	+	-	v/v	v	v	B, A, N	
Kurthia	Chains, plump rods	+	-	+	-	-	-/-	v	+/-	N	Strict aerobe; feathery growth; grow best at 20° to 30° C
Listeria monocytogenes	Small rods, coccobacilli	+	-	+	+	-	-/-	-	-	B	Umbrella motility
Oerskovia	Coccoid, branching filaments	+	-	+	+	-	+/+	v	v	N, A	Yellow pigment
Brevibacterium	Coccoid, short rods	+	-	+	+	-	+/+	v	-	v	Golden yellow
Rothia dentocariosa	Coccoid, diphtheroid, branching filaments	+	-	-	+	-	+/+	+	-	N	Coccoid in broth
Mycobacterium fortuitum	Slender rods	+	-	-	-	-	-/-	+	v	N	Acid-fast
Rhodococcus equi	Coccoid, branching filaments	+	-	-	v	-	-/-	v	v	N	Pink, coral pigment, acid fast
Corynebacterium	Diphtheroid, curved, pleomorphic	+	-	-[c]	-	-	v/v	v	v	v	
Arcanobacterium	Diphtheroid curved, pleomorphic, slender	-	+/-[d]	-	v	-	+/+	-	-	B	
Arachnia	Diphtheroid, pleomorphic	-	+	-	-	-	+/+	v	-	N	
Actinomyces	Diphtheroid, branching filaments	-[e]	+	-	+	-	+/+	+/-[d]	-	N	
Lactobacillus	Thin rods, thick rods, chains	-	+/-[d]	-	v	-	+/+	-	-	N, A	Some grow on tomato juice agar
Erysipelothrix	Pleomorphic, chains, small rods	-	-	-	-	+	+/+	-	-	N, A	
Propionibacterium	Diphtheroid	+	+	-	v	-	+/+	-	-	B, A, N	

SYMBOLS: +, >90% of strains positive   A, Alpha-hemolytic   N, Nonhemolytic
 −, <10% of strains positive   B, Beta-hemolytic

Modified from Clarridge, J.E., and Weissfeld, A.S.: Clin. Microbiol. Newsletter. vol. 6, p. 115. Copyright 1984 by Elsevier Science Publishing Co., Inc.
[a]Small is <0.5 μm in diameter; medium is 0.5 to 0.9 μm; large is >0.9 μm.
[b]+reaction indicates acid production.
[c]Some species are positive.
[d]There is discrepancy in literature as to whether reaction is positive or negative.
[e]*A. viscosus* is positive.

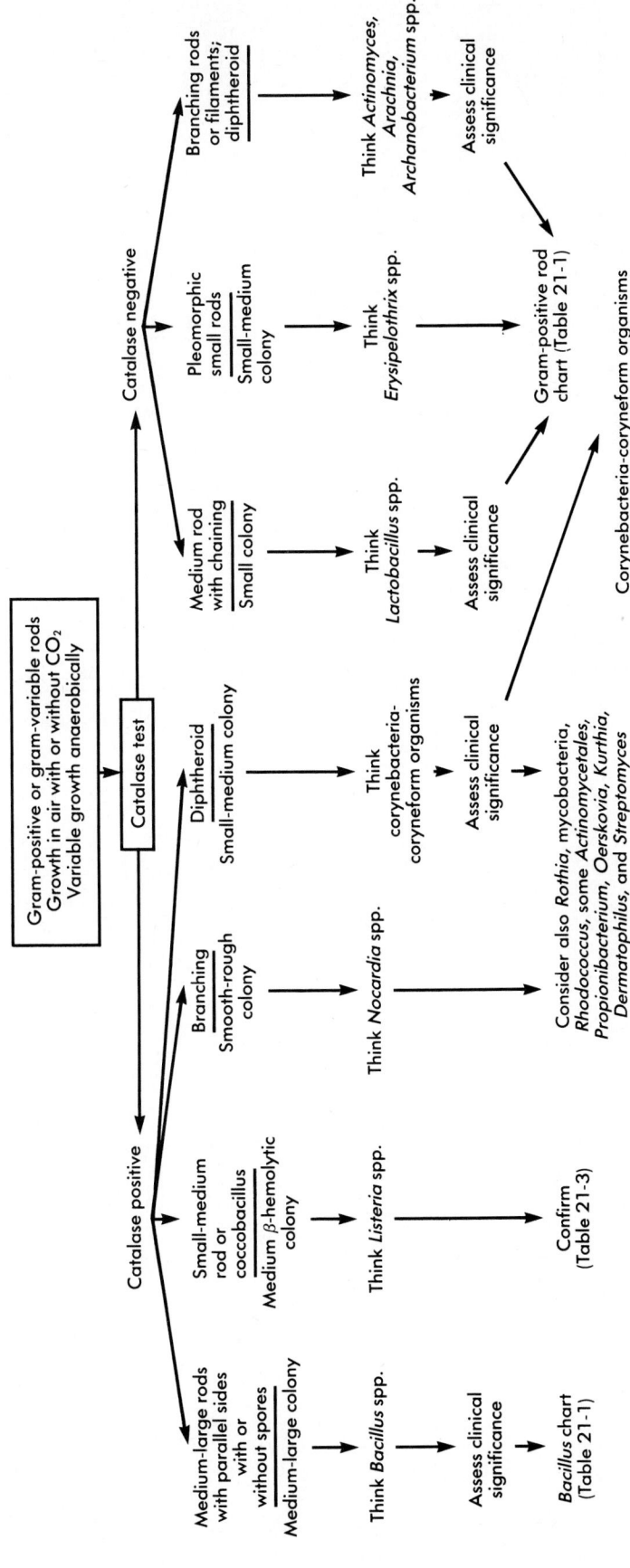

FIGURE 21-1. First-stage identification of gram-positive rods. Small rod is less than 0.5 μm in diameter, medium rod 0.5 to 0.9 μm, and large rod greater than 0.9 μm. Large colony is greater than 3 mm in diameter, and small colony less than 1 mm. "Assess clinical significance" means that, for organisms that can exist as normal flora, identification beyond genus or group level may not be useful. Organisms that are seen on an original Gram stain in presence of inflammatory cells and grow as predominant isolate should be identified. Genus *Dermatophilus* is an aerobic actinomycete that is responsible for dermatitis in a variety of animals and occasionally humans. (Modified from Clarridge, J.E., and Weissfeld, A.S.: Clin. Microbiol. Newsletter, vol. 6, p. 115. Copyright 1984 by Elsevier Science Publishing Co., Inc.)

TABLE 21-2. Identification of *Corynebacterium* and Other Coryneform Organisms

Genus and Species	Tinsdale Halo	Glucose Utilization	Nitrate Reduction	Urease Production	Glucose	Maltose	Sucrose	Beta-Hemolysis	Motility	Comments
C. diphtheriae	100[a]	F	91[b]	0	99	94	1	67	−	Respiratory pathogen
C. ulcerans	100	F	0	100	100	94	19	50	−	Respiratory pathogen
C. pseudotuberculosis (ovis)	100	F	77	96	100	100	79	62	−	Associated with horses
C. xerosis		F	100	0	100	100	100	ND	−	
C. striatum		F	100	0	100	0	100	58	−	
C. matruchotii		F	83	6	83	67	88	0	−	
C. kutscheri		F	100	100	100	93	100	20	−	Associated with rats
C. renale		F	100	90	90	0	0	36	−	Associated with cattle
C. pseudodiphtheriticum (hofmannii)		O	100	100	0	0	0	29	−	
C. minutissimum		F	0	0	100	100	100/0[c]	−	−	
Coryneform groups										
A3[e]		F	100	0	100	100	100	33	100	
A4[e]		F	13	0	100	100	100	28	58	Yellow
A5[e]		F	29	4	100	100	100	32	48	Yellow
ANF-1		O	0	0	0	0	0	20	−	
ANF-3		O	100	0	0	0	0	13	−	
B-1		O	16	0	100	33	42	25	−	
B-3		O	0	8	0	0	0	19	−	
D-2 (*C. urealyticum*)		O	0	100	0	0	0	16	−	
F-1		F	48	100	100	82	100	ND	−	Isolated from humans, especially genitourinary tract
F-2		F	39	88	100	100	0	ND	−	
G-1		F[d]	100	0	100	25	100	25	−	
G-2		F[d]	0	0	100	49	100	14	−	
I-1		F	100	0	100	0	0	44	−	
I-2		F	100	0	100	100	0	ND	−	
J-K		F	2	0	100	43	0	−	−	May need serum; antibiotic resistant
C. bovis[e] (unassigned)		F	−	−	+	v	−	−	−	May need serum
C. aquaticum[e] (unassigned)		O	16	6	94	92	90		66	Yellow
Actinomyces pyogenes		F	0	0	100	87	68	100	−	Catalase negative
Arcanobacterium haemolyticum		F	7	0	71	100	31	100	−	Catalase negative
Rhodococcus equi		O	43	76	28	13	2	−	−	Pink, acid fast

> **SYMBOLS:** +, >90% positive
> −, <10% positive
> v, 10% - 90% positive
> ND, No data available

Modified from Hollis, D.G., and Weaver, R.E.: Identification of gram positive bacilli, Atlanta, 1981, Centers for Disease Control.
[a]Numbers throughout table represent percent positive reactions. Reactions may be delayed up to 7 days.
[b]*C. diphtheriae*, ssp. *mitis* var. *belfanti* is nitrate negative.
[c]One biotype is positive, and the other biotype is negative.
[d]May require added serum.
[e]Does not conform to definition of genus.[19]

Loeffler medium contains serum and egg, which stimulate growth and the distinctive morphology of *C. diphtheriae*. The tellurite-containing media inhibit most gram-negative organisms while supporting the growth of corynebacteria and some other gram-positive organisms. Colonies of *C. diphtheriae* appear gray or black on tellurite-containing media.

Environmental requirements

The media are incubated at 35° C with or without additional CO_2 and examined at 24 and 48 hours for growth of colonies demonstrating the typical Gram stain (see below).

Cultural Characteristics

Staining reaction

The morphology of the organism is influenced by the biotype, media, and stain used.[104] A Gram stain of the organisms grown on Loeffler agar shows them to be pleomorphic and beaded, with some having pointed or rounded ends. Most are rather long rods (2 μm), but some are coccoid. If the organisms are stained with methylene blue, in addition to the irregular staining pattern, reddish metachromatic granules can be seen, often at the ends of the rods (Plate 18, *B*). These granules contain stored polymerized polyphosphate. The organisms can take the Gram stain more evenly if grown on media other than Loeffler medium, making them indistinguishable from some of the other species of *Corynebacterium* (Plate 18, *C*).

Colonial morphology

Three major types of *C. diphtheriae* have been distinguished by their cultural characteristics and named because of originally, but not invariably, observed differences in the severity of the associated disease. The *gravis* type produces the largest colonies on blood agar or cystine-tellurite plates (1 to 2 mm at 24 hours). The *mitis* type produces colonies that on tellurite are black and on blood agar are translucent with white centers (fried egg). The *intermedius* type produces small colonies (0.5 mm at 24 hours) that are colorless on blood agar and black with gray borders on cystine-tellurite.[104] The black color of the colonies on cystine-tellurite results from the reduction of tellurite (TeO_2), which is colorless, to TeO or Te, which are black. Although identification of *C. diphtheriae* types cannot reliably be made from this description, is not necessary for treatment, and should be confirmed by a reference laboratory, the clinical laboratory should be aware of these strain differences. Besides *C. diphtheriae*, other species of *Corynebacterium*, *Staphylococcus aureus*, and species of *Listeria* grow as black colonies on tellurite media.

Colonies of *C. diphtheriae* appear white or gray on Loeffler slants.

Biochemical Identification

Although the cellular and colonial morphology may suggest *C. diphtheriae*, the organism cannot be identified by these criteria alone. Table 21-2 shows the percentage of positive biochemical reactions of *C. diphtheriae* and other clinically important species of *Corynebacterium* and coryneform groups when tests are performed by standard methods, which may take up to 7 days.[43] A more rapid method for determining carbohydrate reactions, which does not require growth of the organisms, has been developed.[42]

Only two species besides *C. diphtheriae* form a brown halo

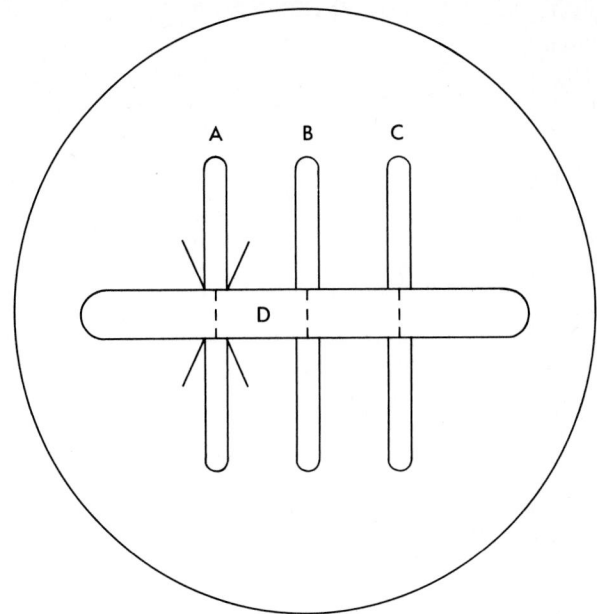

FIGURE 21-2. Elek plate for determination of toxin production of *Corynebacterium diphtheriae*. **A,** Positive control. **B,** Unknown isolate that is nontoxigenic. **C,** Negative control. **D,** Filter paper strip impregnated with antitoxin.

on Tinsdale medium: *C. pseudotuberculosis* and *C. ulcerans*. (The brown halo is caused by the action of cysteine sulfhydrolase with the formation of ferric sulfide in the medium.) *C. ulcerans* and *C. pseudotuberculosis* are closely related to *C. diphtheriae* and are the only other species capable of making a diphtheria-like toxin.[46] These species can be distinguished from *C. diphtheriae* and from each other by the urease and nitrate reactions. Note that *C. diphtheriae* ssp. *mitis* var. *belfanti* is nitrate negative.

Other Identification Procedures

To prove that an isolate can cause diphtheria, one must demonstrate toxin production. Not all *C. diphtheriae* strains are toxinogenic. The property is phageborne and can be lost. Nontoxinogenic *C. diphtheriae* (those without the bacteriophage) can reside in human mucous membranes or skin without causing diphtheria; in some cases they cause a mild sore throat. In any event demonstration of toxin production is necessary to confirm the isolate as the etiologic agent in a case of diphtheria. In some cases both toxinogenic and nontoxinogenic strains have been isolated from the same patient,[15] indicating that several colonies should be tested for toxinogenicity.

Determination of toxin production can be done on an Elek plate.[28] Organisms to be tested are streaked on media of low iron content (which will stimulate toxin production), perpendicular to a strip impregnated with antibody to the toxin (Figure 21-2). The plate is incubated in CO_2 at 35° C for 24 to 48 hours. As organisms grow, toxin diffuses into the medium. The antitoxin diffuses from the strip, and a thin line of precipitate appears where the antibody and antigen (toxin) meet in proper concentration. Controls of toxin-producing and non-toxin-producing *C. diphtheriae* must be applied at the same time.

The toxinogenicity of strains can also be determined by

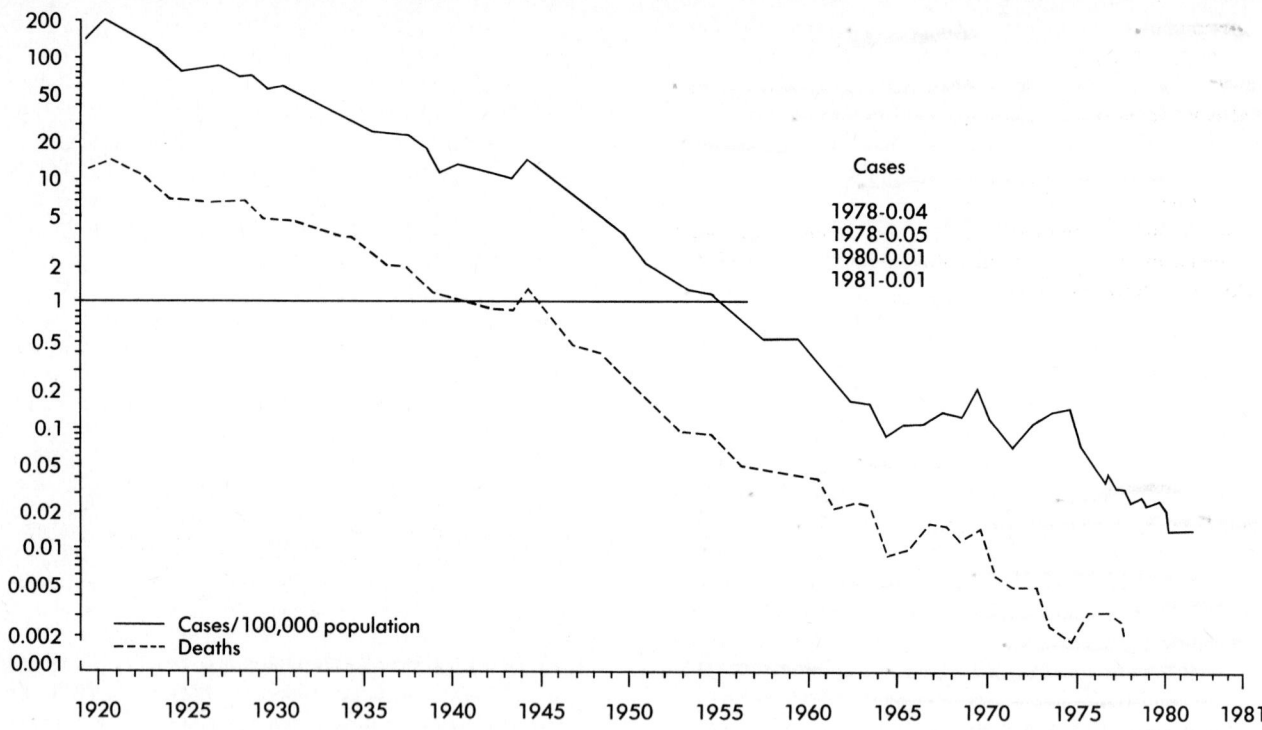

FIGURE 21-3. Decrease in diphtheria from the 1920s to 1980s in United States. Cases and deaths are per 100,000 population. (Data from Centers for Disease Control: MMWR **26:**1978, and **31:**553, 1982.)

measuring the effect of the toxin on tissue culture cells.[63] Toxin production can be assayed by testing susceptible animals such as guinea pigs. Since all methods of testing for toxin are difficult, and some require special materials, they probably should be expected and performed only in a reference laboratory.

Clinical Significance

The most common disease caused by *C. diphtheriae* is diphtheria, an acute communicable disease manifested by both local infection of the upper respiratory tract and the systemic effects of the toxin that are most notable on the heart and peripheral nerves. The signs and symptoms of the disease are a pharyngeal membrane, sore throat, malaise, headache, and nausea. Death can result from respiratory obstruction by the membrane or myocarditis caused by toxin. Since active immunization became available around the 1920s, the number of cases in the United States has decreased (Figure 21-3) from about 60,000 cases in 1932 to five cases in 1982.[12,13] Diphtheria in the United States is now seen only in nonimmunized or partially immunized persons.[13]

Another form of the disease caused by *C. diphtheriae* is cutaneous diphtheria. There are some reports of this disease in the northwest United States,[56] but it is more common in tropical and subtropical areas. The lesions appear necrotic and black with occasional formation of a membrane. Although the organisms are present in high numbers, they can be confused with species of *Corynebacterium* that are normally found on the skin. Pure or predominant cultures of *Corynebacterium* organisms from a well-taken purulent specimen should be speciated.

On rare occasions *C. diphtheriae* can cause endocarditis[60]

without the patient having the symptoms of classical diphtheria.

Mechanisms of Pathogenicity

The bacteria generally do not spread beyond the local lesions, where they multiply in the mucous membranes and cause necrosis and accumulation of inflammatory cells. These combine with the bacteria to form the diphtheritic membrane. From this site a potent extracellular protein (an exotoxin) of molecular weight 62,000 is elaborated. Only strains of *C. diphtheriae* that are infected with a bacteriophage carrying the *tox* gene are able to make the toxin and cause diphtheria.

The toxin is comprised of two components. Fragment A inhibits protein synthesis by catalyzing the transfer of the adenosine-diphosphoribose (ADPR) part of the nicotinamide adenine dinucleotide (NAD) molecule to elongation factor 2 (EF-2) (a protein found in human cells that is responsible for the elongation of the protein chain). When EF-2 is covalently linked to ADPR, it is nonfunctional and the subsequent disruption of protein synthesis causes cell necrosis. Fragment B facilitates the entry of fragment A into the cells. The toxin can enter any cell that has a receptor for fragment B.

Antimicrobial Susceptibility

C. diphtheriae is usually sensitive to penicillin, ampicillin, erythromycin, tetracycline, and clindamycin but is resistant to cephalothin and oxacillin.

Prevention and Treatment of Diphtheria

Diphtheria can almost always be prevented by immunization. A common immunization schedule is vaccination at 2, 3, and 4 months of age, usually given with the pertussis and tetanus vaccines (DPT), with a booster dose at 1 year and another booster before entering school. The vaccine is made from purified inactivated diphtheria toxin. The material used for vaccination is a toxoid prepared by inactivation of the toxin with formaldehyde.

Treatment for diphtheria is twofold. First, the toxin is inactivated by use of diphtheria antitoxin and its further production prevented by the elimination of the organism, usually by penicillin or erythromycin. Second, supportive therapy is instituted to minimize congestive heart failure, suppress arrhythmias, and regulate respiration. Airway obstruction by the membrane may be prevented by tracheostomy. Treatment should be initiated on the basis of clinical suspicion and should not be delayed while awaiting test results.

OTHER *CORYNEBACTERIUM* SPP. AND CORYNEFORM GROUPS
Specimen Collection and Handling

No special specimen handling is required. Because *Corynebacterium* organisms are a significant part of the normal flora of skin and upper respiratory tract, distinguishing commensal from disease-associated organisms is a major problem. Care must be taken in collecting the specimen. A Gram stain of the original specimen should be prepared and examined.

Growth Requirements
Media

The listed *Corynebacterium* spp. and coryneform groups grow on blood agar plates. Some strains grow poorly on chocolate agar.

Environmental requirements

These organisms grow in air, in a candle jar, or in a CO_2 incubator. However, some strains, such as the CDC groups ANF-1 and ANF-3, do not grow well anaerobically.

Several organisms grow slowly, requiring 3 or more days to become visible on agar. Therefore cultures and subcultures from specimens that may contain these organisms (for example, from patients with endocarditis or a prosthesis infection, especially those that have not grown other organisms) should be incubated at least 3 days. There have been reports of blood cultures not becoming positive for 3 weeks,[98] but this might reflect suboptimal culturing technique.

Cultural Characteristics
Staining reactions

The diphtheroid shape is not unique to the genus *Corynebacterium*, and neither are all of the *Corynebacterium* spp. diphtheroid in shape.[2] Some are short rods that may be confused with the genera *Streptococcus* and *Listeria*, and others are slightly curved and have rudimentary branching. *Corynebacterium* spp. and coryneform groups other than *C. diphtheriae* are also gram positive. Most take the stain evenly and demonstrate the typical club shapes and palisade arrangements. The metachromatic granules are often not as conspicuous as those found in *C. diphtheriae*. *Corynebacterium matruchotii*, previously known as *Bacterionema matruchotii*,[18] usually appears as regular gram-positive rods but can assume a "whip with handle" shape, as well as branching and fragmenting filaments.

Plate 18, *D* and *E*, shows the colony morphologies typical for many isolates from skin and sputum. Some are translucent and small; others are larger and white. Other colony morphologies can also be seen.

Biochemical Identification

Table 21-2 lists the biochemical test reactions, given as the percent positive, for *Corynebacterium* spp. and other coryneform organisms. Although many species can be uniquely identified with this information, other organisms are not alone in their biochemical group. For example, *C. xerosis* might be confused with corynebacteria CDC group G1, G2, or B1. Even with an expanded battery of biochemical tests, some isolates do not fit into the described species. This emphasizes the biochemical diversity and problems in classifying these organisms.

If older texts (for example, the eighth edition of *Bergey's Manual*[75]) are used for classifying the organisms, not only are many more organisms unnamed, but the same name might be given to several groups that have since been classified as different species. This has led to confusion in documenting the significance of various species. Because the repeated isolation of a strain of *Corynebacterium* is often the clue to its association with disease, it is important that sufficient biochemical tests be performed to suggest the identity of the isolates. Often a clinically important identification must be confirmed by a reference laboratory. However, note that some identifications are straightforward. With just three simple tests (Tinsdale halo, nitrate reduction, and urea hydrolysis), an organism can be designated as either *C. diphtheriae* or *Corynebacterium* other than *C. diphtheriae*. With the nine tests listed, most isolates can be placed in unique or small groups. The newly described CDC group J-K is relatively inactive and difficult to distinguish from *C. bovis* and the group ANF-1.[73] However, ANF-1 is oxidative and does not utilize glucose, and *C. bovis* colonies are larger than the small gray colonies expected of the group J-K.

Other Identification Procedures

Other methods of analysis that have proved useful in identifying *Corynebacterium* and related genera are gas-liquid chromatography and mass spectrophotometry to determine the mycolic acid profile.[23] Genera can be distinguished by cell wall analysis using thin-layer chromatography. Ninety-two structural and biochemical characteristics have been used[36] to provide a classification scheme for the coryneform bacteria and related organisms of the family *Actinomycetaceae*.[80] In addition, DNA homologic studies have been used to show relatedness among coryneform bacteria.[90] These methods are beyond the needs of the clinical laboratory but underscore the complexity of the group.

Clinical Significance

General infections caused by *Corynebacterium* spp. other than *C. diphtheriae* have been reviewed.[45,50,59,98] Most of these cases involved bacteria that have been removed from the genus *Corynebacterium* (*Propionibacterium* spp., *Rhodococcus* [C.] *equi*,[10,40] *Actinomyces* [C.] *pyogenes*,[20] *Arcanobacteria* [C.] *hemolyticum*[31,101]) or were unnamed and without sufficient description. However, disease caused by valid *Corynebacterium* spp. or coryneform groups other than *C. diphtheriae* has been documented.

C. ulcerans is a well-described species that is closely related to *C. diphtheriae*. It can elaborate a toxin identical to the diphtheria toxin but does so infrequently and at lower levels.

Although the organism can exist as a commensal in both humans and animals (cattle), it can cause mastitis in animals and pharyngitis in humans.[71] Cases of diphtheria caused by *C. ulcerans* have been reported.[62]

C. pseudotuberculosis is almost never isolated from humans who have not had exposure to animals. Infections caused by this organism include lymphadenitis and pneumonia.[34,52,59,98] *C. pseudotuberculosis*, previously called *C. ovis*, can produce an exotoxin,[46] but it is not the same as that produced by *C. diphtheriae*.

Endocarditis, often in patients who have prosthetic heart valves, and infection of pacemakers or other prostheses are the most commonly reported diseases caused by corynebacteria other than *C. diphtheriae* or coryneform groups.[45,59,95,98] The etiologic agents are usually part of the normal flora, including *C. xerosis*, *C. pseudodiphtheriticum*, group J-K, and the ill-defined "skin" bacteria. Similarly bacteremia, often in immunocompromised hosts, can be caused by these organisms, particularly group J-K.[41,106] Urinary tract colonization and stone formation have been reported with group D2.[86]

C. pseudodiphtheriticum was isolated in pure culture from a bronchial wash from a patient with pneumonia.[27] Endophthalmitis caused by group A-4 and breast abscess caused by *C. minutissimum* have been reported.[5,24,42] *C. matruchotii* has been associated with opportunistic infections.[102] *C. bovis*, although presumably not normal human flora, has been isolated from patients with endocarditis, prosthesis infection, and septicemia. *C. bovis*, *C. kutscheri*, *C. pseudotuberculosis*, *C. renale*, and *R. (C.) equi* are primarily animal pathogens. *C. renale* can cause cystitis in cattle.

Antimicrobial Susceptibility

Susceptibility testing must be performed on the isolates because the resistance patterns vary considerably. Penicillin, ampicillin, erythromycin, vancomycin, and an aminoglycoside should be tested. A Mueller-Hinton plate with blood or the addition of serum to the Autobac media is sometimes needed for sufficient growth. Because of the slow growth, incubation times may be extended slightly longer than 18 to 24 hours. Plates should be read with oblique light.

The group J-K was initially reported to be highly resistant to antimicrobial agents,[41,106] but more recent reports have shown variability.[73,98] Erythromycin or ampicillin is the usual drug of choice for all corynebacterial infections except for the group J-K, which has been uniformly susceptible only to vancomycin.[73]

Clinical isolates of group D2 have a highly resistant susceptibility pattern like that of group J-K.[86]

CORYNEFORM ORGANISMS PREVIOUSLY INCLUDED IN THE GENUS *CORYNEBACTERIUM*

At least five species or genera that were previously classified as corynebacteria have been removed from the group *(Actinomyces (C.) pyogenes, Arcanobacteria (C.) hemolyticum, Rhodococcus (C.) equi, Gardnerella (C.) vaginalis,* and *Propionibacterium,* spp.). *Actinomyces pyogenes* (formerly *C. pyogenes*) is generally associated with cattle, sheep, and pigs. On rare occasions it may act opportunistically to produce a variety of diseases in humans.[59,98] It is closely related to the genus *Actinomyces* by cell wall, fatty acid, and respiratory quinone composition.[20] As shown in Table 21-1, it is catalase negative. *Arcanobacterium hemolyticum*[21] has been frequently isolated

from humans. The isolates are beta-hemolytic on blood agar, are isolated from throat cultures, and can cause a pharyngitis[31,101] or abscess.[57] They can be confused with group A beta-hemolytic streptococci because they are also catalase negative. *A. hemolyticum*, however, is not susceptible to bacitracin. *A. hemolyticum* forms delicate, slightly curved, branching gram-positive rods.

Rhodococcus (C.) equi has been associated with respiratory disease in humans and with pneumonia and abortion in equines. Infections are usually seen in immunosuppressed hosts,[40] but soft tissue infections, arthritis, and osteomyelitis have been reported in normal hosts.[10] *R. equi* is frequently isolated from animal feces and soil.[3] It has been removed from the genus *Corynebacterium* because of its biochemical and cell wall characteristics.[35] The organisms grow well, form a light pink or coral colony on most media, and are acid fast in some portions of the life cycle. They are gram positive, sometimes appearing as cocci and sometimes as branching gram-positive rods (Plate 18, *F*). They are also capsulated, with the colonies becoming large and mucoid after about 3 days. *Propionibacterium* organisms have been called "anaerobic diphtheroids," although some species can grow under aerobic conditions (for example, *P. avidum* can grow in a CO_2 incubator) and thus can be confused with *Corynebacterium* spp. *Propionibacterium* spp. differ, however, in that propionic acid is a major metabolic end product.

Gardnerella vaginalis is discussed in Chapter 25.

UNUSUAL GRAM-POSITIVE ASPOROGENOUS AEROBIC BACILLI—*ROTHIA, KURTHIA, AND OERSKOVIA*

Rothia organisms may be isolated from the normal human mouth. *R. dentocariosa* resembles *Actinomyces viscosus* in biochemical characteristics and in forming catalase-positive branching filaments (Plate 19, *A*). They can be distinguished because *R. dentocariosa* can have a positive Voges-Proskauer reaction (that is, produce acetoin) and form spherical cells in broth, whereas *A. viscosus* cannot. *A. viscosus* usually ferments lactose.[2,44] The genus *Rothia* has been associated with abscess and endocarditis.[9,76,77] It is distinguished by having high levels of valine aminopeptidase.[53] A presumed mode of infection is that organisms, inoculated from the mouth into the blood by trauma to the gums, adhere to the heart valves and initiate disease.

The genera *Kurthia* and *Oerskovia* are generally associated with soil. Both are opportunistic pathogens reported to cause endocarditis,[51,67,68,72] or other infections.[26] *Oerskovia* spp. grow well on nutrient and blood agars as branching filaments that fragment into coccobacilli on prolonged incubation. The organisms are usually motile, and colonies are bright yellow.[26,43] *Kurthia* organisms are gram-positive, regular rods. On the basis of Gram stain and colony morphology, *Kurthia* spp. may be confused with *Bacillus* spp., especially *B. mycoides*. Both are motile, sometimes chaining, large (0.8 μm by 3 to 8 μm) rods that form medusa-head colonies.[51] However, *Kurthia* organisms do not form spores or grow anaerobically. A "bird feather" type of growth in stabbed gelatin agar is said to be typical.

LISTERIA

The genus *Listeria* tentatively comprises five species. *Listeria monocytogenes*, the most commonly isolated pathogenic member, is associated with a wide spectrum of human and animal diseases.

L. monocytogenes was first described in 1926 as causing a bacteremia in rabbits, which was characterized by an excess of mononuclear leukocytes in the blood. Subsequently it has been isolated from over 40 mammals and other vertebrates, often from the gastrointestinal tract of a healthy animal. *L. monocytogenes* can cause severe disease in animals, particularly meningoencephalitis and abortion in ruminants. It has been estimated to be the eleventh most economically damaging disease of animals.[7] Animals, soil, and plants that have been contaminated with animal products are presumed to be the source of adult human exposure. Human disease with high morbidity and mortality may occur in a fetus or infant who is infected transplacentally or at birth by the mother.

CLASSIFICATION

Bergey's Manual of Systematic Bacteriology[82] recognizes five species of *Listeria: L. monocytogenes, L. innocua, L. welshimeri, L. seeligeri,* and *L. ivanovii.* The previous *Bergey's Manual* recognized the four species *L. monocytogenes, L. grayi, L. murrayi,* and *L. denitrificans.* Several studies have resulted in this reclassification of the genus.

The subcommittee of the International Committee on Systematic Bacteriology suggested that *L. denitrificans* be removed from the genus *Listeria* and designated as *nomen generum perplexum.*[100] *L. murrayi* and *L. grayi* are closely related and have been assigned to a new genus, *Murraya.*[89] *L. innocua,* which has been cultivated from environment sources, is considered nonpathogenic, although under special conditions an encephalitis has been produced in animals.[81] Two additional species, *L. welshimeri* and *L. seeligeri,* formerly classified as nonpathogenic *L. monocytogenes,* have been recognized on the basis of DNA-relatedness studies.[74] *L. ivanovii,* formerly called *L. monocytogenes* serovar 5 or *L. bulgarica,* is a species associated with disease in sheep.[83] It produces a pronounced beta-hemolysis on blood agar. Among the current serovars of *L. monocytogenes,* serovars la, lb, and 4b account for over 90% of the clinical isolates in humans.

SPECIMEN COLLECTION AND PROCESSING

Although blood and cerebrospinal fluid are the specimens from which *L. monocytogenes* is most commonly isolated, the organism has been recovered from brain, liver, soft tissue, and spinal cord abscesses and from vaginal secretions, amniotic fluid, feces, synovial fluid, respiratory secretions, and the conjunctiva. Fluids should be plated directly in adequate amounts (0.1 ml plate), and tissues should be ground and plated. Pus and biopsy material from skin lesions are suitable for culture.

GROWTH REQUIREMENTS
Media

Most conventional media support growth. *Listeria* organisms grow on Mueller-Hinton agar with or without added blood. A sheep blood agar plate should be used on primary isolation to demonstrate the characteristic hemolysis. For specimens that may be contaminated by other organisms, a Columbia colistin–nalidixic acid plate (Appendix A) is recommended. Enrichment of the organism from a contaminated specimen, particularly fecal, tissue, and animal sources, by incubating at 4° C in tryptose broth with subcultures weekly for a month has also been recommended.[6,37]

Environmental Requirements

Listeria spp. grow at 35° C in air with or without additional CO_2.

CULTURAL CHARACTERISTICS
Staining Reactions

Contrary to the situtation in other types of bacterial meningitis, the Gram stain of cerebrospinal fluid in meningitis caused by *L. monocytogenes* fails to demonstrate the organism in the majority of cases. In the smear from the original tissue, *L. monocytogenes* may appear as gram-positive coccobacilli that may be confused with *Streptococcus agalactiae* (group B), enterococci, or *Corynebacterium* spp. The appearance of organisms grown on solid media is coccoid (Plate 19, *B*), but in broth the organisms are more rodlike. Flagella stains of this peritrichous organism show one to five flagella.

Colonial Morphology

The colonies of *L. monocytogenes* isolated from human or sheep blood agar are small (less than 1 mm at 24 hours), smooth, translucent whitish, and moist. The beta-hemolysis of *L. monocytogenes* is best seen after removal of the colony (Plate 19, *C*).[16]

BIOCHEMICAL IDENTIFICATION

As shown in Table 21-1, the positive tests for catalase production, motility, esculin hydrolysis, and acetoin production (Voges-Proskauer test) separate *Listeria* organisms from most of the gram-positive asporogenous bacilli. The small size of the organisms differentiates *L. monocytogenes* from most species of *Bacillus* and *Oerskovia.*

Listeria is differentiated from the streptococci by a positive catalase test, growth in 6% NaCl, positive Gram stain reaction from a broth culture, and motility. Motility can be demonstrated by incubating the organisms at room temperature in heart infusion or tryptic soy broth and viewing microscopically with a wet mount or hanging drop preparation. The organisms show a tumbling, generally nondirectional type of motility. Alternatively, colonies may be inoculated by a straight stab into a tube of semisolid motility medium. Because of their flagella-mediated chemotactic response, *L. monocytogenes* sometimes establish themselves along the stab line and in a narrow band or hemisphere below the surface of a motility agar tube. This can look like an umbrella (Plate 19, *D*) and is easier to demonstrate in motility media that contain 0.5% agar than in those that contain 0.3% agar.

Although xylose, rhamnose, and hemolysis are used to distinguish among the *Listeria* spp. (Table 21-3),[39,74] the most valuable test to distinguish *L. monocytogenes* from all the other species, except *L. seeligeri* (which has never been isolated in a clinical laboratory), is a test for augmentation of hemolysis. This can be demonstrated with *Staphylococcus aureus* and the unknown strain of *Listeria* inoculated perpendicularly as in the CAMP test (Appendix A) or by using *Rhodococcus (C.) equi* in place of the *S. aureus.*[84,85] As can be seen in Plate 19, *E* and *F,* the test with *R. equi* may be more dramatic. However, *S. aureus* (the same strain used in the CAMP test—for example, ATCC 25923) grows faster than *R. equi,* which usually takes 2 days to exhibit enough growth for a valid test. Skalka and Smola[84] have developed a diagnostic medium using *R. equi* extract that can distinguish *L. innocua, L. monocytogenes,* and *L. ivanovii* by their increasing hemolytic reactions.

TABLE 21-3. Distinctive Biochemical Reactions of the Genus *Listeria* and Related Genera

Organisms	Hemolysis on Sheep Blood Agar	Hemolysis with *S. aureus*	Hemolysis with *R. equi*	Fermentation		Comments
				Xylose	Rhamnose	
L. monocytogenes	+ (Narrow beta)	Augmented	Augmented	−	+	Only confirmed human pathogen
L. innocua	−	−	−	−	v	Isolated from plants, soil, and human and animal feces
L. ivanovii	+ (Two zones)	−	Arrow shaped	+	−	Pathogenic for mice, sheep, and possibly humans
L. welshimeri	−	−	−	+	v	Isolated from plants and soil
L. seeligeri	−	+	−	+	−	Isolated from plants, soil, sheep feces, and possibly humans
Nomen genereum perplexum (*L. denitrificans*)	−	−	−	+	−	Reduces nitrate
Murraya murrayi	−	−	−	−	v	Ferments mannitol
Murraya grayi	−	−	−	−	−	Ferments mannitol

> **SYMBOLS:** +, >90% positive
> −, <10% positive
> v, 10%-90% positive

Modified from Clarridge, J.E., and Weissfeld, A.S.: Clin. Microbiol. Newsletter, vol. 7, p. 59. Copyright 1985 by Elsevier Publishing Co., Inc.

CLINICAL SIGNIFICANCE

L. monocytogenes is the only species of the genus *Listeria* that has been clearly documented as a pathogen for humans. The forms of disease caused by this organism are myriad and age related.[6,7,37] The most common clinical manifestations are meningitis and septicemia. *L. monocytogenes* accounts for 12% to 14% of all cases of meningitis in persons under 1 month and over 50 years of age.[6]

Adults may become exposed to the organisms through contaminated food or animal products.[39] The organisms are thought to be ingested rather than inhaled. Direct cutaneous inoculation has been demonstrated in veterinarians. The disease in healthy adults is generally mild, evidenced as flulike illness or possibly gastrointestinal distress. In 1985, however, over 30 deaths were associated with eating cheese contaminated with *L. monocytogenes.*

Like animals, humans may be healthy carriers of *L. monocytogenes.* From 1% to 5% of the population shows fecal or vaginal carriage of this organism.[6,37,79] Pregnancy[37,61] or immunosuppression, such as that following kidney transplantation,[64,88] renders the patient more susceptible to infection. In an immunosuppressed patient this can manifest as meningitis, septicemia, or pneumonia, all of which have a high mortality. The effect of disease during pregnancy is minimal for the mother, as for other healthy adults, but is devastating to the child, to whom organisms are transmitted either transplacentally or at birth. In these neonates, who account for 50% of all human disease caused by *L. monocytogenes,* there are three major syndromes. If the fetus is exposed prenatally, the disease is characterized by high mortality (abortions and stillbirths) and multiple necrotic granulomata. Neonates who become ill in the first 3 days of life generally have sepsis and other organ involvement with about 30% mortality; those with later onset disease have meningitis with less than 10% mortality. Some of the survivors have sequelae such as mental retardation.

MECHANISMS OF PATHOGENICITY[16]

The hemolytic properties of *L. monocytogenes* have been circumstantially correlated with pathogenicity. Essentially, only the isolates displaying hemolysis on sheep blood agar plates and showing augmentation of hemolysis with *Staphylococcus aureus* or *R. equi* have been associated with disease. In mice, hemolysis is a lethal cardiotoxin, causing damage to myocardial tissue. Recent experimental evidence using chicken embryos also links the level of hemolysis production with the severity of disease.[4]

The hemolysin may not be correlated with pathogenicity of other species of *Listeria. L. ivanovii* is more hemolytic than *L. monocytogenes,* yet it rarely causes disease.[83] Furthermore, an experimentally produced encephalitis with *L. innocua* and animal disease from *L. seeligeri* have been reported.[74,81] (Infection with *L. innocua* seems protective against challenge from virulent *L. monocytogenes.*[97])

Other factors that may be involved in the disease process are a soluble lipase and the listeric polysaccharide, which is antiphagocytic. The tropism toward central nervous system tissue may also be a factor in virulence.

Because the genus *Listeria* is an intracellular parasite, infection depends in part on the organisms' successful entry and growth in the cells of the mononuclear phagocyte system, an action that can be modulated by both host and parasite. Resistance to *L. monocytogenes* is thought to be mediated by macrophages that are activated by T lymphocytes. Alteration of humoral and cellular immune function is associated with pregnancy. Pregnancy has been shown to decrease both resistance to *L. monocytogenes* and the capacity to develop immunity to this organism.[61]

ANTIMICROBIAL SUSCEPTIBILITY

L. monocytogenes demonstrates in vitro susceptibility to penicillin, ampicillin, gentamicin, erythromycin, tetracycline, and chloramphenicol.[92] However, chloramphenicol appears to be ineffective in vivo.[87] Penicillin or ampicillin with or without an aminoglycoside is usually recommended.[64] Adults allergic to penicillins may be treated with tetracycline. Erythromycin is preferred for the treatment of children with a penicillin allergy and pregnant women. Although potentially useful, trimethoprim-sulfamethoxazole and rifampin must be studied more thoroughly before they can be recommended.[78]

ERYSIPELOTHRIX

The genus *Erysipelothrix* (from the Greek *erysipelas,* red skin, and *thrix,* thread) has a single member, its type species *E. rhusiopathiae*[47] (*rhusio,* red, and *pathia,* disease). It is a catalase-negative, pleomorphic, gram-positive, nonsporeforming rod. The most common manifestation of human disease is erysipeloid, a localized inflammation of the skin. *Erysipelothrix* organisms can also cause disseminated infection.

Infection with *Erysipelothrix* organisms is a zoonosis. Fish, cattle, horses, mice, fowl, and especially turkeys and swine can carry or be infected with *Erysipelothrix* spp. The organism can survive for years in the soil,[14] and it is thought that human infection is acquired by inoculation of soil or animal products, usually into a wound. Some of the names (often reflective of the host) that previously have been given to this organism are *E. insidiosa, E. muriseptica,* and *E. porci.* Good reviews on the genus *Erysipelothrix* are provided by Woodbine,[105] Klauder,[55] and Ewald.[29]

CLASSIFICATION

As with other gram-positive rods, the lines of relatedness between the genera *Listeria* and *Erysipelothrix* are not well defined, but these organisms can be easily distinguished by

biochemical means. The characteristics of both organisms can be seen in Table 21-1.

SPECIMEN COLLECTION AND PROCESSING

To examine the erysipeloid infection, biopsy or aspirated material from the leading edge of the lesion is cultured and Gram stained. It is important that subcutaneous skin be sampled. Long, slender, gram-positive rods in Gram stains of tissue from a person with a compatible history would be suggestive for erysipeloid. In disseminated disease the organism can be isolated from blood and infected organs.

Routine blood cultures with subcultures to a blood-containing agar plate, which is incubated in CO_2 and held for at least 48 hours, are adequate for isolation of *Erysipelothrix* organisms.

GROWTH REQUIREMENTS
Media

Tissue should be ground and inoculated to blood, chocolate, and Columbia colistin–nalidixic acid agars. *E. rhusiopathiae* grows on these media, but colonies might be barely visible at 48 hours. A broth such as Schaedler or trypticase soy should also be inoculated and subcultured to blood or chocolate agar plates at 2 and 7 days.

Environmental Requirements

Media should be incubated at $35°C$ in a CO_2 incubator, although the organism does not require additional CO_2.

CULTURAL CHARACTERISTICS
Staining Reactions

In the blood or in blood culture bottles, the gram-positive organisms can assume a variety of shapes, suggesting a polymicrobial infection (Plate 19, *G*). In tissue the organisms do not have this pleomorphism.

Colonial Morphology

Several colonial forms may be observed on solid media: the larger rough colony is composed of long thin filaments (Plate 20, *A*), and the smaller clear colony contains both rods and coccobacilli. All are gram positive but decolorize easily. Although some investigators have associated the rough form with chronic disease and the smooth form with acute disease,[29] others have disagreed.[99] At 48 hours the colonies are small (1 mm) or medium (2 mm), and gray or translucent, sometimes with alpha-hemolysis. Growth is better on blood agar plates than on chocolate agar and better anaerobically or in CO_2 than in air. Two colony types are shown in Plate 20, *B.*

BIOCHEMICAL IDENTIFICATION

The major biochemical characteristics of *E. rhusiopathiae* are compared with those of other gram-positive rods in Table 21-1. *E. rhusiopathiae* is the only catalase-negative organism in this group that produces H_2S in the butt of a triple sugar iron agar slant. Some species of the genus *Bacillus* can do this, but they are catalase positive. *Erysipelothrix* organisms have no flagella and are nonmotile.

CLINICAL SIGNIFICANCE

Erysipelothrix organisms are widespread in nature[14,105] and can cause economically significant disease in swine, turkeys, and sheep. Many other fish, birds, and mammals can carry the organism, some without apparent disease. In swine the most common form of the disease, called diamond-skin disease, follows ingestion of the organisms and is characterized by reddish rhomboid spots on the skin. Acute septicemia and chronic infection with arthritis and endocarditis are more rarely seen.

Human disease also has multiple forms. The localized skin infection, called erysipeloid because of the similarity to streptococcal erysipelas, occurs at the site of inoculation, often following trauma to the hands. It is an occupation-associated disease found in slaughterhouse workers, fish handlers, veterinarians, and others who have animal exposure. The lesion, found 2 to 7 days after inoculation, is characterized by a sharply defined, painful, purplish red zone that advances peripherally with central fading.[54] The organisms are found at the leading edge in the deeper cutaneous layers. Occasionally the organisms disseminate, causing septicemia, endocarditis, and arthritis.[33,38,55] The mortality accompanying endocarditis is high.[96]

MECHANISMS OF PATHOGENICITY

Virulence factors of *Erysipelothrix* spp. are not well defined, although the ability to adhere to heart valves[8] and to produce neuraminidase[65] or hyaluronidase[29] has been investigated.

ANTIMICROBIAL SUSCEPTIBILITY

In disk diffusion tests, *Erysipelothrix* organisms are usually sensitive to penicillin, cephalosporins, erythromycin, tetracyclines, and chloramphenicol and invariably resistant to aminoglycosides, sulfonamides, and vancomycin. Treatment with penicillin is usually recommended.

BACILLUS

The genus *Bacillus*, the group of gram-positive, sporeforming, aerobic bacilli, includes over 40 species. The natural habitat of these organisms is soil and the environment. The most virulent human pathogen in this genus is *B. anthracis*, the etiologic agent of anthrax. However, *B. cereus* is the most frequently isolated pathogen. *B. cereus* and other *Bacillus* spp. are also commonly isolated as contaminants. The genus *Bacillus* also includes insect pathogens, plant pathogens, and thermophilic bacteria that grow best at temperatures over 55° C.

CLASSIFICATION

In the eighth edition of *Bergey's Manual of Determinative Bacteriology*,[32] the genus *Bacillus* is classified in the family *Bacillaceae,* which includes the anaerobic genus *Clostridium* among other sporeforming organisms. The genera *Clostridium* and *Bacillus* are morphologically similar but usually *Bacillus* spp. grow better in air, whereas *Clostridium* spp. grow only anaerobically. Some species of *Clostridium,* however, are aerotolerant, growing in air with added CO_2, and could be confused with *Bacillus* spp.

Bacillus spp. are diverse in their metabolic capabilities. Almost all species except *B. anthracis* are motile by means of peritrichous flagella. Endospore formation, an essential characteristic for inclusion in the group, is a taxonomically useful property. The spores are either large, causing the vegetative cell to swell, or small enough to be entirely contained in the normal cell wall. They can be located centrally or subterminally (toward the ends of the cell) and can be round or oval or have

appendages. Characteristics of selected *Bacillus* spp. that might be isolated in a clinical laboratory are listed in Table 21-4.

SPECIMEN COLLECTION AND HANDLING

Specimens must be carefully collected from patients with suspected disease caused by *Bacillus* organisms because these organisms also exist in the environment and are often isolated as contaminants.

Blood cultures should be obtained for any suspected case of anthrax. For cases of cutaneous anthrax, fluid should be taken from the vesicle with a syringe or swab. Gram stains should be made from the original specimen.

Recovery of *B. anthracis* from contaminated animal products such as hair, rugs, wool, or skins can be accomplished after processing. The material is added to a detergent solution (such as Tween 80) and shaken in a covered jar for 1 hour. Large particles are allowed to settle for 5 minutes, and the supernatant is centrifuged at 2000 rpm for 15 minutes. The supernatant is discarded, and the pellet resuspended in distilled water, heat shocked at 65° C for 10 minutes, and inoculated to sheep blood agar.

All work with *B. anthracis* must be performed in a biologic safety cabinet to avoid aerosols. The working area must be washed with 5% phenol or other suitable disinfectant such as 5% sodium hypochlorite.

GROWTH REQUIREMENTS
Media

Bacillus anthracis and the other *Bacillus* spp. grow well on all commonly used blood culture media and on most nutrient laboratory media. In contrast to most gram-positive organisms, *Bacillus* organisms usually do not grow on Columbia colistin–nalidixic acid (CNA) medium. Although *Bacillus* spp. are usually resistant to colistin (polymyxin B), some strains are sensitive to nalidixic acid. Sheep blood agar is recommended for isolation of *Bacillus* organisms from sterile sites, and phenyl ethyl alcohol (PEA) agar is recommended for contaminated sites. Bicarbonate agar may be used to induce capsule formation.

Environmental Requirements

All media should be incubated at 35° C in air or in a CO_2 incubator.

CULTURAL CHARACTERISTICS
Staining Reactions

Most *Bacillus* spp. in tissue and in young cultures are gram positive (Plate 20, *C*). With age, they can become gram variable or negative (Plate 20, *D*).[22] The spores appear clear with a Gram stain and green with the spore stain. As previously mentioned, the spores may be located entirely within the vegetative cell wall or may swell the cell wall. *B. anthracis* usually grows as short chains in tissue or blood. The measured diameter of the gram-positive organisms is an important identification aid. Only organisms that stain gram positive should be measured; organisms that do not retain the gentian violet stain appear narrower because the cell wall is not apparent.

Colonial Morphology

The *Bacillus* organisms commonly isolated in the clinical laboratory form large colonies (4 to 6 mm) on blood agar plates

TABLE 21-4. Identification of *Bacillus* Spp.[a]

	Usual Cell Diameter (μm)	Penicillin (10 Units)	Motility	Wide Zone Lecithinase	Beta-Hemolysis	Spores Swell Cells	Voges-Proskauer	Nitrate Reduction	Starch	Distinguishing Characteristics
GROUP I										
B. anthracis	≥0.9	S	0	27	–	–	85	100		Produces capsule
B. cereus	≥0.9	R	99	100	+	–	84	89		
B. mycoides	≥0.9	R	63	100	–	–	50	100		Rhizoid colony
B. megaterium	≥0.9	V	42	0	–	–	0	10		
B. thuringiensis	≥0.9	R	+	+	+	–	V	+		Insect pathogen that produces toxin crystals
GROUP II										
B. subtilis	<0.9	S	84	–	V	–	71	89	80	
B. pumilus	<0.9	S	100	–	V	–	78	0	6	
B. licheniformis	<0.9	S	80	–	+	–	83	100	100	
B. firmus	<0.9	S	90	–	V	–	0	70	50	
B. coagulans	<0.9	S	+	–	V	–	V	0		Grows at 55° and 35° C
GROUP III										
B. circulans	<0.9		+	–	–	+	6	76		Colonies may migrate on agar
B. sphaericus	<0.9		+	–	–	+	0	26		Produces spherical spores
B. laterosporus	<0.9		+	V	–	+	0	90		Produces canoe-shaped spores
B. brevis	<0.9		+	–	–	+	–	26		
B. polymyxa	<0.9		+	–	–	+	100	0		
B. alvei (H₂S + *Bacillus*)	<0.9		+	–	V	+	V	+		
B. stearothermophilus	<0.9		+	–	–	+	V	0		Grows at 65° C, no growth at 35° C

SYMBOLS: +, >90% positive
−, <10% positive
V, 10%-90% positive

Data from references 32 and 69.
[a]Percentages are given when available.

after 24 hours of incubation. Under anaerobic conditions the colonies are usually smaller or inapparent. On blood agar, *B. anthracis* and *B. cereus* can form large, rough colonies with swirling projections (Plate 20, *E*). *B. anthracis* produces a copious polypeptide capsule* when grown on bicarbonate agar in a CO₂ environment. As a result the colonies on this media are large and mucoid. *B. mycoides* (*B. cereus* var. *mycoides*) grows rapidly, forming a colony that superficially resembles a fungus (Plate 20, *F*).

BIOCHEMICAL IDENTIFICATION

Tests to differentiate some of the *Bacillus* spp. are shown in Table 21-4. Historically, the most important step in identification has been to distinguish between *B. anthracis* and the rest of

the *Bacillus* spp., which were considered nonpathogenic. The production of a capsule on bicarbonate agar distinguishes *B. anthracis* from other *Bacillus* spp.; however, this capacity may be lost on subculture. It is more difficult to identify *B. anthracis* strains that do not produce capsules.

For simplicity the genus *Bacillus* can be divided into three groups. In group I the cell width is usually greater than 0.9 μm and the spores do not extend the vegetative cell wall. DNA homology studies show that the members of group I—*B. anthracis, B. cereus, B. thuringiensis,* and *B. megaterium*—are as closely related as strains of a single species.[49] However, as shown in Table 21-4, these species can usually be separated. Note that *B. thuringiensis* is distinguished by the presence of toxin crystals, *B. mycoides* by its rhizoid colony form, and the other organisms by a combination of characteristics. *Bacillus* spp. that produce spores that do not swell the vegetative cell and are penicillin sensitive, nitrate positive, and negative for

*The capsule is unique in that it is formed from a polypeptide and not from a polysaccharide.

motility, beta-hemolysis, and growth in 6% NaCl should be sent to a reference laboratory for further identification as possible *B. anthracis*. *B. cereus* and *B. anthracis* can be distinguished in reference laboratories by antigenic differences in the spores.[70]

Organisms in group II are smaller than those in group I, do not have fat granules, and have spores that do not swell the vegetative cell. Group III comprises the organisms in which the spores swell the cell. There are more species in groups II and III than are listed in Table 21-4, and it is probably not useful to distinguish them on a routine basis. It is common to identify the organisms in group I to species level and to assign other organisms to a group.

Serologic and Immunoserologic Identification

Because *B. anthracis* and *B. cereus* are so closely related,[49] serologic identification has been hampered by extensive cross-reactions. Since spore antigens seem to cross-react less then vegetative cell antigens, scientists[70] have used fluorescent antibodies raised against *B. anthracis* spores that had been adsorbed with *B. cereus* spore antigens for specific identification of most strains of these two organisms. This type of testing is available at only a few reference laboratories and still needs to be perfected.

A stain using fluorescent antibodies against the cell wall or capsule of *B. anthracis* can be employed in the direct examination of tissue from a cutaneous lesion. A presumptive diagnosis of anthrax can be made if bacilli are seen occurring in short chains or if two or three bacilli have positive fluorescence in both cell wall and capsule. Again, the diagnosis is presumptive because other bacilli can cross-react.

Acute and convalescent samples of patient serum can be examined in reference laboratories by indirect hemagglutinin agar gel and complement fixation tests for the presence of specific antibodies to *B. anthracis*. A rise in titer constitutes evidence for disease. A single infection with *B. anthracis* confers lifelong immunity.

Clinical Significance[103]

Anthrax is most often seen in ruminants (cattle, sheep, and goats) but can also occur in humans, horses, birds, guinea pigs, mice, and other animals. *B. anthracis* spores reside in soil and on plants and may remain viable for decades. Animals can become infected via the alimentary tract by eating contaminated food or cutaneously by traumatic inoculation. The disease usually terminates with a fulminant septicemia, sometimes just a few hours after the first symptoms appear. Urine, feces, and eventually the blood and carcass of the infected animal contain organisms that recontaminate the environment.

Most human infections follow exposure to infected animals or animal products. However, exposure does not usually result in disease. There are three forms of anthrax: pulmonary, cutaneous, and gastrointestinal. Pulmonary anthrax can occur subsequent to the inhaling of massive numbers of spores. Because this form of disease was first observed in workers in the woolen mills of England, it was called wool-sorter's disease. The most common form of anthrax in humans is malignant pustule, which is caused by cutaneous inoculation of spores. The initial lesion is small and red, resembling an insect bite. The resulting lesion becomes necrotic with many bacilli seen in the vesicular fluid. Eventually a black eschar develops. Gastrointestinal infection, the rarest manifestation, is the result of ingestion of contaminated food. Early symptoms include nausea, abdominal pain, and vomiting and are followed by bloody diarrhea, toxemia, and shock. In all these forms of the disease the organisms can invade the bloodstream and also, infrequently, the meninges, resulting in overwhelming septicemia and death. Overall mortality is about 20%.

Anthrax is enzootic in areas of South America, Asia, and Africa where it causes serious economic losses of animals. There are many more human infections in these countries than in North America or Europe. Only one case of anthrax was reported in the United States in 1980.

Bacillus cereus can cause serious disease[11,30,93] such as septicemia, endocarditis, wound infections, and pulmonary infections including pneumonia[48] in humans and bovine mastitis in animals. In addition, it causes especially fulminant eye infections, which often terminate with enucleations of the eye or loss of vision.[66] If gram-positive rods are seen in a Gram stain of the vitreous fluid of the eye, the physician should be notified immediately. *B. cereus* is also associated with outbreaks of food poisoning characterized by vomiting 1 to 5 hours after ingestion of the contaminated food. The role of *B. cereus* in diarrheal food poisoning is not known.

Early reports associated *B. subtilis* with disease; however, the organisms would probably now be classified as *B. cereus*. Nevertheless, there are some well-documented reports of *B. subtilis*, *B. laterosporus*, and *B. sphaericus* infections,[30,91,93] generally of an opportunistic nature.

Mechanisms of Pathogenicity

Toxins produced by *B. cereus* include a dermonecrotic and lethal toxin, two hemolysins, lecithinase, and an emetic toxin. Other products that might affect virulence are penicillinase, cephalosporinase, proteases, and nucleases.[94] The role of these products in diseases of the eye and systemic infections has not been clearly delineated.

Death ensues not from the presence of the organisms but from the effects of the toxins they produce. Three separate proteins, the lethal factor (LF), protective antigen (PA), and edema factor (EF), comprise the anthrax toxins. The LF and PA together cause death of rats, whereas EF and PA together cause edema in the skin of rodents. The EF has adenylate cyclase activity.[58] The PA presumably allows the EF and perhaps the LF access to the mammalian cell.

Antimicrobial Susceptibility

B. anthracis is susceptible to penicillin, cephalosporins, chloramphenicol, and aminoglycosides. Penicillin is essentially 100% effective against cutaneous anthrax and early systemic disease. However, because the pathologic effects of anthrax result from the toxin, antimicrobial agents do not alter the course of disease once the critical level of toxin is produced in the patient. Thus deaths can be attributed to late diagnosis related to a low index of suspicion resulting from the rarity of the disease.

B. cereus is generally resistant to penicillin and cephalosporin.[22] Clindamycin with or without gentamicin has been suggested as treatment.[48,66] Other species have variable susceptibilities. All strains involved in a disease process need to be tested for susceptibility to antimicrobial agents by standard methods.

VACCINES

A vaccine made from alum-precipitated protective antigen has been used to protect workers at high-risk industrial plants. Another vaccine type, prepared from living spores, has been used in cattle in South Africa to reduce the incidence of anthrax by over 99%.

REFERENCES

1. Barksdale, L.: Identifying *Rothia dentocariosa*, Ann. Intern. Med. **91**:786, 1979.
2. Barksdale, L.: The genus *Corynebacterium*. In Starr, M.P., et al., editors: The prokaryotes: a handbook on habitats, isolation, and identification of bacteria, Berlin, 1981, Springer-Verlag.
3. Barton, M.D., and Hughes, K.L.: Comparison of three techniques for isolation of *Rhodococcus (Corynebacterium) equi* from contaminated sources, J. Clin. Microbiol. **13**:219, 1981.
4. Basher, H.A., et al.: Pathogenesis and growth of *Listeria monocytogenes* in fertile hens' eggs, Zentralbl. Bakteriol. Hyg. [A] **256**:497, 1984.
5. Berger, S.A., et al.: Recurrent breast abscesses caused by *Corynebacterium minutissimum*, J. Clin. Microbiol. **20**:1219, 1984.
6. Bojsen-Moller, J.: Human listeriosis, Acta Pathol. Microbiol. Scand. [B] Suppl. **229**:1, 1972.
7. Bowmer, E.J., Conklin, R.H., and Steele, H.J.: Listeriosis. In Steele, H.J., editor: CRC handbook series in zoonoses, Boca Raton, Fla., 1979, CRC Press, Inc.
8. Bratberg, H.M.: Selective adherence of *Erysipelothrix rhusiopathiae* to heart valves of swine investigated in an in vitro test, Acta Vet. Scand. **22**:39, 1981.
9. Broeren, S.A., and Peel, M.M.: Endocarditis caused by *Rothia dentocariosa*, J. Clin. Pathol. **37**:1298, 1984.
10. Broughton, R.A., et al.: Septic arthritis and osteomyelitis caused by an organism of the genus *Rhodococcus*, J. Clin. Microbiol. **13**:209, 1981.
11. Burdon, K.L., Davis, J.S., and Wende, R.D.: Experimental infection of mice with *Bacillus cereus*: studies of pathogenesis and pathologic changes, J. Infect. Dis. **117**:307, 1967.
12. Centers for Disease Control: Annual summary, MMWR **26**:1978, 1977.
13. Centers for Disease Control: Fatal diphtheria: Wisconsin, MMWR **31**:553, 1982.
14. Chandler, D.S., and Craven, J.H.: Persistence and distribution of *Erysipelothrix rhusiopathiae* and bacterial indicator organisms on land used for disposal of piggery effluent, J. Appl. Bacteriol. **48**:367, 1980.
15. Chang, D.N., Laughren, G.S., and Chalvardjian, N.E.: Three variants of *Corynebacterium diphtheriae* subsp. *mitis (belfanti)* isolated from a throat specimen, J. Clin. Microbiol. **8**:767, 1978.
16. Clarridge, J.E., and Weissfeld, A.S.: *Listeria monocytogenes*, Clin. Microbiol. Newsletter **17**:59, 1985.
17. Clarridge, J.E., and Weissfeld, A.S.: Aerobic asporogenous gram-positive bacilli, Clin. Microbiol. Newsletter **6**:115, 1984.
18. Collins, M.D.: Reclassification of *Bacterionema matruchotii* (Mendel) in the genus *Corynebacterium* as *Corynebacterium matruchotii* comb. nov., Zentralbl. Bakteriol. Hyg., I. Abt. Orig. C **3**:364, 1982.
19. Collins, M.D., and Cummins, C.: *Corynebacterium*. In Krieg, N.R., editor (Holt, J.G., editor-in-chief): Bergey's manual of systematic bacteriology, vol. 2, Baltimore, 1986, Williams & Wilkins Co.
20. Collins, M.D., and Jones, D.: Reclassification of *Corynebacterium pyogenes* (Glage) in the genus *Actinomyces*, as *Actinomyces pyogenes* comb. nov., J. Gen. Microbiol. **128**:901, 1982.
21. Collins, M.D., Jones, D., and Schofield, G.M.: Reclassification of '*Corynebacterium haemolyticum*' (MacLean, Liebow & Rosenberg) in the genus. nov. as *Arcanobacterium haemolyticum* nom. rev. comb. nov., J. Gen. Microbiol. **128**:1279, 1982.
22. Coonrod, J.D., Leadley, P.J., and Eickhoff, T.C.: Antibiotic susceptibility of *Bacillus* species, J. Infect. Dis. **123**:102, 1971.
23. Corino, D.L., and Sesardic, D.: Profile analysis of total mycolic acids from skin corynebacteria and from named *Corynebacterium* strains by gas-liquid chromatography and spectrometry, J. Gen. Microbiol. **116**:61, 1980.
24. Coudron, P.E., et al.: Two similar but atypical strains of coryneform group A-4 isolated from patients with endophthalmitis, J. Clin. Microbiol. **22**:475, 1985.
25. Coyle, M.B., Hollis, D.G., and Groman, N.B.: *Corynebacterium* spp. and other coryneforms. In Lennette, E.H., et al., editors: Manual of clinical microbiology, ed. 4, Washington, D.C., 1985, American Society for Microbiology.
26. Crickshank, J.G., Gawler, A.H., and Shaldon, C.: *Oerskovia* species: rare opportunistic pathogens, J. Med. Microbiol. **12**:513, 1979.
27. Donaghy, M., and Cohen, J.: Pulmonary infection with *Corynebacterium hofmannii* complicating systemic lupus erythematosus, J. Infect. Dis. **147**:962, 1983.
28. Elek, S.D.: The plate virulence test for diphtheria, J. Clin. Pathol. **2**:250, 1949.
29. Ewald, E.: The genus *Erysipelothrix*. In Starr, M.P., et al.: The prokaryotes: a handbook on habitats, isolation, and identification of bacteria, Berlin, 1981, Springer-Verlag.
30. Farrar, W.E.: Serious infections due to "non-pathogenic" organisms of the genus *Bacillus*, Am. J. Med. **34**:134, 1963.
31. Fell, H.W.K., Nagington, J., and Naylor, G.R.E.: *Corynebacterium haemolyticum* infections in Cambridgeshire, J. Hyg. Camb. **79**:269, 1977.
32. Gibson, T., and Gordon, R.E.: *Bacillus*. In Buchanan, R.E., and Gibbons, N.E., editors: Bergey's manual of determinative bacteriology, ed. 8, Baltimore, 1974, Williams & Wilkins Co.
33. Goldberg, J.W., Clarridge, J.E., and Weiman, E.: *Erysipelothrix* septicemia and glomerulonephritis. In preparation.
34. Goldberger, A.C., Lipsky, B.A., and Plorde, J.J.: Suppurative granulomatous lymphadenitis caused by *Corynebacterium ovis (pseudotuberculosis)*, Am. J. Clin. Pathol. **76**:486, 1981.
35. Goodfellow, M., and Alderson, G.: The actinomycete-genus *Rhodococcus*: a home for the rhodochrous complex, J. Gen. Microbiol. **100**:99, 1977.
36. Goodfellow, M., Weaver, C.R., and Minnikin, D.E.: Numerical classification of some rhodococci, corynebacteria and related organisms, J. Gen. Microbiol. **128**:731, 1982.
37. Gray, M.L., and Killinger, A.H.: *Listeria monocytogenes* and listeric infections, Bacteriol. Rev. **30**:309, 1966.
38. Grieco, M.H., and Sheldon, B.S.: *Erysipelothrix rhusiopathiae*, Ann. N.Y. Acad. Sci. **174**:523, 1970.
39. Groves, R.D., and Welshimer, H.J.: Separation of pathogenic from apathogenic *Listeria monocytogenes* by three *in vitro* reactions, J. Clin. Microbiol. **5**:559, 1977.
40. Haburchak, D.R., et al.: Infections caused by Rhodochrous, Am. J. Med. **65**:298, 1978.
41. Hande, K.R., et al.: Sepsis with a new species of *Corynebacterium*, Ann. Intern. Med. **85**:423, 1976.
42. Hanscom, T., and Maxwell, W.A.: *Corynebacterium* endophthalmitis: laboratory studies and report of a case treated by vitrectomy, Arch. Ophthalmol. **97**:500, 1979.
43. Hollis, D.G., and Weaver, R.E.: Identification of gram positive bacilli, Atlanta, 1981, Centers for Disease Control.
44. Hollis, D.G., et al.: Use of the rapid fermentation test in determining carbohydrate reactions of fastidious bacteria in clinical laboratories, J. Clin. Microbiol. **12**:620, 1980.
45. Johnson, W.D., and Kaye, D.: Serious infections caused by diphtheroids, Ann. N.Y. Acad. Sci. **174**:568, 1970.
46. Jolly, R.D.: The pathogenic action of the exotoxin of *Corynebacterium ovis*, J. Comp. Pathol. **75**:417, 1965.

47. Jones, D.: *Erysipelothrix*. In Krieg, N.R., editor (Holt, J.G., editor-in-chief): Bergey's manual of systematic bacteriology, vol. 2, Baltimore, 1986, Williams & Wilkins Co.

48. Jonsson, S., Clarridge, J., and Young, E.J.: Necrotizing pneumonia and empyema by *Bacillus cereus* and *Clostridium bifermentans*, Am. Rev. Respir. Dis. **127:**357, 1983.

49. Kaneko, T., Nozaki, R., and Aizawa, K.: DNA relatedness between *Bacillus anthracis, Bacillus cereus,* and *Bacillus thuringiensis,* Microbiol. Immunol. **22:**639, 1978.

50. Kaplan, K., and Weinstein, L.: Diphtheroid infections of man, Ann. Intern. Med. **70:**919, 1969.

51. Keddie, R.M.: *Kurthia.* In Starr, M.P., et al., editors: The prokaryotes: a handbook on habitats, isolation, and identification of bacteria, Berlin, 1981, Springer-Verlag.

52. Keslin, M.H., et al.: *Corynebacterium pseudotuberculosis:* a new cause of infectious and eosinophilic pneumonia, Am. J. Med. **67:**228, 1979.

53. Kilian, M.: Rapid identification of *Actinomycetaceae* and related bacteria, J. Clin. Microbiol. **8:**127, 1978.

54. King, P.F.: Erysipeloid: survey of 115 cases, Lancet **2:**196, 1946.

55. Klauder, J.V.: *Erysipelothrix rhusiopathiae* infection in animals and in human beings, Ann. N.Y. Acad. Sci. **48:**535, 1947.

56. Koopman, J.S., and Campbell, J.: The role of cutaneous diphtheria infections in a diphtheria epidemic, J. Infect. Dis. **131:**239, 1975.

57. Kovatch, A.L., Schmit, K.E., and Michaels, R.H.: *Corynebacterium haemolyticum* peritonsillar abscess mimicking diphtheria, JAMA **249:**1757, 1983.

58. Leppla, S.H.: Anthrax toxin edema factor: a bacterial adenylate cyclase that increases cyclic AMP concentration of eukaryotic cells, Proc. Natl. Acad. Sci. U.S.A. **79:**3162, 1982.

59. Lipsky, B.A., et al.: Infections caused by nondiphtheria corynebacteria, Rev. Infect. Dis. **4:**1220, 1982.

60. Love, J.W., et al.: Infective endocarditis due to *Corynebacterium diphtheriae:* report of a case and review of the literature, Johns Hopkins Med. J. **148:**41, 1981.

61. Luft, B.J., and Remington, J.S.: Effect of pregnancy on resistance to *Listeria monocytogenes* and *Toxoplasma gondii* infection in mice, Infect. Immun. **38:**1164, 1982.

62. Meers, P.D.: A case of classical diphtheria, and other infections due to *Corynebacterium ulcerans,* J. Infect. **1:**139, 1979.

63. Murphy, J.R., Bacha, P., and Teng, M.: Determination of *Corynebacterium diphtheriae* toxigenicity by a colorimetric tissue culture assay, J. Clin. Microbiol. **7:**91, 1978.

64. Nieman, R.E., and Lorber, B.: Listeriosis in adults: a changing pattern; report of eight cases and review of the literature, 1968-1978, Rev. Infect. Dis. **2:**207, 1980.

65. Nikolov, P., Valerianov, T.S., and Abrashev, I.: Neuraminidase as a factor in the pathogenicity of *Erysipelothrix rhusiopathiae,* Acta Microbiol. Virol. Immunol. (Sofiia) **6:**15, 1977.

66. O'Day, D.M., et al.: The problem of *Bacillus* species infection with special emphasis on the virulence of *Bacillus cereus,* Ophthalmology **88:**833, 1981.

67. Pancoast, S.J., et al.: Endocarditis due to *Kurthia bessonii,* Ann. Intern. Med. **90:**936, 1979.

68. Pape, J., et al.: Infective endocarditis caused by *Oerskovia turbata,* Ann. Intern. Med. **91:**746, 1979.

69. Parry, J.M., Turnbull, P.C.B., and Gibson, J.R.: A color atlas of *Bacillus* species, Wolfe Medical Atlases #19, London, 1983, Wolfe Medical Publication, Ltd.

70. Phillips, A.P., Martin, K.L., and Broster, M.G.: Differentiation between spores of *Bacillus anthracis* and *Bacillus cereus* by a quantitative immunofluorescence technique, J. Clin. Microbiol. **17:**41, 1983.

71. Porschen, R.K., Goodman, Z., and Rafai, B.: Isolation of *Corynebacterium xerosis* from clinical specimens, Am. J. Clin. Pathol. **68:**290, 1977.

72. Reller, L.B., et al.: Bacterial endocarditis caused by *Oerskovia turbata,* Ann. Intern. Med. **83:**664, 1975.

73. Riley, P.S., et al.: Characterization and identification of 95 diphtheroid (group JK) cultures isolated from clinical specimens, J. Clin. Microbiol. **9:**418, 1979.

74. Rocourt, J., and Grimont, P.A.D.: *Listeria welshimeri* sp. nov. and *Listeria seeligeri* sp. nov., Int. J. Syst. Bacteriol. **33:**866, 1983.

75. Rogosa, M., et al.: Coryneform group of bacteria. In Buchanan, R.E., and Gibbons, N.E., editors: Bergey's manual of determinative bacteriology, ed. 8, Baltimore, 1974, Williams & Wilkins Co.

76. Schaal, K.P., and Pulverer, G.: The genera *Actinomyces, Agromyces, Arachnia, Bacterionema* and *Rothia.* In Starr, M.P., et al., editors: The prokaryotes: a handbook on habitats, isolation, and identification of bacteria, Berlin, 1981, Springer-Verlag.

77. Schafer, F.J., Wing, E.J., and Norden, C.W.: Infectious endocarditis caused by *Rothia dentocariosa,* Ann. Intern. Med. **91:**747, 1979.

78. Scheld, W.M.: Evaluation of rifampin and other antibiotics against *Listeria monocytogenes,* Rev. Infect. Dis. **5**(suppl. 3):S593, 1983.

79. Schlech, W.F., III, et al.: Epidemic listeriosis: evidence for transmission by food, N. Engl. J. Med. **308:**203, 1983.

80. Schofield, G.M., and Schaal, K.P.: A numerical taxonomic study of members of the *Actinomycetaceae* and related taxa, J. Gen. Microbiol. **127**(Pt. 2):237, 1981.

81. Seeliger, H.P.R.: Apathogene Listerien: *L. innocue* sp. n. (Seeliger et Schoofs, 1977), Zentralbl. Bakteriol. Mikrobiol. Hyg. I. Abt. Orig. A. **249:**487, 1981.

82. Seeliger, H.P.R., and Jones, D.: *Listeria.* In Krieg, N.R., editor (Holt, J.G., editor-in-chief): Bergey's manual of systematic bacteriology, vol. 2, Baltimore, 1986, Williams & Wilkins Co.

83. Seeliger, H.P.R., et al.: *Listeria ivanovii* sp. nov., Int. J. Syst. Bacteriol. **34:**336, 1984.

84. Shalka, B., and Smola, J.: Selective media for pathogenic *Listeria* spp., J. Clin. Microbiol. **18:**1432, 1983.

85. Shalka, B., Smola, J., and Elischerova, K.: Routine test for *in vitro* differentiation of pathogenic and apathogenic *Listeria monocytogenes* strains, J. Clin. Microbiol. **15:**503, 1982.

86. Sorario, F., et al.: In vitro and in vivo study of stone formation by *Corynebacterium* group D2 *(Corynebacterium urealyticum),* J. Clin. Microbiol. **23:**691, 1986.

87. Stamm, A.M.: Chloramphenicol: ineffective for treatment of *Listeria* meningitis, Am. J. Med. **72:**830, 1982.

88. Stamm, A.M., et al.: Listeriosis in renal transplant recipients: report of an outbreak and review of 102 cases, Rev. Infect. Dis. **4:**665, 1982.

89. Stuart, S.E., and Welshimer, H.J.: Taxonomic reexamination of *Listeria pirie* and transfer of *Listeria grayi* and *Listeria murrayi* to a new genus *Murraya,* Int. J. Syst. Bacteriol. **24:**177, 1974.

90. Suzuki, K., Kaneko, T., and Komagata, K.: Deoxyribonucleic acid homologies among coryneform bacteria, Int. J. Syst. Bacteriol. **31:**131, 1981.

91. Tabbara, K.F., Juffale, F., and Motossin, R.M.: *Bacillus laterosporus* endophthalmitis, Arch. Ophthalmol. **95:**2187, 1977.

92. Tuazon, C.V., Shamsuddin, D., and Miller, H.: Antibiotic susceptibility and synergy of clinical isolates of *Listeria monocytogenes,* Antimicrob. Agents Chemother. **21:**525, 1982.

93. Tuazon, C.V., et al.: Serious infection from *Bacillus* sp., JAMA **241:**1137, 1979.

94. Turnbull, P.C.: *Bacillus cereus* toxins, Pharmacol. Ther. **13:**435, 1981.

95. Van Scoy, R.E., et al.: Coryneform bacterial endocarditis, Mayo Clin. Proc. **52:**216, 1977.

96. Volmer, J., and Hasler, G.: *Erysipelothrix*-Endokarditis, Dtsch. Med. Wochenschr. **101:**1672, 1976.

97. Von Koenig, C.H.W., et al.: Course and development of immunity in experimental infections of mice with *Listeria* serotypes, Infect. Immun. **40:**1170, 1983.

98. Washington, J.A., II: Bacteriology, clinical spectrum of disease, and therapeutic aspects of coryneform bacterial infection. In Remington, J.S., and Swartz, M.N., editors: Current clinical topics in infectious diseases, vol. 2, New York, 1981, McGraw-Hill Book Co.

99. Watts, P.S.: Studies on *Erysipelothrix rhusiopathiae*, J. Pathol. Bacteriol. **50:**535, 1940.

100. Welshimer, H.J.: The genus *Listeria* and related organisms. In Starr, M.P., et al, editors: The prokaryotes: a handbook on habitats, isolation, and identification of bacteria, Berlin, 1981, Springer-Verlag.

101. Wickremeinghe, R.S.B.: *Corynebacterium haemolyticum* infections in Sri Lanka, J. Hyg. Camb. **87:**271, 1981.

102. Wilhelmus, K.R., Robinson, N.M., and Jones, D.B.: *Bacterionema matruchotii* ocular infections, Am. J. Ophthalmol. **87:**143, 1979.

103. Wilson, G.: *Bacillus:* the aerobic spore-bearing bacilli. In Wilson, G., Miles, A., and Parker, M.T., editors: Topley and Wilson's principles of bacteriology, virology, and immunity, vol. 2, ed. 7, London, 1983, Edward Arnold.

104. Wilson, G.: *Corynebacterium* and other coryneform organisms. In Wilson, G., Miles, A., and Parker, M.T., editors: Topley and Wilson's principles of bacteriology, virology, and immunity, vol. 2, ed. 7, London, 1983, Edward Arnold.

105. Woodbine, M.: *Erysipelothrix rhusiopathiae:* bacteriology and chemotherapy, Bacteriol. Rev. **14:**161, 1950.

106. Young, V.M., et al.: The emergence of coryneform bacteria as a cause of nosocomial infections in compromised hosts, Am. J. Med. **70:**646, 1981.

</>

CHAPTER 22

Miscellaneous Gram-Negative Coccobacilli

Pasteurella, Francisella, Bordetella, and *Brucella*

Jill E. Clarridge

Organisms of the genera *Brucella, Bordetella, Francisella,* and *Pasteurella* are small, gram-negative, aerobic coccobacilli. In this chapter the genus *Pasteurella* is considered separately from the other three genera because it is fermentative and grows more readily than the other organisms.[7,8,26]

BRUCELLA, BORDETELLA, AND *FRANCISELLA*

The taxonomic relationships of these genera are not yet determined. They are listed in *Bergey's Manual of Systematic Bacteriology* in the section on gram-negative aerobic rods and cocci, under other genera not assigned to any family.

BRUCELLA
Classification

Members of the genus *Brucella* are intracellular organisms that normally parasitize mammals. There are six recognized species of *Brucella: B. abortus, B. melitensis, B. suis, B. canis, B. ovis,* and *B. neotomae.*[7] The most common natural habitats of these organisms are, respectively, cattle, sheep and goats, swine, dogs, and desert wood rats. Although the animal reservoir of each *Brucella* sp. is distinct, overlap does occur; *B. melitensis, B. suis,* and *B. abortus* all have been isolated from cattle. The organisms can exist in these animals without apparent disease, although infection by some species (*B. abortus* and *B. melitensis* particularly) can result in economically serious losses. The species that infect humans—*B. abortus, B. melitensis, B. suis,* and *B. canis*—are discussed here.

Specimen Collection and Processing

Most of the isolates of *Brucella* organisms come from the blood. Because they are the most dependable source of isolation, blood cultures should always be taken in cases of suspected infection by members of the genus *Brucella.* Organisms can also be isolated from special sites such as bone marrow, liver, spleen, or even cerebrospinal fluid depending on the course of disease. Because infections with *Brucella* are easily transmitted in the laboratory (30% of the cases in a recent review were laboratory acquired[36]), care must be taken not to aerosolize the specimen or allow it to come in contact with the skin, conjunctiva, or mucous membranes. Specimens to be cultured for *Brucella* organisms should be so labeled not only because of the special care required, but because of the special culturing techniques needed.

Growth Requirements
Media

Most blood culture bottles (brain-heart infusion and trypticase soy broth [TSB] are satisfactory) support growth of *Bru-*

cella organisms if a continuous vent is added and the bottles are placed in a CO_2 incubator. However, because the culture bottles may not become turbid and colonies will not be visible from subcultures for 2 to 7 days, blind subcultures should be performed at 2, 7, and 14 days. The subculture plates should be held for a week. Chocolate and blood agar plates can be used for subculturing. Affected tissue, fluid, and bone marrow can also be inoculated to blood culture bottles, in addition to blood and chocolate agar plates. Subculture of these specimens should be done as if they were blood cultures. Although most stains grow in unsupplemented Brucella broth or TSB, blood or serum can stimulate growth.

Castañeda bottles, which have both solid and liquid media in the same container (biphasic), may also be used for culture of *Brucella* organisms. The agar slant in the bottle allows direct observation of colonies developing from the broth culture.

Environmental requirements

Because the species of *Brucella* involved in a particular disease cannot be determined on solely clinical grounds, all specimens must be cultured for the most fastidious organism. *B. melitensis, B. suis,* and *B. canis* generally do not require elevated CO_2, but *B. abortus* usually does; therefore all specimens should be incubated initially in air with 8% to 10% CO_2 at 35° C.

Cultural Characteristics
Staining reactions

Brucella organisms are small (about 0.5 by 0.3 to 0.9 μm) gram-negative coccobacilli. In tissue they are usually intracellular. Because *Brucella* spp. are small and may not retain the safranin counterstain sufficiently, easier visualization may be achieved by substituting carbol-fuchsin for the counterstain in the Gram stain procedure. Organisms usually stain more intensely red with this method. A direct fluorescent antibody technique is available at reference laboratories.

Colonial morphology

On agar plates, growth usually is not apparent at 24 hours. At 48 hours, *B. melitensis, B. suis,* and *B. canis* are pinpoint colonies. At 72 hours, *B. abortus* shows pinpoint colonies, and the other species are larger. All the species begin as translucent colonies and become gray with age. The colonies of *B. abortus, B. melitensis,* and *B. suis* are usually smooth, and *B. canis* colonies are usually rough, although both colony types can be formed by all species. Rough colonies are less translucent and more friable or sticky than smooth colonies. None are hemolytic.

TABLE 22-1. Characteristics of Some Small Gram-Negative Bacilli

Genus	Fermentation of Glucose	Oxidase	Motility	Growth on MacConkey Agar	Urease	Needed Growth Factors	Mol% G+C of DNA
Francisella	−	−	−	−	−	Cysteine or cystine	33-36
Bordetella	−	v	v	+[a]	v	Nicotinamide	66-70
Brucella	−	+	−	v	+	Thiamine	55-58
Pasteurella	+	+	+	v	v	—	40-45
Actinobacillus	+	+[b]	−	+[b]	v	—	40-43
Haemophilus	+	+/−	−	−	v	X and/or Y	38-44
Yersinia	+	−	+	+	v	—	46-50

> **SYMBOLS:** +, ≥ 90% positive
> −, ≤ 10% positive
> v, 10%-90% positive

[a] *B. pertussis* does not grow on MacConkey agar.
[b] *A. actinomycetemcomitans* is usually negative.

TABLE 22-2. Characteristics of *Brucella* Spp.

Species	Urease[a]	H₂S Produced[b]	CO₂ Required
B. abortus	1-2 hr	+	v
B. melitensis	v	−	−
B. suis	<30 min	−	−
B. canis	<30 min	−	−

> **SYMBOLS:** +, 90% positive
> −, <10% positive
> v, 10%-90% positive

[a] Warm the urea slant and inoculate heavily.
[b] Detected by a lead acetate strip above a slant, such as brain heart infusion, inoculated with *Brucella* organisms.

Biochemical Identification

The genus *Brucella* is characterized as gram-negative, non-motile, usually oxidase-positive, catalase-positive, glucose-oxidizing or nonutilizing organisms that do not have capsules or form spores. Differential characteristics distinguishing *Brucella* organisms from other small, gram-negative coccobacilli are given in Table 22-1.

Biochemical characteristics of the genus *Brucella* sufficient for presumptive identification are shown in Table 22-2. There are three recognized biotypes of *B. melitensis*, nine biotypes of *B. abortus*, and four biotypes of *B. suis*. Definitive species and biotype identification can be done at reference laboratories and is based, in addition to biochemical characterization, on growth in the presence of fuchsin and thionine, lysis by phage, and serotyping.

Serologic and Immunoserologic Identification[22]

The serum agglutination test uses a *Brucella abortus* strain as the antigen to detect circulating antibodies to *Brucella* spp. This antigen detects antibody against *B. abortus*, *B. melitensis*, and *B. suis* but not against *B. canis*. A separate test must be requested for *B. canis*. Sera should be obtained as early in the disease course as possible and again after 2 to 3 weeks. Immunoglobulin M antibody is produced initially and, in chronic disease, for an extended period. A titer of at least 1:320 allows a presumptive diagnosis of brucellosis, and absence of antibody makes the diagnosis unlikely.

Clinical Significance

In 1887, while he was working in Malta, the English scientist David Bruce isolated a small microorganism from the livers and spleens of patients dying of undulant fever. The organism was subsequently named *Brucella melitensis*. Undulant fever is so called because of the irregular temperature curve seen during the illness; often there are several weeks of high temperature followed by several days of abatement. A series of scientists discovered that the goat was the natural reservoir for *B. melitensis*, that goats do not have to appear ill to have the infection, that organisms are passed in the goats' milk, and that consumption of goats' milk or cheese is the primary mode of infection for humans. Similarly, *B. abortus* causes infection in cattle and can be passed to humans through the consumption of milk products or contact with the cattle. Human disease caused by *B. suis* and *B. canis* is usually related to exposure to swine and dogs, respectively.

Infection with *Brucella* organisms produces symptoms including fever, malaise, weakness, possibly enlarged spleen and lymph nodes, weight loss, and arthritis. The clinical and epidemiologic aspects of brucellosis have been reviewed.[3-5,36]

Mechanisms of Pathogenicity

The pathogenicity of the genus *Brucella* seems related to its ability to enter and grow in mammalian host cells. With *B. abortus* the bacteria tend to localize in tissue of the reticuloendothelial and genitourinary systems. This may be because of their higher content of erythritol, which stimulates growth.[17] Cattle have higher levels of erythritol, which may explain the susceptibility of this species to *B. abortus*.

Antimicrobial Susceptibility[15]

Because of the intracellular localization of *Brucella* organisms and difficulties in growing the organisms, in vitro susceptibility testing may not predict clinical response to treatment. Therapy with tetracycline with or without streptomycin has usually been recommended,[3] although no synergy between these drugs has been shown in vitro.[23] Rifampin and trimethoprim-sulfamethoxazole may also be used for treatment.[23]

BORDETELLA
Classification

In the sixth edition of *Bergey's Manual of Determinative Bacteriology* the *Bordetella* spp. were listed in separate genera (*Haemophilus pertussis*, *Bacillus parapertussis*, and *Brucella bronchiseptica*). The seventh and eighth editions of *Bergey's Manual of Determinative Bacteriology* and the first edition of *Bergey's Manual of Systematic Bacteriology*[26] listed the three species as members of the genus *Bordetella*, named for Bordet, who with Gengou first isolated the agent of whooping cough. DNA homology studies have confirmed that these three species—*B. pertussis*, *B. parapertussis*, and *B. bronchiseptica*—are closely related.[19] Recently a new species that affects birds, *B. avium*, was described.[18]

Specimen Collection and Processing

Specimens should be collected by a calcium alginate or Dacron swab inserted through the nose to the posterior nasopharynx. The swab is left in place for up to 30 seconds, preferably during a cough. Two swabs should be collected, one for immediate plating or transport and one for smears (two smears for the fluorescent antibody stain and one for the Gram stain).

Growth Requirements
Media

On initial isolation, *Bordetella pertussis* requires special media with additional nutrients for growth and absorbants to remove the toxins found in complex media. The standard Bordet-Gengou medium with potato infusion and sheep blood (Appendix A) is adequate but generally inferior to Bordet-Gengou medium with methicillin or cephalexin (to inhibit normal nasopharyngeal organisms) or Regan-Lowe medium, which contains charcoal, horse blood, and cephalexin.[27] The Regan-

Lowe medium is recommended for transport.

B. parapertussis and *B. bronchiseptica* grow on sheep blood agar.

Environmental requirements

Bordetella organisms grow at 35° C in air or with added (3% to 8%) CO_2.

Cultural Characteristics
Staining reactions

Members of the genera *Bordetella* and *Brucella* resemble each other in being small (0.3 by 0.3 by 1 μm), gram-negative coccobacilli. During the Gram stain procedure the safranin should be left on at least 2 minutes; otherwise the organisms may retain too little stain and be difficult to see. A carbol-fuchsin counterstain may also be used.

Because of the difficulty in growing *Bordetella pertussis* in a clinical laboratory, that is, because fresh, properly quality-controlled plates must be ready at the needed time, two smears for fluorescent antibody stain should always be made at the time of culture. The two air-dried and heat-fixed slides should be sent to a reference laboratory. There one slide is stained with fluorescein-labeled antipertussis rabbit serum and the other (the control) with fluorescein-labeled normal rabbit serum. The antipertussis antibody conjugate attaches specifically to the *B. pertussis* organisms, allowing them to be seen as small fluorescent coccobacilli. The test depends on the quality of antiserum. The rate of false-negative reports is under 10%, and the rate of false-positive reports varies from under 10% to 40%. Direct fluorescent antibody stains should also be used to confirm isolates of suspected *B. pertussis*.

Colonial morphology

The appearance and growth characteristics of the species of *Bordetella* are summarized in Table 22-3.

When *B. pertussis* is isolated from clinical specimens, it grows as smooth colonies (phase 1). With extensive subculturing the colonies tend to become rough (phase 4). Phases 1 to 4 are antigenic types described by Leslie and Gardner in 1936. Because the phase 1 organisms are more sensitive to fatty acids and sulfides, phase 4 organisms are not adequate for quality control of media. In changing from phase 1 to phase 4, the organisms become less virulent as they lose the ability to form pertussis toxin, hemolysis hemagglutinin, and pili, among other factors.[33]

Biochemical Identification

The biochemical characteristics that are useful in distinguishing the species of *Bordetella* are given in Table 22-3. The tests to separate Bordetella from other similar genera are given in Table 22-1.

Serologic and Immunoserologic Identification

Immunoserologic study is of little use for the evaluation of individual clinical cases[20]; however, a new enzyme-linked immunosorbent assay (ELISA) using the fimbrial hemagglutinin as antigen is reported to be more sensitive than culture.[14]

Clinical Significance

Whooping cough (pertussis) is generally acquired by the inhalation of droplets containing *Bordetella pertussis* that have

TABLE 22-3. Characteristics of *Bordetella* Spp.

| Characteristic | B. pertussis | | B. bronchiseptica | B. parapertussis |
	Phase 1	Phase 4		
Time to grow on Bordet-Gengou plates	3-4 days	1-2 days	1-2 days	1-2 days
Appearance on Bordet-Gengou plates at 3-4 days	Half pearl, entire, <1 mm (Plate 21, *A*)	Larger than phase 1, rougher	Pitted; larger than phase 1 of *B. pertussis*	Larger and duller than phase 1 of *B. pertussis*
Growth on blood agar	−	+	+	+
Inhibited by fatty acids and sulfides	+	−	−	−
Urease	−	−	+ (4 hr)	+ (24 hr)
Nitrate	−	−	+	−
Pigment, brown soluble	−	−	−	+
Exotoxin	+	−	−	−
Pili	+	−	−	−
Filamentous hemagglutinins	+	−	−	−
Occurrence	Human respiratory tract	Laboratory	Animals (respiratory and wound); rarely from humans	Humans

> SYMBOLS: +, 90% positive
> −, <10% positive

been aerosolized during a cough by a person in the early stages of the disease. The organism attaches to the respiratory epithelial cells of the nasopharynx and from that site elaborates an exotoxin with a molecular weight of about 120,000 daltons. (This molecule is used for a vaccine and stimulates natural immunity after disease.) At this stage of disease the patient has a mild cough and upper respiratory symptoms. Subsequently, with increasing secretions and irritations to the nasotrachea, the coughs are typically so close in sequence that there is no time to take a breath. When the series of coughs stops, the air is taken in so rapidly that a "whooping" sound results. The symptoms of the disease, which can vary from a mild cough to death resulting from airway obstruction or neurologic complications, seem to depend not only on the age and state of immunity of the host, but also on the quantity of organisms colonizing the nasopharynx. *B. pertussis* rarely spreads to other sites. After the exotoxin is excreted and attached to its receptor cells, eliminating the organism by antimicrobial agents does not alter the course of disease. Immunity subsequent to infection is generally lifelong. *B. parapertussis* can cause a mild form of whooping cough.

B. bronchiseptica is widespread in animal populations, caus-

ing both respiratory and wound infections.[13] Several cases of human infection have been reported. Bordetellosis in swine, dogs, and laboratory animals inflicts great economic losses.

Mechanisms of Pathogenicity

The pathogenesis of whooping cough is not well understood. Research in this area with the goal of making a safer pertussis vaccine has led to identification of a variety of virulence factors. These include pertussin toxin, extracytoplasmic adenylate cyclase, filamentous hemagglutinin, dermonecrotic toxin, and hemolysin.[33,34]

Antimicrobial Susceptibility

Bordetella pertussis is not amenable to standard susceptibility testing,[9] but tests using a special broth and Bordet-Gengou medium have shown the organism to be sensitive to erythromycin and resistant to ampicillin, clindamycin, and trimethoprim.[37] Erythromycin is the drug of choice for whooping cough when antimicrobial treatment is indicated. Chloramphenicol and tetracycline have been used in treatment, but in vitro data are not definitive. All three *Bordetella* spp. have similar sensitivity patterns.

Vaccination

Vaccination is the best protection against pertussis. Outbreaks of disease occur in the unvaccinated segments of the population of both developed and undeveloped countries.[25] There have been rare complications subsequent to the vaccine, but sequelae from the disease are more common. Vaccines prepared from the whole organism are currently being used; however, research is under way to develop safer vaccines from an antigenic protein.

FRANCISELLA
Classification[8]

The genus *Francisella* has one pathogenic species, *Francisella tularensis*, the causative agent of tularemia. The name derives from Edward Francis, who studied these organisms in Tulare County, California, where tularemia was first observed. A second described species, *F. novicida*, has been isolated from water; it is not known to infect humans.

Specimen Collection and Processing[8]

F. tularensis is highly contagious. Care should be taken during collection not to aerosolize the specimen or allow contact with skin or mucous membranes. Inflammatory material from the infected site (exudate from lesions, tissue from lymph nodes, respiratory secretions, conjunctival scrapings) is the preferred specimen. Part of the sample should be frozen at $-30°$ to $-70°$ C for subsequent work.

Growth Requirements
Media

A recommended medium for isolation of *F. tularensis* is glucose-cysteine blood agar with added thiamine, although it has been shown that chocolate agar with added IsoVitaleX (the medium used for the culture of *Neisseria gonorrhoeae*) and Thayer-Martin medium can also support growth. Furthermore, isolation with the charcoal–yeast extract agar used for the genus *Legionella* has been reported.[35] Occasional strains have also been reported to grow on regular sheep blood agar.[32] Specimens from contaminated sites, such as respiratory specimens, are best cultivated on the selective Thayer-Martin medium.

F. novicida grows on ordinary media such as sheep blood agar or MacConkey agar.

Environmental requirements

Both *Franciscella* spp. can be grown at 35° C in air with or without added CO_2.

Cultural Characteristics
Staining reactions

F. tularensis is an extremely small (0.2 by 0.3 to 0.5 μm), nonmotile, unencapsulated, gram-negative rod. Because the organisms are so small and do not retain stain well, Gram stains of specimens often appear negative. The examination of specimens is best done by direct or indirect fluorescent antibody technique.

Colonial morphology

When grown on recommended media, isolated colonies of *F. tularensis* are pinpoint, gray, smooth colonies at 24 hours, growing to about 1 mm at 48 hours and 3 to 4 mm by 96 hours.

Biochemical Identification

The genus *Francisella* is distinguished from other similar genera in that it is oxidase negative and not stimulated by CO_2, requires cysteine or cystine for growth, may not grow on ordinary laboratory blood agar, is obligately aerobic, and is nonmotile (Table 22-1). The *F. tularensis* biotypes and *F. novicida* may be distinguished by oxidation of maltose, sucrose, and glycerol. Biochemical identification is usually done in reference laboratories.

Serologic and Immunoserologic Identification[29]

Serologic examination for tularemia is reliable and may be the most useful diagnostic test when culture findings are negative. Serum is obtained as soon as the diagnosis is considered, and a second serum is obtained 2 to 3 weeks later. With the agglutination test, titers of 1:40 and 1:80 may be significant or may indicate previous disease, since titers of circulating antibody can remain elevated for years after exposure.

Clinical Significance[16,35]

Tularemia is a zoonosis that is most often associated with exposure to rodents (rabbits, hares, moles) or to ticks that have fed on the rodents. Inoculation can occur through abrasions in the skin during the handling of infected animals or by tick bites. Because exposure is associated with an outdoors setting, the number of reported cases of tularemia goes up during hunting season. About 48 hours after inoculation, a lesion appears at the infected site and progresses to an ulcer over the next few days with accompanying enlargement of the adjacent lymph nodes. Pulmonary tularemia, a serious form of the disease, can result from inhaling an aerosol of the organisms. Such an aerosol can be created by improper handling of the organism in the laboratory or when skinning a rabbit. The oculoglandular form of the disease may occur after the eyes are wiped with a contaminated hand.

Antimicrobial Susceptibility

Streptomycin, tetracycline, and chloramphenicol have been used to treat tularemia. Sensitivity testing can be performed on chocolate agar plates with added IsoVitaleX.

PASTEURELLA
Classification

There are six recognized species in the genus *Pasteurella*: *P. multocida*, *P. pneumotropica*, *P. ureae*, *P. gallinarum*, *P. haemolytica*, and *P. aerogenes*.[6] In addition, a group variously called *Pasteurella* spp. (new species 1), *Pasteurella* "gas," or Henriksen type of *P. pneumotropica* has been described.[10] The lines of demarcation between the genera *Actinobacillus*, *Haemophilus*, and *Pasteurella* are still not clear, but further studies may indicate a shift of species among them.[1,21]

Pasteurella organisms are small, gram-negative, fermentative, nonmotile, oxidase-positive bacilli. The majority of strains are catalase positive. Although *P. multocida* is the most common clinical isolate of the group, *P. pneumotropica*, *P. ureae*, and *P. haemolytica* have been reported to cause human disease. Members of the genus *Pasteurella* are usually associ-

TABLE 22-4. Characteristics of *Pasteurella* Spp.

Species	Hemolysis	Ornithine Decarboxylase	Arginine Decarboxylase	Urease	Indole	Glucose Fermentation	Gas from Glucose	Acid from Maltose	Growth on MacConkey Agar	Comments
P. multocida	Alpha (60)[a]	+	−	−	+	+	−	−	−	Many animals, cats and dogs especially
Pasteurella new species 1	Alpha (33)	−	−	v	+	+	v	+	−	Associated with dogs and cats
P. pneumotropica	Alpha (33)	+	−	+	+	+	−	+	v	Usually isolated from rodents
P. gallinarum	Nonhemolytic	−	+	−	−	+	−	+	v	Associated with poultry; usually commensal
P. hemolytica	Beta (72)	−	−	−	−	+	−	+	v	Infections in sheep and cattle
P. ureae	Alpha (16)	−	−	+	−	+	−	+	−	Human respiratory tract, usually commensal
P. aerogenes	Alpha (56)	v	−	+	−	+	+	+	+	Associated with swine, usually commensal

> **Symbols:** +, 90% positive
> −, < 10% positive
> v, 10%-95% positive

[a]Number in parentheses: percent positive.

ated with animals and fowl; however, *P. ureae* has been isolated only from humans.

Growth Requirements
Media

Pasteurella organisms are often isolated with other flora from numerous sites, including wounds, abscesses, blood, and respiratory specimens. No special transport or plating media are needed because the organisms grow well on blood and chocolate agar plates. Most strains, except *P. aerogenes* and *P. haemolytica*, do not grow on MacConkey agar.

Environmental requirements

Pasteurella spp. grow in air temperatures of 22° and 44° C with an optimum of 37° C. Colonies are usually visible at 24 hours.

Cultural Characteristics
Staining reactions

In Gram-stained smears from tissue, *P. multocida* usually appears as tiny coccobacilli that are 0.3 to 0.5 μm by about 1 μm. The organisms can become pleomorphic with rods up to 5 μm long after growth on solid media. The other species of *Pasteurella* are larger than *P. multocida*, being 0.5 to 1.0 by 1 to 2 μm, with some having a tendency to form fila-

ments. *P. multocida* and *P. haemolyticum* can produce a capsule. Although bipolar staining can be seen in some stains under special circumstances, it is not a reliable characteristic.

Colonial morphology

Clinical isolates of *P. multocida* are often smooth and gray (Plate 21, *B*), although rough and mucoid variants can occur. *P. multocida* and all other species except *P. haemolytica* are nonhemolytic on sheep blood agar. Many strains of the genus *Pasteurella* produce a brownish discoloration on blood agar.

Biochemical Identification[6,30]

Characteristics that separate *Pasteurella* spp. are shown in Table 22-4. All of the species ferment glucose, but only *P. aerogenes* and some strains of *Pasteurella* new species 1 form gas. *P. multocida* is distinguished from the other species by its ornithine decarboxylase, indole, and urease reactions. All of the species are oxidase positive when tested by the tetramethyl-*p*-phenylenediamine dihydrochloride reagent, and all reduce nitrates. All except some strains of *P. ureae* and *P. haemolytica* are catalase positive.

P. multocida can be separated into at least five biotypes on the basis of sugar fermentations. The species can also be separated into four capsular types (A, B, D, and E) and about 20 somatic antigen (lipopolysaccharide) serotypes (numbered 1 to 20). Some biochemical and serologic types tend to be associated with certain animals and diseases. For example, A:1 and A:3 are the causative agents of fowl cholera. Knowledge of the biotypes and the serotypes is useful for epidemiologic studies.

P. haemolytica also has biotypes and serotypes that are distinguished in part by their reactions for esculin hydrolysis and fermentation of xylose, mannose, and mannitol.

Clinical Significance[6,30,31]

P. multocida is found as normal respiratory flora in a wide variety of wild and domestic animals including cats, dogs, lynx, rats, rabbits, panthers, and some fowl. However, it can cause hemorrhagic septicemia in cattle and buffalo and avian cholera in waterfowl, as well as a myriad of other primary and opportunistic infections in animals.

The most common manifestation of human *P. multocida* disease is a localized infection such as cellulitis or abscess subsequent to a cat or dog bite or scratch. The localized infection can progress to osteomyelitis or arthritis. *P. multocida* is reported to be isolated from half of all infections subsequent to dog or cat bites.[12] Less common forms of disease are chronic pulmonary infection and bacteremia. Although *P. multocida* can cause serious respiratory tract infections including pneumonia, emphysema, and lung abscess, it may also be found as a colonizing organism in healthy people and in those with underlying pulmonary disease. The connection with animals has not been defined in the latter two types of infection.

Humans seem to be the only host for *P. ureae*. The connection with disease is tenuous. Most isolates come from the respiratory tract of healthy individuals; however, there are reports of septicemia and meningitis caused by *P. ureae*.[30]

P. haemolytica is both a commensal and a respiratory pathogen in sheep, cattle, and chickens. An occasional human isolate is found.

P. pneumotropica is a normal inhabitant of the oropharynx of mice, rats, cats, and dogs. Most of the rarely reported cases of human infections have been associated with cat or dog bites. The infection can spread to contiguous bone or joints.[11]

P. aerogenes is part of the normal intestinal flora of swine. There are rare reports of human infection subsequent to swine exposure.

P. gallinarum has not yet been associated with human disease. It is part of the normal respiratory flora of poultry but can also cause respiratory disease in these birds.

Mechanisms of Pathogenicity

The mucoid capsule of *P. multocida* has been shown to be a virulence factor by its interference with phagocytic cell function. Neutrophils ingest the bacteria more easily when they are unencapsulated. The portion of the capsule that causes the interference has not been fully defined but does not seem to be hyaluronic acid.[28]

The role in disease of the several soluble toxins produced by *P. haemolytica* is still speculative. The proteolytic enzyme that cleaves the sialoglycoprotein of the erythrocyte membrane may render cells more susceptible to other cytotoxins produced by the bacteria.[24]

Antimicrobial Susceptibility

Pasteurella multocida has been found to be uniformly susceptible to penicillin G and its derivatives (including ampicillin, carbenicillin, and piperacillin). The semisynthetic, antistaphylococcal drugs such as nafcillin are not as strong against the organisms. Other drug groups that are active in vitro are the tetracyclines, the second- and third-generation cephalosporins, and chloramphenicol. Ninety-five percent of the strains in one study were resistant or intermediate to the aminoglycosides.[1] The organisms are resistant to clindamycin and vancomycin and intermediate to erythromycin.

P. aerogenes has been reported to be resistant to penicillin G but susceptible to other beta-lactam antibiotics. The nine strains tested were also susceptible to sufonamides, resistant to the macrolides, and mostly intermediate to the aminoglycosides.[2] Other *Pasteurella* spp. are presumed to have susceptibility patterns similar to that of *P. multocida*.

REFERENCES

1. Bercovier, H., Escande, F., and Grimont, P.A.: Biological characteristics of *Actinobacillus* species and *Pasteurella ureae*, Ann. Microbiol. **135**:203, 1984.
2. Bercovier, H., et al.: Characterization of *Pasteurella aerogenes* isolated in France. In Kilian, M., Frederiksen, W., and Biberstein, E.L., editors: *Haemophilus, Pasteurella,* and *Actinobacillus,* New York, 1981, Academic Press, Inc.
3. Buchanan, T.M., Faber, L.C., and Feldman, R.A.: Brucellosis in the United States, 1960-1972: an abattoir associated disease. I. Clinical features and therapy, Medicine **53**:403, 1974.
4. Buchanan, T.M., et al.: Brucellosis in the United States, 1960-1972: an abattoir associated disease. II. Diagnostic aspects, Medicine **53**:415, 1974.
5. Buchanan, T.M., et al.: Brucellosis in the United States, 1960-1972: an abattoir associated disease. III. Epidemiology and evidence for acquired immunity, Medicine **53**:427, 1974.
6. Carter, G.R.: *Pasteurella.* In Krieg, N.R., editor (Holt, J.G., editor-in-chief): Bergey's manual of systematic bacteriology, Baltimore, 1984, Williams & Wilkins Co.
7. Corbel, M.J., and Brindley-Morgan, W.J.: Genus *Brucella.* In Krieg, N.R., editor (Holt, J.G., editor-in-chief): Bergey's manual of systematic bacteriology, Baltimore, 1984, Williams & Wilkins Co.
8. Eigelsbach, H., and McGann, V.G.: *Francisella tularensis.* In Krieg, N.R., editor (Holt, J.G., editor-in-chief): Bergey's manual of systematic bacteriology, Baltimore, 1984, Williams & Wilkins Co.
9. Field, L.H., and Parker, C.D.: Antibiotic susceptibility testing of *Bordetella pertussis,* Am. J. Clin. Pathol. **74**:312, 1980.
10. Frederiksen, W.: Gas-producing species within *Pasteurella* and *Actinobacillus.* In Kilian, M., Frederiksen, W., and Biberstein, E.L., editors: *Haemophilus, Pasteurella,* and *Actinobacillus,* New York, 1981, Academic Press, Inc.
11. Gadberry, J.L., et al.: *Pasteurella pneumotropica* isolated from bone and joint infections, J. Clin. Microbiol. **19**:926, 1984.
12. Goldstein, E.J., Citron, D.M., and Finegold, S.M.: Role of anaerobic bacteria in bite-wound infections, Rev. Infect. Dis. **6**:S177, 1984.
13. Goodnow, R.A.: Biology of *Bordetella bronchiseptica,* Microbiol. Rev. **44**:722, 1980.
14. Granstrom, M., et al.: Serologic diagnosis of whooping cough by an enzyme-linked immunosorbent assay using fimbrial hemagglutinin as antigen, J. Infect. Dis. **146**:741, 1982.
15. Hall, W.E., and Manion, R.E.: *In vitro* susceptibility of *Brucella* to various antibiotics, Appl. Microbiol. **20**:600, 1970.
16. Hornick, R.: Tularemia. In Braude, A.I., editor: Medical microbiology and infectious disease, Philadelphia, 1981, W.B. Saunders Co.

17. Keppie, J., et al.: The role of erythritol in the tissue localization of the brucellae, Br. J. Exp. Pathol. **46:**104, 1965.

18. Kersters, K., et al.: *Bordetella avium* sp. nov. isolated from the respiratory tracts of turkeys and other birds, Int. J. Syst. Bact. **34:**56, 1984.

19. Kloos, W.E., et al.: Deoxyribonucleotide sequence relationships among *Bordetella* species, Int. J. Syst. Bacteriol. **31:**173, 1981.

20. Manclark, C.R.: Serological response to *Bordetella pertussis.* In Rose, N.R., and Friedman, H., editors: Manual of clinical immunology, ed. 2, Washington, D.C., 1980, American Society for Microbiology.

21. Mannheim, W.: *Pasteurellaceae.* In Krieg, N.R., editor (Holt, J.G., editor-in-chief): Bergey's manual of systematic bacteriology, Baltimore, 1984, Williams & Wilkins Co.

22. McCullough, N.B.: Immune response to *Brucella.* In Rose, N.R., and Friedman, H., editors: Manual of clinical immunology, ed. 2, Washington, D.C., 1980, American Society for Microbiology.

23. Mortensen, J.E., et al.: Antimicrobial susceptibility of clinical isolates of *Brucella,* Diagn. Microbiol. Infect. Dis. **5:**163, 1986.

24. Otulakowski, G.L., et al.: Proteolysis of sialoglycoprotein by *Pasteurella haemolytica* cytotoxic culture supernatant, Infect. Immun. **42:**64, 1983.

25. Pertussis—England and Wales, MMWR **31:**629, 1982.

26. Pittman, M.: Genus *Bordetella.* In Krieg, N.R., editor (Holt, J.G., editor-in-chief): Bergey's manual of systematic bacteriology, Baltimore, 1984, Williams & Wilkins Co.

27. Regen, J., and Lowe, F.: Enrichment media for the isolation of *Bordetella,* J. Clin. Microbiol. **6:**303, 1977.

28. Ryu, H., et al.: Effect of type A *Pasteurella multocida* fractions on bovine polymorphonuclear leukocyte functions, Infect. Immun. **43:**66, 1984.

29. Snyder, M.J.: Immune response to *Francisella.* In Rose, N.R., and Friedman, H., editors: Manual of clinical immunology, ed. 2, Washington, D.C., 1980, American Society for Microbiology.

30. Weaver, R.E., Hollis, D.G., and Bottone, E.J.: Gram-negative fermentative bacteria and *Francisella tularensis.* In Lennette, E.H., et al., editors: Manual of clinical microbiology, ed. 4, Washington, D.C., 1985, American Society for Microbiology.

31. Weber, D.J., et al.: *Pasteurella multocida* infections, Medicine **63:**133, 1984.

32. Weber, M.L., et al.: Oculoglandular tularemia, Clin. Microbiol. Newsletter **6:**36, 1984.

33. Weiss, A.A., and Falkow, S.: Genetic analysis of phase change in *Bordetella pertussis,* Infect. Immun. **43:**263, 1984.

34. Weiss, A.A., et al.: Tn5-induced mutation affecting virulence factors of *Bordetella pertussis,* Infect. Immun. **42:**33, 1983.

35. Westerman, E.L., and McDonald, J.: Tularemia pneumonia mimicking legionnaires' disease: isolation of the organism on CYE agar and successful treatment with erythromycin, South, Med. J. **76:**1169, 1983.

36. Young, E.J.: Human brucellosis, Rev. Infect. Dis. **5:**821, 1983.

37. Zackrisson, G., et al.: *In vitro* sensitivity of *Bordetella pertussis,* J. Antimicrob. Chemother. **11:**407, 1983.

CHAPTER 23

Campylobacter

Alice S. Weissfeld
Raymond L. Kaplan

Campylobacter organisms are curved, oxidase-positive, nonsporeforming, microaerophilic, gram-negative rods; they are motile by means of a single polar flagellum. They were originally classified in the genus *Vibrio* but were removed from this genus because (1) unlike the *Vibrio* spp., they are nonfermentative, and (2) their DNA base ratios are lower (29% to 35%) than those of *Vibrio* organisms (45%).[38]

Although *Campylobacter* spp. were recognized as a possible cause of human gastroenteritis as early as the late 1950s,[19] they were not recognized as a common human pathogen until the 1970s, when selective techniques for isolation of the organisms from stool were introduced.[7,34] Today, the genus *Campylobacter* is recognized as one of the leading causes of bacterial diarrhea worldwide.[5,25,29]

CLASSIFICATION

The genus *Campylobacter* is listed in section 2 of *Bergey's Manual of Systematic Bacteriology* with the "Aerobic/Microaerophilic, Motile, Helical/Vibroid Gram Negative Bacteria."[35] The genus is not assigned to any family but is grouped with other organisms that have similar morphologic and physiologic characteristics. The name is derived from the Greek *campylo*, curved, and *bacter*, rod. Five different species are listed in *Bergey's Manual: C. fetus, C. jejuni, C. coli, C. sputorum,* and *C. consisus. C. fetus* is divided into two subspecies, *C. fetus* ssp. *fetus* and *C. fetus* ssp. *venerealis. C. jejuni* and *C. coli* were also previously considered subspecies of *C. fetus,* but DNA hybridization studies have shown those organisms to be two separate species.[24] *C. jejuni* and *C. coli* are identical except in the ability to hydrolyze hippurate; *C. jejuni* is hippurate positive and *C. coli* is hippurate negative.[11] *C. sputorum* is divided into three subspecies, *C. sputorum* ssp. *sputorum, C. sputorum* ssp. *bubulus,* and *C. sputorum* ssp. *mucosalis.* Table 23-1 lists the current nomenclature from *Bergey's Manual* as well as previous designations. Table 23-2 lists other *Campylobacter* spp. and their previous designations. These organisms are not commonly found in clinical specimens.

C. fecalis, C. sputorum ssp. *bubulus, C. sputorum* ssp. *mucosalis,* and *C. fetus* ssp. *venerealis* are principally recovered from animals and are not normally isolated in the clinical microbiology laboratory. *C. sputorum* ssp. *sputorum* is part of the normal human oral flora. *C. fetus* ssp. *fetus, C. jejuni,* and *C. coli* are the major human pathogens. *C. fetus* ssp. *fetus* is principally a bloodborne pathogen that causes a variety of diseases in immunocompromised hosts, and *C. jejuni* and *C. coli* cause gastroenteritis. *C. pylori* has been isolated from human gastric biopsy specimens.

SPECIMEN COLLECTION AND PROCESSING

Blood for culture of *C. fetus* ssp. *fetus* may be collected into any standard blood culture medium. Stool specimens or rectal swabs should be obtained from individuals with diarrhea for isolation of the enteric campylobacters (*C. jejuni, C. coli,* and *C. laridis*).

Stool specimens or rectal swabs can be plated as they arrive in the laboratory or refrigerated for several hours. Rectal swabs are an adequate alternative when a stool specimen cannot be obtained. Stools may be passed through a 0.65 μm filter that retains larger fecal organisms, and the filtrate than can be cultured on a nonselective medium.[7]

If a stool specimen or rectal swab cannot be processed within 4 hours of collection, it should be placed in Cary-Blair transport medium.[32] Although enteric *Campylobacter* (EC) spp. survive in stool for up to 2 weeks at 4° C, *Shigella* organisms do not maintain their viability at this temperature. When the stool is placed in Cary-Blair medium, the viability of the majority of bacterial pathogens in the specimen is ensured. Buffered-glycerol saline, which is a common stool transport medium, is toxic for EC and should not be used.

GROWTH REQUIREMENTS
MEDIA

Campylobacter fetus ssp. *fetus* grows in most blood culture broth media. When the Gram stain suggests *Campylobacter* spp. (see "Cultural Characteristics"), the broth medium should be subcultured to a blood-containing medium and incubated in an appropriate atmosphere (see "Environmental Requirements"). Growth is usually apparent within 48 hours.

Ideally, routine processing of stool or rectal swabs for EC should include direct inoculation onto a selective agar medium (if the more cumbersome and time-consuming filtration technique is not used), as well as inoculation into Campy Thio[2] for the indirect method. Campy Thio (Appendix A) is thioglycolate broth with 0.16% agar and the antimicrobics found in a Campy BAP. It is not an enrichment broth, but it enhances recovery of EC by reducing competitive enteric flora and perhaps by concentrating EC into a narrow layer in the Campy Thio where the oxygen concentration suits the isolate. Specimens should be inoculated into the upper inch of the Campy Thio which should be subcultured to a selective agar medium after overnight incubation at 4° C.[15] This method has been shown to increase the recovery of EC from clinical specimens.[31] Two recently developed enrichment broths increased EC recovery from feces[6,22]; field trials with these new media will be necessary, however, before their utility can be confirmed.

TABLE 23-1. Species of the Genus *Campylobacter*

Bergey's Manual	Previous Designations and Synonyms
C. fetus ssp. *fetus*	*Vibrio fetus* var. *intestinalis*; *Campylobacter fetus* ssp. *intestinalis*
C. fetus ssp. *venerealis*	*Vibrio fetus* var. *venerealis*; *Campylobacter fetus* ssp. *fetus*
C. jejuni	"Related vibrios"; *Vibrio jejuni*; *Campylobacter fetus* ssp. *jejuni*
C. coli	"Related vibrios"; *Vibrio jejuni*; *Campylobacter fetus* ssp. *jejuni*
C. sputorum ssp. *sputorum*	*Vibrio sputorum*
C. sputorum ssp. *bubulus*	*Vibrio bubulus*; *Campylobacter bubulus*; *Vibrio sputorum* var. *bubulum*
C. sputorum ssp. *mucosalis*	None
C. consisus	None

TABLE 23-2. Other *Campylobacter* Organisms

Current Designation	Previous Designation
C. fecalis	None
C. laridis	NARTC[a]
C. cinaedi	CLO-1[b]
C. fennelliae	CLO-2[b]
C. pylori[c]	Pyloric campylobacters
C. hyointestinalis	None

[a]Nalidixic acid–resistant thermophilic campylobacters.
[b]*Campylobacter*-like organisms.
[c]*Campylobacter pylori* was originally named *Campylobacter pylordis*. However, this original nomenclature was a linguistic error and the name was revised.

Several selective agar media are available for the cultivation of EC. The most commonly used medium in the United States is Campy BAP (Appendix A). This medium is a Brucella agar base containing 10% sheep red blood cells and the five antimicrobial agents vancomycin, trimethoprim, polymyxin B, amphotericin B, and cephalothin.[2] Campy BAP and Campy Thio are available from most commercial manufacturers. Two other selective media that have been used successfully are Butzler medium and Skirrow medium.[5] Skirrow medium contains lysed defibrinated horse blood and only three antimicrobics (vancomycin, polymyxin B, and trimethoprim) in Oxoid Blood Agar Base No. 2 (Oxoid, U.S.A., Columbia, Md.). Butzler medium contains 10% sheep blood in a fluid thioglycolateum to which agar is added; it contains five different antimicrobial agents (bacitracin, novobiocin, actidione, colistin, and cefazolin). Recently Butzler[4] reported the development of a new selective medium (medium V) containing cefoperazone, rifampin, colistin, and amphotericin B; this medium more effectively suppressed competing normal fecal flora than the original formulation. A larger inoculum can be used on Butzler and Campy BAP plates, because they are more inhibitory than Skirrow medium.

To isolate C. *pylori*, biopsy specimens should be inoculated onto chocolate agar, incubated as for EC (see "Environmental Requirements") at 37° C, and examined daily for 7 days.

ENVIRONMENTAL REQUIREMENTS

Enteric *Campylobacter* organisms are microaerophilic and capnophilic. Most isolates do not grow anaerobically. Exposure of specimens or inoculated plates to ambient air for a short period of time does not harm them. Ideally the atmosphere

should contain 5% to 10% O_2 and 10% CO_2. Several methods are available to create this environment:

1. Campy Pak II System (BBL, Cockeysville, Md.) or Gas Generating Kit Systems BR 56 (Oxoid, U.S.A., Columbia, Md.). Both systems employ special gas-generating envelopes that are activated by the addition of water. No more than eight plates should be placed in a jar. There is approximately a 1-hour delay between the time an envelope is activated and suitable atmospheric conditions are achieved.

2. Evacuation replacement system. A torbal jar is evacuated twice to a pressure of 15 inches of mercury and refilled each time with one of several gas mixtures, which are (a) 10% CO_2, 90% N_2, (b) 5% CO_2, 10% H_2, and (c) 10% CO_2, 10% H_2, 80% N_2.

3. Bio-Bag Type CFJ (Marion Scientific, Kansas City, Mo.). A single plate and a generator ampule are placed into each bag, and the bag is heat sealed. After the generator ampule is crushed, an atmosphere of 5% to 10% O_2 and 8% to 10% CO_2 is achieved in the bag. An advantage of this system is that a plate can be examined at any time without removal from the bag.

4. Poly Bag system.[15] Polyethylene bags (Levin Bros. Paper Co., Chicago, Ill.) are filled with six to eight agar plates. The bag is then inflated (with a gas mixture containing 5% O_2, 10% CO_2, and 85% N_2), deflated, reinflated, and tied off with a rubber band. The Poly Bag system is cost effective (approximately 10 cents per bag), and the bag may be opened and regassed at any time without affecting the growth of any organisms already incubating. An 8 by 15 inch bag should not be filled with more than eight plates, however, because organisms growing on the plates deplete the oxygen content to an unsuitable level.

5. Bacti-Gas Station (Scott Laboratories, Inc., Fiskeville, R.I.). A small countertop or wall-mounted model Campy gas cylinder (5% O_2, 10% CO_2, 85% N_2) is used to fill single or multiple plate environmental double zip-locked bags. The environmental bags may be reused, and the system is easy and economical to use.

6. Fortner principle.[17] A Campy BAP and a plate inoculated with a facultative organism such as *Proteus* spp. or

Escherichia coli are placed inside a plastic zip-locked bag. As the facultative organism grows, it reduces the oxygen content inside the bag to a level that is acceptable for growth of EC. Cultures should be held at least 72 hours if this system is used, because EC organisms do not grow until the facultative organism has grown and lowered the oxygen tension.

7. Candle extinction jar. A candle jar is probably the least satisfactory system because it relies on the presence of facultative breakthrough organisms growing on the selective Campylobacter medium to reduce the oxygen tension below that initially produced when the candle is extinguished. Total incubation time should be extended to 72 hours with this system to detect all *Campylobacter* organisms.

The enteric *Campylobacter* spp. are isolated best at 42° C for two reasons: (1) this is their optimal growth temperature and (2) other organisms that may be present in stool do not grow readily at this higher temperature. *C. fetus* ssp. *fetus* does not grow at this temperature but grows well at 37° C. Because *C. fetus* ssp. *fetus* is a rare isolate from stool,[10] stools and rectal swabs are usually incubated at 42° C. Subcultures of blood should be incubated at 37° C to ensure the isolation of both EC and *C. fetus* ssp. *fetus*.

Cultures for EC should be examined daily for 48 hours. Blood culture subculture plates should be held a minimum of 48 hours before discarding.

CULTURAL CHARACTERISTICS
STAINING REACTIONS

Campylobacter spp. are gram-negative, thin, curved rods, 0.2 to 0.8 by 0.5 to 5 μm. They do not stain well with the conventional Gram stain. Carbol-fuchsin is a better counterstain; if safranin is used, it should be applied for 2 to 3 minutes. ECs are pleomorphic in smears at 18 to 24 hours and may appear as short curves, S shapes, gull-wing shapes, and long spirals (Plate 21, *C*); in older cultures, organisms may appear coccoid.[16] Both the standard Gram stain[14] and a Gram stain using carbol-fuchsin as a counterstain[33] have been used to rapidly diagnose *Campylobacter* enteritis from direct stool smears (Plate 21, *D*). Darkfield microscopy of feces for presumptive diagnosis of *Campylobacter* enteritis[26] has also been attempted; diarrheic stools containing ECs show characteristic darting motility.

COLONIAL MORPHOLOGY

Colonies of *C. fetus* ssp. *fetus* and ECs are 1 to 2 mm in diameter, smooth, convex, and translucent. Two colony types of EC may be seen. The first is nonhemolytic, round, and raised, and the second is nonhemolytic, flat, and spread along the streak line (Plate 21, *E*). A small percentage of ECs are tan or slightly pink.[15]

BIOCHEMICAL IDENTIFICATION

Campylobacter spp. may be divided on the basis of whether they produce catalase. Differentiation of the catalase-positive species is shown in Table 23-3. The catalase-negative species (*C. sputorum*) are not usually isolated in the clinical microbiology laboratory.

Presumptive identification of EC from stools or rectal swabs may be made if the isolate displays characteristic Gram stain

TABLE 23-3. Differentiation of Catalase-Positive *Campylobacter* Spp.

Species	Oxidase	Motility	H₂S (Lead Acetate Strips)	H₂S (Iron-Containing Media)	Nalidixic Acid (30 μg Disk)	Cephalothin (30 μg Disk)	Nitrate Reduction	Growth in 1% Glycine	Growth at 3.5% NaCl	Growth at 1% Bile	Growth at 25° C	Growth at 35° C	Growth at 42° C
C. jejuni/coli	+	+	+	−	S	R	+	+	−	+	−	+	+
C. laridis	+	+	+	−	R	R	+	+	−		−	+	+
C. fetus ssp. *fetus*	+	+	v	−	R	S	+	+	−	+	+	+	−ᵃ
C. fetus ssp. *venerealis*	+	+	−	−	v	S	+	−	−	+	+	+	−
C. fecalis	+	+	+	+	v	S	+	+	v	v	−	+	+
C. pylori	+	+	+	−	R	S	−	v	−		−	+	v

SYMBOLS: +, >90% strains positive
−, >90% strains negative
v, 10%–90% strains positive
a, Rare strains grow at 42° C
R, Resistant
S, Sensitive

morphology, is oxidase positive (using a heavy inoculum and the tetramethyl-*p*-phenylenediamine dihydrochloride reagent), and is catalase positive. The importance of performing a Gram stain on all suspected *Campylobacter* isolates cannot be over-emphasized because other oxidase-positive bacteria (such as *Aeromonas* spp., *Bordetella bronchiseptica*, *Pseudomonas* spp., *Achromobacter* spp., CDC group EF-6, and *Bacillus* spp.) grow on selective media at 42° C under microaerophilic conditions.[3,23] Isolates may also be examined for characteristic darting motility using phase contrast or darkfield microscopy. The isolate should be suspended in Brucella or tryptic soy broth, since distilled water and saline appear to inhibit motility.

A McFarland no. 1 standard suspension of the organism in sterile distilled water may be used to inoculate the biochemical tests necessary to differentiate *C. fetus* ssp. *fetus* and EC. An 0.5 ml aliquot can be added to Brucella broth to test for growth at 25°, 35°, and 42° C; the suspension can also be used to swab a blood agar plate for the determination of the sensitivity of the isolate to nalidixic acid and cephalothin.

C. pylori can be identified presumptively by the presence of strong urease activity. In Christensen medium a color change is usually observed in as little as 10 minutes.[22b]

SEROLOGIC AND IMMUNOSEROLOGIC IDENTIFICATION

Antibodies in patient sera can be detected using agglutination or fluorescent antibody tests. Serologic tests are rarely used diagnostically; however, they can be of value in investigation of an outbreak of gastroenteritis caused by an EC.

Several investigators have developed reagents for serotyping EC (for epidemiologic purposes) but these are not routinely available.[13,20,27] Despite the existence of approximately 55 serotypes of EC, only a few serotypes have been recovered from human infections.

OTHER IDENTIFICATION METHODS

Because serotyping of isolates is not practical for most clinical microbiologists, a biotyping schema has been developed to subdivide EC.[12] Strains of EC have been placed into eight biotypes on the basis of hippurate hydrolysis, DNA hydrolysis, and growth on charcoal yeast extract agar.

CLINICAL SIGNIFICANCE

C. fetus ssp. *fetus* has a predilection for infecting debilitated, immunosuppressed, or elderly patients[10] and is most commonly isolated from the blood of these patients. This species is rarely the cause of enteritis.

C. jejuni is currently one of the leading causes of bacterial diarrhea worldwide. The disease begins with vague abdominal discomfort following an incubation period of 2 to 10 days. Symptoms progress to crampy abdominal pain, bloody diarrhea, chills, and fever; nausea and vomiting are uncommon. The illness is self-limiting for most patients, and symptoms usually resolve in 3 to 6 days. Untreated patients may excrete the organism for up to several months.[25]

Epidemics of *Campylobacter* enteritis have been linked to milk[30] and water[36]; chickens are also a major source of the organism.[9] The incidence of infection appears to be greatly increased during the summer months.[5] Children under 1 year of age and adults 20 to 29 years old seem most affected. *Campy-*

lobacter spp. are also transmitted sexually.[21,28]

Campylobacter pylori is associated with gastritis and probably also associated with gastric ulcers, although its significance in causing these diseases has not been resolved.[3a]

MECHANISMS OF PATHOGENICITY

The exact mechanism(s) of pathogenicity of the genus *Campylobacter* has yet to be established. Currently there is a lack of suitable in vitro or in vivo models of pathogenesis. An animal model is essential for the assessment of virulence factors. At the Third International Workshop on Campylobacter Infections (July 1985) several animal models and mechanisms of pathogenicity were presented. (The proceedings of the workshop is titled *Campylobacter III* and is published by the Public Health Laboratory Service, England and Wales, through PSG, Inc., Littleton, Mass.) The animal models included marmosets, ferrets, mice, and rabbits. *Campylobacter* spp. were shown to have the following attributes: positive chemotaxis or motility to mucin, the ability to adhere to cells, the ability to produce an enterotoxin, the ability to produce a cytotoxin, the ability to penetrate cells, and the ability to survive intracellularly after phagocytosis.

The development of immunity to some isolates of *C. jejuni* has been proposed. Black and his colleagues[1] have performed volunteer studies in which 20 adults ingested approximately 10^8 or 10^9 *C. jejuni* in milk; nine subjects developed diarrhea. Seven of the ill volunteers were rechallenged with 10^9 of the same strain, along with 12 new volunteers. None of the original group became ill, although six of the 12 new volunteers developed diarrhea. This study shows the existence of at least short-term homologous protective immunity in humans.

ANTIMICROBIAL SUSCEPTIBILITY

In vitro sensitivity testing of *Campylobacter* organisms is not standardized and is usually not performed routinely. Most patients have a spontaneous recovery without antimicrobial agents. Only a small percentage of *C. jejuni* strains are resistant to erythromycin, the drug of choice in treating diarrhea. It appears that *C. coli* may be slightly more resistant to erythromycin than *C. jejuni*.[8] A 15 μg erythromycin disk may be placed on the same plate used to test sensitivity to nalidixic acid and cephalothin.

C. jejuni is also susceptible to tetracycline, gentamicin, chloramphenicol, and clindamycin and resistant to ampicillin, penicillin, cephalothin, and metronidazole.[37]

Systemic *Campylobacter* spp. infections are usually treated with gentamicin, but tetracycline, erythromycin, and chloramphenicol are good alternatives.

REFERENCES

1. Black, R.E., et al.: Studies of *Campylobacter jejuni* infections in volunteers, Abstracts of Second International Workshop on *Campylobacter* Infections, Abstract #20, p. 9, London, 1983, Public Health Laboratory Service.
2. Blaser, M.J., et al.: *Campylobacter* enteritis: clinical and epidemiologic features, Ann. Intern. Med. **91**:179, 1979.
3. Borczyk, A., Chang, D., and Hodge, D.: *Bacillus* species mimicking *Campylobacter jejuni* on selective plating medium, Clin. Microbiol. Newsletter **5**:38, 1983.
3a. Buck, G.E., et al.: Relation of *Campylobacter pylordis* to gastritis and peptic ulcer, J. Infect. Dis. **153**:664, 1986.

4. Butzler, J.P., De Boeck, M., and Goossens, H.: New selective medium for isolation of *Campylobacter jejuni* from faecal specimens, Lancet **2**:818, 1983.

5. Butzler, J.P., and Skirrow, M.B.: *Campylobacter* enteritis, Clin. Gastroenterol. **8**:737, 1979.

6. Chan, F.T.H., and Mackenzie, A.M.R.: Enrichment medium for isolation of *C. fetus* ss. *jejuni* from stools, J. Clin. Microbiol. **15**:12, 1982.

7. Dekeyser, P., et al.: Acute enteritis due to related vibrio: first positive stool cultures, J. Infect. Dis. **125**:390, 1972.

8. Fliegelman, R.M., et al.: Comparative *in vitro* activities of twelve antimicrobial agents against *Campylobacter* species, Antimicrob. Agents Chemother. **25**:504, 1985.

9. Grant, I.H., Richardson, N.J., and Bokkenheuser, V.D.: Broiler chickens as potential source of *Campylobacter* infections in humans, J. Clin. Microbiol. **11**:508, 1980.

10. Guerrant, R.L., et al.: Campylobacteriosis in man: pathogenic mechanisms and review of 91 bloodstream infections, Am. J. Med. **65**:584, 1978.

11. Harvey, S.M.: Hippurate hydrolysis by *Campylobacter fetus*, J. Clin. Microbiol. **11**:435, 1980.

12. Hébert, G.A., et al.: 30 years of campylobacters: biochemical characteristics and a biotyping proposal for *Campylobacter jejuni*, J. Clin. Microbiol. **15**:1065, 1982.

13. Hébert, G.A., et al.: Serogroups of *Campylobacter jejuni*, *Campylobacter coli* and *Campylobacter fetus* defined by direct immunofluorescence, J. Clin. Microbiol. **17**:529, 1983.

14. Ho, D.D., Ault, M.J., and Murata, G.H.: *Campylobacter* enteritis: early diagnosis with Gram's stain, Arch. Intern. Med. **142**:1858, 1982.

15. Kaplan, R.L.: *Campylobacter*. In Lennette, E.H., et al., editors: Manual of clinical microbiology, ed. 3. Washington, D.C., 1980, American Society for Microbiology.

16. Kaplan, R.L., and Barrett, J.E.: Monograph: *Campylobacter* 1981, Kansas City, Mo., 1981, Marion Scientific.

17. Karmali, M.A., and Fleming, P.C.: Application of the Fortner principle to isolation of campylobacter from stools, J. Clin. Microbiol. **10**:245, 1979.

18. Karmali, M.A., et al.: The serotype and biotype distribution of clinical isolates of *Campylobacter jejuni* and *Campylobacter coli* over a three-year period, J. Infect. Dis. **147**:243, 1983.

19. King, E.O.: Human infections with *Vibrio fetus* and a closely related vibrio, J. Infect. Dis. **101**:119, 1957.

20. Leor, H., et al.: Serotyping of *Campylobacter jejuni* by slide agglutination based on heat-labile antigenic factors, J. Clin. Microbiol. **15**:761, 1982.

21. Lichtenberger, C.J., and Perlino, C.A.: *Campylobacter* and pelvic inflammatory disease, Ann. Intern. Med. **97**:147, 1982.

22. Martin, W.T., et al.: Selective enrichment broth medium for isolation of *Campylobacter jejuni*, J. Clin. Microbiol. **17**:853, 1983.

22a. Marshall, B.J., and Goodwin, C.S.: Revised nomenclature of *Campylobacter pylordis*, Int. J. Syst. Bacteriol. **37**:68, 1987.

22b. Megraud, F., et al.: Characterization of "*Campylobacter pylordis*" by culture, enzymatic profile, and protein content, J. Clin. Microbiol. **22**:1007, 1985.

23. Moskowitz, L.B., and Chester, B.: Growth of non-*Campylobacter*, oxidase-positive bacteria on selective *Campylobacter* agar, J. Clin. Microbiol. **15**:1144, 1982.

24. Owen, R.J., and Leaper, S.: Base composition, size and nucleotide sequence similarities of genome deoxyribonucleic acids from species of the genus *Campylobacter*, Fed. Eur. Microbiol. Soc. Lett. **12**:395, 1981.

25. Pai, C.H., et al.: *Campylobacter* gastroenteritis in children, J. Pediatr. **94**:589, 1979.

26. Paisley, J.W., et al.: Darkfield microscopy of human feces for presumptive diagnosis of *Campylobacter fetus* subsp. *jejuni* enteritis, J. Clin. Microbiol. **15**:61, 1982.

27. Penner, J.L., and Hennessy, J.N.: Passive hemagglutination technique for serotyping *Campylobacter fetus* subsp. *jejuni* on the basis of soluble heat-stable antigens, J. Clin. Microbiol. **12**:732, 1980.

28. Quinn, T.C., et al.: *Campylobacter* proctitis in a homosexual man, Ann. Intern. Med. **93**:458, 1980.

29. Rettig, P.J.: *Campylobacter* infections in human beings, J. Pediatr. **94**:855, 1979.

30. Robinson, D.D., et al.: *Campylobacter* enteritis association with consumption of unpasteurized milk, Br. Med. J. **1**:1171, 1979.

31. Rubin, S.J., and Woodard, M.: Enhanced isolation of *Campylobacter jejuni* by cold enrichment in Campy-thio broth, J. Clin. Microbiol. **18**:1008, 1983.

32. Sack, R.B., Tilton, R.C., and Weissfield, A.S.: Cumitech 12. In Rubin, S.J., coordinating editor: Laboratory diagnosis of bacterial diarrhea, Washington, D.C., 1980, American Society for Microbiology.

33. Sazie, E.S.M., and Titus, A.E.: Rapid diagnosis of *Campylobacter* enteritis, Ann. Intern. Med. **96**:62, 1982.

34. Skirrow, M.B.: *Campylobacter* enteritis: a "new" disease, Br. Med. J. **2**:9, 1977.

35. Smibert, R.M.: Genus *Campylobacter* Sebald and Veron 1963, 907. In Krieg, N.R., editor (Holt, J.G., editor-in-chief): Bergey's manual of systematic bacteriology, vol. 1, Baltimore, 1984, Williams & Wilkins Co.

36. Tiehan, W., and Vogt, R.: Waterborne *Campylobacter* gastroenteritis: Vermont, MMWR **27**:207, 1978.

37. Vanhoof, R., et al.: Bacteriostatic and bactericidal activities of 24 antimicrobial agents against *Campylobacter fetus* subsp. *jejuni*, Antimicrob. Agents Chemother. **18**:118, 1980.

38. Veron, M., and Chatelain, R.: Taxonomic study of the genus *Campylobacter* Sebald and Veron and designation of the neotype strain for the type species *Campylobacter fetus* (Smith and Taylor) Sebald and Veron, Int. J. Syst. Bacteriol. **23**:122, 1973.

39. Warren, J.R., and Marshall, B.: Unidentified curved bacilli on gastric epithelium in active chronic gastritis (letter), Lancet **1**:1273, 1983.

CHAPTER 24

Legionella

A. William Pasculle
Alice S. Weissfeld

Species of the genus *Legionella* are fastidious, aerobic, gram-negative, nonsporeforming, motile rods. There are currently 22 recognized species, which contain 35 recognizable serologic variants. *Legionella pneumophila*, the Legionnaires' disease bacterium, is the most commonly isolated member of this group of organisms. Legionnaires' disease, the common name for pulmonary infection with *L. pneumophila*, is the prototype of a group of infections, caused by the legionellae, that are often referred to collectively as legionellosis. Although *L. pneumophila* was first recognized as an etiologic agent of human infections in 1977, an unidentified "rickettsia-like" organism isolated in 1947 from a guinea pig injected with whole blood from a patient with a febrile illness of unknown cause has since been shown to be *L. pneumophila*.[2] The earliest known outbreak of Legionnaires' disease occurred among employees of a meat packing plant in Austin, Minnesota, in 1957.[33]

The legionellae are unique among gram-negative bacteria in that greater than 80% of their cellular fatty acids are branched-chain acids. In this respect they more closely resemble gram-positive bacteria such as the corynebacteria and mycobacteria, which contain similar compounds (mycolic acids) with somewhat longer carbon chains. They do not grow on ordinary laboratory media; artificial media must be supplemented with iron and cysteine. At present a confirmed diagnosis of legionellosis is made by isolation of the agent from clinical specimens, demonstration of the organisms in clinical specimens by direct fluorescent antibody staining, or demonstration of a rise in antibody titer against a specific organism. The greatest proportion of cases will be diagnosed when all three tests are performed.

CLASSIFICATION

The organism isolated from lung tissue obtained at autopsy from patients who had died during the epidemic at the 1976 American Legion Convention in Philadelphia was named *Legionella pneumophila* and is the type genus for a new family, *Legionellaceae,* and a new genus, *Legionella*.[4] There are currently 11 serogroups of *L. pneumophila*. In addition, 22 other species that belong in this genus have been discovered. The *Legionellaceae* are gram-negative rods that are catalase positive and require cysteine for growth. Most are motile by means of one to a few polar to subpolar flagella. The flagella of all *Legionella* spp. thus far examined appear to be antigenically similar. The legionellae do not ferment carbohydrates, reduce nitrates, or hydrolyze urea. Most species produce a soluble brown pigment from tyrosine, and all species liquefy gelatin.[5]

Garrity, Brown, and Vickers[18] proposed that the family *Legionellaceae* be divided into three genera, *Legionella, Tatlockia,* and *Fluoribacter*. This proposal was based solely on the determination of the degree of DNA homology between a small number of isolates of the first five recognized *Legionella* spp. These authors suggested that organisms that are 25% or more related belong in the same species. As additional species and serotypes have been discovered, it has become clear that continued use of this artificial scheme of classification would be highly confusing. Almost all workers prefer to consider these organisms as members of a single genus that reflects the phenotypic, antigenic, pathologic, therapeutic, and environmental similarities of these bacteria.[5]

SPECIMEN COLLECTION AND PROCESSING

Specimens of respiratory secretions or lung tissue are required for the cultural diagnosis of legionellosis. Expectorated sputum is often submitted for culture and immunofluorescent staining. The value of sputum as a diagnostic specimen is quite variable because patients with legionellosis usually do not produce large amounts of sputum. Respiratory secretions that may be contaminated with oropharyngeal flora, for example, sputum or bronchial washings, should not be accepted for culture unless a special semiselective medium and decontamination techniques are used. For best recovery and when necessary, respiratory secretions should be collected by the physician using techniques such as transtracheal aspiration or bronchoalveolar lavage. These techniques eliminate or reduce the contamination of the specimen by normal oral bacteria.

Special transport media are not required. If inoculation of the specimen is to be delayed for several hours, refrigeration appears to be a satisfactory method for preservation and transport. If culture is to be delayed for longer than 24 hours, the specimen should be transported in the frozen state ($-70°$ C).

Sputum specimens should be inoculated onto both nonselective and semiselective media. These media, buffered charcoal–yeast extract (BCYE-alpha) and BMPA-alpha, are described in more detail later in the chapter. In addition, sputum specimens should be treated with acid to selectively kill contaminating bacteria before inoculation on both selective and semiselective media.[1,3]

Aseptically collected specimens can usually be inoculated only onto BCYE-alpha agar. However, it should be borne in mind that legionellosis can occasionally be present concurrently with other recognized pulmonary pathogens, which may overgrow the legionellae on nonselective media.

One fourth to one half of the plate is usually spot inoculated with a liquid specimen and the other half streaked with a loop to obtain isolated colonies on the remaining half of the plate. Tissue specimens may be slid across the surface of the medium, or a suspension may be made emulsifying the tissue in phosphate-buffered saline, pH 7.2.[2]

Although only one laboratory-acquired case of legionellosis has been documented, all work that would cause an aerosol, such as homogenization of tissue, should be performed in a biologic safety cabinet. Centrifugation should be done with safety carriers containing an O-ring seal.[2] In addition, it must be noted that other important pathogens, such as *Coccidioides immitis* and *Francisella tularensis,* may grow on these media. Although it is generally safe to work with inoculated plates on the open laboratory bench, workers in areas where cases of tularemia or coccidioidomycosis have been reported should exercise caution and work in a biologic safety cabinet when white fungal or yeastlike colonies or unrecognized bacterial colonies requiring cysteine are present on these media.

Blood for culture should be inoculated into charcoal yeast extract–diphasic blood culture medium.[13,17] *L. pneumophila* has also been isolated from an aerobic radiometric blood culture bottle[8,39]; the organism was recovered following subculture to BCYE-alpha. However, current blood culture methods are not sufficiently sensitive to be relied on solely for diagnosis.

DIRECT EXAMINATION

Direct fluorescent antibody (DFA) staining is now most often used to demonstrate the legionellae in clinical specimens.[7] Although antibody conjugates for all of the known species and serotypes are not yet available, staining of specimens with conjugates for *L. pneumophila* and *L. micdadei* should detect over 85% of all *Legionella* infections. The DFA stain may be used to examine respiratory secretions such as sputum or other specimens and fresh or formalin-fixed lung tissue when available.[31] *Legionella* organisms appear as short, apple-green rods either free or in phagocytes against an easily identified histologic background. The diagnostic sensitivity of this procedure will vary according to the type of specimen. It is about 50% when sputum is employed and about 70% when deep lung specimens such as bronchoalveolar lavage specimens or lung tissue are used.[2,14] Because antibody conjugates are not available for all species, DFA testing should, when possible, be performed in conjunction with cultural techniques because this is the most sensitive diagnostic procedure. The Dieterle silver stain[6] may be useful for detecting the organism in tissue sections; however, this stain is not specific and stains other bacteria as well.

A polyvalent antibody conjugate that contains antibody against the first six serotypes of *L. pneumophila* is available from several commercial manufacturers. When a specimen gives a positive test with such a conjugate, the result should be confirmed using monovalent conjugates, which are available from the same manufacturers. The specificity is excellent, but rare strains of *Pseudomonas fluorescens, Pseudomonas aeruginosa,* and *Bacteroides fragilis* cross-react with the polyclonal DFA conjugates. Recently a monoclonal antibody reagent that reacts with all 10 known serogroups of *L. pneumophila* has been produced. Preliminary studies indicate that this reagent is as sensitive as the polyclonal reagent but perhaps more specific because the just described cross-reactions are eliminated.[15] More important, ''false-positive'' DFA reactions have been reported to occur when tap water was used to prepare DFA reagents. Because the plumbing systems of many large buildings, including hospitals, may be contaminated with *Legionella* organisms, the reagents (phosphate buffer, buffered neutral formalin, and so on) used for DFA staining should be sterilized by membrane filtration to remove these bacteria. This should be done even if deionized water is used because the possibility always exists that bacteria may pass through a deionizing system.

GROWTH REQUIREMENTS
MEDIA

The legionellae do not grow on ordinary laboratory media. *Legionella pneumophila* and several other species were originally isolated using guinea pigs and embryonated hens' eggs. The first artificial medium to be employed was Mueller-Hinton agar supplemented with IsoVitaleX and hemoglobin (MH-IH)[2]; Feeley-Gorman (F-G) agar,[16] CYE agar,[17] and BCYE agar[34] were developed later. Currently, the preferred medium for primary inoculation of tissue, pleural fluids, or transtracheal aspirates is BCYE that has been supplemented with alpha-ketoglutarate[10]; this medium, BCYE-alpha (Appendix A), is now available commercially from several sources. A semiselective medium for culture of sputum and other potentially contaminated specimens has been developed by the addition of cefamandole, polymyxin, and anisomycin to BCYE-alpha. This medium, BMPA-alpha, is also commercially available.

ENVIRONMENTAL REQUIREMENTS

Legionella spp. (except *L. gormanii*) grow in ambient air, particularly when plated on BCYE-alpha agar. Growth is enhanced, however, in a candle extinction jar or in an atmosphere containing 2.5% CO_2. These organisms do not grow anaerobically. Although the legionellae can survive exposure to temperatures ranging from 4° to about 55° C, the optimal incubation temperature for clinical specimens is 35° C.

Legionellae often grow within 3 to 5 days, although plates should be held at least 7 days before the culture is reported as negative. Plates should be examined daily. Maintenance of proper humidity is essential to prevent drying of the plates during prolonged incubation. Many workers prefer to keep inoculated plates in CO_2-permeable polyethylene bags to conserve moisture during incubation.

CULTURAL CHARACTERISTICS
STAINING REACTIONS

Legionellae in clinical specimens do not stain well by the standard Gram stain. They may be stained, however, by several modified techniques such as (1) using just crystal violet and Gram iodine without decolorization (the so-called half a Gram stain); (2) applying the safranin counterstain longer, for example, for 2 minutes; or (3) using a carbol-fuchsin counterstain instead of safranin.[2] The organisms are gram-negative, pleomorphic rods, 0.3 to 0.7 by 2 to 50 μm. Nevertheless, the Gram stain is not sufficiently sensitive to be relied on for diagnosis; direct fluorescent antibody staining is recommended for this purpose. Agar-passaged bacteria are much more readily stained. After passage on agar the bacteria often appear quite pleomorphic, with both filamentous and bacillary forms present. Many of the cells also appear vacuolated, and when stained with Sudan black B the vacuoles appear black and are thought to contain lipids.

L. micdadei, L. bozemanii, and *L. dumoffii* have been reported to stain weakly acid fast in tissue specimens,[43] but these organisms lose this characteristic on agar passage.

COLONIAL MORPHOLOGY

Growth usually appears in 2 to 4 days on BCYE-alpha and in 3 to 5 days on semiselective BMPA-alpha agars. Colonies are initially pinpoint in size but may reach 3 to 4 mm in 5 to 7 days. Colonies are convex, circular, gray, and glistening with an entire edge; they are usually described as having a characteristic cut-glass or ground-glass appearance when illuminated from the side and viewed with a dissecting microscope (Plate 22, *A*).[2] Incubated plates should be examined daily with the dissecting microscope because colonies will be detected about 24 hours sooner than by examination with the naked eye and because *Legionella* colonies exhibit their typical appearance even when they are visible only microscopically.

BIOCHEMICAL IDENTIFICATION

Because the therapy of all infections with *Legionella* spp. is identical, it is of primary importance only that the laboratory be able to identify an organism as a member of the genus *Legionella.* Speciation and serogrouping of isolates are primarily of epidemiologic importance.

Colonies suspected of being *Legionella* should be subcultured to BCYE-alpha agar and a medium that does not contain L-cysteine, such as 5% sheep blood agar; an organism that grows only on BCYE agar may be presumptively identified as a species of *Legionella. L. jordanis* and *L. oakridgensis* are the only species that lose their requirement for L-cysteine on subculture.[32] The legionellae are relatively biochemically inert, and there is not sufficient phenotypic variation among the various species to permit their identification by biochemical testing (Table 24-1). To some degree, however, biochemical testing can be used to separate the legionellae into several groups. A scheme for such testing is depicted in Figure 24-1. Fortunately, all of the required tests are rapid ones for which results are available within 4 hours or less. None of the *Legionella* spp. reduce nitrate, hydrolyze urea, or utilize carbohydrates; all liquefy gelatin, and all are catalase positive. All of the species except *L. oakridgensis* are motile. *L. pneumophila, L. spiritensis,* and *L. feeleii* are the only species that hydrolyze hippurate. Final confirmation of the identity of an organism may be obtained by direct fluorescent antibody staining.

SEROLOGIC AND IMMUNOSEROLOGIC IDENTIFICATION

The diagnosis of legionellosis may also be made by serologic testing. The indirect fluorescent antibody (IFA) test is currently the test of choice.[42] Demonstration (by IFA) of a fourfold or greater rise in antibody titer to at least 1:128 between acute and convalescent phase sera is considered diagnostic. Acute phase specimens should be drawn within 7 days of onset; convalescent phase specimens should be drawn 3 to 5 weeks after onset (rather than 2 weeks after onset, as would be the case for convalescent phase sera for other infectious diseases.) Single or standing titers of 1:256 or greater simply provide presumptive evidence of infection with *Legionella* organisms at an undetermined time and must be interpreted cautiously because titers in asymptomatic individuals are sometimes high[2] and elevated titers may persist for many years after infection.[27] In addition, a large number of antigens would be required to detect antibody against all of the possible species and serogroups of the genus *Legionella.* Again, however, serologic testing for *L. pneumophila* serogroups 1 through 6 will detect a great majority of *Legionella* infections.

Recently several investigators were able to detect *L. pneumophila* antigens in urine and sputum by radioimmunoassay

TABLE 24-1. Phenotypic Properties of the Legionellae

Species	Oxidase	Catalase	Motility	Beta-Lactamase	Fluorescence	Hippurate	Brown Pigment	Gelatin	Number of Serotypes
L. pneumophila	v	+	+	+	Y	+	+	+	10
L. feeleii	−	+	+	−	Y	v	+^w	−	2
L. spiritensis	+	+	+	+	Y	+^w	+	+	1
L. longbeachae	+	+	+	V	Y	−	+	+	2
L. jordanis	+	+	+	+	Y	−	+	+	1
L. oakridgensis	−	+	−	+^w	Y	−	+	+	1
L. wadsworthii	−	+	+	+	Y	−	−	+	1
L. sainthelensi	+	+	+	+	Y	−	+	+	1
L. hackeliae	+	+^w	+	+	Y	−	+	+	1
L. maceachernii	+	+	+	−	Y	−	+	+	2
L. jamestowniensis	−	+	+	+	Y	−	+	+	1
L. santicrucis	+	+	+	+	Y	+	+	+	1
L. micdadei	+	+	+	−	Y	−	−	−	1
L. bozemanii	V	+	+	V	BW	−	+	+	2
L. dumoffii	−	+	+	+	BW	−	v	+	1
L. gormanii	−	+	+	+	BW	−	+	+	1
L. anisa	+	+	+	+	V^a	−	+	+	1
L. cherrii	+	+	+	+	BW	−	+	+	1
L. steigerwaltii	−	+	+	+	BW	−	+	+	1
L. parisiensis	+	+	+	+	BW	−	+	+	1
L. rubrilucens	−	+	+	+	R	−	+	+	1
L. erythra	+	+	+	+	R	−	+	+	1

> **SYMBOLS:** +, Positive
> −, Negative
> +^w, Some strains may be only weakly positive
> V, Variable
> Y, Yellow
> BW, Blue-White
> R, Red

Modified from Brenner, D.J., et al.: Int. J. Syst. Bacteriol. **35:**50, 1985.
[a]Most strains of *L. anisa* fluoresce blue-white.

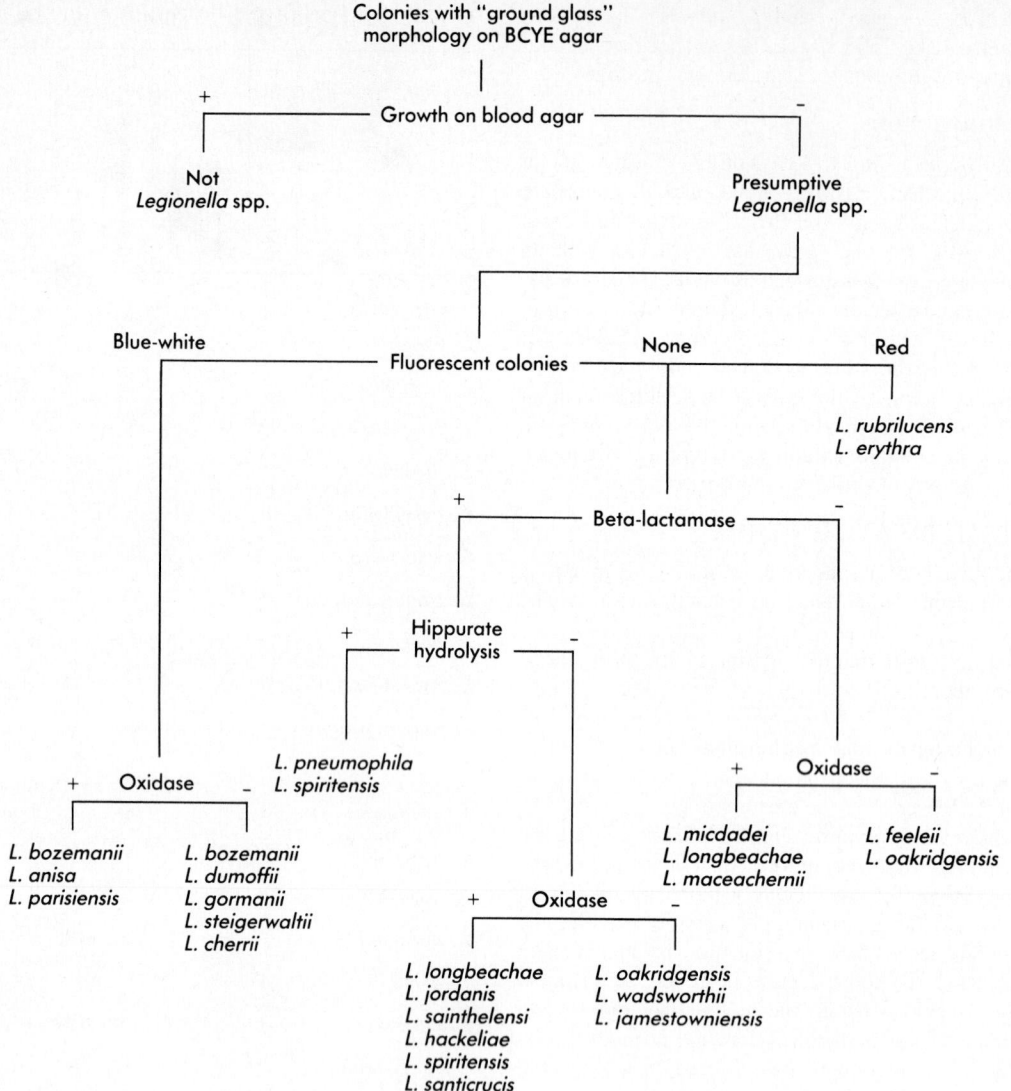

FIGURE 24-1. Presumptive identification of *Legionella* spp. Species and serotype should be confirmed by direct fluorescent antibody testing.

and enzyme-linked immunosorbent assay.[40] These techniques have been shown to be capable of detecting antigen as soon as 3 days after the clinical onset of the disease.[26] At present, however, they are limited to a few research laboratories.

DEFINITIVE IDENTIFICATION METHODS

At present, because specific DFA conjugates for the majority of *Legionella* spp. are unavailable, isolates that cannot be speciated with available reagents must be forwarded to a reference laboratory for identification. DNA hybridization studies and high-pressure or gas-liquid chromatography of branched-chain fatty acids are often used by reference laboratories to aid in the speciation of the legionellae.

CLINICAL SIGNIFICANCE

L. pneumophila infection has two clinical forms[2]: acute pneumonia and an acute, self-limited, nonpneumonic, febrile illness (Pontiac fever). Pneumonic legionellosis is manifested by fever, chills, malaise, and myalgia following an incubation period of 2 to 10 days. This is a multisystem disease of which cough, dyspnea, pleuritic and abdominal pain, vomiting, diarrhea, and delirium are notable clinical features. Hospitalization is frequently required within 3 to 5 days after onset, and the illness is fatal in approximately 15% of cases in the absence of antibiotic therapy. The disease occurs more frequently in males than females and is rarely found in children. The risk of pneumonic legionellosis is higher among cigarette smokers, middle-aged and elderly men, and persons who drink alcohol, receive immunosuppressive medications, or have an underlying disease. It is estimated that 4% to 10% of community-acquired pneumonias in the United States are caused by *Legionella* spp.

Nonpneumonic legionellosis manifests as an acute febrile illness characterized by high fever, chills, myalgias, malaise, and headaches following an incubation period of 24 to 36 hours. This form is remarkable for the absence of pneumonia or fatalities. The first recognized outbreaks of Pontiac fever were caused by *L. pneumophila,* but one outbreak caused by *L. feeleii* has also been described.[20] That both Pontiac fever and Legionnaires' disease can result from exposure to the same environmental source of bacteria has been demonstrated in a case report involving two workers who cleaned an air-conditioning cooling tower. One mechanic developed nearly fatal Legionnaires' disease, but the other developed Pontiac fever.[19]

Most, but not all, of the newly recognized species of *Legionella* have been associated with life-threatening human disease that is virtually identical to Legionnaires' disease. Many of the patients were immunocompromised by their underlying disease or by immunosuppressive therapy before the development of their infection.

Legionella infections can occur in large common-source epidemics, in smaller clusters in presumed hyperendemic areas, or sporadically in isolated cases. Increasing numbers of nosocomial infections have been described. Both epidemic and sporadic cases occur most frequently in summer and early fall. Legionellae have been isolated from water cooling towers or evaporative condensers in air-conditioning systems, from contaminated plumbing fixtures, and from soil. The primary mode of transmission is thought to be airborne, but the isolation of legionellae from a particular environmental source is not in itself evidence that cases of legionellosis are occurring or will occur in association with that source.

MECHANISMS OF PATHOGENICITY

The legionellae are facultative intracellular pathogens. Pulmonary infection most commonly results from inhalation of aerosols containing the organism. Phagocytosis of the invading bacilli, most likely by resident alveolar macrophages, occurs, and many of the invading bacilli are removed from the lung.[9] A few organisms, however, survive and multiply within host phagocytic cells. The survival and multiplication of the bacteria within host phagocytes appear to be related to their ability to inhibit most of the antibacterial defense mechanisms of such cells. Legionellae, for example, appear to inhibit the fusion of lysosomes with phagosomes.[21,22,24]

Studies also suggest that the legionellae may be protected from killing because they are able to inhibit the generation of bactericidal substances within host phagocytic cells. In vitro the legionellae have been found to be susceptible to hydrogen peroxide and to various reactive oxygen intermediates such as superoxide and hydroxyl radicals, which can be generated by phagocytic cells.[29,30] However, treatment of phagocytic cells with legionellae or with certain products of these bacteria has been shown to inhibit the intracellular generation of some of these compounds.[28]

Humoral immunity does not appear to play a major role in defense against *L. pneumophila,* because antibody fails to promote effective killing by polymorphonuclear leukocytes and monocytes and does not inhibit the growth of the organism in monocytes.[24,25] Cell-mediated mechanisms do appear to play an important role in immunity to legionellosis. Lymphocytes from patients who have recovered from legionellosis or mitogen-stimulated cells from normal individuals appear to produce lymphokines, which stimulate the activation of monocytes. These activated cells subsequently inhibit the intracellular rep-

lication of legionellae even though the bacteria are not killed.[23,37]

ANTIMICROBIAL SUSCEPTIBILITY

Susceptibility testing of clinical isolates is not easily performed and need not be done routinely. The legionellae have been shown to be very susceptible to a variety of antimicrobial agents when tested by either agar-diffusion or dilution methods.[12,35,41] However, these in vitro tests do not correctly predict the choice of in vivo chemotherapy because only antimicrobial agents capable of penetrating the cells in which the legionellae multiply are therapeutically effective.[11,36] Most legionellae except *L. micdadei* produce a beta-lactamase. All *Legionella* spp. infections are treated with erythromycin alone or in combination with rifampin. Doxycycline is also sometimes used in place of erythromycin. In addition, studies in model animals suggest that cotrimoxazole (the combination of sulfamethoxazole with trimethoprim) may be effective.[11,36,38]

REFERENCES

1. Beuschling, W.J., Hicklin, R.A., and Ayers, L.W.: Enhanced primary isolation of *Legionella pneumophila* from clinical specimens by low-pH treatment, J. Clin. Microbiol. **17:**1153, 1983.
2. Blackmon, J.A., et al.: Legionellosis, Am. J. Pathol. **103:**429, 1981.
3. Bopp, C.A., et al.: Isolation of *Legionella* species from environmental water samples by low-pH treatment and use of a selective medium, J. Clin. Microbiol. **13:**714, 1981.
4. Brenner, D.J., Steigerwalt, A.G., and McDade, J.E.: Classification of Legionnaire's bacterium: *Legionella pneumophila,* genus novum, species nova, of the family *Legionellaceae,* family nova, Ann. Intern. Med. **90:**656, 1979.
5. Brenner, D.J., et al.: Ten new species of *Legionella,* Int. J. Syst. Bacteriol. **35:**50, 1985.
6. Chandler, F.W., Hicklin, M.D., and Blackmon, J.A.: Demonstration of the agent of Legionnaires' disease in tissue, N. Engl. J. Med. **297:**1218, 1977.
7. Cherry, W.B., et al.: Detection of Legionnaries' disease bacteria by direct immunofluorescent staining, J. Clin. Microbiol. **8:**329, 1978.
8. Chester, B., et al.: Isolation of *Legionella pneumophila* serogroup 1 from blood with nonsupplemental blood culture bottles, J. Clin. Microbiol. **17:**195, 1983.
9. Davis, G.S., et al.: The kinetics of early inflammatory events during experimental pneumonia due to *Legionella pneumophila* in guinea pigs, J. Infect. Dis. **148:**823, 1983.
10. Edelstein, P.H.: Improved semi-selective medium for isolation of *Legionella pneumophila* from contaminated clinical and environmental specimens, J. Clin. Microbiol. **14:**298, 1981.
11. Edelstein, P.H., Calarco, K., and Yasui, V.K.: Antimicrobial therapy of experimentally induced Legionnaires' disease in guinea pigs, Am. Rev. Respir. Dis. **130:**849, 1984.
12. Edelstein, P.H., and Meyer, R.D.: Susceptibility of *Legionella pneumophila* to twenty antimicrobial agents, Antimicrob. Agents Chemother. **18:**403, 1980.
13. Edelstein, P.H., Meyer, R.D., and Finegold, S.M.: Isolation of *Legionella pneumophila* from blood, Lancet **1:**750, 1979.
14. Edelstein, P.H., Meyer, R.D., and Finegold, S.M.: Laboratory diagnosis of Legionnaires' disease, Am. Rev. Respir. Dis. **121:**317, 1980.
15. Edelstein, P.H., et al.: Utility of a monoclonal direct fluorescent antibody reagent specific for *Legionella pneumophila,* J. Clin. Microbiol. **22:**419, 1985.

16. Feeley, J.C., et al.: Primary isolation media for the Legionnaires' disease bacterium, J. Clin. Microbiol. **8:**320, 1978.

17. Feeley, J.C., et al.: Charcoal-yeast extract agar: primary isolation medium for *Legionella pneumophila,* J. Clin. Microbiol. **10:**437, 1979.

18. Garrity, G.M., Brown, A., and Vickers, R.M.: *Tatlockia* and *Fluoribacter:* two new genera of organisms resembling *Legionella pneumophila,* Int. J. Syst. Bacteriol. **30:**609, 1980.

19. Girod, J.C., et al.: Pneumonic and nonpneumonic forms of legionellosis: the result of a common-source exposure to *Legionella pneumophila,* Arch. Intern. Med. **142:**547, 1982.

20. Herwaldt, L.A., et al.: A new *Legionella* species, *Legionella feeleii* species nova, causes Pontiac fever in an automobile plant, Ann. Intern. Med. **100:**333, 1984.

21. Horwitz, M.A.: The Legionnaires' disease bacterium *(Legionella pneumophila)* inhibits phagosome-lysosome fusion in monocytes, J. Exp. Med. **158:**2108, 1983.

22. Horwitz, M.A., and Silverstein, S.C.: The Legionnaires' disease bacterium *(Legionella pneumophila)* multiplies intracellularly in human monocytes, J. Clin. Invest. **66:**441, 1980.

23. Horwitz, M.A., and Silverstein, S.C.: Activated human monocytes inhibit the intracellular multiplication of Legionnaires' disease bacteria, J. Exp. Med. **154:**1618, 1981.

24. Horwitz, M.A., and Silverstein, S.C.: Interaction of the Legionnaires' disease bacterium *(Legionella pneumophila)* with human phagocytes. I. *L. pneumophila* resists killing by polymorphonuclear leukocytes, antibody and complement, J. Exp. Med. **153:**386, 1981.

25. Horwitz, M.A., and Silverstein, S.C.: Interaction of the Legionnaires' disease bacterium *(Legionella pneumophila)* with human phagocytes. II. Antibody promotes binding of *L. pneumophila* to monocytes but does not inhibit intracellular multiplication, J. Exp. Med. **153:**398, 1981.

26. Kohler, R.B., Winn, W.C., and Wheat, W.J.: Onset and duration of urinary antigen excretion in Legionnaires' disease, J. Clin. Microbiol. **20:**605, 1984.

27. Lattimer, G.L., et al.: The Philadelphia epidemic of Legionnaires' disease: clinical, pulmonary and serologic findings two years later, Ann. Intern. Med. **90:**522, 1979.

28. Lochner, J.E., Bigley, R.H., and Iglewski, B.H.: Defective triggering of polymorphonuclear leukocyte oxidative metabolism by *Legionella pneumophila* toxin, J. Infect. Dis. **151:**42, 1985.

29. Lochner, J.E., et al.: Effect of oxygen-dependent antimicrobial systems on *Legionella pneumophila,* Infect. Immun. **39:**487, 1983.

30. Locksley, R.M., et al.: Susceptibility of *Legionella pneumophila* to oxygen-dependent microbicidal systems, J. Immunol. **129:**2192, 1982.

31. Lowry, B.S., Vega, F.G., and Hedlund, K.W.: Localization of *Legionella pneumophila* in tissue using FITC-conjugated specific antibody and a background stain, Am. J. Clin. Pathol. **77:**601, 1982.

32. Orrison, L.H., et al.: *Legionella oakridgensis:* unusual new species isolated from cooling tower water, Appl. Environ. Microbiol. **45:**536, 1983.

33. Osterholm, M.T., et al.: A 1957 outbreak of Legionnaires' disease associated with a meat packing plant, Am. J. Epidemiol. **117:**60, 1983.

34. Pasculle, A.W., et al.: Pittsburgh pneumonia agent: direct isolation from human lung tissue, J. Infect. Dis. **141:**727, 1980.

35. Pasculle, A.W., et al.: Susceptibility of *Legionella micdadei* and other newly recognized members of the genus *Legionella* to nineteen antimicrobial agents, Antimicrob. Agents Chemother. **20:**793, 1981.

36. Pasculle, A.W., et al.: Antimicrobial therapy of experimental *Legionella micdadei* pneumonia, Antimicrob. Agents Chemother. **45:**730, 1985.

37. Plouffe, J.F., and Baird, I.M.: Lymphocyte blastogenic response to *L. pneumophila* in acute legionellosis, J. Lab. Clin. Immunol. **7:**43, 1982.

38. Plouffe, J.F., Para, M.F., and Bollin, G.E.: Sulfamethoxazole-trimethoprim treatment of guinea pigs infected with *Legionella pneumophila,* J. Infect. Dis. **150:**780, 1984.

39. Rihs, J.D., et al.: Isolation of *Legionella pneumophila* from blood with the BACTEC system: prospective study yielding positive results, J. Clin. Microbiol. **22:**422, 1985.

40. Sathapatayavongs, B., et al.: Rapid diagnosis of Legionnaires' disease by urinary antigen detection, Am. J. Med. **72:**576, 1982.

41. Thornsberry, C., Baker, C.N., and Kirven, L.A.: In vitro activity of antimicrobial agents on Legionnaires' disease bacterium, Antimicrob. Agents Chemother. **13:**78, 1978.

42. Wilkinson, H.W., et al.: Indirect immunofluorescence test for Legionnaires' disease. In Jones, G.L., and Hebert, G.A., editors: "Legionnaires": the disease, the bacterium, and the methodology, Atlanta, 1979, Centers for Disease Control.

43. Winn, W.C., and Myerowitz, R.L.: The pathology of the *Legionella* pneumonias, Hum. Pathol. **12:**401, 1981.

CHAPTER 25

Miscellaneous Pathogenic Organisms

Alice S. Weissfeld
Barbara J. Howard
Rebecca D. Almazan
John F. Keiser

GARDNERELLA VAGINALIS

Gardnerella vaginalis is associated with bacterial vaginosis, a polymicrobial infection also involving anaerobic bacteria. This infection, which is characterized by a malodorous discharge, acid pH (5 to 6), presence of clue cells, and minimal or no inflammation of the vaginal epithelium, was previously known as nonspecific vaginitis. The term "bacterial vaginosis" is preferred because the disease shows minimal or no signs of inflammation in the vagina and because of the polymicrobial etiology.[64] It has been suggested that *G. vaginalis* may be sexually transmitted, but most of the supporting evidence is circumstantial.[101]

CLASSIFICATION

Several changes have been made in the taxonomy of *Gardnerella vaginalis* during the last 30 years. In 1955, Gardner and Dukes[49] isolated this small, gram-negative rod from the vaginal secretions of women with nonspecific vaginitis, an infection characterized by the presence of a grayish white malodorous discharge. Because of its morphology and need for certain growth factors present in blood, the organism was named *Haemophilus vaginalis*. Subsequent studies, however, showed that X and V factors were not absolutely necessary for growth, although they did stimulate growth. Zinnemann and Turner[163] studied the *H. vaginalis* isolates of Dukes and other individuals in 1963. The fact that the organisms were pleomorphic and occasionally gram positive and gram variable, like the corynebacteria, led the authors to propose that the organism be reclassified as *Corynebacterium vaginale*. In 1980 Greenwood and Pickett[56] reported DNA hybridization studies and biochemical analyses of the cell wall that revealed the organism to be unique and thus worthy of a new genus. The name *Gardnerella vaginalis* was proposed. The studies of Piot and co-workers[102] supported the suggestion of Greenwood and Pickett. *G. vaginalis* is included in *Bergey's Manual of Systematic Bacteriology*, volume 1, section 5, "Facultatively Anaerobic Gram Negative Rods."[57]

SPECIMEN COLLECTION AND PROCESSING

Cervical, urethral, or vaginal specimens from infected women or urethral specimens from male sexual contacts of these women may be submitted for culture. Vaginal secretions should be collected in duplicate on calcium alginate or cotton-tipped swabs. One swab is plated directly onto the isolation medium (or placed in Amies or Stuart transport medium), and the second swab is used to prepare a wet mount and smear for Gram stain.[100]

G. vaginalis may also be recovered from blood of women with postpartum fever (discussed later) or from neonates with sepsis. Sodium polyanethol sulfonate (SPS) inhibits the growth of *G. vaginalis* in blood culture media, but the inhibition can be overcome by supplementation of most media with gelatin.[108] Bactec 6B and Bactec 7C are not satisfactory for recovery of *G. vaginalis* from blood.[108] *G. vaginalis* may also be recovered from blood by the quantitative direct plating method, which involves direct inoculation of blood onto agar.[77]

DIRECT EXAMINATION

A wet mount examination of vaginal secretions in saline reveals the characteristic "clue cells," which are large desquamated epithelial cells with numerous attached small organisms. A Gram-stained smear of the discharge shows the attached organisms to be gram-negative and gram-variable coccobacilli (*G. vaginalis*) (Figure 25-1). Also of significance in the Gram-stained smear of patients with bacterial vaginosis is the lack of large numbers of gram-positive rods, which represent the lactobacilli that comprise the normal vaginal flora. This is in contrast with normal vaginal smears, which reveal large numbers of large gram-positive rods and few if any gram-variable coccobacilli.

GROWTH REQUIREMENTS
Media

Although *G. vaginalis* is isolated from virtually all women with bacterial vaginosis, it may also be isolated from up to 40% of healthy women.[34] Thus the Gram-stained smear and other clinical features that are discussed below provide a more practical means for diagnosis than culture.[34,100] When laboratory confirmation is desired, the organism may be recovered on semiselective human blood bilayer agar with Tween 80[147] (HBT) or on nonselective vaginalis agar (V agar).[58] Both of these media contain human blood, on which *G. vaginalis* produces beta-hemolysis. The organism also grows well on Columbia–colistin–nalidixic acid (CNA) agar, but it is nonhemolytic on this medium. *G. vaginalis* does not grow on MacConkey agar.

Environmental Requirements

Media are incubated at 35°C in 5% to 10% CO_2 or in a candle jar for 48 hours.

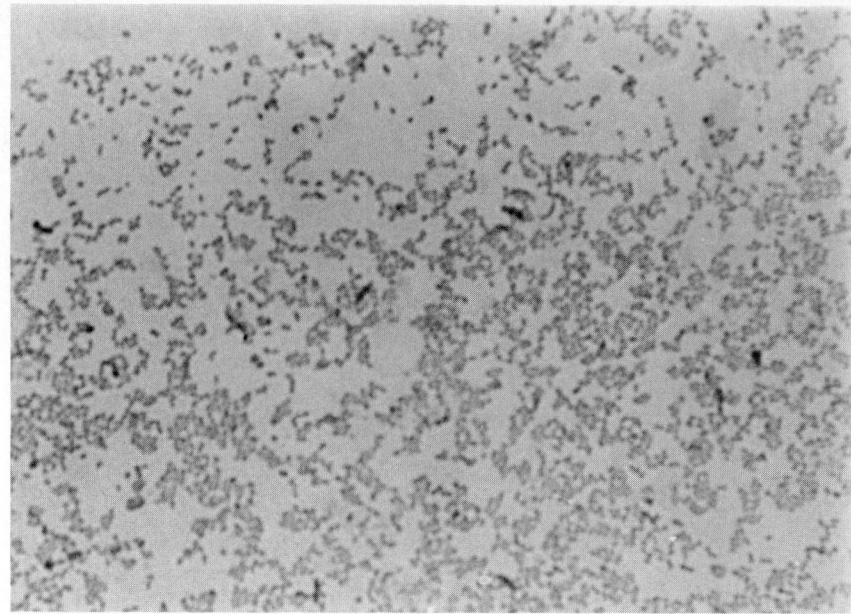

FIGURE 25-1. Gram stain of *Gardnerella vaginalis*. (Photograph by Dr. Leon J. LeBeau, Department of Biocommunication Arts, Medical Center, University of Illinois at Chicago.)

CULTURAL CHARACTERISTICS
Staining Reactions

A Gram stain of colonies of *G. vaginalis* reveals small, gram-negative to gram-variable pleomorphic coccobacilli, some of which have pointed ends (Figure 25-1).

Colonial Morphology

Isolates on HBT medium are beta-hemolytic, opaque, gray, convex, and 0.3 to 0.5 mm in diameter. On V agar, colonies appear opaque, entire, and domed, are approximately 0.5 mm in diameter, and are surrounded by diffuse beta-hemolysis.

BIOCHEMICAL IDENTIFICATION

Observation of beta-hemolytic colonies in HBT medium in combination with a negative catalase test and the presence of thin gram-negative or gram-variable short rods or coccobacilli in a Gram-stained smear allow presumptive identification of *G. vaginalis*.[55,103] Further identification and differentiation of this organism from other catalase-negative, small, gram-variable rods or coccobacilli may be accomplished with hippurate hydrolysis, starch hydrolysis, and the presence of alpha- and beta-glucosidase.[55,103]

Reimer and Reller[109] have recently suggested the combination of susceptibility to a sodium polyanethol sulfonate (SPS) disk and inhibition to alpha-hemolytic streptococci for excellent identification of *G. vaginalis*.

SEROLOGIC AND IMMUNOSEROLOGIC IDENTIFICATION

Fluorescent antibody tests have been used for the identification of *G. vaginalis* in some studies, but these reagents are not routinely available.[100]

CLINICAL SIGNIFICANCE

As mentioned previously, *G. vaginalis* is present in the normal flora of many women, with concomitant problems in the interpretation of culture results. Therefore diagnosis of bacterial vaginosis on the basis of clinical criteria is more practical than diagnosis through culture.[34] According to Amsel and coworker[3] the presence of three of the following four signs signifies the presence of *G. vaginalis* in 98% of cases: (1) vaginal pH above 4.5; (2) characteristic thin, homogeneous vaginal discharge of milklike consistency; (3) liberation of a fishy smell when a drop of 10% potassium hydroxide (KOH) is added to the vaginal discharge; and (4) the presence of clue cells.

Current evidence suggests that *G. vaginalis* and anaerobic bacteria act synergistically to cause bacterial vaginosis.[19,139] *G. vaginalis* generates large amounts of amino acids, and the anaerobic bacteria produce amines such as cadaverine and putrescine from these amino acids, raising the pH to a level that favors the growth of *G. vaginalis*.[19,101] The fishy smell produced when KOH is added to the vaginal secretions (criterion no. 3 above) is attributed to the volatilization of these amines on alkalinization. Numerous anaerobic bacteria, including species of the genera *Morbiluncus* (anaerobic curved rods), *Peptostreptococcus*, and *Bacteroides*, have been recovered from women with bacterial vaginosis.[6] Several studies suggest that mycoplasmas may also play a role in this condition.[64]

G. vaginalis has also been associated with maternal and neonatal septicemia. In fact a recent study suggests that this organism may be a more common cause of postpartum bacteremia, often in association with predisposing conditions such as cesarean section or abortion, than has been previously recognized.[107] The inability of certain blood culture media to support the growth of *G. vaginalis* may be responsible for this underreporting. Bacterial vaginosis has also been associated with premature labor and postpartum endometritis.[35]

ANTIMICROBIAL SUSCEPTIBILITY

Metronidazole is effective in treating bacterial vaginosis, although the organism is often resistant to this drug in vitro.

Because of these inconsistent results, antimicrobial susceptibility testing is not recommended.[100] The efficacy of metronidazole in treating bacterial vaginosis lends support to the theory that anaerobes may play a major role in infection.[110]

MYCOPLASMA

Mycoplasma spp. are the smallest organisms capable of self-reproduction. They are members of the class Mollicutes (from the Latin *mollis*, soft, and *cutis*, skin) and are characterized by the absence of a cell wall. All *Mycoplasma* spp. require sterols for growth; this requirement is usually fulfilled by including horse serum (which contains cholesterol) in the growth medium. Mycoplasmas replicate on artificial media and form typical small colonies embedded in the agar. They are able to pass through filters that retain bacteria (as viruses do), but with the exception of a cell wall, they possess all the cellular constituents of bacteria. Unlike L-forms (bacteria with a defective cell wall), mycoplasmas do not revert to bacteria under appropriate culture conditions. They are susceptible to antibiotics (although not penicillin) and reproduce by binary fission.

Three *Mycoplasma* spp. cause disease in humans; *M. pneumoniae* is principally a pathogen of the respiratory tract, and *M. hominis* and *Ureaplasma urealyticum* are primarily pathogens of the genitourinary tract. *Mycoplasma* spp. frequently contaminate tissue culture cells and can interfere with either cell or viral growth.[61]

CLASSIFICATION

Mycoplasma organisms are included in section 10 of *Bergey's Manual of Systematic Bacteriology*, volume 1.[106] They are members of the family *Mycoplasmataceae*, in the order *Mycoplasmatales*. The family *Acholeplasmataceae* (which does not require sterols for growth) is also in the order *Mycoplasmatales* and contains one genus, *Acholeplasma*. The family *Mycoplasmataceae* contains two genera, *Mycoplasma* (which utilizes arginine and glucose) and *Ureaplasma* (which utilizes urea). There are 51 species in the genus *Mycoplasma* and two species, *U. urealyticum* and *U. diversum*, in the genus *Ureaplasma*. Members of the genus *Ureaplasma* were formerly called T-mycoplasma ("T" for *tiny*) strains because of their small colony size when grown on solid media.

Mycoplasma species that may be encountered in the clinical laboratory include *M. pneumoniae*, *M. salivarium*, *M. fermentans*, *M. genitalium*, *M. orale*, *M. faucium*, *M. baccale*, *M. hominis*, *M. lipophilum*, *M. primatum*, and *U. urealyticum*.[145] *Acholeplasma laidlawii*, formerly *Mycoplasma laidlawii*, may also be isolated.[16]

SPECIMEN COLLECTION AND PROCESSING

Nasopharyngeal or oropharyngeal swabs, sputum, and tracheal aspirates are the specimens of choice for isolation of *Mycoplasma pneumoniae*.[150] Patients may carry the organism in the nasopharynx for 2 to 3 months after infection. Throat swabs, whole blood, urethral discharge, and cervical swabs may be submitted for isolation of *M. hominis*.[143] Specimens likely to contain *Ureaplasma urealyticum* include urethral or vaginal swabs, voided urine, and fetal membranes or tissues.[143]

Blood should be collected in routine blood culture bottles; *M. hominis* will grow in most blood culture media without changing its appearance but is isolated on blind subculture.

Swab specimens should be obtained without the application of any disinfectants, analgesics, or lubricants.[143] Cotton, rayon, or calcium alginate swabs on aluminum or plastic shafts can be used, but wooden shafts cannot. Swabs should be placed immediately into transport media. Fetal membranes and tissue (or other specimens) need not be submitted in transport medium but should not be allowed to dry. Sputum, body fluids, and tissues should be diluted 1:10 or 1:100 with transport medium before inoculation to remove inhibitory substances. Urine should be transported at a temperature of 4°C, centrifuged at 600 × g to deposit epithelial and other cells, and reconstituted in a small amount of supernatant before testing.

GROWTH REQUIREMENTS
Media

A number of different media have been used to propagate the mycoplasmas. Inoculation of both broth and plated media improves the isolation rate[143]; liquid and solid media differ only in that Noble agar is added to the latter. Media are inoculated with a 0.1 ml sample of transport medium (or suitable body fluid). Differential agar medium A7 has been used successfully to isolate the genital mycoplasmas[124]; this medium is available commercially (Remel, Lenexa, Kan.; Gibco Diagnostics, Madison, Wis.). New York City medium, originally described for the isolation of *Neisseria gonorrhoeae*, can also be used to isolate the genital mycoplasmas.[37] Modified New York City medium has been used for growth of *M. pneumoniae*.[54] SP-4 medium,[151] first employed to cultivate *Spiroplasma* organisms, has been used to cultivate newly described glucose-fermenting genital *Mycoplasma* strains,[153] now termed *M. genitalium*, as well as *M. pneumoniae*.[152] Diphasic SP-4 broth cultures prepared in small screw-capped glass vials and SP-4 agar plates are both inoculated. Modified SP-4 broth with arginine and SP-4 broth with urea are especially useful in the recovery of *M. hominis*[154] and *U. urealyticum*, respectively, and provide optimal recovery when used in combination with A7.[41] (These media are discussed in Appendix A.)

Quality control of all media components is extremely important; new lots of media should be tested in parallel fashion, using satisfactory lots and freshly thawed reference strains.

Conventional Mycoplasma broth containing 10% fresh yeast extract, 20% agamma horse serum, and 500 to 1000 units/ml penicillin G is an effective transport medium for *M. pneumoniae* and other mycoplasmas. Sucrose-phosphate transport medium containing 10% heat-activated (56°C for 30 minutes) fetal calf serum but *without antibiotics* may also be used as a good transport medium for *M. hominis* and *Ureaplasma urealyticum*.[143] This medium with antibiotics is usually used for transport of *Chlamydia* organisms, and, as long as antibiotics are not added, mycoplasmal and chlamydial examination can be performed on the same specimen. Adding nystatin to inhibit the growth of fungi is acceptable. Trypticase soy broth with 0.5% bovine albumin has also been used successfully to cultivate both the genital and respiratory mycoplasmas.

Environmental Requirements

Broth culture vials are incubated with the caps tight; agar plates are usually incubated anaerobically. *M. pneumoniae* grows aerobically, although almost none of the other oral species can be isolated under these conditions. *U. urealyticum* is indifferent to the atmosphere in which it is incubated as long as the agar medium is well buffered at pH 6.2. All *Mycoplasma* cultures are incubated at 35° to 37° C. *M. pneumoniae* colonies appear usually after 5 to 14 days of incubation, those of *M. hominis* within 2 to 4 days on solid media, and those of *U. urealyticum* within 24 to 48 hours. Diphasic SP-4 cultures or plain broth cultures should be observed carefully for pH or turbidity changes; when these occur, 0.2 ml of the supernatant medium should be transferred to solid medium. *U. urealyticum* organisms die rapidly in broth cultures after attaining maximum growth, so cultures should be subcultured to agar either every day or immediately on observation of pH changes.

Cultural Characteristics
Staining reactions

Mycoplasmas are too small to visualize with ordinary light microscopy, and they fail to react with organic dyes such as those used in the Gram stain procedure. Thus *M. hominis* septicemia might be suspected when nonhemolytic, pinpoint colonies isolated on blood agar subculture plates incubated anaerobically fail to stain using Gram reagents. These colonies stain, however, when the Dienes stain is used[27]; this is the preferred method for staining mycoplasmas.

Fluorescent dyes that specifically stain DNA[20] or immunoperoxidase staining techniques[63] have been used to identify mycoplasmas in continuous tissue culture cell lines; these stains are actually preferred to culture for preliminary identification of contaminated cells. The Hoescht 33258 stain is available from Flow Laboratories, McLean, Va.

Colonial morphology

The inoculated plates are examined daily by light microscopy using the 10× objective. Colonies of *M. pneumoniae* on primary isolation do not have the typical "fried egg" appearance. Instead, they are usually spherical and slightly granular with a faint lemon-yellow color. Colonial characteristics vary, however, depending on the medium used and the number of colonies on the plate. Other species of large colony–forming mycoplasmas have a dense center of growth that is more deeply embedded in the agar and a more translucent peripheral growth on the surface; colonies are said to resemble fried eggs (Plate 22, *B*). Colonies of *M. pneumoniae* and *M. hominis* vary between 50 and 500 μm in diameter. *U. urealyticum* colonies are very small (15 to 30 μm in diameter) and granular. Characteristic brown accretion colonies form on A7 agar, which contains manganese sulfate ($MnSO_4$) (Plate 22, *C*). If $MnSO_4$ is not incorporated into the agar, the plates must be flooded with urease reagent (which contains $MnSO_4$) before the brown precipitate forms on the *Ureaplasma* colony.

Artifacts (pseudocolonies) must be distinguished from true colonies. Pseudocolonies are composed of magnesium and calcium soap crystals, water droplets, air bubbles, or tissue cells. The Dienes stain can be used to differentiate mycoplasmal from nonmycoplasmal colonies; mycoplasmal colonies stain blue, but most artifacts do not pick up the stain. Bacteria stain blue but usually decolorize within one-half hour.

M. pneumoniae does not produce visible turbidity in broth, but refractile "spherules" can be seen attached to culture vessel surfaces when viewed microscopically. *M. hominis* produces a faint homogeneous turbidity in liquid media, which is best observed with oblique fluorescent light. *U. urealyticum* does not produce turbidity in liquid media. Growth in liquid media is usually detected by a pH change (acid for *M. pneumoniae*, which utilizes glucose, and alkaline for *M. hominis* and *U. urealyticum*, which utilize arginine and urea, respectively). Frankly turbid cultures are probably contaminated by bacteria or fungi.

IDENTIFICATION

Presumptive identification of *Mycoplasma pneumoniae* is made on the basis of colonial morphology and its ability to hemolyze guinea pig red blood cells. The hemolysis test is carried out by overlaying colonies with a layer of 8% guinea pig red blood cells in saline agar and incubating the plate at 35° C for 18 to 24 hours. Colonies of *M. pneumoniae* are surrounded by a clear zone of beta-hemolysis. Identification is confirmed either on subculture using the growth inhibition test with specific antisera or directly from the primary plate using an immunofluorescent antibody test.[150] *M. hominis* does not hemolyze guinea pig red blood cells and is definitely identified using the growth inhibition test. *Ureaplasma urealyticum* is usually identified from the primary plate by virtue of the formation of characteristic brown accretion colonies in the presence of manganese sulfate. If necessary, the identity of the organism is confirmed by the metabolism inhibition test.[143]

SEROLOGIC AND IMMUNOSEROLOGIC IDENTIFICATION

Several serologic tests are available in lieu of culture for the diagnosis of *Mycoplasma pneumoniae*, but not for *M. hominis* or *Ureaplasma urealyticum* infections. For the cold agglutinin test, serial dilutions of the patient's serum are mixed with a suspension of human group O red blood cells and incubated overnight at 4° C. *M. pneumoniae* IgM antibodies react with the I antigen on the red blood cell membrane at 4° C; hemagglutination disappears on warming to 37° C. A single titer of greater than 1:128 is considered significant.

Blood for the cold agglutinin test should be allowed to clot at 22° to 37° C before the serum is removed. Antibodies appear during the first and second week and disappear by the sixth week of illness. However, only one half of patients with proven infections develop cold agglutinins, and these antibodies have also been reported in some nonmycoplasmal diseases, including infectious mononucleosis, rubella, influenza and adenovirus infections, hemolytic anemias, blood dyscrasias, liver diseases, certain allergic conditions, and peripheral vascular disorders.[33] A significant number of patients also develop nonspecific antibodies to *Streptococcus MG-intermedius* (Strep MG test).

Two serologic tests, complement fixation (CF) and metabolism inhibition, are available to demonstrate specific antibodies. Most clinical laboratories perform the CF test with a commercially available lipid antigen. CF antibodies develop during the second and third weeks of illness and persist for 6 to 12 months. A fourfold rise (or fall) in titer between acute and convalescent sera is diagnostic of *M. pneumoniae* infection. The metabolism inhibition test measures the ability of the patient's serum to inhibit growth of *M. pneumoniae*. Unfortunately, the presence of antibiotics in serum may give false-positive results.

The enzyme-linked immunosorbent assay has also been used for serodiagnosis of *M. pneumoniae* infections.[14] A microimmunofluorescence technique has been used to detect antibodies to *M. genitalium*.[48]

CLINICAL SIGNIFICANCE

Mycoplasma pneumoniae (formerly called the Eaton agent) is the major cause of primary atypical pneumonia.[16] *M. pneumoniae* infections are commonly observed in fall and winter and are transmitted from person to person by the droplet route. The peak incidence of infection occurs in late childhood and adolescence, and the organism may account for up to 50% of all cases of pneumonia in college students. The incubation period is 2 to 3 weeks, and the disease begins as a mild upper respiratory infection and progresses to fever, headache, malaise, and persistent dry cough (the most distinct feature of the illness). A chest x-ray film reveals a patchy bronchopneumonia involving one or both lower lobes. The illness is usually mild and self-limited; complications are rare although patients may manifest a skin rash, pleural effusion, otitis media, myringitis, empyema, pericarditis, myocarditis, acute hemolytic anemia, or a neurologic problem.[45]

The association of the genital mycoplasmas with human disease is complicated by the fact that *M. hominis* and *Ureaplasma urealyticum* may be found as part of the normal genitourinary tract flora. *M. hominis* occurs mainly in neonates and sexually active adults. It has been isolated from tissue abscesses and hematomas following severe trauma,[13,97] from women with postpartum fever,[104] from the blood of an infant with severe burns,[25] from neonates with central nervous system infections,[126] and from men following multiple trauma, urinary obstruction, and surgery or catheterization of the urinary tract.[87,146] *M. hominis* has also been associated with acute and chronic pyelonephritis and is a likely cause of pelvic inflammatory disease.[89,144]

U. urealyticum is listed as a cause of nongonococcal urethritis and has been associated with, but not proved to be a cause of, infertility, habitual spontaneous abortion, stillbirth, low birth weight, and the acute urethral syndrome in women.[144] About one third of healthy infants are colonized at birth with *U. urealyticum*, presumably acquired during passage through the birth canal. *Ureaplasma* organisms split urea and may also play a role in the formation of urinary calculi.

Two strains of *M. genitalium*, G-37 and M-30, were isolated originally from urethral specimens obtained from two men with nongonococcal urethritis[145,153]; this *Mycoplasma* sp. may play a role[89] in this disease and also in pelvic inflammatory disease.[88]

All three mycoplasma species known to be pathogenic in humans have been isolated directly from joints of patients with acute arthritis,[16] particularly those suffering from hypogammaglobulinemia.

Attachment, the essential first step in the pathogenicity of *M. pneumoniae,* is mediated by a surface protein designated P1.[67] The organism attaches to a sialoglycoprotein on host cells. The exact mechanism of the subsequent cell injury is unknown, but it has been suggested that the adhering mycoplasmas produce superoxide anions or induce the cells to produce superoxide anions, which lead to oxidative damage of many cell components.[68] Inherent to the pathogenicity of *M. pneumoniae* (and certain other mycoplasmas) is their ability to modulate host immunity.[21,40] These organisms are able to nonspecifically activate B cell production, suppress the initiation of the immune response, and stimulate the production of autoantibodies against host tissues (see Chapter 2).[21,40] The hydrolysis of urea to produce ammonia by *Ureaplasma* spp. may contribute to the pathogenicity of these organisms.[125] Ammonia has been shown to be toxic for several cell lines.[125]

ANTIMICROBIAL SUSCEPTIBILITY

Mycoplasma organisms are sensitive to most broad-spectrum antimicrobial agents (for example, tetracycline and chloramphenicol), but, because they have no cell wall, they are resistant to antimicrobial agents, such as penicillin, that specifically inhibit bacterial cell wall synthesis. Left untreated, acute illness with *M. pneumoniae* usually resolves within 2 to 3 weeks; symptoms disappear or are markedly reduced more rapidly with appropriate therapy, that is, erythromycin or tetracycline.[33] Antimicrobial treatment does not necessarily eradicate the organisms from the respiratory tract, however.

Tetracycline has been used successfully to treat the genital mycoplasmas. Erythromycin inhibits the multiplication of ureaplasmas but does not affect *M. hominis*. Treatment before conception will not necessarily eliminate the genital mycoplasmas for the duration of pregnancy.

In vitro antimicrobial susceptibility testing is not usually performed, although tetracycline-resistant strains of *U. urealyticum* and erythromycin-resistant strains of *M. pneumoniae* have been reported.[10] No standardized procedure is currently available, although a broth disk method has been developed for testing *U. urealyticum*.[138] Urine sediments should be used as the inocula with this method.[76] Modifications of standard agar disk diffusion and agar and broth dilution methods have also been used.

STREPTOBACILLUS

The genus *Streptobacillus* has a single member, its type species, *S. moniliformis*. This organism is one of two agents of rat-bite fever (the other being *Spirillum minor*, discussed later). *S. moniliformis* spontaneously forms L-forms or cell wall–defective variants.

CLASSIFICATION

The genus *Streptobacillus* is included in section 5 of *Bergey's Manual of Systematic Bacteriology*, volume 1, with the gram-negative facultatively anaerobic rods.[119] The organism takes its name from the Latin *moniliformis*, "necklace-shaped." It was named because the distinctive, beaded, necklace-shaped forms that are seen in Gram-stained smears from cultures. The organism is unencapsulated, nonmotile, and nonsporeforming. Synonyms include *Actinomyces muris, Actinobacillus multiformis, Haverhillia moniliformis, Streptothrix muris ratti,* and *Actinobacillus murix*.

SPECIMEN COLLECTION AND PROCESSING

Blood, joint fluid (or other body fluid), and pus and exudate from a cutaneous eruption may be submitted for laboratory examination. Ideally, equal volumes of blood and sterile 2.5% sodium citrate should be mixed,[113] and three separate smears prepared and stained by the Gram, Wayson, and Giemsa procedures. The blood is then centrifuged for 30 to 40 minutes to pack the red cells, and 0.1 ml of the sedimented cells and 0.1 ml of Rogosa broth are mixed and distributed onto the surface of a fresh Rogosa agar plate by gently tilting the plate in several directions. Two tubes of Rogosa broth are also inoculated with 0.1 ml of the sediment. Blood for isolation of *S. moniliformis* can also be inoculated into routine commercial blood culture media, although the concentration of sodium polyanethol sulfonate (SPS) should not exceed 0.025% because this compound has been shown to inhibit growth of the organism when present at higher concentrations.[79]

Joint fluid or other body fluids should be mixed with an equal volume of 2.5% sterile sodium citrate to prevent clotting. Two tubes of broth should be inoculated with at least 1 ml of fluid, an agar medium should be inoculated, and three smears should be prepared and stained as described for blood cultures.

Swabs of pus or exudate from the rash should be inoculated into one tube of broth and one agar plate; again, three smears should be prepared and examined.

GROWTH REQUIREMENTS
Media

Blood, serum, or ascitic fluid is required for growth of *S. moniliformis*. Bacterial-phase organisms (organisms with normal cell walls) can be isolated on any of the common basal media enriched with 15% sterile defibrinated rabbit blood or 20% horse serum; L-forms are preferentially recovered from a clear medium, however. Rogosa medium has been developed for this purpose.[113] Thioglycolate and cooked meat broths support the growth of the organism, although Rogosa medium is preferred if available.

Environmental Requirements

Plates and tubes are incubated at 35° C in a CO_2 incubator or candle jar. Tubes are examined daily for typical fluff balls. If no growth is apparent, 1 ml of broth is transferred to fresh broth tubes daily for at least 3 successive days. Colonies develop on solid media within 3 days of incubation.

CULTURAL CHARACTERISTICS
Staining Reactions

The morphology of the organism is influenced by the media, cultural conditions, and age of the culture. Under optimal conditions, cells appear rodlike and uniform (less than 1 μm by 1 to 5 μm) with occasional short filaments. Under less favorable conditions the organism is highly pleomorphic and may form long, curved, looped filaments. These filaments may consist of a series of oval or elongated bulbous swellings (resembling chlamydospores of yeast) that look like a string of beads; these forms account for the organism's name. *S. moniliformis* is gram negative. However, Giemsa or Wayson stains may be better than the Gram stain in detecting organisms. Bacteria from L-phase colonies exhibit bipolar staining and appear as tiny, gram-negative coccoid or coccobacillary forms.

Colonial Morphology

Bacterial-phase colonies are 1 to 2.5 mm in diameter, round with a discrete edge, low convex or slightly raised, and glistening with a butyrous consistency. On a clear medium, microscopic L-form colonies may be seen beneath or adjacent to bacterial forms. L-phase variants are embedded into the agar and have a "fried egg" appearance (relatively dark center surrounded by a translucent zone containing swollen bodies and what appear to be oil globules); these colonies are observed microscopically using the same techniques as are used to examine *Mycoplasma* colonies. As previously mentioned, L-phase variants are thought to occur naturally.

Growth in liquid medium appears as fluffy balls resembling breadcrumbs and may be confined to the bottom of the tube; bacteria may also settle on the surface of sedimented red cells and stroma.

BIOCHEMICAL IDENTIFICATION

Bacterial-phase inocula are prepared by swabbing colonies from a pure young culture and suspending the growth in 2 ml 0.85% saline; 1 drop of this suspension is then added to each biochemical tube. Testing of L-phase colonies is somewhat more difficult because agar blocks must be cut out and used to inoculate biochemical tests.

Typical biochemical reactions of *S. moniliformis* are shown in Table 25-1. Fermentation reactions are best performed in cystine tryptic agar (CTA) base (BBL, Cockeysville, Md., or Difco Laboratories, Detroit) containing a 1% carbohydrate solution and a drop of ascitic fluid[36] or rabbit serum.[79]

SEROLOGIC AND IMMUNOSEROLOGIC IDENTIFICATION

Agglutinins against *S. moniliformis* appear in patients' serum and are of diagnostic value. Although the test is not routinely available, sera can be titered using the tube agglutination method; a formalin-treated cell suspension of *S. moniliformis* (ATCC 14647) is used as the antigen. Titers higher than 1:80 are usually considered diagnostic. However, a fourfold rise in titer between acute and convalescent sera (drawn at 5- to 10-day intervals) is necessary to confirm a recent infection because titers of 1:80 may persist for at least 2 years.

Specific fluorescent antibody staining using a fluorescein-conjugated anti–*S. moniliformis* reagent has been used to identify colonial isolates.[79] These reagents are not commercially available, however.

OTHER IDENTIFICATION METHODS

Unlike diagnosis of infection caused by *Spirillum minor*, animal inoculation is usually not necessary to make the diagnosis of rat-bite fever caused by *S. moniliformis*. Mice inoculated intraperitoneally with 0.5 to 1 ml of the patient's citrated blood develop either acute infection with septicemia and early death or chronic infection with arthritis or conjunctivitis. Because laboratory animals may be naturally infected with *S. moniliformis*, animals used for diagnostic studies must be carefully screened before inoculation.

CLINICAL SIGNIFICANCE

S. moniliformis is part of the normal flora of the oropharynx of wild or laboratory rats, mice, or other rodents. Human infection is usually acquired following the bite of a rat, mouse, or cat. (Weasels, squirrels, dogs, and pigs have also been associated with human disease.) Human cases resulting from ingestion of milk contaminated with rat feces were first reported in Haverhill, Massachusetts, in 1926; thus the term "Haverhill fever" is used to describe cases of human infection for which no history of a rat bite can be found. "Rat-bite fever" is used to describe cases in which a bite can be documented. Infection can also occur in persons working or living in rat-infested buildings with no evidence of direct animal contact.[36]

Illness caused by *S. moniliformis* begins abruptly after an incubation period of less than 10 days. Clinical manifestations include chills, fever, vomiting, and severe headache; alternate remissions and febrile episodes may persist for weeks or months. A rash, frequently affecting the palms and soles, is usually seen; the rash may resemble that seen in Rocky Mountain spotted fever. More than one half of patients develop polyarthritis involving the elbows, wrists, knees, or ankles. The arthritic symptoms are a hallmark of the disease, which is also known as erythema arthriticum epidemicum. Individuals with cardiovascular defects and immunocompromised patients are prone to sequelae of endocarditis or pneumonia.[86] Mortality may be as high as 10% in untreated cases.

ANTIMICROBIAL SUSCEPTIBILITY

Bacterial-phase cells are susceptible to penicillin, which is the drug of choice.[32] Antimicrobial susceptibility testing can be performed using the agar diffusion method.[32] L-phase cells are resistant to penicillin but can be treated with tetracycline, erythromycin, streptomycin, chloramphenicol, or gentamicin.[116] Combination therapy has been used successfully, as has clindamycin therapy.[17] Patients usually improve rapidly following initiation of antimicrobial therapy.

ACTINOBACILLUS

The genus *Actinobacillus* is composed of fastidious, slow-growing, facultatively anaerobic gram-negative rods; they are nonmotile and nonsporeforming, and they ferment carbohydrates without gas production. *A. actinomycetemcomitans* is the most frequently isolated species but *A. lignieresii, A. equuli,* and *A. suis* are also recovered from clinical specimens. *A. actinomycetemcomitans* is a rare cause of endocarditis and focal infections and is a possible copathogen in actinomycosis. *A. lignieresii, A. equuli,* and *A. suis* are primarily of veterinary significance but have caused localized purulent granulomata and abscesses and septicemia in humans.

CLASSIFICATION

The genus *Actinobacillus* is included in section 5 of *Bergey's Manual of Systematic Bacteriology,* volume 1, with the gram-negative facultatively anaerobic rods; it is listed in the family *Pasteurellaceae.*[99] The genus name is derived from the Greek *actinis,* "ray," which reflects the characteristic morphology of sulfur granules. *A. lignieresii, A. equuli, A. actinomycetemcomitans, A. capsulatus,* and *A. suis* are listed as species of the genus. *A. capsulatus* is strictly a veterinary pathogen and is not discussed in this chapter. *A. actinomycetemcomitans* was formerly called *Bacterium actinomycetemcomitans;* this designation reflected the fact that the organism is found together with *Actinomyces israelii* in actinomycotic lesions.

SPECIMEN COLLECTION AND PROCESSING

Pus (with or without sulfur granules) and blood are usually submitted for isolation of *Actinobacillus* organisms, although other specimens are also acceptable. The effects of various transport media on *Actinobacillus* spp. are unknown.

GROWTH REQUIREMENTS
Media

Actinobacillus spp. grow best on blood or chocolate agars. The organisms grow poorly on ordinary peptone media, may show only light growth on MacConkey agar, and do not grow on Salmonella-Shigella or eosin–methylene blue agars. Most commercial blood culture media support growth; subculture should be on blood or chocolate agar in 5% to 10% CO_2.

TABLE 25-1. Biochemical Characteristics of *Streptobacillus moniliformis*

Characteristic	Reaction
Triple sugar iron agar (TSI)	No change/no change
H_2S (butt/paper)	$-/2+$
Catalase	−
Oxidase	−
Motility	−
Growth on MacConkey agar	−
Growth on Salmonella-Shigella agar	−
Cetrimide	−
Simmons citrate	−
Urea hydrolysis	−
Gelatin liquefaction	−
Litmus milk	−
Indole	−
Nitrate reduction	−
Lysine decarboxylase	−
Ornithine decarboxylase	−
Arginine dihydrolase	−
Esculin hydrolysis	+ weak
Gas from glucose	−
Acid from:	
Adonitol	−
Arabinose	−
Cellobiose	−
Dulcitol	−
Fructose	+
Galactose	+
Glucose	+
Glycerol	−
Inositol	−
Inulin	v
Lactose	−
Maltose	+
Mannitol	−
Mannose	+
Melezitose	−
Melibiose	−
Raffinose	−
Rhamnose	−
Salicin	v
Sorbitol	−
Sorbose	−
Starch	+
Sucrose	−
Trehalose	−
Xylose	v

SYMBOLS: v, Variable; more than 10% but less than 90% strains positive; reaction may be delayed
+, 90% or more strains positive
−, 90% or more strains negative

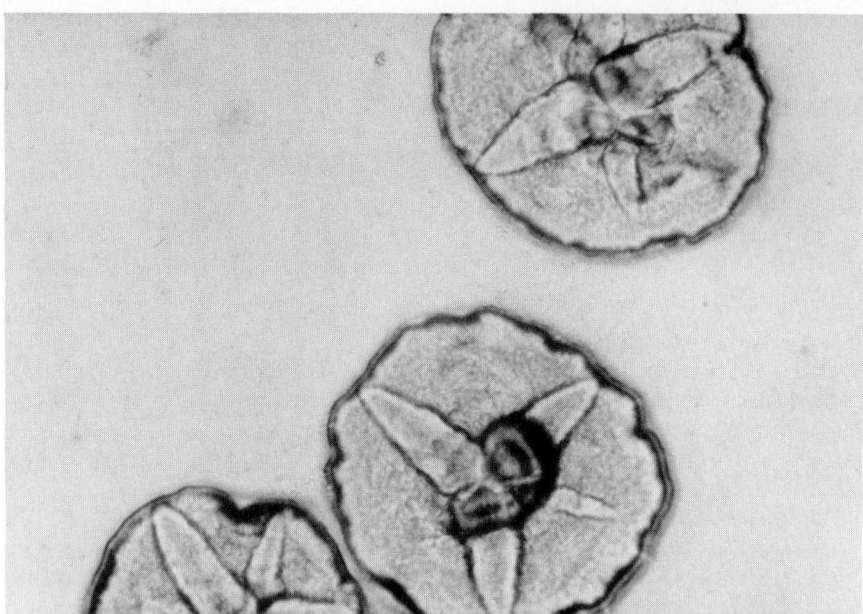

FIGURE 25-2. Star-shaped configuration may be observed in colonies of *Actinobacillus actinomycetemcomitans.* (Courtesy Dr. Edward J. Bottone, Mt. Sinai Hospital, New York.)

Environmental Requirements

Actinobacillus spp. are microaerophilic and grow best in the presence of elevated moisture and CO_2. *Actinobacillus* spp. may be recovered on solid media after 24 to 48 hours' incubation at 35° to 37°C. Blood cultures may require a week of incubation before growth is apparent.

CULTURAL CHARACTERISTICS
Staining Reactions

Actinobacillus spp. are gram-negative coccobacilli or bacilli that are about 0.3 to 0.5 μm by 0.6 to 1.4 μm in size. They occur singly, in pairs, and in chains and have a tendency toward bipolar staining. Sulfur granules of *A. lignieresii* contain a central detritus with a few gram-negative rods and radially extending gram-negative clubs. In actinomycotic granules, *A. actinomycetemcomitans* is seen as densely packed gram-negative coccobacilli.

Colonial Morphology

After 24 hours at 37°C, colonies of *A. lignieresii* and *A. equuli* are 0.5 to 1.5 mm in size, nonhemolytic, and smooth or rough, and they stick to the surface of the blood agar. *A. suis* is beta-hemolytic on sheep blood agar but otherwise resembles *A. lignieresii* and *A. equuli*. Colonies of *A. actinomycetemcomitans* are also adherent; after 24 hours at 35°C, colonies on blood agar range from punctate to 0.5 mm in diameter (Plate 22, *D*). On continued incubation a four- to six-pointed star structure is often seen in the center of the colony growing into the agar (Figure 25-2).

Growth of *A. actinomycetemcomitans* in blood culture broths may be first seen as delicate granules in the sedimented blood; granules may also adhere to the sides of the bottle near the surface of the broth.

BIOCHEMICAL IDENTIFICATION

A. lignieresii, A. equuli, and *A. suis* are oxidase-positive, urease-positive glucose fermenters; this distinguishes them from *Bordetella bronchiseptica* and *Pseudomonas pickettii,* which are oxidase-positive, urease-positive nonfermenters. *A. actinomycetemcomitans* is similar to *Cardiobacterium* spp., *Eikenella* spp., *Haemophilus aphrophilus,* and *Kingella kingae* in its slow growth and requirement for elevated CO_2 and humidity. It may be differentiated from *E. corrodens* by a negative ornithine decarboxylase test and fermentation of carbohydrates and from *H. aphrophilus* by a positive catalase test and negative *o*-nitrophenyl-beta-D-galactopyranaside (ONPG) and lactose fermentation tests. *A. actinomycetemcomitans* differs from *C. hominis* in being indole negative and catalase positive; the catalase test is also important in differentiating *K. kingae* (which is negative) and *A. actinomycetemcomitans.*

Fermentation tests are best performed in liquid peptone media with Andrade indicator. Interestingly, *A. actinomycetemcomitans* produces an acid slant and acid butt in triple sugar iron agar even though it does not ferment sucrose or lactose; this probably occurs because the organism does not grow well enough to produce sufficient alkaline products to revert the slant to an alkaline pH. Biochemical characteristics of the species of *Actinobacillus* most commonly isolated from clinical specimens are shown in Table 25-2.

SEROLOGIC AND IMMUNOSEROLOGIC IDENTIFICATION

No routine serologic tests are available for antibody detection or for identifying the organisms. Slots and co-workers[135] recently reported the use of species-specific rabbit antibodies against the three serotypes of *A. actinomycetemcomitans* to identify the organism in subgingival smears by the indirect fluorescent antibody technique.

TABLE 25-2. Biochemical Characteristics of *Actinobacillus* Spp.

Characteristic	Reaction			
	A. lignieresii	*A. equuli*	*A. suis*	*A. actinomycetemcomitans*
Triple sugar iron agar (TSI)	Acid/acid	Acid/acid	Acid/acid	Acid/acid
H_2S (butt/paper)	−/−	−/−	−/−	−/−
Kligler iron agar (KIA)	Acid/acid	Acid/acid	Acid/acid	Acid/acid
Catalase	v	v	v	+
Oxidase	+	+	+	v
Motility	−	−	−	−
Growth on MacConkey agar	v	v	+	−
Growth on Salmonella-Shigella agar	−	−	−	−
Simmons citrate	−	−	−	−
Urea hydrolysis	+	+	+	−
Gelatin liquefaction	−	v	−	−
Indole	−	−	−	−
Nitrate reduction	+	+	+	+
Lysine decarboxylase	−	−	−	−
Ornithine decarboxylase	−	−	−	−
Arginine dihydrolase	−	−	−	−
Esculin hydrolysis	−	−	+	−
ONPG (production of beta-galactosidase)	+	+		−
Gas from glucose	−	−	−	v
Acid from:				
Arabinose	+	v		−
Dulcitol	v	−		−
Fructose	+	+		+
Galactose	+	+		v
Glucose	+	+	+	+
Lactose	v	+	+	−
Maltose	+	+	+	+
Mannitol	+	+	v	v
Melibiose	−	+	+	−
Raffinose	v	+	+	−
Rhamnose	−	v		−
Salicin	−	v		−
Sucrose	+	+	+	−
Trehalose	−	+	+	−
Xylose	+	+	+	v

> **SYMBOLS:** v, Variable; > 10% but < 90% positive; reaction may be delayed
>   +, 90% or more strains positive
>   −, 90% or more strains negative

CLINICAL SIGNIFICANCE

A. lignieresii, A. equuli, and *A. suis* are principally animal pathogens that have rarely been recovered from human infections. *A. lignieresii* produces granulomatous lesions in the upper alimentary tract of cattle and suppurative lesions in the skin and lungs of sheep. *A. equuli* causes septicemia, arthritis, and nephritis in foals and pigs. *A. suis* causes septicemia and a variety of lesions of piglets. *A. lignieresii, A. equuli,* and *A. suis* have been isolated from animal bite wounds, other wounds, blood, sputum, and cerebrospinal fluid.[26,94]

A. actinomycetemcomitans is part of the normal human oral flora, and human infections are endogenous. The organism was

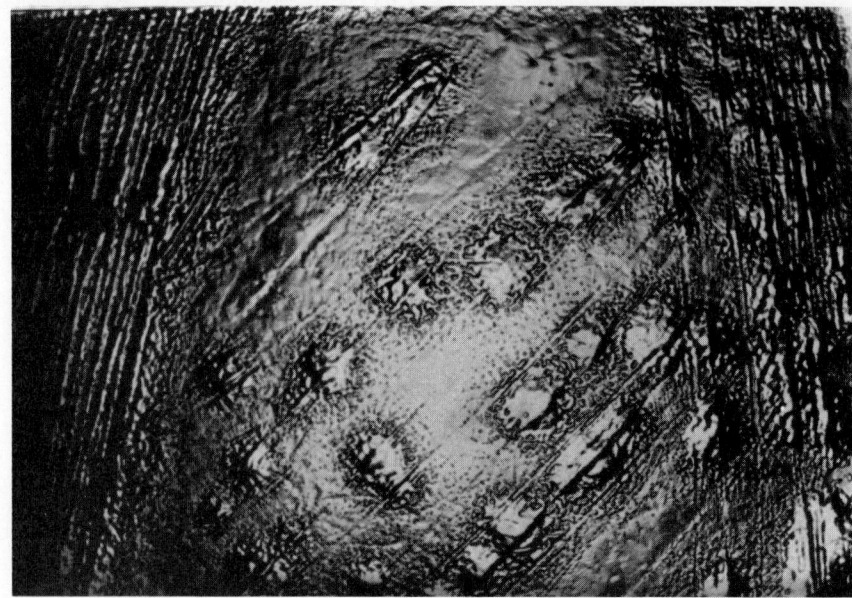

FIGURE 25-3. *Capnocytophaga* on blood agar. Spreading occurs concentrically and is flat with fingerlike edge. (Photograph by Dr. Leon J. LeBeau, Department of Biocommunication Arts, Medical Center, University of Illinois at Chicago.)

originally isolated from actinomycotic lesions and is thought to strengthen the comparatively low invasive power of the *Actinomyces* organisms either by providing reduced conditions in tissue or by supporting the bacteria through production of extracellular enzymes and toxins.[66] *A. actinomycetemcomitans* is frequently associated with subacute bacterial endocarditis[8,50,120] and has also been isolated from patients with brain abscess,[83] thyroid gland abscess,[12] oral abscess,[98] urinary tract infection,[148] and vertebral osteomyelitis.[90] *A. actinomycetemcomitans* has also been implicated as a cause of localized juvenile periodontitis.[133,161,162] The organism produces numerous virulence factors including leukotoxin, a polymorphonuclear leukocyte chemotaxis–inhibiting factor, lymphocyte-suppressing factor, endotoxin, acid and alkaline phosphatases, collagenase, a fibroblast-inhibiting factor, and an epitheliotoxin.[132,161]

ANTIMICROBIAL SUSCEPTIBILITY

Organisms of the genus *Actinobacillus* do not have predictable susceptibilities, and all clinical strains should be tested; susceptibility testing has been performed using both the agar disk diffusion and agar dilution techniques.

The antimicrobial susceptibility patterns of *A. lignieresii, A. equuli,* and *A. suis* have not been systemically studied, but the organisms are usually sensitive to chloramphenicol, resistant to penicillin, and variably resistant to tetracycline, streptomycin, and erythromycin. Studies on *A. actinomycetemcomitans*[65,134] indicate that the organism is sensitive to chloramphenicol, tetracycline, trimethoprim-sulfamethoxazole, gentamicin, tobramycin, and amikacin, variably sensitive to penicillin, ampicillin, cephalothin, and erythromycin, and resistant to clindamycin. Combination therapy with ampicillin and gentamicin has been recommended for treatment of endocarditis.[8] The variable sensitivity of *A. actinomycetemcomitans* to penicillin may account for the persistence of actinomycotic lesions even when the penicillin-sensitive *Actinomyces* spp. are eliminated.

CAPNOCYTOPHAGA

Microorganisms of the genus *Capnocytophaga* are capnophilic, microaerophilic, gliding, gram-negative, fusiform bacilli.[96] These organisms are normal inhabitants of the oral cavity and have most commonly been associated with juvenile periodontitis, as well as with bacteremia in immunocompromised granulocytopenic patients.[43,96]

CLASSIFICATION

The genus *Capnocytophaga* consists of three species—*C. ochracea, C. sputigena,* and *C. gingivalis*—and was formerly identified as *Bacteroides ochraceus* or CDC biogroup DF-1. This genus will be included in volume 3 of *Bergey's Manual of Systematic Bacteriology,* to be published in 1987.

GROWTH REQUIREMENTS
Media and Environmental Requirements

Capnocytophaga spp. grow on 5% sheep blood agar and on chocolate agar[42,43]; these organisms do not grow on MacConkey agar. A selective medium containing bacitracin and polymyxin B has also been described.[84] *Capnocytophaga* organisms grow under anaerobic conditions or under aerobic conditions in the presence of 5% to 10% CO_2. Growth is slow and may not be apparent until 48 to 72 hours of incubation at 35° to 37° C.

CULTURAL CHARACTERISTICS

A Gram stain of *Capnocytophaga* spp. reveals fusiform, gram-negative bacilli. Colonies are yellow, nonhemolytic, spreading, and usually 2 to 3 mm in diameter by 2 to 4 days. The spreading occurs concentrically and is flat with a fingerlike edge (Figure 25-3). The spreading or gliding motility of *Capnocytophaga* organisms is similar to that of *Proteus* spp., but, unlike *Proteus,* is not associated with the presence of peritrichous flagella.[47]

TABLE 25-3. Key Biochemical Characteristics of *Capnocytophaga* Spp.

Characteristic	*C. ochracea*	*C. sputigena*	*C. gingivalis*
Anaerobic growth	+	+	+
Aerobic growth in 5% to 10% CO_2	+	+	+
Growth in air	−	−	−
Starch hydrolysis	v	−	−
Nitrate reduction	−	+	−
Oxidase production	−	−	−
Catalase production	−	−	−
Indole production	−	−	−
Urease production	−	−	−
Acid production from:			
Glucose	+	+	+
Lactose	v	v	v
Maltose	+	+	+
Mannitol	−	−	−
Sucrose	+	+	+
Xylose	−	−	−

> **SYMBOLS:** +, ≥ 90%
> −, ≤ 10%
> v, Variable reactions

Data from references 47, 74, 137, and 159a.

BIOCHEMICAL IDENTIFICATION

Presumptive identification can be made in the presence of a yellow, fusiform, gram-negative bacillus that exhibits gliding motility on 5% sheep blood agar or on chocolate agar and grows only under anaerobic conditions or under aerobic conditions with 5% to 10% CO_2. The organism produces acid fermentatively from glucose and sucrose and is negative for oxidase, catalase, indole, and urease. Major metabolic end products are succinic and acetic acids.[137] Other key biochemical characteristics are indicated in Table 25-3. Differentiation of *Capnocytophaga* spp. from phenotypically similar genera and species is included in Table 25-4.

CLINICAL SIGNIFICANCE

Organisms of the genus *Capnocytophaga* are rare human pathogens. Of clinical importance to dentists is the association of increased bacterial counts of *Capnocytophaga* spp. in diseased periodontal pockets of patients with localized juvenile periodontitis and Papillon-Lefévre syndrome.[91,92] Diagnostic techniques as suggested by Bartlett[7] can be useful. More sensitive techniques recommended by Newman and co-workers[93] may also be used for culturing organisms from oral lesions.

In addition to localized dental disease, this group of bacteria has been shown to be an important pathogen in a number of additional clinical situations. A review by Parenti and Snydman[96] has demonstrated this genus as being clinically signifi-

TABLE 25-4. Differentiation of *Capnocytophaga* Spp. and Phenotypically Similar Genera and Species

Genus and Species	Catalase	Oxidase	Indole	Urease	Fermentation of Glucose	Nitrate Reduction	Motility
Capnocytophaga spp.	−	−	−	−	+	v	+
Cardiobacterium hominis	−	+	+	−	+	−	−
Chromobacterium spp.	+	v	v	v	+	+	+
Actinobacillus actinomycetemcomitans	+	v	−	−	+	+	−
Pasteurella spp.	+	+	v	v	+	+	−
Eikenella corrodens	−	+	−	−	−	+	−
Kingella spp.	−	+	v	−	+	v	−
Haemophilus aphrophilus	−	v	−	−	+	+	−

> **SYMBOLS:** +, ≥ 90%
> −, ≤ 10%
> v, Variable reactions

Data from references 78, 157, and 158.

cant in the following nonimmunocompromised disease entities: empyema, lung abscess, sinusitis, conjunctivitis, subphrenic abscess, osteomyelitis, bacteremia, and infected wounds. Most of the infections were polymicrobial and presumably were acquired from defects in the oral cavity. The immunocompromised patients had leukemia, possessed solid tumors, or had received a kidney transplant. All had positive blood cultures, and 75% had evidence of oral disease. Warren and Allen[156a] have called attention to a higher incidence in the pediatric age group. Five of seven of their bacteremic patients were younger than 20 years of age. Additional reports indicate that *Capnocytophaga* spp. are involved in congenital bacteremias,[38] soft tissue swellings,[60] arthritis,[160] and endocarditis.[22]

ANTIMICROBIAL SUSCEPTIBILITY

In vitro antimicrobial susceptibility studies show that achievable serum concentrations of penicillin, erythromycin, clindamycin, tetracycline, and ampicillin adequately inhibit growth.[44,142] Reports of varying susceptibilities to vancomycin, metronidazole, and the second- and third-generation cephalosporins necessitate individual analysis of encountered strains.[44,60,115,142] A recent study has demonstrated susceptibility to the quinolone antimicrobial agents, as well as to the antipseudomonal penicillins.[60a] *Capnocytophaga* spp. have shown consistent resistance to the aminoglycosides.

CARDIOBACTERIUM

The genus *Cardiobacterium* has a single member, its type species, *C. hominis*. The organism was first recognized as a human pathogen in 1962.[149]

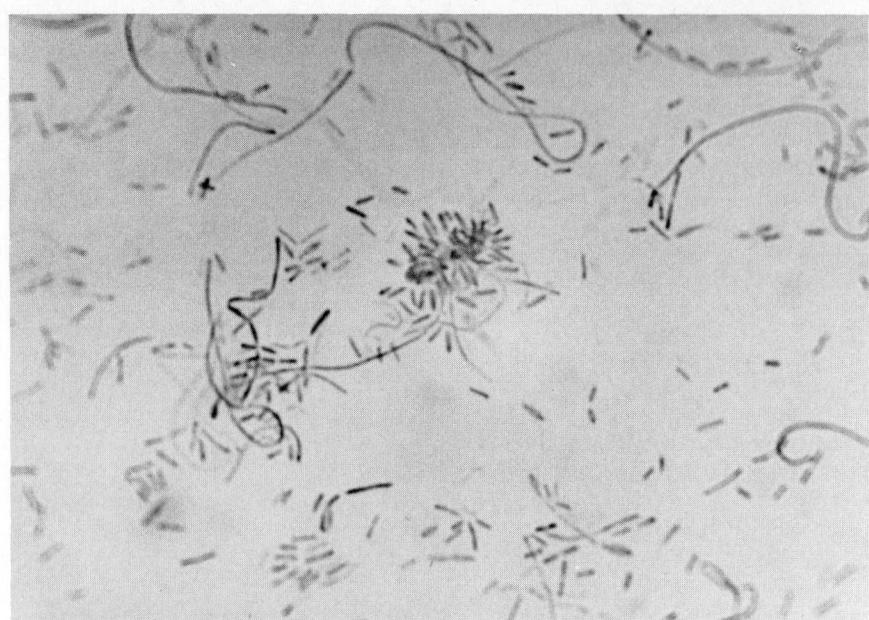

FIGURE 25-4. Gram stain of *Cardiobacterium hominis*. Note rosette formation. (Courtesy Dr. Edward J. Bottone, Mt. Sinai Hospital, New York.)

CLASSIFICATION

The genus *Cardiobacterium* is included in section 5 of *Bergey's Manual of Systematic Bacteriology,* volume 1, with the gram-negative facultatively anaerobic rods.[157] The genus name is derived from the Greek *cardia,* "heart," and reflects the isolation of the type species from cases of endocarditis. *C. hominis* is a gram-negative, fermentative rod; the organism was originally called CDC Group II D and was given its present name by Slotnick and Dougherty.[130]

SPECIMEN COLLECTION AND PROCESSING

Blood for culture of *C. hominis* may be inoculated into any of the conventional blood culture broths that have an atmosphere of 5% to 10% CO_2 and contain 0.025% sodium polyanethol sulfonate (SPS) as the anticoagulant. Bottles are incubated at 35° C for a minimum of 7 days.

Aliquots of body fluids, exudates, and tissue for culture should be streaked onto three blood agar plates; one plate is then incubated in air, one in a CO_2 incubator (or candle jar), and one in an anaerobic jar (or glove box). Plates are held at 35° C for a minimum of 4 days.

GROWTH REQUIREMENTS
Media

C. hominis grows well on trypticase soy agar (BBL) or tryptose blood agar (Difco) with or without the addition of 5% blood. Chocolate agar, brain-heart infusion agar, and cystine heart agar also support its growth, although growth is poor on nutrient agar. The bacteria will not grow on MacConkey agar, Salmonella-Shigella (SS) agar, eosin–methylene blue (EMB) agar, or Endo agar.

C. hominis remains viable for several years when stored at −70° C in a nutrient broth to which 15% glycerol has been added.

Environmental Requirements

C. hominis is a facultative anaerobe that grows best in an atmosphere containing 3% to 5% CO_2. The organism is a humidiphile (lover of high humidity). Growth in a candle jar is often used to satisfy the requirement for increased CO_2 and moisture; filter paper strips or paper towels saturated with water are placed in the bottom of the jar before the candle is lit to provide extra moisture. Colonies of *C. hominis* attain maximum size after 48 to 72 hours at 35° C.

CULTURAL CHARACTERISTICS
Staining Reactions

C. hominis is a gram-negative rod (0.5 μm by 1 to 2.2 μm in size) with one rounded and one tapered end (resembling a teardrop). Bacteria are arranged singly, or in pairs, short chains, or clusters. The tendency to form clusters resembling rosettes is more pronounced in Gram-stained preparations from blood agar (Figure 25-4); pleomorphism is less marked from media containing yeast extract.[118]

Colonial Morphology

Colonies on blood agar are punctiform after 24 hours and attain maximum size of 1 to 2 mm between 48 and 72 hours; mature colonies are circular, convex, smooth, entire, glistening, opaque, and butyrous. A slight greening of the blood agar may develop in 48 to 72 hours around areas containing the heaviest growth; a brownish color develops on further incubation. Some strains may produce colonies that "pit" the agar.

In blood culture broths, colonies appear as small, discrete, grayish puff balls superimposed on settled red blood cells.

BIOCHEMICAL IDENTIFICATION

C. hominis may be differentiated from *Haemophilus aphrophilus,* *Actinobacillus actinomycetemcomitans,* *Streptobacillus*

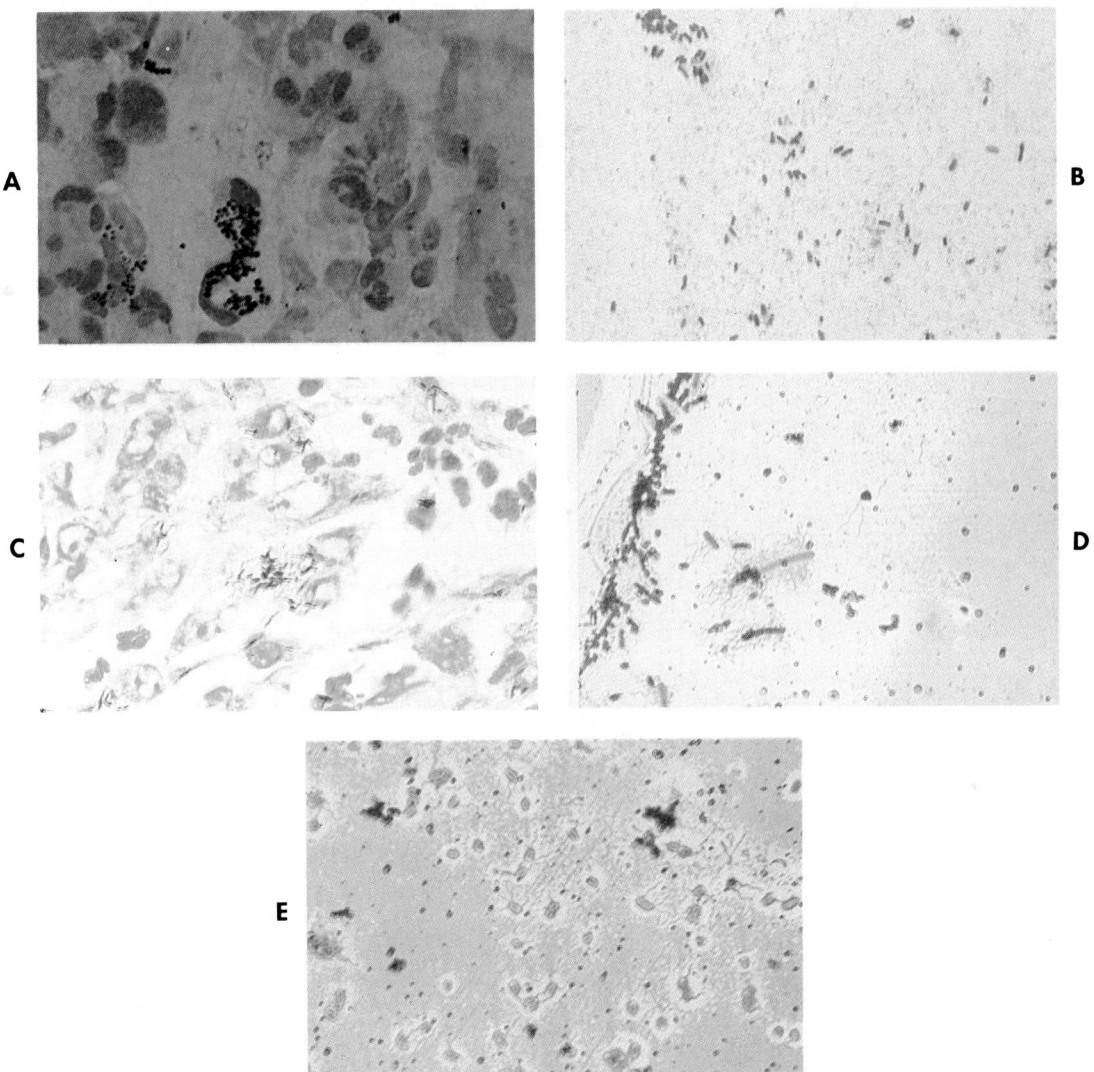

PLATE 1. **A,** Gram stain showing clusters of gram-positive cocci *(Staphylococcus aureus)* in sputum. **B,** Gram stain showing gram-negative rods of *Yersinia enterocolitica* in fluid. **C,** Ziehl-Neelsen stain of tissue. Acid-fast organisms of *Mycobacterium kansasii* stain red against blue background. (Courtesy Carol Ormes, Washington Hospital Center, Washington, D.C.) **D,** Flagella stain of *Proteus mirabilis.* Flagella are distributed across entire cell surface; this is called peritrichous flagellation. **E,** Flagella stain of *Aeromonas hydrophila.* This organism demonstrates polar flagellation; that is, flagella are present only at poles.

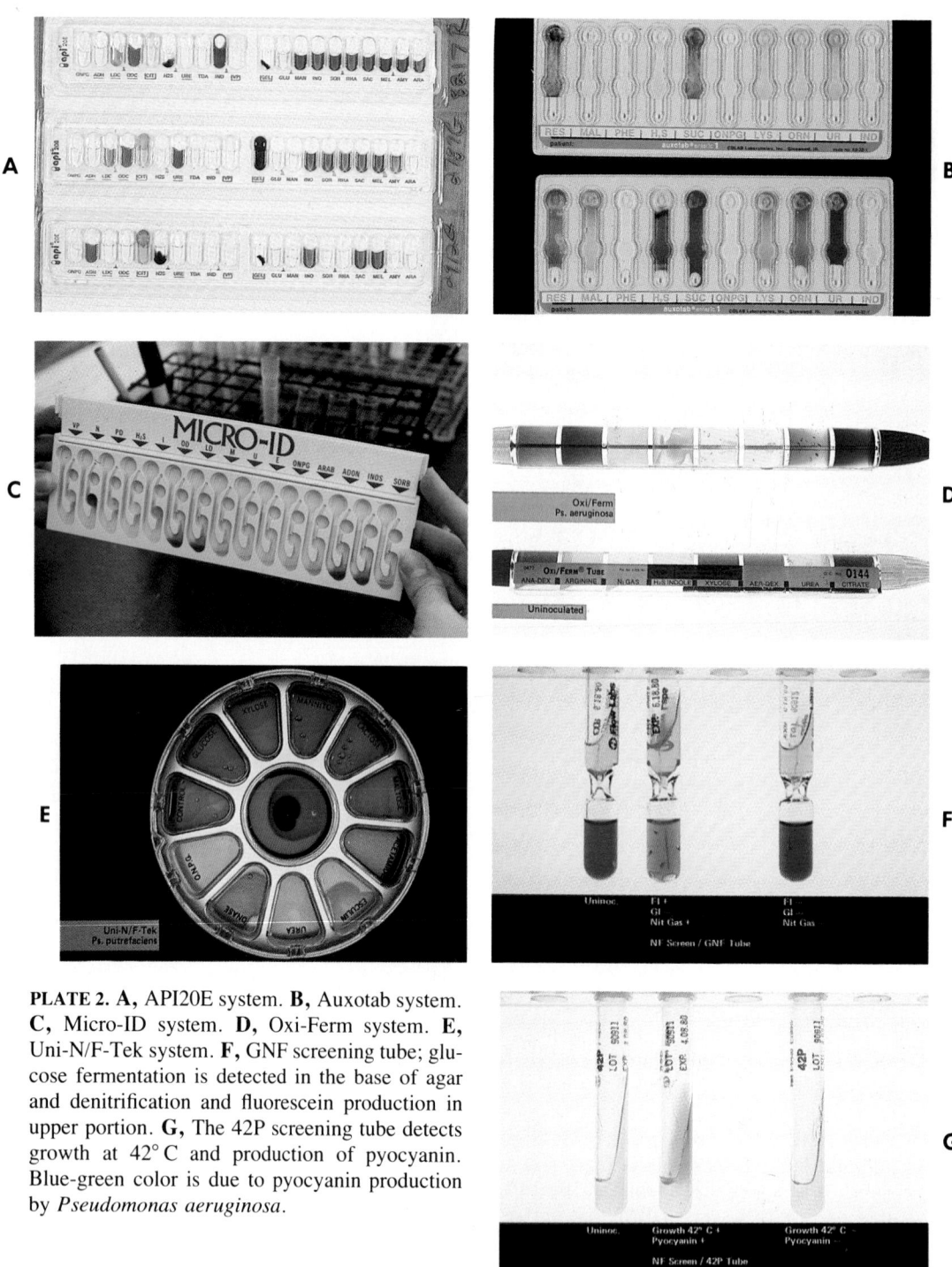

PLATE 2. A, API20E system. **B,** Auxotab system. **C,** Micro-ID system. **D,** Oxi-Ferm system. **E,** Uni-N/F-Tek system. **F,** GNF screening tube; glucose fermentation is detected in the base of agar and denitrification and fluorescein production in upper portion. **G,** The 42P screening tube detects growth at 42° C and production of pyocyanin. Blue-green color is due to pyocyanin production by *Pseudomonas aeruginosa*.

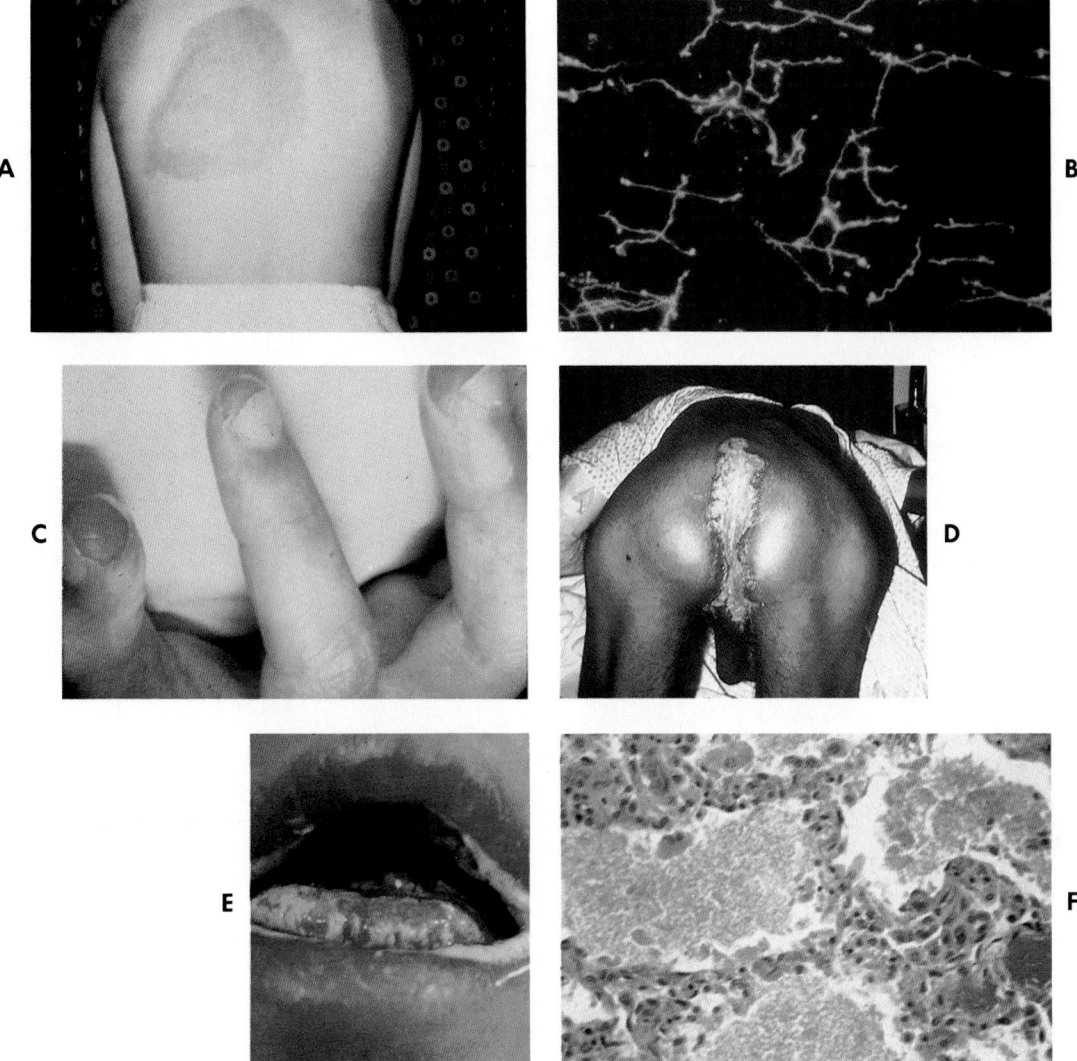

PLATE 3. A, Erythema chronicum migrans: characteristic skin lesion of Lyme disease. (From Steere, A.C., et al.: Ann. Intern. Med. **86:**685, 1977.) **B,** Indirect immunofluorescence stain of *Borrelia burgdorfii,* the Lyme disease spirochete. (×1000.) (From Barbour, A.G., et al.: Infect. Immun. **41:**795, 1983.) **C,** Characteristic desquamation of fingertips in toxic shock syndrome. **D,** Perianal herpes. **E,** Oral candidiasis (thrush). Note cream-white pseudomembranes, which are composed of masses of yeast and pseudohyphae of *Candida albicans.* **F,** *Pneumocystis carinii* in lung biopsy stained with hematoxylin and eosin (H & E). Alveolar spaces are filled with intensely acidophilic honeycombed material, which is composed of masses of *Pneumocystis carinii* cysts. Alveolar septa are broadened by epithelial hyperplasia and inflammatory cell infiltration, mainly macrophages and eosinophils.

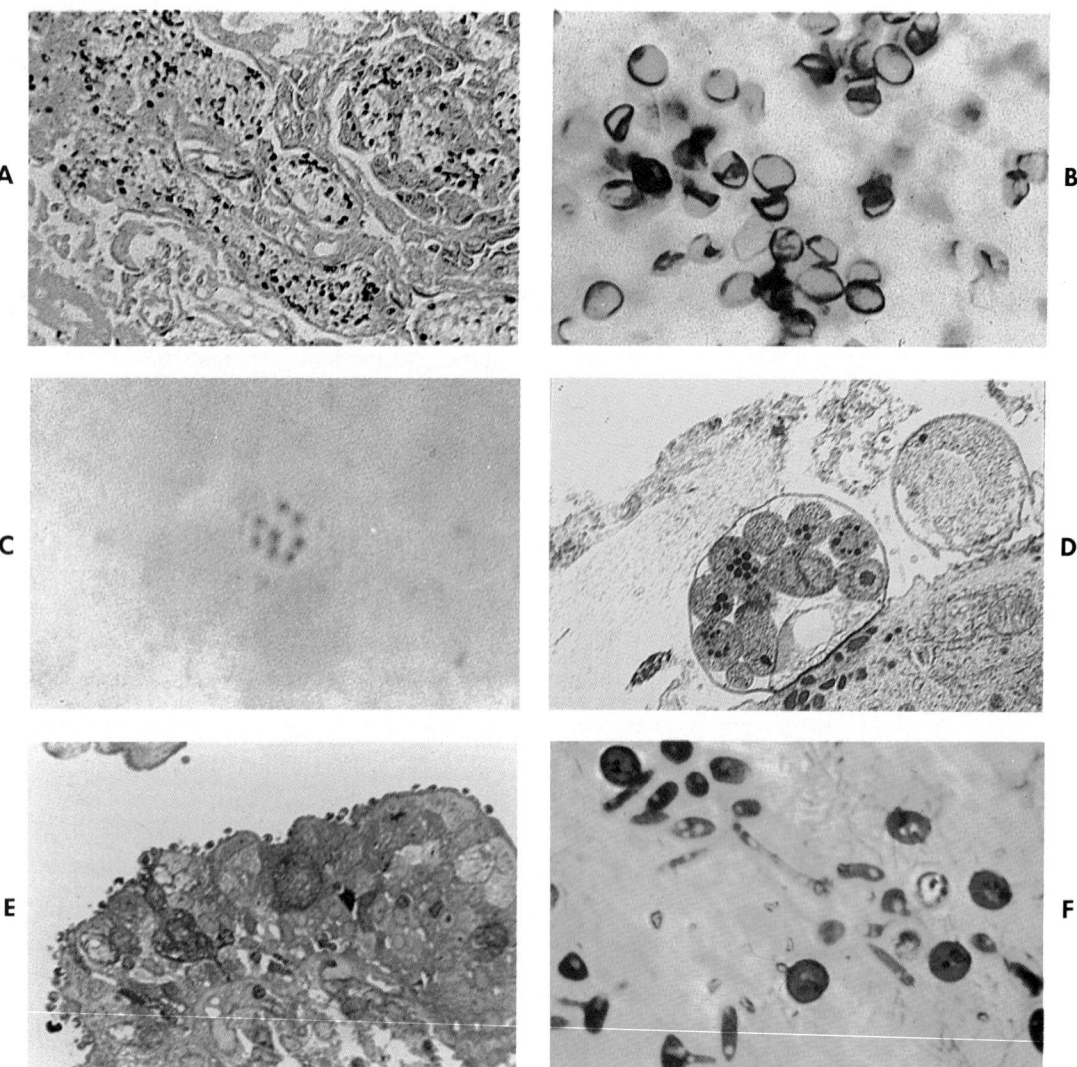

PLATE 4. A, Cysts of *Pneumocystis carinii* in exudate of alveoli. Walls stain black with Grocott-Gomori methenamine–silver nitrate stain. **B,** Cysts of *Pneumocystis carinii* stained with Grocott-Gomori methenamine–silver nitrate stain. In some cases wall of cyst collapses, evolving into characteristic crescent-shaped structures. **C,** Cyst of *Pneumocystis carinii* containing eight sporozoites. Giemsa stain of impression smear of lung. **D,** Electron microscopy of *Cryptosporidium* schizont with eight merozoites. Note electron-dense plate at interface between organism and host cell. **E,** Intestinal biopsy specimen stained with toluidine blue. *Cryptosporidium* can be seen on surface of epithelium. **F,** *Cryptosporidium*. In acid-fast stain of stool sample, *Cryptosporidium* oocysts stain red whereas everything else stains blue.

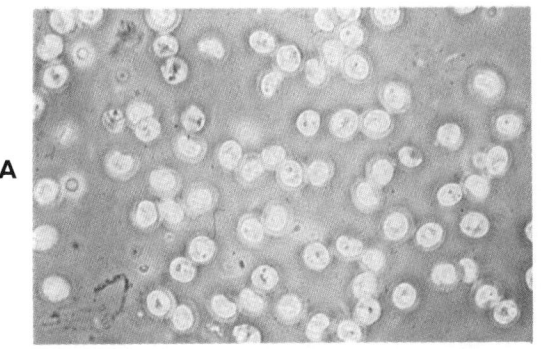

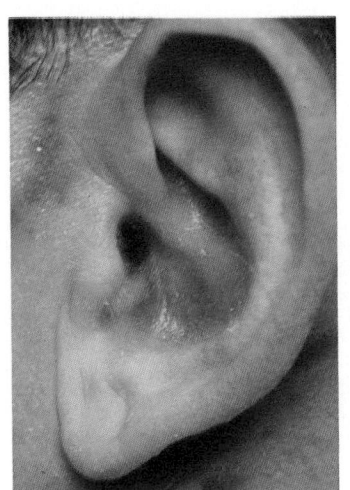

PLATE 5. A, *Cryptosporidium* cysts. Sheather sugar flotation technique. **B,** Kaposi's sarcoma of skin.

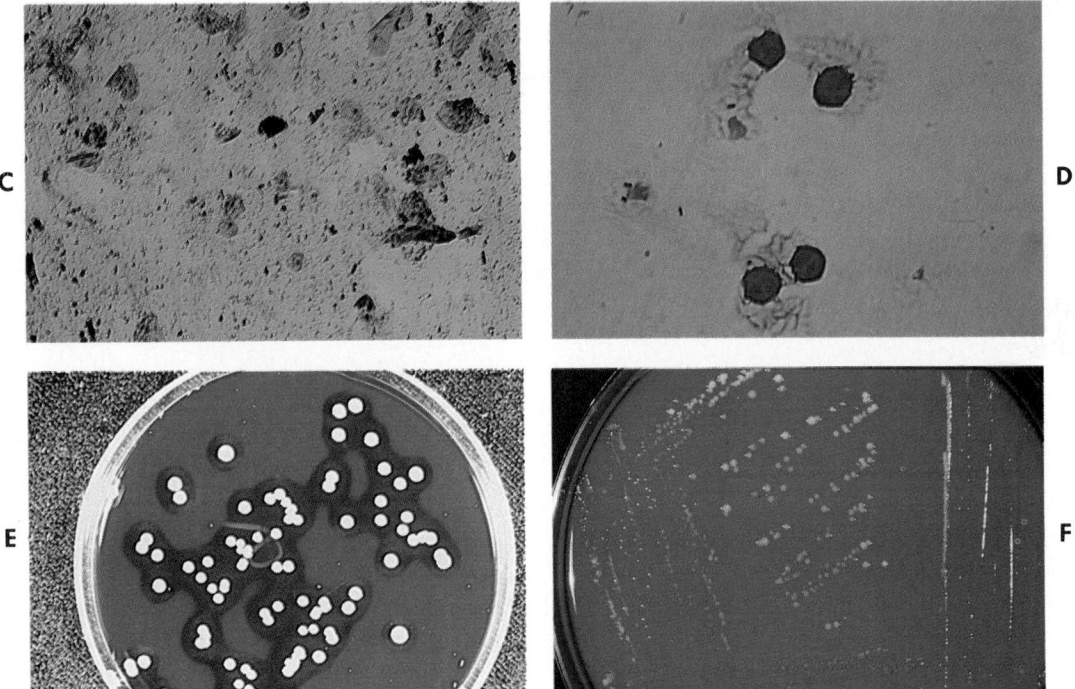

PLATE 5, cont'd. C, Gram-stained sputum smear with greater than 25 squamous epithelial cells per low power field. **D,** Gram stain of cerebrospinal fluid with *Streptococcus pneumoniae*. **E,** Beta-hemolytic colonies of *Staphylococcus aureus* on sheep blood agar. **F,** Colonies of *Staphylococcus epidermidis* on sheep blood agar (1:4.5). (Photograph by Dr. Leon J. LeBeau, Department of Biocommunication Arts, Medical Center, University of Illinois at Chicago.)

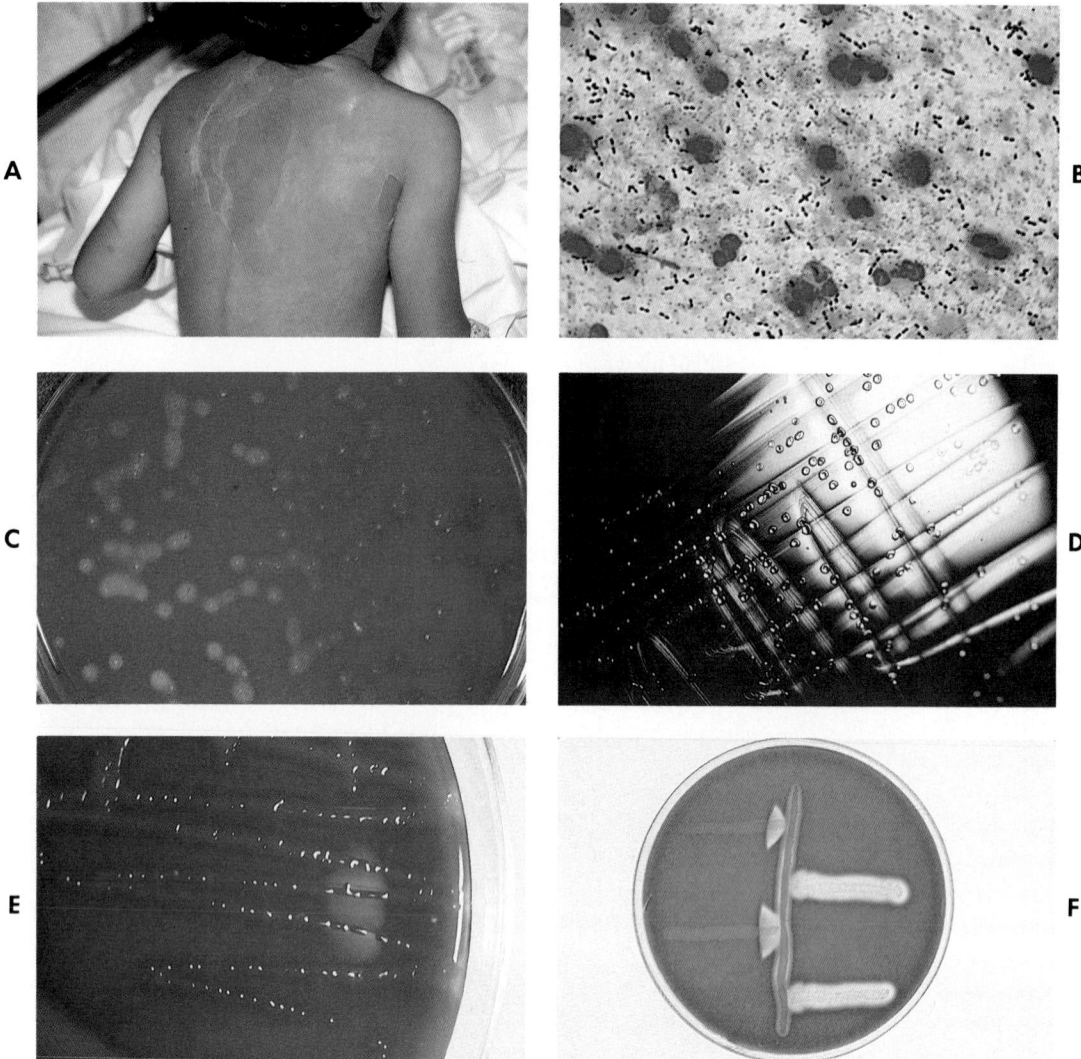

PLATE 6. A, Scalded skin syndrome. (Courtesy Dr. Marian Melish, Kapiolami Children's Medical Center, Honolulu.) **B,** Gram stain of sputum showing gram-positive, lancet-shaped diplococci of *Streptococcus pneumoniae* and gram-negative, short, slender rods of *Haemophilus influenzae*. (Courtesy Carol Ormes, Washington Hospital Center, Washington, D.C.) **C,** Group A beta-streptococcus on sheep blood agar (1:4.5). Note large zone of hemolysis in relation to size of colony. **D,** Umbilicated colonies of *Streptococcus pneumoniae*. (Courtesy Carol Ormes, Washington Hospital Center, Washington, D.C.) **E,** Watery-appearing mucoid colonies of *Streptococcus pneumoniae*. (Courtesy Carol Ormes, Washington Hospital Center, Washington, D.C.) **F,** CAMP test. Arrowhead hemolysis demonstrated by two strains on left is positive reaction and is presumptive identification of group B beta-streptococcus. Isolates on right are negative for CAMP test. (Courtesy Carol Ormes, Washington Hospital Center, Washington, D.C.)

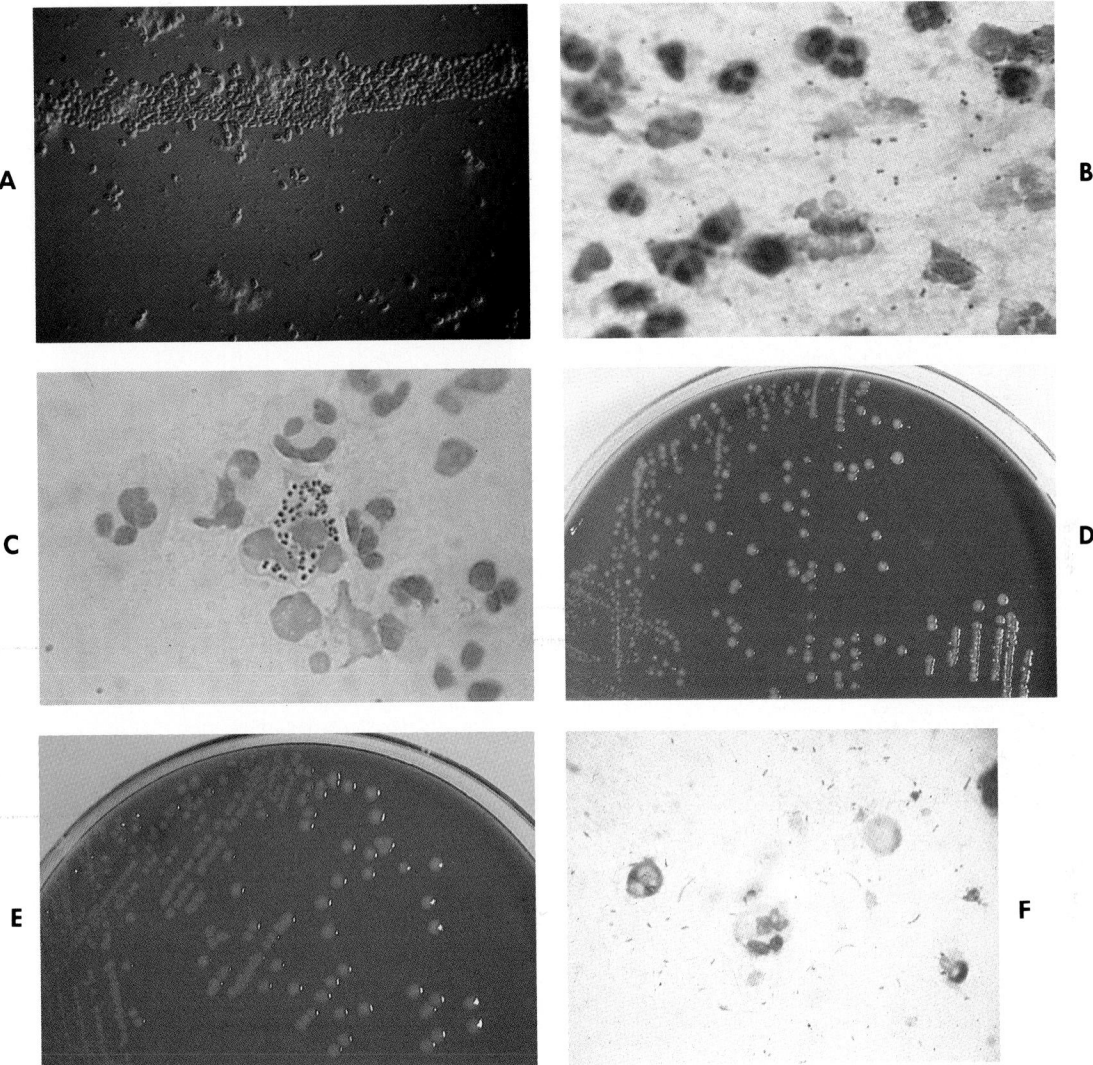

PLATE 7. A, Neufeld quellung reaction. (×1000.) Combination of capsule of *Streptococcus pneumoniae* with its specific antiserum results in formation of clearly defined capsular halo around organism. (Photograph by Dr. Leon J. LeBeau, Department of Biocommunication Arts, Medical Center, University of Illinois at Chicago.) **B,** Gram stain of sputum with *Branhamella catarrhalis*. This organism typically appears as gram-negative diplococci with adjacent sides flattened. **C,** Typical intracellular, gram-negative, kidney bean–shaped diplococci of *Neisseria gonorrhoeae* in exudate from male. **D,** Colonies of *Neisseria gonorrhoeae* on chocolate agar. (Courtesy Carol Ormes, Washington Hospital Center, Washington, D.C.) **E,** Colonies of *Neisseria meningitidis* on chocolate agar. (Courtesy Carol Ormes, Washington Hospital Center, Washington, D.C.) **F,** Gram stain of cerebrospinal fluid showing typical short and slender gram-negative rods of *Haemophilus influenzae*. Organisms stain very lightly and may be mistaken for debris.

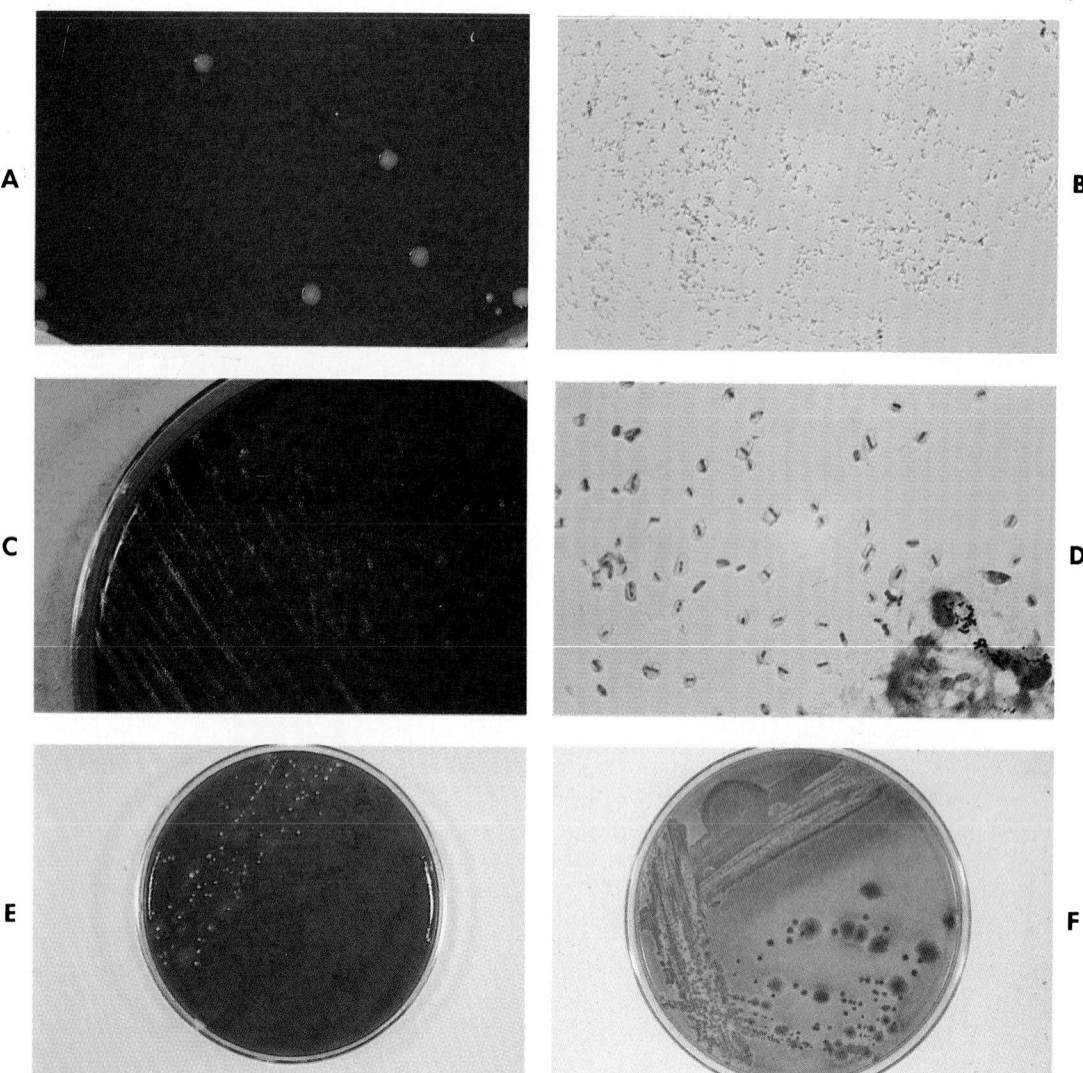

PLATE 8. A, *Haemophilus influenzae* satelliting staphylococci on blood agar. (Courtesy Carol Ormes, Washington Hospital Center, Washington, D.C.) **B,** Gram stain of *Haemophilus influenzae* from chocolate agar. (Courtesy Carol Ormes, Washington Hospital Center, Washington, D.C.) **C,** Small, smooth, translucent, gray colonies of *Haemophilus influenzae* on chocolate agar. (Courtesy Carol Ormes, Washington Hospital Center, Washington, D.C.) **D,** Direct smear of sputum showing encapsulated *Klebsiella pneumoniae*. (Courtesy Carol Ormes, Washington Hospital Center, Washington, D.C.) **E,** *Proteus mirabilis* swarming on blood agar. (Courtesy Carol Ormes, Washington Hospital Center, Washington, D.C.) **F,** Two types of *Escherichia coli* on MacConkey agar.

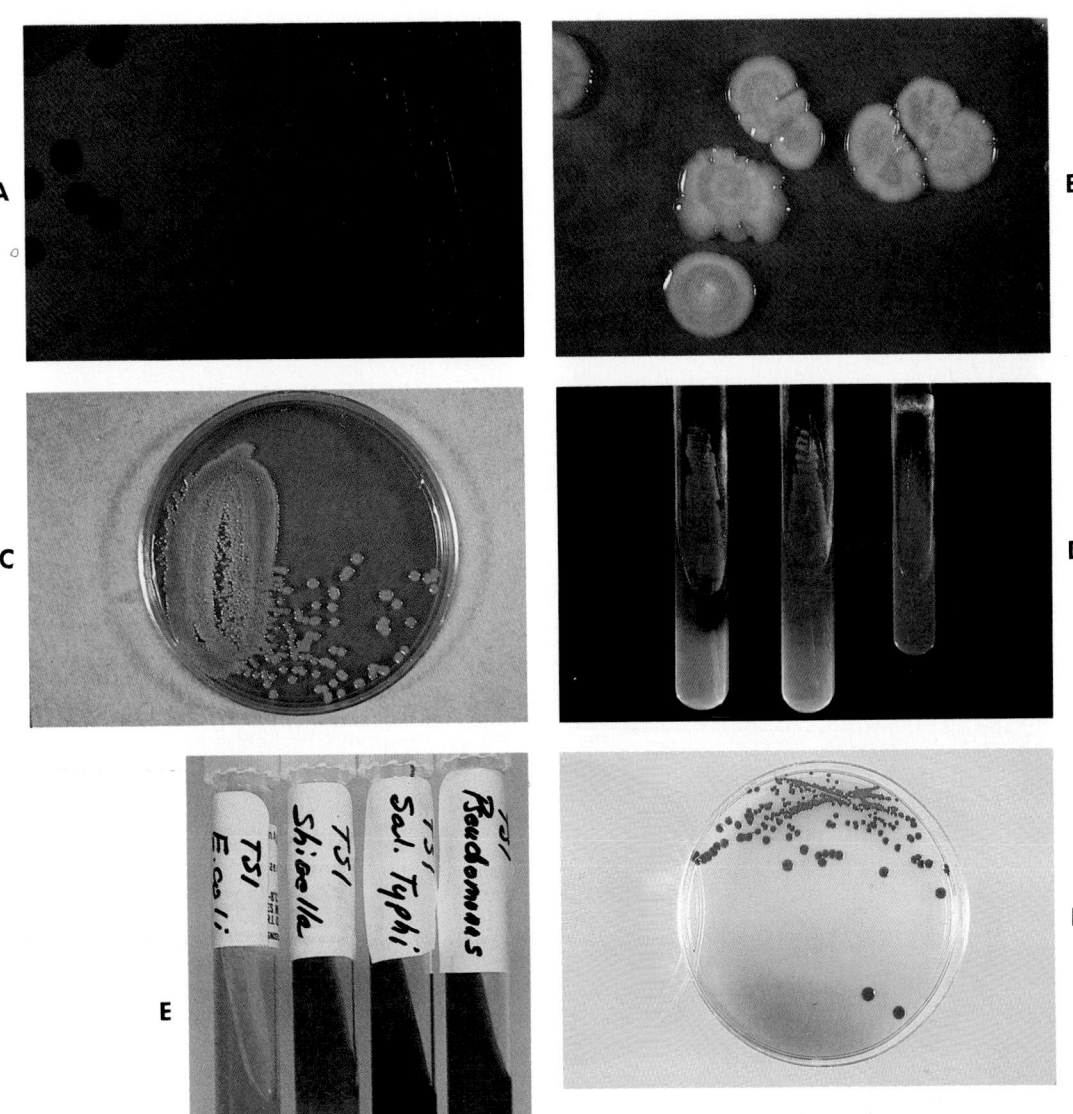

PLATE 9. A, Metallic sheen of *Escherichia coli* on eosin–methylene blue agar (1:2.5). (Photograph by Dr. Leon J. LeBeau, Department of Biocommunication Arts, Medical Center, University of Illinois at Chicago.) **B,** Pink, mucoid colonies of *Klebsiella pneumoniae* on MacConkey agar. (Courtesy Carol Ormes, Washington Hospital Center, Washington, D.C.) **C,** Pink colonies of *Enterobacter* on MacConkey agar. (Courtesy Carol Ormes, Washington Hospital Center, Washington, D.C.) **D,** Triple sugar iron, lysine iron agar, and urea screen of *Proteus*. (Photograph by Dr. Leon J. LeBeau, Department of Biocommunication Arts, Medical Center, University of Illinois at Chicago.) **E,** Triple sugar iron reactions *(left to right): Escherichia coli,* A/A +/−; *Shigella,* K/A −/−; *Salmonella typhi,* K/A −/+; *Pseudomonas,* K/NC. **F,** Pigmented *Serratia marcescens* on MacConkey agar. (Courtesy Carol Ormes, Washington Hospital Center, Washington, D.C.)

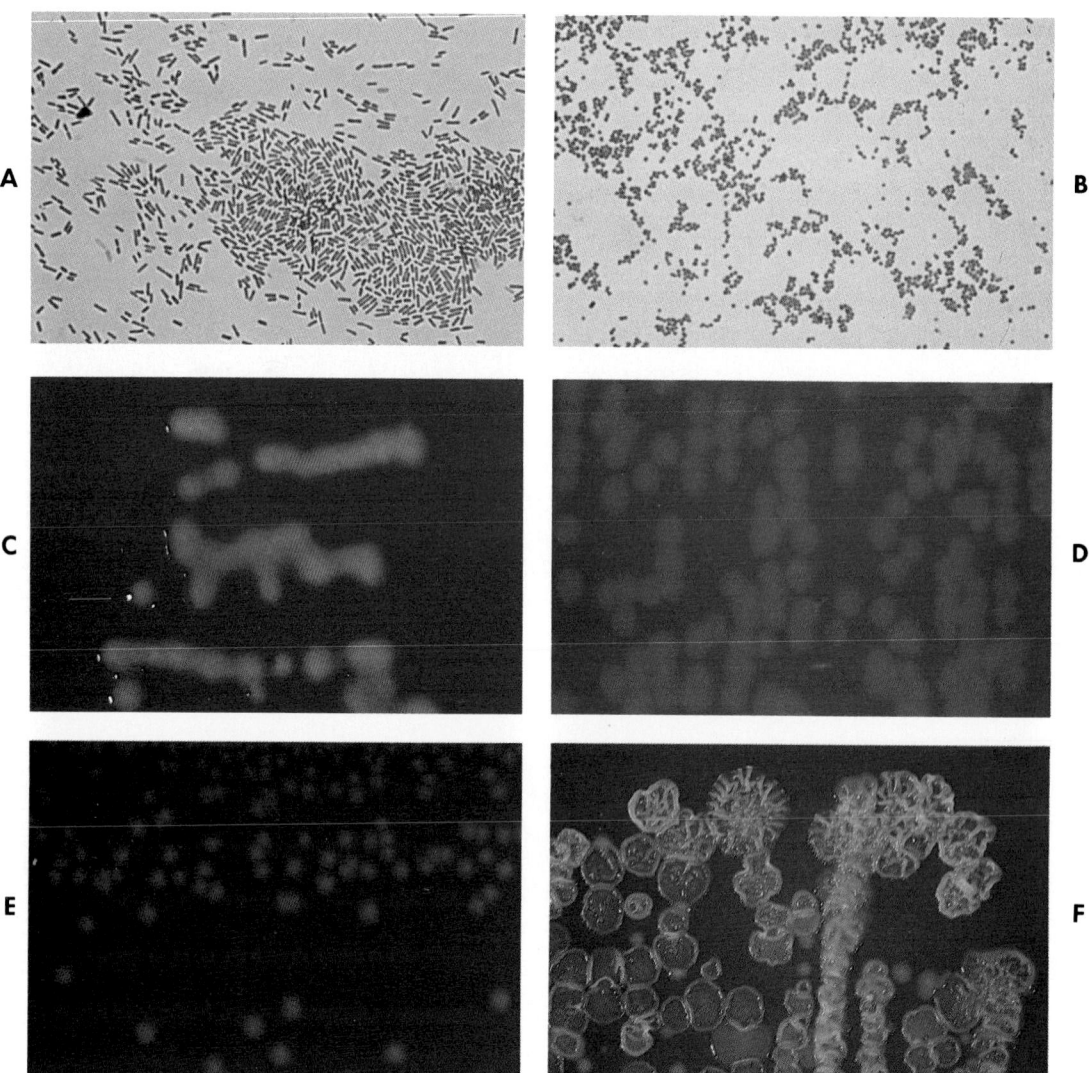

PLATE 10. A, Long, thin, gram-negative rods of *Pseudomonas aeruginosa*. **B,** Gram-negative coccobacilli of *Acinetobacter anitratus*. **C,** Mucoid forms of *Pseudomonas aeruginosa* on blood agar after 24 hours' incubation. **D,** Typical colonies of *Pseudomonas aeruginosa* with ground-glass appearance. Blood agar after 24 hours' incubation. **E,** Smooth colonies of *Pseudomonas aeruginosa* on blood agar after 24 hours' incubation. **F,** Mixed smooth and wrinkled colonies of *Pseudomonas stutzeri* after 48 hours' incubation.

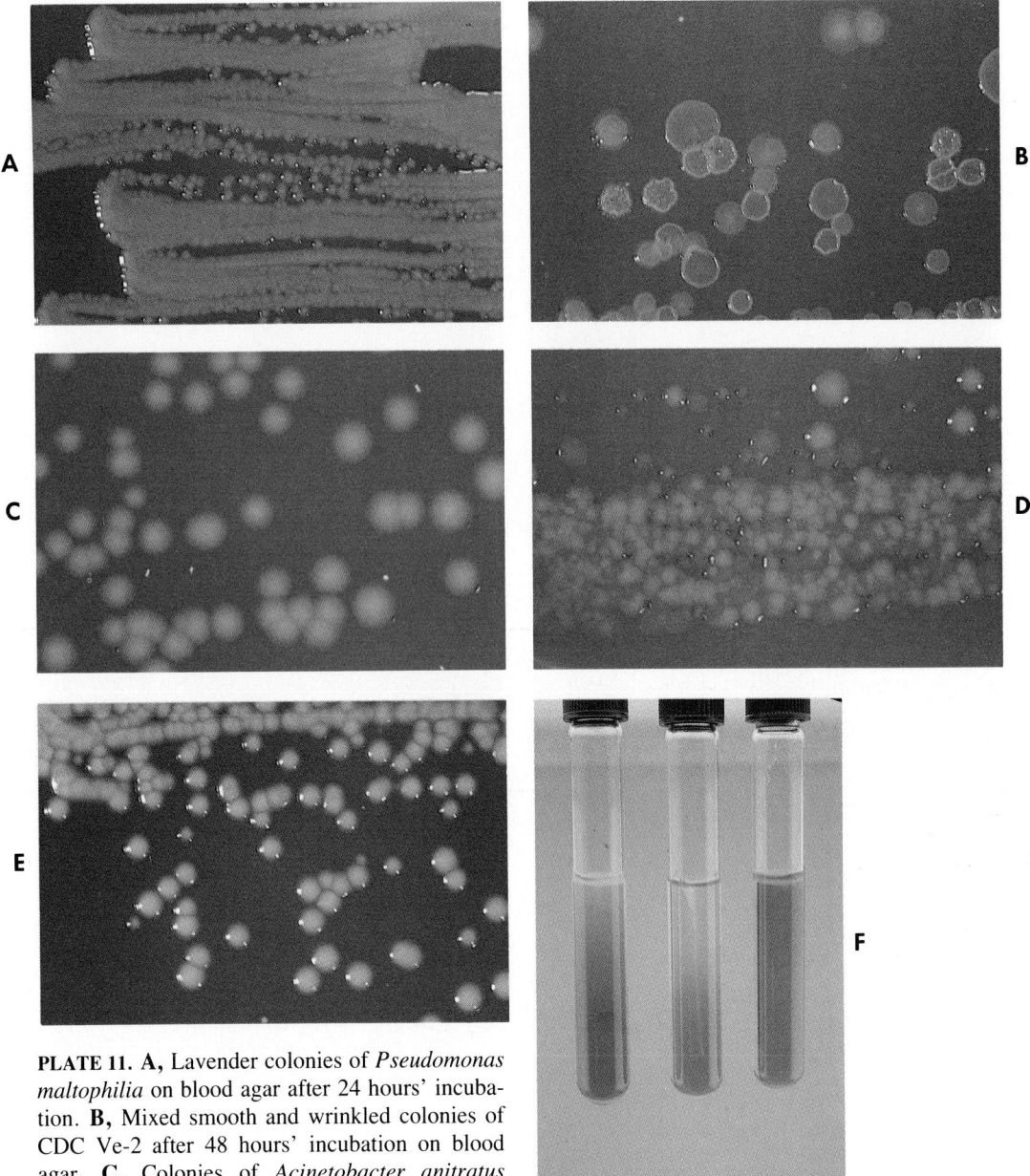

PLATE 11. A, Lavender colonies of *Pseudomonas maltophilia* on blood agar after 24 hours' incubation. **B,** Mixed smooth and wrinkled colonies of CDC Ve-2 after 48 hours' incubation on blood agar. **C,** Colonies of *Acinetobacter anitratus* resemble those of *Enterobacteriaceae*. **D,** Mixed large and small yellow-orange colonies of *Flavobacterium* sp. group IIb. **E,** Yellow colonies of *Pseudomonas paucimobilis* on blood agar after 48 hours' incubation. **F,** Motility-glucose medium (MGM). *Left,* Motile, glucose positive; *center,* nonmotile, glucose positive; *right,* uninoculated control.

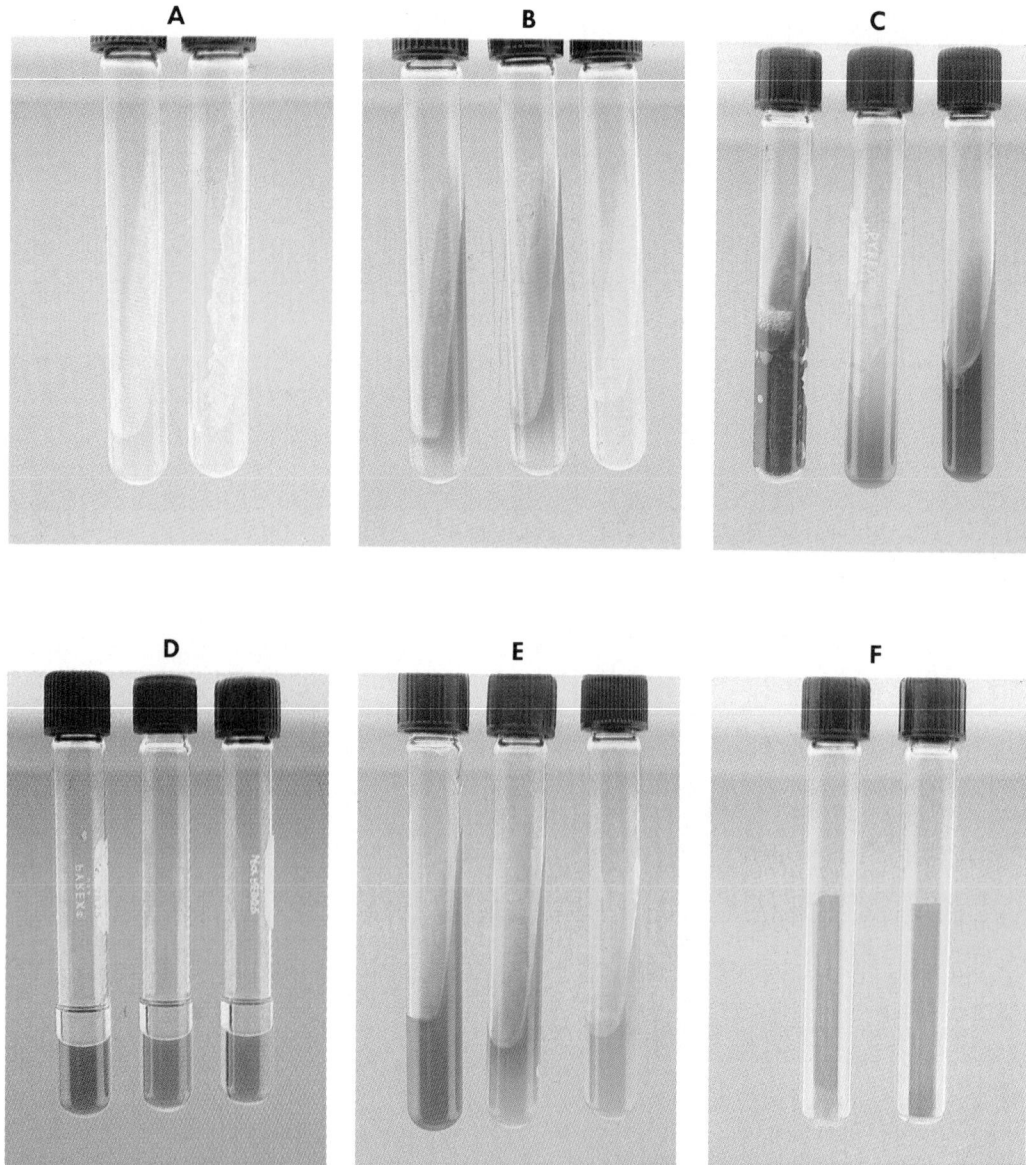

PLATE 12. A, Fluorescein medium. *Left,* Fluorescein production; *right,* no fluorescein. **B,** Pyocyanin medium. *Left,* Strong pyocyanin; *center,* weak pyocyanin; *right,* no pyocyanin. **C,** Fluorescein-denitrification-lactose (FDL) medium. *Left,* Nitrogen gas production; *center,* lactose oxidation; *right,* no change. **D,** Rapid decarboxylase medium. *Left,* Lysine decarboxylase positive; *center,* arginine dihydrolase negative; *right,* ornithine decarboxylase negative. **E,** Urea hydrolysis. *Left,* Strong positive; *center,* positive; *right,* negative. **F,** Gelatin (film strip) liquefaction. *Left,* Positive; *right,* negative.

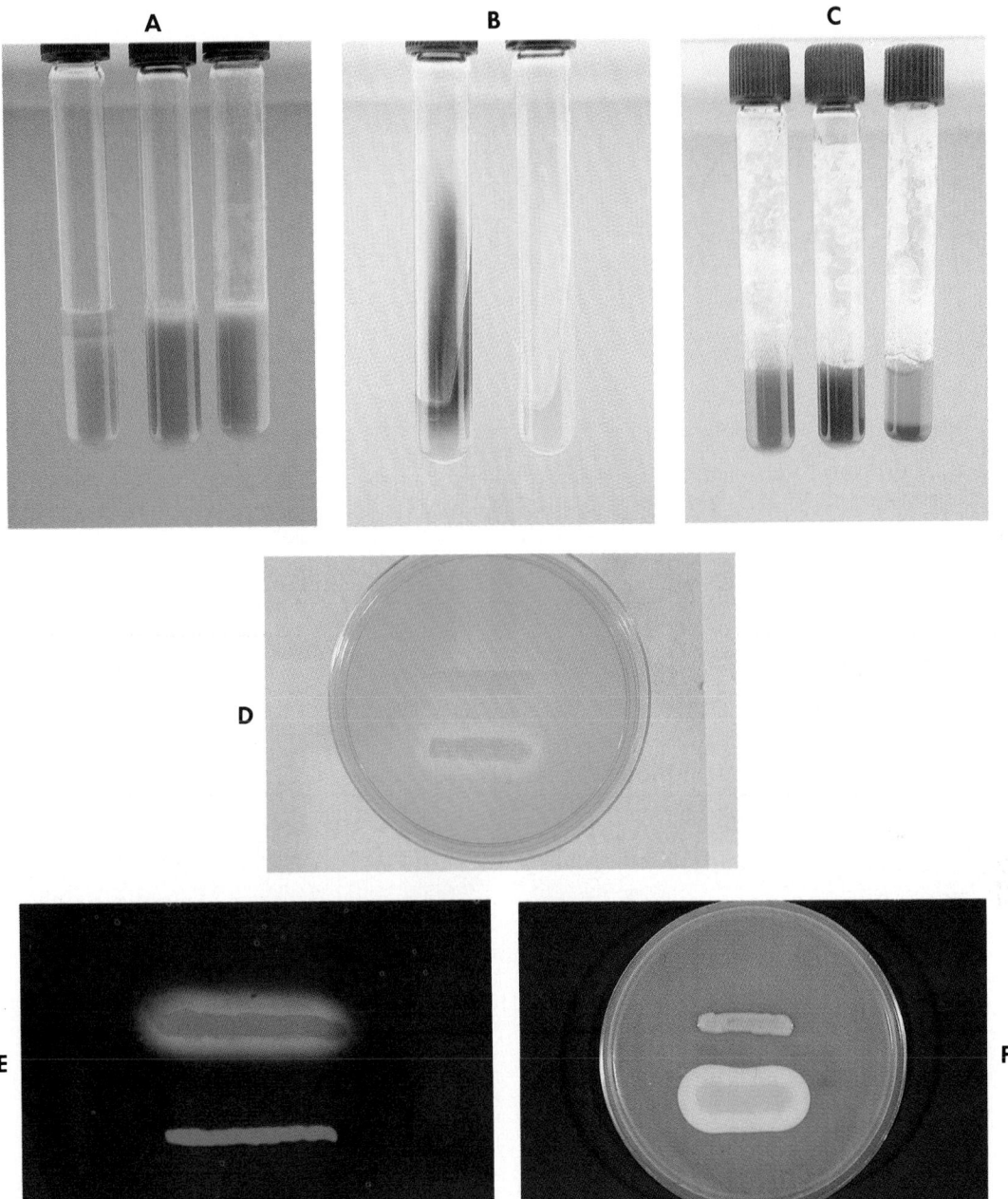

PLATE 13. A, Litmus milk peptonization. *Left,* Peptonization; *center,* alkaline; *right,* no change. **B,** Bile-esculin agar. *Left,* Positive (esculin hydrolyzed); *right,* negative. **C,** Gluconate oxidation. *Left,* Strong positive (4+); *center,* weak positive (1+); *right,* negative. **D,** Deoxyribonuclease. *Top,* Negative; *bottom,* positive. **E,** Starch hydrolysis. *Top,* Positive; *bottom,* negative. **F,** Lecithinase (egg yolk reaction). *Top,* Negative; *bottom,* positive.

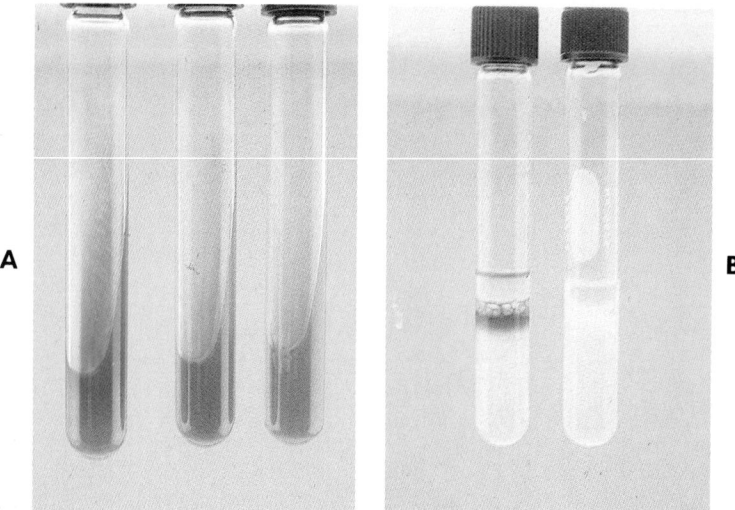

PLATE 14. A, Acetamide alkalinization. *Left,* Positive; *center and right,* negative. **B,** Indole (xylene extraction). *Left,* Positive; *right,* negative.

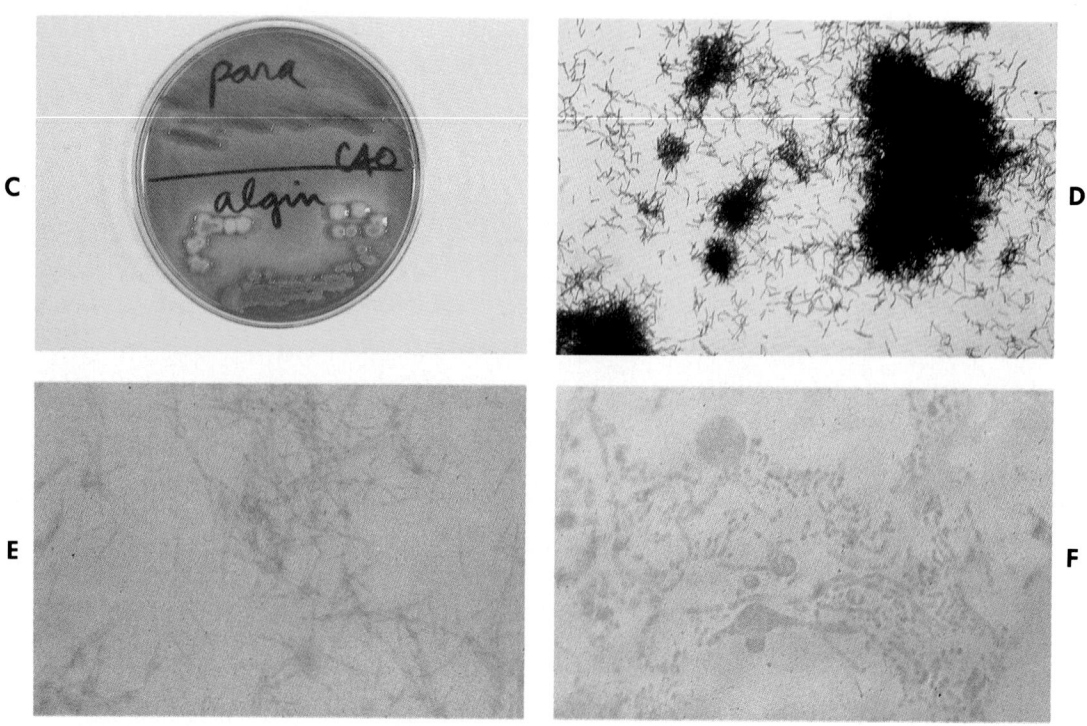

PLATE 14, cont'd. C, Colonies of *Vibrio parahaemolyticus (top),* and *Vibrio alginolyticus* on thiosulfate–citrate–bile salts–sucrose (TCBS) agar. (Courtesy Carol Ormes, Washington Hospital Center, Washington, D.C.) **D,** Gram stain of *Actinomyces israelii.* **E,** Gram stain of *Fusobacterium nucleatum* showing long, spindle-shaped bacilli. **F,** Gram stain of *Fusobacterium necrophorum.* Note pleomorphic gram-negative bacilli with swollen areas, filaments, and large round bodies.

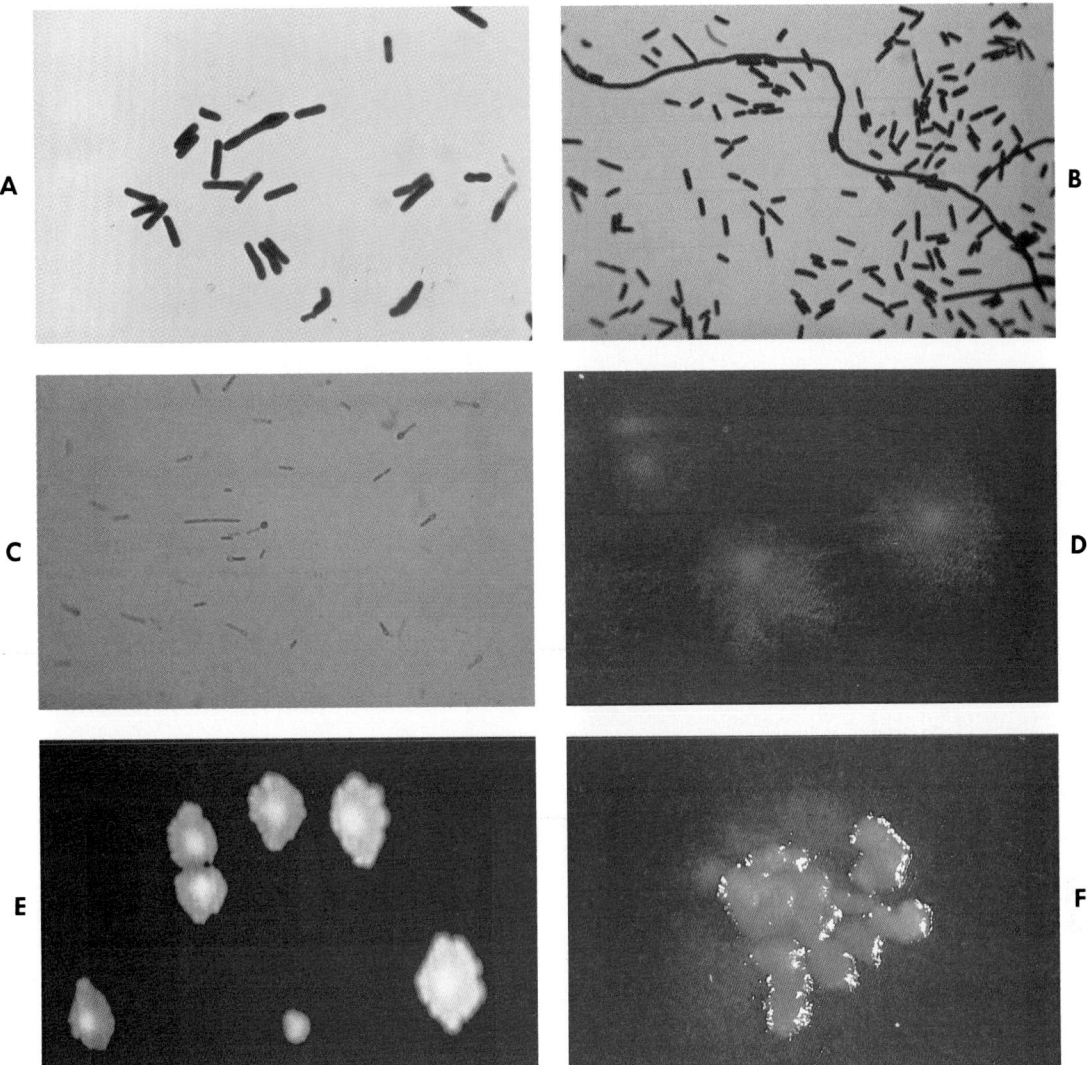

PLATE 15. A, *Clostridium novyi* B. Gram stain of thioglycolate broth. (Courtesy Dr. William J. Brown, Hutzel Hospital, Detroit.) **B,** Gram stain of *Clostridium perfringens* from 24-hour thioglycolate broth. Note boxcar-shaped, gram-positive rods. (From CDC Slide Collection.) **C,** Gram stain of *Clostridium tetani* from 48-hour blood agar plate. Note ''drumstick'' or ''tennis racket'' appearance. (From CDC Slide Collection.) **D,** Colonies of *Clostridium difficile* on blood agar after 48 hours' incubation. (Courtesy Dr. William J. Brown, Hutzel Hospital, Detroit.) **E,** Colonies of *Clostridium histolyticum* on blood agar after 48 hours' incubation. (Courtesy Dr. William J. Brown, Hutzel Hospital, Detroit.) **F,** Colonies of *Clostridium novyi* B on blood agar after 72 hours' incubation. (Courtesy Dr. William J. Brown, Hutzel Hospital, Detroit.)

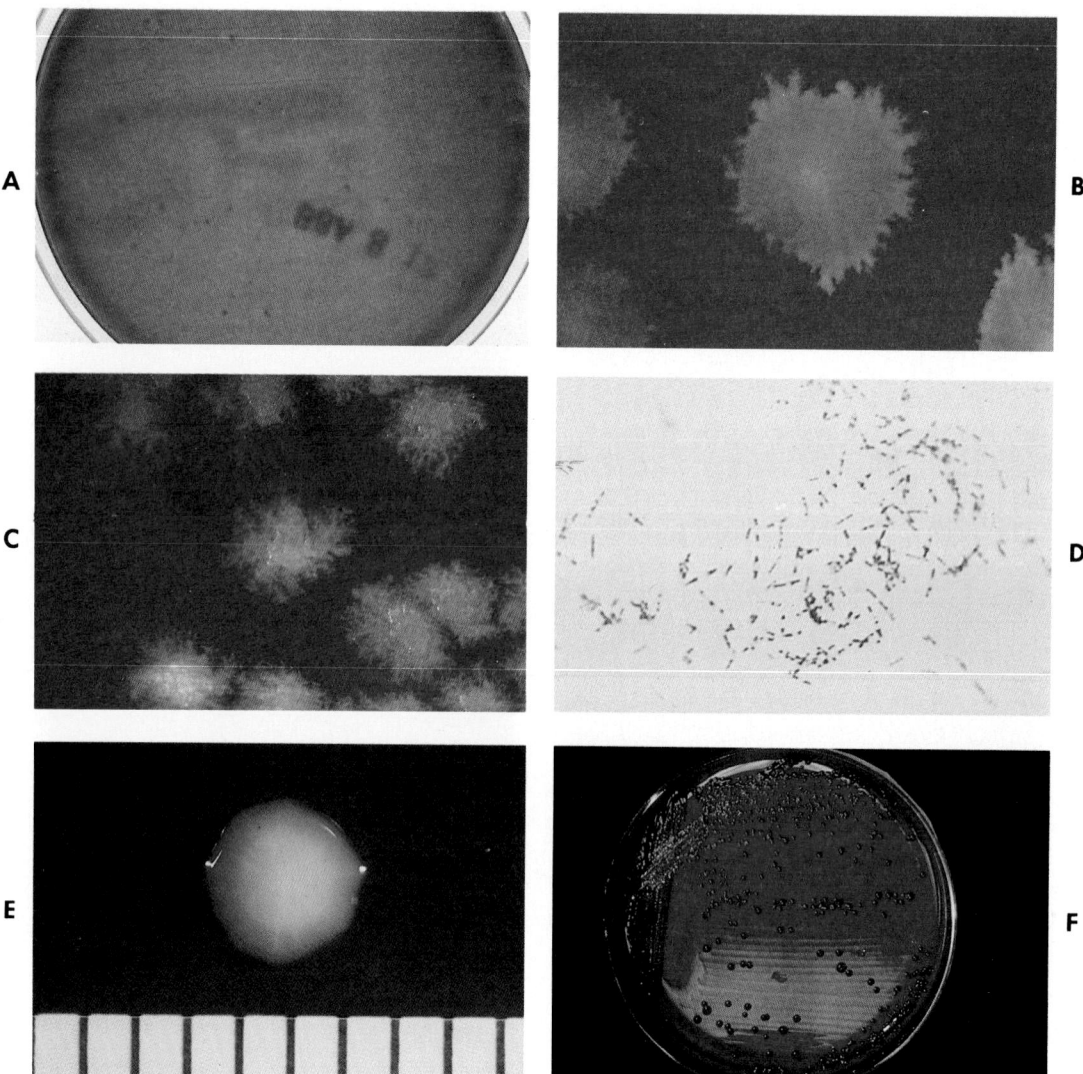

PLATE 16. A, Double zone of hemolysis of *Clostridium perfringens* on blood agar. **B,** Colonies of *Clostridium sordellii* on blood agar after 48 hours' incubation. (Courtesy Dr. William J. Brown, Hutzel Hospital, Detroit.) **C,** Colonies of *Clostridium sporogenes* on blood agar after 48 hours' incubation. (Courtesy Dr. William J. Brown, Hutzel Hospital, Detroit.) **D,** Gram stain of *Bacteroides fragilis*. Note pale-staining, pleomorphic gram-negative rods with round ends, vacuoles, and bipolar staining. **E,** Colonies of *Bacteroides fragilis* on Columbia blood agar. Distance between bars = 1 mm. (Courtesy Dr. William J. Brown, Hutzel Hospital, Detroit.) **F̄,** Black-pigmented *Bacteroides melaninogenicus* on Brucella blood agar.

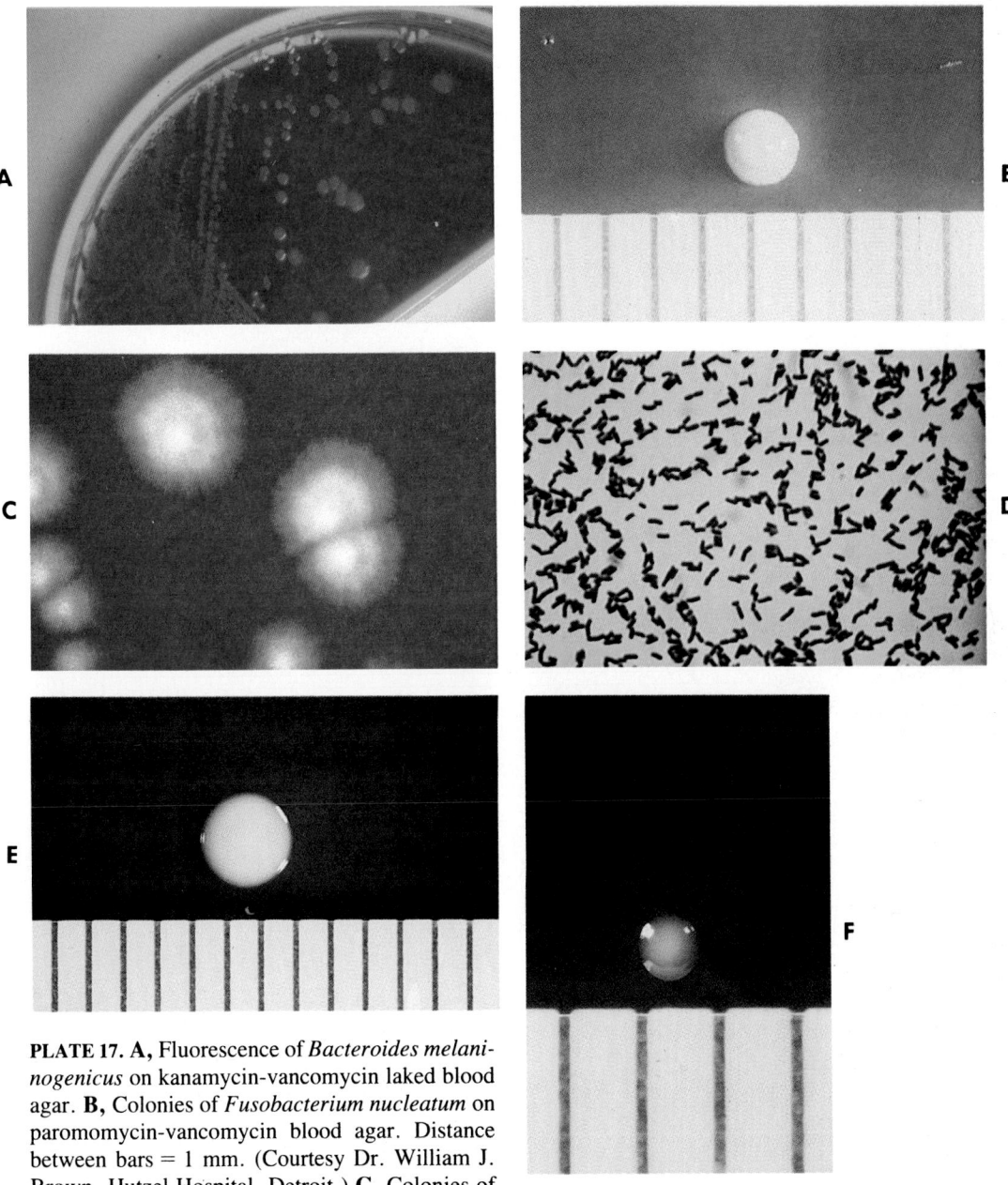

PLATE 17. A, Fluorescence of *Bacteroides melaninogenicus* on kanamycin-vancomycin laked blood agar. **B,** Colonies of *Fusobacterium nucleatum* on paromomycin-vancomycin blood agar. Distance between bars = 1 mm. (Courtesy Dr. William J. Brown, Hutzel Hospital, Detroit.) **C,** Colonies of *Fusobacterium necrophorum* on blood agar after 48 hours' incubation. (Courtesy Dr. William J. Brown, Hutzel Hospital, Detroit.) **D,** Gram stain of *Eubacterium limosum*. (Courtesy Dr. William J. Brown, Hutzel Hospital, Detroit.) **E,** Colonies of *Peptostreptococcus anaerobius* on blood agar. Distance between bars = 1 mm. (Courtesy Dr. William J. Brown, Hutzel Hospital, Detroit.) **F,** Colonies of *Veillonella parvula* on paromomycin-vancomycin blood agar. Distance between bars = 1 mm. (Courtesy Dr. William J. Brown, Hutzel Hospital, Detroit.)

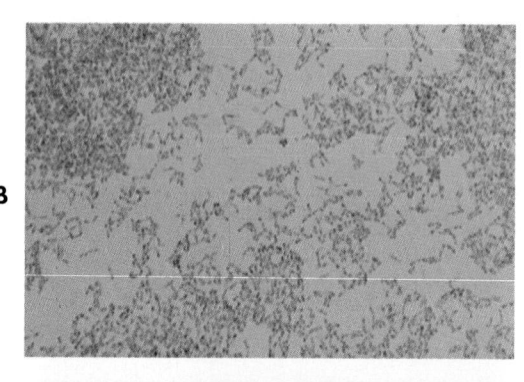

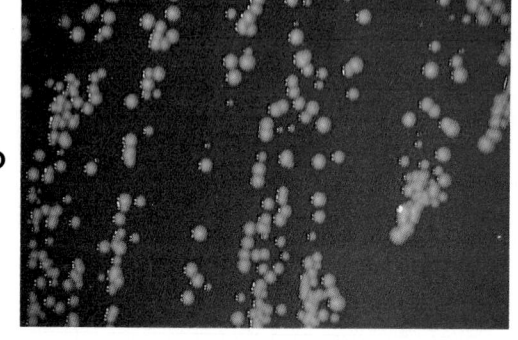

PLATE 18. A, *Actinomyces israelii* in thioglycolate medium. No growth occurs at surface of medium. (Courtesy of Dr. William J. Brown, Hutzel Hospital, Detroit.)

PLATE 18, cont'd. B, Methylene blue stain of *Corynebacterium diphtheriae* showing metachromatic granules. **C,** Gram stain of *Corynebacterium diphtheriae* grown on medium other than Loeffler's. **D** and **E,** Various colonial morphologies of *Corynebacterium* species isolated from skin and sputum. **F,** Gram stain of *Rhodococcus equi.*

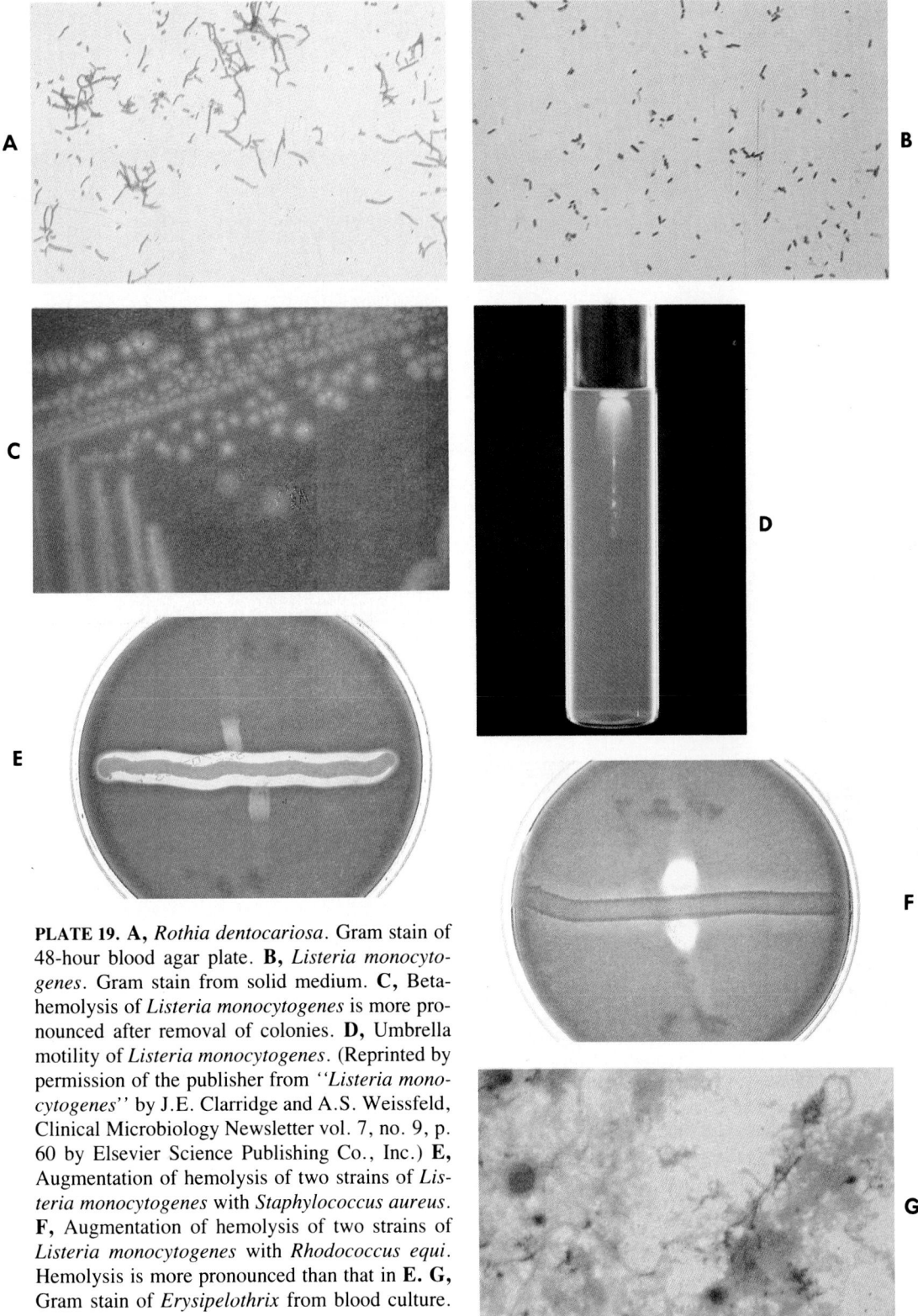

PLATE 19. A, *Rothia dentocariosa.* Gram stain of 48-hour blood agar plate. **B,** *Listeria monocytogenes.* Gram stain from solid medium. **C,** Beta-hemolysis of *Listeria monocytogenes* is more pronounced after removal of colonies. **D,** Umbrella motility of *Listeria monocytogenes.* (Reprinted by permission of the publisher from *"Listeria monocytogenes"* by J.E. Clarridge and A.S. Weissfeld, Clinical Microbiology Newsletter vol. 7, no. 9, p. 60 by Elsevier Science Publishing Co., Inc.) **E,** Augmentation of hemolysis of two strains of *Listeria monocytogenes* with *Staphylococcus aureus.* **F,** Augmentation of hemolysis of two strains of *Listeria monocytogenes* with *Rhodococcus equi.* Hemolysis is more pronounced than that in **E. G,** Gram stain of *Erysipelothrix* from blood culture. Note pleomorphism.

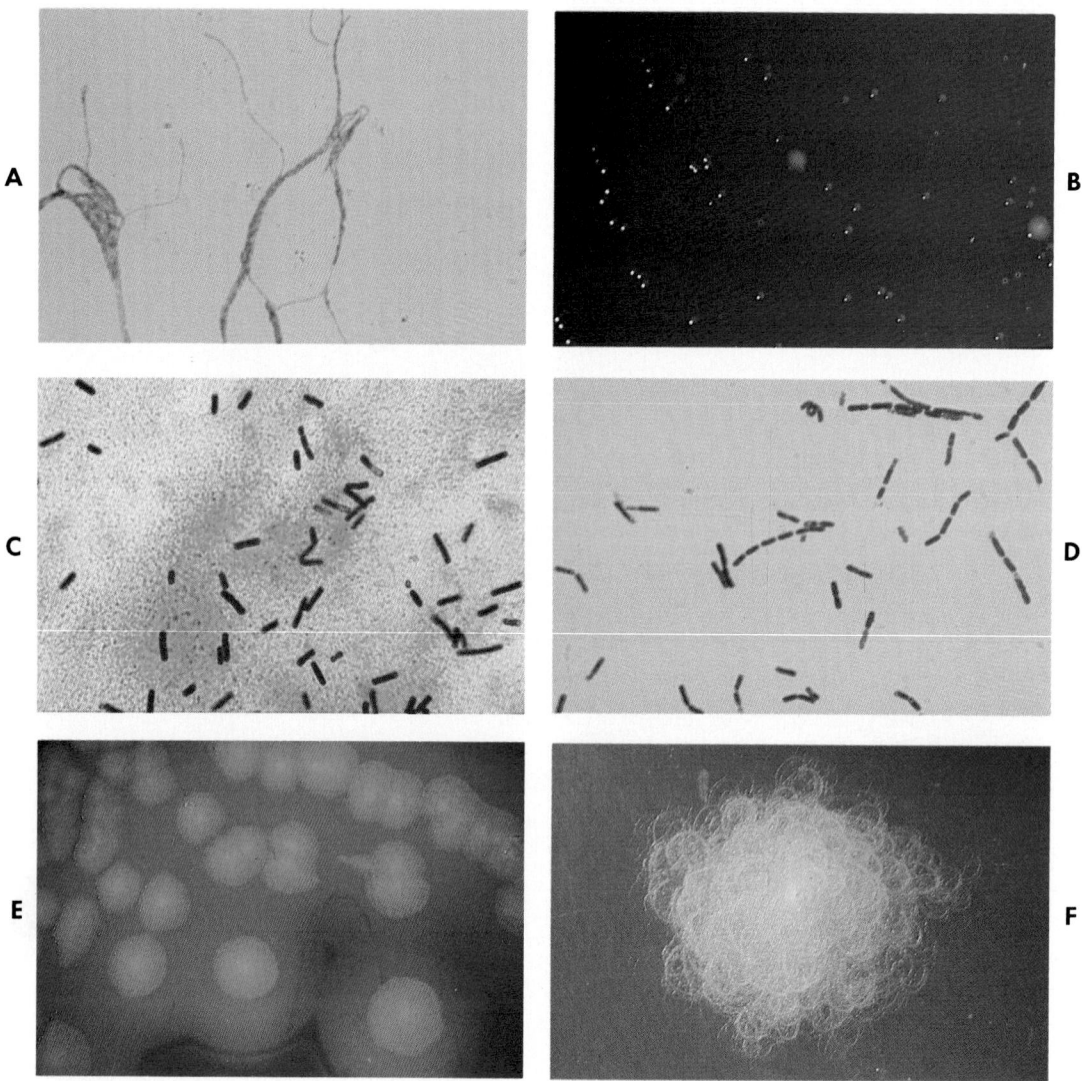

PLATE 20. A, Gram stain of rough colony of *Erysipelothrix*. Note long, thin filaments. **B,** Colonial forms of *Erysipelothrix*. Note rough colonies in upper left, middle, and lower right. Other colonies are smooth forms. **C,** Gram stain of *Bacillus cereus* from young culture. Note large gram-positive rods with spores. **D,** Gram stain of *Bacillus cereus* from older culture. Organisms appear gram variable. **E,** Colonies of *Bacillus cereus*. **F,** Funguslike colony of *Bacillus mycoides*.

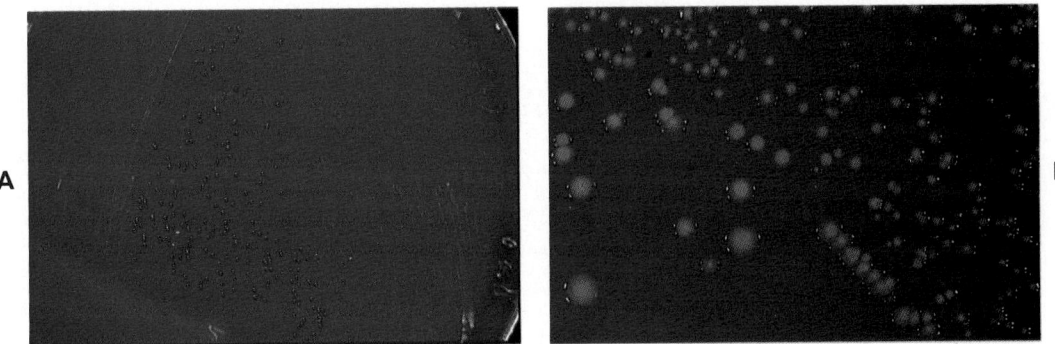

PLATE 21. A, Colonies of *Bordetella pertussis* on Bordet-Gengou agar (1:4). (Photograph by Dr. Leon J. LeBeau, Department of Biocommunication Arts, Medical Center, University of Illinois at Chicago.) **B,** Colonies of *Pasteurella multocida* on blood agar (1:2). (Photograph by Dr. Leon J. LeBeau, Department of Biocommunication Arts, Medical Center, University of Illinois at Chicago.)

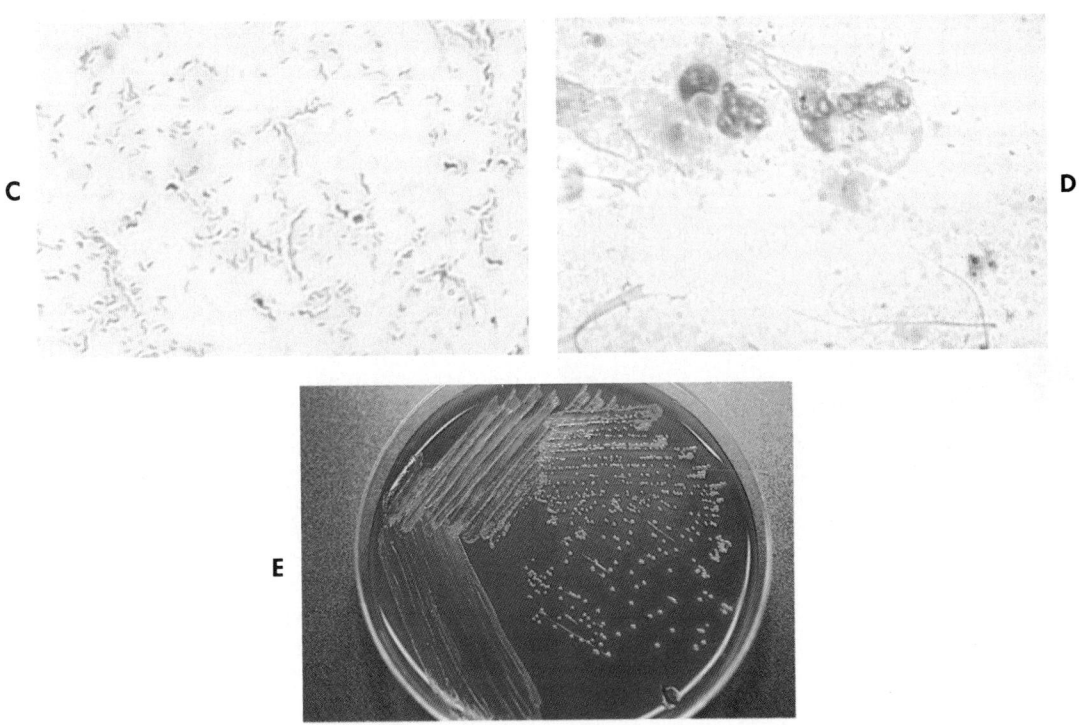

PLATE 21, cont'd. C, Gram stain of colony of *Campylobacter jejuni*. **D,** Gram stain of stool with *Campylobacter jejuni*. Note its gull-wing and S shapes. **E,** Typical colonial morphology of *Campylobacter jejuni*. Note spreading colony.

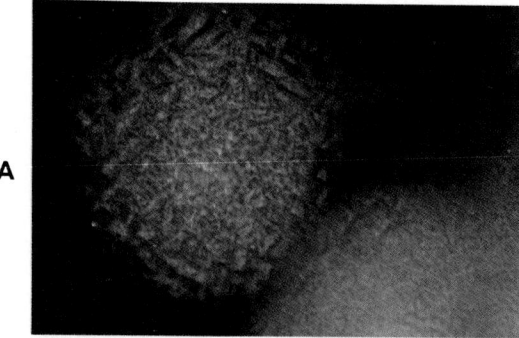

PLATE 22. A, Colonies of *Legionella pneumophila* on BCYE-alpha agar. Other *Legionella* spp. are morphologically similar. (×40.)

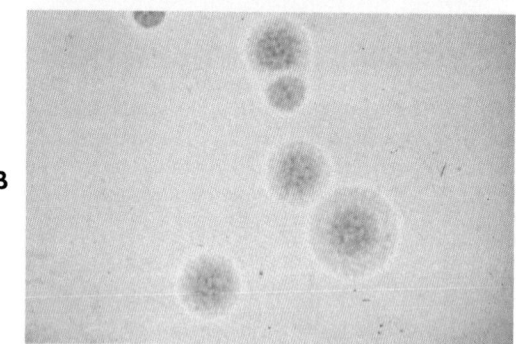

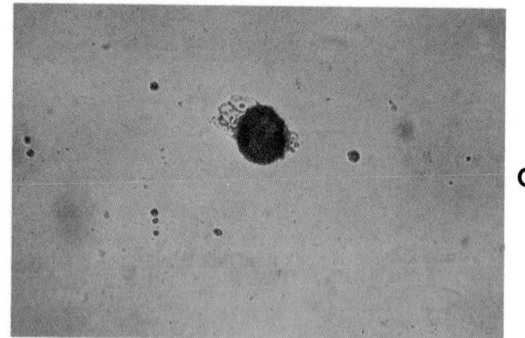

PLATE 22, cont'd. B, Colonial morphology of *Mycoplasma pneumoniae* on SP-4 agar with glucose. Dense central growth surrounded by more translucent peripheral growth gives appearance of fried eggs. **C,** Colonial morphology of *Ureaplasma urealyticum* on A7 agar. Colony of *Ureaplasma* is surrounded by epithelial cells.

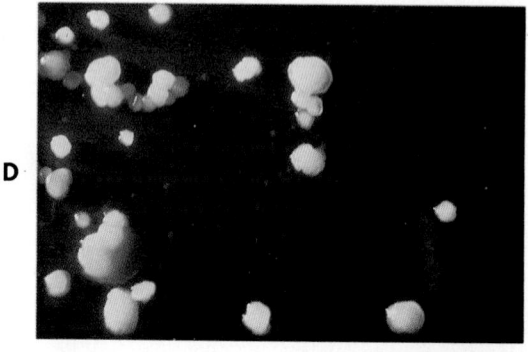

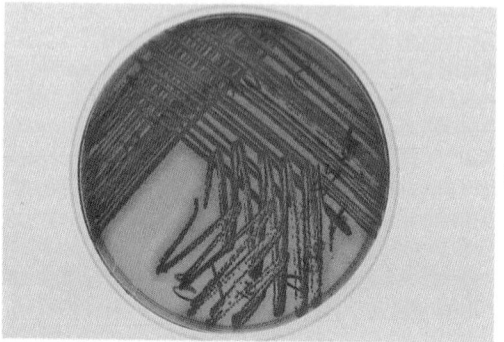

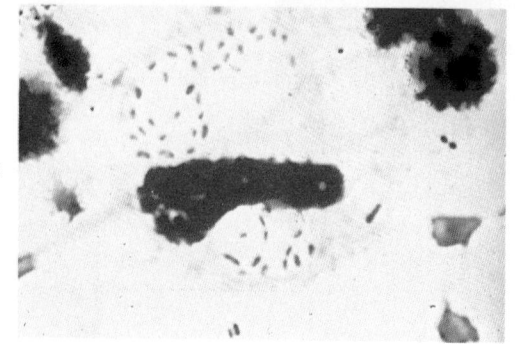

PLATE 22, cont'd. D, Colonial appearance of *Actinobacillus actinomycetemcomitans* (small colonies) in association with molar tooth colonies of *Actinomyces israelii* on blood agar. **E,** Striking purple pigment of *Chromobacterium violaceum* on DNAse agar. **F,** Gram stain of Donovan bodies of *Calymmatobacterium granulomatis*. (×1000.)

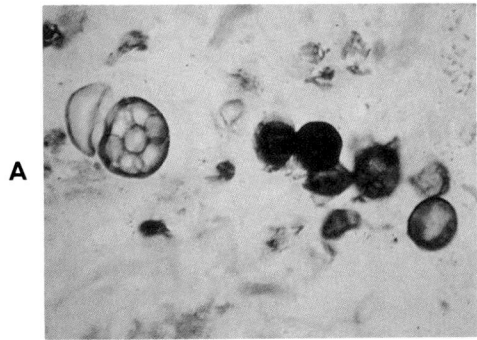

PLATE 23. **A,** Grocott-Gomori methenamine–silver nitrate stain of *Prototheca wickerhamii* in tissue biopsy. (From Arch. Dermatol. **112:**1751, 1976, Copyright © AMA.)

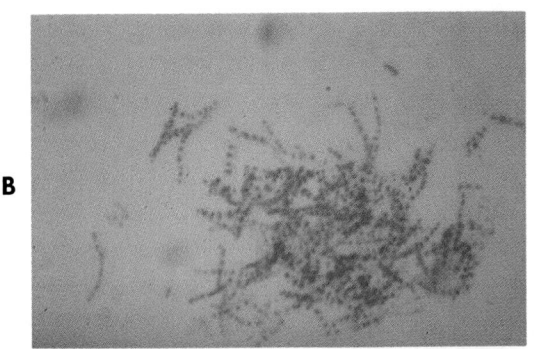

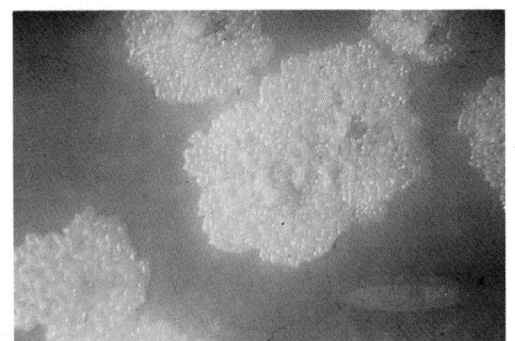

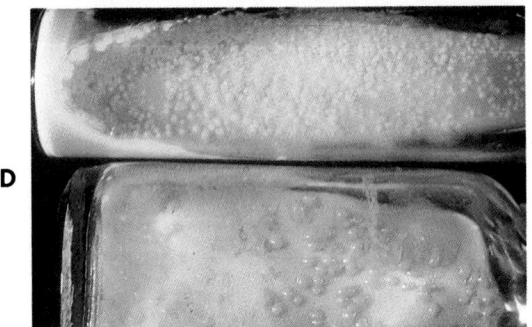

PLATE 23, cont'd. **B,** Ziehl-Neelsen stain of *Mycobacterium tuberculosis*. Alternating dark-staining areas (beads) and clear sections make organisms appear banded. (From CDC Slide Collection.) **C,** Colonies of *Mycobacterium tuberculosis* on Lowenstein-Jensen agar after 8 weeks' incubation. (From CDC Slide Collection.) **D,** Yellow colonies of *Mycobacterium kansasii* after light exposure.

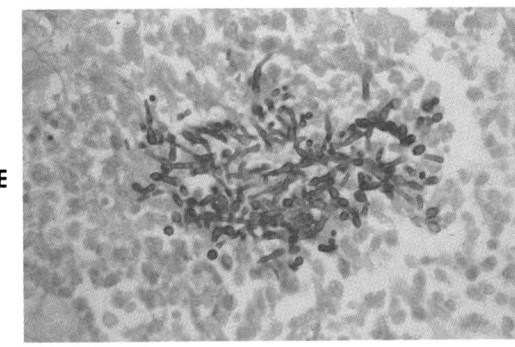

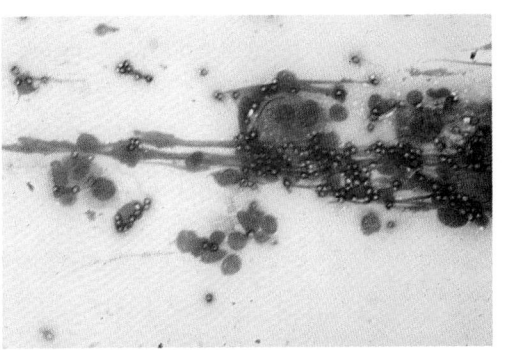

PLATE 23, cont'd. **E,** Periodic acid–Schiff stain of kidney tissue showing magenta yeast cells of *Candida albicans*. (×400.) **F,** Giemsa stain of *Histoplasma capsulatum*. (×400.)

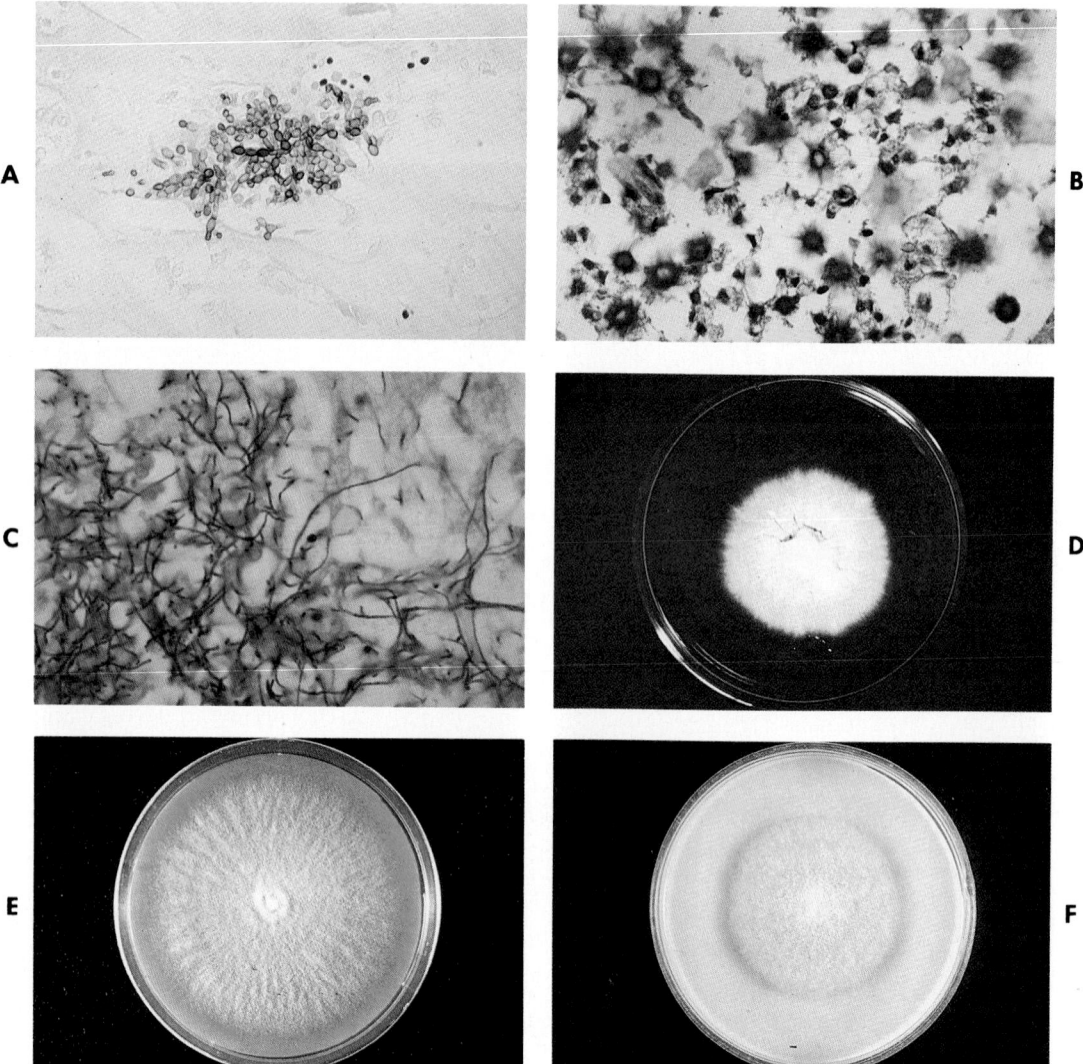

PLATE 24. A, Grocott-Gomori methenamine–silver nitrate stain of *Candida albicans* in kidney. (×400.) **B,** Mayer mucicarmine stain of *Cryptococcus neoformans* in brain tissue. Note ''starburst'' rose-colored capsules of this organism. **C,** Brown and Brenn stain of specimen from patient with nocardiosis. Note gram-positive branching filaments approximately 0.5 μm in diameter. **D,** Colony of *Epidermophyton floccosum;* Sabouraud dextrose agar. (Courtesy L. Ajello, Centers for Disease Control, Atlanta.) **E,** Colony of *Microsporum audouinii*, Sabouraud dextrose agar. (Courtesy L. Ajello, Centers for Disease Control, Atlanta.) **F,** Colony of *Microsporum canis;* Sabouraud dextrose agar. (Courtesy L. Ajello, Centers for Disease Control, Atlanta.)

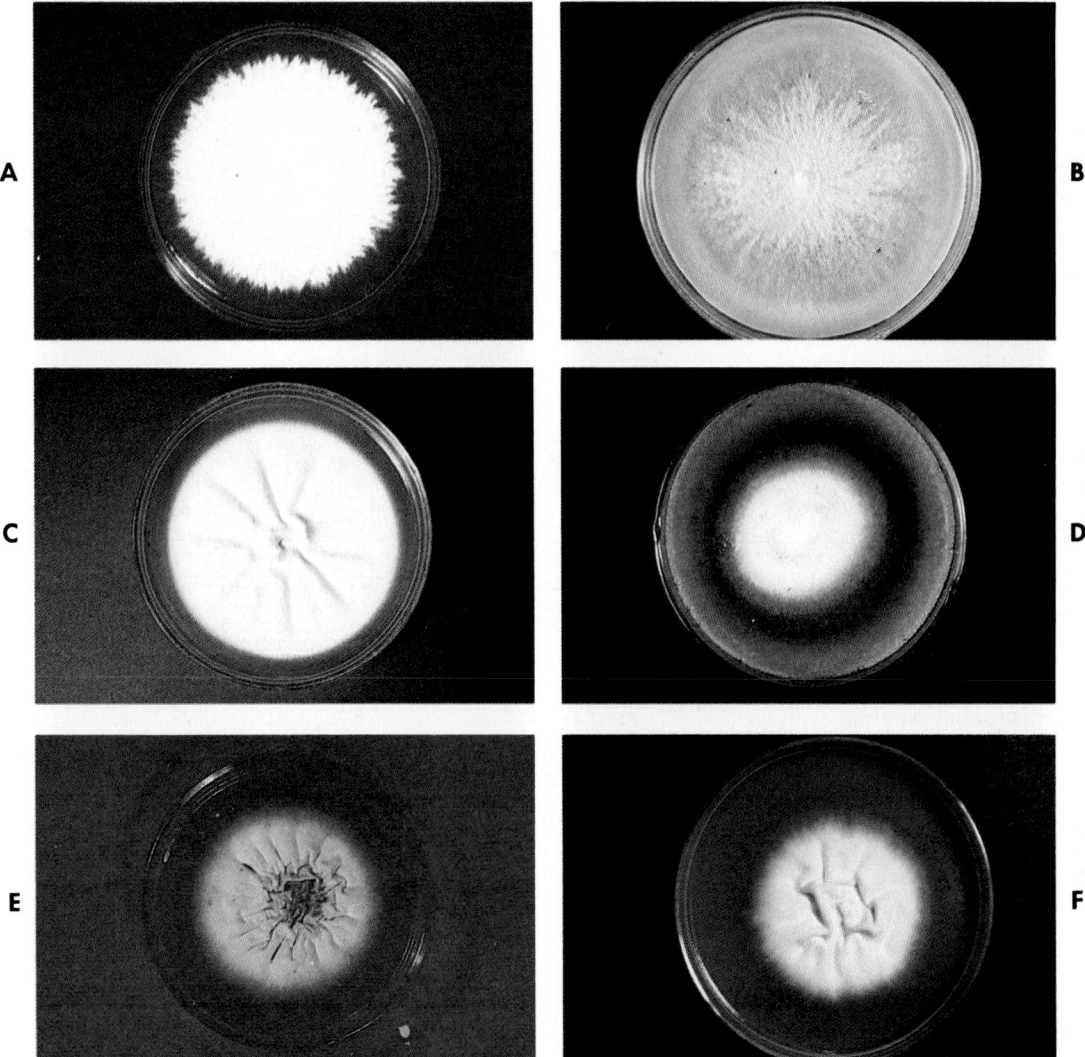

PLATE 25. A, Colony of *Microsporum gypseum;* Sabouraud dextrose agar. (Courtesy L. Ajel-lo, Centers for Disease Control, Atlanta.) **B,** Colony of *Microsporum nanum;* Sabouraud dextrose agar. (Courtesy L. Ajello, Centers for Disease Control, Atlanta.) **C,** Colony of *Tri-chophyton mentagrophytes* (var. *quinckeanum*); Sabouraud dextrose agar. (Courtesy L. Ajello, Centers for Disease Control, Atlanta.) **D,** Colony of *Trichophyton rubrum,* Sabouraud dextrose agar. (Courtesy L. Ajello, Centers for Disease Control, Atlanta.) **E,** Colony of *Trichophyton schoenleinii;* Sabouraud dextrose agar. (Courtesy L. Ajello, Centers for Disease Control, Atlanta.) **F,** Colony of *Trichophyton tonsurans;* Sabouraud dextrose agar. (Courtesy L. Ajello, Centers for Disease Control, Atlanta.)

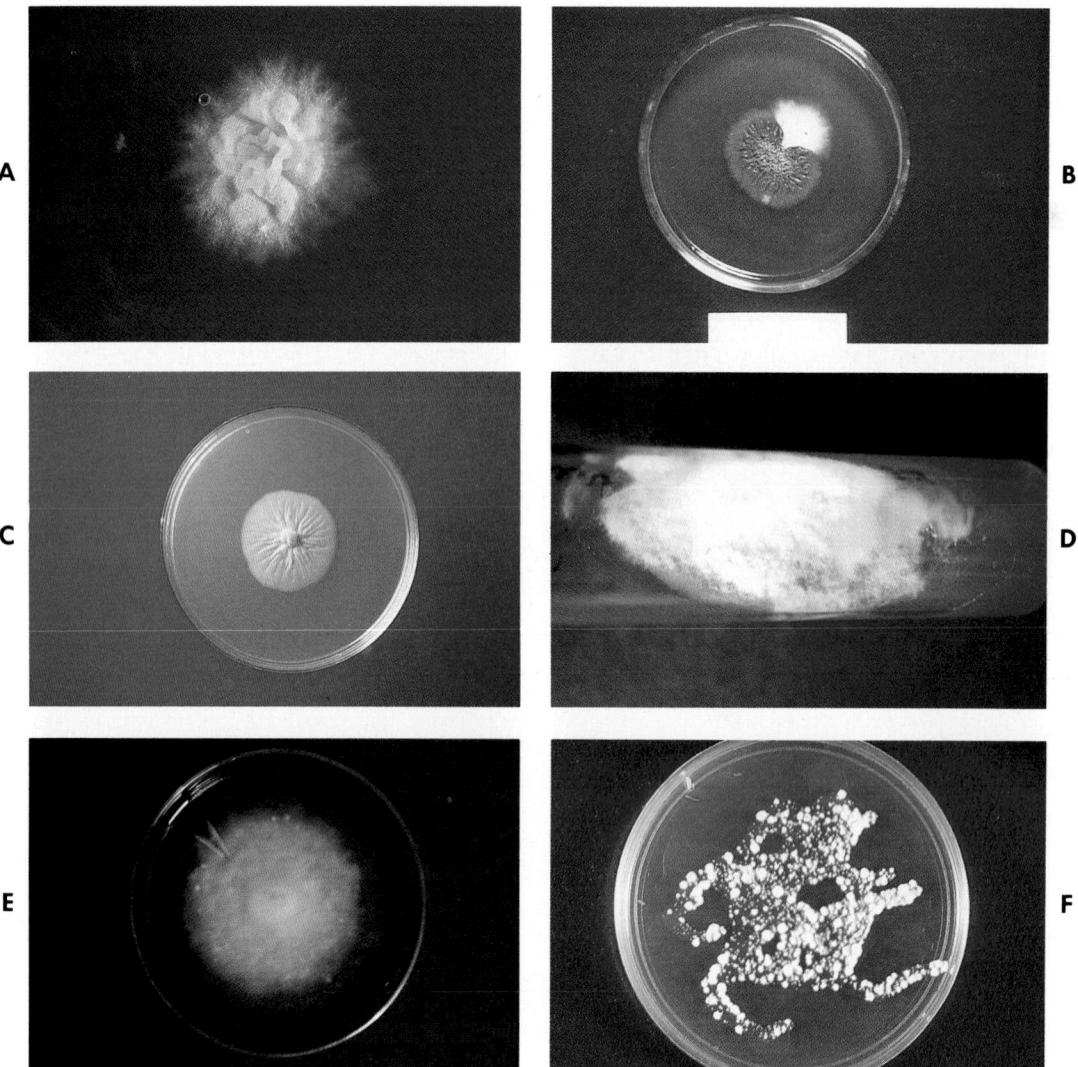

PLATE 26. A, Colony of *Trichophyton verrucosum;* Sabouraud dextrose agar. (Courtesy L. Ajello, Centers for Disease Control, Atlanta.) **B,** Colony of *Trichophyton violaceum;* Sabouraud dextrose agar. (Courtesy L. Ajello, Centers for Disease Control, Atlanta.) **C,** Colony of *Blastomyces dermatitidis;* Sabouraud dextrose agar. (Courtesy L. Ajello, Centers for Disease Control, Atlanta.) **D,** *Coccidioides immitis;* Sabouraud dextrose agar. (From Kern-Singer, M.: Basic medical mycology, Philadelphia, 1985, F.A. Davis Co.) **E,** Colony of *Histoplasma capsulatum* (soil isolate); Sabouraud dextrose agar. (Courtesy L. Ajello, Centers for Disease Control, Atlanta.) **F,** *Paracoccidioides brasiliensis* on Sabhi agar.

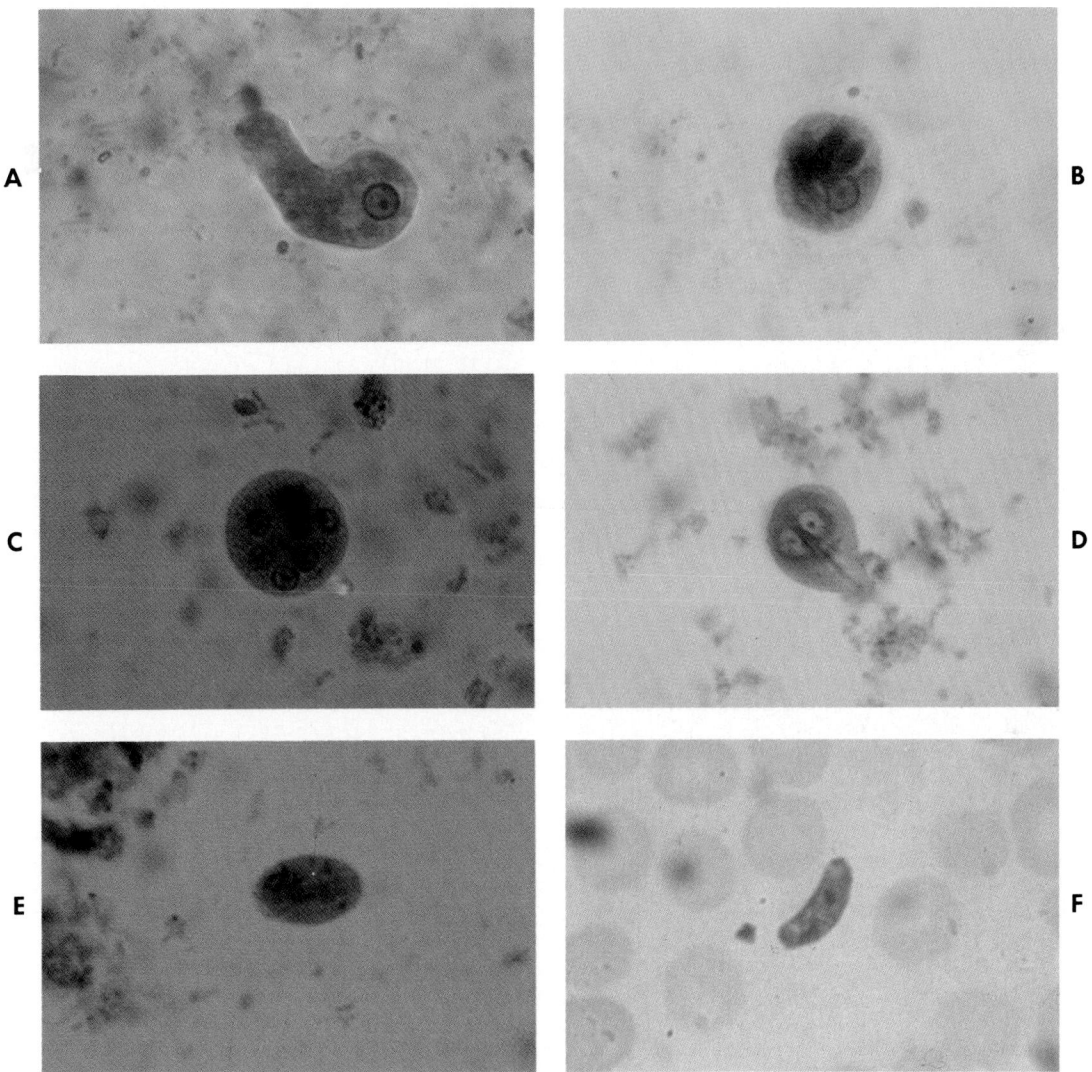

PLATE 27. A, Trophozoite of *Entamoeba histolytica* (trichrome stain). **B,** Cyst of *Entamoeba histolytica* (trichrome stain). **C,** Cyst of *Entamoeba coli* (iron-hematoxylin stain). **D,** Trophozoite of *Giardia lamblia* (trichrome stain). **E,** Cyst of *Giardia lamblia* (trichrome stain). **F,** Gametocyte of *Plasmodium falciparum* (Giemsa stain).

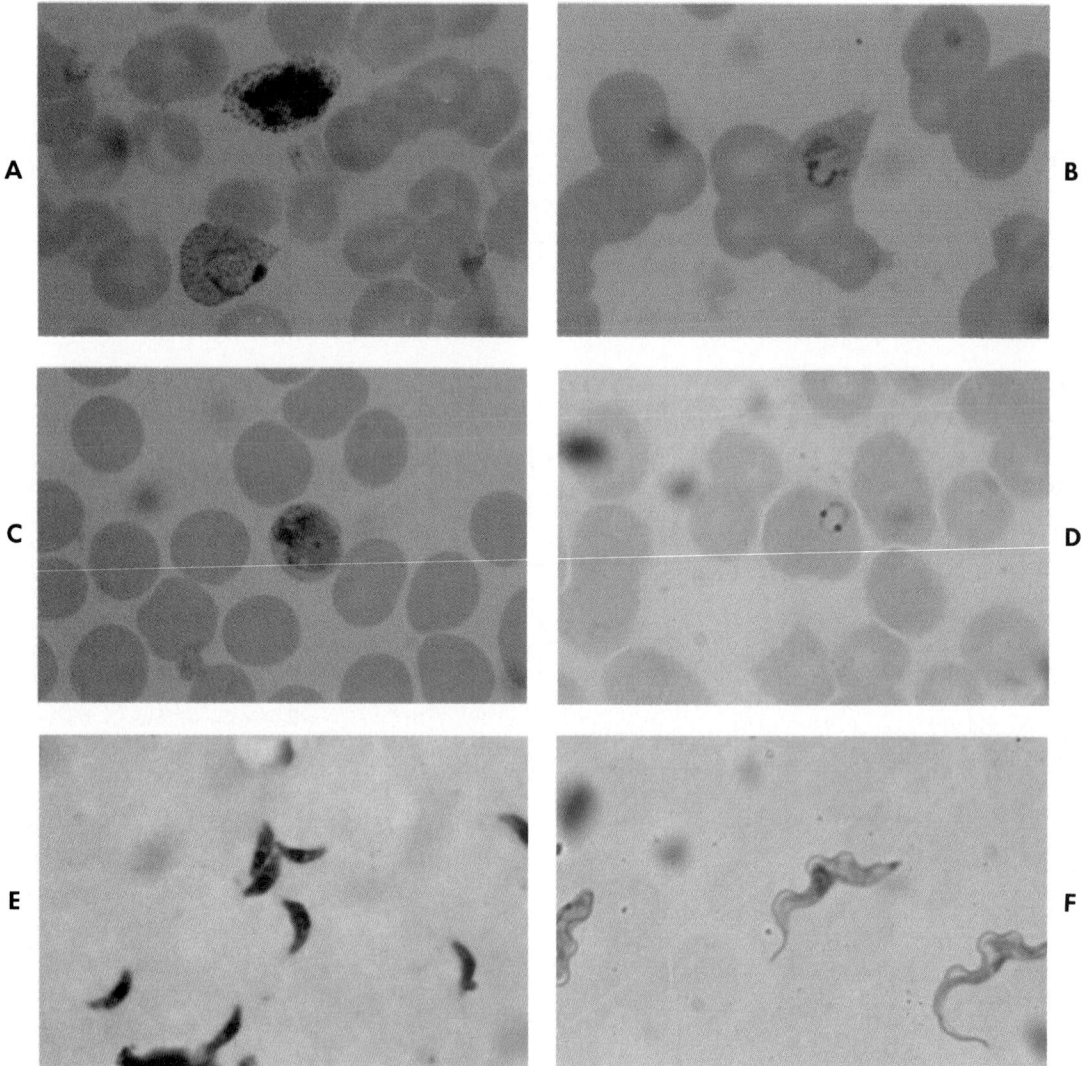

PLATE 28. A, Trophozoite with Schuffner's dots *(lower)* and schizont *(upper)* of *Plasmodium vivax* (Giemsa stain). **B,** Trophozoite of *Plasmodium ovale* (Giemsa stain). **C,** Trophozoite of *Plasmodium malariae* (Giemsa stain). **D,** Ring of *Plasmodium falciparum* (Giemsa stain). **E,** Trophozoites of *Toxoplasma* (Giemsa stain). **F,** Trypomastigote of *Trypanosoma brucei* (Giemsa stain).

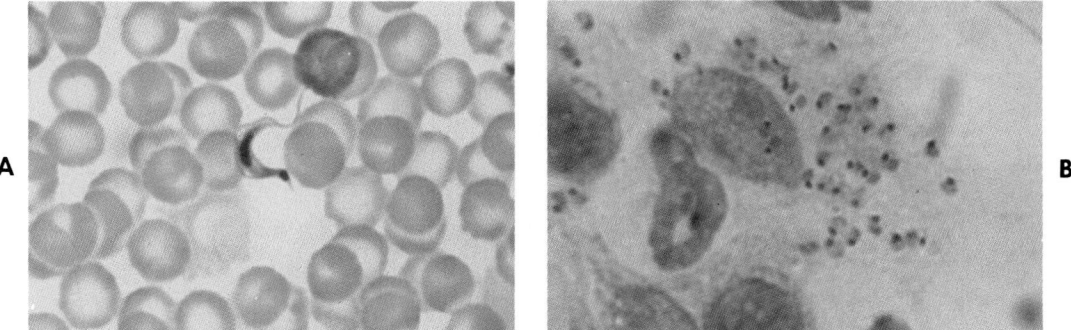

PLATE 29. A, Trypomastigote of *Trypanosoma cruzi* (Giemsa stain). **B,** Intracellular amastigotes of *Leishmania* (Giemsa stain).

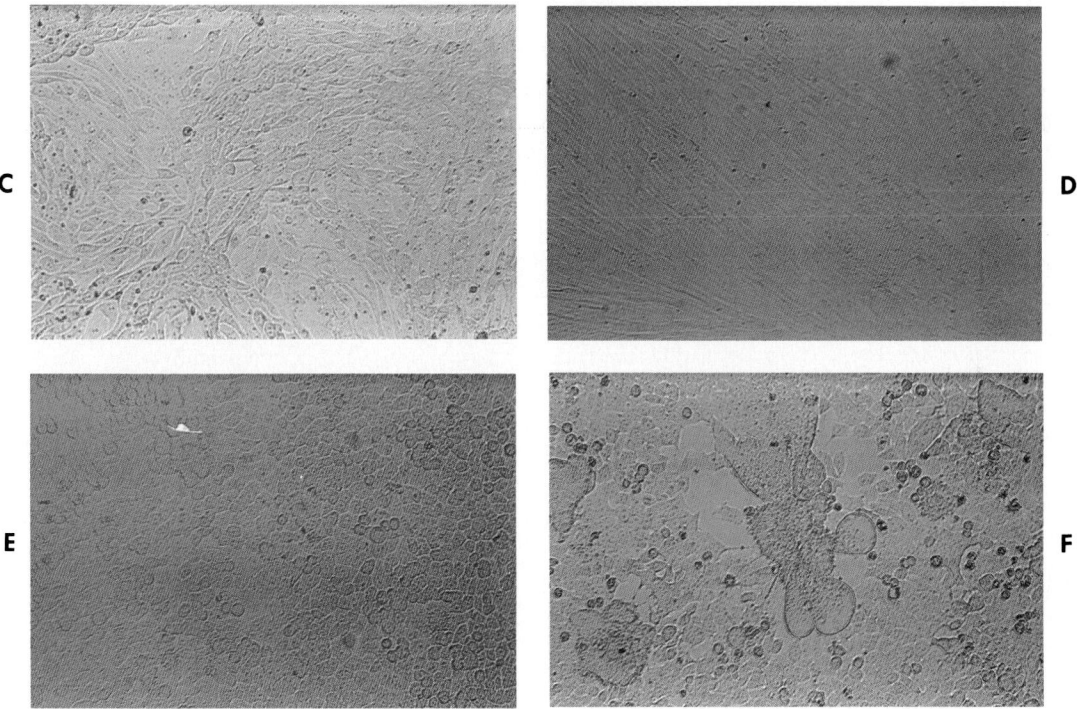

PLATE 29, cont'd. C, Uninfected primary monkey cell culture. Cells are mixed population with polygonal epithelial cells predominating. (From CDC Slide Collection.) **D,** Uninfected human diploid fibroblast cell culture (WI-38). Cells are elongated and oriented in common direction. (From CDC Slide Collection.) **E,** Uninfected HEp2 cell culture. This heteroploid cell line was derived from a human epidermoid carcinoma. Cells are short, polygonal-shaped epithelial cells. (From CDC Slide Collection.) **F,** Example of viral cytopathic effect in cell culture: respiratory syncytial virus in HEp2 cells. (From CDC Slide Collection.)

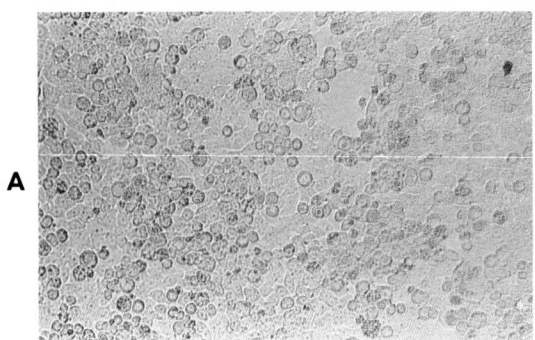

A

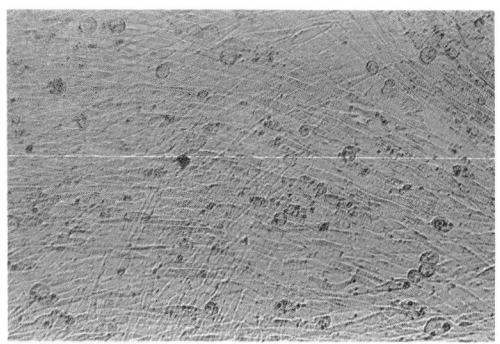

B

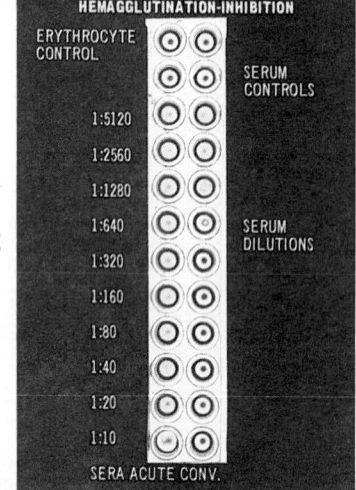

C

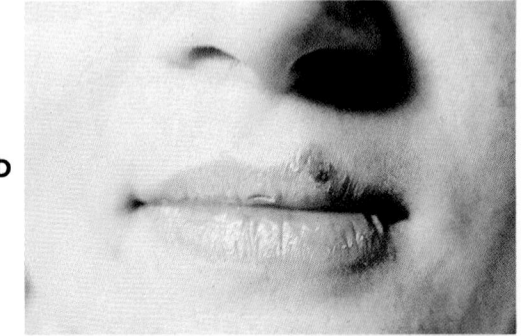

D

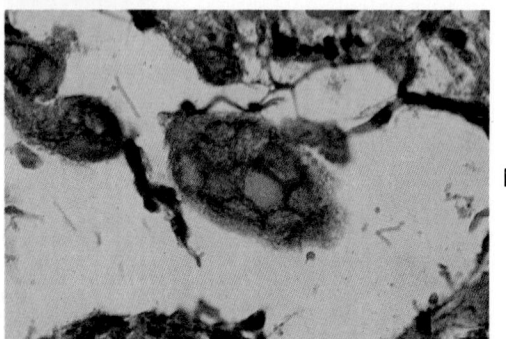

E

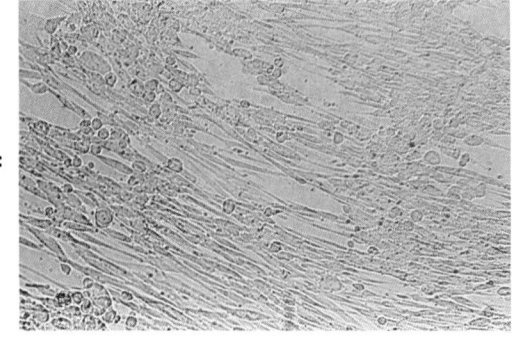

F

PLATE 30. A and **B,** Examples of viral cytopathic effect in cell culture: **A,** Adenovirus in HEp2 cells and, **B,** cytomegalovirus in WI-38 cells. (From CDC Slide Collection.) **C,** Hemagglutination inhibition showing acute titer of < 1:10 and convalescent titer of 1:320. **D,** Recurrent herpes simplex virus oral infection—a ''cold sore.'' **E,** Herpes virus inclusions. Herpes esophagitis (Papanicolaou stain; ×400). **F,** Herpes simplex virus cytopathic effect in human diploid fibroblast cells showing extensive cell rounding. (From CDC Slide Collection.)

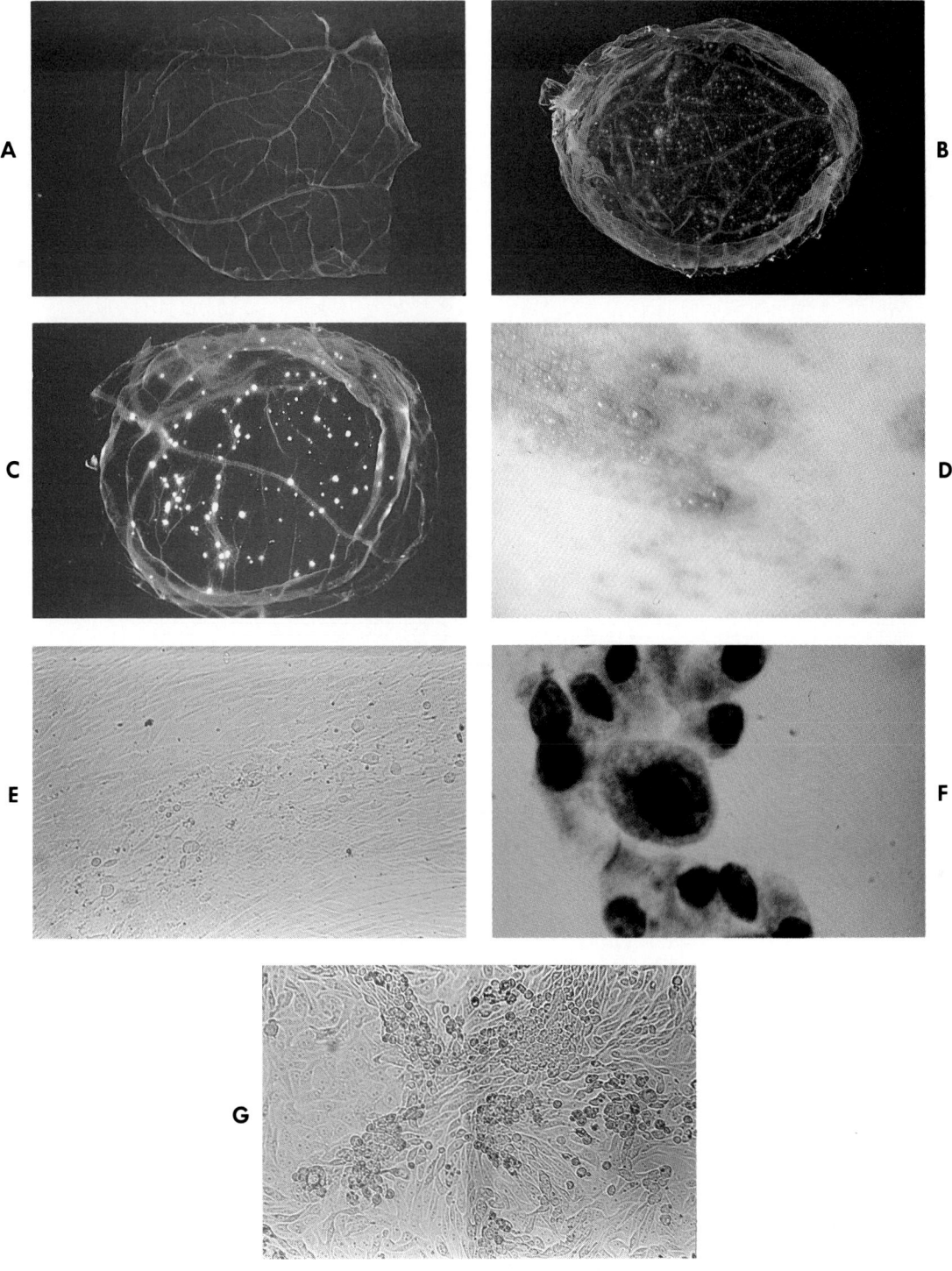

PLATE 31. A to **C,** Herpes simplex–infected chorioallantoic membrane (CAM): **A,** Uninfected CAM. (From CDC Slide Collection.) **B,** HSV-1 infection of CAM results in small pocks. (From CDC Slide Collection.) **C,** HSV-2 infection of CAM results in large pocks. (From CDC Slide Collection.) **D,** Typical vesicular lesions of varicella-zoster virus. **E,** Cytopathic effect (rounded cells in large cytopathic lesion) of varicella-zoster virus in human diploid fibroblasts. (From CDC Slide Collection.) **F,** Cytomegalovirus inclusions in lung (Papanicolaou stain). **G,** Primary rhesus monkey kidney cell culture infected with echovirus. General rounding of cells is seen. (From CDC Slide Collection.)

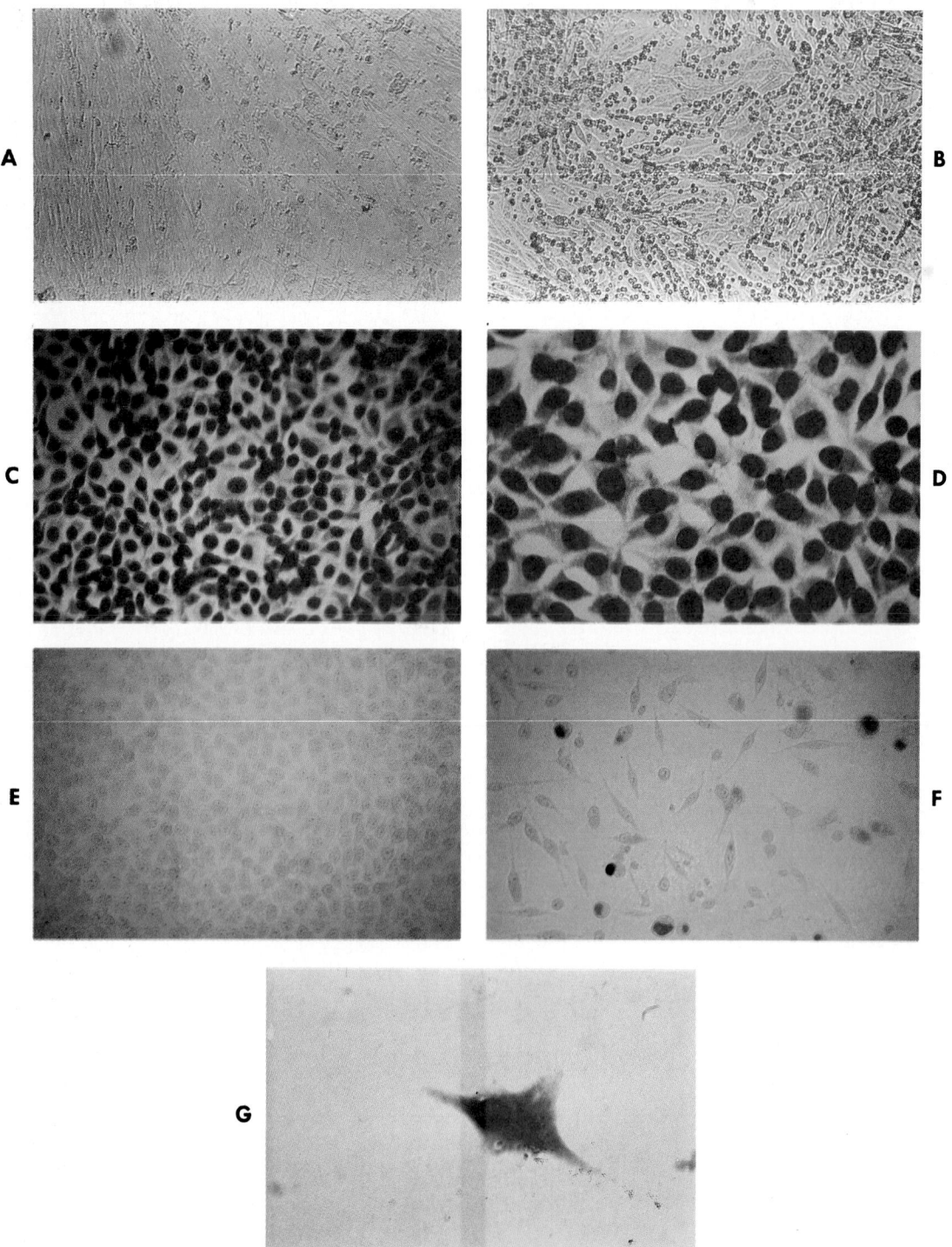

PLATE 32. **A,** Human diploid fibroblasts infected with poliovirus showing large areas of cell rounding and cell degeneration. (From CDC Slide Collection.) **B,** Hemadsorption of guinea pig red blood cells to influenza virus–infected primary rhesus monkey kidney cell culture. (From CDC Slide Collection.) **C,** Uninfected McCoy cell monolayer (Giemsa stain). **D,** *Chlamydia trachomatis* inclusions in McCoy cell monolayer (Giemsa stain). **E,** Uninfected McCoy cell monolayer (iodine stain). **F,** *Chlamydia trachomatis* inclusions in McCoy cell monolayer (iodine stain). **G,** Giemsa stain of *R. tsutsugamushi* in resident peritoneal macrophage of mice. (Courtesy Dr. Carol Nacy, Walter Reed Army Institute of Research, Washington, D.C.)

TABLE 25-5. Biochemical Characteristics of *Cardiobacterium hominis*

Characteristic	Reaction
Triple sugar iron (TSI) agar	Acid/acid
H$_2$S (butt/paper)	−/+ weak
Kligler iron agar (KIA)	Alkaline/acid
Catalase	−
Oxidase	+
Motility	−
Growth on MacConkey agar	−
Growth on Salmonella-Shigella agar	−
Simmons citrate	−
Urea hydrolysis	−
Gelatin liquefaction	−
Indole	+ weak
Nitrate reduction	−
Lysine decarboxylase	−
Ornithine decarboxylase	−
Arginine dihydrolase	−
Esculin hydrolysis	−

TABLE 25-5. Biochemical Characteristics of *Cardiobacterium hominis*—cont'd

Characteristic	Reaction
ONPG (production of beta-galactosidase)	−
Hippurate hydrolysis	−
Gas from glucose	−
Acid from:	
Adonitol	−
Arabinose	−
Dulcitol	−
Fructose	+
Galactose	−
Glucose	+
Inositol	−
Lactose	−
Maltose	+
Mannitol	+
Raffinose	−
Rhamnose	−
Salicin	−
Sorbitol	+
Sucrose	+
Trehalose	−
Xylose	−

SYMBOLS: +, 90% or more strains positive
−, 90% or more strains negative

moniliformis, Eikenella corrodens, and EF-4 on the basis of positive indole test results. Differentiation from *Kingella indologenes* may be more of a problem because both organisms are oxidase positive, catalase negative, and indole positive; however, *C. hominis* ferments mannitol and sorbitol and *K. indologenes* does not.[11] These two organisms may also be distinguished by differences in enzyme production.[11] *C. hominis* also ferments various other sugars without the production of gas. Carbohydrate utilization test media may need to be supplemented with serum or ascitic fluid to obtain sufficient growth (2 drops of rabbit serum per 3 ml of liquid peptone medium). Detection of indole production may require extraction with xylene and addition of Ehrlich reagent. Typical biochemical characteristics of *C. hominis* are shown in Table 25-5.

SEROLOGIC AND IMMUNOSEROLOGIC IDENTIFICATION

Specific fluorescent antibody staining with fluorescein-conjugated anti–*C. hominis* antibody has been used to detect the organism,[131] but this reagent is not available commercially.

CLINICAL SIGNIFICANCE

C. hominis is primarily a causative agent of endocarditis in patients with preexisting cardiovascular defects[118] but has also been involved in a case of fatal septicemia in an immunocompromised patient with no known preexisting heart disease.[114] The organism is part of the normal human respiratory flora and has also been found in stool and as part of genital tract flora.

ANTIMICROBIAL SUSCEPTIBILITY

Penicillin and streptomycin, singly or in combination, are the drugs of choice in treating *C. hominis* infections. The organism is also susceptible to tetracycline, chloramphenicol, erythromycin, cephalothin, colistin, trimethoprim-sulfamethoxazole, and the aminoglycosides. Susceptibility has been determined by both disk diffusion and minimum inhibitory concentration procedures.

CHROMOBACTERIUM

Organisms in the genus *Chromobacterium* are gram-negative, fermentative, motile, nonsporeforming rods that usually produce violet colonies. They are soil and water bacteria that occasionally cause serious infections in humans. Human infections have usually been reported from areas with tropical or subtropical climates.

CLASSIFICATION

The genus *Chromobacterium* is included in section 5 of *Bergey's Manual of Systematic Bacteriology,* volume 1, with the gram-negative facultatively anaerobic rods; it is listed along with several "other genera."[136] The genus consists of two species, *C. violaceum* (the type species) and *C. fluviatile. C. violaceum* is the only species isolated from human specimens. *C. fluviatile* (a psychrophile) does not grow at 37° C; it has been isolated from river water in England. The genus name derives from the Greek *chroma,* "color," referring to the characteristic violet pigment (violacein); the species name *violaceum* is from the Latin word meaning violet-colored.

Specimen Collection and Processing

Specimens submitted for isolation of *C. violaceum* include pus, blood, and autopsy tissues. The effects of various transport media on the recovery of *C. violaceum* are not known.

Growth Requirements
Media

C. violaceum grows on most ordinary laboratory media including blood agar, MacConkey agar, and eosin–methylene blue agar; growth on Salmonella-Shigella agar is delayed. For long-term storage the isolates should be lyophilized or stored frozen at −70° C in nutrient broth with 15% glycerol.

Environmental Requirements

C. violaceum grows both aerobically and anaerobically at 30° to 35° C. Colonies are seen after 24 to 48 hours of incubation.

Cultural Characteristics
Staining Reactions

C. violaceum is a 0.8 to 1.2 μm by 2.5 to 6 μm gram-negative rod with rounded ends. The organism may be pleomorphic and usually occurs singly. The unique flagellar arrangement (both unipolar and usually with one to four subpolar or lateral flagella) is best seen in smears from young cultures grown on solid media; the lateral flagella are rare in broth cultures.

Colonial Morphology

After 24 hours, colonies of *C. violaceum* are 1 to 2 mm in size, round, smooth, and low and convex on blood agar; beta-hemolysis may be observed on rabbit blood. Most colonies exhibit the typical violet pigment (optimally produced at 22° C), which is not water soluble and thus does not readily diffuse into the culture medium (Plate 22, *E*). Colonies on blood agar may appear to be black. Nonpigmented strains do occur and are pathogenic.[129] *C. violaceum* produces hydrogen cyanide, and cultures smell of cyanide. Broth cultures show uniform turbidity and a violet pellicle.

Biochemical Identification

Nonpigmented strains of *C. violaceum* may be confused with the genera *Aeromonas*, *Pseudomonas*, or *Vibrio* or the family *Enterobacteriaceae*. *C. violaceum* may be differentiated from *Aeromonas hydrophila* on the basis of negative tests for indole and mannitol and maltose fermentation. It may be differentiated from *Plesiomonas shigelloides* on the basis of negative tests for lysine and ornithine decarboxylase and lactose fermentation and a positive test for gelatin liquefaction. *C. violaceum* may be differentiated from *Vibrio* spp. on the basis of negative tests for lysine and ornithine decarboxylase, indole, and mannitol and maltose fermentation. *C. violaceum* is a glucose fermenter and thus may be differentiated from the *Pseudomonas* spp., which utilize glucose oxidatively. *C. violaceum* is usually oxidase positive using the Kovacs test and thus may be differentiated from the *Enterobacteriaceae*.

The key reactions for identification of *C. violaceum* are a positive catalase test (although the organism is highly sensitive to hydrogen peroxide); fermentation of glucose, but not mannitol and lactose; growth on MacConkey agar; arginine dihy-

drolase positivity; and absence of growth at 4° C. Care must be taken during performance of the oxidase test; if the violet pigment interferes with reading the test, the test should be repeated from an anaerobic culture (because oxygen is necessary for pigment production). Liquid peptone basal medium with Andrade indicator should be used for carbohydrate fermentation studies. Typical biochemical characteristics of *C. violaceum* are shown in Table 25-6.

Serologic and Immunoserologic Identification

No routine serologic tests are available for antibody detection or for identifying the organism.

Clinical Significance

The natural habitat of *C. violaceum* is soil and natural water sources in tropical and semitropical climates (Southeast Asia and southeastern United States). This organism rarely causes infections in humans, but when it does it usually is manifest as skin abscesses or as overwhelming septicemia with pulmonary, liver, and subcutaneous abscesses; the eye may also be involved.[39,82,127] The portal of entry of human infections is probably the skin, although organisms may also gain entrance through ingestion of contaminated material.[140] The portal of entry in one recently reported case was the eye; the patient fell into muddy water and the eye was contaminated with mud.[39,127] Septicemia may occur in previously healthy individuals and in patients with chronic granulomatous disease of childhood. Most cases are fatal. Fourteen cases of septicemia have been reported in the United States; 12 from Florida and two from Louisiana.[39,82,127] Skin infections have been reported in immunosuppressed patients with leukemia.[31]

Antimicrobial Susceptibility

Once generalized septicemia has become established, treatment is usually ineffective, although a few cases of systemic chromobacteriosis have been successfully treated.[39,82,127,156] Susceptibility testing of most clinical strains has been performed using the agar disk diffusion test. Isolates are typically susceptible to ampicillin, carbenicillin, chloramphenicol, tetracycline, gentamicin, tobramycin, and trimethoprim-sulfamethoxazole and resistant to cephalothin.[140]

AGROBACTERIUM

Microorganisms of the genus *Agrobacterium* rarely occur in clinical specimens. They are gram-negative, nonsporeforming rods usually found in soil. *A. radiobacter* has been isolated from blood, urine, sputum and wounds, although the clinical significance of most of these isolates is uncertain.[80,105,111]

Classification

The genus *Agrobacterium* is listed in section 4 of *Bergey's Manual of Systematic Bacteriology*, volume 1, with the gram-negative aerobic rods and cocci.[71] It is included in the family *Rhizobiaceae*. The genus derives its name from the Greek *agrus*, "field," and *bakterion*, "small rod." Four species are included in this genus: *A. tumefaciens*, *A. rhizogenes*, *A. rubi*, and *A. radiobacter*. The first three species are plant pathogens. *A. radiobacter* (also called CDC group Vd-3) is not a phytopathogen and is the only species isolated in the clinical microbiology laboratory.

TABLE 25-6. Biochemical Characteristics of
  C. violaceum

Characteristic	Reaction
Triple sugar iron (TSI) agar	Alkaline/acid, no gas[a] *or* acid/acid, no gas[a]
H$_2$S (butt/paper)	$-/-$
Kligler iron agar (KIA)	Alkaline/acid, no gas[a]
Catalase	+
Oxidase	v
Motility	+
Growth on MacConkey agar	+
Growth on Salmonella-Shigella agar	v
Simmons citrate	v
Urea hydrolysis	v
Gelatin liquefaction	v
Indole	$-$[b]
Nitrate reduction	$+$[c]
Lysine decarboxylase	$-$
Ornithine decarboxylase	$-$
Arginine dihydrolase	+
Esculin hydrolysis	$-$
ONPG (production of beta-galactosidase)	$-$
Acetylmethylcarbinol production (Voges-Proskauer test)	$-$

TABLE 25-6. Biochemical Characteristics of
  C. violaceum—cont'd

Characteristic	Reaction
Growth in potassium cyanide (KCN)	+
Gas from glucose	$-$[a]
Acid from:	
Adonitol	$-$
Arabinose	$-$
Dulcitol	$-$
Fructose	+
Galactose	$-$
Glucose	+
Inositol	$-$
Lactose	$-$
Maltose	$-$
Mannitol	$-$
Mannose	v
Raffinose	$-$
Rhamnose	v
Salicin	$-$
Sorbitol	v
Sucrose	v
Trehalose	+
Xylose	$-$

> **SYMBOLS:** v, Variable; >10% but <90% positive; reaction may be delayed
> +, ≥90% positive
> −, ≤90% negative

[a] Rare strains are aerogenic.[128]
[b] Nonpigmented strains may be indole positive.
[c] Some strains reduce nitrite also.

GROWTH REQUIREMENTS
Media

A. radiobacter grows on rabbit and sheep blood agars and on MacConkey agar.

Environmental Requirements

A. radiobacter is an aerobic organism. Colonies can be observed after 24 hours' incubation at 35° C.

CULTURAL CHARACTERISTICS
Staining Reactions

A. radiobacter is a gram-negative rod, 0.4 to 0.8 μm by 1.3 to 2.5 μm in size, that has parallel sides and rounded ends.[111]

Colonial Morphology

Colonies of *A. radiobacter* are punctate, circular, and convex with an entire edge after 24 hours' growth on 5% blood agar at 35° C.

BIOCHEMICAL IDENTIFICATION

The production of 3-ketolactonate is a key test that differentiates *A. radiobacter* from other oxidase-positive glucose oxidizers that grow on MacConkey agar.[111] If the 3-ketolactose test is not performed, the oxidation of mannitol, lactose, and maltose will separate *A. radiobacter* from CDC groups Vd and Va-1, *Pseudomonas pickettii, Pseudomonas stutzeri, Achromobacter xylosoxidans,* and *Pseudomonas fluorescens.* A flagella stain can separate *A. radiobacter* from *P. cepacia* and *P. pseudomallei; A. radiobacter* is peritrichously flagellated. A list of biochemical characteristics of *A. radiobacter* is shown in Table 25-7.

CLINICAL SIGNIFICANCE

A. radiobacter has been associated with one case each of prosthetic valve endocarditis[3] and septicemia[46] and was probably the cause of urinary tract infection.[2] All of these conditions occurred in debilitated patients. Usually, organisms isolated from clinical specimens are thought to occur either as incidental inhabitants in the patient or as contaminants introduced during sample processing.[80,111]

ANTIMICROBIAL SUSCEPTIBILITY

Little information is available on the antimicrobial susceptibility of *A. radiobacter.* Isolates from the three cases cited previously showed variable susceptibility patterns.

TABLE 25-7. Biochemical Characteristics of *Agrobacterium radiobacter*

Characteristic	Reaction
Oxidase	+
Catalase	+
Growth on MacConkey agar	+
Growth on Salmonella-Shigella agar	v
Motility	+
Urease	+
Phenylalanine deaminase	+
Nitrate reduction	+
Nitrate to gas	–
Cetrimide	–
Growth at 42° C	v
Esculin hydrolysis	+
Pyocyanine	–
Pyoverdin	–
Indole	–
Simmons citrate	+
Gelatin liquefaction	–
Arginine dihydrolase	–
Lysine decarboxylase	–
Ornithine decarboxylase	–
3-Ketolactose production	+
Acid from[a] :	
Glucose	+
Lactose	+
Maltose	+
Mannitol	+
Sucrose	+
Xylose	+

> **SYMBOLS:**   +, >90% strains positive
> –, >90% strains negative
> v, >10% but <90% strains positive

[a] Oxidative-fermentative (OF) medium.

CALYMMATOBACTERIUM

Calymmatobacterium granulomatis is the causative agent of granuloma inguinale (also called donovanosis and granuloma venereum), a chronic, progressive granulomatous disease that generally involves the skin and subcutaneous tissue of the genital, inguinal, and anal regions. The bacteria are encapsulated, nonmotile, nonsporeforming, gram-negative, pleomorphic rods that exhibit bipolar staining.

CLASSIFICATION

The genus *Calymmatobacterium* is included in section 5 of *Bergey's Manual of Systematic Bacteriology,* volume 1, with the gram-negative facultatively anaerobic rods; it is listed along with other genera of uncertain affiliation.[28] The genus has a single member, its type species, *C. granulomatis*. The organism takes its name from the Greek *calymma* ("mantle, sheath"), which describes its distinct capsule. The bacterium was previously known as *Donovania granulomatis,* named after Charles Donovan, who discovered it in 1905.

SPECIMEN COLLECTION AND PROCESSING

Scrapings or biopsy specimens may be submitted for the diagnosis of granuloma inguinale. Before the specimen is obtained, the lesion should be swabbed with sterile saline; material is then gathered by scraping or curetting rather deeply between the actively extending border of the ulcer. If scrapings are nonproductive, a punch biopsy should be obtained from the edge of the lesion; the clean underside of the tissue is then used to make smears.

GROWTH REQUIREMENTS
Media and Environmental Requirements

Routine culture in embryonated eggs is neither practical nor highly successful, and the diagnosis of granuloma inguinale is usually based on finding typical intracellular organisms, known as Donovan bodies, within large mononuclear cells (histiocytes) on stained smears of tissue from the lesion (see below).[75] Coagulated egg yolk slants (Dulaney slants) and semidefined media in which the growth factors in egg yolk are replaced by either lactalbumin hydrolysate or Phytone (BBL, Cockeysville, Md.) have been used to cultivate the organism.[51] A low oxidation-reduction potential is necessary for growth.

CULTURAL CHARACTERISTICS

Donovan bodies are better observed in freshly prepared smears stained with Wright or Giemsa stain than in formalin-fixed, hematoxylin and eosin–stained material.[75] With the Wright stain, Donovan bodies appear as clusters of safety pin–shaped rods surrounded by well-defined, dense, pinkish capsules in the cytoplasm of histiocytes (Plate 22, *F*). Intracellular organisms must be observed to confirm the diagnosis. The safety pin forms result from single or bipolar condensation of chromatin.

CLINICAL SIGNIFICANCE

C. granulomatis is the cause of granuloma inguinale, a chronic granulomatous disease that usually affects the genitalia. The disease is more commonly reported in men, blacks, and persons of low socioeconomic status. It is rare in Western countries and occurs mainly in New Guinea, India, central Australia, Africa, the Caribbean, and other tropical or subtropical areas. The clinical presentation is highly suggestive of the diagnosis in most cases. In males, lesions most commonly occur on the prepuce or glans, and in females lesions are usually on the labia. The disease begins as a single or multiple subcutaneous nodule that eventually erodes the skin surface to produce a clear, granulomatous, sharply defined lesion. Constitutional symptoms are absent, and the lesions are not painful unless secondarily infected. The disease progresses by extension to adjacent skin and frequently spreads along the groin folds. The involvement of the subcutaneous tissue of the inguinal region without involvement of the inguinal lymph nodes can resemble the lymphadenopathy seen with lymphogranulo-

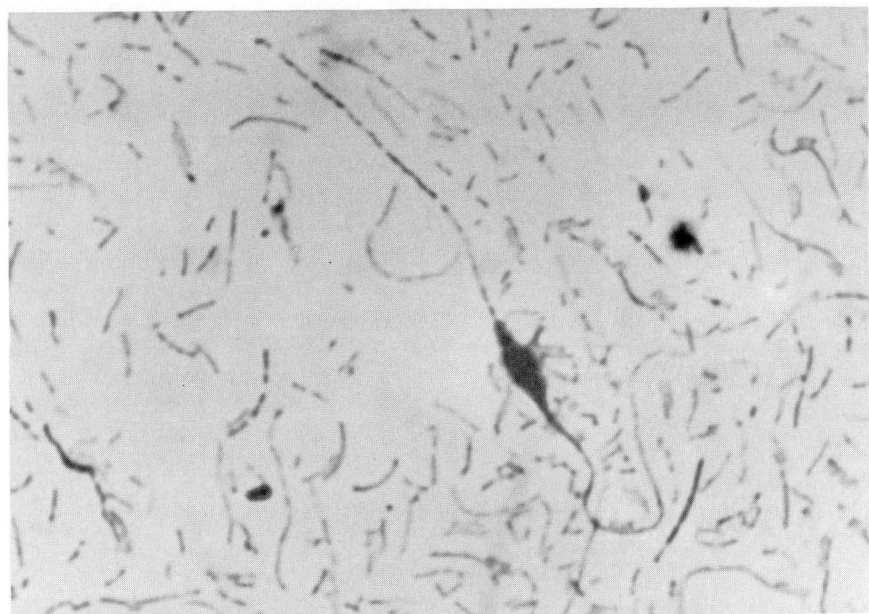

FIGURE 25-5. Gram stain of DF-2. (Courtesy Dr. Edward J. Bottone, Mt. Sinai Hospital, New York.)

ma venereum. The "pseudobuboes" seen in granuloma inguinale commonly break down to form inguinal ulcers. Untreated lesions are progressive and mutilating.

Granuloma inguinale is thought to be sexually transmitted, although several findings are incompatible with this mode of transmission.[75] These findings include the fact that the disease occurs in sexually inactive individuals (including young children), there is a low incidence of disease in prostitutes and conjugal partners, the organism can be recovered from feces,[52] the disease is autoinoculable, and the frequency of nongenital lesions (involving the mouth, lips, throat, and face) is high. Several unanswered questions remain about this disease, specifically its incubation period, mechanism of transmission, mode of infection, and factors governing the susceptibility of the host.[70]

ANTIMICROBIAL SUSCEPTIBILITY

C. granulomatis is susceptible to tetracycline, chloramphenicol, gentamicin, and trimethoprim-sulfamethoxazole, variably susceptible to ampicillin and erythromycin, and resistant to penicillin.[75] Chloramphenicol and erythromycin are probably the most effective drugs but are not widely used because of their toxicity.[59] Tetracycline is probably the most widely used antimicrobial agent.[59]

DF-2

DF-2 is the designation given by the Centers for Disease Control to an unclassified gram-negative rod that has been isolated from human blood and frequently associated with dog bites. The organism is nonflagellated, nonsporeforming, and fastidious. Its slow growth on laboratory media is reflected in its name, that is, DF for dysgonic (poor growth) fermenter. In some cases DF-2 organisms have been seen in peripheral blood smears.

GROWTH REQUIREMENTS
Media and Environmental Requirements

DF-2 grows slowly on 5% sheep blood or chocolate agars; the bacterium does not grow at all on MacConkey or SS agars. Heart infusion agar with 5% rabbit blood is recommended for growth of the organism.[15] Although this medium is more nutritive than ordinary sheep blood agar, it is not routinely available in most clinical microbiology laboratories.

The organism has been isolated from a variety of conventional blood culture media, including radiometric Bactec bottles.[121] Occasionally initial subcultures on agar media grow only under anaerobic conditions, but after a few transfers growth can be obtained in a candle jar atmosphere. Plates should be incubated for at least 5 days.[117]

CULTURAL CHARACTERISTICS
Staining Reactions

DF-2 is a long, thin, gram-negative rod, 1 to 3 μm long, with tapering ends. It may resemble *Fusobacterium* spp. on Gram stain (Figure 25-5).

Colonial Morphology

Colonies of DF-2 are punctate after 24 hours at 35° C and 1 to 2 μm in size after 48 hours. Colonies are convex, smooth, and circular. On rabbit blood agar growth is smooth and has a purplish cast in the area of confluent growth.[15]

BIOCHEMICAL IDENTIFICATION

DF-2 is a fastidious fermenter that does not grow on MacConkey agar. It is usually oxidase positive, but the reaction may be weak. Long, thin, slowly growing, oxidase-positive, catalase-positive, gram-negative rods that do not grow on MacConkey agar are suggestive of DF-2.[117] Other biochemical tests are listed in Table 25-8.[15] The tetramethyl-*p*-phenylenediamine

TABLE 25-8. Biochemical Characteristics of DF-2

Characteristic	Reaction
Oxidase	$+^a$
Catalase	+
Triple sugar iron agar (TSI)	No growth or poor growth
Kligler iron agar (KIA)	No growth or poor growth
Growth on MacConkey agar	−
Growth on Salmonella-Shigella agar	−
Simmons citrate	−
Christensen urea	−
Nitrate reduction	−
Gas from nitrate	−
Indole	−
Motility	$-^b$
Cetrimide	−
Methyl red	+
Acetylmethylcarbinol production (Voges-Proskauer test)	−
Esculin hydrolysis	v
Gelatin liquefaction	−
Lysine decarboxylase	−
Arginine dihydrolase	v
Ornithine decarboxylase	−
Acid from:	
Glucose	+
Lactose	+
Maltose	+
Mannitol	−
Sucrose	−
Xylose	−

> **SYMBOLS:** +, ≥ 90% strains positive
> −, ≥ 90% strains negative
> v, 10%–90% strains positive

[a]Oxidase reaction may be weak and sometimes negative.
[b]Nonflagellated.

dihydrochloride reagent should be applied to growth on an 18- to 24-hour blood agar plate for determination of the oxidase reaction. Three percent hydrogen peroxide should be added to growth on a heart infusion slant to determine the catalase reaction. The indole test should be performed from 4 ml heart infusion broth containing 0.1 ml sterile rabbit serum; the culture should be incubated for 4 days at 35° C, extracted with xylene, and tested with Ehrlich reagent. Nitrate reduction should be tested from 4 ml heart infusion broth containing 0.2% potassium nitrate and 0.1 ml sterile rabbit serum; tubes should be incubated 4 days before performing the test. Carbohydrate fermentation tests should be performed in 3 ml broth base with Andrade indicator containing 0.3 ml filter-sterilized 10% car-

bohydrate solution and 0.1 ml sterile rabbit serum; oxidation-fermentation (OF) media should not be used. Attention must be paid to using the specified reduced amounts of liquid media because the organism may not grow in the regular volumes of broth. The rapid fermentation test is very useful for the carbohydrate characterization of this organism.

DF-2 may be distinguished from other slow-growing, oxidase-positive fermenters on the basis of a few key tests. A positive catalase finding distinguishes it from *Capnocytophaga* spp., *Cardiobacterium hominis*, *Kingella* spp., HB-5, and *Eikenella corrodens*, which are all catalase negative. A negative indole reaction separates DF-2 from *Pasteurella multocida*, which is indole positive. A negative nitrate test distinguishes DF-2 from *P. multocida*, *Pasteurella haemolytica*, and EF-4. Finally, DF-2 is resistant to colistin, whereas all these other organisms are sensitive.

CLINICAL SIGNIFICANCE

The clinical syndromes most commonly caused by DF-2 are septicemia, meningitis, endocarditis, and cellulitis.[9,15,18,117,121] Infection may be severe and potentially fatal, especially in patients with underlying diseases, chronic alcoholism, or a prior splenectomy.[69,117] Most patients have a dog bite or a history of recent animal exposure. The presence of an eschariform lesion at the bite site may serve as an early clue to infection with DF-2.[69] This organism has been isolated from dog saliva.[5]

ANTIMICROBIAL SUSCEPTIBILITY

Antimicrobial susceptibility testing has been performed by an agar-dilution method using Schaedler medium with 5% lysed horse blood.[15] Plates were incubated in 5% CO_2 for 48 hours. The organism is susceptible to penicillin, ampicillin, carbenicillin, cephalothin, erythromycin, clindamycin, chloramphenicol, tetracycline, and the combination trimethoprim-sulfamethoxazole. It is resistant to gentamicin, kanamycin, and colistin.

Penicillin is the drug of choice in cases of dog bites because both DF-2 and *P. multocida* are sensitive to this antibiotic.

PROTOTHECA

Prototheca spp. are aerobic algaelike organisms similar to achlorophyllic strains of the green alga *Chlorella*. They reproduce asexually by endosporulation. *Prototheca* species produce hyaline yeastlike colonies on most mycologic media. Three species are currently recognized: *P. stagnora*, *P. zopfii*, and *P. wickerhamii*.[141] *P. wickerhamii* is most commonly isolated from human infections.

The diagnosis of protothecosis may be made by demonstration of protothecal cells in tissue or by isolation of *Prototheca* spp. in culture.

EXAMINATION OF TISSUE

In histologic sections *Prototheca* spp. stain well with fungal stains such as periodic acid–Schiff (PAS) or Grocott-Gomori methenamine–silver nitrate (Plate 23, *A*). In tissue sections *Prototheca* spp. are ovoid or spherical and range in size from 3 to 15 μm (*P. wickerhamii*) or from about 7 to 30 μm (*P. zopfii*). Single cells of *Prototheca* spp. may resemble *Blastomyces dermatitidis* or *Cryptococcus neoformans;* mature sporangia may resemble small spherules of *Coccidioides immitis*.[155]

TABLE 25-9. Biochemical Characteristics of *Prototheca* Spp.

Characteristic	*P. wickerhamii*	*P. zopfii*	*P. stagnora*
Assimilation of:			
Cellobiose	−	−	−
Galactose	+	+	+
Glucose	+	+	+
Propanol	−	+	−
Sucrose	−	−	+
Trehalose	+	−	−
Xylose	−	−	−
Urease	−	−	−
KNO₃	−	−	−

SYMBOLS: +, Positive
−, Negative

GROWTH REQUIREMENTS
Media and Environmental Requirements

Protothecae grow on Sabouraud dextrose agar; they do not grow on Mycosel (BBL Microbiology Systems, Cockeysville, Md.), however, because of the presence of cycloheximide in this medium. The organisms also grow on ordinary blood agar. *P. wickerhamii* and *P. zopfii* grow at 30° C.[95]

Colonies on Sabouraud dextrose agar are smooth, yeastlike, and white to cream in color.

CULTURAL CHARACTERISTICS

Microscopic examination of lactophenol cotton blue wet mounts is necessary to differentiate *Prototheca* spp. from *Candida* and *Cryptococcus* spp. Production of endospores and the absence of budding cells are characteristic of the genus *Prototheca*. Cells are hyaline, thick-walled, and globose to oval and range in size from 1.3 by 13.4 μm to 1.3 by 16.1 μm. Colonies on Sabouraud dextrose agar are smooth, yeastlike, and white to cream in color.

BIOCHEMICAL IDENTIFICATION

Prototheca organisms are nonfermentative and do not hydrolyze urea or reduce nitrates. Key biochemical characteristics are shown in Table 25-9. The API 20C systems (Analytab Products, Inc., Plainview, N.Y.) may also be used to speciate the *Prototheca* spp.[95] Identification should not rest on the API 20C assimilation pattern alone because many of the assimilation profiles of *Prototheca* spp. are identical to those of commonly isolated yeasts.

CLINICAL SIGNIFICANCE

Prototheca spp. are usually found in soil, marine water, and sewage. Most human cases involve trauma and environmental contamination. There are three forms of human infections: skin lesions on exposed body surfaces,[85] olecranon bursitis,[1] and disseminated visceral disease.[23] The majority of case reports are from tropical areas (Panama, Africa, China, and Vietnam); a few cases have been reported from temperate climates of New Zealand and the southern United States. A total of 23 cases of protothecosis have been reported in the literature.[53,62,155]

ANTIMICROBIAL SUSCEPTIBILITY

The minimal inhibitory concentration (MIC) and minimal algacidal concentration (MAC) of clinical isolates of *Prototheca* spp. have been tested.[85,123] The organisms are susceptible to amphotericin B and nystatin, variably susceptible to miconazole, and resistant to 5-fluorocytosine and griseofulvin.

Amphotericin B has been used successively in several instances.[23,85] The combination of amphotericin B and tetracycline is the treatment of choice[62] and is used to improve serum algacidal activity.[155] Lesions involving the olecranon bursa have generally been cured by simple bursectomy.

SPIRILLUM MINUS

Spirillum minus is the causative agent of a form of rat-bite fever named soduku by the Japanese. Although the disease was first reported from India and Japan, its distribution is probably worldwide.

CLASSIFICATION

Spirillum minus is included in section 2, "Aerobic/Microaerophilic, Motile, Helical/Vibrioid Gram-Negative Bacteria," of volume 1 of *Bergey's Manual of Systematic Bacteriology*.[73] Although the organism has historically been included in the genus *Spirillum*, it is not included in this genus in *Bergey's Manual* but rather is indicated as *S. minus* and described under *species incertae sedis*. It is similar to the genus *Spirillum* because of its shape (small spiral) and the arrangement of its flagella (bipolar tufts). However, because of its morphology, pathogenicity, and sources, it has been suggested that *S. minus* might be more closely related to the genus *Campylobacter* than to the saprophytic spirilla.[72,73] *S. minus* stains gram negative with the Gram stain and to date has not been cultivated on artificial media. The organism has also been called *Spirochaeta morsus muris* and *Spirillum minor*.

DIAGNOSIS

Diagnosis of *S. minus* infection is made by (1) microscopic demonstration of the organism in blood from the patient or in exudates from the initial bite wound, adjacent lymph nodes, or cutaneous eruption (rash) or (2) by animal inoculation studies. Wet mounts are best examined by darkfield or phase contrast microscopy; blood films can also be stained with the Giemsa or Wright stain. Cells of *S. minus* are short and thick (0.5 μm by 1.7 to 5 μm) with two to six spirals. The organism possesses bipolar tufts of flagella, and active motility is usually seen on direct microscopic examination.

Animal studies are undertaken when microscopy fails to demonstrate the organism. Four mice are injected intraperitoneally with 1 ml of patient blood, and one guinea pig is injected intraperitoneally with 2 ml of blood.[113] The organism can be demonstrated in mouse or guinea pig blood within 1 to 3 weeks after inoculation using darkfield or phase contrast microscopy or by Giemsa stain; in addition, wet mounts and smears of mouse peritoneal fluid are examined weekly for 4 weeks. The blood of laboratory animals must be examined carefully before inoculation for the presence of naturally occurring organisms.

CLINICAL SIGNIFICANCE

S. minus causes soduku, the spirillary form of rat-bite fever. Infection follows the bite of a rat, a mouse, or an animal that has ingested a rodent; the incubation period is longer than for streptobacillary rat-bite fever (usually 2 weeks). Several major clinical features differentiate the two types of rat-bite fever. Disease caused by *S. minus* is distinguished by inflammation, induration, and occasional chancrelike ulceration at the original bite site; associated lymphangitis and regional lymphadinitis; a dark-purple rash that spreads from the initial lesion; and an absence of arthritic symptoms. Complement fixation tests for syphilis have been reported to give biologic false-positive results. The mortality is 6% to 10% in untreated cases. However, in the past two decades all reported cases have been successfully treated with streptomycin or, preferably, penicillin.

ANTIMICROBIAL SUSCEPTIBILITY

Antimicrobial susceptibility testing of *S. minus* is not possible because the organism does not grow on artificial media. However, spirillary rat-bite fever has been successfully treated with the combination of penicillin and streptomycin and with tetracycline.[116]

BARTONELLA

Bartonella bacilliformis is the causative agent of bartonellosis or Carrión's disease. The organism is a small coccobacillus that parasitizes red blood cells. It is named for Dr. A.L. Barton who first described its association with Carrión's disease.

The genus *Bartonella* is listed in section 9 of *Bergey's Manual of Systematic Bacteriology,* volume 1, in the order *Rickettsiales* and the family *Bartonellaceae.*[112] The organism can be cultivated from blood in leptospira medium, but bartonellosis is most often diagnosed by demonstration of the etiologic agent in peripheral blood films or skin biopsies. Carrión's disease is strictly limited to the western Andes and is rarely seen in the United States; a history of residence in an endemic area is important diagnostically.

DIAGNOSIS

Thick and thin blood films should be examined after staining with Giemsa or Wright stain. Fresh drops of blood are preferred for preparing films. The organism is reddish, pleomorphic, rod or ring shaped, and approximately 1 to 3 μm by 0.5 to 0.75 μm.[29,159] In cutaneous nodules, bacteria appear within endothelial cells.

In cultures the organisms are gram negative and motile with a tuft of one to 10 unipolar flagella. No acid is detected from glucose, xylose, mannitol, lactose, sucrose, or maltose. Subcultures grow slowly in a container with a beaker of water at room temperature or 25° C.

CLINICAL SIGNIFICANCE

Human bartonellosis occurs only in certain mountainous regions of Peru, Colombia, and Ecuador. The insect vector, the sandfly of the genus *Phlebotomus,* transmits the disease to humans during nocturnal feeding; the insects survive only in the limited ecosphere in which the disease is found.[122]

Bartonellosis is a diphasic illness. Oroya fever, the initial phase of the infection, appears as a severe, febrile, hemolytic anemia. It is frequently complicated by superinfection with *Salmonella,* and if it is untreated the mortality is approximately 40%.[24] *B. bacilliformis* may infect more than 90% of the red blood cells during this stage.

The second stage of infection is verruga peruana, or Peruvian warts. During this period, bartonellae disappear from the

blood, and the patient develops multiple, disfiguring, cranberry-like skin eruptions. Bartonellae may be demonstrated in Giemsa-stained biopsy specimens from lesions during this stage. The tumorlike growths of verruga peruana may persist for up to 1 year, but this phase of illness is rarely fatal.

ANTIMICROBIAL SUSCEPTIBILITY

Antimicrobial agents restrict the growth of *B. bacilliformis* but do not necessarily eradicate the organism; patients who have recovered from Oroya fever may still have positive blood cultures and may still develop verruga peruana. Chloramphenicol is the therapeutic agent of choice because it is effective against both bartonellae and salmonellae. Penicillin, streptomycin, and tetracycline are also effective.

MOROCOCCUS

Morococcus cerebrosus is the only species in the new genus *Morococcus.*[81] The bacterium was originally isolated from pus obtained from a brain abscess. It is a small (less than 1 μm in diameter), oxidase-positive, gram-negative, spherical organism that forms tightly bound, mulberry-like aggregates of 10 to 20 colonies. This characteristic Gram stain appearance is responsible for the isolate's name, *Morococcus,* the mulberry coccus. The genus *Morococcus* is a new member of the family *Neisseriaceae. M. cerebrosus* closely resembles the neisseriae (especially *N. mucosa*). Adjacent sides of both species are often flattened; however, *M. cerebrosus* does not occur singly or in pairs or tetrads. Acid is produced from glucose, fructose, sucrose, and maltose but not lactose. The organism is susceptible to kanamycin, gentamicin, streptomycin, penicillin, ampicillin, erythromycin, nalidixic acid, chloramphenicol, and tetracycline.

HEMOTROPIC BACTERIA

Bartonellosis was once considered the only human infection caused by a hemotropic bacterium. There have been several recent reports, however, of individuals with acute febrile anemia in whom rare erythrocyte-associated (that is, hemotropic) bacteria were found in peripheral blood or bone marrow.[30] Most of these isolates (from patients in Thailand, the Sudan, Niger, Connecticut, and Illinois) were gram-negative rods. Gram-positive rods were observed, however, in peripheral blood films from a 49-year-old splenectomized man from Virginia.[4]

The diagnosis of infection with one of these hemotropic bacteria is usually made in the hematologic rather than clinical microbiologic laboratory from Wright- or Wright-Giemsa-stained smears of peripheral blood or bone marrow; organisms also stain with Gomori methenamine-silver stain. Organisms are seen in close association with red blood cells and seem to adhere to them.

Some of the strains have been grown in nonliving media, and some have been grown in tissue culture cells. Isolation attempts should be made only at reference laboratories, however. The bone marrow has been postulated as the reservoir of the organism in at least one case.[4] The patient was apparently cured (following three relapses) after chloramphenicol therapy.

Although human infections caused by agents that parasitize erythrocytes are rare in the continental United States, careful examination of bone marrow aspirates and peripheral blood smears may be helpful in patients with severe hemolytic anemia.

REFERENCES

1. Ahbel, D.E., et al.: Prototheal olecranon bursitis: a case report and review of the literature, J. Bone Joint Surg. **62**:835, 1980.

2. Alos, J.I., et al.: Urinary tract infection probably caused by *Agrobacterium radiobacter*, Eur. J. Clin. Microbiol. **4**:596, 1985.

3. Amsel, R., et al.: Nonspecific vaginitis: diagnostic criteria and microbial and epidemiologic associations, Am. J. Med. **74**:14, 1983.

4. Archer, G.L., et al.: Human infection from an unidentified erthyrocyte-associated bacterium, N. Engl. J. Med. **301**:897, 1979.

5. Bailie, W.E., Stowe, E.C., and Schmitt, A.M.: Aerobic bacterial flora of oral and nasal fluids of canines with reference to bacteria associated with bites, J. Clin. Microbiol. **7**:223, 1978.

6. Baron, E.J., Wexler, H.M., and Firegold, S.M.: Biochemical and polyacrylamide gel electrophoretic analyses of vaginosis-associated anaerobic curved rods, Scand. J. Urol. Nephrol. **86**(suppl.):65, 1984.

7. Bartlett, R.C.: Laboratory diagnostic techniques. In Topazian, R.G., and Goldberg, M.H., editors: Management of infections of the oral and maxillofacial regions, Philadelphia, 1981, W.B. Saunders Co.

8. Blair, T.P., et al.: Endocarditis caused by *Actinobacillus actinomycetemcomitans*, South. Med. J. **75**:559, 1982.

9. Bobo, R.A., and Newton, E.J.: A previously undescribed gram negative bacillus causing septicemia and meningitis, Am. J. Clin. Pathol. **65**:564, 1976.

10. Brunner, H., and Weidner, W.: Chemotherapy of human mycoplasma diseases, Isr. J. Med. Sci. **17**:656, 1981.

11. Bruun, B., et al.: Phenotypic differentiation of *Cardiobacterium hominis*, *Kingella indologenes*, and CDC group EF-4, Eur. J. Clin. Microbiol. **3**:230, 1984.

12. Burgher, L.W., Lommis, G.W., and Ware, F.: Systemic infection due to *Actinobacillus actinomycetecomitans*, Am. J. Clin. Pathol. **60**:412, 1973.

13. Burke, D.S., and Madoff, S.: Infection of a traumatic pelvic hematoma with *Mycoplasma hominis*, Sex. Transm. Dis. **5**:65, 1978.

14. Busolo, F., and Meloni, G.A.: Serodiagnosis of *M. pneumoniae* infections by enzyme-linked immunosorbent assay (ELISA), Yale J. Biol. Med. **56**:517, 1983.

15. Butler, T., et al.: Unidentified gram-negative rod infection: a new disease of man, Ann. Intern. Med. **86**:1, 1977.

16. Cassell, G.H., and Cole, B.C.: Mycoplasmas as agents of human disease, N. Engl. J. Med. **304**:80, 1981.

17. Centers for Disease Control: Rat-bite fever in a college student: California, MMWR **33**:318, 1984.

18. Chaudhuri, A.K., Hartley, R.B., and Maddocks, A.C.: Waterhouse-Friderichsen syndrome caused by a DF-2 bacterium in a splenectomised patient, J. Clin. Pathol. **34**:172, 1981.

19. Chen, K.C.S., et al.: Amine content of vaginal fluid from untreated and treated patients with nonspecific vaginitis, J. Clin. Invest. **63**:828, 1979.

20. Chen, T.R.: *In situ* detection of mycoplasma contamination in cell cultures by fluorescent Hoechst 33258 stain, Exp. Cell Res. **104**:255, 1977.

21. Clyde, W.A., Jr., and Fernald, G.W.: Mycoplasmas: the pathogens' pathogens, Cell. Immunol. **82**:88, 1983.

22. Coignard, S., et al.: Endocardite à *Capnocytophaga ochracea*, Nouv. Presse Med. **11**:1338, 1982.

23. Cox, G.E., Wilson, J.D., and Brown, P.: Prototheosis: a case of disseminated algal infection, Lancet **2**:379, 1974.

24. Cuadra, M.: Salmonellosis complication in human bartonellosis, Tex. Biol. Med. **14**:97, 1956.

25. Dan, M., et al.: *Mycoplasma hominis* septicemia in a burned infant, J. Pediatr. **99**:743, 1981.

26. Dibb, W.L., Digranes A., and Tonjum, S.: *Actinobacillus lignieresii* infection after a horse bite, Br. Med. J. **283**:583, 1981.

27. Dienes, L. and Weinberger, H.J.: The L forms of bacteria, Bacteriol. Rev. **15**:245, 1951.

28. Dienst, R.B., and Brownell, G.H.: *Calymmatobacterium*. In Krieg, N.R., editor (Holt, J.G., editor-in-chief): Bergey's manual of systematic bacteriology, vol. 1, Baltimore, 1984, Williams & Wilkins Co.

29. Dooley, J.R.: Bartonellosis. In Binford, C.H., and Connor, D.H., editors: Pathology of the tropical and extraordinary diseases: an atlas, vol. I, Washington, D.C., 1976, Armed Forces Institute of Pathology.

30. Dooley, J.R.: Haemotropic bacteria in man, Lancet **2**:1237, 1980.

31. Dreizen, S., et al.: Unusual mucocutaneous infections in immunosuppressed patients with leukemia: expansion of an earlier study, Postgrad. Med. **79**:287, 1986.

32. Edwards, R., and Finch, R.G.: Characterization and streptococcal antibiotic susceptibilities of *Streptobacillus moniliformis*, J. Med. Microbiol. **21**:39, 1986.

33. Embree, J.E., and Embil, J.A.: Mycoplasmas in diseases in humans, Can. Med. Assoc. J. **123**:105, 1980.

34. Eschenbach, D.A., Pollock, H.M., and Schacter, J.: Laboratory diagnosis of female genital tract infections. In Rubin, S.J., editor: Laboratory diagnosis of female genital tract infections, Cumitech 17, American Society for Microbiology, 1983, Washington, D.C.

35. Eschenbach, D.A., et al.: Bacterial vaginosis during pregnancy: an association with prematurity and postpartum complications, Scand. J. Urol. Nephrol. **86**(suppl.):213, 1984.

36. Faro, S., Walker, C., and Pierson, R.L.: Amnionitis with intact amniotic membranes involving *Streptobacillus moniliformis*, Obstet. Gynecol. **55**:9S, 1980.

37. Faur, Y.C., Weisburd, M.H., and Wilson, M.E.: A comparison of horse, cow, and sheep blood in NYC medium: effect on recovery of *N. gonorrhoeae* and urogenital mycoplasmas, Health Lab. Sci. **13**:194, 1976.

38. Feldman, J.D., Kontaxis, E.N., and Sherman, M.P.: Congenital bacteremia due to *Capnocytophaga*, Pediatr. Infect. Dis. **4**:415, 1985.

39. Feldman, R.B., Stern, G.A., and Hood, I.: Chromobacterium violaceum infection of the eye: a report of two cases, Arch. Ophthalmol. **102**:711, 1984.

40. Fernald, G.W., and Clyde, W.A., Jr.: Immune responses to *Mycoplasma pneumoniae* infection. In Bienenstock, J., editor: Immunology of the lung and upper respiratory tract, New York, 1984, McGraw-Hill Book Co.

41. Fiacro, V., et al.: Comparison of media for isolation of *Ureaplasma urealyticum* and genital *Mycoplasma* species, J. Clin. Microbiol. **20**:862, 1984.

42. Forlenza, S.W.: *Capnocytophaga*: an opportunistic pathogen, Clin. Microbiol. Newsletter **7**:17, 1985.

43. Forlenza, S.W., and Newman, M.G.: *Capnocytophaga*. In Bottone, E.J., editor: Unusual microorganisms, New York, 1983, Marcel Dekker, Inc.

44. Forlenza, S.W., et al.: Antimicrobial susceptibility of *Capnocytophaga*, Antimicrob. Agents Chemother. **19**:144, 1981.

45. Foy, H.M., Nolan, C.M., and Allan, I.D.: Epidemiologic aspects of *M. pneumoniae* disease complications: a review, Yale J. Biol. Med. **56**:469, 1983.

46. Freney, J., et al.: Septicemia caused by *Agrobacterium* sp., J. Clin. Microbiol. **22**:683, 1985.

47. Fung, J.C., Berman, M., and Fiorentino, T.: *Capnocytophaga*: a review of the literature, Am. J. Med. Technol. **49**:589, 1983.

48. Furr, P.M., and Taylor-Robinson, D.: Microimmunofluorescence technique for detection of antibody to *Mycoplasma genitalium*, J. Clin. Pathol. **37**:1072, 1984.

49. Gardner, H.L., and Dukes, C.D.: *Haemophilus vaginalis* vaginitis: a newly defined specific infection previously classified nonspecific vaginitis, Am. J. Obstet. Gynecol. **69**:962, 1955.

50. Geraci, J.E., Wilson, W.R., and Washington, J.A., II: Infective endocarditis caused by *Actinobacillus actinomycetemcomitans*: report of four cases, Mayo Clin. Proc. **55**:415, 1980.

51. Goldberg, J.: Studies on granuloma inguinale. IV. Growth requirements of *Donovania granulomatis* and its relationship to the natural habitat of the organism, Br. J. Vener. Dis. **35**:266, 1959.

52. Goldberg, J.: Studies on granuloma inguinale. V. Isolation of a bacterium resembling *Donovania granulomatis* from the faeces of a patient with granuloma inguinale, Br. J. Vener. Dis. **38**:99, 1962.

53. Goldstein, G.D., Bhatia, P., and Kalivas, J.: Herpetiform protothecosis, Int. J. Dermatol. **25**:54, 1986.

54. Granato, P.A., Paepke, J.L., and Weiner, L.B.: Use of modified New York City medium for growth of *Mycoplasma pneumoniae,* Am. J. Clin. Pathol. **73**:702, 1980.

55. Greenwood, J.R., and Pickett, M.J.: Salient features of *Haemophilus vaginalis,* J. Clin. Microbiol. **9**:200, 1979.

56. Greenwood, J.R., and Pickett, M.J.: Transfer of *Haemophilus vaginalis* Gardner and Dukes to a new genus, *Gardnerella: G. vaginalis* (Gardner and Dukes) comb. nov., Int. J. Syst. Bacteriol. **30**:170, 1980.

57. Greenwood, J.R., and Pickett, M.J.: Genus *Gardnerella,* Greenwood and Picket 1980, 170 VP. In Krieg, N.R., editor (Holt, J.G., editor-in-chief): Bergey's manual of systematic bacteriology, vol. 1, Baltimore, 1984, Williams & Wilkins Co.

58. Greenwood, J.R., et al.: *Haemophilus vaginalis (Corynebacterium vaginale):* method for isolation and rapid biochemical identification, Health Lab. Sci. **14**:102, 1977.

59. Hart, G.: Donovanosis. In Holmes, K.K., et al., editors: Sexually transmitted diseases, New York, 1984, McGraw-Hill Book Co.

60. Hawkey, P.M., et al.: *Capnocytophaga ochracea* infection: two cases and a review of the published work, J. Clin. Pathol. **37**:1066, 1984.

60a. Hawkey, P.M., et al.: In vitro susceptibility of *Capnocytophaga* species to antimicrobial agents, Antimicrob. Agents Chemother. **31**:331, 1987.

61. Hayflick, L.: Cell cultures and mycoplasmas, Tex. Rep. Biol. Med. **123**(suppl.):285, 1965.

62. Heitzman, H.B., Brooks, T.J., Jr., and Phillips, B.J.: Prototothecosis, South. Med. J. **77**:1477, 1984.

63. Hill, A.C.: Demonstration of mycoplasmas in tissue by the immunoperoxidase technique, J. Infect. Dis. **137**:152, 1978.

64. Hill, G.B., Eschenbach, D.A., and Holmes, K.K.: Bacteriology of the vagina, Scand. J. Urol. Nephrol. **86**(suppl.):23, 1984.

65. Hoffler, U., Niederau, W., and Pulverer, G.: Susceptibility of *Bacterium actinomycetem comitans* to 45 antibiotics, Antimicrob. Agents Chemother. **17**:943, 1980.

66. Holm, P.: Studies on the aetiology of human actinomycosis. II. Do the ''other microbes'' of actinomycosis possess virulence? Acta Pathol. Microbiol. Scand. **28**:391, 1951.

67. Hu, P.C., et al.: *Mycoplasma pneumoniae* infection: role of a surface protein in the attachment organelle, Science **216**:313, 1982.

68. Kahane, I.: In vitro studies of the mechanism of adherence and pathogenicity of mycoplasmas, Isr. J. Med. Sci. **20**:874, 1984.

69. Kalb, R., et al.: Cutaneous infection at dog bite wounds associated with fulminant DF-2 septicemia, Am. J. Med. **78**:687, 1985.

70. Kampmeier, R.H.: Granuloma inguinale, Sex. Transm. Dis. **2**:318, 1984.

71. Kersters, K., and Key, J.D.: *Agrobacterium.* In Krieg, N.R., editor (Holt, J.G., editor-in-chief): Bergey's manual of systematic bacteriology, vol. 1, Baltimore, 1984, Williams & Wilkins Co.

72. Krieg, N.R.: Biology of the chemoheterotrophic spirilla, Bacteriol. Rev. **40**:55, 1976.

73. Krieg, N.R.: Other spirilla possibly belonging to the genus *Aquaspirillum.* In Krieg, N.R., editor (Holt, J.G., editor-in-chief): Bergey's manual of systematic bacteriology, vol. 1, Baltimore, 1984, Williams & Wilkins Co.

74. Kristiansen, J.E., et al.: Rapid identification of *Capnocytophaga* isolated from septicemic patients, Eur. J. Clin. Microbiol. **84**:236, 1984.

75. Kuberski, T.: *Granuloma inguinale* (donovanosis), Sex. Transm. Dis. **7**:29, 1980.

76. Kundsin, R.B., and Paulin, S.A.: *Ureaplasma urealyticum:* subcultures invalid for antibiotic susceptibility tests, Diagn. Microbiol. Infect. Dis. **3**:329, 1985.

77. La Scolea, L.J., Jr., Dryja, D.M., and Dillon, W.P.: Recovery of *Gardnerella vaginalis* from blood by the quantitative direct plating method, J. Clin. Microbiol. **20**:568, 1984.

78. Laboratory Methods in Special Medical Bacteriology Course #8390-C, U.S. Dept. of Health and Human Services, Public Health Service, April, 1984, Bacteriology Training Section, Div. of Laboratory Training and Consultation, Laboratory Program Office.

79. Lambe, D.W., et al.: *Streptobacillus moniliformis* isolated from a case of Haverhill fever: biochemical characterization, Am. J. Clin. Pathol. **60**:854, 1973.

80. Lautrop, H.: *Agrobacterium* spp. isolated from clinical specimens, Acta Pathol. Microbiol. Scand. **187**(suppl.):63, 1967.

81. Long, P.A., et al.: Characterization of *Morococcus cerebrosus* gen. nov., sp. nov. and comparison with *Neisseria mucosa,* Int. J. Syst. Bacteriol. **31**:294, 1981.

82. Macher, A.M., Casale, T., and Fauci, A.S.: Chronic granulomatous disease of childhood and *Chromobacterium violaceum* infections in the southeastern United States, Ann. Intern. Med. **97**:51, 1982.

83. Martin, B.F., et al.: Brain abscess due to *Actinobacillus actinomycetemcomitans,* Neurology **17**:833, 1967.

84. Mashimo, P.A., et al.: Selective recovery of oral *Capnocytophaga* species with sheep blood agar containing bacitracin and polymycin B, J. Clin. Microbiol. **17**:187, 1983.

85. Mayhall, C.G., et al.: Cutaneous prototothecosis, Arch. Dermatol. **112**:1749, 1976.

86. McCormack, R.C., Kaye, D., and Hook, E.W.: Endocarditis due to *Streptobacillus moniliformis,* JAMA **200**:77, 1967.

87. Mokbat, J.E., et al.: Peritonitis due to *Mycoplasma hominis* in a renal transplant recipient, J. Infect. Dis. **146**:713, 1982.

88. Moller, B.R., Taylor-Robinson, D., and Furr, P.M.: Serological evidence implicating *Mycoplasma genitalium* in pelvic inflammatory disease, Lancet **1**:1102, 1984.

89. Moller, B.R., et al.: Serological evidence that chlamydiae and mycoplasmas are involved in infertility of women, J. Reprod. Fert. **73**:237, 1985.

90. Muhle, I., Rau, J., and Ruskin, J.: Vertebral osteomyelitis due to *Actinobacillus actinomycetemocomitans,* JAMA **142**:1824, 1979.

91. Newman, M.G., and Socransky, S.S.: Predominant cultivable microbiota in periodontosis, J. Periodont. Res. **12**:120, 1977.

92. Newman, M.G., et al.: Bacterial studies of the Papillon-Lefévre syndrome, J. Dent. Res. **56**:545, 1977.

93. Newman, M.G., et al.: The effect of dietary Gantrisin® supplements in the flora of periodontal pockets in four beagle dogs, J. Periodont. Res. **12**:129, 1977.

94. Orda, R., and Wiznitzer, T.: *Actinobacillus lignieresii* human infection, J. R. Soc. Med. **73**:295, 1980.

95. Padhye, A.A., Baker, J.G., and D'Amato, R.F.: Rapid identification of *Prototheca* species by the API 20C system, J. Clin. Microbiol. **10**:579, 1979.

96. Parenti, D.M., and Snydman, D.R.: *Capnocytophaga* species: infections in nonimmunocompromised and immunocompromised hosts, J. Infect. Dis. **151**:140, 1985.

97. Payan, D.G., Seigal, N., and Madoff, S.: Infection of a brain abscess by *Mycoplasma hominis,* J. Clin. Microbiol. **14**:571, 1981.

98. Peel, M.M., Rich, A.M., and Reade, P.C.: *Actinobacillus actinomycetemcomitans* infection in the oral cavity, Oral. Surg. **52**:591, 1981.

99. Phillips, J.E.: *Actinobacillus.* In Krieg, N.R., editor (Holt, J.G., editor-in-chief): Bergey's manual of systematic bacteriology, vol. 1, Baltimore, 1984, Williams & Wilkins Co.

100. Piot, P.: *Gardnerella vaginalis.* In Lennette, E.H., et al., editors: Manual of clinical microbiology, ed. 3, Washington, D.C., 1985, American Society for Microbiology.

101. Piot, P., and Vanderheyden, J.: *Gardnerella vaginalis* and nonspecific vaginitis. In Holmes, K.K., et al.: Sexually transmitted diseases, New York, 1984, McGraw-Hill.

102. Piot, P., et al.: A taxonomic study of *Gardnerella vaginalis (Haemophilus vaginalis)* Gardner and Dukes, 1955, J. Gen. Microbiol. **119**:373, 1980.

103. Piot, P., et al.: Identification of *Gardnerella (Haemophilus) vaginalis,* J. Clin. Microbiol. **15**:19, 1982.

104. Platt, R., et al.: Infection with *Mycoplasma hominis* in postpartum fever, Lancet **2**:1217, 1980.

105. Plotkin, G.R.: *Agrobacterium radiobacter* prosthetic valve endocarditis, Ann. Intern. Med. **93**:839, 1980.

106. Razin, S., and Freundt, E.A.: The mycoplasmas. In Krieg, N.R., editor (Holt, J.G., editor-in-chief): Bergey's manual of systematic bacteriology, vol. 1, Baltimore, 1984, William & Wilkins Co.

107. Reimer, L.G., and Reller, L.B.: *Gardnerella vaginalis* bacteremia: a review of thirty cases, Obstet. Gynecol. **64**:170, 1984.

108. Reimer, L.G., and Reller, L.B.: Effect of sodium polyanetholesulfonate and gelatin on the recovery of *Gardnerella vaginalis* from blood culture media, J. Clin. Microbiol. **21**:686, 1985.

109. Reimer, L.G., and Reller, L.B.: Use of a sodium polyanetholesulfonate disk for the identification of *Gardnerella vaginalis,* J. Clin. Microbiol. **21**:146, 1985.

110. Rice, P.A., and Dale, P.A.: Infections of the genitourinary tract in women: selected aspects, Adv. Intern. Med. **30**:53, 1984.

111. Riley, P.S., and Weaver, R.E.: Comparison of thirty-seven strains of Vd-3 bacteria with *Agrobacterium radiobacter:* morphological and physiological observations, J. Clin. Microbiol. **5**:172, 1977.

112. Ristie, M., and Kreiger, J.P.: *Bartonellaceae.* In Kreig, N.R., editor (Holt, J.G., editor-in-chief): Bergey's manual of systematic bacteriology, vol. 1, Baltimore, 1984, Williams & Wilkins Co.

113. Rogosa, M.: *Streptobacillus moniliformis* and *Spirillum minus.* In Lennette, E.H., et al., editors: Manual of clinical microbiology, ed. 4, Washington, D.C., 1985, American Society for Microbiology.

114. Ronnevik, P.K., and Neess, H.C.: Septicaemia caused by *Cardiobacterium hominis,* Acta Pathol. Microbiol. Scand. **89**:243, 1981.

115. Rostner, H.: *Capnocytophaga* sepsis in an immunocompromised host, Clin. Microbiol. Newsletter **6**:10, 1984.

116. Roughgarden, J.W.: Antimicrobial therapy of rat-bite fever: a review, Arch. Intern. Med. **116**:39, 1965.

117. Rubin, S.J.: A fastidious fermentative gram-negative rod, Eur. J. Clin. Microbiol. **3**:253, 1984.

118. Savage, D.D., et al.: *Cardiobacterium hominis* endocarditis: description of two patients and characterization of the organism, J. Clin. Microbiol. **5**:75, 1977.

119. Savage, N.: *Streptobacillus.* In Kreig, N.R., editor (Holt, J.G., editor-in-chief): Bergey's manual of systematic bacteriology, vol. 1, Baltimore, 1984, Williams & Wilkins Co.

120. Schack, S.H., et al.: Endocarditis caused by *Actinobacillus actinomycetemcomitans,* J. Clin. Microbiol. **20**:579, 1984.

121. Schlossberg, D.: Septicemia caused by DF-2, J. Clin. Microbiol. **9**:297, 1979.

122. Schultz, M.G.: A history of bartonellosis (Carrion's disease), Am. J. Trop. Med. Hyg. **17**:503, 1968.

123. Segal, E., Padhye, A.A., and Ajello, L.: Susceptibility of *Prototheca* species to antifungal agents, Antimicrob. Agents Chemother. **10**:75, 1976.

124. Shepard, M.C., and Lunceford, C.D.: Differential agar medium (A7) for identification of *Ureaplasma urealyticum* (human T mycoplasmas) in primary cultures of clinical material, J. Clin. Microbiol. **3**:613, 1976.

125. Shepard, M.C., and Masover, G.K.: Special features of ureaplasmas. In Barile, M.F., and Razin, S.: The mycoplasmas, vol. 1, New York, 1979, Academic Press, Inc.

126. Siber, G.R., et al.: Neonatal central nervous system infection due to *Mycoplasma hominis,* J. Pediatr. **90**:625, 1977.

127. Simo, F., et al.: *Chromobacterium violaceum* as a cause of periorbital cellulitis, Pediatr. Infect. Dis. **3**:561, 1984.

128. Sivendra, R.: Unusual *Chromobacterium violaceum:* aerogenic strains, J. Clin. Microbiol. **5**:75, 1976.

129. Sivendra, R., and Tan, S.H.: Pathogenicity of non-pigmented cultures of *Chromobacterium violaceum,* J. Clin. Microbiol. **5**:514, 1977.

130. Slotnick, I.J., and Dougherty, M.: Further characterization of an unclassified group of bacteria causing endocarditis in man: *Chromobacterium hominis* gen. et sp. n., Anton van Leeuwenhoek, J. Microbiol. Serol. **30**:261, 1964.

131. Slotnick, I.J., Mertz, J.A., and Dougherty, M.: Fluorescent antibody detection of human occurrence of an unclassified bacterial group causing endocarditis, J. Infect. Dis. **114**:503, 1964.

132. Slots, J., and Genco, R.J.: Black-pigmented *Bacteroides* species, *Capnocytophaga* species, and *Actinobacillus actinomycetemcomitans* in human periodontal disease: virulence factors in colonization, survival, and tissue destruction, J. Dent. Res. **63**:412, 1984.

133. Slots, J., Reynolds, H.S., and Genco, R.G.: *Actinobacillus actinomycetemcomitans* in human periodontal disease: a cross-sectional microbiological investigation, Infect. Immun. **29**:1013, 1980.

134. Slots, J., et al.: *In vitro* antimicrobial susceptibility of *Actinobacillus actinomycetemcomitans,* Antimicrob. Agents Chemother. **18**:9, 1980.

135. Slots, J., et al.: Detection of *Actinobacillus actinomycetemcomitans* and *Bacteroides gingivalis* in subgingival smears by the indirect fluorescent-antibody technique, J. Periodont. Res. **20**:613, 1985.

136. Sneath, P.H.A.: *Chromobacterium.* In Kreig, N.R., editor (Holt, J.G., editor-in-chief): Bergey's manual of systematic bacteriology, vol. 1, Baltimore, 1984, Williams & Wilkins Co.

137. Socransky, S.S., et al.: *Capnocytophaga:* new genus of gram-negative gliding bacteria. III. Physiological characterization, Arch. Microbiol. **122**:29, 1979.

138. Spaepen, M.S., and Kundsin, R.B.: Simple direct broth-disk method for antibiotic susceptibility testing of *Ureaplasma urealyticum,* Antimicrob. Agents Chemother. **112**:267, 1976.

139. Spiegel, C.A., et al.: Anaerobic bacteria in nonspecific vaginitis, N. Engl. J. Med. **303**:601, 1980.

140. Starr, A.J., et al.: *Chromobacterium violaceum* presenting as a surgical emergency, South. Med. J. **74**:1137, 1981.

141. Sudman, M.S.: Protothecosis, a critical review, Am. J. Clin. Pathol. **61**:10, 1974.

142. Sutter, V.L., Watt, P., and Kwok, X.Y.: In vitro susceptibility of *Capnocytophaga* strains to 18 antimicrobial agents, Antimicrob. Agents Chemother. **20**:270, 1981.

143. Taylor-Robinson, D., and Furr, P.M.: Recovery and identification of human genital tract mycoplasmas, Isr. J. Med. Sci. **17**:648, 1981.

144. Taylor-Robinson, D., and McCormack, W.H.: The genital mycoplasmas, N. Engl. J. Med. **302**:1003, 1063, 1980.

145. Taylor-Robinson, D., et al.: Urogenital mycoplasma infections of man: a review with observations on a recently discovered mycoplasma, Isr. J. Med. Sci. **17**:524, 1981.

146. Ti, T.Y., et al.: Isolation of *Mycoplasma hominis* from the blood of men with multiple trauma and fever, JAMA **247**:60, 1982.

147. Totten, P.A., et al.: Selective differential human blood bilayer media for isolation of *Gardnerella (Haemophilus) vaginalis,* J. Clin. Microbiol. **15**:141, 1982.

148. Townsend, T.R., and Gillenwater, J.Y.: Urinary tract infection due to *Actinobacillus actinomycetemcomitans,* JAMA **210**:558, 1969.

149. Tucker, D.N., et al.: Endocarditis caused by a *Pasteurella*-like organism: report of four cases, N. Engl. J. Med. **267**:913, 1962.

150. Tully, J.G.: Laboratory diagnosis of *Mycoplasma pneumoniae* infections, Isr. J. Med. Sci. **17**:644, 1981.

151. Tully, J.G., et al.: Pathogenic mycoplasmas: cultivation and vertebrate pathogenicity of a new spiroplasma, Science **195**:892, 1977.

152. Tully, J.G., et al.: Enchanced isolation of *Mycoplasma pneumoniae* from throat washing with a newly modified culture medium, J. Infect. Dis. **139**:478, 1979.

153. Tully, J.G., et al.: A newly discovered mycoplasma in the human urogenital tract, Lancet **1**:1288, 1981.

154. Tully, J.G., et al.: Evaluation of culture media for the recovery of *Mycoplasma hominis* from the human urogenital tract, Sex. Transm. Dis. **10**:256, 1983.

155. Venezio, F.R., et al.: Progressive cutaneous protothecosis, Am. J. Clin. Pathol. **77:**485, 1982.

156. Victoria, B., Baer, H., and Ayoub, E.M.: Successful treatment of systemic *Chromobacterium violaceum* infection, JAMA **230:**578, 1974.

156a. Warren, J.S., and Allen, S.D.: Clinical, pathogenetic, and laboratory features of *Capnocytophaga* infections, Am. J. Clin. Pathol. **86:** 513, 1986.

157. Weaver, R.E.: *Cardiobacterium*. In Krieg, N.R., editor (Holt, J.G., editor-in-chief): Bergey's manual of systematic bacteriology, vol. 1, Baltimore, 1985, Williams & Wilkins Co.

158. Weaver, R.E., Hollis, D.G., and Bottone, E.J.: Gram-negative fermentative bacteria and *Francisella tularensis*. In Lennette, E.H., editors: Manual of clinical microbiology, ed. 4, Washington, D.C., 1985, American Society for Microbiology.

159. Weinman, D.: Bartonellosis and anemias associated with *Bartonella*-like structures. In Balows, A., and Hausler, W.J., editors: Diagnostic procedures for bacterial, mycotic and parasitic infections, ed. 6, Washington, D.C., 1981, American Public Health Association, Inc.

159a. Williams, B.L., Hollis, D., and Holdeman, L.V.: Synonymy of strains of Center for Disease Control group Df-1 with species of *Capnocytophaga*, J. Clin. Microbiol. **10:**550, 1979.

160. Winn, R.E., et al.: Septic arthritis involving *Capnocytophaga ochracea*, J. Clin. Microbiol. **19:**538, 1984.

161. Zambon, J.J.: *Actinobacillus actinomycetemcomitans* in human periodontal disease, J. Clin. Periodontol. **12:**1, 1985.

162. Zambon, J.J., Christersson, L.A., and Slots, J.: *Actinobacillus actinomycetemcomitans* in human periodontal disease: prevalence in patient groups and distribution of biotypes and serotypes within families, J. Periodontol. **54:**707, 1983.

163. Zinnemann, K., and Turner, G.C.: The taxonomic position of *Haemophilus vaginalis (Corynebacterium vaginale)*, J. Pathol. Bacteriol. **85:**213, 1963.

Barbara J. Howard
James J. Damato

Mycobacteria

Mycobacterium tuberculosis was discovered by Robert Koch in 1882. Subsequent studies have found that mycobacteria are aerobic, nonsporeforming, slow-growing bacilli. These bacteria have a generation time of approximately 20 hours, and thus their isolation and identification may take up to 6 weeks. The mycobacteria include numerous pathogens and saprophytic organisms.

Of all the afflictions that have beset human beings, few have produced more death and suffering than tuberculosis and related mycobacterial infections. As civilization emerged and grew, so did the depredation of this disease until it received the epithet "Captain of All Men of Death."[25] Although significant progress has been made in the control of mycobacterial disease, only the highly industrialized nations of the world have been spared major morbidity and mortality; even among these nations, a resurgence of mycobacterial disease is occurring in segments of the population sustaining immune system abnormalities. For the developing nations the circumstances are grim, with *M. tuberculosis* and *M. bovis* producing widespread disease.[82] An estimated 20 million persons in the world today have active disease and will subsequently infect an additional 50 to 100 million persons annually. Of approximately 3 million persons who die each year from mycobacterioses, 80% reside in developing nations.[60,66] It should also be noted that disease produced by mycobacteria is not limited to humans and that the incidence of disease in the animal population parallels and often exceeds that noted in the human community.[28,111,112]

In the early part of this century tuberculosis was treated in large sanatoriums and "TB" hospitals. The drastic decline in prevalence of the disease resulted in the closing of most of these institutions in the 1950s to the 1970s. Consequently treatment was transferred to local hospitals or clinics, and laboratory mycobacteriology services became decentralized; however, many of the laboratories now receive only a small number of specimens and it is more difficult to maintain quality diagnostic work in all areas of mycobacteriology. In trying to resolve this problem levels of service or areas of proficiency for the mycobacteriology laboratory have been suggested.[42,59,129] The College of American Pathologists has proposed four levels of service[129] and the American Thoracic Society, three levels.[42] The latter are indicated in the following outline. Levels I, II, and III in this outline are roughly equivalent to levels 2, 3, and 4, respectively, of the College of American Pathologists[42]:

1. Level I
   a. Collect adequate clinical specimens, including aerosol-induced sputa
   b. Transport specimens to a higher-level laboratory for isolation and identification
   c. May prepare and examine smears for presumptive diagnosis or as a means of following the progress of diagnosed patients receiving chemotherapy
2. Level II
   a. Perform functions of level I laboratories
   b. Process specimens as necessary for culture on standard egg-base media or egg- and agar-base media
   c. Identify *Mycobacterium tuberculosis*
   d. May perform drug susceptibility studies against *M. tuberculosis*
   e. Retain mycobacterial cultures for additional or repeat tests
3. Level III
   a. Perform functions of laboratories at lower levels
   b. Identify all *Mycobacterium* spp. from clinical specimens
   c. Should perform drug susceptibility studies against mycobacteria
   d. May conduct research and provide training

Based on the number of specimens received, the resources, and the needs of the community, each laboratory must assess which mycobacterial procedures it can continue to perform competently. Procedures that are completed so infrequently that it is impossible to maintain the necessary technical expertise should be referred to a laboratory offering a higher level of service.

CLASSIFICATION

The mycobacteria are included in Section 16 of volume 2 of *Bergey's Manual of Systematic Bacteriology*. *Mycobacterium* is the only genus of the family *Mycobacteriaceae*. The distinguishing characteristics of this genus include slow growth, acid fastness, and possession of large amounts of lipids in their cell walls. Fifty-one species are recognized in *Bergey's Manual of Systematic Bacteriology;* only 31 species were recognized in the eighth edition of *Bergey's Manual of Determinative Bacteriology*.[91] The species that are isolated from humans and thus must be identified in the clinical laboratory are indicated in Table 26-6. Species found in other animals are reviewed by Gillespie and Timoney[28] and Thoen, Karlson, and Hines.[112] Because some of these species share similar biochemical, serologic, and pathogenic characteristics, they are often grouped and identified as a complex. An example is the *M. avium-intracellulare* (MAI) complex consisting of the species *M. avium* and *M. intracellulare*. Several workers have also suggested that *M. scrofulaceum* be included with these two species to form the *M. avium-intracellulare-scrofulaceum* (MAIS) complex.[139]

479

M. tuberculosis, M. africanum, and *M. bovis* are collectively referred to as the tubercle bacillus complex because these organisms cause tuberculosis, a disease characterized by the formation of tubercles and caseous necrosis in tissues. *M. tuberculosis* is the primary etiologic agent of human tuberculosis in the United States. Until the early 1900s *M. bovis* was responsible for numerous cases of tuberculosis in cattle. Ingestion of milk from these infected animals resulted in many human cases of tuberculosis. Tuberculosis caused by *M. bovis* is now rare in the United States because of the widespread pasteurization of milk and the institution of public health measures, which have virtually eradicated tuberculosis in cattle.[137] *M. africanum* occasionally produces pulmonary tuberculosis in Africa and possesses biochemical characteristics that are intermediate between *M. tuberculosis* and *M. bovis.*

Mycobacteria species other than *M. tuberculosis, M. bovis,* and *M. africanum* have been referred to by several names, including pseudotubercle bacilli, unclassified, anonymous, atypical, nontuberculous, mycobacteria other than tubercle bacilli (MOTT), and others.[16] The term "MOTT" is preferred. Some of these species (*M. kansasii, M. avium, M. malmoense,* and *M. intracellulare*) may produce a pulmonary syndrome indistinguishable from that produced by the tubercle bacilli.[36,123]

In the late 1950s Runyon[89] proposed that these species be divided into four groups based on growth rate and pigmentation. Group I was designated photochromogens, group II scotochromogens, group III nonphotochromogens, and group IV rapid growers (see p. 487 for definitions). Today mycobacterial isolates may be preliminarily assigned to one of these four groups, but it must be kept in mind that these groups are not taxonomic designations and that each group consists of several species. Rather than using the Runyon groupings[16,56,119] it is preferable to use the correct species designation when referring to mycobacteria.

In 1979 and 1980 the Centers for Disease Control in collaboration with the Association of State and Territorial Public Health Laboratory Directors completed a study to determine the distribution and frequency of mycobacteria.[31,32] The most commonly encountered pathogen was *M. tuberculosis,* followed by the *M. avium* complex, the *M. fortuitum* complex, *M. kansasii,* and *M. scrofulaceum* in order of frequency. Among the saprophytic species, *M. gordonae* was the most frequent isolate. More recently, however, the rate of isolation of MOTT had increased and in fact in some areas has surpassed that of *M. tuberculosis.*[137a]

SAFETY[119]

M. tuberculosis is transmitted primarily through the inhalation of airborne droplet nuclei. As a result, laboratory safety procedures are aimed at preventing the spread of potentially infective aerosols, which in addition to endangering workers' health may contaminate other patient samples, rendering them falsely positive. The careful control of aerosols and other forms of mycobacterial contamination is achieved by the use of appropriate biologic safety hoods, centrifuges with safety carriers, and meticulous processing techniques. All personnel must be thoroughly trained and a baseline chest x-ray study and PPD skin test performed before employment. The PPD skin test should also be performed at regular intervals thereafter, and a chest x-ray examination as necessary. In addition, when processing or working with open cultures, all personnel should be properly attired in protective gowns with masks and gloves.

Laboratories should be designed with proper ventilation and exhaust systems. A recommended layout for the mycobacteriology laboratory is discussed by Vestal.[119] All laboratories must have a certified biologic safety cabinet (BSC). These units must be maintained according to the manufacturers' guidelines, and all manipulations of infected materials or viable cultures must be handled in this cabinet. Before and after use the BSC working surfaces must be wiped with appropriate germicide. In addition, a germicide-soaked gauze or towel should cover the work area, excluding airflow grids, during specimen processing. Effective germicides include 5% phenol, 3% to 8% formaldehyde, 1:200 to 1:1000 sodium hypochlorite, 70% ethanol, and phenolic soaps. Seventy percent ethanol and dilute phenolic solutions may also be used on the skin. Ultraviolet light (Ultra-Violet Products, Inc., San Gabriel, Calif.) is a useful adjunct for surface decontamination. Such lights may be mounted in the BSC and turned on for a minimum of 2 hours after work has been completed. If this system is used regularly, ultraviolet light output should be evaluated monthly.

Containers that are subject to shaking or other forceful manipulations are sealed with O-rings and plastic- or rubber-lined caps. For example, all tissue homogenizing equipment should be used with aerosol-free seals and all centrifuges with aerosol-free safety carriers. An alcohol sand flask (a 250 to 500 ml Erlenmeyer flask half filled with washed sand and then filled with 95% ethanol) should be used to clean large clumps of bacilli from inoculating wires, loops, or spades before sterilization. This eliminates the possibility of spattering of the waxy mycobacteria during flaming.

SPECIMEN COLLECTION AND PROCESSING
Collection

All specimens for mycobacterial culture must be collected in sterile, disposable containers before the initiation of therapy and promptly transported to the laboratory. If unavoidable delays are anticipated, these specimens must be refrigerated (0° to 4° C) to prevent the overgrowth of contaminating flora.

Sputum

Although numerous specimen types may be submitted, sputum is by far the principal specimen obtained for evaluation. It is important that the patient be instructed to cough deeply to produce the desirable thick exudate and not saliva. If saliva is received, it should not be processed and another suitable specimen should be requested. Three to five early morning specimens (5 to 10 ml) collected on 3 consecutive days are usually sufficient. Pooled specimens are to be avoided because of increased contamination and lower test sensitivity.[49]

Induced Sputa

If patients are unable to produce suitable specimens, sputa may be induced with nebulization techniques, specifically inhalation of warm (45° C), aerosolized, sterile 10% NaCl or the use of ultrasonic nebulizers. These techniques should be performed by qualified personnel in an enclosed area to minimize risk from infectious aerosols. Induced sputa appear watery and much like saliva; these specimens must be properly labeled to prevent the unnecessary rejection of the specimen by the laboratory.

Gastric Lavage

Gastric lavage is best performed early in the morning before the patient arises. The patient should have fasted for 8 hours before collection. A disposable gastric tube is moistened with sterile water and inserted into the nostril or mouth. The patient slowly swallows small sips of sterile water as he or she swallows the tube. When the tube reaches the stomach, gastric contents are aspirated with a sterile 50 ml syringe and transferred to a sterile flask. Sterile water, 20 to 30 ml, is then given the patient by mouth or by injection through the gastric tube. Gastric washings are then aspirated and added to the first specimen.

Gastric lavage may be necessary for infants or very young children, adults who cannot induce sputa, uncooperative patients, patients who are comatose or have mental disorders, patients with radiologic evidence of tuberculosis but a negative sputum culture, and patients who are suspected of submitting sputa other than their own.[56] This procedure is especially valuable when used in conjunction with sputum induction. When sputum induction is performed 20 minutes after gastric lavage, the combined procedures yield more positive results than either method alone.[11]

It is strongly recommended that gastric lavage specimens be collected in containers without preservatives and processed immediately or at least within 4 hours of collection. When this time requirement is difficult to achieve because of patient and workflow considerations, the specimens should be collected in sterile disposable containers with 100 mg powdered sodium carbonate. Gastric lavage specimens may also be neutralized by adding 1.5 ml of 40% disodium phosphate/50 ml of specimen, or another alkaline buffer salt. However, a fresh unbuffered specimen is still preferred because the buffer may interfere with the decontamination process.

PROCESSING
Sterile Specimens[57]

Sterile tissues or body fluids usually do not require the digestion-decontamination procedures used with contaminated specimens. Sterile tissue may be ground in sterile 0.85% saline or 0.2% bovine albumin and then inoculated directly onto both solid and liquid media. Because large quantities of body fluids commonly contain small numbers of organisms, they should be concentrated before inoculation. These fluids are centrifuged at 3000 × g, and the sediment is inoculated to liquid and solid media. Smaller volumes (5 to 25 ml) of fluids and anticoagulated blood may be added directly to liquid media such as Middlebrook 7H9 in a ratio of one part specimen to five parts broth. Middlebrook 7H9 is an enrichment medium and will promote the growth of the few organisms that may be present. All liquid media should be incubated at 35° to 37° C, screened weekly, and subcultured to solid media as soon as growth is evident. If changes in the turbidity are impossible to detect because of the nature of the specimen (for example, blood), the broth should automatically be smeared at least weekly. If organisms are observed, the broth should be subcultured to solid media.

A recent study[50] showed that the Isolator system (DuPont Co., Wilmington, Del.) (see Chapter 11) is a sensitive method for detecting and quantitating the *M. avium* complex in blood.

Contaminated Specimens

Most specimens for mycobacterial culture contain large amounts of organic debris and are contaminated with a variety of organisms that rapidly outgrow the mycobacteria. Such specimens mandate the use of digestion-decontamination procedures to liquefy the debris and kill the undesirable contaminating organisms. Although the high lipid content of their cell walls renders the mycobacteria more resistant than other organisms to the harsh decontaminating agents, strict adherence to the processing procedures is mandatory because overexposure to these strong acid or alkaline substances also kills the mycobacteria.

The most widely used digestion-decontamination procedure is the *N*-acetyl-L-cysteine NaOH method.[58] The critical reagents used in this procedure include *N*-acetyl-L-cysteine (NALC), the mucolytic agent; sodium hydroxide, the decontaminating reagent; and sodium citrate, which stabilizes the acetylcysteine. The *N*-acetyl-L-cysteine NaOH method may be used to process sputum, gastric lavage specimens, tissue, urine, and other body fluids. The recommended procedures follow.[58,119]

Sputum

Sputum is decontaminated by the following procedure:
1. Prepare NALC-NaOH solution. For each 100 ml desired combine:
   50 ml sterile 4% NaOH
   50 ml sterile 2.9% sodium citrate
   0.5 g *N*-acetyl-L-cysteine powder
   This solution must be used within 24 hours of preparation because the mucolytic activity of NALC is inactivated on exposure to air. It should be noted that Sputolysin (Calbiochem-Behring, La Jolla, Calif.) may be used as a substitute for NALC. This product is not inactivated by exposure to air and provides a more stable digested preparation.
2. Transfer a maximum of 10 ml sputum to a sterile 50 ml screw-capped centrifuge tube (Falcon Plastics). The volume of sputum should not exceed one fifth of the volume of the tube.
3. Add an equal volume of NALC-NaOH solution to the specimen.
4. Tighten the caps of the centrifuge tubes and mix each specimen on the Vortex mixer for 5 to 20 seconds or until liquefied. Avoid extreme agitation because this oxidizes and inactivates the NALC. Set the timer for 15 minutes as soon as one or two specimens have been liquefied.
5. Organize work flow so that the specimens remain in contact with the decontaminating agent for only 15 minutes. Failure to time this step properly results in reduced recovery of mycobacteria.
6. Fill each tube to the 40 ml level with sterile distilled water or preferably with sterile pH 6.8 phosphate buffer (0.67 M). Tighten cap and swirl by hand to mix.
7. Centrifuge at 3000 × g for 15 minutes. NOTE: It has been suggested that this speed be increased to 3800 × g. With increased speed the sensitivity of acid-fast smears is increased, and more viable acid-fast bacilli (AFB) are present in the sediment for inoculation onto culture media. This results in earlier growth and more rapid identification of organisms.[86]
8. Decant the supernatant into a splash-proof can containing a disinfectant. Be careful not to cross-contaminate

patient specimens during the decanting process. Wipe the lip of the tube with a pledget soaked in 5% phenol or 70% alcohol. Use only one pledget per specimen, and do not allow the germicide to contact the specimen.

9. Using a sterile pipette, add 1 or 2 ml of 0.2% bovine fraction V albumin (pH 6.8) to each sediment. Shake the tube gently by hand to resuspend the sediment. Because this solution is well buffered at this point, it does not need to be neutralized. Prepare a smear of the undiluted sediment by spreading 1 drop over a 1 × 2 cm area on a microscope slide. Discard the pipette and place the smears on an electric slide warmer at 65° to 75° C for 2 hours.

10. With a sterile pipette, mix the sediment and prepare a 1:10 dilution by adding 0.5 ml (10 drops) to 4.5 ml sterile water or saline. Mix the 1:10 dilution with the pipette.

   a. Place 0.1 ml (2 drops) of the 1:10 dilution on the surface of one half of a biplate of 7H10 or 7H11 medium, and place 0.1 ml on the surface of each of two tubes of Lowenstein-Jensen medium.

   b. Place 2 drops of the undiluted sediment on the other half of the biplate of 7H10 or 7H11 medium, and place 2 drops on the surface of each of two tubes of Lowenstein-Jensen medium.

   c. With a bent glass rod spread the inoculum over the surface of the 7H10 or 7H11 plates. The plates with the 1:10 dilution should be spread first. (Inocula on plates may be left without spreading provided 3 drops per half plate are used.)

11. All inoculated plates should be placed in CO_2-permeable polyethylene bags and incubated in an incubator containing 5% to 10% CO_2. Candle jars should not be used because of the toxic combustion products.

Gastric lavage specimens

Fluid gastric lavage specimens should first be centrifuged at 3000 × g for 30 minutes. The supernatant should then be decanted and the sediment resuspended in 2 to 5 ml of sterile distilled water. Add an equal volume of NALC-NaOH and proceed as for sputum.

For mucoid gastric lavage specimens the following procedure should be followed.

1. Add 50 to 100 mg (a "pinch") of NALC powder to 20 to 50 ml gastric lavage.
2. Mix until liquefied.
3. Centrifuge at 3000 × g for 15 minutes.
4. Decant supernatant fluid into a splash-proof can containing a disinfectant and resuspend sediment in 2 to 5 ml of sterile distilled water.
5. Add an equal volume of NALC-NaOH and proceed with step 4 above.

Tissue

Tissue that is not collected aseptically should be placed in a tube, homogenized by vortexing, and processed as for sputum.

Urine

Clean-catch, first morning urines are the specimen of choice. Approximately 50 ml of urine should be centrifuged at 3000 ×

g for 30 minutes. The supernatant fluids are discarded and the sediments combined and resuspended in 2 to 5 ml of sterile water. Add an equal volume of NALC-NaOH and proceed as for sputum. Pooled urines are not satisfactory.

Feces

Although processed feces are not routinely cultured, processing may be especially useful in detecting *M. avium* complex in AIDS patients.[50] When acid-fast organisms are detected in a smear of unprocessed fecal material, a suspension of feces (1 g in 5 ml of Middlebrook 7H9) may be prepared and processed like sputum using the NALC-NaOH method discussed previously.[50]

Other body fluids

Body fluids of 10 ml or less should be processed as for sputum. Specimens containing more than 10 ml should be handled as fluid gastric lavage specimens unless the specimen is mucopurulent, in which case it should be treated as a mucoid gastric lavage specimen.

Other Processing Methods

Other processing procedures, including the trisodium phosphate–benzalkonium chloride (Zephiran, Winthrop Laboratories, New York) and sodium hydroxide methods, are also satisfactory for the recovery of mycobacteria from sputum.

In the trisodium phosphate–benzalkonium chloride (Zephiran)[119,126] procedure, the trisodium phosphate serves as the digestant and the benzalkonium chloride (Zephiran) acts as the decontaminating reagent. Since Zephiran is not as harsh as sodium hydroxide, this method may be useful for laboratories that find timed procedures difficult to follow precisely. The procedure follows.

1. Prepare reagent by dissolving 1 kg trisodium phosphate ($Na_3PO_4 \cdot 12H_2O$) in 4 L of hot distilled water. Add 7.5 ml concentrated (17%) benzalkonium chloride. After mixing, store at room temperature.
2. To a specimen contained in a 50 ml disposable centrifuge tube add an equal volume of trisodium phosphate–benzalkonium chloride. Tighten cap.
3. Shake vigorously on a shaking machine for 30 minutes.
4. Allow tube to stand for 20 to 30 minutes without further shaking.
5. Centrifuge at 3000 × g for 20 minutes.
6. Decant supernatant into a splash-proof container of disinfectant.
7. Resuspend sediment in 20 ml of pH 6.6 neutralizing buffer.
8. Recentrifuge for 20 minutes. Decant supernatant.
9. Inoculate the sediment onto isolation media.

In the sodium hydroxide method, sodium hydroxide serves as both the digestant and the decontaminant. Because of the toxicity of this substance to mycobacteria as well as to contaminating organisms, the time limits for processing must be strictly adhered to. The procedure is as follows.

1. Add an equal volume of 2% to 4% NaOH (select lowest concentration necessary for effective digestion and decontamination) to sputum contained in a Teflon-lined, screw-capped tube. Tighten cap securely.
2. Shake tube vigorously in a Vortex mixer for 15 to 20 minutes.

3. Centrifuge the tubes at 3000 × g for 20 minutes.
4. Decant supernatant fluid into a splash-proof container with disinfectant.
5. Neutralize the sediment with 2 N HCl. First add 1 drop of phenol red pH color indicator solution; then add HCl drop by drop until a definite yellow endpoint is obtained. (Alternatively a hydrochloric acid–phenol red indicator may be used. To prepare, combine 30 ml of phenol red [0.4% in 4% NaOH] and 85 ml concentrated HCl with enough distilled water to make 1000 ml.)
6. Back titrate with 4% NaOH until a faint pink color is achieved.
7. Inoculate sediment onto LJ and 7H10 or 7H11 media.

The use of special processing procedures may sometimes be necessary. The oxalic acid method, for example, is recommended for treating sputum specimens that are consistently contaminated with *Pseudomonas* spp., whereas the sulfuric acid method may be used to process urine.

Another special processing procedure is the cetylpyridinium chloride (CPC) method,[102] which has been proposed for the decontamination, liquefaction, and concentration of sputum specimens that will be in transport for more than 24 hours. An equal volume of a solution of 1% cetylpyridinium chloride and 2% NaCl is added to sputum contained in a 50 ml screw-capped centrifuge tube. The tubes are capped and shaken until the sputum appears liquid. The mycobacteria remain viable for 8 days in this solution.

It is important that the person receiving the specimen be informed that no further processing is necessary. On receipt, tubes should be filled with sterile distilled water and centrifuged at 3000 × g. After the supernatant is decanted, the sediment is resuspended in 1 to 2 ml of sterile distilled water, physiologic saline, or 0.2% bovine albumin fraction V and plated onto LJ media. Agar-base media are unacceptable for inoculation because, unlike egg media, they do not contain phospholipids, which neutralize the bacteriostatic effect of the CPC on the growth of the mycobacteria. However, if Neutralizing Buffer (Difco Laboratories, Detroit) is used to resuspend the centrifugate, agar-base media may be used. All specimens containing CPC should be marked clearly to ensure that the CPC is suitably neutralized either by use of egg-base media or by washing with Neutralizing Buffer.

STAINING ACID-FAST BACILLI

The examination of direct smears for mycobacteria is important for several reasons. Although the smear is not as sensitive as culture techniques and requires approximately 10⁴ bacilli/ml sputum to be positive, smear examination provides an easy, rapid, presumptive diagnosis of mycobacterial disease. Microscopic examination can also be used to monitor the progress of patients receiving chemotherapy. Finally, it is imperative to detect the likely presence of mycobacterial disease as rapidly as possible because these patients are considered infectious reservoirs or those most likely to spread tuberculosis.[56]

The large amounts of lipids present in the cell walls of mycobacteria render them impermeable to the dyes used in the Gram stain. In fact, when stained with the Gram stain, the mycobacteria vary from gram positive to ''gram-ghost'' or ''gram-neutral'' bacilli.[43] Mycobacteria are able to form stable complexes with certain arylmethane dyes (dyes with aromatic methane rings) such as fuchsin and auramine O. Once these complexes

are formed, they are very resistant to decolorization with acid alcohols or strong mineral acids and are thus termed acid fast.

Although the exact mechanism responsible for the acid fastness of mycobacteria is unknown, it is largely attributed to the presence of mycolic acids in the outer cell wall. Mycolic acids are long, branched fatty acids up to 90 carbons in length. When stained, intact mycobacterial cell walls take the dye such as fuchsin into their interior and also bind it to the mycolic acid residues of the outer cell wall. The brilliance of acid fastness depends on the trapped fuchsin, which is ensured by the fuchsin–mycolic acid binding of the cell wall.[6]

The Ziehl-Neelsen, Kinyoun, and fluorochrome acid-fast staining techniques are used in mycobacteriology. Careful quality control procedures should be used with these techniques for maximum reliability of results.[76]

The Ziehl-Neelsen and Kinyoun methods employ a carbol-fuchsin stain and a methylene blue counterstain. Carbol-fuchsin contains the dye fuchsin in combination with phenol, which allows the fuchsin to penetrate the cell wall. Fluorochrome techniques employ fluorescent dyes such as auramine O or rhodamine B in combination with phenol. (It should be noted that fluorochrome stains do not represent fluorescent antibody techniques but simply acid-fast stains.) The fluorochrome procedure is preferred over the carbol-fuchsin techniques because of its sensitivity and ability to detect nonviable organisms. Furthermore, the Ziehl-Neelsen and Kinyoun methods may not stain nonviable tubercle bacilli, especially if they are killed during treatment with isoniazid. These organisms stain with auramine O, however. Thus with fluorochrome methods a few more positive smear and negative culture results may be seen at the time of culture conversion to negative.

SMEAR PREPARATION[101]

The first step in any staining technique is proper preparation of the smear. In laboratories that routinely culture for mycobacteria, smears are usually prepared after concentration of the specimen. In situations when rapid evaluation of a clinical specimen is needed, a direct smear may be prepared from the purulent material of the specimen. This latter procedure must be performed under a biologic safety cabinet. Acid-fast stains may be prepared directly from unprocessed fecal material for detection of *M. avium* complex in AIDS patients.[50]

Laboratories that do not culture mycobacteria and do not possess a biologic safety cabinet but must examine smears for AFB should use the sodium hypochlorite procedure for processing the specimen. This procedure, which follows, liquefies the sputum and kills most if not all mycobacteria.[119]

1. Add an equal volume of 5% or 6% sodium hypochlorite (Clorox) to the specimen.
2. Tighten cap. Shake until liquefied and let stand for 15 minutes.
3. Centrifuge at 3000× g for 15 minutes.
4. Decant immediately, draining off excess liquid.
5. Smear sediment and stain.

Sodium hypochlorite causes disintegration of the bacilli if allowed to act too long; therefore smears should be prepared, stained, and examined promptly. Treatment with glutaraldehyde has been suggested as an alternative to sodium hypochlorite.[30]

For preparation of a smear, the specimen should be spread

with an applicator stick or a 3 mm bacteriologic loop over an area of 1×2 cm on a new, clean, unscratched, properly labeled slide. The used applicator stick should be discarded and the wire loop dipped into 70% to 95% ethanol and sand before sterilization in a Bunsen burner flame or incinerator. It is important that the smear be of the proper thickness; although many smears appear cloudy, one should still be able to read newspaper print through them from a distance of 5 to 10 cm. After air drying, the smear is heat fixed on an electric slide warmer (65° to 75° C) for 2 hours or passed three times through the flame of a Bunsen burner. Slides and specimens should not be exposed to ultraviolet light, direct sunlight, or overheating during fixing or autoclaving because this alters the staining characteristics of the mycobacteria.

STAINING PROCEDURES

Smears should be stained on a level staining rack. Staining dishes are unacceptable because they may permit the transfer of acid-fast bacilli from a positive smear to a negative one. If a delay occurs between preparation of smear and staining, it has been recommended that the smears be given additional treatment such as immersion in glutaraldehyde to prevent the survival of tubercle bacilli.[1] The Ziehl-Neelsen, Kinyoun, and auramine-rhodamine fluorochrome staining procedures are outlined in Chapter 6.

READING AND REPORTING OF SMEARS[101]
Ziehl-Neelsen-Stained and Kinyoun-Stained Smears

With the carbol-fuchsin stains, the AFB stain red and the background material stains blue when counterstained with methylene blue (Plate 1, *C*). The mycobacteria are usually rod shaped but may appear as cocci or filaments. They may contain heavily stained areas called beads and often have alternating stained and clear sections, making them appear banded (Plate 23, *B*). The mycobacteria other than *M. tuberculosis* (MOTT) tend to be very pleomorphic, ranging from short organisms to long, banded forms. *M. kansasii* characteristically appears in long, broad, banded forms.

Smears stained with these methods are examined with the oil immersion objective (100×) of a brightfield microscope. Since the field of view seen in the microscope covers only a very small area of the smear and the smear represents a very small portion of the total specimen, the technologist must examine an area of the slide large enough to be truly representative of the specimen. This is best accomplished by making three long longitudinal sweeps of the stained area parallel to the length of the slide. At a total magnification of 1000×, the technologist should be able to view about 100 fields per sweep for a total of 300 fields per slide.

Because acid-fast artifacts may also be present in the smear, it is essential to view cell morphology carefully. Most artifacts show considerable pleomorphism and varied staining, whereas mycobacterial cells exhibit greater uniformity in size, arrangement, and staining. The positive and negative control slides should be used as a guide to establish baseline characteristics. If in spite of these actions, doubts persist concerning the presence of acid-fast organisms, the physician should be contacted to discuss the findings and to determine other relevant clinical information that may help resolve the problem. The acquisition of additional specimens may also be helpful in establishing the possibility of mycobacterial infection. The number of AFB

TABLE 26-1. Suggested Method for Reporting Acid-Fast Bacilli in Fuchsin-Stained Smears

Number of Bacilli[a]	Report
0	No acid-fast bacilli found
1-2/300 fields	±
1-9/100 fields	1+
1-9/10 fields	2+
1-9/field	3+
>9/field	4+

From Kent, P.T., and Kubica, G.P.: Public health mycobacteriology: a guide for the level III laboratory, Atlanta, 1985, Centers for Disease Control.
[a]All observations are made using 800× to 1000×. All reports should state staining method used and actual number of organisms observed.

observed should be reported according to the scheme in Table 26-1.

Fluorochrome-Stained Smears

Fluorochrome-stained smears should be scanned with a fluorescence microscope (for recommended equipment see Chapter 6) at lower magnifications (250× to 630×). The use of lower magnification permits the examination of a larger area of the smear per unit of time than does the oil immersion lens of the brightfield microscope. To equate the numbers of organisms observed at magnifications less than 800× with those seen under oil immersion, the counts must be adjusted. This is discussed by Kent and Kubica.[48a]

The acid-fast bacilli appear bright yellow to orange in fluorochrome-stained smears. If a potassium permanganate counterstain is used, the background appears dark and nonspecific fluorescing debris appear pale yellow. With the acridine orange counterstain, the background appears red to orange.

PROBLEMS WITH STAINING TECHNIQUES[101]

The technologist should be aware of the following potential problems that may arise when staining.
1. False-positive results may occur as a result of the contamination of tap water or distilled water with saprophytic AFB or the transfer of positive flakes from thick slides. Contaminated oil may also give false-positive results.
2. The debris in smears that are too thick may mask the presence of AFB.
3. Too thin smears may give false-negative results.
4. Specimen containers that are free of waxes and oils must be used; these substances may appear on the smear as acid-fast artifacts or they may react with non-acid-fast bacteria and cause them to appear acid fast.
5. Factors that may interfere with staining or reduce fluorescence include excessive exposure of the stained smear to potassium permanganate, exposure of fluorescent stains to solutions of heavy metal ions, high chlorine content of rinse water, and use of absorbent paper during staining.
6. Many strains of rapidly growing mycobacteria are not stained with the auramine-rhodamine stain. All, however, are stained with the Ziehl-Neelsen stain.[48]

TABLE 26-2. Nonselective Mycobacterial Isolation Media[a]

Medium	Components	Inhibitory Agent
Lowenstein-Jensen	Coagulated whole eggs, defined salts, glycerol, potato flour	0.025 g/100 ml malachite green
Petragnani	Coagulated whole eggs, egg yolks, whole milk, potato, potato flour, glycerol	0.052 g/100 ml malachite green
American Thoracic Society	Coagulated fresh egg yolks, potato flour, glycerol	0.02 g/100 ml malachite green
Middlebrook 7H10	Defined salts, vitamins, cofactors, oleic acid, albumin, catalase, glycerol, dextrose	0.0025 g/100 ml malachite green
Middlebrook 7H11	Defined salts, vitamins, cofactors, oleic acid, albumin, catalase, glycerol, 0.1% casein hydrolysate	0.0025 g/100 ml malachite green

From Youmans, G.P., editor: Tuberculosis, Philadelphia, 1979, W.B. Saunders Co.

GROWTH REQUIREMENTS
MEDIA

Although most mycobacteria grow on simple synthetic media once they have adapted to in vitro growth, more complex media should be included for primary isolation.[57] Nonselective, selective, and liquid media should be used.

Mycobacterium leprae cannot be cultivated in vitro. Because the laboratory diagnosis of this organism differs considerably from that of other mycobacteria, it is discussed separately at the end of this chapter.

Nonselective Culture Media

Nonselective media may be egg based or agar based (Table 26-2). One egg-base medium and one agar-base medium should be used in primary isolation.[57] All nonselective media include malachite green, which suppresses the growth of contaminating bacteria.

Egg-base media contain whole eggs, potato flour, salts, and glycerol and are solidified by inspissation. Advantages of the egg media include the greater number of positive cultures obtained and the neutralization by the egg of traces of toxic material in the inoculum.[129] Among the egg-base media, Lowenstein-Jensen (LJ) is the most commonly used. The increased content of the malachite green in Petragnani agar makes this medium more suitable for highly contaminated specimens. Conversely, because of its low concentration of malachite green, the American Trudeau Society medium is more acceptable for specimens less likely to be contaminated, for example, spinal fluids and pleural fluids.

The agar-base media are based on the early formulations of Middlebrook and Cohn. As indicated in Table 26-2, the 7H11 medium differs from the 7H10 medium only in the addition of 0.1% enzymatic casein hydrolysate. Incorporation of this substance stimulates the growth of difficult-to-grow drug-resistant strains of *M. tuberculosis*.[15]

The agar media are transparent and are especially useful because they allow easier and more rapid microscopic detection of colonies. Colonies may be observed in 12 to 14 days, in contrast to 18 to 24 days with the egg-base media. Microscopic examination at 100× can be performed by simply turning the plate medium over and examining it from the reverse side. However, extreme caution must be exercised in the preparation and use of these media. Excessive exposure to light or heat will result in the formation of formaldehyde and subsequent inhibition of growth.[68]

It should be noted that one species of mycobacteria, *M. haemophilum*,[105] requires hemin for growth. Satisfactory isolation media include chocolate agar, 7H10 agar containing hemolyzed sheep erythrocytes or an X factor (hemin) strip,[117] and LJ media with 1% ferric ammonium citrate.[104] Furthermore, for isolation of *M. paratuberculosis* the medium must be supplemented with 2 µg/ml of mycobactin.

Selective Culture Media

The addition of antimicrobial agents to LJ, 7H10, or 7H11 media may help eliminate the growth of contaminating organisms, the major problem in the recovery of the mycobacteria. Although some of these selective media may also inhibit the growth of certain mycobacterial species, overall they result in an increased recovery. One of the selective media from Table 26-3 should be included with the egg-base and agar-base nonselective media during primary isolation.

The selective 7H11 medium in Table 26-3 is McClatchy's modification[65] of the selective 7H10[71] and selective 7H11[70] media of Mitchison. All three of these media may be used to isolate mycobacteria from nondecontaminated specimens. McClatchy modified Mitchison selective 7H11 medium by decreasing the concentration of carbenicillin from 100 to 50 µg. The lower concentration was reportedly less inhibitory to *M. intracellulare*, *M. kansasii*, and *M. scrofulaceum*. The modified medium is useful for the inoculation of heavily contaminated specimens (sputa) after NaOH-NALC treatment or for direct plating of sterile specimens such as spinal fluids without decontaminating processing. This medium has also been used for the direct plating of sputum specimens.

Although the selective 7H10 and 7H11 media are very effective, they should be used only in conjunction with the nonselective media and not as the sole media for the isolation of mycobacteria.[65,71,88]

TABLE 26-3. Selective Mycobacterial Isolation Media

Medium	Components	Inhibitory Agents	
		Agent	Amount
Gruft modification of Lowenstein-Jensen	Coagulated whole eggs, defined salts, glycerol, potato flour, RNA—17 mg/100 ml	Malachite green Penicillin Nalidixic acid	0.025 g/100 ml 50 units/ml 35 µg/ml
Mycobactosel[a] Lowenstein-Jensen	Coagulated whole eggs, defined salts, glycerol, potato flour	Malachite green Cycloheximide Lincomycin Nalidixic acid	0.025 g/100 ml 400 µg/ml 2 µg/ml 35 µg/ml
Middlebrook 7H10	Defined salts, vitamins, cofactors, oleic acid, albumin, catalase, glycerol, and dextrose	Malachite green Cycloheximide Lincomycin Nalidixic acid	0.0025 g/100 ml 360 µg/ml 2 µg/ml 20 µg/ml
Selective 7H11 (Mitchison medium)	Defined salts, vitamins, cofactors, oleic acid, albumin, catalase, glycerol, dextrose, and casein hydrolysate	Carbenicillin Amphotericin B Polymyxin B Trimethoprim lactate	50 µg/ml 10 µg/ml 200 units/ml 20 µg/ml

From Youmans, G.P., editor: Tuberculosis, Philadelphia, 1979, W.B. Saunders Co.

[a]Mycobactosel is the registered trademark of BBL, Cockeysville, Md.

Liquid Media

Liquid media are used to prepare inocula for various identification procedures. Middlebrook 7H9 and Dubos-Middlebrook Tween albumin medium, the most commonly used liquid media, contain the detergent Tween 80 (polyoxyethylene derivative of sorbitan mono-oleate) and albumin. Tween 80 allows dispersed growth of the hydrophobic mycobacteria, and albumin binds excess quantities of the toxic oleate released by the spontaneous hydrolysis of Tween 80.

ENVIRONMENTAL REQUIREMENTS

The mycobacteria grow best in 5% to 10% CO_2. The 7H10 and 7H11 media *must* be incubated initially in an atmosphere containing increased CO_2. The Petri dishes of agar-base media should be placed medium side down into clear, CO_2-permeable, polyethylene bags before incubation. Each bag should contain one plate; no more than six bags should be placed in a single stack in the incubator. The LJ slants should be incubated in a slanted position with the screw caps loose for at least 1 week. This allows even distribution of the inoculum and permits sufficient exposure to CO_2. At the end of 1 week the tubes may be incubated upright if space is a problem.

All cultures except those from skin lesions may be incubated at 35° to 37°C. Cultures of skin lesions must be incubated at 30° to 33°C.

All cultures should be examined after 5 to 7 days of incubation and weekly thereafter for 6 to 8 weeks before being discarded as negative. Skin lesions should be incubated a minimum of 8 weeks; up to 12 weeks' incubation may be required. This is necessary because of the extremely slow growth rate of *M. ulcerans*.[119] (Areas of endemic disease caused by this organism include Zaire, Uganda, Nigeria, Ghana, Cameroon, Malaysia, New Guinea, Guyana, Mexico, and Australia.[137a]) Negative cultures should be examined microscopically before discarding. Depending on the individual laboratory isolation rates, preliminary negative culture reports may be issued after 4 weeks' incubation.

RAPID DETECTION OF MYCOBACTERIA

The Bactec 460 (Johnston Labs) system automatically and rapidly detects the presence of mycobacteria in clinical specimens by monitoring the amount of CO_2 produced when the organisms metabolize specifically labeled substrates. Specimens are prepared by standard procedures and then inoculated into Bactec 7H12 Middlebrook TB medium.[67] This medium is an enriched Middlebrook 7H9 broth base supplemented with bovine serum albumin (fraction V), catalase, casein hydrolysate, and 14C-labeled palmitic acid. An antimicrobial mixture called PANTA (polymyxin B, amphotericin B, nalidixic acid, trimethoprim, and azlocillin) is added to the medium before use to reduce bacterial contamination. (PANTA has replaced the previously used PACT.) The mycobacteria metabolize the radioactive palmitic acid during growth and release radioactive CO_2. The amount of CO_2 produced reflects the rate and amount of growth and is recorded quantitatively as a growth index (GI).

A number of studies have shown more rapid detection using the Bactec as compared with conventional media.[74,87] One study reported average detection times of 8.3 days for *M. tuberculosis* and 5.2 days for MOTT with the Bactec, as compared with 19.4 and 17.8 days, respectively, when conventional means were used.[87] Studies performed by Damato and others[19] indicated that early detection and maximum recovery of mycobacteria may be achieved by using a combination of radiometric and selective and nonselective media. The use of McClatchy's modification of Mitchison 7H11 agar with undecontaminated specimens and radiometric 7H12 media successfully detected 100% of the mycobacteria present; 78% of the slow-growing mycobacteria and 100% of the rapid-growing mycobacteria were detected within 3 to 7 days. This combined use of selective, nonselective, and radiometric media appears to hold significant promise for decreasing detection time and enhancing test sensitivity. The variety of media and methodologies is sufficient to permit technologists to select the optimal *Mycobacterium* isolation system as dictated by their patient and administrative requirements.

CULTURAL CHARACTERISTICS
STAINING REACTIONS

The staining reactions of the mycobacteria are discussed on p. 484.

COLONIAL MORPHOLOGY

Colony morphology should be observed on individual colonies with a hand lens (3× to 10×) or a dissecting microscope (10× to 50×). If growth is confluent, a subculture should be made to obtain well-isolated colonies. An acid-fast smear should be made to ensure that the colony being examined is indeed a species of *Mycobacterium* and that no contaminating organisms are present. The microbiologist should note several colonial characteristics: texture (roughness), shape (flat, umbonate, curved), and pigment.

The texture of *M. tuberculosis* colonies has a characteristic roughness, which on close examination reveals long stacked chains of bacilli described as serpentine cords (Plate 23, *C*). The formation of serpentine cording and concurrent rough colonial texture has generally been attributed to the presence of a cell surface glycolipid (trehalose-6,6'-dimycolate), the so-called cord factor, although this relationship has been questioned.[6] Colonial characteristics of mycobacteria are summarized in Table 26-4. Runyon[90] provides a detailed review.

IDENTIFICATION
PRESUMPTIVE IDENTIFICATION

The observation of rate of growth and pigment production and photoreactivity discussed below facilitates the separation of the mycobacteria into preliminary subdivisions (Figure 26-1). Furthermore, the use of these criteria in combination with other data such as frequency of isolation and clinical diagnosis may permit a presumptive identification of the organism.[77]

RATE OF GROWTH AND GROWTH IN RELATION TO TEMPERATURE

The growth rate refers to the amount of time required to form mature colonies that are visible without magnification. Organisms forming such colonies within 7 days are termed rapid growers, whereas those requiring longer periods of time are called slow growers.

Because certain rapid growers, such as *M. chelonae*,[36] may require several weeks for their primary isolation, the growth rate for all slow-growing organisms should be confirmed with a subculture as follows[56]:

1. Prepare the inoculum by diluting a 7-day broth culture or a saline suspension of organisms from a freshly grown slant so it will yield isolated colonies.
2. Inoculate several 10-fold dilutions of the test organism onto either an egg-base or agar-base medium (or both) and incubate at 35° to 37° C. Isolates suspected of containing *M. ulcerans, M. marinum,* or *M. haemophilum* require incubation at 30° to 32° C.

3. Observe cultures 5 to 7 days and then weekly thereafter for visible colonies.

Growth in relation to temperature can usually be adequately determined by observing the primary cultures or subcultures at 37° or 30° C. When more definitive identification is needed, isolates should be incubated at 24°, 30°, 37°, and 42° C. Growth at these temperatures is interpreted as in Table 26-5.

PIGMENTATION AND PHOTOREACTIVITY

Some mycobacteria produce carotenoid pigments without light, whereas others require light (photoactivation) for pigment production. The terms "photochromogen," "scotochromogen," and "nonphotochromogen" are used to distinguish the MOTT based on their pigmentation and photoreactivity.

Photochromogens are organisms that appear nonpigmented when grown in the dark but produce photoactivated carotenoid pigments (chromogenic) when exposed to light and reincubated. When exposed to continuous light for 2 weeks, some of the photochromogens, notably *M. kansasii*, form orange crystals of beta-carotene within isolated colonies (Plate 23, *D*).

Scotochromogens produce a deep yellow to orange pigment when grown in either dark or light. The deep yellow to orange pigment deepens to orange or dark red when exposed to continuous light for 2 weeks.

Nonphotochromogens may possess pigmentation ranging from white to buff, tan, or pale yellow; however, the pigment does not intensify on light exposure.

If nonpigmented colonies are observed during the routine examination of a culture, the cap of the culture should be loosened and the culture exposed to a bright light (fluorescent or incandescent) for 1 hour. The culture should then be reincubated overnight with the cap remaining loose. Development of pigmentation is indicative of photochromogenicity. The loosened cap is vital in permitting exposure to air,[124] since the induction of the soluble beta-carotene pigment is controlled by a rapidly active, oxygen-dependent, photoinducible enzyme.[6]

Since observation of pigment production and photochromogenicity, like growth rate, depends on the presence of isolated colonies, a more precise and methodical procedure for determination of photochromogenicity is as follows[104]:

1. Sufficiently dilute a broth culture of the test organism to obtain isolated colonies.
2. Inoculate three tubes containing Lowenstein-Jensen medium.
3. Wrap two of the tubes in aluminum foil and leave the third uncovered so it will be exposed to ambient light in the incubator.
4. Cultures thought to be photochromogenic should be incubated at 30° and 37° C, and those thought to be scotochromogenic should be incubated at 24° and 37° C. *M. szulgai* is commonly scotochromogenic when grown at 37° C but photochromogenic when grown at 24° C.
5. Several days after growth is noted on the control tube, examine the foil-wrapped tube for growth.
6. If growth is present, loosen the cap of one of the foil-wrapped tubes and expose it to a 100-watt tungsten bulb or fluorescent equivalent for 3 to 5 hours.
7. Return the tube to the incubator and inspect it after 24 and 48 hours for the development of a yellow or orange pigment.

TABLE 26-4. Morphologic Characteristics of Clinically Significant Mycobacteria

Organism	Colonial Morphology on Lowenstein-Jensen (LJ) Medium	Colonial Morphology on 7H10 Agar
M. avium-intracellulare	Colonies usually smooth, dome shaped, and buff colored; rough, wrinkled colonies sometimes seen; cultures sometimes appear impure, since more than one colony type may appear on same culture	Colonies usually smooth, circular, thin, transparent, and pyramid shaped or hemispheric; as on LJ medium, rough colonies may be seen and more than one colony type may appear on same culture
M. bovis	Low, smooth, colorless, pyramid-shaped colonies	Thin, nonpigmented, wrinkled, rough colonies; cording may be present but is much more pronounced on pyruvate-supplemented media
M. chelonae	Colonies usually rounded, smooth, colorless, and hemispheric; rough colonies occasionally seen, especially on prolonged incubation	As on LJ medium
M. fortuitum	Colonies soft, butyrous, hemispheric, and multilobate or rough with heaped centers; although nonpigmented, may appear green owing to absorption of malachite green	One- to 2-day-old colonies show branching filaments, although older colonies do not; on cornmeal agar branching filaments are conspicuous on both young and old colonies
M. haemophilum	Colonies nonpigmented, predominantly rough with smooth variants occurring frequently	As on LJ medium
M. kansasii	Colonies smooth or rough; although nonpigmented when grown in the dark, become lemon yellow when exposed to light for 1 hour; on continuous light exposure, characteristic orange-red crystals of beta-carotene appear (Plate 23, D)	Colony centers appear elevated and thickened; when observed microscopically thinner peripheral portions show stranding of bacilli; colonies vary in roughness and are most often intermediate between fully smooth and fully rough but may be completely rough, or rarely, completely smooth; pigmentation characteristics as on LJ medium
M. malmoense[76]	Growth observed only after 6 weeks of incubation; colonies dysgonic, smooth, and colorless even after light exposure	Smooth, glistening, grayish white, opaque, domed circular colonies 0.5 to 1.5 mm in diameter with entire margins or, less often, umbonate colonies 0.6 to 2.7 mm in diameter with compact, raised centers and flattened, irregular edges
M. marinum	Similar to M. kansasii	Similar to M. kansasii, although rhizoids more commonly seen
M. paratuberculosis	Initial growth smooth but with continued incubation becomes rough, dry, umbonated, and heaped	Smooth yellow colonies; appear domed with entire margin or flattened irregular periphery; rough colonies rarely seen
M. simiae	Colonies appear smooth and although nonpigmented when grown in the dark, become yellow-orange when exposed to light	As on LJ medium
M. szulgai	Smooth to rough pyramid-shaped colonies with somewhat irregular periphery; scotochromogenic (orange) when incubated at 37° C and photochromogenic at 25° C; continuous light exposure may result in formation of red crystals	As on LJ medium
M. tuberculosis	Nonpigmented, dry, rough, with nodular surface and irregular thin periphery	Nonpigmented, flat, dry, rough, and corded
M. ulcerans	After 4 weeks appear as transparent, minute, domed colonies but with further incubation become rough and low convex to flat with an irregular edge	Colonies rough and corded
M. xenopi	Small, smooth, dysgonic, dome-shaped nonpigmented colonies that become yellow on aging	Small yellow colonies with compact centers surrounded by fringe of branching filaments visible on microscopic examination; resemble bird's nest

TABLE 26-5. Growth of Mycobacteria

Growth Rate	Temperature	Organism
Slow (2 or more weeks)	Growth at 35° to 37° C but none at 24° or 42° C	*M. tuberculosis* or *M. bovis*
	Growth at 35° to 37° C and 42° but none at 24° C	*M. xenopi*, some *M. avium* complex strains
	Growth at 35° to 37° C, slower at 24° C, negative at 42° C	*M. kansasii*
	Growth at 32° and 24° C in 2 weeks, none or poorly at 35° to 37° C	*M. marinum*
	Growth at 32° C in 2 to 4 weeks, at 25° or 35° C in 4 to 8 weeks, no growth at 37° C	*M. haemophilum*
Slow (3 or more weeks)	Growth at 32° C, but none at 24° C or 35° to 37° C	*M. ulcerans*

Modified from Sommers, H.M., and Good, R.C.: Mycobacterium. In Lennette, E.H., et al., editors: Manual of clinical microbiology, ed. 4, Washington, D.C., 1985, American Society for Microbiology.

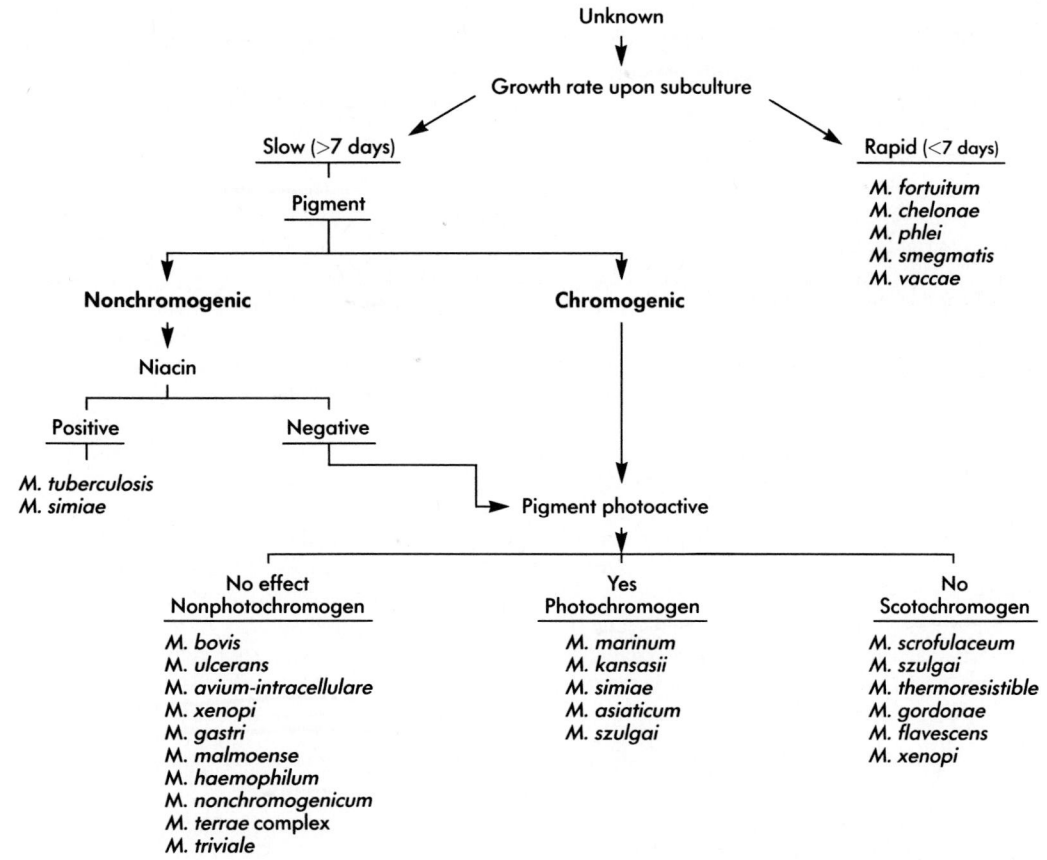

FIGURE 26-1. Preliminary subdivision of the mycobacteria. (Modified from Kubica, G.P., and David, H.L.: The mycobacteria. In Sonnenwirth, A.C., and Jarett, L., editors: Gradwohl's clinical laboratory methods and diagnosis, ed. 8, vol. 2, St. Louis, 1980, The C.V. Mosby Co.)

DEFINITIVE IDENTIFICATION[56,57]

After an isolate has been assigned to a preliminary subgroup (Figure 26-1), further biochemical testing permits identification to species or complex level. The studies of the International Working Group on Mycobacterial Taxonomy[127,128] and various individuals[55] have enabled the establishment of several standard reproducible biochemical tests and key tests for the speciation of the mycobacteria. These standard procedures serve as reference points against which other modified procedures can be evaluated.[122]

The standard biochemical tests most often used in the mycobacteriology laboratory (Table 26-6) are discussed in detail in Appendix A. All biochemical tests in Table 26-6 should be performed on each isolate at the same time that the tests for pigment production, photoreactivity, and speed of growth are being determined.[56] Although selected key tests discussed here are of greatest value in differentiating among the species, all tests should be performed and used in identification.

Identification within each of the subgroups from Figure 26-1 is considered next.

RAPID GROWERS

Organisms of the *M. fortuitum* complex are the only potentially pathogenic members of the rapid growers. Isolation of these organisms, however, does not necessarily imply a pathogenic process, since they may also appear as saprophytes. The *M. fortuitum* complex is distinguished from other rapid growers on the basis of a positive arylsulfatase test and growth on MacConkey agar without crystal violet. Because infections caused by these organisms are more prevalent than was originally thought and because *M. fortuitum* is more sensitive to antimycobacterial agents than *M. chelonae*, it is important to distinguish these two species so preliminary drug therapy can be initiated.[98] Nitrate reduction and iron uptake (Table 26-6) allow differentiation. David, Traore, and Feuillet[24] have also suggested the use of nitrate reduction, beta-glucosidase, and acid production from fructose. Finally, susceptibility to pipemidic acid may be used to differentiate these two organisms.[12] *M. chelonae* is resistant to pipemidic acid, whereas *M. fortuitum* is susceptible.

M. chelonae may be further subdivided into the subspecies *chelonae* and *abscessus* and *M. fortuitum* into the biovars *fortuitum* and *peregrinum* on the basis of growth on sodium citrate, mannitol, and inositol.[98] *M. chelonae* ssp. *chelonae* is found mainly in Europe, whereas *M. chelonae* ssp. *abscessus* predominates in Africa and America.[35]

Differentiation of *M. vaccae*, *M. smegmatis*, and *M. phlei* requires special procedures, and such definitive identification is rarely necessary. In the majority of cases the laboratory can safely report "Rapid grower, not in *M. fortuitum* complex" for isolates that are negative for the arylsulfatase and MacConkey tests.[56]

NIACIN-POSITIVE NONPHOTOCHROMOGENS

The presence of a slow-growing, dry, rough, granular buff-colored organism that is also niacin positive is strong presumptive evidence of *M. tuberculosis*. Since other organisms are also niacin positive, however, additional biochemical tests including nitrate reduction and catalase at 68° C are needed to confirm this organism. If an isolate is rough, niacin positive, nitrate positive, and catalase negative at 68° C and grows in 7

days, the probability that it is *M. tuberculosis* is 0.957; the probability that it is another mycobacterial species is 0.005.[108] Not all strains of *M. tuberculosis* are niacin positive. Multiply drug-resistant strains may be niacin negative.[116]

M. simiae, previously known as *M. habana*,[131] has been recovered from monkeys and humans. *M. tuberculosis* and most stains of *M. simiae* are niacin positive, urease positive, and Tween negative. However, *M. tuberculosis* is nitrate positive and catalase negative at 68° C, and *M. simiae* is nitrate negative and strongly catalase positive at 68° C. The photoreactivity of *M. simiae* is unstable and is often delayed. Some strains may require at least 8 hours of exposure to light to initiate pigment production and, subsequently, more than 24 hours to demonstrate the photoactivated pigment.

NIACIN-NEGATIVE NONPHOTOCHROMOGENS

M. bovis is characterized by its lack of reactivity in all tests in Table 26-6 except urease and sensitivity to thiophen-2-carboxylic acid hydrazide (TCH). The occasional niacin-positive strain of *M. bovis* may be differentiated from *M. tuberculosis* by the pyrazinimidase, nitrate reduction, and TCH sensitivity tests.

Since *M. xenopi* may be nonpigmented, as well as produce a yellow pigment of variable intensity, it is included with both nonphotochromogens and scotochromogens (Figure 26-1). It is biochemically very similar to the *M. avium* complex. Differentiation of *M. xenopi* is best accomplished by observation of the specific filament-like colonies produced on clear agar media and its more rapid growth at 41° to 43° C than at 37° C.[57]

The *M. avium* complex is niacin negative, nitrate negative, urease negative, and Tween hydrolysis negative at 10 days. These organisms produce pyrazinamidase and reduce tellurite in 3 days. The semiquantitative catalase, urease, and niacin tests help distinguish the *M. avium* complex from the biochemically similar *M. simiae*.

M. haemophilum has been isolated from skin lesions and not from sputum. As previously mentioned, it grows at 25° to 30° C and not at 37° C. Other distinguishing characteristics include its growth requirement for hemin, positive reactions for pyrazinamidase and nicotinamidase, and negative reactions for catalase, urease, tellurite, and nitrate reductase. Media must be supplemented with 60 μg of hemin to recover the organism from clinical specimens.

M. malmoense hydrolyzes Tween 80, produces pyrazinamidase, and is nitrate, niacin, and arylsulfatase negative. It does not produce a heat-stable catalase. The ability to hydrolyze Tween 80 is an unusual property of this organism; this characteristic is usually not associated with pathogenic mycobacteria.[93]

M. gastri, *M. nonchromogenicum*, *M. terrae*, and *M. triviale* are nonpathogenic saprophytes. These organisms differ from most of the other niacin-negative nonphotochromogens by hydrolyzing Tween after 5 days. *M. malmoense* also hydrolyzes Tween 80 but is easily differentiated, as previously discussed.

PHOTOCHROMOGENS

The mycobacteria with photoactivated carotenoid pigments include *M. kansasii*, *M. marinum*, *M. simiae*, *M. asiaticum*, and *M. szulgai*. *M. szulgai* is usually scotochromogenic and is discussed below. The other species produce orange carotene

TABLE 26-6. Distinctive Properties of Mycobacteria Encountered in Clinical Specimens

Runyon Group	Complex Name[a]	Species Name	45°C	37°C	31°C	24°C	Usual Colony Morphology	Pigmentation	Niacin	Susceptibility to TZH (5 µg/ml)	Nitrate Reduction	Semiquantitative Catalase (<45 mm)	68°C Catalase	Tween Hydrolysis (5 Days)	Tellurite Reduction (3 Days)	Tolerance to 5% NaCl	Iron Uptake	Arylsulfatase (3 Days)	MacConkey Agar	Urease	Pyrazinamidase (4 Days)	Agglutination Tests Available
I		M. ulcerans	−	−	S	−	r	N	−	−	−	−	+	−			−			+	+	−	
	TB	M. tuberculosis	−	S	S	−	r	N	+	+	+	−	−	−			−				+	+	+
	TB	M. bovis	−	S	S	−	r, t	N	−	+	−	−	−	−			−		−[b]/+		+	+	+
		M. marinum	−	I	M	M	s/sr	P	±	+	−	+	+	+			−		+		+	−	+
		M. kansasii	−	S	S	S	sr/s	P	−	−	+	+	+	+			−	−			+	−	−
		M. simiae	−	S	S	S	s	P	+		−	+	+	−			−	−		−	−	+	+
		M. asiaticum	S	S	S	S	s/r	P	−		−	+	+	+			−				+	−	−
II	Scrofulaceum	M. scrofulaceum		S	S	S	s	Sc	−		−	+	+	−[d]	−	−	−	−	−[b]	−	+	±[d]	+
	Scrofulaceum	M. szulgai		S	S	S	s/r	Sc/P[c]	−		+	+	+	+[d]			−	−	±[b]		+	±	−
III		M. gordonae		S		S	s	Sc	−		−	+	+	+	−	−	+	−		−	−	+	+
		M. flavescens		M		M	s, f	Sc	−		+	+	+	+	−	+	+	−			+	+	+
		M. xenopi	S	S		S	s, f	Sc[e]	−		−	−	+	−		−	−		−[b]		−	+	+
	Avium	M. avium	±	S		±	s, t/r	N	−		−	+	+	−	+	−	−	−			−	+	+
	Avium	M. intracellulare	±	S		±	s, t/r	N	−	−	−	+	+	−	+	−	−	−		−	−	+	
		M. gastri		S		S	s/sr/r	N	−		−	−	−	+		−	−				+	−	
		M. malmoense		S	S	S	s	N	−		−	+	+	+	v	−	−				−	v	
		M. haemophilum	−	−	S[f]	S	r	N	−		−	−	−	−	v	−	−					+	
		M. nonchromogenicum		S		S	sr	N	−		−	+	+	+		−	−				+	±	
IV	Terrae	M. terrae		S		S	sr	N	−		+	+	+	+	−	+		−			−	±[d]	
	Terrae	M. triviale		S		S	r	N	−		+	+	+	+	−	+					−		
	Fortuitum	M. fortuitum	−	R		R	s, f/r, f	N	−		+	+	+	±	v	+	+	−	+	+	+	+	+
	Fortuitum	M. chelonae	−	R		R	s/r	N	v		−	+	+	+	v	v[g]	−	+	+	+	+		+
		M. phlei	R	R		R	r	Sc			+	+	+	+	+	+	+	−	−				
		M. smegmatis	R	R		R	r/s	N			+	+	+	+	+	+	+	−	−	+			
		M. vaccae	R	R		R	s	Sc			+	+	+	+	+	v	+	−	−	+			

SYMBOLS:

+ Present	
− Absent	
v Variable	
Blank, Information unavailable or property unimportant	

S, Slow, ≥21 days	s, Smooth	Sc, Scotochromogenic
M, Moderate, ≅12 days	sr, Intermediate in roughness	N, Nonphotochromogenic
R, Rapid, <7 days	t, Thin or transparent	
I, Intermediate	f, Filamentous extensions	
r, Rough	P, Photochromogenic	

From McClatchy, J.K., and Tsang, A.Y.: Nontuberculous mycobacteria: laboratory and clinical aspects, workshop sponsored by the American Society for Microbiology. Percentages for many of these reactions are available in Wayne.[130] Reference cultures for these organisms are available from the Mycobacterial Culture Collection.[78]

a For most clinical laboratories, designation to "complex" is usually sufficient.

b Positive after 14 days.

c Scotochromogenic at 37° C, photochromogenic at 25° C.

d Positive after 10 days.

e Young cultures may be nonchromogenic or possess only pale pigment that may intensify with age.

f Requires hemin as growth factor.

g Absent in M. chelonae ssp. chelonae; present in M. chelonae ssp. abscessus.

crystals after exposure to light for 2 weeks. Strains of *M. kansasii* may rarely be scotochromogenic or nonchromogenic.

M. asiaticum is a rare isolate. The organism has been isolated from the pulmonary material of five individuals in Australia; two of these isolates were responsible for pulmonary mycobacteriosis.[8] Four isolates were reported in the United States in 1980.[32] All isolates were seen in Florida and were pathogens.[32] *M. asiaticum* can be distinguished from *M. simiae* with the niacin test and from *M. kansasii* with urease and nitrate reduction. Urease, pyrazinamidase, semiquantitative catalase, and growth at 45° C are used to differentiate *M. asiaticum* and *M. marinum* (Table 26-6).

The large majority of clinical isolates of *M. kansasii* produce bubbles larger than 45 mm in the semiquantitative catalase test. These strongly catalase-positive organisms are more frequently associated with disease than the rare strains with low catalase activity.[121] *M. kansasii* is also niacin and pyrazinamidase negative and strongly catalase positive after heating to 68° C at pH 7.

M. marinum is isolated from superficial wounds and never from sputum. In addition to this distinction, *M. marinum* can be differentiated from *M. kansasii* on the basis of its optimal growth at 30° to 32° C, with little or no growth at 37° C, negative results of a nitrate reduction test, and lower catalase activity.

SCOTOCHROMOGENS

Among the scotochromogens, *M. scrofulaceum, M. szulgai,* and *M. xenopi* are potentially pathogenic. Although not absolute, the Tween 80 hydrolysis test may be used to differentiate these organisms from the saprophytic scotochromogens. *M. scrofulaceum, M. szulgai,* and *M. xenopi* are negative in the 5-day test, whereas the saprophytic *M. gordonae* and *M. flavescens* are positive. *M. szulgai,* however, is Tween 80 positive after 7 to 10 days.

Further differentiation among *M. scrofulaceum, M. szulgai,* and *M. xenopi* may be accomplished with the catalase, urease, nitrate reductase, and arylsulfatase tests. Among these three species, only *M. szulgai* is nitrate reductase positive.

SEROLOGIC IDENTIFICATION

Serologic testing is not suitable for routine identification of the mycobacteria, but it has been useful in epidemiologic studies, especially of the *M. avium-intracellulare-scrofulaceum* (MAIS) complex.[64] The seroagglutination tests used at present are based on the original method of Schaefer,[92] and cultures may be sent to the Serotyping Laboratory, National Jewish Center for Immunology and Respiratory Medicine, 3800 E. Colfax Ave., Denver, CO 80206.

OTHER IDENTIFICATION PROCEDURES

Among the developmental procedures used for the identification of mycobacteria are gas-liquid chromatography, thin-layer chromatography, pyrolysis mass spectrometry,[133,134] and radiometric identification with the Bactec system and enzyme-linked immunosorbent assay. The use of nucleic acid probes for identification of mycobacteria was discussed in Chapter 9. Probes are currently available for *M. tuberculosis, M. avium-intracellulare,* and the genus *Mycobacterium* (Gen-Probe, San Diego, Calif.).

GAS-LIQUID CHROMATOGRAPHY

Gas-liquid chromatography (GLC) was used by Ohashi[81] to identify the various species of mycobacteria based on the uniqueness of their cell wall lipids. The principles of GLC are discussed in Chapter 20.

The lipids of the mycobacteria must be extracted from the organisms to be analyzed. Tisdall, Roberts, and Anhalt[113] accomplished this by saponifying the organisms in methanolic NaOH, treating with BF_3 in methanol, and extracting with a hexane-chloroform mixture. A study comparing identification made with the GLC profile with that using conventional biochemicals showed GLC to be an easy, rapid, and reliable method for mycobacterial identification when used in conjunction with cultural characteristics and reasoning.[114]

Guerrant, Lambert, and Moss[39] reported that acid methanolysis was a faster and more reproducible method for extracting lipids for GLC analysis. Furthermore, better separation patterns could be achieved by using higher injection temperatures.

Other studies have substantiated the value of GLC in the identification of mycobacteria.[53,73] Results can be obtained days to weeks faster than conventional biochemical testing. When definitive identification cannot be made, GLC may be used to direct supplemental biochemical testing.[73,114]

THIN-LAYER CHROMATOGRAPHY

Thin-layer chromatography (TLC) directs and separates various substances using a thin layer of sorbent and a selected solvent system. TLC may be used to identify mycobacteria based on the separation and analysis of specific lipids known as methyl mycolates. These lipids are much larger than the fatty acids identified by GLC.

In TLC a thin sorbent layer (0.2 mm) composed of substances such as silica gel, microcellulose, alumina, or Sephadex (Pharmacia Fine Chemicals, Piscataway, N.J.) is applied uniformly to a glass or plastic plate. With the use of various solvents the lipids are extracted from the sample to be analyzed. The extract is applied at a precise spot at the edge of the plate. The plate is then placed in a closed container or tank so the bottom edge is in an appropriate solvent. As the solvent front advances, it separates the components of the sample based on their characteristics in the solvent and sorbent plates. After the solvent front has reached the desired location, the plate is removed from the container and dried, and the sample component is visualized by using ultraviolet light, reagent sprays, or autoradiography. The separated sample may be removed for further study by simply scraping off the desired sorbent area. The TLC method provides sharp separation and is fast, inexpensive, sensitive, and efficient to use with small samples.

The early studies[61] showing the value of TLC in identification of mycobacteria have been confirmed by several more recent studies.[10,33,47,53,115] Of special interest is TLC's ability to identify specific serovars of the MAIS complex that are not amenable to seroagglutination or for which antisera are not available.[10]

Combined use of TLC and GLC for identification of mycobacteria has also been reported. TLC is initially used to group the mycobacteria, and GLC is used to differentiate species within the groups. In a double-blind study of 100 unknown cultures by Knisely and others,[53] the combined TLC and GLC correctly distinguished all of the *M. tuberculosis–M. bovis* isolates from 13 other species of mycobacteria. Of the 39 nontuberculous mycobacteria, 28 could also be speciated. An additional five species were tentatively identified as belonging to either of two species, *M. malmoense* or *M. terrae*. Although definitive differentiation of these two species was impossible, both organisms belonged to the same Runyon group. Six nonmycobacterial species were also differentiated from the mycobacterial species.

Lipid analysis by TLC or GLC is not intended for routine use in a typical microbiology laboratory or even in a national reference laboratory. Rather, these methods provide supplementary evidence when the cultural and biochemical tests are equivocal. With additional studies, however, the use of TLC and GLC will almost certainly expand.

BACTEC INSTRUMENT

Radiometric methods may be used to differentiate *M. tuberculosis* from MOTT. Siddiqi and co-workers[97] reported 100% agreement with the Centers for Disease Control in the differentiation of these two groups. They identified the organisms based on their rate of growth as determined by $^{14}CO_2$ evolution, Bactec niacin, *O*-nitro-l-aceytl amino-beta-hydroxy-propiophene (NAP) susceptibility, and colony morphology. The NAP test is performed by incorporating the agent into 7H12 media.[37] A decrease or no increase in CO_2 production is considered growth inhibition or susceptibility to NAP. The growth of *M. tuberculosis* and *M. bovis* is inhibited by NAP, whereas the growth of the MOTT is not.

ENZYME-LINKED IMMUNOSORBENT ASSAY

As discussed in Chapter 9, the emerging technology of enzyme-linked immunosorbent assay (ELISA) will have a dramatic effect on the ability of laboratories to perform rapid diagnostic procedures. ELISA is a highly sensitive and specific method for detection of antigen-antibody complexes. This test system has been used to provide differentiation of a variety of mycobacteria such as the MAIS complex, *M. simiae,* and *M. chelonae.*[9,138] As the antigenic compositions of additional species of mycobacteria are determined and appropriate antibodies isolated, ELISA will become a useful tool for the rapid identification of mycobacteria.[9,26,46]

CLINICAL SIGNIFICANCE
PRIMARY TUBERCULOSIS[21,40,118,137]

Although *M. tuberculosis* may enter a susceptible host by several routes, including the skin, genitourinary tract, and alimentary tract, the respiratory tract is by far the most common and important portal of entry. The tubercle bacilli are acquired from individuals with active tuberculosis who excrete the organisms when talking, singing, or coughing. Airborne droplet nuclei of 1 to 10 μm enter the respiratory tract and are deposited in the alveoli of the lung. Here the bacilli are phagocytized by alveolar macrophages but are still able to multiply both intracellularly and extracellularly. Although a cellular exudative reaction consisting primarily of polymorphonuclear leukocytes ensues, the organisms generally encounter little host resistance and are disseminated by way of the lymphatics to the lymph nodes. In some cases the organisms escape from the lymph nodes and traverse the thoracic duct to enter the blood-

stream. Blood dissemination results in the production of metastatic foci in various body organs.

The subsequent development of cell-mediated immunity (CMI) over a period of 4 to 6 weeks accounts for the histologic changes characteristic of tuberculosis, as well as the host's response to the disease. Macrophages enter the initial pulmonary lesion to phagocytize the tubercle bacilli and begin to surround the invading organisms, forming elongated epitheloid cells. These cells become arranged in more or less concentric layers to form granulomatous tubercles, the primary pathologic hallmark of tuberculosis. Some of the cells in the center of the tubercles fuse to form giant cells. Lymphocytes and fibroblasts surround the tubercles.

The second hallmark of tuberculosis, caseation, subsequently develops. The center of the tubercles disintegrates to form a coagulated, homogeneous, cheeselike mass. Although the reason for this is not known for certain, it has largely been attributed to delayed hypersensitivity. This phenomenon represents the damaging effect of the cell-mediated immune response. The host becomes sensitized to the tuberculoprotein, and an allergic response resulting in tissue damage ensues.

Up to this point the patient has a tuberculosis infection. Whether the infection progresses to disease depends on the adequacy of the CMI response (see Chapter 2); however, the humoral response may also assist in the containment or destruction of the organisms.[51] If the response is sufficient, multiplication of the organisms markedly decreases, dissemination ceases, and the lesions begin to heal by fibrosis and calcification. These healed calcified primary complex lesions are referred to as the Ghon complex and may be apparent in chest x-ray studies for the remainder of the person's life.

Because of variations in host resistance attributed to both genetic and physiologic factors (malnutrition, overcrowding, and stress), the immune response of a few individuals is insufficient to contain the infection, and disease follows. The caseous mass of the lungs begins to liquefy in a process termed liquefaction, which is often attributed to the actions of the hydrolytic enzymes of the macrophages. During liquefaction the tubercle bacilli multiply extracellularly in large numbers. The enclosed lesions rupture, and the organisms are spread to other parts of the lung and to the environment. This large outpouring of bacilli accounts for the highly contagious nature of tuberculosis.

SECONDARY TUBERCULOSIS

Secondary or reactivation disease occurs in individuals who have been previously infected. It is most commonly caused by recrudescence of dormant foci from the primary infection and is associated with a local breakdown in the host's cellular immune system by factors such as age, diabetes mellitus, immunosuppressive therapy, or obstructive pulmonary disease. Because of the host's hypersensitivity reaction to the tuberculoprotein, the localized lesion becomes necrotic and undergoes liquefaction. If a lesion ruptures into a pulmonary vein, tuberculosis may be disseminated to other body parts. This is known as miliary tuberculosis.

DISEASE CAUSED BY MOTT[13,41,135]

Most disease associated with the MOTT (Table 26-7) occurs in immunosuppressed patients, although life-threatening dis-

TABLE 26-7. Clinical Significance of Atypical Mycobacteria

Species	Environmental Sources	Clinical Significance
M. avium-intracellulare complex	Soil, water (including drinking water), birds and other animals (especially chicken, swine, and cattle), foods such as meat, milk, and eggs	Chronic pulmonary disease, local lymphadenitis, bone and joint diseases, disseminated disease, skin and soft tissue infections including abscesses and corneal infections, rarely genitourinary disease; recently shown to be pathogen of patients with acquired immunodeficiency syndrome; also responsible for the most important mycobacterial diseases in animals
M. fortuitum-chelonae	*M. fortuitum* found almost everywhere in environment including water, soil, and dust; habitat of *M. chelonae* not known for certain, although water may be possible source	Disseminated disease, cutaneous lesions, pulmonary disease and variety of miscellaneous infections; infection often preceded by traumatic or surgical events
M. haemophilum	Unknown	Skin lesions
M. kansasii	Natural reservoir unknown; has been recovered from tap water and rarely from tissues of cattle and swine; has not been recovered from soil or dust	Chronic pulmonary disease, bone and joint disease, disseminated disease, cervical lymphadenitis, rarely genitourinary disease
M. malmoense	Unknown	Chronic pulmonary disease
M. marinum	Found in fresh and salt water as a result of contamination from infected fish and other marine life; has been cultivated from water of natural and constructed swimming pools and aquariums; also recovered from rough surface of swimming pools	Cutaneous disease
M. scrofulaceum	Soil, water (including tap water), raw milk, other dairy products, oysters	Cervical lymphadenitis in children, less commonly chronic pulmonary disease in adults, occasionally disseminated disease in children
M. simiae	Found in monkeys imported from India (*Macaeus rhesus*) and isolated from tap water in hospital in Tucson, but these isolates not associated with disease	Only rarely associated with chronic pulmonary disease, osteomyelitis, and disseminated disease with renal involvement
M. szulgai	Although distribution of organism appears widespread, little information is available in regard to its epidemiology	Chronic pulmonary disease; extrapulmonary disease uncommon but has included infections of elbow, cervical lymphadenitis, and cutaneous infections
M. ulcerans	Environmental source seems likely, but has not been recovered outside human body	Bairnsdale ulcer, Buruli ulcer
M. xenopi	Hot and cold water taps, hot water generators and storage tanks of hospitals, birds	Chronic pulmonary disease

Data from references 2, 13, 100, 112, 134, and 137a.

seminated disease has occurred in previously healthy individuals. These organisms are found throughout the environment, which is assumed to be the source of infection. Person-to-person transmission has rarely been suggested but not proved.

Because MOTT are common environmental saprophytes, they may contaminate mycobacterial cultures. Furthermore, they frequently colonize the body, especially the respiratory tract, without producing overt disease. Distinguishing these colonizers from potential pathogens is important to prevent unnecessary and perhaps toxic therapy. Although this distinction is not an easy one, several factors should aid the microbiologist and clinician in assessing the clinical significance of isolates of MOTT.[3,7,136] The source of the specimen is an important consideration. MOTT frequently colonize the respiratory, gastrointestinal, and urinary tracts, but they are unlikely colonizers of normally sterile body sites. Furthermore, repeated isolation of the same organism from the same source is suggestive of invasive disease, whereas sporadic isolation and recovery of small numbers of organisms suggest colonization. The species of *Mycobacterium* is also important. The species of *Mycobacterium* that are considered saprophytic and rarely cause disease in humans include *M. gordonae, M. asiaticum, M. terrae, M. triviale, M. nonchromogenicum, M. smegmatis, M. vaccae,* and *M. phlei.*[137a] Isolation of one of these species is rarely significant; *M. kansasii, M. avium-intracellulare, M. scrofulaceum, M. fortuitum,* and *M. chelonae,* however, are frequently associated with disease. Other factors that favor a diagnosis of disease are compatible roentgenographic changes such as pulmonary infiltrates or cavitation or isolation of the mycobacteria from a closed lesion.[137a] The presence of certain predisposing conditions discussed in the sections on diseases increases the likelihood of the clinical significance of the isolate.

The majority of disease caused by MOTT is manifested as chronic pulmonary disease, local lymphadenitis, bone and joint disease, and diseases of the skin and soft tissue. Overwhelming disseminated disease caused by MOTT has occurred in patients with the acquired immunodeficiency syndrome (AIDS). These conditions are discussed in the following sections. (AIDS is discussed in detail in Chapter 10.) Woods and Washington[137a] recently reviewed the clinical significance of MOTT.

ACQUIRED IMMUNODEFICIENCY SYNDROME

As noted previously, cell-mediated immunity is essential for the containment and destruction of mycobacteria. Patients with AIDS have a marked dysfunction of T cell–mediated immunity, and not surprisingly, mycobacteria are isolated with increased frequency from these patients (see Chapter 10).[50,94]

In countries where *M. tuberculosis* is endemic, this organism is a significant problem for AIDS patients.[83] In the United States, however, profound infections caused by MOTT have predominated. Although *M. avium-intracellulare* isolates have been of primary importance, disease has also been associated with *M. fortuitum* and *M. kansasii.*[29]

AIDS patients with *M. avium-intracellulare* infection have high numbers of organisms in their blood and stool. Laboratory diagnosis of mycobacterial infection in these patients should include culture of both sites.[50]

CHRONIC PULMONARY DISEASE

Chronic pulmonary disease resembling tuberculosis is the most important clinical problem associated with MOTT. It usually occurs in middle-aged men with chronic lung disease, although it may occur in women and in young or middle-aged men without apparent lung disease. Common predisposing conditions include pneumoconiosis (for example, silicosis or coal miner's pneumoconiosis), previous tuberculosis, chronic bronchitis, chronic obstructive lung disease, bronchiectasis, chronic aspiration from esophageal diseases, and malignant disease.

Although *M. kansasii* and *M. avium-intracellulare* are the most common species associated with disease, the pathogenesis of such disease is obscure. Whether chronic pulmonary disease represents a primary infection of previously damaged lung after inhalation of infected aerosols or a reactivation of previously acquired dormant bacilli is unknown. Both organisms are present in the environment, which presumably serves as the source of the infection. *M. intracellulare* has been isolated from freshwater sources in the southeastern United States as well as from aerosols of these waters. Possibly the organisms are washed into the waters from the soil. They multiply in the waters and flow slowly toward the coast. Droplets formed by bursting bubbles may be released into the air and are blown inland. These droplets containing *M. intracellulare* are small enough to penetrate the alveoli of the human lung and may be inhaled by a susceptible host.[38,132]

CHRONIC LYMPHADENITIS

Cervical lymphadenitis is associated with *M. scrofulaceum* and with *M. avium-intracellulare.* The large majority of patients are 1½ to 5 years of age. Nodal enlargement most commonly appears in the submandibular or submaxillary nodes. Lymphadenitis of peripheral nodes of the feet and hands may also be seen. Without treatment the nodes may soften, rupture, and form draining sinuses. Although there is strong circumstantial evidence that cervical lymph nodes become infected by way of contaminated mouth and throat tissues, only rarely has this portal of entry been proved. However, infected splinters or other breaks in the skin of the hands and feet have led to involvement of these body areas.

SKIN AND SOFT TISSUE INFECTIONS

Skin and soft tissue infections, including localized abscesses, cutaneous granulomas, and ulcers, are frequently associated with *M. fortuitum, M. chelonae, M. marinum,* and *M. ulcerans.* Generally a mycobacterial etiology should be suspected whenever a chronic cutaneous lesion occurs at a traumatized site.[20]

M. fortuitum and *M. chelonae* may cause local abscesses at the site of injections or after trauma and surgical wounds. Outbreaks of infections have occurred following diphtheria-pertussis-tetanus-polio vaccinations, whereas sporadic cases have occurred as a result of injections of penicillin, bacille Calmette-Guérin (BCG), histamine, and iron compounds. The abscesses appear a few days after the injection as warm, firm, palpable masses beneath the skin.

M. fortuitum and *M. chelonae* have been responsible for corneal infections after penetrating injury such as that produced by metal fragments from machinery. These organisms have also been responsible for osteomyelitis as a complication of cutaneous disease or endocarditis after heart surgery; this has become a serious problem in hospitals in recent years.[41]

M. marinum,[17] an organism found naturally in both fresh and salt water, is responsible for cutaneous granulomas and ulcers. Most infections are associated with water; the two aquatic sources most often involved are swimming pools and aquariums. The diseases associated with *M. marinum,* swimming pool granuloma and fish tank granuloma, are named after these sources. Swimming pool granuloma is associated with the infection of a minor injury or abrasion commonly of the elbows or knees; most minor injuries probably occur as children climb out of the swimming pool by lifting themselves up on their knees and elbows.[17] Fish tank granuloma occurs on the fingers and hands of fish fanciers following infection of minor injuries of these sites while they are handling fish or cleaning or maintaining an aquarium. Interestingly, *M. marinum* has also been associated with a number of injuries that did not appear to be related to aquatic activities. In all these conditions the lesions initially appear as groups of papules but subsequently progress to shallow ulceration and scab formation. Cutaneous disease caused by *M. marinum* may also resemble cutaneous sporotrichosis.

Another type of cutaneous ulcer is Bairnsdale ulcer or Buruli ulcer. The pathogenesis of both of these conditions is similar, and both are caused by *M. ulcerans;* the former occurs in Australia and the latter in Africa.

OTHER DISEASES

Mycobacteria possibly play a role in Crohn's disease. An unclassified *Mycobacterium* sp. has been isolated from patients with this disease.[14] This organism is mycobactin dependent and appears to be related to the *M. avium-intracellulare* and *M. paratuberculosis* groups.[14]

MECHANISMS OF PATHOGENICITY[110,139]

Cord factor, a cell surface glycolipid, has received the most attention as a potential virulence factor for the tubercle bacilli. Early studies showed this substance to be toxic for laboratory animals. More recent studies have shown that cord factor plays a major role in the development and persistence of the granulomatous lesions produced by the tubercle bacilli.[99]

Among the other factors that may play a role in the virulence of *M. tuberculosis* are its ability to acquire iron from the host and the presence of oxygen. The high oxygen content of the lung probably accounts for the organism's predilection for this site. Studies have shown that pulmonary disease progresses more rapidly and more extensively in animals maintained in an atmosphere containing increased concentrations of oxygen.

The ability to survive intracellularly is a virulence factor for the mycobacteria. In some cases this ability has been associated with the presence of certain lipids in the cell wall or capsule. Sulfolipids (sulfur-containing lipids) of *M. tuberculosis* may promote intracellular survival by inhibiting lysosome-phagosome fusion and subsequent exposure to lysosomal hydrolases.[34] Recent studies[72] have shown that *M. marinum* is able to multiply within phagolysosomes despite the presence of lysosomal enzymes; the mechanism or cellular component allowing this resistance has not been defined.

Among the other MOTT, there appears to be a relationship between catalase activity and clinical significance in *M. kansasii,* although this relationship has not been defined.[121] Two studies have reported the isolation of a toxin from *M. ulcerans.*[54,85] The toxin reported in the first study was heat labile,[85] whereas that reported in the second study was heat stable.[54]

ANTIMICROBIAL SUSCEPTIBILITY
GENERAL PRINCIPLES[63,104,119]

Routine susceptibility testing of all isolates of *M. tuberculosis* is not advised[5] because of the usual susceptibility of these organisms to the drugs discussed below. As a general rule there is little need to perform routine susceptibility tests in communities having less than a 5% incidence of primary drug-resistant tuberculosis.[5] Tests should be performed, however, in the presence of life-threatening illness, when therapy has failed, or in cases of recurrent tuberculosis when the patient has previously been treated (that is, retreatment cases).[5]

Because of their growth rate the conventional diffusion techniques discussed in Chapter 8 are not suitable for testing *M. tuberculosis* and the other slow-growing mycobacteria. (A modified conventional disk diffusion test[120] has been used for susceptibility testing of the rapidly growing *M. fortuitum* and *M. chelonae,* although problems may be encountered with this method.[106] A broth microdilution procedure may be used for determination of minimum inhibitory concentrations [MICs] of *M. fortuitum* and *M. chelonae.*[109]) The standardized methods used for the slow-growing mycobacteria are based on several principles.[104,119] First, clinical studies of *M. tuberculosis* have shown that, if 1% or more of the organisms are resistant to the drug in vitro, the drug will be ineffective in vivo. Thus susceptibility tests are based on determining this critical proportion of resistant cells. Second, the size of the inoculum is critical in determining the percentage of resistant cells. To avoid confluent growth on the control, which renders the test invalid, two dilutions of the inoculum are used in the testing procedure. Third, all tests must employ a critical concentration of drug in the test media, that is, the concentration of drug that will inhibit growth of the susceptible parent organism but allow growth of the resistant organism. Because the drugs may lose their stability if subjected to drying or prolonged storage, all drug-containing media should be stored in plastic bags in a refrigerator. Media should be used within 4 weeks of preparation.

METHODOLOGY[63,119]

Drug susceptibility tests may be performed by the direct or indirect method. In the direct method, digested concentrated specimens demonstrating acid-fast bacilli in the stained smear are used as the inoculum. In the indirect method a subculture from the primary culture is used as the inoculum. The direct method is preferred because it provides results more rapidly and eliminates the possibility that in vitro subculture will modify the proportion of susceptible to resistant organisms.[104]

Felson quadrant plates containing critical concentrations of drugs in 7H10 or 7H11 media are used for testing in both the direct and indirect methods. The drugs may be prepared in stock solutions and added directly to the medium (Table 26-8). A simpler and much more practical procedure is the use of commercially available disks (BBL, Cockeysville, Md.) containing standardized amounts of drug.[125] The disks are placed in the center of each quadrant as designated in Table 26-9. A 5 ml amount of drug-free 7H10 or 7H11 agar enriched with oleic acid–albumin–dextrose–catalase (OADC) is then drawn by

TABLE 26-8. Drug Concentrations for Susceptibility Testing Using 7H10 or 7H11 Agar

	Drug Concentration (µg/ml)	
Drug	7H10	7H11
Isoniazid	0.2, 1	0.2, 1
p-Aminosalicylic acid (PAS)	2	8
Streptomycin	2	2
Rifampin	1	1
Ethambutol	2	7.5
Ethionamide	5	10
Kanamycin	5	6
Capreomycin	10	10
Cycloserine	20	30
Pyrazinamide	25[a]	

Modified from McClatchy, J.K.: Lab. Med. **9:**47, 1978.
[a]Rather than the 50 µg/ml previously recommended, 25 µg/ml is now recommended.[63] Final pH must be adjusted to 5.5 because pyrazinamide is active only at acid pH. Special problems encountered in determining susceptibility to this drug are discussed by McClatchy.[63]

suction into each quadrant. (The control quadrants contain only medium and no drug.) After the media have solidified, the quadrant plates are incubated overnight at 4° C to allow diffusion of the drug. Commercially prepared drug-containing media are also available.

DIRECT TEST PROCEDURE[63,119]

1. Based on the number of organisms observed in the stain, the digested concentrated specimen should be diluted as follows:

Acid-Fast Stain	Fluorochrome Stain	Dilutions to Inoculate
<1	<25	Undiluted and 10^{-2}
1-10	25-250	10^{-1} and 10^{-3}
>10	>250	10^{-2} and 10^{-4}

2. With a capillary pipette, inoculate 3 drops of the highest dilution onto each control and drug-containing quadrant. Inoculate a second set of quadrant plates with the lower dilution. For patients who have been under treatment, it is recommended that one set of media be inoculated with the undiluted inoculum, since some of the organisms appearing on the smear may represent dead or noncultivable bacteria.

3. Incubate the plates in individual polyethylene bags in an atmosphere of 5% to 10% carbon dioxide at 35° to 37° C and read the plates weekly for 3 weeks. Record the amount of growth as follows: confluent (more than 500 colonies), 4+; almost confluent (200 to 500 colonies), 3+; 100 to 200 colonies, 2+; 50 to 100 colonies, +; fewer than 50 colonies, actual number.

4. Report susceptibility results after 3 weeks unless definite resistance is seen before this time, in which case the results should be reported immediately.

TABLE 26-9. Distribution of Drug-Containing Disks for Susceptibility Tests

Plate No.	Quadrant No.	Drug	Drug in Disk (µg)	Final Drug in Medium (µg/ml)
1	I	(Control #1)	—	0
	II	Isoniazid	1	0.2
	III	Isoniazid	5	1
	IV	Ethambutol	25	5
2	I	(Control #2)	—	0
	II	Streptomycin	10	2
	III	Streptomycin	50	10
	IV	Rifampin	5	1

Modified from Vestal, A.L.: Procedures for the isolation and identification of mycobacteria, Public Health Service, Pub. No. (CDC) 81-8230, Atlanta, 1981, Centers for Disease Control.

5. As previously mentioned, if more than 1% of the organisms are resistant, the drug is not considered clinically useful. In most instances it is not necessary to use the 1% criterion because almost every culture tested can be identified as susceptible or resistant by mere visual inspection.[63] If necessary the percentage of resistance may be calculated as follows:

$$\frac{\text{Number of colonies on drug quadrant}}{\text{Number of colonies on control quadrant}} \times 100 = \begin{array}{c}\text{Percentage of}\\\text{resistance}\end{array}$$

If the proportion of resistant organisms appears to approach the 1% level, it is often better to repeat the test or to report the results as questionable.[63]

6. The final report should include:
   a. Type of test (direct or indirect)
   b. Organism isolated
   c. Percentage of resistant organisms
   d. Actual colony counts according to formula in no. 3 above

INDIRECT TEST PROCEDURE[63,119]

1. Scrape approximately 2 to 5 mg of growth from the subculture. All parts of the culture and preferably a portion of each colony should be sampled.

2. Suspend the growth in a screw-capped tube containing 3 ml of Tween albumin medium and six or eight glass or plastic beads.

3. Homogenize the mixture on a Vortex mixer for 5 to 10 minutes. Exercise caution to prevent aerosol formation.

4. Let the tube stand for several minutes to allow sedimentation of the larger particles.

5. Remove the supernatant and dilute the turbidity of a McFarland no. 1 standard with sterile distilled water or saline.

6. Prepare additional 10^{-2} and 10^{-4} dilutions in distilled water or saline.

7. Proceed with steps 2 through 6 in the direct test procedure just described.

RAPID DRUG SUSCEPTIBILITY TESTING

The Bactec instrument has been used for rapid indirect and direct drug susceptibility testing of *M. tuberculosis.*[96,103] In the indirect Bactec method[96] the test drugs are incorporated into Middlebrook 7H12 medium, and Middlebrook 7H12 without medium serves as the control. The inoculum is adjusted to equal the McFarland no. 1 standard. The test broth is inoculated with 0.1 ml of this suspension, and the control is inoculated with 0.1 ml of a 1:100 dilution of the test inoculum. The significance of the 100-fold dilution of the control broth is that it is representative of a 1% mycobacterial population. The organisms in the vials containing drugs that grow faster than the control are considered to be greater than 1% resistant to the drug. The organisms in the vials containing drugs that grow more slowly or show no increase when compared with the control are considered to be less than 1% resistant and thus susceptible.

The principle of the direct drug susceptibility method is like that of the indirect method. The inoculum, however, is prepared directly from the concentrated specimen and inoculated into drug containing Middlebrook 7H12 medium plus PANTA.

Resistance and Treatment[22,63]

Drug resistance in mycobacteria may occur as a result of inadequate treatment or of spontaneous mutation independent of exposure to the drug. Plasmids have been isolated from some of the saprophytic mycobacteria, but their role in resistance is unknown. Additional factors, perhaps cell wall components, are thought to play a role in the widespread resistance of MOTT.[23,75,84]

Spontaneous mutations occur at low measurable frequencies as a result of random errors during DNA replication. For example, approximately one in 10^5 tubercle bacilli is resistant to isoniazid, whereas one in 10^6 is resistant to streptomycin. Because an open pulmonary cavity in a patient with tuberculosis may contain 10^7 to 10^9 bacteria,[103] there is a strong probability that a streptomycin- or isoniazid-resistant mutant is present. On exposure to the drug to which they are resistant, these resistant organisms rapidly outgrow the susceptible organisms, resulting in treatment failure. To circumvent this possibility, multiple drugs are used to treat tuberculosis. The incidence of resistance to multiple drugs is the product of the incidences of resistance to the individual drugs; for example, the incidence of resistance to both isoniazid and streptomycin is one in every 10^{11} organisms. In theory at least, the simultaneous use of two drugs should eliminate the emergence of resistant organisms, since one drug would prevent the growth of mutants to the other drug.[69] Because of cross-resistance between the two drugs, however, total protection by two drugs may not always be achieved.[69] Thus more than two drugs may be employed to treat tuberculosis.

Isoniazid and rifampin are generally prescribed for treatment of newly diagnosed tuberculosis.[63] Ethambutol, p-aminosalicylic acid, pyrazinamide, and streptomycin may be used in combination with these two agents to help prevent development of resistance, although they are somewhat more toxic and less efficacious.[63] When these six agents cannot be used because of toxicity or drug resistance, capreomycin, cycloserine, ethionamide, and kanamycin are used.[63] The mechanisms of action of these drugs are discussed in Chapter 8. The simplest regimen for treatment of tuberculosis is the administration of isoniazid and rifampin for 9 months; ethambutol or streptomycin is usually added for the first 2 to 8 weeks.[4]

In vitro susceptibility data of the MOTT may not correlate with in vivo results. Some of these organisms respond favorably to antituberculosis drugs whereas others respond poorly. M. kansasii responds favorably to the drugs used for treatment of tuberculosis. The initial treatment of disease caused by this organism should always include rifampin; an additional drug or two, specifically isoniazid and ethambutol or streptomycin, should be administered concomitantly.[4] Some studies emphasize the importance of including streptomycin in the M. kansasii treatment regimen.[63]

The M. avium-intracellulare complex is highly resistant to antituberculosis drugs in vivo and in vitro. However, some studies have shown multiple drug combinations of kanamycin, ethambutol, ethionamide, isoniazid, and cycloserine to be effective in vivo.[63] Studies are under way to determine the susceptibility of these organisms to drugs other than antituberculosis ones.[79,80] Recommendations for treatment of M. intracellulare disease have recently been reported.[46a]

M. fortuitum and M. chelonae are usually resistant to antituberculosis drugs but may be susceptible to traditional antimicrobial agents. These organisms have shown variable susceptibility to various cephalosporin derivatives, sulfonamides, amikacin, doxycycline, norfloxacin, ciprofloxacin and gentamicin.[18,27,63,106,120]

Susceptibility patterns and treatment of the other MOTT species are discussed by Bailey,[3] Bass and Hawkins,[7] Hartley and Yeager,[41] McClatchy,[63] and Wolinsky.[135]

MYCOBACTERIUM LEPRAE

Mycobacterium leprae is the cause of leprosy or Hansen's disease, a disease of the skin and peripheral nerves. Approximately 10 to 20 million people throughout the world are thought to have this disease; it is most prevalent in the developing nations of the Southern Hemisphere, especially India and countries in South America (Brazil), Africa, and Southeast Asia. The disease virtually has been eradicated from Western countries, but recently the incidence of disease in southern California has increased because of immigration from Southeast Asia.

The manifestations of leprosy depend on the adequacy of the host's cell-mediated response.[94] Most infected individuals do not manifest any clinical symptoms. However, in individuals who are unable to mount a sufficient immune response, the form of the disease ranges from tuberculoid (higher resistance) to lepromatous (lower resistance). In the former, patients characteristically have a single, erythematous plaque with raised outer edges and a flattened clearing center. Peripheral nerves are frequently invaded, and loss of sensation occurs in areas of the skin because of myelin damage. In lepromatous disease skin involvement is extensive and of an infiltrative or edematous nature. Nasal mucous membranes are infected and serve as a source of shedding of large numbers of organisms. Nodules are also often present; however, involvement of the peripheral nerves is less severe.

To date, M. leprae has not been cultivated on artificial media. Diagnosis is based on the clinical presentation and the presence of auramine or acid-fast organisms in tissue. The organism grows in selected animal models,[95] the classic model being the footpads of normal mice or thymectomized irradiated mice and more recently the nine-banded armadillo (Dasypus novemcinctus) and the hedgehog (Erinaceus europaeus).[52,107]

A procedure for determining the susceptibility of *M. leprae* to dapsone has been reported. This technique involves the inoculation of mouse peritoneal macrophages with skin biopsy specimens.

Studies are under way to find the appropriate medium and environment for the in vitro cultivation of *M. leprae*. Significant advances have been made in characterizing the antigenic and lipid composition of this organism.[44,45] These studies may ultimately result in rapid detection and identification systems and may pave the way for a useful vaccine.

REFERENCES

1. Allen, B.W.: Survival of tubercle bacilli in heat-fixed sputum smears, J. Clin. Pathol. **34:**719, 1981.
2. Azadian, B.S., et al.: Disseminated infection with *Mycobacterium chelonei* in a haemodialysis patient, Tubercle **62:**281, 1981.
3. Bailey, W.C.: Treatment of atypical mycobacterial disease, Chest **5:**625, 1983.
4. Bailey, W.C., et al.: Treatment of tuberculosis and other mycobacterial diseases (official statement of American Thoracic Society), Am. Rev. Respir. Dis. **127:**790, 1983.
5. Bailey, W.C., et al.: Drug susceptibility testing for mycobacteria, ATS News **10:**9, 1984.
6. Barksdale, L., and Kim, K.S.: *Mycobacterium,* Bacteriol. Rev. **41:**217, 1977.
7. Bass, J.B., and Hawkins, E.L.: Treatment of disease caused by nontuberculous mycobacteria, Arch. Intern. Med. **143:**1439, 1983.
8. Blacklock, Z.M., et al.: *Mycobacterium asiaticum* as a potential pulmonary pathogen for humans: a clinical and bacteriologic review of five cases, Am. Rev. Respir. Dis. **127:**241, 1983.
9. Brennan, P.J., Aspinall, G.O., and Nam Shin, J.E.: Structure of the specific oligosaccharides from the glycopeptidolipid antigens from serovars in the *Mycobacterium avium–Mycobacterium intracellulare–Mycobacterium scrofulaceum* complex, J. Biol. Chem. **256:**6817, 1981.
10. Brennan, P.J., Heifets, M., and Ullom, B.P.: Thin-layer chromatography of lipid antigens as a means of identifying nontuberculous mycobacteria, J. Clin. Microbiol. **15:**447, 1982.
11. Carr, D.T., Karlson, A.G., and Stilwell, G.G.: A comparison of cultures of induced sputum and gastric washings in the diagnosis of tuberculosis, Mayo Clin. Proc. **42:**23, 1967.
12. Casal, M.J., and Rodriguez, F.C.: Simple, new test for rapid differentiation of the *Mycobacterium fortuitum* complex, J. Clin. Microbiol. **13:**989, 1981.
13. Chapman, J.S.: The atypical mycobacteria and human mycobacteriosis, New York, 1977, Plenum Medical Book Co.
14. Chiodini, R.J., et al.: Characteristics of an unclassified *Mycobacterium* species isolated from patients with Crohn's disease, J. Clin. Microbiol. **20:**966, 1984.
15. Cohn, M.L., Waggoner, R.F., and McClatchy, J.K.: The 7H11 medium for the cultivation of mycobacteria, Am. Rev. Respir. Dis. **98:**295, 1968.
16. Collins, C.H., Yates, M.D., and Grange, J.M.: Names for mycobacteria, Br. Med. J. **288:**463, 1984.
17. Collins, C.H., et al.: *Mycobacterium marinum* infections in man, J. Hyg. (Camb.) **94:**135, 1985.
18. Dalovisio, J.R., et al.: Clinical usefulness of amikacin and doxycycline in the treatment of infection due to *Mycobacterium fortuitum* and *Mycobacterium chelonei,* Rev. Infect. Dis. **3:**1068, 1981.
19. Damato, J.J., et al.: Detection of mycobacteria by radiometric and standard plate procedures, J. Clin. Microbiol. **17:**1066, 1983.
20. Damsker, B., and Bottone, E.J.: Nontuberculous mycobacteria as unsuspected agents of dermatological infections: diagnosis through microbiological parameters, J. Clin. Microbiol. **11:**569, 1980.
21. Dannenberg, A.M., Jr.: Pathogenesis of pulmonary tuberculosis, Am. Rev. Respir. Dis. **125:**25, 1982.
22. David, H.L.: Bacteriology of the mycobacterioses, DHEW Pub. No. (CDC)76-8316, Washington, D.C., 1976, Dept. of Health, Education and Welfare.
23. David, H.L.: Basis for lack of drug susceptibility of atypical mycobacteria, Rev. Infect. Dis. **3:**878, 1981.
24. David, H.L., Traore, I., and Feuillet, A.: Differential identification of *Mycobacterium fortuitum* and *Mycobacterium chelonei,* J. Clin. Microbiol. **13:**6, 1981.
25. Dubos, R., and Dubos, J.: The white plague, Boston, 1952, Little, Brown & Co.
26. Fujiwara, T.J., et al.: Chemical synthesis and serology of disaccharides and trisaccharides of phenolic glycolipid antigens from the leprosy bacillus and preparation of a disaccharide protein conjugate for serodiagnosis of leprosy, Infect. Immun. **43:**245, 1984.
27. Gay, J.D., DeYoung, D.R., and Roberts, G.D.: In vitro activities of norfloxacin and ciprofloxacin against *Mycobacterium tuberculosis, M. avium* complex, *M. chelonei, M. fortuitum,* and *M. kansasii,* Antimicrob. Agents Chemother. **26:**94, 1984.
28. Gillespie, J.H., and Timoney, J.F.: Hagan and Bruner's infectious diseases of domestic animals, ed. 7, Ithaca, N.Y., 1981, Cornell University Press.
29. Gold, W.M., and Armstrong, D.: Infectious complications of the acquired immunodeficiency syndrome, Ann. N.Y. Acad. Sci. **437:**383, 1984.
30. Goldfogel, G.A., and Sewell, D.L.: Preparation of sputum smears for acid-fact microscopy, J. Clin. Microbiol. **14:**460, 1981.
31. Good, R.C.: Isolation of nontuberculous mycobacteria in the United States, 1979, J. Infect. Dis. **142:**779, 1980.
32. Good, R.C., and Snider, D.E., Jr.: Isolation of nontuberculous mycobacteria in the United States, 1980, J. Infect. Dis. **146:**829, 1982.
33. Goodfellow, M., and Minnikin, D.E.: Identification of *Mycobacterium chelonei* by thin-layer chromatographic analysis of whole-organism methanolysates, Tubercle **62:**285, 1981.
34. Goren, M.B., and Brennan, P.J.: Mycobacterial lipids: chemistry and biologic activities. In Youmans, G.P. editor: Tuberculosis, Philadelphia, 1979, W.B. Saunders Co.
35. Grange, J.M.: *Mycobacterium chelonei,* Tubercle **62:**273, 1981.
36. Grange, J.M.: Koch's tubercle bacillus—a centenary reappraisal, Zentralbl. Bakteriol. Mikrobiol. Hyg. (A)**251:**297, 1982.
37. Gross, W.M., and Hawkins, J.E.: Radiometric selective inhibition tests for differentiation of *Mycobacterium tuberculosis, Mycobacterium bovis,* and other mycobacteria, J. Clin. Microbiol. **21:**565, 1985.
38. Gruft, H., Falkinham, J.O., III, and Parker, B.C.: Recent experience in the epidemiology of disease caused by atypical mycobacteria, Rev. Infect. Dis. **3:**990, 1981.
39. Guerrant, G.O., Lambert, M.A., and Moss, C.W.: Gas chromatographic analysis of mycolic acid cleavage products in mycobacteria, J. Clin. Microbiol. **13:**899, 1981.
40. Harris, H.W., and McClement, J.H.: Pulmonary tuberculosis. In Hoeprich, P.D., editor: Infectious disease, ed. 3, Hagerstown, Md., 1983, Harper & Row, Publishers.
41. Hartley, C.B., and Yeager, H., Jr.: Nontuberculous mycobacteria, Am. Fam. Phys. **29:**207, 1984.
42. Hawkins, J.E., et al.: Levels of laboratory services for mycobacterial diseases, Am. Rev. Respir. Dis. **128:**213, 1983.
43. Hinson, J.M., Jr., Bradsher, R.W., and Bodner, S.J.: Gram-stain neutrality of *Mycobacterium tuberculosis,* Am. Rev. Respir. Dis. **123:**365, 1981.
44. Hunter, S.W., and Brennan, P.J.: Further specific extracellular phenolic glycolipid antigens and a related diacylphthiocerol from *Mycobacterium leprae,* J. Biol. Chem. **258:**7556, 1983.
45. Hunter, S.W., Fujiwara, T., and Brennan, P.J.: Structure and antigenicity of the major specific glycolipid antigen of *Mycobacterium leprae,* J. Biol. Chem. **257:**15072, 1982.

46. Hunter, S.W., et al.: Trehalose containing lipooligosaccharides: a new class of type specific antigens from *Mycobacterium*, J. Biol. Chem. **25**:10481, 1983.

46a. Iseman, M.D.: Disease due to *Mycobacterium avium-intracellulare*, Chest 87:1395, 1985.

47. Jenkins, P.A.: Lipid analysis for the identification of mycobacteria: an appraisal, Rev. Infect. Dis. **3**:862, 1981.

48. Joseph, S.W., Vaichulis, E.M.K., and Houk, V.N.: Lack of auramine-rhodamine fluorescence of Runyon group IV mycobacteria, Am. Rev. Respir. Dis. **95**:114, 1967.

48a. Kent, P.T., and Kubica, G.P.: Public health mycobacteriology: a guide for the level III laboratory, Atlanta, 1985, Centers for Disease Control.

49. Kestle, D.G., and Kubica, G.P.: Sputum collection for cultivation of mycobacteria, Am. J. Clin. Pathol. **48**:347, 1967.

50. Kiehn, T.E., et al.: Infections caused by *Mycobacterium avium* complex in immunocompromised patients: diagnosis by blood culture and fecal examination, antimicrobial susceptibility tests, and morphological and seroagglutination characteristics, J. Clin. Microbiol. **21**:168, 1985.

51. Kinnman, J., Link, H., and Fryden, A.: Characterization of antibody activity in oligoclonal immunoglobulin G synthesized within the central nervous system in a patient with tuberculous meningitis, J. Clin. Microbiol. **13**:30, 1981.

52. Klingmüller, G., and Sobich, E.: Uberfragung menschlicher Leprabakterien auf den Igel, Naturwissenschaften **64**:645, 1977.

53. Knisley, C.U., et al.: Rapid and sensitive identification of *Mycobacterium tuberculosis*, J. Clin. Microbiol. **22**:761, 1985.

54. Krieg, R.E., Hockmeyer, W.T., and Connor, D.H.: Toxin of *Mycobacterium ulcerans*, Arch. Dermatol. **110**:783, 1974.

55. Kubica, G.P.: Differential identification of mycobacteria VII: key features for identification of clinically significant mycobacteria, Am. Rev. Respir. Dis. **107**:9, 1973.

56. Kubica, G.P., and David, H.L.: The mycobacteria. In Sonnenwirth, A.C., and Jarett, L., editors: Gradwohl's clinical laboratory methods and diagnosis, vol. 2, ed. 8, St. Louis, 1980, The C.V. Mosby Co.

57. Kubica, G.P., and Good, R.C.: The genus *Mycobacterium* (except *M. leprae*). In Starr, M.P., et al., editors: The prokaryotes, vol. 2, New York, 1981, Springer-Verlag.

58. Kubica, G.P., Kaufmann, A.J., and Dye, W.E.: Comments on the use of the new mucolytic agent, *N*-acetyl-L-cysteine, as a sputum digestant for the isolation of mycobacteria, Am. Rev. Respir. Dis. **89**:284, 1964.

59. Kubica, G.P., et al.: Laboratory services for mycobacterial diseases, Am. Rev. Respir. Dis. **112**:773, 1975.

60. Mahler, H.T.: Tuberculosis in the world today, Bull. Int. Union Tuberc. **43**:19, 1970.

61. Marks, J., and Szulga, T.: Thin-layer chromatography of mycobacterial lipids as an aid to classification, Tubercle **46**:400, 1965.

62. McClatchy, J.K.: Susceptibility testing of mycobacteria, Lab. Med. **9**:47, 1978.

63. McClatchy, J.K.: Antimycobacterial drugs: mechanisms of action, drug resistance, susceptibility testing, and assays of activity in biological fluids. In Lorian, V., editor: Antibiotics in laboratory medicine, ed. 2, Baltimore, 1986, Williams & Wilkins Co.

64. McClatchy, J.K.: The seroagglutination test in the study of nontuberculous mycobacteria, Rev. Infect. Dis. **3**:867, 1981.

65. McClatchy, J.K., et al.: Isolation of mycobacteria from clinical specimens by use of selective 7H11 medium, Am. J. Clin. Pathol. **65**:412, 1976.

66. Middlebrook, G., Dubos, R.J., and Pierre, C.: Virulence and morphology characteristics of mammalian tubercle bacilli, J. Exp. Med. **86**:175, 1947.

67. Middlebrook, G., Reggiardo, Z., and Tigertt, W.D.: Automatable radiometric detecting growth of *Mycobacterium tuberculosis* in selective media, Am. Rev. Respir. Dis. **115**:1066, 1977.

68. Miliner, R.A., Stottmeier, K.D., and Kubica, G.P.: Formaldehyde: a photothermal activated toxic substance produced in Middlebrook 7H10 medium, Am. Rev. Respir. Dis. **99**:603, 1969.

69. Mitchison, D.A.: Drug resistance in mycobacteria, Br. Med. Bull. **40**:84, 1984.

70. Mitchison, D.A., Allen, B.W., and Lambert, R.A.: Selective media in the isolation of tubercle bacilli from tissues, J. Clin. Pathol. **26**:250, 1973.

71. Mitchison, D.A., et al.: A selective oleic acid albumin agar medium for tubercle bacilli, J. Med. Microbiol. **5**:165, 1972.

72. Mor, N.: Multiplication of *Mycobacterium marinum* within phagolysosomes of marine macrophages, Infect. Immun. **48**:850, 1985.

73. Morgan, M.A.: The radiometric detection and identification by gas liquid chromatography of mycobacteria from clinical specimens, Ann. N.Y. Acad. Sci. **428**:230, 1984.

74. Morgan, M.A., et al.: Comparison of a radiometric method (BACTEC) and conventional culture media for recovery of mycobacteria from smear-negative specimens, J. Clin. Microbiol. **18**:384, 1983.

75. Moulding, S.M.: Need to define colonial morphology of *M. avium-intracellulare* when reporting susceptibility results, Tubercle **64**:142, 1983.

76. Murray, P.R., Elmore, C., and Krogstad, D.J.: The acid fast stain: a specific and predictive test for mycobacterial disease, Ann. Intern. Med. **92**:512, 1980.

77. Murray, P.R., and Krogstad, D.J.: Preliminary identification of mycobacteria isolated from clinical specimens, J. Clin. Microbiol. **13**:468, 1981.

78. Mycobacterial culture collection, Denver, 1980, National Jewish Center for Immunology and Respiratory Medicine.

79. Nozawa, R.T., Kato, H., and Yokota, T.: Intra- and extracellular susceptibility of *Mycobacterium avium-intracellulare* complex to aminoglycoside antibiotics, Antimicrob. Agents Chemother. **26**:841, 1984.

80. Nozawa, R.T., et al.: Susceptibility of intra- and extracellular *Mycobacterium avium-intracellulare* to cephem antibiotics, Antimicrob. Agents Chemother. **27**:132, 1985.

81. Ohashi, D.K., Wade, T.J., and Mandle, R.J.: Characterization of ten species of mycobacteria by reaction-gas-liquid chromatography **6**:469, 1977.

82. Okada, H.A., Ohno, Y., and Kodama, K.: Global epidemiology of tuberculosis, Nugoya, Japan, 1967, Department of Preventive Medicine, Nugoya University School of Medicine.

83. Pitchenik, A.E., et al.: Tuberculosis, atypical mycobacteriosis, and the acquired immunodeficiency syndrome among Haitian and non-Haitian patients in south Florida, Ann. Intern. Med. **101**:641, 1984.

84. Rastogi, N., et al.: Multiple drug resistance in *Mycobacterium avium*: is the wall architecture responsible for the exclusion of antimicrobial agents? Antimicrob. Agents Chemother. **20**:666, 1981.

85. Read, J.K., et al.: Cytotoxic activity of *Mycobacterium ulcerans*, Infect. Immun. **9**:1114, 1974.

86. Rickman, T.W., and Moyer, N.P.: Increased sensitivity of acid fast smears, J. Clin. Microbiol. **11**:618, 1980.

87. Roberts, G.D., et al.: Evaluation of the BACTEC radiometric method for recovery of mycobacteria and drug susceptibility testing of *Mycobacteria tuberculosis* from acid-fast smear-positive specimens, J. Clin. Microbiol. **18**:689, 1983.

88. Rothlauf, M.V., Brown, G.L., and Blair, E.B.: Isolation of mycobacteria from undercontaminated specimens with selective 7H10 medium, J. Clin. Microbiol. **13**:76, 1981.

89. Runyon, E.H.: Anonymous mycobacteria in pulmonary disease, Med. Clin. North Am. **43**:273, 1959.

90. Runyon, E.H.: Identification of mycobacterial pathogens utilizing colony characteristics, Am. J. Clin. Pathol. **54**:578, 1970.

91. Runyon, E.H., Wayne, L.G., and Kubica, G.P.: Family II *Mycobacteriaceae.* Part 17. Actinomycetes and related organisms. In Buchanan, R.E., and Gibbons, N.E., editors: Bergey's manual of determinative bacteriology, Baltimore, 1974, Williams & Wilkins Co.

92. Schaefer, W.B.: Serologic identification and classification of the atypical mycobacteria by their agglutination, Am. Rev. Respir. Dis. **92:**85, 1965.

93. Schröder, K.H., and Juhlin, I.: *Mycobacterium malmoense* sp. nov., Int. J. Syst. Bacteriol. **27:**241, 1977.

94. Shelhamer, J.H., et al.: Infections due to *Pneumocystis carini* and *Mycobacterium avium-intracellulare* in patients with acquired immune deficiency syndrome, Ann. N.Y. Acad. Sci. **437:**394, 1984.

95. Shepard, C.C.: *Mycobacterium leprae.* In Starr, M.P., et al., editors: The prokaryotes, vol. 2, New York, 1981, Springer-Verlag.

96. Siddiqi, S.H., Libonati, J.P., and Middlebrook, G.: Evaluation of a rapid radiometric method for drug susceptibility testing of *Mycobacterium tuberculosis,* J. Clin. Microbiol. **13:**908, 1981.

97. Siddiqi, S.H., et al.: Rapid radiometric methods to differentiate *M. tuberculosis* from other mycobacterial species, Abstract C188, Abstracts of the Annual Meeting of the American Society for Microbiology, 1982.

98. Silcox, V.A., Good, R.C., and Floyd, M.M.: Identification of clinically significant *Mycobacterium fortuitum* complex isolates, J. Clin. Microbiol. **14:**686, 1981.

99. Silva, C.L., Ekizlerian, S.M., and Fazioli, R.A.: Role of cord factor in the modulation of infection caused by mycobacteria, Am. J. Pathol. **118:**238, 1985.

100. Smith, M.J., and Citron, K.M.: Clinical review of pulmonary disease caused by *Mycobacterium xenopi,* Thorax **38:**373, 1983.

101. Smithwick, R.W.: Laboratory manual for acid-fast microscopy, ed. 2, Atlanta, 1976, Centers for Disease Control.

102. Smithwick, R.W., Stratigos, C.B., and David, H.L.: Use of cetylpyridinium chloride and sodium chloride for the decontamination of sputum specimens that are transported to the laboratory for the isolation of *Mycobacterium tuberculosis,* J. Clin. Microbiol. **1:**411, 1975.

103. Snider, D.E., Jr., et al.: Rapid drug susceptibility testing of *Mycobacterium tuberculosis,* Am. Rev. Respir. Dis. **123:**402, 1981.

104. Sommers, H.M., and Good, R.C.: *Mycobacterium.* In Lennette, E.H., et al., editors: Manual of clinical microbiology, ed. 4, Washington, D.C., 1985, American Society for Microbiology.

105. Sompolinsky, D., et al.: *Mycobacterium haemophilum* sp. nov., a new pathogen of humans, Int. J. Syst. Bacteriol. **28:**67, 1978.

106. Stone, M.J., et al.: Agar disk elution method for susceptibility testing of *Mycobacterium marinum* and *Mycobacterium fortuitum* complex to sulfonamides and antibiotics, Antimicrob. Agents Chemother. **24:**486, 1983.

107. Storrs, E.E.: The nine-banded armadillo: a model for leprosy and other biomedical research, Int. J. Lepr. **39:**703, 1971.

108. Strong, B.E., and Kubica, G.P.: Isolation and identification of *M. tuberculosis,* U.S. Dept. of Health and Human Services Pub. No. (CDC) 81-8390, 1981.

109. Swenson, J.M., Thornsberry, C., and Silcox, V.A.: Rapidly growing mycobacteria: testing of susceptibility to 34 antimicrobial agents by broth microdilution, Antimicrob. Agents Chemother. **22:**186, 1982.

110. Thoen, C.O.: Microbiology 1979, Washington, D.C., 1979, American Society for Microbiology.

111. Thoen, C.O., Jarnagin, J.L., and Richards, W.D.: Isolation and identification of mycobacteria from porcine tissues: a three year summary, Am. J. Vet. Res. **36:**1383, 1975.

112. Thoen, C.O., Karlson, A.G., and Himes, E.M.: Mycobacterial infections in animals, Rev. Infect. Dis. **3:**960, 1981.

113. Tisdall, P.A., Roberts, G.D., and Anhalt, J.P.: Identification of clinical isolates of mycobacteria with gas-liquid chromatography alone, J. Clin. Microbiol. **10:**506, 1979.

114. Tisdall, P.A., et al.: Identification of clinical isolates of mycobacteria with gas-liquid chromatography: a 10-month follow-up study, J. Clin. Microbiol. **16:**400, 1982.

115. Tsang, A.Y., et al.: Use of serology and thin layer chromatography for the assembly of an authenticated collection of serovars within the *Mycobacterium avium–Mycobacterium intracellulare–Mycobacterium scrofulaceum* complex, Int. J. Syst. Bacteriol. **33:**285, 1983.

116. Tsukamura, M.: Niacin-negative *Mycobacterium tuberculosis,* Am. Rev. Respir. Dis. **110:**101, 1974.

117. Vadney, F.S., and Hawkins, J.E.: Evaluation of a simple method for growing *Mycobacterium haemophilum,* J. Clin. Microbiol. **22:**884, 1985.

118. Vandiviere, H.M., Smith, C.E., and Sunkes, E.J.: An evaluation of four methods of collecting and mailing gastric washings for tubercle bacilli, Am. Rev. Tuberculosis **63:**617, 1952.

119. Vestal, A.L.: Procedures for the isolation and identification of mycobacteria, Public Health Service, Pub. No. (CDC)81-8230, Atlanta, 1981, Centers for Disease Control.

120. Wallace, R.J., Jr., Dalovisio, J.R., and Pankey, G.A.: Disk diffusion testing of susceptibility of *Mycobacterium fortuitum* and *Mycobacterium chelonei* to antibacterial agents, Antimicrob. Agents Chemother. **16:**611, 1979.

121. Wayne, L.G.: Two varieties of *Mycobacterium kansasii* with different clinical significance, Am. Rev. Respir. Dis. **86:**651, 1962.

122. Wayne, L.G.: Numerical taxonomy and cooperative studies: roles and limits, Rev. Infect. Dis. **3:**822, 1981.

123. Wayne, L.G.: Microbiology of tubercle bacilli, Am. Rev. Respir. Dis. **125:**31, 1982.

124. Wayne, L.G., and Doubek, J.R.: The role of air in the photochromogenic behavior of *Mycobacterium kansasii,* Am. J. Clin. Pathol. **42:**431, 1964.

125. Wayne, L.G., and Krasnow, I.: Preparation of tuberculosis susceptibility testing mediums by means of impregnated discs, Am. J. Clin. Pathol. **45:**769, 1966.

126. Wayne, L.G., Krasnow, I., and Kidd, G.: Finding the ''hidden positive'' in tuberculosis eradication programs, Am. Rev. Respir. Dis. **86:**537, 1962.

126a. Wayne, L.G., and Kubica, G.P.: Genus *Mycobacterium* Lehmann and Neumann 1896, 363[AL]. In Sneath, P.H.A., et al., editors (Holt, J.G., editor-in-chief): Bergey's manual of systematic bacteriology, vol. 2, Baltimore, 1986, Williams & Wilkins Co.

127. Wayne, L.G., et al.: Highly reproducible techniques for use in systematic bacteriology in the genus *Mycobacterium:* tests for pigment, urease, resistance to sodium chloride, hydrolysis of Tween 80, and β-galactosidase, Int. J. Syst. Bacteriol. **24:**412, 1974.

128. Wayne, L.G., et al.: Highly reproducible techniques for use in systematic bacteriology in the genus *Mycobacterium:* tests for niacin and catalase and for resistance to isoniazid, thiophene 2-carboxylic acid hydrazide, hydroxylamine, and *p*-nitrobenzoate, Int. J. Syst. Bacteriol. **26:**311, 1976.

129. Wayne, L.G., et al.: Referral without guilt or how far should a good lab go? ATS News **2:**8, 1976.

130. Wayne, L.G., et al.: Diagnostic probability matrix for identification of slowly growing mycobacteria in clinical laboratories, J. Clin. Microbiol. **20:**722, 1984.

131. Weiszfeiler, J.G., and Karasseva, E.: Synonymy of *Mycobacterium simiae* Karavsseva et. al. 1965 and *Mycobacterium habana* Valdivia et. al. 1971, Int. J. Syst. Bacteriol. **26:**474, 1976.

132. Wendt, S.L., et al.: Epidemiology of infection by nontuberculous mycobacteria. III. Isolation of potentially pathogenic mycobacteria from aerosols, Am. Rev. Respir. Dis. **122:**259, 1980.

133. Wieten, G., et al.: Application of pyrolysis mass spectrometry to the classification and identification of mycobacteria, Rev. Infect. Dis. **3:**871, 1981.

134. Wieten, G., et al.: Pyrolysis mass spectrometry: a new method to differentiate between the mycobacteria of the 'tuberculosis complex' and other mycobacteria, J. Gen. Microbiol. **122:**109, 1981.

135. Wolinsky, E.: Nontuberculous mycobacteria and associated diseases, Am. Rev. Respir. Dis. **119:**107, 1979.

136. Wolinsky, E.: When is an infection disease? Rev. Infect. Dis. **3:**1025, 1981.

137. Wolinsky, E.: Mycobacteria. In Davis, B.D., et al., editors: Microbiology, ed. 3, Hagerstown, Md., 1983, Harper & Row, Publishers.

137a. Woods, G.L., and Washington, J.A., II: Mycobacteria other than *Mycobacterium tuberculosis:* review of microbiologic and clinical aspects, Rev. Infect. Dis. **9:**275, 1987.

138. Yanagahara, D.L., et al.: Enzyme-linked immunosorbent assay of glycolipid antigens for identification of mycobacteria, J. Clin. Microbiol. **21:**569, 1985.

139. Youmans, G.P., editor: Tuberculosis, Philadelphia, 1979, W.B. Saunders Co.

CHAPTER 27

Spirochetes

Russell C. Johnson

Spirochetes, members of the order *Spirochaetales,* have a number of common morphologic features and a unique type of motility that distinguishes them from other bacteria. These flexible, helically shaped bacteria possess a flexuous form of motility that occurs in the absence of external flagella. Spirochetes share the following structural features: (1) a helically shaped protoplasmic cylinder made up of the peptidoglycan layer, cytoplasmic membrane, and the enclosed cytoplasmic components; (2) a multilayered outer membrane or outer envelope surrounding the protoplasmic cylinder; (3) periplasmic flagella positioned in the periplasmic space between the outer membrane and the protoplasmic cylinder and flagella attached to each end of the protoplasmic cylinder at a subterminal position with the free ends extending toward the opposite cell end (Figure 27-1). Although spirochetes have similar morphologic features, they are heterogeneous in regard to physiology and habitat. The order *Spirochaetales* consists of two families. The family *Spirochaetaceae* contains the genera *Cristispira, Spirochaeta, Treponema,* and *Borrelia,* and the family *Leptospiraceae* contains a single genus, *Leptospira.* Spirochetes of medical importance are in the genera *Leptospira, Borrelia,* and *Treponema.*[14]

LEPTOSPIRA
CLASSIFICATION

Members of the genus *Leptospira* are very thin, tightly coiled (0.1 μm), aerobic spirochetes characterized by active flexuous motility, resulting from rapid oscillating movements of the cell ends (Figure 27-2). A single periplasmic flagellum is inserted at each cell end. Genetic studies indicate that at least seven distinct groups exist within the genus.[4] However, only two species, *L. interrogans* and *L. biflexa,* are currently recognized because of a lack of differential phenotypic characteristics.[16] Members of each species are arranged into serovars on the basis of antigenic composition. In the case of *L. interrogans,* serovars of similar antigenic composition are arranged into serogroups for diagnostic convenience. The term "serogroup" has no taxonomic significance.

L. interrogans is responsible for leptospirosis in humans and animals. Approximately 180 serovars have been isolated from 160 mammalian species. The number and types of serovars associated with human leptospirosis vary according to geographic area. Serovars most commonly encountered in human leptospirosis in the United States include *icterohaemorrhagiae, canicola, pomona, grippotyphosa,* and *hardjo.*

L. biflexa are nonpathogenic, free-living spirochetes. They are widely distributed in fresh surface water and associated soil. Several serovars have been isolated from marine environments. The ability of *L. biflexa* to pass through sterilizing fil-

ters, in combination with their ubiquitous distribution in water, has resulted in their contamination of tissue culture and other filter-sterilized media.[3]

SPECIMEN COLLECTION AND PROCESSING

During the first week of leptospirosis, leptospires are present in the blood and spinal fluid. After this time they enter the kidneys where they multiply and are shed in the urine. In fatal cases of leptospirosis the kidneys and the liver are the best specimens for recovery of the organisms.

DIRECT EXAMINATION

Blood, spinal fluid, and urine may be examined directly by darkfield examination. The examination can be facilitated by concentrating the organisms present in the specimens by high-speed centrifugation. Sodium oxalate– or heparin-treated blood is initially centrifuged at low speed to remove blood cells and then at high speed to concentrate the leptospires. The concentrated sediment is distributed between a coverslip and a glass slide. It must be spread thinly to distribute cellular particles. Clumps of particles may reflect large amounts of light and interfere with observation of the typical morphology and motility of the leptospires.

Although direct examination may provide a rapid diagnosis of leptospirosis, misdiagnosis is likely to occur. Inexperienced microbiologists often identify cellular extrusions and fibrils as spirochetes. Furthermore, leptospires are rarely seen on direct examination because they are usually present in small numbers and detection by direct examination requires approximately 10^3 organisms/ml. Thus a negative direct examination does not rule out leptospirosis. Diagnosis by direct examination requires serologic or cultural confirmation.

Direct microscopic examination of stained preparations[22] of blood, urine, and tissues has the same restrictions as those encountered with the darkfield technique. The silver-deposition technique (Fontana stain in Chapter 6) is useful for demonstrating leptospires in tissues. Only limited studies of the fluorescent antibody technique for detecting leptospires are available, and therefore this technique cannot be recommended.

GROWTH REQUIREMENTS
Media

The diagnosis of leptospirosis requires the demonstration of *L. interrogans* in clinical specimens or a fourfold or greater rise in agglutinating antibody titer. Most leptospires are readily cultivated in the laboratory, so specialized training is not necessary for their isolation.

Two types of media may be used for culture of *Leptospira:* those enriched with rabbit serum (for example, Fletcher or Stu-

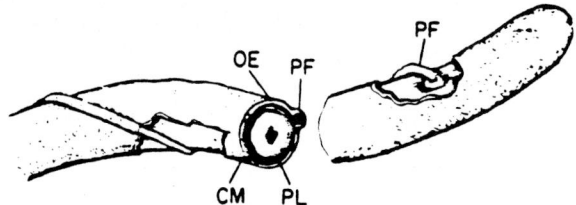

FIGURE 27-1. Structural features of spirochetes. *OE,* Outer envelope; *PF,* periplasmic flagellum; *CM,* cytoplasmic membrane; *PL,* peptidoglycan layer. (From Johnson, R.C., Hyde, F.W., and Rumpel, C.M.: Yale J. Biol. Med. **57**:529, 1984.)

art) and those enriched with bovine serum albumin (BSA)–Tween 80.[17] A 5x BSA–Tween 80 medium, PLM-5 (Armour Pharmaceutical Co., Kankakee, Wis.) and Leptospira Medium 5x (Scientific Protein Laboratories, Waunakee, Wis.), and a lx BSA–Tween 80, EMJH (Difco Laboratories, Detroit) are commercially available. These media are stable for at least 1 year at refrigerator temperatures. Although all media may be used in liquid, solid, or semisolid form, semisolid (0.2% agar) media are recommended.

Media are dispensed in 5 ml volumes in screw-capped tubes. The selective agent, 5-fluorouracil (100 to 200 μg/ml), is added when potentially contaminated specimens such as urine are cultured.[18] Neomycin (5 to 25 μg/ml) has been suggested as a selective agent for the isolation of leptospires. Several laboratories, however, have found this antimicrobial agent to inhibit leptospiral growth.

During the first week of illness, leptospires are most frequently recovered from blood. Daily blood cultures are recommended. If possible, blood is collected before antimicrobial therapy, and 1 to 2 drops are inoculated into 5 ml of media. (A small inoculum of blood is used because blood may contain growth-inhibiting substances.) A minimum of two tubes of semisolid media should be inoculated. If media cannot be inoculated at the time blood is drawn, an anticoagulant is added and the specimen cultured within 1 week.

Spinal fluid may also contain leptospires during the first week of illness and is processed in the same way as blood.

After the first week of illness, leptospires are shed in the urine. The organisms are most frequently present during the second week of the disease but may persist for 1 month or longer. Leptospires have a very short survival time in acid urine. Thus urine should be cultured as soon after collection (within 1 hour) as possible. Clean-voided, midstream, or bladder urine is diluted 1:10 and 1:100 in semisolid media containing 100 to 200 μg/ml 5-fluorouracil. Several isolation attempts on different days should be made because the shedding of leptospires is frequently intermittent.

ENVIRONMENTAL REQUIREMENTS

Leptospires are aerobic organisms that grow in the dark at 30° C. Growth of most leptospires is usually detectable after 7 to 14 days but may require 6 weeks or longer.

CULTURAL CHARACTERISTICS

Growth in semisolid media commonly occurs as a dense ring of cells several millimeters below the surface, but the growth may also be diffuse. The presence of leptospires is confirmed

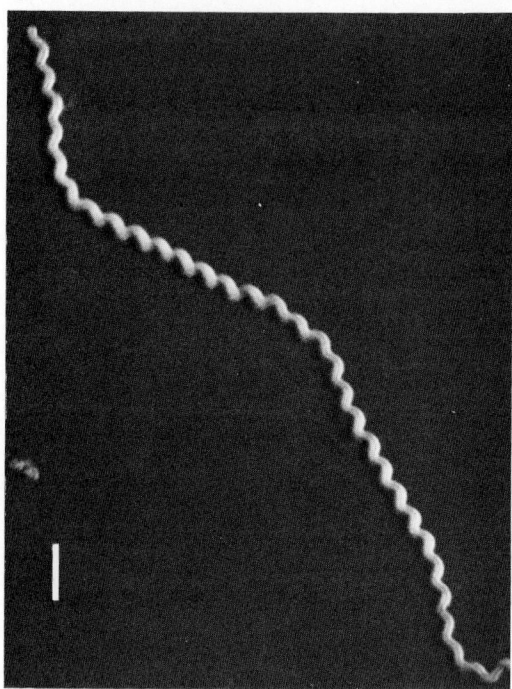

FIGURE 27-2. Electron micrograph of *Leptospira interrogans* ssp. *icterohaemorrhagiae.* (Bar = 0.5 μm.) (From Baron, S., editor: Medical microbiology, ed. 2, Menlo Park, Calif., 1985, Addison-Wesley Publishers.)

by placing a small drop of culture material on a slide, covering it with a coverslip, and examining it by darkfield microscopy for the characteristic tightly coiled cells with hooked ends and an active flexuous motility. When transitional movement occurs in liquid media, one cell end is straight and the other is hooked, with movement in the direction of the straight end. A serpentine-type movement is observed in semisolid media.

The isolated leptospires should be transferred to fresh medium using a 5% to 10% vol/vol inoculum. Stock cultures are maintained in semisolid medium, and transfers are made at 2- to 6-month intervals. Liquid cultures should be transferred every 3 to 4 weeks. Long-term storage of cultures is accomplished by maintaining them at liquid nitrogen temperatures with the use of cryoprotective agents such as glycerol (10%) or dimethyl sulfoxide.[2]

The following methods can be used to purify contaminated cultures: (1) preparation of serial 10-fold dilutions of culture in 5-fluorouracil-containing media; (2) filtration of cultures through 0.22 to 0.45 μm pore size filters; (3) isolation on 1% agar plating medium by streaking or placing a drop of culture in the center of a plate (leptospires will migrate through the agar, and a plug of agar containing leptospires can be removed with a capillary pipette); and (4) intraperitoneal injection of weanling hamsters and leptospire isolation from the heart blood. After 14 days the surviving animals are sacrificed and the kidneys cultured. The latter method can also be used to isolate pathogenic leptospires from soil and water.

BIOCHEMICAL IDENTIFICATION

Although the characteristic tightly coiled cells with hooked ends and active flexuous motility distinguishes leptospires from other spirochetes, the free-living *L. biflexa* and the pathogenic *L. interrogans* are indistinguishable morphologically. Several tests are available for differentiating these two species. *L. interrogans* does not grow at 13° C[17] or in the presence of 225 μg/ml 8-azaguanine,[19] whereas *L. biflexa* does grow under these conditions. Also, serovars of *L. interrogans* are rapidly converted to spherical forms in hypertonic environments (1 M NaCl), whereas *L. biflexa* is relatively resistant to this morphologic change.

SEROLOGIC AND IMMUNOSEROLOGIC IDENTIFICATION[1]

Definitive identification of *L. interrogans* to serogroup and serovar is accomplished by microscopic agglutination and absorption tests. The isolate is first screened against antisera to serovars representative of serogroups present in the geographic area. Antisera to most serovars are commerically available or may be prepared in rabbits. Agglutination of the isolate in a titer range of two twofold dilutions below to one twofold dilution above the homologous titer of the antiserum indicates that it belongs in the same serogroup represented by that antisera. The isolate may be a different or new serogroup if it does not react with any of the antisera used.[1] After the serogroup of the isolate is established, antisera to the serovars within that serogroup are tested. On the basis of the reaction of the isolate with these antisera, representative serovars and antisera are chosen for use in a reciprocal agglutinin-absorption test. After cross-absorption with adequate amounts of heterologous antigen, if 10% or more of the homologous titer remains in at least one of the two antisera in repeated tests, the two strains are different serovars.[1] The identification of an isolate as to serovar is time consuming and requires experience. World Health Organization (WHO) Leptospirosis Reference Laboratories such as the one at the Centers for Disease Control, Atlanta, Georgia, have this capability.

Serodiagnosis of leptospirosis requires the demonstration of seroconversion or a fourfold or greater rise in titer of agglutinating antibodies. The microscopic agglutination (MA) test using live or formalin-inactivated cells is the standard serologic procedure used. This test has excellent sensitivity for the diagnosis of recent and past infections, but it is limited by its high serologic specificity. To ensure detection of antibodies that may be provoked by any of the large number of serovars, a battery of different serovar antigens covering most of the known cross-reactions of leptospires must be tested. Eight serovars (*copenhageni, canicola, pomona, autumnalis, grippotyphosa, wolffi, djatzi, patoc*) detect all but rare cases of leptospirosis. Sera that are negative with these antigens may be retested with a large antigen battery if leptospirosis is highly suspected.

The test is performed by preparing serial twofold dilutions of serum in phosphate-buffered saline (pH 7.2). Equal volumes of diluted serum and antigens are mixed, incubated at 30° C for 2 to 4 hours, and examined by darkfield microscopy for agglutination. The serum dilution that shows 50% of the cells agglutinated is the endpoint.

Antibodies usually reach titers of 100 to 1000 by the sixth to tenth day of illness, rising to maximal titers of 25,000 or more by the third or fourth week of the disease. Agglutination reactions that are higher with heterologous serovars than with the infecting serovar are not uncommon. Thus definitively identifying the infecting serovar on the basis of this test is impossi-

ble. To identify the infecting serovar the organism must be isolated and typed by the MA test as described previously.

Commercial macroscopic agglutination tests are also available for detection of leptospirosis; however, they lack the sensitivity of the MA test. "Genus-specific" complement fixation, sensitized erythrocyte lysis, and hemagglutination tests have been useful, particularly in areas where a number of different serovars exist. The "genus-specific" tests are unsatisfactory for epidemiologic surveys because they detect only antibodies produced early in the disease.

CLINICAL SIGNIFICANCE[10]

Leptospirosis, a zoonosis, is distributed worldwide. Numerous wild animals including rats and other rodents, bats, mongooses, jackals, foxes, opossums, and raccoons are *Leptospira* organism carriers, but they do not exhibit any signs of infection. Leptospires are transmitted from these animals to a wide variety of domestic animals such as sheep, dogs, goats, cattle, swine, and horses. Leptospirosis in domestic animals may be severe, causing serious economic losses in the livestock industry because of abortion and infertility. Death may also occur in livestock or dogs.

Specific serovars of *L. interrogans* are often associated with certain animals but can infect a variety of animals. Serovar *pomona* is frequently associated with swine and cattle, *canicola* with dogs, and *icterohaemorrhagiae* with rats. The proximal convoluted tubule of the mammalian kidney is the normal habitat for *L. interrogans*. Shedding of leptospires in the urine (leptospiruria) may persist for extended periods throughout the lifetime of rodents and other wild animals. Domestic animals commonly shed leptospires for a few months to a year with decreasing intensity.

Rodents associated with human habitation and domestic animals are the most important reservoirs and sources of human leptospirosis.[10,15] Humans contract the disease by direct or indirect contact with the urine of leptospiruric animals. Direct exposure to leptospiruric urine occurs most frequently among pet owners, farm workers, and veterinarians. Indirect exposure, that is, exposure to urine-contaminated soil or water, is the most common method of transmission. Leptospires may survive in moist soil for at least 14 days and in natural waters for several months. The organisms enter the body through mucous membranes of the eye, mouth, or genital tract or through abraded skin. Human-to-human transmission occurs rarely.

The clinical manifestations of leptospirosis are not sufficiently characteristic to be diagnostic, and it is frequently initially misdiagnosed as meningitis, hepatic disease, fever of unknown origin, or influenza. Infections vary from asymptomatic to fulminant. Three organ systems most commonly involved are the central nervous system, kidney, and liver. The virulence, infecting dose of the organism, and portal of entry largely determine the severity of the disease.

Even though patient response to leptospirosis varies, it is often a biphasic disease, consisting of the leptospiremic, or acute, phase and the leptospiruric, or immune, phase. Symptoms such as fever, chills, severe headache, myalgia, malaise, and conjunctival suffusion develop acutely after an incubation period of 1 to 2 weeks (ranges from 2 to 20 days). The leptospiremic phase usually lasts 4 to 8 days, during which time leptospires may also be found in the spinal fluid. Fever is usually 39° to 40° C (102° to 104° F) but may be as high as 41.1° C (106° F). Headache is intense with muscle tenderness of the calf, back, and abdomen frequently experienced. In addition, anorexia, nausea, and vomiting are usually observed. Inflammatory exudates do not accompany the conjunctival suffusion of leptospirosis. In severe leptospirosis cases jaundice occurs during the first week, attaining maximal intensity 7 days after onset.

The leptospiruric, or immune, phase begins during the second week of the disease and correlates with an increasing antibody titer. The antibodies are leptospiricidal in the presence of complement and, as a result, leptospires are eliminated from the host with the exception of the kidney, eye, and possibly the brain where they may persist for extended periods.[14] Symptoms are variable, but usually short febrile relapses often associated with signs of meningeal irritation are observed. Leptospiruria is present but it is not associated with renal dysfunction in milder cases of the disease. Uveitis can occur in up to 10% of cases and is usually transient and self-limited.

Most cases (over 90%) are anicteric and self-limited with an uneventful recovery in 2 to 3 weeks. Convalescence, however, may be extended for several months with the more severe cases. Severe icteric cases are often referred to as Weil's disease and are frequently associated with the serovar *icterohaemorrhagiae* but can be caused by a number of serovars. (Infections with *icterohaemorrhagiae* may also be anicteric or asymptomatic.) Renal failure is responsible for the mortality of 5% to 30% that occurs in untreated, jaundiced patients.

MECHANISMS OF PATHOGENICITY

Leptospiral toxin(s) responsible for the pathologic conditions associated with the disease have been theorized but not identified. Precise mechanisms of pathogenicity of the organisms have not been defined.

TREATMENT

Even though leptospires are susceptible to most commonly used antimicrobial agents in vitro, the therapeutic efficacy of these drugs remains unclear. Antimicrobial therapy appears to be effective only if initiated during the first 2 to 4 days of illness. Subsequently, symptomatic and supportive care seems to be most important. High doses of penicillin G or tetracycline for 7 to 10 days are most frequently recommended. For severe cases control of hydration, electrolyte balance, and kidney and liver function is important. Peritoneal dialysis or hemodialysis should be considered in patients with uremia.

TREPONEMA
CLASSIFICATION[25]

Members of the genus *Treponema* are host-associated spirochetes and can be found in the oral cavity, intestinal tract, rumen, and genitals of humans and animals. There are currently 13 species of *Treponema*. Ten of these are anaerobic organisms; most are found in the oral cavity and on the genitals of man. Only one pathogenic member of the anaerobic treponemes has been identified; *T. hyodysenteriae* is the etiologic agent of swine dysentery. Many of the other anaerobic treponemes have been found in certain human skin ulcers, periodontal disease, and diarrheal illness; however, their role as causative agents of these diseases remains undefined.

The remaining species of *Treponema* include *T. pallidum, T.*

carateum, and *T. paraluis-cuniculi.* The last organism is responsible for diseases in rabbits. *T. pallidum* and *T. carateum* are human pathogens. There are three subspecies of *T. pallidum: T. pallidum* ssp. *pallidum,* the etiologic agent of venereal and congenital syphilis; *T. pallidum* ssp. *pertenue,* the cause of yaws; and *T. pallidum* ssp. *endemium,* the etiologic agent of nonvenereal endemic syphilis. *T. carateum* causes pinta.

The pathogenic treponemes have an average diameter and length of 0.13 to 0.15 μm and 10 to 13 μm, respectively. The cells are not as tightly coiled as in leptospires (Figure 27-3). Three periplasmic flagella are inserted at each cell end. Cytoplasmic tubules are located under the cytoplasmic membrane, and six to eight of these tubules originate at each cell end with the free ends extending toward the cell center. With few exceptions, cytoplasmic tubules are not present in other spirochetes. *T. pallidum* is considered to be a microaerophile requiring low concentrations of oxygen (1.5% to 3%). It has not been cultured for more than one transfer in a cell culture system and is currently propagated by intratesticular inoculation of rabbits.

The four treponemes pathogenic for humans (three subspecies of *T. pallidum* and *T. carateum*) are indistinguishable serologically and morphologically. Yaws, pinta, and endemic syphilis are distinguished from venereal syphilis on the basis of clinical and epidemiologic characteristics. Yaws is largely restricted to rural populations of tropical countries and is characterized by destructive lesions of the skin and bone. Pinta, which is present in Central and South America, causes dyschromic skin lesions that eventually become depigmented. Nonvenereal endemic syphilis is a milder form of syphilis occurring in childhood. This disease is found almost solely in less-developed tropical and subtropical areas. The nonvenereal treponematoses (yaws, pinta, and endemic syphilis) are chronic diseases that may last many years if not properly treated. With the exception of yaws, the nonvenereal treponematoses are of low incidence and are disappearing with improved hygienic living conditions.

Venereal syphilis is distributed worldwide and remains a major public health problem. The remainder of the discussion of *Treponema* organisms will be restricted to the laboratory diagnosis of *T. pallidum* ssp. *pallidum* and venereal and congenital syphilis.

SPECIMEN COLLECTION AND PROCESSING[12]

Material from moist lesions and lymph nodes is examined for the presence of *T. pallidum* by darkfield microscopy, providing an immediate diagnosis of primary, occasionally secondary, and early congenital syphilis. Phase microscopy may also be used, but spirochetes are more readily visualized by darkfield microscopy. Oral lesions usually are not examined by darkfield microscopy because oral treponemes are part of the normal oral flora and cannot be distinguished from *T. pallidum.*

To collect specimens for darkfield examination,[9] first clean the surface of the lesion with saline. Gently abrade the lesion with dry gauze until serous fluid appears. Care must be taken to avoid causing much bleeding because erythrocytes interfere with the darkfield examination. Wipe away the initial fluid that appears and then touch a glass slide to the exudate. Cover material with a coverslip and examine immediately. If an adequate amount of exudate is not produced, a drop of saline may be placed on the lesion and collected with a glass slide as above.

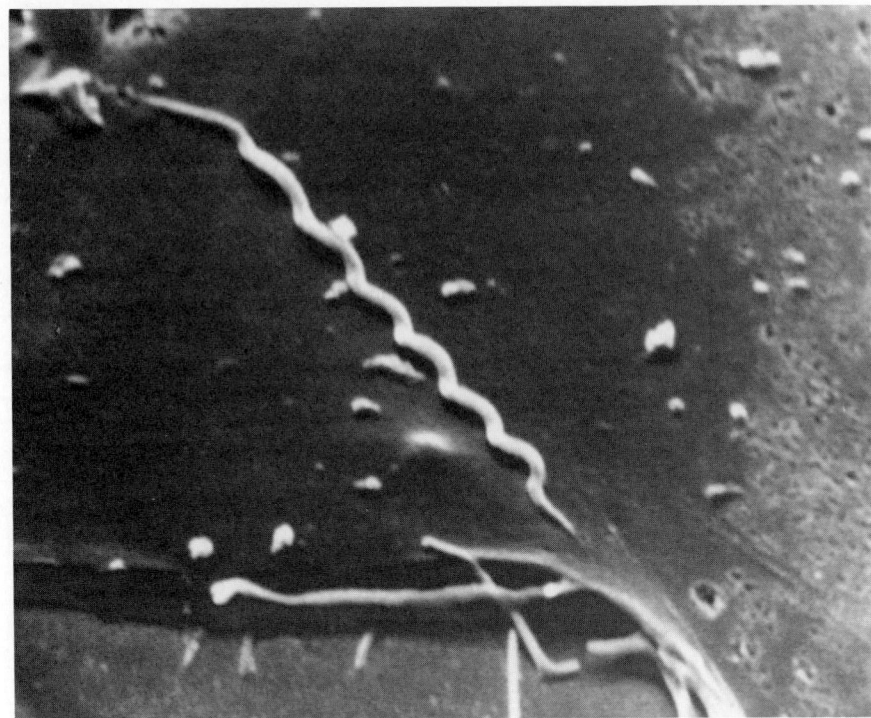

FIGURE 27-3. Electron micrograph of *Treponema pallidum* ssp. *pallidum* (Nichols strain). (Bar = 1 μm.) (From Fitzgerald, T.J., et al.: Scanning electron microscopy of *Treponema pallidum* [Nichols strain] attached to cultured mammalian cells, J. Bacteriol. **130**:1333, 1977.)

Because treponemal lesions and exudates are usually infectious, gloves should be worn by the examiner and the materials used should be appropriately discarded. Since treponemes are very sensitive to adverse conditions such as drying and oxygen concentration, lesion material must be examined as soon as possible after collection.

Serum or plasma samples for serologic examination are stored at −20° C.

GROWTH REQUIREMENTS

T. pallidum cannot be satisfactorily cultivated in vitro. This organism can be propagated by intratesticular injection of rabbits that are free of *T. paralius-cuniculi*, the etiologic agent of rabbit syphilis.

IDENTIFICATION

Diagnosis of syphilis depends on the observation of the organisms in lesions by darkfield examination or the detection of antibodies by serologic tests. Patients with syphilis produce two types of antibodies—nonspecific nontreponemal antibodies that are detected by nontreponemal serologic tests and specific treponemal antibodies detected by treponemal tests. These tests vary in their sensitivity and specificity (Table 27-1).

Nontreponemal Tests

Nontreponemal antibodies, also known as reaginic antibodies (these differ from the reagins of immediate hypersensitivity) or Wassermann antibodies, react with cardiolipin, a normal tissue constituent. The three widely used nontreponemal tests are the Venereal Disease Research Laboratory (VDRL) slide test,

TABLE 27-1. Frequency of Positive Results with Different Serologic Techniques in Known Cases of Syphilis

Method	Percent of Positive Results in Infection		
	Primary	**Secondary**	**Latent**
SCREENING			
VDRL	50-70	99[a]	60-75[b]
RPR	50-80	99	60-75
CONFIRMATORY			
FTA-ABS	80-90	99-100	98
MHA-TP	70-82	99-100	95

From Eschenbach, D., Pollock, H.M., and Schachter, J.: Laboratory diagnosis of female genital tract infections. Cumitech 17, Washington, D.C., 1983, American Society for Microbiology.
[a]Usually high titer.
[b]Usually low titer.

Rapid Plasma Reagin (RPR) card test, and Automated Reagin test (ART). These tests depend on the reaction of the nontreponemal antibodies with a cardiolipin-lecithin antigen.

Nontreponemal tests are quite sensitive but are not specific. Because cardiolipin is present in many tissues, patients with a variety of febrile illnesses, chronic diseases, and immunologic disorders may form antibodies to this antigen and thus give biologic false-positive reactions. The nontreponemal tests are quite suitable for screening because of their low cost, high sensitivity, and ease of performance. Because of their low specificity, however, positive nontreponemal tests must be confirmed with treponemal tests that measure specific antibody.

Nontreponemal tests may be used to evaluate the effectiveness of antimicrobial therapy. These tests will decline in titer over a 6- to 8-month period following adequate treatment. The specific FTA-ABS test discussed below may remain positive for years. The VDRL test may also be used to test spinal fluid for neurologic syphilis.

Treponemal Tests

Treponemal antibodies react with specific *T. pallidum* antigens. Several treponemal tests have been used to detect these antibodies. The *Treponema pallidum* immobilization (TPI) test was one of the first treponemal tests used but now is performed only in research laboratories because of its technical difficulty and expense. The most widely used treponemal test is the fluorescent treponemal antibody absorption (FTA-ABS) test. The patient's serum is absorbed with sorbent, a preparation of a nonpathogenic treponemal antigen (*T. phagedenis* biotype Reiter), to remove cross-reacting antibodies. The absorbed serum is placed on a slide containing a preparation of *T. pallidum* (the Nichols strain). After incubation the slide is washed and reacted with fluorescein-labeled antihuman globulin conjugate. The presence of antibodies in the patient's serum is indicated by the fluorescent staining of the treponemes.

The FTA-ABS (IgM) test has been suggested as an aid in the diagnosis of congenital syphilis. The interpretation of this test assumes that, if the blood of a newborn contains IgM reactive with *T. pallidum,* it was formed by the infant because this class of immunoglobulins does not cross the placenta, whereas maternal IgG does. The results obtained with this test have not been satisfactory, and its use is not recommended.

The microhemagglutination–*Treponema pallidum* (MHA-TP) test may also be used for the detection of anti-*Treponema* antibodies. This simple, sensitive, and specific indirect hemagglutination test uses sheep or turkey erythrocytes that are sensitized with *T. pallidum* antigens. Extensive evaluations of this assay have shown that it is a suitable substitute for the FTA-ABS as a confirmatory test for the diagnosis of syphilis with the exception of first infection primary syphilis. Since these antibodies are more difficult to detect than antibodies formed during the later stages of syphilis, a primary syphilis serum should be included as a test control.

CLINICAL SIGNIFICANCE[21]

The normal course of untreated syphilis is divided into several phases on the basis of clinical manifestations of the disease. After the spirochetes penetrate the mucous membranes or broken skin, they enter the lymphatics and become disseminated throughout the body by the blood. However, the treponemes preferentially multiply at the portal of entry, which results in the formation of the characteristic primary lesion, the hard chancre. The presence of the chancre marks the primary phase of syphilis. The chancre usually occurs about 3 weeks after infection and is teeming with treponemes. After several weeks the chancre heals with little if any detectable scar tissue remaining.

After the chancre has healed, or sometimes as it is healing, the secondary phase of syphilis ensues. The lesions of secondary syphilis are widespread and contain many spirochetes. They are most commonly found on the mucous membranes and skin (including the palms of the hands and soles of the feet), but any organ of the body may be involved. Within a 2- to 4-week period the lesions disappear and the disease appears to be latent. During the subsequent 3 to 4 years approximately one third of the patients with secondary syphilis spontaneously get well. One third of patients with secondary syphilis develop a latent infection characterized by the presence of specific treponemal antibodies but no symptoms of the disease. The remaining one third develop late (tertiary) syphilis.

Late syphilis may occur within 3 to 20 years after the initial infection. The typical granulomatous lesions of late syphilis are known as gummata. These lesions may involve the skin, mucous membranes, soft tissues, bone, eyes, central nervous system, and cardiovascular system. Lesions in the central nervous system may lead to general paralysis, and lesions in the cardiovascular system may result in aortic aneurysms. Late syphilis is also referred to as neurosyphilis, cardiovascular syphilis, or gummatous syphilis.

Syphilis is most commonly transmitted by sexual contact with an infected individual. Refractory endemic foci of syphilis remain in the South and in large cities, especially among lower socioeconomic groups and homosexual communities.[5]

MECHANISMS OF PATHOGENICITY[11]

The mechanisms by which *T. pallidum* damages the host remain unclear. No endotoxin or exotoxins have been identified. Immune complexes and hypersensitivities may play an important role in the pathologic effects of this disease.

TREATMENT[13]

Treponema pallidum is highly susceptible to penicillin. Benzathine penicillin G, crystalline penicillin G in 2% aluminum monostearate, and aqueous procaine penicillin G are the preparations used for the treatment of syphilis. Patients allergic to penicillin are treated with erythromycin and tetracycline.

BORRELIA
CLASSIFICATION[7]

Borrelia organisms are arthropod-transmitted spirochetes that cause relapsing fevers (Figure 27-4). *B. recurrentis* is the species responsible for louseborne or epidemic relapsing fever. This disease is transmitted by the louse *Pediculus humanus* ssp. *humanus.* Several *Borrelia* spp. may be responsible for tickborne or endemic relapsing fevers (Table 27-2). Many of these *Borrelia* spp. have been named after the species of *Ornithodoros* ticks by which they are transmitted (see Table 27-2). *Borrelia burgdorferi* is a recently named species that is responsible for Lyme disease (see Chapter 10).

SPECIMEN COLLECTION AND PROCESSING[7]

Borrelia organisms are present in the blood during the febrile periods of relapsing fever. They can be detected by examining a drop of blood by darkfield microscopy. The blood must be diluted adequately so the red blood cells do not interfere with the examination.

Borrelia organisms may also be observed in stained smears. Thick and thin blood smears may be stained with Giemsa or Wright stain and examined by brightfield microscopy. Thick films should be used for initial diagnosis, since a few spirochetes may be present. A thick film is prepared by placing a drop of blood on a slide and then spreading the blood with a toothpick in a circular motion until it evenly covers an area approximately 1 cm in diameter. After air drying for 30 minutes the preparation is stained with Giemsa stain for 15 to 30 minutes. The spirochetes stain blue. Relapsing fever has often been diagnosed by the laboratory technologist during a differential blood count.

The most sensitive method of detecting *Borrelia* organisms is by inoculation of the patient's blood into suckling Swiss mice or rats. Usually 0.05 to 0.2 ml of a 1:1 dilution of blood in sodium citrate is injected intramuscularly or intraperitoneally, and the animal's blood is examined daily for spirochetes for at least 14 days.

GROWTH REQUIREMENTS

The *Borrelia* organisms are microaerophilic and appear to have fairly complex nutritional requirements. Although several species of *Borrelia* have been cultured in Kelly medium,[20] this procedure is not currently recommended for the diagnostic laboratory.

IDENTIFICATION

Suitable biochemical or serologic tests are not available for identification of the various *Borrelia* spp. The development of a satisfactory test has been complicated by the antigenic variability of the organisms.

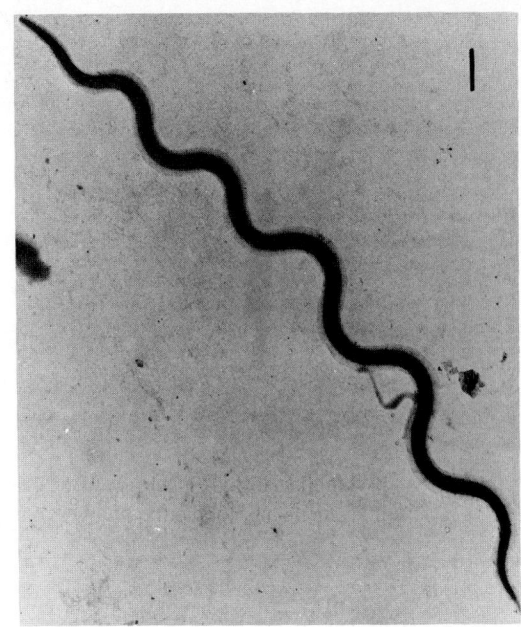

FIGURE 27-4. Electron micrograph of *Borrelia hispanica.* (Bar = 1 μm.) (From Baron, S., editor: Medical microbiology, ed. 2, Menlo Park, Calif., 1985, Addison-Wesley Publishers.)

TABLE 27-2. Characteristics and Distribution of Louseborne and Tickborne Borreliae[a]

Species	Arthropod Vector	Animal Reservoir	Distribution	Disease
B. recurrentis (syn. *B. obermeyeri, B. novyi*)	*Pediculus humanus humanus*	Humans	Worldwide	Louseborne, epidemic relapsing fever
B. duttonii	*Ornithodoros moubata*	Humans	Central, eastern, southern Africa	East African tickborne, endemic relapsing fever
B. hispanica	*O. erraticus* (large variety)	Rodents	Spain, Portugal, Morocco, Algeria, Tunisia	Hispano-African tickborne relapsing fever
B. crocidurae, B. merionesi, B. microti, B. dipodilli	*O. erraticus* (small variety)	Rodents	Morocco, Libya, Egypt, Iran, Turkey, Senegal, Kenya	North African tickborne relapsing fever
B. persica	*O. tholozani* (syn. *O. papillipes, O. crossi?*)	Rodents	From West China and Kashmir to Iraq and Egypt, U.S.S.R., India	Asiatic-African tickborne relapsing fever
B. caucasica	*O. verrucosus*	Rodents	Caucasus to Iraq	Caucasian tickborne relapsing fever
B. latyschewii	*O. tartakovskyi*	Rodents	Iran, Central Asia	Caucasian tickborne relapsing fever
B. hermsii	*O. hermsi*	Rodents, chipmunks, tree squirrels	Western United States	American tickborne relapsing fever
B. turicatae	*O. turicata*	Rodents	Southwestern United States	American tickborne relapsing fever

Continued.

TABLE 27-2. Characteristics and Distribution of Louseborne and Tickborne Borreliae[a]—cont'd

Species	Arthropod Vector	Animal Reservoir	Distribution	Disease
B. parkeri	O. parkeri	Rodents	Western United States	American tickborne relapsing fever
B. mazzottii	O. talaje (O. dugesi?)	Rodents	Southern United States, Mexico, Central and South American	American tickborne relapsing fever
B. venezuelensis	O. rudis (syn. O. venezuelensis)	Rodents	Central and South America	American tickborne relapsing fever
B. anserina	Argas spp. (mites?)	Fowl	Worldwide	Avian borreliosis
B. theileri	Rhipicephalus spp., probably other ixodid ticks	Cattle, horses, sheep	South Africa, Australia	Tick spirochetosis
B. burgdorferi nov. sp.	Ixodes dammini	Rodents	Eastern United States	Lyme disease
	I. pacificus	?	Western United States	Lyme disease
	I. ricinus	?	Europe	Lyme disease and related disorders
	?	?	Australia	Lyme disease
B. brasiliensis	O. brasiliensis	?	South America (Brazil)	?[a]
B. graingeri	O. graingeri	?	East Africa (Kenya)	One laboratory case[a]
B. tillae	O. zumpti	Rodents	South Africa	?[a]
B. queenslandica	O. gurneyi	Rodents	Australia	?[a]
B. armenica	O. alactagalis	Rodents	Armenia	?[a]

From Burgdorfer, W.: *Borrelia.* In Lennette, E.H., et al., editors: Manual of clinical microbiology, ed. 4, Washington, D.C., 1985, American Society for Microbiology.
[a]Spirochete-tick association of unknown or little human health significance.

Identification of borreliae is based primarily on the arthropod vector and the geographic distribution of the disease. For example, if endemic relapsing fever is contracted in a geographic area where the tick *Ornithodorus hermsi* is present, the spirochete should be identified as *B. hermsii*. All louseborne relapsing fevers are caused by *B. recurrentis*.

CLINICAL SIGNIFICANCE[23]

Clinical forms of the relapsing fevers are not diagnostic and resemble those of other febrile diseases. Louseborne (epidemic) relapsing fevers are generally more severe diseases than are the tickborne (endemic) infections. However, both types of relapsing fevers follow the same general clinical pattern. Approximately 2 to 15 days after infection, there is an abrupt onset with fever, headache, and myalgia that lasts for 4 to 10 days and is associated with a spirochetemia. As the host responds with specific antibody, the borreliae decrease to undetectable numbers in the peripheral blood followed by an afebrile period of a few days to several weeks. An antigenic variant of the spirochete then appears and multiplies, and another febrile period occurs. Subsequent relapses are usually milder and of shorter duration. Generally a single relapse is observed in louseborne relapsing fever, whereas as many as 10 relapses can occur in untreated cases of tickborne relapsing fevers.

Myocarditis is probably the most common cause of death in fatal cases of relapsing fever.

Humans are the only reservoir of *B. recurrentis*. Louseborne relapsing fever has disappeared from the United States, with the exception of imported cases. Occurring primarily in African countries such as Ethiopia and Sudan, the prevalence of relapsing fever depends on environmental conditions favoring heavy infestation by *Pediculus humanus humanus*.[6] Spirochetes are primarily limited to the hemolymph of lice; therefore transmission is by contamination of the bite wound by infectious hemolymph released from lice crushed or injured by scratching.[6]

Tickborne relapsing fevers are zoonoses with rodents (mice, rats, squirrels) and rabbits serving as the major sources of spirochetal infections of arthropods. The tickborne relapsing fevers are widespread throughout the world. *Ornithodoros hermsi* and *O. turicata* (soft ticks) most commonly transmit the disease in the United States. All tissues of the tick are infected, and transovarial transmission occurs in many ticks. *Ornithodoros* ticks are mainly nocturnal fast feeders (5 to 20 minutes) that live in the soil of rodent burrows, in crevices of old tree stumps, or between logs of rodent-infested cabins. Spirochetes in the tick saliva and coxal secretions enter the host through the bite wound.

Mechanisms of Pathogenicity

Although fever is a hallmark of the relapsing fevers, borreliae do not contain endotoxin. Endotoxin-like activity is present in the plasma of febrile patients but is not present in the spirochete cells. No toxins of *Borrelia* organisms have been identified that might be responsible for the pathologic effects associated with the disease.

The persistence and cyclic nature of borrelial infections are due to the antigenic variability of these organisms. Although antibody selects for antigenic variants, antigenic variation appears to be an inherent property of the spirochete and occurs in the absence of antibody. See Chapter 2 for further details.

Treatment[24]

Tetracycline is the drug of choice for the treatment of the relapsing fevers. For children less than 7 years old and pregnant women, erythromycin is a satisfactory alternative. Antimicrobial treatment provokes a Jarisch-Herxheimer reaction in most patients with louseborne relapsing fever and in some tickborne relapsing fever. This reaction, which consists of abrupt chills, fever, headache, extreme apprehension and malaise, and nausea and vomiting, is best controlled by providing intensive nursing care and intravenous fluid support during the first day of treatment.

References

1. Alexander, A.D.: Serological diagnosis of leptospirosis. In Rose, N.R., and Friedman, H., editors: Manual of clinical immunology, ed. 2, Washington, D.C., 1980, American Society for Microbiology.
2. Alexander, A.D., et al.: Preservation of leptospiras by liquid-nitrogen refrigeration, Int. J. Syst. Bacteriol. **22**:165, 1972.
3. Brendle, J.J., and Alexander, A.D.: Contamination of bacteriological media by *Leptospira biflexa,* Appl. Microbiol. **28**:505, 1974.
4. Brendle, J.J., Rogul, M., and Alexander, A.D.: Deoxyribonucleic acid hybridization among selected leptospiral serotypes, Int. J. Syst. Bacteriol. **24**:205, 1974.
5. Blount, J.H., and Holmes, K.K.: Epidemiology of syphilis and the nonvenereal treponematoses. In Johnson, R.C., editor: The biology of parasitic spirochetes, New York, 1976, Academic Press, Inc.
6. Burgdorfer, W.: The epidemiology of the relapsing fevers. In Johnson, R.C., editor: The biology of parasitic spirochetes, New York, 1976, Academic Press, Inc.
7. Burgdorfer, W.: *Borrelia.* In Lennette, E.H., et al., editors: Manual of clinical microbiology, ed. 4, Washington, D.C., 1985, American Society for Microbiology.
8. Coffey, E., and Bradford, L.: Serodiagnosis of syphilis. In Rose, N.R., and Friedman, H., editors: Manual of clinical immunology, ed. 2, Washington, D.C., 1980, American Society for Microbiology.
9. Eschenbach, D., Pollock, H.M., and Schachter, J.: Laboratory diagnosis of female genital tract infections, Cumitech 17, Washington, D.C., 1983, American Society for Microbiology.
10. Feigen, R.D., and Anderson, D.C.: Human leptospirosis, CRC Crit. Rev. Clin. Lab. Sci. **5**:413, 1975.
11. Fitzgerald, T.J.: Pathogenesis and immunology of *Treponema pallidum,* Annu. Rev. Microbiol. **35**:29, 1981.
12. Fitzgerald, T.J.: *Treponema.* In Lennette, E.H., et al., editors: Manual of clinical microbiology, ed. 4, Washington, D.C., 1985, American Society for Microbiology.
13. Fiumara, N.J.: Treatment of syphilis. In Johnson, R.C., editor: The biology of parasitic spirochetes, New York, 1976, Academic Press, Inc.
14. Johnson, R.C. The spirochetes, Annu. Rev. Microbiol. **31**:89, 1977.
15. Johnson, R.C.: Introduction to the spirochetes: the genus *Leptospira.* In Starr, M.P., et al., editors: The prokaryotes, a handbook on habitats, isolation, and identification of bacteria, vol. 1, New York, 1981, Springer-Verlag.
16. Johnson, R.C., and Faine, S.: *Leptospira.* In Krieg, N., editor (Holt, J.G., editor-in-chief): Bergey's manual of systematic bacteriology, vol. 1, Baltimore, 1984, Williams & Wilkins Co.
17. Johnson, R.C., and Harris, V.G.: Differentiation of pathogenic and saprophytic leptospires. I. Growth at low temperatures, J. Bacteriol. **94**:27, 1967.
18. Johnson, R.C., and Rogers, P.: 5-Fluorouracil as a selective agent for the growth of leptospirae, J. Bacteriol. **88**:422, 1964.
19. Johnson, R.C., and Rogers, P.: Differentiation of pathogenic and saprophytic leptospires with 8-azaguanine, J. Bacteriol. **88**:1618, 1964.
20. Kelly, R.T.: Cultivation and physiology of relapsing fever borreliae. In Johnson, R.C., editor: The biology of parasitic spirochetes, New York, 1976, Academic Press, Inc.
21. Knox, J.M., Musher, D., and Guzick, N.: The pathogenesis of syphilis and related treponematoses. In Johnson, R.C., editor: The biology of parasitic spirochetes, New York, 1976, Academic Press, Inc.
22. Ryu, E.: A simple method for staining *Leptospira,* Can. J. Microbiol. **9**:423, 1963.
23. Sanford, J.P.: Relapsing fever—pathogenesis. In Johnson, R.C., editor: The biology of parasitic spirochetes, New York, 1976, Academic Press, Inc.
24. Sanford, J.P.: Relapsing fever—treatment and control. In Johnson, R.C., editor: The biology of parasitic spirochetes, New York, 1976, Academic Press, Inc.
25. Smibert, R.M.: *Treponema.* In Krieg, N., editor (Holt, J.G., editor-in-chief): Bergey's manual of systematic bacteriology, vol. 1, Baltimore, 1984, Williams & Wilkins Co.

PART THREE

FUNGI AND ACTINOMYCETES

CHAPTER 28

Fundamentals of Mycology

Richard C. Tilton
Michael R. McGinnis

There are approximately 50,000 to 100,000 "accepted" species of fungi.[8] Of these, about 180 species have been shown to be pathogenic under some circumstances. Because concepts of pathogenicity for all microorganisms have become more clearly defined in the past decade, we are beginning to understand why only a very small portion of the fungi that humans encounter may cause disease. Notwithstanding the advances in cancer chemotherapy, which often lowers the normal host defenses, several factors are necessary for the fungi to invade human tissue. Many of these factors were discussed in Chapter 2 and typically include the abilities to grow at temperatures of 35° to 37° C, to bridge the specific and nonspecific defense barriers of the host, and to utilize available in vivo substrates as sources of nutrients and energy for growth.

The ability of fungi to invade plant and animal tissue was observed in the early nineteenth century. The first documented account of fungal invasion of animals was by Bassi, who in 1835 studied the disease of silkworms called muscardine. Bassi proved that the infection was caused by the fungus *Beauveria bassiana*. Shortly thereafter many of the fungi that cause ringworm were described.[8] In 1910 Sabouraud[19] published his classic book *Les Teignes*, which was a comprehensive study of the dermatophytic fungi. The discovery of many of the principal human fungal infections in the early twentieth century paralleled the "golden age of bacteriology" when the majority of bacterial diseases were also discovered.

Fungi are eukaryotic organisms with absorptive nutrition. They synthesize lysine by the L-alpha-adipic acid biosynthetic pathway, have microtubules composed of the protein tubulin, possess ergosterol in their cell membranes, and have centrioles, 80S ribosomes, and mitochondria. It is essential to recognize the differences between fungi and bacteria, plants, and animals. Unlike bacteria, which are prokaryotes, fungi are eukaryotes. Eukaryotes are structurally and functionally more sophisticated than prokaryotes. Fungi contain a nucleus bound by a membrane, an endoplasmic reticulum, and mitochondria. Prokaryotes do not contain these structures. The prokaryotic bacteria known as the actinomycetes were once thought to be fungi because of their filamentous nature.

Like animals, fungi are heterotrophic and must obtain preformed organic substances from the environment. However, fungi have an absorptive type of nutrition, whereas animals have an ingestive type. Fungi release hydrolytic enzymes into their immediate surroundings; these enzymes degrade the substrate into smaller subunits, which the fungus then absorbs. Human pathogenic fungi possess the enzymes necessary to obtain nutrients directly from the living host.

For years mycologists have recognized that fungi are very different from plants. All fungi possess a cell wall composed of chitin, that is, an unbranched polymer of beta-1,4-linked *N*-acetylglucosamine. In contrast, plant cell walls are composed of cellulose. Furthermore, as previously mentioned, fungi synthesize lysine by the L-alpha-adipic acid biosynthetic pathway, whereas plants synthesize lysine by the meso-alpha-diaminopimelic acid pathway. Unlike plants, fungi do not have chloroplasts and thus are not photosynthetic.

VEGETATIVE STRUCTURES OF FUNGI

Fungi are identified in the laboratory according to the vegetative or growth structures they produce, as well as their reproductive structures. The fungi most commonly seen in the laboratory exist in one or both of two vegetative forms, yeasts or molds.

MOLDS

Molds form dry, fluffy, filamentous colonies consisting of branching hyphae. Hyphae, the primary element of the vegetative form of a mold, are cylindric, tubelike structures that elongate by growth at the tip or apical end. The hyphae are responsible for the fluffy filamentous nature of the mold. They range in diameter from approximately 3 to 20 μm, depending on the species.

Hyphae usually have cross-walls called septa that divide the hyphae into numerous cells. Septa have tiny pores, so the cytoplasm is continuous throughout the hypha. Hyphae that contain septa are referred to as septate. Hyphae lacking septa have in the past been called aseptate or nonseptate. Because all hyphae may have some septa, however, the term "sparsely septate" is more accurate.

A mass of hyphae is called mycelium. Because the term "mycelium" may be singular or collective, the term "mycelia" is inappropriate. There are three basic types of mycelium: vegetative mycelium, which penetrates the surface of the medium and absorbs nutrients; the aerial mycelium that grows above the agar surface; and the fertile mycelium that bears conidia or spores for reproduction and may be located anywhere in the colony. The mycelium composing the colony gives it its texture, tenacity, topography, and color. To subculture a fungus, it is necessary to remove a portion of the colony and transfer it to a new nutrient agar.

The vegetative mycelium of a fungus may produce several unique structures that aid in identification. For example, favic chandeliers, which are clusters of hyphal tips that collectively resemble a chandelier or the antlers of a buck deer, may be produced by some of the dermatophytes (see Chapter 32), especially *Trichophyton schoenleinii*. *Trichophyton* spp. may also

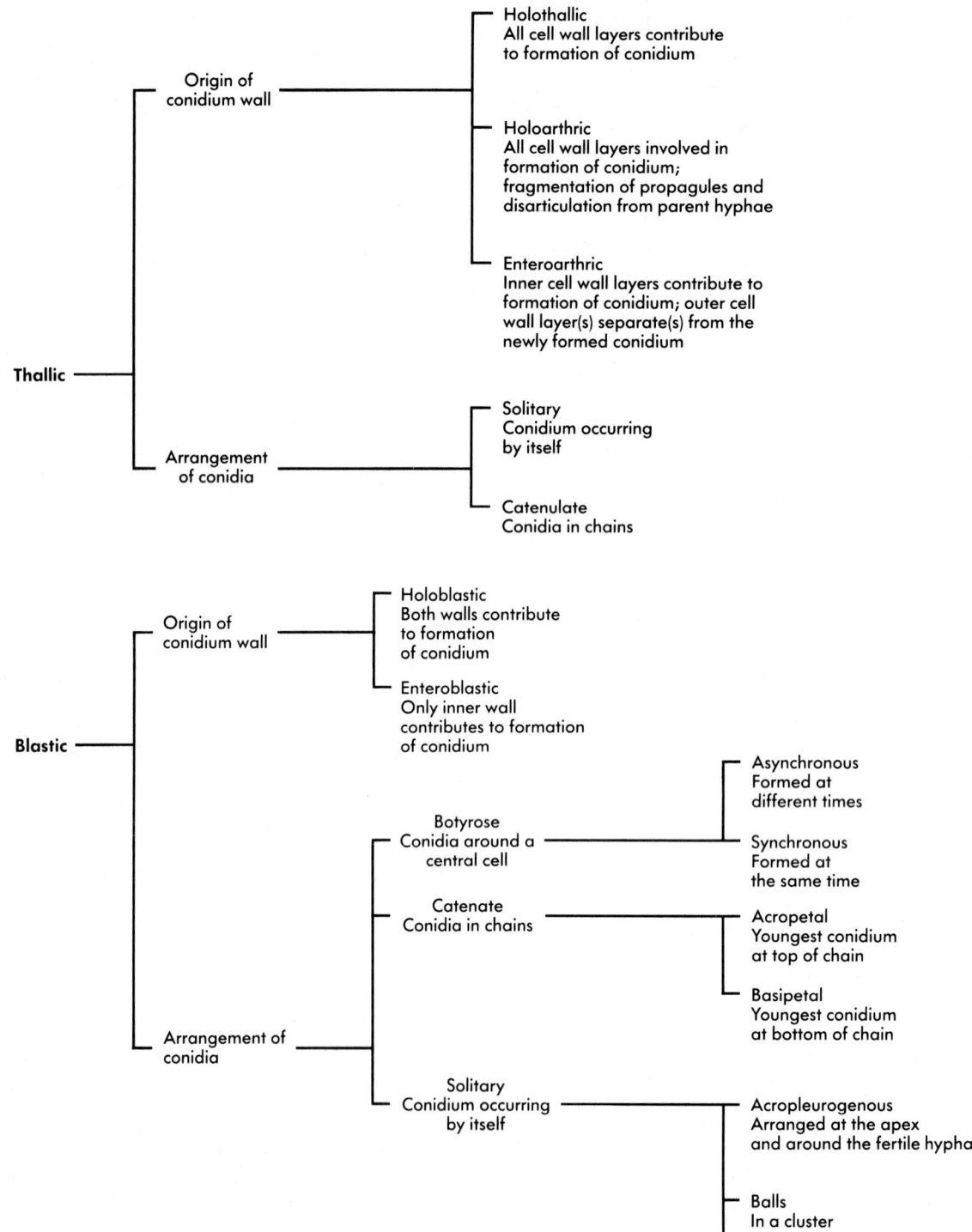

FIGURE 28-1. Ontogeny of blastic and thallic conidia.

TABLE 28-1. Differentiation between Hyphae and Pseudohyphae

Characteristic	Hyphae	Pseudohyphae
Growth	Occurs at hyphal apex by linear elongation with subsequent formation of septa	Results from blowing-out process and subsequently appearing basal constriction of each new blastoconidium, without separation of each blastoconidium from its parent cell
Terminal cell	Typically longer than preceding cell just behind first septum; usually cylindric	Typically shorter than or equal to preceding cell just behind first septum; usually rounded
Walls	Typically parallel with no invagination at septa	Typically contain marked constrictions at septa
Septa	Refractive and straight	Often difficult to discern and usually curved
Side branches	Not constricted at their point of origin; first septum typically some distance from main hypha	Constricted at their point of origin; septum at origin of branch

Modified from McGinnis, M.R.: Laboratory handbook of medical mycology, New York, 1980, Academic Press, Inc.

form tightly or loosely coiled filaments known as spiral hyphae. Dermatophytes sometimes form clusters of swollen cells called nodular bodies; these are mats of twisted hyphae.

A portion of the vegetative hyphae of some zygomycetes may consist of rootlike structures known as rhizoids. Rhizoids may arise from stolons, which are runners similar to those of higher plants.

YEASTS

Yeasts form discrete, smooth, moist colonies consisting of spherical to ellipsoidal cells (3 to 15 μm in diameter), which reproduce by budding. Unlike molds, which are identified on the basis of morphology alone, yeasts are identified by the combination of morphology and physiologic testing. Some yeasts are very small *(Torulopsis glabrata)*, whereas others are large *(Cryptococcus neoformans)*. *C. neoformans* produces a polysaccharide envelope or capsule.

Yeasts reproduce by budding, which typically results in blastoconidia. Conidia are asexual reproductive propagules; blastoconidia are conidia that are formed by the softening of the cell wall and a subsequent blowing-out process (Figure 28-1). Conidial production is initiated when localized enzymatic lysis of the parent yeast cell wall weakens the wall and permits a swelling to occur at that site.[6] The swelling or new blastoconidium increases in size as new cell wall material is deposited. Chitin synthetase, which is located in the chitosomes in the cytoplasm, is important in the regulation of chitin and chitosan biosynthesis, which results in new cell wall fibrils. Before a septum is formed between the parent and daughter cells, the nucleus of the mother cell divides by mitosis and one nucleus passes into the developing daughter yeast cell. A septum is then formed at the base of the daughter cell, which permits it to break free. As the daughter cell enlarges, a constriction becomes evident between the parent cell and the developing daughter cell (blastoconidium) at their common septum. If the yeast cells do not separate, a chain of blastoconidia may form. Some of the blastoconidia composing the chains occasionally elongate to form a hyphalike filament called a pseudohypha. These structures are commonly produced by fungi such as *Candida albicans* (see Figure 35-2). Table 28-1 describes the differences between hyphae and pseudohyphae.[14]

When a yeast cell of *C. albicans* produces a filament by apical elongation without a constriction at the origin of the filament from the parent cell, the filament is called a germ tube (see Figure 35-4). The germ tube is the beginning of the formation of a hypha. Most mycologists consider a germ tube to be a hypha once the first septum is laid down. This typically occurs some distance from the origin of the germ tube from the parent cell. Germ tube formation is a useful method of recognizing *C. albicans* in the clinical laboratory.

DIMORPHIC FUNGI

Fungi that are able to grow in two different forms are considered to be dimorphic. This ability is usually temperature dependent. For example, the fungus that causes blastomycosis, *Blastomyces dermatitidis*, grows as a yeast at 37° C and in tissue but as a mold at room temperature (23° to 25° C). Another dimorphic fungus, *Coccidioides immitis*, forms spherules in tissue and produces hyphae at room temperature.

REPRODUCTIVE STRUCTURES OF FUNGI

Fungi reproduce by asexual, sexual, and parasexual means. For the clinical microbiologist the asexual mode is the most important one because most pathogenic fungi do not reproduce sexually in the laboratory.

ASEXUAL REPRODUCTION
Sporogenesis

Asexual reproduction may involve the formation of spores or more frequently conidia. Only the zygomycetes typically reproduce asexually by forming spores; other medically important fungi reproduce asexually by conidia. Spores may be produced sexually as well as asexually. Sexual spores are produced following meiosis, whereas asexual spores are produced following mitosis.

The asexual spores, or sporangiospores, of zygomycetes form within a saclike structure known as a sporangium. The sporangiospores form as a result of the cleavage of the cytoplasm in the sporangium. The number of spores that are formed within a sporangium varies considerably, from one in the genus *Cunninghamella* to many in the genera *Rhizopus* and *Mucor*. A merosporangium is a special type of sporangium in which all of the sporangiospores are aligned in a single row.

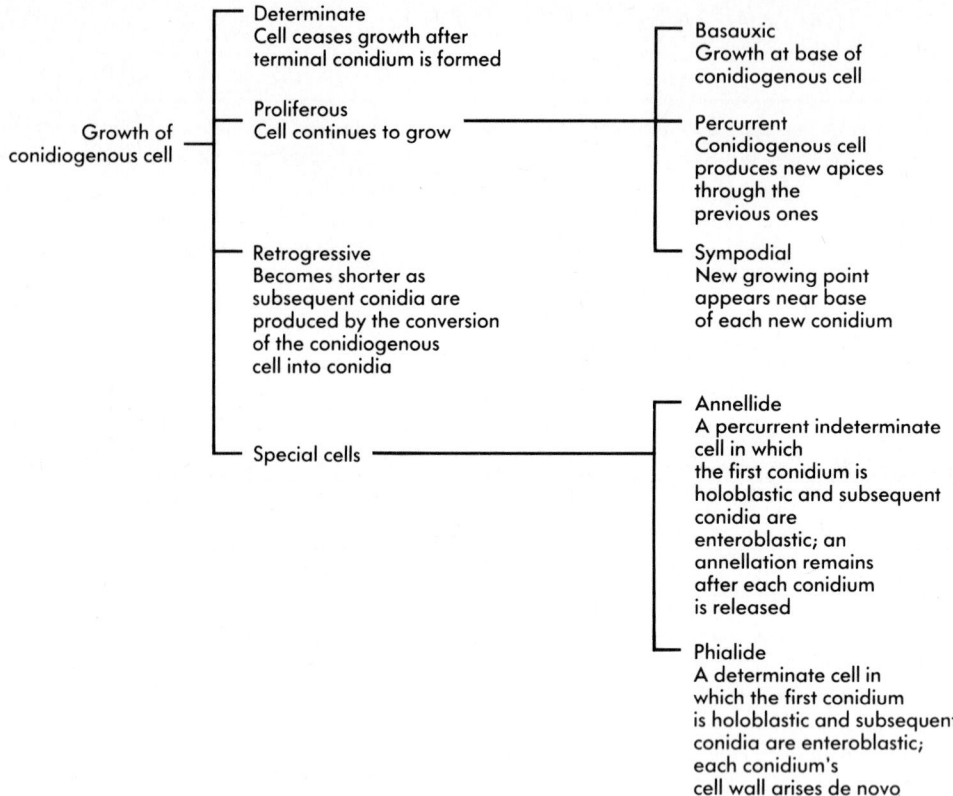

FIGURE 28-2. Growth of conidiogenous cell.

Sporangia are typically produced on specialized hyphae known as sporangiophores. During the development of sporangia in fungi such as *Rhizopus arrhizus,* a sterile dome at the apex of the sporangiophore is formed with the sporangium occurring around it; this sterile domelike structure is called a columella. In some species of zygomycetes a swelling may occur immediately below the columella in the upper portion of the sporangiophore; this swelling is called an apophysis. Identification of the zygomycetes is based on the presence or absence of these reproductive structures and the vegetative structures such as rhizoids mentioned previously, as well as the location of these structures, that is, whether sporangiophores occur opposite rhizoids or between rhizoids (see Chapter 37).

Conidiogenesis

Conidia are nonmotile, asexual, reproductive propagules that result after mitosis has occurred and are formed in any manner except one involving cytoplasmic cleavage in a sporangium. Conidia are typically produced on aerial hyphae.

Conidia are formed by conidiogenesis, a process that occurs in both yeasts and molds. Although somewhat outdated, Barron's classification[3] for the hyphomycetes based on conidiogenesis is discussed in many contemporary mycology books. It includes the following series:

1. Aleuriosporae. Blown-out conidia are released by rupture of parent hypha. Examples are *Blastomyces and Microsporum.*
2. Arthrosporae. Conidia are produced by fragmentation of a hypha. An example is *Coccidioides.*

3. Blastosporae. Conidia are produced by budding. An example is *Candida.*
4. Botryoblastosporae. Conidia develop simultaneously from swollen apex of conidiogenous cell on denticles. An example is *Botrytis.*
5. Meristem Arthrosporae. Arthroconidia in basipetal chains are formed from conidiophore, which increases in length by growth at its base. An example is *Trimmatostroma.*
6. Meristem Blastosporae. Blastoconidia are formed from a conidiophore, which increases in length by growth at its base. An example is *Arthrinium.*
7. Phialosporae. Conidia are produced by phialides. An example is *Acremonium.*
8. Porosphorae. Conidia are produced through pores in wall of conidiophore. An example is *Curvularia.*
9. Sympodulosporae. Conidia are produced on denticles from sympodial conidiogenous cell. An example is *Sporothrix.*
10. Annellosporae. Conidia are produced by annellides. An example is *Exophiala.*

The primary difference between Barron's system and the one used today[11,14] is that now asexual reproduction is defined more clearly with respect to ontogeny of the conidium and the development of the conidiophore as separate processes (Figures 28-1 and 28-2). In regard to ontogeny of the conidium, conidia production may be either thallic or blastic. As discussed on p. 517, in blastic development the conidium begins to enlarge and a septum is formed, which differentiates the developing conidium from its parent cell (Figure 28-3). The conidium originates

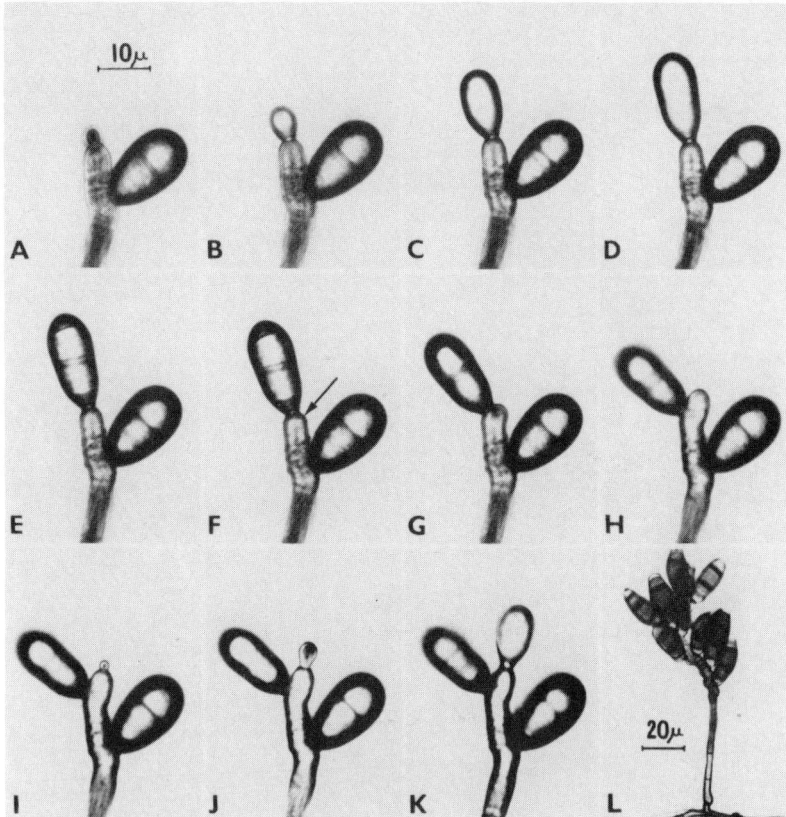

FIGURE 28-3. Blastic conidiogenesis in *Curvularia* organism. Cell wall begins to soften and young conidium (**A**) enlarges. As process continues (**B** and **C**), basal septum is formed. Conidium originates from part of parent cell (**A** to **D, I** to **K**). Conidiophore in this time-lapse sequence is developing sympodially. Arrow in **F** indicates new growing point. (From Cole, G.T.: The sympodula and the sympodioconidium. In Kendrick, B., editor: Taxonomy of Fungi Imperfecti, Toronto, 1971, University of Toronto Press.)

from part of the parent. In the thallic mode of development the conidium is differentiated by a septum before its differentiation commences. Thus the conidium results from the conversion of the entire parent cell into the conidium (Figure 28-4). Conidia may be characterized by differences in the mode of conidiogenesis and by other criteria such as size. Examples of various types of conidia are listed in Table 28-2.

The cell that gives rise to a conidium is called a conidiogenous cell. Some fungi produce conidiophores, which are specialized hyphae that bear conidia. Conidiogenous cells and conidiophores are different. For example, *Acremonium* spp. form cylindric conidiogenous cells called phialides that arise directly from the vegetative hyphae. In this case the conidiogenous cell is the phialide and the supporting hypha is the conidiophore (Figure 28-5). *Aspergillus* spp. have flask-shaped conidiogenous cells (phialides) on a special hypha that has a swollen apical portion (Figure 28-6). The special hypha is a conidiophore on which the conidiogenous cells develop.

The rapid and precise identification of fungi requires a understanding of conidiogenesis, which includes (1) conidium ontogeny (thallic or blastic), (2) conidiogenous cell development, (3) conidial septation, color, and arrangement, (4) conidiophores, and (5) site of conidial development. During the past several years a number of medically important fungi have been either reclassified or better defined because of a clearer understanding of conidiogenesis.

Figure 28-7 summarizes the key characteristics used for identification of the common clinically encountered fungi.[16]

SEXUAL REPRODUCTION

Sexual reproduction in the fungi involves meiosis. Before meiosis can occur, two compatible nuclei must unite. In the first step plasmogamy, or fusion, of two protoplasts but not their nuclei must occur. Occurring next is karyogamy, which is the actual fusion of the two haploid (n) nuclei to produce a diploid (2n) or zygote nucleus. Meiosis now takes place, resulting in four haploid (n) nuclei. There may be a long time period between plasmogamy, karyogamy, and meiosis. Sometimes the two haploid nuclei do not fuse but behave as if they were a single nucleus. Such a condition is called dikaryotic (n + n).

Most fungi are heterothallic, that is, sexually self-sterile. For sexual reproduction to occur, two compatible isolates are required. In some instances only a specific isolate of one mating type crosses with only a specific isolate of the second mating type. Sexual compatibility systems help explain why sexual spores are not typically seen in clinical isolates. These isolates usually represent only one mating type. The presence of sexual spores typically means that the isolate is homothallic, or sexually self-fertile. Each isolate of a homothallic species is able to reproduce sexually under the appropriate conditions.

The chytrids (primitive fungi) form sexual spores called oospores. These develop within a cell known as an oogonium

Text continued on p. 527.

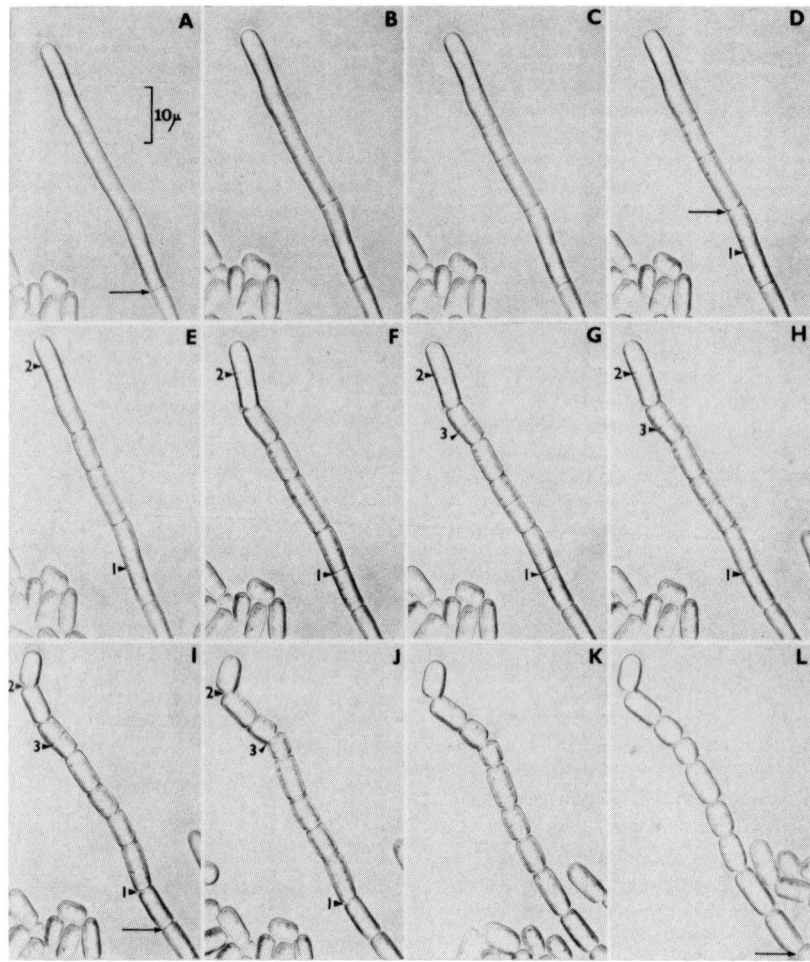

FIGURE 28-4. Thallic conidiogenesis in *Geotrichum* organism. Septum *(arrows)* is formed before conidium is differentiated from its parent cell. All of the parent cells become conidia. Numbers indicate that sequence of septum formation is random in *Geotrichum* organisms. (From Cole, G.T., and Kendrick, W.B.: Can. J. Botany **47:**1773, 1969.)

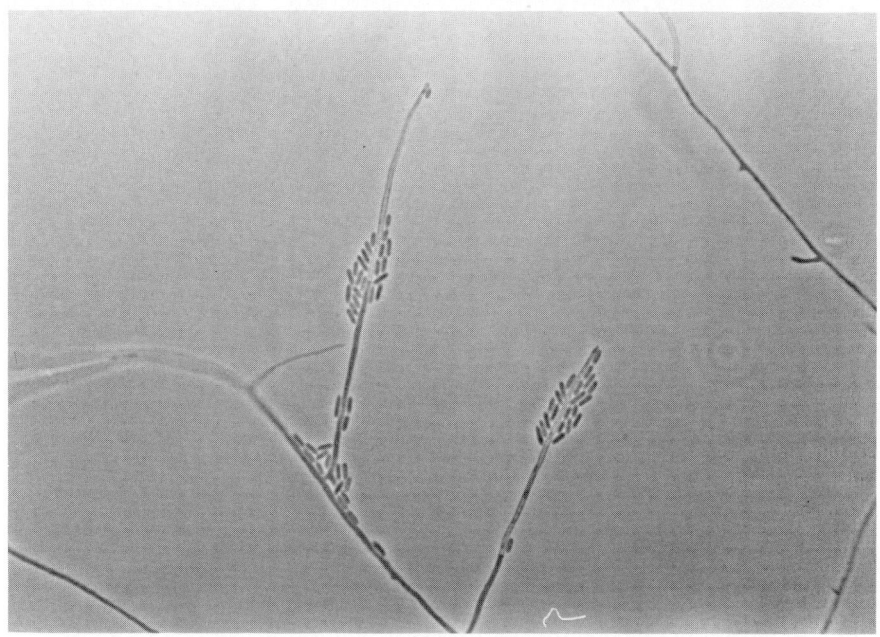

FIGURE 28-5. *Acremonium* organism. Phialides bear conidia at their apices.

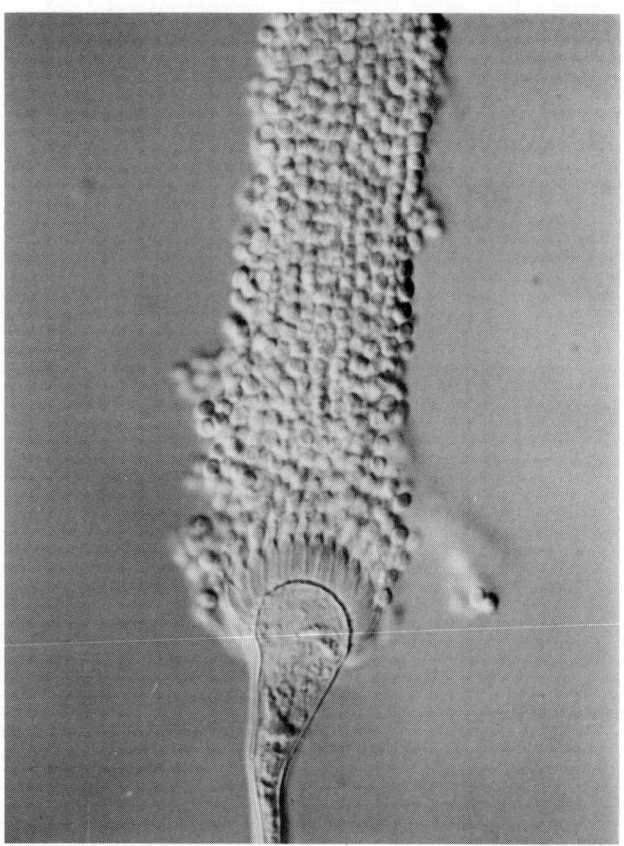

FIGURE 28-6. *Aspergillus fumigatus*. Note swollen vesicle at apex of conidiophore. Upon vesicle are flask-shaped conidiogenous cells (phialides) producing conidia.

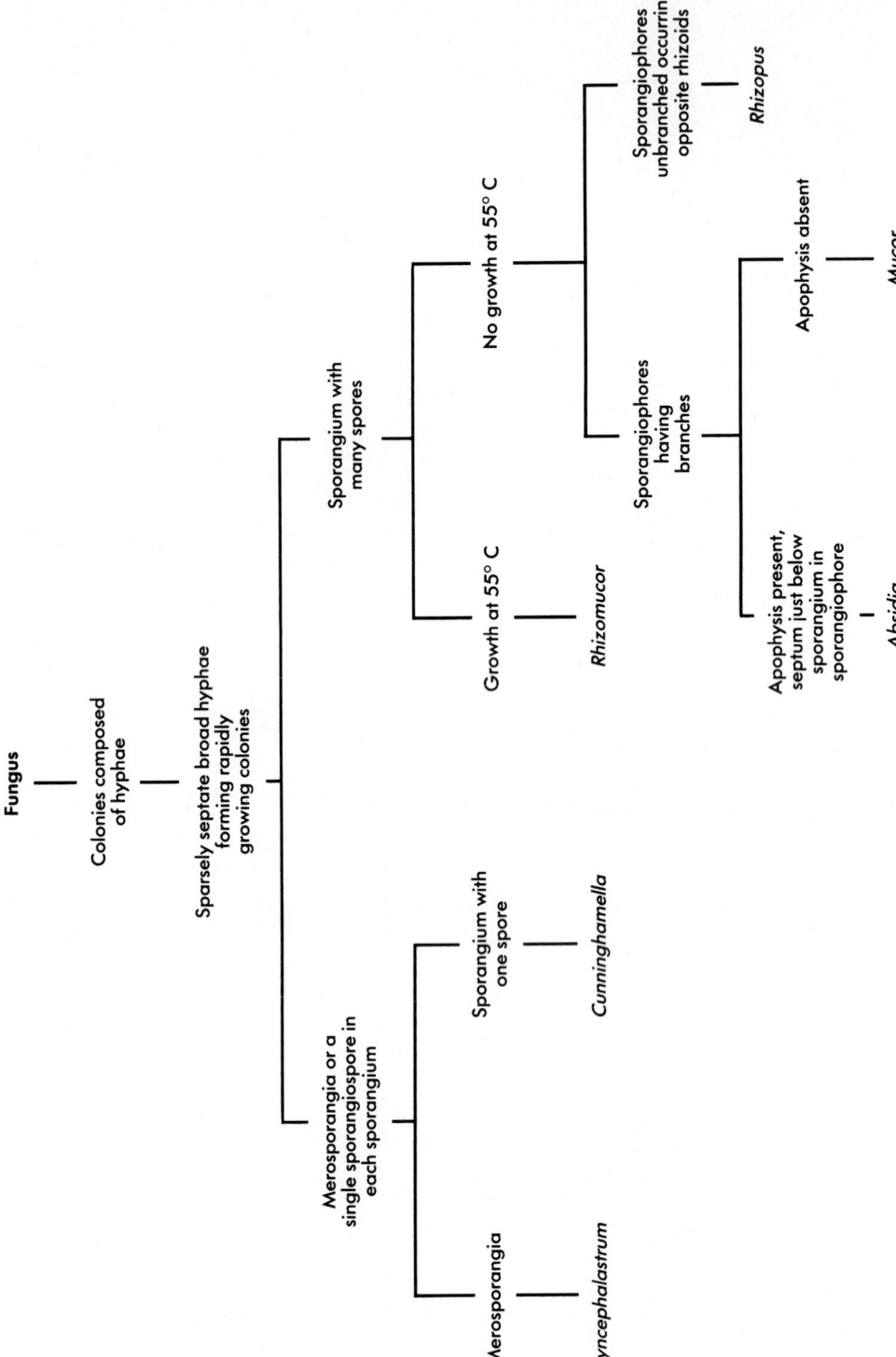

FIGURE 28-7. Key features for identification of most commonly encountered fungi.

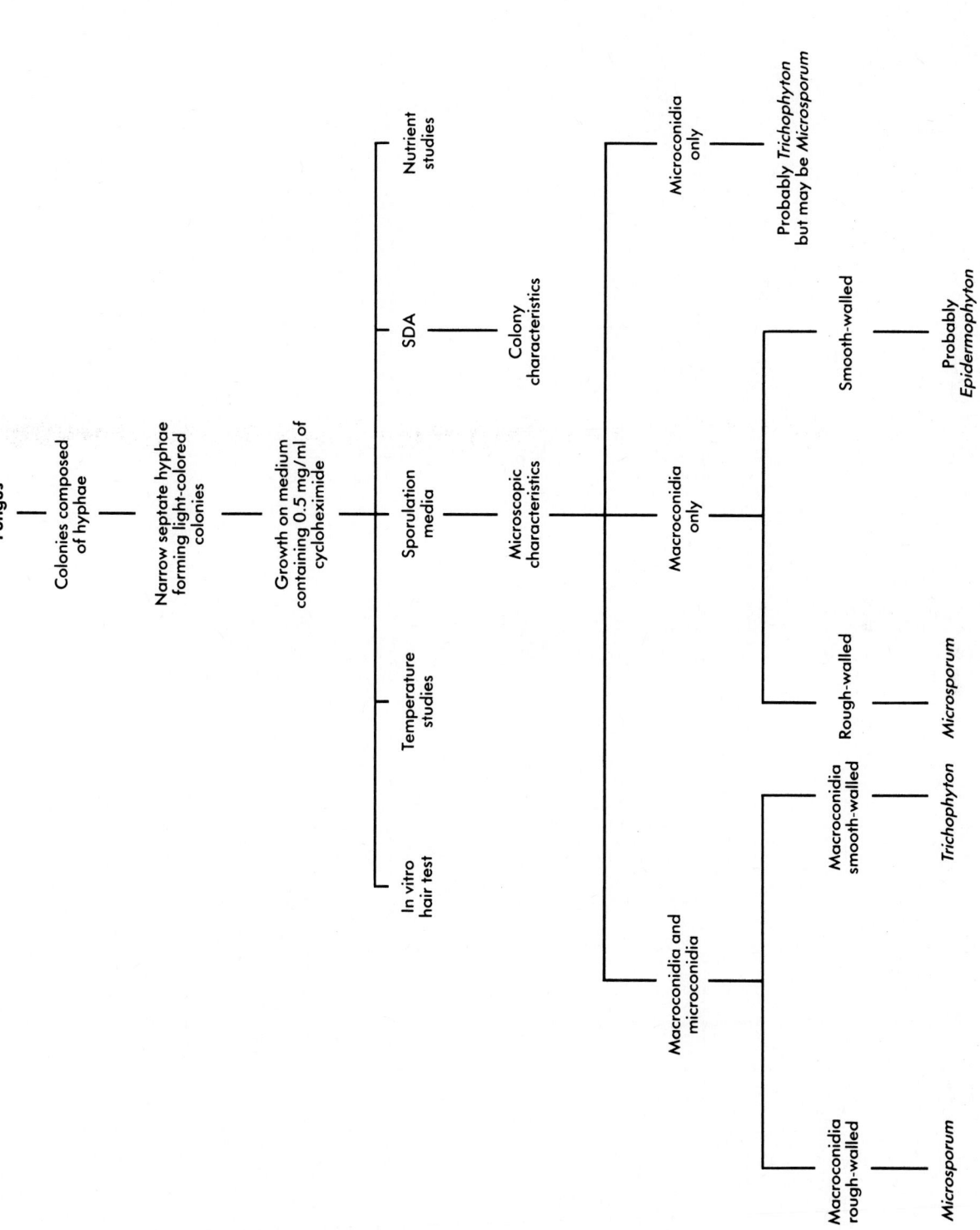

FIGURE 28-7, cont'd. Key features for identification of most commonly encountered fungi.

Continued.

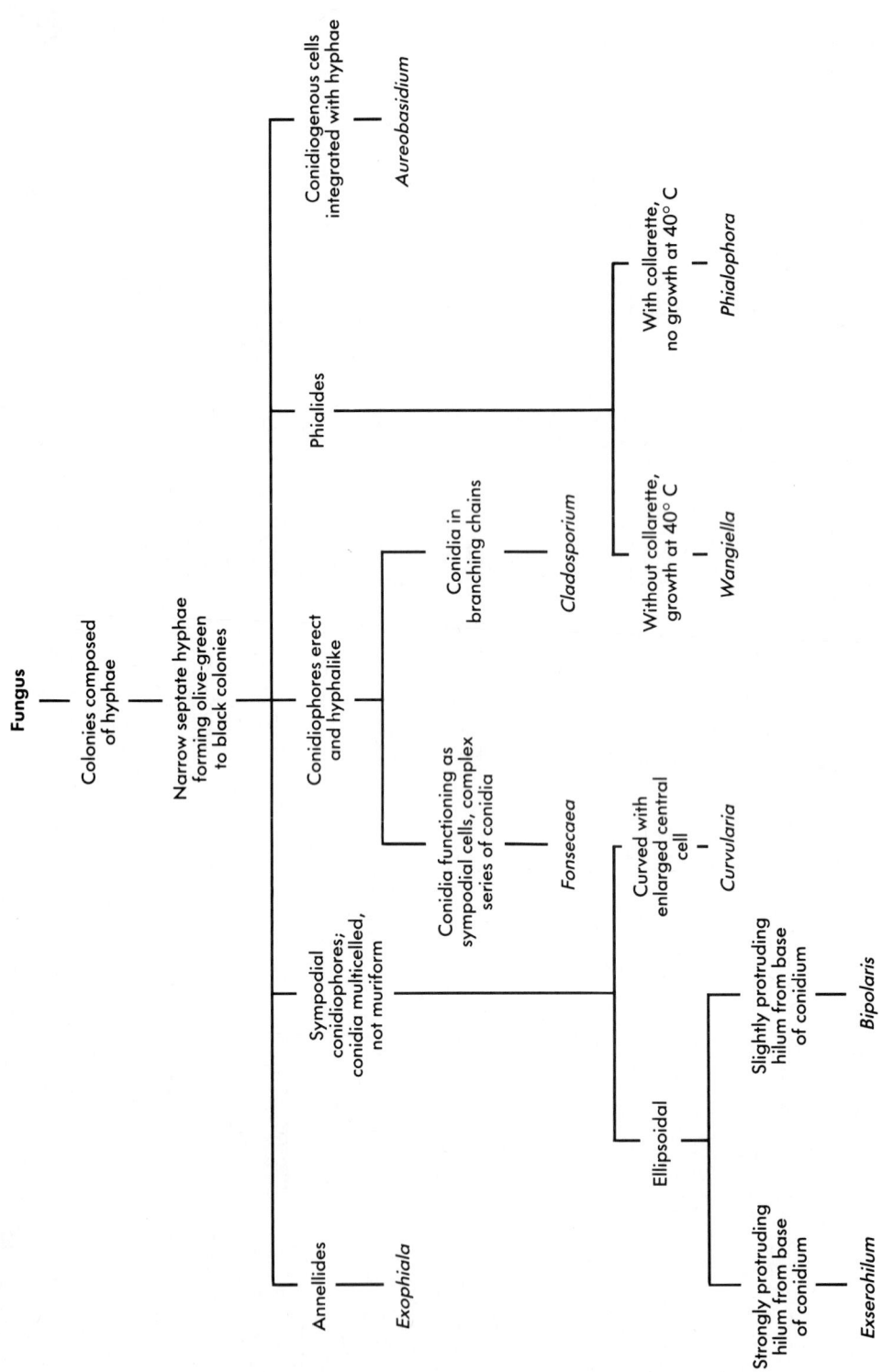

FIGURE 28-7, cont'd. Key features for identification of most commonly encountered fungi.

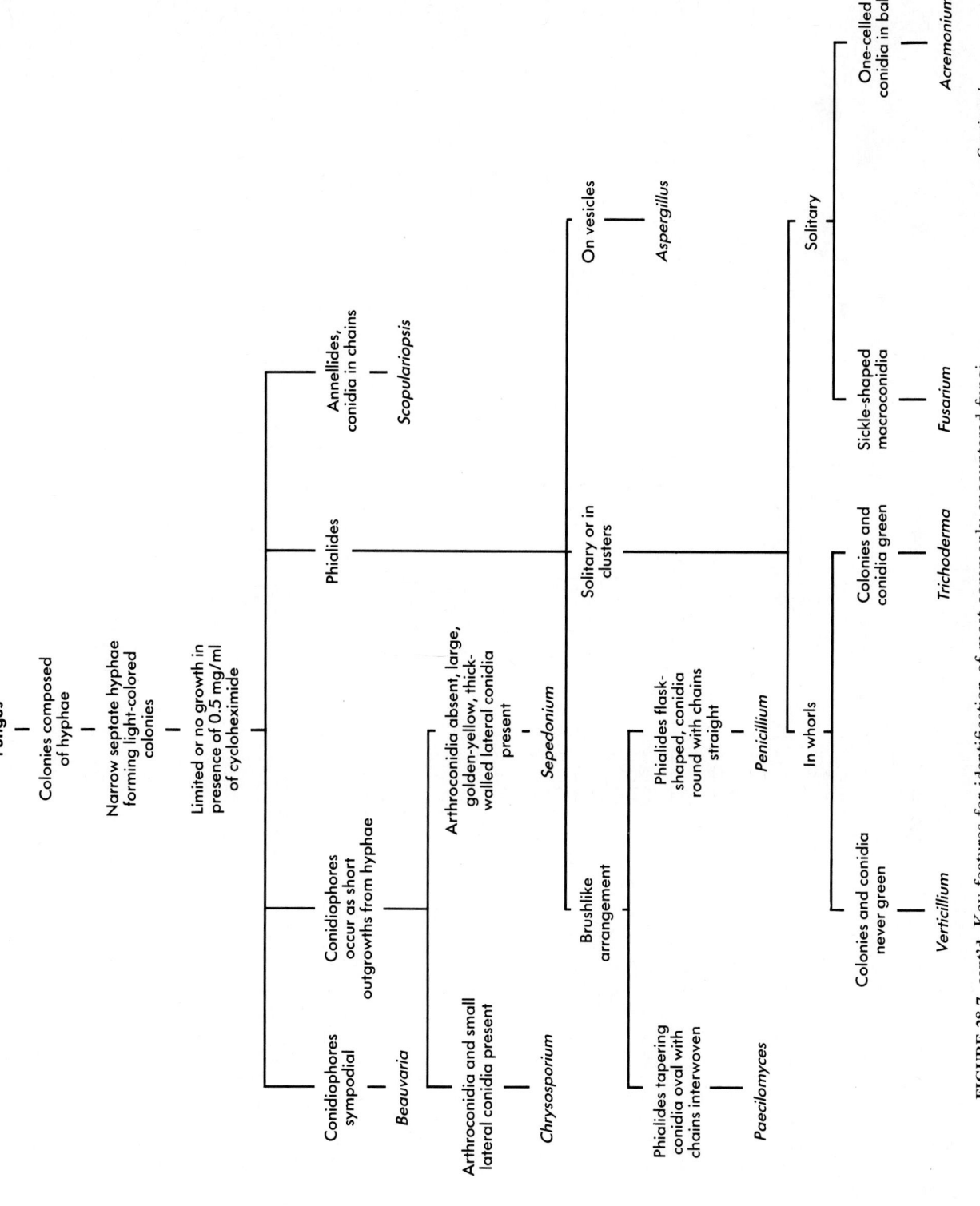

FIGURE 28-7, cont'd. Key features for identification of most commonly encountered fungi.

Continued.

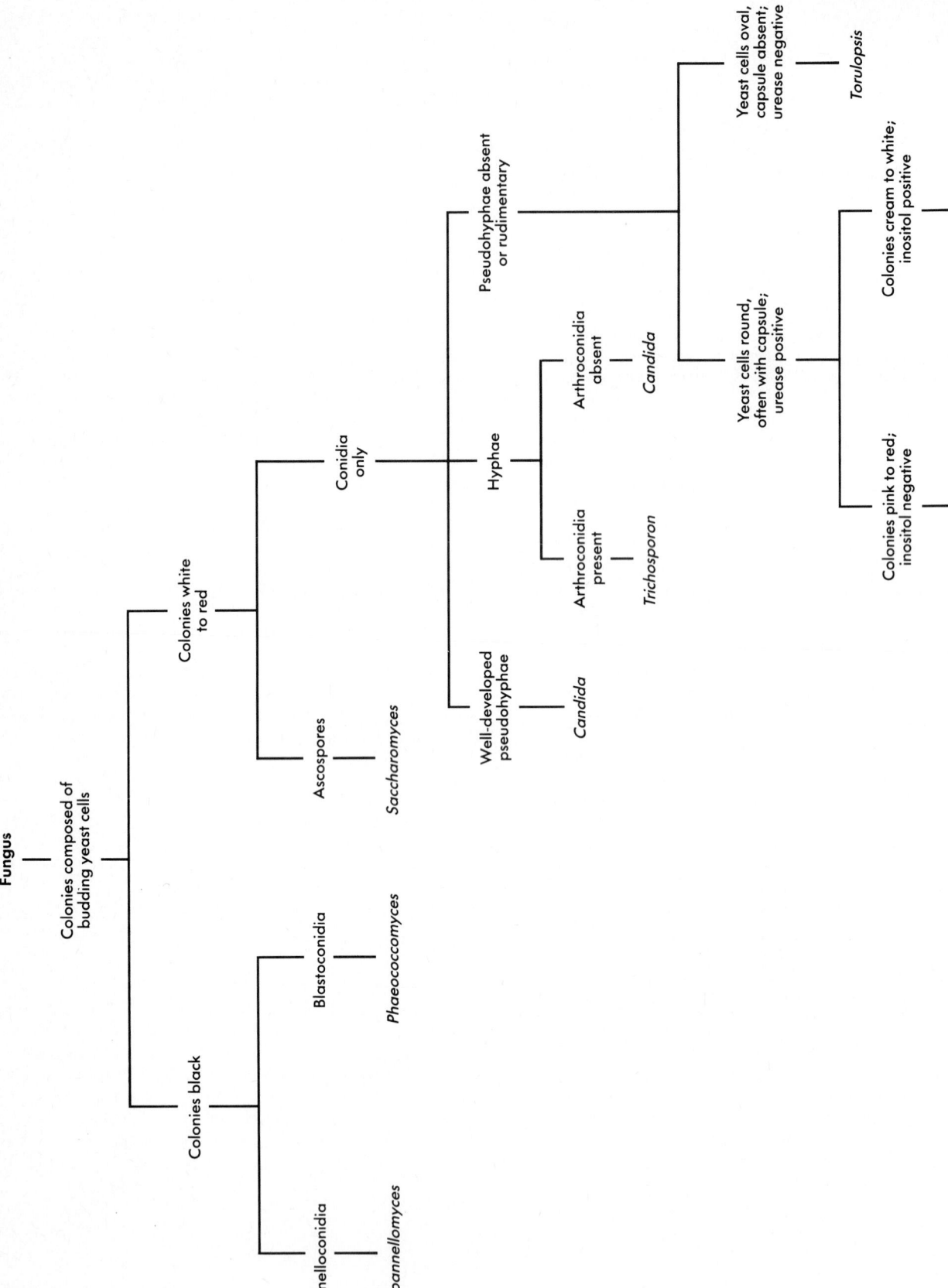

FIGURE 28-7, cont'd. Key features for identification of most commonly encountered fungi. (Modified from McGinnis, M.R., and Salkin, I.F.: Lab. Med. **17**:138, 1986.)

TABLE 28-2. Characterization of Conidia

Type	Definition	Examples of Fungi Forming These Structures
Annelloconidia	Conidia formed by annellide	*Phaeoannellomyces werneckii* (see Figure 31-1)
Arthroconidia	Conidia produced by fragmentation of fertile hypha	*Chrysosporium* spp. (see Figure 37-8) *Coccidioides immitis* (see Figure 34-7) *Geotrichum* spp. (see Figure 37-12) *Trichosporon beigelii* (see Figure 31-3)
Blastoconidia	Conidia formed by softening of cell wall and subsequent blowing-out process	*Aureobasidium* spp. (see Figure 37-7) *Blastomyces dermatitidis* (see Figure 34-2) *Candida albicans* (see Figure 35-5) *Cladosporium* spp. (see Figure 33-4) *Cryptococcus neoformans* (see Figure 29-1) *Fonsecaea pedrosoi* *Trichosporon beigelii* *Xylohypha bantiana*
Chlamydoconidia	Conidia often enlarged with thick walls that serve as survival propagules during adverse environmental conditions	*Fusarium* spp. (see Figure 37-11) *Trichophyton verrucosum* (37° C) (see Figure 32-10)
Macroconidia	Larger of two conidia of different sizes produced in same manner by fungus	Dermatophytes (see Figures 32-3 through 32-7)
Microconidia	Smaller of two conidia of different sizes produced in same manner by fungus	Dermatophytes (see Figures 32-3 through 32-7)
Phialoconidia	Conidia formed by phialide	*Acremonium* spp. (see Figure 28-5) *Penicillium* spp. (see Figure 37-14) *Wangiella dermatitidis*

following fertilization of an oosphere. Because the chytrids are not medically important, the reader is referred to Alexopoulos and Mims[2] for additional information.

The zygomycetes are characterized by the production of sexual spores called zygospores. (Zygomycetes may form sexual and asexual spores.) These spores are round, thick-walled reproductive structures that result from the union of two gametangia, cells containing nuclei that are involved in sexual reproduction. Two hyphal tips from either homothallic or heterothallic isolates contact each other. Plasmogamy, the fusion of cytoplasm but not nuclei, occurs; this results in an area of enlargement. The area increases in size and then is separated from the progametangia by septa. As the young zygospore increases in size, karyogamy takes place, resulting in many diploid nuclei. At the time of germination meiosis occurs, resulting in many haploid nuclei.

Ascomycetes produce sexual spores called ascospores in a special saclike structure known as an ascus. Clinically important ascomycetes usually form antheridia (cells that will fuse with ascogonia to provide them with nuclei for sexual reproduction) and ascogonia (cells that will receive nuclei for sexual reproduction from antheridia). A nucleus (n) is passed from the antheridium into the ascogonium. Ascogenous hyphae having a

dikaryotic (n + n) nuclear condition develop from the ascogonium. In the dikaryotic condition, two nuclei behave as if they were one even though they have not fused with each other. The tip of the ascogenous hypha may bend over to form a structure called a crozier. Karyogamy occurs in the apical cell or ascus mother cell, resulting in a diploid (2n) nucleus. As the ascus mother cell becomes an ascus, meiosis occurs, which results in four haploid (n) nuclei. If mitosis were to occur involving the four haploid nuclei before ascospore formation, the ascus would contain eight ascospores. Most ascomycetes produce asci that contain eight or more ascospores. The protoplasm in the ascus cleaves by free-cell formation into ascospores, each spore containing a single haploid nucleus.

Asci may be either naked or formed within a special fruiting body called an ascocarp. The five types of ascocarps—gymnothecia, cleistothecia, perithecia, apothecia, and ascostromata—are distinguished by differences in the development of the central area of the ascocarp and by differences in the asci. Naked asci are typically produced by yeasts such as *Saccharomyces cerevisiae*.

Basidiomycetes are unique because their vegetative cells are typically dikaryotic (n + n). Theoretically, only one of these cells could give rise to sexual spores. To maintain the dikaryotic hyphal condition, many basidiomycetes have clamp connections (hyphal bridges) that permit the simultaneous mitosis of the two nuclei to occur in such a manner that the n + n nuclei are duplicated. Usually the terminal cell of a dikaryotic hypha becomes a basidium. The basidium enlarges and karyogamy occurs, resulting in a diploid (2n) nucleus. Meiosis then occurs, resulting in four haploid (n) nuclei. Each of the haploid nuclei migrate through one of the sterigmata (tubelike extensions from the basidium) into a basidiospore. The uninucleate basidiospore is then forcibly discharged from the sterigma.

PARASEXUAL REPRODUCTION

Pontecorvo[18] first demonstrated parasexual reproduction in the genus *Aspergillus*. It has been shown to occur in basidiomycetes, ascomycetes, and some of the fungi imperfecti. The process imparts the advantages of sexual reproduction, that is, genetic recombination without the requirement for specific sexual stuctures. Hyphae fuse, and different haploid nuclei coexist in a common cytoplasm. This heterokaryon is stable, and the nuclei continue to divide. Occasionally, nuclear fusion occurs to form a diploid heterozygote, which then divides at about the same rate as the other haploid nuclei in the cell. Somatic recombination occurs when homologous chromosomes pair up. The diploid cell becomes haploid, the original chromosome number is restored, and the haploid recombinant is isolated.[13]

TAXONOMY OF FUNGI[14,15]

In 1969 Whittaker[22] proposed the classification of organisms into five kingdoms, based on three levels of organization. The kingdom Monera, representing the lowest level of organization, includes prokaryotic cells and is represented by bacteria, blue-green algae, and the filamentous bacteria known as actinomycetes. The kingdom Protista includes eukaryotic unicellular organisms; this kingdom represents the second level of organization. The third level of organization is represented by the kingdoms Plantae, Fungi, and Animalia. Members of these kingdoms are multicellular and multinuclear eukaryotes. Fungi, plants, and animals are distinguished on the basis of their type of nutrition, that is, photosynthetic for plants, absorptive for fungi, and ingestive for animals, as well as by the other characteristics previously discussed. Whether five kingdoms are necessary can be argued, although many biologists accept Whittaker's classification.

Several schemes have been proposed to further classify members of the kingdom Fungi. The taxonomic levels of the kingdom as defined by the International Code of Botanical Nomenclature are outlined in Table 28-3. Alexopoulos and Mims[2] separate the kingdom Fungi (Myceteae) into the divisions Mastigomycota and Amastigomycota. The Mastigomycota consists of organisms with flagellated cells such as the chytrids and the oomycetes, and the Amastigomycota consists of fungi without motile cells. This group includes the classes Ascomycetes, Zygomycetes, Basidiomycetes, and Fungi Imperfecti. Ainsworth, Sparrow, and Sussman[1] proposed the division Eumycota with the subphyla Mastigomycotina, Zygomycotina, Ascomycotina, Basidiomycotina, and Deuteromycotina. Inclusion of a fungus in one of the first four subphyla was based on the type of sexual spores produced. The fifth subphylum Deuteromycotina, or Fungi Imperfecti, accommodated fungi in which sexual reproduction was unknown.

The list below presents another widely accepted classification scheme for the kingdom Fungi[14] and the one that is used in this book. Even though the International Code of Botanical Nomenclature uses the term "division," we believe the term "phylum" is more acceptable[12] and thus use it here.

Phylum I: Chytridiomycota (Chytrids)
Class: Harpochytridiomycetes
Class: Chytridiomycetes
Class: Blastocladiomycetes
Class: Monoblepharidiomycetes
Phylum II: Zygomycota (Zygomycetes)
Class: Zygomycetes
    Genera: *Absidia*
      Basidiobolus
      Conidiobolus
      Cunninghamella
      Mucor
      Rhizopus
      Rhizomucor
      Saksenaea
Class: Trichomycetes
Phylum III: Ascomycota (Ascomycetes)
Class: Hemiascomycetes
    Genera: *Saccharomyces*
      Schizosaccharomyces
Class: Loculoascomycetes
    Genus: *Piedraia*
Class: Plectomycetes
    Genus: *Pseudallescheria*
Class: Laboulbeniomycetes
Class: Pyrenomycetes
Class: Discomycetes
Phylum IV: Basidiomycota (Basidiomycetes)
Class: Teliomycetes
    Genus: *Filobasidiella*
Class: Hymenomycetes
Class: Gasteromycetes
Phylum V: Fungi Imperfecti (Asexual fungi)
Class: Blastomycetes
    Genera: *Blastoschizomyces*
      Candida
      Cryptococcus
      Malassezia
      Phaeoannellomyces
      Rhodotorula
      Sporobolomyces
      Torulopsis
      Trichosporon
Class: Coelomycetes
Class: Hyphomycetes
    Genera: *Acremonium*
      Arthrinium
      Aspergillus
      Beauveria
      Bipolaris
      Blastomyces
      Botrytis
      Cladosporium
      Coccidioides
      Curvularia
      Epidermophyton
      Exophiala

TABLE 28-3. Classification Scheme for the Kingdom Fungi

Group	Group Ending
Kingdom	No specific ending
Phylum[a]	-mycota
Subphylum	-mycotina
Class	-mycetes
Subclass	-mycetidae
Order	-ales
Family	-aceae
Genus	No specific ending
Species	No specific ending

Modified from McGinnis, M.R.: Laboratory handbook of medical mycology, New York, 1980, Academic Press, Inc.
[a]We prefer the term ''phylum'' rather than ''division.''

Fonsecaea
Fusarium
Histoplasma
Madurella
Microsporum
Paracoccidioides
Penicillium
Phialophora
Scedosporium
Scopulariopsis
Sporothrix
Trimmatostroma
Wangiella

One of the confusing facets of mycologic nomenclature is the practice of giving the sexual stage of a fungus one name and the asexual stage another name. The sexual form of a fungus is called the teleomorph, the asexual form is called the anamorph, and the entire fungus including its teleomorph and anamorphs is called the holomorph. For example, *Cryptococcus neoformans* consists of an asexual budding yeast, which is an anamorph. When the appropriate isolates (mating types) of *C. neoformans* are placed together under the correct environmental conditions, basidia-bearing basidiospores are formed. This sexual form, or teleomorph, is called *Filobasidiella neoformans*. Just as the name *C. neoformans* is used for the asexual budding yeast, *F. neoformans* is used for the form consisting of basidia and basidiospores, which resulted from a sexual reproductive process. The entire fungus, including its sexual (teleomorph) and asexual (anamorph) form, is called *F. neoformans*. The name *F. neoformans* is used for the whole fungus (holomorph) because it is used for the sexual form (teleomorph). The sexual form of all organisms is the basis of determining phylogenetic relationships, which is the goal of all classification systems.

If sexual reproductive structures are present in a fungus, we believe they should be used for the name of that fungus. In most cases, because fungi that can reproduce sexually are heterothallic and only one mating type is isolated from a particular clinical specimen, sexual spores such as zygospores, ascospores, and basidiospores are absent. In this case the name for the fungus is based on the anamorph(s) produced by the isolate. For example, *Pseudallescheria boydii* (teleomorph) is characterized by cleistothecia, which are frequently present because the fungus is homothallic. In addition to cleistothecia, isolates of *P. boydii* have conidiophores and conidia that are classified as *Scedosporium apiospermum* (anamorph). When cleistothecia and conidia are present, the name *P. boydii* (holomorph) is appropriate. When isolates are recovered that contain only conidia and annellides typical of *S. apiospermum,* the name *P. boydii* should not be used because there are several species of *Pseudallescheria* that have identical *S. apiospermum* anamorphs. Without the cleistothecia (teleomorph) being present, it is not possible to determine if the *S. apiospermum* anamorph belongs to *P. boydii* or one of the other species in the genus. For the classification to be practical, we believe the name used for the fungus should be based on the forms it produces when it is being identified and not the forms it may produce. Even though *Filobasidiella neoformans* is the sexual form of *Cryptococcus neoformans,* the yeast should be called *C. neoformans* when recovered in the clinical laboratory because basidia and basidiospores are not produced unless mating studies are conducted.

Of the fungi listed earlier, the average clinical mycology laboratory encounters the more common Zygomycetes, Ascomycetes, and Fungi Imperfecti. Rarely, organisms of the phylum Basidiomycetes will be recovered. These groups are discussed in the following sections.

ZYGOMYCETES

Zygomycetes, which are often referred to as black bread molds because they commonly grow on bread, contain two medically important orders called the Mucorales and Entomophthorales. As discussed above, the zygomycetes are characterized by sexual spores called zygospores. In the order Mucorales, which contains such genera as *Mucor* and *Rhizopus,* sporangia are produced that contain one to many asexual sporangiospores. From a practical perspective, sporangia and other asexual structures such as rhizoids are used to identify zygomycetes. Zygospores are typically not produced by clinical isolates because they consist of only one mating type. Most zygomycetes require two different mating types for sexual reproduction to occur. The various zygomycetes can be readily identified using the characteristics of sporangia and other structures because these structures are so unique and stable.

Members of the order Entomophthorales produce asexual spores that are forcibly discharged. These are actually sporangia that are so reduced that they contain a single spore. Both groups of fungi have coenocytic hyphae; that is, there are many nuclei in each cell.

ASCOMYCETES

As discussed previously, the members of the phylum Ascomycota produce ascospores within an ascus following sexual reproduction. Sometimes the asci may be enclosed in an ascocarp. The classes Hemiascomycetes, Plectomycetes, Pyrenomycetes, and Loculoascomycetes contain the sexual forms of several medically important pathogens. Like zygomycetes, sexual stages are typically absent in clinical isolates because they are heterothallic. Two different mating types are required for sexual reproduction to occur. When an isolate is homothallic, that is, sexually self-fertile as in *Pseudallescheria boydii*, ascocarps containing asci and ascospores are usually formed.

FUNGI IMPERFECTI

The phylum Fungi Imperfecti, or Deuteromycetes, includes fungi that do not reproduce sexually. This phylum contains the majority of the human pathogens. The name ''Fungi Imperfecti'' is preferred because it means fungi that are imperfect only in the sense that sexual reproduction is unknown or absent. ''Imperfect form'' and ''anamorph'' refer to the concept because they refer to asexual reproduction. The name ''Deuteromycetes'' is not recommended because it implies that these fungi (anamorphs) are classified using the same conceptual basis as those that reproduce sexually (teleomorphs).

There are three classes of Fungi Imperfecti. The class Blastomycetes includes asexual budding yeasts such as *Cryptococcus, Candida, Torulopsis,* and *Rhodotorula.* Blastomycetes may be either dematiaceous or nondematiaceous depending on the presence of melanin in their cell walls. Hyphomycetes vegetatively produce septate hyphae. Some of the members of this class are *Trichophyton, Aspergillus, Exophiala,* and *Histoplasma.* Members of the class Coelomycetes produce acervuli, which are tightly bound mats of hyphae upon which conidia are produced.

BASIDIOMYCETES

Basidiospores are produced by the members of the phylum Basidiomycota by special cells called basidia. The process of meiosis occurs within the basidium as discussed earlier. These spores are frequently produced on sterigmata, which arise from the basidium. The term ''sterigmata'' has been inappropriately used to describe the special cells that form conidia in the genera *Aspergillus* and *Penicillium.* These are not sterigmata because they give rise to asexual propagules called conidia. Only basidiospores are formed upon sterigmata following the sexual process of meiosis. *Filobasidiella neoformans,* the sexual stage of *Cryptococcus neoformans,* is an example of a basidiomycete.

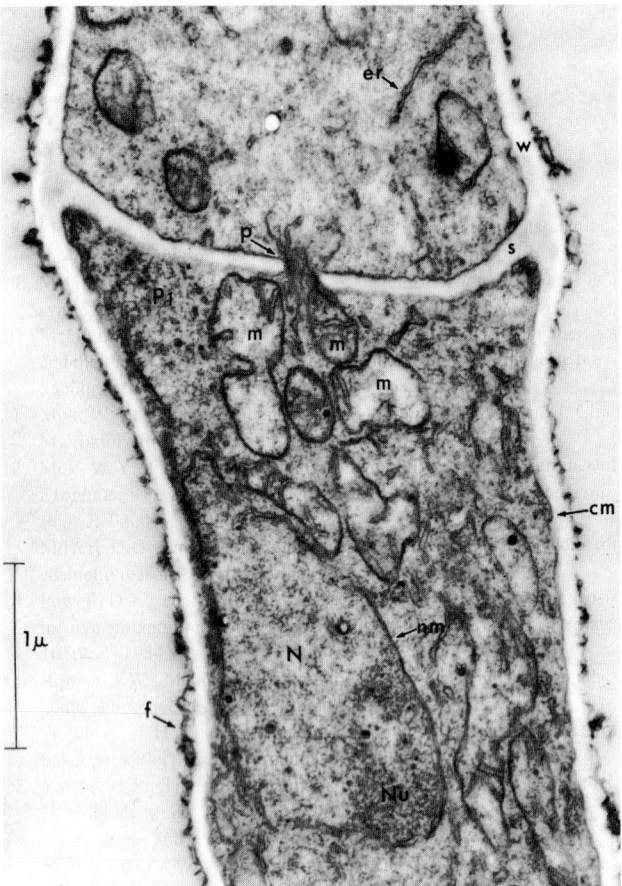

FIGURE 28-8. Coenocytic nature of hyphae. Electron micrograph of longitudinal section through two cells of *Neurospora crassa* partially separated by septum *(s).* Note streaming of mitochondria *(m)* through septal pore *(p). w,* Cell wall; *f,* outer frayed coat of cell wall; *cm,* cell membrane; *N,* nucleus; *Nu,* nucleolus; *nm,* nuclear membrane; *p₁,* ribosomal particles; *er,* endoplasmic reticulum. (Fixed with OsO_4 and stained with uranyl nitrate; ×47,000, reduced.) (Reproduced from Shatkin, A.J., and Tatum, E.L.: J. Biophys. Biochem. Cytol. **6:**423, 1959. By copyright permission of The Rockefeller University Press.)

FUNGAL ULTRASTRUCTURE[9]

Figure 28-8 shows a cross section of a fungal cell. The characteristic nuclear membrane can be seen. It comprises two parallel membranes with many nuclear pores where the membranes join. The endoplasmic reticulum, also a complex membrane system, is closely associated with the nucleus. On the endoplasmic reticulum the ribosomes and the Golgi apparatus can be seen. The mitochondria in fungi are about 1 to 1.5 μm in diameter. (This is the approximate size of some bacteria.) These are the respiratory and metabolic energy organelles of the fungus.

The fungi also contain vacuoles, which are membrane bound. These vacuoles contain hydrolytic or digestive enzymes for the breakdown of substrates. Lipid and glycogen granules may also be present in the fungal cell.

The cytoplasmic membrane is a typical eukaryotic bilayered

membrane. This membrane controls the diffusion of solutes and nutrients, as well as the energy-dependent and energy-independent transport of amino acids and sugars. The cytoplasmic membrane is composed of phospholipids, proteins, glycoproteins, and sterols. The most prevalent lipids are phospholipids and sphingolipids. The major sterol is ergosterol, in contrast to cholesterol in mammalian cells. The greater affinity of amphotericin B for ergosterol rather than cholesterol is at least partially responsible for its effectiveness as an antifungal antibiotic. Amphotericin B binds to the membrane sterols and causes a rapid leakage of potassium, which inhibits metabolic processes such as glycolysis and respiration.

The amount of DNA present in a single fungal cell is approximately four to 10 times that of a bacterium,[11] but only $\frac{1}{1000}$ to $\frac{1}{10,000}$ of that found in a plant or animal cell.[9]

FUNGAL CELL WALL

Fungal walls are complex structures that serve multiple purposes for the cell. The wall imparts rigidity, acts as an osmotic barrier, determines the shape of the organism, and is a primary factor in fungal morphogenesis.[9] The fungal cell wall also mediates the contact of the organism with its environment. Fungi can exist as spheroplasts without cell walls after the wall has been removed by lytic enzymes. As in bacterial cells, these fungal protoplasts are osmotically unstable. No free-living fungi devoid of cell walls exist.

The cell wall comprises 90% of the dry weight of the fungus. Generally yeast cell walls are thicker than mold walls. Walls of old cells appear thicker and more resistant to hydrolytic enzymes. Under light microscopy the cell wall appears as a thick, refractile covering. Electron photomicrographs reveal a structure that is smooth on the outside but fibrillar on the inside. These fibrils may be linear or crosshatched.[4,5] Polysaccharides make up 80% to 90% of the dry weight of isolated cell walls. These polysaccharides include chitin, glucans, chitosan, galactans, and mannans. The remaining 10% to 20% is protein and glycoprotein. The wall polysaccharides are specific for particular fungal groups[4,5,9]:

Fungus Group	Predominant Cell Wall Polysaccharide(s)
Zygomycetes	Chitin, chitosan
Ascomycetes (yeasts)	Beta-glucan, mannan
Basidiomycetes (yeasts)	Chitin, mannan
Ascomycetes, Basidiomycetes, and Fungi Imperfecti	Chitin, beta-glucan
Chytridiomycetes	Chitin, beta-glucan
Trichomycetes	Galactan, polygalactosamine

The remaining 10% to 20% of the cell wall dry weight, the proteins and glycoproteins, may play an active role in contact with host cell surfaces. Costerton, Geesey, and Cheng[7] postulated that glycoproteins and polysaccharides comprise the glycocalyx, which mediates attachment of most microbial cells to animate or inanimate surfaces. These glycoprotein complexes are antigenic and probably explain the observation that virtually all adults with a normal cell-mediated immune response react to *Candida* antigens or antigens of dermatophytes. Yeast mannan, specifically that of *C. albicans,* has been used as a marker for

disseminated *Candida* infection.[21] Yeast mannan consists of a polymannose backbone and mannosyl residues, which are linked via diacetyl chitobiose to an asparagine residue on the protein. Gas chromatography has been used to detect this specific glycoprotein in patients with *Candida* infection.[17] Beta-1,3-glucan is a widespread polysaccharide in fungal cell walls. Some fungi, such as the dimorphic pathogens *Histoplasma capsulatum, Blastomyces dermatitidis,* and *Paracoccidioides brasiliensis,* have an alpha-1,3-glucan in the yeast cell wall. This alpha-glucan is important in pathogenesis because macrophages are unable to digest the alpha-glucan layer of cell walls. The yeast cell wall has alpha-glucans, whereas the mold cell wall has beta-glucans.[20]

CAPSULES

Only a few fungi have capsules. The most common encapsulated clinically significant fungus is *Cryptococcus neoformans.* As in most bacteria, the capsule is a complex polysaccharide that is both antigenic and antiphagocytic. The cryptococcal capsule is a branched glucurono-xylo-mannan polymer and can be readily observed with special stains in tissue such as mucicarmine. Its role in the diagnosis of crytococcosis is described in Chapter 11.

FUNGAL METABOLISM

Fungi require carbon, nitrogen, and many other elements. Carbon is used for the synthesis of compounds such as carbohydrates, proteins, lipids, and nucleic acids. Their oxidation provides energy required by the fungus. Fungi secrete extracellular enzymes such as amylase, protease, and lipase, which degrade organic macromolecules into smaller subunits that can be transported into the fungus. Various systems move these subunits across the membrane. Some transport systems are always present, and some are inducible. Simple diffusion may occur with certain lipids. Most carbon sources are taken up by either diffusion or active transport. Environmental factors such as temperature, pH, and inhibitors are important in these processes.

Nitrogen is required for the synthesis of cellular constituents including amino acids, proteins, purines, pyrimidines, nucleic acids, glucosamine, chitin, and various vitamins. Either inorganic nitrogen sources or organic sources such as amino acids can be used by most fungi. Most sources, except protein, enter the cell directly by diffusion. Their utilization is governed by metabolism other than transport.[10]

Most fungi are aerobic but some—the yeasts and molds such as *Mucor*—are facultative; that is, they can grow in a reduced oxygen environment. None are strict anaerobes.

Fungi are able to tolerate a wide variation in pH values (2 to 10), although they grow best at a pH of approximately 7. Fungi prefer a moist environment; however, the conidia and spores can survive in a dry atmosphere. Although the optimal growth temperature for many fungi is 25° to 37° C, even the casual observer will note that some fungi grow in the refrigerator and others such as *Aspergillus fumigatus,* which is associated with piles of decomposing leaves, grow at 45° C.

CLINICAL CLASSIFICATION SCHEME

Medically important fungi can be classified into disease-causing groups. This approach occasionally helps in the task of identification. No single clinical scheme is inclusive because

TABLE 28-4. A Clinical Classification of Fungal Infections

Nature of Infection	Body Sites	Mycosis	Representative Etiologic Agents
Superficial	Hair	Black piedra	*Piedraia hortae*
	Hair	White piedra	*Trichosporon beigelii*
	Skin	Pityriasis versicolor	*Malassezia furfur*
	Skin (thick) or palms, feet	Tinea nigra	*Phaeoannellomyces*[a] *werneckii*
Cutaneous	Keratinized tissue (hair, nail, skin)	Dermatophytosis	*Epidermophyton floccosum, Microsporum canis, Trichophyton rubrum*
	Skin, nails	Candidiasis	*Candida albicans*
	Nails	Onychomycosis	*Aspergillus fumigatus, C. albicans, Scopulariopsis brevicaulis*
	Eye	Keratomycosis	*Aspergillus flavus, Bipolaris spicifera, C. albicans, Fusarium solani*
	Ear	Otomycosis	*Aspergillus niger, C. albicans*
Subcutaneous	Skin and lymph nodes	Sporotrichosis	*Sporothrix schenckii*
	Skin and subcutaneous tissue and bone (often feet and hands)	Mycetoma	*Madurella mycetomatis, Pseudallescheria boydii*
	Skin and subcutaneous tissue (often legs)	Chromoblastomycosis	*Cladosporium carrionii, Fonsecaea pedrosoi, Phialophora verrucosa*
	Skin and subcutaneous tissue	Zygomycosis	*Basidiobolus ranarum, Conidiobolus coronatus*
	Mucosa of nose	Rhinosporidiosis	*Rhinosporidium seeberi*
	Skin and subcutaneous tissue	Lobomycosis	*Loboa loboi*
	Skin and subcutaneous tissue	Phaeohyphomycosis	*Exophiala jeanselmei, Wangiella dermatitidis*
Systemic	Any organ system may be affected	Blastomycosis	*Blastomyces dermatitidis*
		Coccidioidomycosis	*Coccidioides immitis*
		Cryptococcosis	*Cryptococcus neoformans*
		Histoplasmosis	*Histoplasma capsulatum*
		Paracoccidioidomycosis	*Paracoccidioides brasiliensis*
Opportunistic mycoses	All organs	Disseminated candidiasis	*C. albicans*
	Lung	Aspergillosis	*A. fumigatus*
	Nasal sinuses, lungs, gastrointestinal tract	Zygomycosis	*Rhizopus arrhizus*
	Brain	Phaeohyphomycosis	*Xylohypha*[b] *bantiana*
	Any organ, deep tissue, blood	Systemic fungal disease	*Bipolaris hawaiiensis, Penicillium marneffei, Pseudallescheria boydii, Torulopsis glabrata, Trichosporon beigelii*, virtually any other fungus

[a]Previously classified as *Exophiala werneckii*.
[b]Previously classified as *Cladosporium bantianum*.

some fungi may cause more than one type of disease. One clinical classification scheme is presented in Table 28-4.

IMPORTANCE OF FUNGI

Virtually every inhabitant of earth has been exposed to fungi. Virtually no organic substance is free from fungal attack.

Such substances range from phenolic plastic to marble figures and from bone to wax. Some fungal infections such as athlete's foot, diaper rash, and yeast vaginitis are among the world's most prevalent infectious diseases.

On the other hand, positive contributions of fungi to the world's economy may be greater than most people realize.

Mushrooms are consumed throughout the world. Some of these, such as truffles (an ascomycete), are prized by gourmets and command extremely high prices. Yeast, aside from its important role in the production of alcoholic beverages and in fermentation, is a popular food supplement that provides vitamins and other cofactors. The mold *Penicillium,* in addition to its obvious contributions to medicine by providing penicillin, adds flavor to Roquefort and Camembert cheeses.

The ability of some fungi, mainly yeasts, to produce alcohol and CO_2 from a carbohydrate-containing substrate has given these organisms great importance. Some of the earliest accounts of the history of humanity refer to the fermentation process. Products include bread, alcoholic beverages, soy sauce, and a variety of other foods and drinks. Industrial processes still rely on the fermentation ability of fungi to make industrial alcohol, fats, and citric, oxalic, gluconic, and itaconic acids.

The contributions of fungi to medicine as synthesizers of antimicrobial agents are numerous. The chance discovery of penicillin by Fleming has led to advances in antimicrobial therapy that have had a profound effect on the life span of the world's citizens.

REFERENCES

1. Ainsworth, G.C., Sparrow, F.K., and Sussman, A.S., editors: The fungi: an advanced treatise, vols. 4A and 4B, New York, 1973, Academic Press, Inc.
2. Alexopoulos, C.J., and Mims, C.W.: Introductory mycology, ed. 3, New York, 1979, John Wiley & Sons, Inc.
3. Barron, G.L.: The genera of hyphomycetes from soil, Baltimore, 1968, Williams & Wilkins Co.
4. Bartnicki-Garcia, S.: Cell wall chemistry, morphogenesis, and taxonomy of fungi, Annu. Rev. Microbiol. **22:**87, 1968.
5. Bartnicki-Garcia, S.: Cell wall composition and other biochemical markers in fungal phylogeny. In Hasburne, J.B., editor: Phytochemical phylogeny, New York, 1970, Academic Press, Inc.
6. Cabib, E., and Farkas, V.: The control of morphogenesis: an enzymatic mechanism for the initiation of septum formation in yeast, Proc. Natl. Acad. Sci. USA **68:**2052, 1971.
7. Costerton, J.W., Geesey, G.G., and Cheng, K.-J.: How bacteria stick, Sci. Am. **238:**86, 1978.
8. Emmons, C.W., et al.: Medical mycology, ed. 3, Philadelphia, 1977, Lea & Febiger.
9. Farkas, V.: Morphology and structure of fungi. In Braude, A.I., Davis, C.E., and Fierer, J., editors: Infectious diseases and medical microbiology, Philadelphia, 1986, W.B. Saunders Co.
10. Garraway, M.O., and Evans, R.C.: Fungal nutrition and physiology, New York, 1984, John Wiley & Sons, Inc.
11. Kendrick, B., editor: The whole fungus, vols. 1 and 2, Ottawa, 1979, National Museums of Canada.
12. Kendrick, B.: The fifth kingdom, Waterloo, Ontario, Canada, 1985, Mycologue Publications.
13. Kobayashi, G.S.: Fungi. In Davis, B.D., et al.: Microbiology, ed. 3, Hagerstown, Md., 1980, Harper & Row, Publishers.
14. McGinnis, M.R.: Laboratory handbook of medical mycology, New York, 1980, Academic Press, Inc.
15. McGinnis, M.R.: Recent taxonomic developments and changes in medical mycology, Annu. Rev. Microbiol. **34:**109, 1980.
16. McGinnis, M.R., and Salkin, I.F.: Identification of moulds commonly used in proficiency tests, Lab. Med. **17:**138, 1986.
17. Miller, G.G., et al.: Rapid identification of *Candida albicans* septicemia in man by gas liquid chromatography, J. Clin. Invest. **54:**1235, 1974.
18. Pontecorvo, G.: The parasexual cycle in fungi, Annu. Rev. Microbiol. **10:**393, 1956.
19. Sabouraud, R.: Les Teignes, Paris, 1910, Masson et Cie.
20. San-Blas, G.: *Paracoccidioides brasiliensis:* cell wall glucans, pathogenicity and dimorphism. In McGinnis, M.R., editor: Current topics in medical mycology, vol. 1, New York, 1985, Springer-Verlag.
21. Weiner, M.H., and Yount, W.J.: Mannan antigenemia in the diagnosis of invasive *Candida* infections, J. Clin. Invest. **58:**1045, 1976.
22. Whittaker, R.H.: New concepts of kingdoms of organisms, Science **163:**150, 1969.

CHAPTER 29

General Approaches to the Isolation and Identification of Clinically Significant Fungi

Richard C. Tilton
Michael R. McGinnis

This chapter discusses general principles for the collection and transport of clinical specimens, the direct microscopic examination of specimens, and the isolation and recognition of fungi. Details relating to the identification of fungi are covered in other chapters.

Because fungi tend to grow more slowly than other microorganisms, such as bacteria, a great deal of emphasis is placed on the direct examination of clinical specimens. Direct examination of specimens may provide important information regarding diagnosis, appropriate therapy, and the use of special media or conditions for recovery of the suspected pathogen. Since mycology is a morphology-based science, important decisions regarding the identification of many pathogenic fungi can be made by detecting their presence in specimens.

Many media and techniques have proved useful for the isolation of pathogenic fungi. No universal agreement exists on how fungi should be recovered. It is our intention to provide helpful guidelines based on our and others' experiences.

LABORATORY SAFETY

Because many fungi produce airborne conidia and spores, the possibility of conidia- and spore-containing aerosols is a major concern in the clinical laboratory. The following guidelines for the clinical microbiologist in the mycology laboratory are essential. They should be an important component of the laboratory procedure manual and, when appropriate, should be posted in a conspicuous location.

1. Never smell a fungus culture! Fungus colonies typically release airborne conidia and spores when exposed to slight air currents. Simply opening a culture plate containing fungi may be enough to create dangerous aerosols. Although yeast colonies are smooth, moist, and glistening, they should never be smelled. While many people have been exposed naturally to systemic fungi, such as *Coccidioides immitis,* a technologist who inhales a heavy inoculum of arthroconidia of *C. immitis* probably faces a severe pulmonary infection and possibly death. In animal studies a single arthroconidium could initiate an infection. Sputum cultures, even if they do not harbor pathogenic fungi, may contain *Mycobacterium tuberculosis.* The clinical presentation of tuberculosis is similar to some fungal infections.

2. A biologic safety cabinet (BSC) is essential. The Centers for Disease Control recommends that either a class 1 or a class 2 BSC be used. We prefer a class 2 laminar flow cabinet vented to the outside of the building. The air entering and leaving the cabinet is filtered through high-efficiency particulate air (HEPA) filters, which protects both the microbiologist and the specimen. The BSC also minimizes the possibility of contaminating the environment with fungal reproductive propagules. For example, one hospital's air-handling system was so badly contaminated with an *Acremonium* sp. that diagnostic mycologic and bacteriologic examinations were curtailed; the *Acremonium* organisms were found growing in all of the nutrient agar–containing plates.

The class 2 BSC exchanges approximately 75 to 100 linear feet of air per minute. Although the BSC may be equipped with an ultraviolet (UV) light, which should be left on when the cabinet is not in use, its effectiveness is questionable. The UV light should always be off while the cabinet is in use because it can cause severe eye damage. When the output of the light is checked, special glasses must be worn to protect the eyes. The cabinet should be certified annually for proper operation. The inspection should include an evaluation of the airflow rate, UV light output, and the HEPA filters for damage. The cabinet must be professionally decontaminated before inspection.

3. All media, reagents, and tissue or fluid specimens should be autoclaved before leaving the mycology laboratory. Bagging of such hazardous material and transportation to an incinerator or a landfill before decontamination is not safe. It is important to remember that some of these specimens may also contain mycobacteria.

4. Petri dishes should not be used for fungal cultures unless they are sealed with Parafilm or an oxygen-permeable tape. Petri dishes must always be opened in a BSC and never at the open bench.

5. The mycology laboratory benchtops should be disinfected daily with a good disinfectant. A quaternary ammonia, halogen, or phenolic compound may be used. These same compounds can decontaminate spills or broken culture containers.

6. If test tubes or bottles are used for either fungus cultures or primary isolation, they should have screw-type caps and not cotton, plastic foam, or loose metal closures. Such materials are easily removed from the top of a tube or bottle, increasing the potential for the release of an airborne aerosol.

7. Smoking, drinking, eating, or makeup application should not be allowed. Fingernail biting and insertion of contact lenses in the laboratory should be discouraged.

8. Personnel who are receiving chemotherapy, radiation therapy, or systemic steroids or who are diabetics or pregnant

should not work in the mycology laboratory. These conditions can predispose an individual to a fungal infection.

9. Microbiologists using scalpel blades, tweezers, and needles must be careful. Needles should not be recapped or broken before disposal. Wounds caused by these kinds of objects can lead to accidental fungal infection, hepatitis, and exposure to HIV.

10. When fungi are transferred within the cabinet, a disinfectant-soaked pad should be used as a work surface. This provides a safe and handy way to disinfect the area once the work has been completed.

SPECIMEN COLLECTION AND TRANSPORT

A good rule of thumb is that all fungal specimens should be processed as soon as possible. This prevents fungal and bacterial overgrowth that might hinder the recovery of a pathogen. When delay cannot be avoided, the specimens, with the exception of blood, cerebrospinal fluid, and dermatologic specimens, can be refrigerated for a short time.

Clinical specimens should not be mailed to a reference laboratory unless absolutely necessary. Although there is anecdotal evidence that *Histoplasma* organisms may survive extensive transport delay, the increased growth of normal flora resulting from delayed processing compromises the recovery of pathogenic fungi. We recommend one of the air-express services if the specimen must be shipped over a distance. If fungus cultures are mailed, a U.S. Public Health Service permit, which can be obtained from the Centers for Disease Control in Atlanta, is required. Cultures must be sent in taped, capped tubes and not in plastic culture dishes. The culture tube must be placed in a container, which is then placed in a second one. The outside label must include a biohazard label as well as an etiologic agent label.* If transport is for only a short distance, hand carriage is preferred.

Table 29-1 summarizes specimens that should be collected when various fungal diseases are suspected. Included also are recommendations for specimen containers. It is extremely important that specimens from patients with hepatitis, AIDS, and other infectious diseases be labeled with a precaution label.

DIRECT MICROSCOPIC EXAMINATION OF CLINICAL SPECIMENS

Direct microscopic examination of clinical specimens submitted for mycologic analysis is performed for several reasons. Because long periods of time are often required before some of the pathogenic fungi are recovered from clinical specimens, it is important to provide the physician with rapid information that can assist with the diagnosis and choice of therapy. A clinical specimen can be examined within minutes by direct microscopy, and in many instances the observed morphology of the fungus can provide valuable clinical information. The second purpose of the direct examination is to provide the laboratory technologist with information that could be helpful in more effectively isolating the suspected etiologic agent. For example, if hyphae of a zygomycete are seen, a portion of the specimen should be inoculated to sterile bread or to malt agar

*Details are published in *Interstate Shipment of Etiologic Agents,* Federal Register vol. 45, no. 141, July 21, 1980, Atlanta, Centers for Disease Control, 42 CFR, Part 72.

containing antibacterial agents, such as penicillin and streptomycin. Furthermore, in this situation the specimen should not be homogenized because this processing technique may kill too much of the potential viable inoculum needed for plating. The information gained from the direct detection of fungi in clinical specimens also permits the laboratory technologist to check the adequacy of the isolation procedures. Fungi that are observed on direct examination should be isolated in the laboratory. Regardless of what is seen in a clinical specimen, the routine isolation media are always used. Supplemental media are used as necessary.

Several methods are available for direct microscopic examination. The principles of these methods are considered in the following section. Specific procedures are included in Appendix B.

Table 29-2 summarizes structures most likely to be seen in direct microscopic observation of clinical specimens.

POTASSIUM HYDROXIDE PREPARATION[10,19,25]

The potassium hydroxide (KOH) preparation is frequently used for direct examination. KOH digests protein debris and clears keratinized tissue so fungi present in specimens can be seen more readily. The chitinous cell walls of fungi are somewhat resistant to the action of KOH at the concentration that is used in the clinical laboratory; however, with time, the fungi do dissolve. KOH preparations may be made on virtually all types of clinical specimens.

Cellufluor (Polyscience, Inc.), a brightener, can be added to the KOH solution. When this is examined with a fluorescence microscope, the fungi fluoresce. The cellufluor binds to the chitin of the fungal cell wall.[9,24] Dimethyl sulfoxide (DMSO) may be added for thick specimens of nail and skin. Addition of DMSO permits a more rapid analysis of the slide without warming.[23]

Because of several variable factors, a KOH preparation may not reveal fungi even when they are present. The collection of the specimen by the physician, the selection of the portion of the specimen to be examined by the technologist, the size of the etiologic agent, and the number of organisms present are extremely important. For example, if a biopsy specimen from a cutaneous lesion caused by *Blastomyces dermatitidis* is taken from the center rather than at the edge, the yeast cells of *B. dermatitidis* may not be seen.

PERIODIC ACID–SCHIFF STAIN

Most microbiologists read KOH preparations less reliably than stained preparations. Haley and Callaway[10] recommend that a periodic acid–Schiff (PAS) stain be performed on all negative KOH preparations, as well as on cerebrospinal fluid (CSF) and urine.

In the PAS staining technique, the carbon–carbon (C–C) bonds in the carbohydrates of the cell walls of the fungi are oxidized by the periodic acid to form aldehydes. These aldehyde groups combine with the basic fuchsin dye to form a brilliant magenta (pink-purple) complex that cannot be removed with the decolorizing agent sodium metabisulfite (see Plate 23, *E*). Differentiation of fungi in tissues may be facilitated if a counterstain is also used; light green (fast green) is recommended. With this counterstain the hyphae or yeast cells should stain a brilliant magenta, and the background should stain green.

TABLE 29-1. Specimen Collection Procedures for Isolation of Fungi

Fungal Infection Suspected	Specimen	Collection Procedure	Comments
Pityriasis versicolor or piedra	Skin, scalp, hair (piedra)	Disinfect skin surface with 70% alcohol; scrape edge of lesion; place material in sterile Petri dish; pluck hair with forceps; collect in sterile Petri dish	Skin and hair may be collected in paper envelopes; stopper tubes should not be used because moisture accumulation may result in contamination of specimen
Cutaneous	Skin	As for pityriasis versicolor	Periphery of skin lesion should yield largest number of viable fungal elements
	Nails	Scrape discolored or hyperkeratotic areas; place in sterile Petri dish; infected nails may also be clipped with nail clipper	
	Hair	Remove or pluck hair with forceps	Examine hair with Wood's lamp; selectively culture hairs that fluoresce
	Mucous membranes	Remove some plaque material from mouth with tongue depressor; prepare microscope slide preparation with portion of material, and place remainder in sterile tube containing saline or transport medium; remove mucoid material from vagina with two swabs; send directly to laboratory	Potassium hydroxide (KOH) preparation can help make diagnosis of thrush or *Candida* vaginitis
	Corneal ulcer	Physician collects corneal scrapings; inoculate onto appropriate media at site of collection; prepare microscope slides for Giemsa staining	Suspected pathogens are on streak lines
	Ear	Unless on external ear, physician collects debris from ear canal for direct transport to laboratory	Ensure that enough material is collected for both microscopy and culture
Subcutaneous	Skin and subcutaneous tissue	Biopsy, aspirates, or curettings; examine specimen grossly for presence of granules; biopsy specimens must be immediately transported to laboratory for processing	Agents of mycetoma, chromoblastomycosis, and phaeohyphomycosis are typically seen microscopically; direct microscopy for *Sporothrix schenckii* is unrewarding
Systemic	Sputum	Collect early morning specimen on each day for 3 successive days; have patient expectorate into sterile sputum container; bring immediately to laboratory; specimen may be divided and a portion concentrated for both *Mycobacterium* organisms and aerobic actinomycetes	12-hr or 24-hr sputum specimens unsatisfactory, since overgrowth occurs; do not leave container for specimen collection in patient's room
	Transtracheal aspiration; bronchial brushing; bronchoscope specimen; percutaneous lung biopsy	Specimens are procured by invasive means and must be handled properly to avoid necessity of second collection; specimen may be aspirate (fluid), brush bristle, or small piece of tissue; bring to laboratory without delay; if tissue specimens are too small to macerate, place specimen in small amount of sterile saline and then homogenize	All specimens must be prepared for microscopic examination and culture; do not let specimens dehydrate

Continued.

TABLE 29-1. Specimen Collection Procedures for Isolation of Fungi—cont'd

Fungal Infection Suspected	Specimen	Collection Procedure	Comments
Fungal abscess	Abscess fluid or drainage	If only small portion of aspirate is collected, add small amount of sterile saline; aspirate may be delivered to laboratory in syringe	All specimens must be prepared for direct microscopic examination
Invasion of tissue	Lymph node	Macerate or grind tissue; add 2 to 3 ml saline	
	Other organs	Inspect tissue grossly for necrotic and caseous material and areas with blood, granules, pus, or exudate before grinding; if present, culture and examine microscopically	If zygomycete is suspected, mince tissue and use media to enhance recovery of organisms
Central nervous system	Cerebrospinal fluid	Collect in sterile tube	Culture by membrane filtration if specimen is large; directly plate all small volume specimens; 5 ml of CSF is optimal; cryptococcal latex test should be done on supernatant
Urinary (kidney, bladder)	Urine	Collect clean-catch specimen in a sterile urine cup; place urine from catheter or percutaneous bladder aspiration into sterile container	Specimen must be transported to laboratory within 2 hours to prevent overgrowth by contaminating bacteria
Fungemia	Blood	Several methods may be used; Isolator System (DuPont) is superb for recovery of fungi from blood[25]	Fungi may be seen within 12 to 24 hours of incubation; *Candida, Cryptococcus,* and *Histoplasma* spp. may be seen in Wright or Gram stain of peripheral blood if large number of cells are present in blood such as in AIDS patients
Miscellaneous	Bone marrow	Collect in sterile syringe with added anticoagulant; inoculate media at bedside or bring immediately to laboratory	If sufficient material is available, make slides; ensure that syringe is capped during transport

Data from references 18 and 25.

Deterioration of periodic acid results in the absence of staining of hyphae because the cell wall C–C groups are not oxidized to aldehydes. Similarly, old metabisulfite results in heavy background staining because of its inability to bleach or decolorize the stain. Staining procedures must be controlled. A known positive clinical specimen should be used.

In our judgment equally satisfactory results can be obtained by using a phase contrast microscope in place of the PAS stain. Each laboratory must adopt procedures and techniques based on their own specific levels of service provided.

ACID-FAST STAIN

Acid-fast stains are used primarily in bacteriology for the detection of mycobacteria. *Mycobacterium* and, to a lesser extent, *Nocardia* organisms have cell walls with a high lipid content, which is approximately 40% of the total dry weight.[28] Mycobacteria are resistant to most stains, but once stained with basic fuchsin, they resist decolorization with an acid-alcohol mixture, hence the description ''acid-fast.'' Acid fastness is variable in *Nocardia asteroides, N. brasiliensis,* and *N. caviae.* The Ziehl-Neelsen, the Kinyoun, or the Hank's procedure may be used, but the period of decolorization should not exceed 5 to 10 seconds. These procedures are included in Chapter 6 and Appendix B.

With any of these acid-fast stains, *Nocardia* and *Mycobacterium* cells appear pink and the background a pale blue. The stain is controlled by the use of premade slides of *Nocardia* organisms that are grown on Middlebrook and Cohn 7H10 agar. One of the facultative actinomycetes (*Actinomyces viscosus*) can be used as a negative control. Ascospores of yeasts and the spores of *Streptomyces* may be acid fast. The modified Kinyoun stain may be used to detect the presence of ascospores in yeast cultures. After cultivation, *N. asteroides* often looses its acid fastness.

INDIA INK PREPARATION

India ink is used to highlight the hyaline capsules of *Cryptococcus neoformans.* India ink does not stain the capsular

TABLE 29-2. Actinomycete and Fungal Elements Observed in Clinical Specimens

Element	Specimen	Suggested Infection or Organism	Diagram
Gram-positive, branched, filaments 1 to 1.5 μm; tangled elements typically acid fast	Respiratory secretions, pus, tissue	Nocardiosis	Plate 18, *A*
Hyphae organized into granules; some cells often swollen	Pus, tissue biopsy	Mycetoma; suspect *Pseudallescheria boydii* in United States	Figure 29-2
Large (5 to 20 μm), sparsely septate, irregularly branching, hyaline hyphae	Lesion drainage, pus, tissue, respiratory secretions	Zygomycosis	Figure 29-3
Septate, dichotomous branching, hyaline, 2 to 3 μm, septate hyphae	Lesion drainage, pus, tissue, ear debris, respiratory secretions	Aspergillosis; possibly *P. boydii*	Figure 29-4
Oval hyaline yeast cells, pseudohyphae, hyphae, or any combination; cells 5 to 7 μm	Urine, respiratory secretions, blood, skin, mucocutaneous lesions	Candidiasis; may represent invasion or colonization	Plates 23, *E,* and 24, *A*
Round, hyaline yeasts; capsules typically present; blastoconidia attached by narrow neck; cells 8 to 10 μm	Cerebrospinal fluid, blood, lung biopsy, bone marrow, pus, respiratory secretions, urine	Cryptococcosis	Figure 29-1
Round, hyaline, thick-walled yeast cells; broad-based budding cells 8 to 15 μm	Tissue, draining pus, respiratory secretions	Blastomycosis	Figure 29-5
Spherules (20 to 60 μm), containing endospores	Respiratory secretions, tissues, pus	Coccidioidomycosis	Figure 29-6
Oval, hyaline, intracellular yeast (3 to 5 μm)	Respiratory secretions, bone marrow	Histoplasmosis	Figure 29-7
Thick-walled, brown cells with cross-walls in two planes (10 to 12 μm); hyphae may be present	Subcutaneous tissue, skin	Chromoblastomycosis	Figure 29-8
Arthroconidia in and around hair shaft; cuticle destroyed (ectothrix)	Hair	Tinea capitis	Figure 29-9
Arthroconidia only inside hair shaft; cuticle intact (endothrix)	Hair	Tinea capitis	Figure 29-10
Hyphae, occasionally arthroconidia in keratinized tissue	Skin, nails	Dermatophytosis	Figure 29-11
Carbonaceous, black, hard, hyphal nodules	Hair	Black piedra	Figure 29-12
Short, hyaline hyphae and clusters of bottle-shaped unicellular yeast cells (3 to 7 μm)	Skin	Pityriasis versicolor	Figure 29-13
White to tan nodular masses composed of hyphae and arthroconidia	Hair	White piedra	Figure 29-14

polysaccharide but provides a dark background against which the capsular polysaccharide may be seen (Figure 29-1).

Other yeasts and patient cells may also be observed in the india ink preparation. *C. neoformans,* unlike other yeasts, possesses a narrow tubular neck between the parent cell and its blastoconidium. Occasionally red and white blood cells mimic yeasts. To distinguish *C. neoformans* from human cells, two approaches can be considered. Morphologically, *C. neoformans* possesses a rigid cell wall of chitin, whereas human cells are membrane bound. The examiner can simply look for the presence of a cell wall. Second, a drop of KOH can be added to another preparation. The KOH disrupts the human cell membrane but not the cell wall of *C. neoformans.*

We do not recommend that CSF be examined on either an

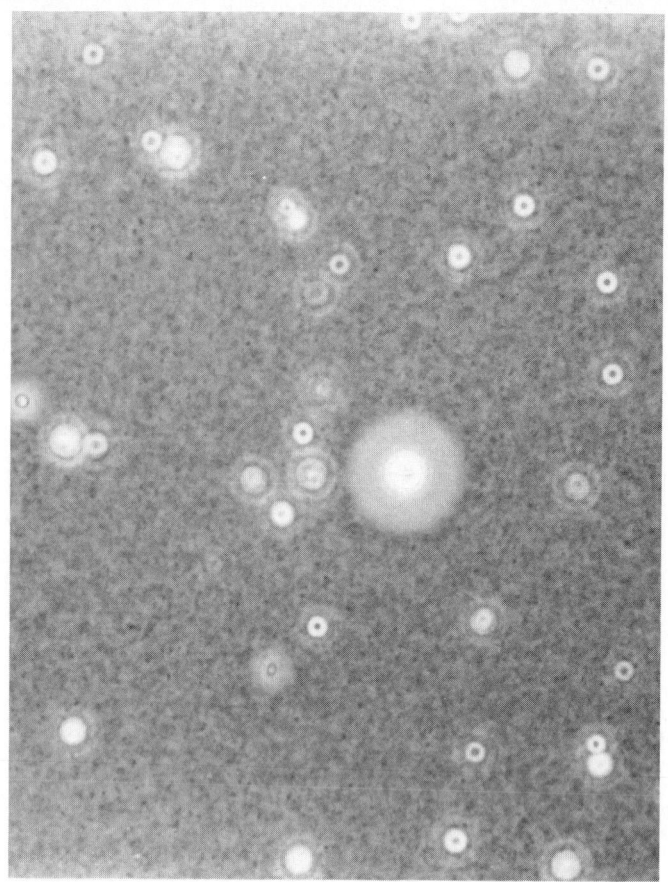

FIGURE 29-1. India ink preparation showing capsule surrounding round yeast cells of *Crypto-coccus neoformans*. Note how ink has created dark background that highlights colorless (hyaline) polysaccharide capsule.

emergency or a routine basis with india ink for the detection of *C. neoformans*. In patients with cryptococcosis involving the meninges, only approximately 50% of these patients have at least one positive india ink examination of their CSF.[18] Both culture and the cryptococcal latex test for polysaccharide should be requested. The cryptococcal latex serodiagnostic test should be the emergency procedure of choice.

The india ink preparation is often used to help physicians monitor therapy for crytococcosis but has limited value in this situation. Yeast cells may be detected for years in the CSF of patients with no indications of infection.[4] If yeast cells are killed by antifungal agents during the budding process, blastoconidia can remain attached to their parent cells. Thus the presence or absence of attached blastoconidia at the end of therapy cannot be used as a reliable indicator of biologic cure. Cultures and serologic tests are needed. The india ink preparation is solely a method of observation; it cannot be used for specific identification.

GIEMSA STAIN

The Giemsa stain can be used for the detection of *Histoplasma capsulatum* in bone marrow smears or other specimens (Plate 23, *F*). Wright stain may be used for the same purpose. Quality control slides must be included whenever the Giemsa stain is used.

HISTOPATHOLOGIC STAINS

The microbiologist should not overlook the cytology laboratory as a source of stained smears. The same specimens received in the microbiology laboratory are also submitted to the cytology laboratory for examination. The cytology, surgical pathology, and microbiology laboratories must work closely together.

Many stains are available for histopathologic identification of fungi. The PAS stain previously discussed is an example. Other common stains include the following:

1. Gomori methenamine–silver nitrate stain sharply outlines fungi in black because silver is precipitated on their cell walls.[8] The internal parts of hyphae are deep rose to black, and the background is light green (Plate 24, *A*). If the fungus is dark black, the section was not stained properly.
2. Gridley stain stains hyphae and yeasts dark blue or rose, tissues deep blue, and backgrounds yellow.[7]
3. Mayer mucicarmine stain stains capsules of *Cryptococcus neoformans* a deep rose.[17] Capsules often appear in a starburst shape (Plate 24, *B*).

FLUORESCENT ANTIBODY STAINS

Immunofluorescence microscopy, or fluorescent antibody (FA) staining, can be effectively used to detect fungi and acti-

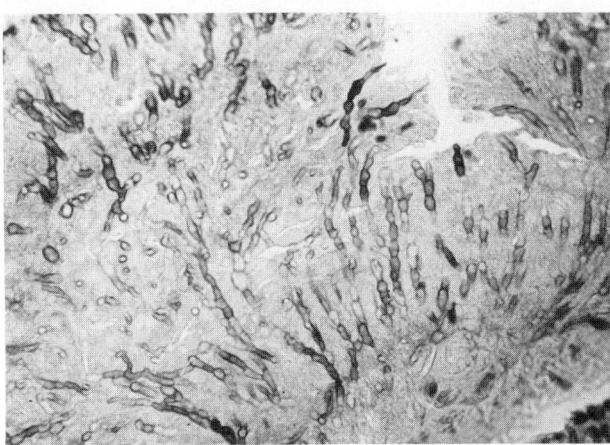

FIGURE 29-2. Gomori methenamine-silver stain of biopsy specimen from foot of patient with mycetoma. Some of the mycelial strands of *Madurella mycetomatis,* the etiologic agent, contain vesicles.

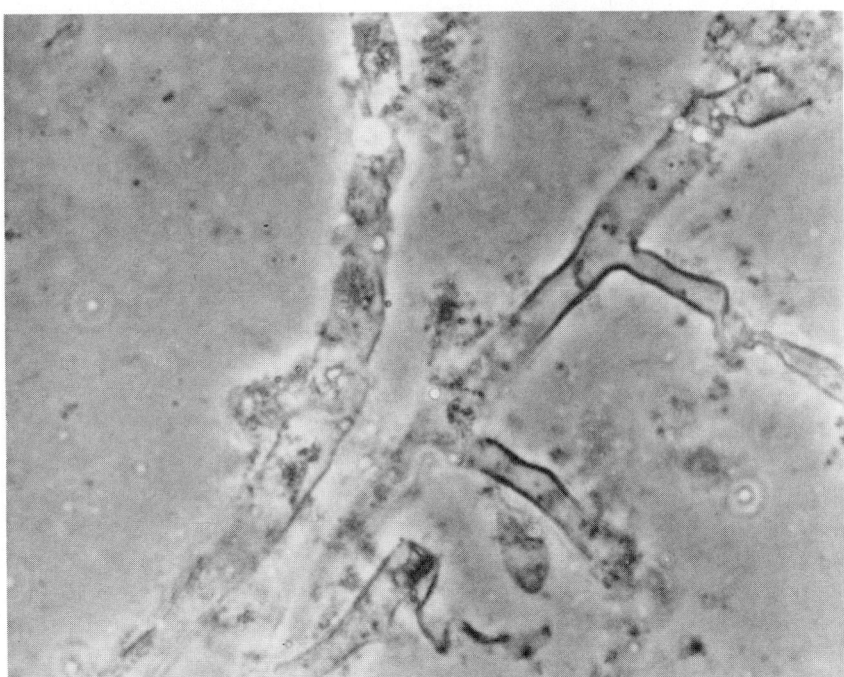

FIGURE 29-3. Large branching hyphae of *Cunninghamella* (a zygomycete) in sputum of patient with zygomycosis. (Potassium hydroxide preparation.)

nomycetes directly in tissue or fluids. The technique is simple, sensitive, and extremely specific. FA staining has been used to detect *Actinomyces* spp., *Histoplasma capsulatum, Coccidioides immitis, Cryptococcus neoformans, Pseudallescheria boydii, Blastomyces dermatitidis, Sporothrix schenckii, Aspergillus* spp., *Candida* spp., and *Paracoccidioides brasiliensis,* as well as several other fungi.[13]

PAPANICOLAOU SMEAR

The Papanicolaou (Pap) smear, particularly on sputum, can provide a good initial differentiation of the dimorphic fungi.

SPECIMEN PROCESSING

Appropriate processing of clinical specimens (Table 29-3) is important to ensure the recovery of potential pathogenic fungi. Processing should not be delayed because the viability of fungi decreases with time.

It is not necessary to concentrate most mycologic specimens. However, if respiratory secretions such as sputum are highly viscous, mucolytic agents such as *N*-acetyl-L-cysteine, dithiothreitol (sputolysin), or sterile saline with L-cysteine may be added. These agents liquefy the secretions and facilitate plating. There is little evidence, however, to suggest that concen-

Text continued on p. 547.

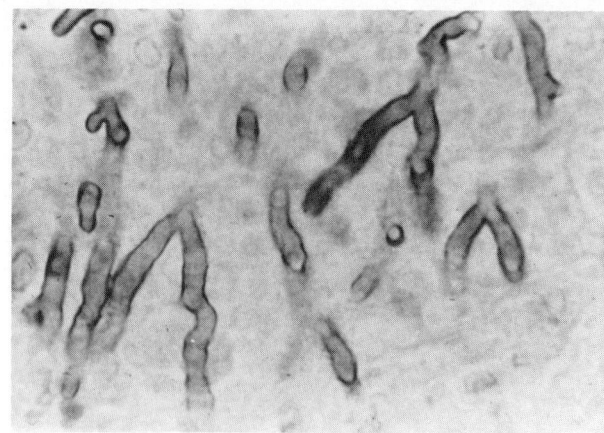

FIGURE 29-4. Septate, dichotomous branching hyphae of *Aspergillus* in lung tissue.

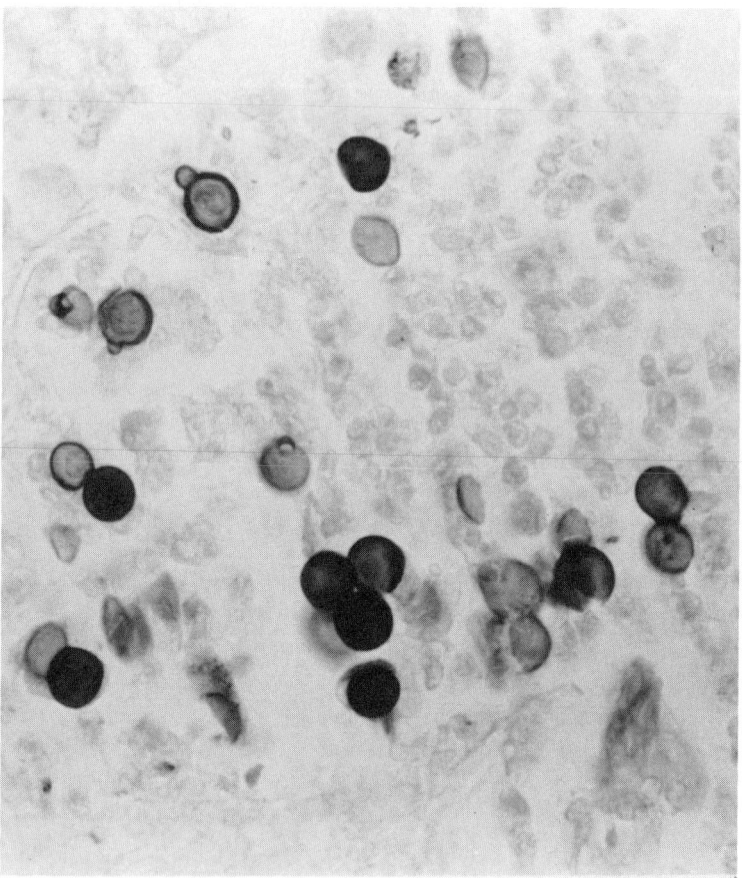

FIGURE 29-5. Gomori methenamine-silver stain of lung tissue of patient with blastomycosis. Note broad base of attachment of blastoconidia of *Blastomyces dermatitidis*.

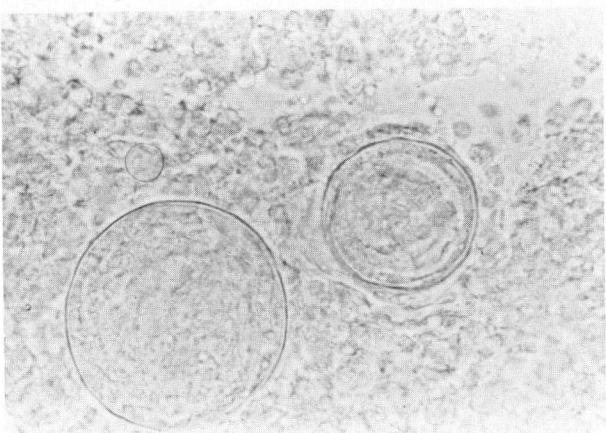

FIGURE 29-6. Thick-walled spherules of *Coccidioides immitis* in sputum. (From CDC Mycology Collection C-73780.)

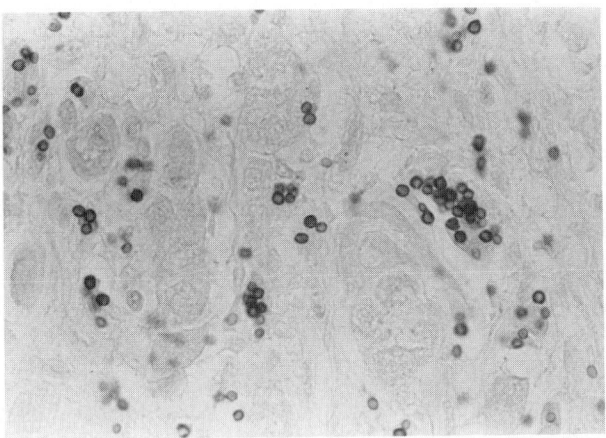

FIGURE 29-7. Small intracellular oval yeast cells of *Histoplasma capsulatum* in Gomori methenamine-silver-stained tissue.

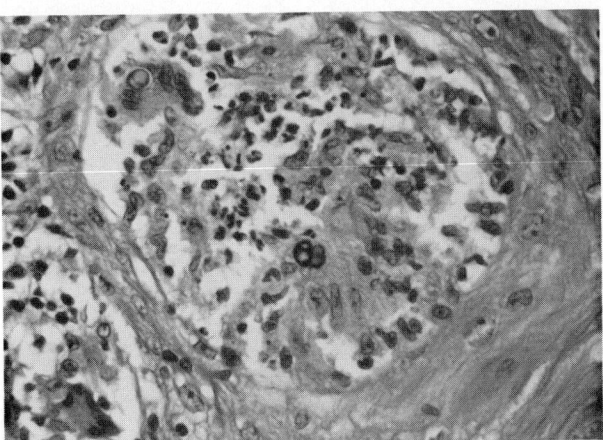

FIGURE 29-8. Hematoxylin and eosin stain of subcutaneous microabscess showing thick-walled chestnut brown spherical cells and sclerotic bodies of *Fonsecaea pedrosoi*.

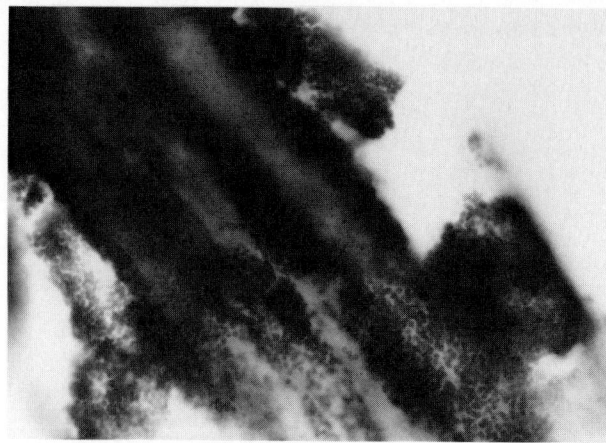

FIGURE 29-9. Periodic acid–Schiff (PAS) stain of ectothrix hair invasion by *Microsporum canis*. Note that arthroconidia are within and outside hair shaft. Cuticle of hair is damaged.

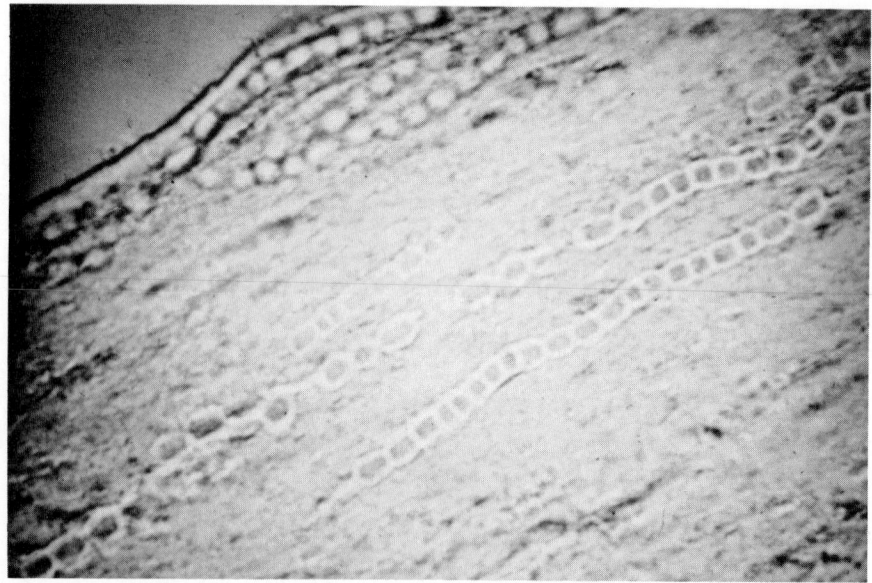

FIGURE 29-10. Endothrix hair invasion of *Trichophyton tonsurans*. Note arthroconidia within hair shaft. (Courtesy L. Ajello.)

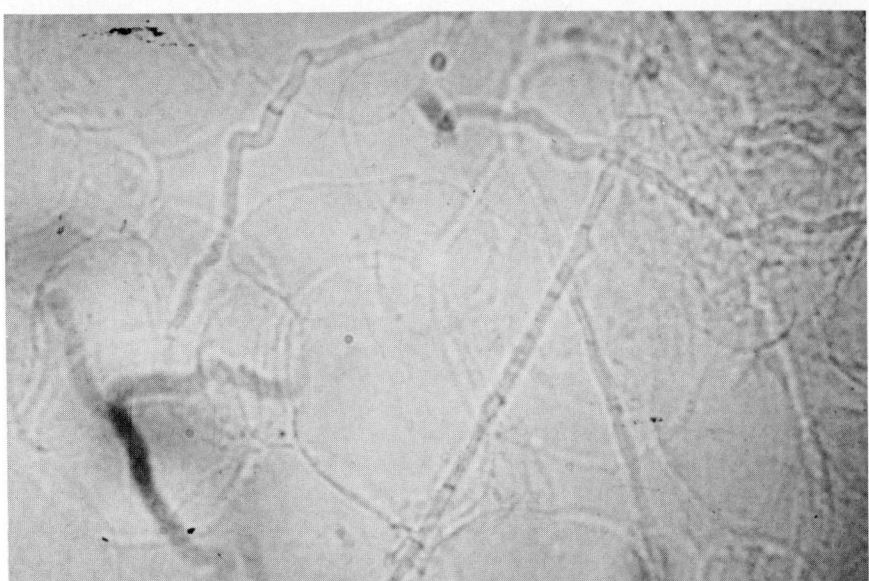

FIGURE 29-11. Hyaline hyphae of *Epidermophyton floccosum* in skin scrapings mounted in 15% potassium hydroxide.

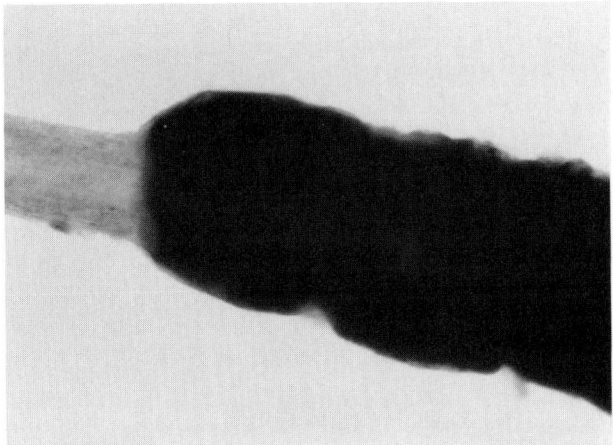

FIGURE 29-12. Hard carbonaceous nodule of *Piedraia hortae* surrounding hair shaft.

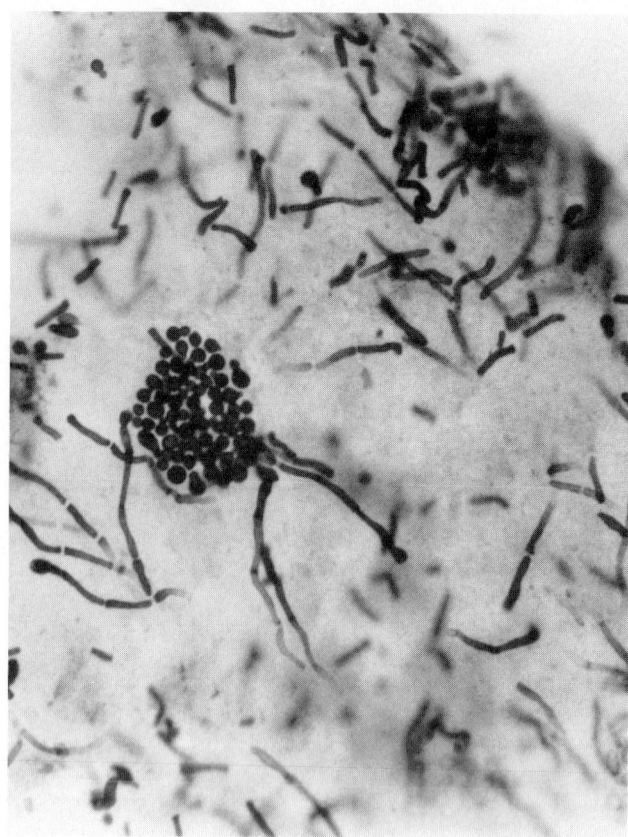

FIGURE 29-13. Periodic acid–Schiff (PAS) stain of skin showing bottle-shaped yeast cells of *Malassezia furfur*, indicative of pityriasis versicolor.

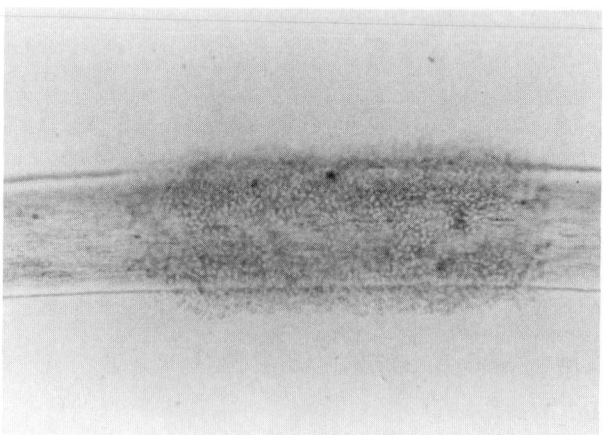

FIGURE 29-14. White piedra. Note white to tan nodular masses produced by *Trichosporon beigelii*. (Courtesy L. Ajello.)

TABLE 29-3. Guidelines for Processing Clinical Specimens

Clinical Specimen	Processing
Blood	Blood specimens may be inoculated directly to biphasic vented culture bottles or Bactec 6A bottles, or concentrated by lysis-centrifugation with the DuPont Isolator; Isolator is recommended because it increases detection of fungemia and decreases recovery time
Bone marrow	Directly inoculate aspirate to isolation media; if specimen is small, inoculate to nutrient broth
Cerebrospinal fluid	Filter through 0.45 μm membrane, and place filter on medium (inoculated side up); may concentrate specimen by centrifugation at 1000 × g for 15 min and culture sediment; can inoculate small quantities directly to nutrient broth or agar
Ear	Directly inoculate to isolation media
Eye	Directly inoculate ocular aspirates to isolation media; scrapings are plated in operating room as C-shaped cuts on medium surface
Hair, nail, and skin	Grind nail in mortar or nail-pulverizing mill before inoculating isolation media; directly inoculate hair and skin
Oral cavity scrapings	Directly inoculate scrapings to isolation media

TABLE 29-3. Guidelines for Processing Clinical Specimens—cont'd

Clinical Specimen	Processing
Respiratory secretions (sputum, aspirates, and washings)	Concentrate bronchoscopy specimens by centrifugation, and inoculate 0.5 ml of sediment to each medium; viscous specimens can be liquefied with small amount of N-acetyl-L-cysteine or dithiothreitol; NALC-NaOH is not used; areas that are caseous, necrotic, bloody, and so on are directly inoculated to isolation media
Sterile fluids (peritoneal, pleural, synovial)	Concentrate by centrifugation and inoculate at least 0.5 ml of sediment to each medium
Tissue	Selectively inoculate areas that are caseous, necrotic, or bloody directly to isolation media; mince or homogenize tissue; homogenize with tissue homogenizer, Stomacher, or mortar and pestle; if tissue is homogenized, small amount of saline or nutrient broth can be added to prepare 20% tissue solution; if zygomycete infection is suspected, mince tissue
Urine	Concentrate by centrifugation and inoculate 0.5 ml of sediment to each isolation medium
Vaginal	Directly inoculate specimens to isolation media

tration and decontamination of respiratory specimens improve the yield of fungi. Furthermore, some of the harsh treatments (for instance, NALC-NaOH) used for concentration of sputum for mycobacteria significantly reduce the yield of fungi. We do not recommend concentrating respiratory specimens for the recovery of fungi.

Heavily contaminated specimens, such as sputum, urine, and tissue, may be decontaminated by direct addition of antimicrobials or by plating on an antimicrobial-containing agar. Cycloheximide, penicillin, chloramphenicol, and streptomycin are frequently used, but some fungi are sensitive to cycloheximide, and the yeast form of *Histoplasma* spp. is sensitive to chloramphenicol. Yeast extract–phosphate agar is an excellent medium for contaminated respiratory specimens because bacteria and saprophytic yeasts are inhibited, whereas the systemic fungi are not.[27] The actinomycetes are also susceptible to most cell wall–active antimicrobial agents. These microorganisms are usually recovered in the mycobacteriology laboratory.

CULTURAL PROCEDURES

Although, with few exceptions, the direct examination of patient specimens rapidly yields important data, specimens must be cultured to identify the fungus. As in bacteriology, several types of media have been proposed for a variety of

purposes. The selection of isolation media is based primarily on personal choice.

PRIMARY ISOLATION MEDIA

As discussed in Chapter 28, fungi require carbon and nitrogen, as well as many other elements. The carbon source provided in many media is glucose because all fungi seem able to use this compound. Major nitrogen sources may include nitrate, nitrite, ammonium, urea, amino acids, and other compounds. Frequently the nitrogen source in the culture medium must be converted by the fungus into an amino acid to be used.

Other essential vitamins, minerals, and amino acids are included in the peptone of the medium. Although a number of solidifying agents are used in microbiology (agar, agarose, gelatin, and polyacrylamide and silica gels), most solid media for fungi contain agar.

Media may be enriched, selective, or differential. An enrichment medium is usually nonselective and is designed to promote the growth of microorganisms. Blood products or other body fluids, such as ascitic fluid, are often added to enrichment media. Enrichment media must not be confused with transport media, which are designed to maintain the specimen in its original condition but not to promote growth of microorganisms.

Maintenance media, on the other hand, usually do not stimulate optimal growth but are designed to maintain microorganisms in a static state. Selective agents are not included in maintenance media. When sugars must be added to maintenance media, buffers are also added to prevent pH shifts that might prove harmful.

Sabouraud Dextrose Agar

This medium was developed by Sabouraud in the late 1800s and initially used crude peptone as a nitrogen source and either maltose or honey as a carbon source. Growth of most fungi was adequate, and bacteria were inhibited by the low pH (4.5 to 5). These natural ingredients have been replaced by refined peptone and dextrose. Emmons and co-workers[5] noted that the carbohydrate content (4%) of Sabouraud's medium was too high and the pH (5.6) was too low for optimal growth of many fungi. The Emmons modification of the Sabouraud dextrose agar (SDA) medium reduced the dextrose content to 2%, and the final pH of the medium was raised to 6.8 to 7.[5] Because many bacteria can grow at the neutral pH of the medium, a selective medium is formed by the inclusion of cycloheximide and chloramphenicol in the medium. The cycloheximide in SDA suppresses saprophytic fungi, many of which may be opportunistic pathogens, and chloramphenicol inhibits most but not all bacteria. Cycloheximide also inhibits *Cryptococcus neoformans* and some species of *Candida*. Kobayashi and Pappagianis[14] reported that, in addition to *Cryptococcus* and *Candida* spp., *Aspergillus fumigatus*, *Trichosporon beigelii*, and *Pseudallescheria boydii* do not grow on media containing cycloheximide. Sabouraud dextrose agar (pH 6.8 to 7) containing these two antimicrobic agents is available commercially as Mycosel agar (BBL Diagnostics, Cockeysville, Md.) or Mycobiotic agar (Difco Laboratories, Detroit).

SDA with 4% dextrose and low pH is still used for studying colonial morphology of dermatophytes. Haley and Callaway[10] recommend the low pH SDA for the isolation and identification of dermatophytes if their keys are to be used.[10] Growth of dermatophytes at a neutral pH alters the gross morphology, as well as the pigment.

Brain Heart Infusion Agar

Some laboratories prefer brain heart infusion (BHI) agar over SDA as a general isolation medium for fungi. It may also be used for conversion of the dimorphic fungi *Blastomyces dermatitidis* and *Sporothrix schenckii* from mold form to yeast form. BHI agar is also commercially available. Antimicrobial agents and blood products may be added to the medium.

Inhibitory Mold Agar

Inhibitory mold agar (IMA) is used for the primary recovery of fungi from clinical specimens. It is commercially available from BBL. The medium is effective in preventing the growth of bacteria because it contains chloramphenicol. It is called IMA because it inhibits bacterial but not fungal growth.

SPECIAL MEDIA
Caffeic Acid Agar[11]

Caffeic acid agar is used to recognize *Cryptococcus neoformans*. On this medium *C. neoformans* produces melanin, which results in black colonies. The medium can be used to help selectively recover *C. neoformans* in mixed cultures. Caffeic acid agar is light sensitive and must be protected.

Birdseed Agar

Birdseed agar is useful for the isolation of *C. neoformans* from contaminated specimens, such as sputum. *C. neoformans* forms a brown melanin pigment on the medium, resulting from phenol oxidase activity.[2] However, other cryptococci may produce pigmentation after extended incubation.[19] Other fungi may grow on this medium but do not form a brown color.

KT Medium

KT medium (a Tween-albumin-niacin medium supplemented with 0.3% casamino acids) is used for the conversion of *Blastomyces dermatitidis* to its yeast form.[12]

Kelley Agar

Kelley agar is used for the conversion of the mycelial form of *Blastomyces dermatitidis* to its yeast form.[19]

Modified Converse Liquid Medium (Levine Modification)

Converse liquid medium[3] (Levine's modification[16]) promotes spherule production by *Coccidioides immitis* when incubated at 40° C in a candle jar. At 40° C, spherules containing endospores are produced but arthroconidia are not. To ensure that the isolate is not a species of *Malbranchea*, endospores must be present in the spherules. At elevated temperatures, *Malbranchea* spp. may produce vesicles that superficially resemble spherules because of their size and shape. The vesicles do not contain endospores.

OTHER MEDIA

Additional media that are used for the isolation and identification of fungi are summarized in Table 29-4.

Table 29-5 outlines general guidelines for media selection for isolation of fungi from clinical specimens. It should be remembered that the choice of media varies depending on geographic location, endemicity of specific fungal diseases, and personal choice. For example, yeast extract–phosphate agar may not be used routinely by laboratories on the East Coast of the United States but would be used in states such as Kentucky because of the prevalence of the dimorphic fungus *Histoplasma capsulatum*. In summary, no single set of media is universal.

ENVIRONMENTAL REQUIREMENTS FOR FUNGAL ISOLATION

Cultures for fungi are incubated at either 30° C or at room temperature (22° to 25° C). A temperature of 30° C is recommended because nearly all of the pathogenic fungi grow better and more rapidly at this temperature. Incubation of primary isolation media at 35° to 36° C should not be used, since it may actually inhibit or greatly retard the growth of some pathogenic fungi. However, incubation of supplemental media at higher temperatures may be useful in some situations. *Aspergillus fumigatus*, for example, is thermotolerant and may be distinguished from other *Aspergillus* spp. by growth at 45° C.

As discussed in Chapter 28, dimorphic fungi may grow as yeasts or as spherules at 37° C or in tissue and as molds at

TABLE 29-4. Supplemental Media for Isolation and Identification of Fungi

Medium	Purpose or Interpretation
Cornmeal agar[5]	Enhances production of distinctive chlamydospores by *Candida albicans;* generally useful for conidiation of fungi[a]
Cornmeal agar with 1% dextrose[10]	Enhances pigment production by *Trichophyton rubrum*
Potato dextrose agar[5]	Enhances conidiation of fungi
Sabhi medium[10]	Isolation medium for *Histoplasma capsulatum;* not satisfactory for mold to yeast conversion; recommended for isolation primarily from sputum
Yeast extract–phosphate agar[27]	Isolation of *Blastomyces dermatitidis* and *H. capsulatum* from contaminated respiratory specimens
18% V-8 juice agar[21]	Induces conidiation of dematiaceous molds
Rice extract agar	Enhances chlamydospore production by *Candida albicans* and studying yeast morphology
Serum[18]	Production of germ tubes by *C. albicans*
Christensen urea agar[19]	Used for the detection of urease activity
Trichophyton agars[6]	Used for selective identification of specific *Trichophyton* spp.

TABLE 29-4. Supplemental Media for Isolation and Identification of Fungi—cont'd

Medium	Purpose or Interpretation
Cottonseed agar[10] and KT medium[12]	Excellent medium for mold to yeast conversion of *B. dermatitidis*
Auxanographic agar for nitrogen assimilation tests[10]	Basal medium lacking source of nitrogen; peptone disk is used as positive control because all yeasts can utilize peptone as nitrogen source; medium is used to test ability of yeast to use nitrate as sole nitrogen source
Dermatophyte test medium (DTM)[26]	Designed to recover dermatophytes from keratinized clinical specimens heavily contaminated with bacteria and fungi; either Mycosel Agar or Mycobiotic Agar is equivalent to DTM[20]; we do not recommend this medium because it is expensive and morphology of recovered fungi is generally atypical
Aspergillus differential medium[1]	Used for identification of *Aspergillus flavus;* enhances reverse pigment production
Malt extract agar[19]	Good for isolation of zygomycetes and identification of *Aspergillus* spp.

[a]Conidiation refers to the making of conidia, whereas conidiogenesis is the method of conidia formation.

TABLE 29-5. Guidelines for Media Selection for Primary Isolation of Fungi from Clinical Specimens[a]

Clinical Specimens	Brain Heart Infusion Agar			Inhibitory Mold Agar	Mycosel or Mycobiotic	Sabhi Agar	Yeast Extract–Phosphate Agar[27]
	Plain	Blood	Antimicrobics				
Blood[b]	+	+		+			
Bone marrow[c]	+	+		+			
Cerebrospinal fluid	+			+			
Ear	+			+			
Eye	+		+	+			
Hair, nail, skin				+	+		
Oral cavity scrapings	+			+			
Respiratory secretions (sputum, aspirates, and washings)	+			+		+	+

Continued.

TABLE 29-5. Guidelines for Media Selection for Primary Isolation of Fungi from Clinical Specimens[a]—cont'd

| Clinical Specimens | Brain Heart Infusion Agar | | | Inhibitory Mold Agar | Mycosel or Mycobiotic | Sabhi Agar | Yeast Extract–Phosphate Agar[27] |
	Plain	Blood	Antimicrobics				
Sterile fluids (peritoneal, pleural, and synovial)	+	+		+			
Tissue	+			+			
Urine	+			+			
Vaginal	+			+			

SYMBOL: +, Appropriate choice

[a]These are general guidelines only. Specific choice of medium is based on types of fungi recovered, which varies depending on geographic area, types of patients, and so on.
[b]Blood processed with DuPont Isolator.
[c]Nutrient broth for small specimen.

25° C. This ability to grow in two different forms at two different temperatures is used to distinguish dimorphic fungi from other morphologically similar fungi. Although these organisms do grow at 37° C, they often grow slowly at this temperature. Thus it is preferable to isolate them initially at 30° C. Initial isolation, incubated at 35° to 36° C, is not cost effective because it does not provide an isolation advantage over media incubated only at 30° C.

Although isolation plates should be sealed and tubes capped, they can dry out after extended incubation if humidity is not high enough. Either incubators should be humidity controlled or water should be placed in a pan in the incubator.

IDENTIFICATION OF FUNGI
OBSERVATION OF COLONIAL MORPHOLOGY

Fungal cultures should be incubated for at least 4 weeks before they are discarded as negative. Because yeasts grow faster than molds, yeast colonies are usually evident within 2 to 3 days after inoculation. The yeast colony should be transferred to another medium and the original isolation plates reincubated to ensure that no other fungi are present. An inoculated primary isolation plate should *never* be discarded until the initial plate has been incubated for the maximum time period.

During the observation of a fungal colony, several items should be noted, including colony size, topography, pigment, color, and texture. The color of a colony can vary depending on media, temperature, and time of incubation, as well as the inherent biologic characteristics of the fungus. Colors range from gray-black to bright yellow, green, and red. Dematiaceous refers to colonies that are olive, brown, or black. All other colors are considered nondematiaceous. The dark color is a result of melanin in the cell walls of the hyphae, conidia, or both. Fungi, such as *Penicillium* spp., may form colored droplets of exudate on the colony surface. Some fungi produce diffusible pigments that color the growth medium.

MICROSCOPIC EXAMINATION

Once colonial observations have been made and recorded, the identification of the fungus can usually be narrowed to one of several groups. At this point microscopic examination is necessary. A lactophenol cotton blue teased preparation, a slide culture, a coverslip culture, or a transparent tape preparation is used.

Teased Preparation

For the adequate study of conidia and conidiophores, portions of their colonies must be "teased" apart with a bent dissecting needle or small insect-mounting pins in a needle holder.[19] A safety cabinet should *always* be used. Usually a sample is taken midway between the center and the edge of the colony. Then if no structures are seen, additional samples are collected closer to the center of the colony. The material is transferred to a drop of lactophenol cotton blue (LPCB) on a clean slide and teased apart with two needles. With a phase contrast microscope, lactophenol without cotton blue is used. A coverslip is applied and the preparation observed microscopically under both low and high power. Fungal elements that have taken up the cotton blue are readily visible. Although the LPCB kills the fungi, the slides should still be autoclaved before disposal. The slides may be preserved, however, by sealing the edges of the coverslip with clear nail polish around the edge of the coverslip.

Slide Culture

The slide culture is used when it is necessary to see how the conidia or spores are produced. Because a tease mount involves teasing the hyphae apart, conidiogenesis is often difficult to study. The slide culture permits the technologist to see clearly how and where the conidia and spores are produced. All procedures involving slide cultures should be performed in a biologic safety cabinet. Either lactophenol cotton blue or lactophenol without cotton blue is used as the mounting medium. Potato dextrose agar, cornmeal agar, or V-8 juice agar should be used as the growth medium.

1. Cover the bottom of a Petri dish with a piece of filter paper.
2. Place a bent V-shaped glass rod or bent V-shaped wooden applicator sticks on the filter paper.
3. Place a clean glass microscopic slide on the V-shaped rod.
4. Sterilize this setup by autoclaving at 121° C for 15 minutes. (If disposable plastic Petri dishes are used, the components are sterilized separately and then added to the Petri dish.)
5. Cut a sterile agar square (1 cm) out of the growth medium and place on a sterile glass slide on the side opposite the frosted edge. More than one kind of medium can be placed on a single sterile glass slide.
6. Inoculate the four sides of agar square with isolate.
7. Using sterile forceps, place a sterile coverslip on top of the agar square. The forceps is sterilized by passing through a flame.
8. Moisten the filter paper with 2 to 3 ml of sterile distilled water.
9. Incubate the slide culture in the dark at 22° to 25° C for approximately 2 weeks. It may be helpful to expose the setup to light for a day or so.
10. Add sterile water to the Petri dish if the culture begins to dry out.
11. When the slide culture has matured, remove the coverslip and quickly pass it through a flame to fix the structures. Add a drop of mounting medium to a clean microscope slide and place the coverslip at the edge of the drop of mounting fluid. Carefully lower the coverslip.
12. Discard the agar block from the microscope slide used in the slide culture setup. The microscope slide may be used as a second mount.
13. Gently heat the microscope slide, add a drop of mounting medium, and cover with a clean coverslip.
14. Seal both slide preparations by placing clear fingernail polish around the edges of the coverslips. Label the slides.

Transparent-Tape Preparation

The transparent-tape preparation should never be used for suspected dimorphic fungi. For other isolates, however, it is a rapid method for observing the undisturbed arrangement of conidia. Because the tape is not sterile, the isolate may become contaminated. The tape preparation should be made using a duplicate culture. The procedure follows:

1. Place a drop of LPCB on a slide.
2. Press transparent tape, sticky side down, on the surface of the mold colony and then onto the slide containing the LPCB.
3. Observe the slide microscopically and then discard it. This is a temporary preparation, and great care must be taken to avoid contamination of the fingers.

USE OF NONMORPHOLOGIC TESTS FOR IDENTIFICATION OF ACTINOMYCETES AND YEASTS

An organism cannot always be identified on a morphologic basis alone. Nutritional, physiologic, biochemical, and envi-

TABLE 29-6. Nonmorphologic Tests for Identification of Aerobic Actinomycetes

Test	Interpretation
Casein hydrolysis	*Streptomyces* positive; *Nocardia* negative
Growth on 0.4% gelatin	*Nocardia brasiliensis* positive; *Nocardia asteroides* negative
Gelatin liquefaction	Determines proteolytic ability by actinomycetes (see Chapter 30)
Litmus milk test	Determines peptonization and clot formation (see Chapter 30)
Paraffin bait[22]	Suggests *N. asteroides; N. asteroides* utilizes paraffin
Starch hydrolysis	*Actinomadura* spp. and *Streptomyces* spp. hydrolyze starch
Urease detection	*Nocardia* spp. and some *Streptomyces* spp. synthesize urease
Xanthine and tyrosine hydrolysis	Patterns of xanthine and tyrosine decomposition are of differential value (see Chapter 30)
Lysozyme resistance	*Nocardia* spp. is resistant to the lytic action of lysozyme
Cell wall analysis of sugars[15] and diaminopimelic acid (DAP)	Identification of aerobic actinomycetes is facilitated by determining cell wall sugars and isomers of DAP by thin-layer or paper chromotography

ronmental tolerance tests may be required. Table 29-6 lists non-morphologic tests used in the identification of the aerobic actinomycetes.

Whereas molds are identified primarily on the basis of morphology, yeasts are identified by a combination of morphologic and physiologic tests. Yeast morphology is studied on cornmeal agar or yeast morphology agar that is inoculated by the Dalmau method. Physiologic data are typically obtained by using a commercial yeast identification system. The traditional auxanographic technique and the Wickerham method are not the most appropriate methods for the clinical laboratory because of the time, expense, and experience required. The identification of yeasts is discussed in detail in Chapter 35.

IMMUNOLOGY

An extensive variety of serologic tests exists for the diagnosis of fungal disease. These include tests for antibodies, antigens, delayed hypersensitivity (skin tests), detection of fungal antigens in culture filtrates (exoantigens), and fluorescent antibody microscopy for fungal identification in tissue. A discussion of fungal immunology is presented in Chapter 36.

ANIMAL INOCULATION

The exoantigen test for the identification of fungi has virtually replaced the need for animal studies as a means of identifying clinical isolates. Animal inoculation is used in some reference centers primarily for isolation of fungi from environmental specimens, such as soil. Small laboratory animals, such as rats, mice, guinea pigs, and hamsters, are inoculated by one of a number of methods: intraperitoneal, intracerebral, intraocular, or intravenous. Necropsy studies are performed on the animals that die, as well as those that survive. The liver, spleen, lymph nodes, and lungs are cultured on appropriate media, and gross lesions are examined histopathologically. Extreme care should be taken when working with infected animals because the potential for laboratory-acquired infection exists.

Susceptibility Testing

Unless a large number of opportunistic infections are seen in the institution, susceptibility testing may not be a valuable procedure to offer. There is no standard method for testing antifungal agents, and furthermore there is no standard clinical correlation and interpretation of the data generated. Each institution tends to develop its own modified procedure, and the clinicians develop experience in using the minimal inhibitory concentration (MIC) values provided by the laboratory. Susceptibility testing is recommended for large medical centers and reference laboratories.

REFERENCES

1. Bothast, R.J., and Fennell, D.I.: A medium for rapid identification and enumeration of *Aspergillus flavus* and related organisms, Mycologia **66**:365, 1974.
2. Chaskes, S., and Tyndall, R.L.: Pigment production by *Cryptococcus neoformans* and other *Cryptococcus* species from aminophenols and diaminobenzenes, J. Clin. Microbiol. **7**:146, 1958.
3. Converse, J.L.: Effect of physico-chemical environment on spherulation of *Coccidioides immitis* in a chemically defined medium, J. Bacteriol. **72**:784, 1956.
4. Diamond, R.D., and Bennett, J.E.: Prognostic factors in cryptococcal meningitis: a study of 111 cases, Ann. Intern. Med. **80**:176, 1974.
5. Emmons, C.W., et al.: Medical mycology, ed. 3, Philadelphia, 1977, Lea & Febiger.
6. Georg, L.K., and Camp, L.B.: Routine nutritional tests for the identification of dermatophytes, J. Bacteriol. **74**:113, 1957.
7. Gridley, H.F.: A stain for fungi in tissue sections, Am. J. Clin. Pathol. **23**:303, 1953.
8. Grocott, R.G.: A stain for fungi in tissue sections and smears using Gomori's methenamine-silver nitrate technique, Am. J. Clin. Pathol. **25**:975, 1955.
9. Hageage, G.J., and Harrington, B.J.: Use of calcofluor white in clinical mycology, Lab. Med. **15**:109, 1984.
10. Haley, L.D., and Callaway, C.S.: Laboratory methods in medical mycology, ed. 4, Atlanta, 1978, U.S. Department of Health, Education and Welfare, HEW Pub. No. (CDC) 78-8361, Centers for Disease Control.
11. Hopfer, R.L., and Blank, F.: Caffeic-acid containing medium for identification of *Cryptococcus neoformans*, J. Clin. Microbiol. **2**:115, 1975.
12. Kane, J.: Conversion of *Blastomyces dermatitidis* to the yeast form at 37 degrees C and 26 degrees C, J. Clin. Microbiol. **20**:594, 1984.
13. Kaufman, L., and Reiss, E.: Serodiagnosis of fungal diseases. In Lennette, E.H., et al., editors: Manual of clinical microbiology, ed. 4, Washington, D.C., 1985, American Society for Microbiology.
14. Kobayashi, G.S., and Pappagianis, D.: Methods for study of medically important fungi. In Sonnenwirth, A.C., and Jarret, L., editors: Gradwohl's clinical laboratory methods and diagnosis, vol. 2, ed. 8, St. Louis, 1980, The C.V. Mosby Co.
15. Lechevalier, M.P., and Lechevalier, H.: Chemical composition as a criterion in the classification of aerobic actinomycetes, Int. J. Syst. Bacteriol. **20**:435, 1970.
16. Levine, H.B., Cobb, J.M., and Smith, C.E.: Immunity to coccidioidomycosis induced in mice by purified spherule, arthrospore, and mycelial vaccines, Trans. N.Y. Acad. Sci. **22**:436, 1960.
17. Mallory, F.B.: Pathological technique, Philadelphia, 1942, W.B. Saunders Co.
18. McGinnis, M.R.: Laboratory handbook of medical mycology, New York, 1980, Academic Press, Inc.
19. McGinnis, M.R.: Detection of fungi in cerebrospinal fluid, Am. J. Med. **75**(suppl. 1B):129, 1983.
20. McGinnis, M.R., and Kane, J.: Dermatologic mycology, Semin. Dermatol. **4**:227, 1985.
21. McGinnis, M.R., Rinaldi, M.G., and Winn, R.: Emerging pathogens of phaeohyphomycosis: the genera *Bipolaris* and *Exserohilum*, J. Clin. Microbiol., **24**:250, 1986.
22. Mishra, S.K., and Randhawa, H.S.: Application of paraffin bait technique to the isolation of *Nocardia asteroides* from clinical specimens, Appl. Microbiol. **18**:686, 1969.
23. Moore, G.S., and Jaciow, D.M.: Mycology for the clinical laboratory, Reston, Va., 1979, Reston Publishing Co., Inc.
24. Rico, H., Miragall, F., and Sentandreu, R.: Abnormal formation of *Candida albicans* walls produced by calcofluor white: an ultrastructural and stereologic study, Exp. Mycol. **9**:241, 1985.
25. Roberts, G.D., et al.: Detection and recovery of fungi in clinical specimens. In Lennette, E.H., et al.: Manual of clinical microbiology, ed. 4, Washington, D.C., 1985, American Society for Microbiology.
26. Rosenthal, S.A., and Furnari, D.: Efficacy of "dermatophyte test medium," Arch. Dermatol. **104**:486, 1971.
27. Smith, C.D., and Goodman, N.L.: Improved culture method for the isolation of *Histoplasma capsulatum* and *Blastomyces dermatitidis* from contaminated specimens, Am. J. Clin. Pathol. **63**:276, 1975.
28. Tilton, R.C.: The laboratory approach to the detection of bacteremia, Annu. Rev. Microbiol. **36**:467, 1982.

CHAPTER 30

Pathogenic Aerobic Actinomycetes

Richard C. Tilton
Michael R. McGinnis

Actinomycetes are bacteria, not fungi. They are susceptible to antibacterial antimicrobics but not to antifungal agents. They are included in the mycology section of this book because their morphology superficially resembles that of fungi and they cause similar diseases. Actinomycetes are either aerobic or anaerobic. The anaerobic actinomycetes are discussed in Chapter 20. The most recent classification of the aerobic actinomycetes (Table 30-1) has been proposed by Goodfellow and Minnikin[7] and Mishra, Gordon, and Barnett.[18] The genus *Mycobacterium* is discussed in Chapter 26; the other genera are discussed in this chapter.

Aerobic actinomycetes form gram-positive, filamentous elements that tend to branch. These filaments are 0.5 to 1 μm in diameter and thus are smaller in diameter than fungal hyphae. Multiplication is by binary fission, sporulation, or fragmentation. The primary constituents of the cell wall are LL-diaminopimelic acid (DAP) and glycine; meso-DAP, arabinose, and galactose; and lysine, aspartic acid, and galactose. Because the composition of the actinomycete cell wall is extremely stable, analysis of the cell wall is a reliable means of identification.[15]

Some of the aerobic actinomycetes may be acid fast (*Nocardia* spp.), whereas others (*Streptomyces* spp.) may only have spores that are acid fast. Not all clinical isolates of *Nocardia* are acid fast. Acid fastness is a useful characteristic for identification of organisms in clinical specimens but is variable in work with cultures.

Micropolyspora, Micromonospora, and *Saccharopolyspora* spp. are thermophilic actinomycetes; that is, their optimal growth temperature is approximately 50° to 55° C. Members of these genera are rarely isolated in the clinical laboratory and can be only when special procedures and media are used. Diagnosis is most often made by detection of specific antibodies (IgE) to these organisms in patients' serum specimens. Lacey[14] has recently reviewed the characteristics of these organisms.

PATHOLOGY AND CLINICAL SIGNIFICANCE

The aerobic actinomycetes normally occur in the soil and are associated with plant material. Possibly they may be found in the dust of the hospital environment. These organisms cause a variety of diseases, including mycetoma and nocardiosis.

MYCETOMA

Several species of aerobic actinomycetes are responsible for mycetoma, a localized infection involving bone and cutaneous and subcutaneous tissue, and characterized by three features: swelling (tumefaction), draining sinuses, and granules.[21] Mycetoma can be caused by fungi as well as by actinomycetes;

disease associated with fungi is designated eumycotic mycetoma, and that associated with actinomycetes is designated actinomycotic mycetoma or actinomycetoma.

Actinomycotic mycetomas are chronic, granulomatous tumors containing granules composed of filaments that are approximately 1 μm in diameter. The tumor enlarges and penetrates deeper into the muscles between the laminae. Tumefaction occurs as suppurative and fibrotic reactions that take place in the subcutaneous tissue. Abscesses form and communicate with the surface, resulting in sinus tracts. When bone is involved, damage is frequently extensive. The process can spread to adjacent tissues by dissemination of filaments or granules or because of improper surgical management. Actinomycete granules are white, red, or yellow, ranging from 5 μm to 2 mm; they can be with or without cement and are soft to hard in texture. They are easily seen in hematoxylin and eosin (H and E) or Gomori methenamine-silver (GMS) stained tissue sections. An actinomycotic mycetoma must be differentiated from botryomycosis, which is caused by nonfilamentous bacteria (such as *Pseudomonas aeruginosa, Actinobacillus lignieresii,* and *Staphylococcus aureus*) and is a chronic, localized bacterial infection of the skin and subcutaneous tissues. When botryomycosis is suspected, tissue should be stained with a tissue Gram stain so the individual coccoid and bacillary forms can be seen more clearly.

The aerobic actinomycetes typically responsible for actinomycetoma are *Actinomadura madurae, Actinomadura pelletieri, Nocardia brasiliensis, Nocardia asteroides, Nocardia caviae,* and *Streptomyces somaliensis.*[17] Although the disease is distributed worldwide, various organisms may be associated with disease in different parts of the world.[17,21] *A. pelletieri* and *S. somaliensis* are most commonly associated with disease in Sudan and other African countries. *N. brasiliensis* and *A. madurae* are most common in Mexico.

The organisms causing actinomycetoma enter the body via trauma through breaks in the skin, most frequently on the feet. One of the aminoglycosides (streptomycin, gentamicin, or tobramycin) is used to treat actinomycotic mycetoma.[1]

NOCARDIOSIS

Members of the genus *Nocardia* may cause nocardiosis,[13] a localized or disseminated disease that usually originates in the lungs after inhalation of the organism. *N. asteroides* is the most common species causing nocardiosis; *N. caviae* and *N. brasiliensis* have also been associated with infection.[2,5,17] The pulmonary infection, which resembles tuberculosis, can remain confined to the lungs, or it may disseminate to various tissues, especially the brain and meninges.

TABLE 30-1. Classification of Aerobic Actinomycetes

Family	Genus	Representative Species
Dermatophilaceae	*Dermatophilus*	*D. congolensis*
Mycobacteriaceae	*Mycobacterium*	*M. tuberculosis*
Nocardiaceae	*Nocardia*	*N. asteroides, N. brasiliensis, N. caviae*
	Rhodococcus	*R. rhodochrous*
Streptomycetaceae	*Streptomyces*	*S. somaliensis*
Thermomonosporaceae	*Actinomadura*[a]	*A. madurae, A. pelletieri*
	Nocardiopsis[a]	*N. dassonvillei*[b]
	Micropolyspora	*M. faeni*
	Micromonospora	*M. chalcea*
	Saccharopolyspora	*S. viridis*

[a]Mishra, Gordon, and Barnett[18] have included *Actinomadura* and *Nocardiopsis* as members of the genus *Nocardia*. However, *Actinomadura* and *Nocardiopsis* are listed in the "Approved Lists of Bacterial Names"[22] as separate taxa.
[b]Previously classified as *Actinomadura dassonvillei*.

Nocardiosis is characterized by multiple and confluent abscesses and intense suppuration. The tissue response is typically an inflammatory reaction that is purulent and at times necrotizing. When the lungs are involved, the infection may extend to the pleura, which can result in empyema. Organisms tend to be more numerous in purulent and necrotic areas and predominantly intracellular in areas of granulomatous inflammation and fibrosing granulomatous tissue associated with abscesses.

In tissue the bacterium forms gram-positive branching filaments. Bacillary forms have been seen in nocardiosis and probably result from fragmentation of filaments.[6] The branching filaments and bacillary bodies in tissue can be demonstrated by histopathologic stains such as the Brown and Brenn stain (Plate 24, *C*) or GMS stain. Stains such as the periodic acid–Schiff (PAS) and H and E are not satisfactory. The organisms are also typically acid fast when stained with the modified Kinyoun or the CDC modified Fite-Faraco procedures. Non-acid-fast filaments in tissue, however, cannot be differentiated from *Actinomyces* spp. unless fluorescent antibody (FA) conjugates for *Actinomyces* spp. are used.

Nocardiosis is usually a disease of compromised hosts. Pulmonary and generalized infections are increasing in incidence, especially in patients receiving intensive chemotherapy, such as steroids and antineoplastic drugs. Among the underlying diseases are leukemia and lymphoma. Other predisposing conditions include pulmonary alveolar proteinosis, chronic lung disease, chronic ileitis and colitis, and cirrhosis.

Approximately 75% of nocardiosis cases occur in men. Fatality rates vary between 40% and 80%, depending on whether the disease is localized or disseminated and on the status of the patient and underlying disease. Sulfonamides or trimethoprim-sulfamethoxazole is the treatment of choice for nocardiosis.[16]

OTHER DISEASES

Members of the genus *Rhodococcus* are usually saprophytes; however, the organisms have been isolated from skin lesions and patients with pneumonia, bronchitis, and pericarditis.[11] Their role as causative pathogens is questionable.

Dermatophilus congolensis is the etiologic agent of dermatophilosis. This is primarily a disease of animals; however, humans may be accidental hosts through contact with diseased animals. The disease in humans resembles eczema and results in the formation of pustular lesions.[10] *D. congolensis* is unique because its fertile hyphae divide into compartments, in which motile zoospores are formed. The zoospores are then released into the environment.

Micropolyspora, Micromonospora, and *Saccharopolyspora* spp. are often implicated in allergic processes, such as farmer's lung (see Chapter 2) and chronic alveolar pneumonitis.

Several comprehensive reviews have been published on actinomycotic diseases,[4,8] and the reader is referred to them for details of the diseases.

LABORATORY DIAGNOSIS
SPECIMEN COLLECTION AND PROCESSING

The laboratory is aided in their isolation and identification of aerobic actinomycetes if clinical information is available that suggests a diagnosis of either nocardiosis or actinomycotic mycetoma. Whether or not such information is available, the tissue or biopsy specimens must be grossly searched for granules. Their presence indicates a mycetoma. If granules are noted in the specimen, they are teased from it and crushed for microscopic examination. If granules are not observed macroscopically, the tissue should be teased apart and macerated in sterile saline before direct examination and culture. Tissue specimens to be examined for *Nocardia* organisms may be very small, especially if they are collected by needle biopsy. Sterile saline, 0.25 to 0.5 ml, should also be added to these specimens before maceration.

The decision whether to concentrate respiratory specimens as for mycobacterial specimens (see Chapter 26) depends on the practices of the laboratory. In our experience the actinomycetes have been recovered from both concentrated and nonconcentrated specimens. If the volume is sufficient, cerebrospinal fluid specimens should be concentrated by centrifugation. Small volumes may be plated directly. Concentration of urine specimens by centrifugation makes recovery of organisms more probable.

TABLE 30-2. Direct Microscopic Appearance of Specimens in Which Aerobic Actinomycetes May Be Present

Specimen	Appearance	Possible Cause
Pus and respiratory secretions (suspected nocardiosis)	Granules absent; variably acid-fast, gram-positive, irregularly stained, beaded, branched filaments (0.5-1 μm in diameter); filaments may be clumped or scattered	*Nocardia asteroides, Nocardia brasiliensis, Nocardia caviae*
Tissue (suspected mycetoma)	Granules present; when crushed, reveal clumped, intertwined, branching, variably acid-fast, gram-positive filaments; description of granules:	
	0.5-5 mm, white, soft	*Actinomadura madurae*
	0.3-0.5 mm, red, soft to hard	*Actinomadura pelletieri*
	0.5-2 mm, yellow, hard	*Streptomyces somaliensis*
	15-200 mm, white, soft	*N. brasiliensis, N. caviae, Nocardiopsis dassonvillei*

In general, specimens should be fresh and not an accumulation of several specimens. Specimens should not be collected with swabs, since they rarely contain enough clinical material for appropriate microscopy and culture procedures. Furthermore, tissue or organisms may become entangled in the swab fibers. If specimens cannot be plated immediately, they should be refrigerated.

DIRECT EXAMINATION OF SPECIMENS

All specimens should be examined under wet mount as well as stained by the Gram method. All actinomycetes are gram positive, but some actinomycetes, such as *Nocardia* spp., may stain irregularly with more deeply staining granules observed in the filaments. This gives the filament a beaded appearance. *N. brasiliensis* may occur as gram-positive cocci or rods in clinical specimens.

An acid-fast stain should be performed on all specimens from which *Nocardia* spp. are suspected. Because *Nocardia* spp. are weakly acid fast or not acid fast, a weak decolorizing agent must be used with acid alcohol and should not be left in place for more than 10 seconds.

Table 30-2 describes granules and other structures that are seen in direct examination and may be of diagnostic significance.

CULTURE AND ISOLATION

Specimens should be inoculated onto 7H10 agar, Lowenstein-Jensen agar, and brain heart infusion (BHI) agar. Agar containing chloramphenicol should *not* be used because it inhibits the actinomycetes. The plates should be well sealed with parafilm. One 7H10 plate and a BHI plate without antibiotics are incubated at 35° C.[12] The other plates and slants are incubated at room temperature (22° to 25° C). The cultures are held for 4 weeks before discarding.

The paraffin-baiting technique is an enrichment culture method for initial isolation of *N. asteroides* from selected clinical specimens.[19] After homogenization of the specimen (sputum, gastric washings) is performed, 2 ml of the homogenate is mixed with 5 ml of sterile yeast nitrogen base broth (BBL, Cockeysville, Md.). A glass rod is coated with paraffin and

sterilized by immersion in 95% ethanol overnight. The rod is then placed in the diluted sample and incubated at 35° C. *N. asteroides* organisms use the paraffin as a carbon source and grow on the side of the glass rod. The specimen should be incubated for 6 weeks before being discarded.

The colonial morphology of the aerobic actinomycetes is summarized in Table 30-3. An acid-fast stain should be performed on all isolates suspected to be from the genus *Nocardia*. It should be noted, however, that acid fastness is variable among *Nocardia* isolates, and although the presence of acid fastness is highly suggestive of this organism, a negative result from an isolated colony has little value. Acid fastness may be enhanced if the organism is grown in litmus milk or on Lowenstein-Jensen agar.

PHYSIOLOGIC TESTING

Morphology alone does not distinguish the aerobic actinomycetes, especially members of the genera *Nocardia*, *Actinomadura*, and *Streptomyces*. Physiologic testing is necessary.

Physiologic tests that may be used to differentiate these genera and that are within the capabilities of many laboratories include hydrolysis of casein, xanthine, hypoxanthine, and tyrosine, fermentation of carbohydrates, and resistance to lysozyme (Table 30-4).[18]

Physiologic tests using carbohydrates to test for the production of acid should be performed by the method of Mishra, Gordon, and Barnett.[18]

Resistance to lysozyme is determined by inoculating both quality control and test lysozyme broths. *Streptomyces* spp. may be used as a control to ensure that the lysozyme is active. All tubes should be incubated at room temperature. Growth of the *Nocardia* spp. is usually in pellicle form but occasionally is granular in the bottom of the tube. Procedures for the preparation of the differential media listed in Table 30-4 are included in Appendix B.

Other tests, such as analysis of diaminopimelic acid isomers and cell wall sugars, require greater sophistication and are usually performed in large university laboratories, reference centers, and laboratories specializing in the actinomycetes. For

TABLE 30-3. Colonial Appearance of Aerobic Actinomycetes[a]

Genus and Species	Macroscopic Appearance[b]	Microscopic Appearance[c]
Actinomadura		Fine, intertwining, branched filaments with delicate aerial hyphae; nonfragmenting and may form short chains of spores
A. madurae	Waxy, heaped, folded, membranous, and tough; white, tan, pale orange, pink, or red	
A. pelletieri	Heaped, irregular, waxy, and granular; areas of bright and dark red; sparse aerial hyphae	
Mycobacterium		Do not show aerial filaments
Nocardia (N. asteroides, N. brasiliensis, N. caviae)	Orange colonies, glabrous, heaped, and folded; may also be white to pink with aerial hyphae; dry, crumbly, and adherent (Figure 30-1)	Fine, intertwining, branched filaments with delicate aerial hyphae; may have hyphal fragmentation to produce spores from aerial hyphae
Nocardiopsis dassonvillei	Orange colonies, glabrous, heaped, and folded; may also be white to pink with aerial hyphae; dry, crumbly, and adherent	
Rhodococcus		Do not show aerial filaments
Streptomyces somaliensis	Leathery, heaped, and folded; wide range of pigmentation from cream to brown-black; white aerial hyphae	Fine, intertwining, branched filaments with delicate aerial hyphae; nonfragmenting and often forms chains of spores

[a]On Sabouraud dextrose agar at 25° to 37° C.
[b]A dissecting microscope is best for macroscopic observation.
[c]Slide cultures must be set up if the original culture shows no aerial hyphae.

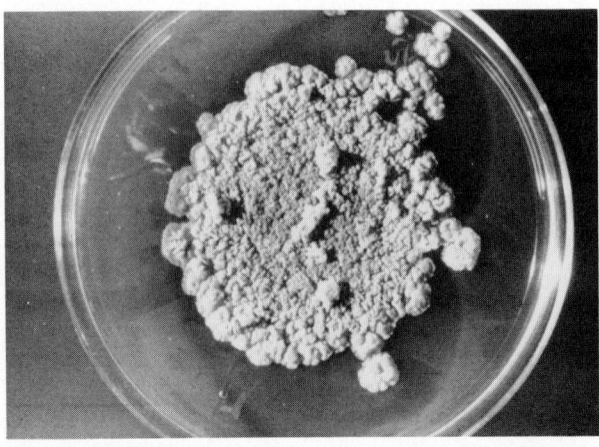

FIGURE 30-1. Dry, crumbly colonies of *Nocardia asteroides* on Sabouraud dextrose agar.

TABLE 30-4. Physiologic Characteristics of Certain Aerobic Actinomycetes

Test	*Actinomadura madurae*	*Actinomadura pelletieri*	*Nocardia asteroides*	*Nocardia brasiliensis*	*Nocardia caviae*	*Nocardiopsis dassonvillei*	*Streptomyces griseus*	*Streptomyces somaliensis*	*Streptomyces* Spp.[a]
Acid from:									
Arabinose	+	−	−	−	−	v	+[b]	−	v
Cellobiose	+	−	−	−	−	+	+	−	v
Inositol	v	−	−	+	+	−	v	−	v
Mannitol	+	−	−	+	+[c]	+	+	−	v
Xylose	+	−	−	−	−	v	+	−	v
Hydrolysis of:									
Casein	+	+	−	+	−	+	+	+	+
Gelatin	+	+	−	+	−	+	+	+	+
Hypoxanthine	+	+[b]	−	+	+	+	+	+	+
Tyrosine	+	+	−	+	v	+	+	+	+
Urea	−	−	+	+	+	v	+	−	v
Xanthine	−	−	−	−	+	+	+	−	+[d]
Lysozyme									
resistance	−	−	+	+	+	−	−	−	v
Cell wall type	IIIB	IIIB	IV	IV	IV	IIIC	I	I	I

> **Symbols:**   +, ≥90% of strains positive except where indicated
> −, ≥90% of strains negative
> v, Variable
> I, LL-diaminopimelic acid (DAP) plus glycine
> III, Meso-DAP
> IIIB, Meso-DAP plus 3-*O*-methyl-D-galactose (madurose)
> IIIC, Same as IIIB, except madurose is absent
> IV, Meso-DAP plus arabinose and galactose

Modified from Mishra, S.K., Gordon, R.E., and Barnett, D.A.: J. Clin. Microbiol. **11**:728, 1980.
[a]Includes *S. albus, S. lavendulae,* and *S. rimosus.*
[b]≥75% of strains positive.
[c]81% of strains positive.
[d]≥90% of *S. lavendulae* and *S. rimosus* positive; 86% of *S. albus* positive.

descriptions of these methods, one can refer to Becker and co-workers,[3] Haley and Callaway,[12] and the Lechevaliers.[15]

IMMUNOLOGY

The immunologic features of the aerobic actinomycetes are not well defined.[17] The aerobic actinomycetes, anaerobic actinomycetes, and mycobacteria share some common antigens in immunodiffusion and immunofluorescence tests.[9] All species have immunologically active polysaccharides, proteins, glycoproteins, and polypeptides, but none of these components has proved useful for either disease diagnosis or identification of the organism. Pier and Fichtner[20] separated *Nocardia* spp. on the basis of extracellular antigens into types I to IV; *N. asteroides* possessed antigen types I to III, and *N. brasiliensis* and *N. caviae* had type IV.

REFERENCES

1. Bach, M.C., Sabath, L.D., and Finland, M.: Susceptibility of *Nocardia asteroides* to 45 antimicrobial agents "in vitro," Antimicrob Agents Chemother. **3**:1, 1973.

2. Beaman, B.L., et al.: Nocardial infections in the United States, 1972-74, J. Infect. Dis. **134**:286, 1976.

3. Becker, B., et al.: Rapid differentiation between *Nocardia* and *Streptomyces* by paper chromatography of whole-cell hydrolysates, Appl. Microbiol. **12**:421, 1964.

4. Berd, D.: Laboratory identification of clinically important aerobic actinomycetes, Appl. Microbiol. **25**:665, 1973.

5. Causey, W.A.: *Nocardia caviae:* a report of 13 new isolations with clinical correlation, Appl. Microbiol. **28**:193, 1974.

6. Chandler, F.W., Kaplan, W., and Ajello, L.: Color atlas and textbook of the histopathology of mycotic diseases, London, 1980, Wolfe Medical Publications, Ltd.

7. Goodfellow, M., and Minnikin, D.E.: Nocardioform bacteria, Annu. Rev. Microbiol. **31**:159, 1977.

8. Goodman, J.S., and Koenig, M.G.: *Nocardia* infections in a general hospital, Ann. N.Y. Acad. Sci. **174**:552, 1970.

9. Gordon, M.A.: Aerobic pathogenic Actinomycetaceae. In Lennette, E.H., et al., editors: Manual of clinical microbiology, ed. 4, Washington, D.C., 1985, American Society for Microbiology.

10. Gordon, M.A., and Perrin, U.: Pathogenicity of *Dermatophilus* and *Geodermatophilus,* Infect. Immun. **4**:29, 1971.

11. Haburchak, D.R., et al.: Infections caused by *Rhodochrous,* Am. J. Med. **65**:298, 1978.

12. Haley, L.D., and Callaway, C.S.: Laboratory methods in medical mycology, ed. 4, U.S. Department of Health, Education and Welfare, Pub. No. (CDC) 78-8361, Atlanta, 1978, Centers for Disease Control.

13. Kurup, P.V., Randhawa, H.S., and Gupta, N.P.: Nocardiosis: a review, Mycopathol. Mycol. Appl. **40:**193, 1970.

14. Lacey, J.: Thermophilic actinomycetes: characteristics and identification, J. Allergy Clin. Immunol. **61:**231, 1978.

15. Lechevalier, M.P., and Lechevalier, H.: Chemical composition as a criterion in the classification of aerobic actinomycetes, Int. J. Syst. Bacteriol. **20:**435, 1970.

16. Maderazo, E.G., and Quintiliani, R.: Treatment of nocardial infection with trimethoprim and sulfamethoxazole, Am. J. Med. **57:**671, 1974.

17. Mishra, S.K., and Gordon, R.E.: *Nocardia* and *Streptomyces*. In Braude, A.I., Davis, C.E., and Fierer, J., editors: Infectious diseases and medical microbiology, ed. 2, Philadelphia, 1986, W.B. Saunders Co.

18. Mishra, S.K., Gordon, R.E., and Barnett, D.A.: Identification of nocardiae and streptomycetes of medical importance, J. Clin. Microbiol. **11:**728, 1980.

19. Mishra, S.K., and Randhawa, H.S.: Application of paraffin bait technique to the isolation of *Nocardia asteroides* from clinical specimens, Appl. Microbiol. **18:**686, 1969.

20. Pier, A.C., and Fichtner, R.E.: Serologic typing of *Nocardia asteroides* by immunodiffusion, Am. Rev. Respir. Dis. **103:**698, 1971.

21. Rippon, J.W.: Medical mycology: the pathogenic fungi and the pathogenic actinomycetes, ed. 2, Philadelphia, 1982, W.B. Saunders Co.

22. Skerman, V.D.B., McGowan, V., and Sneath, P.H.A.: Approved lists of bacterial names, Washington, D.C., 1980, American Society for Microbiology.

CHAPTER 31

Agents of Superficial Mycoses

Richard C. Tilton
Michael R. McGinnis

Superficial fungal infections involve the outer keratinized tissues (stratum corneum) of the skin and hair. Typically no inflammatory response or tissue destruction is present. The fungi grow in the outer layers of the skin or as masses of hyphae around hair shafts. The principal agents of superficial mycoses and their associated diseases include *Malassezia furfur*, the cause of pityriasis versicolor (tinea versicolor), *Phaeoannellomyces werneckii*, the cause of superficial phaeohyphomycosis (tinea nigra), *Trichosporon beigelii*, the cause of white piedra, and *Piedraia hortae*, the cause of black piedra.

PATHOLOGY AND CLINICAL SIGNIFICANCE
PITYRIASIS VERSICOLOR

Pityriasis versicolor, or tinea versicolor, as it was previously called, is a chronic superficial skin infection that occasionally involves the hair follicle. *M. furfur* causes other infections than just pityriasis versicolor. The yeast has been associated with folliculitis, which resembles cutaneous lesions of systemic candidiasis in compromised patients, seborrheic dermatitis, pityriasis capitis, pityriasis simplex, blepharitis, peritonitis, and fungemia in infants receiving fat emulsions intravenously.[14]

Pityriasis versicolor is characterized by spreading red or yellow to brown, slightly raised, scaly patches on the smooth skin of the arms, abdomen, and face.[7] The lesions are papular, nummular, or confluent, cosmetically disfiguring, and often itchy. On white-skinned individuals the lesions usually appear brownish, whereas on dark-skinned people they are lighter than the normal skin. These lesions fluoresce pale yellow under a Wood's lamp. It has been suggested that dicarboxylic acids produced by *M. furfur* may have a cytotoxic effect on melanocytes and subsequently are responsible for hypopigmentation.

Pityriasis versicolor occurs worldwide, but its incidence is highest in the tropics. Burke[2] and others have noted that excessive perspiration, malnutrition, poor hygiene, and pregnancy may predispose a person to this infection, which most often occurs in young adults. Other predisposing factors include high environmental temperature, high relative humidity, use of palm oils and other lipids on the body (especially in tropical areas), defects in production of lymphokines, genetic defects, hyperhidrosis, systemic corticosteroid therapy, and immunosuppressive therapy.[6]

Therapy for pityriasis versicolor can be approached in several ways. The simplest therapy is to wash the infected and adjacent areas with selenium disulfide or zinc pyrithione shampoo. Propylene glycol and the antifungal agents ketoconazole and itraconazole are also effective. Itraconazole seems to be a little less effective in studies of animals.[5]

The genus *Malassezia* includes two species, *M. furfur* and *M. pachydermatis*. *M. furfur* is a lipophilic yeast that requires exogenous fatty acids with C_{12} to C_{24} carbon chains. *M. pachydermatis*, an animal pathogen, does not require exogenous lipids and may be recovered on routine mycology media.

M. furfur is currently the accepted name for this species, as well as for the organisms previously designated *Pityrosporum orbiculare* and *Pityrosporum ovale*. The three names reflect different morphologic forms of the single yeast *M. furfur*. Indirect fluorescent antibody microscopy has revealed that these organisms are identical.[16] The name *Malassezia* is used rather than *Pityrosporum* because it is the earlier name for this yeast.

SUPERFICIAL PHAEOHYPHOMYCOSIS (TINEA NIGRA)

Superficial phaeohyphomycosis (tinea nigra) is an infection of the stratum corneum consisting of brown to black macules that are not scaly. *Phaeoannellomyces werneckii*,[10] which was previously known as either *Cladosporium werneckii* or *Exophiala werneckii*, is the principal cause of this infection. Superficial phaeohyphomycosis may rarely be caused by *Stenella araguata*. The early taxonomy of *Phaeoannellomyces* and *Cladosporium* is confusing. For additional information consult the publications of McGinnis[8] and McGinnis and Padhye.[9]

Superficial phaeohyphomycosis is characterized clinically by a sharply marginated single lesion that increases centrifugally in size. The lesion begins as a light brown macule that becomes darker as it grows larger. Palmar surfaces and the fingers are most commonly infected, but other areas—such as plantar surfaces, neck, and thorax—can be involved. Most patients are less than 19 years old, and females outnumber males 3 to 1. Superficial phaeohyphomycosis must be differentiated from melanoma, contact dermatitis, pigmentation of Addison's disease, and other conditions that it resembles.[4,17]

The infection is generally associated with tropical areas such as Africa, Central and South America, and Asia. Cases that have been reported in North America and Europe in many instances can be traced to visits to tropical areas. Most cases occur in people who live in or near warm coastal areas. The normal habitat and route of transmission to humans is unknown. Mok and co-workers have recovered *P. werneckii* from salted Amazonian fish[12] and showed that the fungus could withstand high salt conditions.[11]

Superficial phaeohyphomycosis caused by *P. werneckii* readily responds to keratolytic agents as Whitfield's ointment. Imidazoles such as miconazole and ketoconazole are also effective. If the infection recurs, it is believed that there was a new exposure.

PIEDRA

Piedra is a fungal infection of hair shafts. Depending on its appearance and cause, the disease is classified as either white piedra caused by *Trichosporon beigelii* or black piedra caused by *Piedraia hortae*.

White piedra occurs in tropical and, occasionally, temperate areas.[3] The hairs of the axilla, beard, scalp, and genital areas have white to tan nodular growths consisting of hyphae and arthroconidia (see Figure 29-14). The mycelium of *T. beigelii* grows inward and through the shaft to form irregularly spaced nodular swellings,[15] where the hair may break. The nodules are soft and can be easily stripped off the hair shaft by pulling the hair through two tightly pressed fingers. Several nodules may coalesce to form a large mass around the hair. White piedra must be differentiated from lice infestations and trichomycosis axillaris, which is caused by *Corynebacterium tenuis*. *T. beigelii* forms hyphae 2 to 4 μm in diameter, in contrast to 1 μm or less for *C. tenuis*. Management of the infection involves shaving or cutting the infected hair. Topical fungicides have proved helpful at times.

Black piedra[13] is caused by *P. hortae*, a dematiaceous loculoascomycete* that infects scalp hairs and is usually seen in tropical areas such as South America, the Pacific islands, and eastern Asia. Adherent, hard, black masses develop on the distal end of the hair shaft, causing it to become weak and break off. In contrast to *T. beigelii*, the hard, carbonaceous nodules of *P. hortae* are tightly attached to the hair shaft (see Figure 29-12). If the nodules of *P. hortae* attached to a hair are pulled through two tightly pressed fingers, the nodules do not separate from the hair. The infection starts under the hair cuticle. The hair is then enveloped by the nodule, which consists of aligned hyphal strands. As discussed later, the nodules contain cavities (locules) that contain ascospores. Black piedra is resolved with a haircut.

LABORATORY DIAGNOSIS
DIRECT EXAMINATION AND CULTURE

Laboratory diagnosis of the agents of the superficial mycoses is accomplished after direct microscopic examination of skin scrapings or hair and the culture of these specimens when necessary.

Skin Scrapings

A potassium hydroxide (KOH) preparation should be made from skin scrapings. If *M. furfur* is present, short, truncate, unbranched hyphae and clusters of round to bottle-shaped yeast cells are present (see Figure 29-13). *P. werneckii* appears as pale brown to olivaceous hyphae and budding yeast cells. The hyphae are septate and branched and often have thickened cell walls.

Culture is not required and generally is not recommended for *M. furfur* because of the lipophilic nature of this organism. For situations in which a culture is necessary, however, the organisms can be isolated on a medium such as Mycosel or Mycobiotic agar. The scrapings are mixed in a very small drop of sterile olive oil and then spread on the agar surface; the oil

---

*A loculoascomycete is an ascomycete that produces a special type of fruiting body, in which asci containing ascospores develop within a lysed cavity called a locule.

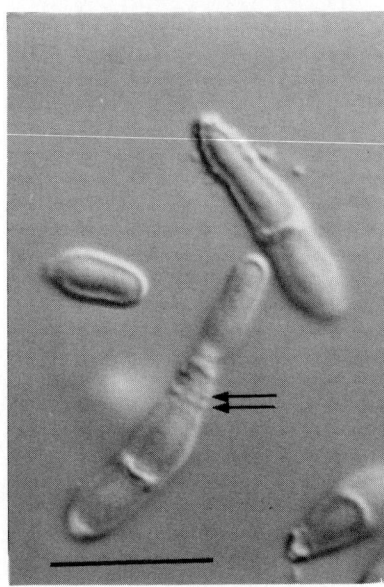

FIGURE 31-1. *Phaeoannellomyces werneckii.* Note cylindric to spindle-shaped two-celled yeast forms. Arrows show annellations that resulted when conidia separated from parent cell. Bar equals 10 μm.

serves as a lipid source. The inoculated medium is incubated at 35° to 37° C.[18] Immature colonies are cream colored, glossy, and raised. They later become dull, dry, and beige.

Skin scrapings suspected to contain *P. werneckii* are inoculated onto the surface of Mycosel or Mycobiotic agar and then incubated at 30° C. *P. werneckii* is not sensitive to 0.5 g/L of cycloheximide.[8] The colonies are initially moist, flat, pasty, black, and yeastlike. With age they become black to gray or olivaceous with some aerial hyphae. The predominant and distinctive form of this yeast consists of cylindric to spindle-shaped cells having a septum. The yeast cells are annellides that produce new annelloconidia from one end, which becomes long, narrow, and tapering. With careful observation annellations can be seen (Figure 31-1). Initially the septum of the yeast cell is central, but as annelloconidia are produced, the elongating conidiogenous area results in a yeast cell with one side longer than the other. Intercalary annellides within the hyphae may also form. This form is the basis for the older name *Exophiala werneckii*. We prefer to use the genus name *Phaeoannellomyces* because the most stable, unique, and characteristic form is the two-celled annellidic yeast cells.

Hair

As previously discussed, the hard carbonaceous nodules of *P. hortae* are tightly attached to the hair shaft, and if the hair is pulled through two tightly pressed fingers, the nodules do not separate from the hair. The nodules of *T. beigelii*, however, are easily stripped off the hair.

Infected hairs should be examined using a KOH preparation. Microscopic examination of the crushed nodules of *T. beigelii* reveal hyphae and many arthroconidia. Within the nodules of hair infected by *P. hortae* are locules that contain asci with eight fusoid ascospores having terminal appendages (Figure 31-2). The ascospores range from 35 to 55 μm in length and 5 to 8 μm in width.[1]

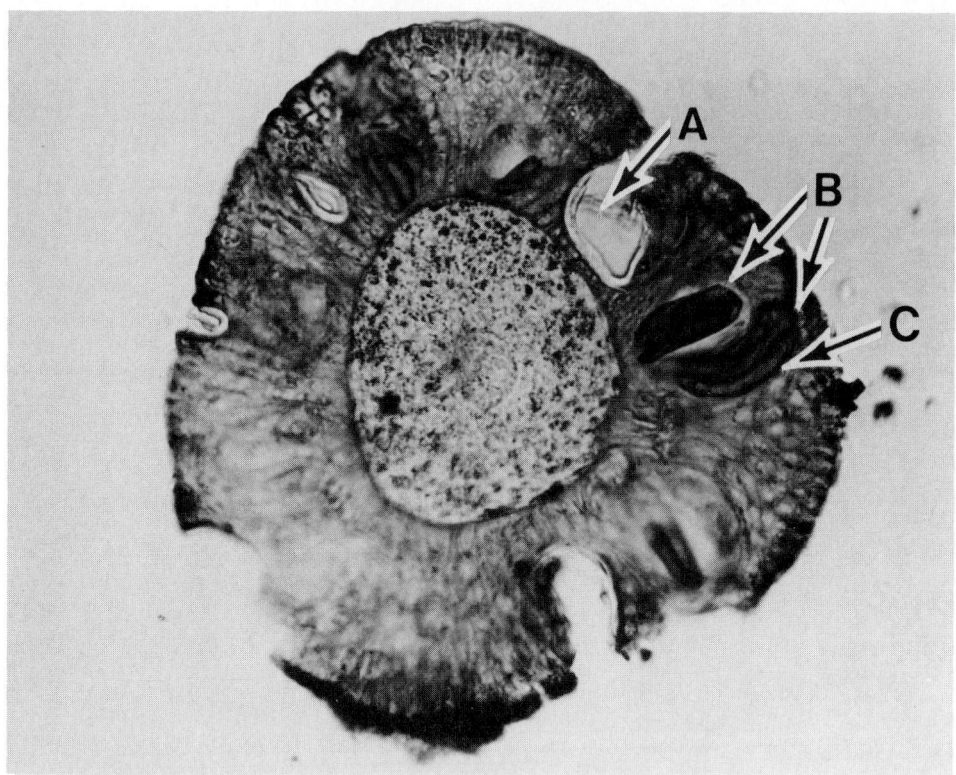

FIGURE 31-2. Cross section of hair infected by *Piedraia hortae*. Locule (*A*) containing asci (*B*) with ascospores (*C*) is formed in ascomycete fruiting body, which surrounds hair shaft. Fruiting body of *P. hortae* is hard and black. (From Mycopathol. Mycol. Appl. **45:**269, 1971.)

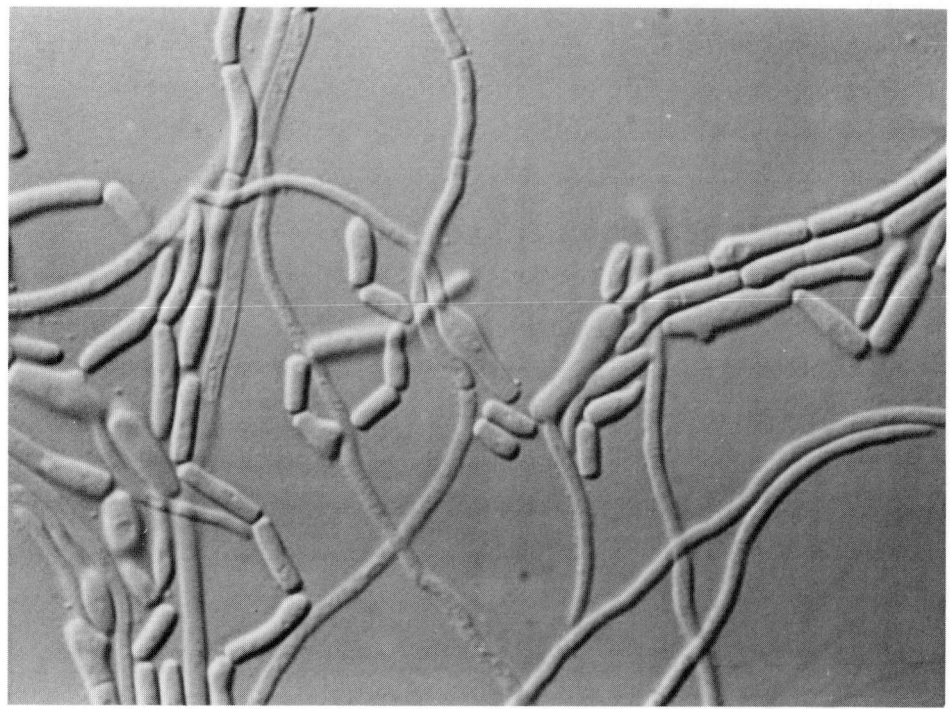

FIGURE 31-3. Septate hyphae of *Trichosporon beigelii* fragmenting to form arthroconidia.

Hairs infected with *T. beigelii* should be cultured on Sabouraud dextrose agar (SDA) with chloramphenicol but without cycloheximide because *T. beigelii* is sensitive to it. Although the direct microscopic examination of *P. hortae* is definitive, this organism may also be recovered on SDA with chloramphenicol.

T. beigelii grows in 3 or 4 days and produces a raised, heaped, creamy, yeastlike colony. In 1 to 2 weeks it becomes yellowish gray. Microscopically *T. beigelii* is characterized by septate hyphae that fragment to form arthroconidia (Figure 31-3). Blastoconidia are common and often form pseudohyphae.

The colonies of *P. hortae* grow slowly and are black to dark brown with a velvety appearance. The cultured fungus usually fails to produce asci or ascospores.

IMMUNOLOGY

There is no evidence that antibodies are produced to the fungi that cause superficial fungal infections. Immunologic diagnosis is unavailable.

REFERENCES

1. Ajello, L., and Padhye, A.: Dermatophytes and the agents of superficial mycoses. In Lennette, E.H., et al.: Manual of clinical microbiology, ed. 4, Washington, D.C., 1985, American Society for Microbiology.
2. Burke, R.C.: Tinea versicolor: susceptibility factors and experimental infection in human beings, J. Invest. Dermatol. **36**:389, 1961.
3. Daly, J.F.: Piedra in Vermont, Arch. Dermatol. **75**:584, 1957.
4. Emmons, C.W., et al.: Medical mycology, ed. 3, Philadelphia, 1977, Lea & Febiger.
5. Faergemann, J.: In vitro and in vivo activities of ketoconazole and intraconazole against *Pityrosporum orbiculare,* Antimicrob. Agents Chemother. **26**:773, 1984.
6. Faergemann, J., and Fredriksson, T.: Tinea versicolor: some new aspects on etiology, pathogenesis, and treatment, Int. J. Dermatol. **21**:8, 1982.
7. Gordon, M.: Lipophilic yeast-like organisms associated with tinea versicolor, J. Invest. Dermatol. **17**:267, 1951.
8. McGinnis, M.R.: Taxonomy of *Exophiala werneckii* and its relationship to *Microsporum mansonii,* Sabouraudia **17**:145, 1979.
9. McGinnis, M.R., and Padhye, A.A.: *Cladosporium castellanii* is a synonym of *Stenella araguata,* Mycotaxon **7**:415, 1978.
10. McGinnis, M.R., Schell, W.A., and Carson, J.: *Phaeoannellomyces* and the Phaeococcomycetaceae: new dematiaceous blastomycete taxa, Sabouraudia **23**:179, 1985.
11. Mok, W.Y.: Nature and identification of *Exophiala werneckii,* J. Clin. Microbiol. **16**:976, 1982.
12. Mok, W.Y., Castelo, F.P., and Barreto da Silva, M.S.: Occurrence of *Exophiala werneckii* on salted freshwater fish *Osteoglossum bicirrhosum,* J. Food Technol. **16**:505, 1981.
13. Moyer, D.G., and Keeler, G.: Note on culture of black piedra for cosmetic reasons, Arch. Dermatol. **89**:436, 1964.
14. Powell, D.A., et al.: Broviac catheter–related *Malassezia furfur* sepsis in five infants receiving intravenous fat emulsions, J. Pediatr. **105**:987, 1984.
15. Rippon, J.W.: Medical mycology: the pathogenic fungi and the pathogenic actinomycetes, ed. 2, Philadelphia, 1982, W.B. Saunders Co.
16. Sternberg, T.H., and Keddie, F.M.: Immunofluorescence studies of tinea versicolor, Arch. Dermatol. **84**:999, 1961.
17. Yaffee, H.S.: Tinea nigra palmaris resembling malignant melanoma, N. Engl. J. Med. **283**:1112, 1970.
18. Wilde, P.F., and Stewart, P.S.: A study of the fatty acid metabolism of the yeast *Pityrosporum ovale,* Biochem. J. **108**:225, 1968.

CHAPTER 32

Dermatophytes

Richard C. Tilton
Michael R. McGinnis

Dermatophytosis is an infection of hair, nail, or skin on a living host, caused by a fungus classified in the genus *Epidermophyton*, *Microsporum*, or *Trichophyton*. Species of these three genera that attack the keratinized tissue of the living host are called dermatophytes.[13] These fungi produce keratinases, proteolytic enzymes that enable them to hydrolyze keratin, the major protein constituent of hair, nail, and skin. Occasionally the terms "tinea" and "ringworm" are used to refer to dermatophytoses. A number of other fungi that are not included in the genera *Epidermophyton*, *Microsporum*, or *Trichophyton* also invade, colonize, and grow in the keratinized tissues of a living host. The infection caused by these fungi is called dermatomycosis.

The major species of dermatophytes are *T. rubrum*, *T. mentagrophytes*, *T. tonsurans*, *E. floccosum*, and *M. canis*.[14] They are anamorphs characterized by the production of distinctive conidia and colonies. When the appropriate mating types are brought together, sexual reproduction can occur. The teleomorphic genus for all of the dermatophytes is *Arthroderma* (Table 32-1). Until recently two teleomorphic genera were recognized; *Arthroderma* was considered the teleomorph for species of *Trichophyton*, and *Nannizzia* for species of *Microsporum*. Weitzman and co-workers[23] concluded that the teleomorphic genera *Arthroderma* and *Nannizzia* were not different enough to be maintained as separate genera. A sexual form for *E. floccosum* is unknown.

PATHOLOGY AND CLINICAL SIGNIFICANCE

No human population is free of the dermatophytes. These organisms may infect humans (anthropophilic) or animals (zoophilic) or grow in soil (geophilic). The following list of the natural habitats of some dermatophytes gives these three reservoirs and the species commonly recovered from each:

1. Anthropophilic (native to humans)
   a. *Microsporum audouinii*
   b. *Epidermophyton floccosum*
   c. *Trichophyton mentagrophytes* var. *interdigitale*
   d. *T. rubrum*
   e. *T. tonsurans*
   f. *T. violaceum*
   g. *T. schoenleinii* } Rarely seen in United States[8]
   h. *T. soudanense*
2. Zoophilic (native to animals)
   a. *Microsporum canis* (cats and dogs)
   b. *M. nanum* (pigs)
   c. *M. gallinae* (chickens)
   d. *Trichophyton mentagrophytes* var. *mentagrophytes* (rodents, cats, dogs, cattle, and sheep)
   e. *T. verrucosum* (cattle and horses)

f. *T. equinum* (horses)
3. Geophilic (native to soil)
   a. *Microsporum gypseum*
   b. *M. fulvum*
   c. *T. ajelloi*
   d. *T. terrestre*

Dermatophytes acquired by humans from either soil or animals typically produce lesions that are acute, highly inflammatory, rapidly developing, and accompanied by pain and pruritus. The identification of these fungi may pose problems for the clinical microbiology laboratory because of the rare occurrence of some of the dermatophytes in clinical specimens. For example, Rippon and Andrews[18] reported the isolation of *Microsporum racemosum*, a zoophilic dermatophyte, from a human patient. The rapidly spreading 5 cm lesion was on the hand. The organism was first isolated from the Venezuelan rat[3,5] and subsequently from normal rat hair.[19] Rippon suggested that human disease represented accidental infection from rat-infested material.

Dermatophytoses are clinically categorized according to the body area affected. For example, tinea barbae refers to infections of the bearded area of the face, whereas tinea pedis is an infection of the foot. Table 32-2 contains a list of the major dermatophytoses and the organisms that cause them, as well as a brief clinical description. Generally, *Microsporum* spp. attack hair and skin but not nails; *Trichophyton* spp. attack hair, skin, and nails; and *Epidermophyton* spp. infect skin and occasionally nails but not hair. It should be noted that each of the body areas may be infected by more than one species of dermatophyte. In some instances, more than one species of dermatophyte may be isolated from the same lesion.[14]

The pathogenesis of dermatophytic infection is complicated; it is not a static process that takes place in a dead layer of tissue. The first contact between the fungus and its human host is on the top layer of the stratum corneum; here, a variety of sweat-derived chemical agents and fatty acids from the microbial degradation of triglycerides can retard the growth of some dermatophytes. The soles of the feet do not have sebaceous glands, which may explain why the foot often has chronic infections. Nonspecific resistance factors include serum dermatophyte–inhibiting factor, complement activation, chemotaxis, and increased cell turnover in the epidermis. Maceration of tissue, hydration of the stratum corneum, and other factors, such as sex hormones and atopic dermatitis, predispose humans to the infectious process. While the production of keratinases appears to be advantageous to the fungus, it is clearly not the only factor in the disease-causing process. Other proteolytic enzymes may also be involved.

Cell-mediated immunity (CMI) is important in the eradication of dermatophyte infections. Delayed hypersensitivity can be measured by the use of the intradermal skin test. Hypersensitivity indicates a previous or current dermatophyte infection. During the course of the infection, results of the skin test become positive, peak, and diminish as a sign of clinical immunity. CMI, as determined by the skin test, indicates the capacity of the individual being tested to eradicate the infection.[9] Some of the characteristics of the immune response to acute and chronic dermatophyte infections are listed in Table 32-3.

Humoral immunity is also important in human dermatophyte infections. In acute and chronic infections, IgG antibodies are present. In chronic infections, IgM, IgA, and IgE antibodies are also present. Antibodies are present during the first month of infection. They usually disappear within 3 months after an acute inflammatory infection but may persist for 6 to 12 months.[22]

LABORATORY DIAGNOSIS

Isolation and identification of dermatophytes is one of the most common cultural procedures in most clinical microbiology laboratories. Isolation can be accomplished without specialized media. Identification is primarily morphologic.

DIRECT EXAMINATION

The Wood's lamp (ultraviolet [UV] light) may be useful for clinical differentiation of the dermatophytoses. Hair that is infected with a dermatophyte may fluoresce under UV light. Fluorescing hairs should be selectively examined (as discussed in this section) and cultured because they contain the fungi. The UV light is also useful for differentiating ringworm of the skin from erythrasma, an infection caused by *Corynebacterium minutissimum;* dermatophyte lesions do not fluoresce, whereas *Corynebacterium* infections do.

In addition to culture, a portion of the clinical specimen consisting of skin, nail, or hair is placed into a drop of 20% potassium hydroxide (KOH) preparation on a clean microscope slide. The slide is gently warmed and then examined with both the low- and high-power objectives of the microscope. If the result is negative, the specimen should be reexamined after the tissue has been cleared for some additional time. Skin and pulverized nail scrapings typically contain septate, branched, hyaline hyphae. Occasionally chains of arthroconidia are present. If the hair is invaded, the invasion may be favic, endothrix, or ectothrix.

Favic hair invasion is caused by *T. schoenleinii.* Invasion of the hair by the fungus produces hyphae that are parallel to the long axis of the hair shaft (Figure 32-1). The hyphae degenerate, leaving tunnels within the hair shaft. These tunnels are best observed by examining the hair immediately after placing it in the KOH solution. The fluid fills the tunnels, and in the process air bubbles can be seen rushing down the hair shaft. This is characteristic of *T. schoenleinii.*

Endothrix hair invasion is caused by *T. tonsurans, T. soudanense,* and *T. violaceum.* The hyphae grow down the hair follicle and then penetrate the hair shaft. The fungus grows within the hair, and the cuticle of the hair remains intact. The hyphae within the hair are converted into arthroconidia (see Figure 29-10).

Ectothrix hair invasion is usually associated with *M. audouinii, M. canis, M. gypseum, M. nanum,* and *T. verrucosum* infections. The arthroconidia can be seen both inside and

TABLE 32-1. Taxonomy of the Asexual and Sexual Forms of Some Dermatophytes

Asexual Form (Anamorph)	Sexual Form (Teleomorph)
Microsporum amazonicum	*Arthroderma borellii*
M. canis (syn., *M. distortum*)	*A. otae*
M. cookei	*A. cajetani*
M. fulvum	*A. fulvum*
M. gypseum	*A. gypseum, A. incurvatum*
M. nanum	*A. obtusum*
M. racemosum	*A. racemosum*
M. vanbreuseghemii	*A. grubyi*
M. persicolor	*A. persicolor*
Trichophyton ajelloi	*A. uncinatum*
T. flavescens	*A. flavescens*
T. georgiae	*A. ciferrii*
T. gloriae	*A. gloriae*
T. mentagrophytes	*A. benhamiae, A. vanbreuseghemii*
T. simii	*A. simii*
T. terrestre	*A. insingulare, A. lenticularum, A. quadrifidum*
T. vanbreuseghemii	*A. gertleri*

Data from references 2, 12, and 15.

outside the hair shaft. The arthroconidia surrounding the hair look like a sheath. Ectothrix hair infection develops in a manner similar to endothrix, except that the hyphae destroy the hair cuticle and also grow around the hair shaft (see Figure 29-9). The hyphae are then converted into arthroconidia. In animal studies these arthroconidia are virulent infective propagules.

A KOH preparation that does not contain fungal elements does not rule out a dermatophyte infection. On the other hand, a positive result for the KOH preparation only confirms that an infection exists. Because the hyphae of different dermatophytes are morphologically similar in keratinized tissues, identification of the particular species involved requires the isolation of the fungus.

CULTURE AND ISOLATION

Clinical specimens, including skin, hair, and nails, that are suspected of containing dermatophytes are inoculated onto media with and without 0.5 g/ml of cycloheximide. In rural areas where *T. verrucosum* may be present, bromcresol purple (BCP) casein–yeast extract agar should be used in addition to the other routine media.[11] Hydrolysis of this medium around a colony is characteristic of *T. verrucosum.* All media are incubated at 30° C. All cultures are held for 3 weeks before being discarded as negative.

TABLE 32-2. Clinical Summary of Dermatophytoses

Disease	Agent	Clinical Characteristics
Tinea barbae	*Trichophyton mentagrophytes,*[a] *T. rubrum,*[a] *T. verrucosum, T. violaceum, Microsporum canis*	Pustular folliculitis in beard hair of face and neck or a superficial infection resembling tinea corporis
Tinea capitis	*M. canis, Trichophyton tonsurans*[a]	Infection of scalp, eyebrows, and eyelashes; inflamed, scaly lesions on scalp; hair loss; ulcerations of skin; either endothrix or ectothrix invasion of hair common; some *Microsporum* spp. infections fluoresce bright green under Wood's lamp
Tinea corporis	*T. rubrum,*[a] *T. mentagrophytes,*[a] *M. canis*	Infection of glabrous skin; scaling, inflammation, erythema, and vesicles to granulomata
Tinea cruris	*Epidermophyton floccosum, T. rubrum, T. mentagrophytes*	Erythematous, pruritic, raised lesion in groin or perineal area; may spread to buttocks and upper thighs; acute or chronic, usually pruritic, well-demarcated, raised lesion with epidermal scaling and a raised erythematous margin
Tinea imbricata	*T. concentricum*[a]	Form of tinea corporis characterized by polycyclic, papulosquamous patches of scales over bodies of populations carrying a recessive autosomal gene marker; occurs in tropical areas in South America, Southeast Asia, and South Pacific
Tinea manuum	*T. rubrum,*[a] *T. mentagrophytes*[a]	Scaly to vesicular lesions on palmar surfaces of hands and between fingers
Tinea pedis (athlete's foot)	*T. mentagrophytes,*[a] *T. rubrum,*[a] *E. floccosum*	Scaly, erythematous, lesions involving toe webs and soles of foot; may be vesicular and inflammatory
Tinea unguium	*T. rubrum,*[a] *T. mentagrophytes,*[a] *E. floccosum*	Invasion of nail plate; may be restricted to patches on surface of nail or may be invasive, beginning at edges and then resulting in infection under nail plate

Data from references 2, 6, 8, and 12.
[a]Most commonly observed species.

TABLE 32-3. Immune Response to Acute and Chronic Dermatophyte Infections

Feature	Acute Infection	Chronic Infection
Source of dermatophyte	Geophilic or zoophilic	Anthropophilic
Histopathologic features	Severe tissue response	Mild tissue response
Course of infection	Weeks	Months to years
IgG antibody response	High	High
Type I immediate hypersensitivity	Low	High
Type IV delayed-type hypersensitivity	High	Low
Frequency of atopy or elevated IgE	Normal	High
Lymphocyte response to trichophytin (in vitro)	High	Usually low
Lymphokine production to trichophytin (in vitro)	Normal to high	Low
Serum-mediated inhibitors of cell-mediated immunity	Absent	Present
T helper/T suppressor ratio	Normal	Normal or low
Response to therapy	Good	Poor
Incidence	High	Low

Modified from Kaaman, T.: Dermatophyte antigens and cell-mediated immunity in dermatophytosis. In McGinnis, M.R., editor: Current topics in medical mycology, New York, 1985, Springer-Verlag.

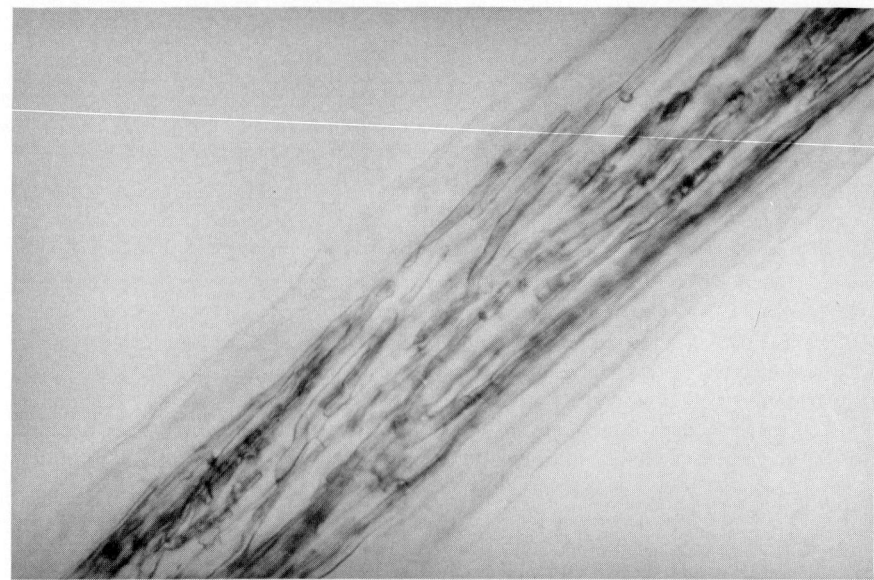

FIGURE 32-1. Favic hair invasion by *Trichophyton schoenleinii.* Note tunnels within hair shaft.

When colonies appear on primary media, they should be immediately transferred to Sabouraud dextrose agar (SDA), incubated at 25° to 30° C, and checked to ensure their purity. Molds, yeasts, and bacteria may contaminate dermatophyte cultures. In some instances a dermatophyte culture may contain two different dermatophytes. For techniques to purify mixed cultures, McGinnis[12] should be consulted. The original isolation plates should be reincubated while purification is being formed.

Pure colonies of suspicious dermatophytes are examined grossly and then microscopically in either slide culture or teased preparations. Table 32-4 contains information regarding the colonial and microscopic features of the dermatophytes most commonly isolated. The descriptions for fungi are based on isolates grown on SDA.

PHYSIOLOGIC TESTS

In some species of dermatophytes, microconidia and macroconidia may be produced or may be produced only infrequently. Furthermore, some species, such as *T. verrucosum* and *T. schoenleinii,* are so morphologically similar that differentiation on this basis alone is difficult. In these cases physiologic testing is necessary.

Trichophyton

Members of the genus *Trichophyton* may be differentiated from similar fungi on the basis of their requirement for certain vitamins. Georg and co-workers[7] devised an identification scheme for these organisms based on absolute or partial growth requirements for six individuals or combinations of vitamins and amino acids. These nutrients in agar are available commercially (Difco Laboratories, Detroit) as Trichophyton agars no. 1 to 7. (Trichophyton agar no. 1 is a basal medium used for comparison with growth on the other agars.) Haley and co-workers[8] suggest that the routine mycology laboratory need use only four of the seven Trichophyton agars. Table 32-5 describes the growth responses of some *Trichophyton* spp. to

these media. As in any nutritional assay, extreme care must be taken not to cross-contaminate reagents or basal media. The fungal inoculum used should be tiny so as not to carry over nutrients from the growth medium. Details of physiologic testing for dermatophytes are presented in McGinnis' *Laboratory Handbook of Medical Mycology.*[12]

Other tests may be required for the differentiation of *T. rubrum* and *T. mentagrophytes,* since colonial appearance, microscopic morphologic features, and nutritional requirements of these two species overlap. Differentiation of these organisms is accomplished with the following three tests:

1. *Urease production test. T. mentagrophytes* typically splits urea in 3 to 7 days when grown on Christensen urea agar.[17] *Trichophyton rubrum* rarely hydrolyzes urea, but when it does, it typically requires at least 7 days. (Rare isolates of *T. mentagrophytes* occur that do not hydrolyze urea.) Kane and Smitka[10] recommend the use of urea broth rather than urea agar. They point out that it is extremely important to purify isolates of *T. rubrum* and *T. mentagrophytes* before testing.
2. *Pigment production test. T. rubrum* produces a deep red pigment on cornmeal agar with 1% dextrose in 2 to 4 weeks at 25° C.[4] *T. mentagrophytes* does not produce this cherry-red pigment.
3. *In vitro hair perforation test.*[1,16,20] When sterile human hair filaments, preferably from blond children, are incubated with *T. mentagrophytes* and *T. rubrum, T. mentagrophytes* perforates the hair in a wedge shape. *T. rubrum* does not perforate hair. Three to five sterile hairs are placed in glass Petri dishes containing 25 ml of sterile distilled water and a few drops of 10% sterile yeast extract. The fungi to be tested are inoculated and the plates incubated at 25° C for up to 4 weeks. The hairs may be removed and placed in lactophenol cotton blue mounting solution for better visualization.

A recent report evaluated the use of urease activity (broth and agar), urea assimilation (filtered and autoclaved urea), hair

Text continued on p. 572.

TABLE 32-4. Colonial and Microscopic Morphology of Commonly Isolated Dermatophytes

Organism	Colonial Appearance[a]	Microscopic Appearance
Epidermophyton floccosum	Mature colonies become yellow or mustard yellow to tan; surface is flat with radial folding; reverse colony is deep orange; white, cotton tufts of sterile mutants may appear on surface of colony (Plate 24, *D*)	Numerous, club-shaped, two- to four-septate conidia (6 to 12 μm × 20 to 40 μm) that occur singly or in groups of two or three (Figure 32-2); cell walls are smooth and thick; microconidia are absent
Microsporum audouinii[b]	Colony is cream or tan to light brown; reverse colony is orange-tan to salmon pink; colony is flat, velvety, and slightly raised in center (Plate 24, *E*)	Terminal, swollen cells occasionally present; hyphae usually sterile; microconidia may be formed; macroconidia infrequent, but when present, they are large, irregularly spindle shaped, and thick walled with roughened surface (Figure 32-3)
Microsporum canis	Colony initially white, becoming bright yellow at edge; reverse colony is yellow, becoming orange to brown; colonies silky, becoming cottony with irregular tufts or concentric rings (Plate 24, *F*)	Macroconidia are spindle shaped, large (35 to 110 μm × 12 to 25 μm); thick outer wall; thin inner cell wall; microconidia one celled, clavate, and smooth walled (Figure 32-4)
Microsporum fulvum	Colony is flat, light tan to medium brown or cinnamon brown, powdery to velvety; reverse colony is rosy buff to cinnamon	Macroconidia and microconidia similar to *M. gypseum*
Microsporum gypseum	Same as *M. fulvum* (Plate 25, *A*)	Macroconidia numerous (25 to 60 μm × 8 to 15 μm); thick walled with four to six septa of similar thickness to outer cell wall; microconidia one celled, clavate, smooth walled (Figure 32-5)
Microsporum nanum	Flat colonies, powdery, cream to buff to medium brown; reverse colony is orange at first, becoming dark red to brown; similar to *M. gypseum* (Plate 25, *B*)	Numerous small (12 to 18 μm × 5 to 7 μm) macroconidia, oval to elliptic, rough walled with one to three septa; microconidia one celled, clavate, smooth walled (Figure 32-6)
Trichophyton mentagrophytes	Colony is flat and may be velvety or powdery (*T. mentagrophytes* var. *interdigitale*) and even granular (*T. mentagrophytes* var. *mentagrophytes*); white to creamy tan; reverse of colony is white to reddish brown (Plate 25, *C*)	Microconidia are round to subglobose, one celled, and hyaline (Figure 32-7); they occur in clusters, along the hyphae, or both; macroconidia typically absent, but may be produced on Sabouraud dextrose agar containing 5% NaCl; when present, they have one to four septa, are cylindric to clavate, and are smooth walled; spirals and nodular bodies may be present
T. rubrum	Mature colonies grown in 1 to 2 weeks and are white and granular to cottony; reverse of colony is white, light brown, or dark red; bright red reverse may be produced when isolate is grown on cornmeal agar (Plate 25, *D*)	Microconidia similar to *T. mentagrophytes*, except they are clavate; in cottony isolates, microconidia rare or absent; macroconidia typically absent, but when present, are cylindric, have two to seven septa, and are smooth walled
T. schoenleinii	Colony is white and becomes tan with age; colony is raised and folded, leathery, glabrous, waxy, granular to velvety; agar tends to crack; reverse of colony is buff to light brown (Plate 25, *E*)	Conidia typically absent; favic chandeliers common (Figure 32-8); mycelium have irregular diameter; numerous chlamydoconidia typically present
T. tonsurans	Colony is flat, compact, and glabrous to granular, becoming heaped and folded with maturity; may be cream or yellow to rose, buff, or brown; reverse colony yellow to mahogany red; growth enhanced by thiamine (Plate 25, *F*)	Numerous microconidia, varying in size; globose, elongate to bulging, borne at right angle to hyphae; macroconidia are rare, but when produced they are cylindric and smooth walled and have one to six septa; fertile hyphae are broader than vegetative hyphae (Figure 32-9)

Continued.

TABLE 32-4. Colonial and Microscopic Morphology of Commonly Isolated Dermatophytes—cont'd

Organism	Colonial Appearance[a]	Microscopic Appearance
T. verrucosum	Surface of colony is dull white or gray to yellowish tan; glabrous to waxy, becoming powdery; aerial hyphae may develop in old colonies; growth more rapid at 37° C (Plate 26, *A*)	Characteristic chains of chlamydoconidia (Figure 32-10) seen at 37° C; on thiamine-rich media, microconidia are present along sides of hyphae; macroconidia are rarely seen
T. violaceum	Heaped and folded colonies with smooth, waxy, or velvety surface; buff to lavender but with a deep purple, diffusible, reverse pigment (Plate 26, *B*)	Microconidia and macroconidia very rare; thiamine often stimulates conidial production

[a]Colonial characteristics based on growth at 25° to 30° C on Sabouraud dextrose agar with 4% sugar and 2 weeks' incubation.
[b]Rarely seen in North America.

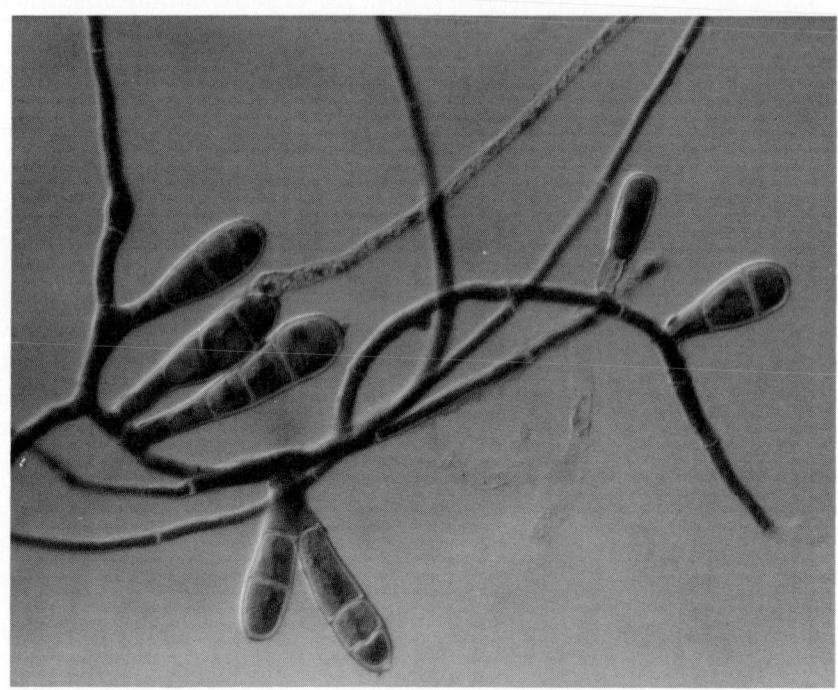

FIGURE 32-2. *Epidermophyton floccosum.* Club-shaped conidia with two to four septa produced singly or in groups.

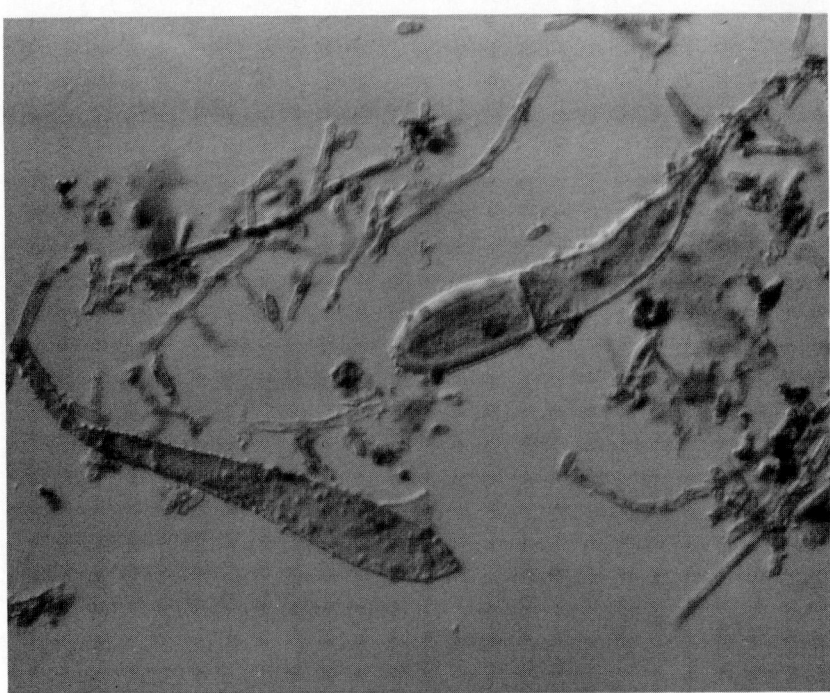

FIGURE 32-3. *Microsporum audouinii.* Large spindle-shaped macroconidia with roughened surface.

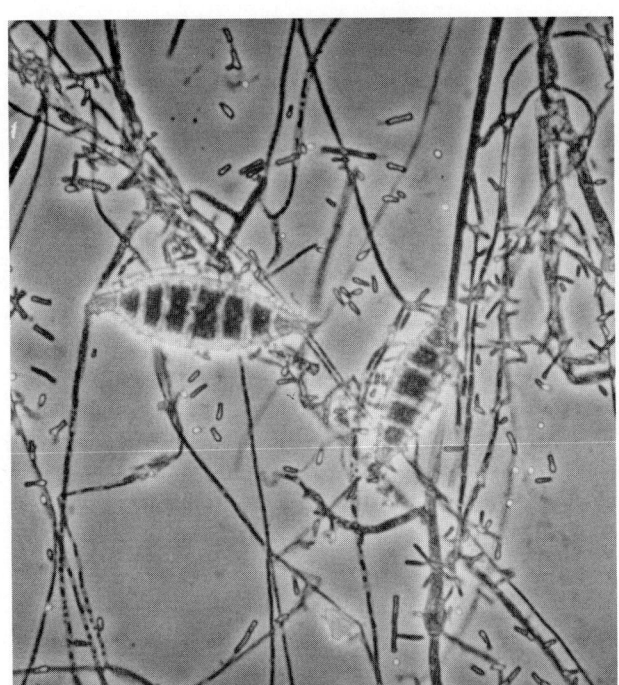

FIGURE 32-4. *Microsporum canis.* Spindle-shaped macroconidia typically have septa that are thinner than outer conidial wall. Note extremely roughened texture of outer cell wall.

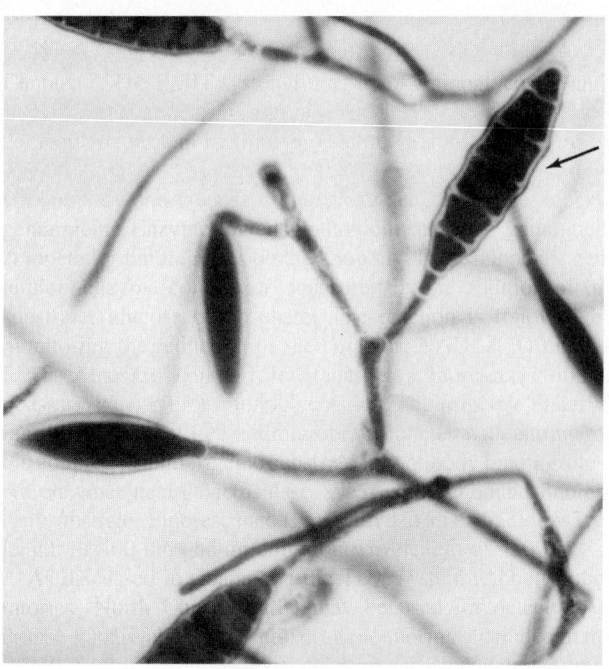

FIGURE 32-5. *Microsporum gypseum*. Various developmental stages of thallic macroconidia are present. In mature macroconidium *(arrow)* outer cell wall tends to collapse slightly.

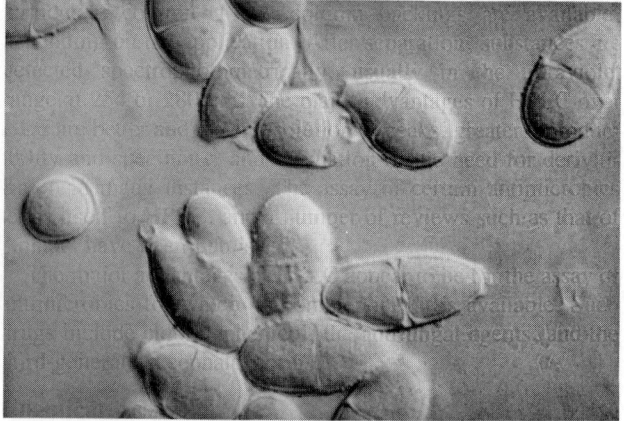

FIGURE 32-6. *Microsporum nanum*. Most clinical isolates produce two-celled roughened macroconidia with flattened bases (truncate).

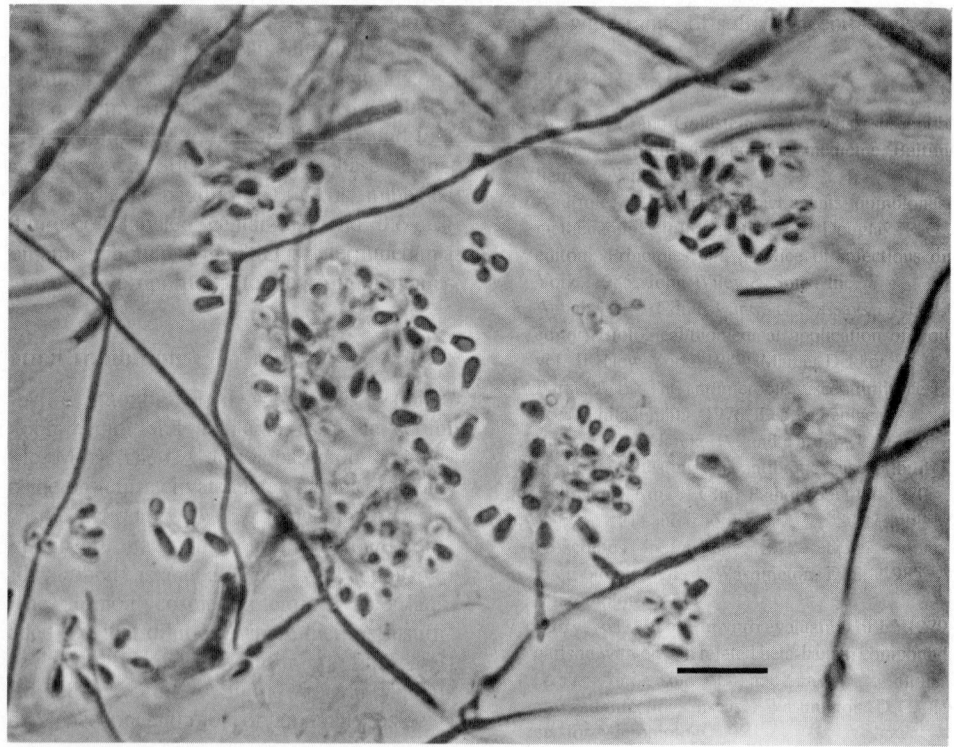

FIGURE 32-7. *Trichophyton mentagrophytes*. Microconidia are one celled and round (globose) to nearly round (subglobose). (From McGinnis, M.R., et al.: Pictorial handbook of medically important fungi and aerobic actinomycetes, New York, 1982, Praeger Publishers.)

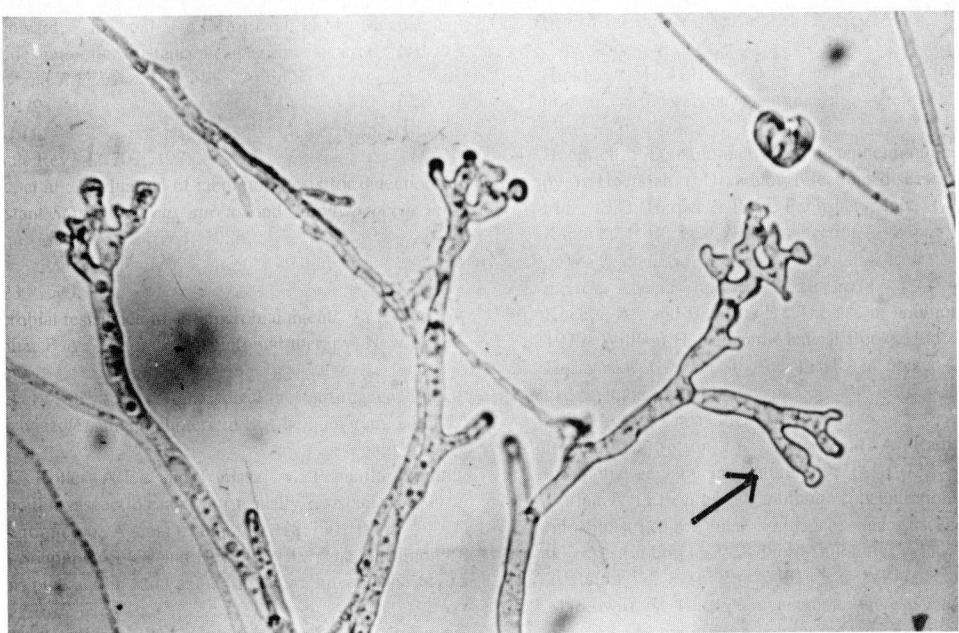

FIGURE 32-8. Characteristic favic chandeliers *(arrow)* of *Trichophyton schoenleinii*. (Courtesy L. Ajello.)

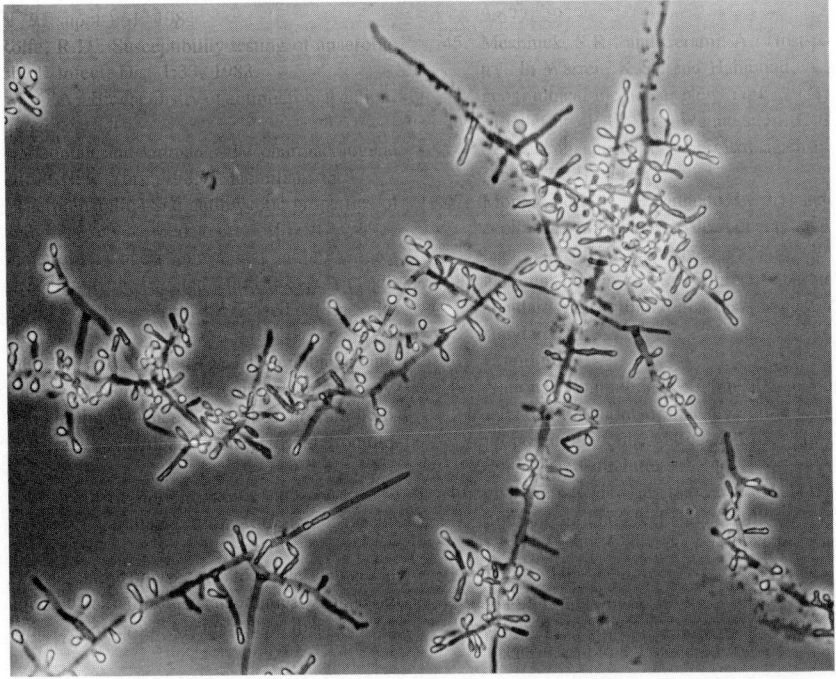

FIGURE 32-9. *Trichophyton tonsurans*. Conidia that vary from round (globose) to elongate resembling matchsticks characterize this dermatophyte. (From McGinnis, M.R.: Laboratory handbook of medical mycology, New York, 1980, Academic Press, Inc.)

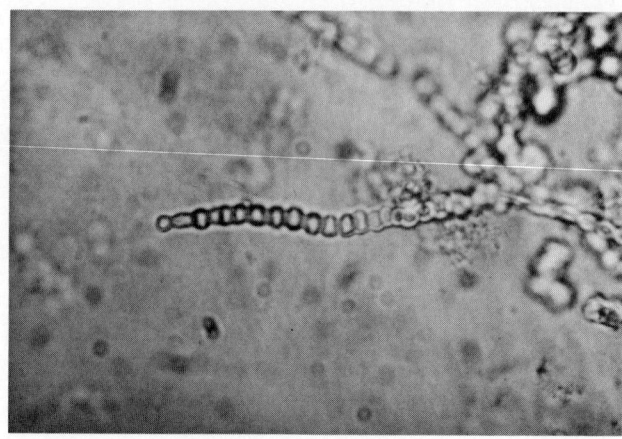

FIGURE 32-10. Typical chains of chlamydoconidia of *Trichophyton verrucosum*. (Courtesy J. Kane.)

TABLE 32-5. Response of Some *Trichophyton* Spp. to Trichophyton Agars 1 to 4

Organism	No. 1 (Basal)[a]	No. 2 (Inositol)	No. 3 (Thiamine and Inositol)	No. 4 (Thiamine)
T. verrucosum	NG	G(+1)[b] (84%)[c] NG (16%)	G(+4)	NG (84%) G(+4) (16%)
T. schoenleinii	G(+4)	G(+4)	G(+4)	G(+4)
T. concentricum	G(+4) (50%) (+2) (50%)	G(+4) (50%) (+2) (50%)	G(+4)	G(+4)
T. tonsurans	G(±)	NG-G(±)	G(+3)	G(+4)
T. violaceum	G(±)	ND	ND	G(+4)
T. rubrum	G(+4)	G(+4)	G(+4)	G(+4)
T. mentagrophytes	G(+4)	G(+4)	G(+4)	G(+4)
T. terrestre	G(+4)	G(+4)	G(+4)	G(+4)

> **SYMBOLS:** NG, No growth
> G, Growth
> ND, Not done

Modified from Haley, L.D., and Callaway, C.S.: Laboratory methods in medical mycology, ed. 4, U.S. Dept. of Health, Education and Welfare Pub. No. (CDC) 78-8361, Atlanta, 1978, Center for Disease Control.
[a]Number is Trichophyton agar number; nutrients are in parentheses.
[b]Growth is rated as 1+ to 4+ as compared with the amount of growth on the basal medium for each test.
[c]The percentage indicates approximate percentage of isolates responding.

perforation (agar block, dip slide, and microperforation), pigment production in potato dextrose agar, and potato-carrot agar for the differentiation of *T. mentagrophytes* and *T. rubrum*.[21] Results indicated that no single test or combination of tests was able to differentiate the two species better than the standard in vitro hair perforation test.[20] The development of microconidia on potato-carrot agar by the majority of isolates of *T. mentagrophytes* did complement the hair perforation results.

The temperature test also may be used to confirm *T. verrucosum* or to distinguish *T. mentagrophytes* from *T. terrestre*.[12] Suspected isolates should be subcultured to two slants of SDA. One is incubated at 25° C and the other at 37° C. Better growth

of *T. verrucosum* occurs at the higher temperature. *T. mentagrophytes* grows at 37° C, whereas *T. terrestre* does not.

Microsporum

Those isolates of *Microsporum canis* and *Microsporum audouinii* organisms that do not produce macroconidia should be transferred from SDA to the surface of sterile rice grains in a glass Petri dish. The culture is incubated at 25° C for 8 to 10 days and examined for the presence of growth. *M. audouinii* does not grow on polished, unfortified rice grains, whereas *M. canis* and other fungi do. If growth of *M. audouinii* is present, a brown discoloration is seen on rice grains under the colony.

IMMUNOLOGY

No procedures are available for immunologic diagnosis of dermatophytoses.

REFERENCES

1. Ajello, L., and Georg, L.K.: In vitro hair cultures for differentiating between atypical isolates of *Trichophyton mentagrophyes* and *Trichophyton rubrum,* Mycopathol. Mycol. Appl. **8:**3, 1957.
2. Ajello, L., and Padhye, A.: Dermatophytes and the agents of superficial mycoses. In Lennette, E.H., et al., editors: Manual of clinical microbiology, ed. 4, Washington, D.C., 1985, American Society for Microbiology.
3. Alteras, I., and Evolceanu, R.: First isolation of *Microsporum racemosum* Dante Borelli 1965 from Romanian soil, Mykosen **12:**223, 1969.
4. Bocobo, F.C., and Benham, R.W.: Pigment production in the differentiation of *Trichophyton mentagrophytes* and *Trichophyton rubrum,* Mycologia **41:**291, 1949.
5. Borelli, D.: *Microsporum racemosum* nova species, Acta Med. Venezol. **12:**148, 1965.
6. Campbell, M.C., and Stewart, J.L.: The medical mycology handbook, New York, 1980, John Wiley & Sons, Inc.
7. Georg, L.K., and Camp, L.B.: Routine nutritional tests for the identification of dermatophytes, J. Bacteriol. **74:**113, 1957.
8. Haley, L.D., and Callaway, C.S.: Laboratory methods in medical mycology, ed. 4, Dept. of Health, Education and Welfare Pub. No. (CDC) 78-8361, Atlanta, 1978, Center for Disease Control.
9. Kaaman, T.: Dermatophyte antigens and cell-mediated immunity in dermatophytosis. In McGinnis, M.R., editor: Current topics in medical mycology, New York, 1985, Springer-Verlag.
10. Kane, J., and Smitka, C.: Early detection and identification of *Trichophyton verrucosum,* J. Clin. Microbiol. **8:**740, 1978.
11. Kane, J., and Smitka, C.: A practical approach to the isolation and identification of members of the *Trichophyton rubrum* complex, PAHO Sci. Pub. No. 396, p. 121, 1980.
12. McGinnis, M.R.: Laboratory handbook of medical mycology, New York, 1980, Academic Press, Inc.
13. McGinnis, M.R., Ajello, L., and Schell, W.A.: Mycotic diseases: a proposed nomenclature, Int. J. Dermatol. **24:**9, 1985.
14. McGinnis, M.R., and Kane, J.: Dermatologic mycology, Semin. Dermatol. **4:**227, 1985.
15. Padhye, A.A., and Carmichael, J.W.: The genus *Arthroderma* Berkeley, Can. J. Bot. **49:**1525, 1971.
16. Padhye, A.A., Young, C.N., and Ajello, L.: Hair perforation as a diagnostic criterion in the identification of *Epidermophyton, Microsporum,* and *Trichophyton* species, PAHO Sci. Pub. No. 396, p. 115, 1980.
17. Philpot, C.: The differentiation of *Trichophyton mentagrophytes* from *T. rubrum* by a simple urease test, Sabouraudia **5:**189, 1967.
18. Rippon, J.W., and Andrews, T.W.: Zoophilic dermatophytosis: a second clinical isolation of *Microsporum racemosum* from the Chicago area, Clin. Microbiol. Newsletter **1:**5, 1979.
19. Rush-Munro, F.M., Smith, J.M.B., and Borelli, D.: The perfect state of *Microsporum racemosum,* Mycologia **62:**856, 1970.
20. Salkin, I.F., et al.: Evaluation of human hair sources for the *in vitro* hair perforation test, J. Clin. Microbiol. **22:**1048, 1985.
21. Sinski, J.T., Avermaete, D.V., and Kelley, L.M.: Analysis of tests used to differentiate *Trichophyton rubrum* from *Trichophyton mentagrophytes,* J. Clin. Microbiol. **13:**62, 1981.
22. Svejgaard, E.: Immunologic investigations of dermatophytes and dermatophytosis, Semin. Dermatol. **4:**201, 1985.
23. Weitzman, I., et al.: The genus *Arthroderma* and its later synonym *Nannizzia,* Mycotaxon **25:**505, 1986.

CHAPTER 33

Agents of Subcutaneous Mycoses

Richard C. Tilton
Michael R. McGinnis

The fungal infections chromoblastomycosis, phaeohyphomycosis, sporotrichosis, mycetoma, lobomycosis, and subcutaneous zygomycosis are similar in that they result from traumatic implementation of the etiologic agent into the skin, with the subsequent development of a subcutaneous infection that is often chronic. In some cases infection may become more widespread, involving multiple organ systems. Subcutaneous mycoses affect the deep layers of skin where there is a host cellular response. In contrast, dermatophytoses affect the keratinized tissues, resulting in cutaneous infections. The numerous agents of subcutaneous mycoses are listed in Table 33-1.

PATHOLOGY AND CLINICAL SIGNIFICANCE

CHROMOBLASTOMYCOSIS

Chromoblastomycosis begins after the implantation of a dematiaceous fungus into the skin, usually as a result of trauma, such as a wound.[29] The lesions develop slowly and usually first appear as small, slightly discolored, scaly papules. The papules gradually increase in size to form a subcutaneous nodule. If untreated the lesions may become larger, raised, and dull red, violet, or gray. Eventually, cauliflower or wartlike lesions, often 1 to 3 cm in diameter, may develop (Figure 33-1). The wartlike or verrucous lesions often have black dots on their surfaces, which have been described as resembling cayenne pepper. The process of dermoepidermal transmigration results in these dots, which contain the sclerotic bodies of the fungus, clotted blood, damaged connective tissue, and foreign matter. The etiologic agents located in the dermis are expelled through the epidermis as the wounds are healed during this transepithelial elimination process.

Patients with chromoblastomycosis experience little if any pain. Only rarely does chromoblastomycosis involve the central nervous system.[29,37,45] Secondary bacterial infections may occur, often resulting in lymphadenitis.

The tissue response in chromoblastomycosis is similar to that in other mycoses, such as blastomycosis, coccidioidomycosis, paracoccidioidomycosis, and sporotrichosis. The epidermis is typically thickened and folded and shows irregular growths that penetrate into the dermis. In the dermis a granulomatous tissue response occurs with abscesses frequently developing. Chromoblastomycosis is characterized by pseudoepitheliomatous hyperplasia, dermal granulomata, intraepidermal microabscesses, fibrosis, and dematiaceous sclerotic bodies 5 to 12 μm. The sclerotic bodies appear to represent an intermediate vegetative form that is phenotypically arrested between a yeast and a mold. Budding from sclerotic bodies in human tissue has been occasionally reported.

The diagnosis of chromoblastomycosis is complicated by the fact that a number of diseases, including blastomycosis, mycetoma, sporotrichosis, leprosy, leishmaniasis, tertiary syphilis, and tropical lymphangitis, can be confused with it. The two clinical features of chromoblastomycosis are the distinctive lesion margins and the satellite lesions that result from autoinoculation. A recent review of both chromoblastomycosis and phaeohyphomycosis presents contemporary clinical, pathologic, and mycologic features of these infections.[29]

The organisms that cause chromoblastomycosis include the dematiaceous fungi, *Fonsecaea pedrosoi*, *Fonsecaea compacta*, *Phialophora verrucosa*, *Cladosporium carrionii*, and *Rhinocladiella aquaspersa*.[27,30,34] These agents have been isolated from soil, wood, and vegetable debris.

Although the infection is centered in the tropics, the mycosis is found throughout the world.[29] Some species are predominant in specific geographic areas. For example, a common cause of chromoblastomycosis is *C. carrionii* in Venezuela, South Africa, and Australia, *F. pedrosoi* in Central and South America and Japan, and *P. verrucosa* in the temperate climates.[7] The increased mobility of people may lead to the isolation of these organisms in unlikely locales. A recent isolate of *F. pedrosoi* from a patient in Hartford, Connecticut, is a case in point.[48] *F. pedrosoi* is the most common etiologic agent worldwide.

Although most patients are between 30 to 50 years old, all ages are susceptible. In most studies the largest group of patients are Caucasians; blacks are the second most frequently attacked group. More males are reported among cases, but this is probably a reflection of occupation rather than the sex of patients.

The early stages of chromoblastomycosis can be treated surgically by excising the lesions. Advanced cases require eradication of the fungus with one or more antifungal agents, such as amphotericin B,[15] 5-fluorocytosine,[40] or thiabendazole.[3]

Chromoblastomycosis has been reported in dogs, frogs, horses, and toads. Unfortunately, not all of these infections have been adequately documented.

LOBOMYCOSIS

Lobomycosis is a chronic subcutaneous infection caused by *Loboa loboi*[22] and occurs only in the New World. The hard, nodular lesions appear primarily on exposed body sites, such as the arms, legs, face, and ears.[38,44] The infection gradually spreads, developing as large verrucous nodular plaques. The lesions are characteristically nodular and keloidal. Satellite lesions often occur and are probably a result of autoinoculation rather than lymphatic or hematogenous spread. The fungus apparently grows in skin because it prefers cool body sites.

In tissue *L. loboi* consists of chains of spherical, hyaline,

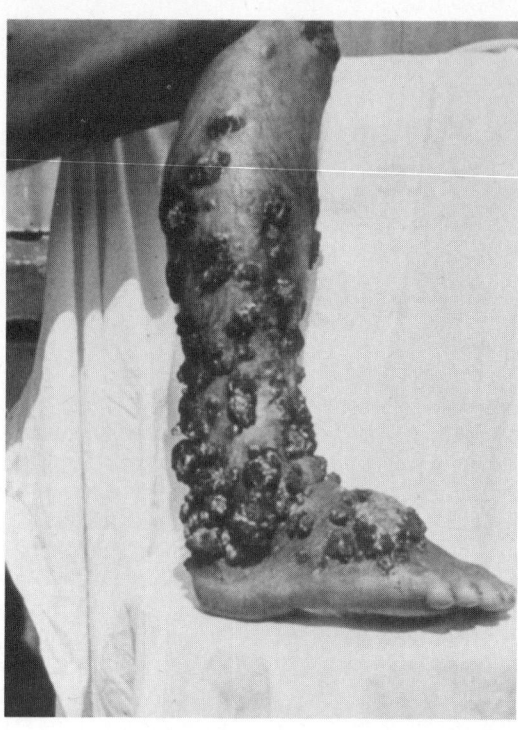

FIGURE 33-1. Typical advanced lesions of chromoblastomycosis.

TABLE 33-1. Direct Microscopic Appearance of Some Clinical Specimens Containing Agents of Subcutaneous Mycoses

Disease	Representative Fungi	Direct Microscopic Appearance
Chromoblastomycosis	*Fonsecaea pedrosoi, Phialophora verrucosa, Cladosporium carrionii*	Pigmented hyphal elements at skin surface; sclerotic bodies thick walled, muriform, chestnut brown structures, approximately 10 μm in diameter, and often are covered with crusty layer of refractile material (Figure 29-8); in crusts, dematiaceous, septate, branched hyphae often present
Lobomycosis	*Loboa loboi*	Large, hyaline, thick walled, spherical to oval yeasts (10 μm), occurring in short chains with tubular connections between each cell of the chain
Mycetoma	*Pseudallescheria boydii, Exophiala jeanselmei, Madurella mycetomatis*	Examine specimen for granules; composed of hyphae
Phaeohyphomycosis	*Bipolaris spicifera, E. jeanselmei, Xylohypha bantiana*	Pale brown to brown yeastlike cells, hyphae, or both; hyphae regular to irregular, often with swollen cells
Sporotrichosis	*Sporothrix schenckii*	Direct microscopic examination not recommended
Subcutaneous zygomycosis	*Basidiobolus ranarum, Conidiobolus coronatus*	Broad, irregularly branching hyphae (5 to 18 μm), sparsely septate; surrounded by eosinophilic material

thick-walled cells, 5 to 12 μm in diameter, that multiply by budding. The cells making up a chain are attached to one another by a tubular isthmus.

Lobomycosis is a tropical disease. Most human infections occur in the state of Mato Grosso in the Amazon valley of west central Brazil. The disease occurs almost exclusively in male agricultural workers.

L. loboi has not been cultivated in vitro in the laboratory. It has been passed in mouse footpads where it can be studied.

Rippon suggests that the inability to culture the organism and its clinical restriction to the cooler extremities of the body might indicate that it is a parasite of a lower animal form.[45] The organism has been recovered from dolphins, but the source of infection in humans is unknown.

MYCETOMA

The term ''mycetoma'' encompasses a clinical syndrome of localized, indolent, tumorous lesions in cutaneous and subcu-

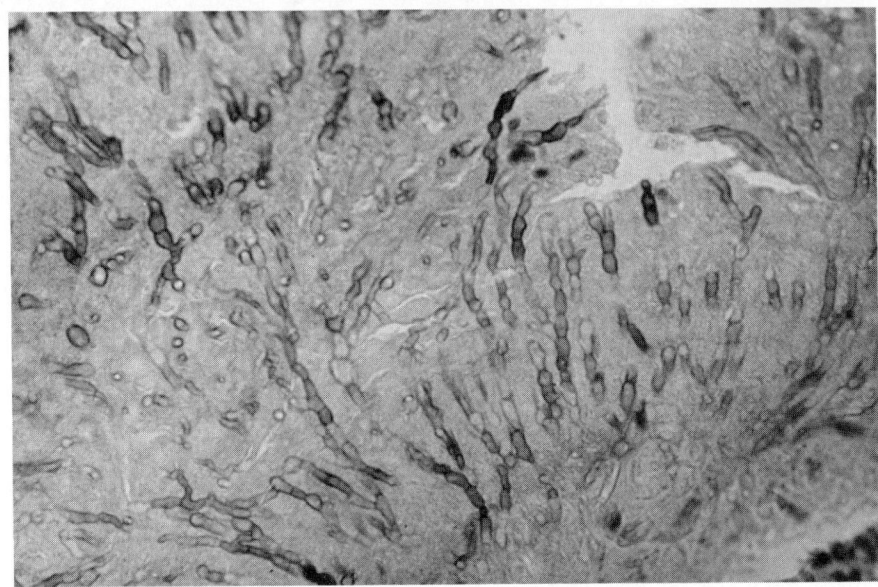

FIGURE 33-2. Granule in toe tissue of *Madurella mycetomatis* composed of moniliform hyphae held together by cement.

taneous tissue, fascia, and bone.[31] Histologically the lesions are composed of suppurative abscesses, draining sinuses, and granulomata. The draining sinus tracts within the lesions discharge pus, containing granules, to the surface of the skin. Granules consist of interwoven masses of hyphae that may be held together by cement (Figure 33-2). The cement is produced by the fungus.

Approximately one half of mycetoma cases are caused by fungi, and the remainder by actinomycetes.[44] Actinomycotic mycetoma is described in Chapter 30. Eumycotic mycetoma follows the traumatic inoculation of the fungus into the skin, usually with an object or thorn that is contaminated with soil containing the fungus. The hands, arms, lower legs, and feet are most commonly involved. Approximately 70% of mycetomas involve feet.

All of the fungi responsible for mycetoma are indigenous to the soil or to plants and are distributed worldwide. In areas where shoes are not worn, the incidence of foot infections tends to be high. Certain countries, such as the Sudan, have high rates of mycetoma; the disease is rare in the United States.[26]

Mahgoub concluded that mycetoma affects males more than females in a 5:1 ratio.[25] In many of the endemic areas, females and males are involved to the same degree in outdoor activities. Why the infection predominantly occurs in males is not known. Mycetoma does not appear to be restricted to any particular occupation.

In some degree individual susceptibility to the agents of mycetoma seems to be correlated with cell-mediated immunity. Some patients become reinfected at different sites with either the same or a different etiologic agent. For example, in Africa and the Arabian Peninsula, where the disease is prevalent, affected persons tend to grow up in poverty conditions characterized by low protein uptake and multiple infections. Possibly these conditions affect cell-mediated immunity.[25]

Mycetomas are difficult to treat medically because the fungi are resistant to drugs and because of bone involvement and the presence of fibrous tissue. Unfortunately, some physicians amputate without first trying medical treatment. The distinction between actinomycotic and eumycotic mycetomas is critical because their chemotherapy differs significantly. Mahgoub[25] recommends careful surgery to remove the swollen tissue and then administration of ketoconazole. Chemotherapy usually requires 9 to 12 months. Therapy is continued until an immunoserologic test such as counterimmunoelectrophoresis indicates that the problem has been resolved.

Species of *Madurella, Aspergillus, Pseudallescheria, Acremonium,* and *Leptosphaeria* are the most common agents of mycetoma. In the United States *Pseudallescheria boydii* or its asexual form *Scedosporium apiospermum* is the most common cause. *P. boydii* may also be responsible for other diseases that mimic infections such as aspergillosis.[44] In fact, *P. boydii* is characterized by Rippon[43] as "the great imitator." This fungus has been implicated in virtually all of the diseases in which *Aspergillus* spp. have been implicated, including allergic bronchopulmonary disease, fungus balls, invasive pulmonary disease, keratitis, endocarditis, endophthalmitis, and meningitis.[9,43]

PHAEOHYPHOMYCOSIS

Ajello[1] recommends that infections caused by fungi having septate, darkly pigmented hyphae or yeast cells in tissue be called phaeohyphomycosis. McGinnis[29] has expanded the description of phaeohyphomycosis to include dematiaceous pathogens that might not always have dematiaceous fungal elements in tissue but still meet all of the criteria Ajello formulated for phaeohyphomycosis. The clinical presentation of phaeohyphomycosis is similar to some forms of chromoblastomycosis.

Phaeohyphomycosis ranges from superficial to systemic infections. Tissue responses to the etiologic agents of phaeohyphomycosis vary greatly because of the wide spectrum of tissues and organisms involved. Unlike chromoblastomycosis, sclerotic bodies are absent in phaeohyphomycosis, regardless of the agent involved. Excision is appropriate at times, but when systemic infections are being controlled, antifungal drugs such as amphotericin B must be used.

The number of etiologic agents of phaeohyphomycosis is rapidly increasing and includes species of *Alternaria, Aureobasidium, Bipolaris, Curvularia, Exophiala, Phialophora, Wangiella,* and numerous others. (*Bipolaris* is the currently accepted genus for some species previously identified as *Drechslera* or *Helminthosporium.*[33]) These agents are soil saprophytes and phytopathogens. Because they are often laboratory contaminants and can be found transiently on skin surfaces, a definitive etiologic diagnosis may be difficult without clinical information, histopathologic examination, and the detection of fungal elements in clinical specimens. Because of the tremendous spectrum of infections and etiologic dematiaceous fungi, it is not possible to discuss the epidemiology of phaeohyphomycosis in this text. The reader should consult the works by McGinnis,[28-30] Rippon,[44] Ellis,[12] and others.

RHINOSPORIDIOSIS

Rhinosporidiosis is caused by *Rhinosporidium seeberi,* an organism that is suspected to be an aquatic fungus. The fungus has not yet been cultured, and its taxonomic placement is in doubt.

The infection is a chronic granulomatous process that involves primarily the mucous membranes of the nose, eyes, and sometimes other body sites. The mucous membranes of the mouth, genital areas, and rectum are rarely affected. Rhinosporidiosis characteristically occurs as polyps involving the nose, eyes, larynx, trachea, bronchi, and sometimes the ears, rectum, and genitals. The polyps are red, soft, and friable and readily bleed if traumatized. Careful surgical excision is the treatment of choice. Microscopic examination of the lesions reveals sporangia approximately 6 to 300 μm in diameter and spores 6 to 7 μm in diameter.

Karunaratne reported approximately 2000 cases of rhinosporidiosis up to 1964.[18] Of these, the great majority were from India and Ceylon. In South America most cases are seen in Brazil and Argentina. Although there is no strict age predilection, most patients are between 20 and 40 years of age.

SPOROTRICHOSIS

The etiologic agent of sporotrichosis[44] is the dimorphic fungus *Sporothrix schenckii.*[4,21,31] The five clinical types of sporotrichosis are lymphocutaneous, fixed cutaneous in which the primary infection is restricted to the inoculation site, mucocutaneous, extracutaneous or disseminated, and pulmonary.

Three fourths of sporotrichosis cases are lymphocutaneous and characterized by ulcerated cutaneous lesions and regional lymphadenopathy. The infection typically develops following trauma, such as pricking of the fingers or feet by thorny plants. Initially a small nodule appears, usually on the arms or legs. These nodules develop into buboes. As the organisms grow within the lesion, the nodule becomes discolored and eventually breaks down, penetrating the skin to form an ulcer. Local or regional lymphadenopathy also develops.

The primary lesion may heal spontaneously, but unless it is treated, chronic infection may develop. In chronic infection new lesions develop particularly along the lymphatic system that drains the area of the initial ulcer.

Extracutaneous or disseminated infection is usually secondary to a cutaneous lesion. Dissemination of the organism to the mucocutaneous areas results in mucocutaneous sporotrichosis. The skeletal system is most commonly involved. Disseminated disease involving other organ systems, such as the central nervous system, is quite rare.[13]

Fixed cutaneous sporotrichosis is seen in highly endemic areas where the population has become sensitized to the organism (that is, they have positive results of sporotrichin skin tests but no infection). The fixed cutaneous lesions are verrucous and ulcerative or appear as a scaly macular or papular rash. Lesions are most commonly seen on the face, neck, and trunk. Lymphadenopathy does not occur.

Primary pulmonary sporotrichosis follows inhalation of the organism.[39] The disease, which resembles tuberculosis, begins as an acute pneumonitis and progresses to a chronic pneumonitis characterized by fibrosis and pleural effusions.

Sporotrichosis is treated with orally administered potassium iodide (KI), but amphotericin B is the drug of choice for disseminated, recurrent, or pulmonary sporotrichosis.

S. schenckii is frequently isolated from woody plants, plant debris, wood, and soil rich in organic matter. In a review of *S. schenckii,* Travassos and co-workers[48] indicated that the organism can also be found in insects, hair, water, and air, as well as in domestic animals and rodents.[2,5,23,46] One of the phytopathogenic ascomycetous fungi, *Ceratocystis stenoceras* (teleomorph), is found in the same habitat and has an anamorph that resembles *Sporothrix* organisms in culture. DNA base composition shows a close relationship between these fungi.[10]

Sporotrichosis occurs worldwide and in all age groups. Most infections are in men, but this may indicate an occupational disease of foresters, gardeners, and horticulturists rather than differences in sex. The cultivation of roses is often associated with the disease, probably resulting from penetrating wounds caused by rose thorns and subsequent infection.[20]

The largest epidemic of sporotrichosis was among gold miners in South Africa and involved 3000 cases. It was finally discovered that miners contracted the disease as they rubbed against mine timbers colonized with *S. schenckii.*[14] Infections have also been observed in clusters on bulb farms,[47] in people exposed to sphagnum moss,[16] and in a Vermont tree nursery.[8] Armadillo hunting in Uruguay has also been associated with this disease.[24]

SUBCUTANEOUS ZYGOMYCOSIS

Subcutaneous zygomycosis is a chronic infection restricted to either subcutaneous tissue or the nasal submucosa. This infection is caused by the zygomycetous fungi *Basidiobolus ranarum*[38] and *Conidiobolus coronatus.*[44]

Infections caused by *B. ranarum* typically begin as a subcutaneous nodule on any portion of the body. As the mass increases in size, it is freely moveable because it is attached to the overlying skin but not to the underlying muscle fascia. The buttocks, thighs, trunk, and perineum are most commonly involved. The mass may become extremely large and involve an entire arm or shoulder. Involvement of underlying tissues, including muscles and thoracic, abdominal, and pelvic viscera, may occur as the infection spreads laterally. The tissue form of *B. ranarum* and *C. coronatus* consists of sparsely septate, broad mycelium. Metastatic lesions seldom occur, and in comparison with the other zygomycetes, there is less tendency for these fungi to invade blood vessels. Often Splendore-Hoeppli material exists around the hyphae. This appears as an antigen-antibody complex that radiates from the fungal elements. The disease primarily involves children, with boys being more commonly infected. Orally administered potassium iodide is the therapy of choice. Amphotericin B is used for infections that do not respond to potassium iodide.

Subcutaneous zygomycosis caused by *B. ranarum* is prevalent primarily in Africa, India, and Indonesia, although it has recently been reported in Southeast Asia and Brazil.[6] The natural reservoir appears to be decaying vegetation, dung from reptiles, and insects such as beetles. At least one case has been reported in the United States.[11]

Infections caused by *Conidiobolus coronatus* begin in the nasal mucosa and then involve the sinuses, pharynx, and subcutaneous areas of the nose and face. *C. coronatus* is more prevalent in warmer climates, especially in the rain forest areas of Africa. Infections have been reported throughout the world, typically in tropical and subtropical regions. The fungus is usually associated with decaying leaves. In contrast to subcutaneous zygomycosis caused by *B. ranarum*, infections caused by *C. coronatus* more frequently involve adults. Most infections occur in farm workers.[44] Treatment for infection caused by *C. coronatus* is the same as for *B. ranarum*.

LABORATORY DIAGNOSIS

The laboratory diagnosis of the subcutaneous mycotic infections depends on astute clinical observations and comprehensive cultural and microscopic examination. Many fungi, such as the dematiaceous fungi, are difficult to identify. These fungi are often sent to a reference laboratory for precise identification.

Pure cultures must be used because many of these fungi are polymorphic, that is, a single isolate may form more than one type of anamorph. Working with isolates that have more than one asexual form, all of which probably have their own genetic names, can cause a great deal of confusion and controversy. We recommend that the most stable, distinctive, and unique anamorph present be used as the basis for identification.

DIRECT EXAMINATION

Specimens such as skin scrapings, exudates, biopsy material, lesion crusts, pus, and aspirated debris are examind in 10% potassium hydroxiode (KOH) after gentle heating of the slide to dissolve the clinical material. Tissue specimens should be homogenized or macerated but only after a search for purulent or necrotic areas that can be examined directly. McGinnis recommends the use of brightfield optics rather than phase contrast when examining specimens for dematiaceous fungi.[30] Since

TABLE 33-2. Microscopic and Macroscopic Morphology of Some Fungi Causing Subcutaneous Infections

Organism	Microscopic Morphology	Macroscopic Morphology
Bipolaris spicifera	Erect, pale brown, sympodial conidiophores giving rise to ellipsoidal conidia with three septa and slightly protruding hila (Figure 33-3) (hila [sing. *hilum*] are scars at base of conidium)	Rapid growing; first white, rapidly becoming olive green to black; texture velvety to woolly
Cladosporium carrionii	Erect, dematiaceous conidiophores giving rise to acropetally branched chains of one-celled, pale brown blastoconidia (Figure 33-4); chains are fragile; conidia close to conidiophore apex, often resembling shields; termed "shield cells" (*Cladosporium carrionii* resembles *Xylohypha bantiana* but is differentiated as discussed under *X. bantiana*)	Rapidly growing, dark-olive to black colony; black submerged hyphae[45]; woolly to cottony; slightly raised
Exophiala jeanselmei	Conidiophores are pale brown, giving rise to cylindric to flask-shaped annellides; conidia are one celled, hyaline to pale brown, and accumulate in a cluster at the apex of the annellide (Figure 33-5)	Moderately fast growing, moist, glistening, gray to black colony, becoming woolly as colony matures
Fonsecaea pedrosoi	Form primary one-celled conidia arising from sympodial conidiophores; primary conidia function as sympodial conidiogenous cells to form secondary one-celled conidia; some conidia occur as branched chains of blastoconidia; may also produce phialides with collarettes and clusters of one-celled conidia; *Fonsecaea* organisms produce three types of anamorphs: (1) those similar to that seen in *Rhinocladiella* spp. (incorrectly called *Acrotheca*-like), (2) those similar to that found in *Cladosporium* spp., and (3) those similar to that found in *Phialophora* spp.	Slow growing, black-brown, gray-black, olive-gray, or black colony; texture velvety to cottony; *F. pedrosoi* and *P. verrucosa* indistinguishable macroscopically

Continued.

TABLE 33-2. Microscopic and Macroscopic Morphology of Some Fungi Causing Subcutaneous Infections—cont'd

Organism	Microscopic Morphology	Macroscopic Morphology
Madurella mycetomatis	Isolates typically sterile, but some fresh isolates on potato dextrose agar (PDA) may produce phialides with collarettes having conidia in balls at their apices; better growth observed at 35° than 30° C	Most isolates form slow-growing, raised to heaped, woolly, olive to gray, yellow, or brown colonies
Phialophora verrucosa	Conidiophores short when present; conidiogenous cells dematiaceous, cylindric to flask-shaped phialides having collarettes; conidia ovoid to cylindric, one celled, hyaline, and occur in balls at the apices of the phialides (Figure 33-6)	Moderately fast growing, dark olive-gray to black colony; initially dome-shaped but becomes woolly to cottony
Pseudallescheria boydii	Cleistothecia are black, spherical (140 to 200 μm in diameter) structures that occur in medium below colony surface and its junction with agar (Figure 33-7); ascospores one celled, ovoid to ellipsoidal, pale brown to copper, with eight ascospores per ascus; anamorphs *Scedosporium apiospermum*, *Graphium* spp.; produce one-celled, hyaline to pale brown, subglobose to elongate conidia; borne on synnemata[41]	Colony initially white, becoming gray; rapid growing, cottony
Sporothrix schenckii	Dimorphic fungus; at 25° C, two kinds of conidia present: (1) hyaline, globose to clavate, one-celled conidia on denticles that develop along hyphae or laterally from sympodial conidiophores, and (2) dark, one-celled, thick-walled conidia along hyphae; identity confirmed by conversion of mold form to yeast form at 37° C (Figure 33-8) (procedure for conversion discussed in Chapter 34)	Fast growing; young colonies may be white, glabrous, yeastlike, becoming cream to dark brown; at first moist, becoming wrinkled; leathery to velvety in texture
Wangiella dermatitidis	Conidiophores hypha like; conidiogenous cells are phialides without collarettes; phialoconidia are one celled, smooth, hyaline to pale brown, forming in clusters at apices of phialides; isolates also commonly produce yeast forms; *W. dermatitidis* readily grows at 40° C, which helps to distinguish it from most other dematiaceous fungi	Rapidly growing; on initial isolation, moist, glistening, olive to black, becoming velvety and olive gray
Xylohypha bantiana	Previously known as *Cladosporium bantianum* or *C. trichoides*, fungus was reclassified as *X. bantiana* because its conidiophores are hypha like and extremely long chains of blastoconidia are sparsely branched[36]; it is differentiated from *C. carrionii* by lacking erect, distinct conidiophores, having longer conidia, and ability to grow at 42° to 43° C; *C. carrionii* does not grow at the latter temperature	Moderately fast growing, like *C. carrionii*

Modified from McGinnis, M.R., et al.: Pictorial handbook of medically important fungi and aerobic actinomycetes, New York, 1982, Praeger Publishers.

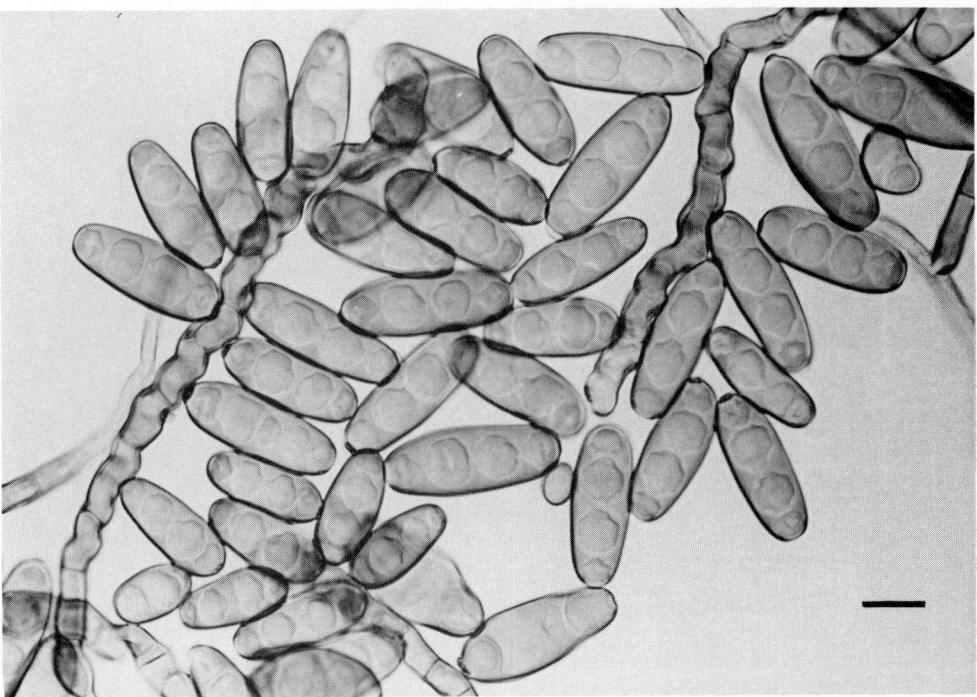

FIGURE 33-3. *Bipolaris spicifera*. Note septate conidia with slightly protruding hila on sympodial conidiophores. (Bar = 10 μm.)

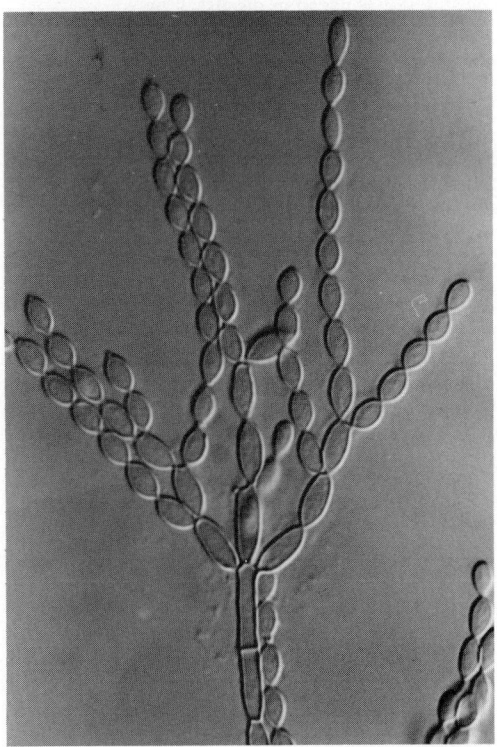

FIGURE 33-4. *Cladosporium carrionii* forms erect conidiophores that bear blastoconidia in branched chains.

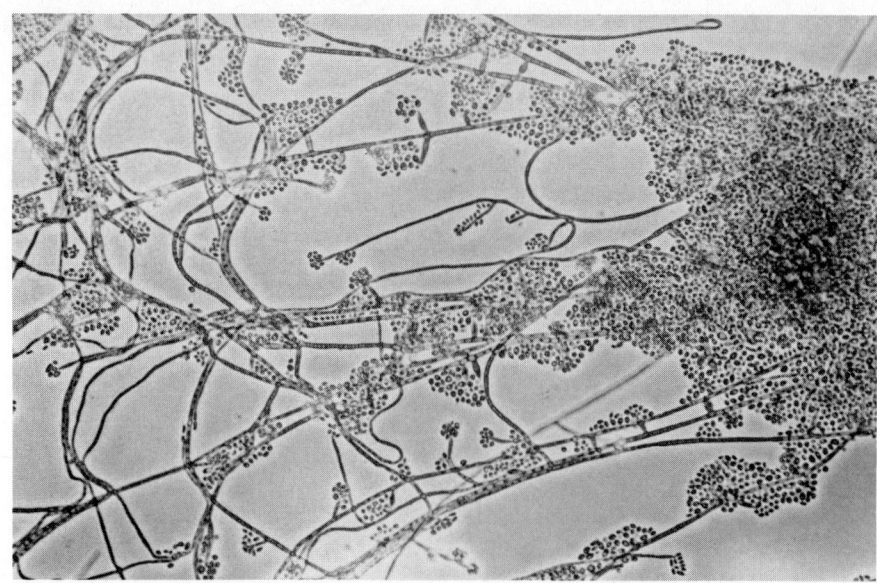

FIGURE 33-5. One-celled annelloconidia accumulating at tips of annellides is characteristic of *Exophiala jeanselmei*.

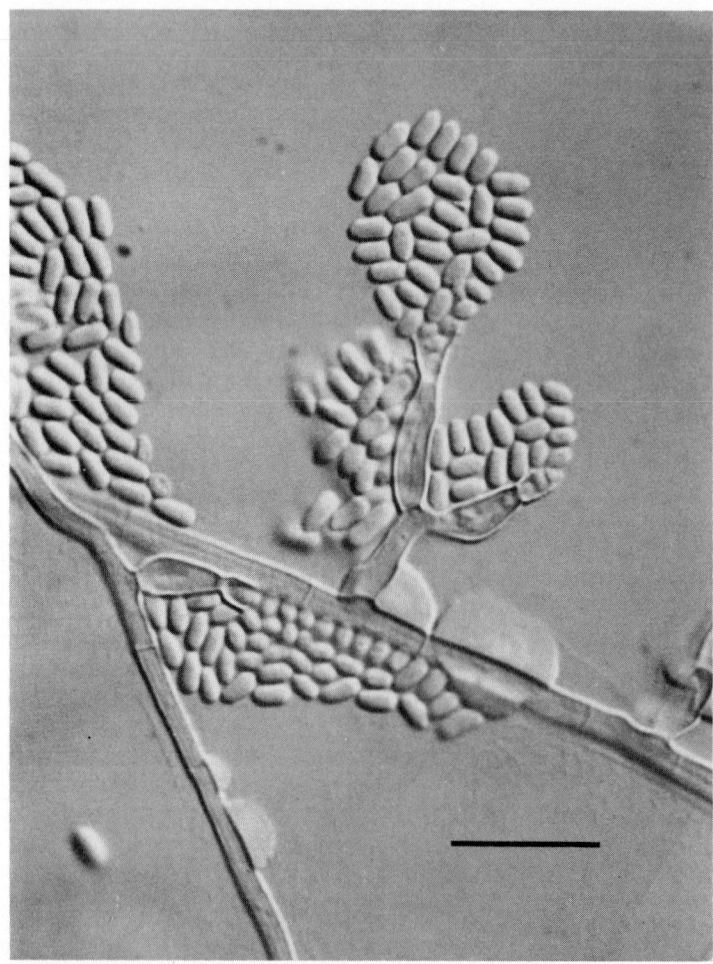

FIGURE 33-6. *Phialophora verrucosa.* Flask-shaped phialides with collarettes give rise to cylindric one-celled conidia that occur in balls. (Bar = 10 μm.) (From McGinnis, M.R., D'Amato, R.F., and Land, G.A.: Pictorial handbook of fungi and aerobic actinomycetes, New York, 1982, Praeger Publishers.)

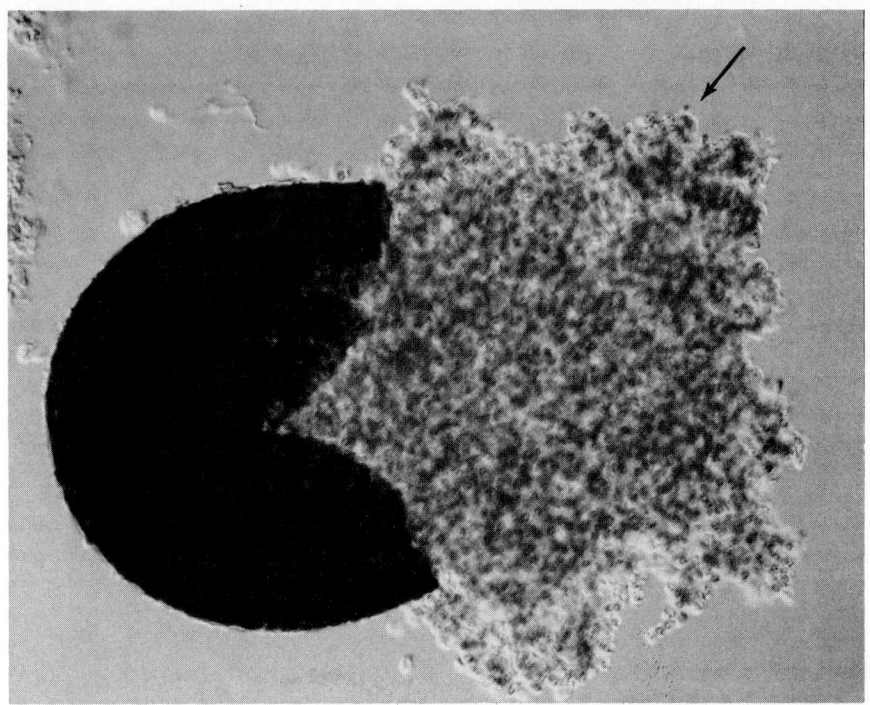

FIGURE 33-7. Ascospores *(arrow)* have been released from mature cleistothecium of *Pseudallescheria boydii*. Many asci, which cannot be seen because their walls have dissolved within cleistothecium as it matured, are randomly dispersed within structure.

demonstrating *Sporothrix schenckii* in a clinical specimen by a KOH preparation is difficult, stained tissue sections or fluorescent stained material should be examined. The differential microscopic appearance of clinical specimens is described in Table 31-1.

CULTURE AND ISOLATION

Specimens for the recovery of fungal agents of subcutaneous infections should be cultured on media with and without antimicrobial agents. Some of the dematiaceous fungi are sensitive to 0.5 mg/ml of cycloheximide. All of these fungi grow well at 30° C, and viable colonies are present in 1 to 2 weeks. Some do not grow at 37° C. Plates should not be discarded for at least 4 weeks. In cases of mycetoma the granules should be cultured on media with and without antimicrobial agents. When actinomycetes are involved, they are sensitive to antibacterial agents such as chloramphenicol.

When colonies appear on the isolation media, they must be purified before identification. McGinnis[30] recommends that dematiaceous fungi be subcultured to potato dextrose agar or cornmeal agar because these stimulate conidial formation. McGinnis also suggests that an isolate resembling *Sporothrix schenckii* be subcultured to a blood agar plate (BAP), which is incubated at 36° C, to confirm its dimorphic nature. One BAP is incubated at 22° to 25° C, and the other in a candle jar at 35° C. Yeast forms should be present at 35° C. It is not necessary for the entire colony to be converted to a yeast to demonstrate dimorphism.

Table 33-2 describes the macroscopic and microscopic morphology of commonly isolated fungi. As with other fungi, all cultural and microscopic preparation should be performed in a biologic safety cabinet.

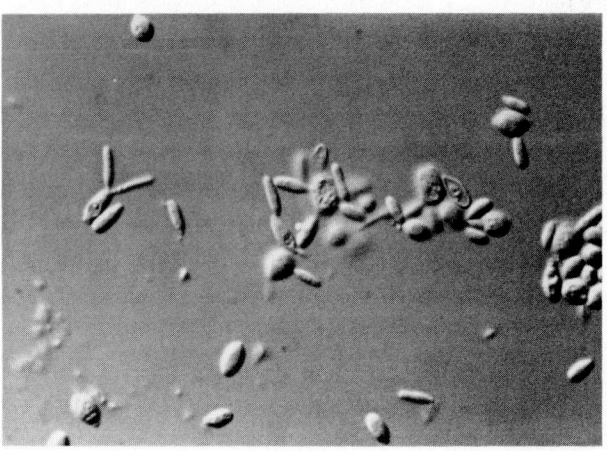

FIGURE 33-8. Yeast form of *Sporothrix schenckii* at 37° C.

IMMUNOLOGY

With the exception of *Sporothrix schenckii, Pseudallescheria boydii,* and *Madurella mycetomatis,* mycoserology is not helpful.

Specific antibodies are usually absent in the early stages of sporotrichosis. The rare yeastlike cells of *S. schenckii* in tissues can be readily visualized with fluorescent antibody conjugants.[17] Skin tests using sporotrichin are also available. A positive result from a skin test indicates past or present infection, whereas a negative result indicates the absence of infection. More recently, immunologic tests have been developed to detect the extracutaneous or systemic form of sporotrichosis. These include latex agglutination and tube agglutination.[19,42]

The details of these tests are discussed in Chapter 38.

Pseudallescheria antibodies can be detected by immunodiffusion. Patients with the disease elicit multiple precipitin bands to the antigens used. The test is similar to the immunodiffusion tests for *Aspergillus* spp.[44] Exoantigens are available for *P. boydii, Cladosporium carrionii, Xylohypha bantiana, Exophiala jeanselmei, Wangiella dermatitidis,* and *S. schenckii* at the Centers for Disease Control.[19]

REFERENCES

1. Ajello, L.: Phaeohyphomycosis: definition and etiology. In Mycoses, PAHO Sci. Publ. **304:**126, 1975.
2. Balabanoff, V.A., and Stoynovski, V.: Sporotrichose bei arbeiten in einer papierfabrik, Berufsdermatosen. **16:**261, 1968.
3. Bayles, M.A.H.: Chromomycosis: treatment with thiabendazole, Arch. Dermatol. **104:**476, 1971.
4. Becker, F.T., and Young, H.R.: Sporotrichosis: a report of 21 cases, Minn. Med. **53:**851, 1970.
5. Beurmann, L., and Gougerot, H.: Decouverte du *Sporotrichum beurmanni* dans la nature, Bull. Mem. Soc. Hosp. Paris **16:**733, 1908.
6. Bittercourt, A.L., et al.: Occurrence of subcutaneous zygomycosis caused by *Basidiobolus haptosporus* in Brazil, Mycopathologia **68:**101, 1979.
7. Carrion, A.L.: Chromoblastomycosis, Ann. N.Y. Acad. Sci. **50:**1255, 1950.
8. D'Alessio, D.J., et al.: An outbreak of sporotrichosis in Vermont associated with sphagnum moss as the source of infection, N. Engl. J. Med. **272:**1054, 1965.
9. Davis, W.A., and Isner, J.M.: Disseminated *Petriellidium boydii* and pacemaker endocarditis, Am. J. Med. **69:**929, 1980.
10. de Bievre, C., and Mariat, F.: Etude de la composition en bases de l'acide desoxyribonucleique de souches de *Sporothrix schenckii* et de *Ceratocystis,* Ann. Microbiol. **132B:**281, 1981.
11. Dworzack, D.L., et al.: Zygomycosis of the maxillary sinus and palate caused by *Basidiobolus haptosporus,* Arch. Intern. Med. **138:**1274, 1978.
12. Ellis, M.B.: Dematiaceous hyphomycetes, Kew, England, 1971, Commonwealth Mycological Institute.
13. Fetter, B.F., et al.: Mycoses of the central nervous system, Baltimore, 1967, Williams & Wilkins Co.
14. Helm, M.A.F., and Berman, C.: The clinical, therapeutic, and epidemiological features of the sporotrichosis infection on the mines, Proc. Transvaal Mine Med. Off. Assoc. **22:**59, 1947.
15. Hughes, W.T.: Chromoblastomycosis: successful treatment with topical amphotericin B, J. Pediatr. **71:**351, 1967.
16. Ingrish, F.M., and Scheidau, J.D.: Cutaneous hypersensitivity to sporotrichin in Maricopa County, Arizona, J. Invest. Dermatol. **49:**146, 1967.
17. Kaplan, W.: Practical application of fluorescent antibody procedures in medical mycology. In Mycoses, PAHO Sci. Pub. **304:**178, 1975.
18. Karunaratne, W.A.E.: Rhinosporidiosis in man, London, 1964, The Athlone Press, Ltd.
19. Kaufman, L., and Reiss, E.: Serodiagnosis of fungal diseases. In Lennette, E.H., et al., editors: Manual of clinical microbiology, ed. 4, Washington, D.C., 1985, American Society for Microbiology.
20. Kedes, L.H., Siemski, J., and Braude, A.I.: The syndrome of the alcoholic rose gardener: sporotrichosis of radial tendon sheath—report of a case with amphotericin B, Ann. Intern. Med. **61:**1139, 1964.
21. Lavalle, P., and Mariat, F.: Sporotrichosis, Bull. Inst. Pasteur **81:**295, 1983.
22. Lobo, J.: Um caso de blastmicose produzida por uma especie nara, encontrada em recife, Rev. Med. Pernambuco **1:**763, 1931.
23. Londer, A.T., Castro, R.M., and Fishman, O.: Two cases of sporotrichosis in dogs in Brazil, Sabouraudia **3:**273, 1964.
24. Mackinnon, J.E.: Ecology and epidemiology of sporotrichosis. In International symposium on mycoses, PAHO Sci. Pub. **205:**169, 1970.
25. Mahgoub, S.E.: Mycetoma, Semin. Dermatol. **4:**230, 1985.
26. Mariat, F., Destomes, P., and Segretain, G.: The mycetomas: clinical features, pathology, etiology, and epidemiology, Contrib. Microbiol. Immunol. **4:**1, 1977.
27. McGinnis, M.R.: Human pathogenic species of *Exophiala, Phialophora,* and *Wangiella.* In The black and white yeasts, PAHO Sci. Publ. **356:**37, 1978.
28. McGinnis, M.R.: Laboratory handbook of medical mycology, New York, 1980, Academic Press, Inc.
29. McGinnis, M.R.: Chromoblastomycosis and phaeohyphomycosis: new concepts, diagnosis, and mycology, J. Am. Acad. Dermatol. **8:**1, 1983.
30. McGinnis, M.R.: Dematiaceous fungi. In Lennette, E.H., et al., editors: Manual of clinical microbiology, ed. 4, Washington, D.C., 1985, American Society for Microbiology.
31. McGinnis, M.R., Ajello, L., and Schell, W.A.: Mycotic diseases: a proposed nomenclature, Int. J. Dermatol. **24:**9, 1985.
32. McGinnis, M.R., D'Amato, R.F., and Land, G.A.: Pictorial handbook of medically important fungi and aerobic actinomycetes, New York, 1982, Praeger Publishers.
33. McGinnis, M.R., Rinaldi, M.G., and Winn, R.: Emerging agents of phaeohyphomycosis: pathogenic species of *Bipolaris* and *Exserohilum,* J. Clin. Microbiol. **24:**250, 1986.
34. McGinnis, M.R., and Schell, W.A.: The genus *Fonsecaea* and its relationship to the genera *Cladosporium, Phialophora, Ramichloridium,* and *Rhinocladiella.* In Superficial, cutaneous, and subcutaneous infections, PAHO Sci. Publ. **396:**215, 1980.
35. McGinnis, M.R., Schell, W.A., and Carson, J.: *Phaeoannellomyces* and the Phaeococcomycetaceae, new dematiaceous blastomycete taxa, Sabouraudia **23:**179, 1985.
36. McGinnis, M.R., et al.: Reclassification of *Cladosporium bantianum* in the genus *Xylohypha,* J. Clin. Microbiol. **23:**1148, 1986.
37. Middleton, F.G., et al.: Brain abscess caused by *Cladosporium trichoides,* Arch. Intern. Med. **136:**444, 1976.
38. Mitchell, T.G.: Subcutaneous mycoses. In Joklik, W.K., Willett, H.P., and Amos, D.B., editors: Zinsser microbiology, ed. 18, New York, 1984, Appleton-Century-Crofts.
39. Mohr, J.A., et al.: Primary pulmonary sporotrichosis, Am. Rev. Respir. Dis. **106:**260, 1972.
40. Nsanzumuhire, H., Vollum, D., and Potera, A.A.: Chromomycosis due to *Cladosporium trichoides* heated with 5-fluorocytosine, Am. J. Clin. Pathol. **61:**257, 1974.
41. Padhye, A.A., and Ajello, L.: Fungi causing eumycotic mycetoma. In Lennette, E.H., et al., editors: Manual of clinical microbiology, ed. 4, Washington, D.C., 1985, American Society for Microbiology.
42. Palmer, D.F., et al.: Serodiagnosis of mycotic diseases, Springfield, Ill., 1977, Charles C Thomas, Publisher.
43. Rippon, J.W.: Petriellidiosis: the great imitator, Clin. Microbiol. Newsletter **3:**57, 1981.
44. Rippon, J.W.: Medical mycology: the pathogenic fungi and the pathogenic actinomycetes, ed. 2, Philadelphia, 1982, W.B. Saunders Co.
45. Rippon, J.W., and Carmichael, J.W.: Petriellidiosis (allescheriosis): four unusual cases and review of the literature, Mycopathologia **58:**117, 1976.
46. Rogers, A.L., and Beneke, E.S.: Human pathogenic fungi recovered from Brazilian soil, Mycopathologia **22:**15, 1964.
47. Singer, J.I., and Muncie, J.E.: Sporotrichosis: etiologic considerations and report of additional cases from New York, N.Y. State J. Med. **52:**2147, 1952.
48. Travassos, L.R., and Lloyd, K.O.: *Sporothrix schenckii* and related species of *Ceratocystis,* Microbiol. Rev. **44:**683, 1980.
49. Welsh, R.D., and Dolan, C.T.: *Sporothrix* whole yeast agglutination test, Am. J. Clin. Pathol. **59:**82, 1973.

CHAPTER 34

Agents of Systemic Mycoses

Richard C. Tilton
Michael R. McGinnis

The four classic agents of systemic mycoses are *Blastomyces dermatitidis*, the cause of blastomycosis, *Paracoccidioides brasiliensis*, the cause of paracoccidioidomycosis, *Coccidioides immitis*, the cause of coccidioidomycosis, and *Histoplasma capsulatum*, the cause of histoplasmosis. These four fungi are grouped together in this chapter for a number of reasons: (1) they share similar epidemiologic features, (2) the procedures for collection, processing, isolation, and identification are similar for all four organisms, (3) they are all dimorphic, and (4) they are traditionally grouped together.

It should be noted that citing these four organisms as the only causes of systemic mycoses may be too restrictive. In the last decade it was recognized that many fungi have the capacity to cause systemic disease, especially in compromised hosts. For example, in Chapter 37, systemic diseases caused by *Rhizopus arrhizus* and *Aspergillus fumigatus* are discussed. *Candida albicans* and *Cryptococcus neoformans* (see Chapter 35) are also etiologic agents of nonlocalized multiorgan infection.

The reader should recall from Chapter 29 that dimorphism is a characteristic feature of *H. capsulatum*, *C. immitis*, *P. brasiliensis*, *B. dermatitidis*, and *Sporothrix schenckii*. (*Sporothrix schenckii* is discussed in Chapter 33). These fungi are dimorphic because they are able to grow in one morphologic form at room temperature (25° C) and in an entirely different morphologic form in tissue or in the laboratory at 37° C. At 37° C they grow as yeasts (or spherules, in the case of *C. immitis*), and at 25° C they appear as molds. Temperature is the most important external factor for dimorphism, even though other factors are required in varying degrees by some species.[25,29,31] Before the use of exoantigens for the identification of cultures, the identification of dimorphic fungi was confirmed by converting the mold form to its corresponding tissue form either in vivo or in vitro, using laboratory animals.

A sixth dimorphic fungus, *Penicillium marneffei*, is being seen more frequently in southern China and Southeast Asia.[7,18] This fungus is a typical *Penicillium* at room temperature. At body temperature it forms yeast cells indistinguishable in size and shape from those of *H. capsulatum*, except that they divide by fission rather than budding.

PATHOLOGY AND CLINICAL SIGNIFICANCE
HISTOPLASMOSIS

Histoplasmosis is a major disease of both humans and animals.[5,27] Infections may range from self-limited, asymptomatic processes to disseminated processes resulting in the death of the patient. Milder infections most frequently occur in the uncompromised host, whereas disseminated disease is most commonly seen in patients having impaired or compromised cellular immunity, for instance, patients with cancer or patients receiving chemotherapy with immunosuppressive drugs.

If the exposure to *H. capsulatum* is light, pulmonary histoplasmosis may be totally asymptomatic in uncompromised hosts. Heavier exposure may result in an influenza-like illness. Even in asymptomatic cases, chest x-ray films may show patchy areas of pneumonitis, usually involving the lower lobes. After heavy exposure more diffuse pulmonary involvement may occur. Necrotic lesions may form, which are healed by fibrous encapsulation and later infiltrated by calcium salts, resulting in calcified lesions. The yeast cells of *H. capsulatum* are usually seen in the centers of the sectioned and stained lesions. Histoplasmosis can become chronic in middle-aged male smokers, and portions of their lung tissue contain cavitary lesions. These patients almost always have a chronic cough. Histoplasmosis may spread to other organs, particularly in babies or immunosuppressed patients. The most common sites of dissemination are the spleen, liver, lymph nodes, and bone marrow. The spread of the organisms may be benign, but in other cases it may be acute and overwhelming, particularly for infants or patients being treated with steroids.[6] If antimicrobial therapy is necessary, amphotericin B is recommended.

Histoplasmosis is an infection of the reticuloendothelial system, where it grows within macrophages and giant cells. Once the conidia of *H. capsulatum* are inhaled, a patchy bronchopneumonia containing yeast-laden phagocytic cells develops in the alveolar spaces. If disease occurs, there is a proliferation of histiocytes or a development of epitheloid and giant cells, forming granulomata with or without central caseation.[3] The yeast cells multiply within giant cells. The fungus can disseminate to many tissues by hematogenous means. In patients with acquired immunodeficiency syndrome (AIDS) *H. capsulatum* was the third most common fungal pathogen in 3170 cases reported to the Centers for Disease Control.[2] Opportunistic infections in the AIDS population occur because cell-mediated immunity cannot limit the proliferation of the fungus in tissue. At times there is little or no apparent host response. The multiplication of the yeast may be so profuse that large extracellular clusters of yeast cells occur, resulting in tissue necrosis. In three AIDS patient we have seen, the yeast cells of *H. capsulatum* were abundant and easily seen in peripheral blood smears. Even though phagocytic cells are important in histoplasmosis, the mechanism they use to kill the yeast is essentially unknown, as is the process whereby immunity assists the intracellular destruction of *H. capsulatum*.[8] It is known that *H. capsulatum* elicits both cellular and humoral immune responses, with both specific IgG and IgM antibodies being produced.

Histoplasmosis is of worldwide distribution. It is endemic in the Mississippi, Missouri, St. Lawrence, and Ohio river valleys and can be cultured from soil that has been enriched with manure from birds, bats, and some animals in endemic areas. Histoplasmosis is often associated with chicken coops and caves in which bats live. The fungus cannot survive in pure chicken manure but requires soil that has been enriched by chicken manure. Its growth is also limited to specific zones within the enriched soil. Even though the fungus grows in this kind of environment, chickens, starlings, and other birds that tend to roost together are not infected by *H. capsulatum*. In contrast, bats are naturally infected and may serve as carriers. They often have intestinal lesions containing viable yeast cells. Disturbances of sites such as starling and chicken roosts, sites inhabited by pigeons, and bat manure in caves can produce infective aerosols. In the United States approximately 40 million people have been exposed, with 500,000 new cases of histoplasmosis per year. Of these, 55,000 to 200,000 patients are symptomatic, 1500 to 4000 may require hospitalization, and 25 to 100 die.[21]

COCCIDIOIDOMYCOSIS

Coccidioidomycosis is usually an asymptomatic or mildly symptomatic, self-limited upper respiratory tract infection, but it may become disseminated and fatal. The infection results from inhalation of arthroconidia and remains asymptomatic in about 60% of patients. The remaining 40% of patients may have a mild to severe acute upper respiratory process.

In the self-limited, symptomatic pulmonary form of the infection, symptoms include cough, pleuritic pain, loss of appetite, malaise, and fatigue. Some patients with x-ray findings of cavities may have chest pains, cough, and hemoptysis.

Approximately 0.2% of patients with pulmonary coccidioidomycosis develop a disseminated form of the infection. Disseminated coccidioidomycosis is serious and may involve cutaneous and subcutaneous tissues, meninges, and visceral organs. Dark-skinned individuals are more likely to develop disseminated coccidioidomycosis. Like histoplasmosis, residual pulmonary coccidioidomycosis may be diagnosed after cavities are observed in the lungs. Amphotericin B is the drug of choice.

The infectious arthroconidia responsible for coccidioidomycosis are produced from fertile septate hyphae that grow in soil in the lower Sonoran Life Zone.* The alternate cells between the arthroconidia undergo autolysis to release the intervening arthroconidia (see Figure 34-7). These arthroconidia are inhaled by the human host and undergo conversion to spherules. Various investigators have suggested that viable leukocytes and CO_2 may be involved in regulating this morphologic change. The spherules rapidly increase in size and undergo segmentation to form peripheral compartments surrounding a central cavity. Endospores, approximately 2 to 4 μm in diameter, develop in packets within these peripheral compartments.

---

*An ecologic classification for an area characterized by being semiarid, with high summer temperatures and mild winters and plants such as creosote brush, cacti, yuccas, and agaves.

The packets are approximately 10 μm in diameter and are surrounded by a thin membranous layer. As the endospores increase in size, some fill the central cavity and eventually rupture the spherule wall. These endospores may be distributed locally or disseminated throughout the body.[4,10,22]

Several factors are thought to contribute to the virulence of *Coccidioides immitis*.[10] First, the cell walls of the infectious arthroconidia are antiphagocytic. Moreover, studies have shown that even when the cell wall is stripped away, polymorphonuclear leukocytes (PMNs) and macrophages are able to phagocytize the arthroconidia but are unable to kill them effectively. In vitro studies have shown that macrophages are able to kill the organisms in the presence of lymphocytes from *C. immitis*–immune mice,[1] thus attesting to the major role of cell-mediated immunity in the control of coccidioidomycosis. Other interesting studies have shown that PMNs and macrophages are much more effective in killing *B. dermatitidis* than *C. immitis*, which may help explain why coccidioidomycosis is a much more common clinical problem than blastomycosis.[9]

The spherule and endospore forms of *C. immitis* also provide major barriers to host defense.[10] The spherule is remarkably thick (see Figure 34-3) and is difficult to digest. The spherules are also too large to be ingested by single phagocytes. Similarly, the endospores are covered by remnants of the antiphagocytic inner spherule cell wall. The large numbers of endospores that are released provide yet another virulence mechanism for *C. immitis*. Each spherule releases hundreds of endospores, overwhelming the defense mechanisms of the nonimmune host.

Several host factors also contribute to virulence.[10] Disseminated disease occurs more frequently in blacks than in whites, in the very young and very old, in patients who are immunosuppressed, and in pregnant women. The propensity of pregnant women to develop disease has been attributed to the depressed cell-mediated immune response and the increased levels of estradiol and progesterone occurring during pregnancy.[10] These two hormones directly stimulate the growth of *C. immitis*.[11]

Coccidioidomycosis is endemic in North, Central, and South America. In the United States the disease occurs primarily in the Southwest, especially in Arizona and California. As already noted, *C. immitis* grows in the alkaline, sandy soil of these areas, which correspond to the lower Sonoran Life Zone. An epidemic of coccidioidomycosis occurred in the San Joaquin Valley in 1978 as a result of airborne dissemination of the organism during a severe dust storm.[12] Coccidioidomycosis occurs in several animals other than humans.

PARACOCCIDIOIDOMYCOSIS

Paracoccidioidomycosis is a primary pulmonary disease in which the etiologic agent—*Paracoccidioides brasiliensis*—disseminates to mucous membranes and other tissues. Paracoccidioidomycosis appears as (1) an asymptomatic pulmonary infection, (2) a mucocutaneous-lymphangitic disease, and (3) a systemic infection.[13] The asymptomatic infection may be benign or progressive, with symptoms like those of respiratory infections in general: cough, weight loss, fever, lethargy, dyspnea, and hemoptysis. Dissemination from the lungs occurs via the lymphatics or blood vessels to the oral cavity, skin, mucous membranes of the mouth, lymph nodes, spleen, liver, or bone. In older patients the infection is chronic, and skin and mucosal lesions are typically present.[13] Mucocutaneous lesions usually involve the oral mucosa, gums, and the nasal and anal mucosa. Lymphadenopathy may occur, with the cervical lymph nodes becoming enlarged. In patients under 30 years of age the reticuloendothelial system is severely affected. The clinical course is acute, and death may occur. For therapy, ketoconazole appears to be the drug of choice.

The source and type of inoculum that reaches the lungs are unknown.[23] The initial lung infection is asymptomatic. The fungus may remain in the lungs or disseminate. Of special interest is the role of alpha-1,3-glucan of the yeast cell wall as a modulator of host-parasite interactions. Macrophages are unable to digest this component of the outer cell wall, which helps to protect the fungus in tissue.[26] The yeast form consists of large cells (10 to 60 μm in diameter) with many daughter cells attached by narrow necks. The expression ''multiple budding'' is often used to characterize this process. The histopathologic features of paracoccidioidomycosis are similar to those of coccidioidomycosis and blastomycosis. The textbook by Chandler, Kaplan, and Ajello[3] should be consulted for further details.

It is thought that the habitat of *P. brasiliensis* might be soil from Central and South America, but this has not been conclusively proved. Endemic zones are associated with warm temperatures (10° to 28° C), rainfall (500 to 2500 mm/year), elevations from 47 to 1300 meters, abundant forests, short winters, rainy summers, and mostly acidic soils.[21,24] Men 30 to 60 years old are most commonly infected. Restrepo and coworkers[23] have shown that a *P. brasiliensis* hormone receptor site recognizes mammalian estrogens. It has been postulated that estrogen's ability to inhibit the transformation of mycelium to yeast form is responsible for the marked resistance of women to paracoccidioidomycosis. (The yeast form must be produced for disease to occur.) The incidence of infection is related to poor nutrition and inadequate public health measures. The skin test has been extremely helpful in epidemiologic studies.

BLASTOMYCOSIS

Blastomycosis is a chronic granulomatous infection of the lungs that may disseminate to other tissues. The fungus is inhaled into the lungs. As with *Paracoccidioides brasiliensis,* the inoculum form is unknown. Like the other systemic infections, most blastomycosis infections are probably clinically inapparent. Symptomatic disease usually appears as a mild respiratory infection, which results in fever, weight loss, malaise, and productive cough. Because of the lack of a skin test, the attack rate is unknown. If the fungus disseminates, tissues such as skin, bones, joints, prostate gland, and testes are most frequently involved. At one time it was thought that blastomycosis developed after inhalation of the fungus or direct inoculation into the skin. It is currently known that the skin lesions result from hematogenous dissemination from the lungs. The lesions are ulcerated, verrucose, granulomatous processes that may become extensive with scar tissue replacing the skin (Figure 34-1). Patients with diabetes have an increased risk of developing blastomycosis.

The tissue response varies depending on the type of infection in the patient. The fungus usually incites a mixed granulomatous and purulent inflammatory reaction. Initially the reaction is purulent, later becoming localized with confluent epithelioid cell granulomata. Cutaneous blastomycosis initially occurs as

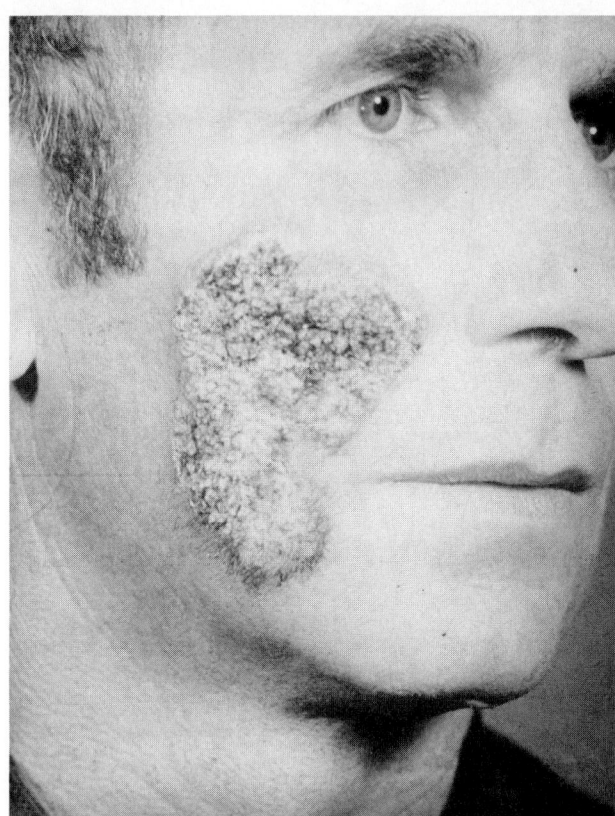

FIGURE 34-1. Characteristic granulomatous lesions of blastomycosis. (From Utz, J.P.: Blastomycosis. In Hoeprich, P.D., editor: Infectious diseases, ed. 3, Philadelphia, 1983, Harper & Row, Publishers.)

microabscesses in the dermis and subcutis. As the skin lesions progress, granulomata are formed and fibrosis occurs. When yeast cells are seen, they are primarily located at the edge of the lesions. Hyperplasia of the epidermis can occur above the inflammatory reaction. In tissue, *B. dermatitidis* can resemble *H. capsulatum* var. *duboisii* and the immature endospores of *C. immitis,* and the small form of *B. dermatitidis* is similar to *H. capsulatum* var. *capsulatum.* Large, round, thick-walled hyaline yeast cells with broadly attached blastoconidia are characteristic of *B. dermatitidis.*

B. dermatitidis is found worldwide. Native infections have been reported in England, Africa, Mexico, Europe, and elsewhere. The disease is endemic in the Mississippi, Ohio, and Missouri river valleys, southern Canada, the Great Lakes area, and the mid-Atlantic coastal states. Blastomycosis is more common in rural than in urban areas. The fungus is suspected to live in soil or wood, but instances of isolation from nature have been rare and sometimes questionable. Studies have shown that some of the aerobic actinomycetes in soil readily lyse *B. dermatitidis* when it is placed in soil. *B. dermatitidis* is not transmitted from person to person or from animal to human. It is more common in men than in women, with the most severe infections in patients 20 to 50 years of age. There is no marked racial predilection, but blacks are more commonly infected than whites. The treatment for blastomycosis, as for all of the systemic mycoses, is amphotericin B.

LABORATORY DIAGNOSIS
SAFETY

The fungi discussed in this chapter are dangerous microorganisms that must be handled with care. All manipulations involving clinical specimens and cultures must be performed in a biologic safety cabinet (BSC). The technologist should *never smell a fungus culture*. If a colony bears a resemblance to a systemic fungus, it should be handled as if it were one. Controversy exists whether to culture specimens initially in screw-capped tubes with slanted agar or in agar-containing Petri dishes. We prefer plastic Petri dishes because they have more surface on which one can isolate and view isolated colonies. However, the plates *must* be sealed with Parafilm or oxygen-permeable tape that permits gas exchange. All contaminated material—slides, tubes, and so forth—must be autoclaved before disposal.

SPECIMEN COLLECTION AND TRANSPORT

Because the systemic fungal diseases described are primarily pulmonary, many of the specimens are sputum and other respiratory secretions. The optimal respiratory secretion specimen is one that originates in the lower lung. Saliva is totally unacceptable. Often the allegedly good specimen is contaminated with saliva; the microbiologist must inspect the specimen grossly for purulent portions before culturing. Because the systemic fungi may also be found in other tissues and multiple organ systems, the lymph nodes, cerebrospinal fluid, synovial fluid, prostatic secretions, skin, tissue biopsy specimens, and bone marrow can also be used for isolation and detection of systemic fungi through direct examination. Specific instructions for processing can be found in Chapter 29.

Specimens for mycologic examination (in particular, the systemic fungi) should be delivered to the laboratory and processed as soon as possible after collection. This is especially true for *Histoplasma capsulatum* because the yeast cells are extremely sensitive to contaminants and environmental conditions. For example, Thompson, Kaplan, and Phillips[30] report that *H. capsulatum* does not survive for long periods of time in the refrigerator or on dry ice. Most fungi, with this exception, survive refrigeration. If left at room temperature or placed in an incubator, *H. capsulatum* becomes overgrown by contaminating bacteria and yeasts. In fact, yeasts such as *Candida albicans* may lower the pH of the environment and become toxic to *H. capsulatum*.[30]

In practice the laboratory worker might have little control over the transport of an individual specimen. If the specimen is delayed in transport and the collection of another specimen is impossible or poses a risk to the patient, the specimen should be processed. The report should state "delayed in transit, specimen may be unreliable." A repeat specimen should be requested.

DIRECT EXAMINATION OF SPECIMENS

All specimens for systemic fungi should be examined at the time of their receipt. In some instances a specific diagnosis can be made rapidly; this may influence the therapeutic regimen or alert the laboratory worker to use additional media or techniques for isolation. If specimens must be concentrated, microscopy should be performed as soon as possible after concentration. The sediment can be examined directly. It is sometimes necessary to clear the specimen with potassium hydrox-

TABLE 34-1. Microscopic Appearance in Clinical and Tissue Specimens

Organism	Microscopic Appearance
Blastomyces dermatitidis	Large spherical yeast cells 8 to 12 μm, with thick walls; blastoconidia attached to parent cell by broad base (Figure 34-2)
Coccidioides immitis	Spherules round, hyaline, large, 30 to 60 μm, thick-walled structures filled with one-celled, hyaline, small, 2 to 5 μm endospores (Figure 34-3)
Histoplasma capsulatum	Rarely seen in sputum; may be evident in touch preparations of lymph nodes, bone marrow, and blood smears of patients with AIDS; small (2 to 5 μm) oval yeasts resembling *Torulopsis glabrata* (Figure 34-4); oil immersion is recommended; in tissue sections the small yeasts are intracellular in polymorphonuclear leukocytes, giant cells, or macrophages
Paracoccidioides brasiliensis	Multiple budding blastoconidia around large one-celled, hyaline, thick-walled cells; blastoconidia are variable in size and arranged radially around the parent cells, attached by narrow tubular denticles; they are often described as a "pilot's wheel" (Figure 34-5)

ide (KOH) before evaluation. KOH preparations, use of Celluflor, Gram stains, periodic acid–Schiff (PAS) stain, phase-contrast microscopy, and fluorescent antibody (FA) stains can provide useful and important data.

Table 34-1 describes structures seen on direct smears of specimens for systemic fungi.

CULTURE AND ISOLATION

Media with and without antimicrobial agents must be used when culturing for systemic fungi. *Cryptococcus neoformans, Pseudallescheria boydii, Aspergillus* spp., and some zygomycetes are sensitive to cycloheximide. *H. capsulatum* is inhibited by high concentrations of gentamicin and chloramphenicol, especially when incubated at 37° C. *Actinomyces* spp. and the aerobic actinomycetes, such as *Nocardia asteroides,* are susceptible to chloramphenicol and other antimicrobics, such as penicillin.

Yeast extract–phosphate medium[28] should be used to recover *H. capsulatum* from contaminated respiratory specimens, such as sputum. In AIDS patients the Isolator blood culture system (DuPont) is useful for the detection of histoplasmosis fungemia.

Isolation plates or slants are incubated at 30° C and inspected every 2 to 4 days for evidence of growth. Plates should be sealed entirely around their edges with oxygen-permeable tape. The lids of the Petri dishes should not be removed during the inspection, to prevent accidental contamination of workers and the environment. Plates are inspected within a BSC. When oxygen-permeable tape is used to seal the entire dish, the

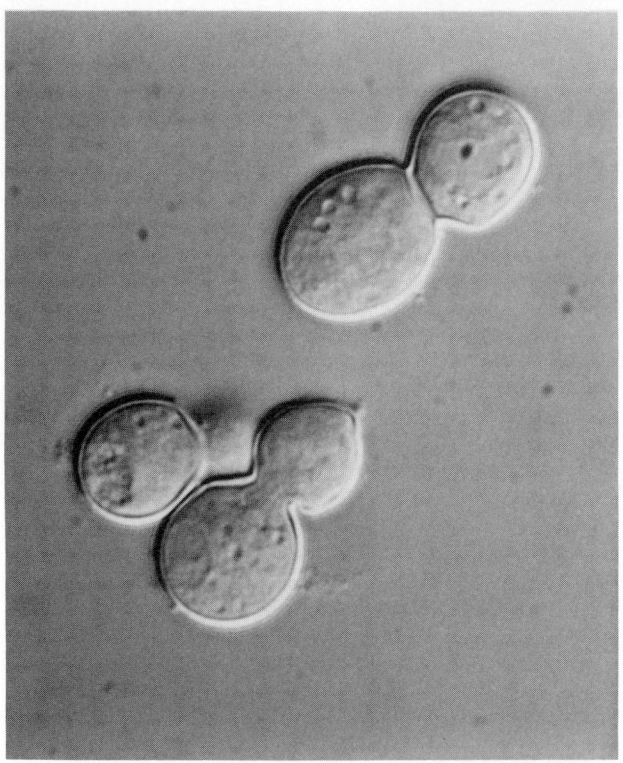

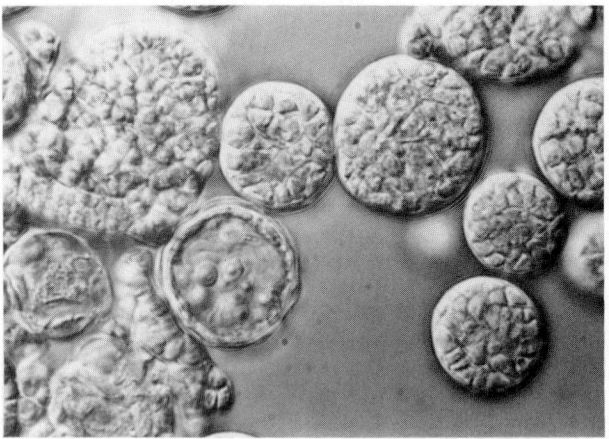

FIGURE 34-2. *Blastomyces dermatitidis* in its yeast form. Note broad base of attachment of blastoconidium to parent cell.

FIGURE 34-3. Thick-walled spherules of *Coccidioides immitis*.

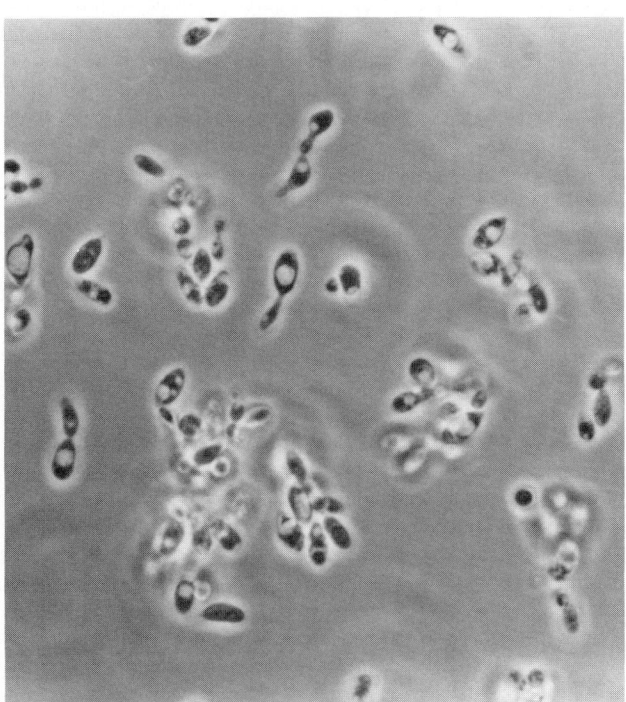

FIGURE 34-4. *Histoplasma capsulatum*. Small oval yeast cells producing blastoconidia.

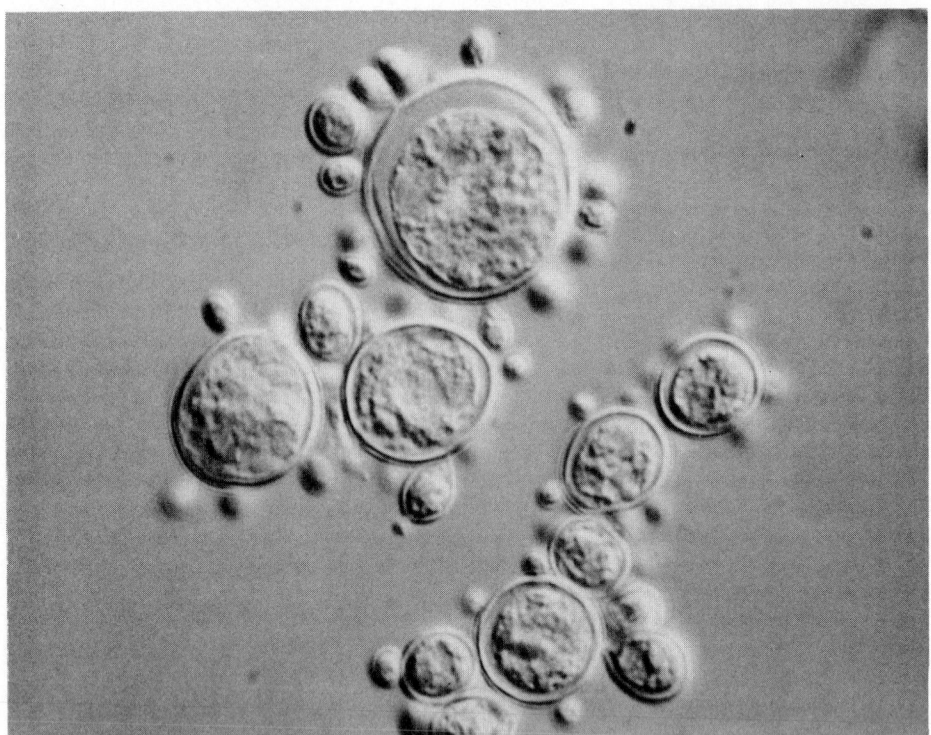

FIGURE 34-5. *Paracoccidioides brasiliensis*. Yeast cells are round with multiple blastoconidia attached to parent cell by narrow necks.

unopened dish can be examined under a good light source.

Of the four dimorphic fungi described in this chapter, *Coccidioides immitis* grows the most quickly (4 to 5 days), and *H. capsulatum* and *Paracoccidioides brasiliensis* grow the most slowly (2 to 3 weeks). The microbiologist cannot assume that a saprophytic fungus is present simply because colonial growth appears in a few days.

Lactophenol cotton blue (LCB) preparations should be made on all colonies to evaluate the nature of conidiogenesis. Contaminated cultures must be purified before their identification.

MORPHOLOGY

At 30° C *H. capsulatum* grows as a white to brownish mold. Other morphologic characteristics are summarized in Table 34-2. At 37° C on special media the colony is slow growing and consists of yeastlike cells. At room temperature, both one-celled microconidia and macroconidia are typically produced on short, hyphalike conidiophores. The macroconidia are round (7 to 12 μm in diameter), with thickened cell walls that are typically tuberculate. The microconidia are 2 to 5 μm, round, and smooth walled. The conidia of some *Chrysosporium* and *Sepedonium* spp. are similar to those of *Histoplasma*, but neither genus contains species that are dimorphic. However, because of the morphologic similarity of these two genera to *H. capsulatum*, suspected isolates of *H. capsulatum* must be confirmed as such by exoantigen testing.

Kwon-Chung[16] discovered the sexual stage (teleomorph stage) of *H. capsulatum* and proposed the name *Emmonsiella capsulatum*. The sexual form consisted of gymnothecia with radiating spirals and secondary peridial hyphae. A careful study

of *E. capsulatum* by McGinnis and Katz[20] showed that *E. capsulatum* should be classified in the genus *Ajellomyces*. As a result of their study the sexual stage of *H. capsulatum* was renamed *A. capsulatus*. The genus *Ajellomyces* contains the sexual forms of *B. dermatitidis* and *H. capsulatum*.

There are actually two varieties of *H. capsulatum*. The variety isolated in the United States is *H. capsulatum* var. *capsulatum*. *H. capsulatum* var. *duboisii* is the cause of African histoplasmosis. These two varieties are morphologically indistinguishable in culture. When their isolates are crossed with each other, *A. capsulatus* is produced. Clinically the infections are different, and in tissue *H. capsulatum* var. *duboisii* is much larger.

The colonial and microscopic morphology of *C. immitis* is described in Table 34-2. The arthroconidia of *C. immitis* are similar to those produced by species of *Malbranchea*. As with other systemic fungi, all suspected isolates of *C. immitis* must be confirmed. We recommend the exoantigen test.

As just mentioned, the genus *Ajellomyces* also contains the sexual form of *B. dermatitidis*. The teleomorph of *B. dermatitidis* is called *Ajellomyces dermatitidis*. Colonies of *B. dermatitidis* growing at room temperature may be membranous, smooth, and cream-colored with no aerial hyphae, or they may be woolly with a white to tan color. This mold form of *B. dermatitidis* produces oval, smooth-walled, one-celled conidia (3 to 5 μm) borne on short lateral hyphal branches. Some isolates of *B. dermatitidis* produce echinulate conidia. At 35° C the colonies are yeastlike in appearance. The yeast are thick walled, spherical, one celled, and hyaline and produce a single blastoconidium attached to the parent cell by a wide base. The yeast cells are 10 to 15 μm in diameter. The conidia of *B.*

TABLE 34-2. Colonial Appearance and Microscopic Morphology of the Systemic Fungi at Room Temperature

Organism	Colonial Appearance	Microscopic Morphology
Blastomyces dermatitidis	Young colonies may be thin and membranous; older colonies may be glabrous to woolly; color varies from dirty white to tan; slow to moderate growing (Plate 26, *C*)	Small, oval, smooth-walled conidia borne on short, lateral, hyphalike conidiophores (Figure 34-6)
Coccidioides immitis	Young colonies glabrous and grayish, becoming white and cottony; with age, becoming white to brown to dark gray; rapid growing (Plate 26, *D*)	Alternating one-celled, thin-walled, barrel-shaped arthroconidia and disjunctor cells (Figure 34-7)
Histoplasma capsulatum	Colonies woolly, cottony, or granular; initially white, becoming brown in color; slow growing (Plate 26, *E*)	Macroconidia one celled, round (7-12 μm), and tuberculated; microconidia small, one celled (2-5 μm), round, smooth walled (Figure 34-8); hyphalike conidiophores
Paracoccidioides brasiliensis	Colonial forms vary and may be glabrous, leathery, flat to wrinkled, folded, or velvety; color of colony white to beige; slow growing (Plate 26, *F*)	Hyphae are typically sterile; fresh isolates may produce one-celled, hyaline conidia similar to those produced by *B. dermatitidis*

Data from references 14 and 19.

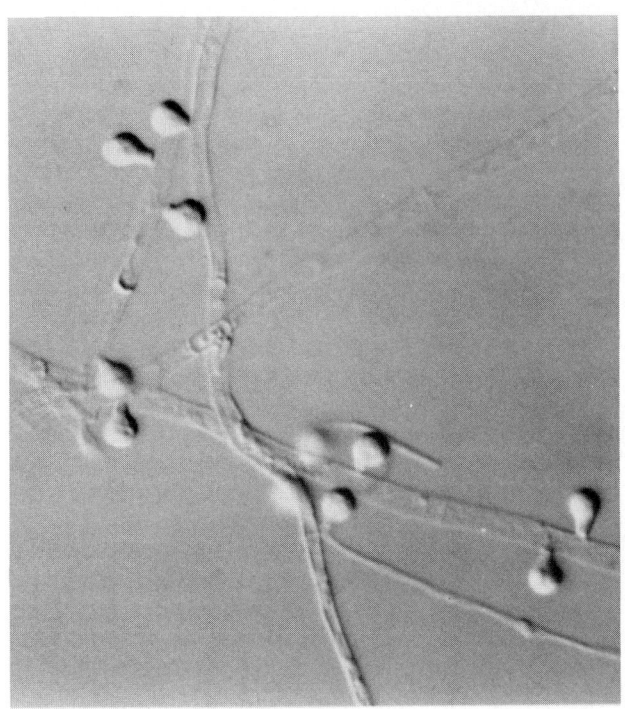

FIGURE 34-6. *Blastomyces dermatitidis* in its mold form. Hyphalike conidiophores give rise to small, one-celled conidia.

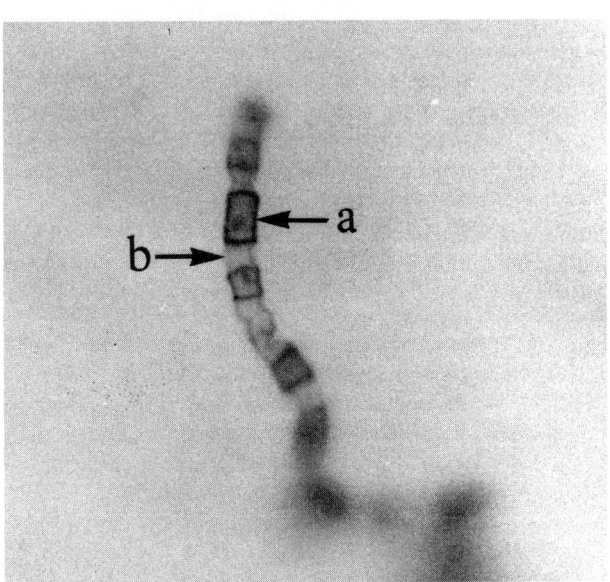

FIGURE 34-7. Arthroconidium (*a*) and disjunctor cell (*b*) of *Coccidioides immitis*. (From Mycopathol. Mycol. Appl. **45:**269, 1971.)

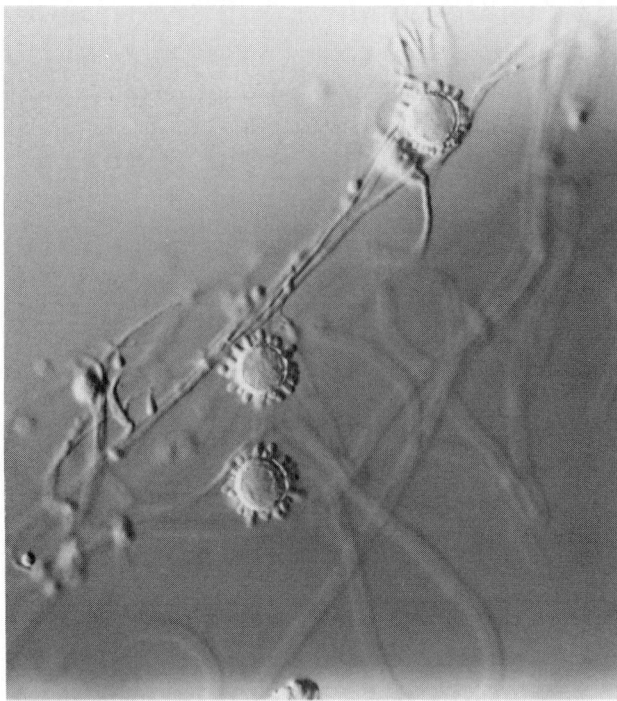

FIGURE 34-8. *Histoplasma capsulatum.* Large, single, thick-walled macroconidia with robust projections from the cell wall develop on hyphalike conidiophores.

dermatitidis resemble those produced by some species of *Chrysosporium* and must be confirmed. *Blastomyces dermatitidis* readily converts from mold to yeast form at 37° C on enriched media. The exoantigen procedure is also an excellent method to confirm its identification.

Isolates of *P. brasiliensis* are slow growing, and its hyphae are typically sterile. Some fresh isolates produce one-celled, hyaline, smooth-walled, small conidia laterally from the hyphae on short hyphaelike conidiophores. When grown at 37° C the fungus produces large, one-celled, thick-walled yeast cells that have multiple blastoconidia attached by narrow tubular necks. This is often referred to as multiple budding. Some of the yeast cells may be as large as 30 μm in diameter. Because isolates may either be sterile or resemble isolates of *Chrysosporium*, their identification must be confirmed. We recommend the exoantigen procedure because of its accuracy and speed.

CONFIRMATION OF SYSTEMIC FUNGI

As already discussed, identification of the systemic fungi must be confirmed by converting the mold form to either the corresponding yeast form *(H. capsulatum, B. dermatitidis, P. brasiliensis)* or the spherule form *(C. immitis)* on conversion media or by use of specific antigens obtained from culture filtrates in the exoantigen test. With the advent of good conversion media and the exoantigen tests, animal inoculation is unnecessary. We recommend the use of exoantigens.

Mold-to-Yeast and Mold-to-Spherule Conversion

The following procedures for mold-to-yeast conversion and mold-to-spherule conversion are extracted from McGinnis[17]:

1. Procedure for mold-to-yeast conversion
   a. Perform all procedures in a BSC.
   b. With a long-handled inoculating needle, remove a small portion of the isolate to be examined and transfer it to two tubes containing the appropriate medium (Table 34-3) for the suspected dimorphic fungus. Incubate one tube at 37° C and one tube at 25° C.
   c. Examine the yeastlike areas for the presence of typical yeast cells, conversion of hyphae to yeast growth, or both. If the results are questionable, rapidly subculture the isolate to fresh media. Several weeks may be required for complete conversion. The conversion is considered positive when typical yeast cells are present, regardless of their number. If the suspected conversion does not occur, exoantigen studies are necessary.
2. Procedure for mold-to-spherule conversion
   a. Perform all procedures in a BSC.
   b. Prepare a standard slide culture preparation using the Levine modification of Converse medium in 1% ion agar no. 2.
   c. Add approximately 2 ml of Levine modification of Converse medium to an actively growing isolate suspected to be *C. immitis*.
   d. With a sterile loop, transfer a loopful of the floating arthroconidia to the agar block in the slide culture setup.
   e. Place a sterile cover glass on the inoculated agar block, and then moisten the filter paper with sterile water.
   f. Transfer the slide culture to a candle jar, light the candle, and incubate at 40° C for 4 to 5 days.
   g. After 5 days add 10 ml of formalin for each liter of

TABLE 34-3. Mold-to-Tissue Conversion of the Dimorphic Fungi

Fungus	Media and Conditions	Morphologic Form Obtained	Some Similar Fungi at 25° C
Blastomyces dermatitidis	KT medium, Kelley agar, or blood agar, 37° C	Yeast	*Chrysosporium* spp.
Coccidioides immitis	Modified Converse medium, 40° C, 5% to 10% CO_2	Spherules containing endospores	*Malbranchea* spp.
Histoplasma capsulatum	Pines medium or glucose-cysteine-blood (GCB) agar,[a] 37° C	Yeast	*Sepedonium* spp., *Chrysosporium* spp.
Paracoccidioides brasiliensis	BHI agar, 37° C	Yeast	*Chrysosporium* spp., Mycelia Sterilia
Sporothrix schenckii	BHI agar, 37° C, 5% to 10% CO_2	Yeast	*Acrodontium* spp., *Sporothrix* spp.

[a]GCB agar is 1% glucose, 0.1% cysteine, and 10% rabbit or sheep blood.

volume to the candle jar, and then incubate for an additional 24 hours at 37° C. The formalin kills the fungus.

h. Examine the preparation microscopically for the presence of spherules containing endospores. Fungi similar to *C. immitis* may produce large vesicles, but they do not form spherules with endospores.

i. Autoclave the preparation, slide culture, and candle jar when the test is completed.

The mold-to-spherule conversion can also be made on the Levine modification of Converse medium with 1.5% agar in small disposable plastic dishes. The isolate is inoculated on the medium surface in the plastic dish. The conversion occurs in the Petri dish rather than in a slide-culture setup. After inoculation of the medium all the remaining steps are identical to those outlined above. Later a small amount of growth must be transferred to a microscope slide for examination. These setups can be incubated at 37° C, but this is not recommended because hyphae and arthroconidia are also formed at this temperature. Arthroconidia are not formed at 40° C.

Exoantigen Techniques

The five systemic fungi can be identified immunologically through detection of cell-free antigens[15] from culture filtrates. A 10-day-old (or older) Sabouraud dextrose agar slant culture is extracted with an aqueous merthiolate solution for 24 to 48 hours at 25° C. The extract is concentrated by ultracentrifugation or a disposable microconcentrator (Minicon, Amicon, Inc., Danvers, Mass.) and tested by immunodiffusion with a homologous antibody for each of the fungi.[15]

IMMUNOLOGY

Several techniques are used routinely to evaluate the patient's immunologic response to infection by the dimorphic systemic fungi, especially histoplasmosis and coccidioidomycosis. They include skin testing for delayed hypersensitivity reactions, as well as the detection of circulating antibodies by complement fixation, immunodiffusion, tube precipitin, latex

agglutination, and counterimmunoelectrophoresis. Specific descriptions of these tests and their applications are discussed in Chapter 38.

REFERENCES

1. Beaman, L., Benjamini, E., and Pappagianis, D.: Role of lymphocytes in macrophage-induced killing of *Coccidioides immitis* in vitro, Infect. Immun. **34:**347, 1981.
2. Chandler, F.W.: Pathology of the mycoses in patients with the acquired immunodeficiency syndrome (AIDS). In McGinnis, M.R., editor: Current topics in medical mycology, vol. 1, New York, 1985, Springer-Verlag.
3. Chandler, F.W., Kaplan, W., and Ajello, L.: A colour atlas and textbook of the histopathology of mycotic diseases, London, 1980, Wolfe Medical Publications, Ltd.
4. Cole, G.T., and Sun, S.H.: Arthoconidium-spherule-endospore transformation in *Coccidioides immitis*. In Szaniszlo, P.J., editor: Fungal dimorphism, New York, 1985, Plenum Publishing Corp.
5. Darling, S.T.: A protozoön general infection producing pseudotubercles in the lungs and focal necroses in the liver, spleen, and lymph nodes, JAMA **46:**1283, 1906.
6. Davies, S.F., Khan, M., and Sarosi, G.A.: Disseminated histoplasmosis in immunologically suppressed patients: occurrence in a nonendemic area, Am. J. Med. **64:**94, 1978.
7. Deng, Z., and Connor, D.H.: Progressive disseminated penicilliosis caused *Penicillium marneffei:* report of eight cases and differentiation of the causative organism from *Histoplasma capsulatum*, Am. J. Clin. Pathol. **84:**323, 1985.
8. Domer, J.E., and Moser, S.A.: Histoplasmosis, a review, Rev. Med. Vet. Mycol. **15:**159, 1980.
9. Drutz, D.J., Frey, C.L., and Huppert, M.: Pleomorphism: adaptation of fungal pathogens to host tissue. In Schlessinger, D., editor: Microbiology—1983, Washington, D.C., 1983, American Society for Microbiology.
10. Drutz, D.J., and Huppert, M.: Coccidioidomycosis: factors affecting the host-parasite interaction, J. Infect. Dis. **147:**372, 1983.
11. Drutz, D.J. et al.: Human sex hormones stimulate the growth and maturation of *Coccidioides immitis*, Infect. Immun. **32:**897, 1981.
12. Flynn, N.M., et al.: An unusual outbreak of coccidioidomycosis, N. Engl. J. Med. **301:**358, 1979.

13. Giraldo, R., et al.: Pathogenesis of paracoccidioidomycosis: a model based on the study of 46 patients, Mycopathologia **58**:63, 1976.

14. Haley, L.D., and Callaway, C.: Laboratory methods in medical mycology, ed. 4, Dept. of Health, Education and Welfare Pub. No. 78-8361, Atlanta, 1978, Centers for Disease Control.

15. Kaufman, L., and Reiss, E.: Serodiagnosis of fungal diseases. In Lennette, E.H., et al., editors: Washington, D.C., 1985, American Society for Microbiology.

16. Kwon-Chung, K.J.: Studies on *Emmonsiella capsulata*. I. Heterothallism and development of the ascocarp, Mycologia **65**:109, 1973.

17. McGinnis, M.R.: Laboratory handbook of medical mycology, New York, 1980, Academic Press, Inc.

18. McGinnis, M.R.: Progressive disseminated penicilliosis caused by *Penicillium marneffei* (letter), Am. J. Clin. Pathol. **85**:529, 1986.

19. McGinnis, M.R., D'Amato, R.F., and Land, G.A.: Pictorial handbook of medically important fungi and aerobic actinomycetes, New York, 1982, Praeger Publishers.

20. McGinnis, M.R., and Katz, B.: *Ajellomyces* and its synonym *Emmonsiella*, Mycotaxon **8**:157, 1979.

21. Mitchell, T.G.: Systemic mycoses. In Joklik, W.K., Willett, H.P., and Amos, D.B., editors: Zinsser microbiology, ed. 18, Norwalk, Conn., 1984, Appleton-Century-Crofts.

22. Miyaji, M., Nishimura, K., and Ajello, L.: Scanning electron microscope studies on the parasitic cycle of *Coccidioides immitis*, Mycopathologia **89**:51, 1985.

23. Restrepo, A., et al.: Estrogens inhibit mycelium-to-yeast transformation in the fungus *Paracoccidioides brasiliensis:* implications for resistance of females to paracoccidioidomycosis, Infect. Immun. **46**:346, 1984.

24. Restrepo, A.: The ecology of *Paracoccidioides brasiliensis:* a puzzle still unsolved, Sabouraudia **23**:323, 1985.

25. Rippon, J.W.: Dimorphism in pathogenic fungi, CRC Crit. Rev. Microbiol. **8**:49, 1980.

26. San-Blas, G.: *Paracoccidioides brasiliensis:* cell wall glucans, pathogenicity, and dimorphism. In McGinnis, M.R., editor: Current topics in medical mycology, New York, 1985, Springer-Verlag.

27. Sarosi, G.A., and Davies, S.F.: Histoplasmosis. In Braude, A.I., Davis, C.E., and Fierer, J., editors: Infectious diseases and medical microbiology, ed. 2 Philadelphia, 1986, W.B. Saunders Co.

28. Smith, D.C., and Goodman, N.L.: Improved culture method for isolation of *Histoplasma capsulatum* and *Blastomyces dermatitidis* from contaminated specimens, Am. J. Clin. Pathol. **63**:276, 1975.

29. Szaniszlo, P.J., Jacobs, C.W., and Geis, P.A.: Dimorphism: morphologic and biochemical aspects. In Howard, D.H., editor: Fungi pathogenic for humans and animals. Part A, Biology, New York, 1983, Marcel Dekker, Inc.

30. Thompson, D.W., Kaplan, W., and Phillips, B.J.: The effect of freezing and the influence of isolation medium on the recovery of pathogenic fungi from sputum, Mycopathologia **61**:105, 1977.

31. Vanden Bossche, H., editor: Workshop on fungal dimorphism, Beerse, Belgium, 1984, Janssen Research Foundation.

CHAPTER 35

Yeasts

Richard C. Tilton
Michael R. McGinnis

In the past, *Candida albicans* and *Cryptococcus neoformans* were considered the only true pathogenic yeasts. Indeed, in many laboratories these are still the only yeasts identified to the species level. The advent of cancer chemotherapy, radiotherapy, steroids, and antimicrobial agents has contributed to a milieu in which not only are cellular and humoral immune functions compromised, but the normal microbial flora is altered or destroyed. One result of this complex change in the human biosphere is an environment in which opportunistic microorganisms thrive without competition. *C. albicans* and *C. neoformans* are still major yeast pathogens, but the so-called nonpathogenic yeasts are being implicated with greater frequency as opportunistic pathogens in the compromised host.

Yeasts can be our friends and our enemies. Yeasts have numerous applications in food preparation. Yet yeast infections of the mucous membranes, such as thrush and *Candida* vaginitis, afflict millions worldwide. Although localized yeast infections may be merely a nuisance, other yeast infections can be deadly. Yeasts in the bloodstream (fungemia) are often a result of intravenous catheterization or parenteral nutrition (hyperalimentation). Invasion of the heart valves by yeasts can follow the installation of artificial valves, resulting in endocarditis. Overwhelming disseminated yeast infections can contribute to the death of cancer patients[14,36] and, more recently, patients with acquired immmunodeficiency syndrome (AIDS).[17]

Because yeasts are a part of the normal human microflora, their isolation from clinical specimens that originate from nonsterile sites may create misunderstanding about their significance. Yeasts in mixed culture and in small numbers from a site contiguous to mucous membranes (sputum, urine, feces, and vagina) are not usually treated as pathogens without additional clinical information. Yet their isolation from a sterile body fluid or tissue specimen is cause for concern. The presence of yeasts in pure culture and in large numbers from any body site is highly suspect. As in all areas of clinical microbiology, effective and rapid communication with the physician should be used to determine the significance of an isolate.

CLASSIFICATION

Yeasts typically occur as unicellular, budding microorganisms under the growth conditions provided in the clinical microbiology laboratory. The colonies are smooth, pasty to creamy in texture, and moist. Under conditions of reduced oxygen tension or in tissue, some yeasts may form hyphae, pseudohyphae, or both. Yeasts form a variety of reproductive structures that identify the various genera and species. These structures, including germ tubes, pseudohyphae, blastoconidia, chlamydospores, arthroconidia, ballistoconidia, annellides, phialides, and capsules, are discussed in Chapter 28. Yeasts are identified by a combination of morphologic characteristics (genus level) and physiologic profiles (species level).

The teleomorphs of some yeasts are known and are occasionally seen in the clinical laboratory. McGinnis[21] indicates that yeasts have traditionally been divided into two groups based on their ability or inability to reproduce by sexual means.[21] One group is the true, or perfect, yeasts, which reproduce sexually and develop ascospores or basidiospores. The second group consists of the imperfect, or yeastlike, yeasts, which reproduce only by asexual means. The term "anamorph" is applicable to the various asexual forms produced. For convenience the term "yeast" is used to encompass all unicellular, budding fungi, regardless of whether sexual reproduction is known or unknown.

Representative genera of medically important yeasts are indicated in the following list:

Class: Ascomycetes
    Genus: *Saccharomyces*
              Endomycopsis
              Pichia
Class: Basidiomycetes
    Genus: *Leucosporidium*
              Filobasidiella
              Filobasidium
Class: Fungi Imperfecti
  Nondematiaceous yeasts
    Genus: *Blastoschizomyces*
              Candida
              Cryptococcus
              Rhodotorula
              Torulopsis
              Trichosporon
  Dematiaceous yeasts
    Genus: *Phaeoannellomyces*
              Phaeococcomyces

There is currently some controversy regarding the genus *Candida* and its relationship to the genus *Torulopsis*. Yarrow and Meyer[37] proposed that these two genera be merged because they believed that the presence or absence of pseudohyphae is not a characteristic that should be used to separate yeast genera. Because the name *Candida* is better known, they consider it to be the correct name. As a result of their study, they transferred species such as *T. glabrata* to the genus *Candida*. McGinnis and co-workers[24] also reevaluated the genera *Candida* and *Torulopsis*. They concluded that the absence of well-developed pseudohyphae was an acceptable characteristic for maintaining these two genera as separate groups. They also pointed out that the genus *Torulopsis* is a valid, published name, which means, if the taxonomic recommendation of Yarrow and Meyer is accepted, all of these yeasts would become species of *Torulopsis* and not *Candida*. We think that the genera *Candida* and *Torulopsis* are separate and distinct groups of yeasts.

The black, or dematiaceous, yeasts represent a unique group having darkly pigmented cell walls that result in brown to black colonies. Many of the black yeasts are anamorphs associated with filamentous fungi, like *Exophiala jeanselmei* and *Wangiella dermatitidis*. Some black yeasts occur solely as yeasts and are not associated with other anamorphs. McGinnis and Schell[23] have proposed that the black yeasts be classified in the family Phaeococcomycetaceae. Currently they recognize two genera of black yeasts, *Phaeococcomyces* and *Phaeoannellomyces*, which are distinguished from each other on the basis of conidiogenesis. Members of the genus *Phaeoannellomyces* produce yeast cells that function as annellides. Distinct annellated zones are visible with the 100× oil objective of a microscope. *Phaeococcomyces* spp. produce yeast cells that form phialoconidia or blastoconidia.

The genus *Blastoschizomyces* contains only the species *B. capitatus*, which was previously known as *Trichosporon capitatum*.[31] Isolates of *B. capitatus* form annellides and annelloconidia. The annelloconidia subsequently undergo division by fission and then form blastoconidia.

PATHOLOGY AND CLINICAL SIGNIFICANCE
BLASTOSCHIZOMYCES

The fungus *Blastoschizomyces* is an unusual opportunistic pathogen that is recovered from infections involving compromised hosts.

CANDIDA

Candida albicans is part of the normal microflora of both the gastrointestinal tract and mucocutaneous areas.[19] It is also present in the vagina of about 5% of females.[19]

The term "candidiasis" is used for any infection caused by a member of the genus *Candida*. *Candida* organisms can infect virtually all organ systems, leading to an extensive array of clinical manifestations, as given in the following outline:

I. Mucocutaneous involvement
  A. Oral
    1. Thrush (Figure 35-1)
    2. Glossitis
    3. Stomatitis
    4. Cheilitis
    5. Perlèche
  B. Vaginitis and balanitis
  C. Bronchial and pulmonary
  D. Alimentary: esophagitis, enteric, and perianal disease
  E. Chronic mucotaneous candidiasis
II. Cutaneous involvement
  A. Intertriginous and generalized candidiasis
  B. Paronychia and onychomycosis
  C. Diaper disease
  D. Candidal granuloma
III. Systemic involvement
  A. Urinary tract
  B. Endocarditis
  C. Meningitis
  D. Septicemia
  E. Iatrogenic candidemia (barrier-break candidemia)
IV. Allergic diseases
  A. Candidid
  B. Eczema
  C. Asthma
  D. Gastritis

Adherence of *C. albicans*, which is probably mediated by the interaction of glycoproteins on the yeast's surface with those on the host epithelial cells, is an important first step toward colonization and invasion of mucocutaneous tissues. It appears that the germ tube or the hyphae of *C. albicans* directly penetrate the epithelial cells following adherence achieved with hydrolytic enzymes, such as proteinases, phosphatases, and phospholipases.[28] Once within the epithelial cells, the fungus proliferates. Generally, nonadherent species of *Candida* are nonpathogenic.[16] A similar adherence process may be needed before other tissues are invaded.[29,33] Guentzel, Cole, and Pope[9] should be consulted for a review of the adherence mechanisms of *C. albicans*.

As the yeast infection develops, an inflammatory reaction occurs, showing a predominance of neutrophils. Neutrophil function, that is, chemotaxis and phagocytosis, and the ability to attach hyphae can be impaired by a substance originating from the yeast. It has been suggested that the substance is a low-molecular-weight protein from the cell wall. Certain glycoproteins have been demonstrated to be responsible for fever, chemotaxis of leukocytes, release of histamine from mast cells, alterations of hemodynamics, generation of suppressor T cells, and other effects on humoral and cell-mediated immunity observed in candidiasis.[9]

C. albicans causes infection when the normal host defenses are compromised. Predisposing conditions include the following[26,33]:

1. Skin barriers that have been damaged by maceration of tissue, wounds and abrasions, thermal or chemical burns, and intravascular catheters
2. Mucosal barriers that have been altered by diabetes, antimicrobial agents, irradiation, smoking, cytotoxic drugs, corticosteroids, cimetidine, vagotomy resulting in an increased gastric pH, and foreign bodies, such as dentures, nasogastric tubes, and diaphragms
3. Hormonal or nutritional imbalances resulting from diabetes, oral contraceptives, pregnancy, menses, malnutrition, and uremia
4. Decreased numbers of phagocytic cells as a result of leukemia, irradiation, cancer chemotherapy, and agranulocytosis
5. Intrinsic defects in the function of phagocytic cells as the result of chronic granulomatous diseases and myeloperoxidase deficiency
6. Alterations in phagocyte functions caused by uremia, viral infections, and the use of corticosteroids and antimicrobics, such as the aminoglycosides and sulfonamides
7. Cell-mediated immunity problems arising from defects such as chronic mucocutaneous candidiasis and DiGeorge syndrome, from using corticosteroids, irradiation, cancer chemotherapy, and immunosuppression for transplantation, and from collagen vascular diseases.

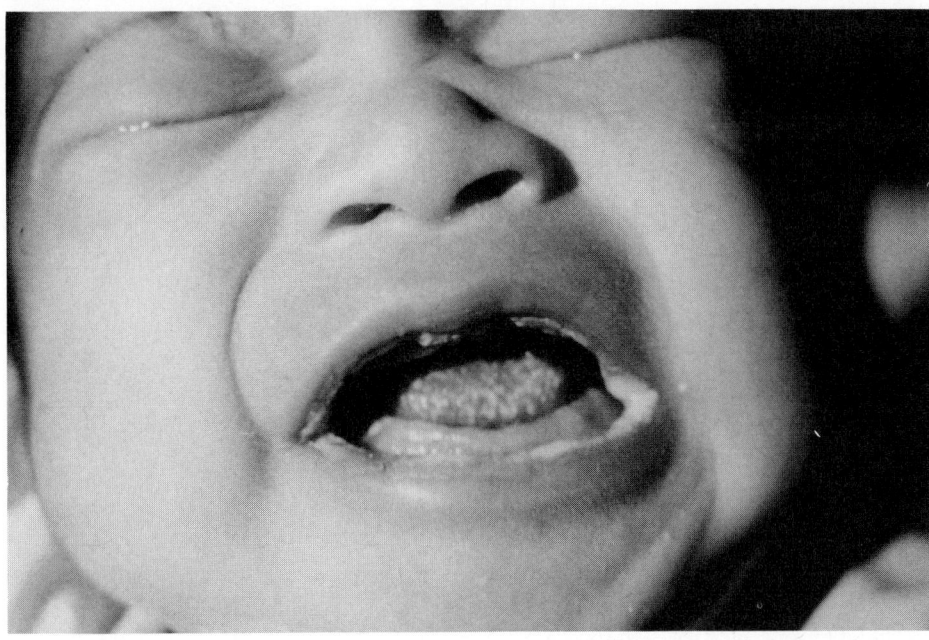

FIGURE 35-1. Oral thrush. Note *Candida albicans* around mouth. (Courtesy C. Halde.)

The association of these conditions with infection is related to their predisposition to increased colonization by *C. albicans*. Antimicrobial agents, for example, inhibit the growth of the normal flora, the presence of which is probably the most important environmental factor affecting the degree of colonization.[33] (The importance of the normal flora in the host-parasite relationship is discussed in Chapter 2.) In the healthy host the normal flora are able to inhibit *C. albicans* through competitive inhibition for binding sites and nutrients, but in the presence of antimicrobial agents, such as tetracycline and aminoglycosides (which inhibit gram-negative enteric organisms), the less susceptible *C. albicans* proliferate.[31]

Despite the mechanisms of pathogenicity cited previously, *C. albicans* has inherently low pathogenicity. Generally hormonal imbalances or the use of antimicrobial agents is associated with superficial candidiasis.[31] Disseminated disease is associated with severe defects in the functions of phagocytic cells or cell-mediated immunity.[31] An example of the latter is AIDS patients; candidal oropharyngitis (41.8% of cases) and candidal esophagitis (9.4% of cases) are the two most common fungal infections observed in these patients.[4]

CRYPTOCOCCUS

Cryptococcosis, which is caused by *Cryptococcus neoformans,* is a multisystem disease, although the primary portal of entry is the lung. The six clinical types of cryptococcosis include pulmonary, central nervous system (CNS), visceral, osseous, cutaneous, and mucocutaneous. In all cases of cryptococcosis the infection is first pulmonary with subsequent dissemination.

Cryptococcosis may be either benign or acute. In the general population cryptococcosis is primarily pulmonary and is asymptomatic or very mild. The CNS cryptococcal infections, such as meningitis or brain abscess, are most commonly seen in the acute clinical setting. Why *C. neoformans* has a predilec-

tion for the CNS is unknown. The differentiation of CNS cryptococcal infection is made through isolation of the organism or detection of cryptococcal polysaccharide, or both, from the brain or cerebrospinal fluid. Cutaneous and mucocutaneous cryptococcosis is the result of disseminated disease and occurs in about 10% to 15% of cases.[30] Bone may be involved in 5% to 10% of cases of cryptococcosis, with bony prominences, cranial bones, and vertebrae most commonly affected.[30] Visceral cryptococcosis follows the dissemination of the fungus to any organ or tissue of the body, most commonly the heart, testis, prostate, and eye.[30]

In tissue the host response may range from little or no inflammation to a granulomatous reaction with necrosis. When a tissue response is difficult to detect, large numbers of yeast cells tend to be present. This is especially true in patients with AIDS. In tissue the cells of *C. neoformans* are pleomorphic and are approximately 8 to 10 μm in diameter but may range from 2 to 20 μm or more.

Patients with AIDS, carcinoma, leukemia, collagen vascular disease, Hodgkin's disease, or sarcoid are at risk for cryptococcosis, as are patients undergoing organ transplantation and systemic corticosteroid therapy. The alteration of cell-mediated immunity in all of these conditions predisposes patients to cryptococcosis. Suppressor T cells are activated, at least in animal studies.[11]

Cryptococcal meningitis occurs in about 5.3% of AIDS cases.[4] Of 27 AIDS patients, 18 had meningitis; of 26 patients, 18 had positive blood cultures; of 18 patients with meningitis, all had positive CSF cultures; and of 16 patients with meningitis, all had a positive cryptococcal antigen test (geometric mean titer of 294).[17]

C. neoformans is distributed worldwide. There is no age, race, geographic, or occupational predilection. Pigeon excreta appears to be the chief source for the distribution and maintenance of the organism.[18,30] *C. neoformans* may remain viable

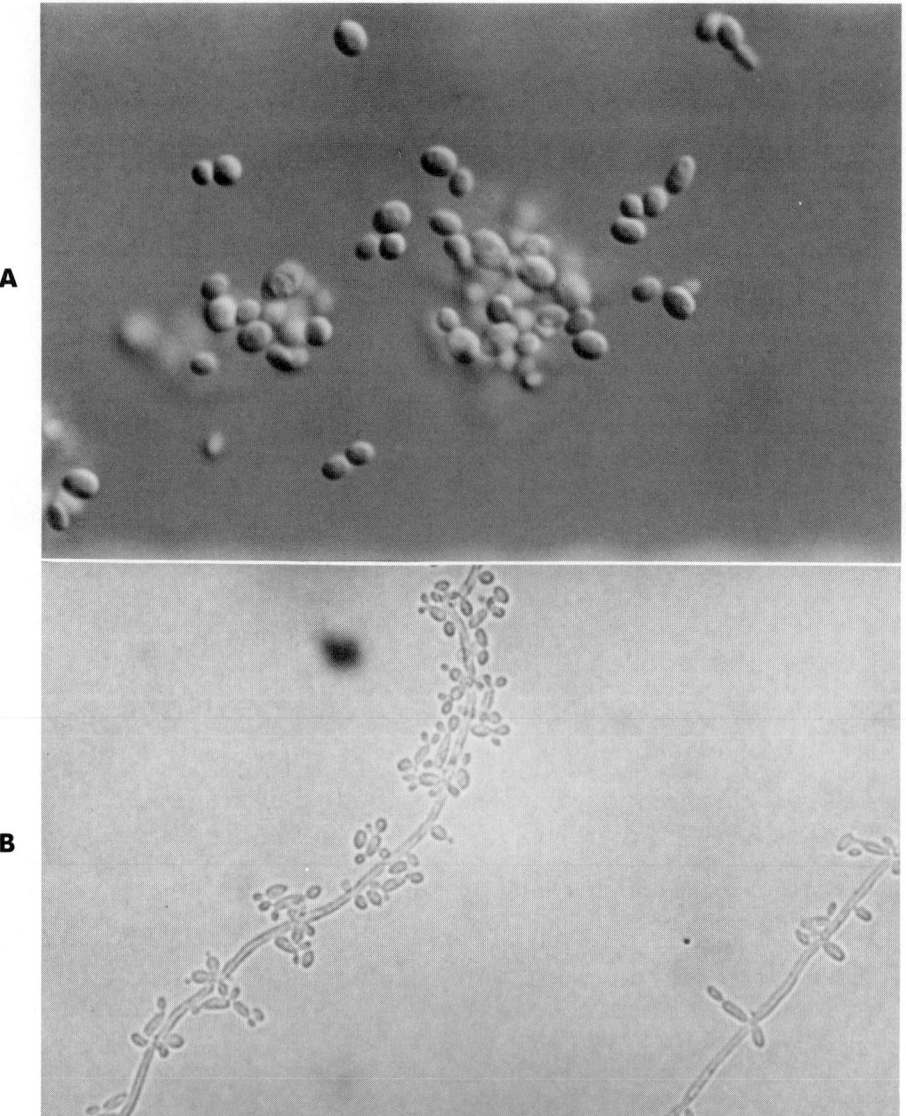

FIGURE 35-2. Lack of pseudohyphae in, **A,** *Torulopsis* distinguishes this genus from, **B,** *Candida*.

in large numbers in desiccated pigeon excrement for prolonged periods.[18] Weathering does appear to reduce the degree of contamination.[18] Although one might assume that pigeon breeders and racers are more susceptible to infection, they are not; however, they do appear to have increased antibody.[6] The actual incidence of cryptococcosis is unknown, but the number of confirmed cases in the United States rose from 24 in 1965 to 338 in 1976.[15] The latter figure was based on a Centers for Disease Control study in which serologic techniques were used to confirm cases of cryptococcosis. Because only 40% of the hospitals and physicians contacted participated in this study, the actual number of cases of cryptococcosis in the United States was probably greater.[15]

The capsule of *C. neoformans* is an important feature of this organism. The capsule, which is polysaccharide in nature, protects the yeast from phagocytosis. The capsule is composed of (1 → 3)-alpha-linked D-mannose residues attached to single-unit side branches of both xylose and glucuronic acid residues.

Four serotypes of *C. neoformans* may be distinguished according to differences in their capsule, specifically differences in the proportions of xylose and glucuronic residues, in the degree of mannose substitution, and in the percentage of O-acetyl attachments.[7] The four serotypes are designated A, B, C, and D.

Serotypes A and D are usually isolated from environmental sources, such as bird nests, fruits, vegetables, and dairy products. Serotype A is the most common type isolated from clinically important infections and some natural habitats. It accounts for over 95% of the clinical isolates seen in the United States. Serotype D is clinically important and is common in Denmark and Italy. Serotypes B and C have been isolated only from clinical specimens and may be clinically significant. Serotypes A and D are associated with *C. neoformans* var. *neoformans* and serotypes B and C with *C. neoformans* var. *gattii*. Both of these varieties have the same teleomorph, *Filobasidiella neoformans*.

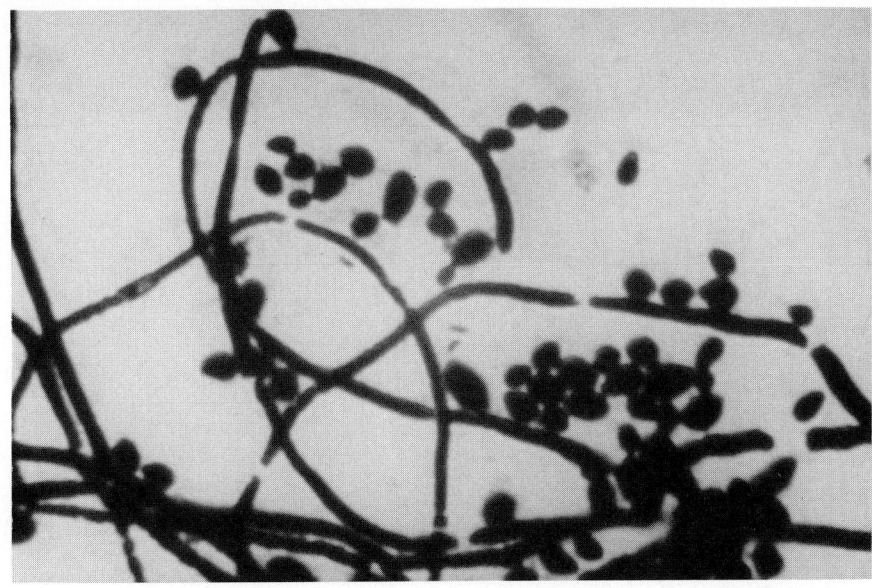

FIGURE 35-3. Gram stain of sputum showing budding yeast cells and pseudohyphae of *Candida albicans.*

TORULOPSIS

The genus *Torulopsis* is distinguished from *Candida* by the absence of well-developed pseudohyphae; if pseudohyphae are produced, they are only rudimentary (Figure 35-2). The major opportunistic pathogen classified in this genus is *T. glabrata.* This yeast is part of the normal flora of the gut, skin, and upper respiratory tract.

The most common types of infections caused by *T. glabrata* include fungemia and genitourinary tract infections. The lungs, kidneys, heart, and central nervous system are the organs most commonly involved in fungemia. Inflammation may be present, ranging from mild levels to purulent, necrotizing, granulomatous tissue responses. Factors that predispose to fungemia include the presence of intravenous catheters, malignancy, immunosuppressive drugs, diabetes, and antimicrobial therapy.[12,32]

T. glabrata may resemble *Histoplasma capsulatum* in clinical specimens and tissue sections. The two can be readily distinguished in tissue by the use of fluorescent antibody specific conjugates. The yeast cells are 2 to 3 μm in diameter and oval in shape.

TRICHOSPORON

Trichosporon beigelii (*T. cutaneum*), which produces hyphae, arthroconidia, blastoconidia, and pseudohyphae, may cause either white piedra (see Chapter 31) or various kinds of opportunistic mycoses, primarily in immunosuppressed patients. The fungus occurs widely in nature and is occasionally isolated from normal skin and nails, especially from the foot.[27] As an opportunistic pathogen, it occurs primarily in patients with acute leukemia. *T. beigelii* is reported to cause disseminated infections, endocarditis, fungemia, and infections involving the brain, eye, and stomach. When tissue is examined histologically, arthroconidia often can be observed.

LABORATORY IDENTIFICATION
SPECIMEN PROCESSING

Yeasts are most frequently recovered from sputum, urine, and cerebrospinal fluid.

Sputum

Sputum may be liquefied with a number of mucolytic agents before processing (see Chapter 29), although this is usually unnecessary. In most cases sputum is processed for either bacteriologic or mycobacteriologic studies, and yeasts are seen on the Gram stain (Figure 35-3), by the acid-fast stain, or growing on microbiologic media (Figure 35-3).

Although yeasts are routinely isolated from sputum, they usually reflect normal flora, candidiasis of the oral cavity and esophagus, or improper handling of the specimen. For example, *C. albicans,* which is a normal inhabitant of the mouth of healthy adults, is frequently recovered from sputum because the sputum must pass through the oral cavity. Thus the role of *C. albicans* in bronchopulmonary infection is difficult to determine. People with poor oral hygiene or those treated with antibacterial agents, even for a short period of time, show a significant increase in the number of yeasts in the mouth, but infection rarely occurs. In disseminated candidiasis yeasts are sometimes cultured from multiple body sites, including sputum.

Urine

Urine should be plated quantitatively for yeasts, as it is for bacteria. The isolation of small numbers of yeasts from urine is probably insignificant. However, with the isolation of *Cryptococcus neoformans, Blastomyces dermatitidis, Histoplasma capsulatum,* or other systemic fungi a single colony is significant. There is a great deal of disagreement about the significance of the specific number of colony-forming units (CFU) of yeasts per milliliter of urine. Goldberg and co-workers[8] suggest that greater than 1000 CFU/ml may indicate pyelonephritis.

A Gram stain, potassium hydroxide (KOH) preparation, or india ink preparation of urine often reveals yeasts with pseudohyphae. Some believe that this is indicative of colonization or invasion of tissue. In our experience this observation has not been substantiated.

Cerebrospinal and Other Body Fluids

Cerebrospinal fluid (CSF) and other body fluids should be concentrated by centrifugation or filtration. The concentrate is then plated directly onto the isolation media. The supernatant can be used for fungal serologic tests. The yeast of greatest importance in CSF is *C. neoformans*. One of the preparations demonstrating capsules for this yeast is the india ink preparation (see Chapter 29). Artifacts such as fat globules, starch granules, and red or white blood cells in CSF or other fluids may superficially resemble *C. neoformans*. As discussed in Chapter 29, cerebrospinal fluid should not be routinely examined for *C. neoformans* by the india ink method because yeasts are detected in the CSF of only approximately 50% of patients with cryptococcal meningitis.[21] If cryptococcosis is suspected, the latex agglutination (LA) test for cryptococcal capsular polysaccharide and culture should be requested. The LA test is far more sensitive and accurate. The CSF must always be cultured because this provides the highest sensitivity and specificity. In AIDS patients, in whom the numbers of *C. neoformans* are so great, an india ink examination of CSF may be appropriate.

DIRECT EXAMINATION

Material from the vagina, mouth, or other mucous membranes can be stained by the Gram stain, although this stain distorts the morphology and size of the yeast. Yeasts, when present, are typically gram positive. If histopathologic stains, such as periodic acid–Schiff (PAS) stain, are used, yeasts can readily be seen. KOH is an ideal mounting medium for direct examination of specimens because it dissolves cells and clears material so fungal cells can be seen more readily. As discussed in Appendix A, when examining these mounts, it is important to reduce the amount of light by stopping down the iris diaphragm. Contrast can be enhanced by lowering the substage condensor.

CULTURE AND ISOLATION

A variety of media are available for the initial isolation of yeasts. In practice, yeasts are most commonly isolated on either mycology media without antimicrobial agents or enriched bacteriologic media, such as brain heart infusion agar, trypticase soy agar, or Columbia agar. Media with cycloheximide (0.5 mg/ml) are never used alone because yeasts such as *C. neoformans* are inhibited by cycloheximide. Caffeic acid agar is a good isolation medium for *C. neoformans*.[13] This yeast produces a characteristic brown-black pigmented colony because of the enzymatic deposition of melanin in the cell wall.

Most pathogenic yeasts grow well at both 25° and 35° C. The inability of some yeasts to grow at 35° C typically denotes a saprophytic nature.

PRACTICAL APPROACH TO THE IDENTIFICATION OF YEASTS

Many have asked how far to go with yeast identification.[25] The notion that identification of *C. albicans* by a germ-tube test

or of *C. neoformans* by demonstration of a capsule is sufficient is not in consonance with the expanding role of yeasts in infectious disease. New rapid tests for yeast identification (see Chapter 9) allow virtually any microbiology laboratory to be more proficient in yeast identification.

The following approach should be used in the identification of yeasts:

1. Observe microscopic morphologic structure using a wet mount in water.
2. Determine the presence of a capsule using an india ink preparation.
3. Inoculate sheep blood agar to check for purity.
4. Use a germ-tube test to presumptively identify *C. albicans*.
5. Inoculate cornmeal agar, rice extract agar, or yeast morphology agar by the Dalmau technique to determine chlamydospore production and other morphologic features.
6. Use physiologic tests to identify organisms.

The details for performing these steps are discussed in the following sections.

Microscopic Morphology

The microscopic morphologic structure of the yeast is evaluated by using a wet mount. The presence of capsules and ascospores and the purity of the culture can be determined in a wet mount. Capsule formation can be confirmed with an india ink preparation. If capsules are seen, a rapid swab urease test may be performed to presumptively confirm the identity of *C. neoformans*.[38] The presence of ascospores suggests ascosporogenous yeasts, such as *Saccharomyces* and *Pichia*. Because special media and physiologic tests are required for identification of these organisms, ascomycetous yeasts are usually sent to a mycology reference laboratory.

Purification of Isolate

Yeasts are purified by streaking them on blood agar for colony isolation to ensure that the isolate is not contaminated by a bacterium, mold, or second yeast.

Germ-Tube Test

A rapid screening test for *C. albicans* is the germ-tube test (Figure 35-4). A light suspension of yeast is added to 0.5 ml of bovine, sheep, or human serum. (If human serum is used, it must be hepatitis B surface antigen [Hb$_s$Ag] free.) The inoculated serum is incubated in a water bath at 35° C for 2 to 3 hours. If germ tubes are present, they can be seen readily with the 40× high-dry objective. A germ tube is recognized by having parallel walls at its origin from the yeast cell. Because germ tubes are the beginning of the formation of hyphae, they grow by linear elongation from the yeast cell. Hence their walls at the union of the cell are parallel and not constricted, as in elongated blastoconidia. Virtually all *C. albicans*, as well as rare isolates of *C. stellatoidea*, produce germ tubes. Martin[20] has reported that *C. tropicalis* may rarely produce germ tubes.

Chlamydospore Production

If the germ-tube test is negative, more extensive morphologic analysis, such as for chlamydospore production, is required. Using the Dalmau technique,[21] the culture is inoculated to either cornmeal agar with 0.3% Tween-80, rice extract agar, or yeast morphology agar. The yeast inoculum is diluted on the medium in the form of streak lines on the surface. A cover glass

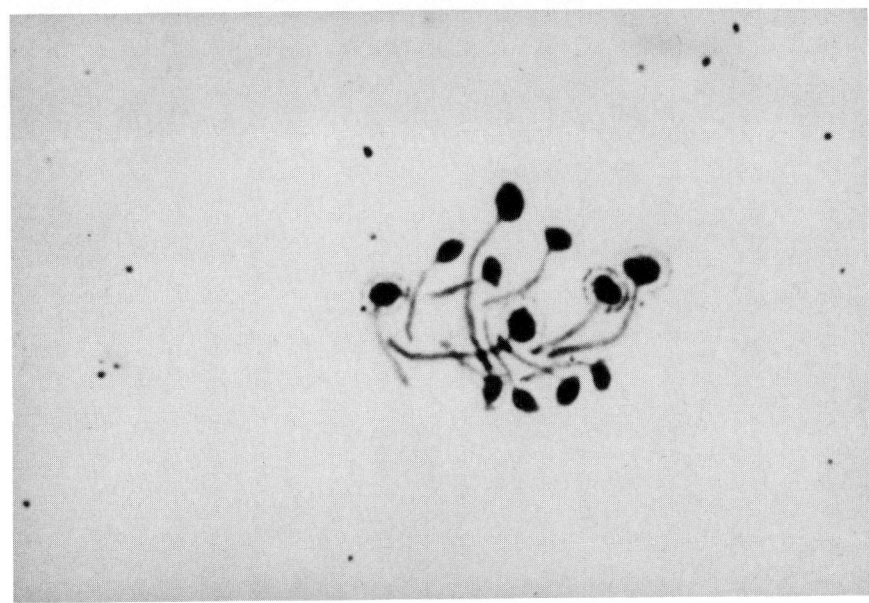

FIGURE 35-4. Germ tubes of *Candida albicans*. (Courtesy L. Ajello.)

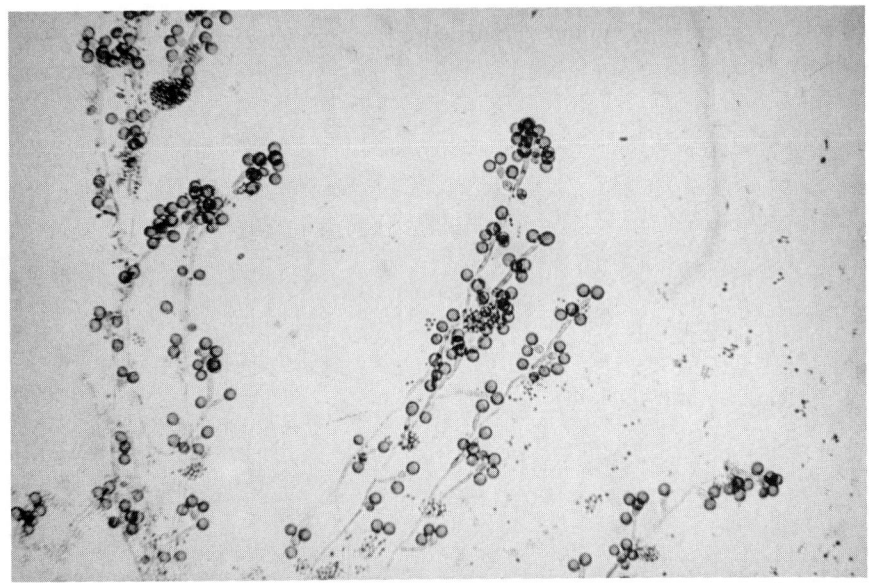

FIGURE 35-5. Typical thick-walled chlamydospores produced by *Candida albicans* on cornmeal agar. (Courtesy L. Ajello.)

through which the fungus can be microscopically observed is placed on the agar surface. The agar plates are incubated at 22° to 25° C for 1 to 2 days. *C. albicans* and *C. stellatoidea* produce thick-walled chlamydospores (Figure 35-5). *Cryptococcus, Rhodotorula,* and *Torulopsis* organisms are unicellular, nonfilamentous yeasts. Figure 35-6 outlines the typical morphologic forms observed on cornmeal agar.

Physiologic Tests

Precise identification of yeasts to the species level cannot be made on the basis of morphology alone. Tests for carbohydrate assimilation, alcohol assimilation, nitrate utilization, urease

production, and, occasionally, carbohydrate fermentation must be performed.

Assimilation is the aerobic utilization of a carbon source by a yeast. Glucose, for example, is oxidized to carbon dioxide and water. Assimilation can be measured by observing growth in the presence of the assimilable carbon substrate. Carbohydrate assimilation is typically measured by one of three techniques. The auxanographic technique, as first proposed by Beijerinck,[3] was an agar method and was performed by adding carbohydrates in powdered form to a carbohydrate-free agar. A zone of growth around the carbohydrate indicated assimilation. The Wickerham[34,35] technique was similar but incorporated the

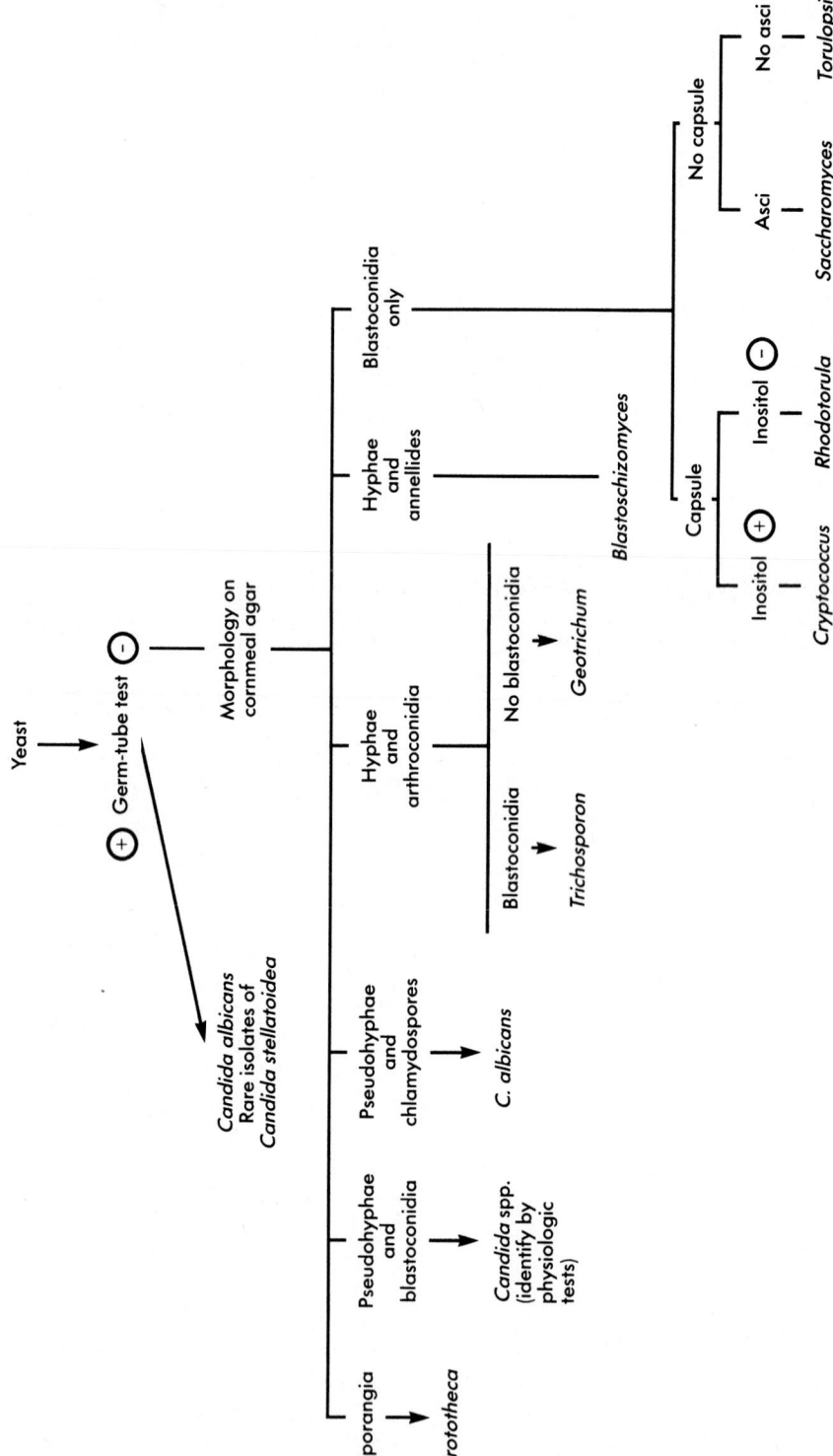

FIGURE 35-6. Practical approach to initial identification of yeasts and yeastlike fungi.

assimilable carbohydrates into a broth medium. The assimilation agar technique, which was modified from the Wickerham technique, uses agar slants containing yeast nitrogen base to which are added the various carbohydrates to be tested.[1]

Haley and Calloway[10] recommend a modification of the Beijerinck technique. This procedure, as follows, can be read in 24 hours compared with the 14 to 28 days required for the Wickerham method:

1. Melt a tube of yeast nitrogen base (see Appendix B) and cool to 47° to 48° C.
2. Make a suspension of 24- to 72-hour yeast inoculum in 4 ml of sterile distilled water and adjust to a McFarland no. 4 or no. 5 standard.
3. Pour the inoculum into the tube of molten agar and mix by inversion.
4. Pour the molten mixture into a 15 × 150 mm plastic Petri dish and cool at room temperature.
5. Using flamed forceps, place the following carbohydrate disks (Minitek, BBL, Cockeysville, Md.) on the surface of the plate: dextrose, maltose, sucrose, lactose, galactose, cellobiose, raffinose, D-xylose, trehalose, inositol, and meliobiose.

6. Incubate the plate at 30° C for 18 to 24 hours, and then examine for growth around the disk. No growth indicates that sugar was not assimilated. The zone size is insignificant. Minitek disks contain phenol red, which may turn the medium yellow. This color does not indicate growth.

Alternatively, one of the commercial assimilation systems, such as the API 20C yeast identification kit or the Uni-Yeast-Tek identification system may be used (see Chapter 9). We recommend a commercial identification system for the diagnostic laboratory.

Fermentation is the anaerobic utilization of a carbohydrate, resulting in the production of CO_2 and ethanol. Detection of fermentation therefore is by gas production (CO_2) and not by pH change. The sugars used for yeast fermentation differ from those used for testing bacterial fermentation and include the sugars indicated in Table 35-1. The recommended, traditional fermentation method, if necessary, is based on Wickerham's method, as modified by Haley and Callaway[10] and as discussed by McGinnis.[21] Some of the kits for rapid yeast identification incorporate fermentable substrates (see Chapter 9). Fermentation tests are rarely necessary for the identification of yeasts.

TABLE 35-1. Physiologic Patterns of the Various Yeasts

Genus and Species	Assimilation of											Germ-Tube Production	Growth at 37° C	KNO₃ Utilization	Urease Production
	Cellobiose	Galactose	Glucose	Inositol	Lactose	Maltose	Meliobiose	Raffinose	Sucrose	Trehalose	Xylose				
Blastoschizomyces capitatus	−	+/v	+	−	−	−	−	−	−	−	−	−	+	−	−
Candida albicans	−	+	+	−	−	+	−	−	−	−	−	+	+	−	
Candida guilliermondii	+	+	+	−	−	+	+	+	+	+	+	−	+	−	−
Candida krusei	−	−	+	−	−	−	−	−	−	−	−	−	+	−	+/v
Candida parapsilosis	−	+	+	−	−	+	−	−	+	+	+	−	+	−	−
Candida pseudotropicalis	+	+	+	−	+	−	−	+	+	−	+/v	−	+	−	−
Candida rugosa	−	−	+	−	−	−	+	−	−	−	−	−	−	−	−
Candida stellatoidea	−	+	+	−	−	+	−	−	−	+/v	+	+	+	−	
Candida tropicalis	+/v	+	+	−	−	+	−	−	+	+	+	−	+	−	−
Cryptococcus albidus var. *albidus*	+	−/v	+	+	+/v	+	−/v	+	+	+	+	−	+	+	+
Cryptococcus albidus var. *diffluens*	+	−/v	+	+	−	+	+/v	+	+	+	+	−	+	+	+
Cryptococcus gastricus	+	+	+	+	+	+	−	−	−/v	+	+	−	−	−	+

Continued.

TABLE 35-1. Physiologic Patterns of the Various Yeasts—cont'd

| Genus and Species | Assimilation of | | | | | | | | | | | Germ-Tube Production | Growth at 37° C | KNO₃ Utilization | Urease Production |
	Cellobiose	Galactose	Glucose	Inositol	Lactose	Maltose	Melibiose	Raffinose	Sucrose	Trehalose	Xylose				
Cryptococcus laurentii	+	+	+	+	+	+	+/v	+/v	+	+	+	−	+	−	+
Cryptococcus luteolus	+	+	+	+	−	+	+	−/v	+	+	+	−	−	−	+
Cryptococcus neoformans	+	+/v	+	+	−	+	−	+/v	+	+	+	−	+	−	+
Cryptococcus terreus	+	+/v	+	+	−/v	+/v	+	−	−/v	+	+	−	+	+	+
Cryptococcus unguttulatus	−/v	−/v	+	+	−	+	−/v	+/v	+	+/v	+	−	−	−	+
Geotrichum candidum (not a yeast but may be confused with yeasts)	−	+	+	−	−	−	−	−	−	−	+	−	−	−	−
Rhodotorula glutinis	+/v	+	+	−	−	+	−	+/v	+	+	+/v	+/v	+	+	+
Saccharomyces cerevisiae	−	+	+	−	−	+	−	+	+	−	+	−	+/v	−	−
Trichosporon beigelii	+	+	+	+/v	+	+/v	+/v	+/v	+/v	+/v	+/v	−	+/v	−	+
Torulopsis candida	+	+	+	−	+/v	+	+/v	+	+	+	+	−	+	−	−
Torulopsis glabrata	−	−	+	−	−	−	−	−	−	+	−	−	+	−	−

SYMBOLS:	+, Positive
	−, Negative
	v, Variable reaction

Data from references 2 and 22.

Table 35-1 illustrates the specific physiologic patterns of the various yeasts.

Immunology

Candida precipitins in the serum of patients with invasive candidiasis may be detected by a number of methods.[5] Interpretation of the presence of precipitins remains controversial, and routine use is not recommended. The detection of mannan and arabitol in patients suspected to have invasive candidiasis is discussed in Chapter 38.

Cryptococcus neoformans capsular substance can be detected in body fluids by a latex agglutination test. The same test can also confirm the identity of the *C. neoformans* once growth appears on the plate. These tests are discussed in detail in Chapter 38. The serotypes of *C. neoformans* may be distinguished with specific fluorescent antibody conjugates.

REFERENCES

1. Adams, E.D., and Cooper, B.H.: Evaluation of a modified Wickerham medium for identifying medically important yeasts, Am. J. Med. Technol. **40:**377, 1974.
2. Barnett, J.A., Payne, R.W., and Yarrow, D.: Yeasts: characteristics and identification, Cambridge, Mass., 1983, Cambridge University Press.
3. Beijerinck, M.W.: L'auxanographie, ou le methode de l'hydro diffusion dans la gelatine appliquee aux recherche microbiologiques, Arch. Nierland Sci. Exact. Nat. **23:**367, 1889.
4. Chandler, F.W.: Pathology of the mycoses in patients with the acquired immunodeficiency syndrome (AIDS). In McGinnis, M.R., editor: Current topics in medical mycology, New York, 1985, Springer-Verlag.
5. Dee, T.H., and Rytel, M.W.: Clinical application of counterimmunoelectrophoresis in detection of *Candida* serum precipitins, J. Lab. Clin. Med. **85:**161, 1975.

6. Fink, J.N., Barboriak, J.J., and Kaufman, L.: Cryptococcal antibodies in pigeon breeders' disease, J. Allergy Clin. Immunol. **41:**297, 1968.

7. Fleet, G.H.: Composition and structure of yeast cell walls. In McGinnis, M.R., editor: Current topics in medical mycology, New York, 1985, Springer-Verlag.

8. Goldberg, P.K., et al.: Incidence and significance of candiduria, JAMA **241:**582, 1979.

9. Guentzel, M.N., Cole, G.T., and Pope, L.M.: Animal models for candidiasis. In McGinnis, M.R., editor: Current topics in medical mycology, New York, 1985, Springer-Verlag.

10. Haley, L.D., and Callaway, C.: Laboratory methods in medical mycology, ed. 4, Dept. of Health, Education and Welfare Pub. No. (CDC) 78-8361, Atlanta, 1978, Center for Disease Control.

11. Hay, R.J.: *Cryptococcus neoformans* and cutaneous cryptococcosis, Semin. Dermatol. **4:**252, 1985.

12. Hickey, W.F., Sommerville, L.H., and Schoen, F.J.: Disseminated *Candida glabrata:* report of a uniquely severe infection and a literature review, Am. J. Clin. Pathol. **80:**724, 1983.

13. Hopfer, R.L., and Blank, F.: Caffeic acid–containing medium for identification of *Cryptococcus neoformans*, J. Clin. Microbiol. **2:**115, 1975.

14. Kaplan, M.H., Rosen, P.P., and Armstrong, D.: Cryptococcosis in a cancer hospital: clinical and pathological correlates in forty-six patients, Cancer **39:**2265, 1977.

15. Kaufman, L., and Blumer, S.: Cryptococcosis: the awakening giant. In The black and white yeasts, PAHO Sci. Pub. No. 356, p. 176, 1978.

16. King, R.D., Lee, J.C., and Morris, A.L.: Adherence of *Candida albicans* and other *Candida* species to mucosal epithelial cells, Infect. Immun. **27:**667, 1980.

17. Kovacs, J.A., et. al.: Cryptococcosis in the acquired immunodeficiency syndrome, Ann. Intern. Med. **103:**533, 1985.

18. Littman, M.L., and Walter, J.E.: Cryptococcosis: current status, Am. J. Med. **45:**922, 1968.

19. Marples, M.J.: The ecology of the human skin, Springfield, Ill., 1965, Charles C Thomas, Publisher.

20. Martin, M.V.: Germ tube formation by oral strains of *Candida tropicalis*, J. Med. Microbiol. **12:**187, 1979.

21. McGinnis, M.R.: Laboratory handbook of medical mycology, New York, 1980, Academic Press, Inc.

22. McGinnis, M.R.: Detection of fungi in cerebrospinal fluid, Am. J. Med. **75(1B):**129, 1983.

23. McGinnis, M.R., Schell, W.A., and Carson, J.: *Phaeoannellomyces* and the Phaeococcomycetaceae, new dematiaceous blastomycete taxa, Sabouraudia **23:**179, 1985.

24. McGinnis, M.R., et al.: Taxonomic and nomenclatural evaluation of the genera *Candida* and *Torulopsis*, J. Clin. Microbiol. **20:**813, 1984.

25. Murray, P.R., Van Scoy, R.E., and Roberts, G.D.: Should yeasts in respiratory secretions be identified? Mayo Clin. Proc. **52:**42, 1977.

26. Odds, F.C.: *Candida* and candidosis, Baltimore, 1979, Leicester University Press.

27. Pritchard, R.C., and Muir, D.B.: *Trichosporon beigelii:* survey of isolates from clinical material, Pathology **17:**20, 1985.

28. Pugh, D., and Cawson, R.A.: The cytochemical localization of phospholipase in *Candida albicans* infecting the chick chorio-allantoic membrane, Sabouraudia **15:**29, 1977.

29. Ray, T.L., Digre, K.B., and Payne, C.D.: Adherence of *Candida* species to human epidermal corneocytes and buccal mucosal cells: correlation with cutaneous pathogenicity, J. Invest. Dermatol. **83:**37, 1984.

30. Rippon, J.W.: Medical mycology: the pathogenic fungi and the pathogenic actinomycetes, ed. 2, Philadelphia, 1982, W.B. Saunders Co.

31. Salkin, I.F., et al.: *Blastoschizomyces capitatus:* a new combination, Mycotaxon **22:**375, 1985.

32. Sekhon, A.S.: *Bacteroides fragilis* and *Torulopsis glabrata* septicemia in a patient with gastrointestinal ulcers and chronic renal failure, with review of literature on torulopsosis. In The black and white yeasts, PAHO Sci. Pub. No. 356, p. 167, 1978.

33. Smith, C.B.: Candidiasis: pathogenesis, host resistance and predisposing factors. In Bodey, G.P., and Fainstein, V., editors: Candidiasis, New York, 1985, Raven Press.

34. Wickerham, L.J.: Taxonomy of yeasts, USDA Tech. Bull. no. 29, 1951.

35. Wickerham, L.J., and Burton, K.A.: Carbon assimilation tests for the classification of yeasts, J. Bacteriol. **56:**363, 1948.

36. Williams, D.M., Krick, J.A., and Remington, J.S.: Pulmonary infection in the compromised host. Part I, Am. Rev. Respir. Dis. **114:**359, 1976.

37. Yarrow, D., and Meyer, S.A.: Proposal for amendment of the diagnosis of the genus *Candida* Berkhout nom. cons., Int. J. Syst. Bacteriol. **28:**611, 1978.

38. Zimmer, B.L., and Roberts, G.D.: Rapid selective urease test for presumptive identification of *Cryptococcus neoformans*, J. Clin. Microbiol. **10:**380, 1979.

CHAPTER 36

Mycotic Infections of the Eye and the Ear

Richard C. Tilton
Michael R. McGinnis

INFECTIONS OF THE EYE
PATHOLOGY, CLINICAL SIGNIFICANCE, AND LABORATORY DIAGNOSIS

The three categories of eye infections caused by fungi are mycotic keratitis, endogenous oculomycosis, and extension oculomycosis.[5]

Mycotic keratitis is an opportunistic fungal infection of the cornea resulting from trauma or surgical contamination by soil, plant material, or fomites. The corneal ulcer is raised and white or dirty gray with irregular margins, delicate radiating lines at the perimeter of the anterior stromal infiltrate, satellite lesions, endothelial plaque, hypopyon, and late vascularization if steroid treatment was used earlier. Many different fungi are etiologic agents of mycotic keratitis. Over half of the cases of fungal keratitis in the United States are caused by *Fusarium solani*.[2] Other fungi, such as *Acremonium* spp., *Aspergillus flavus*, *Aspergillus fumigatus*, *Aspergillus niger*, *Bipolaris spicifera*, *Curvularia lunata*, *Curvularia geniculata*, *Fusarium oxysporum*, *Pseudallescheria boydii*, and *Candida albicans*, have also been reported. Mycotic keratitis is influenced by factors such as the sex, age, occupation, and immune status of the host, as well as geographic conditions. In a survey of the literature, Sandhu and Rattan[6] concluded that men between 20 and 40 years of age are more prone to mycotic keratitis, especially if they are farmers or laborers. The most common predisposing factors are trauma caused by accidental injury. Sandhu and Rattan noted that antibacterial agents tend to permit conditions more favorable for fungal growth and that topical steroids interfere with the host's response to the opportunistic fungal pathogen.

The direct examination of corneal scrapings is of critical importance for diagnosis of mycotic keratitis. The scrapings are collected by an ophthalmologist and usually received in the laboratory on either a sterile glass slide or a scalpel blade that has been placed in a sterile container. Swabs are unacceptable because the fungi that are causing keratitis are in the eye tissue, and thus specimens must be obtained by corneal scraping. Part of the scrapings are cleared with a 10% to 20% potassium hydroxide (KOH) preparation, and the remainder is cultured. If *Candida* spp. are present, yeast and pseudohyphae can be seen microscopically. The other fungi cannot be differentiated microscopically; however, the demonstration of fungal elements in the scrapings and the clinical presentation are sufficient for making a diagnosis of fungal keratitis. While it can be argued that fungal culture for mycotic keratitis is of academic importance only, cultural procedures should be attempted for precise identification of the causative organisms and for epidemiologic purposes. Rippon[6] suggests that, because most of the fungi found in eye infections are soil saprophytes, the laboratory approach to mycologic analysis must be different than for other specimens. For example, multiple eye cultures should be processed if material is available. The presence of only one colony on a streak may be highly significant when correlated with the direct microscopic examination of the scrapings and with the clinical presentation. Sabouraud dextrose agar (SDA) without antimicrobial agents or sheep blood agar is the preferred medium because cycloheximide inhibits many of the saprophytic fungi. The plates should be incubated at 22° to 25° C and initially examined after 1 to 2 days of incubation. Identification of these opportunistic pathogens is often difficult, and a reference laboratory should be consulted without delay if an unfamiliar fungus appears to be the etiologic agent of the infection.

Fungal infection of the eyelid is rare but may be caused by *Candida* spp. and occasionally the dermatophytes. Fungal conjunctivitis also is rare but may be caused by *Sporothrix schenckii*, *Rhinosporidium seeberi*, *Coccidioides immitis*, and some of the dermatophytes. Fungal infection of the lacrimal (tear) ducts often follows a stone in the duct. Although *C. albicans* is most commonly isolated, other fungi may be recovered sporadically.

All eye infections are serious and can lead to vision loss. Some infections, however, can lead even to loss of life. Endogenous oculomycosis, that is, infection of the inside of the eye, is most often associated with hematogenous dissemination of fungi such as *A. fumigatus*, *C. albicans*, *Cryptococcus neoformans*, *Histoplasma capsulatum*, and *Blastomyces dermatitidis*. *C. albicans* is the most common. The retina, orbit, sclera, or optic nerves may be involved.

Extension oculomycosis, a special form of rhinocerebral zygomycosis, may occur as the result of trauma, immunosuppression, or extension from paranasal sinuses or the nasal septum.[1,4] The infection may continue to spread to the central nervous system. The zygomycete most often isolated is *Rhizopus arrhizus*.[4] A KOH preparation of the infected material usually reveals large (6 to 15 μm in diameter), sparsely septate, irregularly branched hyphae. Zygomycetes are recovered in only approximately 40% of the cases of rhinocerebral zygomycosis.

Rhinosporidiosis is a mycotic infection of the mucous membranes of the nose (see Chapter 33) and the conjunctiva caused by *R. seeberi*. Polyps, or small tumors, develop on the membranes. These polyps must be removed surgically to eradicate the infection. Sometimes local application of amphotericin B is successful. Large sporangia (300 μm), containing many small sporangiospores, lie beneath the hyperplastic epithelium. These characteristic structures can be seen in a KOH preparation of the epithelial layer. The fungus has never been cultured in vitro.

TREATMENT

Few therapies are completely effective for mycotic keratitis. A new drug, pimaricin, appears to be effective and is the drug of choice.[5] Amphotericin B has been used effectively for infections other than those caused by *Fusarium* spp.; however, permanent eye damage may be associated with its use.[3]

The treatment of endogenous oculomycosis depends on the susceptibility of the disseminated fungus. Often such infections are an end-stage result of extensive fungal metastasis. In addition to intravenous administration of antifungal agents, intraocular injection of amphotericin B, 5-fluorocytosine, and pimaricin has been attempted.

Extension oculomycosis is normally associated with zygomycosis in people with diabetes. Apart from control of the diabetic condition, systemic and local amphotericin B administration is the treatment of choice pending antifungal susceptibility testing.

INFECTIONS OF THE EAR
PATHOLOGY, CLINICAL SIGNIFICANCE, AND LABORATORY DIAGNOSIS

Otomycosis is a fungal infection of the external ear canal. It is characterized by mild irritation, debris in the ear, and some-times, inflammatory pus. Predisposing factors include other infections, medications, trauma, and irritants. The organisms most commonly isolated from this infection are those fungi that also may be isolated from the normal canal, an observation that tends to cast doubt on the role of some of these fungi in otomycosis. The fungi associated with this disease include *A. niger, Penicillium* spp., *R. arrhizus, C. albicans,* and *Candida tropicalis.* Either yeasts or hyphae can be seen in these organisms. *A. niger* is the most common agent of otomycosis.

REFERENCES

1. Binder, P.S.: Ocular fungal and parasitic infections. In Braude, A.I., Davis, C.E., and Fierer, J., editors: Infectious diseases and medical microbiology, Philadelphia, 1986, W.B. Saunders Co.
2. DeVoe, A.G., and Silva-Hutner, M.: Fungal infections of the eye. In Locatcher-Khorazo, D., and Seegal, B.C., editor: Microbiology of the eye, St. Louis, 1972, the C.V. Mosby Co.
3. Jones, D.B., Sexton, R., and Rebell, G.: Mycotic keratitis in South Florida: a review of 39 cases, Trans. Ophthalmol. Soc. U.K. **89:**781, 1970.
4. McGinnis, M.: Laboratory handbook of medical microbiology, New York, 1980, Academic Press, Inc.
5. Rippon, J.W.: Medical mycology: the pathogenic fungi and the pathogenic actinomycetes, ed. 2, Philadelphia, 1982, W.B. Saunders Co.
6. Sandhu, D.K., and Rattan, A.S.: Keratomycosis: a review, Mykosen **24:**503, 1981.

CHAPTER 37

Opportunistic Fungi

Richard C. Tilton
Michael R. McGinnis

Opportunistic pathogenic fungi are our constant companions in the environment. Their ubiquity is demonstrated when bread or fruit is not properly stored for any length of time. These same harmless molds that grow on a variety of complex organic substances flourish equally well on human tissue when the host's natural defense mechanisms have been compromised.

The most common opportunistic fungal infections are zygomycosis, aspergillosis, candidiasis, and cryptococcosis. This chapter summarizes the diseases caused by aspergilli and zygomycetes and the mycologic basis for their identification. The other fungi are discussed in previous chapters. In addition, other saprophytic fungi that are usually contaminants but that may be pathogenic are presented both in tabular form and in photomicrographs. Under the appropriate conditions most of the so-called saprophytic fungi are probably capable of causing opportunistic infection in a compromised host.

PATHOLOGY AND CLINICAL SIGNIFICANCE
ASPERGILLOSIS

Aspergillosis refers to a broad spectrum of diseases caused by members of the genus *Aspergillus*. Diseases associated with *Aspergillus* spp. include allergic bronchopulmonary aspergillosis, saprophytic bronchopulmonary aspergillosis, aspergillomas, and invasive aspergillosis. *Aspergillus* spp. are among the most ubiquitous fungi. They occur throughout the world in soil, organically enriched debris, and decaying vegetation. Only a small number of species are well-documented opportunistic pathogens.[17] The major pathogenic *Aspergillus* spp. are *A. fumigatus*, *A. flavus*, *A. niger*, *A. terreus*, and *A. nidulans*.

Pulmonary aspergillosis varies from pulmonary hypersensitivity to invasive infections that often contribute to the death of immunocompromised patients. Pulmonary hypersensitivity as a result of either colonization or invasion of tissue by the aspergilli is unique because the host's principal reaction is the production of antibody rather than a cell-mediated immune response. Allergic bronchopulmonary aspergillosis (ABPA) results in a markedly elevated serum IgE level. The IgE and probably IgG[4] contribute to the immediate dermal hypersensitivity response of erythema, induration, and wheal and flare and to the immediate bronchial and nasal response.[19] The diagnostic criteria for ABPA include reversible episodic bronchial obstruction, immediate dermal reactivity to the *Aspergillus* antigen, elevated total serum IgE, peripheral blood eosinophilia, antibodies in serum against *Aspergillus* spp., history of pulmonary infiltrates, central bronchiectasis, brown plugs in sputum, and an Arthus reactivity to *Aspergillus* organisms.[5,6,8,19] It is important to differentiate patients with ABPA from those with saprophytic bronchopulmonary aspergillosis (SBPA) in which the *Aspergillus* spp. colonize the airways but do not damage the tissue.

It is believed that in ABPA the conidia of *Aspergillus* organisms are inhaled and then trapped in the viscid secretions produced by asthmatic patients. As the fungus grows, it may produce toxins. The fungus reacts with homocytotrophic IgE that is bound to mast cells, resulting in the release of histamine, eosinophil chemotactic factor, kinins, serotonin, prostaglandins, and slow-reacting substance of anaphylaxis. The prostaglandins cause gland hypersecretion, bronchospasm, increased bronchial mucosa permeability, and pulmonary and peripheral blood eosinophilia. Absorbed antigen forms antigen-antibody immune complexes with the precipitating and complement-fixing IgG and IgM antibodies. Cell-mediated immunity is involved in the pathogenesis of ABPA, but it is not a major component. ABPA is managed with corticosteroids.

Aspergillomas, or fungus balls, consisting of zones of hyphae alternating with layers of cellular debris may be seen in SBPA. These occur within preexisting pulmonary cavities resulting from diseases such as chronic tuberculosis, sarcoidosis, and healed abscess cavities. The conidia of *Aspergillus* spp. are inhaled and grow in the cavity if it communicates with the bronchial tree. The fungus typically remains within the cavity for months or years without invading the cavity well. A recurrent hemoptysis occurs in 50% to 80% of patients. Aspergillomas have a characteristic appearance on x-ray films, consisting of an airspace around the fungus ball in the cavity. Lung scanning with radioactive strontium is helpful in their diagnosis. The strontium accumulates around the aspergilloma in the lung, presumably because of its affinity for calcium oxalate, a product of the fungus. Precipitating antibodies have been found in 92% to 100% of patients.[19] Therapy is antifungal agents, such as amphotericin B, and surgical resection.

Acute invasive bronchopulmonary aspergillosis (AIBPA) is the most serious form of *Aspergillus* infection. In AIBPA the parenchyma is damaged by inflammation or hemorrhagic infarction. Bronchopneumonia or focal abscess formation is often a result. The fungus may also be disseminated to other organs and tissues, such as the central nervous system, heart, gastrointestinal tract, and thyroid gland.[19] Currently amphotericin B is the drug of choice for invasive aspergillosis.

The tissue response in invasive aspergillosis consists of a mixed purulent and necrotizing inflammation. The necrosis is the result of vascular obstruction and possible toxin production. In chronic infections the lesions are often granulomatous with progressive fibrosis. Because of the propensity of the mycelium to invade blood vessels, hematogenous dissemination may occur. Thrombosis can lead to hemorrhage, infarction, and death.[3] Hyphae tend to penetrate the walls of blood vessels. The hyphae have parallel walls and septa and are 3 to 6 μm in diameter. They often branch dichotomously, that is, in two roughly equal parts.

Patients who have leukemia, especially acute lymphocytic and acute myelogenous leukemia, and who are granulocytopenic are especially prone to invasive aspergillosis.[7] Patients with lymphoma are also highly susceptible to invasive aspergillosis. In some studies up to 20% of these patients die.

Other factors predisposing to aspergillosis include aplastic anemia, diabetes mellitus, carcinoma, collagen vascular disease, immunosuppressive drugs, steroids, cytotoxic drugs, and antimicrobics.

Many of the predisposing conditions inhibit the phagocytosis of *Aspergillus* spp. Macrophages are effective in killing conidia of *Aspergillus* spp., and polymorphonuclear leukocytes (PMNs) in handling the hyphae of these organisms. Large doses of cortisone, for example, impair the killing of conidia by macrophages and the mobilization of PMNs around hyphae.[17] There is also evidence that toxins may contribute to the necrosis mentioned earlier in this section and may facilitate the infectious process; a zone of tissue death can sometimes be seen beyond the hyphal tips of *A. fumigatus*. Mycotoxins produced by *Aspergillus* spp. have been found in food. Aflatoxin, for example, may be found in products such as peanut butter and has been linked to cancer in animals although there is no clear indication that similar responses occur in humans. However, Shank[21] reports that strong epidemiologic evidence exists for the association between hepatocarcinoma and aflatoxin ingestion through ingestion of contaminated peanuts, corn, and rice in Africa and Southeast Asia.

Aspergillosis involving the tracheobronchial tree may occur in patients who are not severely compromised and granulocytopenic. This form of invasive aspergillosis is characterized by superficial damage to the mucosa.

ZYGOMYCOSIS

Zygomycosis (mucormycosis) is caused by a number of fungi in the class Zygomycetes. Examples include *Rhizopus arrhizus*, *Rhizomucor pusillus*, *Absidia corymbifera*, *Cunninghamella bertholletiae*, *Basidiobolus ranarum*, and *Conidiobolus coronatus*. These fungi are ubiquitous in the environment. We prefer the term "zygomycosis" to "mucormycosis" because it encompasses all infections caused by members of the class Zygomycetes.[13] Some mycologists designate infections caused by *B. ranarum* and *C. coronatus* as special forms of zygomycosis by using the clinical term "entomophthoramycosis." However, by using descriptive adjectives such as pulmonary, cerebral, rhinocerebral, and subcutaneous before the term "zygomycosis," a useful, logical, and descriptive nomenclature for mycoses caused by zygomycetes is established.

Subcutaneous zygomycosis caused by *B. ranarum* occurs most often in patients living in Africa and Asia. The infections usually involve the trunk and limbs where they begin as small, painless nodules. As the surrounding tissue is invaded, a large, firm mass forms. The fungus often penetrates underlying tissue, including the muscles and the thoracic, abdominal, and pelvic viscera. Compared with zygomycetes classified in the order Mucorales, *B. ranarum* is less likely to invade blood vessels. The hyphae are 6 to 25 μm in diameter with irregular branching and occasional septa. Because Splendore-Hoeppli

material often is present around the hyphae, they are better visualized in tissue sections with the hematoxylin and eosin (H and E) stain. Therapy with iodides is effective.

C. coronatus may cause subcutaneous zygomycosis involving the nasal area, with progressive swelling of the nose, cheeks, and upper lip. For unknown reasons the infection is limited to the nasal mucosa, nasal sinuses, and subcutaneous tissues of the head.[3] In contrast, the buttocks, thighs, trunk, and perineum are commonly infected by *B. ranarum*. Most cases of subcutaneous zygomycosis caused by *C. coronatus* occur in Africa, with a few cases diagnosed in the Caribbean and South America. The lesions caused by *B. ranarum* and *C. coronatus* are essentially identical histologically. If potassium iodide does not resolve the infection, amphotericin B should be considered.

Systemic zygomycosis is caused by *R. arrhizus* (syn. *R. oryzae*), *R. pusillus*, *C. bertholletiae*, and *Saksenaea vasiformis*. The clinical presentations of systemic zygomycosis are variable, depending on the organs involved. Rhinocerebral zygomycosis, typically caused by *R. arrhizus*, is usually associated with acute diabetes accompanied by ketoacidosis. The fungus attacks the nasal turbinates and paranasal sinuses and spreads by direct extension to the nose, eyes, and brain, invading blood vessels and destroying the cranial nerves. The key symptoms include sinusitis with nasal discharge consisting of black and blood-tinged material, necrotic tissue in the nasal septum and turbinates, inflammation of tissue around the eyes, ophthalmoplegia (paralysis of the eye muscles), proptosis (fixed forward position of the eye), and meningoencephalitis signs. In tissue the zygomycetes grow as large (3 to 25 μm in diameter), irregularly branching, sparsely septate hyphae. The zygomycetes are often found in and around blood vessels, resulting in thrombi within the vessel lumen. Management involves control of the acidotic state, surgery, and amphotericin B administration.

Several mechanisms seem to play a role in the pathogenesis of zygomycosis.[1] These mechanisms appear to be related to the ketoacidotic state of the diabetic patient and the resulting low pH. The ability of transferrin to bind iron is pH dependent, and in the ketoacidotic patient a pH-induced reduction of the iron-binding capacity of this plasma protein is present, as is a loss of serum inhibitory activity against the zygomycete. As a result of these conditions the fungus has plenty of available iron and is able to grow profusely in tissue. Some evidence also suggests that zygomycetes can produce and secrete an iron-chelating factor that may be a siderophore. More research is needed to confirm the role of these potential virulence factors.

LABORATORY DIAGNOSIS OF *ASPERGILLUS* AND THE ZYGOMYCETES
DIRECT EXAMINATION

Sputum, other pulmonary specimens, and tissue should be placed on a microscope slide containing a drop of 10% to 20% potassium hydroxide (KOH) and then examined. Tissue is minced in sterile saline. Body fluids, which are usually sterile, should be centrifuged. Austwick[2] recommends that caseous tissue be digested with pepsin before microscopic observation. This procedure breaks down the tissue and allows the microbiologist to see the characteristic structures of the aspergilli, that is, hyaline, dichotomously branched, septate hyphae. In the fungus ball the hyphae may already be dead, and no growth occurs. If debris from the ears or material from the nose is examined directly, conidiophores may be seen. In acute aspergillosis swollen, empty, enlarged hyphae also may be seen.

The zygomycetes are characterized by large (6 to 25 μm), hyaline, broad, irregularly branched, sparsely septate hyphae (see Figure 29-3). Tissue sections may be stained with periodic acid–Schiff (PAS), methenamine-silver, or H and E stain to see the hyphae of both *Aspergillus* organisms and the zygomycetes. H and E–stained sections are often the best.

CULTURE AND ISOLATION

Specimens should be cultured on primary isolation media. Sterile bread without preservatives is also an excellent culture medium for zygomycetes. Cycloheximide should be excluded from the medium because many of the saprophytic fungi are susceptible to it at 0.5 mg/ml. Since the specimens received for mycologic examination are often heavily contaminated with bacteria, gentamicin or streptomycin and polymyxin B can be added to the isolation media. The sealed plates are incubated at 30° C.

Both aspergilli and the zygomycetes form colonies within a few days. The identification of both groups is based on morphologic examination; therefore lactophenol cotton blue preparations of the isolated colonies and slide cultures should be initiated as soon as colonies are evident. Several monographs are excellent sources of information on identification of the species of the class Zygomycetes.[4,15,20,22] The monograph by Raper and Fennell[16] and the book by Domsch, Gams, and Anderson[4] are effective guides in identifying aspergilli.

The box on p. 612 presents a key to the identification of the major *Aspergillus* spp. Table 37-1 summarizes the colonial and microscopic morphology of the zygomycetes.

IMMUNOLOGY

Enzyme-linked immunosorbent assay (ELISA) is available for the diagnosis of zygomycosis. Immunologic methods also play a vital role in the diagnosis of aspergillosis.[10] Patients with ABPA are screened for specific IgE and IgG and *Aspergillus* serum antigens. Patients with invasive aspergillosis may not be detected with a precipitin test because they may be anergic.[18] Minute quantities of specific antibodies can be detected, however, by ELISA or by radioimmunoassay.[11] For immunosuppressed patients serologic diagnosis may not be adequate. Specific fluorescent antibody conjugates are available for distinguishing the hyphae of *Aspergillus* organisms and zygomycetes in tissue.

SAPROPHYTIC FUNGI

Many normally saprophytic fungi can become opportunistic pathogens in compromised hosts. A few of these fungi may be confused with primary fungal pathogens because they have a similar morphologic structure. Table 37-2 summarizes the colonial and microscopic morphology of some of these saprophytes that are isolated from various kinds of clinical specimens. *Text continued on p. 623.*

TABLE 37-1. Colonial and Microscopic Morphology of Some Clinically Significant Zygomycete Genera

Genus	Colonial Morphology	Microscopic Appearance
Absidia	Rapid growing; woolly to cottony; olive gray	Sporangiophores branching, rising from stolons between rhizoids; sporangia pear shaped and contain one-celled, globose to ovoid sporangiospores; columella round, merging with apophysis (Figure 37-1)
Cunninghamella	Rapid growing; cottony; white to dark gray	Elongate branched sporangiophores with terminal vesicle on which one-celled, globose spores form on denticles (Figure 37-2)
Mucor	Rapid growing; woolly to cottony; white to gray brown	No rhizoids; branching or simple sporangiophores arising from hyphae; sporangia round, containing one-celled sporangiospores; columella variable (Figure 37-3)
Rhizomucor	Rapid growing; cottony; white; becoming smoke-gray to brown	Sporangiophores develop from simple or branched aerial hyphae or stolons; rhizoids poorly developed; sporangia round, containing one-celled, round sporangiospores; columella round; thermotolerant; growth at 50° to 55° C (Figure 37-4)
Rhizopus	Rapid growing; cottony; white to brownish gray; colonies tenacious	Sporangiophores long, dark, unbranched, solitary or in clusters; rhizoids at base of sporangiophores; sporangia black, round, containing one-celled, globose sporangiospores; columella hemispheric (Figure 37-5)
Saksenaea	Rapid growing; woolly; white	Flask-shaped sporangia with long necks and rhizoids at base of sporangiophore

Modified from McGinnis, M.R., D'Amato, R.F., and Land, G.A.: Pictorial handbook of medically important fungi and aerobic actinomycetes, New York, 1982, Praeger Publishers.

Key to the More Common Species of *Aspergillus*

1. Heads are uniseriate[a] only   2

1. (1) Heads are biseriate[b] or are both uniseriate and biseriate.   3

    2. Vesicles[c] clavate with phialides covering the entire surface; conidia elliptic and smooth with thick walls . . . .   *A. clavatus*

    2. (1) Vesicles hemispheric with phialides covering the upper half; conidia globose to subglobose, echinulate or delicately roughened, 2 to 3.5 μm in diameter; conidial heads forming compact columns; good growth at 45° C . . . .   *A. fumigatus*

3. Heads are biseriate only   4

3. (1) Uniseriate or biseriate conditions seen in the same isolate or on a single vesicle; conidiophores roughened; conidial heads yellow green, radiating, splitting into several poorly defined columns .   *A. flavus*

    4. Conidial heads black; vesicles globose with large metulae and small phialides; conidial heads radiating around vesicle . . . . . .   *A. niger*

    4. (1) Conidial heads green, cinnamon, or buff to orange brown.   5

5. Conidial heads green; conidiophores sinuous, cinnamon brown, with a hemispheric vesicle; conidial heads as short columns; cleistotheca and hülle cells typically present . . . .   *A. nidulans*

5. (1) Conidial heads cinnamon or buff to orange brown; conidiophores hyaline with a hemispheric vesicle; conidial heads are long, compact columns . . . .   *A. terreus*

From McGinnis, M.R., D'Amato, R.F., and Land, G.A.: Pictorial handbook of medically important fungi and aerobic actinomycetes, New York, 1982, Praeger Publishers.

[a]Uniseriate. Phialides arises directly from vesicle.

[b]Biseriate. Phialides arising from sterile cells that develop directly from vesicle.

[c]Vesicle. Swollen apical portion of the conidiophore.

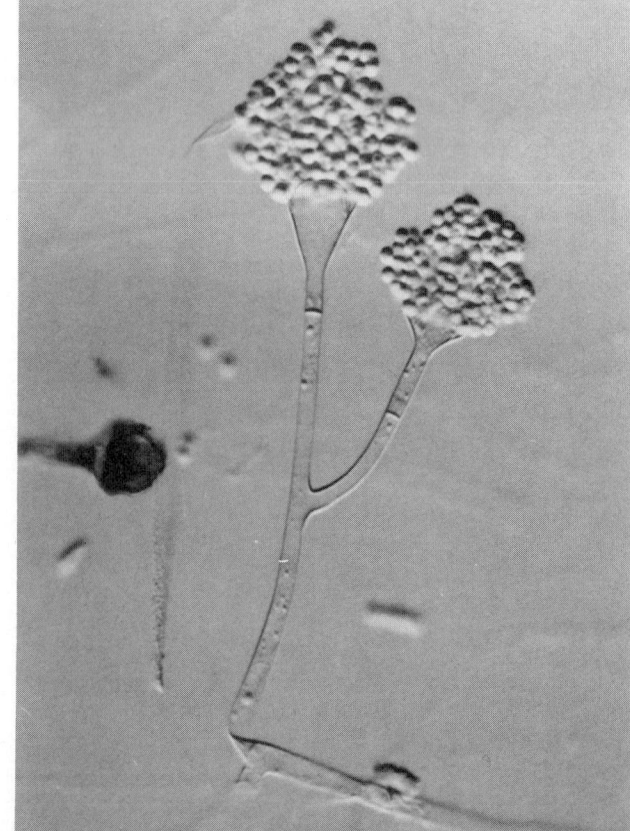

FIGURE 37-1. *Absidia.* Note pear-shaped sporangia on branching sporangiophore. Swelling at junction of sporangium and sporangiophore is apophysis.

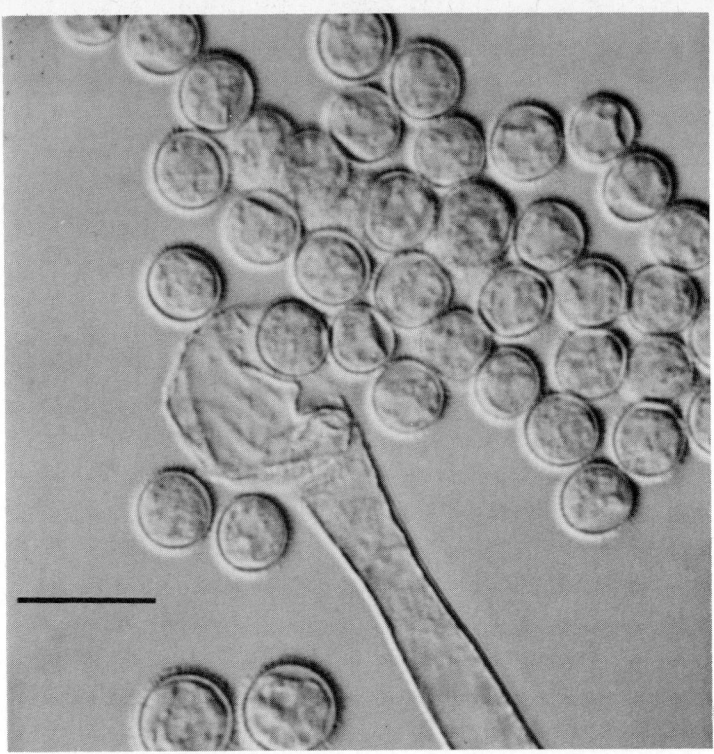

FIGURE 37-2. Terminal vesicles of *Cunninghamella* containing one-celled spores. (Bar = 10 μm.) (From McGinnis, M.R., D'Amato, R.F., and Land, G.A.: Pictorial handbook of fungi and aerobic actinomycetes, New York, 1982, Praeger Publishers.)

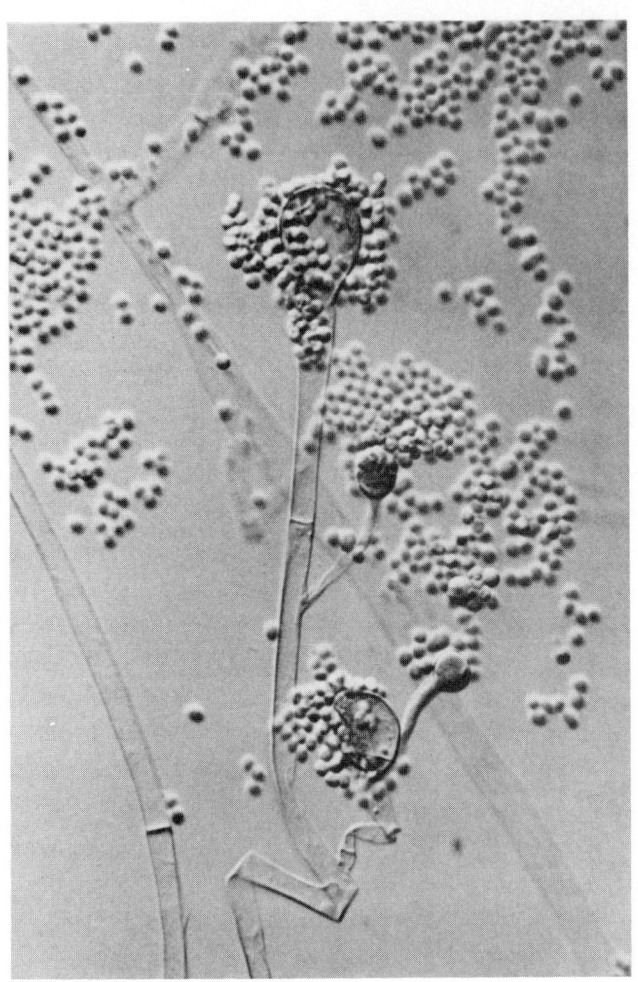

FIGURE 37-3. *Mucor*. Round sporangia containing sporangiospores on branching or simple sporangiophores. (From McGinnis, M.R.: Laboratory handbook of medical mycology, New York, 1980, Academic Press, Inc.)

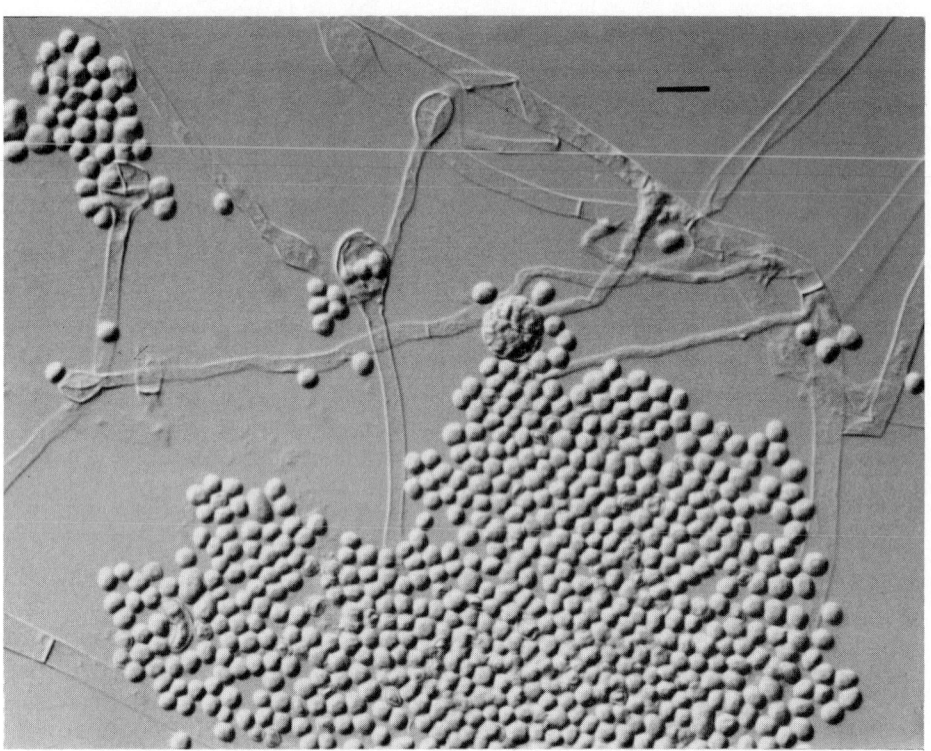

FIGURE 37-4. *Rhizomucor* is thermotolerant mold that produces sporangia and poorly differentiated rhizoids. (Bar = 10 μm.) (From McGinnis, M.R., D'Amato, R.F., and Land, G.A.: Pictorial handbook of fungi and aerobic actinomycetes, New York, 1982, Praeger Publishers.)

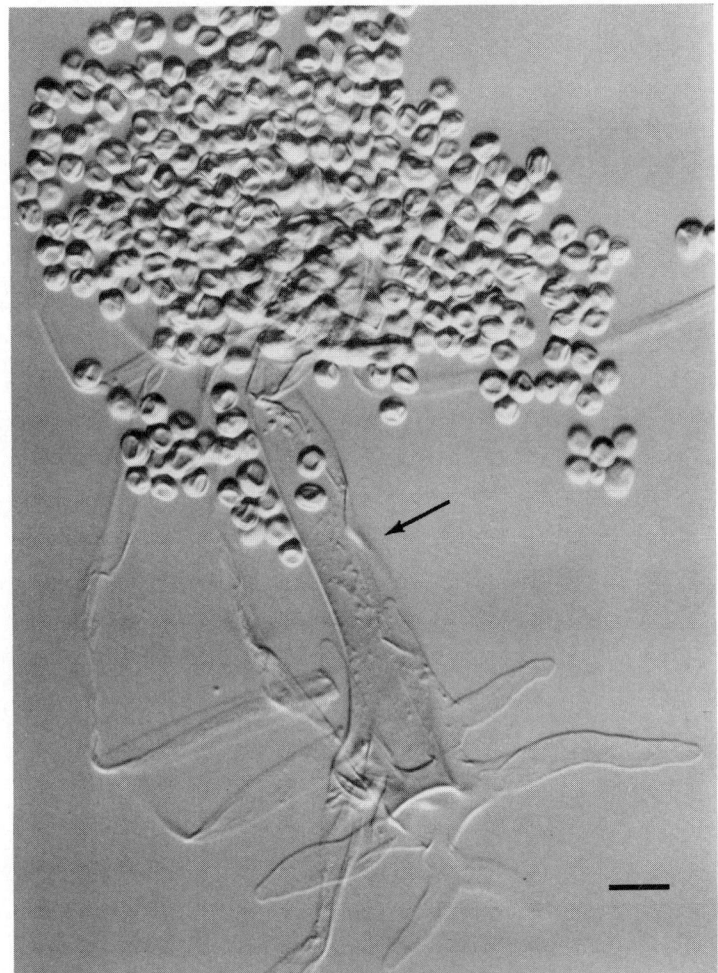

FIGURE 37-5. *Rhizopus*. Rhizoids arise from below unbranched sporangiophore *(arrow)*. (Bar = 10 μm.) (From McGinnis, M.R., D'Amato, R.F., and Land, G.A.: Pictorial handbook of fungi and aerobic actinomycetes, New York, 1982, Praeger Publishers.)

TABLE 37-2. Colonial and Microscopic Morphology of Some Genera of Fungi

Organism	Colonial Morphology	Habitat	Microscopic Appearance	Clinical Aspects
Acremonium	Rapid growing; flat, membranelike; white-yellow-rose; older colonies with aerial hyphae	Soil; decaying organic matter	Conidiophores thin, erect, with tapering phialides; phialoconidia one celled and globose to cylindric, accumulating in balls at tip of phialides (see Figure 28-5)	Mycotic keratitis; mycetoma; opportunistic infections; occasional contaminant
Alternaria	Rapid growing; cottony to woolly; gray-white to olive	Soil; plants; decaying vegetable matter	Conidiophores sympodial, giving rise to branching chains of conidia; conidia acropetal and muriform, having swollen basal portion and terminal beak; walls darkly pigmented, olive brown to black, and smooth or rough (Figure 37-6)	Implicated in allergy; occasional contaminant
Arthrographis	Moderately rapid growing; downy to powdery; cream-white to buff	Soil	Chains of one-celled, hyaline, cylindric arthroconidia on short hyphalike conidiophores	Occasional contaminant
Aureobasidium	Moderately rapid growing; moist and mucoid to pasty; white to pink; occasionally black; colonies become wrinkled	Soil; wood; fruit	One-celled oval to cylindric hyaline conidia developing from hyphae; conidia often bud to produce blastoconidia; thick-walled, dematiaceous arthroconidia often present (Figure 37-7)	Unusual contaminant
Bipolaris	Rapid growing; woolly to cottony; olive green to black	Soil; plants; vegetable matter	Conidiophores sympodial, geniculate, brown; conidia multicelled, fusoid to cylindric, light brown, with slightly protruding dark hila (see Figure 33-3)	Mycotic keratitis and other forms of phaeohyphomycosis, especially sinusitis; unusual contaminant
Chrysosporium	Moderately rapid growing; granular; woolly to cottony; white to pale brown	Soil	Conidia one celled, broader than vegetative hyphae, terminal or along sides of hyphae; annular frill at base of conidium; random arthroconidia that are larger than parent hyphae typically present (Figure 37-8)	Sensitive to cycloheximide; unusual contaminant; morphologically similar to *Blastomyces dermatitidis* and *Histoplasma capsulatum*
Cladosporium	Moderately rapid growing; velvety to woolly; grayish green to olive green	Soil; plants; vegetable matter	Erect conidiophores; septate, pigmented conidia one to four celled, pale brown with dark hila, in branching acropetal chains; conidia near conidiophore often shield shaped (see Figure 33-4)	Allergin but rare pathogen; occasional contaminant
Curvularia	Rapid growing; woolly; olive green to black	Soil; vegetable matter	Conidiophores sympodial, geniculate, brown; conidia several celled, curved, with enlarged central cell and end cells lighter in color than other cells (Figure 37-9)	Mycotic keratitis; endocarditis; other forms of phaeohyphomycosis; unusual contaminant
Exophiala	Slow to rapid growing; often yeastlike; becoming woolly; gray to black	Soil; wood; vegetable matter	Conidiophores hyphalike; annellides cylindric to flask shaped; conidia one celled, hyaline to pale brown, accumulating in balls; *Phaeoannellomyces* yeast anamorph often present (see Figure 33-5)	Occasional agent of phaeohyphomycosis; occasional contaminant
Exserohilum	Rapid growing; woolly to cottony; olive green to black	Soil; plants; vegetable matter	Conidiophores sympodial, geniculate, brown; conidia cylindric, multicelled, light brown, with strongly protruding dark hila (Figure 37-10)	Phaeohyphomycosis, especially sinusitis; unusual contaminant

TABLE 37-2. Colonial and Microscopic Morphology of Some Genera of Fungi—cont'd

Organism	Colonial Morphology	Habitat	Microscopic Appearance	Clinical Aspects
Fusarium	Rapid growing; woolly to cottony; white to purple	Grain; soil; decaying plant matter	Conidia of two types: macroconidia, multicelled, curved or sickle shaped, with foot cell, smooth walled; microconidia typically one celled, in balls or occasionally chains, similar to *Acremonium;* microconidia and macroconidia produced by phialides (Figure 37-11)	Mycotic keratitis; mycetoma; burn infections; other opportunistic mycoses; occasional contaminant
Geotrichum	Rapid growing; cottony; white	Milk; fruit; soil; vegetable matter	Hyaline hyphae; arthroconidia cylindric to globose, one celled, in chains; conidiophores absent; blastoconidia absent (Figure 37-12)	Rare opportunistic pathogen; occasional contaminant
Paecilomyces	Rapid growing; cottony to ropy; white to olive brown	Soil; vegetable matter	Erect, branching, septate conidiophores; phialides with tapering apices, in pairs, groups, or verticils; chains of one-celled, ovoid to fusoid conidia forming entangled chains; conidia may be pigmented (Figure 37-13)	Endocarditis; other opportunistic mycoses; occasional contaminant
Penicillium	Rapid growing; velvety; usually in some shade of green	Soil; decaying organic matter	Conidiophores unbranched or branched; conidiogenous cells flask-shaped phialides produced directly on metulae; phialoconidia one celled, in basipetal, unbranched chains (Figure 37-14)	Common contaminant
Scedosporium	Rapid growing; cottony; white becoming smoky-brown	Soil; vegetable matter	Conidiophores short, hyphalike, giving rise to cylindric annellides that often have swollen area just below apex; conidia one celled, nearly round to elongate, pale brown, accumulating in balls; some conidia solitary along hyphae (Figure 37-15)	Pulmonary infections; mycetoma; other mycoses; occasional contaminant
Scopulariopsis	Moderately rapid growing; granular to powdery white, becoming tan	Soil; organic matter	Branched or unbranched conidiophores; conidiogenous cells annellides; conidia one-celled basipetals in chains, round, rough walled and flattened at basal portion (Figure 37-16)	Nail infection; occasional contaminant
Sepedonium	Rapid growing; woolly to cottony; white to tan	Soil	Large, one-celled, hyaline to golden conidia on slender hyphalike conidiophores (Figure 37-17); phialides occasionally present	Sensitive to cycloheximide; rare contaminant, morphologically similar to *Histoplasma capsulatum*
Syncephalastrum	Rapid growing; cottony; white or gray to black	Soil	Sporangiospores formed in row within long cylindric sporangia (merosporangia) (Figure 37-18); tip of sporangiophore swollen; rhizoids present	Rare contaminant
Verticillium	Rapid growing; velvety to cottony; white to pinkish brown	Soil; plants; vegetable matter	Conidiophores erect, hyaline to pigmented, often branched; phialides long, hyaline, arising in whorls; branches also in whorls; conidia one celled, ovoid to allantoid, accumulating in balls (Figure 37-19)	Rare pathogen; rare contaminant

Data from references 9, 12, and 14.

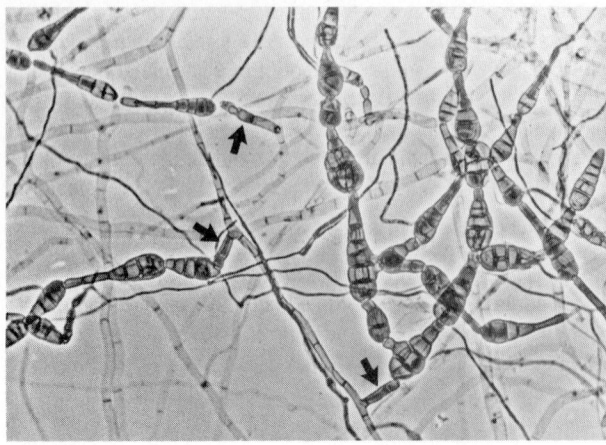

FIGURE 37-6. *Alternaria*. Branched chains of muriform conidia arise from conidiophores *(arrows)*. Note that upper portions of conidia are beak shaped.

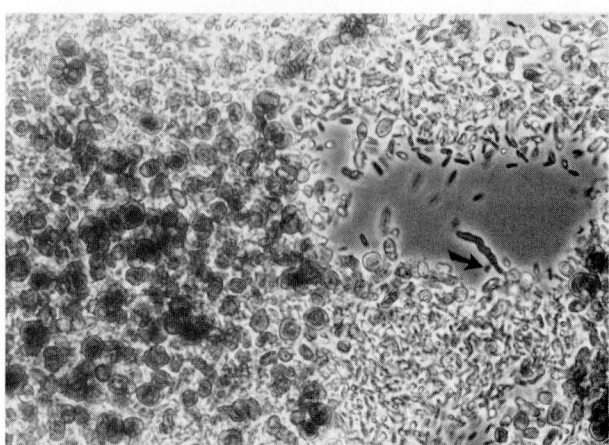

FIGURE 37-7. *Aureobasidium*. Hyphae have fragmented into thick-walled, dematiaceous, one- or two-celled arthroconidia. One-celled hyaline conidium *(arrow)* is arising laterally from hypha.

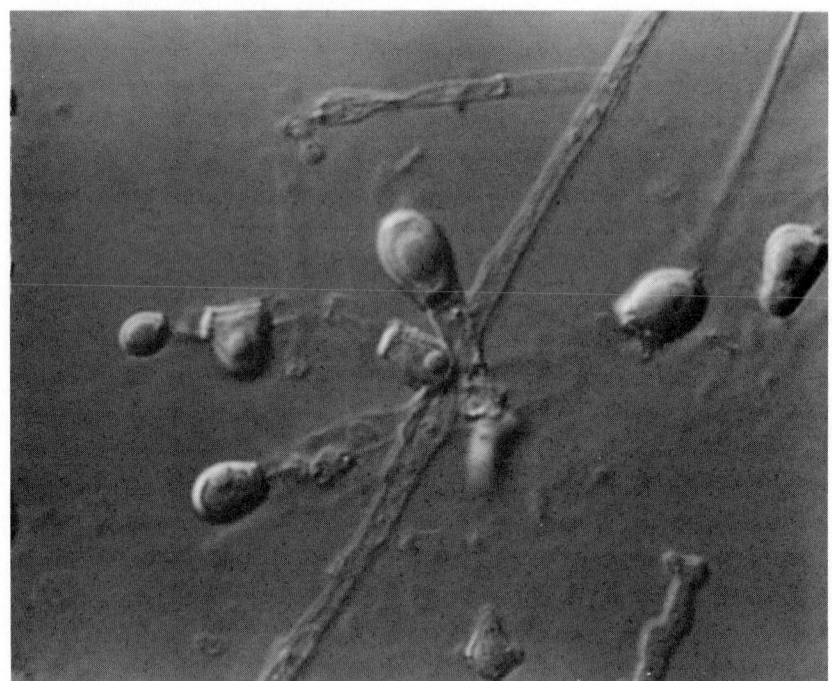

FIGURE 37-8. *Chrysosporium*. Truncate conidia formed on short hyphalike conidiophores.

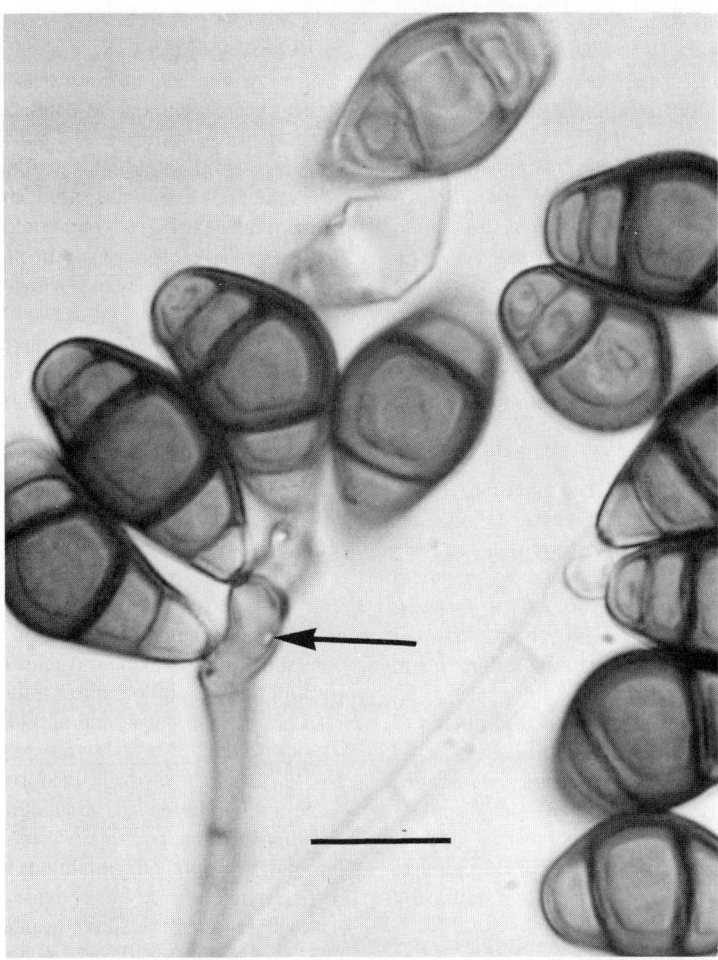

FIGURE 37-9. *Curvularia.* Septate, curved conidia with darkly pigmented swollen central cell. Conidia arise from sympodial conidiophore *(arrow).* (Bar = 10 µm.) (From McGinnis, M.R., D'Amato, R.F., and Land, G.A.: Pictorial handbook of fungi and aerobic actinomycetes, New York, 1982, Praeger Publishers.)

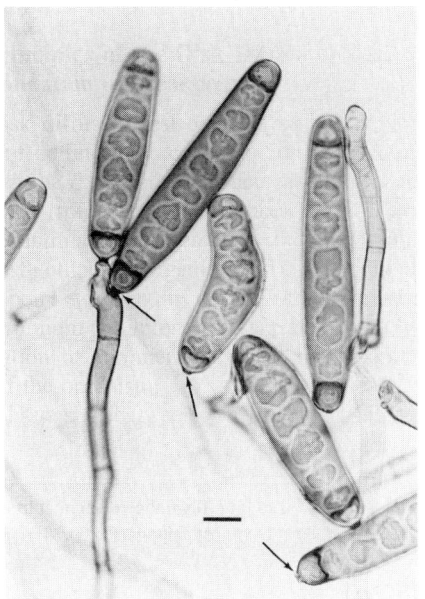

FIGURE 37-10. *Exserohilum.* Cylindric to ellipsoidal septate conidia with strongly protruding hilum *(arrows).* Conidia arise from sympodial conidiophore.

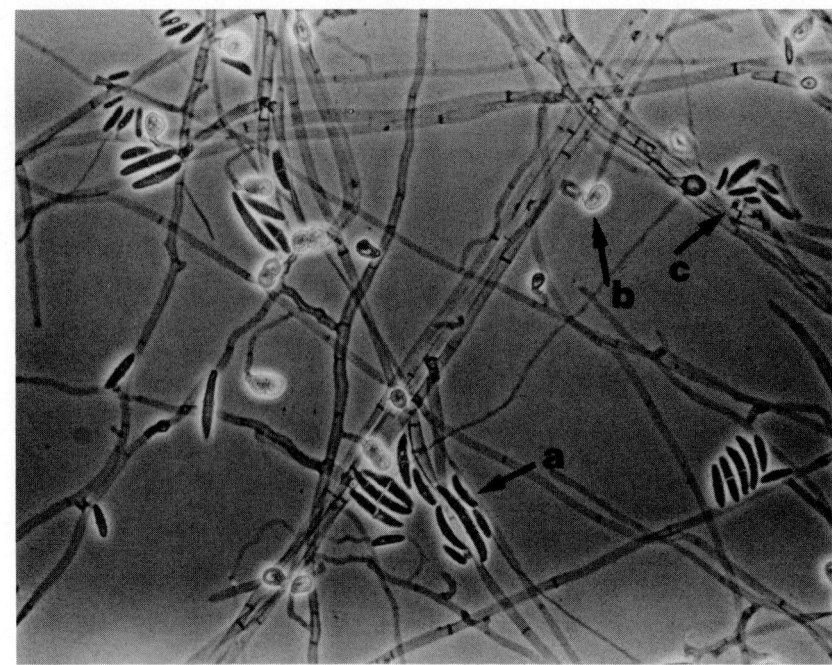

FIGURE 37-11. *Fusarium.* Note sickle-shaped macroconidia *(a)*, chlamydoconidia *(b)*, and one-celled microconidia *(c)*.

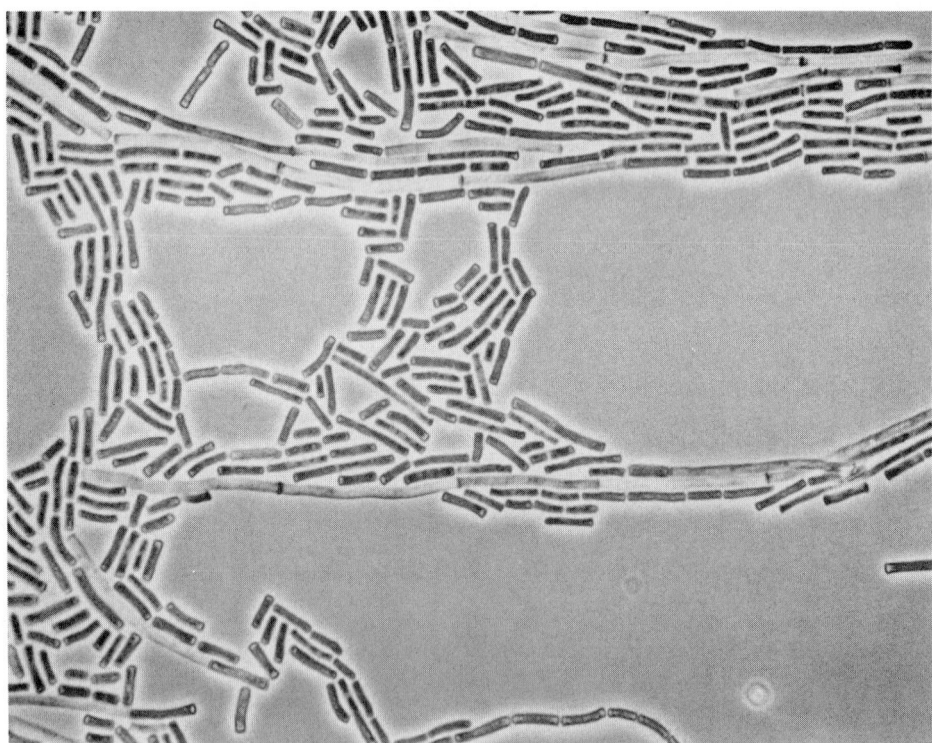

FIGURE 37-12. *Geotrichum.* Cylindric arthroconidia result from fragmentation of fertile hyphae.

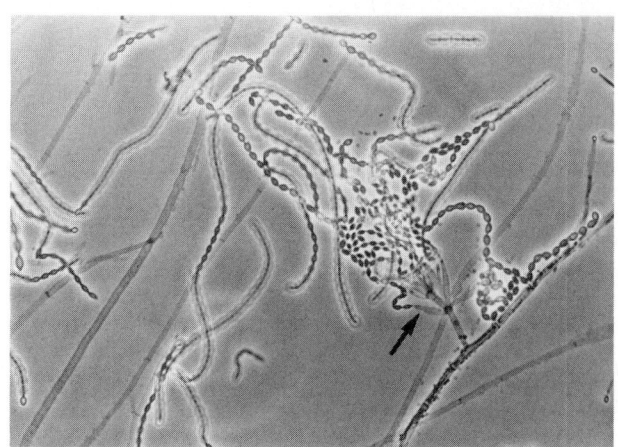

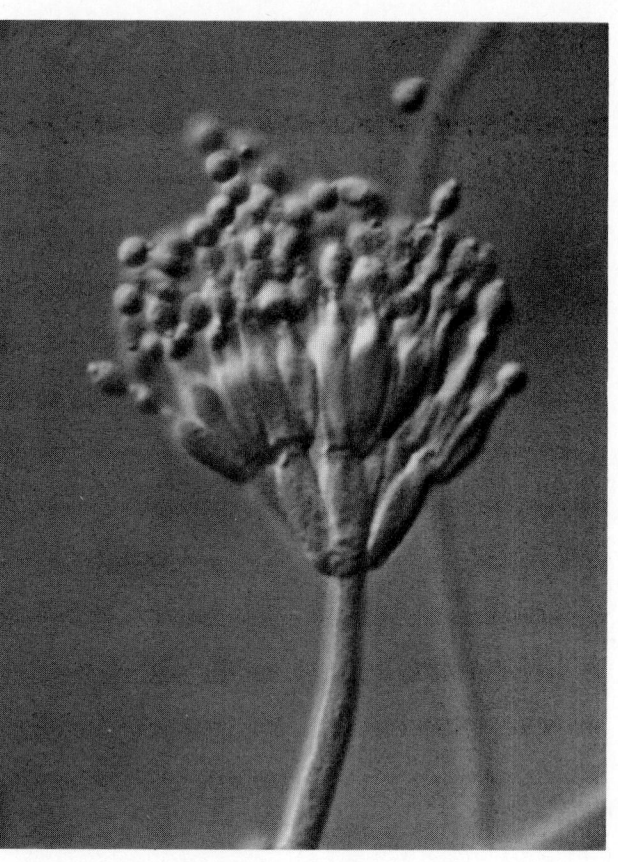

FIGURE 37-13. *Paecilomyces*. Chains of one-celled conidia form entangled chains. Phialides *(arrow)* have long, narrow, tapering necks.

FIGURE 37-14. *Penicillium*. Conidial structure resembles brush.

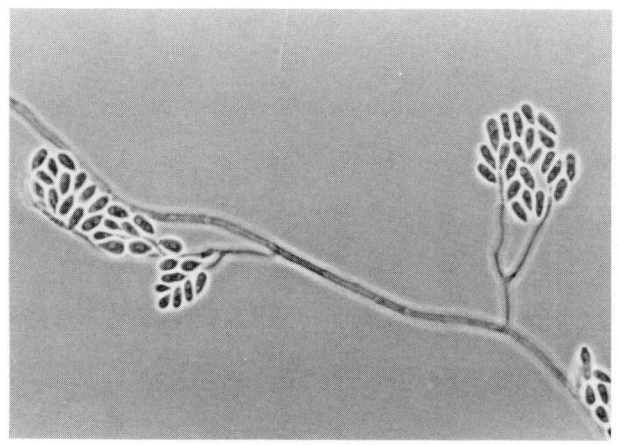

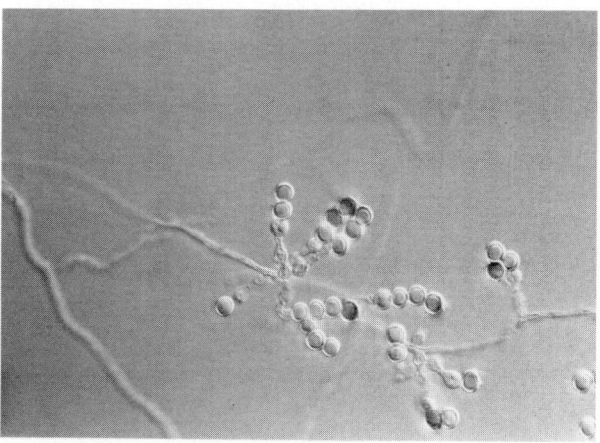

FIGURE 37-15. *Scedosporium*. Annellides with balls of conidia at their tips. Note that bases of conidia are truncate.

FIGURE 37-16. *Scopulariopsis*. Chains of conidia with truncate bases arise from annellides.

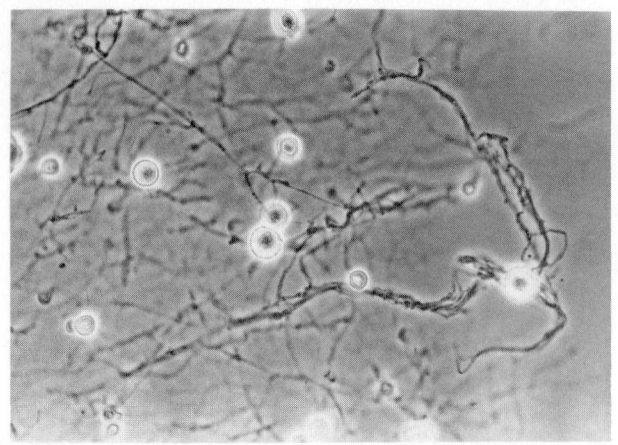

FIGURE 37-17. *Sepedonium*. Large, one-celled, rough-walled conidia form solitarily on slender hyphalike conidiophores.

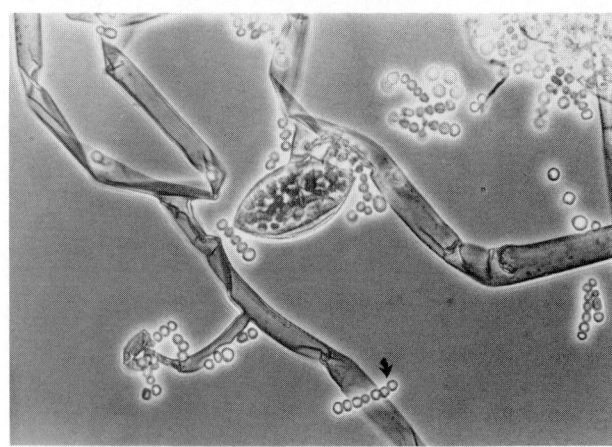

FIGURE 37-18. *Syncephalastrum*. Sporangiospores formed in row within long cylindric merosporangium *(arrow)*.

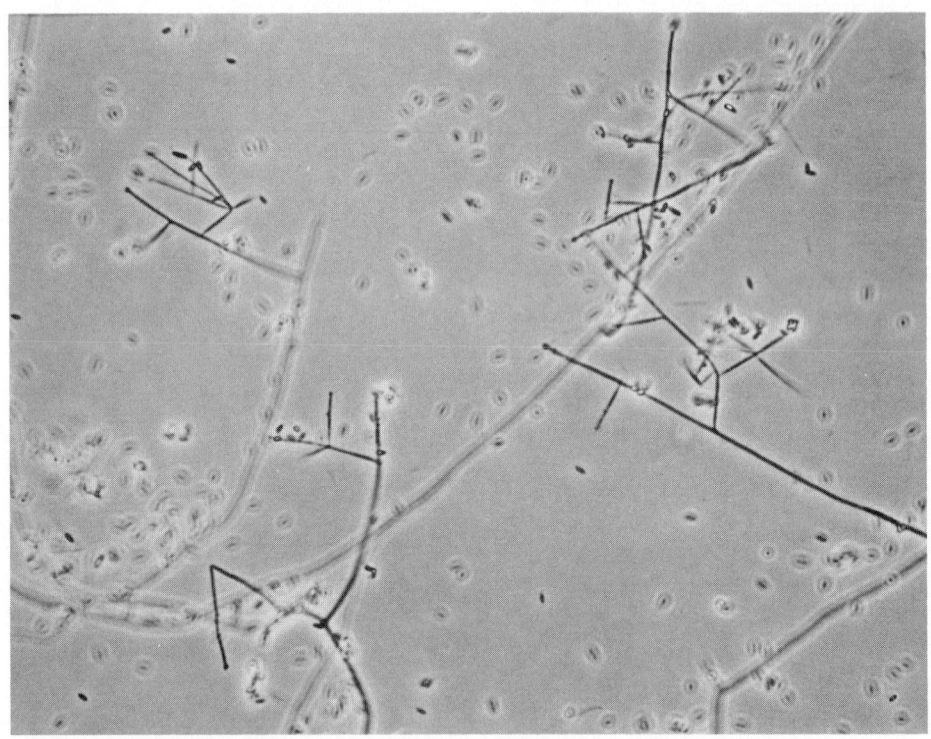

FIGURE 37-19. *Verticillium*. Conidia arise in balls from narrow, tapering, needlelike phialides. Phialides occur in whorls.

REFERENCES

1. Artis W.M., et al.: Mechanism of host defense against fungus infections: transferrin, iron, and fungal siderophores. In Arai, T., et al., editors: Filamentous microorganisms: biomedical aspects, Tokyo, 1985, Japan Scientific Societies Press.

2. Austwick, P.K.C.: Pathogenicity. In Raper, K.B., and Fennell, D.F., editor: The genus *Aspergillus,* Baltimore, 1965, Williams & Wilkins Co.

3. Chandler, F.W., Kaplan, W., and Ajello, L.: A colour atlas and textbook of the histopathology of mycotic diseases, London, 1980, Wolfe Medical Publications, Ltd.

4. Domsch, K.H., Gams, W., and Anderson, T.: Compendium of soil fungi, New York, 1980, Academic Press, Inc.

5. Fink, J.N.: Allergic bronchopulmonary aspergillosis, Chest **87**(suppl. 1):81S, 1985.

6. Fisher, M.R., et al.: Use of linear tomography to confirm the diagnosis of allergic bronchopulmonary aspergillosis, Chest **87**:499, 1985.

7. Gerson, S.L., et al.: Prolonged granulocytopenia: the major risk factor for invasive pulmonary aspergillosis in patients with acute leukemia, Ann. Intern. Med. **100**:345, 1984.

8. Greenberger, P.A.: Allergic bronchopulmonary aspergillosis, J. Allergy Clin. Immunol. **74**:645, 1984.

9. Haley, L.D., and Callaway, C.S.: Laboratory methods in medical mycology, ed. 4, Department of Health, Education and Welfare, Pub. No. (CDC) 78-8361, Atlanta, 1978, Center for Disease Control.

10. Longbottom, J.L., and Pepys, J.: Diagnosis of fungal diseases. In Gill, P.G.H., Coombs, R.R.A, and Lachman, P.J., editors: Clinical aspects of immunology, ed. 3, Oxford, Eng., 1975, Blackwell Scientific Publications, Ltd.

11. Marier, R., et al.: A solid-phase radioimmunoassay for the measurement of antibody to *Aspergillus* in invasive aspergillosis, J. Infect. Dis. **140**:771, 1979.

12. McGinnis, M.R.: Laboratory handbook of medical mycology, New York, 1980, Academic Press, Inc.

13. McGinnis, M.R., Ajello, L., and Schell, W.A.: Mycotic diseases: a proposed nomenclature, Int. J. Dermatol. **24**:9, 1985.

14. McGinnis, M.R., D'Amato, R.F., and Land, G.A.: Pictorial handbook of medically important fungi and aerobic actinomycetes, New York, 1982, Praeger Publishers.

15. O'Donnell, K.L.: Zycomycetes in culture: Palfrey contributions in botany, Athens, 1979, University of Georgia.

16. Raper, K.B., and Fennell, D.L., editors: The genus *Aspergillus,* Baltimore, 1965, Williams & Wilkins Co.

17. Rinaldi, M.G.: Invasive aspergillosis, Rev. Infect. Dis. **5**:1061, 1983.

18. Rippon, J.W.: Medical mycology: the pathogenic fungi and the pathogenic actinomycetes, ed. 2, Philadelphia, 1982, W.B. Saunders Co.

19. Rohatgi, P.K., and Rohatgi, N.B.: Clinical spectrum of pulmonary aspergillosis, South. Med. J. **77**:1291, 1984.

20. Scholer, H.J., Müller, E., and Schipper, M.A.A.: Mucorales. In Howard, D.H., editor: Fungi pathogenic for humans and animals, vol. 3, New York, 1983, Marcel Dekker, Inc.

21. Shank, R.C.: Mycotoxicoses of man: dietary and epidemiological considerations. In Wyllie, T.D., and Morehouse, L.G., editor: Mycotoxic fungi, mycotoxins, mycotoxicoses, vol. 3, New York, 1978, Marcel Dekker, Inc.

22. Zycha, H., Siepmann, R., and Linnemann, G.: Mucorales, Lehre, Federal Republic of Germany, 1969, J. Cramer.

CHAPTER 38

Immunologic Diagnosis of Fungal Infection

Richard C. Tilton
Michael R. McGinnis

Many observations and analyses contribute to the diagnosis of fungal disease. Precise clinical history, characteristic symptoms and signs, suggestive epidemiology, and even the isolation of a clinically significant fungus may provide the key information necessary for the diagnosis. In many instances, however, the patient's symptoms are not specific, there is no apparent history of environmental exposure or travel to an endemic area, and no organism is isolated. In these situations the first suggestion of a fungal infection may be the appearance of specific antibody. Larsh[12] reports that a single sputum specimen from patients with pulmonary disease results in a clinically significant culture less than 5% of the time. However, when appropriate serologic tests are used to detect the suspected mycosis, cultural results may be positive in greater than 50% of the serologically positive patients.

Five types of tests are commonly used in mycoserology: (1) skin tests (delayed or immediate hypersensitivity tests), (2) detection of circulating antibodies, (3) detection of circulating antigens, (4) exoantigen analysis, and (5) visualization of the organism by direct or indirect fluorescence microscopy. (See Kaufman and Reiss[7,8] for procedures for these tests.)

SKIN TESTS

Cutaneous delayed hypersensitivity response is now recognized as an in vivo determination of cell-mediated immunity. A positive skin test result generally signifies an intact cellular immune system. Although a negative result may suggest that the patient has not been exposed to a particular fungal disease, it may also indicate a specific immune dysfunction. In addition, a skin test result may be negative in a very small number of patients who have had fungal infections.

Skin tests are available for the mycoses histoplasmosis, paracoccidioidomycosis, coccidioidomycosis, and sporotrichosis. These tests cannot be employed as one-time tests to diagnose an infection because they cannot discriminate between past and present infection.

A positive skin test finding does have diagnostic value if there is a history of a negative finding before the onset of clinical symptoms. The conversion of a negative test result to a positive result after having a fungal infection is a good prognostic sign. It may be appropriate at times to test several skin test antigens such as coccidioidin or spherulin and histoplasmin to compare their responses. This is necessary because fungi share common antigens that can cross-react in skin testing.[8] The interpretation of the results must be correlated with the clinical presentation and other laboratory data that may be available.

Reversion from a positive skin test finding to a negative one may reflect a poor prognosis and indicate anergy. Reversion is occasionally observed in coccidioidomycosis.[8]

The application of a skin test antigen before some tests for humoral antibody may produce false elevations in titer or cause false-positive immunoprecipitants in the immunodiffusion test. Serum for mycoserology should always be collected before skin testing. The skin test is a reliable epidemiologic tool that has helped to define endemic areas for some of the systemic fungi by screening large populations.

DETECTION OF CIRCULATING ANTIBODY

Complement fixation (CF), immunodiffusion (ID), latex agglutination (LA), counterimmunoelectrophoresis (CIE), enzyme-linked immunosorbent assay (ELISA), and radioimmunoassay (RIA) are often used to detect circulating antibodies to fungal antigens. Of these, CF, ID, and LA are the most commonly used. No one test fulfills all of the necessary attributes of specificity, sensitivity, and speed, although ID is quite sensitive and specific for the serologic diagnosis of histoplasmosis, blastomycosis, and coccidioidomycosis.

Usually a diagnosis cannot be made based on a single serum specimen unless there is a high titer. A rising antibody titer, usually fourfold or greater, is considered suggestive of infection. Samples should be spaced 2 to 3 weeks apart and be collected before skin testing for optimal results. Table 38-1 summarizes the available antibody tests and their interpretation, sensitivity, and specificity.

Rarely have standardized serologic tests for fungal infections been evaluated methodically in a large outbreak. Recently a large urban outbreak of histoplasmosis occurred; 276 of 495 patients affected were studied serologically.[25] Serologic findings were positive in 96% of the patients; positive results were 22% from culture and 19% from direct microscopy of specimens. ID test results were negative in 13% of patients who had positive findings by complement fixation (CF). CF was twice as sensitive as ID for subclinical infections. High mycelial titers were associated with intense exposure, and high yeast titers with youth (less than 36 years old). This one example demonstrates the utility of serologic screening and the limitations of cultural procedures for this type of diagnostic problem.

Some of the problems associated with the detection of circulating antibody, however, can be seen with *Candida* organisms. The presence of circulating *Candida* precipitins is not reliable evidence for candidiasis, since it may reflect only colonization with the organism. The issue is controversial; some claim efficacy and others do not.[11,14,17,18,21] Buckley[1] outlined new methodology that potentially increased the specificity of

TABLE 38-1. Detection of Circulating Fungal Antibody or Antigen

Fungal Infection	Test	Application	Interpretation
Aspergillosis	ID	Patients with allergic bron-chopulmonary disease or aspergilloma; immunosuppressed patients with fever of unknown origin; *A. flavus, A. fumigatus,* and *A. niger* antigens should be used	Must use control sera from patient with positive test result and look for "lines of identity"; when reference sera used, 100% specific and 70%-90% sensitive; may see cross-reactions with C-reactive protein; precipitins can be found in 70% of cases of allergic disease and 90% of aspergillomas but are less common in invasive disease
	CF	Some report CF is as sensitive but less specific than ID; others indicate that CF is less sensitive and less specific	Should be used to test a battery of antigens
	CIE	Good screening test for aspergillosis	Also used to detect antigenemia; sensitivity and specificity similar to ID
Blastomycosis	ID	Patients with respiratory symptoms, purulent sputum, or skin lesions; useful when CF cross-reaction is suspected	"A" precipitin line is indicative of blastomycosis when yeast phase antigen is used; 100% specific, 80% sensitive; tests for histoplasmosis and coccidioidomycosis should also be performed
	CF	Widely used but inferior to ID; 50% of patients with culturally proven blastomycosis have CF antibody; lacks both sensitivity and specificity	≥1:8 is "positive" titer, but fourfold increase in titer over 4-6 wk is necessary for confirmation of diagnosis; negative CF result has little value, but positive result may have prognostic value
Candidiasis	CF	Systemic candidiasis; patients with candidemia and can-diduria; patients receiving immunosuppressive therapy; sensitivity 90%; cross-reaction with *Torulopsis glabrata* for CIE and ID; LA less specific; tests useful in immunologically intact host	CF unreliable because of false-positive titers
	LA, ID, CIE		Presence of *Candida* precipitins, 4-fold titer rise or titer of 1:8 or greater may signify disease, but because of colonization, precipitins may be seen in absence of disease; serologic conversion or rapid increase in titer is strong evidence for candidiasis; tests for antigenemia may be helpful
Coccidioidomycosis	CF	Useful for patients with pulmonary or meningeal symptoms who live in endemic area and patients with positive coccidioidin or spherulin skin tests; CF will appear later in disease than precipitating antibody	Any CF titer presumptive; CF titers of 1:2 and 1:4 indicate early residual or meningeal disease; titers 1:2 to 1:8 plus ID Ab highly suggestive of recent or active coccidioidomycosis; CF >1:16 indicative of dissemination; CF titer in CSF diagnostic for central nervous system (CNS) disease; sensitivity about 95%
	TP	Effective for detection of early pulmonary infection; not useful for meningitis	Positive finding diagnostic but not prognostic; in 80% of patients finding is positive within 2 weeks of symptoms; 90% sensitive and specific
	ID, LA	Good screening tests; ID has greater sensitivity than TP but less sensitivity than LA	LA lacks specificity (6%-10% false-positive results)
Cryptococcosis	IFA, TA	Patients with symptoms of pulmonary cryptococcosis or cryptococcal meningitis; antibody detection less sensitive and more time consuming than antigen detection	IFA and TA antibody tests' sensitivity 50% with extrameningeal infections; specificity about 77% and 89%, respectively

TABLE 38-1. Detection of Circulating Fungal Antibody or Antigen—cont'd

Fungal Infection	Test	Application	Interpretation
	LA, EIA	Used to detect antigen	LA titer of 1:2 suggestive; titer diagnostic and prognostic; sera showing weak reaction should be treated with pronase
Histoplasmosis	CF	Paired specimens (serum, cerebrospinal fluid, peritoneal fluid) from patients with suspected acute, chronic, disseminated, and meningeal infection; CF using yeast form antigen is more sensitive (96%) than CF antibody to mycelial filtrate (83%) (histoplasmin); CF yeast-form antibodies appear earlier in disease	Cross-reactions may occur with blastomycosis and coccidioidomycosis; antibody to yeast form appears in 4 weeks; when CF cross-reactions occur, titers usually range from 1:8 to 1:32, Titers (CF) > 1:32 strongly suggestive of histoplasmosis; fourfold increase above 1:32 is highly significant; direction of titer change has prognostic value; anergy may exist in disseminated histoplasmosis
	ID, CIE	More specific than CF; 90% agreement with CF; may be used on cerebrospinal fluid if meningeal involvement is suspected; CIE uses histoplasmin as antigen	One band, H, seen in active infections, is uninfluenced by skin tests; M band seen in acute and chronic histoplasmosis and in skin test–sensitized patients; if patient has *not* had skin test, M band indicates early disease because it usually is first band to appear; M band occurs as result of active disease, inactive disease, skin testing; both M and H bands highly suggestive of infection; Y precipitin band, in absence of M and H, indicates acute histoplasmosis
	LA	Good for anticomplementary sera; useful for early detection of acute histoplasmosis; may be negative in chronic histoplasmosis	Significant titer is ≥1:32; false-positive results may occur if titer is low
Paracoccidioidomycosis	CF, ID	Patients with chronic lung disease, ulcerative mucosal lesions, and skin lesions; history of travel in Latin America	CF antibodies are diagnostic, but infrequent cross-reactions may be observed at 1:8 dilution level; sensitivity is 80%-96%; ID test with yeast antigen is more specific and equally sensitive; combination of ID and CF yields diagnosis in >98% of cases[7]
Sporotrichosis	TA, LA	Useful for extracutaneous sporotrichosis; greater sensitivity and specificity than CF and ID; LA tests rapid (5 min); TA may show false-positive results in patients with leishmaniasis	1:4 LA titers presumptive evidence of infection; false-positive titers of 1:4 to 1:8 seen; rising titer indicative of sporotrichosis; 80%-90% sensitivity, but cross-reactions with *Leishmania* antibodies may occur; LA titer 1:32 or greater in CSF is evidence of meningeal infection
Zygomycosis	ID, ELISA	Antigens of *Absidia, Rhizopus,* and *Rhizomucor* organisms used; sensitivity 70%; specificity unknown but cross-reactions with other zygomycetes occur	Available from Centers for Disease Control

SYMBOLS:	ID,	Immunodiffusion	IFA,	Indirect fluorescent antibody
	CF,	Complement fixation	TA,	Tube agglutination
	CIE,	Counterimmunoelectrophoresis	EIA,	Enzyme immunoassay
	LA,	Latex agglutination	ELISA,	Enzyme-linked immunosorbent assay
	TP,	Tube precipitin		

Data from references 7 to 9.

the *Candida* precipitin test. Sera were screened for antibodies using double immunodiffusion and then tested by crossed immunoelectrophoresis (XIE) according to the method of Axelson and Svendsen. Two precipitin bands were seen, one to cell wall antigens and the other to nonmannan (non–cell wall) antigens. Syverson, Buckley and Gibian[20] further increased the specificity of the test by precipitating out the mannan antigens with concanavalin A. Kaufman[6] stated that carbohydrates or mannan antigens contribute to the lack of specificity of the *Candida* precipitin test but also reported that the mannan antigens are the only ones reactive in certain cases of invasive candidiasis. He concluded that both protein and mannan antigens should be used to detect *Candida* precipitins and that a crude cell homogenate was better than purified antigens.

DETECTION OF FUNGAL ANTIGENS

A disadvantage of antibody detection for diagnosis is that only rarely are single titers reliable, and, in most cases, paired sera are drawn 2 to 3 weeks apart. Second, immunocompromised hosts usually are not producing antibody. If antigen can be detected in body fluid, an immediate provisional diagnosis could be made. Confirmation still rests, however, on recovery and isolation of the fungus. The two fungal diseases cryptococcosis and candidiasis can be rapidly diagnosed by detection of their antigens in vivo.

Several commercial kits exist for the identification of cryptococcal polysaccharide in body fluids by latex agglutination (LA). The two most useful fluids are cerebrospinal fluid (CSF) and blood, but the titers in CSF and blood are essentially independent of each other. The test is sensitive and simple to perform. Nonspecific cross-reactions are seen primarily with rheumatoid factor. Eng and Person[4] used ethylenediaminetetra-acetic acid (EDTA) extraction and heat treatment (boiling water for 5 minutes) to remove rheumatoid factor (RF) from the sera of nine patients with cryptococcal infection and four patients with rheumatoid arthritis with positive RF. They reported that the sensitivity of the cryptococcal antigen latex test improved and that RF was completely removed. The 9% false-positive results observed in CSF[15] could also be eliminated by boiling CSF without extraction by EDTA. Stockman and Roberts[19] described the use of a protease for the elimination of interfering RF. The method requires only 20 minutes and makes the LA test for cryptococcal antigen highly specific. All weakly positive CSF specimens should be treated with protease. When properly performed, the LA test is quantitative. A titer of 1:2 is suggestive of cryptococcosis, and a titer of 1:8 is indicative of active cryptococcosis. A rising titer denotes a poor prognosis. In our laboratories, tests for cryptococcal capsular material are performed routinely on all CSF for which an india ink preparation is requested. We do not recommend the use of the india ink preparation because the LA test and culture are both superior to microscopy. LA approaches 92% to 100% sensitivity, and it is 100% specific when the appropriate controls are run.

Circulating metabolic and structural components of *Candida albicans* have been detected in the blood of patients with candidiasis. Kiehn and co-workers[10] have proposed that the presence of arabinitol, a major metabolite of *C. albicans,* might be predictive of invasive candidiasis. Eng, Chmel, and Buse,[3] using gas-liquid chromatography, noted that patients with invasive candidiasis did not show elevated levels of arabinitol, but

patients in renal failure with or without candidiasis did have elevated levels of arabinitol. Thus the value of serum arabinitol concentrations in serum of patients having invasive candidiasis is controversial.[2,5,16,26]

It has been reported that the detection of mannan, another polysaccharide constituent of the *Candida* organism cell wall, is suggestive of invasive candidiasis.[23,24] Meckstroth and co-workers[13] used ELISA to detect mannan in the blood of 92 leukemic patients. In 82 patients without candidiasis, false-positive results of tests for antigenemia were seen in 9%. However, up to 35% of those patients had *Candida* antibodies determined by either ID or CIE. Of the 10 patients with clinical evidence of disseminated candidiasis, seven were antigenemic. Nine of 10 had no *Candida* antibodies. Meckstroth and co-workers concluded that measuring mannan antigen by ELISA was feasible for the detection of disseminated candidiasis. It has been recently suggested that serial assays for mannan in serum, plus fungal blood cultures, should be used to diagnose invasive candidiasis.[2] Fung and co-workers[4a] reported on the value of a commercially available latex agglutination test (CAND-TEC, Ramco Laboratories, Inc., Houston, Tex.) for diagnosing invasive candidiasis.

Both CIE and radioimmunoassay[22] have been used to detect antigenemia in patients suspected to have aspergillosis before cultures became positive. Although the results are promising, it remains to be seen whether the tests have sufficient sensitivity to distinguish colonization from infection.

EXOANTIGEN ANALYSIS

When fungi fail to produce conidia or other distinguishing morphologic features, the microbiologist's ability to make a precise identification is compromised. Kaufman and Standard[9] have developed an exoantigen test using an immunodiffusion technique that detects cell-free antigens in the supernatant of fungal growth media. Exoantigen tests are available for *B. dermatitidis, Coccidioides immitis, Paracoccidioides brasiliensis, Histoplasma capsulatum, Pseudallescheria boydii, Sporothrix schenckii, Exophiala jeanselmei, Wangiella dermatitidis, Xylohypha bantiana,* and several other fungi. For the dimorphic fungi a 10-day-old Sabouraud dextrose agar (SDA) slant culture is extracted with 8 to 10 ml of aqueous merthiolate solution for 24 to 48 hours at 25° C. The extract is concentrated by ultrafiltration. The antisera used in the test are specific for the mycelial forms of the fungi to be identified. The exoantigen technique is not technically difficult, but it relies on the availability of sensitive and specific antisera. At present only a few of these reagents are commercially available. However, we believe that these methods are among the most exciting in mycology today.

FLUORESCENCE ANTIBODY MICROSCOPY

The technical aspects and immunologic basis for immunofluorescence microscopy are discussed in Chapter 7.

Immunofluorescence using fluorescein-labeled antiglobulins provides a valuable approach to the specific and sensitive recognition of several medically important fungi and actinomycetes. FA procedures can be used to detect either viable or dead fungal elements in tissue sections. The technique has application for the detection of fungal antigens in pus, exudates, CSF, and other clinical specimens.[8] FA reagents are available from the Centers for Disease Control for staining *Actinomyces israe-*

lii, Actinomyces naeslundii, Actinomyces viscosus, hyphae of *Aspergillus* spp., *Arachnia propionica,* yeast form of *Blastomyces dermatitidis, Candida* spp., spherules and endospores of *Coccidioides immitis,* four serotypes of *Cryptococcus neoformans,* yeast-form of *Histoplasma capsulatum* (*H. capsulatum* var. *capsulatum* and *H. capsulatum* var. *duboisii* cannot be distinguished), yeast form of *Paracoccidioides brasiliensis, Pseudallescheria boydii,* yeast form of *Sporothrix schenckii,* and the zygomycetes.

REFERENCES

1. Buckley, H.R.: Advances in the immunoserology of *Candida* infections. In Friedman, H., Linna, T.J., and Prier, J.E., editors: Immunoserology in the diagnosis of infectious diseases, Baltimore, 1979, University Park Press.
2. de Repentigny, L., et al.: Comparison of enzyme immunoassay and gas-liquid chromatography for the rapid diagnosis of invasive candidiasis in cancer patients, J. Clin. Microbiol. **21:**972, 1985.
3. Eng, R.H.K., Chmel, H., and Buse, M.: Serum levels of arabinitol in the detection of invasive candidiasis in animals and humans, J. Infect. Dis. **143:**677, 1981.
4. Eng, R.H.K., and Person, A.: Serum cryptococcal antigen determination in the presence of rheumatoid factor, J. Clin. Microbiol. **14:**700, 1981.
4a. Fung, J.C., Donta, S.T., and Tilton, R.C.: *Candida* detection system (CAND-TEC) to differentiate between *Candida albicans* colonization and disease, J. Clin. Microbiol. **24:**542, 1986.
5. Gold, J.W.M., et al.: Serum arabinitol concentrations and arabinitol/creatinine ratios in invasive candidiasis, J. Infect. Dis. **147:**504, 1983.
6. Kaufman, L.: Immunoserology of fungal infections. In Tilton, R.C., editor: Rapid methods and automation in microbiology, Washington, D.C., 1982, American Society for Microbiology.
7. Kaufman, L., and Reiss, E.: Serodiagnosis of fungal diseases. In Rose, N.R., and Friedman, H., editors: Manual of clinical immunology, ed. 3, Washington, D.C., 1985, American Society for Microbiology.
8. Kaufman, L., and Reiss, E.: Serodiagnosis of fungal diseases. In Lennette, E.H., et al., editors: Manual of clinical microbiology, ed. 4, Washington, D.C., 1985, American Society for Microbiology.
9. Kaufman, L., and Standard, P.: Immuno-identification of cultures of fungi pathogenic to man, Curr. Microbiol. **1:**135, 1978.
10. Kiehn, T.E., et al.: Candidiasis: detection by gas liquid chromatography of D-arabinitol, a fungal metabolite, in human serum, Science **206:**577, 1979.
11. Kozinn, P.J., et al.: The precipitin test in systemic candidiasis, JAMA **235:**628, 1976.
12. Larsh, H.W.: Blastomycosis: a world-wide problem, Mycology Memo **2:**1, 1981.
13. Meckstroth, K.L., et al.: Detection of antibodies and antigenemia in leukemic patients with candidiasis by enzyme-linked immunosorbent assays, J. Infect. Dis. **144:**24, 1981.
14. Preisler, H.D., Hasenclever, H.F., and Henderson, E.S.: Anti-*Candida* antibodies in patients with acute leukemia: a prospective study, Am. J. Med. **51:**352, 1971.
15. Prevost, E., and Newell, R.: Commercial latex kit: clinical evaluation in a medical center hospital, J. Clin. Microbiol. **8:**529, 1978.
16. Reiss, E., and de Repentigny, L.: Author's reply, J. Clin. Microbiol. **21:**479, 1985.
17. Remington, J.S., Gaines, J.D., and Gilmer, M.A.: Demonstration of *Candida* precipitins in human sera by counterimmunoelectrophoresis, Lancet **1:**413, 1972.
18. Stallybrass, F.C.: *Candida* precipitins, J. Pathol. Bacteriol. **87:**89, 1964.
19. Stockman, L., and Roberts, G.D.: Specificity of the latex test for cryptococcal antigen: a rapid, simple method for eliminating interference factors, J. Clin. Microbiol. **16:**965, 1982.
20. Syverson, R.E., Buckley, H.R., and Gibian, J.: Increasing the predictive value positive of the precipitin test for the diagnosis of deep-seated candidiasis, Am. J. Clin. Pathol. **70:**826, 1978.
21. Taschdjian, C.C., et al.: Serodiagnosis of systemic candidiasis, J. Infect. Dis. **117:**180, 1967.
22. Weiner, M.H.: Antigenemia detected by radioimmunoassay in systemic aspergillosis, Ann. Intern. Med. **92:**793, 1980.
23. Weiner, M.H., and Coats-Stephen, M.: Immunodiagnosis of systemic candidiasis: mannan antigenemia detected by radioimmunoassay in experimental and human infections, J. Infect. Dis. **140:**989, 1979.
24. Weiner, M.H., and Yount, W.J.: Mannan antigenemia in the diagnosis of invasive *Candida* infections, J. Clin. Invest. **58:**1045, 1976.
25. Wheat, J., et al.: The diagnostic laboratory tests for histoplasmosis: analysis of experience in a large urban outbreak, Ann. Intern. Med. **97:**680, 1982.
26. Wong, B., et al.: Evaluation of the aldononitrile peracetate method for measuring arabinitol in serum, J. Clin. Microbiol. **21:**478, 1985.

PART FOUR

PARASITES

CHAPTER 39

Introduction to Parasitology

John Klaas II

A complete understanding of any infectious disease requires a knowledge of how the three major factors of infectious disease epidemiology—host, agent, and environment—interact to produce the pathologic changes that ultimately result in the signs and symptoms of infection. In this context the goals of parasitologists are not unlike those of bacteriologists, virologists, or mycologists. The only real difference is that medical parasitologists have traditionally focused their studies on the invertebrate animals that are pathogenic for humans.

The invertebrate animal parasites of humans can be divided into two major categories: the unicellular organisms (protozoans) and the multicellular organisms (metazoans). Among the unicellular organisms, parasitologists are concerned with parasitic members of the phylum Protozoa. Within this phylum organisms are classified into four major subdivisions according to their methods of locomotion and reproduction. Thus the amoebae (superclass Sarcodina, class Rhizopodea) move by means of pseudopodia (''false feet'') and reproduce exclusively by asexual binary division. The flagellates (superclass Mastigophora, class Zoomastigophorea) typically move by means of long, whiplike flagella and reproduce by binary fission. A third group, the ciliates (subphylum Ciliophora, class Ciliatea), are typically propelled by rows of cilia that beat with a synchronized, wavelike motion. Normally ciliates reproduce by asexual binary division, but they also possess the ability to multiply by a specialized type of sexual reproduction called conjugation, which involves an exchange of nuclear material between two separate individuals. The final group of protozoans, the sporozoans (subphylum Sporozoa), lack specialized organelles of motility but have a unique type of life cycle. Among these protozoans a regular alternation of sexual and asexual reproductive cycles occurs; this is termed alternation of generations.

The multicellular parasites of humans are distinct from other infectious agents in that they possess specialized organ systems that perform functions such as digestion, excretion, and locomotion. These multicellular parasites are generally divided into two major subgroups: the helminths, also commonly called worms, and the arthropods, which are often incorrectly referred to as insects. (True insects belong to only one class of arthropods, the Insecta, which are characterized by three pairs of legs and three distinct body regions—head, thorax, and abdomen. Other arthropods such as spiders, mites, and ticks lack these characteristics and thus are not true insects.)

The majority of medically important helminths belong to two major phyla, the Nematoda, or roundworms, and the Platyhelminthes, or flatworms. As their common names suggest, the most obvious difference between the two groups is that the body of a nematode is round in cross section, whereas a platy-

helminth has a flattened body. The nematodes are further characterized by the presence of a complete digestive system and usually have separate adult males and females. On the other hand, platyhelminths have, at most, a saclike digestive cavity with no anal opening and are usually hermaphroditic (both male and female reproductive structures present in any one adult organism).

Flatworms are further divided into two readily recognized classes, the Cestoidea, or tapeworms, and the Trematoda, or flukes. The obvious difference between these two classes is that the cestodes have long bodies that consist principally of a series of individual segments, or proglottids, each containing separate sets of male and female reproductive organs. Adult trematodes lack these individual segments and may have either separate male and female organisms or may be hermaphrodites like the cestodes. Another major difference is that the cestodes have no discernible digestive tract and absorb their nutrients directly through the body surface. Adult trematodes, on the other hand, have the rudimentary saclike digestive tract mentioned previously. Among the many subdivisions (that is, subclasses, orders, and so forth) of Trematoda one distinction often helps in the understanding of the life cycles of these parasites. All the common parasitic trematodes of humans belong to the subclass Digenea. All the members of this group of trematodes have multiple hosts during their life cycles that include at least one species of mollusk (for example, snails) in which the parasite multiplies by asexual reproduction and a vertebrate host (for example, humans) in which the parasites multiply by sexual reproduction. Thus the typical trematode parasites of humans have alternation of generations similar in principle to that found in the protozoan parasites of the subphylum Sporozoa.

Certainly the largest and most diverse group of invertebrates of interest to parasitologists is the arthropods. Members of this group often constitute a necessary part of the life cycle of human parasites, and understanding their role in the life cycle of human parasites often leads to the formulation of methods that may be used to prevent infection or to control the spread of disease. Moreover, arthropods such as ticks, mites, fleas, and venomous spiders and scorpions may act as direct agents of human disease, producing diseases such as the skin infections caused by the mite *Sarcoptes scabiei* and chiggers of *Eutrombicula alfreddugesi*, myiasis caused by the larval stage of flies, and necrotic arachnidism caused by bites of the brown recluse spider *Loxosceles reclusus*.

The traditional perspective that medical parasitologists are concerned only with invertebrate animals pathogenic in humans ignores the fact that the term ''parasitology'' actually refers to the study of any plant or animal that lives on or within and at the expense of another living organism. In this broader context parasitologists do not limit their studies to specific taxonomic groups but rather focus on the interaction between any two different organisms that are bound together in an intimate association. This concept of parasitology suggests that all medical microbiologists are ultimately parasitologists who recognize that clinically manifest disease results from a unique series of events that can be described in terms of the interaction between host, agent, and environment. For example, the routes of infection or exposure to invertebrate parasites are not especially different from those of other pathogenic agents and include such mechanisms as ingestion of contaminated food or water, penetration of the skin by an infective stage, respiratory transmission, injection of an arthropod-borne infective stage, sexual transmission, or transplacental infection. One of the few differences between infections with invertebrate animals and with other pathogens is the relative number of agents transmitted by the different routes and not the differences in the routes of transmission. Where many bacterial and viral infections are acquired by the airborne route and very few by penetration of the agent through unbroken skin, the opposite is true for invertebrate parasites of humans.

Other factors that influence the development of clinical manifestations in animal parasite infections (such as host susceptibility, virulence or pathogenicity of the infecting agent, and the types of pathologic changes) are similar, if not identical, to those of other types of microbial infections.

CHAPTER 40

Laboratory Methods in Medical Parasitology

John Klaas II

The three basic laboratory techniques—direct microscopic examination of clinical specimens, cultivation, and serologic tests—used for the detection and identification of animal parasites are similar to those used for other groups of human pathogens. However, the relative importance of each of these techniques for the detection and definitive identification of animal parasites differs from the other subdisciplines of microbiology.

BASIC MATERIALS AND METHODS
MICROSCOPY

The compound microscope is the single most important tool in diagnostic parasitology. In general, the standard compound microscopes used for diagnostic bacteriology are satisfactory for parasitology provided they are fitted with a mechanical stage and a calibrated ocular micrometer. However, having the proper microscope is but one small part of proficient diagnostic parasitology. Obtaining proper illumination of any diagnostic preparations and religiously using the ocular micrometer to measure any suspect objects are probably more important.

Methods for adjusting compound microscopes to provide optimal illumination are described in most standard laboratory references and need not be discussed in detail here. One excellent monograph on the subject has been written by Brandt.[13] The importance of routinely using a calibrated ocular micrometer to measure helminth eggs and protozoan trophozoites and cysts cannot be overemphasized. Not only is this an important identification aid for technologists who have limited experience in diagnostic parasitology, but it is also an essential part of making the distinction between certain parasites that are identical except for their size. One specific example of this type of situation is the distinction between the pathogenic amoeba *Entamoeba histolytica* and the smaller but identical appearing nonpathogen *E. hartmanni*. Another situation where size differences can prove of value is the detection of zoonotic parasites that occasionally infect humans and have diagnostic stages similar to those of the indigenous parasites of humans.[68]

CENTRIFUGATION[94]

Since centrifugation is a key step in most procedures for concentrating the diagnostic stages of intestinal and blood parasites, a few points about the selection and use of a centrifuge need to be emphasized. First, the centrifuge should be equipped with a swinging bucket-type rotor, not an angle-head rotor. The principle of operation of these two types of rotors is different, and the centrifugation techniques employed in diagnostic parasitology are based on the use of the swinging bucket rotor.

Laboratory personnel should be cautious about following protocols from the literature that express centrifuge speeds only as revolutions per minute (rpm). In fact, the gravitational force (g) applied to any specimen depends on both the rpm and the rotating radius of the specimen. Thus, with different centrifuges, rpm readings can be considered equivalent only when the rotating radii and the rotation speed of the specimens are identical.

A final and often overlooked concern about centrifuge use is the potential hazard of procedures that require centrifugation of flammable reagents such as ether. This problem has several possible solutions. The most direct and safest approach is to use one of the specially designed explosion-proof centrifuges that are commercially available. As an alternative, one might consider operating a standard table-top centrifuge inside an explosion-proof fume hood. The latter procedure should not pose any additional expense, since an explosion-proof fume hood is essential equipment for any parasitology laboratory using toxic, volatile substances such as xylene in staining procedures.

COLLECTION, PROCESSING, AND EXAMINATION OF DIAGNOSTIC SPECIMENS

The basic types of diagnostic specimens and the methods for their collection, processing, and examination can be divided into two major groups: (1) specimens and methods for the lumen-dwelling parasites of the gastrointestinal, pulmonary, and genitourinary tracts and (2) specimens and methods for the blood and tissue parasites. Infections with lumen-dwelling parasites are usually confirmed by direct examination of diagnostic stages in natural body secretions and excretions such as feces, sputum, or urine. In vitro cultivation and immunodiagnostic methods are used only infrequently for these infections and with varying degrees of success, depending on the parasite. Infections with blood and tissue parasites are also usually confirmed by direct examination of diagnostic stages in primary specimens. However, the in vitro cultivation and immunodiagnostic techniques available for blood and tissue parasites are more reliable than those for intestinal parasites and are often invaluable methods for the diagnosis of these infections.

LUMEN-DWELLING PARASITES
Fecal Specimens
Collection

Since the most common habitat of lumen-dwelling parasites is the intestinal tract, feces is the specimen most commonly submitted to the laboratory. Certain basic guidelines govern the collection of fecal specimens, regardless of whether they are submitted as fresh specimens collected at the hospital or as preserved specimens collected by outpatients. First, the patient should not have received medications containing antimicrobial agents, bismuth, barium, mineral oil, kaolin, or any antidiarrheal or laxative preparations during the 10 days before collection of the sample.[61] These substances interfere with detection of intestinal parasites by reducing visibility in diagnostic preparations or by causing a temporary reduction in the number of diagnostic stages. Second, the specimens must not become contaminated with urine, water, or dirt during collection. These substances may destroy protozoan trophozoites or may contain free-living protozoans that can be mistaken for parasites. The easiest way to avoid such contamination is to collect the specimen directly in a clean, detergent-free, wide-mouth container (for example, a half-pint ice cream container of waxed cardboard) that can also be used for specimen transport. Alternatively, the specimen may be collected on clean, dry newspaper and then transferred to an appropriate transport container.

The best results are obtained when a fresh specimen can be examined within 30 minutes to 1 hour after it is collected. If the specimen is soft or liquid, it may contain the trophozoite stage of protozoan parasites, and early processing permits observation of the organism's characteristic motility. When the specimen is formed and thus more likely to contain the cyst stage of protozoans, rapid examination is less critical. In any case, if the fecal specimen cannot be quickly delivered to the laboratory or the examination of the specimen may be delayed after receipt by the laboratory, some type of preservation technique must be used.[18,112]

The accepted preservation methods include (1) holding the specimen at room temperature if it can be examined within 2 or 3 hours, (2) holding the specimen at refrigerator temperature for a maximum of 2 to 3 days, or (3) placing the specimen in one or more of the various types of preservation solutions if examination will be delayed for an indeterminate time. The most serious error in attempting to preserve a fecal specimen is to hold the specimen at an elevated (incubator) temperature in the belief that this will promote survival of any parasites that may be present. In fact, this technique commonly has the opposite effect; it promotes bacterial overgrowth and pH changes that will destroy the trophozoite stages of protozoan parasites.[142]

In selecting a chemical preservation method the ideal choice would be a single chemical that (1) preserves the diagnostic stages of all possible intestinal parasites and (2) is compatible with all the techniques that may be required for complete examination of the specimen. Unfortunately, development of a reagent that meets both of these requirements has been difficult. Two preservatives that probably come closest are the merthiolate-iodine-formalin (MIF) preservative described by Sapero and Lawless[121] and the sodium acetate–acetic acid (SAF) preservative described by Yang and Scholten.[156] These preservatives provide reasonably good fixation of helminth eggs and larvae and protozoan cysts and trophozoites. In addition, both methods are compatible with at least one concentration method and one method of preparing permanent stained smears. The major criticism of these methods is the difficulty in preparing high-quality, permanent stained smears.[113,124] Specifically, albumin must be smeared on the slide as an adhesive for the specimen, and the quality of preservation and subsequent staining of protozoan parasites may not be as good as with preservation methods that employ separate chemicals to preserve the diagnostic stages of different parasites.

The most widely used of the multiple chemical systems is probably the so-called two-vial or PVA fixative/formalin sys-

tem. This system is designed to improve preservation by using two different solutions, each intended to provide optimal preservation of different diagnostic stages. One portion of the specimen is added to a vial containing 5% to 10% formalin that acts as a preservative for helminth eggs and larvae and protozoan cysts and is used for preparation of direct wet mounts and for concentration procedures. Another portion of the specimen is added to a vial containing a PVA fixative (prepared from polyvinyl alcohol and Schaudinn fixative) that is intended to preserve protozoan cysts and trophozoites for permanent staining. In a modification of this system Garcia[42] has developed a procedure that permits the preparation of concentrates and permanent smears from specimens preserved in PVA fixative. This reportedly eliminates the need for the formalin preservative.

A third method of chemical preservation that may be employed in laboratories processing large numbers of fresh specimens is to use Schaudinn fixative without PVA for preparing permanent stained slides. With this method fresh specimens are fixed and permanent smears are prepared shortly after the specimen is received by the laboratory. Obviously this would pose difficulties for laboratories that receive specimens when there are not sufficient personnel to process specimens immediately on receipt. The alternative is to add a portion of the fresh specimen to a vial of Schaudinn fixative and use this preserved material to prepare the smear at a later, more convenient time.[125] The remainder of the specimen could be held at room temperature or refrigerated until final processing.

Probably the best method for handling fresh specimens when the final processing of fresh specimens may be delayed is to preserve a portion of the specimen by the same method the laboratory uses for collecting outpatient specimens. The remainder of the fresh specimen could then be held at room temperature or refrigerated. If the laboratory is using the two-vial system of preservation and there is only a small amount of specimen, the entire specimen could be added to the vial of PVA fixative. Later, if additional specimens cannot be obtained, the laboratory could use this preserved material to prepare both concentrates and permanent stained slides as described by Garcia.[42]

When fresh fecal specimens are collected, the entire passage should be submitted for examination. This permits the laboratory to make a thorough macroscopic examination for diagnostic stages such as tapeworm proglottids or small adult nematodes that might be overlooked if only a small portion of the specimen were examined.

When specimens are to be chemically preserved for later delivery or examination, representative portions from the beginning, middle, and end of the passage should be added to the preservative. Any portions that contain blood, mucus, or suspect objects should also be placed in the preservative. Since collection and initial preservation of fecal specimen are often the responsibility of patients or allied medical personnel not trained in parasitology, it is important that complete instructions be provided with each collection kit. These instructions should include both written directions (if necessary, in languages other than English) and diagrams.

The number of fecal specimens required to detect an intestinal infection varies with the individual case. In severe infections a single specimen may suffice: in other cases multiple specimens may be required. In general, three normally passed specimens, each spaced 2 or 3 days apart, permits detection of most infections.* If complete examination of these specimens does not reveal an infection and the physician's suspicion of a parasitic infection remains high, either additional specimens or special collection and processing techniques may be required. One of these special techniques is to administer to the patient a saline cathartic of buffered phosphosoda or sodium sulfate to purge the intestine. This procedure, however, should be restricted to situations in which rapid processing of all the bowel movements can be guaranteed, since it is most effective when all bowel movements immediately following the purge can be processed as fresh specimens. If a delay occurs in transport or in laboratory processing, a portion of each bowel movement should be appropriately preserved. In addition, the order of collection of purged specimens should be indicated on the specimen containers, since diagnostic stages in the earlier specimens are often distorted and not as easily identified as stages found in the later portions.[88]

The use of a saline enema to improve recovery of diagnostic stages is, in general, less effective than a purge because only a few species of animal parasites routinely inhabit the lower colon. Moreover, if this type of specimen is accepted by the laboratory, rapid examination or preservation is essential.

Other special techniques for detecting intestinal parasites, such as in vitro cultivation, immunodiagnosis, sigmoidoscopy, tissue biopsies, and examination of aspirates, are usually intended for specific infections and are discussed in later sections.

In addition to the usual requirements for accepting any diagnostic specimen, such as a properly labeled specimen and a matching requisition, the exact date and time of specimen collection must be indicated. If there has been undue delay in delivering a fresh specimen, it may be either rejected as unacceptable or if necessary preserved for later examination after consultation with the physician responsible for the case. Regardless of the circumstances, any laboratory asked to process an otherwise unacceptable specimen should note on the laboratory records and final report to the physician that the results are unreliable because of the condition of the specimen.

Once the laboratory accepts a fecal sample, three general methods are used for examination of the specimen: direct wet mounts, concentration, and permanent stained slides. Whenever possible, all three types of examination should be performed on every fecal specimen. However, if manpower or time is limited, selected procedures may be used for different types of fecal specimens. The particular procedures are chosen according to the type of specimen (either fresh or preserved), and for fresh specimens, the consistency of the specimen (formed, soft, or loose and watery).

Selection of procedures—fresh specimens

The first step in selecting the appropriate procedures for fresh fecal specimens is a macroscopic examination of the specimen. This serves two purposes. First, it is used to "grade" the consistency of the specimen and, in turn, decide the most appropriate methods for subsequent examination of the specimen. Second, macroscopic examination may reveal larger diagnostic stages such as tapeworm proglottids, intact worms, or areas of blood or mucus that should be examined microscopically.

Formed specimens. After macroscopic examination the

processing of formed fresh specimens should include microscopic examination of a direct wet mount and a concentrate of the specimen. Omitting the direct wet mount may be tempting, since this procedure is reportedly of greatest value for observing motile protozoan trophozoites, a diagnostic stage that is unlikely to occur in formed specimens. However, not all diagnostic stages of helminths or protozoans that occur in formed specimens are effectively recovered by concentration procedures. For example, eggs of *Hymenolepis nana* and cysts of *Giardia lamblia* may not concentrate well with the formalin-ether concentration procedure, and certain trematode eggs and infertile eggs of *Ascaris lumbricoides* are not effectively concentrated by the zinc sulfate flotation method. Examination of the direct wet mount ensures that these diagnostic stages are not overlooked.

Some question exists about whether routine examination of permanent stained smears, which are usually intended for detection and identification of protozoan parasites, is needed with each formed specimen. Probably the most practical approach is to routinely prepare permanent smears of formed specimens but proceed with the staining and examination of the smears only when the direct wet mount or concentration procedures fail to reveal any parasites, or when there is doubt about the identity of protozoan parasites detected by other methods of examination.

Soft specimens. Since soft specimens may contain the entire range of diagnostic stages, including helminth eggs and larvae and protozoan cysts and trophozoites, the processing of soft specimens should routinely include the preparation and examination of direct wet mounts, concentrates, and permanent stained smears.

Loose and watery specimens. Diagnostic stages in loose and watery specimens can usually be detected by a combination of direct wet mounts and permanent stained smears. Concentration procedures are usually not required, since they are ineffective for protozoan trophozoites (the stage expected in loose or watery specimens). Moreover, in this type of specimen, helminth eggs or larvae are usually present in sufficient numbers to be detected by the direct wet mount alone. However, if the direct wet mount and permanent stained smear fail to reveal an infection, it is usually advisable to proceed with a concentration procedure.

Selection of procedures—preserved specimens

The use of a chemical preservation system makes it difficult to determine the original consistency of a fecal specimen. In these cases the usual approach is to process the specimen by the same methods used for soft, unpreserved feces, that is, preparation and examination of a direct wet mount, a concentrate, and a permanent stained smear. If a portion of the original specimen is submitted along with the preserved material, the laboratory may choose to "grade" the consistency of the unpreserved portion and process the specimen on that basis. Even this grading based on examination of specimens submitted with preserved material requires some caution; water loss from fresh feces may change the consistency of the specimen, especially if the collection container is not well sealed.

Examination procedures—direct wet mounts

Direct wet mounts are most conveniently prepared on 2×3 inch microscope slides. The large size of these slides allows for sealing of the coverglass to the slide and prevents drying of the mounted specimen, movement of material under the coverglass if it is necessary to use the oil immersion objective, and accidental contamination of the technologists and their work areas with specimen. In addition, the use of this larger slide facilitates the preparation of multiple mounts on a single slide. In fact, two preparations of each specimen are usually made on each slide, one an unstained preparation and the second, a preparation containing a temporary staining solution.

The crucial step in making both the stained and unstained direct wet mount is to prepare a suspension of feces that is just dense enough that newspaper print is still legible through the slide. If the suspension is too thick, diagnostic stages may be obscured by fecal debris; if it is too thin, the diagnostic stages may be too diluted to detect.

With fresh specimens the unstained mount is prepared by mixing on the slide a small amount of the specimen with 1 drop of physiologic saline. Tap or distilled water should not be substituted for the saline, since protozoan trophozoites may be destroyed by the resulting osmotic imbalance. With chemically preserved specimens the unstained wet amount can usually be prepared directly from the preserved feces without further dilution. The ratio of one part feces to three parts preservative, as used in most preservative systems, generally yields a properly diluted fecal suspension. The one restriction on preparing direct wet mounts from chemically preserved feces is that the preservative must be compatible with wet mounts. For example, wet mounts are not usually attempted with material preserved in PVA fixative because PVA begins to harden and turn opaque when exposed to air. These properties of PVA fixative render the material unsuitable for direct wet mounts but do not interfere with preparation of permanent stained smears where the hardening helps the specimen adhere to the slide and the staining chemicals eliminate the opacity.

Although unstained wet mounts are considered essential for detecting motile protozoan trophozoites, certain difficulties may accompany this use of wet mounts. For example, at the end of a parasitology training course Gardner and co-workers[47] found that only 4.8% of the participants recognized motile amoebae in unstained fresh specimens, whereas 58.5% detected the trophozoites in permanent stained smears. Similarly, Krogstad and co-workers[71,72] noted that laboratories frequently mistake white blood cells for trophozoites of *Entamoeba histolytica* in unstained saline mounts. Thus a serious question exists about the value of unstained saline mounts for accurately detecting motile trophozoites in fecal specimens. In addition, it has been recognized that the nuclear structure of intestinal protozoans is usually more visible in formalin-preserved specimens than in fresh specimens mounted in saline.[94]

Stained wet mounts. The value of wet mounts may be improved by preparing a temporary stained wet mount. A small portion of the specimen, either fresh or preserved, is mixed with a small portion of staining solution in a manner similar to that used to prepare the unstained mount. The stain is intended to enhance the morphologic details of protozoan cysts or trophozoites and thus facilitate their recognition and identification.[33]

Several staining solutions have been developed for wet mounts, and the selection of a particular stain depends primarily on whether the specimen is most likely to contain protozoan trophozoites, cysts, or both. For loose, watery specimens, which are most likely to contain trophozoite stages, parasitologists usually choose either Quensel stain[136] or Nair buffered methylene blue.[100] For formed specimens, which are most likely to contain only the cyst stage, the most popular stains are Dobell,[94] Lugol,[94] or D'Antoni[26] iodine stains. Unfortunately, even these widely recommended choices have certain disadvantages. For example, iodine-stained cysts are less refractile than unstained cysts and may be easily overlooked, and the chromatoid bodies characteristically found in immature cysts of *Entamoeba* spp. are not as prominent in iodine-stained mounts as in unstained preparations. Disadvantages of the trophozoite stains include a tendency to cause the organisms to round up and poor staining of certain species, especially flagellates.

After the stained and unstained samples of the specimen are prepared, they should be covered with 22×22 mm, no. 1 thickness coverglasses. Using thin coverglasses on wet mounts is essential because wet mounts that are too thick may prevent the microscopist from focusing on objects in the lower levels of the preparation. To prevent drying and allow the use of the $100\times$ oil immersion objective, the edges of the coverglasses should be sealed with either a heated mixture of 50% paraffin–50% petroleum jelly (vaspar) or clear nail polish. Proper examination of wet mounts requires that the entire unstained mount be examined first, using the $10\times$ objective and low-intensity illumination. This examination must be done systematically, beginning at one corner of the mount and continuing field by field until the entire mount has been examined. Any suspect structures should be measured with a calibrated ocular micrometer and carefully studied using, if necessary, the high dry or oil immersion objectives. If identification of any suspicious object cannot be confirmed by examination of the unstained mount alone, the stained wet mount should be examined for similar objects in an attempt to confirm the identification. If all attempts to confirm the identification from the direct wet mounts are unsuccessful, or if no diagnostic stages are observed in the unstained wet mount, the specimen should be further processed by preparing a concentrate or a permanent stained smear or both as dictated by the protocol for the particular type of specimen.

Concentration methods

The basic purpose of any fecal concentration procedure is to increase the probability of detecting and identifying any diagnostic stages that may be present in a fecal specimen. To meet this objective an ideal concentration procedure should (1) increase the density of all possible diagnostic stages, including protozoan cysts and trophozoites and helminth eggs and larvae, (2) eliminate fecal debris so the diagnostic stages are not hidden, and (3) preserve the key morphologic features of the diagnostic stages. Unfortunately, none of the current methods meet all these requirements. An especially notable shortcoming has been the absence of a method that reliably concentrates protozoan trophozoites.

Depending on the underlying principle, concentration methods can be divided into two major categories, flotation or sedimentation. In the flotation methods, diagnostic stages are "floated" free of fecal debris by mixing the specimen with a solution having a specific gravity greater than the diagnostic stages and less than the fecal debris (Figure 40-1). Methods based on this principle are especially effective in reducing the amount of fecal debris in diagnostic preparations and in con-

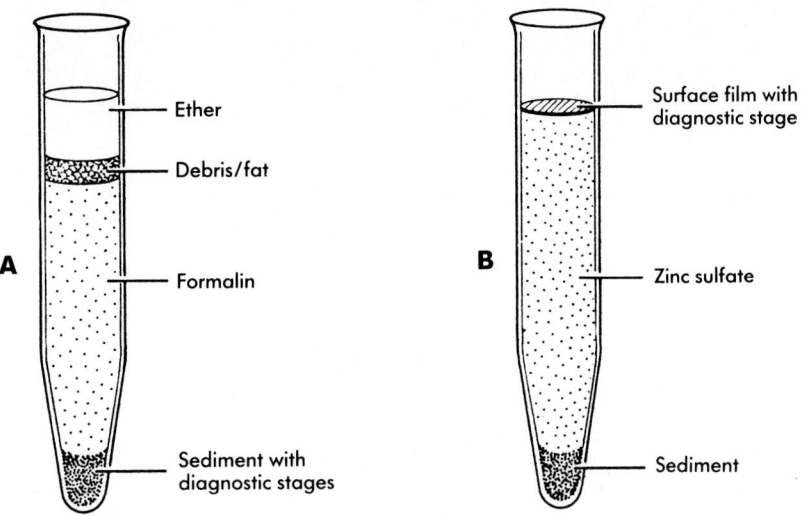

FIGURE 40-1. Fecal concentration procedures: various layers seen in tubes after centrifugation. **A,** Formalin-ether. **B,** Zinc sulfate. (Illustration by Nobuko Kitamura. From Garcia, L.S., and Ash, L.R.: Diagnostic parasitology, clinical laboratory manual, ed. 2, St. Louis, 1979, The C.V. Mosby Co.)

centrating most nematode and cestode eggs and protozoan cysts. However, they frequently fail to concentrate operculated or "heavy" eggs, such as those of *Schistosoma* spp. and infertile *Ascaris* spp., and they often distort the appearance of protozoan cysts and helminth larvae. In addition, if a fecal specimen contains large amounts of fatty material or oils, these substances also rise to the surface and make examination of the final wet mount difficult.

Attempts to overcome some of these problems have resulted in numerous modifications of the basic flotation method using different concentrations of various chemical solutions, including sodium chloride,[76] sugar,[20] and zinc sulfate,[106] as the flotation solution. Another common modification of these methods is the use of centrifugation steps to reduce the amount of fecal debris or fats before adding the flotation solution.

Probably the most widely used flotation procedures are those that employ solutions of zinc sulfate in either a simple flotation without centrifugation as described by Otto, Hewitt, and Strohan[106] or with a preliminary centrifuge washing as originally described by Faust and co-workers[36] and later modified by Melvin and Brooke.[94] A recent study by Bartlett and co-workers[5] suggests that preserving fecal specimens in formalin before concentration with zinc sulfate further improves these methods by reducing the distortion of protozoan cysts and increasing the recovery of operculated eggs.

In sedimentation procedures the diagnostic stages are concentrated as a sediment by simple gravity or centrifugation, whereas the fecal debris and fats or oils remain suspended in the supernatant (see Figure 40-1). The many variations of this basic principle generally involve the use of different chemicals to wash the sediment and decrease the amount of fecal debris and fats in the specimen. For example, hydrochloric acid[84,150] has been employed to reduce the amount of extraneous protein, mucin, phosphates, and calcium salts. Organic solvents such as ether,[83,84,115,150] xylene,[83,84] and ethyl acetate[159] have been used to reduce the amount of fats and oils, and detergents such

as Triton[150] and Calgon[83] have been used to reduce surface tension and promote sedimentation.

Generally, sedimentation methods concentrate the diagnostic stages of a greater variety of parasites than flotation methods. Most of this improved recovery is because sedimentation procedures are more effective in concentrating operculated eggs, schistosome eggs, and the "heavier" eggs such as infertile *Ascaris* spp. Also, diagnostic stages are usually less distorted because these methods do not employ the concentrated salt solutions used in the flotation methods. The disadvantage of sedimentation techniques is that they are usually less effective in reducing extraneous fecal debris and concentrating protozoan cysts than the flotation procedures.[20,45,140]

Probably the most popular sedimentation method is the so-called formalin-ether procedure developed by Ritchie.[115] A recent modification of this method, in which less flammable ethyl acetate is substituted for the ether,[159] appears to be as effective as the original procedure[35,44,140] and at the same time reduces the hazards associated with the storage and handling of ether. Another modification of the traditional Ritchie technique that also appears to be very effective and affords additional protection against infectious agents in fecal specimens is the FPC fecal concentration device (Evergreen Scientific, Los Angeles, Calif.) originally described by Zierdt.[163] This device is a three-part apparatus that permits mixing, filtration, and concentration of the fecal specimen in a closed system of test tubes. In addition, Triton X-100 (a detergent) is added to the specimen to enhance recovery of eggs, larvae, and cysts. One of the major reasons for the recent interest in this procedure is that it appears to be very effective for the concentration of *Cryptosporidium* spp.[161]

Besides the general advantages of a sedimentation procedure, the formalin-ether or ethyl acetate methods have at least one other major advantage that may account for their popularity—they are suitable for processing both fresh specimens and specimens preserved in most of the different chemical preser-

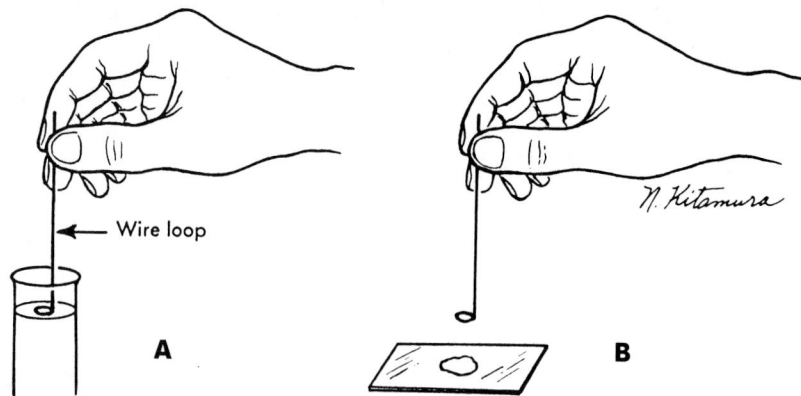

FIGURE 40-2. Method used to remove surface film of zinc sulfate flotation concentration procedure. **A,** Wire loop is gently placed on (not under) surface film. **B,** Loop is then placed on glass slide. (Illustration by Nobuko Kitamura. From Garcia, L.S., and Ash, L.R.: Diagnostic parasitology, clinical laboratory manual, ed. 2, St. Louis, 1979, The C.V. Mosby Co.)

vatives. For example, these methods, or slight modifications, may be used for processing specimens preserved in formalin,[94] merthiolate-iodine-formalin,[10,112] sodium acetate–acetic acid–formalin,[156] or phenol-alcohol-formalin.[20] Unfortunately, even these concentration procedures are not without their limitations. They are less effective in concentrating *Giardia lamblia* and *Iodamoeba butschlii* cysts and *Hymenolepis nana* eggs than some of the other concentration procedures.

In selecting a particular concentration technique for routine laboratory use it is important to evaluate several factors carefully. First, the advantages of any method depend on careful attention to details of the method. For example, in zinc sulfate flotation procedures the specific gravity of the solution used for unpreserved specimens (1.18) differs from that used for formalin-preserved specimens (1.20), and the specific gravity of these solutions must be checked each day the solution is used. In addition, if the centrifugal modification of this procedure is used, the centrifuge must be allowed to coast to a stop and the tubes removed carefully to prevent agitation of the surface layer containing the concentrated organisms. A wire loop is used to transfer the organisms to a glass slide (Figure 40-2). In the formalin-ether or ethyl acetate methods the amount of feces must be carefully regulated; after the first centrifugation the amount of sedimented material must be between 1 and 1.5 ml for fresh specimens or 0.5 and 0.75 ml for preserved specimens.

A second important consideration is whether the procedure is compatible with the laboratory's workflow. For example, in the zinc sulfate flotation method, eggs and cysts concentrated in the surface layer begin to sink within 30 minutes to 1 hour after the concentration is completed. Moreover, wet mounts of the concentrate should be examined shortly after preparation, since the zinc sulfate begins to distort protozoan cysts within a few hours if the original specimen was not preserved in formalin.[5] In the formalin–ether or ethyl acetate procedures, on the other hand, processing may be interrupted at several points for long periods without any adverse effect, and examination of the final wet mount may be delayed for long periods provided the wet mount is sealed to prevent drying.

Other factors that should be considered are the availability and cost of reagents and supplies and whether the procedure is

to be used in a survey for a particular parasite or for a group of parasites. Generally, the materials required for the common flotation or sedimentation procedures are inexpensive and readily available except in the most remote areas. On the other hand, in surveys for particular parasites, certain specialized concentration procedures may be more effective than the usual zinc sulfate flotation or formalin–ether or ethyl acetate methods. For example, the brine flotation method[153] is particularly efficient for recovery of hookworm eggs, whereas recovery of schistosome eggs is improved by using special variations of the formalin-ether method that include the use of various acids, alcohols, and detergents.[69,150]

In the final analysis no one concentration method is ideal for detection of all possible intestinal parasites, and best results are probably obtained when both flotation and sedimentation methods are used for all fecal specimens.[20,140] However, even using two concentration techniques will not compensate for improper collection or preservation of specimens, failure to collect repeat specimens when the initial specimen is negative, or inadequate preparation and examination of stained permanent fecal smears to detect and identify intestinal protozoa.[43] When a clinical laboratory has limited personnel, it is usually more productive to use a single concentration technique and devote extra effort to ensuring proper collection of an adequate number of stool specimens and regular preparation and examination of stained permanent fecal smears, rather than adding a second concentration procedure. In this context the best concentration techniques are probably the formalin-ether or formalin–ethyl acetate procedures. Despite their limitations, these techniques concentrate the greatest variety of organisms, are compatible with most chemical preservatives, and are easily adapted to the workflow in most clinical laboratories.

Permanent stained fecal smears

The value of permanent stained fecal smears for the detection and identification of intestinal protozoa cannot be overemphasized. Numerous investigations[49,52,102,125] have clearly demonstrated that more intestinal protozoan infections are detected by examining permanent stained fecal smears than by any other method, especially when stool specimens contain primarily the trophozoite stage. For example, in a study by Garcia and co-workers[43] of 855 stools containing the trophozoite stages of *Entamoeba histolytica, Giardia lamblia,* or *Dientamoeba fragilis,* 95% of all the positive specimens were detected only by the stained fecal smear, whereas none were detected by a concentrate alone. This same study also demonstrated that there is considerable advantage in preparing permanent fecal smears even when cysts are the predominant diagnostic stage. In another 975 stools that contained cyst stages of *E. histolytica* or *G. lamblia* (*D. fragilis* does not form cysts), these investigators found that 73% of the *E. histolytica* and 34% of the *G. lamblia* positive results were detected only in the stained smears. In less than 1% of these specimens cysts were detected by the concentration procedure alone.

Although the value of routine preparation and examination of permanent stained fecal smears is widely accepted, opinions vary about the best method of staining the smears. These varied opinions undoubtedly reflect differences in the workload of individual laboratories and the personal experiences and training of the individuals responsible for performing the procedures. At least two staining methods, trichrome stain and iron-hematoxylin stain, have proved popular in clinical laboratories because they provide rapid and reliable results with both fresh and preserved specimens.

Probably the most widely used staining procedure is the Wheatley modification of the Gomori trichrome stain,[151] or as it is commonly called, the trichrome stain. In laboratories where the responsibility for parasitology is rotated among different technologists, this technique offers serveral advantages. First, except for one or two steps, the timing of the different staining stages is less critical than with most other methods. Second, the reagents, especially the stain, are generally stable and can be used repeatedly, provided precautions are taken to prevent the carryover of excess reagent from one step to another. Finally, the normal variation in the color of the stained smear is helpful in distinguishing between background debris and organisms; in a well-fixed, correctly stained fecal smear the background debris is usually blue-green, and protozoa or leukocytes have a blue-green cytoplasm and red or purple-red nuclear structure.

The quality of a trichrome-stained smear may be adversely affected by several factors. For example, if the organisms are not properly fixed before staining, they may fail to stain or may stain predominantly red. Specimens processed in PVA fixative are particularly susceptible to this problem if the specimen was not thoroughly emulsified in the preservative. A less viscous form of PVA, commercially marketed as LV-PVA (Meridian Diagnostics, Cincinnati, Ohio), may alleviate this problem. Another problem common to any of the fixatives that contain mercuric chloride (for example, Schaudinn fixative) is the failure to completely remove the mercuric chloride in the first step of the staining procedure. If the iodine-alcohol reagent used in the first step is too weak to extract the mercuric chloride, the formation of a crystalline residue will make subsequent examination of the stained specimen difficult. Similarly, the final preparation may be hazy or cloudy if there is incomplete dehydration or clearing of the specimen. Finally, at the most critical step in the entire procedure, the destaining with acid-alcohol, the most common error is excessive destaining. The key to success in this step is to destain each slide separately. Usually it is sufficient to dip each slide in and out of the acid-alcohol one time and quickly remove the acid-alcohol by rinsing the slide

thoroughly in 95% alcohol. If the smear is especially thin, the destaining step may be omitted completely. On the other hand, thick smears may need to be dipped in the acid-alcohol three or four times. Destaining for longer than 5 seconds should not be necessary and rarely improves the final result. It is also important to change the 95% alcohol rinse frequently to prevent its becoming acidified by carryover of the destaining reagent.

Another popular stain for permanent fecal smears is the iron-hematoxylin stain. This stain is noted for providing excellent morphologic detail that often makes it possible to identify organisms than cannot be identified by other staining methods. Unfortunately, many of the various methods for staining with iron-hematoxylin are time consuming and demand careful attention to procedural details. Some of these problems may be overcome if the laboratory adopts one of the shorter and slightly less demanding modifications such as the Tompkins-Miller method.[139] One important advantage of this method is that the phosphotungstic acid used as the destaining reagent provides the correct amount of destaining regardless of whether the slide remains in the solution for 2 minutes or 2 hours. This is in contrast to methods that use picric acid for destaining and require microscopic observation of a series of test slides to determine the optimal time for destaining. However, even the shorter methods such as Tompkins-Miller do not resolve all the problems that may limit the usefulness of iron-hematoxylin stains for routine diagnostic use. For example, the entire smear, including the background and any organisms, is stained shades of black to gray, and distinguishing between organisms and background debris may be difficult for inexperienced technologists. In addition, short versions of the iron-hematoxylin procedure often do not provide the same high quality of staining with PVA-fixed specimens as with fresh specimens: a 6-week "ripening" period is required for stock solutions of hematoxylin stain versus 30 minutes for trichrome, and a fresh working solution of the stain must be prepared each day.

Limiting this discussion to the trichrome and iron-hematoxylin methods of staining does not suggest that other staining methods such as Chlorazol Black-E,[48] the Lawless stain,[77] and Celestine Blue-B[155] are inferior. In fact, each of these other methods may provide results superior to trichrome or iron-hematoxylin in certain situations. However, the popularity of trichrome and iron-hematoxylin suggests a balance of versatility, speed, reliability, and quality not matched by other techniques. It is also important to remember that the widespread use of any particular technique provides an extensive base of practical experience that can be invaluable should a laboratory have difficulties with the technique.

In vitro cultivation

Protozoa. In vitro cultivation techniques are available for nearly all the intestinal protozoa of humans. However, the routine use of in vitro cultivation for the diagnosis of intestinal protozoan infections is generally restricted to larger medical centers that receive large numbers of fresh specimens, and where resources and interest are sufficient to develop the proficiency required to prepare and use the special media these organisms require. In these circumstances, in fact, in vitro cultivation detects a significant number of infections not revealed by other methods.[101,116] Cultivation of intestinal protozoa should not, however, be considered an alternative to other methods of detection, since specimens that are positive by microscopic examination are often culture negative.[34,126]

A second consideration for any laboratory contemplating the use of in vitro cultivation is the lack of a single medium that supports the growth of all the pathogenic species of intestinal protozoa. For example, numerous media have been developed for the cultivation of *Entamoeba histolytica*. However, few of these media are satisfactory for the cultivation of *Balantidium coli* or *Giardia lamblia*. Thus most laboratories attempting in vitro cultivation focus their efforts on *E. histolytica* and only rarely use in vitro cultivation for the diagnosis of *B. coli* or *G. lamblia* infections. Among the more popular media for *E. histolytica* are the modified Boeck-Drbohlav medium,[101] Balamuth medium,[3] and Cleveland and Collier medium.[23] If necessary, *B. coli* may be cultivated in a modified version of Barret and Yarbrough medium[114] and *G. lamblia* is a medium developed by Karapetyan.[66]

Helminths. The so-called in vitro cultivation methods for intestinal helminths are actually limited forms of cultivation. Unlike methods for the cultivation of protozoa, the methods used for in vitro cultivation of helminths in diagnostic laboratories are not designed to increase the number of diagnostic stages but are actually simple ''egg-hatching'' techniques. Recovery of larval stages by these techniques can aid in the species identification of organisms that cannot be differentiated by the egg stage (for example, hookworms) or in determining whether eggs are viable (for example, schistosomes). To aid in the differentiation and speciation of *Strongyloides* and *Trichostrongylus* organisms and hookworms, infective (filariform) larval stages may be cultivated from eggs using the so-called Harada-Mori filter paper strip technique.[58,122] In this technique feces containing eggs are smeared on the center of a filter paper strip. One end is then immersed in 3 to 4 ml of distilled water in a loosely capped test tube. Characteristic larvae, which usually develop after about a week of incubation at room temperature, may be identified using the morphologic criteria described by Hsieh.[58]

Another type of ''egg-hatching'' technique may be used to distinguish between active schistosome infections that require treatment and schistosome infections that are inactive by virtue of successful chemotherapy or the host's normal immune responses. Schistosome eggs are suspended in a small Erlenmeyer flask filled nearly to the lip with distilled water and allowed to incubate at room temperature overnight. If the eggs are viable, small, ciliated miracidia emerge from the eggs and swim toward the surface layer in the neck of the flask. The miracidia are readily visible when observed against a black background with the aid of a simple magnifying glass.[22]

Special examination procedures

Certain specialized techniques are occasionally requested by physicians to aid in their selection of therapeutic regimens or in evaluation of the effectiveness of a particular therapy. Typically these methods require estimates of the number of adult worms harbored by a patient or posttreatment examination of fecal specimens for worms expelled by treatment.

The more common methods for estimating the number of adult worms, such as the direct smear technique of Beaver[7] and the Stoll dilution method,[132] are based on counting the number of eggs in a given amount of feces and then using conversion factors to determine the patient's worm burden.[86,91] Since these techniques are most reliable for infections in which the eggs are shed more or less continuously, they are usually restricted to infections with *Ascaris* and *Trichuris* organisms and hookworms.[94,95] In the Beaver direct smear technique a calibrated light source and light meter are used to prepare a fecal wet mount that has a standardized density. The smear is then systematically examined, and all the eggs are counted. The dilution technique of Stoll is, in principle, similar to a standard blood count. A standard volume of feces is thoroughly mixed with a known volume of diluent. A wet mount is then prepared from a known volume of the suspension, and the total number of eggs in the wet mount is counted.

To aid in the identification of parasites that cannot be differentiated by their egg stage (for example, hookworms, *Taenia* spp.), or to ensure that a tapeworm scolex has been expelled after treatment, patients undergoing treatment for these infections may be asked to take a saline cathartic and collect and preserve in formalin all the feces passed within 24 hours. When received by the laboratory, this material can be strained through a narrow (30 to 50 mesh) sieve, carefully rinsed with a gentle stream of water, and thoroughly examined for any intact or fragmented parasites.

A method somewhat similar to this sieve technique may be used to diagnose light infections with *Strongyloides stercoralis* or hookworms.[94,149] With this so-called Baermann technique, feces are placed in a gauze-lined sieve that rests in a funnel closed at the narrow end with a short piece of rubber tubing and pinch clamp and filled with warm water so the water just touches the bottom of the sieve. Within 2 or 3 hours any larvae present in the feces migrate into the water and fall to the bottom of the funnel. The pinch clamp can then be opened and 10 ml of water drained off and centrifuged. The resulting sediment is examined for characteristic larvae of *Strongyloides* organisms or hookworms.

Specimens Other than Feces
Anal swabs for *Enterobius vermicularis*

Unlike most of the other intestinal nematodes, *Enterobius vermicularis* does not usually release its eggs within the intestine. Instead the females migrate out of the anus and deposit their eggs on the skin surrounding the anus. To recover these eggs two basic types of anal swabs are commonly used: the cellophane tape slide preparation[15] and the petroleum jelly–paraffin swab.[89]

In the cellophane tape method one end of a piece of clear cellophane tape is attached firmly to the end of a glass microscope slide. The back of the slide is then held firmly against a wooden tongue depressor and the remainder of the tape is looped over the tongue depressor so the adhesive side of the tape points outward (Figure 40-3). The patient's buttocks are spread apart, and the adhesive side of the tape is pressed firmly against the right and left perianal folds. Once collection is completed the tape is folded back and gently pressed against the slide. When received in the laboratory, the tape is gently peeled back, a small amount of xylene or toluene is placed on the slide, and the tape is pressed back into place over the reagent. The slide is then examined with the low-power microscope objective (10×) for the characteristic eggs.

With the petroleum jelly–paraffin method a cotton swab coated with a mixture of four parts petroleum jelly and one part paraffin is rubbed over the perianal folds and then inserted about ¼ inch into the anus. The swab is then transported to the

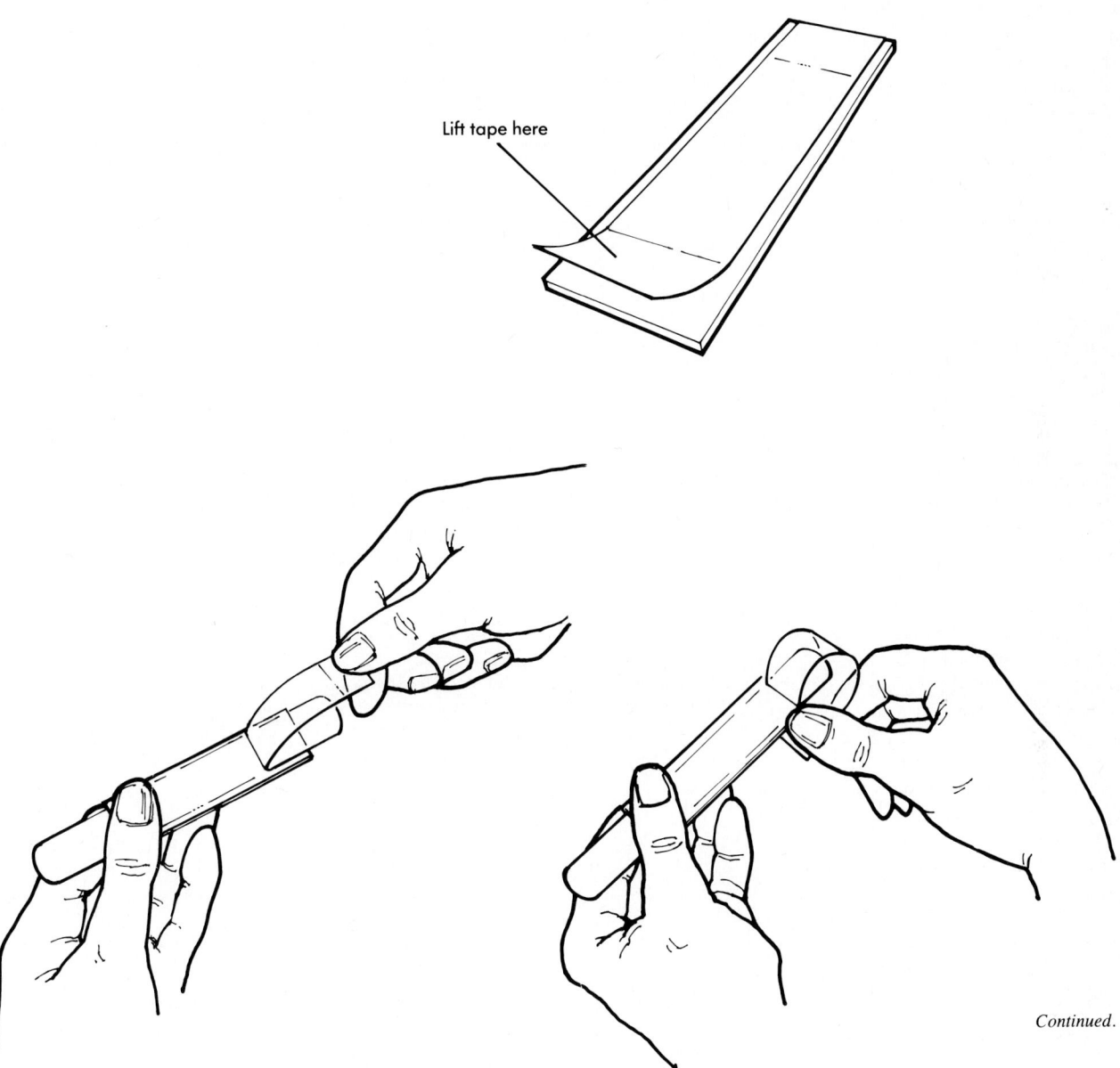

Lift tape here

Continued.

FIGURE 40-3. Cellophane tape procedure for collection of *Enterobius vermicularis* egg. (From Parasitology Training Division, Centers for Disease Control.)

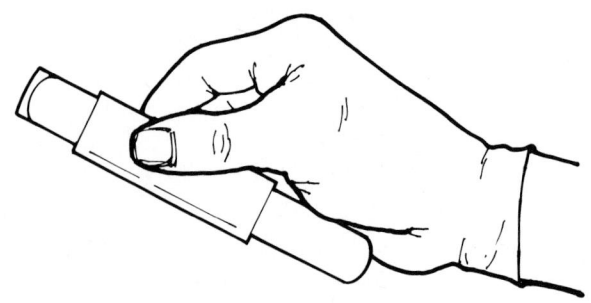

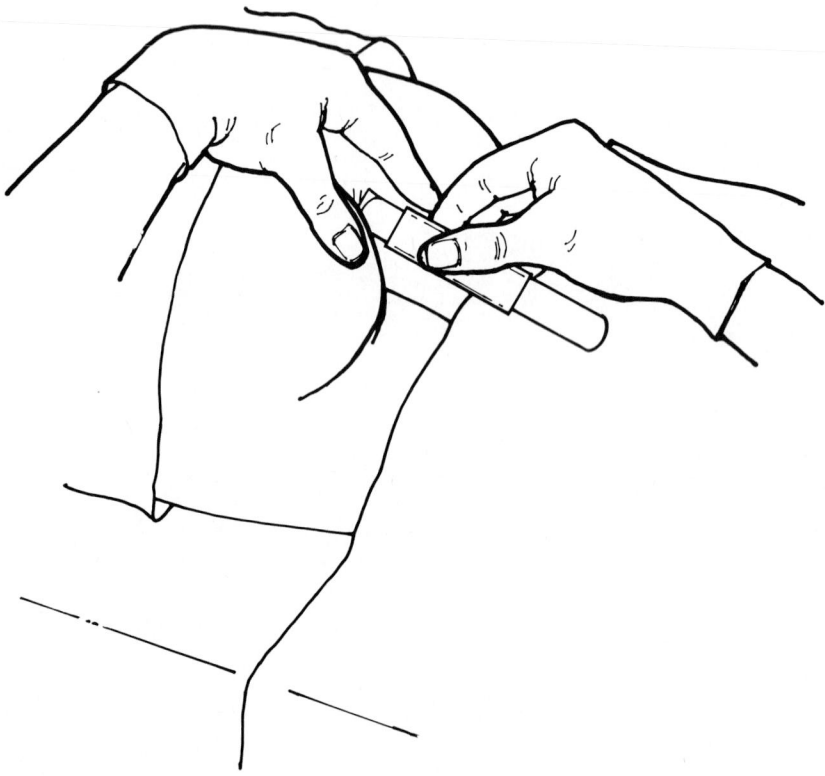

FIGURE 40-3, cont'd. Cellophane tape procedure for collection of *Enterobius vermicularis* egg. (From Parasitology Training Division, Centers for Disease Control.)

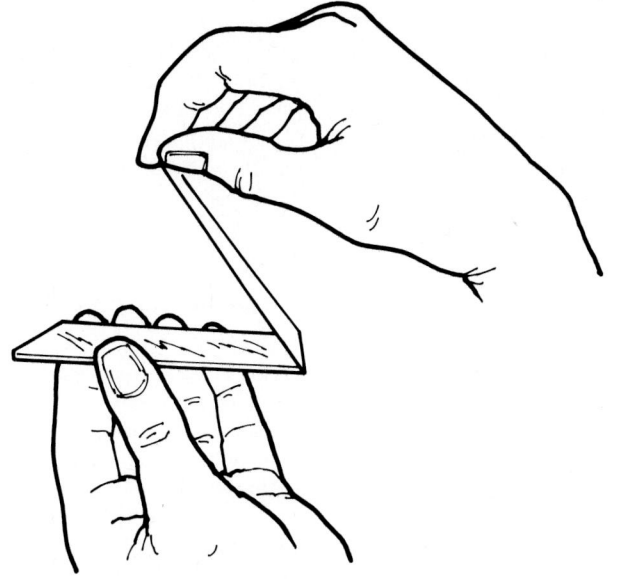

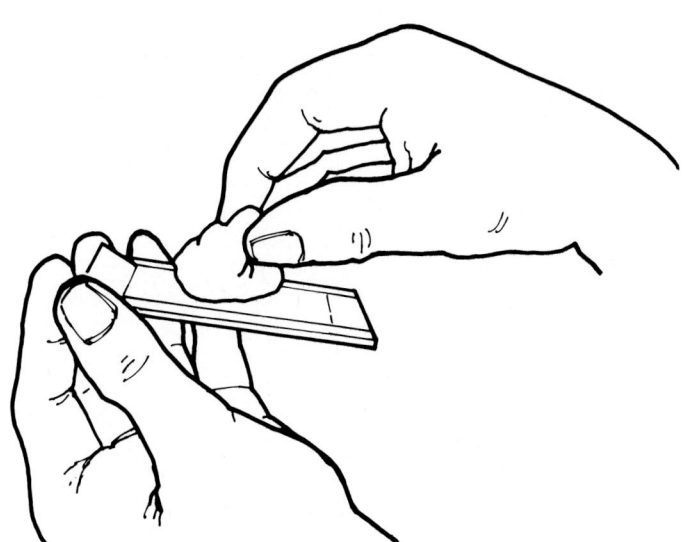

FIGURE 40-3, cont'd. For legend see opposite page.

laboratory in a sealed test tube. When received by the laboratory, the test tube is filled with just enough xylene to cover the swab and allowed to stand for 3 to 5 minutes. The swab is then removed, the xylene centrifuged for 1 minute at 500 × g, and the resulting sediment examined for the characteristic eggs.

Regardless of the collection method employed, maximum egg recovery of *E. vermicularis* eggs requires that the specimen be collected early in the morning before the patient uses the bathroom or toilet. Between three and six such specimens, collected on consecutive days, may be required to detect light infections.[120]

Genital specimens for *Trichomonas vaginalis*[79,85]

The identification of *Trichomonas vaginalis* is usually based on the characteristic jerky motion of the organism in wet mounts of vaginal or urethral discharge or prostatic secretions. If a permanent record is required, permanent stained smears may be prepared using the same trichrome or iron-hematoxylin methods used for permanent stained fecal smears. Other stains such as the Papanicolaou and Gram stains have also been used in some laboratories.[24,108] Unfortunately, the interpretation of these stained smears is so often complicated by the presence of artifacts and distortion of the organism that they cannot be recommended for routine diagnostic purposes.[108] Another staining technique that has been suggested for *Trichomonas* organisms is an acridine-orange fluorescence stain. As with other staining techniques for these organisms, there is no agreement on the value of this technique.[50,79]

In vitro cultivation using a medium such as the Feinberg-Whittington medium[37] or a modified Diamond medium described by Fouts and Kraus[40] can significantly improve detection of *T. vaginalis* infections. Studies by these investigators and others[19,108] have found that as many as 50% more cases are detected by using cultivation techniques.

Urine specimens

Besides genital secretions or discharge, *T. vaginalis* is frequently observed in urine specimens, often during routine urinalysis. Urine specifically submitted for detection of *T. vaginalis* must be fresh and preferably the first portion of the voided urine. The same procedures used to process and examine genital specimens for this organism are also applicable to urine specimens. In addition, a simple centrifugation of the urine and examination of the resulting sediment is useful for improving the detection of this organism in urine specimens.

Probably the single most important indication for examination of urine specimens is detection of *Schistosoma hematobium* infections. Although this parasite actually inhabits the blood vessels around the urinary bladder, the diagnostic egg stage is commonly shed into the bladder and carried from the body in the urine. These eggs are most likely to be detected in the last portion of a voided urine collected at midday.[131] The specimen should be concentrated by simple centrifugation and the resulting sediment examined for the characteristic spined eggs with the low-power (10×) microscope objective.

Sputum specimens

Another tissue-dwelling trematode for which the primary diagnostic specimen is a natural body excretion or secretion is the lung fluke, *Paragonimus westermani*. Even though this parasite resides within the lung tissue, the diagnostic egg stages are shed into the alveoli and are carried up the respiratory tree in the sputum. Since sputum is often swallowed, these eggs are also commonly found in fecal specimens. Larval stages of other parasites such as *Ascaris* and *Strongyloides* organisms and hookworms may also be detected in sputum if the specimen is obtained during the lung migration of these parasites. Similarly, the trophozoites of *Entamoeba histolytica* may be found in the sputum of patients with pulmonary amoebic abscesses.

Examination of sputum should include at least a direct wet mount. A simple centrifugation procedure may also be used in suspected cases of helminth infections. To facilitate detection of helminth eggs, mucoid specimens should be liquefied by mixing with an equal amount of 3% sodium hydroxide or undiluted chlorine bleach. If an amoebic abscess is suspected, a permanent, stained smear should be prepared and examined using procedures similar to those used for fecal samples.

Aspirates and biopsies

Occasionally, invasive techniques such as aspiration and biopsy may be required to diagnose infections with lumen-dwelling parasites if other, more conventional techniques have failed or if the parasite invades deeper tissues of the body (for example, amoebic liver abscess).

Duodenal contents. In some cases of giardiasis and strongyloidiasis repeated fecal examinations may not reveal the infection[60,65,99] and the physician may wish to collect duodenal fluid for examination.

One of two methods, either intubation and suction of duodenal fluid or the so-called Entero-Test,[6,9] may be used to obtain this material. In the Entero-Test one end of a length of nylon yarn, which is coiled in a weighted gelatin capsule, is taped to the side of the patient's face (Figure 40-4). The patient then swallows the capsule and the line uncoils as the capsule is carried into the duodenum. After about 4 hours, the line is retrieved, and the fluid and mucus adhering to the bile-stained region of the yarn are squeezed from the yarn and examined.

Fluid obtained by either intubation or the Entero-Test should be examined immediately as a direct wet mount. If examination must be delayed for more than 1 hour, the material should be preserved in a small amount of formalin and PVA fixative for examination at a later time.

Sigmoidoscopy aspirates. Occasionally, multiple stool examinations fail to reveal organisms in suspected cases of amoebiasis, and the physician may perform a sigmoidoscopy to obtain material directly from the intestinal mucosa.[87] These samples should be aspirated or scraped from at least six representative areas of the mucosa, including any suspicious lesions. Samples obtained on cottom swabs are rarely satisfactory, since any organisms in the sample are likely to be absorbed and trapped within the swab.

Usually only a small sample can be obtained by sigmoidoscopy, and the immediate priority in processing must be the preparation of a permanent smear similar to those prepared for fecal specimens. The quickest technique is to smear the sample on a slide, fix the smear in Schaudinn solution, and then proceed with trichrome staining. Alternatively, 1 or 2 drops of the sample may be mixed directly on a slide with 2 or 3 drops of PVA fixative and allowed to dry for at least 2 hours (preferably overnight) before staining. Any sample remaining after preparation of a permanent smear should be examined in a direct

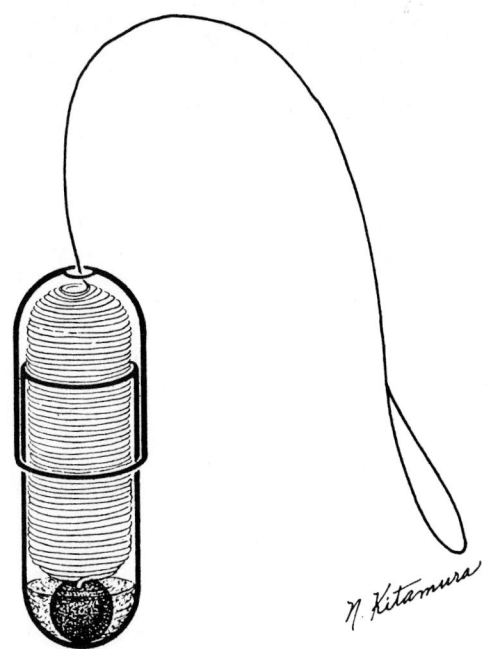

FIGURE 40-4. Entero-Test capsule for sampling duodenal contents. (Illustration by Nobuko Kitamura. From Garcia, L.S., and Ash, L.R.: Diagnostic parasitology, clinical laboratory manual, ed. 2, St. Louis, 1979, The C.V. Mosby Co.)

saline wet mount for the presence of motile trophozoites or added to an in vitro cultivation medium.

Abscess aspirates. In some cases of extraintestinal amoebiasis, involvement of the intestinal mucosa is minimal, and consequently, repeated fecal examinations may fail to reveal the parasite.[126] In such cases physicians often request serologic tests or examination of aspirates from extraintestinal abscesses. However, since serologic tests may remain positive for long periods after treatment of an earlier infection, aspiration of abscesses is the best method for confirming cases of extraintestinal amoebiasis when no parasites are detected by repeated stool examinations.

The basic procedures for the examination of the aspirates are similar to those used for sigmoidoscopy samples. There are, however, some special difficulties in detecting amoebae in aspirates from extraintestinal abscesses. First, the organisms are usually concentrated on the wall of the abscess; very few are found in the necrotic center of the lesion. Thus the ideal sample is the final portion of the aspirate containing material from the wall of the lesion. Second, the organisms are often immobilized in the thick pus of the aspirate and must be freed from this material by treating the sample with a proteolytic enzyme such as streptodornase.[41] Finally, *Entamoeba histolytica* grows poorly, if at all, on primary isolation in the traditional cultivation media if bacteria are not present. Since most amoebic abscesses are bacteriologically sterile, an inoculum of either mixed fecal bacteria or *Clostridium perfringens* should be added to the cultivation medium.

Biopsies. Traditionally, biopsy samples are processed as tissue sections in the histopathology laboratory and the results are interpreted by the pathologist.[87] This is also true for most biopsy specimens obtained in suspected parasitic infections. How-

ever, a simple tissue examination technique that does not require microscopic sections or specialized stains may be performed in the microbiology laboratory. In this technique, which can be used to demonstrate larvae of *Trichinella spiralis* in muscle biopsy samples or schistosome eggs in biopsy samples of intestinal or urinary bladder mucosa, a small piece of tissue is compressed between two glass slides and examined microscopically for the respective larvae or eggs.[80] This technique may in fact be more sensitive than the traditional histologic techniques, since a large amount of tissue may be examined. In addition, the viability of schistosome eggs may be ascertained directly by this method, since viable eggs are typically translucent and contain active miracidia.

Serology

Numerous serologic tests have been developed for detecting antibodies to intestinal parasites, including *Ascaris* spp.,[105] *Clonorchis* spp.,[107] *Entamoeba histolytica*,* *Fasciola* spp.,[57,133] hookworms,[4,129] *Paragonimus* spp.,[157,158] schistosomes,[17,64,154] and *Trichinella* spp.[†] In general, however, serologic tests are rarely used to diagnose infections caused by intestinal parasites. Many of the serologic tests for intestinal parasites require antigens that are often difficult, if not impossible, to obtain from commercial sources in the United States (see reference 146 for a list of sources). In addition, many of these tests do not provide a good balance between sensitivity and specificity. The tests that employ seemingly crude antigens often have the best sensitivity but at the same time tend to suffer from cross-reactions that reduce their specificity. The use of more purified antigens usually has the opposite effect: the specificity is improved, but the sensitivity declines. Other factors known to have a major influence on the value of serologic tests are the method of testing (that is, a complement fixation test, an agglutination test, an indirect immunofluorescence test, and so forth) and the stage of the disease when the test is performed.

Two diseases caused by intestinal parasites for which serologic tests have proved extremely reliable and useful are invasive amoebiasis and trichinosis. Serologic tests for antibodies to *Entamoeba histolytica* are most useful in the more severe forms of the disease.[73] Data compiled by Kagan[63] from published reports on the indirect hemagglutination (IHA), double diffusion (DD), and indirect immunofluorescence tests (IIF) showed that test results were positive from at least one of these three tests for an average of 94% of patients with amoebic abscesses, 71% of patients with amoebic dysentery, and 29% of asymptomatic patients passing only the cyst stage of the organism. Among patients who were otherwise healthy or suffering from other diseases, only 4% had positive test results. These data illustrate the overall value of serologic tests for the different forms of amoebiasis; however, it should be noted that Kagan's data suggest that different tests may be more sensitive for particular forms of the disease. The most dramatic differences are in the ability of the tests to detect asymptomatic cyst passers. For example, the DD test detected 55% of the positive conditions, the IIF 23%, and the IHA only 9%. Despite the low sensitivity of the IHA in detecting the asymptomatic cases, Walls and Smith[148] report that the IHA is probably the most

---

*References 11, 54, 55, 67, 74, 97, and 130.
†References 31, 75, 98, 109, 118, and 119.

popular serologic test for amoebiasis. Another test that correlates well with the IHA[74] is counterimmunoelectrophoresis (CIE). This technique has the advantage of being readily available in kit form and is probably more suitable for laboratories that perform single tests at irregular intervals.

One disadvantage of the more sensitive tests for amoebiasis is that they may remain positive for as long as 2 years after successful therapy.[55] This would seem to limit the usefulness of these tests in areas where the disease is prevalent. However, in such situations a negative test result for a patient with an extraintestinal abscess (for example, liver abscess) may be equally informative; it is strong evidence that *E. histolytica* is not the cause of the patient's abscess.[54,55,97]

Among laboratory methods for the diagnosis of trichinosis, one of the most valuable is the detection of specific antibodies by the bentonite flocculation test.[63,103] This test is extremely sensitive and specific, provided it is performed no earlier than 3 weeks after infection. This 3-week delay may seem excessive; however, the alternative, a muscle biopsy, is rarely successful if attempted before the second week of infection and is certainly a less pleasant diagnostic procedure.

In most infections the antibody titer to *Trichinella* organisms reaches a peak in about 2 months and remains detectable for several years.[63] As is true for many serologic tests, the persistence of these low titers may make it difficult to confirm the infection unless there is a fourfold change in the antibody titer.

BLOOD AND TISSUE PARASITES
Blood Samples[46]

As might be expected, blood is the primary specimen for diagnosis of infections with blood and tissue parasites. Besides permitting the direct detection and identification of most blood and tissue parasites, blood samples are also required when serologic tests are used as primary or secondary methods of diagnosis. For example, in the early (acute) stage of *Trypanosoma cruzi* infections, diagnosis is usually based on finding the characteristic trypomastigote stage in blood smears. In later (chronic) stages of the disease, the number of parasites detectable in the blood is usually small and serologic tests become the principal diagnostic method. In certain other infections, such as toxoplasmosis, serology is the principal diagnostic method in all stages of the disease.

Collection of blood samples

Blood specimens used for permanent stained smears should be collected without anticoagulant. Finger sticks or, in infants, heel or earlobe sticks are the easiest and most reliable method of collecting such samples. If use of an anticoagulant is necessary, ethylenediaminetetra-acetic acid (EDTA) may be used, provided the blood smear is prepared within 1 hour of sample collection.

Larger blood samples, such as those required for concentration or cultivation techniques, are usually collected by venipuncture using a minimal amount of sodium citrate as an anticoagulant. Excessive amounts of anticoagulant often have an adverse effect on the viability or morphologic characteristics of microorganisms.

For serologic tests, blood samples must be collected without anticoagulant using aseptic technique. The sample should be allowed to clot at room temperature for 1 or 2 hours and refrig-

erated overnight to retract the clot. The resulting serum is aseptically transferred to a sterile, tightly sealed test tube, and if testing is delayed, the sample is frozen. To prevent bacterial contamination of serum that must be mailed to a reference laboratory for testing, it is usually desirable to add 0.01 ml of a 1% aqueous solution of sodium azide to each milliliter of serum.

Except for serodiagnosis, which typically requires two samples (acute and convalescent) collected 10 to 14 days apart, the timing and number of blood samples vary with the particular infection. These varying requirements are discussed in the sections on each individual parasite.

Examination of blood samples

Methods for examination of blood samples are basically similar to the methods used for fecal samples, including techniques such as direct wet mounts, stained permanent smears, concentration procedures, and cultivation. The major difference is that detection and identification of the diagnostic stages of most blood and tissue infections require examination of a stained permanent smear and wet mounts have a very limited use, as described below.

Wet mounts. Wet mounts of blood specimens may be used as a screening technique for detecting motile blood parasites such as trypanosomes and the microfilariae of tissue nematodes. In thin blood preparations viewed with reduced microscopic illumination these organisms can be detected by their rapid movement among the red cells. This rapid movement, however, usually serves only to detect the presence of the parasite; permanent stained smears are required for specific identification once the parasites have been detected. Moreover, even if a wet mount appears negative, a permanent stained smear should be examined because false-negative wet mounts may occur if the wet mount is too dense, the blood clots before examination, or the infection is caused by a nonmotile parasite such as *Plasmodium* spp.

Permanent stained smears.[127,146,152] Two types of blood smears are used in parasitology, thin blood smears and thick blood smears. Thin blood smears, which are the best preparations for studying morphologic detail of blood parasites, are prepared in the same manner as blood smears for differential white cell counts; they should have a large area free of streaks or gaps and the erythrocytes should be side by side in a single layer. Problems often arise in preparation of thin smears when laboratories use so-called precleaned slides. Many times these slides are covered with an oily residue that may cause streaks or gaps in the smear. A separate cleaning with alcohol is always best for slides that will be used for parasitology blood smears.

To obtain reliable results, thin smears should first be completely examined with the low-power objective (10×) to detect the larger diagnostic stages such as microfilariae. To detect the smaller parasites such as trypanosomes or malaria the slide must be examined with the oil immersion objective, a procedure that might take several hours if the entire smear had to be examined. For this reason most authorities recommend that a thin smear be examined with the oil immersion objective for a minimum of 30 minutes or until a total of 100 microscopic fields have been studied. This is a *minimum* standard, and a more extensive examination may be indicated before a report of "No parasites found" is issued.

Although thin blood smears can usually reveal moderate to

heavy infections and are the best preparation for identifying blood parasites, they are less than ideal for detecting light infections. Thick smears are much better for detecting light infections, since a larger amount of blood can be examined in a short period of time. One microscopic field of a thick smear contains 15 to 25 times as much blood as a comparable field in a thin smear, and a parasite first detected after examining 25 fields of a thick smear may not be detected in a thin film until hundreds of fields have been examined. With this greater sensitivity, the minimal requirements for thorough examination of a thick smear are less than those for a thin smear. Specifically, a thick smear should first be examined with low power to detect any microfilariae and then examined with the oil immersion objective for a minimum of 5 minutes or until 100 microscopic fields have been studied.

To prepare thick blood smears, 3 or 4 drops of fresh blood (no anticoagulant) are placed close together on a clean slide and mixed together in an area about the size of a dime. If the thick smear is of the proper density, newsprint will be just legible through the center of the wet smear. The smear should be allowed to dry in a horizontal position for 12 to 24 hours at room temperature before staining. Attempts to hasten drying by heating the slide fix the red cells and interfere with removal of hemoglobin from the cells during staining. If necessary, both thick and thin films for a single patient can be prepared on one slide as a so-called combination smear. However, since thick and thin blood films are treated slightly differently in the preliminary steps of staining, it is usually best to use different slides for the two different types of smears. Moreover, since thick smears require longer to dry than thin smears, the diagnosis of a moderate or heavy infection may be unnecessarily delayed if only combination smears are prepared.

The major disadvantage of thick smears is that the morphology of many blood parasites is distorted. In the case of malaria parasites, this distortion requires that different criteria be used to identify the organisms in thick smears. Where malaria is endemic, there is sufficient experience with thick smear examination that most species of malaria (except *Plasmodium vivax* and *P. malariae*) can be identified by a thick smear alone. However, when the speciation is in question or technologists lack the experience to interpret thick smears, thin smears must be used for identification.

Unfortunately, in the United States technologists are not familiar with the interpretation of thick smears and rely on thin smears for both detection and identification of blood parasites. If an infection is light or in the early stages, relying only on thin blood smears may seriously delay or prevent the detection of the infection. Even if the parasite cannot be identified in a thick film, the presence of an unidentified organism in the blood would prompt the physician to review the patient's diagnosis carefully and ensure that laboratory personnel thoroughly examine the thin smear or request assistance from a reference laboratory. In fact, it is a good practice to routinely submit any positive or suspicious blood smears to the state or regional public health laboratory for confirmation and possible epidemiologic investigation of the case.

Most of the stains used for blood smears are modifications of the methylene blue–eosin stain developed by Romanovsky to detect malaria parasites in red cells.[81,111] Four of these stains—Leishmann, Wright, Field, and Giemsa—are still used.[38,39,78] The major distinction among these stains is that the working solutions of the Leishmann and Wright stains are alcohol based, whereas the working solutions of the Giemsa and Field stains are water based. These differences are important because preliminary processing of thick and thin blood smears differs with alcohol- and water-based stains. With an alcohol-based stain thick films must be laked (dehemoglobinized) with either buffered water or a saponin reagent[143] before staining; thin smears do not need special pretreatment. If a water-based stain, such as Giemsa, is used, the thin smears must be fixed in alcohol (that is, absolute methanol) before staining; thick smears do not require pretreatment.

In selecting a stain for routine use these differences in pretreatment are actually minor considerations because any stain would require pretreatment of either thick or thin blood smears. However, other factors, such as quality of staining, availability of commercially prepared stock solutions, and time required for completing the procedure, vary with the different stains and may play a significant role in selecting the most appropriate stain for parasitology blood smears. For example, Giemsa staining is recommended as the best routine method because it provides excellent morphologic detail of blood parasites in both thick and thin films, has excellent resistance to fading, and is generally available as a stock solution from commercial sources. The major disadvantage of Giemsa staining is that it usually requires 20 to 50 minutes for staining versus 10 minutes for Wright and Leishmann stains and less than 1 minute for the Field stain. These other stains may also provide some of the advantages of Giemsa staining such as resistance to fading (Wright), good staining of thin films (Wright and Leishman), good staining of thick films (Field), and commercial availability (Wright), but none offer all the advantages of Giemsa.

If a laboratory selects Giemsa stain for routine use, certain steps require special attention.[152] For example, if combination smears (thick and thin smears on the same slide) are used, care must be taken to prevent fixation of the thick film when alcohol is used to fix the thin film before staining. One effective method of fixing only the thin smear is to hold the slide at an angle with the thick smear at the top and then to use a pipette to dispense a gentle stream of alcohol over the thin film and allow the slide to dry in a nearly vertical position with the thick film at the top. Because even fumes from the alcohol may produce some fixation of the thick film, it is often better to prepare the thick and thin films on separate slides and process the two types of smears separately.

Selection and preparation of reagents used in staining blood smears also require special attention. Stock solutions of Giemsa stain obtained from commercial sources should be carefully evaluated to determine whether they are suitable for staining blood parasites; formulations suitable for routine hematology may not perform satisfactorily when used to stain blood parasites. In evaluating any commercial formulation it is important to note that two types of Giemsa stain, Azure A and Azure B, are recognized by the Commission for the Standardization of Biological Stains. Azure B is preferred for staining blood parasites.[20,152] Even if the formulation of a commercial stock matches published formulations, the laboratory should routinely perform quality control tests on each lot of stock and working stain before use.[111] If a laboratory chooses to make its own stock solutions, it is important that all reagents, not just the stain powder, be reagent grade and that the directions for preparation be followed explicitly.

Since the best results with Giemsa stain are obtained when staining and washing of blood smears are performed in a pH range of 7 to 7.2 (6.8 may be used to enhance Schuffner stippling), a phosphate-buffered water should be used in preparing all working dilutions of stain and rinse solutions. In addition, adding small amounts of the detergent Triton to the buffered water enhances the staining and reduces the possibility of malaria parasites transferring from positive to negative smears when large numbers of smears are stained simultaneously.[14,32] Usually 0.01% Triton X-100 is added to the buffered water used for thin or thick and thin combination films, and 0.1% is added to the buffered water used for thick blood films or tissue and exudate smears.[93] Finally, it is important to prepare fresh working solutions of buffered water and Giemsa stain immediately before use and to check the pH of each solution carefully.

With any of the staining techniques, including Giemsa, blood smears should be stained within 3 days of their preparation. If necessary, the staining may be delayed for 1 or 2 weeks, provided special precautions are used. Specifically, thin smears should be fixed before storage, and thick smears should be laked in buffered distilled water (pH 7 to 7.2) or treated with a buffered solution of methylene blue before storage.[146] The treated slides should be protected from heat and moisture during storage.

Special stains. In addition to Giemsa stain, other stains may be used to enhance the morphologic details of certain species of blood and tissue parasites. One of the more common special stains is Delafield hematoxylin. This stain is used to enhance the morphologic detail of two key diagnostic features of microfilariae, the nuclei and microfilarial sheath.[42] On occasion it may be used in histology laboratories to stain tissue sections of muscle biopsy specimens from patients suspected of having *Trichinella spiralis*.[20]

Concentration techniques. Although thick blood films may be considered a type of concentration procedure, certain blood and tissue parasites, such as hemoflagellates and filarial nematodes, may escape detection if a laboratory relies only on thick and thin blood films.

One technique that may be used to concentrate the trypomastigote stage of *Trypanosoma* infections is fractional centrifugation.[42] Basically this procedure involves repeated centrifugation of a large sample of citrated blood. By using increasing gravitational force with each centrifugation, it is possible to separate the trypomastigotes from most of the erythrocytes and leukocytes. The final sediment is then examined for trypomastigotes by any of several methods, including wet mounts to detect motile organisms, Giemsa-stained smears, or, if the procedure was performed aseptically, inoculation into animals or a cultivation medium.

Microfilariae in the blood of patients suspected to have filariasis may be concentrated by either centrifugation or membrane filtration techniques. Probably the most widely used centrifugation method is the Knott technique,[70] in which blood collected in sodium citrate is mixed with formalin or acetic acid to hemolyze the erythrocytes and then centrifuged to sediment any microfilariae. The resulting sediment may be examined as a permanent smear stained with Delafield hematoxylin or Giemsa stain. Since the chemicals used to hemolyze the red cells in this technique also kill or immobilize any microfilariae, Harris and Summers[53] substituted a weak solution of saponin for the formalin. The advantage of this modification is that the microfilariae remain viable and are readily detected by their motility in wet mounts.

In the membrane filtration method[8,28-30] a sample of citrated blood is first hemolyzed and then forced through a moistened membrane filter (5 μm pore size). The filter is stained with Harris hematoxylin, dried, and mounted on a glass slide for examination. For temporary mounts the filter is simply covered with immersion oil; this makes the filter material transparent and permits examination with the oil immersion objective (100×). If a permanent slide is required, Permount or a similar mounting medium can be used to clear the filter material and seal the preparation with a coverglass.

Quantitation of blood parasites

Enumeration of the number of parasites per cubic millimeter of blood is a valuable technique in certain blood parasite infections.[12,27] These estimates not only provide an indication of the severity of infection and help monitor the effectiveness of a particular therapeutic regimen but may also be an important clue for identification of a parasite. For example, in cases of *Plasmodium falciparum* infection it is not unusual for the parasitemia to reach levels of 100,000 parasites/mm³ of blood; in fatal cases it may exceed 500,000 parasites/mm³. This level of parasitemia is unusual with other species of *Plasmodium*. *P. vivax* rarely exceeds 50,000 parasites/mm³ of blood, *P. malariae* is usually less than 10,000/mm³, and *P. ovale* is probably less than 26,000/mm³ in most cases.[12,59]

One of the simplest methods for approximating the number of parasites is to simultaneously count the number of parasites and the number of leukocytes seen in a thick blood smear until a minimum of 100 leukocytes is counted.[152] Using the value obtained from a total leukocyte count on the same sample of blood, the number of parasites per cubic millimeter of blood can be estimated by the following formula:

$$\frac{\text{No. of parasites per cubic millimeter}}{\text{Total leukocytes per cubic millimeter}} = \frac{\text{No. of parasites counted in thick smear}}{\text{No. of leukocytes counted in thick smear}}$$

Tissue Biopsies and Aspirates[46]

Several blood and tissue infections are routinely identified with tissue biopsies and aspirates. In the United States one of the most common examples is opportunistic pulmonary infections caused by the protozoan *Pneumocystis carinii*.[128] In these infections specimens collected by invasive techniques such as open lung biopsy, bronchial brushing, and transtracheal aspirates are more likely to reveal the parasite than are more easily collected specimens such as sputum.[117] Two types of stains may be used to detect the organism in these samples. One group, represented by Grocott methenamine-silver–toluidine blue and Gram-Weigert stains, stain only the organism's cyst wall; the cyst contents do not stain. Since certain pulmonary fungi such as *Histoplasma capsulatum* may appear similar to cysts of *Pneumocystis* organisms,[160] a second type of stain, Giemsa, may be used to reveal the cyst contents and provide an unequivocal identification. The principal disadvantage of Giemsa staining is the lack of contrast between stained organisms and background material, which often makes locating the organisms difficult. Giemsa staining is also less satisfactory with tissue sections than with impression smears or aspirates. For these reasons some laboratories prefer to use one of the cyst stains for tissue sections or screening of smears and then use Giemsa staining to confirm the identification.

In infections with the filarial nematode *Onchocerca volvulus* the microfilariae are found principally in the skin and only rarely circulate in the blood.[16,51] To diagnose these infections, small skin snips are taken from the scapular region (Central American form of the disease) or the pelvis or upper leg (African form of the disease). When the skin samples are mounted in a drop of physiologic saline under a coverglass, microfilariae usually migrate out of the tissue within 30 minutes to 1 hour. The motile microfilariae can be observed with reduced illumination at low magnification ($10\times$ objective), or the preparation can be allowed to dry and stained with Giemsa stain or Delafield hematoxylin for more detailed examination of the microfilariae. Alternatively, the skin sample may be teased apart in saline to speed release of the microfilariae or processed as traditional tissue sections.

In many of the hemoflagellate infections such as cutaneous and visceral leishmaniasis, detection of the amastigote stage in tissue biopsies or aspirates is the principal method of diagnosing the infection. For example, skin biopsies or aspirates obtained from below the base or edges of cutaneous ulcers are commonly used in the diagnosis of cutaneous leishmaniasis. Solid tissue samples collected in this manner may be processed as stained tissue sections or may be used to prepare impression smears where solid portions of tissue are pressed firmly against the surface of a slide, leaving a thin layer of cells that is dried and processed as a Giemsa-stained thin blood film. Aspirated liquid samples are also easily processed if the aspirate is handled as though it were a blood sample, and a Giemsa-stained thin film is prepared. If care is taken to avoid bacterial contamination during collection, these samples may also be used as inoculum for in vivo or in vitro cultivation.

The diagnosis of visceral leishmaniasis also relies largely on detecting amastigotes in tissue biopsies and aspirates, with the samples being obtained from lymph nodes, spleen, liver, and bone marrow. In all other respects the samples may be processed like those for cutaneous leishmaniasis.

In a third type of hemoflagellate infection, American trypanosomiasis, the trypomastigote stage of the parasite may be detectable in blood smears during the early (acute) stages of the disease. However, in the later stages of the disease the organism may be detectable only as amastigotes in stained aspirates or biopsy specimens obtained and processed like the samples used for visceral leishmaniasis. As with samples for the other hemoflagellate infections, these materials, if handled aseptically, may be used as inoculum for in vitro or in vivo cultures.

Cerebrospinal fluid samples are of value in two types of infections. Wet mounts and hematoxylin- or trichrome-stained smears of spinal fluid are a primary diagnostic tool for detecting cases of amoebic meningoencephalitis (inflammation of the brain and meninges) caused by free-living amoebae of the genera *Naegleria* and *Acanthamoeba*. In the later stages of African trypanosomiasis, trypomastigotes of the two subspecies of African trypanosomes *(Trypanosoma brucei* ssp. *rhodesiense* and *gambiense),* may be found by using wet mounts or Giemsa-stained smears of cerebrospinal fluid.

The diagnosis of human infections with the larval stages of cestodes such as *Echinococcus granulosus* (unilocular hydatid disease), *E. multilocularis* (alveolar hydatid disease), *Taenia solium* (cysticercosis), *Multiceps* spp. (coenurosis), and *Spirometra* spp. (sparganosis) frequently depends on examination of surgically removed larvae. Generally, identification of these larval stages requires expertise found only in reference laboratories. However, in cases of *E. granulosus,* aspirates of cyst contents may be submitted to the laboratory after surgical removal of the cyst. When examined as a wet mount under low magnification ($10\times$ objective), these aspirates are found to contain a mixture of intact and deteriorating scolices and calcified granules. Aspiration of these cysts should be confined to open surgical procedures and not attempted as a blind exploratory procedure because leakage of the cyst contents exposes the patient to possible anaphylaxis and spread of viable cysts within the body.

In Vitro Cultivation[138]

In general, the most reliable in vitro cultivation methods for blood and tissue parasites are those used for the major pathogenic species of hemoflagellates, especially *Leishmania* spp. and *Trypanosoma cruzi*. Like the methods for intestinal protozoa, the methods for cultivation of these parasites often require special media, and it may be difficult for all but the larger laboratories to acquire proficiency and maintain proper quality control with these methods.

Among the more reliable and versatile media that are relatively easy to prepare from materials readily available in most clinical laboratories are blood agar–based media such as Novy, MacNeal, Nicolle (NNN) medium[104] or the medium used in the National Institutes of Health (NIH) method of cultivation.[42] Another medium that may prove particularly attractive to clinical laboratories is the liquid medium described by Hendricks, Wood, and Hajduk.[56] In addition to promoting better growth of a wide variety of *Leishmania* and *Trypanosoma* spp., the Hendricks medium can be freeze dried, stored for up to 2 years, and rehydrated when needed.

Since these methods for cultivation of hemoflagellates are intended to duplicate conditions in the insect vector and not the human host, the culture must be incubated at room temperature ($22°$ to $25°$ C), not at $35°$ to $37°$ C, and the stages recovered from positive cultures are the same stages normally found in the insect vector. Care should also be taken to prevent bacterial contamination during the initial inoculation and subsequent examination of the cultures because bacteria inhibit the development and multiplication of the organisms. If specimens are obtained from contaminated body sites (for example, skin) it is advisable to add a penicillin-streptomycin mixture to the medium. Finally, it is important that cultures not be prematurely reported as negative; in some media such as NNN it may take up to 1 month before organisms can be detected.

Besides the hemoflagellates, cultivation techniques for protozoans may also be of value in detecting central nervous system infections with free-living amoebae of the genera *Naegleria* and *Acanthamoeba*. Culbertson, Ensminger, and Overton[25] have described a simple method in which low-salt, plain agar plates are seeded with cultures of *Escherichia coli*, then spot inoculated with samples of cerebrospinal fluid and incubated at $37°$ C. If amoebae are present, they feed on the bacteria and produce a clear zone that extends out from the point of inoculation and resembles the zone of inhibition around antimicrobial disks in a Bauer-Kirby susceptibility test. Wet mounts can be prepared from the edge of the zone and observed for motile amoebae that can be identified by the techniques described in the section on primary amoebic meningoencephalitis.

In Vivo Cultivation

Many common laboratory animals are susceptible to infections with human blood and tissue parasites. However, the use of animal inoculation as a means of diagnosing human infections is generally limited to larger reference laboratories that have the facilities and trained personnel required to maintain animal colonies and provide for isolation of infected animals. If these conditions are met, a laboratory may occasionally find it useful to use animal inoculation as an aid in the diagnosis of hemoflagellate and *Toxoplasma* and *Babesia* infections. For *Leishmania* and *Babesia* infections hamsters are acceptable host animals. White rats may be used for *Trypanosoma* infections, and white mice are susceptible to *Toxoplasma* spp. and *Trypanosoma cruzi*. The usual procedure is to inoculate intraperitoneally with the same type of specimens that would be used for in vitro cultivation or for direct smears. Depending on the parasite suspected, blood (*Trypanosoma* spp., *Babesia* spp.), spleen (*Lieshmania* spp.), or peritoneal fluid (*Toxoplasma* spp.) smears are prepared from the infected animals at various time intervals. In the case of *Toxoplasma* infections, the parasite may be detected as early as 2 days after inoculation. On the other hand, *Leishmania* infections usually develop slowly and the animal should not be sacrificed for spleen smear before 4 to 6 weeks have elapsed. In addition to the long period required for some infections to develop in an initial host animal, it may occasionally be necessary, as for *Toxoplasma* spp., to make a "blind passage" of tissue or fluid from a previously inoculated animal to another animal before the infection can be detected. A final limitation to animal inoculation is the possibility of strain differences in some parasites (for example, *Babesia* spp.), which means that not all isolates are infectious for the usual animal host; thus negative results do not rule out the possibility of a human infection.

Another rather exotic but effective method of in vivo cultivation, called xenodiagnosis, may be used in infections where an arthropod serves as a vector or intermediate host for a human parasite. In this technique laboratory-reared, disease-free arthropods are allowed to feed on patients suspected of being infected. The arthropods are then maintained under conditions that would promote development of the parasite and are eventually examined to determine whether the arthropod has acquired the infection. Probably the most common application of this method is found in South America where the technique is used to diagnosis American trypanosomiasis. With this infection, laboratory-reared reduviid bugs are allowed to take a blood meal from patients suspected to have the disease. After 1 or 2 months feces of the exposed bugs are examined for the stage of the parasite normally found in the arthropod host.

Serology

Numerous serologic tests have been developed to aid in the diagnosis of infections with blood and tissue parasites. Some of these tests, such as the indirect hemagglutination,[21] indirect immunofluorescence,[21] and direct agglutination[1] tests for *Trypanosoma cruzi,* the indirect immunofluorescence,[134] enzyme-linked immunosorbent,[144,145] and fluorescent immunoassay

"X" test[147] for toxoplasmosis, the bentonite flocculation test[103] for trichinosis, and the enzyme-linked immunosorbent assay for toxocariasis,[110] are both specific and sensitive. Others, such as the indirect immunofluorescence[135] and indirect hemagglutination tests[96] for malaria, are sensitive and specific for a particular genus or closely related genera of parasites, but, depending on the antigen used, may not differentiate among different species or closely related genera. Finally, a third group of tests, such as the indirect hemagglutination and bentonite flocculation test for filariasis,[62,92] vary in sensitivity depending on the clinical history of the individual patient and lack specificity because of extensive cross-reactions with sera from patients with unrelated parasitic infections.

Obviously, results from highly specific and sensitive tests, such as those for *Toxoplasma* and *Trichinella* organisms, may be used as a primary diagnostic tool, whereas results from tests with low sensitivity and specificity, such as those for filariasis, are of limited diagnostic value unless supported by other tests such as positive blood smears. Unfortunately, even the highly specific and sensitive tests may be of limited value in the clinical setting. If such tests are used indiscriminately, that is, as screening tests or when signs and symptoms of the particular disease are nonspecific, the predictive value of a positive test drops significantly. An even more immediate limitation of these tests is the availability of a reliable supply of high-quality reagents. Commercial suppliers are reluctant to undertake the expense of development and government certification of diagnostic reagents that have a limited market; thus reagents for many of these tests are not commercially available in the United States. In this situation, laboratories that cannot produce their own antigens or antisera must rely on commercial, state, and federal reference laboratories to provide serologic testing.

One common blood and tissue parasite infection that is reliably diagnosed by serologic methods using commercial reagents is toxoplasmosis. A variety of tests including indirect hemagglutination, indirect immunofluorescence, and enzyme-linked immunosorbent assay are available from commercial sources (see reference 146 for a partial listing). The traditional test for toxoplasmosis and the one used as a standard to measure the performance of other tests is the so-called Sabin-Feldman or methylene blue dye test. However, because this test is technically demanding and requires the use of live, potentially infectious, organisms, it is rarely used in clinical laboratories. Instead, most laboratories have adopted the commercial systems that employ killed antigens, especially the indirect immunofluorescence and enzyme-linked immunosorbent assays. These assays are not only sensitive and specific, but also readily adapted to testing for IgM antibodies that are indicative of neonatal and acute adult infections.[63] Since serologic testing is the primary diagnostic tool for toxoplasmosis and is often requested by obstetricians as a prenatal screening test in women of childbearing age, it is reasonable to expect that even smaller laboratories can routinely provide reliable results using one of the commercial kits.

REFERENCES

1. Allain, D.S., and Kagan, I.G.: An evaluation of the direct agglutination test for Chagas' disease, J. Parasitol. **60:**179, 1974.
2. Andrews, J.: The diagnosis of intestinal protozoa from purges and normally passed stools, J. Parasitol. **20:**253, 1934.

3. Balamuth, W.: Improved egg yolk infusion for cultivation of *Endamoeba histolytica* and other intestinal protozoa, Am. J. Clin. Pathol. **16**:380, 1946.

4. Ball, P.A.J., and Bartlett, A.: Serologic reactions to infection with *Necator americanus,* Trans. R. Soc. Trop. Med. Hyg. **63**:362, 1969.

5. Bartlett, M.S., et al.: Comparative evaluation of a modified zinc sulfate flotation technique, J. Clin. Microbiol. **7**:524, 1978.

6. Beal, C.B., et al.: A new technique for sampling duodenal contents, Am. J. Trop. Med. Hyg. **19**:349, 1970.

7. Beaver, P.C.: The standardization of fecal smears for estimating egg production and worm burden, J. Parasitol. **36**:451, 1950.

8. Bell, D.: Membrane filters and microfilariae: a new diagnostic technique, Ann. Trop. Med. Hyg. **61**:220, 1967.

9. Bezjak, B.: Evaluation of a new technique for sampling duodenal contents in parasitologic diagnosis, Am. J. Dig. Dis. **17**:848, 1972.

10. Blagg, W., et al.: A new concentration technic for the demonstration of protozoa and helminth eggs in feces, Am. J. Trop. Med. Hyg. **4**:23, 1955.

11. Bos, H.J., Von der Eyk, A.A., and Steerenberg, P.A.: Application of ELISA in the serodiagnosis of amebiasis, Trans. R. Soc. Trop. Med. Hyg. **69**:440, 1975.

12. Boyd, M.F.: Present day problems of malaria mortality, JAMA **124**:1179, 1944.

13. Brandt, W.H.: The student's guide to optical microscopes, Los Altos, Calif., 1976, William Kaufmann, Inc.

14. Brooke, M.M., and Donaldson, A.W.: The use of a surface-active agent to prevent transfer of malarial parasites between blood films during mass staining procedures, J. Parasitol. **36**:84, 1950.

15. Brooke, M.M., Donaldson, A.W., and Mitchell, R.B.: A method of supplying cellulose tape to physicians for diagnosis of enterobiasis, Pub. Health Rep. **64**:879, 1949.

16. Buck, A.A., editor: Onchocerciasis, Geneva, Switzerland, 1974, World Health Organization.

17. Buck, A.A., and Anderson, R.I.: Validation of the complement fixation and slide flocculation tests for schistosomiasis: geographic variations of test capacity, Am. J. Epidemiol. **96**:205, 1972.

18. Buck, A.J., Wells, W.H., and Vail, J.R.: Techniques for differentiating and preserving protozoa in feces, U.S. Armed Forces Med. J. **4**:1195, 1953.

19. Burch, T.A., Rees, C.W., and Reardon, L.: Diagnosis of *Trichomonas vaginitis,* Am. J. Obstet. Gynecol. **27**:309, 1959.

20. Burrows, R.B.: Microscopic diagnosis of the parasites of man, New Haven, Conn., 1965, Yale University Press.

21. Cerisola, J.A.: Immunodiagnosis of Chagas' disease: hemagglutination and immunofluorescence tests, J. Parasitol. **56**:409, 1970.

22. Chernin, E., and Dunavan, C.A.: The influence of host-parasite dispersion upon the capacity of *Schistosoma mansoni* miracidia to infect *Australorbis glabratus,* Am. J. Trop. Med. Hyg. **11**:455, 1962.

23. Cleveland, L.R., and Sanders, E.P.: The production of bacteria-free amoebic abscesses in the liver of cats and observations on the amoebae in various media with and without bacteria, Science **72**:149, 1930.

24. Cree, G.E.: *Trichomonas vaginalis* in Gram stained smears, Br. J. Vener. Dis. **44**:226, 1968.

25. Culbertson, C.G., Ensminger, P.W., and Overton, W.M.: The isolation of additional strains of pathogenic *Hartmanella* sp. *(Acanthamoeba):* proposed culture method for application to biological material, Am. J. Clin. Pathol. **43**:383, 1965.

26. D'Antoni, J.S.: Standardization of the iodine stain for wet preparations of intestinal protozoa, Am. J. Trop. Med. **17**:79, 1937.

27. Denham, D.A., et al.: Comparison of a counting chamber and thick smear methods of counting microfilariae, Trans. R. Soc. Trop. Med. Hyg. **65**:521, 1971.

28. Dennis, D.T., and Kean, B.H.: Isolation of microfilariae: report of a new method, J. Parasitol. **57**:1146, 1971.

29. Desowitz, R.S., and Hitchcock, J.C.: Hyperendemic Bancroftian filariasis in the kingdom of Tonga: the application of the membrane filter concentration technique to an age-stratified blood survey, Am. J. Trop. Med. Hyg. **23**:877, 1974.

30. Desowitz, R.S., Southgate, B.A., and Mataika, J.U.: Studies on filariasis in the Pacific. 3. Comparative efficacy of the stained blood-film, counting chamber, and membrane filtration techniques for the diagnosis of *Wuchereria bancrofti* microfilaremia in untreated patients in low areas of endemicity, Southeast Asian J. Trop. Med. Pub. Health **4**:329, 1973.

31. Despommier, D., et al.: Immunodiagnosis of human trichinosis using counterelectrophoresis and agar gel diffusion techniques, Am. J. Trop. Med. Hyg. **23**:41, 1974.

32. Donaldson, A.W.: Effects of various modifications of a mass staining procedure on the transfer of malarial parasites between blood films, J. Nat. Malaria Soc. **9**:239, 1950.

33. Donaldson, R.: An easy and rapid method for detecting protozoal cysts in faeces by means of wet-stained preparations, Lancet **1**:571, 1917.

34. Edelman, M., and Spingarn, C.: The relation between the number of cysts in the stool inoculum to the incidence of positive cultures of *Endamoeba histolytica* from stools, Am. J. Trop. Med. Hyg. **1**:412, 1954.

35. Erdman, D.D.: Clinical comparison of ethyl acetate and diethyl ether in the formalin-ether sedimentation technique, J. Clin. Microbiol. **14**:483, 1981.

36. Faust, E.C., et al.: Comparative efficiency of various techniques for the diagnosis of protozoa and helminths in feces, J. Parasitol. **25**:241, 1939.

37. Feinberg, J.G., and Whittington, M.J.: A culture medium for *Trichomonas vaginalis,* Donne and species of *Candida,* J. Clin. Pathol. **10**:327, 1957.

38. Field, J.W.: A simple and rapid method of staining malaria parasites in thick blood smears, Trans. R. Soc. Trop. Med. Hyg. **34**:195, 1940.

39. Field, J.W.: Further note on a method of staining malarial parasites in thick blood films, Trans. R. Soc. Trop. Med. Hyg. **35**:35, 1941.

40. Fouts, A.C., and Kraus, S.J.: *Trichomonas vaginalis:* reevaluation of its clinical presentation and laboratory diagnosis, J. Infect. Dis. **141**:137, 1980.

41. Freedman, L., Maddison, S.E., and Elsdon-Dew, R.: Monoxenic culture of *Entamoeba histolytica* derived from human liver abscesses, S. Afr. Med. Sci. **23**:9, 1958.

42. Garcia, L.S., and Ash, L.R.: Diagnostic parasitology: clinical laboratory manual, ed. 2, St. Louis, 1979, The C.V. Mosby Co.

43. Garcia, L.S., Brewer, T.C., and Bruckner, D.A.: A comparison of the formalin-ether concentration and trichrome-stained smear methods for the recovery and identification of intestinal protozoa, Am. J. Med. Technol. **45**:932, 1979.

44. Garcia, L.S., and Shimizu, R.: Comparison of clinical results for the use of ethyl acetate and diethyl ether in the formalin-ether sedimentation technique performed on polyvinyl alcohol–preserved specimens, J. Clin. Microbiol. **13**:709, 1981.

45. Garcia, L.S., and Voge, M.: Diagnostic clinical parasitology. I. Proper specimen collection and processing, Am. J. Med. Tech. **46**:459, 1980.

46. Garcia, L.S., and Voge, M.: Diagnostic clinical parasitology. IV. Identification of the blood parasites, Am. J. Med. Technol. **47**:21, 1981.

47. Gardner, B.B., et al.: Comparison of direct wet mount and trichrome-staining techniques for detecting *Entamoeba* species trophozoites in stools, J. Clin. Microbiol. **12**:656, 1980.

48. Gleason, N.N., and Healy, G.R.: Modification and evaluation of Kohn's one-step staining technic for intestinal protozoa in feces or tissue, Am. J. Clin. Pathol. **43**:494, 1965.

49. Goldman, M., and Brooke, M.M.: Protozoans in stools unpreserved and preserved in PVA fixative, Pub. Health Rep. **68**:203, 1953.

50. Greenwood, J.R., and Kirk-Hillaire, K.: Evaluation of acridine orange stain for detection of *Trichomonas vaginalis* in vaginal secretions, J. Clin. Microbiol. **14:**699, 1981.

51. Hardner, H.I., and Watson, D.: Human filariasis: identification of species on the basis of staining and other morphologic characteristics of microfilariae, Am. J. Clin. Pathol. **42:**333, 1964.

52. Harper, K., Little, M.D., and Damon, S.K.: Advantages of the PVA fixative two-bottle stool collection techniques in the detection and identification of intestinal parasites, Pub. Health Lab. **15:**96, 1957.

53. Harris, J.S., and Summers, W.A.: A concentration method for demonstrating microfilaria in blood, Am. J. Trop. Med. **25:**497, 1945.

54. Healy, G.R.: The use and limitations to the indirect hemagglutination test in the diagnosis of intestinal amebiasis, Health Lab. Sci. **5:**174,

55. Healy, G.R., Visvesvara, G.S., and Kagan, I.G.: Observations on the persistence of antibodies to *Entamoeba histolytica,* Arch. Invest. Med. **5:**495, 1974.

56. Hendricks, L.D., Wood, D.E., and Hajduk, M.E.: Hemoflagellates: commercially available liquid media for rapid cultivation, Parasitology **76:**309, 1978.

57. Hillyer, G.V., and Capron, A.: Immunodiagnosis of human fascioliasis by counterelectrophoresis, J. Parasitol. **62:**1011, 1976.

58. Hsieh, H.C.: A test-tube filter-paper method for the diagnosis of *Ancylostoma duodenale, Necator americanus,* and *Strongyloides stercoralis,* WHO Tech. Rep. Ser. **255:**27, 1963.

59. Jeffrey, G.M., Wilcox, A., and Young, M.D.: A comparison of West African and West Pacific strains of *Plasmodium ovale,* Trans. R. Soc. Trop. Med. Hyg. **49:**168, 1955.

60. Jones, C.A., and Abadie, S.H.: Studies on human strongyloidiasis. II. A comparison of the efficiency of diagnosis by examination of feces and duodenal fluid, Am. J. Clin. Pathol. **24:**1154, 1954.

61. Juniper, K., Jr.: Acute amebic colitis, Am. J. Med. **33:**377, 1962.

62. Kagan, I.G.: A review of immunologic methods for the diagnosis of filariasis, J. Parasitol. **49:**773, 1963.

63. Kagan, I.G.: Serodiagnosis of parasitic diseases. In Lennette, et al., editors: Manual of clinical microbiology, ed. 3, Washington, D.C., 1980, American Society for Microbiology.

64. Kagan, I.G., and Pellegrino, J.: A critical review of immunological methods for the diagnosis of bilharziasis, Bull. WHO **25:**611, 1961.

65. Kamath, K.R., and Murugasu, R.: A comparative study of four methods for detecting *Giardia lamblia* in children with diarrheal disease and malabsorption, Gastroenterology **66:**16, 1974.

66. Karapetyan, A.E.: In vitro cultivation of *Giardia duodenalis,* J. Parasitol. **48:**337, 1962.

67. Keesel, J.F., et al.: Indirect hemagglutination and complement fixation tests in amebiasis, Am. J. Trop. Med. Hyg. **14:**540, 1965.

68. Kenney, M., and Eveland, L.K.: Infection of man with *Trichuris vulpis,* the whipworm of dogs, Am. J. Clin. Pathol. **69:**199, 1978.

69. Knight, W.B., et al.: A modification of the formol-ether concentration technique for increased sensitivity in detecting *Schistosoma mansoni* eggs, Am. J. Trop. Med. Hyg. **25:**818, 1976.

70. Knott, J.: A method for making microfilarial surveys on day blood, Trans. R. Soc. Trop. Med. Hyg. **33:**191, 1939.

71. Krogstad, D.J., Spencer, H.G., and Healy, G.R.: Amebiasis, New Engl. J. Med. **298:**262, 1978.

72. Krogstad, D.J., Spencer, H.C., and Healy, G.R.: Amebiasis: epidemiologic studies in the United States, 1971-1974, Ann. Intern. Med. **88:**89, 1978.

73. Krupp, I.M.: Antibody response in intestinal and extraintestinal amebiasis, Am. J. Trop. Med. Hyg. **19:**57, 1970.

74. Krupp, I.M.: Comparison of counterimmunoelectrophoresis with other serologic tests in the diagnosis of amebiasis, Am. J. Trop. Med. Hyg. **23:**27, 1974.

75. Labzoffsky, N.A., et al.: Immunofluorescence as an aid in the early diagnosis of trichinosis, Can. Med. Assoc. J. **90:**920, 1964.

76. Lane, C.: The mass diagnosis of ankylostome infestation, Trans. R. Soc. Trop. Med. Hyg. **17:**407, 1924.

77. Lawless, D.K.: A rapid permanent-mount stain technic for the diagnosis of the intestinal protozoa, Am. J. Trop. Med. Hyg. **2:**1137, 1953.

78. Leishman, W.B.: A simple and rapid method of producing Romanovsky staining in malarial and other blood films, Br. Med. J. **2:**757, 1901.

79. Levett, P.N.: A comparison of five methods for the detection of *Trichomonas vaginalis* in clinical specimens, Med. Lab. Sci. **37:**85, 1980.

80. Lichtenberg, F., and Valladares, C.: Compression examination of fresh tissue for ova of *Schistosoma mansoni,* Am. J. Clin. Pathol. **25:**1099, 1955.

81. Lillie, R.D.: Romanovsky-Malachowski stains: the so-called Romanovsky stains; Malachowski's 1891 use of alkali polychromed methylene blue for malaria plasmodia, Stain Technol. **53:**23, 1978.

82. Lincicome, D.R.: Fluctuation in numbers of cysts of *Endamoeba histolytica* and *Endamoeba coli* in the stools of rhesus monkeys, Am. J. Hyg. **36:**321, 1942.

83. Loughlin, E.H., and Spitz, S.H.: Diagnosis of helminthiasis, JAMA **139:**997, 1949.

84. Loughlin, E.H., and Stoll, N.R.: An efficient concentration method (AEX) for detecting helminthic ova in feces (modification of the Telemann technic), Am. J. Trop. Med. **26:**517, 1946.

85. Lowe, G.H.: A comparison of culture media for the isolation of *Trichomonas vaginalis,* Med. Lab. Technol. **29:**389, 1972.

86. Maldonado, J.F.: An evaluation of the standardized direct smear for egg counting in parasitological work, Am. J. Trop. Med. Hyg. **5:**888, 1956.

87. Manson-Bahr, P., and Muggleton, W.J.: Rectal biopsy as an aid to the diagnosis of amoebic dysentery and allied diseases of the colon, Lancet **6972:**763, 1957.

88. Markell, E.K., and Voge, M.: Medical parasitology, ed. 5, Philadelphia, 1981, W.B. Saunders Co.

89. Markey, R.L.: A Vaseline swab for the diagnosis of *Enterobius* eggs, Am. J. Clin. Pathol. **20:**493, 1950.

90. Marsden, A.T.H.: Detection of cysts of *E. histolytica* in feces by microscopic examination, Med. J. Aust. **1:**915, 1918.

91. Martin, L.K., and Beaver, P.C.: Evaluation of Kato thick-smear for quantitative diagnosis of helminth infections, Am. J. Trop. Med. Hyg. **17:**382, 1968.

92. McQuay, R.M.: Parasitologic studies in a group of furloughed missionaries. II. Helminth findings, Am. J. Trop. Med. Hyg. **16:**161, 1967.

93. Melvin, D.M., and Brooke, M.M.: Triton X-100 in Giemsa staining of blood parasites, Stain Technol. **30:**269, 1955.

94. Melvin, D.M., and Brooke, M.M.: Laboratory procedures for the diagnosis of intestinal parasites, Department of Health Education and Welfare, Pub. No. (CDC) 75-8282, Washington, D.C., 1974, U.S. Government Printing Office.

95. Melvin, D.M., Sadun, E.H., and Heimlich, C.R.: Comparison of the direct smear and dilution egg counts in the quantitative determination of hookworm infections, Am. J. Hyg. **64:**139, 1956.

96. Meuwissen, J.H.E.T., and Leeuwenberg, A.D.E.M.: Indirect hemagglutination test for malaria with lyophilized cells, Trans. R. Soc. Trop. Med. Hyg. **66:**666, 1972.

97. Milgram, E.A., Healy, G.R., and Kagan, I.G.: Studies on the use of the indirect hemagglutination test in the diagnosis of amebiasis, Gastroenterology **50:**645, 1966.

98. Muraschi, T.F., Bloomfield, N., and Newman, R.B.: A slide latex–particle agglutination test for trichinosis, Am. J. Clin. Pathol. **37:**227, 1962.

99. Naik, S.R., Rau, N.R., and Vinayak, V.K.: A comparative evaluation of examinations of three stool samples, jejunal aspirate and jejunal mucosal impression smears in the diagnosis of giardiasis, Ann. Trop. Med. Parasitol. **72:**491, 1978.

100. Nair, C.P.: Rapid staining of intestinal amoebae on wet mounts, Nature **172**:1051, 1953.

101. Norman, L., and Brooke, M.M.: The use of penicillin and streptomycin in the routine cultivation of amebae from fecal specimens, Am. J. Trop. Med. Hyg. **4**:472, 1955.

102. Norman, L., and Brooke, M.M.: The effectiveness of the PVA-fixative technique in revealing intestinal amebae in diagnostic cultures, Am. J. Trop. Med. Hyg. **4**:479, 1955.

103. Norman, L., and Kagan, I.G.: Bentonite, latex, and cholesterol flocculation tests for the diagnosis of trichinosis, Pub. Health Rep. **78**:227, 1963.

104. Novy, F.G., and McNeal, W.J.: On the cultivation of *Trypanosoma brucei,* J. Infect. Dis. **1**:1, 1904.

105. Oliver-Gonzales, J.P., et al.: Serologic activity of antigen isolated from the body fluid of *Ascaris suum,* J. Immunol. **103**:15, 1969.

106. Otto, G.F., Hewitt, R., and Strahan, D.E.: A simplified zinc sulfate levitation method of fecal examination for protozoan cysts and hookworm eggs, Am. J. Hyg. **33**:32, 1941.

107. Pacheco, G., Wykoff, D.E., and Jung, R.C.: Trial of an indirect hemagglutination test for the diagnosis of infections with *Clonorchis sinensis,* Am. J. Trop. Med. Hyg. **9**:367, 1960.

108. Perl, G.: Errors in the diagnosis of *Trichomonas vaginalis* infection, Obstet. Gynecol. **39**:7, 1972.

109. Plonka, W.S., Gancarz, Z., and Zawadzka-Jedrzejewska, B.: A rapid screening hemagglutination test in the diagnosis of human trichinosis, J. Immunol. Methods **1**:309, 1972.

110. Pollard, Z.F., et al.: ELISA for diagnosis of ocular toxocariasis, J. Ophthalmol. **86**:743, 1979.

111. Power, K.T.: The Romanowsky stains: a review, Am. J. Med. Technol. **48**:519, 1982.

112. Price, D.L.: Comparison of three collection-preservation methods for detection of intestinal parasites, J. Clin. Microbiol. **14**:656, 1981.

113. Price, D.L., and Harvey, A.E.: A method for preparing trichrome-stained slides from MIF-fixed fecal specimens, Abstract No. C 112, Annual Meeting of American Society for Microbiology, Washington, D.C., 1980.

114. Rees, C.W.: Balantidia from pigs and guinea pigs: their viability, cyst production and cultivation, Science **66**:89, 1927.

115. Ritchie, L.S.: An ether sedimentation technique for routine stool examinations, Bull. U.S. Army Med. Dept. **8**:326, 1948.

116. Robinson, G.L.: The laboratory diagnosis of human parasitic amoebae, Trans. R. Soc. Trop. Med. Hyg. **62**:285, 1968.

117. Rosen, P.P., Martini, N., and Armstrong, D.: *Pneumocystis carinii* pneumonia: diagnosis by lung biopsy, Am. J. Med. **58**:794, 1975.

118. Ruitenberg, E.J., et al.: Application of immunofluorescence and immunoenzyme methods in the serodiagnosis of *Trichinella spiralis* infections, Ann. N.Y. Acad. Sci. **254**:296, 1975.

119. Sadun, E.H., Anderson, R.I., and Williams, J.S.: Fluorescent antibody test for the serological diagnosis of trichinosis, Exp. Parasitol. **12**:424, 1962.

120. Sadun, E.H., and Melvin, D.M.: The probability of detecting infections with *Enterobius vermicularis* by successive examination, J. Pediatr. **48**:438, 1956.

121. Sapero, J.J., and Lawless, D.K.: The "MIF" stain-preservation technique for the identification of intestinal protozoa, Am. J. Trop. Med. Hyg. **2**:613, 1953.

122. Sasa, M., et al.: Application of test-tube cultivation method on the survey of hookworm and related human nematode infection, Jpn. J. Exp. Med. **28**:129, 1958.

123. Sawitz, W.G., and Faust, E.C.: The probability of detecting intestinal protozoa by successive stool examinations, Am. J. Trop. Med. Hyg. **22**:131, 1942.

124. Scholten, T.: An improved technique for the recovery of intestinal protozoa, J. Parasitol. **58**:633, 1972.

125. Scholten, T.H., and Yang, J.: Evaluation of unpreserved and preserved stools for the detection and identification of intestinal parasites, Am. J. Clin. Pathol. **62**:563, 1974.

126. Sheehan, D.J., et al.: *Entamoeba histolytica:* efficacy of microscopic, cultural, and serological techniques for laboratory diagnosis, J. Clin. Microbiol. **10**:128, 1979.

127. Shute, P.G.: The staining of malaria parasites, Trans. R. Soc. Trop. Med. Hyg. **60**:412, 1966.

128. Smith, J.W., and Bartlett, M.S.: Diagnosis of *Pneumocystis* pneumonia, Lab. Med. **10**:430, 1979.

129. Sood, P., Prakash, O., and Bhujwala, R.A.: A trial of hemagglutination, circumoval precipitin and gel diffusion tests in hookworm infection, Indian J. Med. Res. **60**:1132, 1972.

130. Stamm, W.P.: The laboratory diagnosis of clinical amoebiasis, Trans. R. Soc. Trop. Med. Hyg. **51**:306, 1957.

131. Stimmel, C.L., and Scott, J.A.: The regularity of egg output of *Schistosoma hematobium,* Texas Rep. Biol. Med. **14**:440, 1956.

132. Stoll, N.R., and Hansheer, W.C.: Concerning two options in dilution egg counting: small drop and displacement, Am. J. Hyg. **6**(suppl.):134, 1926.

133. Stork, M.G., et al.: An investigation of epidemic fascioliasis in Peruvian village children J. Trop. Med. Hyg. **76**:231, 1973.

134. Sulzer, A.J., and Hall, E.C.: Indirect fluorescent antibody tests for parasitic diseases. IV. Statistical study of variation in the indirect fluorescent antibody (IFA) test for toxoplasmosis, Am. J. Epidemiol. **86**:401, 1967.

135. Sulzer, A.J., Wilson, M., and Hall, E.C.: Indirect fluorescent antibody tests for parasitic diseases. V. An evaluation of a thick-smear antigen in the IFA test for malaria antibodies, Am. J. Trop. Med. Hyg. **18**:199, 1969.

136. Svensson, R.: Studies on human intestinal protozoa, Acta Med. Scand. **70**(suppl.):vi, 1935.

137. Swartzwelder, C.: Laboratory diagnosis of amebiasis, Am. J. Clin. Pathol. **22**:379, 1952.

138. Taylor, A.E.R., and Baker, J.R.: The cultivation of parasites *in vitro,* Oxford, Eng., 1968, Blackwell Scientific Publications.

139. Tompkins, V.N., and Miller, J.K.: Staining intestinal protozoa with iron-hematoxylin-phosphotungstic acid, Am. J. Clin. Pathol. **17**:755, 1947.

140. Truant, A.L., et al.: Comparison of formalin-ethyl ether sedimentation, formalin-ethyl acetate sedimentation, and zinc sulfate flotation techniques for detection of intestinal parasites, J. Clin. Microbiol. **13**:882, 1981.

141. Tsuchiya, H.: Observations on "encystment cycle" of *Endamoeba histolytica* in a carrier, Proc. Soc. Exp. Biol. Med. **29**:930, 1943.

142. Tsuchiya, H.: Survival time of trophozoites of *Endamoeba histolytica* and its practical significance in diagnosis, Am. J. Trop. Med. Hyg. **25**:277, 1945.

143. Ulmas, J., and Fallon, J.N.: New thick-film technique for malaria diagnosis: use of saponin stromatolytic solution for lysis, Am. J. Trop. Med. Hyg. **20**:527, 1971.

144. Voller, A., et al.: A microplate enzyme-immunoassay for toxoplasma antibody, J. Clin. Pathol. **29**:150, 1976.

145. Voller, A., et al.: A comparison of isotopic and enzyme-immunoassays for tropical parasitic diseases, Trans. R. Soc. Trop. Med. Hyg. **71**:431, 1977.

146. Walls, K.W.: Serodiagnostic tests for parasitic diseases. In Lennette, E.H., et al., editors: Manual of clinical microbiology, ed. 4, Washington, D.C., 1985, American Society for Microbiology.

147. Walker, A.J.: Manual for the microscopical diagnosis of malaria, ed. 3, PAHO Scientific Pub. No. 161, Washington, D.C., 1968, Pan American Health Organization.

148. Walls, K.W., and Barnhart, E.R.: Titration of human serum antibodies to *Toxoplasma gondii* with a simple fluorometric assay, J. Clin. Microbiol. **7**:234, 1978.

149. Walls, K.W., and Smith, J.W.: Serology of parasitic infections, Lab. Med. **10**:329, 1979.

150. Watson, J.M., and Al-Hafidh, R.: A modification of the Baermann funnel technique and its use in establishing the infection potential of human hookworm carriers, Ann. Trop. Med. Parasitol. **51**:15, 1957.

151. Weller, T.H., and Dammin, G.J.: An improved method of examination of feces for diagnosis of intestinal schistosomiasis, Am. J. Clin. Pathol. **15**:496, 1945.

152. Wheatley, W.B.: A rapid staining procedure for intestinal amoebae and flagellates, Am. J. Clin. Pathol. **21**:990, 1951.

153. Wilcox, A.: Manual for the microscopical diagnosis of malaria in man, Public Health Service Pub. No. 796, Washington, D.C., 1960, U.S. Government Printing Office.

154. Willis, H.H.: A simple levitation method for the detection of hookworm ova, Med. J. Aust., Oct. 29, 1921, p. 375.

155. Wilson, M., Sulzer, A.J., and Walls, K.W.: Modified antigens in the indirect immunofluorescence test for schistosomiasis, Am. J. Trop. Med. Hyg. **23**:1072, 1974.

156. Yang, J., and Scholten, T.: Celestine Blue B stain for intestinal protozoa, Am. J. Clin. Pathol. **65**:715, 1976.

157. Yang, J., and Scholten, T.: A fixative for intestinal parasites permitting the use of concentration and permanent staining procedures, Am. J. Clin. Pathol. **67**:300, 1977.

158. Yogore, M.G., Lewert, R.M., and Madraso, E.D.: Immunodiffusion studies on paragonimiasis, Am. J. Trop. Med. Hyg. **14**:586, 1965.

159. Yokogawa, M.: *Paragonimus* and paragonimiasis, Adv. Parasitol. **7**:375, 1969.

160. Young, K.H., et al.: Ethyl acetate as a substitute for diethyl ether in the formalin-ether sedimentation technique, J. Clin. Microbiol. **10**:852, 1979.

161. Young, R.C., Bennett, J.E., and Chu, E.W.: Organisms mimicking *Pneumocystis carinii*, Lancet **2**:1082, 1976.

162. Zierdt, W.S.: A simple device for concentration of parasite eggs, larvae, and protozoa, Am. J. Clin. Pathol. **70**:89, 1978.

163. Zierdt, W.S.: Concentration and identification of *Cryptosporidium* spp. by use of a parasite concentrator, J. Clin. Microbiol. **20**:860, 1984.

CHAPTER 41

Lumen-Dwelling Helminths

John Klaas II

Each organism included in this chapter has two common characteristics. First, all are helminths (worms); this includes nematodes (roundworms), cestodes (tapeworms), and trematodes (flukes). Second, all these organisms, with one exception (*Schistosoma* spp.), inhabit the lumen spaces of the body, that is, parts of the body that have direct communication with the exterior environment, such as the intestinal tract, genitourinary tract, and lungs. This approach represents an alternative to a traditional taxonomic approach in which each different taxonomic group, such as the nematodes, cestodes, and trematodes, would be discussed in separate chapters, and a diagnostic laboratory approach in which organisms would be divided according to the type of specimen, such as feces, urine, or sputum, that is collected to confirm an infection. As with any system used to categorize organisms, the system used here was not without exceptions. For example, some parasites that do not inhabit lumen spaces as adults are included (for example, *Schistosoma* spp.), whereas others that do inhabit lumen spaces as adults (for example, *Trichinella spiralis)* are included in other chapters. The underlying criterion for all for these decisions was whether the diagnostic stage was passed in one of the natural body secretions or excretions, such as urine or feces, or whether an invasive technique such as drawing blood or obtaining tissue specimens is used to obtain the diagnostic specimen. If the organism's diagnostic stage is shed in a natural body secretion or excretion, it was included in the lumen-dwelling groups; if not, the organism was placed with the blood and tissue groups. This same approach was followed with all the other chapters on parasitology.

Within each chapter the organisms are grouped according to their taxonomic classification and within the classification according the increasing complexity of their life cycles. Thus the nematodes are discussed first, followed by the cestodes and finally the trematodes. The discussion of each organism is divided, in turn, into life cycle, epidemiology, pathology and clinical manifestations, and laboratory diagnosis.

These chapters are not intended to be a comprehensive review of all the various animal parasites that have ever been responsible for human disease. Rather, they are an overview of the major animal parasites of humans that are seen in the United States or have global health implications. Some of the other, less common parasites are included in Chapter 45.

ENTEROBIUS VERMICULARIS (PINWORM)
LIFE CYCLE[78,90]

Normally, infections with *Enterobius vermicularis* are acquired by ingesting eggs containing third-stage larvae (Figure 41-1). The eggs hatch in the upper small intestine, and the liberated larvae migrate to the ileocecal region of the intestine where they develop into adult worms. The adult worms attach themselves to the mucosa where they feed on bacteria and epithelial cells and become sexually mature 15 to 43 days after infection occurs. Shortly after fertilization of the females, the males die and, usually unnoticed, pass out of the body in the feces. When gravid, the female worms detach from the mucosa and begin migrating down the lumen of the intestine toward the anus. At night the females migrate out of the anus, deposit their sticky eggs on the perianal skin, and then die. Each female may deposit between 4000 and 16,000 eggs, which become fully embryonated and infective within about 6 hours of the time they are deposited. The eggs are relatively resistant to drying and may survive as long as 10 days in a humid environment.

In some cases, if the eggs remain in moist perianal folds for several days, the larvae may hatch, migrate into the anus, and mature into adult worms in the intestine. This unusual mode of reinfection is called retrofection. Occasionally, adult worms migrate out of the anus and enter the genitourinary tract of female patients or migrate directly through the intestinal wall into the peritoneal cavity, or up the intestinal tract and then into the lungs via the respiratory tract.[9,20]

EPIDEMIOLOGY[24,25,66,82,89]

Enterobiasis is prevalent throughout the world, particularly in temperate zones and colder climates. In the United States enterobiasis is probably the most prevalent helminth infection. The infection tends to be more common in children and among persons living in close or crowded conditions, such as institutionalized groups or members of the same household. Indeed, when one individual in a household is infected, commonly other family members are also infected.

The most common mode of infection is direct transfer (hand to mouth) of the infective eggs from the perianal region of an infected individual to the same or another host. Infections may also occur if an individual ingests eggs after contaminating the fingers while handling clothing, bedding, or even bathroom fixtures contaminated by an infected individual. So-called dust-borne infections reportedly occur when the lightweight eggs of this parasite become airborne and are subsequently inhaled and swallowed. The widespread contamination of the patient's environment with the resistant eggs and infection of multiple household members makes control of the infection particularly difficult. It has been common practice to encourage careful personal hygiene and a thorough cleaning of living quarters while all the infected members of the household are being treated. A few studies, however, suggest that even the most vigorous sanitary measures have little effect on control of the infection, and the major source of reinfection is from extrafamilial sources.

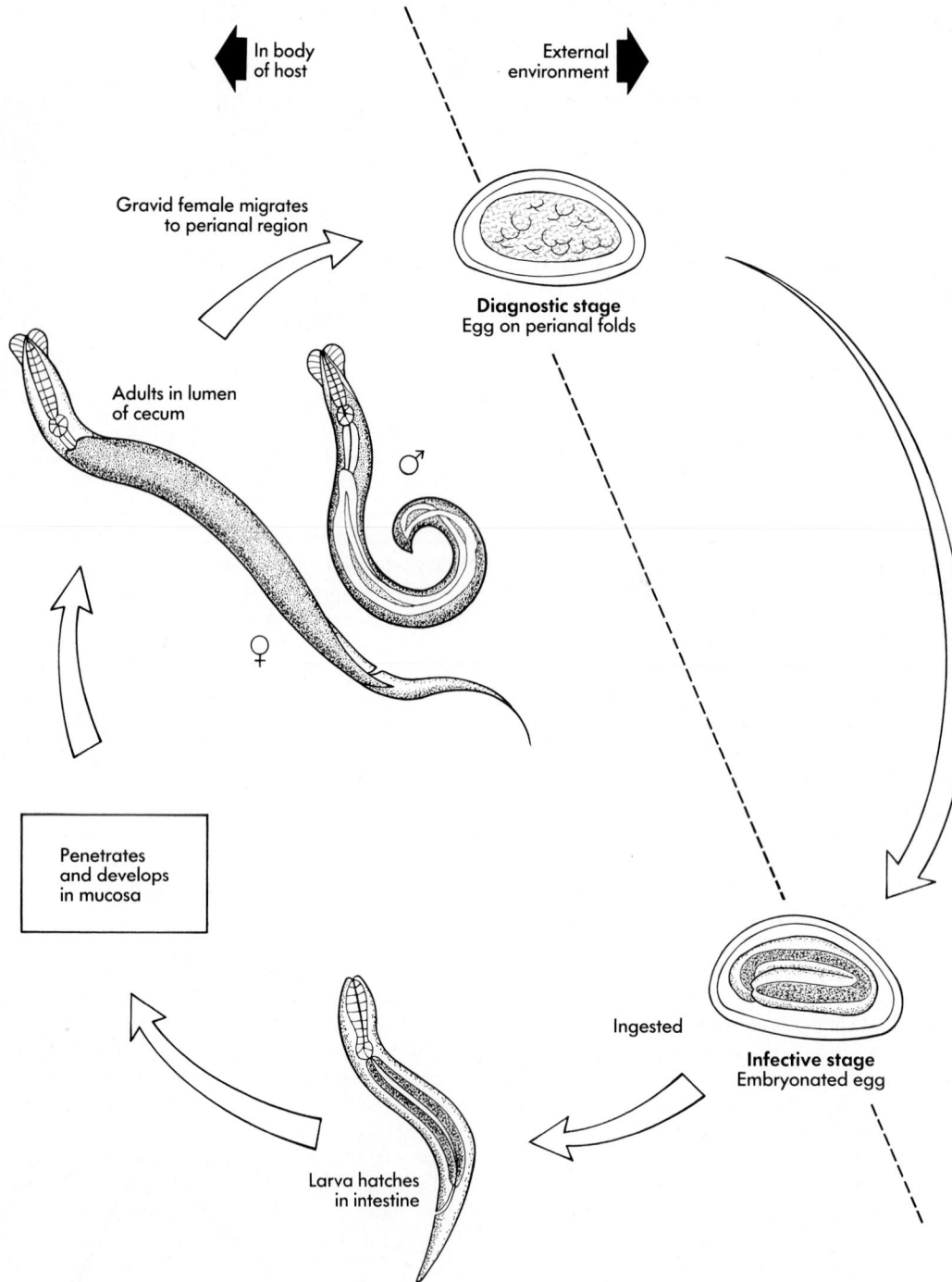

FIGURE 41-1. Life cycle of *Enterobius vermicularis*. (Modified from Melvin, D.M., Brooke, M.M., and Sadun, E.H.: Common intestinal helminths of man—life cycle charts, Atlanta, 1965, PHS Pub. No. 1235, Laboratory Branch of the Communicable Disease Center.)

A common misconception is that pinworm infections may be acquired from pet dogs or cats. These animals are not naturally infected with any species of pinworm and thus are not a source of infection for humans. However, there is at least one report that a natural pinworm of rats and mice (*Syphacia obvelata*) may produce infections in humans.

PATHOLOGY AND CLINICAL MANIFESTATIONS*

In perhaps one third of all pinworm infections the patient is asymptomatic, and in many other cases the symptoms are minimal. In symptomatic cases the most common complaint is a nocturnal perianal and perineal pruritus associated with migration of gravid female worms out of the anus. In severe cases the pruritus may provoke an intense scratching that results in hemorrhage, eczema, and secondary bacterial infections of the affected region. These severe cases are often accompanied by behavioral changes that include insomnia, irritability, nervousness, inattention, lack of cooperation, and poor appetite. Both the pruritus and behavioral changes are probably caused by the absorption of metabolites secreted by the worm and the subsequent development of hypersensitivity to these metabolites.

In young girls the migration of gravid female worms into the genital tract has been reported to cause vulvovaginitis, pelvic inflammatory disease, and granulomata in the fallopian tube or peritoneal cavity. It has also been suggested that worms migrating into the urethra and bladder may carry enteric bacteria that contribute to the development of urinary tract infections or enuresis. Other clinical manifestations occasionally observed are rectal colic when large numbers of worms are in the rectum and upper gastrointestinal disturbance caused by migration of adult worms up to the small intestine.

LABORATORY DIAGNOSIS[6,38,48]

Recovery of the characteristic eggs from the perianal and perineal areas is the most reliable means of confirming the diagnosis of enterobiasis. The so-called Scotch tape technique has proved to be the simplest and most effective method of recovering eggs from these sites. The specimen should be collected immediately after the patient awakens in the morning and before the patient passes a stool or takes a bath. Six specimens, collected on successive mornings, should be examined before eliminating enterobiasis as a possible diagnosis. Since female worms do not oviposit until they migrate onto the perianal skin, eggs are rarely found in the feces of infected individuals.

When seen in diagnostic preparations, the eggs of *Enterobius* organisms are normally embryonated (contain a developed larva), are 50 to 60 μm long and 20 to 32 μm wide, and have a translucent shell that is flattened on one side. If found in the feces, the eggs may not be fully embryonated, but they are still easily recognized by the characteristic size and shape (Figure 41-2).

Although specific recovery of adult worms is rarely attempted or needed to confirm the diagnosis, they may occasionally be seen migrating in the perianal region or in the feces and if properly identified can also be used to confirm the diagnosis of enterobiasis. The adult worms of both sexes are a light yellowish white color and have characteristic winglike extensions of the cuticle (called cephalic alae) at the anterior end.

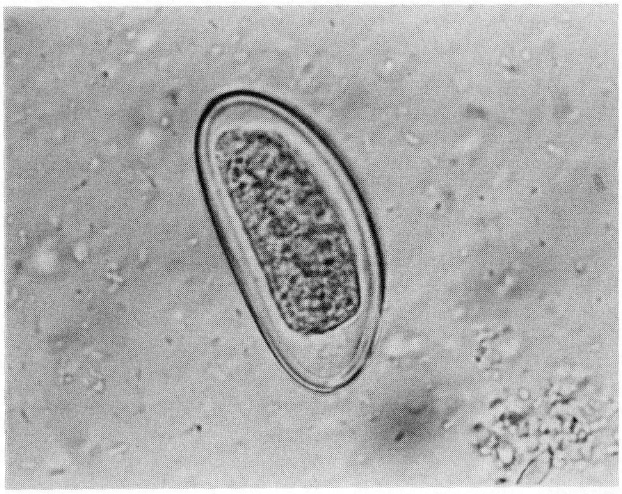

*References 16, 17, 25, 60, 67, 84, 87, 92, 101, and 112.

FIGURE 41-2. Egg of *Enterobius vermicularis*. (Approximately ×1200.)

The male worms are distinguished by their small size, typically 2 to 5 mm long, and a strongly curved posterior end. The females, in contrast, are usually 8 to 13 mm long and have a long, straight, sharply pointed posterior that gives this nematode its common name, pinworm.

TRICHURIS TRICHIURA (WHIPWORM)
LIFE CYCLE[54]

Humans are infected with *Trichuris trichiura* by ingesting eggs containing first-stage larvae (Figure 41-3). When liberated in the duodenum the larvae enter the nearby crypts (Lieberkuhn crypts) of the small intestine, where they grow and develop for about 10 days. The larvae then reenter the lumen of the intestine and migrate to the cecum where they develop into mature adults in about 3 months and may survive for several years. Adult males (30 to 45 mm long) and females (35 to 50 mm long) have a long slender esophageal region that comprises about two thirds of the total body length and a thickened posterior that contains the intestine and reproductive organs. This gives the worms the appearance of a whip and thus their common name, whipworm. In the host this esophageal region is "threaded" into the intestinal mucosa and provides a secure means of attachment within the intestinal tract; the thickened posterior hangs free in the lumen of the intestine. In heavy infections the adults may be found throughout the large intestine, extending as far down as the rectum.

After fertilization the females begin to produce characteristic barrel-shaped eggs that are passed in the feces in the single-cell stage. Estimates of the egg-laying capacity of the female worms vary widely, but the average is probably 5000 to 7000 per female per day. If the feces are deposited on moist soil in warm areas of dense shade and high humidity, the eggs develop to the infective stage in about 3 weeks and remain viable for approximately 2 additional weeks.

EPIDEMIOLOGY[19,55]

Trichuriasis occurs worldwide but is most common in warm, moist climates and areas where sanitation is poor. Because of their similar environmental requirements and mode of infection, *Trichuris* and *Ascaris* infections coexist in many parts of

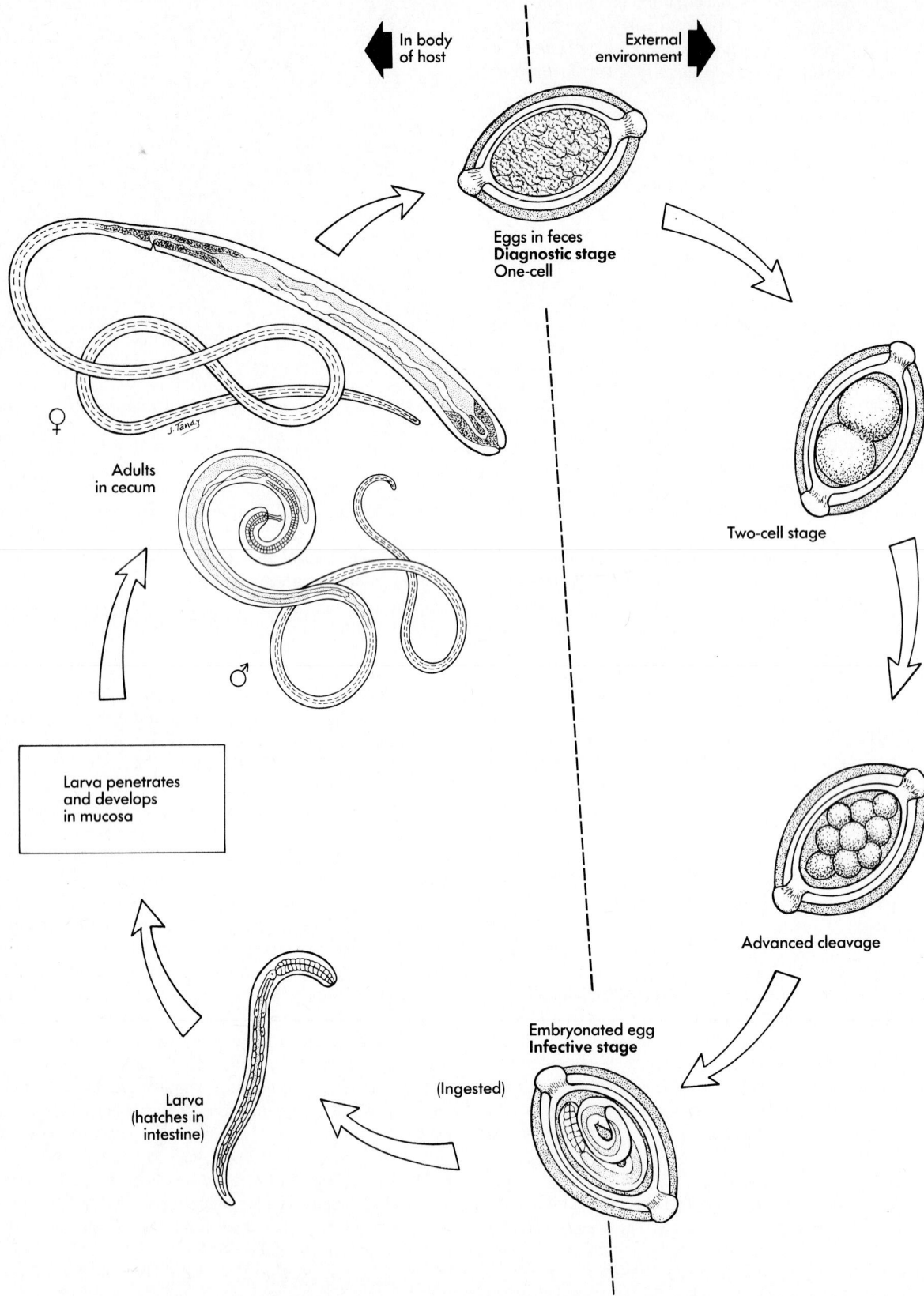

In body of host

External environment

Eggs in feces
Diagnostic stage
One-cell

Two-cell stage

♀

Adults
in cecum

♂

Advanced cleavage

Larva penetrates
and develops
in mucosa

Embryonated egg
Infective stage

(Ingested)

Larva
(hatches in
intestine)

FIGURE 41-3. Life cycle of *Trichuris trichiura*. (Modified from Melvin, D.M., Brooke, M.M., and Sadun, E.H.: Common intestinal helminths of man—life cycle charts, Atlanta, 1965, PHS Pub. No. 1235, Laboratory Branch of the Communicable Disease Center.)

the world. However, since the eggs of *Trichuris* organisms are less resistant to environmental stress such as drying or exposure to direct sunlight, *Trichuris* spp. have a slightly more restricted distribution than *Ascaris* organisms. The Centers for Disease Control reported that in 1978 *Trichuris* organisms were the most commonly identified helminth in fecal specimens submitted to state public health laboratories; they were found in 1.8% of the fecal specimens examined by these laboratories.

As is typical of many intestinal helminth infections, children are more commonly infected than adults, and control of the disease depends on providing facilities and education in the proper methods for handwashing and sanitary disposal of feces.

Although pigs and wild primates harbor species of *Trichuris* morphologically similar to *T. trichiura* and there are reports that *Trichuris vulpis,* the whipworm of dogs, may infect humans, the role of animals as a reservoir for human infections is uncertain.

PATHOLOGY AND CLINICAL MANIFESTATIONS*

Trauma to the intestinal mucosa and allergic responses to the worm and its metabolites are probably the major cause of the pathologic changes and clinical manifestations of trichuriasis. Penetration of the worm into the mucosa leads to superficial erosion of the mucosa and may be followed by invasion of bacteria and subsequent inflammation. The esoinophilia and urticaria occasionally reported in trichuriasis suggest that allergic responses also contribute to the pathogenesis of the disease.

In infections with small numbers of worms (100 to 300) the host usually suffers minimal traumatic damage or allergic reactions and remains asymptomatic unless the infection is complicated by malnutrition or infection with other species of intestinal parasites. Occasionally these light infections are manifest as nervousness, insomnia, anorexia, and a moderate eosinophilia. In more severe cases the clinical manifestations may mimic amoebiasis, hookworm infection, or acute appendicitis. Severe cases are sometimes complicated by obstruction and inflammation of the appendix when the worms become matted together or by prolapse of the rectum caused by severe inflammation and edema of the rectal mucosa.

LABORATORY DIAGNOSIS

Trichuris infections are usually diagnosed by finding the characteristic eggs (Figure 41-4) in the feces. Typically the eggs are barrel shaped with clear ''polar plugs'' at each end, measure 50 to 54 μm long by 22 to 23 μm wide, and are in the one-cell stage of development (nonembryonated). A simple direct fecal smear is usually sufficient for detecting significant infections because infections with fewer than 150 worms are usually asymptomatic and the direct smear can detect as few as five male-female worm pairs.

ASCARIS LUMBRICOIDES (LARGE ROUNDWORM)
LIFE CYCLE

Ascariasis is acquired by ingesting eggs containing second-stage larvae (Figure 41-5). The eggs hatch in the duodenum,

---

*References 30, 41, 54, 59, 61, 99, and 113.

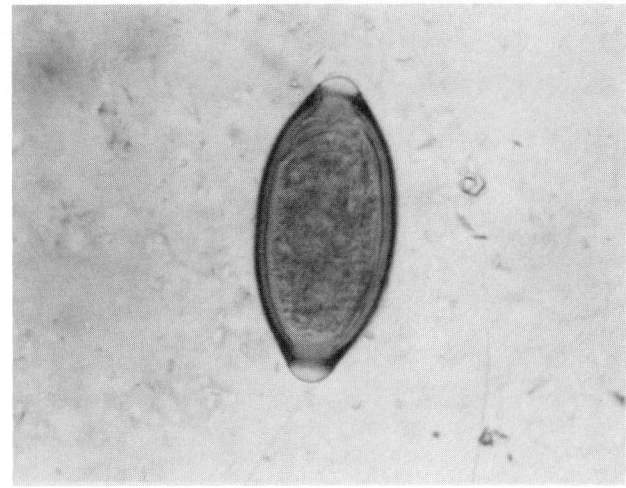

FIGURE 41-4. Egg of *Trichuris trichiura.* (Approximately ×850.)

and the liberated larvae penetrate the intestinal wall and enter lymphatic vessels or venules. Once in the circulatory system the larvae are carried to the right side of the heart and then into the pulmonary circulation where they are filtered out in the pulmonary capillaries. After entering the alveoli the larvae molt twice to become fourth-stage larvae about 10 days after infection. These fourth-stage larvae migrate up the respiratory tree to the pharynx, where they are swallowed, and pass through the stomach into the small intestine. In the small intestine the larvae undergo the final molt to adults about 25 to 30 days after infection. Shortly after fertilization the female worms begin to release embryonated eggs, producing on the average 200,000 per female per day. Over the normal 17-month life span of the adult female this egg production can amount to a total of 26 million eggs per female. If the eggs are deposited in an ideal environment of shaded, warm, moist soil, they can develop to the infective stage in about 10 to 15 days and may remain infective for many months, perhaps even years.

In cases where individuals accidentally ingest a large number of eggs, some of the larvae that reach the pulmonary capillaries may continue through these capillaries, return to the left side of the heart, and be carried into the systemic circulation. Once in the systemic circulation, larvae may be filtered out and eventually die in organs such as the spleen, liver, or brain. On rare occasions larvae undergoing this abnormal migration are also filtered out in the kidneys and passed in the urine or pass through the placenta of pregnant patients and infect the fetus.

EPIDEMIOLOGY[115]

Ascariasis occurs worldwide but is most prevalent in moist tropical climates; in the United States the disease is most prevalent in the South. In the tropics entire populations are commonly infected. However, in most areas infections with this parasite are usually more common in preschool and early school-age children.[11,49]

Infection often follows ingestion of the egg stage in raw foods, especially if human feces (nightsoil) has been used as fertilizer for vegetable crops. Among children, eating dirt (ge-

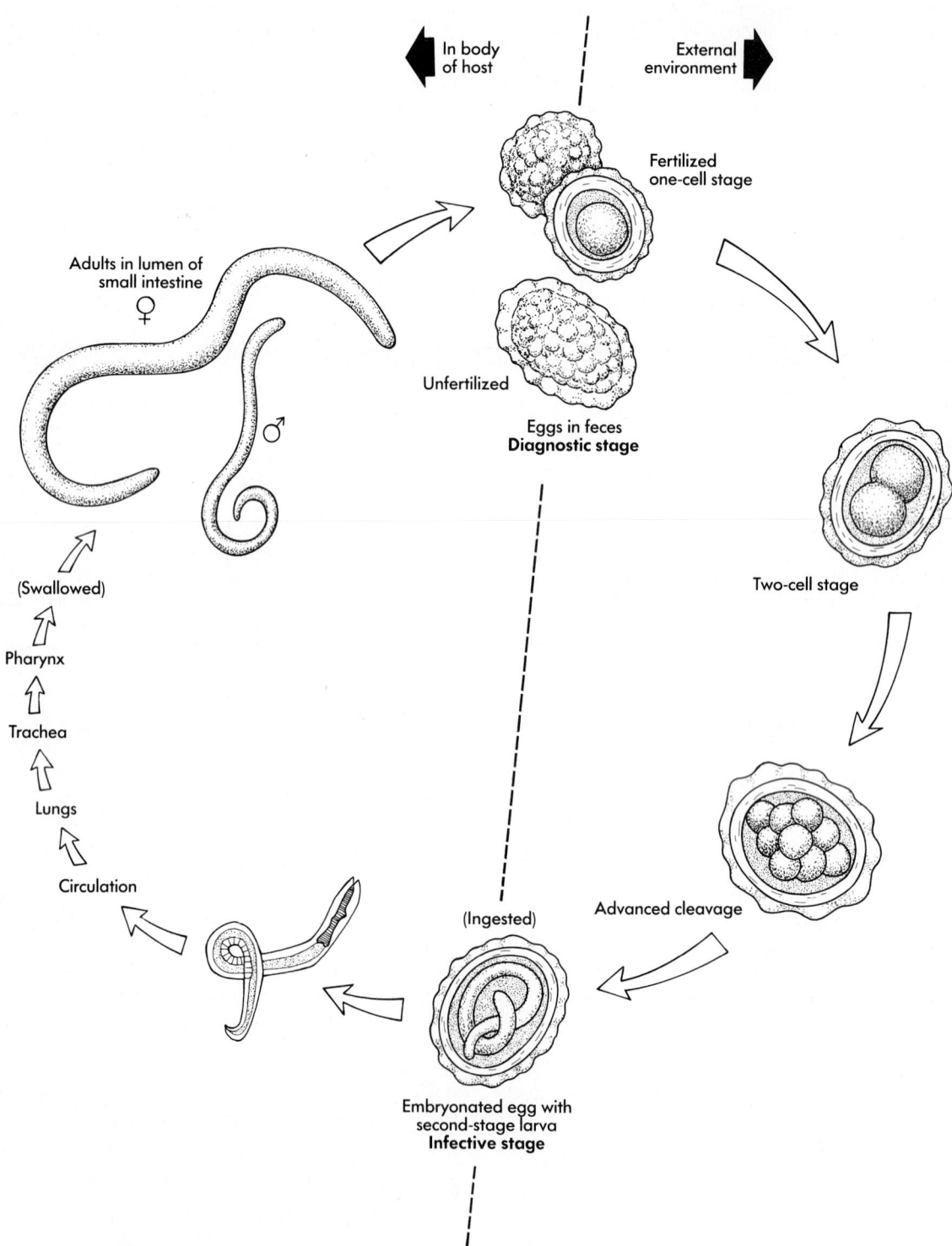

FIGURE 41-5. Life cycle of *Ascaris lumbricoides*. (Modified from Melvin, D.M., Brooke, M.M., and Sadun, E.H.: Common intestinal helminths of man—life cycle charts, Atlanta, 1965, PHS Pub. No. 1235, Laboratory Branch of the Communicable Disease Center.)

ophagia) or placing soiled fingers and toys in the mouth is a common mode of infection.

Although the eggs of *Ascaris* organisms are adversely affected by excessive heat and drying caused by direct exposure to the sun, they are remarkably resistant to most other environmental extremes. Laboratory studies have revealed that the eggs can survive and continue maturation even when immersed in 2% formalin, potassium dichromate, and 50% solutions of acetic, hydrochloric, nitric, and sulfuric acid. Under natural conditions, up to 50% of eggs may remain infective for as long as 10 years. This resistance of eggs to chemicals and their natural longevity make the disease difficult to control even after proper sanitation is initiated.

PATHOLOGY AND CLINICAL MANIFESTATIONS*

The pathologic changes and clinical manifestations brought on by *Ascaris* infections can be divided into two major phases: (1) the pathologic changes and clinical manifestations produced by the migrating larvae and (2) the pathologic changes and clinical manifestations produced by the adult worms.

Larval Migrations

Until the larvae break out of the pulmonary capillaries into the lungs, they generally provoke few pathologic changes or symptoms during their migration. In the lungs, however, small hemorrhages usually occur at each site of larval penetration into the alveoli, and cellular and serous exudate accumulates in the alveolar spaces. These pathologic changes are usually manifest as a fever of 39.5° to 40° C, an asthmatic type of breathing, frequent coughing spasms, and bronchial rales. In severe cases there may be significant pulmonary edema, consolidation of the involved lobules of the lungs, and even complete lobular consolidation and serious respiratory impairment.

In areas where reinfection with *Ascaris* organisms is common, the pulmonary pathologic conditions are often manifest as a more pronounced pneumonia-like syndrome (Loeffler's syndrome). This syndrome is characterized by a slight initial fever and production of abundant yellowish sputum containing eosinophils,[8,95] usually lasts 1 to 3 weeks, and is presumed to be an allergic reaction to larval antigens.

Larvae that pass through the pulmonary circulation and enter the systemic circulation eventually become trapped in small inflammatory nodules. Later these nodules become necrotic and the larvae are destroyed or encapsulated. The clinical manifestations of these abnormal larval migrations depend on the number of migrating larvae and the tissues in which they eventually lodge. The most obvious clinical manifestations of these migrations occur when the larvae lodge in the central nervous system, the eyes, or the kidneys.

Adult Worms

The pathologic changes and clinical manifestations associated with adult worms are related to the ''normal'' metabolism of the adult worms in the small intestine and to ''abnormal'' migrations of the adults.

In the small intestine the adult worms normally feed and metabolize the liquid contents in the lumen of the intestine. The most common reactions to these metabolic activities are colicky epigastric pain and vague abdominal discomfort. However, in

young children harboring large numbers of adult worms, the intensive feeding of the worms may result in malnutrition and retarded development. In patients of all ages, toxemia caused by absorption of metabolic end products of the worms or hypersensitivity to the foreign proteins of the worms or both can result in rashes, restlessness, photophobia, or even conditions resembling meningitis or paraplegia.

Abnormal migrations of adult worms have been associated with administration of certain drugs (for example, tetracycline), disturbances in the host's digestive function, a large ratio of female to male worms, and heavy worm burdens. These abnormal migrations of adult worms produce varied and often serious consequences, including intestinal obstruction if the worms knot together in the lumen of the intestine, appendicitis if worms occlude the appendiceal lumen, perforation of the bowel with subsequent peritonitis, and obstruction of the pancreatic or bile ducts. Adult worms have also been reported to migrate back through the stomach, be vomited, and migrate into the trachea, causing suffocation, or into the eustachian tube and middle ear. Less serious but equally distressing is migration of adult worms out of the nose, mouth, or anus. Because the abnormal migration of even a single worm may have serious consequences, it is imperative that even very light infections be detected and adequately treated.

LABORATORY DIAGNOSIS

The laboratory diagnosis of ascariasis is usually based on finding characteristic fertilized or unfertilized eggs in the feces (Figure 41-6). The typical fertilized eggs found in the feces are unembryonated, measure 60×45 μm, and have a thick, bile-stained shell covered with many small, rounded projections called mamillations. Occasionally, elongate or bizarrely shaped infertile eggs are found in the feces. These infertile eggs usually measure 90×40 μm and may have a distorted mamillated coat. Because each female worm produces an average of 200,000 eggs per day, one or two direct wet mounts are usually sufficient to diagnose an infection with even a small number of worms. If concentration procedures are routinely employed in the laboratory, the flotation type of concentration (for example, zinc sulfate) is not as effective as sedimentation procedures (for example, formalin-ether) in concentrating infertile eggs.

Occasionally a patient recovers adult worms that have migrated out of the nose, mouth, or anus. In such cases the diagnosis can be based on the morphology of the adult worms. The most distinctive features of the adult are its large size (males are 15 to 31 cm long with a ventral curve of the posterior end, and females are 20 to 35 cm long with a straight posterior end) and the presence of three prominent anterior ''lips,'' each with a row of small papillae or teethlike projections.

ANCYLOSTOMA DUODENALE (OLD WORLD HOOKWORM) AND *NECATOR AMERICANUS* (NEW WORLD HOOKWORM)

Two species of hookworms commonly infect humans: *Ancylostoma duodenale* and *Necator americanus*. There are some differences between these two parasites, but their biology, epidemiology, and pathology are sufficiently similar to discuss both as a single topic with notations of major differences.

LIFE CYCLE

Humans are normally infected with hookworms when third-stage filariform larvae penetrate skin exposed to contaminated

---

*References 8, 11-13, 27, 34, 50, 62, 95, 100, 102, 103, and 106.

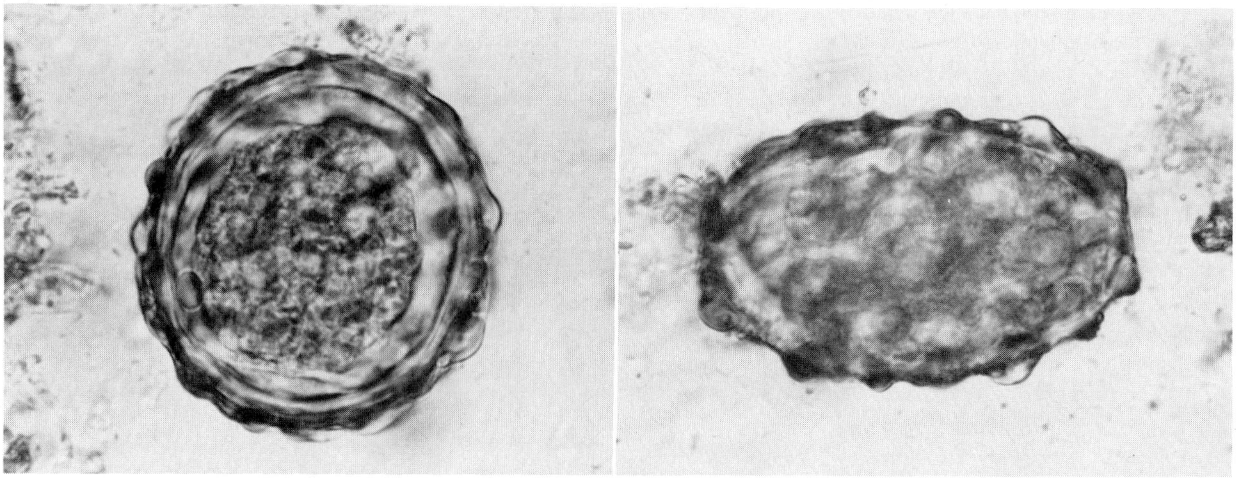

FIGURE 41-6. Eggs of *Ascaris lumbricoides*. **A,** Fertilized. (Approximately ×1200.) **B,** Unfertilized. (Approximately ×850.)

soil (Figure 41-7). A 5- to 10-minute contact with the contaminated soil is usually required for the larvae to penetrate the skin. Penetration may occur at any site on the skin, but the most frequent sites of entry are the areas that normally contact soil: the feet, hands, and buttocks. Filariform larvae may also initiate infection by penetrating the mucous membranes of the oral cavity if they are accidentally ingested. There is also evidence that filariform larvae of *A. duodenale* may be swallowed and complete development to the adult stage without making a lung migration.

By mechanical and lytic action larvae migrate through the epidermis into the dermis and subcutaneous tissues. Once in these deeper tissues larvae find their way into venules and lymphatic vessels, where they are carried to the right side of the heart and then into the capillary beds of the lungs. Larvae that do not reach the circulatory system soon die and are phagocytized.

From the capillary beds of the lungs, the larvae break into the alveoli, migrate up the respiratory tree to the pharynx, are swallowed, and pass down the digestive tract to the small intestine. During this migration or shortly after arrival in the small intestine, the larvae undergo a third molt to become fourth-stage larvae. In the small intestine the fourth-stage larvae attach to the villi and begin to grow, eventually undergoing a final molt to become adults. About 5 weeks after infection the adults reach sexual maturity, fertilization occurs, and the females begin to release eggs. The life span of most adult worms is about 1 year.

If the eggs are deposited on favorable soil—ideally shaded, warm, and moist—embryonation continues and first-stage rhabditiform larvae hatch from the eggs in 24 to 48 hours. These newly hatched larvae feed on organic material and bacteria in the soil for 2 or 3 days and then molt to a second rhabditiform larval stage.* The second-stage rhabditiform larvae feed in the soil for another 2 to 5 days and finally undergo a molt to become infective, nonfeeding, filariform larvae (third-stage larvae).

The filariform larvae, which normally inhabit the thin layer of water that surrounds particles or vegetation in the upper few millimeters of soil, wave in a snakelike fashion in the air while awaiting contact with the bare skin of a suitable host. Under ideal conditions the filariform larvae may survive for several weeks.

EPIDEMIOLOGY[7,11,37,65,96]

Estimates of the prevalence of ancylostomiasis and necatoriasis have been as high as one quarter of the world population. The World Health Organization estimated in 1975 that 450 million people were infected worldwide. The infection is especially common in the tropical farming regions of Africa, Asia, Central and South America, and Caribbean countries where sanitary disposal of feces is poor or absent and soil conditions are optimal for development of the infective larval stage. In the early twentieth century similar conditions existed in the southeastern United States, and it was estimated that 42% of the white population of this region was infected. However, work of the Rockefeller Sanitary Commission between 1910 and 1920 reduced the disease to the present level of 2% to 15%.

Although the geographic distributions of the two species generally overlap, *N. americanus* is generally a more common cause of hookworm infection than is *A. duodenale*. The notable exception is in North America, where *N. americanus* is the predominant, if not the only, species; in Europe and the Mediterranean countries *A. duodenale* predominates.

Susceptibility to the infection varies with race, age, and sex. The infection is more prevalent in whites than in nonwhites, and children and females seem less resistant to infection and development of symptoms than adults or males. Also, as might be expected, the disease is more prevalent in rural areas.

PATHOLOGY AND CLINICAL MANIFESTATIONS*

The pathologic changes and clinical manifestations of hookworm infections can be associated with three phases of the parasite's life cycle: the cutaneous phase associated with penetration of filariform larvae into the skin, the pulmonary phase

---

*Rhabditiform larvae differ from a second larval form, filariform larvae, by being feeding stages with shorter, thicker bodies and a prominent esophagus.

*References 5, 31, 32, 58, 65, 68, and 83.

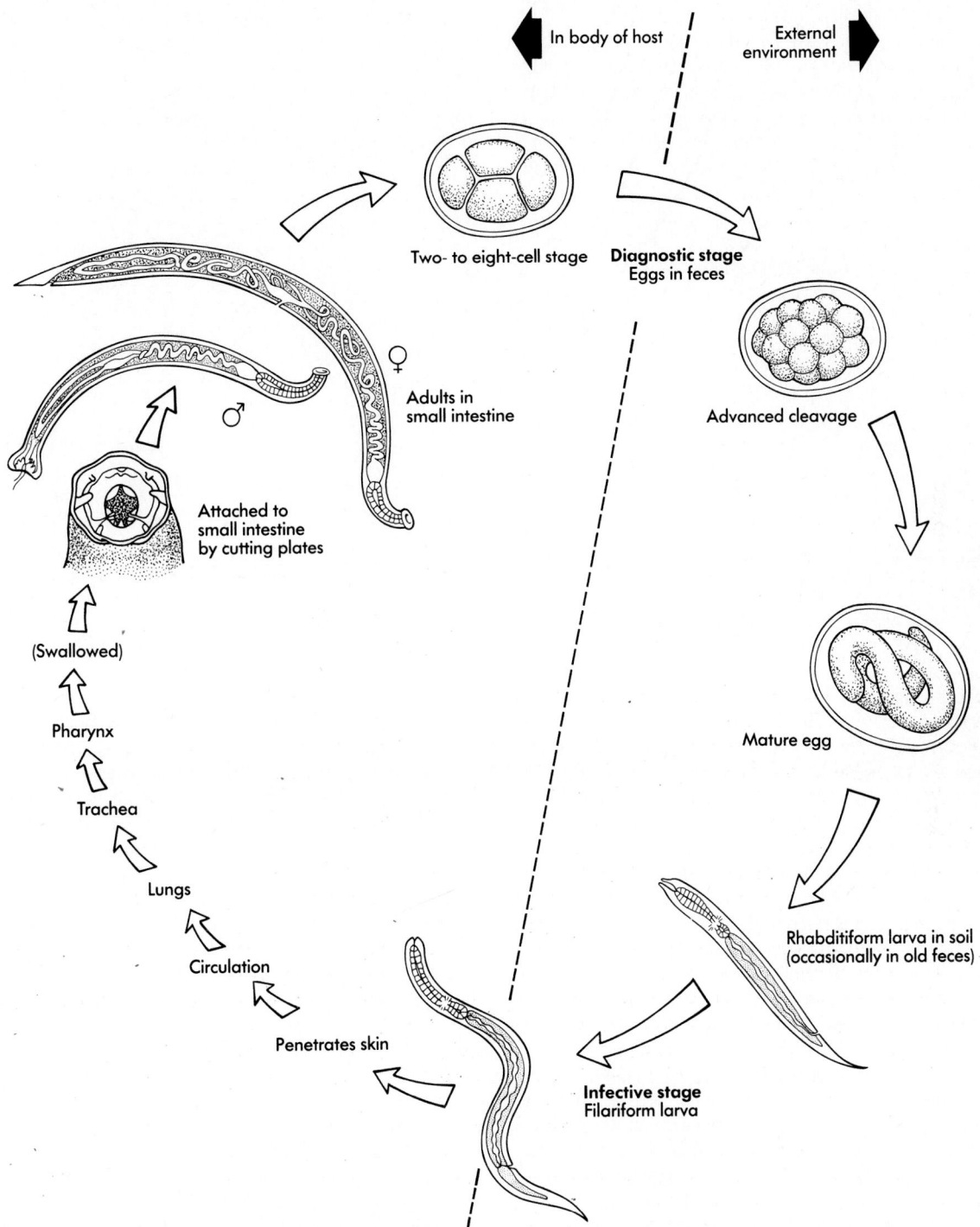

In body of host

External environment

Two- to eight-cell stage

Diagnostic stage
Eggs in feces

Adults in
small intestine

Advanced cleavage

Attached to
small intestine
by cutting plates

Mature egg

(Swallowed)

Pharynx

Trachea

Lungs

Circulation

Rhabditiform larva in soil
(occasionally in old feces)

Penetrates skin

Infective stage
Filariform larva

FIGURE 41-7. Life cycle of *Necator americanus*. *Ancyclostoma duodenale* has similar life cycle except structure of adult worms is different. (Modified from Melvin, D.M., Brooke, M.M., and Sadun, E.H.: Common intestinal helminths of man—life cycle charts, Atlanta, 1965, PHS Pub. No. 1235, Laboratory Branch of the Communicable Disease Center.)

associated with migration of larvae through the lungs, and the intestinal phase associated with the feeding activity of the adult worms.

Cutaneous Phase

During the cutaneous phase a localized dermatitis, commonly called ground itch, occurs at the entry sites of the infective filariform larvae. This dermatitis is characterized by intense pruritus, edema, erythema, and a papulovesicular rash and is usually more severe in *Necator* infections and in individuals with repeated exposure or secondary bacterial infections of the affected area.

Pulmonary Phase

In the pulmonary phase the migration of larvae from the capillaries into the alveoli produces minute hemorrhages and an infiltration of leukocytes. This pathologic condition is usually not clinically apparent and is generally much less severe than the pulmonary pathologic finding of *Ascaris* or *Strongyloides* infections. However, if large numbers of larvae simultaneously migrate through the lungs or if there is a secondary bacterial infection of the lungs, the patient may have fever, headache, nausea, dyspnea, a dry or productive cough, and pharyngitis. In more severe cases pneumonia with pulmonary consolidation or bronchitis may develop.

Intestinal Phase

The most significant pathologic changes and clinical manifestations of hookworm infections are associated with the attachment of the adult worms to the villi of the small intestine and their subsequent ingestion of blood and tissue fluids. In heavy infections a total blood loss of 100 ml/day is not unusual.

During the early intestinal phase of the disease the patient may have a low-grade fever and a variety of nonspecific abdominal complaints such as nausea, vomiting, flatulence, diarrhea, or constipation. These symptoms gradually disappear as the disease becomes chronic.

In the chronic phase of the disease the development of clinical manifestations depends on the number of adult worms present in the intestine and the nutritional status of the host. In infections where there are a large number of worms or the host's diet is deficient in iron, the blood loss produced by the worms' feeding may eventually lead to a characteristic hypochromic microcytic anemia. A relatively mild anemia may not produce any obvious clinical symptoms; however, if the anemia progresses to a moderate form, patients commonly complain of fatigue, headache, shortness of breath, palpitations, numbness and tingling sensations, and gastrointestinal symptoms that include indigestion, loss of appetite, and constipation or diarrhea. When the anemia is severe, patients frequently exhibit pallor, tachycardia, systolic murmurs, a slight hepatosplenomegaly, and a normal diastolic pressure but a diminished systolic pressure. If the host's diet is also deficient in protein, hypoalbuminemia caused by protein loss may develop.

An additional characteristic frequently associated with the chronic phase of the disease is a history of pica, especially the ingestion of soil or any bulky material that may serve to relieve the intestinal discomfort. Children may exhibit irritability and behavioral problems, and in prolonged infections they may suffer retarded physical and mental development. Severe untreated

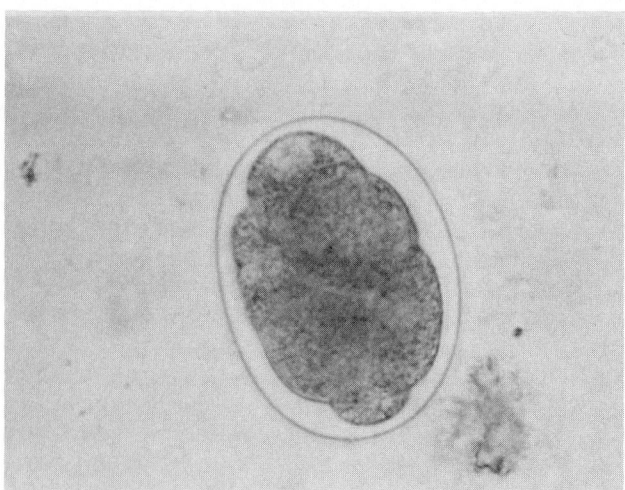

FIGURE 41-8. Egg (unembryonated) of hookworm. (Approximately ×850.)

cases often terminate in physical exhaustion and cardiac failure.

LABORATORY DIAGNOSIS[46]

The definitive diagnosis of hookworm infections is usually based on finding the characteristic unembryonated eggs in the feces (Figure 41-8). Since the eggs of *A. duodenale* and *N. americanus* cannot be distinguished from each other, the appropriate laboratory report on finding eggs in the feces is "hookworm eggs found." Occasionally, if there is a long delay before a fecal specimen is examined or if the specimen is from a constipated patient, the first-stage larvae may develop and hatch from the eggs within the fecal specimen. In such cases it is necessary to distinguish the rhabditiform larvae of hookworms from the rhabditiform larvae of *Strongyloides* and *Trichostrongylus* spp. or the free-living nematodes of the genus *Rhabditis,* any of which may also be found in fecal specimens. The key characteristics in making this distinction are illustrated in Figure 41-9 and include morphology of the buccal cavity (long), size of the genital primordium (small and indistinct), and morphology of the tail (no terminal bulb). An additional clue that may be helpful is that the eggs of *Strongyloides* organisms are rarely if ever seen in fecal specimens. Thus the presence of larvae without any developing eggs or without empty egg shells is strong presumptive evidence that the patient does not have a hookworm or *Trichostrongylus* infection, but rather a *Strongyloides* infection or a stool contaminated with *Rhabditis* organisms.

If definitive identification of the species of hookworm is required, one may use the morphologic characteristics of filariform larvae recovered after in vitro cultivation of the eggs or adults recovered from the feces of patients undergoing therapy. The filariform larvae of *A. duodenale* have a blunt tail and anterior end and measure about 720 μm including the sheath (660 μm without the sheath). The filariform larvae of *Necator* organisms have a rounded anterior and sharply pointed tail and measure about 660 μm including the sheath (590 μm without the sheath). The adult hookworms of both species are characterized by a sharply curved anterior end that gives the worms a hooklike appearance and thus their common name hookworm.

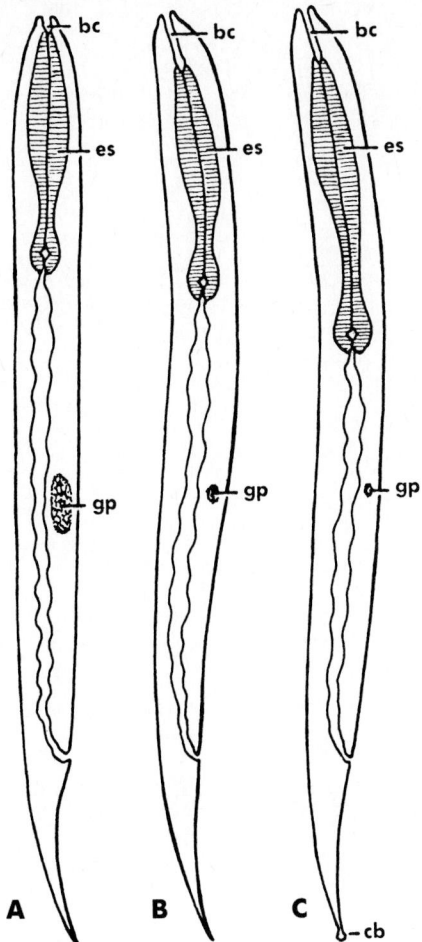

FIGURE 41-9. Rhabditiform larvae. **A,** *Strongyloides*. **B,** Hookworm. **C,** *Trichostrongylus*. *bc,* Buccal cavity; *es,* esophagus; *gp,* genital primordia; *cb,* beadlike swelling of caudal tip. (Illustration by Nobuku Kitamura. From Garcia, L.S.: Laboratory diagnosis of parasitic infections. In Finegold, S.M., et al.: Bailey and Scott's diagnostic microbiology, ed. 5, St. Louis, 1978, The C.V. Mosby Co.)

The two species can be distinguished by a variety of characteristics but most easily by the arrangement and shape of toothlike projections in the buccal (mouth) cavity. The adults of *A. duodenale* can be identified by two pairs of teeth at the anterior margin of the buccal cavity and a small inconspicuous pair of teeth deep in the buccal cavity. The adult *Necator* organisms, on the other hand, have two pairs of "cutting plates" at the anterior margin of the buccal cavity and two pairs of small, inconspicuous teeth near the back of the buccal cavity.

Because a direct fecal smear reliably permits detection of 1200 eggs/ml of feces and each female has a relatively large egg output, most infections can easily be detected at a level well below those likely to produce an anemia. In situations where the patient is likely to be reinfected, specific drug therapy may not be indicated for light infections unless the patient's diet is deficient in iron or protein. Consideration of the patient's diet is often more important in developing countries where generalized malnutrition may exacerbate the development of the anemia, or if the patient has a high-carbohydrate diet, which

can bind and prevent the absorption of any available iron. Even in patients with diets rich in proteins and iron, specific treatment is usually indicated if the worm burden is heavy. Because of these varying indications for treatment, the laboratory may be asked to provide the physician with an estimate of the worm burden. A variety of methods such as the techniques of Stoll and of Beaver and McMaster have been developed for this type of quantitation (see Chapter 40). However, Marcial-Rojas[64] has reported that if an unconcentrated, direct fecal smear contains fewer than 20 eggs per coverglass, treatment is unnecessary unless the patient is malnourished.

Along with the estimates of worm burdens, the hematologic findings are useful for determining the degree of anemia and the necessity for treatment.

STRONGYLOIDES STERCORALIS (THREADWORM)
LIFE CYCLE[36]

Strongyloides stercoralis is one of a unique group of nematodes that have both parasitic and free-living generations and thus appear to bridge the gap between parasitic and free-living modes of existence. The three basic life cycles are the direct, the indirect or heterogonic, and the autoinfection (Figure 41-10).

Direct Life Cycle

The direct life cycle of *Strongyloides* organisms is similar to the life cycle of hookworms. Infection of the host is initiated when third-stage filariform larvae penetrate exposed skin. Once the larvae penetrate the skin, they travel via a route similar to hookworm larvae to the alveoli of the lungs where they reside for several days and molt twice to become juvenile adults. These young adult worms then migrate up the respiratory tree, are swallowed, and complete their development to mature adults in the upper portions of the small intestine.

The only sexually mature stages found in the intestine of humans are females. The female worms, which may survive for as long as a year, burrow into the mucosa of the small intestine and 17 to 28 days after infection begin to release between 30 and 40 embryonated eggs per day.

First-stage rhabditiform larvae hatch from the eggs while they are still in the mucosa, burrow into the lumen of the intestine, and are carried out in the feces. Depending on environmental conditions outside the body, the first-stage larvae may complete a direct type of life cycle by molting into second-stage rhabditiform larvae and then into infective third-stage filariform larvae. Alternatively, the first-stage larvae passed in the feces may initiate the free-living generations of the indirect life cycle by molting through a series of additional rhabditiform stages and finally into free-living males and females.

Indirect Life Cycle

The indirect life cycle is essentially a free-living cycle of the parasite that occurs most frequently in tropical climates where moisture and abundant organic material in the soil support such a cycle. In this cycle rhabditiform larvae passed in the feces develop into free-living males and females in the soil. Once fertilized, the free-living females release partially embryonated eggs, which complete their development to first-stage rhabditiform larvae in the soil and hatch within a few hours. The rhabditiform larvae, which actively feed on organic material in the

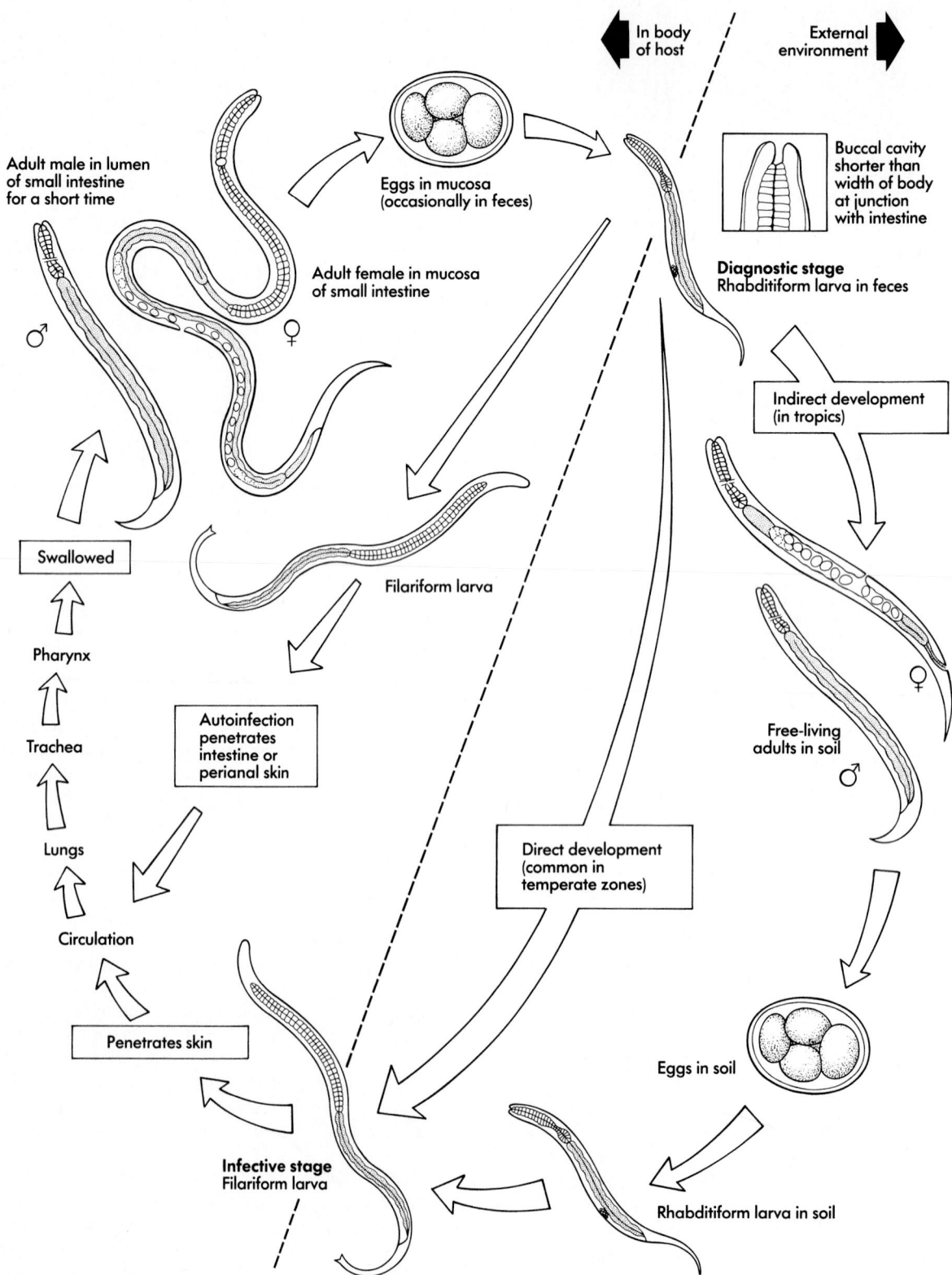

FIGURE 41-10. Life cycle of *Strongyloides stercoralis*. (Modified from Melvin, D.M., Brooke, M.M., and Sadun, E.H.: Common intestinal helminths of man—life cycle charts, Atlanta, 1965, PHS Pub. No. 1235, Laboratory Branch of the Communicable Disease Center.)

soil, in turn develop into more adult male and female worms. Theoretically this cycle could continue as long as the environmental conditions are favorable; however, in most instances it probably continues for only one or two generations. Under conditions that are not clearly defined, free-living rhabditiform larvae in the soil transform into infective filariform larvae that can reinitiate the organism's parasitic cycle.

Autoinfection Life Cycle

Autoinfection occurs when the first-stage rhabditiform larvae in the intestinal tract prematurely molt into filariform larvae that immediately reinfect the host. If this reinfection occurs while the larvae are still within the intestinal tract, it is termed internal autoinfection or hyperinfection. If reinfection occurs when the larvae penetrate perianal skin soiled with feces, it is termed external autoinfection. In either case the larvae undergo the same circulatory-pulmonary-gastrointestinal migration that occurs in the direct cycle.

Autoinfection is particularly significant because it is one of the few situations in which the number of adult helminths harbored by a host can increase in the absence of reexposure to an external source of the parasite or in which a normally short-lived (1 year) infection can persist for many years in the absence of reexposure.

EPIDEMIOLOGY[11,35]

Strongyloidiasis is generally not as prevalent as the other major intestinal nematode infections. Less than 10% of most populations are infected, and the World Health Organization has estimated that there were 35 million cases worldwide in 1975. In general, the disease is more common in tropical and subtropical climates. In rainy areas of some countries, such as Brazil, 85% of the population may be infected. In the southern United States surveys have found a prevalence of 0.4% to 4%. Outside the usual geographic range of infection, strongyloidiasis may also be endemic or epidemic in crowded settings where personal hygiene is poor, especially in mental hospitals.

As would be expected from the similarities in the mode of infection for *Strongyloides* organisms and hookworms, the methods for control of both infections are identical. However, the problem of controlling *Strongyloides* spp. may be complicated by the fact that the parasite occurs in a variety of animals, including dogs and cats; at least one human case has been reportedly contracted from dogs.

PATHOLOGY AND CLINICAL MANIFESTATIONS

The pathologic effects and clinical manifestations of *Strongyloides* infections can be divided into three major phases: cutaneous, pulmonary, and intestinal.

Cutaneous Phase[97]

When there are few invading larvae and the patient has not been previously infected, usually symptoms are absent and the only sign of infection is small papules or macules that develop at the sites of penetration and may be mistaken for insect bites. In cases where large numbers of larvae penetrate the skin, a prominent pruritic erythema develops within 24 hours at the site of infection. If the host is hypersensitive by virtue of previous infections or if a secondary bacterial infection develops at the site of penetration, the cutaneous manifestations are more severe and may include a localized acute inflammatory

response, urticarial rash, petechiae, and edema.

In chronically infected patients the larvae may also produce snakelike tracts in the skin that resemble those seen in patients with cutaneous larval migrans caused by filariform larvae of dog and cat hookworms. Since these tracts advance faster than those seen in cutaneous larval migrans, the condition has been termed larva currens.

Pulmonary Phase

The pathologic findings and clinical manifestations of the pulmonary phase of the disease are highly variable. Generally the penetration of the larvae into the lungs is accompanied by an exudate of neutrophils, lymphocytes, macrophages, and desquamated epithelial cells and a minimal amount of hemorrhage. These pathologic changes usually result in no obvious clinical manifestations. However, if the migration of the larvae up the respiratory tree is delayed by these changes or by underlying pulmonary diseases such as emphysema or bronchiectasis, the larvae may complete their development to the adult stage within the alveoli. This, in turn, can lead to a frank pneumonitis or bronchopneumonia that in the more severe forms may be accompanied by a prominent eosinophilia and resemble the Loeffler's syndrome seen in ascariasis. Other pulmonary manifestations that have been recorded include shortness of breath and coughing up blood. During migration of the worms through the pharynx, patients may have throat irritation and a mild cough.

Intestinal Phase*

The intestinal pathologic changes of strongyloidiasis and in turn the clinical manifestations depend on the severity and duration of the infection and the host's reaction to the parasite. In mild or asymptomatic cases, gross lesions of the intestine are usually absent or minimal. The most common manifestations of the less severe forms of the disease include abdominal pain (93% of cases); diarrhea (78% of cases), which may alternate with constipation; indigestion (66% of cases); and nausea, vomiting, and anorexia (50% of cases).

Intestinal manifestations are particularly severe and may lead to death in patients who are hyperinfected. This type of infection is particularly common in patients who are immunosuppressed by virtue of underlying diseases (for example, hematologic malignancies, autoimmune disorders, or malnutrition) or because of treatment with cytotoxic drugs or corticosteroids. Failure to control the more severe infections may lead to malabsorption or protein-losing enteropathy and ultimately result in the patient's death from intestinal blockage caused by decreased intestinal motility.

LABORATORY DIAGNOSIS[28]

About 70% to 80% of the cases of strongyloidiasis are confirmed by finding characteristic larvae in the feces if the laboratory examines multiple specimens using an appropriate concentration technique. The usual larval stage found in feces is the rhabditiform larva. However, the filariform stage may be present if the patient has been constipated, if internal autoinfection is occurring, or if the fecal specimen has been held at room temperature for 24 to 28 hours before it is examined. Care

---

*References 10, 14, 15, 26, 43, 51, 69, 71, 77, and 81.

in confirming the identity of larvae in feces as *Strongyloides* spp. is essential, since larvae of hookworms or free-living nematodes such as *Rhabditis* organisms occasionally may be found in fecal specimens (see ''Hookworm—Laboratory Diagnosis''). This is most likely to be a problem if the fecal specimen is held at room temperature for an extended period (24 to 48 hours) before examination or if the specimen is contaminated with water or soil.

In patients with very severe infections, the eggs of *Strongyloides* organisms, which are virtually identical to the eggs of the hookworm, may be found in the feces. If an absence of larval stages in these specimens precludes an immediate distinction between a hookworm and a *Strongyloides* infection, larvae can be cultivated from the eggs by the Harada-Mori technique and identified.

If repeated fecal examinations are negative and other likely causes for the patient's condition are ruled out by noninvasive tests, a sample of duodenal contents obtained by intubation and aspiration or the Entero-Test may reveal the larval stage. Similarly, biopsies of duodenal tissue may reveal the adult stage, eggs, and larvae. An associated laboratory finding that may suggest the need for a more invasive procedure is a persistent eosinophilia of up to 40% in the early stages of the disease. In fact, the absence of eosinophils is suggestive of hyperinfection and is a poor prognostic sign.

HYMENOLEPIS NANA (DWARF TAPEWORM) AND *HYMENOLEPIS DIMINUTA* (RAT TAPEWORM)

LIFE CYCLE[2]

Although there are some differences in the life cycle and morphology of *Hymenolepis nana* and *H. diminuta*, these two cyclophyllidean cestodes* are sufficiently similar to warrant their being considered together (Figure 41-11).

In the typical human-to-human cycle of *H. nana*, the infection is acquired by ingestion of infective eggs. In the small intestine the embryo (oncosphere) is released from the egg, penetrates a villus of the small intestine, and develops into a small larval stage known as a cysticercoid. Maturing in 3 or 4 days, the cysticercoid migrates into the lumen of the small intestine where the scolex evaginates and attaches to the wall of the small intestine with the aid of four round suckers and a row of 20 to 30 hooks. About 2 to 3 weeks after infection the adult worm reaches its mature length of 2 to 4 cm and begins to release embryonated eggs as the gravid proglottids (wider than they are long) break off the adult worm and disintegrate while they pass down the intestinal tract.

When passed in the feces, the eggs of *H. nana* not only are immediately infective for humans or rodents but also are infective for numerous species of arthropods, especially rat and mice fleas and grain beetles. If susceptible arthropods ingest infective eggs, they act as intermediate hosts; that is, the oncosphere hatches in the arthropod's intestine and a cysticercoid develops within the body cavity. Should these infected fleas or beetles be ingested by either humans or rodents, the parasite directly transforms into an adult worm in the small intestine of the host; no additional development of the cysticercoid need occur in the intestinal villi of the definitive host.

In contrast to the diverse life cycles possible for *H. nana*, *H. diminuta* has a more restricted life cycle—an arthropod intermediate host is required. One possible explanation for this difference is that the cysticercoids of *H. nana* can develop at a higher temperature (for example, mammal body temperature) than the cysticercoids of *H. diminuta*. Consequently, humans and rodents cannot be infected by ingesting eggs of *H. diminuta;* they must ingest infected arthropods. Among the 90 or more species of arthropods that may act as intermediate hosts, the most common are probably grain or flour beetles of the genus *Tribolium*.

The adult worm of *H. diminuta*, which develops directly from a cysticercoid stage when a rodent (or human) ingests an infected arthropod, is similar to *H. nana* except for its larger size (up to 90 cm long) and the absence of hooks on the scolex. The life cycle is perpetuated when infective eggs are passed in the feces after gravid proglottids break off the adult worm and disintegrate in the feces.

EPIDEMIOLOGY[108,111]

Probably the most common of all the cestode infections of humans, *H. nana* infections occur worldwide and can affect individuals of any age. However, they are most prevalent in warmer climates and in children. The same pattern of infection occurs with *H. diminuta*, although the infection is slightly less common than *H. nana*. In some areas the prevalence of hymenolepiasis may be as high as 25%, but in most areas it is less than 5% of the population. In the United States these infections tend to be more common in the southeastern states with a maximal prevalence of about 3%.

As would be expected with an infection that has a higher prevalence among children, the most common mode of transmission of *H. nana* infections appears to be hand-to-mouth passage of eggs, either from person to person or from play areas contaminated with human or rodent feces. And, although these parasites are normally short lived (2 to 3 weeks), individuals with poor personal hygiene may continually reinfect themselves (autoinfection) with eggs passed in their own feces.

H. diminuta infections, on the other hand, are acquired only by accidental ingestion of infected arthropods because the egg stage is not infective for humans. Thus most of these infections are associated with the consumption of grains, cereals, and similar foodstuffs that have been contaminated by infected grain beetles.

PATHOLOGY AND CLINICAL MANIFESTATIONS[47,111]

Except when adult worms are present in large numbers, no pronounced pathologic changes or clinical manifestations are associated with either *H. nana* or *H. diminuta*. When large numbers of parasites are present, for example, 1000 to 2000 adults of *H. nana*, the patient may have the typical but nonspecific headaches, dizziness, anorexia, diarrhea, and abdominal discomfort presumed to be caused by the absorption of toxic metabolites released by the parasite.

LABORATORY DIAGNOSIS[111]

The recognition and differentiation of these two infections are normally based on detection and identification of the char-

---

*Cyclophyllidean cestodes are characterized by a scolex (head) that has four round suckers; the intermediate host, when present, is a terrestrial animal. A pseudophyllidean cestode is characterized by two lengthwise groovelike suckers on the scolex and has a crustacean as the first intermediate host.

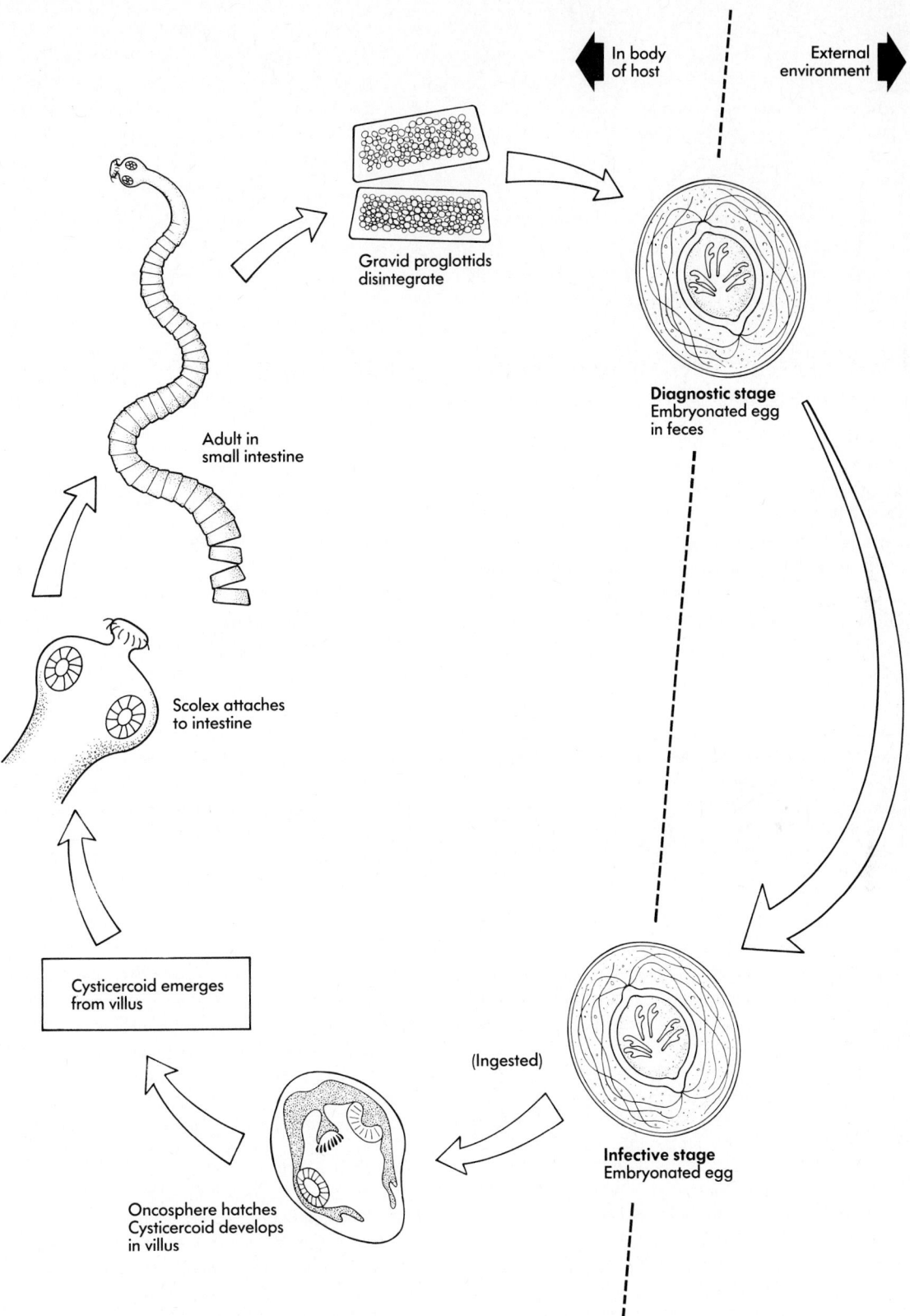

FIGURE 41-11. Life cycle of *Hymenolepis nana*. (Modified from Melvin, D.M., Brooke, M.M., and Sadun, E.H.: Common intestinal helminths of man—life cycle charts, Atlanta, 1965, PHS Pub. No. 1235, Laboratory Branch of the Communicable Disease Center.)

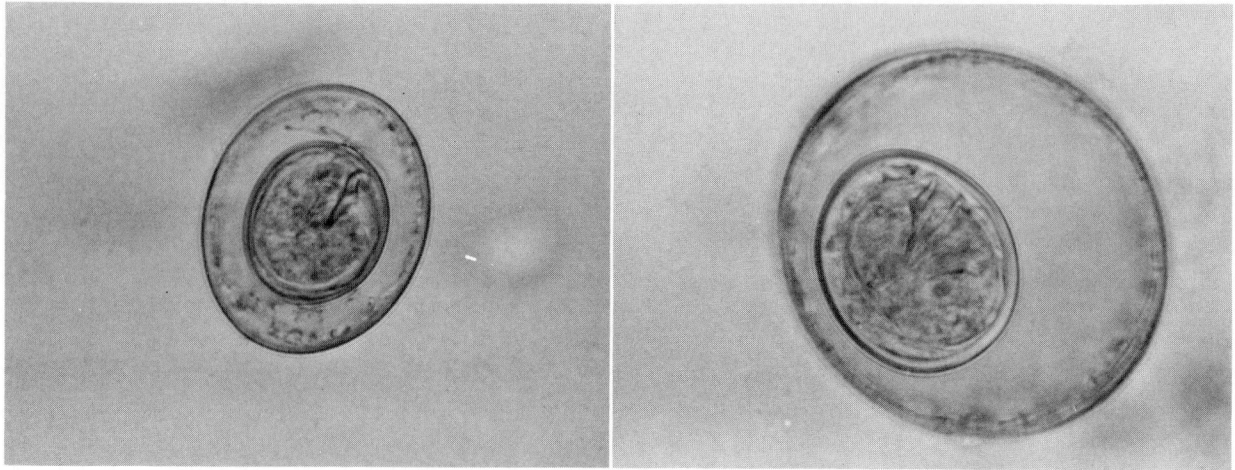

FIGURE 41-12. Eggs. **A,** *Hymenolepis nana.* (Approximately ×850.) **B,** *Hymenolepis diminuta.* (Approximately ×850.)

acteristic eggs passed in the feces. The gravid proglottids of these two parasites usually disintegrate within the intestine and are rarely passed intact in the feces.

The general appearance of the eggs of both species is similar; both have an outer shell surrounding a smaller inner membrane, which encloses the six-hooked oncosphere. The eggs of *H. nana,* however, are smaller (40 to 50 μm in contrast to 50 to 70 μm for *H. diminuta*) and more oval shaped, and they have four to eight filaments attached to thickened areas at the poles of the oncosphere (polar filaments) (Figure 41-12). Because distinguishing the presence of polar filaments and whether an egg is round or oval is often difficult, the difference in size of the two eggs is frequently used as the major criterion for differentiating the two species.

TAENIA SAGINATA (BEEF TAPEWORM) AND *TAENIA SOLIUM* (PORK TAPEWORM)
LIFE CYCLE[72]

The life cycle and morphology of the cyclophyllidean cestodes *Taenia saginata* and *Traenia solium* are similar (Figure 41-13). In both infections the parasite is acquired by ingestion of a larval stage called a cysticercus that is found in the muscle of the intermediate hosts, cattle in the case of *T. saginata* and pigs in the case of *T. solium.*

When a cysticercus of either of these parasites is ingested in raw or improperly cooked meat, the invaginated scolex and neck of the cysticercus evaginate under the influence of bile salts in the small intestine and the scolex attaches to the wall of the small intestine. The scolex of *T. saginata* is attached with only four round suckers; there are no hooks on the scolex. The scolex of T. solium is attached by four round suckers and two rows of hooks located at the anterior end of the scolex (rostellum). At maturity, which occurs 5 to 12 weeks after infection with *T. solium* and 10 to 12 weeks after infection with *T. saginata,* the segmented chain of reproductive structures (proglottids), which stretches behind the scolex, usually measures 2 to 7 meters in *T. solium* and 5 to 10 meters in *T. saginata.*

In both species the embryonated eggs contained in gravid proglottids may be released either (1) within the intestine if the gravid proglottids disintegrate in the intestine or (2) after intact proglottids are passed in the fecal mass or actively migrate out of the anus onto the perianal skin. In either situation the eggs are infective immediately when passed from the body. When the egg is ingested by a suitable intermediate host, the oncosphere is released in the intermediate host's small intestine, penetrates the intestinal wall, and is carried throughout the body by the lymphatics or circulatory system. Most of the oncospheres localize in the muscles and subcutaneous tissues where they transform into the larval cysticercus stage within 2 to 3 months.

Besides being infective for pigs, the eggs of *T. solium* are infective for humans, and the larval cysticerci may develop in human tissue. Known as cysticercosis, this type of infection follows essentially the same development that occurs when the normal intermediate host, the pig, is infected by ingesting the egg stage of the parasite. It is generally believed that the eggs of *T. saginata* are not infective for human, and thus cysticercosis is associated only with *T. solium.*

EPIDEMIOLOGY[80,108,111]

Both *T. saginata* and *T. solium* are found throughout the world, being especially prevalent in areas where there is a combination of improper disposal of human feces and consumption of raw beef or pork. In particular, these parasites are endemic in most of Central and South America and in large parts of the Soviet Union and Africa. In other parts of the world, ethnic or religious customs strongly influence the distribution of the disease. For example, among devout Moslems, who may consume beef but not pork, it is not uncommon to find infections with the adult stage of *T. saginata* but not with the adult stage of *T. solium.* This restriction against the consumption of pork, however, does not protect against the possibility that a person may accidentally ingest the egg stage of *T. solium* and develop cysticercosis. Even in areas where infections with the adult stage of *T. solium* are rare, cysticercosis may be very common if there is poor personal hygiene, which may contribute to a hand-to-mouth transfer of eggs, or improper disposal of feces, which may lead to contamination of food and drink with the infective egg. Individuals infected with the adult stage of *T. solium* have an additional risk of developing cysticercosis. If gravid proglot-

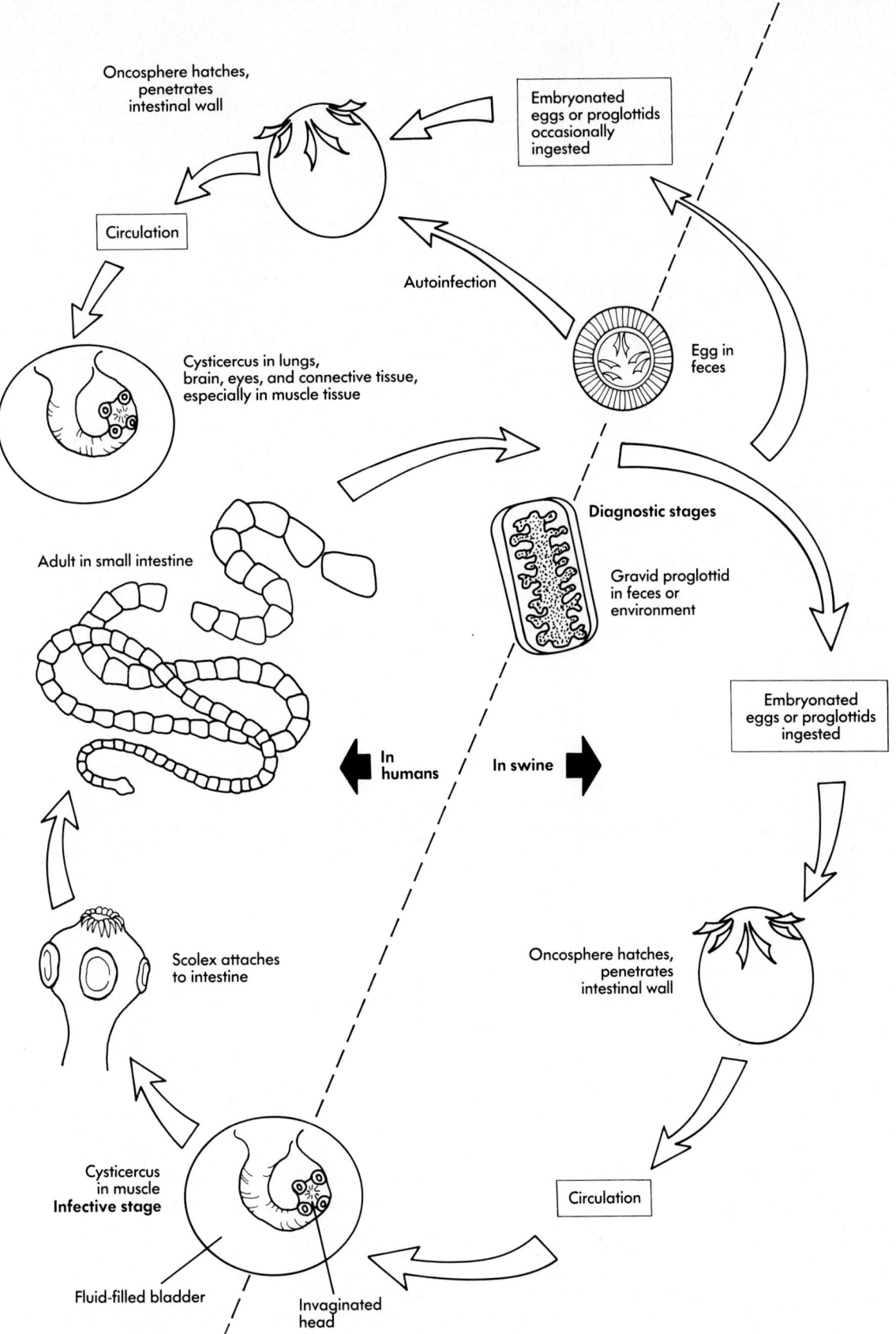

FIGURE 41-13. Life cycle of *Taenia solium*. (Modified from Melvin, D.M., Brooke, M.M., and Sadun, E.H.: Common intestinal helminths of man—life cycle charts, Atlanta, 1965, PHS Pub. No. 1235, Laboratory Branch of the Communicable Disease Center.)

tids either actively migrate or are swept by reverse peristalsis to the upper part of the small intestine in an individual harboring an adult worm, the eggs may hatch, invade the wall of the intestine, and initiate a tissue infection with the larval stage.

Because cysticercosis has serious consequences, it is fortunate that *T. solium* infections are much less common than *T. saginata* infections both worldwide and in the United States. The prevalence of *T. saginata* in the United States is estimated to be 200,000 cases, whereas *T. solium* is much less common and probably accounts for only one of every hundred new human cases of taeniasis.

PATHOLOGY AND CLINICAL MANIFESTATIONS[72,80,111]

Most individuals infected with the adult stage of either of these two tapeworms harbor only a single adult worm and have few if any pathologic changes or clinical manifestations. Despite the traditional folklore that tapeworms deplete the host of a significant amount of nutrients, calculations based on the mass of new proglottids created by the worms during a year suggest that less than 2 pounds of new proglottids are created each year, hardly enough to cause significant malnutrition in an otherwise well-nourished host. The major clinical manifestation and patient complaint (96%) is the passage of motile proglottids. It has been suggested that the vague abdominal complaints and nervous manifestations ascribed to these infections may be psychogenic; that is, patients do not have noticeable abdominal discomfort until they realize that they have a tapeworm infection.

Infections with the larval stages of *T. solium* (cysticercosis) are often more serious than infections with the adult stage alone. In most sites, such as the subcutaneous or muscle tissue, the cysticerci are confined by a fibrous capsule of host origin and do not elicit serious pathologic changes or clinical manifestations unless large numbers die about the same time. However, when cysticerci lodge in the eye, brain, or cardiac muscle, consequences may be serious. For example, cysticerci that lodge in the eye are not confined by the fibrous capsule, and their development may cause irreparable damage to the retina or they may be mistaken for a malignant tumor and result in unnecessary removal of the eye. Those that lodge in the brain may produce a pressure necrosis of the brain tissue and manifestations such as paralysis, disorientation, or most commonly, sudden onset of a parasite-induced epilepsy.

LABORATORY DIAGNOSIS[72,75,85,111]

Infections with the adult of *T. saginata* or *T. solium* can be detected by the passage of eggs or proglottids in the feces (Figure 41-14). However, since the eggs of both species measure 30 to 40 μm in diameter and have thick, radially striated, dark brown shells surrounding developed embryos (oncospheres) containing six small hooklets, the only report that can be made based on egg identification is "*Taenia* sp. found." If definitive identification is required, one must recover and examine either intact proglottids that are being normally passed in the feces or the scolex after treatment has been initiated. Intact proglottids should be gently pressed between two large glass slides (1 × 3 inches) and held to a strong light to determine the uterine structure, specifically the number of major lateral uterine branches. *T. solium* has seven to 13 major branches, whereas *T. saginata* has 15 to 20 branches. If the structure cannot be discerned by simple, direct illumination, injecting the uterus with a small

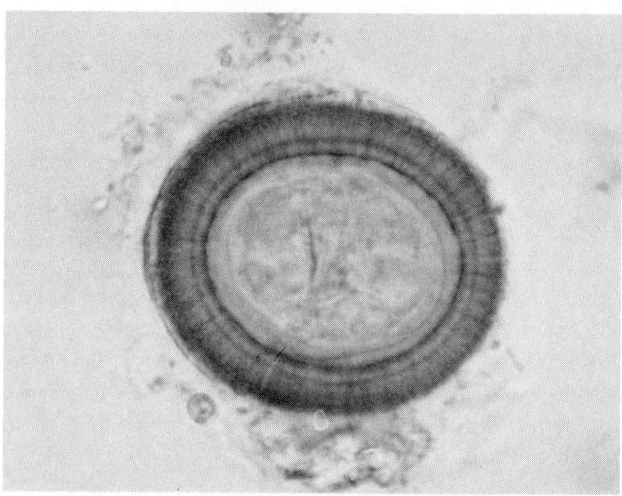

FIGURE 41-14. Egg of *Taenia* spp. (Approximately ×1700.)

amount of india ink to enhance the appearance of the lateral branches is often helpful. If the identification is based on morphology of the scolex, the major criterion is the absence of hooks on the scolex of *T. saginata*.

The diagnosis of cysticercosis is usually based on patient history suggesting probable exposure, recognition of the clinical manifestations, and x-ray films revealing calcified soft tissue lesions that resemble rice grains or puffed rice. Serologic tests such as indirect hemagglutination, counterimmunoelectrophoresis, and indirect immunoelectrophoresis have also proved to be valuable diagnostic tools. For example, the indirect hemagglutination test has been reported to have a sensitivity of 85% and a specificity of 95%. Ultimate confirmation of the diagnosis depends on identification of cysticerci recovered by biopsy.

DIPHYLLOBOTHRIUM LATUM (BROAD TAPEWORM, FISH TAPEWORM)
LIFE CYCLE[105]

The most common pseudophyllidean cestode that infects humans is *Diphyllobothrium latum*. Human infections with this parasite are acquired by eating raw or improperly cooked freshwater fish (second intermediate hosts) infected with the second larval stage (plerocercoid) (Figure 41-15). The adult worm, which reaches maturity in the small intestine about 1 to 2 weeks after infection, typically measures 10 meters (the range is 3 to 15 meters) and is attached to the wall of the intestine by two elongate, groovelike suckers on either side of the tiny, fingerlike scolex; the adult scolex has no hooks. The gravid proglottids, which may constitute as much as 70% of the mature worm, are characteristically broader than they are long (hence the common name, broad tapeworm), and each contains a uterus that resembles the petals of a flower or rosette clustered around a uterine pore or opening in the center of the proglottid. Unembryonated eggs are expelled from the gravid proglottids through this uterine pore and are passed in the feces.

If the eggs reach fresh water, they complete their embryonation to a ciliated embryo (coracidium) in 8 to 14 days, depending on the water temperature. The coracidium emerges from the egg when a tiny lid (operculum) on the top of the egg pops open. The coracidium swims randomly through the water,

SCHISTOSOMA JAPONICUM, SCHISTOSOMA HAEMATOBIUM, AND *SCHISTOSOMA MANSONI*
LIFE CYCLE[53,57,91]

The life cycle and morphology of the three major species of schistosomes that infect humans—*Schistosoma japonicum, Schistosoma haematobium,* and *Schistosoma mansoni* (Figure 41-17)—differ in several significant ways from the life cycles of the other major trematode parasites of humans. The major differences are that (1) schistosome infections are acquired by penetration of exposed skin by infective cercariae rather than by ingestion of metacercariae; (2) the adult worms are not hermaphroditic—they are either male or female; (3) the egg stage is not operculated; and (4) there is only a single intermediate host, a snail.

Infections with all three major species of schistosomes are acquired when cercariae, which measure between 100 and 250 μm in length, depending on the particular species, are released from infected freshwater snails and penetrate exposed skin. On contact with skin the cercariae shed their characteristic forked tails and within 24 hours enter the cutaneous capillaries. Once in the capillaries the cercariae are carried throughout the systemic circulation. However, only cercariae that reach the portal circulation in the liver complete the development to sexually mature adult worms. Even reaching the liver does not ensure final development; once the adult worms have matured in the liver, they must migrate against the venous blood flow to the veins of mesenteries supporting the small or large intestine or the urinary bladder. Generally the adults of *S. japonicum* migrate into veins that drain the small intestine, whereas *S. mansoni* adults usually migrate into the mesenteric veins that drain the large intestine. *S. haematobium* adults migrate into veins of the vesicle plexus near the urinary bladder.

One notable feature of the adult stage of schistosomes is that the adult males, which are 7 to 20 mm long, depending on the species, have a groove (gynecophoral canal) that extends almost the length of the body. During their entire mature life, which may be as long as 25 to 30 years, each male holds one of the slightly larger females in a nearly constant embrace in this canal.

After the worms reach the mesenteric or vesicle plexus veins (about 5 to 6 weeks after infection with *S. japonicum* and *S. mansoni* and 12 weeks for *S. haematobium*), the female worms are fertilized and egg release begins. During egg deposition the female worm leaves the male and migrates into small venules to deposit her eggs. As the female withdraws from the site of egg deposition, the small venules, which are dilated when the female enters them, return to their normal size, leaving the eggs tightly wedged in the venules. The extent to which schistosome eggs become trapped in blood vessels near the wall of the intestine or bladder is directly related to the size of a characteristic spine on the egg. Two of the species have a large spine on each of their eggs; it is more likely that these eggs will be trapped and will penetrate through the adjacent tissues. *S. mansoni* eggs have a large lateral spine, whereas the eggs of *S. haematobium* have a large terminal spine. In contrast, the smaller eggs of *S. japonicum* have a minute lateral spine that may even be missing in some strains of the parasite. Because the eggs of *S. japonicum* are smaller and rounder and lack a large spine, the tendency is greater for its eggs to be swept back into the general circulation and filtered out by the liver, lung, or other organs.

Aided by the action of proteolytic enzymes that are released from the eggs and by the tearing effect of the spines, many of the 3500 eggs released daily by each fertilized female eventually penetrate through the wall of the venule into the adjacent wall of the intestine or bladder and finally into the lumen of the intestine or the urinary bladder. If these embryonated eggs reach fresh water after passing from the body, the eggs hatch, releasing a ciliated embryo (miracidium) that swims about in search of a suitable species of snail to be the intermediate host. If a suitable snail is located, the miracidium penetrates the snail and undergoes a period of development and asexual reproduction (two generations of sporocysts) that ends with the release of infective cercariae 4 to 8 weeks after the snail is infected.

EPIDEMIOLOGY*

Among the three major species of human schistosomes there are significant differences in geographic distribution, importance of reservoir hosts, and species of snail that are suitable intermediate hosts.

S. mansoni is probably the most widely distributed of the three species, with significant foci of infection in South America, Africa, and some of the Caribbean islands. However, the infection is derived almost exclusively from human sources because there are very few reservoir hosts, aside from a few wild primate species and perhaps some rodents. The major intermediate hosts for this species are snails of the genus *Biomphalaria.*

The principal foci of *S. japonicum* infections are parts of Asia, including Japan, China, and the Philippines. Unlike *S. mansoni* infections, reservoir animals play an important role in maintaining this infection in nature because numerous species of wild and domestic animals such as rats, mice, dogs, cats, cattle, horses, pigs, and sheep may be infected. Also, a different genus of snail, *Oncomelania,* serves as the primary intermediate host.

S. haematobium infections are most prevalent in Africa, especially in the Nile Valley. Other foci of infection have been found in parts of the Near East and India. As in *S. mansoni* infections, humans appear to be a major source of infection with this parasite. However, another genus of snail, *Bulinus,* serves as the primary intermediate host.

Fortunately none of these major schistosome infections of humans occurs naturally in North America. However, in many areas of the world where there are natural foci of these infections the prevalence of schistosomiasis has steadily and sometimes dramatically increased. Generally this increasing prevalence can be related to two factors: a lack of proper feces disposal and an increase in the population of susceptible snail hosts as open irrigation systems are extended. In Egypt, for example, development of more extensive irrigation systems after completion of the Aswan High Dam was accompanied by the appearance of *S. haematobium* infections in areas previously free of the disease.

PATHOLOGY AND CLINICAL MANIFESTATIONS†

The pathologic changes and clinical manifestations of schistosome infections can be divided into three major phases: mat-

---

*References 1, 53, 63, 91, 107, and 108.
†References 3, 4, 18, 21-23, 33, 70, 79, 91, 93, 94, 109, 110, and 116.

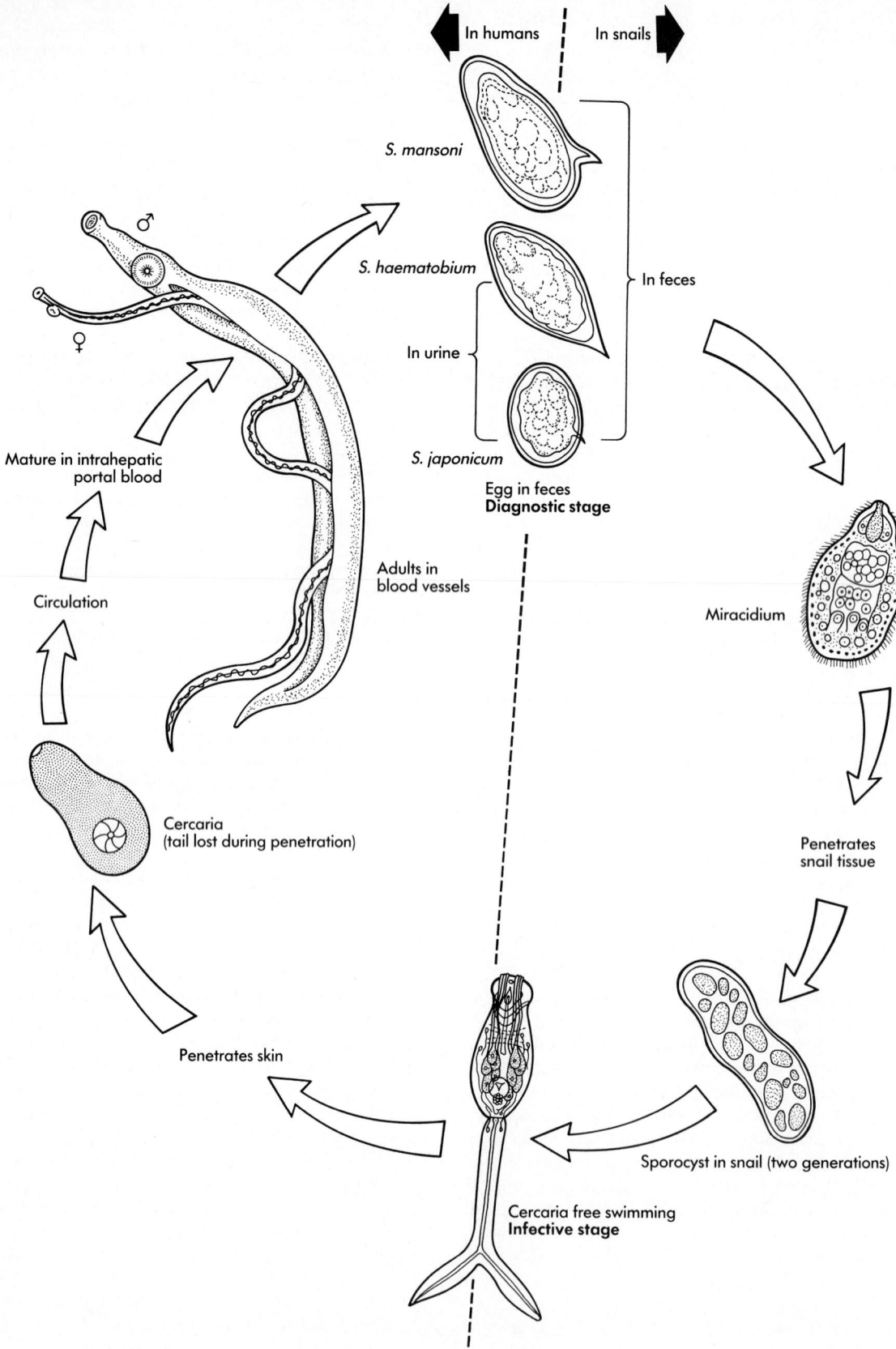

FIGURE 41-17. Life cycle of schistosomes. (Modified from Melvin, D.M., Brooke, M.M., and Sadun, E.H.: Common intestinal helminths of man—life cycle charts, Atlanta, 1965, PHS Pub. No. 1235, Laboratory Branch of the Communicable Disease Center.)

uration of the parasite, especially during the development of the parasite in the liver; the period of egg deposition; and the long-term host tissue reaction. Whereas the first of these three phases represents a reaction of the host to the worm itself, the other two phases, which account for the most serious pathologic changes, are related primarily to the host response to eggs and their metabolites.

During the maturation phase the earliest manifestation is a dermatitis where the cercariae have penetrated the skin. Most prominent about 24 to 36 hours after infection, this so-called schistosome dermatitis may be particularly severe when cercariae of schistosomes for which humans are not hosts penetrate the skin. (In this case the cercariae do not complete their development to adult worms.) Later, as the larvae migrate through the lungs, hemorrhage is common, along with a localized infiltration of eosinophils, epithelioid cells, and giant cells around the pulmonary vessels; this condition is outwardly manifest as a cough with hemoptysis. After the immature worms reach the liver and begin their maturation, the secretion of metabolites often provokes hepatitis syndrome of short duration.

In the second phase of pathologic changes, which are associated with migration of worms to the mesentery veins and the beginning of egg deposition about 1 to 3 months after infection, the host often has a serum sickness–like syndrome (Katayama syndrome or acute schistosomiasis). In *S. japonicum* and *S. mansoni* infections this stage is characterized by allergic manifestations, eosinophilia, fever, abdominal pain, and diarrhea. In *S. haematobium* infections the same general manifestations are present except that frequently hematuria and dysuria are present instead of diarrhea.

The final phase of pathologic changes, the chronic phase, has a more prolonged onset and duration while extensive hyperplasia, infiltration of leukocytes, and eventually fibrosis develop around the sites of egg deposition. With time the continued fibrosis of normal tissue may lead to serious functional impairment and stenosis of the intestine or urinary system.

Equally or even more serious pathologic changes during the chronic stage of the disease result from inflammation and fibrosis around eggs that are swept by the blood from the site of their initial deposition to internal organs such as the liver, lungs, and brain. Because of differences in the shape and site of egg deposition, these manifestations are usually more pronounced in infections caused by *S. japonicum* and least common in *S. haematobium* infections.

In heavy infection, eggs swept back and filtered out in the liver provoke a severe inflammation and fibrosis around branches of the portal vein that characteristically make the liver appear to be studded with clay pipes, a condition commonly called pipe-stem fibrosis. As a consequence of this fibrosis, the blood flow through the liver is slowed, causing a back-pressure hypertension and enlargement of the spleen and liver. As the body attempts to compensate for this reduced blood flow by creating alternate venous pathways, some of which go to the lungs, eggs are sometimes swept into the lungs, where the process of inflammation and fibrosis begins anew. In addition to inducing pathologic changes in the liver and lungs, eggs may also be swept into the brain or spinal cord and induce localized lesions that are manifest as focal neurologic disorders.

One final pathologic change that is still being debated is the possibility that continued irritation of the bladder by eggs of *S. haematobium* may be responsible for inducing cancer of the urinary bladder. A significant relationship between chronic *S. haematobium* infections and squamous cell tumors of the bladder has been noted in Egypt and the Sudan. This relationship, however, does not seem to be as significant in other areas where the infection is also prevalent.

LABORATORY DIAGNOSIS[53,63,91]

The laboratory techniques for diagnosis of schistosomiasis are based primarily on recovery of the egg stage in feces, urine, or biopsy specimens. Serologic techniques may be employed as an alternative in cases where the egg stage cannot be recovered.

In general, the eggs of *S. japonicum* and *S. mansoni* may be detected in fecal specimens or intestinal biopsies, and the eggs of *S. haematobium* may be found in urine specimens or biopsy samples from the urogenital tract. Occasionally there is a "crossover" in this pattern of egg release; eggs of *S. japonicum* or *S. mansoni* are found in the urine, and *S. haematobium* eggs in the feces.

The longer the infection remains, the more difficult it is to demonstrate eggs in simple fecal or urine specimens. Because of the fibrotic reaction that traps the eggs in the walls of the intestine or bladder, usually the eggs are shed at irregular intervals and in low numbers. It is therefore essential that examination of each fecal or urine specimen in cases of suspected schistosomiasis include a sedimentation concentration technique and that numerous specimens be examined over several weeks. If repeated fecal examination is unsuccessful, resorting to biopsies of the intestinal or urinary bladder walls may be necessary in an attempt to discover the eggs in situ. If the biopsies fail to reveal the characteristic eggs, serologic tests may be needed.

The standard formalin–ether or ethyl acetate technique is an acceptable concentration technique for general fecal examination. However, when suspicion of schistosomiasis is strong, a modification of the formalin-ether technique, such as the AMS III technique, may give better results. Most of these modified techniques incorporate the use of weak acid solutions and detergents to help separate the eggs from encapsulating fibrous material.

Essentially the same techniques used for fecal specimens may also be used for urine; however, additional precautions and techniques enhance egg recovery from urine. First, the number of eggs released from the bladder wall varies according to the time of day, and the maximum numbers are usually present in specimens collected between 10 AM and 2 PM. This follows a different pattern from that for bacterial infections of the urinary tract, where the best recovery is from a first morning specimen. The explanation for this difference is that, because the eggs are trapped in the bladder wall, movement of the bladder during early morning urination forces the release of eggs from the wall and the eggs appear in the later specimens.

Urine specimens should be placed in some type of fixative solution if they cannot be examined within 1 or 2 hours after specimen collection. If examination of unpreserved specimens is delayed, the miracidium within the egg may hatch and make identification more difficult.

Finally, concentration techniques other than formalin-ether may prove useful for detecting eggs in urine. One of these techniques, which is similar to the method used to detect the microfilariae of the tissue nematodes, is to filter about 10 ml of the urine through a membrane filter with a porosity of 8 μm and allow the filter to dry face down on a microscope slide. Just before examination the filter is moistened with a drop of immersion oil, which clears the filter and allows examination for the eggs.

If biopsy specimens are submitted to the microbiology laboratory, the simplest method of examination is to press the tissue between two large (2 × 3 cm) glass slides and examine the unstained tissue for trapped eggs.

When recovered in these various specimens, the eggs of all *Schistosoma* spp. are embryonated (contain a developed miracidium) and lack the operculum that is seen in eggs of other species of trematodes. The distinction among the eggs of the different species of schistosomes is based on their overall size and the size and location of spines that project from the egg shell. The typical eggs of *S. japonicum* measure 55 to 85 μm in length and 40 to 60 μm in width and have a tiny lateral spine that may be absent in some strains of the parasite. The eggs of *S. mansoni* are usually 114 to 180 μm long by 45 to 75 μm wide and have a prominent, thorn-shaped lateral spine (Figure 41-18). Eggs of *S. haematobium* are 112 to 170 μm long and 40 to 70 μm wide and have a prominent spine projecting from one end of the egg.

Special tests such as the miracidium hatching test (see Chapter 40) may be used when it is necessary to determine whether the eggs are viable. Usually these tests are required only when there is a question of whether a schistosome infection is still active or is an old "burned-out" infection in which dead eggs are still trapped in the tissue.

FASCIOLOPSIS BUSKI
LIFE CYCLE

The life cycle of *Fasciolopsis buski* (Figure 41-19) is similar to the life cycles of the other major hermaphroditic trematodes infecting humans; that is, there are two intermediate hosts and the first intermediate host is a species of aquatic snail. However, the second intermediate hosts for this parasite are aquatic plants instead of aquatic animals; the infective larval stage (metacercaria) is encysted on the nuts or roots of aquatic plants such as water caltrops, water chestnuts, and bamboo. When nuts or roots of these plants are eaten raw or uncooked, the metacercariae excyst in the small intestine and attach to its wall, where they develop into mature adults in about 3 months. The adults, which are typically 50 to 75 mm long, are the largest of all the major trematode parasites of humans.

For the life cycle to continue, the characteristic operculated eggs, which are passed unembryonated in the feces, must reach fresh water containing snails that are suitable first intermediate hosts and water plants that are suitable second intermediate hosts. In fresh water the eggs complete embryonation to a miracidium in about 3 to 7 weeks, depending on the water temperature. After emerging through the operculum of the egg, the miracidium swims about seeking a suitable snail host (*Hippeutis*, *Segmentina*, or *Planorbis* spp.). Penetrating the tissues of one of these snail hosts, each miracidium transforms through three asexual reproductive stages (a sporocyst and two rediae stages) into the cercarial stage. About 30 to 50 days after infection the cercariae begin to emerge from the infected snail and swim about in search of a suitable water plant host. The cercariae penetrate the tissues of these plants, encyst, and transform into infective metacercariae.

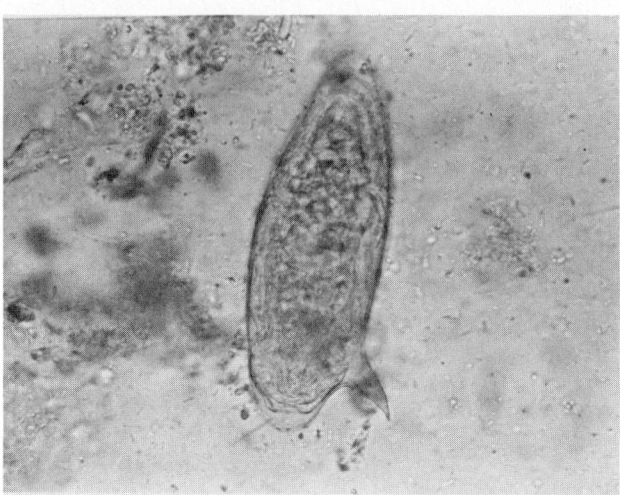

FIGURE 41-18. Egg of *Schistosoma mansoni*. (Approximately ×425.)

EPIDEMIOLOGY[88]

With an estimated prevalence of 10 million human cases worldwide, *F. buski* is particularly prevalent in the Far East. In certain rural areas of Bangladesh, Taiwan, Thailand, and Vietnam, as much as 20% to 40% of the population may be infected. In many areas of high prevalence the infection is maintained by agricultural practices that promote a life cycle in which pigs act as a definitive host. The feces of infected pigs are used to fertilize commercial crops of water plants, which are sold for human consumption and used to feed the pigs. The use of feces from infected humans as fertilizer for commercial crops also maintains an endemic presence of the parasite.

Normally the metacercariae of the parasite cannot survive drying, and thus only freshly harvested plants constitute a source of infection. However, in an effort to present their products as fresh, vendors frequently sprinkle the plants with water, preventing the drying that would naturally destroy the metacercariae.

PATHOLOGY AND CLINICAL MANIFESTATIONS[74]

Most individuals with fasciolopiasis harbor only a small number of worms and are asymptomatic. However, in heavy infections there may be extensive ulceration, localized inflammation, and hemorrhage at the attachment site of each adult worm. These patients most commonly have vague abdominal complaints that include alternating periods of diarrhea and constipation, abdominal pain that may mimic a duodenal ulcer, and a feeling of constant hunger. Severe infections, especially in children, are often accompanied by edema and ascites that are presumably caused by a hypersensitivity to toxic metabolites released by the adult worms.

LABORATORY DIAGNOSIS

The laboratory diagnosis of *F. buski* is usually based on detection and identification of the unembryonated eggs passed in the feces (Figure 41-20). The typical eggs of this parasite, which are operculated and measure 120 to 180 μm (average is 150 μm) in length and 60 to 100 μm (average is 80 μm) in width, are among the largest of all the helminth eggs.

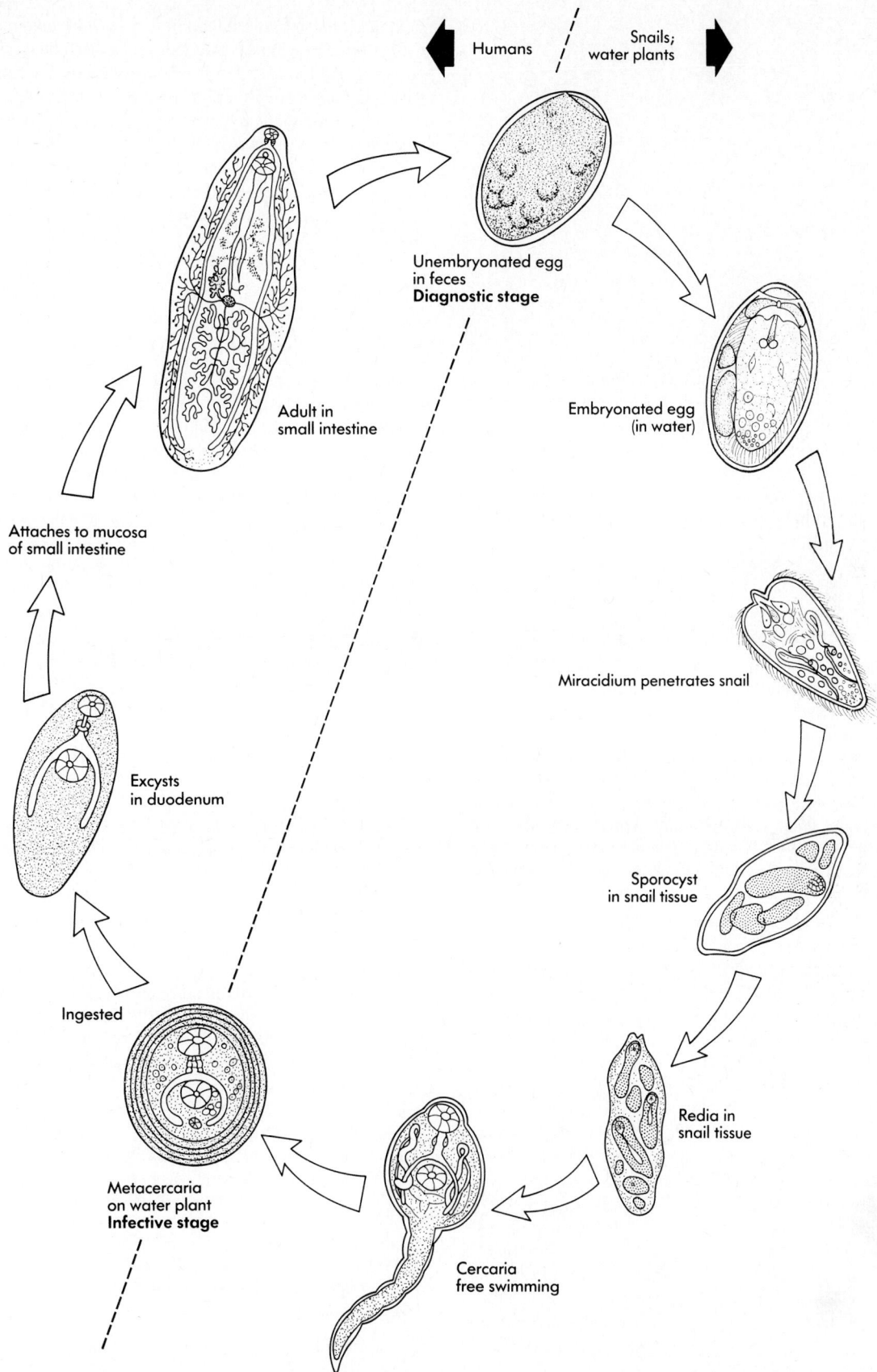

Humans   Snails;
water plants

Unembryonated egg
in feces
Diagnostic stage

Adult in
small intestine

Embryonated egg
(in water)

Attaches to mucosa
of small intestine

Miracidium penetrates snail

Excysts
in duodenum

Sporocyst
in snail tissue

Ingested

Redia in
snail tissue

Metacercaria
on water plant
Infective stage

Cercaria
free swimming

FIGURE 41-19. Life cycle of *Fasciolopsis buski*. (Modified from Melvin, D.M., Brooke, M.M., and Sadun, E.H.: Common intestinal helminths of man—life cycle charts, Atlanta, 1965, PHS Pub. No. 1235, Laboratory Branch of the Communicable Disease Center.)

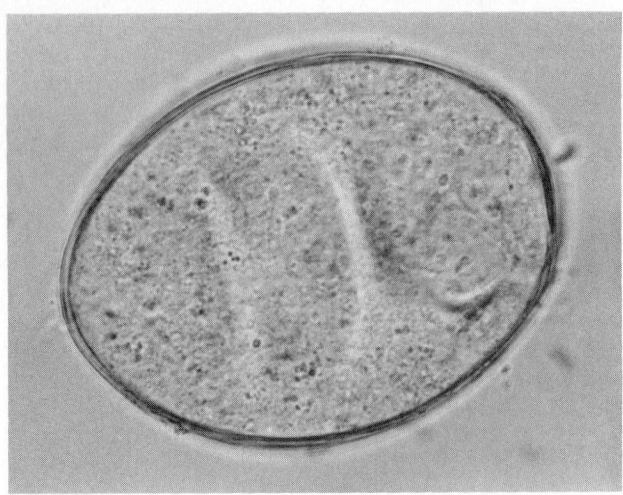

FIGURE 41-20. Egg of *Fasciolopsis buski*. (Approximately ×600.)

The average adult worm produces 25,000 eggs per day, and even a light infection should be readily detectable by direct fecal examination. Unfortunately the definitive identification of *F. buski* based on recovery of the eggs alone is complicated by their similarity to eggs of other species of intestinal trematodes belonging to the genus *Fasciola*, especially *F. hepatica*. The average size of the eggs of these two species differs slightly with *F. buski* eggs measuring, on the average, 150 by 90 μm and *F. hepatica* eggs measuring an average of 150 by 80 μm. The size range of the eggs of these two species overlaps, and it is common practice to report the finding of eggs of these parasites as *"Fasciola/Fasciolopsis."*

Slight differences in the epidemiology of the two infections may provide clues to the correct identification. For example, *F. buski* is generally a more common infection and is more likely to occur in Asian countries where pigs constitute a reservoir for the parasite. *F. hepatica*, on the other hand, is generally rare in humans and is more prevalent in sheepherding countries because sheep are the normal definitive host and humans are considered only an accidental host. The most definitive technique for differentiating the two species is examination of the adult parasite, but this method is rarely employed because it almost always requires surgical removal of the worms.

FASCIOLA HEPATICA
Life Cycle

The life cycle of *Fasciola hepatica* is nearly identical to the life cycle of *Fasciolopsis buski*. The major difference is that when larvae of *Fasciola* organisms emerge from metacercariae in the small intestine, they do not simply attach to the wall of the small intestine and grow to adults as do *Fasciolopsis* larvae. Rather, they penetrate through the intestinal wall and wander in the peritoneal cavity until they locate the surface of the liver. The larvae then penetrate the liver and migrate to the bile ducts where they develop into sexually mature adults. The total time from ingestion of the metacercariae to development of mature adults is about 3 months.

Epidemiology[29,40,52]

F. hepatica infections are widespread and fairly common in ruminant animals such as sheep, goats, cattle, and horses. In humans, however, the infection is relatively uncommon, with Cuba, southern France, Algeria, and other countries in Latin America and the Mediterranean basin the foci of most human cases. In the United States the infection is common in cattle and sheep in the southern and western states, but indigenous human cases are rare. Presumably this low rate of infection is because the U.S. diet rarely includes the raw water plants that harbor the infective metacercarial stage. Aside from these differences in the distribution, the prevalence of animal and human infections, and the different snail intermediate hosts (from the genera *Lymnaea*, *Stagnicola*, and *Fossaria*), most of the epidemiologic characteristics of *F. hepatica* infections are similar to those of *F. buski*.

Pathology and Clinical Manifestations[39]

Fascioliasis in humans is characterized by two distinct clinical phases and very low worm burdens, usually only two worms. The first phase, which occurs as larvae migrate through the liver about 6 to 9 weeks after infection, is associated with necrosis and fibrosis of the liver parenchyma. This liver damage is usually manifest clinically as fever, abdominal pain, diarrhea, and eosinophilia. In more severe infections or in individuals who are particularly sensitive to toxic metabolites secreted by the developing worm, hepatomegaly, urticaria, myalgia, and jaundice may occur.

In the second phase of the infection, which takes place after the larvae migrate to their final development site in the bile ducts, most of the early clinical manifestations of the disease disappear. In the rare instances of a heavy worm burden, however, there may be extensive inflammation, epithelial hyperplasia, and fibrosis around the adult worms and even partial or complete occlusion of the bile ducts.

Laboratory Diagnosis[39]

The laboratory diagnosis of *F. hepatica* infections is usually based on detection and identification of the operculated, unembryonated eggs passed in the feces. However, this presents several difficulties. A major concern is that clinical manifestations of *F. hepatica* infections are most prominent before the adult worms have reached maturity, and by the time eggs are being produced, the clinical manifestations have usually subsided. In this situation, diagnosis usually depends on a strong clinical suspicion of the cause of the early manifestations and persistence by the physician in requesting repeated stool examination even after the early symptoms have subsided.

One final problem is the possibility of a false-positive diagnosis in individuals who have consumed liver from infected animals. In these cases, eggs that are seen during an initial fecal examination would not be present in subsequent fecal specimens, provided the patient has not consumed more infected liver.

CLONORCHIS (OPISTHORCHIS) SINENSIS (CHINESE LIVER FLUKE), *OPISTHORCHIS VIVERRINI*, AND *OPISTHORCHIS FELINEUS*
Life Cycle[42,56]

The trematodes *Clonorchis sinensis*, *Opisthorchis viverrini*, and *O. felineus* have identical life cycles (Figure 41-21), and there are only slight differences in the morphology of the various stages of the parasites. Human infections with these parasites are acquired by ingestion of raw or improperly cooked fish containing cystlike larval states (metacercariae). Once swal-

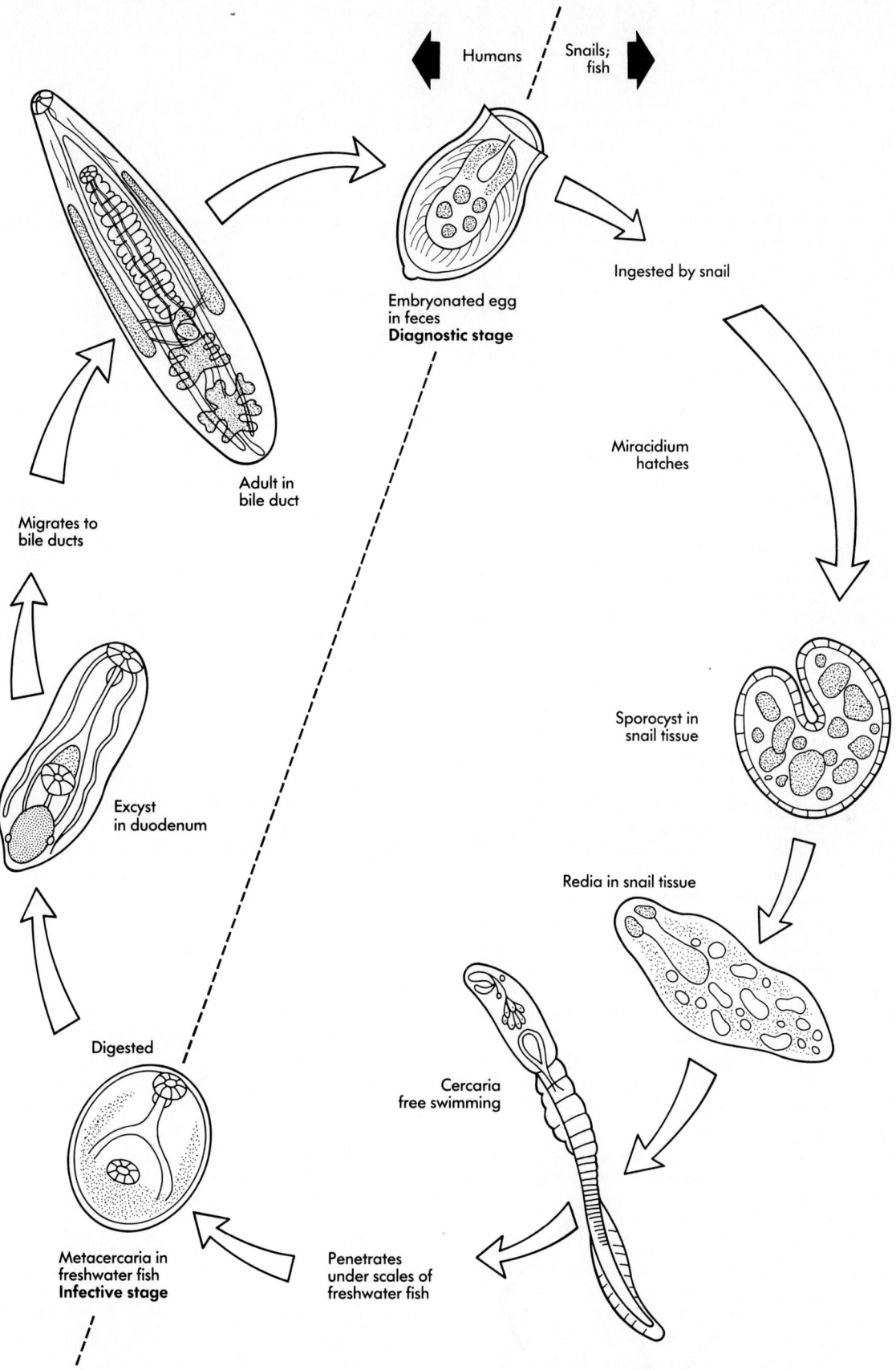

FIGURE 41-21. Life cycle of *Clonorchis sinensis*. (Modified from Melvin, D.M., Brooke, M.M., and Sadun, E.H.: Common intestinal helminths of man—life cycle charts, Atlanta, 1965, PHS Pub. No. 1235, Laboratory Branch of the Communicable Disease Center.)

lowed, the metacercariae excyst in the duodenum, migrate into the bile ducts, and develop into mature adults in about 1 month. The adults of *C. sinensis* measure 1 to 2.5 cm long and 0.3 to 0.5 cm wide. Adults of the two species of *Opisthorchis* are nearly identical to *Clonorchis* organisms: the three species are usually distinguished by the arrangement of the testes and the size of the oral sucker.

For the life cycle to continue, the embryonated eggs passed in the feces must reach fresh water containing species of snails that are suitable first intermediate hosts and fish that are suitable second intermediate hosts. One of the unique features at this point in the life cycle of these parasites is that the embryo (miracidium) does not hatch from the eggs until after the eggs are ingested by suitable snail intermediate hosts (for example, *Parafossarulus*, *Bulimus*, and *Bythnia* spp.). After ingestion by the snail, the miracidia hatch, penetrate the snail's internal tissues, and transform through a series of asexual reproductive stages (sporocysts and rediae). This transformation and asexual reproduction within the snail are complete in 2 to 3 months and result in the formation of large numbers of cercariae. The short-lived cercariae emerge from the snail and swim through the water seeking a suitable second intermediate host, any of 40 species of freshwater fish, especially members of the family *Cyprinidae*.

On contact with a susceptible species of fish, the cercariae penetrate the scales and migrate to the underlying muscles, where they transform into infective metacercariae by rounding up and secreting a cyst wall. This final transformation to the infective stage takes about 3 weeks.

EPIDEMIOLOGY[42,56]

Clonorchiasis and opisthorchiasis may be considered zoonoses in which the principal definitive hosts are domestic (for example, dogs and cats) and wild animals (for example, mink and rats) that feed on fish. However, in areas of the world where raw fish is considered a delicacy, human infections probably number in the millions. The use of human or animal feces as fertilizer in ponds where freshwater fish are commercially harvested increases the probability of human infection.

Given the factors that contribute to human infection, it is not surprising that these infections are most common in the Far East. In particular, *C. sinensis* infections are common in Japan, Korea, China, and Vietnam. *O. felineus* infections also occur in Asia, but they are most prevalent in Eastern Europe and the Soviet Union. *O. viverrini* is found principally in Southeast Asia, especially Thailand, where approximately 90% of the population in the northeastern region is infected. These infections are rarely seen in the United States except among immigrants from Asia or individuals who have eaten raw or improperly cooked fish shipped into the United States from endemic areas.

PATHOLOGY AND CLINICAL SIGNIFICANCE[44,45,56,76,98]

The basic pathologic change in these infections is a parasite-induced inflammation of the lining of the bile ducts and hyperplasia of the endothelial lining of the ducts. In most infections the worm burden is relatively light and the pathologic changes are not sufficiently severe to produce signs or symptoms.

Symptomatic cases are usually associated with long-term infections and a large worm burden. Prolonged tissue inflammation in these cases leads to fibrotic thickening and extensive

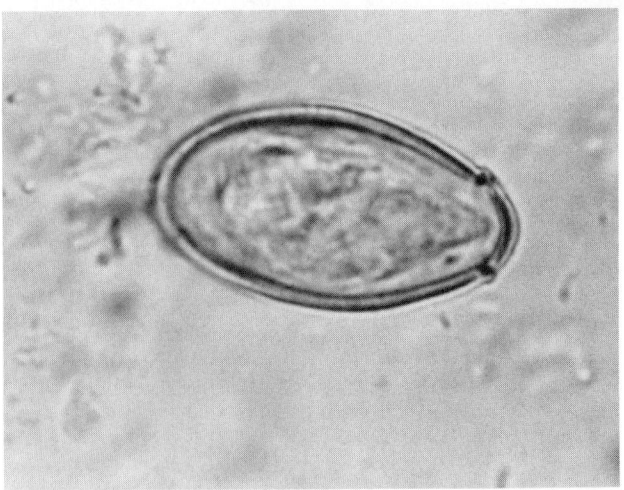

FIGURE 41-22. Egg of *Clonorchis sinensis*. (Approximately ×2100.)

constriction or obstruction of the bile ducts that may be aggravated by the formation of bile stones. At the very least these patients have colicky pain, diarrhea, and abdominal bloating. The more serious manifestations include progressive liver dysfunction manifest as hepatitis, cirrhosis, and even malignancies of the liver.

LABORATORY DIAGNOSIS[40]

The diagnosis of many cases of clonorchiasis or opisthorchiasis is probably based on accidental discovery of the eggs in the stool specimen of a patient suspected to have another type of infection. Most infections with these parasites are asymptomatic, and it is unlikely that a patient with one of these infections would have a fecal examination unless he or she had a concomitant infection with another gastrointestinal parasite. Moreover, these parasites release a relatively small number of eggs (2500 eggs per worm per day, in contrast, for example, to 200,000 per day per female *Ascaris* organism), and light infections may not be readily detected without the use of a fecal concentration procedure.

Beyond discovery of the egg stage, the definitive diagnosis of these infections is complicated by the nearly identical appearance of the eggs of four different genera: *Clonorchis*, *Opisthorchis*, *Heterophyes*, and *Metagonimus* (Figure 41-22). As a general distinction that many parasitologists consider sufficient for routine clinical practice, these parasites are divided into two groups. The *Clonorchis-Opisthorchis* group, as previously discussed, share a similar human-snail-fish-human life cycle, have small operculated eggs with a tiny, comma-shaped knob projection on the end opposite the operculum, and are embryonated when passed in the feces. One feature that may be used to distinguish the eggs of these three species is their size: *C. sinensis* eggs average 35 μm in length by 19.5 μm in width. *O. viverrini* eggs tend to be the shortest of the three, averaging 26.7 μm long by 15 μm wide, and *O. felineus* eggs tend to be the narrowest, averaging 30 μm long by 11 to 12 μm wide. There is also a slight difference in the size of the tiny "shoulder" that protrudes from just below the operculum; it is generally more prominent in *Clonorchis* organisms.

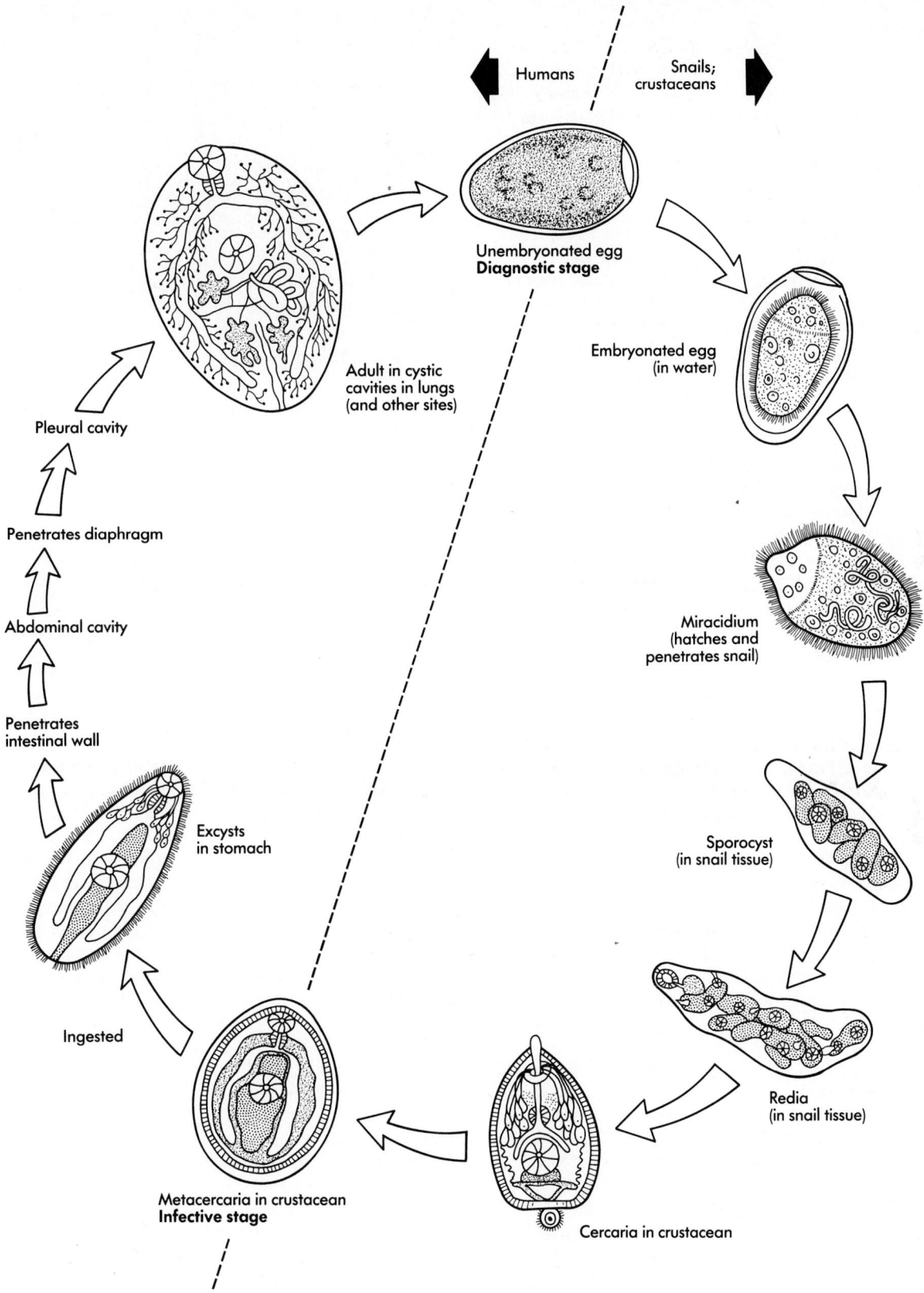

Humans

Snails; crustaceans

Unembryonated egg
Diagnostic stage

Embryonated egg
(in water)

Adult in cystic
cavities in lungs
(and other sites)

Pleural cavity

Penetrates diaphragm

Abdominal cavity

Penetrates
intestinal wall

Excysts
in stomach

Ingested

Metacercaria in crustacean
Infective stage

Cercaria in crustacean

Redia
(in snail tissue)

Sporocyst
(in snail tissue)

Miracidium
(hatches and
penetrates snail)

FIGURE 41-23. Life cycle of *Paragonimus westermani.* (Modified from Melvin, D.M., Brooke, M.M., and Sadun, E.H.: Common intestinal helminths of man—life cycle charts, Atlanta, 1965, PHS Pub. No. 1235, Laboratory Branch of the Communicable Disease Center.)

Similarly, *Heterophyes* and *Metagonimus* organisms share a life cycle that is nearly identical to that of *Clonorchis* and *Opisthorchis* organisms (human-snail-fish-human) and have operculated eggs that are of the same size and general appearance as eggs of *Clonorchis* and *Opisthorchis* organisms. The major differences are that the adults of *Heterophyes* and *Metagonimus* organisms inhabit the small intestine, not the bile ducts, and the eggs of these organisms lack the distinct "shoulder" where the operculum attaches to the egg shell.

PARAGONIMUS WESTERMANI (LUNG FLUKE)
LIFE CYCLE[42,117,118]

Infections with *Paragonimus westermani,* the most common of the human lung flukes, result from the ingestion of infective metacercariae encysted in the tissues of several different genera of freshwater crabs or crayfish (for example, the genera *Cambaroides, Eriocheir, Potamon, Sesarma,* and *Cambarus*) (Figure 41-23). In the small intestine the metacercariae excyst and begin a 3-week migration in which most of the metacercariae penetrate through the intestinal wall into the peritoneal cavity and then migrate through the diaphragm into the pleural cavity and the parenchyma of the lungs. In about 2 to 3 months the metacercariae develop into sexually mature adults that typically measure 10 mm long by 6 mm wide and are surrounded by a fibrous capsule of host origin. Eggs produced by the mature adults are released into the cyst cavity and can pass from the body only if a bronchiolar branch passes directly through the cyst wall or if the cyst ruptures into a bronchiole. Although most metacercariae eventually reach the lungs, a few may wander to abnormal sites in organs of the peritoneal cavity or even to the brain. In these ectopic sites the parasites usually develop in the same manner as those that reach the lungs, complete with a fibrous capsule and egg production. However, the trapped eggs have little if any chance of leaving the body.

Eggs released from pulmonary cysts are carried up the respiratory tree to the mouth where they may be immediately expectorated or may be swallowed and passed out in the feces. If the eggs reach a suitable freshwater environment, the first larval stage, a miracidium, develops and hatches from an egg in about 2 to 6 weeks, depending on the water temperature. Susceptible first intermediate hosts include a variety of snail genera (for example, *Semisulcospira, Thiara, Hua,* and *Brotia*). In these snails the parasite develops through a series of asexual reproductive stages (sporocysts and rediae) that terminate with the production of cercariae 3 to 5 months after the snail is first infected.

Crabs and crayfish that serve as second intermediate hosts may become infected either by ingesting snails that contain the cercarial stage or, more commonly, by cercariae that are released from the snail and crawl about near the bottom with the aid of their tiny, knoblike tails. The cercariae invade the muscles and viscera of the susceptible crabs and crayfish and develop into infective metacercariae in about 6 to 8 weeks.

EPIDEMIOLOGY[42,117,18]

Numerous species of *Paragonimus* infect reservoir animals, especially feline animals, throughout the world. Most of these species are also potentially infective for humans, but human infections are rare outside the Far East and some regions of Africa and Central and South America. The prevalence of human infections in the latter areas is usually related to the

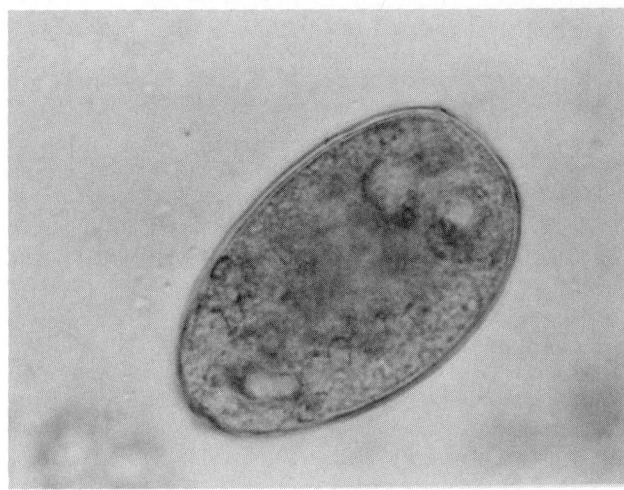

FIGURE 41-24. Egg of *Paragonimus westermani.* (Approximately ×850.)

dietary practice of eating raw or improperly cooked (for example, pickled) freshwater crabs and crayfish. Occasionally infections have been traced to foods other than crabs or crayfish. In these cases it is usually poor food preparation practices, such as improper cleaning of utensils used in preparing crabs and crayfish, that lead to infection.

PATHOLOGY AND CLINICAL MANIFESTATIONS[117,118]

Since the primary pathologic change of paragonimiasis is inflammation and cyst formation around adult worms, the major clinical manifestations depend on the site(s) and number of adult worms in the body. Usually there are only a small number of adults and the primary site of development is the lungs, and the typical signs and symptoms of the infection resemble a chronic bronchitis or bronchiectasis with a productive morning cough. The sputum is usually thick, gelatinous, and brown or reddish tinged. Hemoptysis is also common.

In the rare cases when large numbers of adults become encysted in the abdominal cavity, the patient may complain of vague abdominal pain and tenderness and occasionally bloody, mucoid diarrhea. Worms that accidentally reach the brain produce localized lesions and clinical manifestations that resemble those seen in cysticercosis (see the section on *Taenia solium*).

LABORATORY DIAGNOSIS[117,118]

The diagnosis of paragonimiasis is confirmed by the detection and identification of the typical eggs (Figure 41-24) either in the sputum or in the feces. The eggs passed out by either route typically average 90 μm in length by 55 μm in width and are unembryonated and operculated.

As mentioned previously, these eggs are similar in appearance to those of *Diphyllobothrium latum,* but they may be differentiated by several key characteristics: a thickened shell opposite the operculum (*D. latum* eggs have a knob on the shell); a flattened operculum (*D. latum* eggs have a rounded operculum); and the broadest part of the egg nearer the operculated end (the broadest part of the *D. latum* egg is in the middle).

Ideally the eggs are found in the sputum, since this eliminates possible confusion with the eggs of *D. latum*. In examining a sputum specimen the recommended procedure is first to perform a simple direct wet mount of the specimen. If no eggs are seen in this preparation, a concentrate should be prepared by mixing the sputum with an equal amount of 3% sodium hydroxide and allowing the mixture to stand at room temperature for 30 minutes. The mixture is then centrifuged for 10 minutes at 450 × g, the supernatant decanted, and the sediment examined for eggs.

In many cases, especially in young children who tend to swallow their sputum, eggs cannot be recovered in the sputum. In these circumstances fecal specimens, in addition to sputum, should be collected and examined for eggs by direct wet mount and after formalin–ether or ethyl acetate concentration.

REFERENCES

1. Ansari, N., editor: Epidemiology and control of schistosomiasis (bilharziasis), Baltimore, 1973, University Park Press.
2. Arai, H.P., editor: Biology of the tapeworm *Hymenolepis diminuta*, New York, 1980, Academic Press, Inc.
3. Ariizumi, M.: Cerebral schistosomiasis japonica: report of one operated case and fifty clinical cases, Am. J. Trop. Med. Hyg. **12**:40, 1963.
4. Attah, E.B., and Nkposong, E.O.: Schistosomiasis and carcinoma of the bladder: a critical appraisal of causal relationship, Trop. Geogr. Med. **28**:268, 1975.
5. Banwell, J.G., and Schad, G.A.: Hookworm, Clin. Gastroenterol. **7**:129, 1978.
6. Beaver, P.C.: Methods of pinworm diagnosis, Am. J. Trop. Med. **29**:577, 1949.
7. Beaver, P.C.: Persistence of hookworm larvae in soil, Am. J. Trop. Med. Hyg. **2**:102, 1953.
8. Beaver, P.C., and Danaraj, T.J.: Pulmonary ascaris resembling eosinophilic lung: autopsy report with description of larvae in the bronchioles, Am. J. Trop. Med. Hyg. **7**:100, 1958.
9. Beaver, P.C., Kriz, J.J., and Lau, T.J.: Pulmonary nodule caused by *Enterobius vermicularis*, Am. J. Trop. Med. Hyg. **22**:711, 1973.
10. Berk, J.E., Woodruff, M.T., and Frediani, A.W.: Pulmonary and intestinal changes in strongyloidosis, Gastroenterology **1**:1100, 1943.
11. Blumenthal, D.S.: Intestinal nematodes in the United States, N. Engl. J. Med. **297**:1437, 1977.
12. Blumenthal, D.S., and Schultz, M.G.: Incidence of intestinal obstruction in children infected with *Ascaris lumbricoides*, Am. J. Trop. Med. Hyg. **24**:801, 1975.
13. Blumenthal, D.S., and Schultz, M.G.: Effects of *Ascaris* infection on nutritional status in children, Am. J. Trop. Med. Hyg. **25**:682, 1976.
14. Boyd, W.P., Campbell, F.W., and Trudeau, W.L.: *Strongyloides stercoralis*—hyperinfection, Am. J. Trop. Med. Hyg. **27**:39, 1978.
15. Bradley, S.L., Dines, D.E., and Brewer, N.S.: Disseminated *Strongyloides stercoralis* in an immunosuppressed host, Mayo Clin. Proc. **53**:332, 1978.
16. Brady, F.J., and Wright, W.H.: Studies on oxyuriasis. XVIII. The symptomatology of oxyuriasis as based on physical examination and case histories on 200 patients, Am. J. Med. Sci. **198**:367, 1939.
17. Brooks, T.J., Jr., Goetz, C.C., and Plauche, W.C.: Pelvic granuloma due to *Enterobius vermicularis*, JAMA **179**:492, 1962.
18. Budzilovich, G.N., Most, H., and Feigin, I.: Pathogenesis and latency of spinal cord schistosomiasis, Arch. Pathol. **77**:383, 1964.
19. Center for Diease Control: Intestinal parasite surveillance, annual summary, 1978, Atlanta, 1979, Department of Health, Education and Welfare.
20. Chandrasoma, P.T., and Mendis, K.N.: *Enterobius* in ectopic sites, Am. J. Trop. Med. Hyg. **26**:644, 1977.
21. Cheever, A.W.: A quantitative post-mortem study of schistosomiasis mansoni in man, Am. J. Trop. Med. Hyg. **17**:38, 1968.
22. Cheever, A.W., and Andrade, Z.A.: Pathological lesions associated with *Schistosoma mansoni* infections in man, Trans. R. Soc. Trop. Med. Hyg. **61**:626, 1967.
23. Cort, W.W.: Studies on schistosome dermatitis, Am. J. Hyg. **52**:251, 1950.
24. Cram, E.B.: Studies on oxyuriasis. IX. The familial nature of pinworm infestation, Med. Ann. Dist. Columbia **10**:39, 1941.
25. Cram, E.B.: Studies on oxyuriasis. XXVIII. Summary and conclusions, Am. J. Dis. Child. **65**:46, 1943.
26. Cuni, L.J., Rosner, F., and Chawia, S.K.: Fatal strongyloidiasis in immunosuppressed patients, N.Y. State J. Med. **77**:2109, 1977.
27. Davies, N.J., and Goldsmid, J.M.: Intestinal obstruction due to *Ascaris suum* infection, Trans. R. Soc. Trop. Med. Hyg. **72**:107, 1978.
28. Eveland, L.K., Kenney, M., and Yermakov, V.: Laboratory diagnosis of autoinfection in strongyloidiasis, Am. J. Clin. Pathol. **63**:421, 1975.
29. Facey, R.V., and Marsden, P.D.: Fascioliasis in man: an outbreak in Hampshire, Br. Med. J. **2**:619, 1960.
30. Farhadian, H., and Schneider, E.A.: Trichuriasis in Calcasieu Parish, Southwest Louisiana, J. La. State Med. Soc. **127**:337, 1975.
31. Foster, A.O., and Landsberg, J.W.: The nature and cause of hookworm anemia, Am. J. Hyg. **20**:259, 1934.
32. Foy, H., and Nelson, G.S.: Helminths in the etiology of anemia in the tropics, with special reference to hookworms and schistosomes, Exp. Parasitol. **14**:240, 1963.
33. Garcia-Palmieri, M.R., and Marcial-Rojas, R.A.: The protean manifestations of schistosomiasis mansoni: a clinicopathological correlation, Ann. Intern. Med. **57**:763, 1962.
34. Gelpi, A.P., and Mustafa, A.: *Ascaris* pneumonia, Am. J. Med. **44**:377, 1968.
35. Georgi, J.R., and Sprinkle, C.L.: A case of human strongloidosis apparently contracted from asymptomatic colony dogs, Am. J. Trop. Med. Hyg. **23**:899, 1974.
36. Gill, G.V., and Bell, D.R.: *Strongyloides stercoralis* infection in former Far East prisoners of war, Br. Med. J. **2**:572, 1979.
37. Gloor, R.F., Breylery, E.R., and Martinez, I.G.: Hookworm infection in a rural Kentucky county, Am. J. Trop. Med. Hyg. **19**:1007, 1970.
38. Graham, C.F.: A device for the diagnosis of *Enterobius* infection, Am. J. Trop. Med. **21**:159, 1941.
39. Hadden, J.W., and Pascarelli, E.F.: Diagnosis and treatment of human fascioliasis, JAMA **202**:149, 1967.
40. Hardman, E.W., Jones, R.L.H., and Davies, A.H.: Fascioliasis—a large outbreak, Br. Med. J. **3**:502, 1970.
41. Hartz, P.H.: Histopathology of the colon in massive trichocephaliasis in children, Doc. Med. Geog. Trop. **5**:303, 1953.
42. Healy, G.R.: Trematodes transmitted to man by fish, frogs, and crustacea, J. Wildl. Dis. **6**:255, 1970.
43. Hinman, E.H.: A study of 85 cases of *Strongyloides stercoralis* infection with special reference to abdominal pain, Trans. R. Soc. Trop. Med. Hyg. **30**:531, 1937.
44. Hou, P.C.: The pathology of *Clonorchis sinensis* infestation of the liver, J. Pathol. Bacteriol. **70**:53, 1955.
45. Hou, P.C.: The relationship between primary carcinoma of the liver and infestation with *Clonorchis sinensis*, J. Pathol. Bacteriol. **72**:239, 1965.
46. Hsieh, H.C.: WHO Technical Report Series, No. 255. Geneva, 1963, World Health Organization.
47. Insler, G.D., and Roberts, L.S.: *Hymenolepis diminuta;* parasite or commensal? Abstract No. 78, p. 36. Forty-Ninth Annual Meeting, American Society of Parasitology, 1974.
48. Jacobs, A.H.: Enterobiasis in children: incidence, symptomatology, and diagnosis, with a simplified Scotch cellulose tape technique, J. Pediatr. **21**:497, 1942.

49. Jeffrey, G.M., et al.: Study of intestinal helminth infections in a coastal South Carolina area, Pub. Health Rep. **78:**45, 1963.

50. Jenkins, M.Q., and Beach, M.W.: Intestinal obstruction due to ascariasis: report of thirty-one cases, Pediatrics **13:**419, 1954.

51. Jones, C.A.: Clinical studies in human strongyloidiasis. I. Semeiology, Gastroenterology **16:**743, 1950.

52. Jones E.A., et al.: Massive infection with *Fasciola hepatica* in man, JAMA **214:**519, 1977.

53. Jordan, P., and Webbe, G.: Human schistosomiasis, London, 1969, Heinemann.

54. Jung, R.C., and Beaver, P.C.: Clinical observations on *Trichocephalus trichiurus* (whipworm) infestation in children, Pediatrics **8:**548, 1952.

55. Kenney, M., and Eveland, L.K.: Infection of man with *Trichuris vulpis*, the whipworm of dogs, Am. J. Clin. Pathol. **69:**199, 1978.

56. Koymiya, Y.: *Clonorchis* and clonorchiasis, Adv. Parasitol. **4:**53, 1966.

57. Kuntz, R.E.: Biology of the schistosome complexes, Am. J. Trop. Med. Hyg. **4:**383, 1955.

58. Layrisse, M., et al.: Intestinal absorption tests and biopsy of the jejunum in subjects with heavy hookworm infections, Am. J. Trop. Med. Hyg. **13:**297, 1964.

59. Layrisse, M., et al.: Blood loss due to infection with *Trichuris trichiura*, Am. J. Trop. Med. Hyg. **16:**613, 1967.

60. Little, M.D., Cuello, C.J., and D'Alessandro, A.: Granuloma of the liver due to *Enterobius vermicularis*: report of a case, Am. J. Trop. Med. Hyg. **22:**567, 1973.

61. Lotero, H., Tripathy, K., and Bolanos, O.: Gastrointestinal blood loss in *Trichuris* infection, Am. J. Trop. Med. Hyg. **23:**1203, 1974.

62. Louw, J.H.: Abdominal complications of *Ascaris lumbricoides* infestation in children, Br. J. Surg. **53:**510, 1966.

63. Mahmoud, A.A.F.: Current concepts in parasitology: schistosomiasis, N. Engl. J. Med. **297:**1329, 1977.

64. Marcial-Rojas, R.A., editor: Pathology of protozoal and helminthic diseases with clinical correlation, Baltimore, 1971, Williams & Wilkins Co.

65. Martin, L.K.: Hookworm in Georgia. I. Survey of intestinal helminth infections and anemia in rural school children, Am. J. Trop. Med. Hyg. **21:**919, 1972.

66. Matsen, J.M., and Turner, J.A.: Reinfection in enterobiasis (pinworm infection), Am. J. Dis. Child. **118:**576, 1969.

67. McDonald, G.S.A., and Hourihane, D.O.: Ectopic *Enterobius vermicularis*, Gut **13:**621, 1972.

68. Miller, T.A.: Pathogenesis and immunity in hookworm infection, Trans. R. Soc. Trop. Med. Hyg. **62:**473, 1968.

69. Milner, P.F., et al.: Intestinal malabsorption in *Strongyloides stercoralis* infestation, Gut **6:**547, 1965.

70. Mostofi, K.F., editor: Bilharziasis, New York, 1967, Springer-Verlag.

71. O'Brien, W.: Intestinal malabsorption in acute infection with *Strongyloides stercoralis*, Trans. R. Soc. Trop. Med. Hyg. **69:**69, 1975.

72. Pawlowski, Z., and Schultz, M.G.: Taeniasis and cysticercosis *(Taenia saginata)*, Adv. Parasitol. **10:**269, 1972.

73. Peters, L., Cavis, D., and Robertson, J.: Is *Diphyllobothrium latum* currently present in Northern Michigan? J. Parasitol. **64:**947, 1978.

74. Plaut, A.G., Kamapanart-Sanyakorn, C., and Manning, G.S.: A clinical study of *Fasciolopsis buski* infection in Thailand, Trans. R. Soc. Trop. Med. Hyg. **63:**470, 1969.

75. Proctor, E.M., Powell, S.J., and Elsdon-Dew, R.: The serological diagnosis of cysticercosis, Ann. Trop. Med. Parasitol. **60:**146, 1966.

76. Purtillo, D.T.: Clonorchiasis and hepatic neoplasms, Trop. Geogr. Med. **28:**21, 1976.

77. Purtillo, D.T., Meyers, W.M., and Connor, D.H.: Fatal strongyloidiasis in immunosuppressed patients, Am. J. Med. **56:**488, 1974.

78. Reardon, L.: Studies on oxyuriasis. XVI. The number of eggs produced by the pinworm, *Enterobius vermicularis*, and its bearing on infection, Pub. Health Rep. **53:**978, 1938.

79. Reboucas, G.: Clinical aspects of hepatosplenic schistosomiasis: a contrast with cirrhosis, Yale J. Biol. Med. **48:**369, 1975.

80. Rees, G.: Pathogenesis of adult cestodes, Helm. Abs. **36:**1, 1967.

81. Ribera, E., et al.: Hyperinfection syndrome with *Strongyloides stercoralis*, Ann. Med. **72:**199, 1972.

82. Riley, W.A.: A mouse oxyurid, *Syphacia obvelata*, as a parasite of man, J. Parasitol. **6:**89, 1920.

83. Roche, M., and Lyrisse, M.: The nature and causes of "hookworm anemia," Am. J. Trop. Med. Hyg. **15:**1031, 1966.

84. Royer, A., and Berdknikoff, I.K.: Pinworm infestation in children: the problem and its management, Can. Med. Assoc. J. **86:**60, 1962.

85. Rydzewski, A.K., Chisholm, E.S., and Kagan, I.G.: Comparison of serologic tests for human cysticercosis by indirect hemagglutination, indirect immunofluorescent antibody and agar gel precipitin test, J. Parasitol. **61:**154, 1975.

86. Saarni, M., et al.: Symptoms in carriers of *Diphyllobothrium latum* and in non-infected controls, Acta Med. Scand. **174:**147, 1963.

87. Sachdev, Y.V., and Howards, S.S.: *Enterobius vermicularis* infestation and secondary enuresis, J. Urol. **113:**143, 1975.

88. Sadun, E.H., and Maiphoom, C.: Studies on the epidemiology of the human intestinal fluke, *Fasciolopsis buski* (Lankester), in central Thailand, Am. J. Trop. Med. Hyg. **2:**1070, 1953.

89. Sawitz, W., et al.: Studies on the epidemiology of oxyuriasis, South. Med. J. **33:**913, 1940.

90. Schuffner, W., and Swellengrebel, N.H.: Retrofection in oxyuriasis: a newly discovered mode of infection with *Enterobius vermicularis*, J. Parasitol. **35:**138, 1943.

91. Shookoff, H.C.: Clinical aspects of Manson's schistosomiasis, N.Y. State J. Med. **61:**3864, 1961.

92. Simon, R.D.: Pinworm infestation and urinary tract infection in young girls, Am. J. Dis. Child. **128:**21, 1974.

93. Smith, J.H., et al.: A quantitative post mortem analysis of urinary schistosomiasis in Egypt. I. Pathology and pathogenesis, Am. J. Trop. Med. Hyg. **23:**1054, 1974.

94. Smithers, S.R., and Terry, R.J.: The immunology of schistosomiasis, Adv. Parasitol. **14:**399, 1975.

95. Spillman, R.K.: Pulmonary ascariasis in tropical communities, Am. J. Trop. Med. Hyg. **24:**791, 1975.

96. Stoll, N.R.: On endemic hookworm, where do we stand today? Exp. Parasitol. **12:**241, 1962.

97. Stone, O.J., Newell, G.B., and Mullins, J.F.: Cutaneous strongyloidiosis: larva currens, Arch. Dermatol. **106:**734, 1972.

98. Strauss, W.G.: Clinical manifestations of clonorchiasis: a controlled study of 105 cases, Am. J. Trop. Med. Hyg. **11:**625, 1962.

99. Swartzwelder, J.C.: Clinical *Trichocephalus trichiurus* infection: an analysis of 81 cases, Am. J. Trop. Med. **19:**473, 1939.

100. Swartzwelder, J.C.: Clinical ascariasis: an analysis of 202 cases in New Orleans, Am. J. Dis. Child. **72:**172, 1946.

101. Symmers, W.St.C.: Pathology of oxyuriasis, with special reference to granulomas due to the presence of *Oxyuris vermicularis* (*Enterobius vermicularis*) and its ova in tissues, Arch. Pathol. **50:**475, 1950.

102. Tripathy, K., et al.: Effects of *Ascaris* infection on human nutrition, Am. J. Trop. Med. Hyg. **20:**212, 1971.

103. Tripathy, K., et al.: Malabsorption syndrome in ascariasis, Am. J. Clin. Nutr. **25:**1276, 1972.

104. Von Bonsdorff, B.: *Diphyllobothrium latum* as a cause of pernicious anemia, Exp. Parasitol. **5:**207, 1956.

105. Von Bonsdorff, B.: Diphyllobothriasis in man, New York, 1977, Academic Press, Inc.

106. Waller, C.E., and Othersen, H.B., Jr.: Ascariasis: surgical complications in children, Am. J. Surg. **120:**50, 1970.

107. Warren, K.S.: Regulation of the prevalence and intensity of schistosomiasis in man: immunology or ecology, J. Infect. Dis. **127:**595, 1973.

108. Warren, K.S.: Helminthic diseases endemic in the United States, Am. J. Trop. Med. Hyg. **23:**723, 1974.

109. Warren, K.S.: Schistosomiasis: a multiplicity of immunopathology, J. Invest. Dermatol. **67:**464, 1976.

110. Warren, K.S.: The pathology, pathobiology, and pathogenesis of schistosomiasis, Nature **273:**609, 1978.

111. Warren, K.S., and Mahmoud, A.A.F.: Algorithms in the diagnosis and management of exotic diseases. XIV. Tapeworms, J. Infect. Dis. **134:**108, 1976.

112. Weller, T.H., and Sorenson, C.W.: Enterobiasis: its incidence and symptomatology in a group of 505 children, N. Engl. J. Med. **224:**143, 1941.

113. Whittier, L., Einhorn, N.H., and Miller, J.F.: Trichuriasis in children, Am. J. Dis. Child. **70:**289, 1945.

114. Wolfgang, R.W.: Indian and Eskimo diphyllobothriasis, Can. Med. Assoc. J. **70:**536, 1954.

115. World Health Organization: The control of ascariasis, WHO Tech. Rep. Ser. No. 379, Geneva, Switzerland, 1967.

116. Yeh, S.D.J., McSeeney, J., and Shiu, M.H.: *Schistosoma japonica* of liver, N.Y. State J. Med. **77:**396, 1977.

117. Yokogawa, M.: *Paragonimus* and paragonimiasis, Adv. Parasitol. **7:**375, 1969.

118. Yokogawa, S., Cort, W.W., and Yokogawa, M.: *Paragonimus* and paragonimiasis, Exp. Parasitol. **10:**81, 1960.

CHAPTER 42

Lumen-Dwelling Protozoa

John Klaas II

Along with the lumen-dwelling nematodes (see Chapter 39) the lumen-dwelling protozoa produce some of the most common animal parasite infections seen in the United States. Most of these organisms are traditional pathogens with relatively simple life cycles, such as *Entamoeba histolytica;* others, such as the genus *Cryptosporidium,* are newly recognized pathogens with complex life cycles. All the major groups of protozoa, including the amoebae, flagellates, ciliates, and sporozoa, have at least one member that is a lumen-dwelling pathogen of humans. Some groups, such as the amoebae, have numerous representatives that occur in humans but that are not considered pathogens. Discussion of these nonpathogens has been limited to a review of their major diagnostic characteristics in the sections that pertain to their pathogenic relatives.

ENTAMOEBA HISTOLYTICA
LIFE CYCLE[23]

Infections with *E. histolytica* typically begin with ingestion of mature, quadrinucleate cysts (metacysts; Figure 42-1). In the small intestine the quadrinucleate amoeba is liberated from the cyst and quickly undergoes a series of cytoplasmic and nuclear divisions to form eight tiny metacystic trophozoites. Carried through the small intestine by peristalsis, the metacystic trophozoites enter the cecal region of the large intestine, where they find the crypts of the mucosal lining a suitable environment for establishing a colony. The subsequent course of the infection appears to be influenced by individual variations in the pH, oxidation-reduction (redox) potential, bacterial flora, and nutritional factors of this region. In some individuals the developing colony of trophozoites produces little if any tissue damage, preferring to limit its feeding to starches and mucous secretions on the surface of the mucosa. In other individuals infected under identical circumstances, the trophozoites may lyse and invade the tissue, sometimes extending beyond the confines of the intestine to organs such as the liver.

In any case the life cycle is perpetuated by cysts that develop from trophozoites swept along with feces from the site of their colonization toward the lower areas of the large intestine. As water is withdrawn from the fecal mass, the trophozoites are stimulated to form the cyst stage. Without this stimulus trophozoites do not encyst, and they die quickly once they are outside the body. Thus the cyst stage is found only in formed or semiformed fecal specimens; they are not found in affected tissues or in the stools of patients with diarrhea. As the trophozoites begin to encyst, they expel any undigested food and round up into precysts. In this stage, which frequently contains glycogen vacuoles and bar-shaped particles of condensed ribonucleic acid (known as chromatoid bodies), the organism secretes a thin but tough cyst wall that protects it from the adverse environment outside the body. The rate at which the feces pass out of the body determines whether the precysts have time to complete their transformation to mature cysts. In formed fecal specimens the passage has generally been slow enough that the predominant form is the mature cysts, which are typically recognized by the presence of four nuclei and the absence of either a glycogen vacuole or chromatoid bodies. When fecal passage has been more rapid and the feces is semiformed, the precysts or immature cysts with one or two nuclei and glycogen vacuoles and chromatoid bodies are usually the predominant form.

EPIDEMIOLOGY[23,34,46,58]

Although usually thought of as a tropical disease, amoebic infections occur worldwide. It has been estimated that there are 400 million cases worldwide, but the prevalence of the infection varies from region to region, depending largely on the general level of sanitation in the particular region. These differences in the sanitation levels are usually the explanation for the observation that 40% to 80% of the population may be infected in tropical climates, whereas in more temperate climates, such as the United States, the estimated prevalence is between 3% and 10%.

Within a given geographic region, amoebiasis is usually more common in children older than 5 years and adults, and in males rather than females. The prevalence is also greater among the poor and those in mental hospitals, prisons, and orphanages.

The most common source of infection is food or water contaminated with cysts passed in the formed or semiformed feces of asymptomatic or mildly ill individuals. In a cool, moist environment with low levels of bacteria the cysts may remain viable for as long as 30 days. In dry environments with high temperatures (the thermal death point being 122° F) or in the presence of large numbers of accompanying bacteria, the viability of cysts is considerably reduced. In water supplies the cysts are usually resistant to the normal levels of chlorination but may be destroyed or removed by hyperchlorination, treatment with dilute iodine, or filtration of the water.

Infections acquired from contaminated water are frequently associated with consumption of water supplies or accidental leakage of sewage into treated water supplies. Infections associated with contaminated foods are usually the result of improper food-handling practices by people unaware of their infections, whereas infections in mental hospitals, prisons, and orphanages are often the result of person-to-person transfer among individuals with poor personal hygiene. In regions where there is improper disposal of feces, and foodstuffs are unprotected, flies or cockroaches may transmit cysts from feces

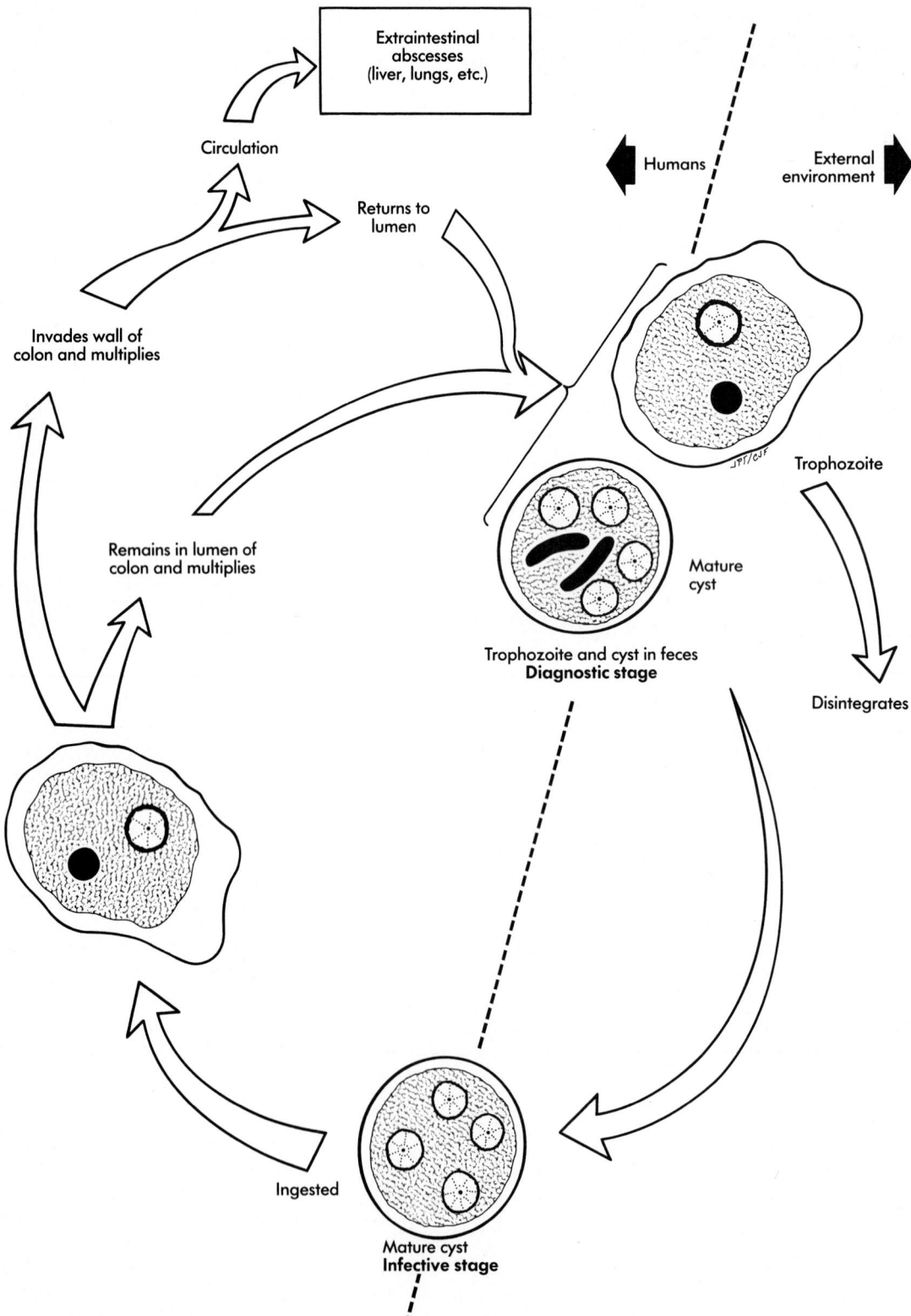

FIGURE 42-1. Life cycle of *Entamoeba histolytica*. (Modified from Brooke, M.M., and Melvin, D.M.: Common intestinal protozoa of man—life cycle charts, Atlanta, 1964, HEW Pub. No. [CDC] 79-8311, Laboratory Branch of the Communicable Disease Center.)

to the food products. In parts of the world where commercial fertilizers are scarce or expensive, infections have been traced to the practice of using human feces as fertilizer for vegetable crops. Finally, in recent years there have been several reports of sexually transmitted *Entamoeba histolytica,* especially (but not exclusively) among the homosexual population.

Several studies have demonstrated that animals such as monkeys may be naturally infected with *E. histolytica,* and that dogs, cats, and pigs can be infected under experimental conditions or may harbor organisms that resemble *E. histolytica.* As a source of human infections, however, cases traced to animal sources are insignificant compared with those traced to human sources.

PATHOLOGY AND CLINICAL MANIFESTATIONS*

The pathologic changes and clinical manifestations of *E. histolytica* infections can be divided into two major categories: intestinal amoebiasis and extraintestinal amoebiasis.

In intestinal amoebiasis the primary lesions are ulcers that develop in the wall of the colon, since trophozoites secrete lytic enzymes that digest the tissue of the intestinal wall (hence the species named *histolytica*). As the trophozoites multiply and advance more deeply into the intestinal mucosa, they encounter increasing tissue resistance. This natural tissue resistance, coupled with the normal regeneration of damaged tissue, may limit the spread of the organisms or even spontaneously eliminate the organisms from the tissue. More frequently, however, the trophozoites penetrate the lamina muscularis mucosae layer and reach the submucosa before their advance is slowed. Once in the submucosa the trophozoites begin to spread laterally in the tissue, producing characteristic flasklike lesions that have tiny openings to the lumen of the intestine. At this stage of infection there is little if any inflammation of the tissue; the mucosal inflammation seen in later stages of the infection occurs only after intestinal bacteria have invaded the ulcer.

If the individual ulcers continue to spread laterally, they eventually undermine large areas of the mucosa. These undermined areas may subsequently slough off, exposing the underlying muscular layers and leading to edema and formation of fibrous membranes. A relatively uncommon form of amoebic lesion that may develop in long-term infections is a benign, granulomatous intestinal tumor called an amoeboma.

Originating from the intestinal ulcers, trophozoites may spread by direct extension or be carried via the blood or lymphatic system to extraintestinal sites. Direct extension of the ulcers may lead to cutaneous ulcers (amoebic cutis). A more serious consequence of the trophozoites' continual erosion of the intestinal wall is peritonitis.

Trophozoites that penetrate the submucosa of the intestinal wall frequently lyse the walls of mesenteric venules and are carried by the intrahepatic portal venules into the liver. If trapped by thrombi in small venules in the liver, the trophozoites may spread into the liver and form a solitary liver abscess. Such liver abscesses, which are the most common form of extraintestinal amoebiasis, may serve as a focus of infection from which trophozoites spread by direct extension or by the bloodstream to other internal organs, such as the lungs or brain.

The clinical manifestations of amoebiasis vary widely, depending on the extent of tissue pathology, which in turn is usually related to the particular strain of *E. histolytica,* the mode of infection, and host's state of health before exposure. The less severe forms of clinically manifest intestinal disease are usually characterized by vague abdominal discomfort, malaise, anorexia, and weight loss. In cases of moderate tissue involvement there is usually a gradual onset of colicky abdominal pain, tenesmus, and frequent bowel movements. In the more severe dysenteric form of the disease there may be 20 or more bowel movements per day, with the feces containing variable amounts of fresh blood and mucus. These patients also typically exhibit constitutional signs such as fever, dehydration, and electrolyte imbalance.

In the extraintestinal forms of amoebiasis the signs and symptoms depend on the particular organ involved and the extent of the tissue damage.

LABORATORY DIAGNOSIS[13,26,30,35,45]

The primary means of confirming suspected cases of amoebiasis is identification of the trophozoite or cyst stage in stool specimens or the trophozoite in aspirates from the wall of the intestine and extraintestinal abscesses. Experienced technologists, especially those who live in areas where the disease is prevalent, can probably provide a reliable identification of both the cyst and the trophozoite stage of the organism in simple wet mounts. In areas such as the United States, where the disease is less common and the technologists are generally less experienced in identification of amoebae, confirmation of amoebic infections should be based on examination of permanent stained smears. This policy should reduce the incidence of one of the most common laboratory errors—misidentifying white cells in the stool as trophozoites or cysts of *E. histolytica.* Other major problems include excessive delay in processing specimens and accepting specimens from patients who have received medications that interfere with examination (including antidiarrheal or antimicrobial medication) or substances used to enhance radiologic examination of the intestinal tract (such as barium and bismuth).

Whenever forms resembling cysts or trophozoites of amoebae are observed in stained smears, the process of identification can be divided into three phases: distinguishing amoebae from white cells, distinguishing members of the genus *Entamoeba* from other genera of amoebae, and finally distinguishing *E. histolytica* from other members of the genus *Entamoeba.*

The distinction between amoebae and white cells is usually based on estimating the amount of nuclear material versus the amount of cytoplasm. In white cells the ratio is typically 1 part nuclear material to 1 to 1.5 parts cytoplasm; in amoebae the ratio is 1 part nuclear material to 3 parts cytoplasm. Once technologists can reliably distinguish between amoebae and the various leukocytes and epithelial cells that are often found in fecal specimens, they may be able to make practical use of the observation that the number and types of white cells found in the stools of patients with amoebic dysentery are noticeably different from those found in patients with bacterial dysentery. In amoebic dysentery the number of white cells is usually small, with a predominance of mononuclear leukocytes, 2% to 5% eosinophils, Charcot-Leyden crystals (in 25% of cases), and large numbers of bacteria. In bacillary dysentery (*Shigella* spp.), however, there is usually a large number of white cells,

---

*References 1, 2, 22, 24, 33, and 51.

TABLE 42-1. Typical Characteristics of Intestinal Amoebic Trophozoites

| Organism | Size (μm) | Nuclear Structure | | Cytoplasm | |
		Peripheral Chromatin	Karyosome	Appearance	Inclusions
Entamoeba histolytica	15-30	Present; fine granules evenly distributed	Small; usually centrally located	Smooth; finely granular; few if any vacuoles	Erythrocytes
Entamoeba hartmanni	5-12	Same as above	Same as above	Same as above	Bacteria but no erythrocytes
Entamoeba coli	10-50	Present; irregular granules unevenly distributed	Large, usually eccentric	Coarse and granular; many vacuoles	Bacteria, yeast, debris
Endolimax nana	6-12	Absent	Very large, irregular shape	Granular; vacuolated	Bacteria
Iodamoeba bütschlii	9-20	Absent	Very large; surrounded by achromatic granules	Coarse and granular; many vacuoles	Bacteria, yeast, debris

Modified from Garcia, L.S., and Ash, L.R.: Diagnostic parasitology: clinical laboratory manual, ed. 2, St. Louis, 1979, The C.V. Mosby Co.

predominantly polymorphonuclear leukocytes, rarely any eosinophils or Charcot-Leyden crystals, and only small numbers of bacteria. In applying these criteria it is important to remember that patients may have amoebic and bacillary dysentery at the same time, and bowel diseases such as ulcerative colitis may have exudates similar to those of either bacillary or amoebic dysentery.

Having distinguished white cells from amoebae, the next step in identification is to determine whether the amoeba is a member of the genus *Entamoeba*. The essential steps in this particular stage of identification require determinations of whether the organism is in the cyst or the trophozoite stage, the size of the organism, and the basic structure of the nucleus. Additional criteria, such as appearance of the cytoplasm and type of ingested food, are useful if the organism is in the trophozoite stage. If, on the other hand, the organism is in the cyst stage, knowledge of characteristics such as the number of nuclei and the appearance of any inclusions (chromatoid bodies[40] or glycogen vacuoles) is particularly useful. The appearance of the cytoplasm and the type of ingested food material are of little use in identifying organisms in the cyst stage, since the cytoplasm in nearly all cysts is identical in appearance: very dense and free of undigested food.

The distinction between amoebae of the genus *Entamoeba* and other genera of amoeba is more often based on the distinctive nuclear structure than on any other single characteristic. The nuclei of *Entamoeba* spp. typically have a layer of dark-staining nuclear material (chromatin) lining the inner surface of the nuclear membrane (Plate 27, *A*). This layer of chromatin, which is not found in the nuclei of other genera of amoebae, may vary from a layer of unevenly distributed, large, irregularly shaped blocks of chromatin to evenly distributed, tiny dots of chromatin, depending on the particular species of *Entamoeba*. One possible error in applying this criterion is that the nuclear structure of some species of flagellates, such as *Chilomastix mesnili*, closely resembles that of *Entamoeba*. Consequently, technologists must carefully examine an organism for other characteristics, such as flagella, cytostomes, and undulating membranes, that suggest the organism is not an amoeba. Another potential source of error in applying this criterion is

that other species of amoebae, such as *Endolimax nana*, may be mistaken for *Entamoeba* spp. if the karyosome of the nucleus is pushed against the nuclear membrane, giving the appearance of peripheral chromatin. In most of these cases the absence of a clearly defined karyosome indicates that what appears to be peripheral chromatin is actually a displaced karyosome.

A second unique characteristic of *Entamoeba* spp. is the presence of rod-shaped chromatoid bodies in the cyst stage (Plate 27, *B*). These inclusions of condensed RNA are not found in all cysts; they are more commonly seen in the immature cysts and may be absent in mature cysts. However, if present, they are a definitive indication of *Entamoeba* spp.

Two amoebae that frequently must be differentiated from *Entamoeba* spp. are the nonpathogens *E. nana* and *Iodamoeba bütschlii* (Tables 42-1 and 42-2). Both of these organisms appear similar in the trophozoite stage, having nuclei that contain large karyosomes and cytoplasm that is often filled with numerous vacuoles and ingested bacteria. They also overlap in size, with the trophozoites of *E. nana* (Figure 42-2) measuring 6 to 12 μm and the trophozoites of *I. bütschlii* (Figure 42-3) measuring 9 to 20 μm. The one major difference in these trophozoites (although in my experience it is difficult to observe) is the presence of glistening achromatic granules around the karyosome of *Iodamoeba*. In the cyst stage these two species are more easily differentiated. Both the immature and mature cysts of *Iodamoeba* (Figure 42-4), which typically are round to oval and measure 5 to 16 μm, contain a large glycogen vacuole that occupies most of the cytoplasmic space and a single nucleus that is identical in structure to the nucleus seen in the trophozoite stage. In contrast, the cysts of *Endolimax* (Figure 42-5) are often irregular in shape, measuring from 4 to 8 μm in width to 8 to 14 μm in length, lack the large glycogen vacuole seen in *Iodamoeba*, and when mature have four nuclei that are identical in appearance to the nuclei seen in their trophozoite stage.

Once an organism has been identified as belonging to the genus *Entamoeba*, the final step is to distinguish among the various intestinal species of *Entamoeba*, specifically *E. histolytica*, *E. coli*, *E. hartmanni*, and *E. polecki* (Tables 42-1 and 42-2).

Trophozoites of *E. histolytica* typically measure between 15

TABLE 42-2. Typical Characteristics of Intestinal Amoebic Cysts

Organism	Size (μm)	Shape of Cyst	Number of Nuclei	Cytoplasm	
				Chromatoid Bodies	**Glycogen**
Entamoeba histolytica	10-30	Commonly spherical	Four in mature cyst	Often present; cigar-shaped, smooth edges, rounded ends	Absent in mature cysts
Entamoeba hartmanni	5-10	Same as above	Same as above	Same as above	Same as above
Entamoeba coli	10-50	Commonly spherical	Eight in mature cyst	Often present; splinterlike with jagged or pointed ends	Absent in mature cysts
Endolimax nana	5-10	Various shapes: oval, ellipsoid, spherical	Four in mature cyst	Absent	Absent
Iodamoeba bütschlii	5-16	Various shapes: oval, ellipsoid, spherical	One	Absent	Present as large compact mass

Modified from Garcia, L.S., and Ash, L.R.: Diagnostic parasitology: clinical laboratory manual, ed. 2, St. Louis, 1979, The C.V. Mosby Co.

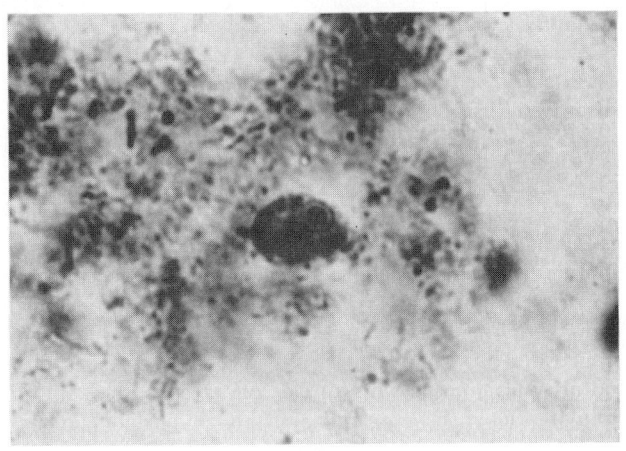

FIGURE 42-2. Trophozoite of *Endolimax nana*. (Approximately ×2000.)

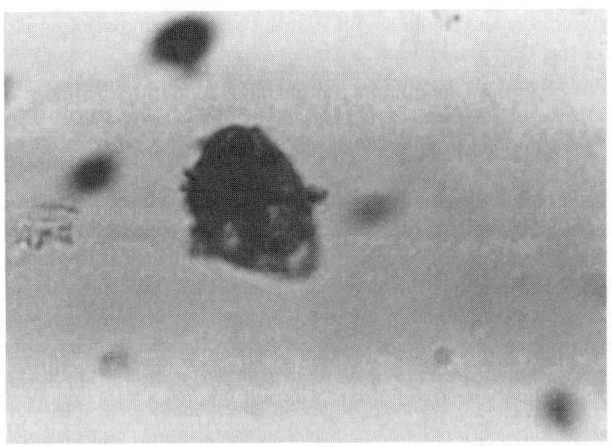

FIGURE 42-3. Trophozoite of *Iodamoeba bütschlii*. (Approximately ×2000.)

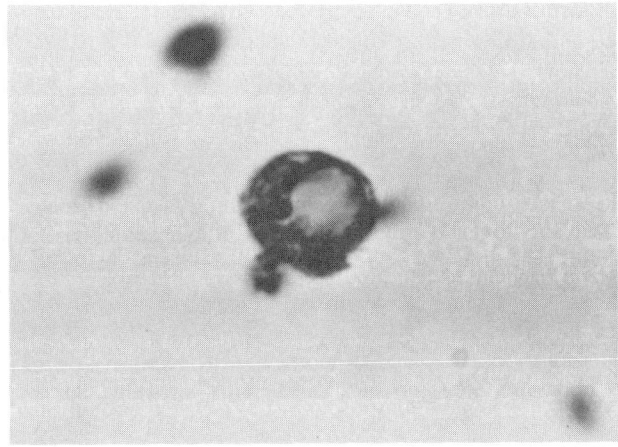

FIGURE 42-4. Cyst of *Iodamoeba bütschlii*. (Approximately ×2000.)

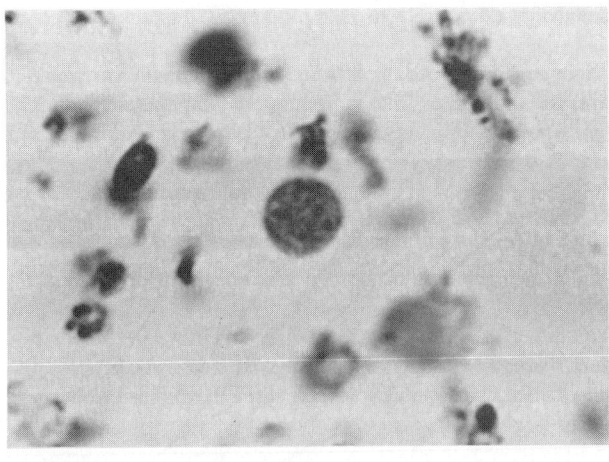

FIGURE 42-5. Cyst of *Endolimax nana*. (Approximately ×2000.)

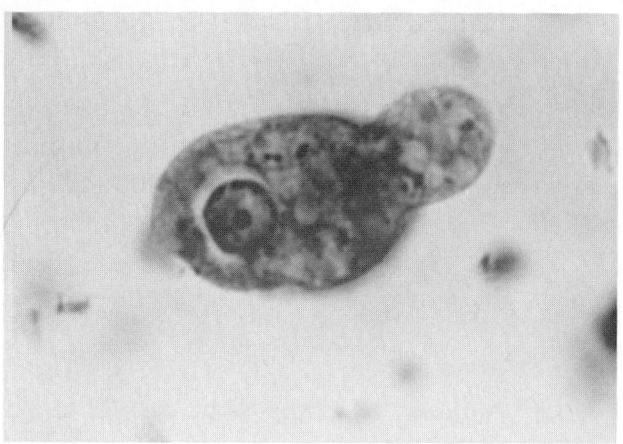

FIGURE 42-6. Trophozoite of *Entamoeba coli*. (Approximately ×2000.)

to 30 μm (sometimes as large as 60 μm) and have a single nucleus with a small central karyosome and an evenly distributed band of peripheral chromatin. The cytoplasm usually has a very smooth, finely granular appearance and is free of vacuoles or ingested bacteria. One characteristic that is considered definitive for *E. histolytica* trophozoites is the presence of ingested erythrocytes; no other species of amoeba is known to ingest red cells. In contrast, the trophozoite stage of the nonpathogenic *Escherichia coli* (Figure 42-6) may measure between 10 and 50 μm and has a single nucleus with a large, commonly off-center karyosome and an unevenly distributed, thick band of peripheral chromatin. The cytoplasm is usually very vacuolated, granular, and filled with ingested bacteria.

Mature cysts of *E. histolytica* typically measure between 10 and 30 μm and contain four nuclei identical in appearance to those found in their trophozoite stage. By comparison, the mature cysts of *E. coli* (Plate 27, *C*) typically measure 10 to 50 μm and have eight nuclei, also identical in appearance to those found in their trophozoite stage. Because of differences in the number of nuclei found in the mature cysts of these two species, it would seem that differentiation is relatively easy; however, special care must be taken to keep from mistaking immature cysts of *E. coli* that contain only four nuclei for mature quadrinucleate cysts of *E. histolytica*. Besides relying on differences in the nuclear structure of the two organisms, examining the chromatoid bodies frequently found in immature cysts of *Entamoeba* spp. is often helpful. In *E. coli* these chromatoid bodies are typically splinterlike with pointed or jagged ends, whereas in *E. histolytica* the chromatoid bodies are usually rodlike with rounded ends (Plate 27, *B*).

In some respects the easiest species of *Entamoeba* to distinguish from *E. histolytica* is the nonpathogenic species *E. hartmanni*. Formerly known as "small race" *E. histolytica*, *E. hartmanni* is virtually identical to *E. histolytica* except that it is smaller (trophozoites typically 12 μm or less in length and cysts 10 μm or less in diameter) and does not ingest red blood cells. The problem in differentiation occurs when an individual organism is at the upper limit of the size range for *E. hartmanni*. In these cases one should not rely on the characteristics of a single organism for identification but instead should examine

the specimen more thoroughly to determine the predominant size of the organisms present. If most of the organisms are small, an identification of *E. hartmanni* is appropriate; if, however, most of the organisms are larger than the upper size limit for *E. hartmanni,* the few small organisms are probably *E. histolytica*. If both species are present, there are usually large numbers of both and the size difference between the two is readily apparent.

The final species of intestinal *Entamoeba* that must be distinguished from *E. histolytica* is *E. polecki*. The latter species, traditionally considered rare in the United States, has been incriminated as a pathogen in a small number of reported infections. However, given the possibility of the organism's pathogenicity and increasing numbers of refugees from the Orient, where the organism appears to be most prevalent, technologists should become familiar with the distinguishing characteristics of *E. polecki*. In general, the trophozoites of *E. polecki* have a cytoplasm (vacuolated, ingested bacteria, and so forth) and motility (nonprogressive) that resembles *E. coli* but a nuclear structure that is more like *E. histolytica* (a small central karyosome, evenly distributed peripheral chromatin). The cyst stage is similar to that of *E. histolytica,* except that when mature it is uninucleate, with a larger karyosome than *E. histolytica*. In the immature cyst stage *E. polecki* has pointed chromatoid bars like those of *E. coli*. The similarity in characteristics often makes *E. histolytica* exceedingly difficult to distinguish from *E. polecki*. As is the case with identification of *E. hartmanni*, it is usually necessary to form an overall impression based on observing many different individual organisms in a single slide. For example, the presence of large numbers of uninucleate cysts and no multinucleate cysts is suggestive of *E. polecki*.

Besides routine examination of fecal specimens for characteristic trophozoites or cysts, serologic tests for specific antibodies to *E. histolytica* often prove a valuable adjunct in severe cases of amoebic dysentery or extraintestinal amoebiasis. Tests such as indirect hemagglutination, indirect immunofluorescence, counterimmunoelectrophoresis, and agar-gel diffusion can provide strong evidence of the infection even in the absence of positive fecal findings.

In vitro cultivation, described in Chapter 40, may also be used in difficult cases, but it is probably effective only in laboratories with the special expertise needed to maintain proper quality control of the system. This requires significant time and skill in preparation and testing of the special media and in inoculation and processing of the cultures.

In any case, where suspicion of amoebiasis is strong, repeated stool examinations, including permanent stained smears, are imperative. If there is any doubt about identification of *E. histolytica*, a properly preserved specimen (with formalin and PVA fixative) and stained slides should be submitted to a qualified reference laboratory for confirmation of the identification.

DIENTAMOEBA FRAGILIS
LIFE CYCLE[14,15,57]

Because of its amoeba-like structure and progressive motility by what appear to be pseudopods, *Dientamoeba fragilis* was originally classified as an amoeba. Within this original classification, however, the organism was unlike most other amoebae in that it has no cyst stage, and as many as 80% of the trophozoites in any population are binucleate. Later investigations, which included careful electron microscopic studies, determined that the organism is actually a flagellate.

The trophozoites of *D. fragilis* do not invade tissue but rather feed on bacteria in the mucosal crypts of the large intestine. Since the organism lacks a cyst stage, it is passed in the feces as a trophozoite.

EPIDEMIOLOGY[14,57]

Since the organism lacks a cyst stage, the mode of infection is uncertain. One hypothesis is that the trophozoite may be carried into the body within the egg of a nematode parasite of humans, particularly *Enterobius vermicularis*.

The prevalence of *D. fragilis* infections is reported to range from 1.5% to 20%. This rate may be even higher when individuals live in crowded institutional conditions or personal hygiene is poor.

PATHOLOGY AND CLINICAL MANIFESTATIONS[57]

Although the pathogenesis of symptomatic infections is not clear, 15% to 27% of infected individuals are symptomatic. Based on data from Yang and Scholten[57] approximately 50% of the clinically manifest infections are characterized by diarrhea and abdominal pain.

LABORATORY DIAGNOSIS

Laboratory diagnosis of *Dientamoeba* infections is generally based on finding a large percentage of binucleate, amoeba-like trophozoites in permanent stained smears. Each of these trophozoites, which vary in diameter from 3 to 18 μm, is distinguished by nuclei that lack peripheral chromatin and karyosomes composed of four to eight separate chromatin granules.

The mononucleate form of *Dientamoeba* is easily confused with trophozoites of *E. nana* or even *I. bütschlii* unless the karyosome is carefully examined to determine whether it is solid *(E. nana, I. bütschlii)* or fragmented *(D. fragilis)*.

GIARDIA LAMBLIA
LIFE CYCLE[12,44]

Infections with *Giardia lamblia* are acquired by ingestion of mature quadrinucleate cysts (Figure 42-7). When the cyst wall is removed by the action of digestive juices in the small intestine, the organism quickly differentiates into two binucleate, teardrop-shaped trophozoites, each propelled by four pairs of flagella. The newly emerged trophozoites attach to epithelium cells in the crypts of the duodenum and upper jejunum by their ventral sucking disk and begin to multiply. Originally it was believed that the trophozoites did not invade the mucosa; however, careful histologic studies, supported by electron microscopy, have revealed that the organism occasionally penetrates the mucosa.

Cyst formation is initiated when trophozoites are displaced from their site of attachment in the small intestine and carried with the fecal mass into the large intestine. If the fecal mass moves slowly thorough the large intestine, the dehydration of feces in the large intestine provokes formation of the cyst stage. If, however, movement of feces through the large intestine is abnormally rapid and dehydration of the feces is not complete, the feces may contain trophozoites or trophozoites and cysts, depending on the extent of dehydration.

EPIDEMIOLOGY*

Giardiasis has been reported worldwide, with a prevalence that varies from 1% to 30% depending on the population studied. The disease often occurs in epidemic proportions when municipal water supplies become contaminated with the organism in its cyst stage. This is a problem that appears to be ongoing in many parts of the Soviet Union and Asia and has been responsible for several outbreaks in New York and the Rocky Mountain states. Historically it was assumed that this water contamination must be from human sources. Recently, however, it has been discovered that human strains of *Giardia* may infect other animals, especially beavers and dogs, and that these animals may constitute a source of infective cysts. Controlling the waterborne spread of the disease is also complicated by the ability of *Giardia* cysts to remain viable for as long as 3 months in fresh water and, like *E. histolytica*, to resist the usual levels of chlorine used in water purification plants. It is therefore imperative that water treatment include adequate sedimentation, flocculation, and filtration, all of which appear effective in removing cysts and preventing the waterborne spread of the disease.

Person-to-person transmission of the disease has been reported among homosexuals[38,47] and in situations of individuals with poor personal hygiene living in close proximity. Of special concern have been the reports of outbreaks among children in day-care centers, since children appear to be more susceptible and have more severe infections than adults. Individuals with malnutrition, achlorhydria, or hypogammaglobulinemia also appear to be particularly susceptible to infection and the development of severe chronic infections.

PATHOLOGY AND CLINICAL MANIFESTATIONS†

The pathologic changes and clinical manifestations associated with *Giardia* infections vary significantly from person to person. Moreover, there does not appear to be a direct correlation between the severity of the illness and the magnitude of the parasite burden; some patients with a large parasite burden show no symptoms, whereas others with a small parasite load manifest severe symptoms.

Approximately 50% or more of *Giardia* infections are asymptomatic. When symptoms exist, giardiasis is often manifest as a short-lived, acute disease characterized by severe attacks of diarrhea with foul-smelling, greasy, mucus-laden stools, flatulence, epigastric pain, nausea, anorexia, and abdominal cramps. In some individuals, especially those with secretory IgA deficiencies, the disease becomes chronic and the patient has intermittent acute attacks, loses weight, and shows evidence of malabsorption of proteins, folic acid, and fat-soluble vitamins.

LABORATORY DIAGNOSIS[48,56]

Usually *Giardia* infections can be confirmed by demonstrating either the cyst or the trophozoite stage of the organism in fecal specimens. Often this requires examination of multiple specimens because the number of organisms in the feces may vary greatly from day to day. If, after comprehensive examination of multiple fecal specimens, the diagnosis is still in

---

*References 6, 9, 11, 18, 21, 32, 42, and 49.
†References 4, 12, 31, 42, 48, 56, and 61.

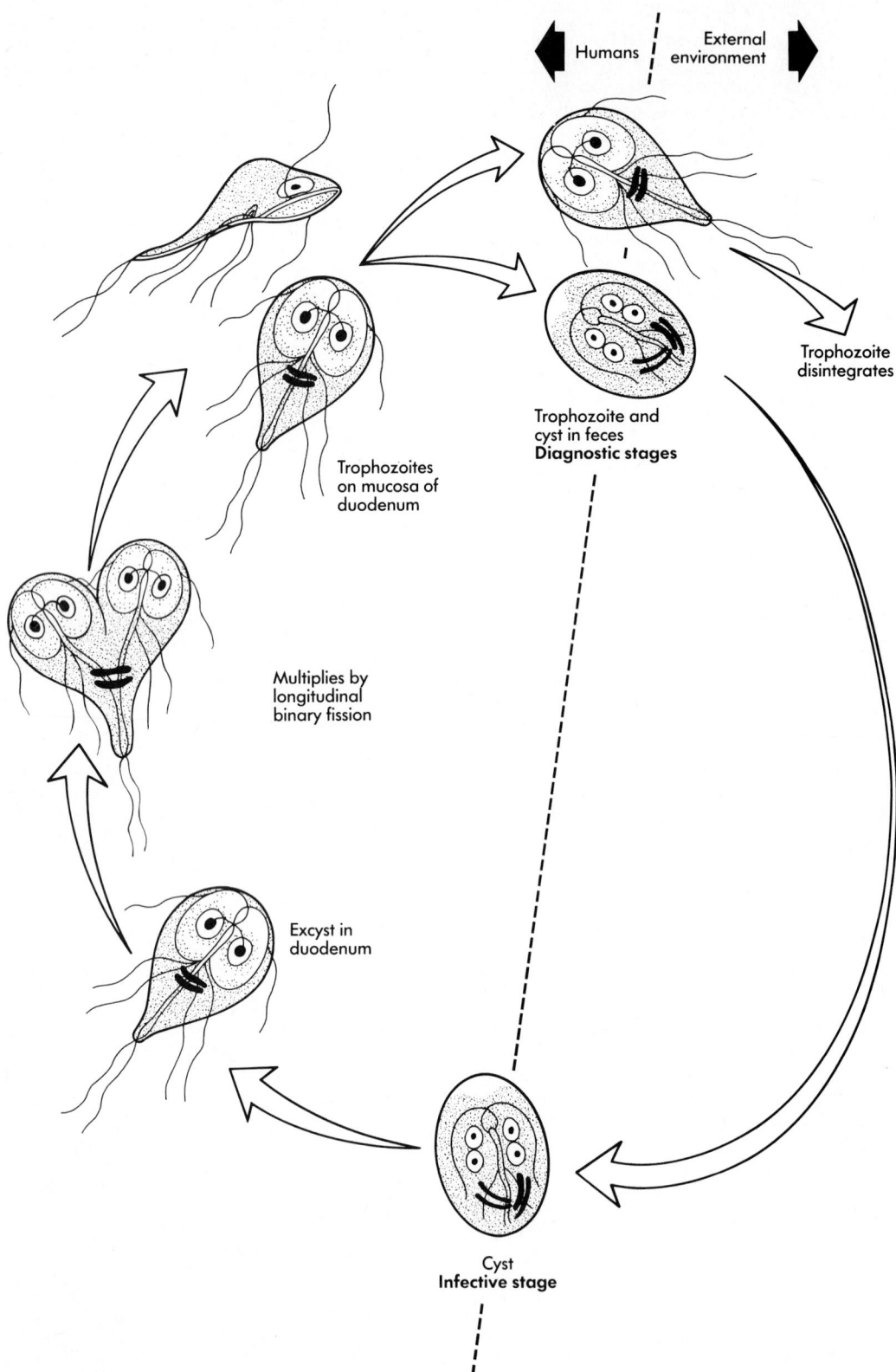

Humans External environment

Trophozoite disintegrates

Trophozoites on mucosa of duodenum

Trophozoite and cyst in feces
Diagnostic stages

Multiplies by longitudinal binary fission

Excyst in duodenum

Cyst
Infective stage

FIGURE 42-7. Life cycle of *Giardia lamblia*. (Modified from Brooke, M.M., and Melvin, D.M.: Common intestinal protozoa of man—life cycle charts, Atlanta, 1964, HEW Pub. No. [CDC] 79-8311, Laboratory Branch of the Communicable Disease Center.)

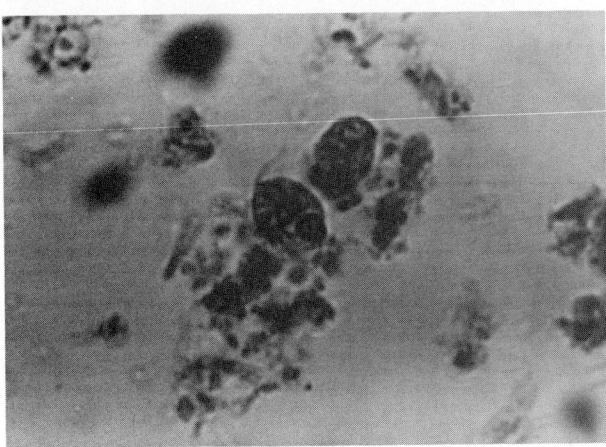

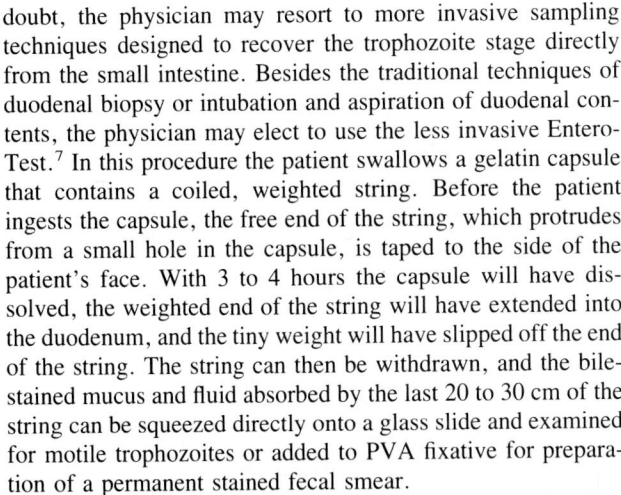

FIGURE 42-8. Trophozoite of *Chilomastix mesnili*. (Approximately ×2000.)

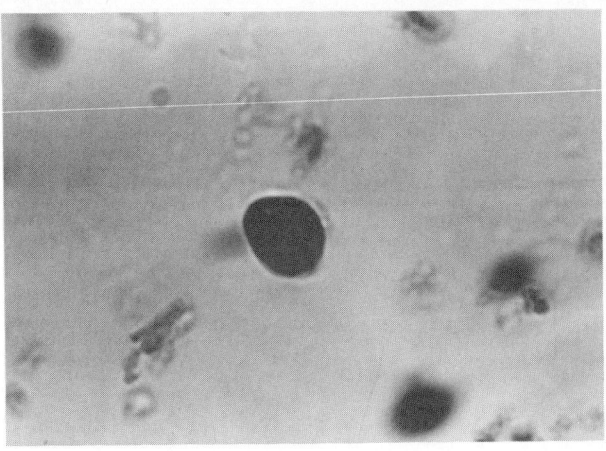

FIGURE 42-9. Cyst of *Chilomastix mesnili*. (Approximately ×2000.)

doubt, the physician may resort to more invasive sampling techniques designed to recover the trophozoite stage directly from the small intestine. Besides the traditional techniques of duodenal biopsy or intubation and aspiration of duodenal contents, the physician may elect to use the less invasive Entero-Test.[7] In this procedure the patient swallows a gelatin capsule that contains a coiled, weighted string. Before the patient ingests the capsule, the free end of the string, which protrudes from a small hole in the capsule, is taped to the side of the patient's face. With 3 to 4 hours the capsule will have dissolved, the weighted end of the string will have extended into the duodenum, and the tiny weight will have slipped off the end of the string. The string can then be withdrawn, and the bile-stained mucus and fluid absorbed by the last 20 to 30 cm of the string can be squeezed directly onto a glass slide and examined for motile trophozoites or added to PVA fixative for preparation of a permanent stained fecal smear.

In wet mounts the trophozoites may be identified by their characteristic ''falling-leaf'' type of motility. A more reliable identification of the trophozoite may be obtained if one examines permanent stained smears for the typical teardrop-shaped, binucleate trophozoite, which resembles a tiny face (Plate 27, *D*).[9] In this stage, which measures 10 to 21 μm long by 5 to 15 μm at its greatest width, the two nuclei are on either side of a pair of rodlike axonemes, which extend from the rounded anterior end of the body to the pointed posterior. There is also usually a pair of sausage-shaped median bodies located in the midbody of the organism, just posterior to the sucking disk and parallel to the axonemes. These median bodies are especially significant, since they are unique to members of the genus *Giardia*. However, a *Giardia* trophozoite so resembles a tiny face that it is not likely to be mistaken for another organism unless the specimen was improperly preserved or stained.

The cyst stage of *Giardia* (Plate 27, *E*) is typically football shaped and measures 8 to 12 μm long by 7 to 10 μm wide. Each cyst typically contain two or four nuclei, depending on the stage of maturity, and fibril-like structures, which are the axonemes and median bodies. An especially distinctive characteristic of preserved *Giardia* cysts is the apparent retraction of the cytoplasm from one end of the cyst wall.

The two major species of nonpathogenic intestinal flagel-

lates, *Chilomastix mesnili* and *Trichomonas hominis*, are more likely to be confused with amoebae than with *Giardia* organisms, especially when seen in stained or improperly preserved fecal specimens. In duodenal aspirates these two nonpathogens are unlikely to be confused with *Giardia* spp., since both organisms inhabit the large intestine and, like the amoebae, are not recovered in duodenal aspirates.

The trophozoite of *Chilomastix* spp. (Figure 42-8), which usually measures 13 to 24 μm long and 6 to 11 μm wide, has a pear-shaped body that is somewhat similar in appearance to *Giardia* organisms, except that the body is twisted lengthwise to form a characteristic spiral groove. When propelled by its four flagella, the organism rotates with a boring motion around the lengthwise axis formed by the spiral grove. The single nucleus of the organism, which has a small central karyosome and no peripheral chromatin, is situated at the rounded anterior end of the body, next to a primitive cleftlike mouth called a cytostome. The cyst of a *Chilomastix* organism (Figure 42-9), which measures 6 to 10 μm long, is shaped like a lemon and has a small, clear nipple at one end; in iodine or permanent stained specimens the single nucleus and cytostome may be visible.

Like other members of the genus *Trichomonas, T. hominis* has no cyst stage. The pear-shaped trophozoite stage, which typically measures 5 to 14 μm long and 7 to 10 μm wide, possesses three characteristics typical of other trichomonads: a single anterior nucleus, a rodlike axostyle that extends the entire length of the body and terminates as a sharply spiked projection outside the body, and a characteristic undulating membrane. Propelled by three to five anterior flagella that impart a quick, jerky motion, the trophozoites of this species differ from those of other species of *Trichomonas* in that the undulating membrane extends the length of the body and terminates in a free flagellum. However, aside from this morphologic difference and provided that the fecal specimen is not contaminated with urine, it is unlikely that *T. hominis* will be confused with the other two species of trichomonads that are found in humans, since each species is restricted to a particular body site: *T. vaginalis* in the urogenital tract, *T. tenax* in the mouth, and *T. hominis* in the large intestine. In improperly preserved specimens *T. hominis* may be mistaken for an amoe-

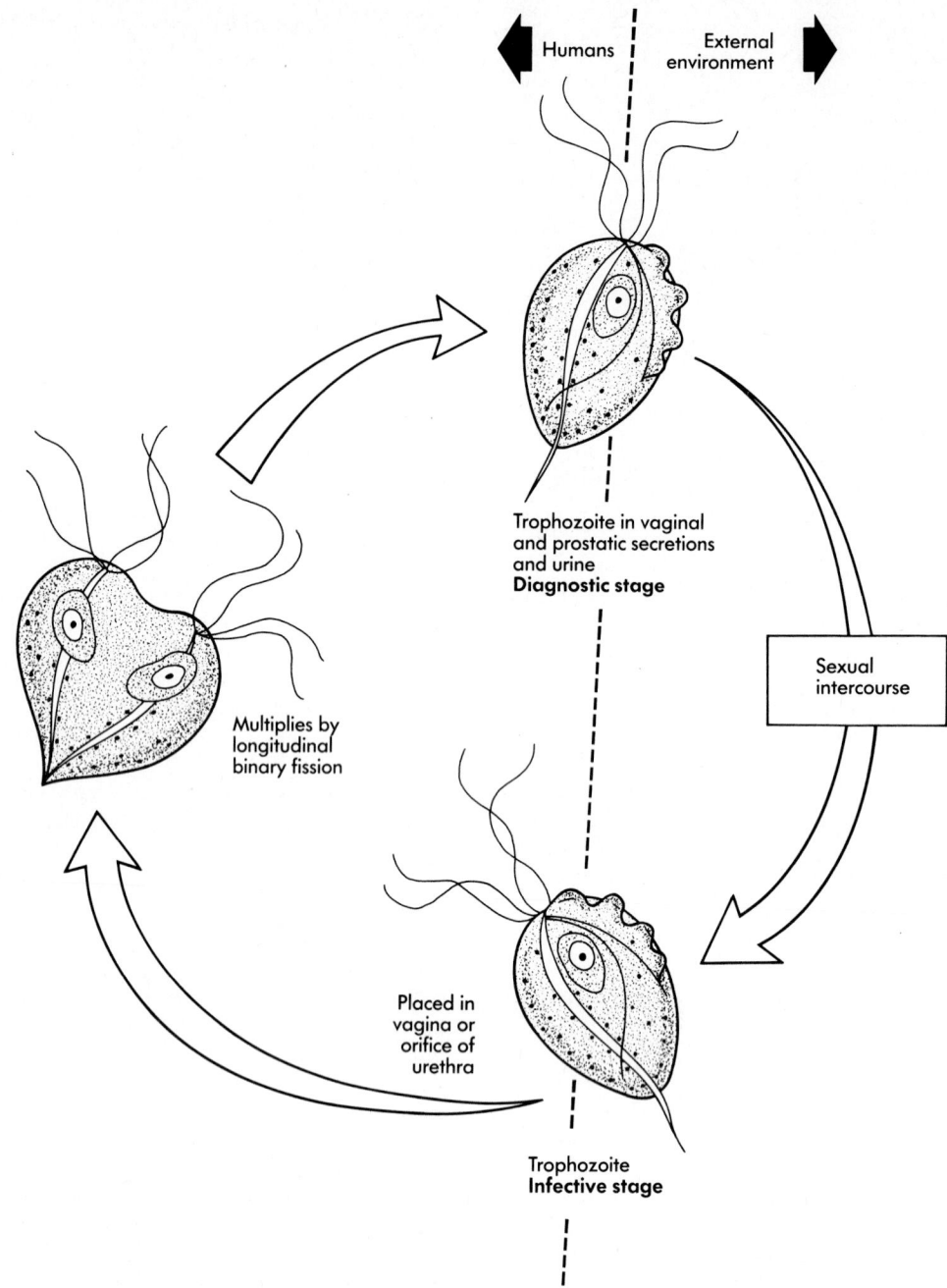

FIGURE 42-10. Life cycle of *Trichomonas vaginalis*. (Modified from Brooke, M.M., and Melvin, D.M.: Common intestinal protozoa of man—life cycle charts, Atlanta, 1964, HEW Pub. No. [CDC] 79-8311, Laboratory Branch of the Communicable Disease Center.)

ba, since it has a tendency to round up and send out portions of cytoplasm that may be mistaken for pseudopods.

TRICHOMONAS VAGINALIS
LIFE CYCLE

Trichomonas vaginalis has all the typical features of the other members of its genus; it exists only in a trophozoite stage and has an axostyle and undulating membrane. *T. vaginalis* is unique, however, not only because it has a short undulating membrane that extends less than half the body length, but

because it is the only pathogenic species of *Trichomonas* regularly found in humans and is the only trichomonad known to inhabit the human urogenital tract.

Infections with *T. vaginalis* are most often acquired when the trophozoite stage is passed to an uninfected sexual partner during intercourse (Figure 42-10). Once in the urogenital tract the organisms divide by longitudinal fission and establish colonies of trophozoites close to or on the surface of epithelial cells in the vagina and urethra of females and the urethra, prostate, and seminal vesicles of males.

Like most sexually transmitted diseases, trichomoniasis is prevalent in the sexually active age groups in all climates and racial groups. Depending on the population examined, estimates of the infection's prevalence range from 5% in males to 50% in females. Newborn girls appear to be at special risk of acquiring trichomoniasis from an infected mother during passage through the birth canal. Although the organism dies rapidly when dried, exposed to direct sunlight, or exposed to water for 35 to 40 minutes, person-to-person transmission may occur where there are a lack of proper toilets or bathing facilities and a sharing of contaminated clothing or washcloths.

PATHOLOGY AND CLINICAL MANIFESTATIONS[29]

Trichomonas infections in males are usually asymptomatic unless there is extensive involvement of the prostate or seminal vesicles or a secondary bacterial infection. When involvement is more extensive, the common manifestations include a thin urethral discharge, dysuria, nocturia, pain in the groin, and an enlarged prostate.

In females the severity of the disease may vary from a mild vaginal itching to an intense vaginal burning accompanied by dysuria, a thick yellow discharge, and severe dermatitis of the inner thighs caused by constant scratching.

LABORATORY DIAGNOSIS

The laboratory diagnosis of trichomoniasis is usually based on finding characteristic motile trophozoites in wet mounts prepared from the vaginal or urethral discharge in females or urethral discharge and prostatic secretions in males. Since the organism has a characteristic jerky, nondirectional motility and no other species of trichomonads are routinely found in the genitourinary tract, preparing permanent stained slides for identification is rarely necessary. The organism is also frequently detected during routine urinalysis and should be reported.

BALANTIDIUM COLI
LIFE CYCLE

Although *Balantidium coli* is a ciliated protozoan with unique cyst and trophozoite stages, its life cycle is similar to that of *E. histolytica* (Figure 42-11). For example, both organisms are infective for humans in the cyst stage, exist in the small intestine, and migrate to the large intestine, where they may simply browse on the mucosal surface or may invade the mucosa and produce extensive ulceration. From a medical standpoint the major difference in the life cycles of these two organisms is that *B. coli* rarely invades beyond the wall of the intestine or produces the extensive extraintestinal disease associated with *E. histolytica* infections.

EPIDEMIOLOGY[5,43,55,59,60]

Based on reported cases, infections with *B. coli* occur worldwide but are apparently rare. Most cases have been reported from tropical and subtropical regions, but the disease has also been reported in temperate climates where there is crowding or poor personal hygiene, such as in mental institutions or penitentiaries.

Besides the possibility of person-to-person transmission, infections may be associated with close contact with any of a number of other animal species, especially pigs and monkeys,

that harbor *Balantidium* spp. remarkably similar to *B. coli*. Whether these are actually different species or are only different strains of *B. coli* is not clear. Except in humans and the lower primates, *Balantidium* spp. do not appear to cause disease, and efforts to transmit the infection from lower animals to humans have not been successful. There is, however, evidence that balantidiasis is more common in individuals closely associated with pigs, and in at least one epidemic outbreak it appears likely that water contaminated with feces from infected pigs was the source of human infection.[55]

PATHOLOGY AND CLINICAL MANIFESTATIONS[5,19,50,55]

Like *E. histolytica*, the trophozoites of *Balantidium* may remain on the surface of the intestinal mucosa, where they feed on undigested starch and bacteria and produce little disease or clinical manifestations of infection. Indeed, most infections with this protozoan are asymptomatic.

In a few individuals, however, the organism begins to feed on host cells of the intestinal mucosa and, with the aid of the enzyme hyaluronidase, burrows into the submucosa of the large intestine producing flasklike ulcers similar to those seen in *E. histolytica* infections. Unlike *E. histolytica*, however, the trophozoites of *B. coli* rarely invade beyond the intestinal mucosa or produce the tumorlike structures (amoebomas) in the intestine.

When the infection is clinically manifest, the typical symptoms are an intermittent diarrhea alternating with periods of constipation. In more severe infections the patient may have dysentery, abdominal pain, nausea, vomiting, and a variety of toxic manifestations, such as fever, headache, and insomnia.

LABORATORY DIAGNOSIS

The laboratory diagnosis of balantidiasis is based on identifying the typical cyst or trophozoite stage of the organism in fecal samples. The trophozoite stage of *B. coli*, which is covered by rows of tiny cilia, ranges from 30 to 120 μm in length and 25 to 120 μm in width. The exact length and width dimensions vary depending on the amount of ingested food material. As a result the trophozoite may appear round, oblong, or very elongate; typically, however, the trophozoite is oblong with a slightly pointed anterior end and a rounded posterior (Figure 42-12). At the anterior end of the body is a distinctive V-shaped groove that constitutes the organism's primitive pharynx (cytopharynx) and mouth (cytostome). As the organism moves forward with the boring type of motility, food material is swept into this cleft and incorporated into food vacuoles that can be seen in the cytoplasm. In addition to the numerous food vacuoles, the trophozoite also contains two usually indiscernible contractile vacuoles and two separate nuclei that control different cellular functions. One nucleus, a large sausage-shaped macronucleus, controls the routine vegetative functions of the cell and asexual reproduction; the other, a tiny, often indiscernible micronucleus, participates in the organism's sexual reproduction by conjugation. The cysts of *B. coli* are typically round and much larger than those of other intestinal protozoa, measuring between 50 and 70 μm in diameter. Each cyst contains only a single organism, which in the early stages may still have active cilia. As the cyst matures, the cilia disappear.

Because of the large size of both the trophozoite and cyst stages and the characteristic boring motility of the trophozoite, the organism can easily be identified simply by use of wet

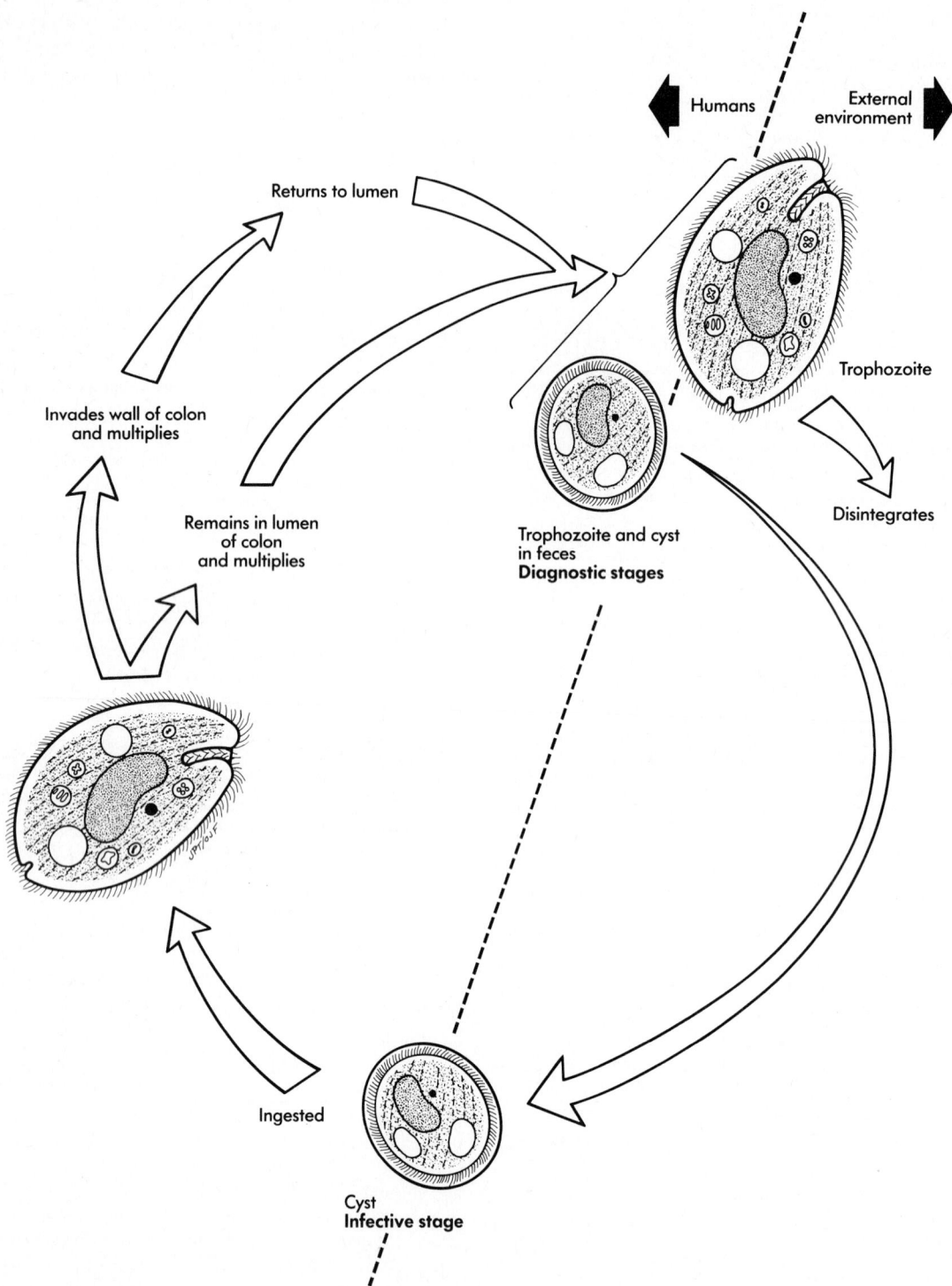

FIGURE 42-11. Life cycle of *Balantidium coli*. (Modified from Brooke, M.M., and Melvin, D.M.: Common intestinal protozoa of man—life cycle charts, Atlanta, 1964, HEW Pub. No. [CDC] 79-8311, Laboratory Branch of the Communicable Disease Center.)

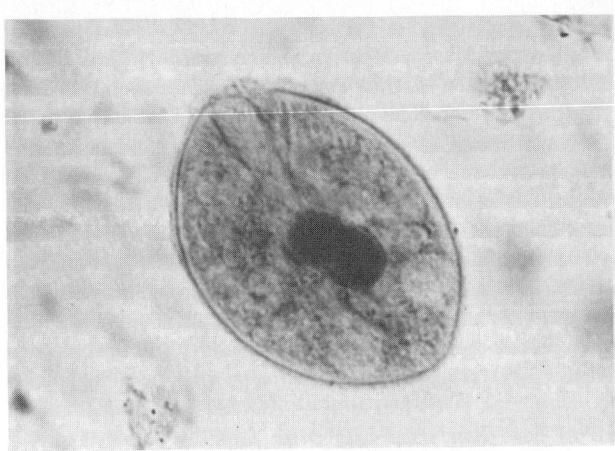

FIGURE 42-12. Trophozoite of *Balantidium coli*. (Approximately ×1000.)

mounts. In fact, a wet mount is probably the preferred method of examination, since the trophozoite is the predominant diagnostic stage in most clinically manifest infections. If necessary, samples can also be directly obtained from intestinal lesions by sigmoidoscopy and examined with a wet mount for the motile trophozoite stage.

ISOSPORA BELLI
LIFE CYCLE[10]

Human infections with *Isospora belli*, an intestinal sporozoan parasite, are acquired by ingestion of the product of the parasite's sexual reproduction—the oocyst (Figure 42-13). Each of the mature, oval oocysts contains two round sporoblasts, which in turn contain four sausage-shaped sporozoites (much like a nested Chinese box). The sporozoites are released when the oocyst wall is digested away in the small intestine, invade the epithelial cells of the small intestine, and develop into trophozoites that multiply intracellularly by a process of asexual binary fission (schizogony). The product of this asexual reproduction, a schizont, is actually a cluster of tiny, immature trophozoites (merozoites) that are released when the infected epithelial cell ruptures. When released, these individual merozoites invade other epithelial cells where they may initiate another cycle of asexual reproduction (most common occurrence) or initiate a cycle of sexual reproduction (sporogony) by transforming into male (microgametocytes) or female (macrogametocytes) sex cells.

In the sexual cycle the microgametocytes ultimately transform into tiny, flagellated, spermlike microgametes that migrate into the intestinal lumen in search of epithelial cells containing mature macrogametocytes. Once fertilized, the macrogametocytes develop into oocysts, which are passed in the feces. The oocysts may be passed in the feces in almost any stage of development, depending on when they rupture from the infected epithelial cell and the rate at which feces are passed from the body. If passed in the immature stage, the oocysts are capable of becoming infective in about 5 days under the proper environmental conditions.

The life cycle of *Isospora* spp., including the alteration of sexual and asexual generations and the terminology of the various stages in the life cycle, is similar to the life cycle of the major sporozoan parasites of humans: *Toxoplasma gondii* and *Plasmodium* spp. The most notable differences are that *Isospora belli* has only a single host—humans—in whom both the sexual and asexual cycles occur, and the infection is confined entirely to one body region, the intestinal tract. Both of the other two organisms have true intermediate hosts, in which only the asexual cycle occurs, and the parasites may be found spread throughout the body.

EPIDEMIOLOGY[25]

Little is known about the exact epidemiology of *Isospora* infection. Presumably the major features of its mode of transmission are similar to those of other intestinal protozoans.

PATHOLOGY AND CLINICAL MANIFESTATIONS[27,39,52,60]

Most infections with *Isospora* are apparently asymptomatic, while clinically manifest cases are generally mild and limited to a few weeks' duration. More serious cases may last for years, and the patient may have severe dysentery accompanied by abdominal pain and weight loss. Many of the clinically manifest cases of *Isospora* have signs and symptoms suggesting a malabsorption syndrome similar to that observed in some cases of giardiasis.

LABORATORY DIAGNOSIS

The laboratory diagnosis of *Isospora* infections is based on finding mature or immature oocysts in fecal specimens. Typically measuring 30 by 12 μm, each oval-shaped mature oocyst (Figure 42-14) contains two spherical, cell-like structures (sporocysts). The immature oocysts are a similar size and shape but contain only a single, round, cell-like structure, the sporoblast. As immature oocysts complete their development in the external environment, the sporoblast divides into two sporocysts.

Because of their relatively large size and distinctive appearance, the oocysts of *Isospora* spp. are easily observed in iodine-stained wet mounts prepared directly from the fecal specimen or after concentration. Permanent stained smears are rarely required.

CRYPTOSPORIDIUM
LIFE CYCLE[8,41,53]

Species of the *Cryptosporidium* genus have long been recognized as sporozoan (coccidia) parasites of the intestinal tract of numerous domestic animals. The normal life cycle of the parasite is similar to that of *Isospora* spp., except that the parasite does not have an intracellular stage; all the development takes place on the surface of the mucosal cells.

EPIDEMIOLOGY*

Human infections with this parasite have recently become of interest because of the serious consequences of the infection in compromised hosts, especially in patients with acquired immunodeficiency syndrome (AIDS). The infection also occurs in immunocompetent individuals with less serious consequences.

The infection is apparently acquired by ingesting the oocyst stage that is passed in the feces of other infected humans or of one of the naturally infected animals such as calves or puppies.

---

*References 16, 17, 20, 41, 53, and 54.

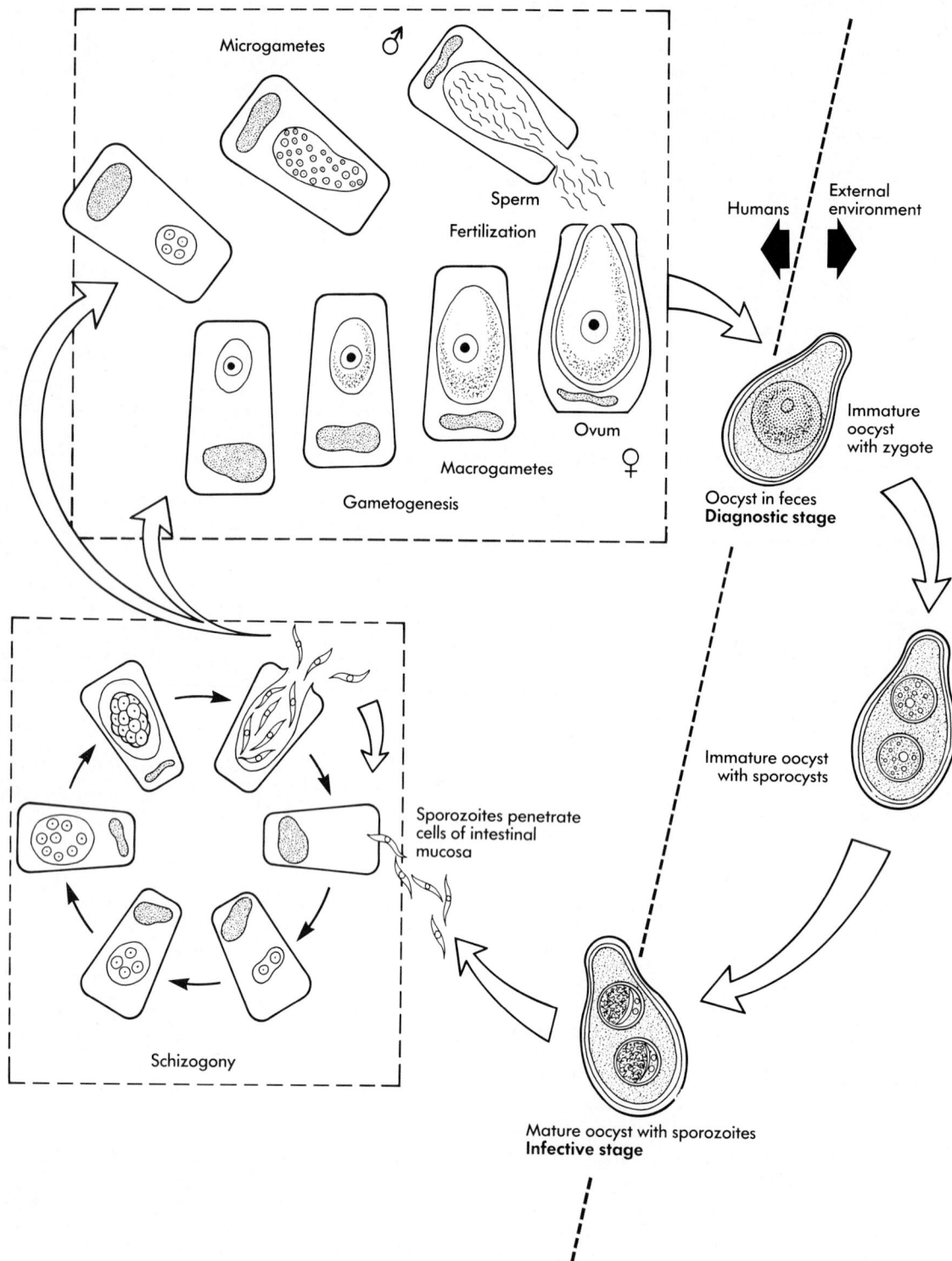

FIGURE 42-13. Life cycle of *Isospora belli*. (Modified from Brooke, M.M., and Melvin, D.M.: Common intestinal protozoa of man—life cycle charts, Atlanta, 1964, HEW Pub. No. [CDC] 79-8311, Laboratory Branch of the Communicable Disease Center.)

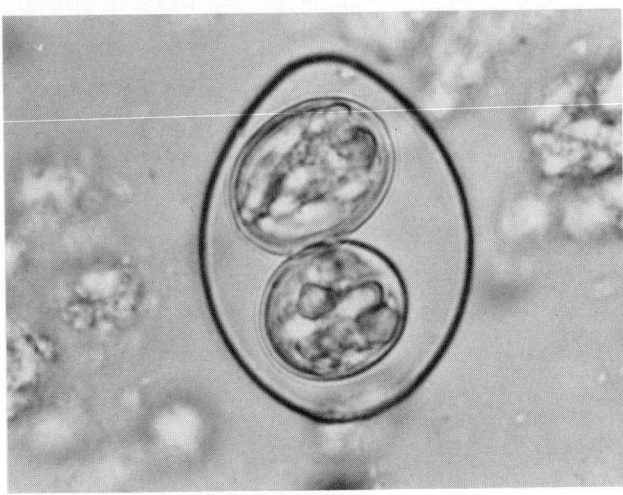

FIGURE 42-14. Oocyst of *Isospora belli.* (Approximately ×2000.)

In the past, most infections have occurred as sporadic isolated cases. Recently there have been reports of epidemic outbreaks among animal handlers, veterinary students, and children in day-care centers.

PATHOLOGY AND CLINICAL MANIFESTATIONS[41,53]

Human infections in individuals who are immunocompetent usually take the form of a self-limited diarrhea, similar to that occurring with *Isospora* spp. However, in immunocompromised individuals the diarrhea may be prolonged, causing large fluid losses and sometimes death. The parasite may even disseminate to internal organs such as the lungs.

LABORATORY DIAGNOSIS[28,37]

Currently, most diagnoses of cryptosporidioses are based on finding the tiny (4 to 6 μm) oocyst stage in fecal specimens rather than on the traditional method of intestinal biopsy, which appears to be a less sensitive technique. However, besides a traditional iodine-stained wet mount, in which the oocyst appears as an unstained yeastlike structure (provided that the smear is examined within 15 minutes, since after that the oocysts begin to stain), special processing and staining techniques are required for optimal detection of the oocysts in fecal specimens. With a modified Ziehl-Neelsen acid-fast stain (see Chapter 6), the oocyst is readily detected as tiny acid-fast bodies in fresh or formalin-preserved stool specimens; specimens processed in PVA fixative do not stain as well. If a concentration technique is used, the best results are obtained with a sugar flotation technique (Sheather's technique), which has long been used in veterinary parasitology.

REFERENCES

1. Adams, E.B., and Macleod, I.N.: Invasive amebiasis. I. Amebic dysentery and its complications, Medicine **56:**315, 1977.
2. Adams, E.B., and Macleod, I.N.: Invasive amebiasis. II. Amebic liver abscess and its complications, Medicine **56:**325, 1977.
3. Al-Salihi, F.L., Curran, J.P., and Wang, J.: Neonatal *Trichomonas vaginalis:* report of three cases and review of the literature, Pediatrics **53:**196, 1974.
4. Ament, M.E., and Rubin, C.E.: Relation of giardiasis to abnormal intestinal structure and function in gastrointestinal immuno-deficiency syndrome, Gastroenterology **62:**216, 1972.
5. Arean, V.M., and Koppisch, E.: Balantidiasis: a review and report of cases, Am. J. Pathol. **32:**1089, 1956.
6. Babb, R.R., Peck, D.C., and Vescia, F.G.: Giardiasis: a cause of traveller's diarrhea, JAMA **217:**1359, 1971.
7. Beal, C.B., et al.: A new technique for sampling duodenal contents, Am. J. Trop. Med. Hyg. **19:**349, 1970.
8. Bird, R.G., and Smith, M.D.: Cryptosporidiosis in man: parasite life cycle and fine structural pathology, J. Pathol. **132:**217, 1980.
9. Black, R.E., et al.: Giardiasis in day-care centers: evidence of person-to-person transmission, Pediatrics **60:**486, 1977.
10. Brandborg, L.L., Goldberg, S.B., and Briendenbach, W.C.: Human coccidiosis: a possible cause of malabsorption—the life cycle in small bowel mucosal biopsies as a diagnostic feature, N. Engl. J. Med. **283:**1306, 1970.
11. Brodsky, R.E., et al.: Giardiasis in American travelers to the Soviet Union, J. Infect. Dis. **130:**319, 1974.
12. Brooks, S.E.H., et al.: Electron microscopy of *Giardia lamblia* in human jejunal biopsies, J. Med. Microbiol. **3:**196, 1970.
13. Burrows, R.B.: *Entamoeba hartmanni,* Am. J. Hyg. **5:**172, 1957.
14. Burrows, R.B., and Swerdlow, M.A.: *Enterobius vermicularis* as a probable vector of *Dientamoeba fragilis,* Am. J. Trop. Med. Hyg. **5:**258, 1956.
15. Camp, R.R., Mattern, C.F.T., and Honigberg, B.M.: Study of *Dientamoeba fragilis* Jeeps ad Dobell. I. Electron microscopic observations of the binucleate stages. II. Taxonomic position and revision of the genus, J. Protozool. **21:**69, 1974.
16. Center for Disease Control: Giardiasis: Vail, Colorado, MMWR **27:**155, 1978.
17. Centers for Disease Control: Cryptosporidiosis: assessment of chemotherapy of males with acquired immune deficiency syndrome (AIDS), MMWR **31:**589, 1982.
18. Centers for Disease Control: Cryptosporidiosis among children attending day-care centers—Georgia, Pennsylvania, Michigan, California, New Mexico, MMWR **33:**599, 1984.
19. Christian, E.C.: Fatal balantidiasis, Ghana Med. J. **13:**86, 1974.
20. Current, W.L., et al.: Human cryptosporidiosis in immunocompetent and immunodeficient persons: studies of an outbreak and experimental transmission, N. Engl. J. Med. **308:**1252, 1983.
21. Davies, R.B., and Hibler, C.P.: Animal reservoirs and cross-species transmission of *Giardia.* In Jakubowski, W., and Hoff, J.C., editors: Waterborne transmission of giardiasis, Environmental Protection Agency Pub. No. 600/9-79-001, Washington, D.C., 1979, U.S. Government Printing Office.
22. Dorrough, R.L.: Amebic liver abscess, South Med. J. **60:**305, 1967.
23. Elsdon-Dew, R.: The epidemiology of amoebiasis. In Kreier, J.P., editor: Advances in parasitology, vol. 6, New York, 1968, Academic Press, Inc.
24. Faust, E.C.: The multiple facets of *Entamoeba histolytica* infection, Int. Rev. Trop. Med. **1:**43, 1961.
25. Faust, E.C., et al.: Human isosporiasis in the Western Hemisphere, Am. J. Trop. Med. **10:**343, 1961.
26. Freedman, L., and Elsdon-Dew, R.: Size as a criterion of species in the human intestinal amebae, Am. J. Trop. Med. Hyg. **8:**327, 1959.
27. French, J.M., Whitby, J.L., and Whitfield, A.G.W.: Steatorrhea in a man infected with coccidiosis *(Isospora belli):* case reports, Gastroenterology **47:**642, 1974.
28. Garcia, L.S., et al.: Techniques for the recovery and identification of *Cryptosporidium* oocysts from stool specimens, J. Clin. Microbiol. **18:**185, 1983.
29. Garcia-Tamayo, J., Nunez-Monteil, J.T., and de Garcia, H.P.: An electron microscopic investigation of the pathogenesis of human vaginal trichomoniasis, Acta Cytol. **22:**447, 1978.

30. Healy, G.R.: Laboratory diagnosis of amebiasis, Bull. N.Y. Acad. Sci. **47:**478, 1971.

31. Hoskins, L.C., et al.: Clinical giardiasis and intestinal malabsorption, Gastroenterology **53:**265, 1967.

32. Jarroll, E.L., Bingham, A.K., and Meyer, E.A.: *Giardia* cyst destruction: effectiveness of six small-quantity water disinfection methods, Am. J. Trop. Med. Hyg. **29:**8, 1980.

33. Kagan, I.G.: Pathogenicity of *Entamoeba histolytica,* Infection **3:**96, 1975.

34. Kean, B.H.: Venereal amebiasis, N.Y. State J. Med. **76:**930, 1976.

35. Levin, R.L., and Armstrong, D.E.: Human infection with *Entamoeba polecki,* Am. J. Clin. Pathol. **54:**611, 1970.

36. Littlewood, J.M., and Kohler, H.G.: Urinary tract infection by *Trichomonas vaginalis* in a newborn baby, Arch. Dis. Child. **41:**693, 1966.

37. Ma, P., and Soave, R.: Three-step stool examination for cryptosporidiosis in 10 homosexual men with protracted watery diarrhea, J. Infect. Dis. **147:**824, 1983.

38. Meyers, J.D., Kuharic, H.A., and Holmes, K.K.: *Giardia lamblia* infections in homosexual men, Br. J. Vener. Dis. **53:**54, 1977.

39. Miller, F.H., Jr., Pizzuto, A.V., and McCauley, H.: Human isosporosis: two cases, Am. J. Trop. Med. Hyg. **20:**23, 1974.

40. Morgan, R.S., and Uzman, B.G.: Nature of the packing of ribosomes within chromatoid bodies, Science **152:**214, 1966.

41. Navin, T.R., and Juranek, D.D.: Cryptosporidiosis: clinical, epidemiologic, and parasitologic review, Rev. Infect. Dis. **6:**313, 1984.

42. Osterholm, M.T., et al.: An outbreak of food-borne giardiasis, N. Engl. J. Med. **304:**24, 1981.

43. Radford, H.J.: Balantidiasis in Papua, New Guinea, Med. J. Aust. **1:**238, 1973.

44. Saha, T.K., and Ghosh, T.K.: Invasion of small intestinal mucosa by *Giardia lamblia* in man, Gastroenterology **72:**402, 1977.

45. Salaki, J.S., Shirey, J.L., and Strickland, T.: Successful treatment of symptomatic *Entamoeba polecki* infection, Am. J. Trop. Med. Hyg. **28:**190, 1979.

46. Schmerin, M.J., Gelston, A., and Jones, T.C.: Amebiasis: an increasing problem among homosexuals in New York City, JAMA **238:**1386, 1977.

47. Schmerin, M.J., Jones, T.C., and Klein, H.: Giardiasis: association with homosexuality, Ann. Intern. Med. **88:**801, 1978.

48. Schultz, M.G.: Giardiasis, JAMA **233:**1383, 1975.

49. Shaw, P.K., et al.: A community-wide outbreak of giardiasis with documented transmission by municipal water, Ann. Intern. Med. **87::**426, 1977.

50. Shookhoff, H.B.: *Balantidium coli* infection with special reference to treatment, Am. J. Trop. Med. **31:**442, 1951.

51. Thomas, J.A., and Anthony, A.J.: Amoebiasis of the penis, Br. J. Urol. **48:**269, 1976.

52. Trier, J.S., et al.: Chronic intestinal coccidiosis in man: intestinal morphology and response to treatment, Gastroenterology **66:**923, 1974.

53. Tzipori, S.: Cryptosporidiosis in animals and humans, Microbiol. Rev. **47:**84, 1983.

54. Tzipori, S., et al.: Experimental infection of lambs with *Cryptosporidium* isolated from a human patient with diarrhoea, Gut **23:**71, 1982.

55. Walter, P.D., et al.: Balantidiasis outbreak in Truk, Am. J. Trop. Med. Hyg. **22:**33, 1973.

56. Wolfe, M.S.: Giardiasis, JAMA **233:**1362, 1975.

57. Yang, J., and Scholten, T.: *Dientamoeba fragilis:* a review with notes on its epidemiology, pathogenicity, mode of transmission, and diagnosis, Am. J. Trop. Med. Hyg. **26:**16, 1977.

58. Ylvisaker, J.T., and McDonald, G.B.: Sexually acquired amebic colitis and liver abscess, West. J. Med. **132:**153, 1980.

59. Young, M.D.: Attempt to transmit human *Balantidium coli,* Am. J. Trop. Med. **30:**70, 1950.

60. Zaman, V.: Observations on human *Isospora,* Trans. R. Soc. Trop. Med. Hyg. **62:**556, 1968.

61. Zinnemann, H.H., and Kaplan, A.P.: The association of giardiasis with reduced intestinal secretory immunoglobulins A, Am. J. Dig. Dis. **17:**793, 1972.

ADDITIONAL READINGS

Binford, C.H., and Connor, D.H.: Pathology of tropical and extraordinary diseases: an atlas, vols. 1 and 2, Washington, D.C., 1976, Armed Forces Institute of Pathology.

Brooke, M.M., and Melvin, D.M.: Intestinal and urogenital protozoa. In Lennette, E.H., et al., editors: Manual of clinical microbiology, ed. 3, Washington, D.C., 1980, American Society for Microbiology.

Committee on Education, American Society of Parasitologists: Procedure suggested for use in examination of clinical specimens for parasitic infection, J. Parasitol. **63:**959, 1977.

Faust, E.C., Russell, P.F., and Jung, R.C.: Craig and Faust's clinical parasitology, ed. 8, Philadelphia, 1970, Lea & Febiger.

Hunter, G.W., Swartzwelder, J.C., and Clyde, D.F.: Tropical medicine, ed. 5, Philadelphia, 1976, W.B. Saunders Co.

Levine, N.D.: Nematode parasites of domestic animals and man, Minneapolis, 1968, Burgess Publishing Co.

Marcial-Rojas, R.A., editor: Pathology of protozoal and helminthic diseases with clinical correlation, Baltimore, 1971, Williams & Wilkins Co.

Markel, E.K., and Voge, M.: Medical parasitology, ed. 5, Philadelphia, 1981, W.B. Saunders Co.

Melvin, D.M., and Smith, J.W.: Intestinal parasitic infections. I. Problems in laboratory diagnosis, Lab. Med. **10:**207, 1979.

Schmidt, G.D., and Roberts, L.S.: Foundations of parasitology, ed. 3, St. Louis, 1985, The C.V. Mosby Co.

Warren, K.S., and Mahmoud, A.A.F., editors: Geographic medicine for the practitioner: algorithms in the diagnosis and management of exotic diseases, Chicago, 1978, The University of Chicago Press.

CHAPTER 43

Blood and Tissue Protozoa

John Klaas II

With the exception of a few diseases, such as toxoplasmosis and pneumocystosis, infections with the major blood and tissue protozoan parasites of humans are not common in the United States. Worldwide, however, this group of organisms constitutes a major continuing threat to human health. For microbiologists and public health officials in the United States, there must be cause for concern. We have repeatedly seen these infections in tourists returning from endemic areas, and many of these infections have the potential to become epidemic in the United States. For example, mosquitoes capable of transmitting malaria are widespread in the southern and western states; in fact, malaria was at one time an endemic disease in the Southeast. Also, because the infections are uncommon in the United States, diagnosis is often delayed, a factor that not only endangers the individual patient but also increases the possibility that the infection may be acquired by some of the natural vectors of the disease.

The taxonomic arrangement of the organisms in this chapter follows the reverse order of that used in Chapter 42 on lumen-dwelling protozoa; that is, the sporozoa are discussed first, followed by the flagellates, and finally the amoebae. (There are no parasitic ciliates in the blood and tissue category.) This arrangement was selected for two reasons. First, in this order the more significant parasites are discussed earlier in the chapter, and second, there is a natural transition from the life cycle of *Isospora* spp. to the life cycle of *Plasmodium* spp.; both are sporozoa, and similar terminology is used to describe the various stages of their life cycles.

PLASMODIUM VIVAX, PLASMODIUM FALCIPARUM, PLASMODIUM MALARIAE, AND PLASMODIUM OVALE
LIFE CYCLE[28,37,58,62,88]

Most human malarial infections are caused by one of four species of the genus *Plasmodium: P. vivax* (benign tertian malaria), *P. falciparum* (subtertian, malignant tertian, or estivoautumnal malaria), *P. malariae* (quartan malaria), and *P. ovale* (ovale malaria). Some species of malaria found in lower primates, most notably *P. cynomolgi* and *P. knowlesi*, have occasionally been reported to cause human infections, but the disease is usually mild.

The life cycles (Figure 43-1) of all the *Plasmodium* spp. that infect humans with malaria are similar, with a cycle of sexual reproduction occurring in female mosquitoes of the genus *Anopheles* (the definitive host) and cycles of asexual reproduction occurring in humans (the intermediate host). The asexual cycles begin with the bite of an infected female anopheline mosquito. When taking the blood meal, the mosquito injects salivary fluids containing infective sporozoites into the wound.

These sporozoites are motile, spindle shaped, and 10 to 15 μm long. The sporozoites enter the circulation and, in about 1 hour, leave the circulation and enter the parenchymal cells of the liver, where they initiate the first phase of the asexual cycle: exoerythrocytic schizogony.

During exoerythrocytic schizogony the parasites divide by binary fission to produce large numbers of daughter cells (merozoites). The duration of the exoerythrocytic phase and the number of daughter cells vary with the particular species of parasite. Specifically, *P. falciparum* usually completes the cycle in 5 to 7 days, and each sporozoite produces about 40,000 merozoites. The figures for the other species are 6 to 8 days and 10,000 merozoites for *P. vivax*, 9 days and 15,000 merozoites for *P. ovale*, and 12 to 17 days and 2000 merozoites for *P. malariae*.

Current evidence suggests that daughter merozoites cannot reinvade the liver cells and repeat the process. However, in infections with *P. vivax* and *P. ovale* some of the invading sporozoites give rise to exoerythrocytic forms (hypnozoites) that may remain dormant in the liver for up to 5 years before beginning exoerythrocytic schizogony. This delayed production of merozoites from hypnozoites is presumably responsible for recurrences of active vivax or ovale malaria long after a patient has recovered from the initial clinical attacks of the disease.

The second phase of the asexual reproduction, erythrocytic schizogony, begins when merozoites released from infected liver cells invade circulating erythrocytes and continue to reproduce asexually (erythrocytic schizogony). When the erythrocytic schizont has matured, the erythrocyte ruptures; the freed merozoites then invade other uninfected erythrocytes, and the cycle of asexual reproduction is repeated. This erythrocytic cycle occurs with a characteristic regularity for each different species and results in schizont stages with a typical number of merozoites. In *P. vivax* infections the typical cycle takes 48 hours and yields 12 to 24 merozoites from each schizont (average 16). In *P. falciparum* and *P. ovale* infections the length of the cycle is the same, 48 hours; however, each schizont of *P. falciparum* yields between eight and 24 merozoites, compared with 12 to 24 merozoites for each schizont of *P. ovale*. In *P. malariae* infections the asexual cycle requires 72 hours and yields six to 12 (average eight) merozoites from each schizont.

The sexual cycle of *Plasmodium* spp., which can be completed only within female anopheline mosquitoes, actually begins during the erythrocytic cycle in a human host. After invading erythrocytes, some of the merozoites differentiate into male (microgametocyte) and female (macrogametocyte) sexual forms instead of trophozoites. When ingested with the blood

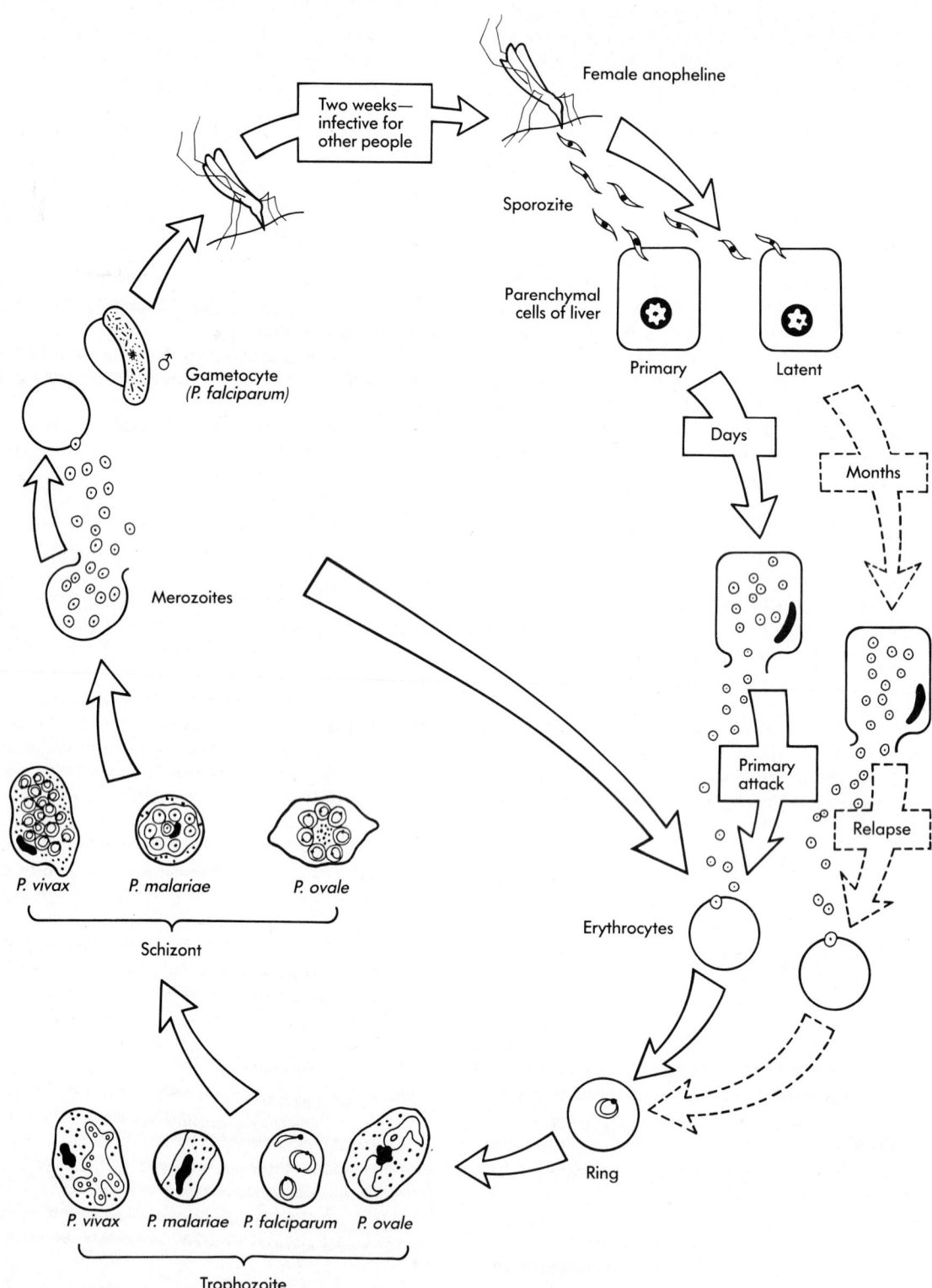

FIGURE 43-1. Life cycle of *Plasmodium* spp.

meal of a female anopheline mosquito the microgametes continue their development within the intestine of the mosquito. The microgametocytes form spermlike microgametes that seek out and fertilize the macrogametes. The fertilized macrogametes then transform into elongate embryos (ookinetes) that penetrate to just under the membrane that covers the mosquito's intestinal tract and mature into round, cystlike structures (oocysts). Within 10 to 14 days the oocyst (diploid number) undergoes a reduction division (sporogony) that results in the formation of thousands of infective sporozoites (haploid number) that burst from the oocyst and migrate to the salivary glands, where they await injection into another human host.

EPIDEMIOLOGY*

Malaria is epidemic in most of the tropical and subtropical regions of the world, with an estimated prevalence of 120 million to 400 million cases among the 1.2 billion persons at risk of the infection. Within this wide geographic region, however, the incidence of the disease varies considerably depending on the prevalence of malaria in the human population, the number of susceptible individuals in the population, the abundance, feeding habits, and susceptibility of the indigenous anopheline mosquitoes, the local climatic and geographic factors that influence the size of the mosquito population, and the characteristics of the particular *Plasmodium* sp. or strain in the endemic area.

The interaction of these various factors appears, in part, to explain why particular species of malaria are more common in some areas and why the disease appears seasonally in some areas and year-round in others. For example, *P. vivax* and *P. malariae* are more common in temperate climates than either *P. falciparum* or *P. ovale*; the latter two species are generally restricted to tropical and subtropical climates. Seasonal variation in the size of the mosquito population may explain the more limited distribution of *P. falciparum* and *P. ovale*. Neither of these species has the dormant liver stage (hypnozoite) that would ensure parasite survival in climates where mosquito breeding occurs only a few times each year. Similarly, wherever there is seasonal variation in temperature or defined wet and dry seasons, the incidence of the disease tends to increase in the warm wet months, which are the major mosquito breeding periods. Even in highly endemic regions, malaria transmission is often limited to rural areas in which proximity to mosquito breeding sites places the human population at greater risk of infection.

Except for partial protection against *P. vivax* infections in blacks with sickle cell trait and *P. falciparum* infections in blacks lacking certain blood group factors (Duffy factors; see Chapter 2), all ages, sexes, and racial groups appear to be equally susceptible to malarial infections. In the United States most cases of malaria are diagnosed in persons who have acquired the infection while traveling in endemic areas overseas. The majority of these U.S. cases are caused by either *P. vivax* (about 50%) or *P. falciparum* (about 25%), which is not surprising because these two species are the most common causes of malaria worldwide. A smaller number of infections may be traced to transmission by blood transfusions and sharing of contaminated needles and syringes among drug addicts.

In very rare instances the infection may be acquired congenitally.

PATHOLOGY AND CLINICAL MANIFESTATIONS*

The major pathologic and clinical manifestations of malaria are associated with the erythrocytic phase of the life cycle; the exoerythrocytic stage in the liver produces few if any pathologic changes. Common to almost all cases of malaria are hemolysis of both infected and uninfected erythrocytes, toxic and antibody responses to the parasite's metabolites, and production of an insoluble brown-black "malaria pigment" (hemozoin) as an end product of the parasite's metabolism of hemoglobin.

In *P. vivax*, *P. ovale*, and *P. malariae* infections, the extent of these pathologic changes tends to be more limited because these species prefer to infect erythrocytes of a particular age. Specifically, *P. vivax* and *P. ovale* prefer to infect younger erythrocytes (reticulocytes), whereas *P. malariae* prefers older erythrocytes. The longer cycle of schizogony (72 hours) in *P. malariae* also tends to limit the degree of disease caused by this species.

Disease associated with *P. falciparum* infections is generally more serious because the parasite readily infects erythrocytes of any age and erythrocytes infected with this species have a greater tendency to adhere to the vascular endothelium of internal organs, especially in the later stages of schizogony (that is, older trophozoites and schizonts). This characteristic of *P. falciparum* is responsible for extensive thrombosis of capillaries and for ischemia and tissue anoxia within affected organs.

Another common feature of malarial infections is hyperplasia of the spleen's reticuloendothelial elements. Darkening of the tissue occurs as fixed phagocytic cells within the spleen destroy both infected and uninfected erythrocytes and ingest circulating hemozoin. Generalized anemia and tissue anoxia are consequences of these pathologic changes and are outwardly manifest as splenomegaly and a normocytic normochromic anemia.

Other organs may also be enlarged and discolored, but the outward manifestations of their involvement are usually less prominent, except when unusually large numbers of erythrocytes infected with *P. falciparum* become sequestered in the capillaries of one particular organ. Among the organs that are particularly prone to *P. falciparum* infections are the brain (cerebral malaria), the liver (bilious remittent fever), the adrenal glands and gastrointestinal tract (algid malaria), the kidney, and the lungs (pneumonic malaria). A generalized intravascular hemolysis (blackwater fever) has also been associated with individuals having repeated infections with *P. falciparum*.

Besides splenomegaly and anemia, the other typical clinical manifestation of malaria is periodic attacks of chills and fever (paroxysms) induced by the toxic metabolites released each time infected erythrocytes rupture. At first the fever may be continuous, or the paroxysms may occur at irregular intervals. This may indicate the presence of two or more groups of parasites maturing at different rates. As the infection continues, however, one group of parasites predominates, and the paroxysms occur at characteristic intervals—approximately every 48 hours for *P. vivax* and *P. ovale* and every 72 hours for *P. malariae*. In *P. falciparum* infections the typical cycle is every

---

*References 1, 15, 17, 35, 39, 58, 73, 78, and 88.

*References 21, 48, 57, 58, 88, 93, and 109.

36 to 48 hours; however, many patients suffer from an unremitting fever caused by the absence of a dominant group of parasites.

Regardless of the particular species, most malarial infections follow a typical course that begins with a prodromal stage of headache, myalgia, anorexia, nausea, and a slight fever before the onset of the first paroxysm. The actual paroxysm begins with a sudden, shaking chill that lasts for 10 to 15 minutes and is accompanied by a rising body temperature, even though the patient typically complains of feeling cold and the skin is pale, cyanotic, and dry. At the end of this chill the fever peaks, the skin becomes flushed, and the patient complains of severe frontal headaches, pain in the back and limbs, and feeling hot. Disorientation and delirium may occur in the fever stage of the paroxysm. Lasting from 2 to 6 hours in *P. vivax* or *P. ovale* infections and as long as 20 hours in *P. falciparum* infections, the fever stage is followed by a sweating stage in which the patient sweats profusely for several hours as the temperature declines. The patient, exhausted at the end of this cycle of chills, fever, and sweating, usually falls asleep and later awakes, feeling normal until the next paroxysm.

In untreated cases that are not fatal, the paroxysms become less severe and more infrequent as the body's immune system begins to control the infection. Latent liver stages (relapses) may activate weeks or even years after apparent well-being following *P. vivax* infections. In infection with *P. ovale*, the other species of malaria with persisting liver stages, most relapses occur within the first year after the primary attack. In *P. malariae* and *P. falciparum* infections there are no persisting liver stages. However, erythrocytic stages may persist in very small numbers and initiate a recrudescence. In general, a recrudescence is identical to a relapse except that new paroxysms are initiated by parasites from within the erythrocytes and not from exoerythrocytic stages. In *P. falciparum* infections, recrudescences usually occur only in the first year; however, in *P. malariae* infections, recrudescences may occur as long as 40 years after the initial infection. Presumably, both relapses and recrudescences are related to a depression of the patient's immune system from such obvious causes as onset of disease or treatment known to depress immunity, or less obviously from stress or the trauma of an accident or surgery.

Mortality from most malaria infections, even if untreated, is very low if the patient is in good health before infection and complications do not develop. On the other hand, *P. falciparum* infections are particularly dangerous, even in otherwise healthy patients, because of the extent of erythrocyte destruction and the tendency of the infected erythrocytes to become sequestered in individual internal organs and produce thrombosis and tissue anoxia of the affected organ.

LABORATORY DIAGNOSIS[37,88,106]

Confirmation of active cases is based on identifying the *Plasmodium* sp. from stages found in Giemsa-stained thick or thin smears of peripheral blood. In most cases the characteristic stages are apparent if peripheral blood samples are collected without anticoagulant (a finger stick should be used) twice a day (morning and afternoon) for 3 consecutive days.

Similar to the stepwise process used to identify *Entamoeba histolytica*, the identification of malarial parasites can be divided into a series of steps, each of which provides the physician with relevant information and leads closer to the final identification.

The first and perhaps most important step is to recognize the presence of malarial parasites. With this information alone, the physician can closely monitor the patient for possible complications and initiate therapy that may prove lifesaving. In thin blood smears the basic clue to the presence of malarial parasites is stained intracellular organisms composed of blue cytoplasm and red nuclear (chromatin) material (Plate 28, *A*). Artifacts such as fragments of the formed elements of the blood and stain debris rarely meet all these criteria; either they are not intracellular or they do not have both blue- and red-staining components. Recognizing the parasites in thick smears is more difficult, because the parasites do not appear intracellular (the erythrocytes are dehemoglobinized and not visible) and their morphology is significantly different from that seen in thin smears. However, the basic staining characteristics of the parasite remain the same, and with practice one can learn to recognize the compressed forms of the parasite that are seen in thick smears.

Once it has been decided that malarial parasites are present, the second step is speciation of the organism. This process is essential, because therapy for species with latent liver stages requires the use of additional drugs to eliminate persisting liver stages and prevent relapses. Moreover, if the organism is *P. falciparum*, there are a high risk of fatal complications and a possibility the parasite may be resistant to certain drugs usually considered part of the standard regimen for malarial infections. The critical questions at this stage are "Is the parasite *P. falciparum* or another species?"; "If not *P. falciparum*, is the parasite either *P. vivax* or *P. ovale* (which will require additional therapy to eliminate persisting liver stages)?"; and "Is the patient infected with more than one species of *Plasmodium*?"

To answer each of these questions, certain stages in the erythrocytic development of the parasite can be considered keys to proper identification (Table 43-1).

Except for *P. falciparum*, the most reliable stage for speciation, in either thick or thin blood smears, is the schizonts, which have a unique number and arrangement of merozoites. In *P. vivax* infections there are 12 to 24 merozoites in an irregular arrangement within the infected erythrocyte, whereas the schizonts of *P. malariae* typically have six to 12 merozoites, often arranged like petals of a flower around a central core of dark brown-black blocks of hemozoin. *P. ovale* has four to 16 merozoites arranged similarly to *P. malariae*. In *P. falciparum* infections the schizont stages are rarely seen in the peripheral blood except when the patient is in the terminal stages of a fatal infection; when present, however, the schizonts consist of eight to 24 randomly arranged merozoites. In *P. falciparum* infections the best criterion for speciation is the distinctive sausage- or banana-shaped gametocytes. These are commonly found in the peripheral blood and may appear to be extracellular even in thin blood smears (Plate 27, *F*).

Other stages, such as older trophozoites, are most helpful in distinguishing *P. vivax* (Plate 28, *A*) from *P. ovale* (Plate 28, *B*) and *P. malariae* (Plate 28, *C*). In *P. vivax* infections the older trophozoites appear very amoeboid, with thin strands of blue-staining cytoplasm extending throughout the infected erythrocyte. In *P. ovale* and *P. malariae* infections the trophozoite stages are similar; both are compact and lack the amoeboid appearance of *P. vivax*. Two of the more distinctive forms of older trophozoites of *P. malariae* are the so-called band and basket forms. In the band form the compact trophozoite appears

TABLE 43-1. Major Diagnostic Characteristics of Malarial Parasites in Erythrocytes

Characteristic	*Plasmodium vivax*	*Plasmodium malariae*	*Plasmodium falciparum*	*Plasmodium ovale*
Appearance of infected erythrocyte	Pale, enlarged; stippling (Schüffner's dots) common	Normal color and size; stippling rare	Normal color and size; stippling rare	Pale, enlarged, majority stippling (Schüffner's dots) common
Appearance of older trophozoite	Very amoeboid; vacuolated cytoplasm; fine, light brown malarial pigment	Very compact; may have band shape; vacuole small or absent; coarse, dark brown malarial pigment	Not normally seen in peripheral blood except in severe cases	Similar to *P. malariae*
Appearance of mature schizont	12 to 24 merozoites that almost fill enlarged red cell	Six to 12 merozoites arranged in rosette with malarial pigment clustered in center of normal-size red cell	Not normally seen in peripheral blood except in severe cases	Four to 16 merozoites arranged similar to *P. malariae* but fills only two thirds of cell
Appearance of gametocytes	Compact, eccentric chromatin in male; diffuse chromatin in female; surrounded by rounded or oval, often pale cytoplasm	Similar to *P. vivax*	Diagnostic banana- or sausage-shaped male and female gametocytes	Similar to *P. vivax* but smaller

Modified from Garcia, L.S., and Ash, L.R.: Diagnostic parasitology: clinical laboratory manual, St. Louis, 1979, The C.V. Mosby Co.

stretched as a band across the infected erythrocyte, and in the basket form the trophozoite has a large eccentric vacuole that is bordered on one side by a thin "handle" of cytoplasm.

In thick blood smears it is more difficult to use the trophozoite stages for identification because all trophozoites basically appear to be compact. One clue that a thick film contains trophozoites of *P. vivax* is that the compacted cytoplasm often appears as a series of separate cytoplasmic masses accompanied by a mass of red-staining nuclear material. In infections with *P. malariae* and *P. ovale* the older trophozoites, normally very compact even in thin blood smears, are even more compact and rarely have separated masses of cytoplasm.

In general, the younger trophozoites are not considered a definitive guide to speciation of malarial parasites because they all resemble tiny rings in thin blood smears and exclamation points or commas in thick blood smears. The one important exception is that ring stages of *P. falciparum* (Plate 28, *D*) are more likely to have multiple chromatin dots than are the other species, and in thin blood smears the parasite may appear as so-called accolé forms, in which the young trophozoite appears as a flattened ring stage (with no vacuole) on the very edge of the infected erythrocyte. In thin blood smears it is also common to observe several parasites within each infected erythrocyte. When these morphologic findings are coupled with an extremely large number of parasites within each microscopic field and the absence of older trophozoites or schizonts, one should immediately suspect a *P. falciparum* infection. If further examination of the blood smear fails to reveal the unique banana-shaped gametocytes that would confirm the identification, a presumptive report of *P. falciparum* should be issued. This warns the physician that a patient may have falciparum malaria and should be monitored closely for possible development of complications and effectiveness of the therapeutic regimen.

Besides the actual morphologic characteristics of the parasite, the appearance of infected erythrocytes, including size,

shape, and presence of cytoplasmic inclusions called stippling, can provide important clues for speciation of malaria. In fact, *P. ovale* can be definitively identified only by observing characteristics of both the organism and the infected erythrocyte in thin blood smears; in thick blood smears *P. ovale* so closely resembles *P. vivax* that the two cannot be reliably differentiated. In thin blood smears and *P. ovale* can be distinguished by the compact older trophozoites, schizonts that resemble those of *P. malariae,* and the enlarged, occasionally oval-shaped or crenated infected erythrocytes that are stippled with tiny red dots called Schüffner's dots (Plate 28, *A*). Interestingly, erythrocytes infected with *P. vivax* are nearly identical to those infected with *P. ovale.* Also, because the trophozoites of *P. ovale* are similar to the trophozoites of *P. malariae,* whereas the infected erythrocytes are similar to those of *P. vivax,* some parasitologists have described *P. ovale* as resembling a *P. malariae* parasite inside a *P. vivax* erythrocyte.

Erythrocytes infected with *P. malariae* or *P. falciparum* are not enlarged and do not usually have visible stippling when treated with Giemsa stain at a pH of 7 to 7.2. When erythrocytes are stained at a more alkaline pH (7.5), however, stippling may be found in the more mature erythrocytic stages of either parasite. Under these conditions the stippling of *P. malariae,* called Ziemann's dots, is very pale and almost indistinct in comparison to the Schüffner's dots seen in erythrocytes infected with *P. vivax* or *P. ovale.* In *P. falciparum* infections the chances of observing stippling, called Maurer dots or clefts, are even more remote. This is because the mature trophozoites and schizonts that usually contain stippling are rarely seen in the peripheral blood unless the patient is gravely ill. When seen, however, Maurer dots have varying sizes and shapes and are much less numerous than Schüffner's dots.

In addition to detecting and identifying malaria parasites in stained smears of peripheral blood, serologic tests such as indirect immunofluorescence can detect antibodies to *Plasmodium* spp. Unfortunately, there is a significant cross-reaction among the different *Plasmodium* spp., and consequently these tests are of little value to clinicians who must make appropriate therapeutic decisions when confronted with active cases of malaria. Serologic tests are of greatest value in detecting asymptomatic infections in which the parasitemia is of a very low level, in tracing the source of blood responsible for transfusion-induced malaria, and in epidemiologic studies of the prevalence and incidence of malaria in endemic areas.

BABESIA
LIFE CYCLE[47,50,107]

Human infections with sporozoan parasites of the genus *Babesia* are transmitted by the bite of hard ticks (family *Ixodidae*). Except for the absence of exoerythrocytic and sexual stages, the life cycle of genus *Babesia* in humans is very similar to that of genus *Plasmodium*. Numerous intraerythrocytic trophozoites, nearly identical to the tiny rings of *P. falciparum*, are the most common form of the parasite found in humans. An asexual reproductive form consisting of two or four daughter cells linked together within infected erythrocytes (''Maltese cross'') may also be found, but are far less common than the trophozoite stage.

The development of the parasite within ticks is not completely understood. However, it appears likely that some of the intraerythrocytic stages ingested when ticks take a blood meal develop in a manner analogous to the development of malarial parasites within mosquitoes. Because ticks may transmit the infection from one stage to another (for example, larva to adult) and from one generation to another (for example, from female tick to the egg), the infection may persist even in the absence of a vertebrate host.

EPIDEMIOLOGY[20,38,86,107]

Babesiosis (piroplasmosis) is a widespread disease that affects many different species of wild and domestic animals and only rarely humans. Among the more than 70 species of *Babesia* known to exist, only three have definitely been incriminated in human infections: *B. bovis*, *B. divergens*, and *B. microti*.

Two of these species, *B. bovis* and *B. divergens*, are maintained by a cattle-tick cycle that has been reported from Europe, Africa, Asia, and the East Indies for *B. bovis* and from Northern Europe and the United Kingdom for *B. divergens*. The few cases (about seven) of well-documented symptomatic human infection with these two species have generally been restricted to splenectomized individuals living in temperate zones of the parasites' geographic distribution and have almost always been fulminant infections terminating in death. In North America approximately six other cases are presumed to have been caused by these bovine species. None of the North American cases were fatal, and only two involved patients who had been splenectomized.

B. microti, on the other hand, is maintained by a rodent-tick cycle that is prevalent in North America and Europe and has been responsible for most human babesiosis (about 100 cases). Very few of the well-documented human infections with *B. microti* species have occurred in splenectomized individuals or resulted in death. Most of the symptomatic cases have occurred in individuals over 48 years of age who contracted the disease on one of the coastal islands of the eastern United States.

Serologic testing for specific antibodies suggests that inapparent or subclinical human infections may also occur.

PATHOLOGY AND CLINICAL MANIFESTATIONS[38,50,85,86,107]

Symptomatic babesiosis produces a malaria-like illness with nonspecific manifestations, including irregular fever, chills, drenching sweats, fatigue, nausea, vomiting, and myalgia. Physical examination typically reveals an enlarged liver and spleen. The more severe cases, usually associated with splenectomized patients, progress rapidly from renal failure, hypotension, and coma to death. In patients with intact spleens the infection is more prolonged, less severe, and rarely fatal. Except for the absence of a brown-black malarial pigment, the pathologic changes of babesiosis and malaria are similar.

LABORATORY DIAGNOSIS[47]

Except during epidemic outbreaks, babesiosis is easily mistaken for malaria. In general, however, babesiosis should be suspected in a patient who has not lived or traveled in an area where malaria is endemic and in whom Giemsa-stained thick or thin blood smears reveal intracellular parasites that resemble malaria. In fact, the typical intraerythrocytic stages of *Babesia* spp. are nearly identical to the tiny-ring stages of *P. falciparum*. Moreover, what are often described as the major distinguishing features of babesiosis, including the absence of gametocytes, schizonts, and the brown-black malarial pigment, may also occur in infections with *P. falciparum*. For example, some strains of *P. falciparum* do not produce large numbers of gametocytes. Also, except in fatal cases, it is unusual to see intermediate stages of *P. falciparum* (for example, stages with pigment or schizonts) in the peripheral blood. Adhering to the rule that it is best not to rely on the absence of morphologic characteristics for identification, the best criterion for distinguishing *Babesia* from *Plasmodium* organisms is to find the pairs or tetrads of *Babesia* daughter cells in an infected erythrocyte. Unfortunately, these unique stages of *Babesia* organisms may easily be overlooked in blood smears, especially if the diagnostician forms a premature impression that the parasite is a species of *Plasmodium*. Such a mistake in identification has not proved to be a fatal error in immunocompetent individuals, because the drugs used to treat the blood stages of *Plasmodium* spp. also provide symptomatic relief to patients with babesiosis. However, these drugs do not significantly reduce the patient's parasitemia; it usually subsides of its own accord, and the patient recovers without ill effect. In immunocompromised patients a correct diagnosis in the early stages is more critical because there are experimental drugs that may be lifesaving.

For these reasons it is imperative that any blood smear suspected of containing either *Plasmodium* or *Babesia* organisms be submitted to a reference laboratory skilled in the identification of these genera. In addition to stained and unstained blood smears, it is generally helpful to submit paired serum samples. Most reference laboratories have access to serologic tests, such as the indirect immunofluorescence test, that are helpful in diagnosing the infection in individuals from areas free of malaria. Finally, attempts may be made to cultivate the parasite in vivo by injecting whole blood samples from patients suspected to be infected into susceptible laboratory rodents. This technique is also generally restricted to reference or larger clinical laboratories because animal inoculation is more likely to succeed when the animals have been rendered susceptible by splenectomy or prior treatment with steroids. Usually only specialized or larger laboratories have the facilities to maintain the necessary animal colonies.

TOXOPLASMA GONDII
LIFE CYCLE[32,34,49,54,99]

The life cycle of the sporozoan parasite *Toxoplasma gondii* has two distinct stages (Figure 43-2). In the first stage, the enteric cycle, the parasite multiplies in the intestinal epithelial cells of the definitive hosts: domestic cats and other felines. The second stage of the life cycle is characterized by multiplication of trophozoites in cells outside the intestinal tract.

The intestinal cycle is essentially identical to the life cycle of *Isospora belli* in humans. Two stages of the parasite's development may infect cats and initiate the enteric cycle—oocysts passed in the feces of another infected cat or pseudocysts found in the tissues of reservoir hosts such as rodents or birds. If the infection begins with ingestion of oocysts, sporozoites are freed from the oocysts in the intestine and invade epithelial cells, where they transform into trophozoites. During the first reproductive cycle in the intestine the trophozoites divide asexually (schizogony) and produce mature schizonts composed of many individual daughter cells (merozoites). When infected epithelial cells rupture, the merozoites invade other epithelial cells and develop into a new generation of trophozoites. In these subsequent generations, individual trophozoites may continue to divide asexually, or they may initiate a cycle of sexual reproduction (sporogony) in which some trophozoites develop into either male (microgametocytes) or female (macrogametocytes) sex cells. This sexual reproduction gives rise to immature oocysts, which are passed in the cat's feces starting about 1 to 2 weeks after infection. In the external environment the oocysts continue to develop and mature in 1 to 5 days.

The second stage of the life cycle, characterized by the multiplication of trophozoites in cells outside the intestinal tract, may occur in cats at the same time as the intestinal cycle. It may also occur in almost any species of bird or mammal, in which it is the only stage of the life cycle; the enteric stage of the life cycle does not occur in these reservoir hosts. In either cats or reservoir hosts the extraintestinal cycle may be initiated by ingestion of the same two stages that initiate the enteric phase in cats: oocysts or pseudocysts. The difference is that the infective stages released from these "cysts" penetrate the intestinal wall and begin to invade cells throughout the body, especially white blood cells. Within the infected cells the parasite transforms into crescent-shaped trophozoites (tachyzoites), 6 to 7 μm by 2 to 4 μm in size. These rapidly multiply by producing two daughter cells inside each tachyzoite (called endodyogeny). Early in the extraintestinal stage of toxoplasmosis, the tachyzoites spread rapidly throughout the body. Infected cells rupture and release eight to 16 tachyzoites, which reinfect other cells and repeat the cycle. Later, as the host's immune system, especially the T cells, responds to the spreading infection, the tachyzoites' rate of division slows. At this slower rate of multiplication, the tachyzoites, now called bradyzoites, begin to accumulate in large numbers within infected host cells. The bradyzoites become encapsulated within structures variously called cysts, pseudocysts, or zoitocytes. These cysts, which measure from 200 to 1000 μm in diameter, generally remain dormant as long as the host's immune system is functioning

properly. However, if the host's immune system is later compromised, viable bradyzoites may be released from the pseudocysts and initiate a new cycle of extraintestinal infection.

EPIDEMIOLOGY*

Human infections with *Toxoplasma* spp. occur throughout the world; however, the prevalence varies widely from one region to another. Based on positive serologic tests, estimates of the prevalence of toxoplasmosis range from 1% to 70% worldwide and 20% to 70% in the United States.

Many if not most human infections with *Toxoplasma* organisms are acquired by ingestion of the cyst stage in raw or improperly cooked meat from domestic animals such as cattle, sheep, pigs, and chickens. Ingestion of oocysts passed in the feces of cats is also a potential mode of infection; however, there are conflicting reports of the risk of infection by contact with pet cats. It is most likely that oocysts, which may survive as long as 18 months in the external environment, are an important source of infection only where personal and environmental sanitation are minimal.

A third mode of transmission, and the one that creates the greatest concern, is the possibility of congenital transmission to the fetus if a woman acquires toxoplasmosis during pregnancy. Congenital transmission appears to occur only in women who become infected during pregnancy; when there are detectable levels of circulating antibody before pregnancy, no risk of fetal infection appears to be present. An estimated 3000 congenital infections occur each year with a mortality of one to four per 10,000 live births.

The risk of congenital transmission increases during each successive trimester of the pregnancy, with the rate of fetal infections increasing from 17% in women infected in the first trimester to 65% in women infected in the third trimester. However, infections acquired in the third trimester generally cause less serious defects than those acquired in the first trimester.

Less commonly, transmission occurs by blood transfusion, leukocyte infusion, and organ transplantation.

PATHOLOGY AND CLINICAL MANIFESTATIONS†

Although toxoplasmosis is a common infection, the number of individuals with clinically manifest disease is small. Because there is no prolonged enteric multiplication of the parasite in humans, the major pathologic and clinical manifestations of the infection are related to dissemination and multiplication of the organism in extraintestinal tissues. The basic pathologic response to tissue invasion is a localized inflammation of lymphocytes and monocytes around the infected cells. Later the inflammatory lesions develop into necrotic foci with minute consolidation and occasionally granulomata. Calcification of the lesions is usually restricted to the brain and is more common in congenital infections.

The inflammatory lesions occur in almost all tissues of the body, but the most prominent clinical manifestations are related to involvement of the reticuloendothelial system (lymph nodes, liver, spleen) and of the lungs, heart, brain, and eyes. In so-called acquired toxoplasmosis, which occurs in immunocompetent individuals who have ingested either oocysts or cysts,

---

*References 22, 32-34, 61, 81, 89, 95, and 100.
†References 44, 55, 56, 65, 77, 81, 87, and 90.

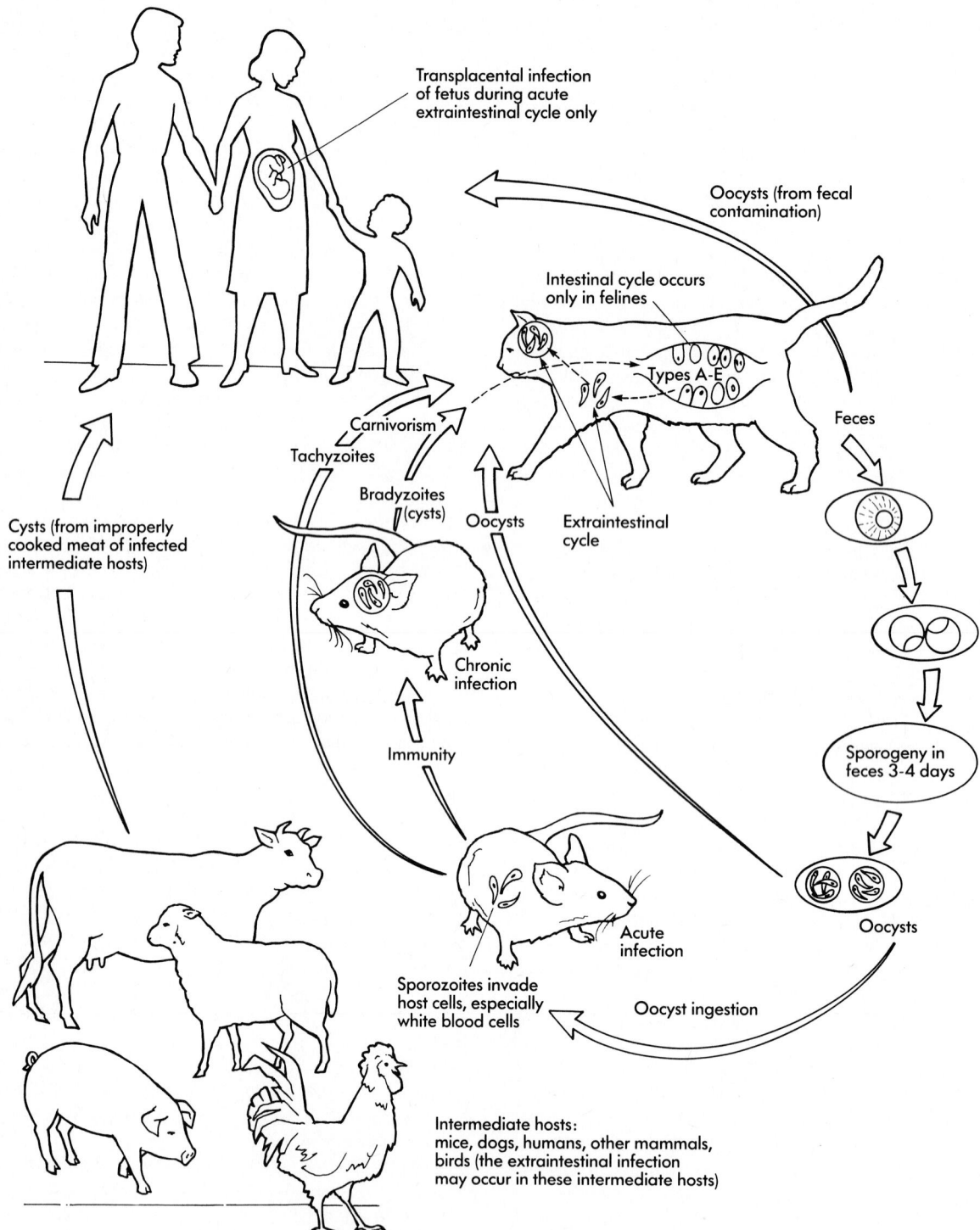

FIGURE 43-2. Life cycle of *Toxoplasma gondii*.

the most common clinical presentation is a localized lymphadenopathy, especially in the cervical region. When accompanied by other typical signs and symptoms, such as fever, fatigue, and hepatosplenomegaly, the acute phase of the disease may be mistaken for infectious mononucleosis. Even examination of the peripheral blood often reveals an absolute lymphocytosis with an occasional atypical lymphocyte. Less common but more serious manifestations include encephalitis, myocarditis, hepatitis, and pneumonia, and in some cases a unilateral inflammation of the choroid and retina of the eye.

Congenital toxoplasmosis need not be a fatal or even serious disease; in fact, fetal infections acquired in the third trimester of pregnancy are often asymptomatic. Severe fetal infections, often associated with early fetal infection, may result in stillbirth or serious tissue damage to the central nervous system, eyes, and viscera. Severe fetal syndromes typically include hydrocephalus, often with microcephaly; encephalitis with diffuse cerebral calcifications and psychomotor disturbances; and bilateral chorioretinitis. In less seriously affected infants the infection may not become apparent until months or even years later, when the infections are recognized by cerebral calcifications or bilateral chorioretinitis in a child with mental retardation or a learning disability.

Immunosuppressed adults, especially those with hematologic malignancies, may develop serious disseminated toxoplasmosis from either a newly acquired primary infection or reactivation of dormant pseudocysts in the tissues. In these cases the disease usually resembles one of the more serious forms of acquired infections, such as encephalitis, myocarditis, and pneumonia. Encephalitis in particular is a common manifestation, occurring in approximately 50% of these patients and accounting for 90% of the fatal cases.

LABORATORY DIAGNOSIS[23,32,87]

Unlike most other infections with animal parasites, the diagnosis of toxoplasmosis depends primarily on the results of serologic testing for specific antibodies. Among the many tests available, including the traditional Sabin-Feldman dye test, the complement fixation test, and the indirect hemagglutination test, the most popular method is probably the indirect immunofluorescence test. The advantages of the indirect immunofluorescence test are that it does not require living organisms, as the Sabin-Feldman test does, and that it has been adapted to the detection of IgM antibodies.

The most reliable criterion for serologic diagnosis of active infections in immunocompetent individuals is either a fourfold rise to a high titer (greater than 1:1000 in the indirect immunofluroescence test) in two sera collected 2 to 3 weeks apart or a single high IgM titer (1:80 or greater in the indirect immunofluroescence test). When interpreting the results from these tests, it is important to note that most of the tests detect IgG antibodies, which rise to a peak and stabilize within 1 to 2 months of the infection. Thus, if a rising titer is to be documented, the conventional tests must be performed early in the infection. This is especially true for the Sabin-Feldman and indirect immunofluorescence tests, which seem to reach a peak titer slightly faster than the indirect hemagglutination or complement fixation test and may remain at levels as high as 1:4000 for more than a year. On the other hand, IgM-specific antibodies are usually detectable earlier, often within the first week, and rise to a peak titer within a month. IgM antibodies

also decline more rapidly than IgG antibodies and are usually undetectable within a few months after infection.

The interpretation of serologic results is slightly more complicated in pregnant women and immunocompromised patients. Women with a documented titer to toxoplasmosis before conception are not at risk of transmitting the infection to the fetus and usually need not be tested during pregnancy. However, pregnant women without a documented titer or development of signs or symptoms of the disease should be tested to establish if there is a potential risk to the fetus. If initial testing with one of the conventional tests is positive at any titer, tests should be performed for IgM-specific antibodies. Conventional tests for IgG should be repeated with sera collected 3 weeks later. If the IgM-specific test is negative and the conventional test reveals a low, stable titer, the probability of a current active infection is very low, and further testing is usually unnecessary. However, when the tests are first performed late in the infection and the IgM test is negative but the conventional tests reveal a high, stable titer, interpretation is more difficult. It would be unlikely in this situation that the infection occurred in the 3 weeks preceding the test for IgM antibodies; however, infection may have occurred during an earlier period in the pregnancy, and more serious consideration would have to be given to the possibility of fetal infection.

The value of serologic testing in immunocompromised patients depends on their ability to mount a humoral immune response. Fortunately, most of these patients have a detectable immune response to the infection. However, patients with antinuclear antibodies or rheumatoid factor often give false-positive reactions in the immunofluorescence tests; they should be tested by one of the other methods.

The best serologic method of establishing the diagnosis of congenital infection in neonates is to test for IgM-specific antibodies in the infant's serum. In the presence of signs and symptoms of congenital infection a single elevated IgM titer may be considered diagnostic. If one of the IgG tests is used, the antibody levels of the infant and the mother must be determined simultaneously. If the infant's titer is significantly (fourfold) higher than the mother's, the infant may be presumed infected. If the titer is the same as the mother's, however, it cannot be assumed that the infant's antibodies were merely transferred passively from the mother. Instead, the infant's test should be repeated at 4 months of age. By this time, passively transferred antibodies will have declined significantly; if there has been no decline or if there has been a rise in the titer the infant may be presumed infected.

Additional methods for diagnosing the infection usually require a biopsy to collect tissue from the lymph nodes, liver, or spleen. This material may be used to inject mice or for histopathologic examination.

Mice free of toxoplasmosis that are injected intraperitoneally with positive tissue samples usually develop toxoplasmosis, which can be detected by testing for specific antibody in 2 to 3 weeks after infection. Histologic examination of the mouse's brain for cysts about a month after injection may also be performed. Lymph node tissue taken directly from the patient may also be examined by a histopathologist for stages of the parasite's development or a typical histiocytic hyperplasia. Unfortunately, it is often difficult to detect the tachyzoites (Plate 28, E) in tissue, and the presence of cysts alone does not confirm an active infection. A histiocytic hyperplasia of the lymphatic tissue is also highly suggestive but, again, does not confirm an active infection with *Toxoplasma* organisms.

PNEUMOCYSTIS CARINII
LIFE CYCLE[45,46,97]

Most current literature suggests that *Pneumocystis carinii* is probably a sporozoan parasite, even though its staining pattern with periodic acid–Schiff and silver methenamine stains are more characteristic of fungi and its apparent lack of intracellular or sexual stages is not typical of the sporozoa. There are only two known stages in the life cycle: (1) a resistant cyst stage that usually measures 5 μm in diameter and contains eight oval-shaped intracystic bodies or "sporozoites" and (2) pleomorphic "trophozoites" that measure 2 to 12 μm in length and are covered with tiny tubular projections. These projections presumably aid in attachment to the epithelial cells and increase the organism's absorptive surface area. Most infections are probably acquired by inhalation of a cystlike stage of the parasite. "Sporozoites" are released from cysts in the alveoli and transform into trophozoites, which multiply asexually on the surfaces of epithelial cells. When exposed to a yet undefined stimulus, the trophozoites round up and form the characteristic cyst stage. None of these stages occurs intracellularly, and there is no known stage of sexual reproduction of the parasite.

EPIDEMIOLOGY*

Pneumocystis carinii is widespread in nature and occurs in many mammals. The organism is especially common in rodents, which have been implicated as a possible reservoir for human infections. However, serologic studies and attempts to infect rodents with human strains suggest that the rodent strains are distinct from the strains found in humans. In most human infections the organism is probably acquired during infancy and, after an asymptomatic infection, remains latent in the tissues as long as the patient is not immunologically compromised.

Symptomatic pneumocystosis occurs in two distinct forms. The earliest recognized form of the disease was seen after World War II in Europe as endemic or epidemic infection among poorly nourished or premature infants. Before specific treatment was available, the mortality was as high as 50% in these infants. More recently, isolated cases of the disease have been seen in older children or adults undergoing immunosuppressive therapy or having serious underlying diseases that compromise the immune system. This form of the disease is especially prevalent in patients with acquired immunodeficiency syndrome (AIDS); in fact, pneumocystosis is the initial clinical manifestation in up to 50% of individuals affected by AIDS. If not treated, these sporadic cases in immunocompromised patients are almost always fatal.

The exact type of immune deficiency that predisposes to pneumocystosis is not clear. In infants with congenital immunodeficiencies the disease is more likely to occur when levels of IgG are depressed. However, in patients with AIDS or malignancies, the diseases may occur even when immunoglobulin levels are normal.

---

*References 6, 13, 40, 53, 79, 102, 103, and 105.

PATHOLOGY AND CLINICAL MANIFESTATIONS*

Active cases of pneumocystosis manifest a diffuse interstitial pneumonia in which the alveolar spaces are distended and filled with a foamy material that consists primarily of desquamated macrophages filled with degenerating organisms. In later stages of the disease the walls of alveoli have a honeycomb appearance, with cysts of the organism interspersed among areas of alveolar fibrosis. It is not clear whether this fibrosis is caused directly by the infection or results from the supportive and drug-specific therapy administered to the patients.

In most cases the organism does invade beyond the lungs. However, a small number of reports suggest that the organism may spread hematogenously to the liver, spleen, myocardium, gastrointestinal tract, bone marrow, adrenal glands, thyroid gland, and eye.

The clinical findings of pneumocystosis are nonspecific and often mimic the interstitial pneumonia caused by some viral agents or *Mycoplasma* organisms. The typical infection is manifested by shortness of breath, a nonproductive cough, and fever (38.8° C). Inspiratory rales may or may not be found on physical examination. As the disease progresses, the patient's breathing becomes rapid, and an obvious cyanosis develops. Although the course of the disease is highly variable among individual patients, there is almost always a significant depression of arterial oxygen tension (35 to 37 mm Hg) and a normal or low arterial carbon dioxide tension and alkaline arterial pH.

LABORATORY DIAGNOSIS[52,72,105]

In active cases the laboratory diagnosis of *Pneumocystis carinii* infection is based on finding cysts or trophozoite stages in secretions or tissue from the lungs. The most dependable method of detecting the organism is by examination of stained impression smears or histologic sections of lung tissue obtained by open biopsy. Unfortunately, this technique is not without risk, especially in immunocompromised patients whose infection is far advanced. For these reasons it is imperative that definitive diagnosis be attempted early in any high-risk patients with signs or symptoms of the disease. Other, less invasive, methods, including needle aspiration through the chest wall, transbronchial biopsy, and bronchial brushings, have also been employed to obtain pulmonary tissue. However, these techniques are slightly less productive in the recovery of organisms and are not without their own risks. The least productive of all methods is examination of stained pulmonary secretions, obtained either as expectorated sputum or by aspiration.

Two basic techniques are used to stain *Pneumocystis* organisms. The toluidine blue O stain and methenamine–silver nitrate stain of Gomori and Grocott are used to stain the thick-walled cyst stage. The trophozoite stage is best detected by using a polychrome stain such as the Giemsa or Gram-Weigert stain. The recommended procedure is first to stain and examine the tissue for cysts and then to confirm the identification using another slide stained with one of the trophozoite stains. This two-step procedure is preferred because the cyst stains, although very sensitive, are not specific for *Pneumocystis* organisms. A variety of normal tissue structures, as well as

---

*References 9, 26, 27, 40, 91, 104, and 105.

yeasts, may easily be confused with the cysts of *Pneumocystis* spp. The polychrome stains are generally less sensitive but more specific. They permit definitive identification of "sporozoites" within the cysts, a characteristic unique to *Pneumocystis carinii*.

TRYPANOSOMA BRUCEI SSP. *GAMBIENSE* AND *TRYPANOSOMA BRUCEI* SSP. *RHODESIENSE*

Life Cycle[42,75]

The life cycle (Figure 43-3) of the two subspecies of *Trypanosoma brucei* responsible for African trypanosomiasis (African sleeping sickness) are essentially identical; these hemoflagellates have the same developmental stages in humans and the insect vectors. The only major differences are that the rhodesian form of the parasite *(T. brucei* ssp. *rhodesiense)* has slightly different species of insect vectors, has a natural animal reservoir besides humans, and invades the central nervous system much more rapidly than the gambian form *(T. brucei* ssp. *gambiense)*.

Both forms of the disease are transmitted by various species of tsetse flies *(Glossina* spp.); however, in the gambian form of the disease the primary vector is *Glossina palpalis,* whereas *Glossina morsitans* is the primary vector for the rhodesian form of the disease. Both male and female flies are capable of transmitting the disease to humans. The infective metacyclic trypomastigotes are slender, spindle-shaped flagellates (15 μm long) with an undulating membrane extending the full length of the body. These trypomastigotes pass from the fly's salivary ducts into the bite wound at the time of a blood meal. Once in the skin the metacyclic trypomastigotes transform into enlongate, more slender trypomastigotes that multiply asexually for 1 or 2 days before entering the peripheral blood and lymphatic circulation. In the peripheral circulation the trypomastigotes continue to divide extracellularly and take a variety of shapes. The predominant forms are long, slender trypomastigotes that average 28 μm long and have a free flagellum extending from the anterior terminus of the undulating membrane; less common are short, stumpy, aflagellate forms that average 15 μm long.

When ingested by a tsetse fly during a blood meal, the trypomastigotes multiply in the midgut of the fly for about 10 days and then migrate to the fly's salivary glands, where they transform into epimastigotes. The parasite continues to divide in the epimastigote stage and eventually transforms into the infective metacyclic trypomastigotes. Development of the infective stage within the fly requires 25 to 50 days, depending on the species of fly, the strain of parasite, and the ambient temperature. Normally the fly remains infective for its entire 2- to 3-month life span.

Epidemiology[24,94,108]

The distribution of African trypanosomiasis is limited by the natural range of the insect vector and extends from about the latitude of 15° N to 15° to 25° S. Within this geographic range the two different forms of African trypanosomiasis often overlap. However, the gambian form of the disease is generally more prevalent and occurs in epidemic proportions, especially in the western and central sectors of the parasite's range. The rhodesian form occurs more often as isolated or sporadic cases in the eastern sections of the range.

Besides the natural type of infection in which *Glossina* organisms inject metacyclic trypomastigotes into a bite wound, infections may also occur if blood forms of trypomastigotes are quickly transmitted to another susceptible host. In nature, this may occur if biting flies are interrupted during their feeding and carry trypomastigote stages on the proboscis to another host. Although there are only a few reports, transfusion of blood from an infected host may also be a possible source of infection.

Pathology and Clinical Manifestations*

Except for differences in the rate at which the two diseases develop, both forms of African trypansomiasis have nearly identical pathologic effects and clinical manifestations. The first sign of infection is usually a hard, painful nodule or chancre that develops within 4 to 10 days at the site of the fly bite and is accompanied by regional lymphadenopathy. Within a few weeks, after the parasites have completed their initial transformation and multiplication and begun to invade the bloodstream, the chancre spontaneously subsides.

As the parasite begins to multiply within the bloodstream, the patient outwardly appears healthy. Occasionally the infection does not progress beyond this stage. In most individuals, however, the parasites invade the reticuloendothelial system and induce a generalized hyperplasia of the lymphoid tissue and intermittent febrile episodes. These febrile episodes, which may last for 1 to 7 days, are commonly manifest as a high, irregular fever, malaise, night sweats, and headache and are followed by a symptom-free period that lasts several weeks before the next episode. Each febrile episode is apparently initiated by separate subgroups of trypanosomes that have slightly different surface antigens (see Chapter 2). In the early period of the disease the host responds to each new subgroup of trypanosomes by producing IgM antibodies specific for the subgroup's surface antigens. The extent of this continuing immunologic response is manifested by a generalized lymphadenopathy, especially by an enlargement of the lymph nodes in the posterior cervical triangle (Winterbottom's sign). As the disease progresses, however, the immune system's ability to mount a response is overwhelmed, and the lymph nodes become atrophied and fibrotic.

In most untreated individuals the later stages of African trypanosomiasis, especially the gambian form of the disease, are marked by progressive inflammation of the brain, meninges, and spinal cord as parasites invade the central nervous system. The onset of this central nervous system involvement is usually insidious and initially manifest as a constant severe headache, insomnia, weakness, and decreased sensory and motor function. Later, there are progressive lethargy and apathy accompanied by changes in personality and behavioral changes, including delusions, hysteria, or even mania. In the classic, final, sleeping sickness stage of the disease, the patient develops an uncontrollable desire to sleep, severe malnutrition, and loss of motor control. If death does not occur first from malnutrition or a secondary bacterial infection, the patient lapses into a true coma before death.

The major clinical differences between the two forms of

---

*References 2, 24, 31, 41-43, 80, and 84.

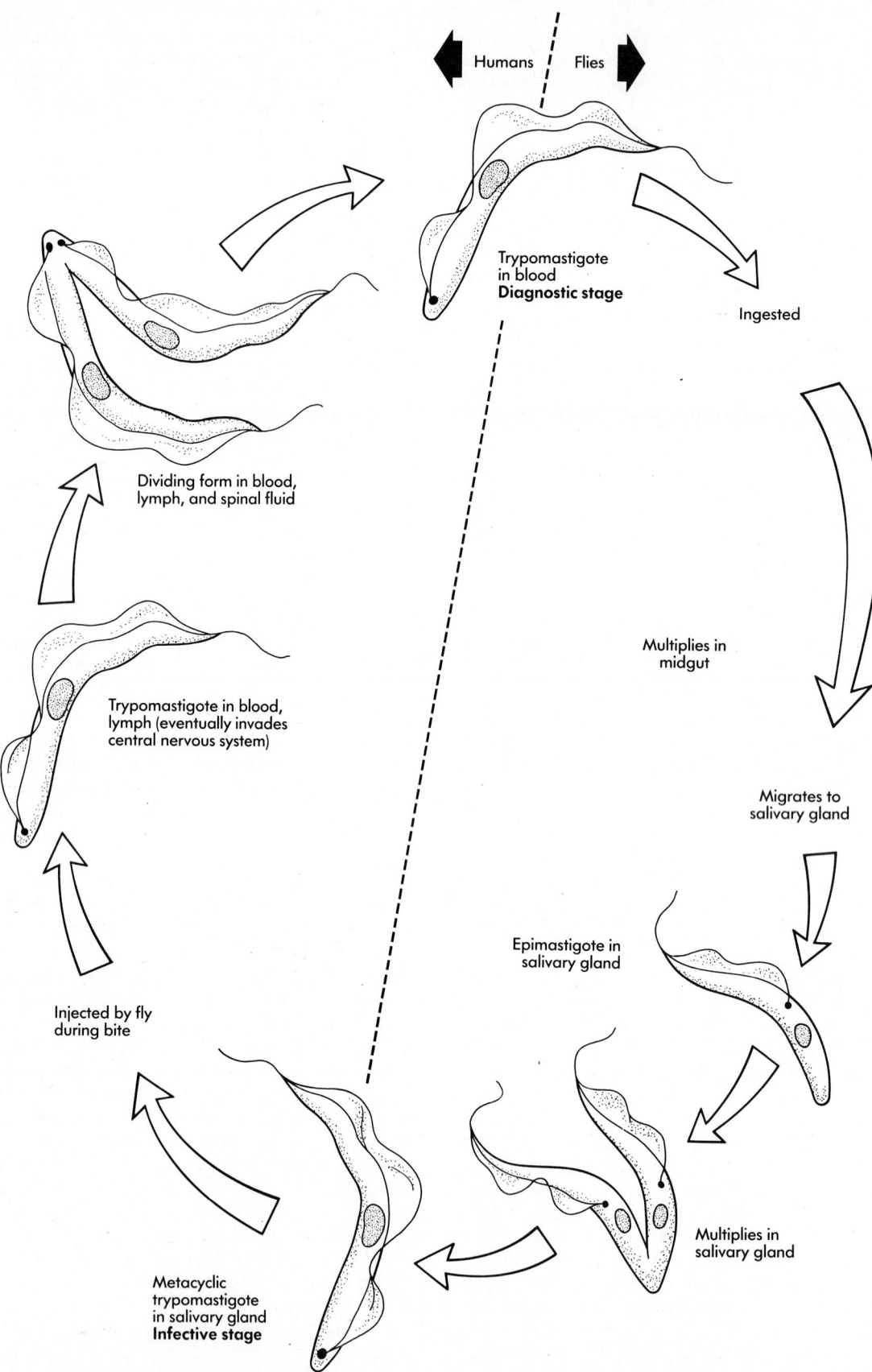

FIGURE 43-3. Life cycle of *Trypanosoma brucei*. (Modified from Melvin, D.M., Brooke, M.M., and Healy, G.R.: Common blood and tissue parasites of man—life cycle charts, Atlanta, 1965, PHS Pub. No. 1234, Laboratory Branch of the Communicable Disease Center.)

African trypanosomiasis are the speed at which the disease develops and the extent of central nervous system involvement before death. In the gambian form of the disease the pathologic changes develop slowly, with an incubation period of several weeks to months and a delay of months or even years before the brain involvement becomes apparent. In contrast, the rhodesian form of the disease follows a more rapid course that begins with an incubation period of 2 to 3 weeks and a more prominent trypanosomal chancre. During the period of lymphatic involvement these patients are more likely to have myocarditis and die of cardiac failure.

LABORATORY DIAGNOSIS[24,41,94]

The usual laboratory procedures for confirmation of African trypanosomiasis cannot differentiate between the two subspecies of *T. brucei* responsible for human infections. The distinction is usually based on differences in the geographic distribution and clinical manifestations of the infections. In this context the primary role of the laboratory is to confirm the presence of trypomastigotes of *T. brucei* and assist the physician in determining the proper therapy based on whether the parasite is restricted to the bloodstream and lymphatics or has invaded the central nervous system.

In the early stages of infection the trypomastigotes may be detected in smears of the peripheral blood or lymph node aspirates. Generally, peripheral blood samples are better for detecting the rhodesian form of the disease, whereas lymph node aspirates are more likely to reveal the gambian subspecies. Once the parasite has invaded the central nervous system, trypomastigotes may also be detected in spinal fluid.

Any of these various specimens may be used to prepare direct wet mounts or Giemsa-stained smears. Wet mounts are particularly sensitive in detecting the faintly visible, snakelike trypomastigotes as they move with a rapid thrashing motion through the mass of red blood cells. Final identification of the organisms, however, should be confirmed with Giemsa-stained smears.

In stained smears the trypomastigotes of both subspecies appear as spindle-shaped flagellates of varying length (12 to 40 μm, average 25 μm) (Plates 28, *F*, and 29, *A*). Unlike *T. cruzi*, C-shaped trypomastigotes are rare in *T. brucei*: instead, most of the trypomastigotes of these two subspecies appear stretched out with a few wavelike curves in the body. An undulating membrane, originating in a small, red-staining kinetoplast near the rounded posterior end, extends the entire length of the body and terminates in a single free flagellum at the pointed anterior end.

If the parasites cannot be detected in simple wet mounts or stained smears, various concentration procedures are available. Blood samples are most easily concentrated in thick smears. Alternatively, the parasites may be concentrated from anticoagulated whole blood by differential centrifugation or, in more sophisticated laboratories, by a special type of column chromatography and membrane filtration. Concentration procedures are rarely required with lymph node aspirates, but if necessary spinal fluid samples may be concentrated by simple centrifugation.

Aside from serologic methods that are generally reserved for mass surveys or epidemiologic studies, and aside from the animal inoculation that may be used in specialized laboratories, at least one other laboratory test may be helpful when organisms cannot be demonstrated in wet mounts or stained smears. Almost all patients with African trypanosomiasis have very high levels of total serum IgM and, later, cerebrospinal IgM. In many cases the total serum IgM exceeds eight times the normal amount, or the ratio of IgM to IgC may equal or exceed 3:1. This elevation of total IgM is considered so characteristic of African trypanosomiasis that its absence suggests the patient has some other disease.

TRYPANOSOMA CRUZI
LIFE CYCLE[70]

Aside from differences in their insect vectors, the most important difference between American and African trypanosomiasis is that in American trypanosomiasis (Chagas' disease) an intracellular, aflagellate stage (amastigote), rather than the circulating trypomastigote, is the stage of the parasite that multiplies in the body and is responsible for the pathologic and clinical manifestations of the disease.

Infections with *Trypanosoma cruzi* occur when infective metacyclic trypomastigotes penetrate the skin of susceptible hosts (Figure 43-4). These metacyclic trypomastigotes are short and stumpy and have an undulating membrane and free flagellum. They are passed onto the host's skin in the feces of insect vectors of the family *Reduviidae* (genus *Rhodnius*, *Triatoma*, or *Panstrongylus*) as they defecate during a blood meal. The trypomastigotes may actively migrate into the bite wound and penetrate mucous membranes contaminated with the insect's feces, or they may be rubbed into the skin when the host scratches the area of the bite wound. In the skin or mucous membranes the metacyclic trypomastigotes enter a variety of cells, especially fixed phagocytic cells. Within these various cells the metacyclic trypomastigotes transform into small (1.5 to 4 μm), round, aflagellate forms (amastigotes) that multiply by asexual division. After 3 or 4 days the infected cells begin to rupture and release daughter amastigotes that may either spread and infect other cells or transform into a trypomastigote that circulates in the peripheral blood.

At first the spreading amastigote stages metastasize to the regional lymph nodes, but later, cells in almost all the internal organs of the body are invaded, especially the fixed phagocytic cells of the reticuloendothelial system, the muscle cells of the heart, and the neuroglial cells of the central nervous system. The circulating trypomastigotes, unlike in African trypanosomiasis, do not divide, and during the later, chronic stages of the disease are in the peripheral blood only in small numbers.

Susceptible insect vectors become infected when they ingest circulating trypomastigotes. In the midgut of the vector the trypomastigotes first transform into epimastigotes (a form with the kinetoplast located just anterior to the nucleus, an undulating membrane extending one half the length of the body, and a single free flagellum). The epimastigotes actively multiply in the posterior region of the midgut by asexual division and, under ideal conditions, transform into infective metacyclic trypomastigotes, which migrate to the hindgut of the insect within 8 to 10 days.

EPIDEMIOLOGY*

Reduviid bugs responsible for the transmission of American trypanosomiasis are widespread throughout the Americas and,

---

*References 7, 30, 66, 70, 74, and 110.

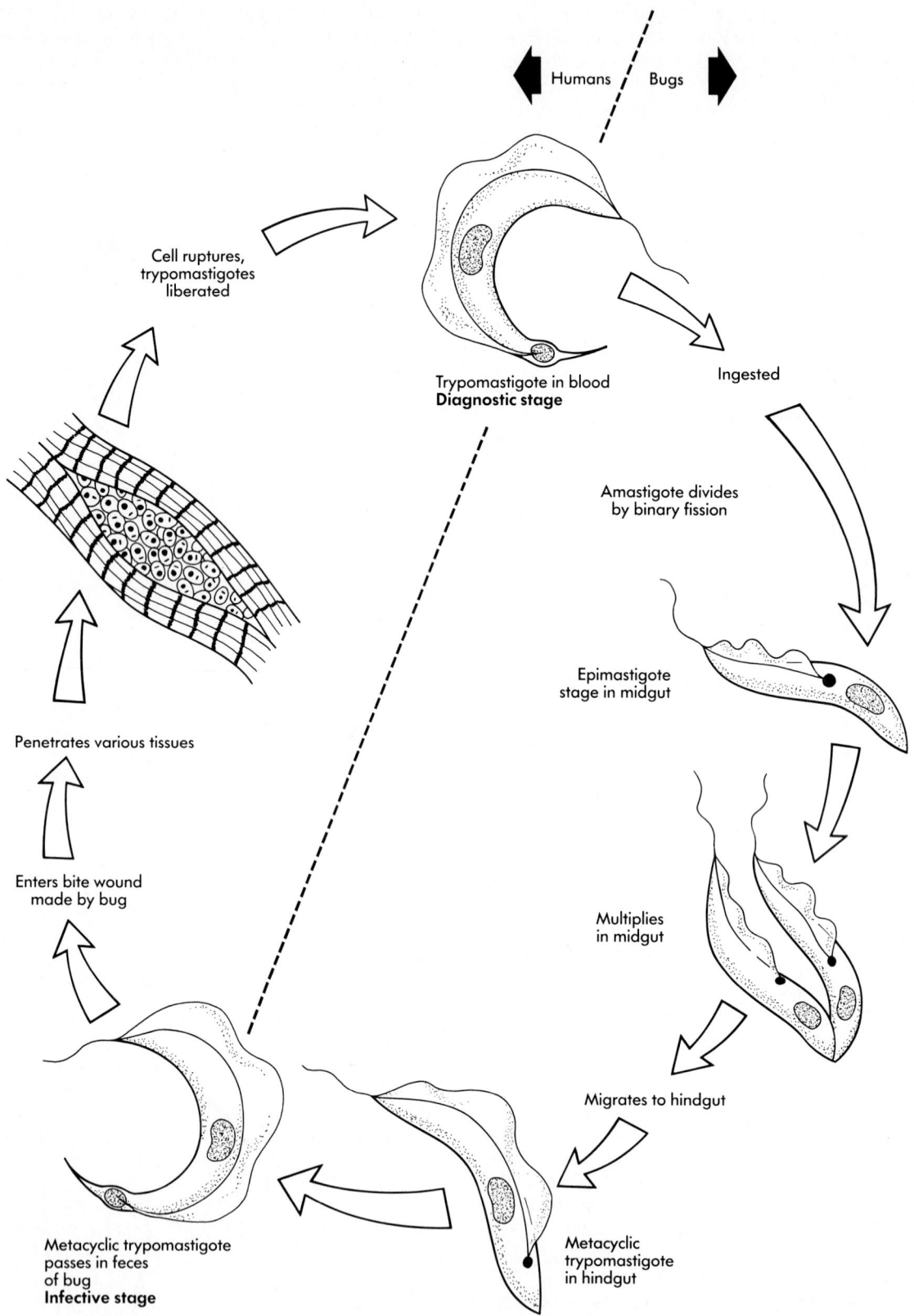

Humans / Bugs

Cell ruptures,
trypomastigotes
liberated

Trypomastigote in blood
Diagnostic stage

Ingested

Amastigote divides
by binary fission

Epimastigote
stage in midgut

Penetrates various tissues

Multiplies
in midgut

Enters bite wound
made by bug

Migrates to hindgut

Metacyclic trypomastigote
passes in feces
of bug
Infective stage

Metacyclic
trypomastigote
in hindgut

FIGURE 43-4. Life cycle of *Trypanosoma cruzi.* (Modified from Melvin, D.M., Brooke, M.M.,
and Healy, G.R.: Common blood and tissue parasites of man—life cycle charts, Atlanta, 1965,
PHS Pub. No. 1234, Laboratory Branch of the Communicable Disease Center.)

depending on the particular region, 20% to 60% may be infected with *T. cruzi*. Besides humans, the parasite infects a variety of wild and domestic mammals such as opossums, raccoons, wood rats, dogs, and cats. However, despite the parasite's widespread distribution, human infections have a limited geographic range; the disease is more prevalent in South America, especially Brazil, Argentina, Uruguay, Chile, and Venezuela, than in Central or North America. In the United States the parasite has been found extensively among reservoir animals throughout the southern states, both eastern and western. However, with the exception of a few isolated infections discovered in the Southwest, most cases of American trypanosomiasis in the United States have occurred in immigrants or travelers from the endemic region of South or Central America. Presumably these differences in incidence of human infections are related to differences in the feeding habits of different species of reduviids, strain differences in the virulence of the parasite, and differences in housing conditions that favor human contact with the reduviids. The single most important factor in determining the distribution of the disease is probably the differences in the housing conditions of populations at risk of acquiring the disease. Individuals living in poorly constructed thatch or mud houses are at particular risk of infection. These structures are prone to reduviid infestation because the crevices of the buildings provide a cool resting place for the insects during the warm daylight hours. They can emerge at night to feed undisturbed on sleeping humans or their domestic pets. Thus, even in areas where the disease is common, it tends to be more prevalent among poor, rural populations than urban populations that have more substantial housing. Domestic pets, which serve as reservoirs of the infection, appear to impose an additional risk. In a serosurvey in Brazil, households with infected reduviids and dogs or cats had twice the rate of positive tests for the antibody to *T. cruzi* as households with infected reduviids but no domestic pets.

Besides natural transmission of the parasite by reduviids, the possibility of acquiring the disease by transfusion is a particularly serious problem in areas where the disease is endemic. Because the organism can remain viable in stored whole blood for as long as 10 days, and because up to 9% of donors may be infected in some areas, it is common practice in many endemic areas to screen potential donors for antibodies to the parasite before accepting blood donations. Other reported modes of transmission include congenital infections and the use of contaminated hypodermic needles and syringes.

Pathology and Clinical Manifestations*

The clinical manifestations of American trypanosomiasis are usually divided into two phases: the acute phase, which occurs soon after infection and may last for 1 to 4 months, and a chronic phase, which may not be clinically manifest until decades after infection.

Development of overt signs and symptoms of the acute stage of the disease varies with the age of the host and from one geographic area to another. In general, the acute stage of the disease is most often symptomatic in children under 2 years of age and begins with facial swelling and a pronounced edema of the eyelids of one eye (Romaña's sign) if the parasite enters the body by being rubbed into the eyes (50% of cases). A less

common (25% of cases) but more circumscribed area of erythema and swelling, called a chagoma, occurs if the parasite enters through an abrasion of the skin. Although chagomas may occur on any part of the body, they are generally more common on the face because reduviids seem to bite the face more often than other areas. As a result of this feeding preference, reduviids are often referred to by their common name—"kissing bugs." About one quarter of all patients have no early lesions.

In patients with overt acute American trypanosomiasis the systemic manifestations that accompany dissemination of the parasite from the initial site of invasion begin about 1 to 2 weeks after the appearance of the primary lesion and last for 1 to 4 months. The typical syndrome, attributed directly to the destruction of parasitized cells and the host's inflammatory response, may include fever, headache, malaise, muscle pain, generalized lymphadenopathy, and hepatosplenomegaly. The most common manifestation of acute American trypanosomiasis is the development of cardiac abnormalities. These may include findings as obvious as tachycardia or subtler findings that are apparent only in electrocardiograms. Together with meningoencephalitis, these cardiac abnormalities cause most deaths that occur during the acute stage of the disease. Deaths during the acute stage are estimated to occur in 5% to 10% of cases and are more likely to occur in children.

Once the acute stage has passed, the infection may enter a chronic stage in which there is slow but continued cellular dysfunction, especially among muscle and nerve cells. The principal manifestations of this stage of the disease are related to damage of the muscles and nerves that control muscle tone of the hollow organs, particularly the heart, esophagus, and intestine. The heart of an affected patient becomes enlarged and flabby, with a resulting cardiac insufficiency that is said to account for 70% of the cardiac-related deaths among young adults in endemic areas. Progressive loss of muscle tone of the esophagus and intestine results in decreased peristalsis and, eventually, a massive distension of the affected organs that is termed megadisease.

Laboratory Diagnosis[30,66,70]

The laboratory techniques appropriate for the diagnosis of *T. cruzi* infections depend primarily on the stage of the disease.

During the acute phase of American trypanosomiasis, trypomastigotes are particularly plentiful in the peripheral blood and may be readily detected by wet mounts or stained thick and thin blood smears. In wet mounts the trypomastigotes are only faintly visible, but their rapid, progressive, snakelike motion among the erythrocytes makes their presence apparent. Confirmation of the identification requires examination of the organism in a Giemsa-stained thick or thin blood smear. In these preparations the trypomastigotes often have a U- or C-shaped body that measures 15 to 20 μm long. There is a large kinetoplast in the pointed posterior end of the body and a undulating membrane that runs the full length of the body to the anterior end, where it terminates in a single free flagellum (Plate 29, *A*). Confirmation with stained blood smears is particularly important because a nonpathogenic trypanosome, *T. rangeli*, may be found in the same geographic range as *T. cruzi*. Fortunately, this distinction is relatively easy because *T. rangeli* is generally more slender and longer (average 31 μm versus 18 μm for *T. cruzi*), is not usually U or C shaped, and has a much smaller kinetoplast. The

---

*References 29, 59, 60, 66, 70, and 110.

possibility of confusing *T. cruzi* with the subspecies of *T. brucei* responsible for African trypanosomiasis should be remote provided there is good communication between the physician and laboratory regarding the patient's clinical history. The geographic distributions of the two diseases are very different, and it is unlikely that international businesspeople would live in conditions that would put them at high risk of infection. One of the more helpful laboratory clues that the infection is American and not African trypanosomiasis is that, unlike in African trypanosomiasis, the total serum IgM is usually within normal limits in American trypanosomiasis.

In the later, chronic stages of the American form of the disease, more elaborate techniques are usually required to demonstrate trypomastigotes in the peripheral blood because they become scarce as the disease progresses. Probably the best technique available to most clinical laboratories is lysis centrifugation, in which the erythrocytes in an anticoagulated sample of whole blood are first lysed, the sample is centrifuged, and sediment is smeared and stained as if it were a blood smear (see Chapter 40). Better-equipped laboratories may attempt either in vitro cultivation using a medium such as Warren or NNN (see Chapter 40) or in vivo cultivation by intraperitoneal injection of blood into mice, rats, or guinea pigs. The most sensitive of all techniques used to recover the organism is probably xenodiagnosis. In this technique, which is generally used only in South and Central America, laboratory-reared, disease-free reduviids are allowed to feed on the patient and, after 30 to 60 days, examined for metacyclic trypomastigotes in their rectal contents.

As an alternative to actually demonstrating the parasite in the chronic phase of American trypanosomiasis, a laboratory may choose to test for specific antibodies in the patient's serum. It must be recognized, however, that these serologic methods, including complement fixation, immunofluorescence, and enzyme-linked immunosorbent assay, generally provide evidence only that the patient was infected at some time in the past. Proof of active infection by these serologic methods would require demonstrating a general fourfold rise in antibody titer, which is difficult in the chronic stages of any disease, or detecting elevated levels of specific IgM antibodies with a modified test procedure. Nevertheless, these tests can be valuable in diagnosing the illness in individuals who normally reside in areas where it is not endemic. The physician must, however, have strong additional evidence for infection and understand how the predictive value of a positive test is adversely affected by low disease prevalence in a test population.

LEISHMANIA TROPICA COMPLEX, *LEISHMANIA MEXICANA* COMPLEX, *LEISHMANIA BRAZILIENSIS* COMPLEX, AND *LEISHMANIA DONOVANI* COMPLEX
LIFE CYCLE*

Although there are differences in the epidemiology, pathology, and clinical manifestations, the life cycles (Figure 43-5) of all the hemoflagellates of the genus *Leishmania* that infect humans are essentially identical. Human infections occur when promastigotes (a stage in which a single anterior flagellum arises from a kinetoplast located at the anterior end of the body

and there is no undulating membrane) are injected into the skin as infected female sandflies take a human blood meal. In the Western Hemisphere ("New World"), the sandflies are typically members of the genus *Lutzomyia*; in the other parts of the world they usually belong to the genus *Phlebotomus*.

In humans the promastigotes are ingested by phagocytic cells and transform into aflagellate amastigotes, which proliferate within the phagocytic cells of the reticuloendothelial system and the endothelial cells of the capillaries. Depending on the particular type of leishmaniasis, the amastigotes, which are essentially identical to those seen in *Trypanosoma cruzi* infections, may remain localized in tissues near the site of the bite (cutaneous leishmaniasis; *L. tropica* and *L. mexicana*), may have a limited spread that involves more extensive areas of the skin and mucous membranes (mucocutaneous leishmaniasis; *L. braziliensis*), or may spread throughout the body and infect cells in many of the internal organs of the reticuloendothelial system, such as the spleen, liver, and bone marrow (visceral leishmaniasis; *L. donovani*).

The female sandflies become infected when they feed on blood or host tissue juices containing cells infected with the amastigote stage of the parasite. In the midgut of the fly the amastigotes are released from the infected host cells and transform into promastigotes, which actively divide by simple binary fission within the gut of the fly. Later the promastigotes migrate to the pharynx and buccal cavity of the fly. From here the promastigotes may be injected into a susceptible host when the fly takes other blood meals during its 2- to 3-week life span.

EPIDEMIOLOGY*

The epidemiology of leishmaniasis is extremely complex. Some of the difficulty arises because of frequent taxonomic reorganization and renaming of the different species of the genus *Leishmania*. Initially the distinction was based on differences in the clinical presentation of the infection, mode of transmission, type of natural animal reservoirs, and ability to cultivate the various species in vitro or in vivo. As newer techniques for identification have been developed, such as analysis of isoenzymes, buoyant density of the kinetoplast DNA, and ultrastructural morphology, there have been further reorganizations of the genus and a proliferation in the number of recognized species and subspecies. Because most of these sophisticated identification techniques are not routinely available in clinical laboratories, and the diagnosis and treatment are usually based on differences in the clinical presentation of the infection, it is probably best to discuss these infections in terms of three major clinical forms: cutaneous leishmaniasis, mucocutaneous leishmaniasis, and visceral leishmaniasis.

Two major groups or complexes of *Leishmania* species are responsible for cutaneous leishmaniasis. Members of the *Leishmania tropica* complex (*L. tropica major*, *L. tropica minor*, *L. aethiopica*) are responsible for cutaneous leishmaniasis (Old World cutaneous leishmaniasis, Oriental sore) throughout urban and rural areas of the Near and Middle East, the Mediterranean basin, India, and Africa. Members of the *Leishmania mexicana* complex (*L. mexicana mexicana*, *L. mexicana pifanoi*, or *L. mexicana amazonensis*) are responsible for most cases of cutaneous leishmaniasis that occur in the rural areas of

---

*References 5, 36, 51, 63, 68, and 71.

*References 3, 5, 36, 51, 63, 64, 68, 69, 71, and 92.

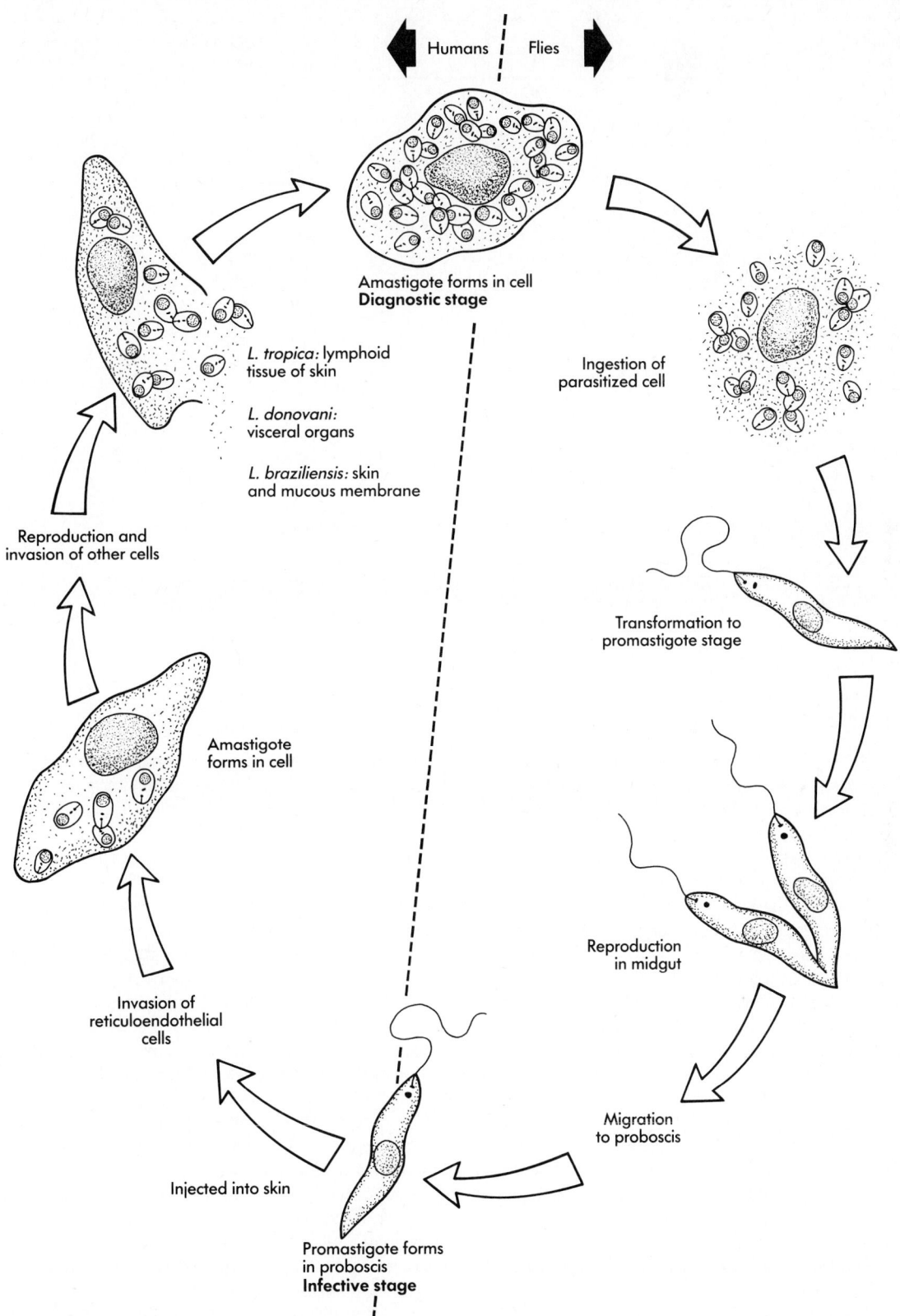

FIGURE 43-5. Life cycle of *Leishmania* spp. (Modified from Melvin, D.M., Brooke, M.M., and Healy, G.R.: Common blood and tissue parasites of man—life cycle charts, Atlanta, 1965, PHS Pub. No. 1234, Laboratory Branch of the Communicable Disease Center.)

TABLE 43-2. Key Epidemiologic Features of *Leishmania* Infections

Disease and Species	Geographic Distribution	Arthropod Vector	Animal Reservoir
CUTANEOUS LEISHMANIASIS			
L. tropica major	Rural areas in Near/Middle East, Mediterranean, India, West Africa	*Phlebotomus papatasi*	Rodents
L. tropica minor	Same as above except in urban areas	*Phlebotomus sergenti*	Humans and dogs
L. aethiopica	Highlands of Ethiopia and Kenya	*Phlebotomus longipes*	Hydrax
L. mexicana ssp. *mexicana, pifanoi, amazonensis*	Rural forested lowlands in Central and South America	*Lutzomyia* spp.	Rodents
L. braziliensis ssp. *peruviana*	Urban areas of the Andes Mountains	*Lutzomyia verrucarum*	Humans and dogs
MUCOCUTANEOUS LEISHMANIASIS			
L. braziliensis ssp. except *peruviana*	Rural forested lowlands in Central and South America	*Lutzomyia* spp.	Rodents
VISCERAL LEISHMANIASIS			
L. donovani complex	Mediterranean (urban areas)	*Phlebotomus perniciosus*	Dogs
	India (urban areas)	*Phlebotomus argentipes*	Humans
	China (urban areas)	*Phlebotomus chinensis*	Dogs
	East Africa (rural areas)	*Phlebotomus martini*	Rodents
	Brazil (urban areas)	*Lutzomyia longipalpis*	Rodents

Modified from Garcia, L.S., and Ash, L.R.: Diagnostic parasitology: clinical laboratory manual, St. Louis, 1979, The C.V. Mosby Co.

South and Central America (New World cutaneous leishmaniasis, chiclero ulcer). One member of the *L. braziliensis* complex, *L. peruviana,* is responsible for a form of cutaneous leishmaniasis that occurs in areas of human habitation in the Andes Mountains of South America. Within these broad geographic areas there are regional differences in the species of parasite, the reservoir host, and the insect vector (Table 43-2).

Although a few locally acquired cases have been reported in the United States, mucocutaneous leishmaniasis (espundia) is generally restricted to South and Central America, where it is primarily a disease of individuals who work in rural, forested lowlands. And, except for *L. peruviana,* which causes a cutaneous form of leishmaniasis, the parasites responsible for this infection are members of the *L. braziliensis* complex that are transmitted to humans from a reservoir in forest-dwelling rodents by anthropophilic sandflies of the genus *Lutzomvia.*

Visceral leishmaniasis (kala azar) is the most widely distributed form of leishmaniasis and is considered endemic in the Mediterranean basin, India, East Africa, Central and South America, and China. Visceral leishmaniasis is essentially a disease of rural areas; however, as with cutaneous forms of leishmaniasis, regional differences exist in the reservoir host and insect vector (see Table 43-2).

PATHOLOGY AND CLINICAL MANIFESTATIONS*

In all forms of cutaneous leishmaniasis the early lesions are usually single or multiple erythematous papules (2 to 5 mm in diameter) that appear at sites of sandfly bites on the face, arms, and legs. As the amastigotes continue their intracellular multiplication and destruction within the skin, the papule slowly increases in diameter (up to 3 cm) through the development of multiple satellite lesions that form and coalesce on the periphery of the primary lesion. Within a few weeks or months the lesion becomes a shallow ulcer, which eventually heals with fibrosis and scarring.

The rate at which the lesion evolves and the appearance of the developed ulcers vary with the *Leishmania* sp. responsible for the infection and the host's response to the infection. Two of the most common clinical patterns of Old World cutaneous leishmaniasis are the so-called moist ulcers associated with *L. tropica major* infections and the dry ulcers associated with *L. tropica minor* infections. The development of moist ulcers typically occurs after an incubation period of a few weeks to months and is followed by the rapid development of weeping ulcers that heal within 6 months. The development and healing of dry ulcers are more prolonged; the incubation period may last for several years before the first appearance of a slowly developing ulcer that is covered with a scaly crust. This lesion may not heal completely for several years. Although the lesions of cutaneous leishmaniasis in the New World are generally caused by different species (*L. mexicana* complex), they resemble the ulcers associated with *L. tropica* infections in the Old World form of the disease.

Healing of the lesions of cutaneous leishmaniasis usually signifies a cell-mediated, species-specific, lifelong immunity against reinfection. However, these infections are not without possible serious complications. One of the most common is

---

*References 3-5, 8, 16, 36, 51, 68, 82, 96, 101, and 111.

secondary bacterial infections of the ulcerated lesion. Another, even more serious complication is the development of diffuse cutaneous leishmaniasis. This form of leishmaniasis, which has been associated with *L. aethiopica* infections in the Old World and *L. mexicana* infections in the New World, occurs in the rare individual with a compromised cellular immune response. In these cases multiple lesions, which do not ulcerate and may be confused with lepromatous leprosy, appear widely disseminated across the skin, especially on the face and lower areas of the body.

Mucocutaneous leishmaniasis (*L. braziliensis*) may actually be considered a complication of an otherwise typical case of cutaneous leishmaniasis. The initial lesions of mucocutaneous leishmaniasis are similar to those seen in Old World cutaneous leishmaniasis, except that the ulcer may extend deeper into the skin. In many cases the localized cutaneous lesions heal with scar formation but no further tissue involvement. If the infection is caused by the subspecies *L. braziliensis braziliensis* the infection tends to spread, presumably via the bloodstream, to other areas of the skin and mucous membranes, especially the mucocutaneous borders and cartilaginous regions of the nose and mouth. Extensive, uncontrolled ulceration and scar formation lead to serious destruction and deformity of the nasal and oral passages. Secondary bacterial infection of the ulcers is common and increases the tissue destruction.

In visceral leishmaniasis the parasites are not restricted to the skin or mucous membranes; in fact, the primary skin lesion of this form of leishmaniasis often goes unnoticed. The parasites of the *L. donovani* complex are viscerotropic; that is, they prefer to multiply in macrophages or other reticuloendothelial cells associated with the spleen, liver, bone marrow, and lymph nodes. In these internal organs, extensive hyperplasia of parasitized tissues eventually impairs the functioning of the organ.

The onset of clinical manifestations in visceral leishmaniasis is usually insidious, coming after an incubation period that may vary from 10 days to 9 years (typically 2 to 6 months). In native populations the disease usually has a gradual onset. The earliest manifestation is a cycle of fever and sweating that first occurs at irregular intervals but later in a pattern that resembles the undulant fever of brucellosis. Besides fever, the common physical findings include splenomegaly, generalized lymphadenopathy, and hyperpigmentation of the skin of the hands, feet, and abdomen. (The term "kala azar" can be translated as "black disease.")

If the host mounts an adequate cell-mediated immune response, the infection may be mild or asymptomatic. However, in untreated persons with an inadequate immune response, jaundice and blood disorders may develop and eventually the host may die of secondary infections such as bacterial pneumonia, tuberculosis, and bacillary or amoebic dysentery. Less than 25% of untreated persons survive once the disease reaches the terminal stages.

LABORATORY DIAGNOSIS[5,36,68,71,76]

Depending on the type of leishmaniasis, laboratory confirmation may require different techniques. In cutaneous leishmaniasis the diagnosis is usually based on demonstrating the intracellular amastigotes (Plate 29, *B*) in Giemsa-stained touch preparations of skin samples obtained from the nonulcerated border of active lesions.

In the early stages of mucocutaneous leishmaniasis the parasites may also be abundant in such skin preparations. Howev-

er, in the later stages of the disease when there is extensive involvement of the mouth and face, demonstrating the organisms in stained smears is more difficult. In these cases in vitro cultivation of the promastigote stages in Novy, MacNeal, Nicolle (NNN) medium incubated at room temperature may be necessary. Unfortunately, because members of the *L. braziliensis* complex do not always grow well in vitro, the physician may need to base the diagnosis solely on the history and physical examination and the results of the Montenegro skin test.

Similar techniques may be employed for the diagnosis of visceral leishmaniasis except that the tissue samples are obtained by biopsy of bone marrow, spleen, liver, and lymph nodes. The best results are usually obtained using tissue from the spleen, but because of the risk of complications many physicians prefer to use bone marrow from sternal puncture. If the parasite cannot be directly demonstrated in stained smears, the same type of samples used for smears may be used in an attempt to cultivate the promastigote stage in NNN medium or to produce a laboratory infection in hamsters. Of these two alternatives, in vitro cultivation in NNN is usually preferred because of a better diagnostic yield and the relative simplicity of the technique.

The Montenegro skin test is probably of little value in the clinical diagnosis of visceral leishmaniasis because findings are usually negative in active cases and become positive only after successful treatment or spontaneous cure. However, in vitro serologic tests for specific antibodies are often helpful, especially the indirect immunofluorescence agglutination tests and agar-gel precipitation tests.

Most clinical laboratories cannot perform the sophisticated techniques required for specific identification of amastigote stages of hemoflagellates (including *Trypanosoma cruzi*), and they must be content to report "Amastigotes of hemoflagellate seen." In this circumstance the physician must rely on the patient's history and physical examination to make the definitive diagnosis. As in all such cases, the laboratory should make every effort to obtain a definitive diagnosis by consulting a qualified reference laboratory.

NAEGLERIA AND *ACANTHAMOEBA*
LIFE CYCLE[11,18,25,98]

Two groups of free-living amoebae that naturally inhabit soil and fresh water have been reported as etiologic agents of primary amoebic meningoencephalitis—*Naegleria* spp. and *Acanthamoeba* spp. Members of the genus *Naegleria* are amoeboflagellates that can exist in their natural habitat in three different forms—trophozoites, flagellates, and cysts. In water and moist soil the trophozoite may reversibly transform into an oval-shaped biflagellate (average 15 μm in length). The spherical to ovoid cysts average 10 μm in diameter and have a smooth cyst wall.

The only vegetative stage of *Acanthamoeba* spp. is a large (20 to 50 μm in length), slow-moving trophozoite that is commonly covered with characteristic spinelike projections called acanthapodia; there is no flagellate stage. The typical cysts of *Acanthamoeba* spp. (10 to 25 μm in length) have double-layered, polygonal walls that give clusters of cysts the appearance of a honeycomb.

Infections with either organism may occur when trophozoites invade the nasal mucosa and migrate to the brain along the route of the olfactory nerve through the cribriform plate. *Acanthamoeba* organisms may also enter the brain by a hematogenous route after trophozoites invade mucous membranes in the lungs, the skin, or the conjunctiva of the eye. In the brain, trophozoites spread by way of the subarachnoid spaces to produce an extensive generalized involvement of the meninges. They then migrate inward to the gray matter, especially the cerebellum and the base of the cerebrum. Clusters of trophozoites are also found in the perivascular spaces of both the cortex and subcortex of the brain. In *Acanthamoeba* infections both cysts and trophozoites may be found in affected tissues; only the trophozoite stage of *Naegleria* is found in the tissue.

Although infections with *Naegleria* spp. appear to be restricted to the central nervous system, *Acanthamoeba* spp. have also been reported to cause corneal and skin ulcerations and ear and pulmonary infections.

EPIDEMIOLOGY[12,14]

A relatively rare disease (fewer than 200 cases worldwide, 68 in the United States), primary amoebic meningoencephalitis occurs worldwide, especially in warmer climates. Almost all the well-documented cases have been attributed to *Naegleria* spp. (50 in the United States). There have been only 30 documented cases worldwide of meningoencephalitis caused by *Acanthamoeba* spp.

Naegleria infections typically occur in previously healthy children or young adults who have been swimming in freshwater pools or ponds during the warmer months. The principal pathogenic species, *Naegleria fowleri,* is present year-round but only in small numbers when the temperature is low or the water is free flowing. When the water is stagnant or at higher temperatures, the number of organisms and consequently the risk of infection increase. Normal chlorination procedures appear to have little effect on the organism's survival. In well-maintained swimming pools with effective water circulation and filtration systems, however, there seems to be little risk of infection.

Perhaps because *Acanthamoeba* meningoencephalitis is exceedingly rare, the exact mechanism of infection is not clearly understood. Most cases have occurred in chronically ill or debilitated patients who gave no history of swimming before the onset of illness. Patients with eye infections caused by this organism usually give a history of trauma and probable soil contamination of the affected area. In other cases the organisms may gain access when airborne cysts are inhaled.

PATHOLOGY AND CLINICAL MANIFESTATIONS*

Naegleria spp. infections characteristically have a fulminant course with signs and symptoms that suggest an acute bacterial meningitis. Lapsing into a deep coma within a week, the patient usually dies from cardiorespiratory failure or brain herniation.

LABORATORY DIAGNOSIS[15,35]

The laboratory diagnosis of primary amoebic meningoencephalitis is based on identifying the trophozoites of *Naegleria* spp. or the trophozoites or cysts of *Acanthamoeba* spp. in the spinal fluid. Specimens of spinal fluid may be prepared as direct wet mounts and examined for motile trophozoites, preferably using phase contrast microscopy. Care must be taken to differentiate the trophozoites of these two amoebae from motile white cells, and perhaps from the trophozoites of *Entamoeba histolytica* if the patient has a brain abscess. One method of differentiation is to add the spinal fluid to a small amount of warm distilled water; the white cells and *E. histolytica* trophozoites generally rupture, whereas *Naegleria* and *Acanthamoeba* spp. remain intact and motile. This same technique can also be used to differentiate between the genera *Naegleria* and *Acanthamoeba.* After several hours' incubation at 37° C the diluted spinal fluid can be reexamined for the presence of flagellated forms that are unique to the genus *Naegleria.* For added assurance in identification, stained slides may be prepared from the spinal fluid using the same methods as for fecal specimens. The typical trophozoites (10 to 20 μm in length) are readily recognized by their large central karyosome and delicate nuclear membrane.

If necessary the organisms may be cultivated by adding a drop of spinal fluid to the center of an agar plate that has previously been seeded with *Escherichia coli.* If *Naegleria* or *Acanthamoeba* organisms are present, the trophozoite stage may be found near the site of inoculation after the plate has been incubated for 1 or 2 days at 37° C.

REFERENCES

1. Allison, A.C.: Protection afforded by sickle-cell trait against subtertian malarial infection, Br. Med. J. 1:290, 1954.
2. Barett-Connor, E., Uroretz, R.J., and Braude, A.I.: Disseminated intravascular coagulation in trypanosomiasis, Arch. Intern. Med. 131:574, 1973.
3. Barlow, D., et al.: American mucocutaneous leishmaniasis, South. Med. J. 70:246, 1977.
4. Barnetson, R.S., Ridley, D.S., and Wheate, H.W.: A form of mucocutaneous leishmaniasis in the Old World, Trans. R. Soc. Trop. Med. Hyg. 72:516, 1978.
5. Bray, R.S.: Leishmania, Annu. Rev. Microbiol. 28:189, 1974.
6. Brazinsky, J.H., and Phillips, J.E.: Pneumocystis pneumonia transmission between patients with lymphoma, JAMA 209:1527, 1969.
7. Bruce-Chwatt, L.J.: Blood transfusion and tropical disease, Trop. Dis. Bull. 69:825, 1972.
8. Bryceson, A.D.: Diffuse cutaneous leishmaniasis in Ethiopia. I. The clinical and histological features of the disease, Trans. R. Soc. Trop. Med. Hyg. 63:708, 1969.
9. Burke, B.A., and Good, R.A.: *Pneumocystis carinii* infection, Medicine 52:23, 1973.
10. Butt, C.G.: Primary amebic meningoencephalitis, N. Engl. J. Med. 274:1473, 1966.
11. Carter, R.F.: Primary amoebic meningoencephalitis: an appraisal of present knowledge, Trans. R. Soc. Trop. Med. Hyg. 66:193, 1972.
12. Centers for Disease Control: Primary amebic meningoencephalitis: California, Florida, New York, MMWR 27:343, 1978.
13. Centers for Disease Control: Acquired immunodeficiency syndrome (AIDS): United States, MMWR 32:465, 1983.
14. Chang, S.H.: Etiological, pathological, epidemiological and diagnostic consideration of primary amoebic meningoencephalitis, CRC Crit. Rev. Microbiol. 3:135, 1974.
15. Coatney, G.R.: The simian malarias: zoonoses, anthroponoses, or both? Am. J. Trop. Med. Hyg. 20:795, 1971.
16. Convit, J., Pinardi, M.E., and Rondon, A.J.: Diffuse cutaneous leishmaniasis: a disease due to an immunological defect of the host, Trans. R. Soc. Trop. Med. Hyg. 66:603, 1972.
17. Covell, G.: Congenital malaria, Trop. Dis. Bull. 47:1147, 1950.
18. Culbertson, C.G.: The pathogenicity of soil amebas, Annu. Rev. Microbiol. 25:231, 1971.

*References 10, 14, 19, 67, 83, and 98.

19. Cursons, R.T.M., Brown, T.J., and Keyes, E.A.: Virulence of pathogenic free-living amebae, J. Parasitol. **64:**744, 1978.

20. Dammin, G.J.: The rising incidence of clinical *Babesia microti* infection, Hum. Pathol. **12:**398, 1981.

21. Deaton, J.G.: Fatal pulmonary edema as a complication of acute falciparum malaria, Am. J. Trop. Med. Hyg. **19:**196, 1970.

22. Desmonts, G., and Courreur, J.: Congenital toxoplasmosis: a prospective study of 378 pregnancies, N. Engl. J. Med. **290:**1110, 1974.

23. Dorfman, R.F., and Remington, J.S.: Value of lymph-node biopsy in the diagnosis of acute acquired toxoplasmosis, N. Engl. J. Med. **289:**878, 1973.

24. Duggan, A.J., and Hutchinson, M.P.: Sleeping sickness in Europeans: a review of 109 cases, J. Trop. Med. Hyg. **69:**124, 1966.

25. Dumas, R.J.: Primary amoebic meningoencephalitis, CRC Crit. Rev. Clin. Lab. Sci. **3:**163, 1972.

26. Durack, D.T.: Opportunistic infections and Kaposi's sarcoma in homosexual men, N. Engl. J. Med. **305:**1465, 1981.

27. Dutz, W.: *Pneumocystis carinii* pneumonia, Pathol. Annu. **5:**309, 1970.

28. Dvorak, J.S.A., et al.: Invasion of erythrocytes by malaria merozoites, Science **187:**748, 1975.

29. Earlam, R.J.: Gastrointestinal aspects of Chagas' disease, Am. J. Dig. Dis. **17:**559, 1972.

30. Farrar, W.E., et al.: Serologic evidence of human infections with *Trypanosoma cruzi* in Georgia, Am. J. Hyg. **78:**166, 1963.

31. Francis, T.I.: Visceral complication of Gambian trypanosomiasis in a Nigerian, Trans. R. Soc. Trop. Med. Hyg. **66:**140, 1972.

32. Frenkel, J.K.: Toxoplasmosis: mechanisms of infection, laboratory diagnosis, and management, Curr. Top. Pathol. **54:**29, 1971.

33. Frenkel, J.K., and Dubey, J.P.: Toxoplasmosis and its prevention in cats and man, J. Infect. Dis. **126:**664, 1972.

34. Frenkel, J.K., and Wallace, G.D.: Transmission of toxoplasmosis by tachyzoites: possibility and probability of a hypothesis, Med. Hypotheses **5:**529, 1979.

35. Friedmann, C.T., et al.: A malaria epidemic among heroin users, Am. J. Trop. Med. Hyg. **22:**302, 1973.

36. Gardener, P.J.: Taxonomy of the genus *Leishmania*, Trop. Dis. Bull. **74:**1069, 1977.

37. Garnham, P.C.C.: Malaria parasites and other haemosporidia, Oxford, Eng., 1966, Blackwell Scientific Publications, Inc.

38. Garnham, P.C.C.: Human babesiosis: European aspects, Trans. R. Soc. Trop. Med. Hyg. **74:**153, 1980.

39. Garvey, G., Neu, H.C., and Katz, M.: Transfusion-induced malaria after open heart surgery, N.Y. State J. Med. **75:**602, 1975.

40. Golden, J.: Pneumocystis lung disease in homosexual men, West. J. Med. **137:**400, 1982.

41. Goodwin, L.G.: The pathology of African trypanosomiasis, Trans. R. Soc. Trop. Med. Hyg. **64:**797, 1970.

42. Gray, A.R.: Antigenic variation in a strain of *Trypanosoma brucei* transmitted by *Glossina morsitans* and *G. palpalis*, J. Gen. Microbiol. **41:**195, 1965.

43. Greenwood, B.M., Whittle, H.C., and Molyneux, D.H.: Immunosuppression in Gambian trypanosomiasis, Trans. R. Soc. Trop. Med. Hyg. **67:**846, 1973.

44. Gump, D.W., and Holden, R.A.: Acquired chorioretinitis due to toxoplasmosis, Ann. Intern. Med. **90:**58, 1979.

45. Hasleton, P.S., and Curry, A.: *Pneumocystis carinii:* the continuing enigma, Thorax **37:**481, 1982.

46. Hasleton, P.S., Curry, A., and Rankin, E.M.: *Pneumocystis carinii* pneumonia: a light microscopical and ultrastructural study, J. Clin. Pathol. **34:**1138, 1981.

47. Healy, G.R., and Ruebush, T.K.: Morphology of *Babesia microti* in human blood smears, Am. J. Clin. Pathol. **73:**107, 1980.

48. Heineman, H.S.: The clinical syndrome of malaria in USA, Arch. Intern. Med. **129:**607, 1972.

49. Hoare, C.A.: The developmental stages of *Toxoplasma*, J. Trop. Med. Hyg. **75:**56, 1972.

50. Hoare, C.A.: Comparative aspects of human babesiosis, Trans. R. Soc. Trop. Med. Hyg. **74:**143, 1980.

51. Hoogstraal, H., and Heyneman, D.: Leishmaniasis in the Sudan Republic: final epidemiologic report, Am. J. Trop. Med. Hyg. **18:**1089, 1969.

52. Hughes, W.T.: Current status of laboratory diagnosis of *Pneumocystis carinii* pneumonia, CRC Crit. Rev. Clin. Lab. Sci. **6:**145, 1975.

53. Hughes, W.T., et al.: Protein-calorie malnutrition: a host determinant for *Pneumocystis carinii* infection, Am. J. Dis. Child. **128:**44, 1974.

54. Hutchinson, W.M., et al.: Coccidian-like nature of *Toxoplasma gondii,* Br. Med. J. **1:**142, 1970.

55. Kean, B.H.: Clinical toxoplasmosis: 50 years, Trans. R. Soc. Trop. Med. Hyg. **66:**549, 1972.

56. Kean, B.H., Kimball, A.C., and Christenson, W.N.: An epidemic of acute toxoplasmosis, JAMA **208:**1002, 1969.

57. Kean, B.H., and Reilly, P.D.: Malaria: the mime—recent lessons from a group of civilian travelers, Am. J. Med. **61:**159, 1976.

58. Keieger, J.P., editor: Malaria, New York, 1980, Academic Press, Inc.

59. Koberle, F.: Chagas' disease and Chagas' syndromes: the pathology of American trypanosomiasis, Adv. Parasitol. **6:**63, 1968.

60. Koberle, F.: The causation and importance of nervous lesions in American trypanosomiasis, Bull. WHO **42:**739, 1970.

61. Krogstad, D.J., Juranek, D.D., and Walls, K.W.: Toxoplasmosis: with comments on risk of infection from cats, Ann. Intern. Med. **77:**773, 1972.

62. Krotoski, W.A.: Relapses in primate malaria: discovery of two populations of exoerythrocytic stages—preliminary note, Br. Med. J. **1:**153, 1980.

63. Lainson, R., and Shaw, J.J.: Leishmaniasis of the New World: taxonomic problems, Br. Med. Bull. **28:**44, 1972.

64. Lainson, R., and Shaw, J.J.: Epidemiology and ecology of leishmaniasis in Latin America, Nature **273:**595, 1978.

65. Lake, K.B., Jr., et al.: Lymphoglandular toxoplasmosis, Postgrad. Med. **65:**110, 1979.

66. Laranja, F.S., et al.: Chagas' disease: a clinical, epidemiologic and pathologic study, Circulation **4:**1035, 1956.

67. Ma, P., et al.: A case of keratitis due to *Acanthamoeba* in New York, New York, and features of 10 cases, J. Infect. Dis. **143:**662, 1981.

68. Manson-Bahr, P.E.C.: Leishmaniasis, Int. Rev. Trop. Med. **4:**123, 1971.

69. Manson-Bahr, P.E.C., and Southgate, B.A.: Recent research on kala-azar in East Africa, J. Trop. Med. Hyg. **67:**79, 1964.

70. Marsden, P.D.: South American trypanosomiasis, Int. Rev. Trop. Med. **4:**97, 1971.

71. Marsden, P.D.: Current concepts in parasitology: leishmaniasis, N. Engl. J. Med. **300:**350, 1979.

72. Meuwissen, J.H.E., et al.: Parasitologic and serologic observations of infection with *Pneumocystis* in humans, J. Infect. Dis. **136:**43, 1977.

73. Miller, L.H., et al.: The resistance factor to *Plasmodium vivax* in blacks, N. Engl. J. Med. **295:**302, 1976.

74. Mott, K.E., et al.: *Trypanosoma cruzi* infection in dogs and cats and household seroreactivity to *T. cruzi* in a rural community in northeast Brazil, Am. J. Trop. Med. Hyg. **27:**1123, 1978.

75. Omerod, W.E., and Venkatesan, S.: An amastigote phase of the sleeping sickness trypanosome, Trans. R. Soc. Trop. Med. Hyg. **65:**736, 1971.

76. Pampiglione, S., et al.: Studies in Mediterranean leishmaniasis. III. The leishmanin test in kala-azar, Trans. R. Soc. Trop. Med. Hyg. **69:**60, 1975.

77. Perkins, E.S.: Ocular toxoplasmosis, Br. J. Ophthalmol. **57:**1, 1973.

78. Peters, W.: Malaria, N. Engl. J. Med. **297:**1261, 1977.

79. Pifer, L.L., et al.: *Pneumocystis carinii* infection: evidence of high prevalence in normal and immunosuppressed children, Pediatrics **61**:35, 1978.

80. Poltera, A.A., Cox, J.N., and Owor, R.: Pancarditis affecting the conducting system and all valves in human African trypanosomiasis, Br. Heart J. **38**:827, 1976.

81. Remington, J.S., Jacobs, L., and Kaufman, H.E.: Toxoplasmosis in the adult, N. Engl. J. Med. **262**:180, 1960.

82. Ridley, D.S.: The pathogenesis of cutaneous leishmaniasis, Trans. R. Soc. Trop. Med. Hyg. **73**:150, 1979.

83. Ringsted, J., et al.: Probable *Acanthamoeba* meningoencephalitis in a Korean child, Am. J. Clin. Pathol. **66**:723, 1976.

84. Robins-Browne, R.M., Schneider, J., and Metz, J.: Thrombocytopenia in trypanosomiasis, Am. J. Trop. Med. Hyg. **24**:226, 1975.

85. Ruebush, T.K., et al.: Human babesiosis on Nantucket Island: clinical features, Ann. Intern. Med. **86**:6, 1977.

86. Ruebush, T.K.: Human babesiosis in North America, Trans. R. Soc. Trop. Med. Hyg. **74**:149, 1980.

87. Ruskin, J., and Remington, J.A.: Toxoplasmosis in the compromised host, Ann. Intern. Med. **84**:193, 1976.

88. Russell, P.F., et al.: Practical malariology, ed. 2, London, 1963, Oxford University Press.

89. Ryning, F.W., et al.: Probable transmission of *Toxoplasma gondii* by organ transplantation, Ann. Intern. Med. **84**:193, 1979.

90. Samuels, B.S., and Rietchel, R.L.: Polymositis and toxoplasmosis, JAMA **235**:60, 1976.

91. Sanyal, S.K., et al.: Course of pulmonary dysfunction in children surviving *Pneumocystis carinii* pneumonia: a prospective study, Am. Rev. Respir. Dis. **124**:161, 1981.

92. Shaw, P.K., et al.: Autochthonous dermal leishmaniasis in Texas, Am. J. Trop. Med. Hyg. **25**:788, 1976.

93. Sitprija, V.: Renal involvement in malaria, Trans. R. Soc. Trop. Med. Hyg. **64**:695, 1970.

94. Spencer, H.C., et al.: Imported African trypanosomiasis in the United States, Ann. Intern. Med. **82**:633, 1975.

95. Teutsch, S.M., et al.: Epidemic toxoplasmosis associated with infected cats, N. Engl. J. Med. **300**:695, 1979.

96. Thornburgh, D.B., Johnson, C.M., and Elton, N.W.: The histopathology of cutaneous leishmaniasis in Panama, Trans. R. Soc. Trop. Med. Hyg. **46**:550, 1962.

97. Varva, J.K., and Kucera, K.: *Pneumocystis carinii* Delanoe, its ultrastructure and intrastructural affinities, J. Protozool. **17**:463, 1970.

98. Visvesvara, G.S., Jones, D.B., and Robinson, N.M.: Isolation, identification, and biological characterization of *Acanthamoeba polyphaga* from a human eye, Am. J. Trop. Med. Hyg. **24**:784, 1975.

99. Wallace, G.D.: The role of the cat in the natural history of *Toxoplasma gondii*, Am. J. Trop. Med. Hyg. **20**:411, 1973.

100. Wallace, G.D.: Experimental transmission of *Toxoplasma gondii* by filth-flies, Am. J. Trop. Med. Hyg. **27**:313, 1974.

101. Walton, B.C., Chinel, L.V., and Eguia y Eguia, O.: Onset of espundia after many years of occult infection with *Leishmania braziliensis*, Am. J. Trop. Med. Hyg. **22**:696, 1973.

102. Walzer, P.D., Powell, R.D., and Yoneda, K.: Experimental *Pneumocystis carinii* pneumonia in different strains of cortisonized mice, Infect. Immun. **24**:66, 1979.

103. Walzer, P.D., and Rutledge, M.E.: Comparison of rat, mouse, and human *Pneumocystis carinii* by immunofluorescence, J. Infect. Dis. **142**:449, 1980.

104. Walzer, P.D., et al.: *Pneumocystis carinii* pneumonia and primary immunodeficiency diseases of infancy and childhood, J. Pediatr. **82**:416, 1973.

105. Walzer, P.D., et al.: *Pneumocystis carinii* pneumonia in the United States: epidemiologic, diagnostic, and clinical features, Ann. Intern. Med. **80**:83, 1974.

106. Wilcox, A.: Manual for the microscopical diagnosis of malaria in man, U.S. Public Health Service Pub. No. 796, Washington, D.C., 1960, U.S. Government Printing Offices.

107. Williams, H.: Human babesiosis, Trans. R. Soc. Trop. Med. Hyg. **74**:157, 1980.

108. Wolfe, M.S.: Parasites other than malaria transmissible by blood transfusion. In Greenwalt, T.J., and Jamieson, G.A., editors: Transmissible disease and blood transfusion, New York, 1975, Grune & Stratton, Inc.

109. Woodruff, A.W., Ansdell, V.E., and Pettitt, L.E.: Cause of anemia in malaria, Lancet **2**:1055, 1979.

110. Woody, N.C., and Woody, H.B.: American trypanosomiasis. I. Clinical and epidemiologic background of Chagas' disease in the United States, J. Pediatr. **58**:568, 1961.

111. Zuckerman, A.: Parasitological review: current status of the immunology of blood and tissue protozoa. I. *Leishmania*, Exp. Parasitol. **38**:370, 1975.

CHAPTER 44

Blood and Tissue Helminths

John Klaas II

With the exception of a few species such as *Trichinella spiralis* and *Echinococcus* spp., most of the major blood and tissue helminths are not naturally transmitted in the United States. However, like the blood and tissue protozoa, many of these species cause a significant amount of disease worldwide and have the potential for being imported and beginning an epidemic focus in the United States.

All the major groups of helminths have representatives that can be considered blood and tissue parasites. The one questionable group is the trematodes; however, even this group is represented if one considers the *Schistosoma* spp. as blood and tissue parasites rather than lumen-dwelling parasites. The approach used in this discussion of parasitic infections places *Schistosoma* organisms with the lumen-dwelling parasites only because their diagnostic stages are passed in natural body excretions. However, based on their site of infection they could as easily be placed with the blood and tissue helminths.

TRICHINELLA SPIRALIS
LIFE CYCLE

Humans are infected with *Trichinella spiralis* by ingesting raw or undercooked meat, most commonly pork, that contains encysted larvae (Figure 44-1). Liberated by the action of the digestive juices, larvae enter the duodenal and jejunal mucosa and within 2 days develop into adult males and females. The males die shortly after copulation and are passed out, usually unnoticed, in the feces. The fertilized females remain in the mucus covering the villi or burrow into the intestinal wall or mesenteric lymph nodes. About 6 or 7 days after infection a new generation of larvae is released from the female worms. This larva positing continues for most of the adult females' 5- to 14-week life span, with each female producing between 1500 and 2000 larvae.

The newly released larvae penetrate the mesenteric lymphatics or venules and are carried by the circulatory system through the heart, the lungs, and all regions of the body by the systemic circulation. The larvae may temporarily lodge in a variety of tissues such as the myocardium and the central nervous system. However, further development of the larvae to the infective stage takes place only in striated muscles, where the larvae slowly grow, molt, and eventually curl into the characteristic spiral form for which the species is named.

About 30 days after muscle penetration, a host reaction has surrounded the larvae with an ellipsoidal capsule (cyst), and the larvae enter a stage of "suspended animation" that continues until they are ingested by a new host or they die and become calcified within the cyst.

EPIDEMIOLOGY*

Cases of trichinosis in humans have been reported from most areas of the world, but the prevalence of the disease varies from region to region, depending in part on the dietary customs of the populace, the use and efficacy of control measures, and the extent to which the disease is recognized and reported. Trichinosis has been frequently reported from the eastern European countries, Russia, Spain, Chile, Mexico, and the United States.

In humans trichinosis is considered an accidental infection that occurs when an individual enters into one of the three natural cycles of transmission among lower animals: the feral cycle, the semidomestic cycle, or the domestic cycle. Trichinosis probably originated in a feral cycle among the carnivorous animals of arctic and subarctic areas. Today in these regions the infection is still common in bears, foxes, and walruses, and humans' accidental entry into this feral cycle has resulted in epidemics in Alaska, Canada, and Vermont, typically following the consumption of bear meat. As civilization evolved, the parasite was apparently transferred from wild to semidomestic animals and then to domestic animal populations.

The semidomestic cycle, which occurs most commonly in the temperate zones, principally involves dogs, cats, rats, and wild mammals. These animals perpetuate a cycle of infection that forms a link between the feral and domestic cycles by eating each other or scraps of infected meat, especially uncooked pork in garbage. In fact, the high incidence of human infection in Poland has been attributed to the practice of feeding hogs the flesh and viscera of wild animals.

The domestic cycle primarily occurs from pig to pig and is commonly perpetuated by feeding uncooked garbage containing meat scraps to pigs. This practice was widespread in the United States until the 1950s. At that time the pork industry was suffering heavy economic losses because of the spread of vesicular exanthema, a viral disease of hogs that is related to the use of raw garbage as feed. To control this spread, the U.S. government adopted regulations and laws to prohibit the use of raw garbage as animal feed. This produced a dramatic decrease not only in the spread of viral exanthema, but also in trichinosis. Despite the reduction of infection in hogs, most infections with *T. spiralis* in the continental United States still result from eating improperly prepared pork or other meat products that are prepared either intentionally or inadvertently with pork. For

---

*References 4, 14, 19, 30, 40, 44, and 50-52.

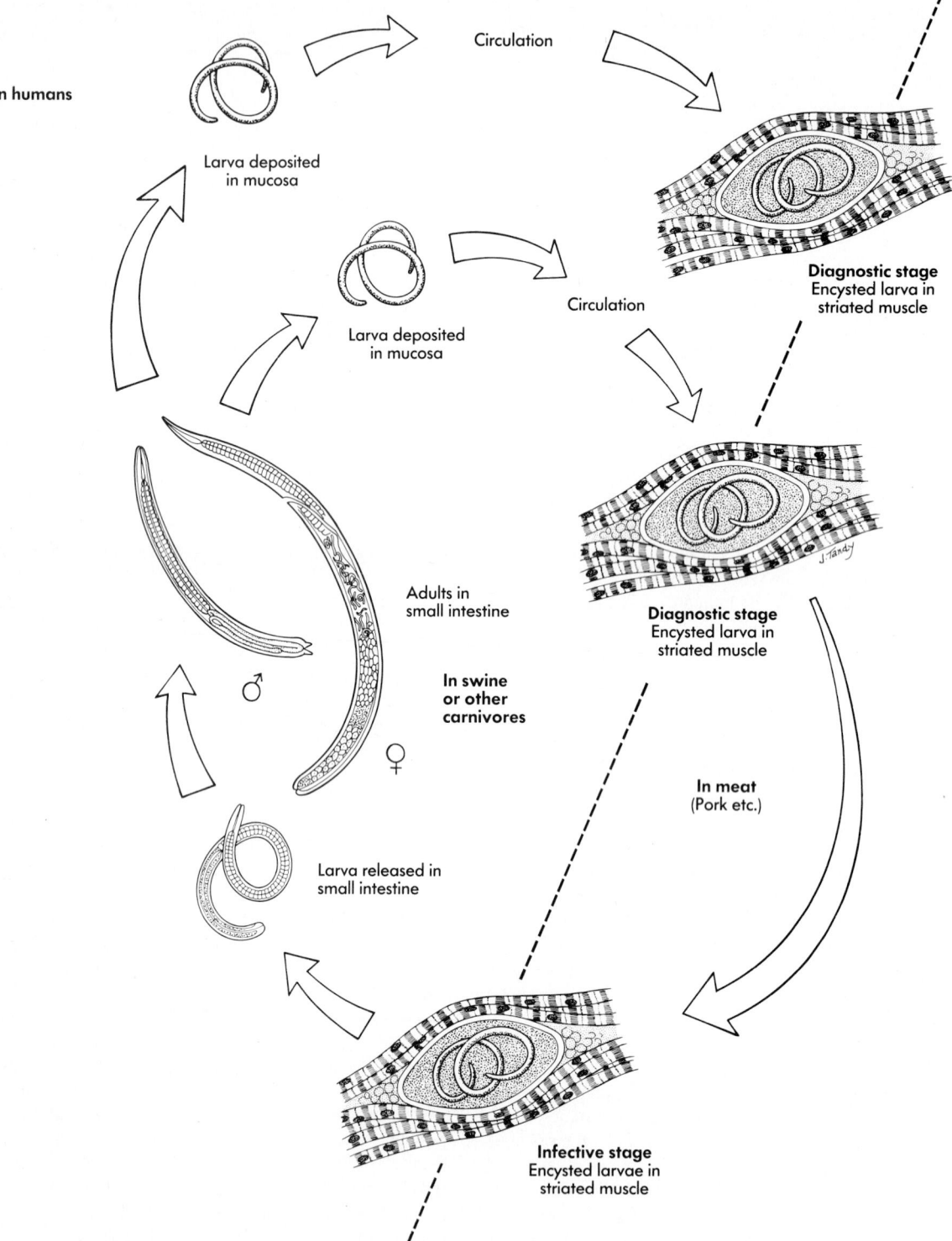

In humans

Circulation

Larva deposited
in mucosa

Diagnostic stage
Encysted larva in
striated muscle

Larva deposited
in mucosa

Circulation

Diagnostic stage
Encysted larva in
striated muscle

Adults in
small intestine

♂

**In swine
or other
carnivores**

♀

In meat
(Pork etc.)

Larva released in
small intestine

Infective stage
Encysted larvae in
striated muscle

FIGURE 44-1. Life cycle of *Trichinella spiralis*. Cycle ends with humans. (Modified from Melvin, D.M., Brooke, M.M., and Healy, G.R.: Common blood and tissue parasites of man—life cycle charts, Atlanta, 1965, PHS Pub. No. 1234, Laboratory Branch of the Communicable Disease Center.)

example, of the 130 cases reported in 1980, 109 were related to consumption of domestic pork products, 12 to the consumption of the meat of wild animals (seven from bear meat, eight from walrus meat, and two from wild pig meat), and the remainder acquired from unknown sources.

PATHOLOGY AND CLINICAL MANIFESTATIONS[2,14,15,21,26]

Trichinosis has a wide variety of clinical manifestations and may mimic many other diseases. Depending on the number of viable larvae that encyst in muscles, the infection may vary from totally asymptomatic to a fulminating fatal disease; usually it is a mild febrile illness. It has been reported that the ingestion of as few as 100 encysted larvae may elicit symptoms; fatal doses are about 300,000 larvae.

The pathologic changes and resulting manifestations of the disease can be divided into three phases that correspond to the three major phases of the life cycle of the parasite: the intestinal phase, the extraintestinal migration and muscle invasion phase, and the convalescent phase. In the intestinal phase of the disease, clinical manifestations occur in only about one half of infected individuals and are typically those of a nonspecific gastroenteritis, for example, diarrhea, abdominal discomfort, and vomiting. These signs and symptoms are associated with a generalized inflammation of the small intestine that is apparently induced by toxic metabolites released by the adult worms and occasionally a secondary bacterial infection of the mucosa. The symptoms of this stage of the disease may begin as early as 24 hours after infection and persist for several weeks.

The second stage of the disease, beginning about 2 weeks after infection, is characterized by fever, headache, acute edema about the eyes, and muscular pain. Later, as the larvae leave the vessels and penetrate striated muscle fibers, the resulting myositis gives rise to myalgias. Often the first muscles affected are the extraocular muscles, followed later by the masseter muscles, neck muscles, tongue, flexor muscles of the extremities, and lumbar muscles. In most patients these symptoms subside about 3 weeks after infection, although malaise and weakness may persist for long periods.

About the time that manifestations of the second stage subside and convalescence begins, cardiac, pulmonary, and neurologic symptoms may develop in some patients as a result of allergic granulomatous reactions and hemorrhage. The most serious complication and the one that usually accounts for the observed 2% case-fatality rate is a myocarditis that usually begins about 4 to 8 weeks after infection.

LABORATORY DIAGNOSIS[14,23]

Because adult and larval stages cannot be reliably recovered in fecal specimens, examination of feces is not recommended for establishing the diagnosis. Instead, the most useful laboratory tests have been serologic examinations and muscle biopsies.

A wide variety of serologic tests have been developed to detect trichinosis. The most widely used and valuable tests are bentonite flocculation, complement fixation, and indirect immunofluorescence. Among these methods, the bentonite flocculation test is generally considered the standard, even though the complement fixation test detects antibodies earlier and the indirect immunofluorescence test is more sensitive in detecting light infections. Studies at the Centers for Disease Control, where bentonite flocculation is the standard test for

trichinosis, have found the test to be 97% sensitive and 100% specific, with positive reactions first occurring about 3 weeks after infection. Maximal reactivity occurs about at about 2 months, and the test remains positive for 2 to 3 years. In equivocal situations in which the patient's signs and symptoms are not compatible with trichinosis or the antibody titer remains positive at a low level, a second serologic test using a different method is recommended.

Definitive diagnosis of active disease may be confirmed by recovery of viable larvae from muscle tissue, although this is usually unnecessary. A positive biopsy from a swollen, tender muscle about 3 weeks after infection is a relatively reliable indicator of infection because of the many larvae that can be expected in the muscles. The viability of larvae can be determined by digesting the muscle with a pepsin–hydrochloric acid mixture and examining the digest for motile larvae. In moderate infections larvae can also be detected microscopically by simply pressing the muscle biopsy specimen between two glass slides or preparing stained histologic sections. These latter procedures, however, are not satisfactory for light infections, and they do not indicate the presence of viable larvae, which is an important clue to distinguishing old, "burned-out" infections from recent ones.

An additional laboratory finding that is suggestive but not unique to trichinosis is eosinophilia, which occurs in about 90% of the symptomatic cases. Typically, the relative number of eosinophils observed in peripheral blood smears increases rapidly in the early stages of the disease. It reaches a peak of 10% to 90% in the third or fourth week of infection and gradually declines thereafter. The absence of eosinophilia in confirmed cases of trichinosis is considered a grave prognostic sign.

WUCHERERIA BANCROFTI
LIFE CYCLE[9,34]

Humans are infected with *Wuchereria bancrofti* when third-stage filariform larvae escape from the proboscis of an infected female mosquito while she is taking a blood meal (Figure 44-2). The larvae, which measure 1.4 to 2 mm long, enter the skin through the puncture wound made by the mosquito, migrate into the peripheral lymphatic vessels, and are carried to the main afferent lymphatics, especially those in the lower half of the body. In the afferent lymphatics the larvae slowly develop into adult worms, which may survive for 6 to 15 years in intertwined, tightly coiled, nodular masses. Between 6 months and 1 year after infection, the adults have matured and mated. The female begins to release thousands of elongate embryos (microfilariae) into the peripheral circulation. Depending on the species of filarial nematode, the microfilariae may or may not remain in the egg membrane (sheath); the microfilariae of *W. bancrofti* are characteristically sheathed.

In most geographic areas, the microfilariae have a daily nocturnal periodicity in the peripheral circulation; the greatest number of microfilariae are found in the peripheral blood between 10 PM and 2 AM. During the day the microfilariae are concentrated in the blood vessels of deep tissues, predominantly the pulmonary vessels. The causes of this periodicity are not clear, but it has been suggested that body temperature and arterial oxygen tension may act as stimuli to synchronize an inherent biologic rhythm of the microfilariae. In certain areas of the Pacific, including Fiji, the Philippines, Samoa, and Tahiti,

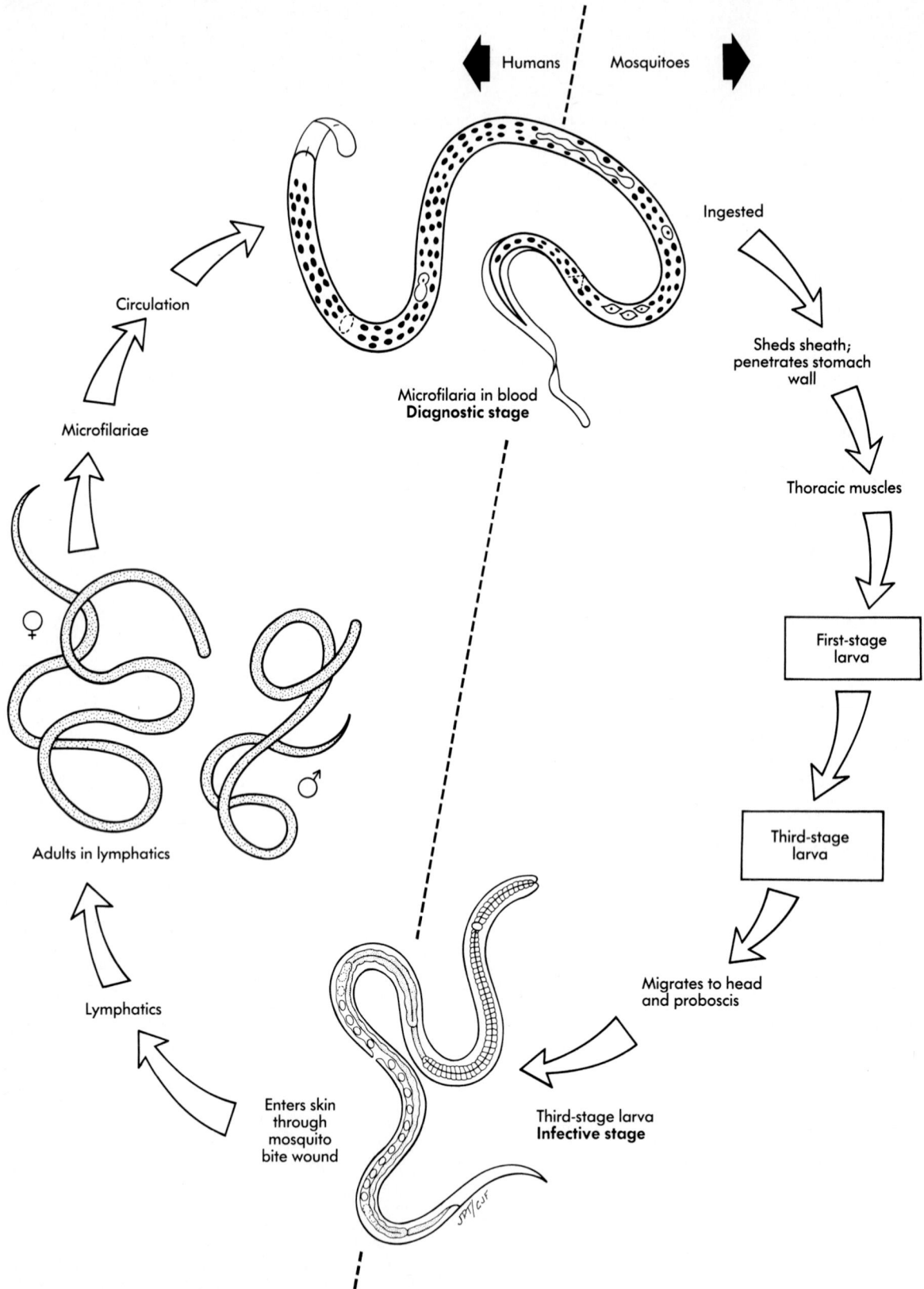

FIGURE 44-2. Life cycle of *Wuchereria bancrofti*. (Modified from Melvin, D.M., Brooke, M.M., and Healy, G.R.: Common blood and tissue parasites of man—life cycle charts, Atlanta, 1965, PHS Pub. No. 1234, Laboratory Branch of the Communicable Disease Center.)

there are other strains of *W. bancrofti* that are either nonperiodic or have a diurnal periodicity, with the greatest numbers appearing in the peripheral blood between noon and 8 PM. Although these so-called subperiodic strains are morphologically identical to strains with a nocturnal periodicity, some authorities consider the strains a separate variety or even a separate species, which they designate *W. pacifica*.

Development of the parasite's larval stages begins when microfilariae are ingested in the blood meal of a susceptible female mosquito. Under ideal conditions of temperature and humidity the microfilariae shed their sheath, penetrate through the mosquito's gut wall into the body cavity, and migrate into the thoracic muscles within 2 to 7 hours after ingestion. The infective third-stage larvae develop in about 10 or 11 days. These larvae migrate into the sheath around the mosquito's proboscis. When the mosquito takes another blood meal, the larvae escape from the proboscis sheath onto the host's skin, and the life cycle begins again.

EPIDEMIOLOGY*

Bancroft's filariasis is principally a disease of the tropics and subtropics. The disease is prominent in the Caribbean, Central Africa, Japan, the Philippines, the East Indies and southwestern Pacific Islands, India, and the eastern and northern coasts of South America. Focal areas of infection occur in Central America, the Mediterranean coasts of Africa and Europe, and the northern coast of Australia. The nocturnal periodic strain of the parasites predominates in all these areas except for the southwestern Pacific islands where the diurnal subperiodic strain is more common.

None of the filarial infections, including *W. bancrofti* infection, is currently endemic in the United States; however, the potential exists for imported cases to give rise to focal areas of infection. In fact, a small focus of *W. bancrofti* infections existed around Charleston, South Carolina, until the 1920s; in 1915 the parasite was found in 20% of 400 hospitalized patients.

Of the many different species of mosquitoes that may act as intermediate hosts, the most important are *Culex* and *Aedes* spp. (for example, *Culex pipiens* and *Aedes aegypti*). These mosquitoes are anthropophilic (prefer human blood) and live near human habitation. The mosquito population must be very large if the natural cycle of infection is to be maintained. The number of larvae developing in the mosquitoes may be only a fraction of the number of microfilariae they ingest. One compensation for this low development rate is that most endemic areas have very large mosquito populations, and individuals receive thousands of bites each year.

PATHOLOGY AND CLINICAL MANIFESTATIONS†

In *W. bancrofti* and most other major filarial infections of humans (the exception being *Onchocerca volvulus*), the pathologic changes are related to damage produced by the adult worms and the host's immune response to these changes; the microfilariae are relatively innocuous.

In natives of endemic areas the disease usually has an asymptomatic incubation period of 1 or more years as the

worms mature in lymphatic spaces close to the site of entry. However, in individuals who have recently entered the endemic area and become infected, there are usually early manifestations of lymphangitis and dilation of the lymph vessels in response to the fluids and castoff body coverings the worms release as they molt in the lymphatic spaces. As the worms mature, there is typically an acute tissue reaction characterized by the infiltration of plasma cells, eosinophils, and macrophages around the affected vessels, damage to the lymph valves, and leakage of fluid from the lymphatics into the surrounding tissue. In symptomatic cases these changes are manifested by lymphangitis with swelling, redness, and pain. Initially these episodes of acute tissue reactions, which are commonly associated with physical exertion, recur once each month or even more frequently. Over time, the frequency and severity of the attacks usually decrease.

As the acute tissue reactions subside, a fibrosis of the regional lymph nodes and lymphatic vessels begins to cause stenosis and obstruction proximal to dead or dying worms. The sites most often affected by the resulting lymph stasis are the groin, lower extremities, and external genitalia. As a result of this lymph stasis there is eventually an accumulation of fibroblasts that leads to the classic picture of elephantiasis: noticeable tissue enlargement caused by accumulation of lymph and fatty tissue in a fibrous matrix that is covered by a tight, thickened skin. Eventually the mass of dead worms and fibrotic tissue becomes calcified.

Development of elephantiasis is not an inevitable consequence of every infection. In fact, severe elephantiasis usually is seen in only a few individuals in endemic areas. The factors said to contribute to these severe manifestations include secondary bacterial infections and an abnormally heightened host response to repeated infections.

LABORATORY DIAGNOSIS[18,20]

The diagnosis of *Wuchereria bancrofti* infections is based on identification of microfilariae circulating in the peripheral blood. Thick blood smears treated with Giemsa stain or Delafield hematoxylin are prepared from blood samples obtained between 10 PM and 2 AM and then examined with the oil immersion objective for the typical microfilariae. The specific identification of these microfilariae, which usually measure between 250 and 300 μm in length and contain parallel rows of cells with stained nuclei, is based on the following characteristics: the presence of a sheath, a cephalic space (the unstained area between the anterior end of the body and the beginning of the rows of nuclei) with a length/width ratio of 1:1, and the absence of cells (nuclei) in the tip of the tail (Figure 44-3).

Microfilariae may not be present in the peripheral blood. In endemic areas, up to 50% of the infections may not be accompanied by the appearance of organisms in the blood. Microfilaremia is even rarer in individuals who become infected in an endemic area and then leave. If examination of the peripheral blood smear fails to reveal microfilariae, they may be detectable in stained slides prepared from the sediment of chylous urine or lymph fluid that has been centrifuged. Slightly more complicated, but certainly warranted in difficult cases, is the use of membrane filtration of venous blood (similar to that which is commonly used by U.S. veterinarians to detect the microfilariae of dog heartworms) or Knott's centrifugal concentration techniques. Both these techniques permit concentra-

---

*References 11, 17, 18, 34, 35, and 42.
†References 8, 9, 11, 16-18, 34, 35, 38, and 46.

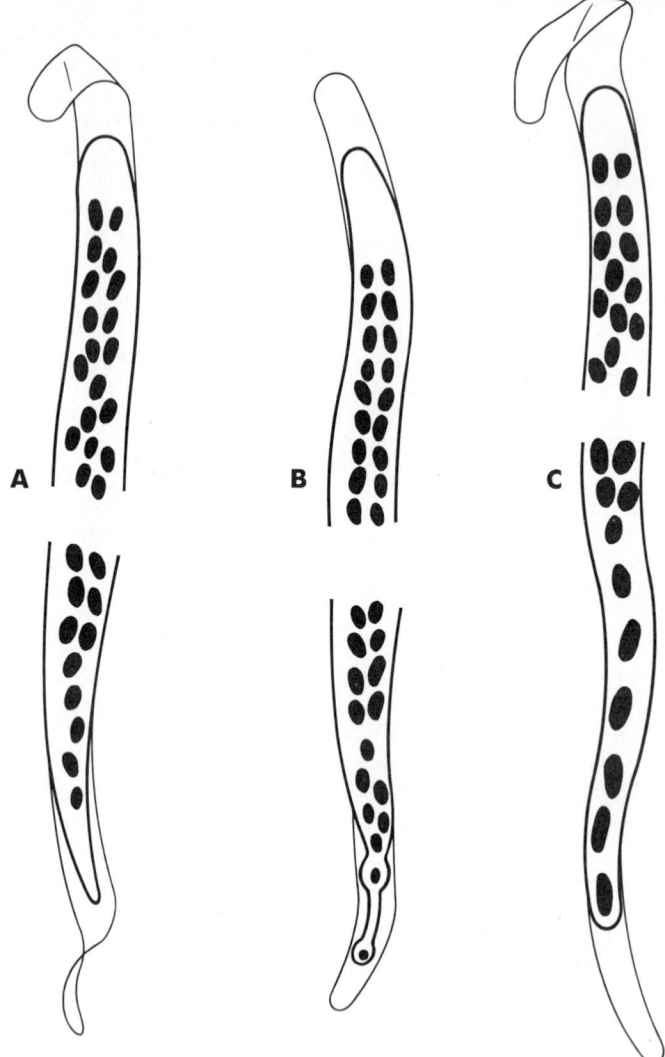

FIGURE 44-3. Sheathed microfilariae of pathogenic filarial nematodes. **A,** *Wuchereria bancrofti.* **B,** *Brugia malayi.* **C,** *Loa loa.* (Modified from Smith, J.W., et al.: Diagnostic medical parasitology: blood and tissue parasites, Chicago, 1976, American Society of Clinical Pathologists.)

tion of small numbers of microfilariae. Finally, it is possible to induce the release of microfilariae into the peripheral blood by administering to the patient a single dose of diethylcarbamazine at a rate of 2 mg/kg body weight. The blood sample should be drawn about 15 to 20 minutes after drug administration and processed immediately.

When microfilariae cannot be demonstrated by any of the methods previously described, the diagnosis must depend on the patient's history or histopathologic examination of tissue from an enlarged node proximal to the involved lymphatic.

BRUGIA MALAYI
LIFE CYCLE[1,10,42]

The life cycle and morphology of *Brugia malayi* are similar to those of *Wuchereria bancrofti.* The major differences are in the morphology of the smaller adult worms of *B. malayi* (females measure 43 to 55 mm long and males 13 to 23 mm). In both species the adult worms live in the lymphatics, and some strains have nocturnal periodic and subperiodic migration of the

microfilariae in the peripheral blood. *B. malayi* also has intermediate mosquito hosts, although the species are different (see "Epidemiology").

EPIDEMIOLOGY[1,7,10,42]

The periodic strain of *B. malayi,* which is responsible for most human cases of the disease, occurs in most areas of Asia and Indonesia. The principal intermediate hosts of this strain are mosquitoes of the genus *Mansonia,* a few species of *Anopheles,* and *Aedes togoi.* There are no natural animal reservoirs for this periodic strain.

The subperiodic strain of *B. malayi* is found primarily in parts of Southeast Asia and the Philippines, where the usual intermediate hosts are also mosquitoes of the genus *Mansonia.* The site of infection, however, is more remote. Most infections occur primarily in swamp-forest environments, where leaf monkeys act as a natural reservoir for the infection. Surprisingly, in leaf monkeys the microfilariae of this strain have a nocturnal periodicity.

PATHOLOGY AND CLINICAL MANIFESTATIONS[42]

The pathologic and clinical manifestations of *B. malayi* infections in humans are essentially identical to those of *Wuchereria bancrofti*.

LABORATORY DIAGNOSIS[42]

The techniques used for confirming the diagnosis of a *B. malayi* infection are identical to those used for the diagnosis of *Wuchereria bancrofti* infections. The morphology of the microfilariae, however, is different; the microfilariae of *B. malayi* are sheathed, as are those of *Wuchereria* spp., but the cephalic space of *B. malayi* has a length/width ratio of 2:1, and there are two distinctive, isolated nuclei in the tip of the tail (Figure 44-3).

LOA LOA (EYE WORM)
LIFE CYCLE[13,42]

Human infections with the filarial nematode *Loa loa* are acquired when the intermediate host—a deer fly (*Chrysops* spp.)—takes a blood meal and injects third-stage larvae into the skin. Maturation of the adult stage occurs in the subcutaneous tissues and requires about 6 months. Surviving as long as 17 years, the adults migrate throughout the subcutaneous tissue, and the females release sheathed microfilariae. These microfilariae enter the bloodstream and have a diurnal periodicity in the peripheral circulation; at other times of the day, microfilariae are found in the capillary beds of the lungs. When ingested by deer flies the microfilariae develop into infective third-stage larvae in about 10 days.

EPIDEMIOLOGY[13,25,42]

At present, *Loa loa* infections occur only in western and central Africa. Within this range the incidence is greatest in small villages near the tropical forests and plantations that are major breeding sites of the primary intermediate hosts of the parasite—*Chrysops silacea* and *C. dimidiata*.

PATHOLOGY AND CLINICAL MANIFESTATIONS[13,41,42]

The pathologic and clinical manifestations associated with *Loa loa* infection are usually more a nuisance than a serious threat to human health. The primary manifestations of the disease are fugitive swellings (Calabar swelling) that occur as the adult worms wander through the subcutaneous tissues. These swellings, which may reach the size of hens' eggs, are temporary areas of inflammation that presumably result from the sudden release of toxic metabolites by the adult worm. In caucasian hosts the allergic reaction to these metabolites may take the form of a more severe, generalized reaction in which there are giant urticarial swellings of the skin, fever, and an eosinophilia of 50% to 70%.

Often the most distressing manifestation for infected individuals occurs when adult worms migrate across the bridge of the nose or across the cornea of the eye. This is usually painless and causes no permanent damage to the eye, however.

LABORATORY DIAGNOSIS

The diagnosis can usually be made on clinical grounds alone by physicians familiar with the disease. However, if laboratory confirmation is required, the microfilariae can be recovered and identified in blood samples obtained during the day, especially between 11 AM and 1 PM.

The same procedures are used for preparing the blood samples of *Loa loa* as for *Wuchereria bancrofti*. Once found, the microfilariae can be identified by their length (250 to 300 μm), the presence of a sheath, a cephalic space that has a length/width ratio of about 1.2 or 1.5:1, and a gradually tapered tail that has nuclei all the way into the tip (see Figure 44-3). One problem for those inexperienced in identifying microfilariae is that these characteristics seem similar to those of *Brugia malayi*. However, once having seen the two isolated nuclei in the tail of *B. malayi* versus the continuous chain of nuclei in the tail of *Loa loa*, it is unlikely that one will confuse the two parasites.

ONCHOCERCA VOLVULUS
LIFE CYCLE[33,42]

Infections with *Onchocerca volvulus* are acquired when blackflies (genus *Simulium*) inject larvae into the wound created when they obtain a blood meal (Figure 44-4). The larvae migrate to the subcutaneous tissues, where they develop into mature adult worms in about 3 to 15 months. At maturity, the females begin to release unsheathed microfilariae.

Although the microfilariae may migrate into the peripheral blood and urine, they are found in largest numbers in the lymphatics of nearby connective tissue and cutaneous layers. They also migrate into the stratum germinativum and the conjunctiva of the eye. Adult females, which may live as long as 15 years, continue to produce microfilariae for 9 to 10 years.

The feeding pattern of blackflies is ideally suited to ingesting the microfilariae. Unlike mosquitoes, whose proboscises function much like a hypodermic needle, blackflies feed with a slashing action that produces a pool of blood and tissue fluids just below the skin surface. Microfilariae ingested during this feeding migrate through the gut wall of the fly, into the hemocele, and then into the fly's thoracic muscles, where they develop into infective third-stage larvae in about 1 week. The infective larvae migrate to the blackfly's mouthparts, where they wait until the fly takes its next blood meal.

EPIDEMIOLOGY[6,42]

Onchocerciasis (''river blindness'') occurs in many countries in South and Central America, where there are active breeding sites for blackflies. Because these flies have a short flight range and their larvae and pupae develop only in highly oxygenated water, most infections occur in individuals who live or work close to rapidly flowing streams.

Natural infections have been found in some nonhuman primates such as the spider monkey and gorilla, but there is no conclusive evidence that these animals constitute an important reservoir of human infection.

PATHOLOGY AND CLINICAL MANIFESTATIONS*

The adults of *Onchocerca volvulus* live singly or in coiled masses in the subcutaneous tissue or fascia. Many of these adults appear to live free in the tissue without provoking a detectable tissue response, although others provoke an inflammatory response that leads to encapsulation in a fibrous capsule or nodule called an onchocercoma. The nodules are readily detectable when they lie where large bones, such as the scalp,

---

*References 3, 5, 6, 12, 33, 36, and 49.

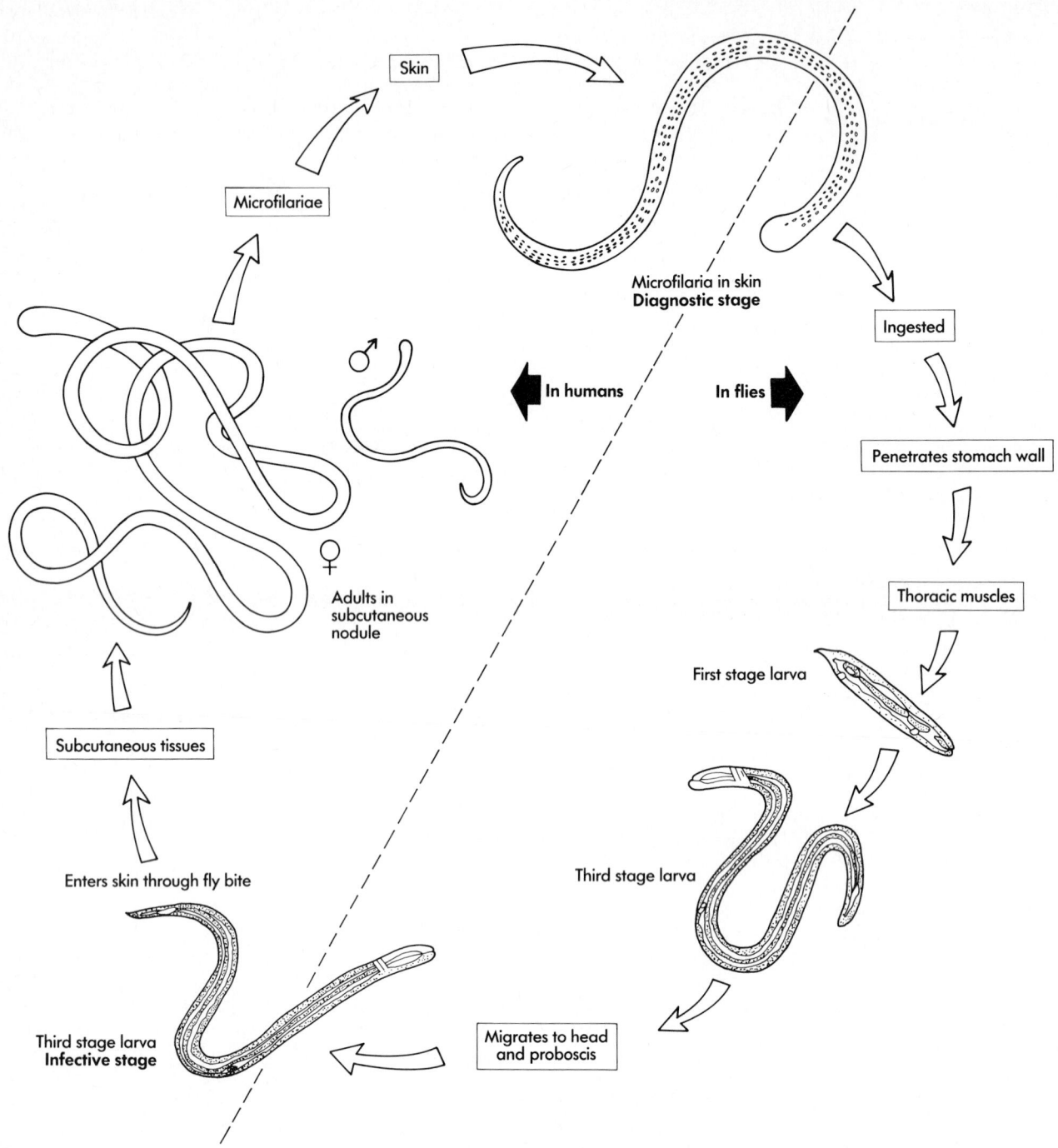

FIGURE 44-4. Life cycle of *Onchocerca volvulus*. (Modified from Melvin, D.M., Brooke, M.M., and Healy, G.R.: Common blood and tissue parasites of man—life cycle charts, Atlanta, 1965, PHS Pub. No. 1234, Laboratory Branch of the Communicable Disease Center.)

ribs, elbows, pelvis, and knees, are close to the surface. Other nodules may be located in deeper tissue and are not palpable. Interestingly, in the African form of onchocerciasis the nodules are most prominent around the pelvis, whereas in Central America the nodules are most prominent in the head. Usually these nodules cause no clinical manifestations other than their effect on the patient's physical appearance. At times, however, deep-seated nodules close to joint capsules or tendon sheaths may produce pain.

Unlike the other filarial infections, in which the major pathologic and clinical manifestations are associated with changes induced by the adult worms, the major manifestations in onchocerciasis are associated with findings induced by the microfilariae, especially in the skin and eyes. Because of variations in the irritation produced by the microfilariae and the host responses to this damage, a variety of clinical patterns are observed.

In the skin, where the major pathologic changes are fibrosis, deposition of an acid mucosaccharide, and phagocytosis of melanin pigment, the major clinical manifestations include an acute pruritus and rash of small papules that is most common on the lower parts of the body in the African form of the disease; hyperpigmented, thickened skin; and in chronic cases atrophy, scaling, drying, and depigmentation of the skin, which cause it to appear prematurely aged and lizardlike.

More serious than skin changes is ocular involvement, which may lead to blindness. Depending on the extent of pathologic changes in the eye, a patient may have no vision impairment, simple photophobia, blurred vision, or total blindness.

LABORATORY DIAGNOSIS[3,31,49]

Because the microfilariae of *Onchocerca volvulus* do not normally circulate in the blood but rather are found in the skin and subcutaneous nodules, confirmation of this infection is based on identification of microfilariae from skin snips or aspirates of subcutaneous nodules. Aspirates may be prepared directly as thick smears and treated with Giemsa stain or Delafield hematoxylin. Skin snips, however, should be placed in a few drops of warm saline on a glass slide, incubated at 35° C in a covered Petri dish for 2 hours, and then examined under low power for the presence of microfilariae that have migrated out of the tissue. If the specimen is positive, a thick smear may be prepared from the saline containing the microfilariae and treated wtih Giemsa stain or Delafield hematoxylin.

The microfilariae of *O. volvulus* may be recognized by their large size (300 to 350 μm in length), absence of a sheath, a sharply pointed tail with no nuclei at the tip, and a cephalic space with a length/width ratio of about 1.5 or 2:1.

ECHINOCOCCUS GRANULOSUS AND *ECHINOCOCCUS MULTILOCULARIS*
LIFE CYCLE[45]

In infection with *Echinococcus* spp., humans are an accidental intermediate host that becomes infected with a cystlike larval stage (hydatid cyst) after ingestion of the parasites' egg stage (Figure 44-5). In the normal life cycle of *E. granulosus* the definitive host may be any of a variety of carnivores, such as dogs, wolves, jackals, and cats, and the intermediate host may be any of a variety of herbivores, such as sheep and cattle. Human infections are commonly related to close association with domestic dogs that harbor the adult stage.

In contrast, the normal life cycle of *E. multilocularis* is usually associated with wild rather than domestic animals; the normal definitive hosts are wild carnivores such as foxes and other wild canids, whereas the intermediate hosts are typically wild rodents such as field mice. In this instance human infections are commonly traced to consumption of fruits or vegetables contaminated with the feces of infected carnivores, or to the handling of contaminated soil. Domestic dogs and cats may also harbor the adult stage and may be a source of infective eggs if they feed on wild rodents.

The adult stage of *E. granulosus* is a small tapeworm, typically 3 to 6 mm long and consisting of a scolex with four round suckers, two row of hooks, and three proglottids—immature, mature, and gravid. The adults of *E. multilocularis* are almost identical to *E. granulosus;* the major difference is that *E. multilocularis* is slightly shorter (1.5 to 4 mm long) and has slightly different reproductive structures (for example, no lateral uterine branches and a smaller number of testes). In both species

the gravid proglottid usually ruptures and releases the infective eggs before detaching from the strobila. The eggs of *E. granulosus* and *E. multilocularis* are indistinguishable from those of *Taenia solium* or *T. saginata*.

When ingested by a susceptible intermediate host, the eggs hatch in the small intestine. The liberated oncospheres penetrate the intestinal wall and are carried by the circulatory system to various internal organs. The most common sites in which the oncospheres become trapped are the liver and the lungs; less frequent sites include the brain, eye, and bones. Oncospheres that survive the host's initial inflammatory response reach maturity in about 5 months. In *E. granulosus* the mature cyst consists of a thick, laminated outer layer that surrounds a thin inner layer of germinal tissue and a fluid-filled interior. Multiple buds of tissue develop from the inner germinal layer toward the fluid-filled interior. These buds, in turn, develop into hollow, fluid-filled capsules known as brood capsules. From the walls of the brood capsules more tissue buds develop; in this instance, however, the buds develop into immature scolices that somewhat resemble the cysticercoids of *Hymenolepis* organisms. Occasionally, so-called daughter cysts appear in the original hydatid cyst. These daughter cysts are simply smaller versions of the parent hydatid cysts, having identical outer and inner layers and brood capsules containing immature scolices. The early mature cysts typically measure about 1 cm in diameter. If the cysts are located in tissue where they can expand freely and not seriously impair the function of the affected tissue (for example, the liver), they may continue to expand for 10 or more years and eventually contain several liters of fluid. As the cysts grow older, the walls of the brood capsules and daughter cysts often rupture and release scolices into the fluid of the parent cyst. These free scolices constitute the so-called hydatid sand, which may be aspirated and sent to the laboratory for confirmation of the diagnosis.

A different type of hydatid cyst, called an alveolar, malignant, or multilocular hydatid cyst, is formed by *E. multilocularis*. In this type of hydatid cyst the outer membrane is very thin, and secondary cysts commonly bud from the *outside* of the primary cyst (exogenous budding), creating a mass of multiple cysts in infected tissue. Moreover, these secondary cysts may metastasize to other tissues, where they again proliferate by exogenous budding: thus the name "malignant hydatid cyst." In most human cases, multilocular hydatid cysts are filled only with purulent material and few if any scolices. As a result, the diagnosis cannot be confirmed by the aspiration of hydatid sand.

EPIDEMIOLOGY*

Most human infections with *E. granulosus* infections are related to close association with dogs that are part of a natural dog-sheep-dog cycle. As a consequence, the highest prevalence of this disease is among sheepherders in areas such as Australia, New Zealand, Argentina, Uruguay, Spain, and Iran, where sheep raising is a major occupation. In the continental United States most infections follow a similar pattern, with the highest prevalence being among the sheepherders of the western states of Arizona, New Mexico, and Utah. In Alaska and northern Canada the normal cycle involves dogs or wolves as the definitive hosts and deer, moose, or reindeer as the intermediate

---

*References 24, 28, 29, 37, 39, and 47.

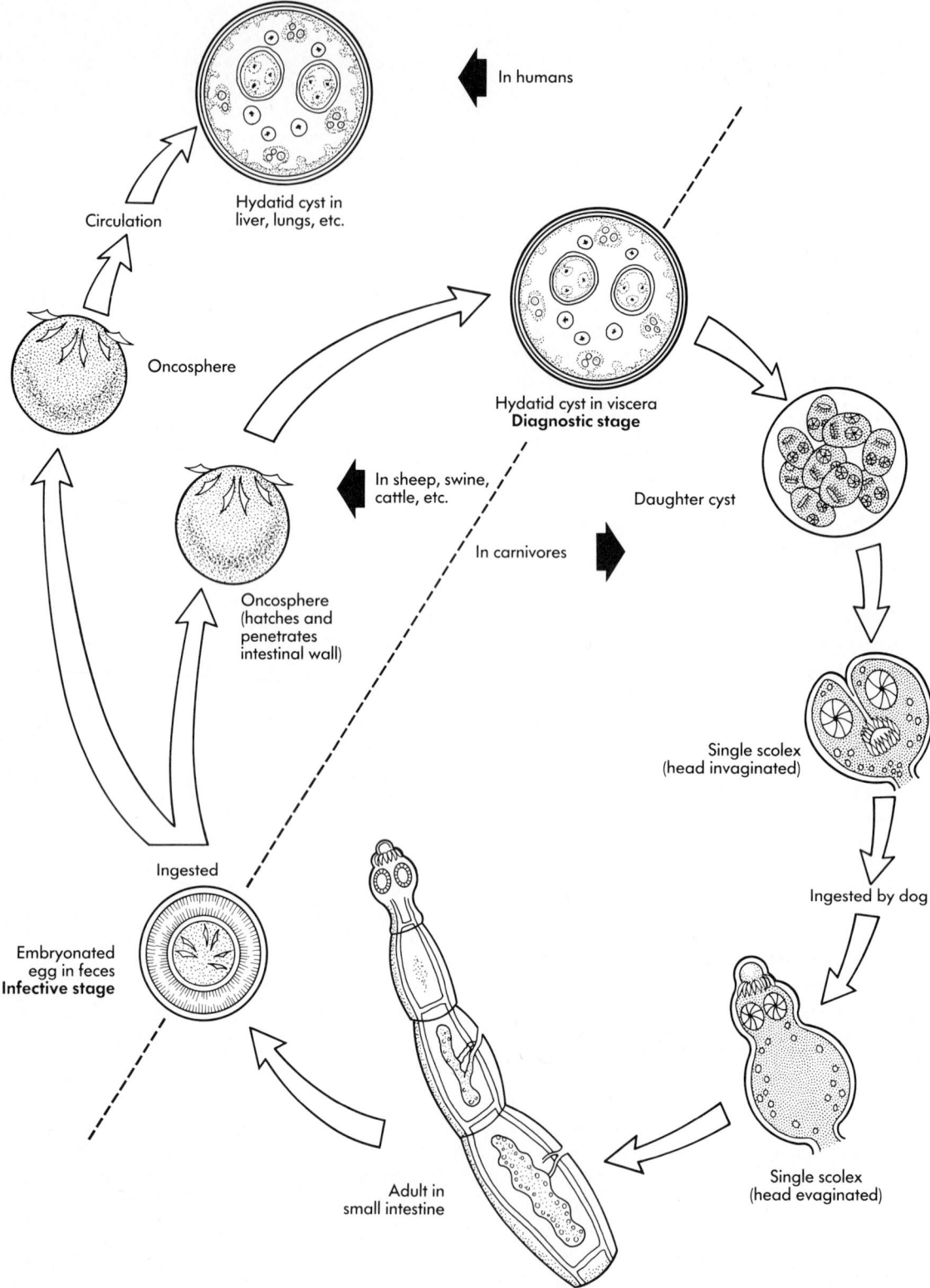

FIGURE 44-5. Life cycle of *Echinococcus granulosus*. (Modified from Melvin, D.M., Brooke, M.M., and Healy, G.R.: Common blood and tissue parasites of man—life cycle charts, Atlanta, 1965, PHS Pub. No. 1234, Laboratory Branch of the Communicable Disease Center.)

hosts. In these more northern climates, the infection is most common in native Indian and Eskimo hunters.

Echinococcus multilocularis infections of humans are presumably less common than *E. granulosus* infections because the parasite has a more limited geographic distribution and the normal life cycle does involve domestic animals. *E. granulosus* occurs principally in temperate and sub-Arctic regions, where the usual cycle is a fox-rodent-fox cycle. In North America human infections have most often been associated with Eskimos and Indians of Alaska and Canada, who apparently become infected when taking fox pelts. The infection is also endemic through much of the European regions of Russian and in Switzerland, France, Germany, Austria, and Belgium. In these latter areas the infection appears to be associated with the consumption of wild fruits that have been contaminated with the feces of infected foxes. Human infections have also been occasionally traced to close contact with domestic cats infected with the adult stage of the parasite.

PATHOLOGY AND CLINICAL MANIFESTATIONS[27,43,48]

The symptoms of both *E. granulosus* and *E. multilocularis* infection depend on the location of the cyst in the body and the extent to which the cyst can enlarge before producing sufficient tissue damage to elicit clinical manifestations. Early in *E. granulosus* infections the major response is an infiltration of mononuclear cells into the tissue, where the oncospheres lodge. This response probably results in the death of many of the invading oncospheres. The oncospheres that survive begin to grow. By the end of the third week the host responds by forming a fibrous capsule around the parasite. The host response to *E. multilocularis* is less likely to confine the growth of the parasite. There is little, if any, development of a fibrous capsule, and most of the response consists of a single zone of eosinophils and giant cells around the cyst.

Most infections with these two parasites remain asymptomatic until growth of the cysts produces sufficient pressure necrosis of surrounding tissues to impair the normal function of the affected organ. In the most commonly affected organ, the liver, the reserve capacity is sufficient that the infection may not become clinically apparent for 5 to 20 years. In other tissues, such as the brain, the onset of clinical manifestations is usually more rapid and the prognosis more serious.

Besides the pathologic and clinical manifestations related to pressure necrosis of affected tissues, there is an additional danger that patients infected with *E. granulosus* may suffer anaphylactic shock (see Chapter 2).

LABORATORY DIAGNOSIS[22,43]

Asymptomatic infections with *E. granulosus* are often detected by chance discovery of the cyst during x-ray studies of the liver or lungs. When a mass lesion is discovered and the patient's occupation, avocation, or history of contact with potential hosts of the adult worm suggests the possibility of echinococcosis, serologic testing may confirm the infection. The usual method for serodiagnosis is to test the patient's sera by an indirect hemagglutination test and at least one other procedure, such as bentonite flocculation or latex agglutination.

Because of the risk of anaphylaxis and spread of the infection by daughter cysts, surgeons should not attempt the diagnosis by percutaneous aspiration of the cyst. If surgical intervention is required for treatment, as is the usual case, the sur-

geon may confirm the diagnosis by submitting hydatid sand to the laboratory after in situ chemical sterilization and removal of the cyst.

With *E. multilocularis* infections the disease is rarely diagnosed until after the patient has died or the cysts have reached a stage in which treatment is unlikely to be successful. If the diagnosis has been confirmed before death, in most cases it has been based on the patient's history, serologic test results, and histopathologic picture. The serologic tests for *E. multilocularis* are identical to those for *E. granulosus*. However, because there is complete serologic cross-reaction between the two species, a definitive diagnosis requires direct examination of material from the cyst.

REFERENCES

1. Ahamed, S.S.: Location of developing and adult worms of *Brugia* sp. in naturally and experimentally infected animals, J. Trop. Med. Hyg. **69**:291, 1966.
2. Andy, J.J., O'Connell, J.P., and Daddario, R.C.: Trichinosis causing extensive ventricular mural endocarditis with superimposed thrombosis: evidence that severe eosinophilia damages endocardium, Am. J. Med. **63**:824, 1977.
3. Buck, A.A., editor: Onchocerciasis: symptomatology, pathology, diagnosis, Geneva, 1974, Switzerland, World Health Organization.
4. Centers for Disease Control: Trichinosis surveillance annual summary, 1980, Atlanta, 1981, Public Health Service, U.S. Department of Health and Human Services.
5. Choyce, D.P.: Onchocerciasis: ophthalmic aspects, Trans. R. Soc. Trop. Med. Hyg. **60**:707, 1966.
6. Connor, D.H.: Current concepts in parasitology: onchocerciasis, N. Engl. J. Med. **298**:379, 1978.
7. Dedham, D.A., and McGreevy, P.B.: Brugian filariasis: epidemiological and experimental studies, Adv. Parasitol. **15**:243, 1977.
8. Dondero, T.J., Jr., et al.: Clinical manifestations of bancroftian filariasis in a suburb of Calcutta, India, Am. J. Trop. Med. Hyg. **25**:64, 1976.
9. Edeson, J.F.B.: Filariasis, Br. Med. Bull. **28**:60, 1972.
10. Edeson, J.F.B., et al.: Experimental transmission of *Brugia malavi* and *B. pahangi* to man, Trans. R. Soc. Trop. Med. Hyg. **54**:229, 1960.
11. Galindo, L., von Lichtenberg, F., and Baldizon, C.: Bancroftian filariasis in Puerto Rico: infection pattern and tissue lesions, Am. J. Trop. Med. Hyg. **11**:739, 1962.
12. Garner, A.: Pathology of ocular onchocerciasis: human and experimental, Trans. R. Soc. Trop. Med. Hyg. **20**:374, 1976.
13. Gordon, R.M.: A brief review of recent advances in our knowledge of loiasis and some of the still outstanding problems, Trans. R. Soc. Trop. Med. Hyg. **49**:98, 1955.
14. Gould, S.E.: Trichinosis in man and animals, Springfield, Ill., 1970, Charles C Thomas, Publisher.
15. Gray, D.F., Morse, B.S., and Phillips, F.: Trichinosis with neurologic and cardiac involvement: review of the literature and report of three cases, Ann. Intern. Med. **57**:230, 1962.
16. Grove, D.I., and Farber, I.J.: Immunosuppression on bancroftian filariasis, Trans. R. Soc. Trop. Med. Hyg. **73**:23, 1979.
17. Grove, D.I., Valeza, F.S., and Cabrera, B.D.: Bancroftian filariasis in a Philippine village: clinical, parasitological, immunological and social aspects, Bull. WHO **56**:975, 1978.
18. Grove, D.I., Warren, K.S., and Mahmoud, A.A.F.: Algorithms in the diagnosis and management of exotic disease. VI. The filariases, J. Infect. Dis. **132**:340, 1975.
19. Harbottle, J.E., English, D.K., and Schultz, M.G.: Trichinosis in bears in northeastern United States, Health Serv. Ment. Health Admin. Rep. **86**:473, 1971.

20. Harder, H.I., and Watson, D.: Human filariasis: identification of species on the basis of staining and other morphologic characteristics of microfilariae, Am. J. Clin. Pathol. **42:**1027, 1964.

21. Jacobson, E.S., and Jacobson, H.G.: Trichinosis in an immunosuppressed human host, Am. J. Clin. Pathol. **68:**791, 1977.

22. Kagan, I.G.: Serodiagnosis of parasitic diseases. In Lennette, E.H., et al., editors: Manual of clinical microbiology, ed. 3, Washington, D.C., 1980, American Society for Microbiology.

23. Kagan, I.G.: Serodiagnosis of parasitic diseases. In Rose, N.R., and Friedman, H., editors: Manual of clinical immunology, ed. 2, Washington, D.C., 1980, American Society for Microbiology.

24. Kahn, J.B., et al.: Echinococcosis in Utah, Am. J. Trop. Med. Hyg. **21:**185, 1972.

25. Kershaw, W.E.: The epidemiology of infections with *Loa loa,* Trans. R. Soc. Trop. Med. Hyg. **49:**143, 1955.

26. Kramer, M.D., and Aita, J.F.: Trichinosis with central nervous system involvement: a case report and review of the literature, Neurology **22:**485, 1972.

27. Lafond, D.J., Thatcher, D.S., and Handeyside, R.G.: Alveolar hydatid disease, JAMA **186:**35, 1963.

28. Leiby, P.C., and Kritsky, D.C.: *Echinococcus multilocularis:* a possible domestic life cycle in central North America and its public health importance, J. Parasitol. **58:**1213, 1972.

29. Loveless, R.M., et al.: *Echinococcus granulosus* in dogs and sheep in central Utah, 1971-1976, Am. J. Vet. Res. **39:**499, 1977.

30. Maynard, J.E., and Pauls, F.P.: Trichinosis in Alaska: a review and report of two outbreaks due to bear meat, with observations on serodiagnosis and skin testing, Am. J. Hyg. **76:**252, 1962.

31. McMahon, J.E.: The examination-time/dose interval in the provocation of nocturnally periodic microfilariae of *Wuchereria bancrofti* with diethylcarbamazine and the practical uses of the test, Tropenmed. Parasitol. **33:**28, 1982.

32. Most, H.: Trichinellosis in the United States: changing epidemiology in the past 25 years, JAMA **193:**871, 1965.

33. Nelson, G.S.: Onchocerciasis, Adv. Parasitol. **8:**173, 1970.

34. Nelson, G.S.: Mosquito-borne filariasis, Trans. R. Soc. Trop. Med. Hyg. **20:**15, 1978.

35. Nelson, G.S.: Current concepts in parasitology: filariasis, N. Engl. J. Med. **300:**1136, 1979.

36. Ngu, J.L.: Immunological studies on onchocerciasis, Acta Trop. **35:**269, 1978.

37. Pappaioanou, M., Schawbe, C.W., and Sard, D.M.: An evolving pattern of human hydatid disease transmission in the United States, Am. J. Trop. Med. Hyg. **26:**732, 1977.

38. Price, E.W.: The mechanisms of lymphatic obstruction in endemic elephantiasis of the lower legs, Trans. R. Soc. Trop. Med. Hyg. **69:**177, 1975.

39. Rausch, R.L.: On the occurrence and distribution of *Echinococcus* spp. (Cestoda: Taeniidae) and characteristics of their development in the intermediate host, Ann. Parasitol. **42:**19, 1967.

40. Roselle, H.A., Schwartz, D.T., and Geer, F.G.: Trichinosis from New England bear meat: report of an epidemic, N. Engl. J. Med. **272:**304, 1965.

41. Sacks, N.H., Williams, D.N., and Eifrig, D.E.: Loiasis: report of a case and review of literature, Arch. Intern. Med. **136:**914, 1976.

42. Sasa, M.: Human filariasis: a global survey of epidemiology and control, Baltimore, 1976, University Park Press.

43. Schiller, C.F.: Complications of *Echinococcus* cyst rupture, JAMA **195:**220, 1966.

44. Schmitt, N., et al.: Trichinosis from bear meat and adulterated pork products: a major outbreak in British Columbia—1971, Can. Med. Assoc. J. **107:**1087, 1972.

45. Smyth, J.D.: The biology of the hydatid organism, Adv. Parasitol. **2:**169, 1964.

46. Wijetunge, H.: Clinical manifestations of early Bancroftian filariasis: a study of 212 cases of microfilariaemia, J. Trop. Med. Hyg. **70:**90, 1967.

47. Williams, J.F., Lopez-Adaros, H., and Trjos, A: Current prevalence and distribution of hydatidosis with special reference to the Americas, Am. J. Trop. Med. Hyg. **20:**224, 1971.

48. Wilson, J.F., Diddams, A.C., and Rausch, R.L.: Cystic hydatid disease in Alaska: a review of 101 autochthonous cases of *Echinococcus granulosus* infection, Am. Rev. Respir. Dis. **98:**1, 1968.

49. Woodruff, A.W., et al.: Onchocerciasis in Guatemala: a clinical and parasitological study with comparisons between the disease there and in East Africa, Trans. R. Soc. Trop. Med. Hyg. **60:**707, 1966.

50. Wright, W.H., Kerr, K.B., and Jacobs, L.: Studies on trichinosis. XV. Summary of the findings of *Trichinella spiralis* in a random sampling and other findings of the population of the United States, Public Health Rep. **58:**1293, 1943.

51. Zimmerman, W.J., Steele, J.H., and Kagan, I.G.: Trichiniasis in the U.S. population, 1966-1970: prevalence and epidemiologic factors, Health Serv. Rep. **88:**606, 1973.

52. Zimmerman, W.J., and Zinter, D.E.: The prevalence of trichiniasis in swine in the United States, 1966-1970, Health Serv. Ment. Health Admin. Rep. **86:**937, 1971.

CHAPTER 45

Miscellaneous Parasites and Drug Therapy

John Klaas II

MISCELLANEOUS PARASITES

This chapter includes brief summary descriptions of animal parasites that occur in humans but are uncommon in the United States. Many of these parasites have limited geographic distribution and unusual life cycles that make human infection less likely, or they may be primary parasites of other animals and only accidental parasites of humans. The organisms described do not by any means represent all those that are found in humans, but many that are common in limited geographic areas or have diagnostic stages that may be confused with the more common animal parasites of humans are included.

INTESTINAL NEMATODES
CAPILLARIA PHILIPPINENSIS
Basic Life Cycle

Adult stages of *Capillaria philippinensis* buried in the mucosa of the large and small intestine shed unembryonated eggs in the feces. Eggs embryonate in fresh water and are eaten by fish. Larvae hatch in the intestine of the fish, migrate to the musculature, and become infective in about 3 weeks.

Epidemiology

The infections found in humans have occurred primarily in the Philippines and Thailand among individuals who have ingested raw or improperly cooked freshwater fish containing the infective larvae. There are no known animal reservoirs.

Major Pathology and Clinical Manifestations

Capillariasis has an autoinfection cycle similar to that of infection with *Strongyloides* spp. Abdominal pain, frequent episodes of diarrhea, fat malabsorption, and severe protein loss are common clinical findings. In severe cases death may result from the malabsorption and protein loss.

Laboratory Diagnosis

Diagnosis is based on finding the *Trichuris*-like eggs in fecal specimens. They are differentiated from eggs of the genus *Trichuris* by their less tapering shape and their flattened polar plugs.

TRICHOSTRONGYLUS
Basic Life Cycle

Adult worms of the genus *Trichostrongylus* buried in the mucosa of the small intestine release eggs that are unembryonated when passed in the feces. With ideal conditions of moisture, shade, and warmth the eggs embryonate. The larvae hatch within 24 hours after passing from the body. During a 4- to 7-day period the larvae grow and molt into infective third-stage

filariform larvae. These larvae must be swallowed to complete their life cycle.

Epidemiology

The genus *Trichostrongylus* is normally a parasite of wild and domestic ruminant animals; most human infections are accidental and occur when infective filariform larvae are ingested. As a human disease, trichostrongyliasis is common in the Middle East and in many parts of Asia; rarely is it acquired in the United States.

Major Pathology and Clinical Manifestations

Mild *Trichostrongylus* infections are usually asymptomatic. Heavier worm burdens are usually manifested by nonspecific complaints such as diarrhea, abdominal pain, and anorexia.

Laboratory Diagnosis

Diagnosis is based on finding the hookwormlike eggs in the feces. They are differentiated from hookworm eggs by their larger size (average 90 by 45 μm) and one end that is more pointed than the other; they resemble chicken eggs. If larvae are found in the feces, they may be differentiated from hookworm and *Strongyloides* larvae by the knob at the end of their tail (see Figure 41-9).

TERNIDENS DEMINUTUS
Basic Life Cycle

Adults of *Ternidens deminutus* attached to the wall of the large intestine release hookwormlike eggs that are passed unembryonated in the feces. The eggs embryonate and hatch in the soil. As with the genus *Trichostrongylus,* the infective filariform larvae that eventually develop must be swallowed for the life cycle to continue. When ingested, the infective larvae burrow into the wall of the small intestine, where they develop into young adults inside nodules formed as a host response to the parasite. The young adult worms leave the nodule and migrate to the large intestine, where they complete their maturation.

Epidemiology

Ternidens infection is primarily a disease of nonhuman primates, especially baboons, in Africa and Southeast Asia. Human infections, which have a similar distribution, are acquired by ingestion of filariform larvae.

Major Pathology and Clinical Manifestations

Ulceration and cystic nodules are seen in the intestinal wall.

Laboratory Diagnosis

The eggs closely resemble hookworm eggs but may be differentiated by their larger size (average 82 by 50 μm) and larger volume (length by width^2), which is greater than 170,000 μm^3 for *T. deminutus* versus less than 150,000 μm^3 for hookworms.

INTESTINAL CESTODES
DIPYLIDIUM CANINUM
Basic Life Cycle

Gravid *Dipylidium caninum* proglottids break off the adult worm and migrate out of the body onto the perianal area, where they break apart and release the eggs. Eggs may also pass in the feces. The larval stages of fleas, which live in the soil or in houses and feed on organic material, ingest the eggs. The oncosphere hatches in the flea's intestine, migrates into the flea's body cavity, and develops into an infective cysticercoid that remains viable during the flea's development to the adult stage. The adult fleas return to the dog or cat and take blood meals. Infection of the dog occurs when it attempts to remove the flea by biting the area of the flea bite. The flea is crushed by the animal's teeth, and the cysticercoid is swallowed.

Epidemiology

D. caninum is a common parasite of dogs and cats worldwide and only accidentally infects humans. Most human infections occur in children who are infected with the cysticercoid while playing with a dog that licks them on the face after biting an infected flea.

Major Pathology and Clinical Manifestations

Most *D. caninum* infections are asymptomatic, but when clinically manifest they have symptoms similar to those caused by pinworm *(Enterobius vermicularis)* infections.

Laboratory Diagnosis

Individual eggs found in the feces are similar to those of *Hymenolepis nana,* except they lack polar filaments. In most cases, however, the eggs (up to 40) are enclosed in a membranous sac or packet.

TISSUE NEMATODES (FILARIAL NEMATODES)
DIPETALONEMA (ACANTHOCHEILONEMA)
PERSTANS
Basic Life Cycle

The adults of the parasite *Dipetalonema perstans* inhabit the peritoneal, the pleural, and occasionally the pericardial cavities of the body. Their microfilariae circulate in the peripheral blood at all hours, but the peak concentration is between 9 AM and 11 PM. The intermediate hosts are the biting midges of the genus *Culicoides.*

Epidemiology

Dipetalonemiasis is primarily a human disease that occurs throughout the tropical regions of Africa and Central and South America. Infection is acquired by the bite of infected midges of the genus *Culicoides.*

Major Pathology and Clinical Manifestations

Traditionally considered to be a nonpathogen, *D. perstans* has been reported to cause transient joint and abdominal pains,

subcutaneous swellings, and allergic phenomena such as rashes.

Laboratory Diagnosis

The diagnosis of dipetalonemiasis is based on identification of the unsheathed microfilariae in stained blood films. These microfilariae usually measure about 200 μm in length and have a pointed tail with no nuclei in the tip.

MANSONELLA OZZARDI
Basic Life Cycle

Adults of the filarial nematode *Mansonella ozzardi* inhabit the peritoneal cavity and the associated mesenteries. Microfilariae released by the female worms circulate in the peripheral blood at all hours, with a peak occurring between 11 AM and 1 PM. The intermediate hosts in which the infective larval stages develop are biting midges of the genus *Culicoides.*

Epidemiology

M. ozzardi is a New World human filaria that occurs in Central and South America and parts of the West Indies.

Major Pathology and Clinical Manifestations

M. ozzardi is generally recognized as nonpathogenic; it does not produce overt clinical manifestations.

Laboratory Diagnosis

The diagnosis of mansonelliasis is based on identifying the unsheathed microfilariae in stained smears of peripheral blood. Measuring about the same size as *Dipetalonema perstans* (200 μm), the unsheathed microfilariae are recognized by their blunt tail that contains nuclei all the way into the tip.

NEMATODES OTHER THAN FILARIAE
DRACUNCULUS MEDINENSIS
Basic Life Cycle

Early in the course of *Dracunculus medinensis* infection, adult worms are found in the lymphatics and connective tissue of the body. Once the female worm is fertilized, the males die and the female begins to wander through the body cavities and connective tissues for about 1 year. During this time the eggs mature, and first-stage larvae hatch from the eggs within the female's uterus. The gravid female then migrates to the subcutaneous tissues, in particular those of the lower extremities. Lying just below the skin surface, the female secretes a substance that induces the formation of a painful, burning blister on the skin. When the host washes or immerses the blister to relieve the pain, the blister bursts and the worm pokes her anterior end through the opening and discharges larvae into the water. For development to continue the larvae must be ingested by tiny crustaceans of the genus *Cyclops.* If ingested by these predatory crustaceans, the larvae develop into the infective stage in 1 or 2 weeks. The definitive host is infected by ingesting water contaminated with infected *Cyclops* organisms. Once freed from the crustacean by the action of digestive juices, larvae penetrate the intestinal wall and enter the lymphatics and connective tissue of the definitive host, humans.

Epidemiology

In addition to humans, dracunculiasis occurs in numerous domestic and wild animals throughout the endemic range: Africa, the Near East, and India. Except for parts of Brazil, the infection is rare in the New World.

Major Pathology and Clinical Manifestations

Dracunculiasis is usually asymptomatic during maturation of the adult worms and the early wanderings of the female worm. However, when the female begins her migration to the subcutaneous tissues, patients often experience a variety of toxic and allergic manifestations, such as rash, fever, vomiting, and diarrhea. If care is not taken to protect the open wound once the blister has broken, secondary bacterial infections may lead to septicemia and gangrene.

Laboratory Diagnosis

The diagnosis of *Dracunculus medinensis* infection rarely requires laboratory confirmation and is usually based on clinical manifestations once the female worm has migrated to the surface.

ANGIOSTRONGYLUS CANTONENSIS
Basic Life Cycle

The adults of the parasite *Angiostrongylus cantonensis* normally inhabit the pulmonary arteries of rodents. Eggs released by the female are trapped in the capillary beds of the rodents' lungs, where the larvae hatch and then migrate into the alveolar spaces. From the lungs the larvae are carried up the bronchial tree into the mouth, swallowed, and passed out in the feces. On reaching water or moist soil that harbors susceptible species of snails, the intermediate hosts, the larvae penetrate a snail and develop into the infective larval stage. The snail may be eaten directly by the final rodent host or by a variety of freshwater crabs and crayfish or free-living platyhelminths (flatworms) that act as paratenic hosts. When an infected snail or paratenic host is eaten by a rodent, the larvae penetrate the intestinal wall and are carried by the circulation to the capillaries of the brain, where they develop into juvenile adults. From the brain the immature adults migrate to the pulmonary artery and complete their development to sexually mature adults.

Epidemiology

Human infections are most common in parts of the world where raw snails or one of the paratenic hosts is considered a dietary delicacy. Consequently, most infections have been reported from the Pacific and Southeast Asia.

Major Pathology and Clinical Manifestations

Humans are an accidental host for *A. cantonensis;* the parasite cannot reach sexual maturity in humans. The final stage of parasite development in humans is the juvenile adults that eventually die in the vessels of the brain.

The usual clinical manifestation of these infections is a meningitis syndrome with its typical fever, irritability, and nuchal rigidity. Later some patients have paralysis of the extremities, exaggerated reflexes, and sensitivity to touch. Except in very heavy infections, these manifestations are transient and the patient survives the infection.

Laboratory Diagnosis

The diagnosis of angiostrongyliasis is usually suspected in endemic areas when the patient has a bacteriologically sterile spinal fluid with a white blood cell count of 200 to 5000 leukocytes/mm^3, of which 25% or more are eosinophils. Aside from detection of the immature adults in brain tissue obtained at necropsy, confirmation of the diagnosis depends on recovery and identification of larvae that may wander into the spinal fluid.

TOXOCARA CANIS
Basic Life Cycle

In the normal life cycle of the parasite *Toxocara canis* the adult worm is found in the lumen of the small intestine of young dogs. The eggs are passed in the feces onto soil, where the eggs embryonate and become infective. When the embryonated eggs are ingested by another dog, the eggs hatch in the small intestine and the larvae penetrate the wall of the intestine, from which they are carried via the circulation throughout the body. In the various body tissues the larvae remain in a state of "suspended animation." The cycle continues only during pregnancy in female dogs when, under the influence of maternal hormones, the larvae become active and migrate across the placenta to infect the unborn fetus. When the puppies are born, they are already infected with juvenile adult parasites in the intestine.

Epidemiology

Humans become accidental hosts of *T. canis* when embryonated eggs in the soil are ingested. Given this setting for infection, it is not surprising that most human infections occur in children who have been playing in soil contaminated with dog feces. Because *T. canis* is found in dogs worldwide, human infections probably have the same cosmopolitan distribution. However, because of differences in degree of interest or availability of medical services, the infection has not been reported from all areas. In the United States, most reports come from the East and South.

Major Pathology and Clinical Manifestations

In humans the clinical manifestations depend on where the larvae migrate once they have hatched from the egg and entered the systemic circulation. There appear to be two basic clinical forms of the disease. In one form, commonly called visceral larva migrans, the earliest manifestations are often pulmonary and include an asthmalike or bronchitic syndrome with coughing, wheezing, and fever. In other cases the manifestations may include hepatomegaly or neurologic abnormalities, if larvae reach the liver or central nervous system. In most of these patients the manifestations disappear without any residual problems.

In a second form of the infection, the only manifestation may be the development of a tumorlike mass that encapsulates larvae that have migrated to the eye. Unfortunately, this form of the infection may have serious consequences, because the ocular mass is easily mistaken for a highly invasive form of cancer that is treated by removal of the eye.

Laboratory Diagnosis

T. canis infection is often difficult to confirm except by serologic tests. Even in many of these tests, there is a cross-reaction between *T. canis* and *Ascaris lumbricoides*. In addition, some of the more reliable tests, which are very sensitive and specific for the visceral form of the disease, do not have the same reliability for the ocular form.

DRUG THERAPY

The information in Table 45-1 is intended as general information about the types of drugs used to treat the more common parasitic infections. *Table 45-1 should not be used by physicians as a specific guide for treatment.* For details on specific treatment regimens and on the availability of drugs, physicians should consult the original or a more recent issue of *The Medical Letter on Drugs and Therapeutics* or contact the Parasitic Diseases Division, Center for Infectious Diseases, Centers for Disease Control, Atlanta, GA 30333.

TABLE 45-1. Primary Drugs of Choice for Parasitic Infections[a]

Organisms and Infections	Drug of Choice
Acanthamoeba spp.	See *Naegleria fowleri*
Ancylostoma duodenale	See Hookworms
Ascaris lumbricoides	Mebendazole or pyrantel pamoate
Babesia spp.	Clindamycin plus quinine
Balantidium coli	Tetracycline
Brugia malayi	See Filarial nematodes
Cestodes	
Adult or intestinal stage	Niclosamide
Larval stages in tissue	
Echinococcus granulosus	Surgery
Taenia solium	Praziquantel
Clonorchis sinensis	See Trematodes
Cutaneous larva migrans	Thiabendazole
Dientamoeba fragilis	Iodoquinol or tetracycline
Diphyllobothrium latum	See Cestodes
Dracunculus medinensis	Niridazole
Echinococcus spp.	See Cestodes
Entamoeba histolytica	
Intestinal disease	
Asymptomatic	Iodoquinol
Symptomatic	Metronidazole plus iodoquinol
Hepatic abscess	Metronidazole plus iodoquinol
Enterobius vermicularis	Pyrantel pamoate or mebendazole
Fasciola and *Fasciolopsis* spp.	See Trematodes
Filarial nematodes for *Onchocerca volvulus*	Diethylcarbamazine, suramin
Giardia lamblia	Quinacrine
Hookworms (*Ancylostoma duodenale* and *Necator americanus*)	Mebendazole or pyrantel pamoate

TABLE 45-1. Primary Drugs of Choice for Parasitic Infections[a]—cont'd

Organisms and Infections	Drug of Choice
Hymenolepis spp.	See Cestodes
Leishmania spp.	Stibogluconate sodium
Loa loa	See Filarial nematodes
Naegleria fowleri	Amphotericin B
Necator americanus	See Hookworms
Onchocerca volvulus	See Filarial nematodes
Opisthorchis spp.	See Trematodes
Paragonimus westermani	See Trematodes
Plasmodium spp.	
P. vivax, ovale, malariae, or *falciparum* not resistant to chloroquine	
Suppression in endemic area	Chloroquine phosphate
Prevention after leaving endemic area (not required for *P. malariae* or *P. falciparum*)	Primaquine phosphate
Treatment of attack	
Uncomplicated	Chloroquine phosphate
Severe	Quinine dihydrochloride or chloroquine
Prevention of relapse (not required for *P. malariae* or *P. falciparum*)	Primaquine phosphate
P. falciparum resistant to chloroquine	
Suppression in endemic area	Pyrimethamine plus sulfadoxine
Treatment of attack	
Uncomplicated	Quinine sulfate plus pyrimethamine and sulfadiazine
Severe	Quinine dihydrochloride
Pneumocystis carinii	Trimethoprim-sulfamethoxazole
Schistosoma spp.	See Trematodes

TABLE 45-1. Primary Drugs of Choice for Parasitic Infections[a]—cont'd

Organisms and Infections	Drug of Choice
Strongyloides stercoralis	Thiabendazole
Taenia spp.	See Cestodes
Toxocara spp.	See Visceral larva migrans
Toxoplasma gondii	Pyramethamine plus trisulfapyrimidines
Trematodes	Praziquantel
Trichinella spiralis	Thiabendazole plus steroids
Trichomonas vaginalis	Metronidazole

TABLE 45-1. Primary Drugs of Choice for Parasitic Infections[a]—cont'd

Organisms and Infections	Drug of Choice
Trichostrongylus spp.	Thiabendazole
Trichuris trichiura	Mebendazole
Trypanosomiasis	
Trypanosoma cruzi	Nifurtimox
Trypanosoma brucei	
Blood-lymphatic stages	Suramin
Central nervous system stage	Melarsoprol
Visceral larva migrans	Diethylcarbamazine or thiabendazole
Wuchereria bancrofti	See Filarial nematodes

Modified from Med. Lett. Drugs Ther. **26**:27, 1984.

[a] This table should not be used as a specific guide for treatment. See the original reference.

PART FIVE

VIRUSES, CHLAMYDIAE, AND RICKETTSIAE

CHAPTER 46

Introduction to Virology

Sally Jo Rubin*

Viruses are obligate intracellular microorganisms that range in diameter from under 30 nm to 300 nm. Several characteristics, including their simpler organization, their mechanism of replication, and their nucleic acid content, distinguish viruses from other microorganisms (Table 46-1). Unlike bacteria, viruses do not multiply by binary fission and contain only a single type of nucleic acid as genetic material rather than both ribonucleic acid (RNA) and deoxyribonucleic acid (DNA). Viruses may be specific for animals, plants, or bacteria (bacteriophage), and within each group individual viruses may infect only certain cell species. Currently 16 different families of animal viruses are known: five contain DNA and 10 contain RNA.

The infectious viral particle, or *virion,* consists of nucleic acid, is capable of autonomous replication, and is surrounded by a protein coat and sometimes a membrane envelope.

The nucleic acid, or core, is either DNA or RNA. The number of genes encoded by the nucleic acids ranges from three or four in small viruses to several hundred in large viruses. The DNA of animal viruses is usually double stranded except for the parvoviruses, which have single-stranded linear DNA. Double-stranded DNA may be circular or linear. More variation is found in nucleic acid configuration among RNA viruses. Many have single-stranded RNA that may be in a single long piece or in segments. Single-stranded RNA that functions in the cell as a messenger RNA is called positive ($+$). RNA that must first be transcribed is designated as a negative ($-$) strand. Reoviruses have double-stranded, segmented RNA.

Viral nucleic acid is surrounded by a protective protein coat, the capsid, which is necessary for attachment to the host cell. The capsid is formed from many identical repeating units. The core and the capsid comprise the nucleocapsid. Most viruses have an icosahedral or helical symmetric structure (Figure 46-1). The icosahedral capsid has 20 equilateral triangular faces, 12 vertices, and 30 edges. Helical viruses are long rods. The repeating protein subunits surround the core in a helical fashion to form a cylindric capsid.

Helical or icosahedral nucleocapsids may be surrounded by a loose membrane envelope (Figure 46-1). The envelope, which is acquired during maturation, is similar to cellular membranes. The envelope is made up of a lipid bilayer, glycoproteins, and matrix proteins. The proteins of the envelope are determined by viral genes, but the lipid and carbohydrate moieties depend on the host cell and sometimes can be different on the same virus grown in different host cells. The glycoproteins are on the outer surface and may look like spikes. The matrix proteins form a layer at the inner surface of the envelope and in some viruses appear to connect the envelope and capsid. The lipid content of the envelope makes these viruses susceptible to inactivation by lipid solvents such as ether or chloroform. Enveloped viruses are also more heat labile.

Viral morphology is determined by the type of symmetry and the presence or absence of an envelope. Nonenveloped (naked) helical viruses appear as long rods, whereas naked icosahedral viruses appear spherical (Figure 46-1). Enveloped viruses are highly pleomorphic because the membrane is not rigid (Figure 46-1). Some viruses, such as poxviruses and some bacteriophages, are more complex morphologically. The poxviruses have several lipoprotein layers and exhibit neither type of symmetry.

VIRAL REPLICATION

Viruses have few or no enzymes and thus must use the host cell's replicative machinery. Separate components are synthesized and then assembled. Viral nucleic acid must enter the cell and specify the synthesis of proteins required for new viral nucleic acid and capsid protein synthesis. This process can take place in a number of ways depending on the virus and the type and configuration of its nucleic acid. Regardless of the nucleic acid, however, the following basic steps are required for progeny virus production:

1. *Attachment and adsorption.* The first step in replication is attachment to the host cell. The host cell has specific receptor sites that depend on both the species and tissue of derivation. Nonenveloped viruses lack specialized attachment organs and probably have attachment sites all over their surface, whereas enveloped viruses such as myxoviruses attach via their glycoprotein spikes. At this stage viruses can still be recovered in infectious form.

2. *Penetration.* Penetration rapidly follows adsorption. Viruses generally enter the cell in one of two ways: fusion or phagocytosis. In most cases the enveloped virus's membrane fuses with the cellular plasma membrane, whereas nonenveloped viruses usually are taken into the cell by phagocytosis. At this point virus can no longer be recovered from the intact cell.

3. *Uncoating.* The viral capsid is removed, probably by host enzymes, and the nucleic acid is released.

4. *Eclipse.* Initiation of intracellular viral synthesis marks the eclipse period. It ends when a mature virus can be demonstrated in disrupted cells. Viral synthesis varies depending on the type and configuration of the nucleic acid. During the eclipse, viral nucleic acid directs the synthesis of proteins required in further synthesis (early

---

*The virology section of this book was updated by Thomas F. Smith.

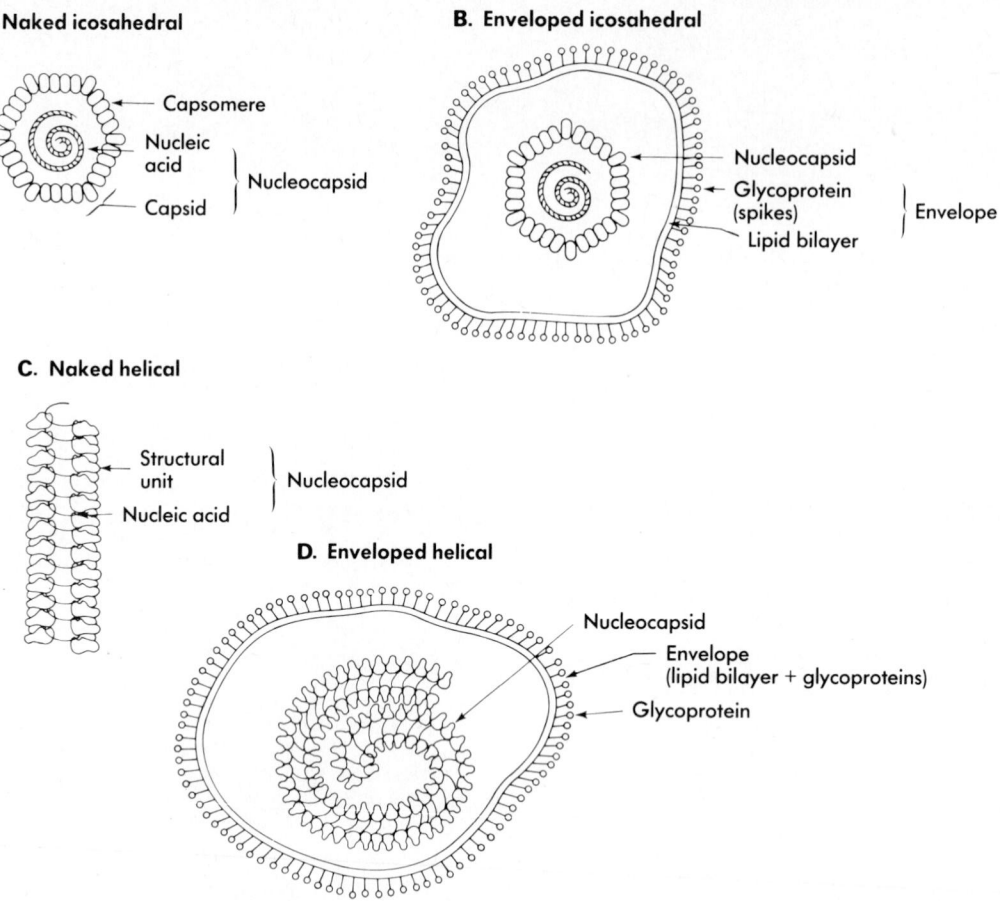

FIGURE 46-1. Schematic representation of morphologic groups of viruses. (From Freeman, B.A.: Burrows textbook of microbiology, ed. 21, Philadelphia, 1979, W.B. Saunders Co.)

TABLE 46-1. Properties of Viruses Compared with Other Microorganisms

Microorganism	Require Living Cells	Divide by Binary Fission	Have Both DNA and RNA	Susceptible to Antimicrobial Agents
Bacteria	−	+	+	+
Mycoplasmas	−	+	+	+
Rickettsiae	+	+	+	+
Chlamydiae	+	+	+	+
Viruses	+	−	−	−

SYMBOLS: +, Positive for property
−, Negative for property

proteins). Viral nucleic acid is duplicated, and viral structural proteins are synthesized, followed by random assembly. Protein synthesis takes place in the cytoplasm, but capsid formation may occur in the cytoplasm or nucleus.

5. *Maturation*. In DNA virus replication, assembly of the capsid and then association with the nucleic acid are clearly separate steps. In naked icosahedral RNA viruses the two steps are almost concurrent, whereas in enve-

loped RNA viruses synthesis of viral RNA clearly precedes assembly.

6. *Release*. Release of naked virions depends on cell type and virus but is usually rapid. The nucleocapsid of enveloped viruses migrates to the nuclear or cytoplasmic membrane depending on the virus. The membrane then surrounds the nucleocapsid to form the envelope. Enveloped virus is detached by a process that is probably the reverse of penetration.

TABLE 46-2. Classification of Important DNA Viruses Infecting Humans

Capsid Symmetry	Envelope	Site of Capsid Assembly	Size (Diameter in nm)	Family	Genus	Common Name
Icosahedral	No	Nucleus	45-55	*Papovaviridae*	*Papovavirus* A *Papovavirus* B	Wart virus BK and JC viruses
Icosahedral	No	Nucleus	18-26	*Parvoviridae*	*Parvovirus*	Possibly Norwalk-like agent
Icosahedral	No	Nucleus	45-55	*Adenoviridae*	*Mastadenovirus*	Adenovirus
Icosahedral	Yes	Nucleus	100	*Herpesviridae*	*Alphaherpesvirinae*	Herpes simplex virus, varicella-zoster virus
					Betaherpesvirinae	Cytomegalovirus
					Gammaherpesvirinae	Epstein-Barr virus
Complex	Complex coats	Cytoplasm	230 × 300	*Poxviridae*	*Orthopoxvirus*	Smallpox virus (variola), vaccinia virus
Complex	Yes	Unknown	42	*Hepadnaviridae*	Not classified	Hepatitis B virus

TABLE 46-3. Classification of Important RNA Viruses Infecting Humans

Capsid Symmetry	Envelope	Site of Capsid Assembly	Size (nm)	Configuration of RNA	Family	Genus	Common Name
Icosahedral	No	Cytoplasm	24-30	SS (+)	*Picornaviridae*	*Enterovirus*	Poliovirus, coxsackie viruses, echovirus, hepatitis A virus
						Rhinovirus	Rhinovirus (cold virus)
	Yes	Cytoplasm	70	DS (segmental)	*Reoviridae*	*Rotavirus*	Rotavirus
			60	SS (+)	*Togaviridae*	*Alphavirus*	Arbovirus (Group A)
			40			*Flavivirus*	Arbovirus (Group B)
			60			*Rubivirus*	Rubella virus
Helical	Yes	Cytoplasm	80-120	SS (−) (segmental)	*Orthomyxoviridae*	*Influenzavirus*	Influenza virus
			150-300	SS (−)	*Paramyxoviridae*	*Pneumovirus*	Respiratory syncytial virus
						Paramyxovirus	Parainfluenza virus, mumps virus
						Morbillivirus	Measles virus
			60 × 180	SS (−)	*Rhabdoviridae*	*Lyssavirus*	Rabies virus
Unknown/unsymmetric	Yes	Cytoplasm	50-300	SS	*Arenaviridae*	*Arenavirus*	Lymphocytic choriomeningitis virus, Lassa fever virus
			80-100	SS (+)	*Coronaviridae*	*Coronavirus*	Human coronavirus
			100	SS	*Bunyaviridae*	*Bunyavirus*	Bunamwera, California encephalitis virus
Icosahedral capsid with probable helical nucleocapsid	Yes	Cytoplasm	100	SS (+)	*Retroviridae* Subfamily *Oncovirinae*	*Oncovirus*	Leukosis, sarcoma, mammary tumor viruses
					Subfamily *Lentivirinae*	*Lentivirus*	Slow-acting viruses

SYMBOLS: SS, Single stranded   +, Positive strand; strand that functions as mRNA
         DS, Double stranded   −, Negative strand; strand that must first be transcribed

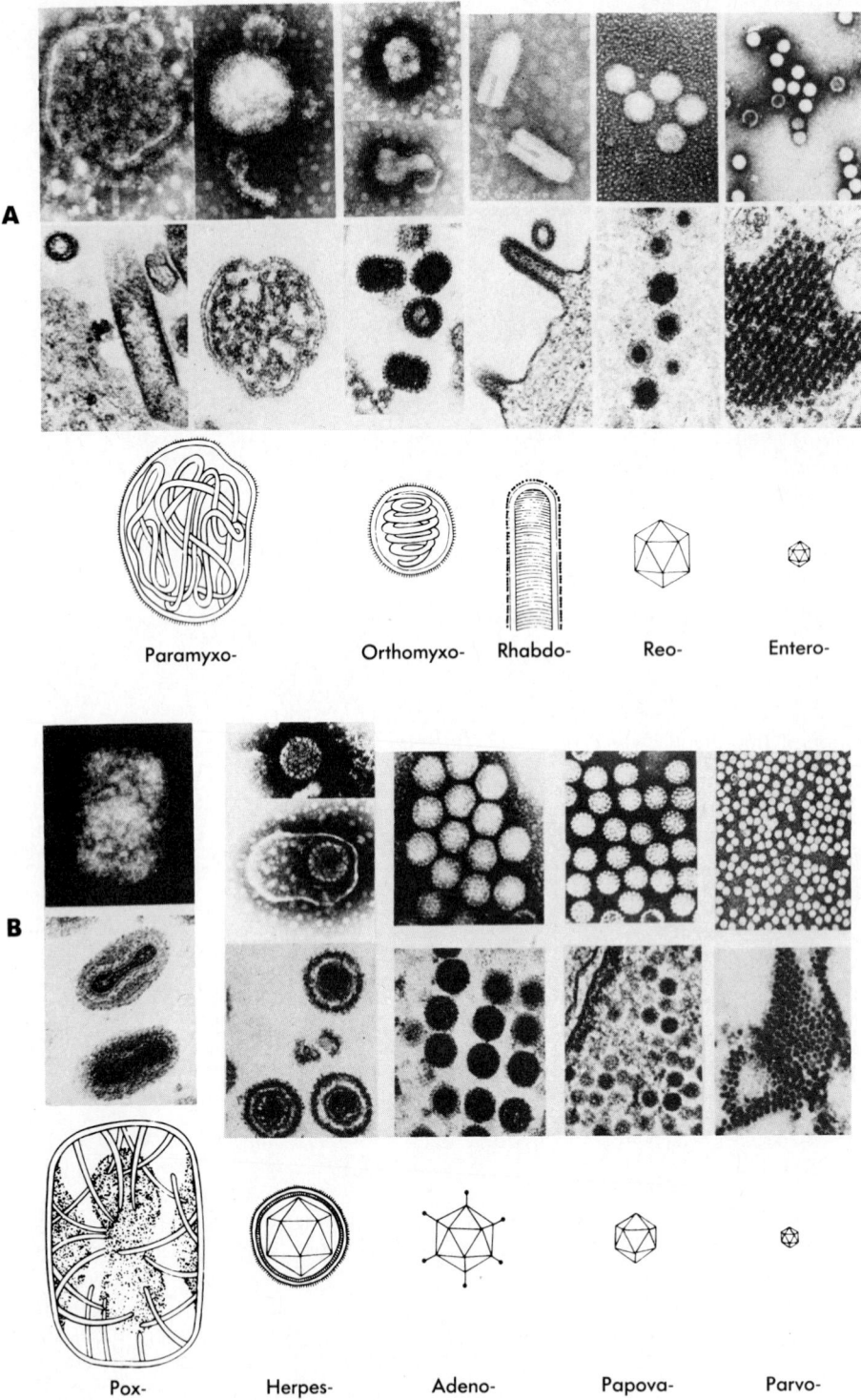

FIGURE 46-2. Electron micrograph of, **A,** RNA viruses and, **B,** DNA viruses in negatively stained preparations *(top row)* and in thin sectioned cells *(middle row)* as compared with schematic drawings *(bottom row).* (From Hsiung, G., Fong, C.K.Y., and August, M.J.: Prog. Med. Virol. **25:**133, 1979.)

VIRUS CLASSIFICATION

Viruses are classified on the basis of their morphology and composition. Some of the characteristics used are size, shape, type, and configuration of nucleic acid and the presence or absence of an envelope. Characteristics of the major viruses infecting humans are listed in Tables 46-2 and 46-3. The relative size and shape of many of these viruses may be seen in Figure 46-2.

Viruses commonly detected in the clinical laboratory are covered in the rest of this section. Readers interested in other viruses should refer to a basic microbiology textbook such as *Microbiology* by Davis and co-workers (see "Suggested Readings").

LABORATORY SAFETY

The hazard of a laboratory infection exists for all laboratory workers and paramedic personnel. Precautions required to prevent these infections vary with the level of risk involved. The risk in the diagnostic virology laboratory can range from about equal to that of the bacteriology laboratory to highly hazardous. As an absolute minimum the basic safety rules of microbiology are to be followed. These include no eating, drinking, or smoking in the laboratory; no mouth pipetting; availability of appropriate disinfectants; and proper disposal of contaminated materials and specimens.

The major sources of laboratory-acquired viral infections are aerosol production, accidents, and contact with animals or their ectoparasites. Many laboratory procedures, including pipetting, sonication, and centrifugation, produce aerosols. All of these procedures should be performed in a biologic safety hood. The class of hood required depends on the agents involved. The most common accidents are spills and needle sticks. Spattering of infected material has resulted in herpes simplex virus and adenovirus eye infections, whereas the greatest hazard of contaminated needles is hepatitis B virus or human immunodeficiency virus (HIV) infection.

Highly dangerous agents, such as Marburg, Ebola, Lassa fever, and rabies viruses, should never be handled in the routine clinical virology laboratory. Work with these viruses should be done only by experienced virologists in appropriate containment facilities. Material from patients with suspected Creutzfeldt-Jakob disease, a subacute spongiform virus encephalopathy, should be autoclaved for 1 hour.

Workers in virology laboratories should receive viral vaccines. Also, their serum should be collected periodically and stored in case a laboratory-related infection occurs.

SUGGESTED READINGS

Braude, A.I., Davis, C.E., and Fierer, J., editors: Infectious diseases and medical microbiology, Philadelphia, 1986, W.B. Saunders Co.

Davis, B.D., et al.: Microbiology, ed. 3, Hagerstown, Md., 1980, Harper & Row, Publishers, Inc.

Lennette, E.H., and Schmidt, N.J.: Diagnostic procedures for viral, rickettsial, and chlamydial infections, ed. 5, Washington, D.C., 1979, American Public Health Association, Inc.

Melnick, J.L.: Taxonomy and nomenclature of viruses, Prog. Med. Virol. **28:**208, 1982.

Patterson, W.B., et al.: Occupational hazards to hospital personnel, Ann. Intern. Med. **102:**658, 1985.

Tierno, P.M., Jr.: Preventing acquisition of human immunodeficiency virus in the laboratory: safe handling of AIDS specimens, Lab. Med. **17:**696, 1986.

CHAPTER 47

Laboratory Diagnosis of Viral Infections

Sally Jo Rubin

Since the first demonstration of in vitro cultivation of a virus in cell culture, diagnostic virologic services have been available only in medical center hospitals, usually as a spinoff of a virus research laboratory. A survey in 1976 showed that only 60% of medical centers had on-site viral diagnostic facilities.[27] Traditionally physicians have believed that viral diagnosis is too expensive and too slow to be clinically useful. Laboratory administrators have hesitated to provide virologic services because of a mystique surrounding viruses and a feeling that working with viruses is too complex for the routine laboratory.[11a] With the introduction of simpler, faster diagnostic techniques this attitude is beginning to change, but the question "Why bother?" is still a common one.[45]

The most obvious answer is that diagnosis of most viral infections cannot be made clinically but requires the aid of the laboratory. The same clinical syndrome can be caused by many viruses, and an individual virus may cause a number of different clinical syndromes. In some cases, such as central nervous system infection in infants, clinical differentiation of viral and bacterial infection is difficult and may not be resolved by cerebrospinal fluid (CSF) cytologic and chemical analysis.[8] Furthermore, a definitive viral diagnosis can affect the community as well as the individual patient because knowledge of which viruses are present in the community is necessary for public health programs such as vaccination.

Although antiviral agent development is still in its infancy, therapy is available for some viruses, and a correct diagnosis is imperative for appropriate treatment. For example, adenine arabinoside (vidarabine) reduces the mortality of herpes simplex virus encephalitis from 70% to 30%, and acyclovir has reduced the effects of this infection even more.[49] Accurate viral diagnosis is also necessary for proper prophylactic treatment, particularly in the use of hyperimmune serum globulins or in the decision to perform a cesarean delivery to prevent herpes simplex virus infection in the newborn or to abort a fetus with possible congenital viral infection. Viral diagnosis is required for infection control because certain viral infections in the hospital setting can lead to outbreaks with serious consequences. Viruses in the respiratory tract, such as respiratory syncytial virus (RSV), are most commonly involved. RSV can cause severe or even fatal disease, particularly in immunocompromised children and premature infants.[26] Less common, but often a major problem, are outbreaks of rubella or varicella.[25] Early detection of primary cases requires viral diagnostic services so preventive measures such as vaccination can be taken.

For both the physician and the patient, a specific diagnosis increases understanding of the disease process and provides prognostic information. Patients feel much more confident with a specific diagnosis than with "It's just a virus" and more comfortable if the physician can provide an accurate prognosis.

The more rapid viral diagnostic methods now in use can provide laboratory data as quickly as bacteriologic methods do. This helps justify the cost of viral diagnostic services, as does the possible decrease in antimicrobial agent use and time of hospitalization.[8]

In making a virologic diagnosis of a viral infection, the most critical step is the selection of the appropriate test followed by correct specimen collection and transport. The patient's clinical symptoms and history are the most important factors in deciding which diagnostic approach(es) will be most helpful. Although a number of viruses can produce the same clinical picture, symptomatologic study narrows the spectrum of possible viruses involved (Tables 47-1 and 47-2). For example, Norwalk agent would not be suspected in a patient with respiratory symptoms, nor would feces be an appropriate specimen. The patient's age is helpful in diagnosis because some viruses (such as rotavirus) are common in infants and young children.

The date of onset of symptoms is also critical because some viruses are difficult to isolate more than 3 to 4 days after onset. Determining whether serologic study will be useful also requires knowledge of the duration of illness. Immunization history is important because the laboratory may isolate vaccine virus (for example, poliovirus) from a recent vaccinee or need the information as a guide to serologic testing. Many viruses, such as enteroviruses and influenza virus, occur seasonally, so the time of year can aid in test selection.

Three approaches are used to make a laboratory diagnosis of a viral infection: direct detection by microscopic, immunologic, or molecular techniques; isolation in cell cultures, embryonated eggs, and animals; and measurement of virus-specific antibody (serology). Deciding which approach to use is based on the factors just cited and on specific attributes of the virus (for example, rotavirus is noncultivable and thus direct examination by electron microscopy or antigen detection by immunologic assays must be used). Materials and reagents are commercially available from a number of sources for immunologic detection of viral antigen, isolation in cell culture, viral antibody detection, and detection by nucleic acid probes.

COLLECTION AND TRANSPORT OF SPECIMENS

Unlike specimens for bacteriologic culture, specimens for virus detection are not necessarily collected from the site of infection because most viruses are shed from the respiratory or gastrointestinal tract. Some viruses (mumps, cytomegalovirus) are also shed in the urine. Although throat and rectal swabs are the usual specimens submitted, in some instances nasopharyngeal swabs or secretions[29] and feces[40] are superior.

TABLE 47-1. Specimens for Direct Examination

Symptoms	Virus	Specimen	Methods
Respiratory (pharyngitis, croup, bronchiolitis, pneumonia)	Adenovirus	NP, throat swab,[a] tissue	FA
	Herpes simplex	NP, throat swab	FA
	Influenza	NP, throat, nasal washing	FA
	Mumps	NP, throat swab, urine sediment	FA
	Parainfluenza	NP, throat swab	FA
	Respiratory syncytial	NP, aspirate/swab	FA, ELISA
Gastrointestinal	Parvovirus (Norwalk agent)	Stool	EM, RIA
	Rotavirus	Stool	EM, ELISA, LA
Rash or vesicle	Herpes simplex	Lesion scraping	FA
	Rubella	Respiratory smear	FA
	Vaccinia	Lesion scraping	FA
	Varicella-zoster	Lesion scraping	FA, EM
Central nervous system (aseptic meningitis, encephalitis)	Herpes simplex	Brain biopsy	FA, EM
	Mumps	Throat, urine	FA
	Rabies	Corneal scraping, tissue	FA
Eye	Adenovirus	Conjunctival scraping	FA
	Herpes simplex	Conjunctival, corneal scraping	FA
	Varicella-zoster	Conjunctival, corneal scraping	FA
Congenital or perinatal	Cytomegalovirus	Urine sediment, tissue	FA, EM
	Herpes simplex	Lesion scraping, throat	FA
	Rubella	Throat, urine sediment, tissue	FA
	Varicella-zoster	Lesion scraping, tissue throat	FA

Symbols: NP, Nasopharyngeal	ELISA, Enzyme-linked immunosorbent assay	
FA, Immunofluorescence	RIA, Radioimmunoassay	
EM, Electron microscopy	LA, Latex agglutination	

[a]Nasopharyngeal and throat swabs may be pooled.

If lesions are present, material should be collected from them for culture and in some cases direct examination (Table 47-1). The same is true for viral infections of the eye. Except for enteroviruses, virus is rarely recovered from CSF. Mumps virus is not difficult to isolate from CSF but is an unusual infection today. Thus many laboratories inoculate CSF specimens only during enterovirus season and under special circumstances such as suspected mumps or varicella encephalitis. Direct examination of CSF by immunofluorescence (FA) is no longer recommended because white blood cells autofluoresce, resulting in false-positive tests.

Virus is isolated from blood only during the acute phase of infection and is more likely to be positive in severe disease; thus blood is usually cultured only from immunosuppressed patients. Documentation of viremia may also be helpful in evaluating enteroviral infection in infants under 3 months old.[46]

Most specimens for viral examination are collected by the same technique as for bacteriologic culture (Table 47-3). Major exceptions are nasal or throat washings and lesion specimens. Swabs may be of any material, although calcium alginate may inactivate herpes simplex virus.[7] Commercial collection

devices include Virocult[51] (Medical Wire and Equipment Co., Cleveland) and Viral Culturettes (Marion Scientific Laboratories, Kansas City, Mo.). Many laboratories use the Culturette (Marion Scientific) system, which was designed for bacteriologic specimens.[35] The Culturette consists of a rayon swab and modified Stuart transport medium.

Swab specimens should be immersed in 2 or 3 ml of transport medium on arrival in the laboratory. After all liquid is expressed, the swab is discarded. If a Culturette is used, the plastic cylinder should be rinsed with 0.5 ml of transport medium. If transport to the laboratory takes more than about 15 minutes, the swab should be placed directly into a tube of cold transport medium.

A number of different transport media have been used. They consist of a base that will not affect the cell culture and often a stabilizer such as serum albumin or gelatin and antimicrobial agents to control bacterial and fungal contamination. Commonly used transport media are Hank's balanced salt solution (BSS) with bovine serum albumin, veal infusion broth, and tissue culture medium with calf serum and antimicrobial agents. Few comparative studies of these media have been done. However,

TABLE 47-2. Specimens for Viral Culture

Symptoms	Common Viruses	Specimen
Respiratory (pharyngitis, croup, bronchitis, pneumonia)	Adenovirus	Throat or NP swab[a]
	Enterovirus	Throat or NP swab
	Herpes simplex	Throat or NP swab
	Influenza	Throat or NP swab/nasal washing
	Mumps	Throat swab (Stensen's duct), NP swab, urine
	Parainfluenza	Throat or NP swab
	Respiratory syncytial	NP aspirate or swab, throat swab
	Rhinovirus	Nasal swab
Gastrointestinal	Adenovirus	Stool/rectal swab
	Parvovirus (Norwalk agent)	Stool for EM or RIA
	Rotavirus	Stool for EM or ELISA
Maculopapular rash	Adenovirus	Throat, stool
	Rubella	Throat, urine
	Enterovirus	Throat, stool
Vesicular	Herpes simplex	Vesicle fluid or swab, cervical-vaginal swab
	Varicella-zoster	Vesicle fluid or swab
	Coxsackievirus A and echovirus	Vesicle fluid or swab
	Vaccinia	Vesicle fluid or swab
Central nervous system (aseptic meningitis, encephalitis)	Arbovirus	Throat, CSF
	Enterovirus	Throat, stool, CSF, vesicle fluid
	Herpes simplex: meningitis	CSF, vesicle fluid
	Herpes simplex: encephalitis	Brain tissue
	Lymphocytic choriomeningitis	CSF, urine, throat
	Mumps	Throat, CSF, urine
	Rabies	Brain biopsy
Eye	Adenovirus	Conjunctival swab or scraping, throat
	Enterovirus	Conjunctival swab or scraping, throat
	Herpes simplex	Conjunctival swab or scraping, throat
	Varicella-zoster	Conjunctival swab or scraping, throat
Congenital or perinatal	Cytomegalovirus	Throat, urine, buffy coat
	Enterovirus	Throat, stool, CSF
	Herpes simplex	Throat, CSF, vesicle swab
	Rubella	Throat, urine, eye
	Varicella-zoster	Lesions

Symbols: NP, Nasopharyngeal	EM, Electron microscopy	RIA, Radioimmunoassay
CSF, Cerebrospinal fluid	ELISA, Enzyme-linked immunosorbent assay	

Data from references 7, 12, 35, and 50.

[a]Throat and nasopharyngeal swabs may be pooled.

TABLE 47-3. Collection of Specimens for Viral Diagnosis

Specimen	Collection Method
Respiratory	
Throat	Collect on Culturette[a] as for bacteriologic culture, or use swab and viral transport medium
Nasopharyngeal	Collect on Calgiswab[b] as for bacteriologic culture; place in viral transport medium
Nasal washing	Use 1-ounce rubber suction bulb with 3-7 ml phosphate-buffered saline; tilt patient's head back to about 70-degree angle; squeeze and release bulb once
Sputum	As for bacteriologic culture
Bronchoalveolar lavage	Flexible fiberoptic bronchoscope[36a]
Gastrointestinal (feces, rectal swab)	As for bacteriologic culture

Continued.

TABLE 47-3. Collection of Specimens for Viral Diagnosis—cont'd

Specimen	Collection Method
Skin or genital lesion	1. Collect vesicle fluid with tuberculin syringe with 26 g needle bevel side up *or* 2. Unroof vesicle and scrape base of lesion with swab or scalpel blade
Cervix	Place swab in endocervix and rotate gently
Vagina	Place swab in vagina and swab vaginal walls
Eye (conjunctiva, cornea)	As for bacteriologic culture
Body fluids	
Urine	Collect two or three specimens (10-20 ml) on successive mornings as for bacteriologic culture
Blood	Collect 5 ml in heparinized Vacutainer[c] tube; isolate lymphocytes and polymorphonuclear leukocytes with Lymphocyte Separation Medium[d] density gradient[30]
Spinal and other fluids	As for bacteriologic culture (1-3 ml)
Tissue	As for bacteriologic culture
Blood for serology	As for bacterial etiology; acute and convalescent sera usually required

Data from references 13, 24, 34, 35, and 50.
[a]Marion Scientific Laboratories, Inc., Kansas City, Mo.
[b]Spectrum Diagnostics, Inc., Glenwood, Ill.
[c]Becton Dickinson, Paramus, N.J.
[d]Litton Bionetics, Kensington, Md.

at 4° C, survival of influenza and parainfluenza viruses is approximately the same in Hank's BSS, veal infusion broth, or charcoal viral transport media.[4] Survival of other viruses in various media has not been evaluated.

Before inoculation, specimens must be kept at 0° to 4° C (refrigerated or held on wet ice). Most viruses retain infectivity for a day or two at 4° C but lose titer rapidly at room temperature. Specimens should not be frozen, especially at −15° to −20° C, before inoculation. Respiratory syncytial virus and most of the enveloped viruses lose infectivity during this freeze-thaw cycle. If freezing is absolutely necessary, specimens should be quick frozen and maintained on dry ice or at −70° C.[36]

PROCESSING VIRAL SPECIMENS (Table 47-4)

After arrival in the laboratory, specimens should be processed as soon as feasible. If there is any delay, specimens should be stored in the refrigerator. In general, specimens for FA are centrifuged to concentrate virus-containing cells. Cells are fixed to slides in cold acetone. The purpose of FA technology is to provide a rapid diagnosis. Therefore slides should be stained and examined on the day received. Preparation of specimens for electron microscopy, enzyme immunoassay, or radioimmunoassay depends on the specimen source. Processing for cell culture inoculation also depends on the specimen type. Some specimens are inoculated directly, and others require antimicrobial treatment or removal of extraneous (and possibly toxic) material. Some laboratory workers like to inoculate a cell culture tube directly from a swab and use the inoculated medium to inoculate other tubes of cell culture, whereas others prefer to mix the swab with transport medium as described previously and use this for the inoculum.

Blood submitted for serologic testing is allowed to clot, and the serum is removed. Sera are stored in the refrigerator unless testing will be delayed more than a few days. These sera are stored frozen.

DIRECT DETECTION OF VIRUS OR VIRAL ANTIGENS
CYTOPATHOLOGY

An experienced observer can detect the presence of virus by examining stained tissue or cells by light microscopy. Location of the lesion, observation of cytologic changes, and the presence and location of inclusions aid in determining a viral etiology. Cytologic changes include intracellular structures called inclusions, necrosis, multinucleate "giant" cells, cytomegaly and cytoplasmic modifications, and vacuolization.[10] Inclusions may be intranuclear or cytoplasmic depending on the virus. For example, herpes simplex virus inclusions are intranuclear, whereas those of rabies and poxviruses are cytoplasmic. Cytologic examination is inexpensive and rapid but is specific only for the virus group (for example, herpes virus), is not very sensitive, requires an experienced observer, and is useful only if the specimen contains intact cells.[43]

ELECTRON MICROSCOPY

Many virologists hoped that laboratory workers would use electron microscopy (EM) for virology as easily as light microscopy is used to examine bacteria. Although EM has not become widespread, some laboratories use it very successfully. Two basic techniques are used: negative staining and thin sectioning. Negative staining is simple and rapid. Clinical material is dropped on a Formvar-carbon-coated copper grid, stained with potassium phosphotungstate, and examined. Stain surrounds the virus particle, and the electron beam cannot pass through this metallic background but can pass through the low electron density of the virus; therefore a light virus is seen against a dark background.[1] Specimens of vesicular fluid, serum, urine, and feces are most suited for negative staining.

Thin sectioning preserves cellular structure and is useful when few virus particles are present. It is the method of choice for tissue[31] but takes 3 to 4 days.

TABLE 47-4. Processing Viral Specimens

Specimen	Direct Examination	Culture
Respiratory	Immerse swab (throat and nasopharyngeal can be combined) in transport medium; centrifuge transport medium or washings to sediment cells; wash with PBS and place on slides; air dry; fix in cold acetone; may be stored at $-70°$ C	Immerse swabs in transport medium or directly into PMK tube (leave in PMK tube 30 min at room temperature); use liquid extract to inoculate other cells Inoculate washings directly
Feces or rectal swab	Emulsify stool in PBS and filter; filtrate is examined by electron microscopy	Make 10% suspension of feces or immerse swab in transport medium; mix well; treat with antibiotics; centrifuge at low speed to deposit debris; inoculate supernatant
Lesion scrapings	Roll swab across slide and air dry, *or* immerse swab in transport medium and centrifuge to sediment cells; apply cells on slides; fix slides in cold acetone; slides may be stored at $-70°$ C	Immerse swab directly into cell culture tube as above or in transport medium
Vesicle fluid	Examine only by electron microscopy, not by immunofluorescence	Rinse syringe with transport medium and inoculate cells
Cerebrospinal fluid	Do not examine	Inoculate directly
Urine	Centrifuge to sediment cells and proceed as for other fluids	Inoculate directly
Tissue	Make tissue imprints on slides; proceed as for lesion scrapings	Mince tissue; prepare 20% suspension; grind; centrifuge and inoculate supernatant
Blood	—	Prepare buffy coat (Table 47-3)
Other fluids	Sediment cells, wash with PBS, and place cells on slides; air dry and fix in cold acetone; slides may be stored at $-70°$ C	Inoculate directly

SYMBOLS: PMK, Primary monkey kidney cells
PBS, Phosphate-buffered saline

Data from references 13 and 24.

For detection of virus particles by EM, the original specimen must contain at least 10^6 and preferably 10^7 to 10^9 virus particles. Although EM is rapid, it is not very sensitive. Various techniques have been devised to improve sensitivity. In one method, immune electron microscopy (IEM), the specimen is first mixed with specific antibody, which aggregates viral particles. Sensitivity is increased about a hundred times.[54] IEM requires a high degree of suspicion of the correct viral cause so the appropriate antiserum is selected. Pseudoreplication and agar gel diffusion also enhance virus detection by EM. In both techniques agar is used to remove specimen by diffusion and thus concentrate the virus.

EM can be used to identify virus groups on the basis of size and shape, but morphologically similar viruses (such as herpes viruses) cannot be differentiated.[29] The major contribution of EM has been in the detection of noncultivable viruses such as hepatitis B virus and rotavirus.[5]

IMMUNOFLUORESCENCE

Immunofluorescence (FA) is discussed in Chapter 7. Direct FA (DFA) is quicker to perform because there is only one incubation period. Nonspecific staining is decreased, but DFA is less sensitive than indirect FA (IFA) because some antibody is destroyed during conjugation with the label,[17] and in IFA the antibody globulin around the viral antigen results in a larger surface area for attachment of labeled antibody. IFA takes longer to perform but is more sensitive, and if all antisera tested are prepared in the same animal species, only one conjugated antiserum is required for all viruses tested. IFA produces more autofluorescence, especially with cells from the superficial layers of skin and white blood cells; counterstains such as naphthelene black or Evans blue reduce autofluorescence.

Specimens examined for viruses by FA must contain intact cells of the type infected by the suspected virus (for example, herpes simplex virus infects epithelial cells, not polymorphonuclear leukocytes). Acceptable specimens include nasopharyngeal secretions, throat gargles, lesion or conjunctival scrapings, tissue, and urine sediments (Table 47-1). Cells in respiratory specimens are concentrated by centrifugation and washed before being placed on a slide. Slides are fixed in cold acetone (10 minutes at $4°$ C) and may be stored at $-70°$ C.

DFA or IFA has been used for essentially every virus group

TABLE 47-5. Staining Reaction in Direct Immunofluorescence Test of Common Viruses

Virus or Virus Group	Appearance of Viral Fluorescence in Infected Cells
Herpes simplex (HSV)	HSV fluorescence is in nucleus and cytoplasm; HSV-1 generally produces strong perinuclear staining; HSV-2 produces homogeneous staining
Varicella	Fluorescence seen in both nucleus and cytoplasm
Cytomegalovirus (CMV)	CMV antigens are found in both nuclear and cytoplasmic inclusions of infected cells; cytoplasmic staining in absence of nuclear staining is probably nonspecific
Adenovirus	Adenovirus fluorescence varies widely; typical fluorescence, however, generally consists of both nuclear and cytoplasmic staining; extracellular staining of soluble antigens is present with some serotypes
Influenza	Fluorescence may be present in nucleus alone, in nucleus and cytoplasm, or in cytoplasm alone
Parainfluenza	Fluorescence in cells infected with parainfluenza virus is cytoplasmic; fine particles, coarse particles, and strands may fluoresce
Mumps	Mumps virus fluorescence is cytoplasmic; fine and coarse fluorescent particles are usually present
Respiratory syncytial (RSV)	RSV fluorescence is entirely cytoplasmic; both large inclusion-like bodies and fine fluorescent particles may be present
Measles	Specific fluorescence appears in cytoplasm or nucleus or both
Rabies	Fluorescence may vary from small particles less than 1 μm to masses 2 to 10 μm in diameter; fluorescence is cytoplasmic
Vaccinia	Specific fluorescence appears first as cytoplasmic inclusions and later becomes diffuse in cytoplasm

From Lyerla, H.C., and Forrester, F.T.: Immunofluorescence methods in virology, Course No. 8231-C, Atlanta, 1979, Centers for Disease Control.

that has a group antigen or only a few serotypes.[11,39,46a,48] Commercial reagents are available for both DFA and IFA. Not all commercial reagents are acceptable or always available, and they must not be used without careful testing and sufficient quality control. The World Health Organization recommends that testing of these reagents include the following:

1. Infected and uninfected control cells must be tested to determine the optimum dilutions to use. The optimal dilution is at least four times greater than the last dilution causing nonspecific fluorescence with uninfected cells. Control cells should be of four different types.
2. Final evaluation should include testing dilutions on clinical material.
3. Noninfected human specimens should be used as negative controls.
4. Cell culture infected with a number of closely related viruses should be tested to determine any cross-reactions.

Interpretation of FA results requires an experienced observer because a positive result must have not only intracellular fluorescence but also the expected fluorescence pattern of the correct cell type and site (Table 47-5).

The greatest problem with the FA technique for examination of clinical specimens is obtaining an acceptable specimen with enough cells. Physicians must be instructed in collecting good specimens for FA. Obtaining high-quality antisera and conjugates is another major obstacle. FA is not practical for virus groups, such as enteroviruses and rhinoviruses, that have many serotypes and no common antigen, and interpretation is subjective and dependent on the examiner's expertise.

However, FA is a rapid technique, relatively inexpensive, and under the best of circumstances a valuable diagnostic tool. It provides an identification of the virus and may detect viral antigen after infectious virus can no longer be isolated. Until better reagents are available, FA should not be used without culture backup.[37]

IMMUNOPEROXIDASE

Immunoperoxidase (IP) techniques are similar to FA techniques except that the label used is an enzyme, horseradish peroxidase, instead of fluorescein isothiocyanate (FITC). After treatment with labeled antiserum, slides are exposed to diaminobenzidine, which reacts with the enzyme to produce a reddish brown color. Slides are examined by light microscopy, which eliminates the need for a fluorescence microscope. Unfortunately, endogenous peroxidases are common, and nonspecific reactions can be difficult to interpret.

ENZYME-LINKED IMMUNOSORBENT ASSAY

The principle of enzyme-linked immunosorbent assay (ELISA) is discussed in Chapter 7. Two methods have been used to detect viral antigen in clinical specimens: double-sandwich ELISA, and indirect ELISA.[2,19] For both, specific viral antibody is bound to a solid phase such as a microtiter well, polystyrene beads, or test tubes. The double-sandwich technique requires enzyme-linked virus specific antibody, whereas the indirect ELISA method uses enzyme-conjugated antispecies immunoglobulins.

As mentioned in Chapter 7, ELISA techniques require careful quality control. Each test run should include a positive and negative control, a substrate control (antibody-coated surface plus substrate), and a conjugate control (antibody-coated surface plus all reagents except the test material).

ELISA procedures can be as sensitive and as specific as radioimmunoassay (discussed later). Expensive equipment is not an absolute requirement because the reaction can be read visually. Reagents are relatively inexpensive, do not pose any biologic hazard, and have a long shelf life. Use of a spectrophotometer eliminates any subjectivity in interpretation.

Compared to FA, ELISA is relatively complicated and time consuming. Major problems include variation in behavior of the plastics used for the solid phase and the production of high-titer antisera. In some viral infections the amount of antigen may be too small to be detected by ELISA.[38] At present the only commercially available ELISA kits are for detecting rotavirus, respiratory syncytial virus, herpes simplex virus, and hepatitis B surface antigen (HB$_s$Ag). ELISA techniques for directly detecting several other viruses in clinical specimens have been reported from research laboratories.[6,41]

Generally the sensitivity of the ELISA test for the direct detection of herpes simplex virus or its antigenic components has been 50% to 70% compared with the recovery of the agents in cell culture.[42] However, the level of detection, at least for herpes simplex virus, may be significantly increased by complexing biotin to the herpes simplex antibody with subsequent detection with alkaline phosphate–labeled streptavidin and appropriate substrate.[44] In addition, incorporation of a spin amplification (centrifugation) step in cell culture in the commercially available ELISA kit (ELISA-SAT, Ortho Diagnostics) has provided a sensitivity of HSV detection of 97.6% 48 hours after inoculation.[38a] In the future, modified ELISA tests, using capillary tubes that require less than 2 hours' reaction time or an immunofiltration staining assay (30 minutes), should be advantageous for the diagnosis and hence treatment and management of patients with herpesvirus infection.[9a,48a]

RADIOIMMUNOASSAY

Radioimmunoassay (RIA) techniques use a radioisotope, usually ^{125}I, to detect antigen-antibody reactions. Methods are similar to those described for ELISA and can be performed with radiolabeled virus-specific antibody or indirectly with radiolabeled antispecies globulins. Solid-phase RIA with radiolabeled virus antibody has been widely used for detection of HB$_s$Ag. The test works well because HB$_s$Ag is usually present in high concentrations and antigen is present in serum rather than in other host tissues.[14] Therefore antigen can be easily purified and used to prepare high-titer antisera. RIA for detecting virus in clinical specimens has been reported for other viruses such as herpes simplex virus and Norwalk agent, but commercial reagents are not available.[15,22]

RIA is highly sensitive and can detect small amounts of virus. Major problems with RIA are the need for expensive equipment and, if multiple specimens are not tested together, high cost per test. The most important drawback is the need for radioisotopes, which are unstable and a hazard to personnel. Disposal of radioactive wastes is expensive and difficult.

DIRECT EXAMINATION: INTERPRETATION OF RESULTS

A positive result is considered significant if the specimen was obtained from the site of disease (lesion scraping) and correlates with the patient's symptoms. Virus detected in specimens collected from sites not involved in the disease are more difficult to assess. Although no viruses are considered "normal flora," some, such as cytomegalovirus, adenovirus, and enteroviruses, can be shed intermittently for a long time. The need for culture confirmation of a positive direct examination result depends on the specificity of the method used.

A negative result never rules out infection with a particular virus because direct methods may not detect small amounts of virus or virus antigen. If a cultivable virus is suspected, a negative direct examination result should be followed by culture for the virus.

VIRUS ISOLATION

The mainstay of diagnostic virology is still the isolation of virus from clinical specimens. Hosts used for the cultivation of human viruses include laboratory animals, embryonated hens' eggs, and cell cultures. No one host system is susceptible to every virus, and each has its advantages and disadvantages. The choice of host systems is based on the viruses to be isolated, cost, and practicality. In the diagnostic laboratory, systems providing the broadest host range are usually chosen.

ANIMALS

Laboratory animals are expensive to produce and maintain in appropriate facilities and may be difficult to handle. Animals have their own indigenous viruses, which may be activated and interfere with laboratory results, as well as cause human infection. The most commonly used laboratory animal is the white Swiss mouse. Suckling mice are used because adult mice are less susceptible. The most common routes of inoculation are intraperitoneal and intracerebral. Animals are observed for signs of illness or death. Suckling mice are used mainly for the isolation of arboviruses, coxsackie A viruses, and rabies virus, and are thus used more often in reference than in hospital laboratories.

EMBRYONATED EGGS

Fertile hens' eggs have a rather narrow host range and are now used more in the research laboratory than the clinical laboratory. Various routes of inoculation and embryo ages are used depending on the agents sought (Table 47-6). After inoculation, eggs are incubated and examined by shining a light through the egg shell and harvesting either when the embryo dies or when evidence of virus would be expected. Virus can be detected serologically or by lesions or pocks on the chorioallantoic membrane. Eggs are particularly useful for producing large amounts of virus antigen and for isolating certain strains of influenza virus.

CELL CULTURE

In diagnostic virology, cell cultures have for the most part replaced animals and eggs. Cultures are inoculated and examined microscopically for virus-induced morphologic changes or cytopathic effect (CPE). Some viruses do not produce CPE, and other detection methods are used (see "Virus Detection in Cell Culture"). Cell cultures are fairly easy to maintain, can have a wide host range, and, most important, can be obtained commercially. The term "cell culture" is used to describe cells growing in vitro that have lost their differentiation. Tissue or organ cultures contain tissue that remains differentiated when growing or maintained in vitro; original architecture and func-

TABLE 47-6. Embryonated Hens' Eggs for Virus, Rickettsia, and Chlamydia Isolation

Route of Inoculation	Embryo Age (Days)	Microbe
Yolk sac	5-7	Chlamydiae, rickettsiae
Amniotic	7-11	Influenza and mumps viruses
Allantoic	7-11	Influenza virus
Chorioallantoic membrane	10-12	Poxviruses, herpes simplex virus

tion may be retained. These cultures are difficult to handle and not widely used in the diagnostic laboratory.

Cells in culture may be grown in a monolayer, a single layer of cells growing on a surface, or in suspension, in which cells multiply while suspended in liquid medium. Suspension cultures are used primarily for growing large volumes of virus, whereas monolayers are used widely in diagnostic virology for virus isolation.

There are three types of cell cultures: primary, diploid, and heteroploid. Most diagnostic laboratories use at least one of each of these types to provide a broad host range. Cell cultures employed include the following:

1. Primary
   a. RMK (from rhesus monkey kidney)
   b. CMK (from cynomolgus monkey kidney)
   c. RK (from rabbit kidney)
   d. AGMK (from African green monkey kidney)
   e. HEK (from human embryonic kidney)
2. Diploid
   a. WI-38 (from human embryonic lung)
   b. MRC-5 (from human embryonic lung)
   c. HEK (from human embryonic kidney)
3. Heteroploid
   a. HeLa (from carcinoma, human cervix)
   b. HEp-2 (from carcinoma, human larynx)
   c. Vero (from African green monkey kidney)

Primary cells are obtained from original tissue. Tissue is minced and treated with a proteolytic enzyme, trypsin, to separate individual cells. Following filtration to remove undigested tissue, a known number of cells is mixed with a nutrient medium and inoculated into a container with a flat surface. The cells multiply and form a monolayer (Plate 29, C). Cells in primary cell cultures have the same karotype as the original tissue and thus have the same chromosome number and retain the sex chromatin.

If a primary cell culture is subcultivated, it becomes a cell line. Subculture is accomplished by removing a monolayer with trypsin, dispersing the cell clusters into individual cells, diluting the cells and mixing them with nutrient medium, and again seeding a container with a flat surface. Cells are incubated until a new monolayer is formed. A diploid cell line (Plate 29, D) has at least 75% of the cells with the same karyotype as the normal cells of the animal from which the cells were derived. Diploid cell lines cannot be serially passed indefinitely but tend to die out by about the fiftieth subculture. The virus spectrum and cell morphology are usually the same as the corresponding primary cell culture. Subcultivated cells with less than 75% of the cells as normal are heteroploid cell lines. Heteroploid cell lines (Plate 29, E) can be subcultured indefinitely,

are called established cell lines, and are often derived from malignant tissue.

CELL CULTURE INOCULATION

In selecting which cell cultures to inoculate, the virologist must first decide which viruses are likely to be isolated and which cells will be susceptible to them. To keep down costs, cells with the broadest host range that are readily available are selected. In practice, most virology laboratories include primary monkey kidney (PMK) cells, diploid cells, and often a heteroploid cell line. The PMK cells are primarily for the isolation of myxoviruses, paramyxoviruses, and enteroviruses. Until a few years ago, rhesus monkey kidneys were used. The Indian government has banned exportation of these animals, so rhesus monkey cells are now expensive and difficult to obtain. It appears that cells prepared from the kidneys of cynomolgus monkeys (*Macaca fascicularis*) are an acceptable substitute.[9,28]

Human diploid fibroblast (HDF) cells have a wide host range and are particularly useful for isolation of herpes viruses (herpes simplex virus, cytomegalovirus, varicella-zoster virus). Until recently most laboratories used WI-38 cells, but the quality of commercial cells has become poor. Friedman and Korophak[16] showed that HDF cells derived from a 14-week fetus (MRC-5) are just as good as WI-38, and most laboratories now use MRC-5.

Depending on the patient population, some laboratories also include heteroploid cells for the isolation of adenoviruses and respiratory syncytial virus. HEp-2 is most commonly used.

Selection of cell cultures for each specimen type and the number of tubes inoculated vary from laboratory to laboratory. To reduce costs, some laboratories inoculate only one tube of each cell type. Others believe that problems with toxicity and bacterial or fungal contamination are reduced if a "backup" culture tube is included. Table 47-7 shows an example of an inoculation chart.

All of these cells are commercially available (Flow Laboratories, Inc., McLean, Va.; M.A. Bioproducts, Walkersville, Md.; Bartels Immunodiagnostic Supplies, Inc., Bellevue, Wash.). Cells obtained commercially are examined when they arrive in the laboratory. If a good monolayer is present, the growth medium is replaced with a maintenance medium. The maintenance medium is changed about once a week depending on the growth and appearance of the cells. Growth media are nutrient media with a high (usually 10%) serum concentration to produce rapid cell growth. Maintenance media are used to maintain the cells in a steady state and are often the same base medium as the growth medium but with a lower serum concentration or in some cases no serum. The most commonly used

13. Drew, W.L., and Stevens, G.R.: How your laboratory should perform viral studies (continued): isolation and identification of commonly encountered viruses, Lab. Med. **11**:14, 1980.

14. Forghani, B.: Radioimmunoassay. In Lennette, E.H., and Schmidt, N.J., editors: Diagnostic procedures for viral, rickettsial, and chlamydial infections, Washington, D.C., 1979, American Public Health Association.

15. Forghani, B., Schmidt, N.J., and Lennette, E.H.: Solid-phase radioimmunoassay for identification of herpes virus hominis types 1 and 2 from clinical materials, Appl. Microbiol. **28**:661, 1974.

16. Friedman, H.M., and Korophak, C.: Comparison of WI-38, MRC-5, and IMR-90 cell strains for isolation of viruses from clinical specimens, J. Clin. Microbiol. **7**:368, 1978.

17. Gardner, P.S.: Rapid virus diagnosis, J. Gen. Virol. **36**:1, 1977.

18. Gershon, A.A.: Problems of infancy: TORCH infections and diagnostic virology. In Lennette, D., Spector, G., and Thompson, K.D., editors: Diagnosis of viral infections: the role of the clinical laboratory, Baltimore, 1979, University Park Press.

19. Gilman, S.C., and Docherty, J.J.: Enzyme-linked immunosorbent assay (ELISA): detection of herpes simplex virus antibody in human sera and other applications. In Lennette, D., Spector, S., and Thompson, K.D., editors: Diagnosis of viral infections: the role of the clinical laboratory, Baltimore, 1979, University Park Press.

20. Gleaves, C.A., et al.: Comparison of standard tube and shell vial cell culture techniques for the detection of cytomegalovirus in clinical specimens, J. Clin. Microbiol. **21**:217, 1985.

21. Gleaves, C.A., et al.: Detection and serotyping of herpes simplex virus in MRC-5 cells by use of centrifugation and monoclonal antibodies 16 h postinoculation, J. Clin. Microbiol. **21**:29, 1985.

22. Greenberg, H.B., et al.: Solid-phase microtiter radioimmunoassay for detection of the Norwalk strain of acute non-bacterial epidemic gastroenteritis virus and its antibodies, J. Med. Virol. **2**:97, 1978.

23. Griffiths, P.D., et al.: Rapid diagnosis of cytomegalovirus infection in immunocompromised patients by detection of early antigen fluorescent foci, Lancet **2**:1242, 1984.

24. Grist, N.R., et al.: Diagnostic methods in clinical virology, ed. 3, Boston, 1979, Blackwell Scientific Publications, Inc.

25. Gustafson, T.L., Shehab, Z., and Brunell, P.A.: Outbreak of varicella in a newborn intensive care nursery, Am. J. Dis. Child. **138**:548, 1984.

26. Hall, C.B.: Nosocomial viral respiratory infections: perennial weeds on pediatric wards, Am. J. Med. **70**:670, 1981.

27. Herrmann, E.C., and Herrmann, J.A.: Survey of viral diagnostic laboratories in medical centers, J. Infect. Dis. **133**:359, 1976.

28. Hollick, G.E., Reichrath, L., and Smith, T.F.: Comparison of primary rhesus and cynomolgus monkey kidney cell cultures for viral isolation from clinical specimens, Am. J. Clin. Pathol. **68**:276, 1977.

29. Horn, M.E.C., Taylor, P., and Yealland, S.J.: Nasopharyngeal secretions as a source of material for identification of respiratory viruses in infants and young children, Arch. Dis. Child. **50**:829, 1975.

30. Howell, C.L., Miller, M.J., and Martin, W.J.: Comparison of rates of virus isolation from leukocyte populations separated from blood by conventional and Ficoll-Paque/Macrodex methods, J. Clin. Microbiol. **10**:533, 1979.

31. Hsiung, G.D., Fong, C.K.Y., and August, M.J.: The use of electron microscopy for diagnosis of virus infections: an overview, Prog. Med. Virol. **25**:133, 1979.

32. Hughes, J.H., and Hamparian, V.V.: Commercial simian virus antisera that inhibit virus replication in primary monkey kidney cell cultures, J. Clin. Microbiol. **13**:824, 1981.

33. Johnson, R.B., Jr., and Libby, R.: Separation of immunoglobulin M (IgM) essentially free of IgG from serum for use in systems requiring assay of IgM-type antibodies without interference from rheumatoid factor, J. Clin. Microbiol. **12**:451, 1980.

34. Jones, D.B., Liesegang, T.J., and Robinson, N.J.: Cumitech 13: laboratory diagnosis of ocular infections, Washington, D.C., 1981, American Society for Microbiology.

35. Lennette, D.A., and Lennette, E.T.: A user's guide to the diagnostic virology laboratory, Baltimore, 1981, University Park Press.

36. Lennette, E.T., and Lennette, D.A.: Immune adherence hemagglutination: alternative to complement-fixation serology, J. Clin. Microbiol. **7**:282, 1978.

36a. Martin, W.J., Jr., and Smith, T.F.: Rapid detection of cytomegalovirus in bronchoalveolar lavage specimens by a monoclonal antibody method, J. Clin. Microbiol. **23**:1006, 1986.

37. McIntosh, K.: Recent advances in viral diagnosis, Arch. Pathol. Lab. Med. **104**:3, 1980.

38. McIntosh, K., et al.: Summary of a workshop in new and useful techniques in rapid viral diagnosis, J. Infect. Dis. **142**:793, 1980.

38a. Michalski, F.J., et al.: Enzyme-linked immunosorbent assay spin amplification technique for herpes simplex virus antigen detection, J. Clin. Microbiol. **24**:310, 1986.

39. Minnich, L.L., and Ray, C.G.: Comparison of direct immunofluorescent staining of clinical specimens for respiratory virus antigens with conventional isolation techniques, J. Clin. Microbiol. **12**:391, 1980.

39a. Minnich, L.L., and Ray, C.G.: Early testing of cell culture for detection of hemadsorbing viruses, J. Clin. Microbiol. **25**:421, 1987.

40. Mintz, L., and Drew, W.L.: Relation of culture site to the recovery of nonpolio enteroviruses, Am. J. Clin. Pathol. **74**:324, 1980.

41. Miranda, Q.R., et al.: Solid-phase immunoassay for herpes simplex virus, J. Infect. Dis. **136**:S304, 1977.

42. Morgan, M.A., and Smith, T.F.: Evaluation of an enzyme-linked immunosorbent assay for the detection of herpes simplex virus antigen, J. Clin. Microbiol. **19**:730, 1984.

43. Moseley, R.C., et al.: Comparison of viral isolation, direct immunofluorescence, and indirect immunoperoxidase techniques for detection of genital herpes simplex virus infection, J. Clin. Microbiol. **13**:913, 1981.

44. Nerurkar, L.S., et al.: Rapid detection of herpes simplex virus in clinical specimens by use of a capture Biotin-Streptavidin enzyme-linked immunosorbent assay, J. Clin. Microbiol. **20**:109, 1984.

45. Osborn, J.E.: Precise viral diagnosis—why bother? In Lennette, D.A., Spector, S., and Thompson, K.D., editors: Diagnosis of viral infections: the role of the clinical laboratory, Baltimore, 1979, University Park Press.

46. Prather, S.L., et al.: The isolation of enteroviruses from blood: a comparison of four processing methods, J. Med. Virol. **14**:221, 1984.

46a. Ray, C.G., and Minnich, L.L.: Efficiency of immunofluorescence for rapid detection of common respiratory viruses, J. Clin. Microbiol. **25**:355, 1987.

47. Reimer, C.B., et al.: The specificity of fetal IgM: antibody or anti-antibody? Ann. N.Y. Acad. Sci. **254**:79, 1975.

48. Schmidt, N.J., et al.: Direct immunofluorescence staining for detection of herpes simplex and varicella-zoster virus antigens in vesicular lesions and certain tissue specimens, J. Clin. Microbiol. **12**:651, 1980.

48a. Shekarchi, I.C., et al.: Capillary enzyme immunoassay for rapid detection of herpes simplex virus in clinical specimens, J. Clin. Microbiol. **25**:320, 1987.

49. Sköldenberg, B., et al.: Acyclovir versus vidarabine in herpes simplex encephalitis, Lancet **2**:707, 1984.

50. Smith, T.F.: Specimen requirements, transport, and recovery of viruses in cell cultures. In Lennette, D., Spector, S., and Thompson, K., editors: Diagnosis of viral infections: the role of the clinical laboratory, Baltimore, 1979, University Park Press.

51. Stanley, T.V., and Leask, B.G.S.: A new virus transport system, Practitioner **225**:204, 1981.

52. Sumaya, C.V., et al.: Use of a simple separation column in detection of immunoglobulin M antibody to Epstein-Barr virus, J. Clin. Microbiol. **20**:298, 1984.

53. Swenson, P.D., and Kaplan, M.H.: Rapid detection of cytomegalovirus in cell culture by indirect immunoperoxidase staining with monoclonal antibody to an early nuclear antigen, J. Clin. Microbiol. **21**:669, 1985.

54. Yunis, E.J., Hashida, Y., and Haas, J.E.: The role of electron microscopy in the identification of viruses in human disease, Pathol. Annu. **12**:311, 1977.

55. Ziegler, D.W.: Determination of IgM antibodies in diagnostic virology. In Lennette, D., Spector, S., and Thompson, K., editors: Diagnosis of viral infections: the role of the clinical laboratory, Baltimore, 1979, University Park Press.

CHAPTER 48

Adenoviruses

Sally Jo Rubin

Adenoviruses were first isolated from human adenoid cell cultures in the early 1950s, and their association with respiratory disease in the military population at Fort Leonard Wood, Missouri, soon followed. *Adenoviridae* are divided into two genera: *Mastadenovirus* (animal viruses) and *Aviadenovirus* (avian viruses). They are generally species specific in that "human" strains infect only humans. Adenoviruses are relatively stable at temperatures from 4° to 36° C and can easily be maintained at −70° C.[3] Adenoviruses share a common complement fixation antigen and are further subdivided into at least 41 distinct serotypes[6] based on neutralization with type-specific antisera. The number of serotypes will likely expand.[1,13a]

Human adenoviruses are divided into four major subgroups on the basis of hemagglutination patterns obtained with rat and rhesus monkey erythrocytes. Hemagglutination inhibition (HI) can be used for serotyping. Serotyping by both neutralization and HI has revealed that human adenoviruses are becoming more complex antigenically.[5] Antigenic variants have been isolated that are one type by neutralization and another by HI.[4,5,12] Such strains are designated as adenovirus x/y where x is the serotype(s) by neutralization and y the serotype(s) by HI.

CLINICAL ASPECTS

Adenoviruses cause infection of the eye, upper and lower respiratory tract, and urinary and gastrointestinal tracts. They are associated primarily with self-limited respiratory and ocular disease occurring mainly in children under 4 and among military personnel. Adenovirus infection is extremely common, and by 5 years of age 75% of the population has antibody. The incubation period varies from 5 to 10 days. Although a relationship between serotype and some clinical syndromes exists (Table 48-1), 95% of adenovirus infections related to illness are caused by types 2, 1, 7, 3, and 5. Rarely, adenoviruses have been implicated in more severe infection including meningitis,[8] but in most of these cases a causal relationship has not been proved.

Noncultivable adenoviruses can be seen by electron microscopy in the feces of infants with diarrhea.[3,11] Antigen of these viruses can also be detected in feces by counterimmunoelectrophoresis or enzyme-linked immunosorbent assay (ELISA) and in inoculated cell culture by fluorescent antibody (FA). Their role in gastroenteritis is not yet clear, but patients do produce antibodies to these viruses, which appear to be a new subgroup of adenovirus. Two serotypes, types 40 and 41, have been characterized.[1,3,7]

The epidemiology of adenovirus infections also varies somewhat with type (see Table 48-1). For example, type 4 occurs in epidemics in the winter among military recruits and is transmitted by aerosols, whereas type 2 infection occurs mainly in infants and young children and is transmitted by the fecal-oral route.

TREATMENT AND CONTROL

Deaths caused by adenovirus are unusual among civilians, and thus vaccine development or testing of any antiviral agents has not been done. In military recruits, however, adult respiratory disease caused by types 4 and 7 can be severe, and fatalities, although rare, do occur. An attenuated oral type 4 and 7 live-virus vaccine is available for this population.[14]

LABORATORY DIAGNOSIS
SPECIMEN TYPES

Adenoviruses are usually isolated from throat swabs, nasal washings, conjunctival swabs or scrapings, and feces. Less commonly, they are isolated from urine, blood, or tissue.

DIRECT EXAMINATION

Respiratory secretions, conjunctival cells, urine, and tissue can be directly examined for viral antigen by electron microscopy or immunofluorescence. Generally, both nuclear and cytoplasmic fluorescence is observed, and for some serotypes, extracellular staining of soluble antigens is seen.[9] In feces, adenovirus antigen of both cultivable and noncultivable strains can be detected by ELISA[7] or by electron microscopy. Commercial systems for detecting fecal antigen are not available.

VIRUS ISOLATION

Human adenoviruses do not grow in embryonated eggs, nor are they pathogenic for most common laboratory animals. Adenoviruses multiply best in cells of the same species they normally infect. Thus human adenoviruses are optimally isolated in primary human embryonic kidney (HEK) cells, but continuous human cell lines of epithelial origin such as HEp-2 or HeLa may be used. Fetal diploid cell cultures (WI-38 or MRC-5) are not as sensitive, and cytopathic effect (CPE) is slower to appear. Typical CPE, at least with the more common serotypes (1 to 7), is usually visible in heteroploid cells in 4 to 6 days. Other serotypes may take longer. FA identification may be attempted when there is 25% to 50% CPE. Complement fixation (CF) requires 75% to 100% CPE.

In HEK, adenovirus infection results in cells that are rounded, enlarged, highly refractile, and aggregated into irregular grapelike clusters. In diploid cells there is less clumping, and CPE usually does not progress to involve the entire monolayer. Rhesus or cynomolgus monkey kidney (CMK) cells are acceptable but less sensitive than HEK for adenovirus isolation.[13] The CPE in CMK infected with adenovirus types 1, 2, 3, and 5 is characterized by increasingly granular and thickened cells.

TABLE 48-1. Clinical Syndromes Caused by Adenoviruses

Syndrome	Population Infected	Primary Symptoms	Comments	Types[a]
Acute febrile pharyngitis	Infants, young children	Exudative pharyngitis, enlarged cervical nodes	Transmission fecal-oral; rectal excretion; many months with no further symptoms	2, 1, 5 (3, 6, 7)[b]
Pharyngoconjunctival fever	Children and young adults	Unilateral conjunctivitis, sore throat, fever	Endemic; close contact; often related to swimming pools; epidemic (discrete outbreaks)	3, 7 (1, 2, 4, 6, 14)
Acute respiratory disease	Military recruits	Fever, nonproductive cough, sore throat, pneumonia in about 10%	January-March epidemic	4, 7 (3, 14, 21)
Pneumonia	Infants, young children, immunocompromised	Pneumonia	Fatality rare; only with types 4, 7	3, 7, 21 (1, 4, 5, 18)
Epidemic keratoconjunctivitis	Any	Follicular conjunctivitis followed by subepithelial corneal keratitis	Shipyards, industrial settings, hand-to-eye transmission	37 (8, 11, 19)
Pertussis-like syndrome	Infants, young children	Indistinguishable clinically from whooping cough	Endemic	5 (1, 2, 3)
Acute hemorrhagic cystitis	Pediatric, occasionally adults	Hematuria, dysuria, frequency, urgency	More common in males	11 (21)

[a]In order of frequency.
[b]Less common types are in parentheses; rarely, infection may occur with other types.

Clumping occurs, and some cells retract from the clusters, giving a weblike appearance.[13]

Adenoviruses are usually cell associated, with little virus released into the medium. Therefore, to pass virus isolates to new uninfected host cells, two or three freeze-and-thaw cycles are necessary to release virus. Virus isolates are confirmed as adenovirus by FA, CF, or neutralization.[3,11] CF is the standard method but is cumbersome, the least sensitive, and requires more extensive CPE. FA can detect antigen as early as 2 days after inoculation, often before CPE is visible, and is simple to perform. Reagents are commercially available.

All human serotypes except type 18 agglutinate either rhesus monkey or rat erythrocytes; thus HI can be used to determine serotype. Since variant types are found, type should be determined by both HI and neutralization.

SIGNIFICANCE OF ISOLATES

Certain adenoviruses (especially types 1, 2, 3, and 5) may cause persistent infection resulting in intermittent virus shedding for as long as 6 months.[2,10] Therefore serologic support is required to confirm that an adenovirus isolated from the stool is the cause of a current infection. Isolation from the respiratory tract is more likely to be significant.[3]

SEROLOGIC DIAGNOSIS

Detecting an antibody rise following adenovirus infection depends on proper specimen timing, patient age, virus serotype, and procedure used. The CF test for antibody to the group antigen is the least sensitive test, with about 60% of patients developing CF antibody.[2] HI is next in sensitivity, and neutralization is most sensitive, with 90% of patients infected with type 1 or 2 having detectable type-specific antibody. Despite its disadvantages, the CF test is the procedure used by most diagnostic laboratories.

REFERENCES

1. deJong, J.C., et al.: Candidate adenoviruses 40 and 41, J. Med. Virol. **11**:215, 1983.
2. Fox, J.P., and Hall, C.E.: Viruses in families: surveillance of families as a key to epidemiology of virus infections, Littleton, Mass., 1980, PSG/Wright Publishing Co., Inc.
3. Gary, G.W., Jr., Hierholzer, J.C., and Black, R.E.: Characteristics of noncultivable adenoviruses associated with diarrhea in infants: a new subgroup of human adenoviruses, J. Clin. Microbiol. **10**:96, 1979.
4. Hierholzer, J.C., and Rodriguez, F.H.: Antigenically intermediate human adenovirus strain associated with conjunctivitis, J. Clin. Microbiol. **13**:395, 1981.

5. Hierholzer, J.C., Torrence, A.E., and Wright, P.F.: Generalized viral illness caused by an intermediate strain of adenovirus (21/H21 + 35), J. Infect. Dis. **141:**281, 1980.

6. Hierholzer, J.C., et al.: New human adenovirus associated with respiratory illness: candidate adenovirus type 39, J. Clin. Microbiol. **16:**15, 1982.

7. Johansson, M.E., et al.: Direct identification of enteric adenoviruses, a candidate new serotype, associated with infantile gastroenteritis, J. Clin. Microbiol. **12:**95, 1980.

8. Kelsey, D.S.: Adenovirus meningoencephalitis, Pediatrics **61:**291, 1978.

9. Lyerla, H.C., and Forrester, F.T.: Immunofluorescence methods in virology, Course No. 8231-C, Atlanta, 1979, Centers for Disease Control.

10. Martone, W.J., et al.: An outbreak of adenovirus type 3 disease at a private recreation center swimming pool, Am. J. Epidemiol. **111:**229, 1980.

11. Retter, M., et al.: Enteric adenoviruses: detection, replication, and significance, J. Clin. Microbiol. **10:**574, 1979.

12. Schoop, G.J.P., et al.: A new intermediate adenovirus type causing conjunctivitis, Arch. Ophthalmol. **97:**2336, 1979.

13. Smith, T.F.: Viruses. In Washington, J.A., editor: Laboratory procedures in clinical microbiology, New York, 1981, Springer-Verlag.

13a. Takiff, H.E., et al.: Detection of enteric adenoviruses by dot-blot hybridization using a molecularly cloned viral DNA probe, J. Med. Virol. **16:**107, 1985.

14. Top, F.H., Jr., et al.: Control of respiratory disease in recruits with type 4 and 7 adenovirus vaccines, Am. J. Epidemiol. **94:**142, 1971.

CHAPTER 49

Herpesviruses

Sally Jo Rubin

The over 70 members of the family *Herpesviridae* are widespread in nature, mainly infecting animals. Human beings serve as the host for five members of this family: herpes simplex viruses (HSV) types 1 and 2, varicella-zoster virus (VZV), cytomegalovirus (CMV), and Epstein-Barr virus (EBV). *Herpes simiae* (herpes B) virus, which naturally infects Asian monkeys, can also infect humans and is usually fatal (mortality 85%). *H. simiae* is found in about 0.1% of monkey kidney cell cultures. People working with these monkey tissues are at risk for *H. simiae* infection.[132]

All herpesviruses are large, contain DNA, have icosahedral symmetry, and are surrounded by a lipid-containing envelope derived from the host cell membrane.[116,132] Herpesviruses are unique in their ability to cause persistent infections. In the latent state HSV and VZV exist in nerve tissue while CMV and EBV persist in lymphoid tissue. Reactivation and subsequent secondary disease may be clinical or subclinical.

HERPES SIMPLEX VIRUS

Clinical syndromes probably resulting from HSV were described as early as Hippocrates. The virus was first isolated in 1919 and 1920 by inoculating specimens from human oral and ocular lesions onto rabbit corneas. The concept of latent virus with subsequent recurrences was not suggested for another 20 years. Serologic differentiation of HSV into two types was accomplished in 1961. HSV-1 and HSV-2 differ in many biologic and biochemical properties (Table 49-1). Their structural polypeptides and DNA nucleotide sequences also differ. The differences in nucleotide sequences have been examined by cleavage of viral DNA with bacterial endonucleases. To date, 80 different HSV strains have been detected, and probably hundreds or even thousands of different strains exist.[140]

HSV is relatively thermolabile at 37° C with a half-life in cell culture medium of 1½ hours.[132] The virus survives at least 48 hours at 4° C in a liquid environment but is rapidly inactivated without moisture.[24] HSV survives a wide pH range (5.5 to 9.5). Organic solvents destroy the virus, as do quaternary ammonium compounds. HSV is inactivated by 5% phenol in 18 hours.

HSV-1 and HSV-2 share cross-reacting antigens as well as type-specific antigens. These antigens are glycoproteins found on the surface of the virus envelope.[111]

CLINICAL SIGNIFICANCE

HSV causes a variety of clinical syndromes ranging from asymptomatic to fatal disseminated disease (Table 49-2). Anatomic sites infected include skin, lips and oral cavity, eyes, genital tract, and central nervous system (CNS).[135] The Greek word *herpes* (''to creep'') is descriptive of the characteristic lesion of HSV infection, which is a fluid-filled vesicle on an erythematous base. These vesicles may coalesce (that is, creep) to form the familiar ''cold sore'' (Plate 30, *D*). Vesicular lesions occur in most HSV infections except for some CNS infections.

Primary HSV infections are acquired by direct contact with secretions containing virus. Autoinoculation from one site to another also occurs.[112] For example, children with oral lesions may transfer virus to the genital tract. Infections occur worldwide, at all times of the year, and most commonly in lower socioeconomic groups. The incubation period of a primary infection is 2 to 11 days followed by several weeks of virus shedding. The period of viral shedding in recurrent infection is shorter (around 3 to 5 days). Various nonspecific factors such as fatigue, stress, menses, fever, trauma, and exposure to sun or cold often precede a recurrence. Lesions in recurrent disease usually appear at the same site with each episode. Host immune status and prior HSV infection with a different serotype affect extent of infection.

The majority of cutaneous infections above the waist are caused by HSV-1 and those below the waist by HSV-2. However, both types have been isolated from both areas.

Primary oral HSV-1 infections range from rhinitis, pharyngitis, or tonsillitis to severe acute gingivostomatitis. Infections are self-limited but may be followed by recurrent episodes of ''cold sores.'' Almost 50% of young adults have recurrent oral herpes, usually involving the mucocutaneous junction of the lip. Prodromal symptoms of tingling, burning, or itching occur in 60% to 75% of cases. Virus can be isolated from 85% to 90% of early lesions, but by 4 days most are culture negative.[155] Most afflicted populations have an average of less than one recurrence every 6 months (10% to 65%), but 5% to 25% have recurrences as frequently as once a month.

Primary herpetic eye infections are seen mainly in infancy and adolescence and like primary oral infections are associated with constitutional symptoms including fever. Herpetic keratitis is almost always caused by HSV-1. About 25% of primary eye infections recur, and about half of patients in this group have a second recurrence within 2 years. Recurrent HSV keratitis can result in visual impairment.[91]

About 80% to 90% of primary genital HSV infections are caused by HSV-2. The clinical course is similar to oral infections in that the primary infection is usually more severe (lesions are present 14 to 19 days) and is accompanied by systemic symptoms and longer viral shedding (8 to 11 days). Primary HSV-2 infection tends to be less severe in people with a previous HSV-1 infection.

The course of recurrent genital infections is also similar to that of recurrent oral infections. The majority of patients expe-

TABLE 49-1. Comparison of Herpes Simplex Viruses 1 and 2

Characteristic	HSV-1	HSV-2	Reference
Primary infection sites	Mouth, face, lips, eyes	Genitals, buttocks, thighs	132
Type of CNS infection	Encephalitis	Meningitis	132
Transmission	Oral, respiratory secretions	Genital secretions, mother to infant	132
Population with primary infection	Prepuberty	Postpuberty	106
Latent site (ganglia)	Trigeminal, superior cervical, vagal	Sacral	174
Temperature sensitivity (40° C)	−	+	111
Guanine + cytosine (moles/100 ml)	67	69	132
Pock size on chorioallantoic membrane	Small	Large	4
Plaques and cytopathic effect (CPE) in chick embryo cells	No	Yes	39
Neurovirulence in mice	Less	More	110
Ocular pathogenicity (rabbit cornea)	Less	More	114
Dermatotropic tendency	Little	Great (disseminated)	115

TABLE 49-2. Clinical Syndromes Associated with Herpes Simplex Viruses

Syndrome	HSV Serotype[a]	Primary or Recurrent	Age
Acute gingivostomatitis	1 (97%)	Primary	1-5 yr, young adults
Pharyngitis	1	Primary	Children, young adults
Herpes labialis	1 (80%-90%)	Recurrent	Children, adults
Genital herpes	2 (80%-90%)	Primary or recurrent	Post puberty
Neonatal herpes	2 (75%)	Primary	Newborn
Encephalitis	1	Primary or recurrent	All
Aseptic meningitis	2	Primary or recurrent	Young adults
Meningoencephalitis	2	Primary	Newborn
Disseminated, generalized	1, 2	Primary or recurrent	All

Data from references 106 and 116.

[a]The HSV serotype most commonly associated with each clinical syndrome is listed.

rience prodromal symptoms; maximum viral shedding and maximal pain occur within the first 2 days, and the duration of lesions is short.[58,142] Recurrences are frequent, although incidence is lower following a primary HSV-1 genital infection than it is following a primary HSV-2 genital infection.[134] Recurrences may be asymptomatic. In women most recurrent lesions are vulvar, but unnoticed cervical lesions may occur, and one third of women with recurrent vulvar lesions shed virus from the cervix.[58,142] Virus may be shed between recurrences.

An unfortunate and serious consequence of female genital infection is virus transmission to the newborn. Most infections in infants are due to HSV-2 and are acquired at birth. The risk of infection is about 10% in infants of mothers who have primary or recurrent genital HSV at 32 weeks' gestation. If virus is present at delivery, the risk is 40% to 60%, with half of infected babies having fatal or severe disease.[77] Only about 18% survive without apparent sequelae. Recent evidence suggests that maternal antibody is protective against perinatal acquisition of HSV.[128a] Risk of infection is greatly reduced if delivery is by cesarean section, so current recommendations for women with a history of genital herpes are to obtain specimens for culture each week from the thirty-sixth week until delivery.[56] Clinical examination alone is insufficient because virus may be shed from the cervix without occurrence of lesions.[77] Vaginal delivery should be considered if HSV culture results are negative in two successive examinations, one of which is within the week of delivery, and if no lesions are present at delivery.[10,19]

HSV infection acquired postnatally has been reported in several instances. These infections, the result of direct contact with active lesions, may have been caused by HSV-1 and had a mortality of 66%.[86] Some clinicians recommend separating infants from anyone with active lesions,[86] whereas others believe that covering any active lesions and not handling infants are sufficient.[104]

HSV infection in the central nervous system (CNS) may be a benign, self-limited aseptic meningitis caused by HSV-2 or a rapidly progressing, severe or even fatal encephalitis caused by HSV-1. Herpes encephalitis has a mortality of 60% to 80%, and less than 10% of patients survive without significant sequelae.[178] HSV-2 may cause severe meningoencephalitis in neonates, and HSV-2 infection can progress from meningitis to encephalitis in immunosuppressed patients. CNS HSV infection may be a consequence of primary or recurrent infection.

Generalized or disseminated HSV infection may occur in compromised hosts such as patients with severe burns, lymphoreticular malignancies, a renal transplant, or inherited immunodeficiency disease. The virus may disseminate to visceral organs such as the liver. Most disseminated disease is fatal.

Pathogenesis and Immune Response

Following primary infection of epithelial cells, HSV establishes a latent infection in sensory neurons including the trigeminal, sacral, thoracic, superior cervical, and vagal ganglia.[43,174] HSV-1 and HSV-2 appear to infect different ganglia (Table 49-1). The virus's latent form in nerve cells is not known nor is the reason for reactivation. Perhaps minimal or apparent trauma to the sensory root activates the latent virus.[121] Current theory suggests that the virus travels centripetally via the neuronal axons to sensory ganglia. Reactivated virus then travels centrifugally along the sensory nerves to the cutaneous site and again infects epithelial cells.

Epidemiologic studies suggest an association between cervical HSV-2 infection and cervical carcinoma.[106,133] Clearly women with a history of genital HSV-2 infection are at increased risk for cervical cancer. This is not true for any other sexually transmitted disease. HSV-2 is also associated with vulvar squamous cell carcinoma in situ.[75] This type of cancer has been increasing, which is perhaps related to increases in genital HSV infection. Although data linking HSV with human cancer strongly suggest a cause-and-effect relationship, research data are not yet conclusive.

Treatment and Control

Effective and safe vaccines against HSV are not yet available. Investigators are reluctant to use attenuated or even killed virus because of HSV's oncogenic potential and the fear of inducing latent infection in immunized persons. In addition, neutralizing antibody does not protect against recurrent disease. The safest and most effective vaccine may involve recombinant DNA–produced proteins or synthetic polypeptide.[159]

Several antiviral agents are effective for the treatment of ocular HSV infections, including iododeoxyuridine, adenine arabinoside, acyclovir,[36a] and trifluorothymidine.[104] Adenine arabinoside (Ara-A, vidarabine) significantly reduces the mor-

tality of herpes encephalitis,[180] especially in those less than 30 years old.[181] Vidarabine also appears to be beneficial for disseminated or CNS HSV infection in neonates.[12,64] A newer, more active antiviral agent, acyclovir, is being tested in clinical trials. Initial results indicate that it is effective for prevention of reactivated HSV in bone marrow transplant patients[144] and for treatment of severe mucocutaneous HSV in heart transplant patients.[16] Acyclovir reduced mortality of patients with HSV encephalitis to 19% compared with 50% in matched individuals treated with vidarabine.[152]

The discomfort and high incidence of recurrent oral and genital HSV have led to suggestions for many "curative" modalities, none of which have been effective when tested in double-blind, placebo-controlled studies. Topical, oral, and intravenous administration of acyclovir has demonstrated efficacy in the treatment of first episode genital HSV infections.[13,21,22] Recurrences, however, were not prevented, nor did the drug have much effect on recurrent lesions. Oral treatment does reduce systemic symptoms such as malaise and fever.

LABORATORY DIAGNOSIS
Specimen Types

Specimens for HSV isolation include vesicular fluid or scrapings from lesions, throat swabs, conjunctival scrapings, tissue (lung, brain, or liver), and spinal fluid. Alginate swabs should not be used for specimen collection if tissue culture is not immediately inoculated.[24] Cotton, rayon, Dacron, and polyester are acceptable. If kept moist, specimens from lesions may be stored at 4°C for 48 hours with little loss in virus titer.[183]

Direct Examination

Direct examination of clinical specimens for HSV detection is widely used (Table 49-3). Lesion or conjunctival scrapings and tissue may be examined. Methods for direct detection of HSV include electron microscopy, Tzanck preparation, Papanicolaou smear (Plate 30, E), direct and indirect immunofluorescence, and immunoperoxidase. Cytologic examination of cell scrapings is inexpensive and fast but is not as sensitive or specific as immunofluorescence or immunoperoxidase.[132,170] Commercial reagents are available for both direct and indirect immunofluorescence[51,52] and immunoperoxidase tests. Immunofluorescence is not as sensitive as virus culture; it detects HSV in about 80% of culture-positive specimens from vesicular lesions.[79a,102,141,146] If tests are properly controlled and high-quality monoclonal reagents are used, false-positive results are not a problem. Obtaining adequate specimens is critical.[102,141] At least 25 exfoliated epithelial cells must be seen to evaluate a specimen.[102]

Indirect immunoperoxidase tests do not require a fluorescence microscope and may be slightly more sensitive than immunofluorescence. Sensitivity of both methods decreases with the age of the lesion.[20,141]

Virus Isolation

Although HSV can infect many laboratory animals, including mice, guinea pigs, rabbits, and hamsters, animals are now used mainly for research rather than for viral isolation. HSV is easily isolated from a number of cell cultures. HSV reportedly grows best in either primary rabbit kidney (RK) cells or human embryonic lung (HEL) fibroblast cells.[14,98] Fetal diploid cell

TABLE 49-3. Appearance of Herpes Simplex Virus–Infected Cells in Direct Preparations

Method	Appearance of HSV-Infected Cells	Comment	References
Tzanck preparation (Giemsa stain)	Giant cells (cell nucleus has diameter three times diameter of a leukocyte, the nucleus/cytoplasm ratio at least 1:1, and cell diameter no greater than one and a half times diameter of nucleus) and intranuclear inclusions	Detects HSV	170
Papanicolaou preparation	Multinucleated giant cells with eosinophilic inclusion bodies	Detects HSV	18, 132
Immunofluorescence Exfoliated epithelial cells	HSV-1: perinuclear, apple-green fluorescence; nucleus clearly distinguishable; HSV-2: homogeneous diffuse staining of entire cell; nucleus not always clearly distinguishable	Detects HSV and indicates stage of infection; patterns of fluorescence vary with conjugate and stage of infection	4, 11, 141, 146, 164
Brain	Fluorescence is usually associated with larger motor neurons and glial cells in cerebral cortex; it is seen in both cytoplasm and nucleus and may extend outward into associated axons		
Immunoperoxidase	Dark red-brown nuclear and cytoplasmic staining to distinct cytoplasmic rimming without nuclear staining	Detects HSV	6, 102

lines, such as WI-38 and MRC-5, are widely used for HSV isolation. Primary HEK, HEp-2, and HeLa cells also support the growth of HSV, although the sensitivity and rate of HSV recovery are low compared with use of RK or HEL cells.

CPE depends on the type of cells infected as well as the strain of HSV. Cell rounding and clumping, as well as syncytia and giant cells, may be seen (Plate 30, F). HSV-2 infection tends to increase syncytial cell formation and piling up of cells. Initially rounded cells or foci of clear areas with a ring of infected cells may appear and later enlarge to cover the entire monolayer.

The time for the first appearance of CPE depends on the cells used and the amount of virus in the specimen. Cell cultures inoculated with specimens of vesicular fluid may show CPE in less than 24 hours, whereas cells inoculated with a throat swab or a cervical swab from an asymptomatic patient may take a week or longer. The vast majority of positive specimens are positive within 7 days. In most laboratories 80% to 90% of positive specimens are detected within 48 hours. Cell culture amplification of virus combined with centrifugation and subsequent staining with monoclonal antibodies provides a diagnosis 16 hours after inoculation with no loss of sensitivity compared with conventional tube cell culture methodology.[52] Cell culture amplification with subsequent fluorescent antibody detection of viral antigens with biotin-avidin or the direct assay of herpes simplex virus with a capture biotin-streptavidin assay have also been used for rapid tests.[108,109] Without cell culture amplification of the virus or detection with a biotin-avidin assay, the sensitivity of viral detection in enzyme-linked immunosorbent assay (ELISA) falls to below 70%.[101]

Although isolates may be confirmed as HSV by a number of methods, most laboratories use immunofluorescence or less commonly immunoperoxidase testing.

The two HSV types can be differentiated biologically (Plate 31, A to C) or serologically. Serologic techniques used include immunofluorescence,[52] radioimmunoassay,[45] immunoperoxidase,[6] mixed agglutination,[71] ELISA,[96,109a] neutralization,[133] and complement-dependent cytotoxicity. Addition of monoclonal antibody to purified HSV glycoprotein antigens has eliminated past problems with cross-reactions between HSV-1 and HSV-2.

Immunofluorescence is the most widely used technique but can be difficult to interpret unless monoclonal antibodies are used. Commercial monoclonal reagents for HSV typing are available. The pattern of fluorescent staining may vary with type (Table 49-3).

Biologic methods, such as the differential susceptibility of HSV-1 and HSV-2 to (E)-5-(2-bromvinyl)-2′deoxyuridine[92] and DNA hybridization,[11] are available only in research laboratories.

Serologic Diagnosis

As in other viral infections, when immune response to a primary HSV infection is measured by complement fixation with whole virus antigens, antibody rises within 10 to 14 days after infection with a peak at 4 to 6 weeks. During a recurrence or reinfection with the same or a different HSV serotype, titers often do not increase.

In children and adults IgM appears early and is not detectable after about 8 weeks. In newborns IgM appears within the first 2 to 4 weeks and may persist for months. An infant's IgG response is dependent on the maternal antibody titer. Generally mother and infant titers at birth are equal. However, in an HSV-infected infant, the titer persists and may increase over time. In a noninfected infant, passively transferred maternal antibody is usually undetectable by 6 months. If the mother's primary HSV infection occurred near delivery, the infected infant has a response similar to an older child's because little maternal antibody is transferred.[107]

Current serologic tests do not differentiate between HSV-1

and HSV-2 because the major antibody response to both viruses is to common rather than type-specific antigens.[94] Vestergaard and others have examined immune response to 10 glycoproteins of HSV-1 and HSV-2. The principal immunogens in human infection are two shared antigenic determinants. Antibodies are formed against type-specific antigens in low amounts.[171] By using these type-specific glycoproteins it should now be possible to develop serologic tests that will measure type-specific immune response. The relationships between antibody to type-specific antigenic determinants and various clinical syndromes, latency, and recurrence are not known.

Serologic diagnosis of HSV currently is useful only for a primary HSV infection. Complement fixation has been commonly used, but new, commercially available procedures are at least as sensitive and are easier to perform. A solid-phase immunofluorescence technique (FIAX) is as sensitive as complement fixation,[7] and an enzyme immunoassay is more sensitive.[25] Antibody may also be detected by neutralization or indirect immunofluorescence. None of these tests clearly distinguishes between HSV-1 and HSV-2 infection.

Some cross-reactivity exists between HSV and varicella-zoster virus, particularly when complement fixation is used to measure antibody response. Patients with a past HSV infection and primary varicella-zoster virus may have an antibody rise to HSV, and vice versa. Usually the homologous titer is higher.

Serologic tests are not acceptable for the diagnosis of HSV encephalitis. Although about 80% of patients seroconvert, so do 15% to 20% of patients with other neurologic diseases.[107] Similar patterns of antibody response are seen in the cerebrospinal fluid (CSF). Many patients have a serum/CSF ratio ≤ 20, but this may not be demonstrable until late in infection.[107] Culture of brain tissue is still the only definitive method of diagnosing HSV encephalitis.

VARICELLA-ZOSTER VIRUS

Herpesvirus varicellae, or varicella-zoster virus (VZV), like all members of the *Herpesviridae* family, is a DNA virus surrounded by a lipid envelope. It causes chickenpox (varicella) as a primary infection and shingles (zoster) when reactivated. Zoster was described in medieval times, but varicella was not differentiated as a disease from smallpox until almost 1900. In 1909, Von Bokay published his postulate that chickenpox and shingles were caused by the same agent. Evidence for the dual role of VZV gradually accumulated until final proof was obtained with the ability to grow the viruses in the laboratory. Antigenic and restriction enzyme analysis[113] clearly show that one strain of VZV causes both chickenpox and shingles. Humans are the only natural hosts for VZV. Antigens of VZV studied to date include a membrane antigen,[184] a soluble complement fixation (CF) antigen in vesicular fluid, and three glycoproteins that are major nucleocapsid polypeptides.[186]

VZV remains in close association with the host cells, and thus the condition of the cell culture greatly influences the laboratory's ability to grow and maintain the virus. VZV is highly labile and is best preserved by using stabilizing agents such as sorbitol or skim milk.

CLINICAL SIGNIFICANCE

Chickenpox is usually a mild, generalized vesicular eruption occurring primarily in children under 10 years of age. Lesions first appear on the scalp or trunk and spread toward the extremities. Crops of lesions appear for several days, so different stages (papules, vesicles, crusts) are present at the same time. In smallpox, which was formerly clinically confused with chickenpox, the lesions at any one time are all at the same stage.

Initial viral replication presumably occurs in the oropharynx and results in a viremia, followed by virus dissemination to the skin. Usually viremia is transient and of low level, but in severe or progressive varicella viremia persists.[103] The virus then establishes a latent infection.

Although chickenpox is normally a mild disease, it can be severe and even fatal in certain circumstances, particularly in immunosuppressed children, especially those with leukemia or a transplanted kidney.[100,126] Primary infection is more severe in adults, and complications such as encephalitis and disseminated fatal disease can occur but are rare.

Because VZV can infect the fetus in utero, chickenpox is of special concern to the 6% to 14% of women of childbearing age who have never had chickenpox.[49] Manifestations of congenital varicella are varied and depend on the time the maternal infection occurs during pregnancy. Severe fetal infection can occur if the virus is contracted during the first trimester or within a few days of delivery.

Chickenpox occurs in epidemic-like fashion in winter and spring. It is highly contagious, with an estimated incidence of about 1500 cases/100,000 population.[125] Although transmission is primarily by droplet and direct contact, airborne transmission has been documented.[82] Patients are probably most infectious from 1 to 2 days before the rash appears to 5 or 6 days later. Virus is shed for 3 to 5 days after onset.

Shingles or zoster is caused by a reactivation of VZV and occurs in about 1% to 2% of people.[175] Vesicular lesions appear unilaterally following a dermatomal distribution (Plate 31, *D*). In order of frequency the ganglia affected are the thoracic, cervical, lumbar, facial, and sacral. Zoster is seen sporadically in all seasons and in all age groups but is much more common and severe in older people, especially those over 60 years of age. Incidence and severity of zoster are higher in immunosuppressed patients, particularly those with lymphoma, leukemia, and organ transplants. The incidence is as high as 7% to 25% in those with Hodgkin's disease.[27] Although zoster is very painful, mortality, even if the disease is disseminated, is very low.[27,93]

Pathogenesis of shingles is unresolved. The site of latency is thought to be the dorsal root ganglia.[70] Reactivation is often associated with surgery or trauma to the ganglia. Presumably the virus then travels back along the nerve to the skin.

Treatment and Control

Treatment is rarely necessary for chickenpox except in immunosuppressed children and neonates exposed in utero. Treatment by passive immunization with varicella-zoster immune globulin (VZIG) or plasma is effective if given within 72 hours of VZV exposure.[15] Passive immunization has no effect on zoster.[57] Vidarabine[179] and acyclovir are effective in treatment of zoster but do not significantly decrease postzoster neuralgia.[3,5,148,176]

Although VZIG is now more easily obtained than in the past, it is expensive. Therefore trials have been initiated in the United States with a varicella vaccine developed by the Japanese that appears to be effective in preventing chickenpox and has few or no side effects. If this vaccine is given within 72 hours after VZV exposure has occurred, susceptible children are also protected.[1]

LABORATORY DIAGNOSIS

Most cases of VZV infection are diagnosed clinically, but laboratory confirmation is sometimes essential. Unusual manifestations of HSV can closely resemble zoster,[87] and varicella must be distinguished from smallpox, vaccinia, or enteroviral infection. HSV and VZV eye infections must be differentiated because their treatment is different.[90]

Specimen Types

The specimen of choice for virus isolation is material from a vesicular lesion. Virus has also been isolated from the buffy coat fraction of the blood of patients with progressive varicella,[93] the spinal fluid, tissue, and joint fluid.[128]

Direct Examination

Lesion scrapings (but not vesicular fluid) can be stained with Giemsa stain and examined for intranuclear inclusions in multinucleated giant cells. Electron microscopy can be used to visualize viral particles but offers no advantage over light microscopy. Neither method is specific for VZV. Fluorescent antibody (FA) staining has proved simple, specific, and more sensitive than virus isolation[28] and is the preferred method for VZV detection. Diagnosis of VZV by ELISA techniques has been shown to be a sensitive assay but is not yet commercially available.[185]

Virus Isolation

Except in immunosuppressed patients or those with disseminated disease, virus isolation should be attempted only if specimens are collected within 72 hours of onset. Patients with severe disease may shed virus for as long as 10 days and may also be viremic.

VZV grows in a number of human cell lines, but the most commonly used are the human fetal diploid cells, WI-38 or MRC-5. CPE is focal and in MRC-5 is characterized by a small group of swollen, refractile cells with spread of infection to adjacent cells (Plate 31, *E*). Extension of CPE depends on the presence of a uniform, healthy monolayer. CPE usually appears by the fourth day but may take longer. To transfer virus to fresh cell culture, cells (not cell culture medium) must be passed because VZV is cell associated. Isolates can be confirmed by CF or FA.

Serologic Diagnosis

Humoral antibody response to primary infection with VZV is characterized by the presence of IgG and IgM antibody at onset of the rash or a few days later. Peak titers are reached in 2 to 3 weeks. IgM declines to undetectable levels within 2 months. IgG antibody probably would be found for life if measured by sensitive methods. CF titers are often negative in 6 to 12 months.[23,48,153]

Antibody may or may not be detectable at the onset of zoster depending on the sensitivity of the test method, but all zoster patients are antibody positive within several days of onset.[48,153]

The CF test is the most widely used procedure for serologic diagnosis of VZV infection. Any titer is evidence of past varicella infection. The CF test is useful only for confirmation of primary infection, and a rise in titer must be demonstrated. Immune status should not be measured by CF because titers are often negative after 1 year.

More sensitive serologic tests have been developed for antibody screening of children before administration of VZIG. The most frequently used is the fluorescent antibody to varicella-induced membrane antigen (FAMA) test.[184] An anticomplement immunofluorescence test using VZV-infected substrate cells (Bion Enterprises, Park Ridge, Ill.) is as sensitive as the FAMA test.[127] Neutralization tests are the most sensitive for antibody detection but are tedious and time consuming.

One problem with all serologic tests for VZV antibody is the heterotypic antibody response that sometimes occurs in persons with a previous HSV infection.[23,44] When infected with VZV they may have a titer rise in complement fixation HSV antibody. Conversely, if VZV IgG is present at the time of a primary HSV infection, a fourfold or greater rise in VZV antibody can occur.[23] Thus serologic tests may be difficult to interpret and are not the method of choice in confirming VZV infection.

CYTOMEGALOVIRUS

Cytomegalovirus (CMV), a member of the *Herpesviridae* family, is widespread in nature, infecting both humans and animals. It is very species specific, although some serologic cross-reactions occur between human CMV and simian CMV. Human CMV, also called "salivary gland virus," was isolated by Smith, Weller, and their co-workers and by Rowe and co-workers in 1955 from tissue and urine of infants with cytomegalic inclusion disease. Association of CMV with adult infection occurred 10 years later.

CMV does not survive well outside the body. Viral titer is decreased substantially by freezing and thawing, and preservation of virus requires low-temperature freezing with 35% sorbitol or glycerol for stabilization. CMV is inactivated by heat (56° C for 30 minutes), acid (pH less than 5), and ultraviolet irradiation, and like other herpes viruses is ether and chloroform sensitive.

CMV's antigenic structure has not been well defined. Antigenic heterogeneity among human isolates occurs with considerable cross-reactivity,[154,172] but no epidemiologic relationship exists among serologically heterogeneous isolates, nor do they fall into antigenic groups.

Results of DNA endonuclease analysis of CMV show many different strains.[26] As with HSV, only strains that are epidemiologically related have identical patterns.[69]

CLINICAL SIGNIFICANCE

CMV infections are very common and may occur in utero, at birth, or later in life. Clinical disease, however, is uncommon, and its occurrence depends on the age and immune competence of the infected individual.

Congenital Infection

About 0.5% to 2.5% of infants are congenitally infected with CMV,[117,157] although the majority are asymptomatic. Symptomatic babies with congenital CMV may have jaundice, hepatosplenomegaly, growth retardation, motor disability, ophthalmologic abnormalities, and hearing loss.[117] Almost all symptomatic babies have serious sequelae, and a substantial number of asymptomatic babies develop neurologic sequelae, with subnormal intelligence or mental retardation and hearing loss the most common.[60,117,120,137] Congenitally infected infants usually are excreting virus at birth and may continue to excrete for months.

Congenital infection is most commonly the result of a primary CMV infection of the nonimmune mother during pregnancy. However, the fetus of an immune mother is not protected from infection. Endogenous CMV appears to be the source of virus in intrauterine infections in immune women.[69] None of the infected babies of these women has been symptomatic at birth.[157]

Perinatal Infection

CMV infection acquired at birth or early in life by normal infants is also rarely clinically apparent. Cervically shed virus is probably the source for most perinatal infections, although CMV is also found in breast milk and can be acquired by ingestion.[117,124] Approximately 3% to 25% of women shed CMV from the cervix consistently or, more commonly, intermittently.[8,124,173] Cervically shed virus is usually reactivated endogenous virus and has never been associated with disease in these women.[8]

When infants are infected with CMV during birth or shortly after, virus is not excreted for 4 to 8 weeks but is then shed in saliva, urine, and the nasopharynx for several months.

Childhood and Adult Infection

Between the ages of 11 and 50 years, the risk of CMV infection is about 0.5% to 1% per year. Almost all infections are asymptomatic[46] except in some young adults and in immunocompromised hosts. In young adults CMV causes about 7% to 8% of infectious mononucleosis–like syndromes.[78] Unlike Epstein-Barr virus (EBV) infection, however, pharyngitis, tonsillitis, lymphadenopathy, and splenomegaly are rare.[46,66]

CMV infection is a major problem in organ and bone marrow transplant recipients and in patients with AIDS. The most common syndromes in these patients are prolonged fever, pneumonitis, hepatitis, and leukopenia associated with a long period of virus excretion.[122,162,169] Retinitis has also been reported.[124] A suppressant effect on host defenses occurs, predisposing the patient to a usually fatal superinfection (see Chapter 2).[122]

Adult infection is usually acquired by close contact with previously infected individuals who may shed virus in the urine and nasopharynx for several months. Sexual contact is also a likely means of transmission.[59] Disease in the compromised transplant patient may be the result of primary infection acquired from the transplanted organ[119] or activation of latent infection.[2]

Latent infection with CMV clearly occurs, although reactivation is not accompanied by disease except in immunosuppressed hosts.[74] Neither the mechanism and site of latency nor the form in which the virus persists is known. During primary infection CMV can be isolated from mononuclear and polymorphonuclear leukocytes,[31] but after clinical recovery virus cannot be isolated from the blood. Viral DNA has been detected in lymphoid cells,[68] and it has been suggested that a small percentage of lymphocytes, which release small amounts of virus,

supports CMV replication and results in long-term persistence.[143]

Treatment and Control

Trials of antiviral drugs such as vidarabine and interferon have been unsuccessful for treatment of CMV.[89,95] A new drug, structurally related to acyclovir, provides promise of effective treatment of CMV infections.[37,149] Immunization trials with live attenuated virus are in progress,[123] although the vaccine is controversial.

Health-care workers are often concerned about acquiring CMV from infected patients, especially infants. The risk of primary infection, however, is no greater among pediatric health-care workers than it is among young women in the community at large.[29] The general precautions taken when handling possibly contaminated materials should provide sufficient protection from CMV infection.

LABORATORY DIAGNOSIS
Specimen Types

Urine is the usual specimen for detection and culture of CMV. Virus may also be isolated from saliva, tears, breast milk, semen, vaginal or cervical secretions, and, in acute disease, blood. For optimal recovery, both urine and oropharyngeal secretions should be cultured. CMV has been isolated from fluid obtained by amniocentesis[182] and from CSF.[72]

CMV is highly susceptible to freezing and thawing; therefore specimens not cultured immediately should be held at 4° C. After a week at 4° C viral titers drop about a half logarithm.[158] For attempted long-term storage, freezing with a stabilizing material (sorbitol or glycerol) is necessary.

Centrifugation of urine has been suggested as a means of increasing virus yield; however, urinary sediment is often toxic. The best yield is obtained by diluting unspun urine 1:2 or 1:3 before inoculation.[84]

Direct Examination

Cytologic examination of urine sediment cells for inclusions may be useful in detecting congenital CMV. Cells with inclusions are large (25 to 35 μm in diameter) and contain a large, basophilic, prominent, central, intranuclear inclusion that is separated from the thickened nuclear membrane by a clear zone (Plate 31, F). These inclusions resemble an owl's eye.

Cytology is about one third to one half as sensitive as culture in detecting congenital CMV and even less sensitive in adult cases.

Electron microscopy is also not specific for CMV, but rapid procedures such as pseudoreplication can provide results within 30 minutes. The yield is very high in specimens from infants less than 6 months old, with at least 10 virus particles per milliliter.[83]

Both direct FA and ELISA techniques may eventually be useful for rapid detection of CMV in clinical specimens, but use of these techniques is currently hampered by the inavailability of appropriate high-titer antisera. Monoclonal antibodies to CMV may alleviate some of these problems in the future.[38]

Virus Isolation

No laboratory animals are susceptible to human CMV. The virus grows in human fibroblast cells (WI-38, MRC-5, neonatal foreskin) producing a cytopathic effect (CPE) in anywhere from 24 hours to a month depending on virus titer. Focal CPE with rounded, refractile cells is characteristic, usually occurring in the center of the monolayer rather than at the edge (Plate 31, *F*).

The foci slowly enlarge but rarely involve the whole monolayer.[136] A rapid test has been developed in which (after centrifugation of specimens onto coverslips) viral amplification occurs, with monolayers of fibroblast cells in shell vials. Early antigens of CMV are detected by staining with monoclonal antibodies in a fluorescence assay 16 hours after inoculation.[150]

Cell culture isolates may be identified by a number of methods including CF, neutralization, and FA. FA examination must be interpreted with care. Prominently staining nuclear inclusions are seen, as well as nonspecific perinuclear cytoplasmic inclusions. CMV-infected cells develop Fc receptors in the cytoplasm, which bind IgG nonspecifically.[177] One way to avoid this nonspecific fluorescence is with an anticomplement immunofluorescence assay.[145] Serologic tests are often used for both diagnosis and epidemiologic studies because virus isolation can take several weeks. In newborns, however, the amount of virus excreted is high, and serologic results are difficult to interpret. Therefore the best way to diagnose congenital CMV is virus isolation from urine.

Serologic Diagnosis

Humoral immune response to CMV infection in young children and adults is similar to the response to other viral infections, with antibody to early antigens appearing first followed by antibody to late antigens. Distinguishing primary infection from reactivation, persistent primary infection, or superinfection by another strain may not be possible.[117] In primary infection CF antibody levels rise before neutralizing antibody levels, and in reactivated infection both rise together. The presence of antibody to early antigen or CMV-specific IgM is not necessarily indicative of a primary infection because people who are shedding CMV frequently have antibody to early antigen.[47,55]

The immune response in congenital CMV is similar to the response seen in other congenitally acquired infections.

The CF test has been the most widely used for measuring antibody response to CMV. Two complement-fixing antigens have been isolated, one by freezing and thawing infected cells and the other by glycine buffer extraction. Procedures using CF antigen prepared by freeze-thaw methods are not as sensitive as those using alkaline glycine buffer–extracted antigen.[9] The indirect fluorescent antibody (IFA) test is rapidly replacing the CF test, since it is simpler to perform and reagents are commercially available. Antibodies detected by IFA appear earlier, and the procedure can be used to determine different classes of antibody as well as antibodies to various types of antigens, such as early antigens.[9]

The incidence of false-positive IFA results for CMV IgM is significant.[158] Some are due to rheumatoid factors and some to EBV infection. CMV IgM is present in about half the cases of acute EBV infection.[8] False-positive results can be reduced by removing the anti–IgG-IgM by sucrose gradient centrifugation[139] or by absorbing sera with antiserum to Fc receptors.[62]

Another problem with the IFA test is nonspecific cytoplas-

mic staining. It can be eliminated by removing the cytoplasm from infected cells before staining,[156,166] by using a simian strain of CMV that cross-reacts with human CMV but does not induce Fc receptors in the infected cell,[163] or by using an anti-complement immunofluorescence assay.[76,97,130] None of these techniques is now available commercially. Other methods available for measuring CMV antibody include ELISA (Abbott Labs, North Chicago, Ill.; M.A. Bioproducts, Walkersville, Md.; Litton Bionetics, Kensington, Md.),[138] and a fluorescence immunoassay (FIAX, International Diagnostic Technology, Santa Clara, Calif.).[7,147] The commercially available IFA, ELISA, and FIA tests appear to be acceptable for detecting CMV antibody.

Unfortunately, even with appropriately timed acute and convalescent sera, results of CMV serologic tests can be difficult to interpret. In immune persons titers can fluctuate as much as fourfold. Viral shedding can occur with minimal or no changes in titer. Compromised hosts usually have a rapid rise in titer and may also have a reappearance of IgM antibody.

EPSTEIN-BARR VIRUS

Epstein-Barr virus (EBV) is the major cause of the syndrome infectious mononucleosis (IM), the ''kissing disease.'' The clinical syndrome of IM was described in 1920, and by 1932 Paul and Bunnell recognized its association with the presence of heterophil antibodies in the serum. In 1967 the viral etiology of heterophil positive IM was confirmed.

EBV was first detected microscopically by Epstein, Achong, and Barr in 1964 when they found herpeslike particles in biopsy cultures from a lymphoma of the head and neck called Burkitt's lymphoma (BL). BL is the most common childhood cancer in Africa. An infectious agent was being sought because BL occurred in clusters in areas where mosquito-transmitted infections such as malaria and yellow fever were common.

In an attempt to clarify the association between EBV and BL, Gertrude and Werner Henle developed an indirect immunofluorescence test to survey BL patients for EBV antibody. To their surprise, not only did patients from Africa with BL have antibody, but so did most African children as well as children from many parts of the world.

The pieces of this puzzle began to fall into place in the winter of 1967 when IM developed in one of the Henles' technicians. A serum specimen collected after her illness contained EBV antibody, whereas a specimen stored in the laboratory before her illness had no antibody. Futher epidemiologic studies have confirmed that EBV is the cause of heterophil-positive mononucleosis. Heterophil-negative, IM-like illness may also be caused by EBV, as well as by CMV and *Toxoplasma gondii*.

In addition to IM and African BL, EBV is associated with nasopharyngeal carcinoma (NPC) in Southern China. Like patients with African BL, those with NPC have high antibody titers to EBV, and virus can be demonstrated in cultured tumor cells.[34] Antibody response to EBV antigens in BL and NPC, however, differs from the pattern seen in patients with a past EBV infection and no malignancy.

High titers of EBV antibodies have also been found in patients with Hodgkin's disease[36] and with rheumatoid arthritis,[165] but no viral particles or EBV genetic material has been demonstrated in cells from these patients. Although it is tempting to conclude that EBV is the cause of all these syndromes, especially BL and NPC, further proof is required. The incidence of EBV-induced B cell lymphoma after renal transplantation, however, strongly supports an etiologic role for this virus in some neoplastic diseases.[61]

Why one virus, EBV, is associated with such different syndromes is not known. The Henles believe that these differences depend on epidemiologic and other factors rather than strain differences in the virus.[63] These variables include age at primary infection, type of primary infection, immune response and antibodies produced, and various cofactors such as malaria, genetic predisposition, and exposure to environmental carcinogens.

Like other herpesviruses, EBV is an enveloped DNA virus that is ubiquitous in humans. Only one strain of EBV is recognized to infect humans.[63]

CLINICAL SIGNIFICANCE

IM is an acute, benign lymphoproliferative disease. In developing countries or among lower socioeconomic groups, infection occurs early in life, and by 10 years of age 70% to 90% of children have been infected.[34] Usually infection in children is asymptomatic or mild and may be associated with minor illnesses such as an upper respiratory infection, pharyngitis, tonsillitis, bronchitis, and otitis media. Lymphadenopathy and skin rashes may occur.[40,131,161]

In developed countries or among higher socioeconomic groups, infection is more likely to be delayed until older childhood or young adulthood. At this age the host response to infection is more likely to be clinically apparent IM.[34] EBV mononucleosis is characterized by sore throat, fatigue, fever, lymph node enlargement, and often an enlarged spleen. Usually patients have mild subclinical liver disease with elevated liver enzyme levels. By their early twenties, about 50% to 60% of Americans show serologic evidence of infection.[34]

The clinical spectrum of infection produced by EBV has been greatly expanded recently with the association of this virus with a chronic or persistent infection. The syndrome has been characterized by profound fatigue, myalgia, mild pharyngitis, tender adenopathy, and low-grade fever. The symptoms have been found to recur one to six times yearly.[73,160]

Rare complications of IM include aplastic anemia,[81] ruptured spleen, and neurologic syndromes, such as encephalitis[80] and Guillain-Bárre syndrome. Most people recover completely from the infection, and fatalities are unusual.

Contrary to its name, EBV IM is not highly contagious and infection probably requires close contact (for example, a family member) with someone shedding EBV in his or her saliva.[42] Virus excreters include people recently infected, who may shed virus up to 18 months, and previously infected normal adults, 15% of whom are virus positive at any one time. EBV has also been spread by blood transfusion[129] and transplantation.[88]

EBV enters the patient's body through the oropharynx, where it probably infects either specialized lymphoid cells or some type of epithelial cell and undergoes a productive replicative cycle.[151] The type of cell that is infected is unknown, but buccal, pharyngeal, palatine mucosa, and tonsillar lymphocytes are all negative for infectious EBV.[99] Dissemination from the oropharynx may occur in two ways: either EBV infects B lymphocytes and produces infectious virus that is spread to other B lymphocytes by the blood; or infected B cells circulate

and release infectious virus that infects other B lymphocytes.[32]

EBV can follow two pathways in the B lymphocyte. It can undergo a productive replicative cycle resulting in the release of mature virus and in cell death, or it can become latent.[33] Both situations are found in infected individuals. In latently infected cells the full cytocidal replicative cycle does not occur and only early antigens are expressed. The early membrane antigen on infected cells is specifically recognized by T killer cells and stimulates their production. The large number of activated T cells causes lymph node hyperplasia and tonsillar and adenoidal changes resulting in the sore throat and atypical lymphocytes seen in patients with EBV IM. The T cells also destroy many of the latently infected B cells, so antigenic stimulation is decreased followed by a decrease in T cells. Unlike B lymphocytes from uninfected people, latently EBV-infected B cells can divide continuously, thereby producing cells carrying the virus genome. A small percentage can be spontaneously activated to a lytic cycle, and thus low levels of virus are produced throughout an individual's life.

Treatment of IM is mainly supportive. Although acyclovir inhibits DNA replication in productively infected cells, it has little effect on viral DNA synthesis in latently infected cells.[17] A vaccine against EBV infection used in people at high risk for development of BL and NPC could provide protection against EBV infection; it might also reduce the incidence of these malignancies and thus support the theory of the role of EBV as their cause. No vaccine is available, but a first step, the isolation of a DNA-free membrane antigen, has been reported. Antibodies to this antigen neutralize EBV infection of lymphocytes in vitro.[167]

LABORATORY DIAGNOSIS

EBV can be detected in cultured B lymphocytes of infected persons by IFA, but this is mainly a research tool. The mainstay of laboratory diagnosis is hematologic and serologic tests. Peripheral blood of patients with EBV IM contains 50% or more lymphocytes of which at least 10% are large atypical cells with deeply basophilic cytoplasm and sequestered nuclei. Diagnosis is confirmed by a heterophil antibody response or by showing the development of specific EBV antibody.

Heterophil Tests

Heterophil tests detect the presence of heterophil antibodies and are the first-line tests for the laboratory diagnosis of IM. Heterophil antibodies, which are mostly IgM, are antibodies that occur in one species but react with antigens of a different species. Heterophil antibodies appear in IM, in serum sickness, and even in the sera of healthy individuals. In the last instance the antibodies are referred to as Forssman antibodies. Forssman antibodies and the heterophil antibodies of IM and serum sickness all agglutinate sheep red blood cells (RBCs) and horse RBCs.

To distinguish the heterophil antibodies of IM, a differential absorption test based on the early work of Davidsohn is used. The test involves two absorption procedures; in the first a portion of the serum is absorbed with guinea pig cells, and in the second a portion is absorbed with beef cells. Sheep (or horse; see below) RBCs are added to each of the absorbed sera. Absorption of serum with guinea pig cells removes the anti–sheep agglutinins of healthy individuals and of patients with

TABLE 49-4. Sensitivity and Specificity of Serologic Tests for EBV Infectious Mononucleosis[35,a]

| | | Positive Sera (%) | | | | | | | |
| | | Weeks after Onset | | | Months after Onset | | | | |
Test	False-Positive before IM (%)	1	2	3	1	2	3	4-6	12
EBV SPECIFIC									
VCA-IgG	0	88	93	100	93	97	100	100	100
VCA-IgM	1.3	82	87	100	85	72	45	15	0
HETEROPHIL									
Sheep RBC	12	69	80	80	75	90	50	35	25
Horse RBC	6.7	86	100	100	95	98	98	85	70
Ox cell hemolysin	0	69	86	100	75	75	10	10	0

[a]The ox cell hemolysin and VCA-IgM determinations are the most sensitive. The most specific are the VCA-IgG and ox cell hemolysin. Heterophil tests using horse cells are often positive 1 year after infection. Ox cell hemolysin and VCA-IgM findings are usually negative in 2 to 3 months.

TABLE 49-5. Antibodies Produced in Response to EBV Infection (IM)

Antigen	Time of Appearance	Method of Detection	Cases Positive (%)	Length of Persistence	Comments
Horse RBC	Usually first week	Agglutination, hemolysis	100	1 yr	Heterophil antibody
Sheep RBC	Usually first week	Agglutination	80	2-4 mo	Heterophil antibody
Viral capsid antigen					
IgG	At onset	IFA	100	Life	Indicates past infection
IgM	At onset	IFA	100	4-8 wk	Indicates present infection
Membrane antigen					
Early		FA, IFA	100	Life	Found in most viral carriers
Late		Blocking FA			Technically difficult
Early antigens					
Diffuse	3-4 wk after onset	IFA	80	Transient	Diffuse staining, nucleus and cytoplasm
Restricted	2 wk to several months after onset	IFA	low	Up to 1 yr	Mass in cytoplasm, usually seen in BL
EB nuclear antigen	3-4 wk	ACIF[a]	100	Life	Absence of EBNA with VCA Ab[b] equals acute infection
Soluble CF (antigens)	3-4 wk	CF	100	Life	
VP (enveloped virus)	3-4 wk	Neutralization	100	Life	

[a]Anticomplement immunofluorescence.
[b]Antibody.

serum sickness but does not remove the anti–sheep agglutinins of patients with IM. Absorption of serum with beef cells removes the anti–sheep agglutinins of patients with IM but may or may not remove the anti–sheep agglutinins of patients with serum sickness or of those with normal sera.

Many commercial slide test kits are available for the diagnosis of IM. All are based on the differential absorption principle and use citrated horse RBCs, formalinized horse RBCs, or formalinized sheep RBCs. All appear to be acceptable,[53] but those using citrated horse cells are more sensitive (Table 49-4).

Sometimes heterophil antibodies are difficult to detect in children; with the commonly used kit procedures only 30% to 60% of findings in children under 5 years old are positive.[40] Less than 1% of positive heterophil tests are false positive; those that are occur with diseases such as rubella, viral hepatitis, leukemia, lymphomas, and malaria. Rarely, false-positive results occur in tests on noninfected persons.[67]

The ox cell hemolysin test measures a more specific but shorter-lived heterophil antibody. The antibody titer is measured by the dilution of antiserum that lyses ox RBCs in the presence of complement. A titer of at least 1:40 is diagnostic. The ox cell hemolysin test may be used to evaluate a possible false-positive slide test.[54] The most sensitive of the heterophil tests is immune adherence hemagglutination,[85] which can be used to demonstrate antibodies in young children.[41]

If there is a strong clinical suspicion of IM in a patient with atypical lymphocytes and negative heterophil test findings, measurement of EBV-specific antibodies may be helpful.[66] This situation is uncommon, and a repeat heterophil test may be more productive (Table 49-4).

Epstein-Barr Virus–Specific Antibodies

Antibodies to many EBV antigens have been detected. The first to appear is anti–viral capsid antigen (VCA) IgM, followed shortly by IgG antibody to the same antigen (VCA). By the third week after onset, all patients are positive for VCA-IgM, which is then undetectable 4 to 8 weeks later whereas VCA-IgG persists for life. The VCA-IgG level rises quickly so that the acute phase serum has high antibody levels, making it difficult to demonstrate a diagnostic titer rise. However, because of the sequence of production of antibody to other EBV antigens, a diagnosis can usually be made with a single serum specimen. Most IM patients also produce VCA-IgA, and about 5% to 30% are VCA-IgA positive years later.[30]

Antibodies to various other antigens (Table 49-5) appear 3 to 4 weeks after infection. Antibodies to the diffuse early antigen are transient; others persist for life. Thus in VCA-IgG-positive patients, the presence of antibody diffuse early antigen is diagnostic for acute infection as is the absence of EBV nuclear antigen (EBNA) antibody. Neutralizing antibodies are directed against a major glycoprotein of the mature virus particle.[65,168] The patterns of EBV antibody response in young children are the same as those in older patients.[50]

The procedures used to detect EBV-specific antibodies are listed in Table 49-5. Measurement of IgM antibodies to VCA is most useful[118] because all patients with IM produce IgM and it is often difficult to demonstrate a rise in VCA-IgG. Tests for detecting VCA-IgM are commercially available, but they are expensive (unless tests can be batched) and have yet to be evaluated. The most common procedure for measuring VCA-IgG is immunofluorescence, and commercial reagents for this are available. Immunoperoxidase tests have also been used.[79]

REFERENCES

1. Asano, Y., et al.: Protection against varicella in family contacts by immediate inoculation with live varicella vaccine, Pediatrics 59:3, 1977.
2. Balfour, H.H.: Cytomegalovirus: the troll of transplantation, Arch. Intern. Med. 139:279, 1979.
3. Balfour, H.H., et al.: Acyclovir halts progression of herpes zoster in immunocompromised patients, N. Engl. J. Med. 308:1448, 1983.
4. Ballew, H.C., Lyerla, H.C., and Forrester, F.T.: Laboratory methods for diagnosing herpes virus infections, Course 8229-C, Atlanta, 1978, Centers for Disease Control.
5. Bean, B., Braun, C., and Balfour, H.H.: Acyclovir therapy for acute herpes zoster, Lancet 2:118, 1982.
6. Benjamin, D.R.: Rapid typing of herpes simplex virus strains using the indirect immunoperoxidase method, Appl. Microbiol. 28:568, 1974.
7. Benjamin, W.R., et al.: Evaluation of solid-phase immunofluorescence for quantitation of antibodies to herpes simplex virus and cytomegalovirus, J. Clin. Microbiol. 12:558, 1980.
8. Betts, R.F.: Syndromes of cytomegalovirus infection, Adv. Intern. Med. 26:447, 1980.
9. Betts, R.F., et al.: Comparative activity of immunofluorescent antibody and complement-fixing antibody in cytomegalovirus infection, J. Clin. Microbiol. 4:141, 1976.
10. Binkin, N.J., Koplan, J.P., and Cates, W., Jr.: Preventing neonatal herpes: the value of weekly viral cultures in pregnant women with recurrent genital herpes, JAMA 251:2816, 1984.
11. Brautigam, A.R., Richman, D.D., and Oxman, M.N.: Rapid typing of herpes simplex virus isolates by DNA:DNA hybridization, J. Clin. Microbiol. 12:226, 1980.
12. Brunell, P.: Antiviral drugs for the neonate: the risk-benefit ledger, J. Pediatr. 86:317, 1985.
13. Bryson, Y.J., et al.: Treatment of first episodes of genital herpes simplex virus infection with oral acyclovir, N. Engl. J. Med. 308:916, 1983.
14. Callihan, D.D., and Menegus, M.A.: Rapid detection of herpes simplex virus in clinical specimens with human embryonic lung fibroblast and primary rabbit kidney cell cultures, J. Clin. Microbiol. 19:563, 1984.
15. Centers for Disease Control, Department of Health and Human Services: Varicella-zoster immune globulin for the prevention of chickenpox, Ann. Intern. Med. 100:859, 1984.
16. Chou, S., Merigan, T., and Gallagher, J.G.: Controlled clinical trial of intravenous acyclovir in heart transplant patients with mucocutaneous herpes simplex, Lancet 2:1392, 1981.
17. Colby, B.M., et al.: Effect of acyclovir (9-[2-hydroxyethoxymethyl] guanine) on Epstein-Barr virus DNA replication, J. Virol. 34:560, 1980.
18. Coleman, D.V.: Cytological diagnosis of virus-infected cells in Papanicolaou smears and its application in clinical practice, J. Clin. Pathol. 32:1075, 1979.
19. Committee on Fetus and Newborn and Committee on Infectious Diseases, American Academy of Pediatrics: Perinatal herpes simplex virus infections, Pediatrics 66:147, 1980.
20. Corey, L., and Holmes, K.K.: Genital herpes simplex virus infections: current concepts in diagnosis, therapy, and prevention, Ann. Intern. Med. 98:973, 1983.
21. Corey, L., et al.: A trial of topical acyclovir in genital herpes simplex virus infections, N. Engl. J. Med. 306:1313, 1982.
22. Corey, L., et al.: Intravenous acyclovir for the treatment of primary genital herpes, Ann. Intern. Med. 98:914, 1983.
23. Cradook-Watson, J.E., Ridehalgh, M.K.S., and Bourne, M.S.: Specific immunoglobulin responses after varicella and herpes zoster, J. Hyg. 82:319, 1979.
24. Crane, L.R., et al.: Incubation of swab materials with herpes simplex virus, J. Infect. Dis. 141:531, 1980.
25. Denoyel, G.A., Gaspar, A., and Nouyrigat, C.: Enzyme immunoassay for measurement of antibodies to herpes simplex virus infection: comparison with complement fixation, immunofluorescent antibody and neutralization techniques, J. Clin. Microbiol. 11:114, 1980.
26. Doerr, H.W., Kuenzler, A. and Schmitz, H.: Cytomegalovirus strain differentiation by DNA restriction analysis, Oncology 36:245, 1979.
27. Dolin, R., et al.: Herpes zoster-varicella infections in immunosuppressed patients, Ann. Intern. Med. 89:375, 1978.

28. Drew, W.L., and Mintz, L.: Rapid diagnosis of varicella-zoster virus infection by direct immunofluorescence, Am. J. Clin. Pathol. **73:**699, 1980.

29. Dworsky, M.E., et al.: Occupational risk for primary cytomegalovirus infection among pediatric health-care workers, N. Engl. J. Med. **309:**950, 1983.

30. Edwards, J.M.B., and Woodroof, M.: EB virus specific IgA in serum of patients with infectious mononucleosis and of healthy people of different ages, J. Clin. Pathol. **32:**1036, 1979.

31. Einhorn, L., and Öst, A.: Cytomegalovirus infection of human blood cells, J. Infect. Dis. **149:**207, 1984.

32. Epstein, M.A., and Achong, B.G.: Pathogenesis of infectious mononucleosis, Lancet **2:**1270, 1977.

33. Epstein, M.A., and Achong, B.G.: Recent progress in Epstein-Barr virus research, Annu. Rev. Microbiol. **31:**421, 1977.

34. Evans, A.S.: Infectious mononucleosis and related syndromes, Am. J. Med. Sci. **276:**325, 1978.

35. Evans, A.S., et al.: A prospective evaluation of heterophil and Epstein-Barr virus—specific IgM antibody tests in clinical and subclinical infectious mononucleosis: specificity and sensitivity of the tests and persistence of antibody, J. Infect. Dis. **132:**546, 1975.

36. Evans, A.S., et al.: A case-control study of Hodgkin's disease in Brazil. II. Seroepidemiologic studies in cases and family members, Am. J. Epidemiol. **112:**609, 1980.

36a. Falcon, M.G.: Acyclovir in herpes simplex keratitis, J. Infect. **6**(suppl. 1):37, 1983.

37. Felsenstein, D., et al.: Treatment of cytomegalovirus retinitis with 9-[2-hydroxy-1- (hydroxymethyl) ethoxymethyl] guanine, Ann. Intern. Med. **103:**377, 1985.

38. Fiacco, V., Bryson, Y.J., and Bruckner, D.A.: Comparison of monoclonal and polyclonal antibody for confirmation of cytomegalovirus isolates by fluorescent staining, J. Clin. Microbiol. **19:**928, 1984.

39. Figueroa, M.E., and Rawls, W.E.: Biological markers for differentiation of herpes-virus strains of oral and genital origin, J. Gen. Virol. **4:**259, 1969.

40. Fleischer, G., et al.: Incidence of heterophil antibody responses in children with infectious mononucleosis, J. Pediatr. **94:**723, 1979.

41. Fleischer, G., et al.: Primary infection with Epstein-Barr virus in infants in the United States: clinical and serologic observations, J. Infect. Dis. **139:**553, 1979.

42. Fleischer, G.R., et al.: Intrafamilial transmission of Epstein-Barr virus infections, J. Pediatr. **98:**16, 1981.

43. Forghani, B., Klassen, T., and Baringer, J.R.: Radioimmunoassay of herpes simplex virus antibody: correlation with ganglionic infection, J. Gen. Virol. **36:**371, 1977.

44. Forghani, B., Schmidt, N.J., and Dennis, J.: Antibody assays for varicella-zoster virus: comparison of enzyme immunoassay with neutralization, immune adherence hemagglutination, and complement fixation, J. Clin. Microbiol. **8:**545, 1978.

45. Forghani, B., Schmidt, N.J., and Lennette, E.H.: Solid phase radioimmunoassay for identification of herpes virus hominis types 1 and 2 from clinical materials, Appl. Microbiol. **28:**661, 1974.

46. Friedman, H.M.: Cytomegalovirus: subclinical infection or disease, Am. J. Med. **70:**215, 1981.

47. Gerna, G., et al.: Immunoglobulin G to virus-specific early antigens in congenital, primary and reactivated human cytomegalovirus infections, Infect. Immun. **22:**833, 1978.

48. Gershon, A.A., and Steinberg, S.P.: Cellular and humoral immune responses to varicella-zoster virus in immunocompromised patients during and after varicella-zoster infections, Infect. Immun. **25:**170, 1979.

49. Gershon, A.A., et al.: Antibody to varicella-zoster virus in parturient women and their offspring during the first year of life, Pediatrics **58:**692, 1976.

50. Ginsburg, C.M., et al.: Infectious mononucleosis in children: evaluation of Epstein-Barr virus-specific serological data, JAMA **237:**781, 1977.

51. Gittzus, J.G., and Rubin, S.J.: Clinical evaluation of commercial conjugates for direct immunofluorescence of herpes simplex virus, J. Clin. Microbiol. **6:**574, 1977.

52. Gleaves, C.A., et al.: Detection and serotyping of herpes simplex virus in MRC-5 cells by use of centrifugation and monoclonal antibodies 16 hour postinoculation, J. Clin. Microbiol. **21:**29, 1985.

53. Goldin, M.: Rapid differential slide tests for the diagnosis of infectious mononucleosis, Am. J. Med. Tech. **40:**317, 1974.

54. Golubjatnikov, R., Koehler, J.E., and Inhorn, S.L.: Absorbed heterophile and ox-cell hemolysis tests in serodiagnosis of infectious mononucleosis, Health Lab. Sci. **12:**201, 1975.

55. Griffiths, P.D., et al.: A longitudinal study of the serological and virological status of 18 women infected with cytomegalovirus, Arch. Virol. **58:**111, 1978.

56. Grossman, J.H., III, Wallen, W.C., and Sever, J.L.: Management of genital herpes simplex virus infection during pregnancy, Obstet. Gynecol. **58:**1, 1981.

57. Groth, K.E., et al.: Evaluation of zoster immune plasma: treatment of cutaneous disseminated zoster in immunocompromised patients, JAMA **239:**1877, 1978.

58. Guinan, M.E., et al.: The course of untreated recurrent genital herpes simplex infection in 27 women, N. Engl. J. Med. **304:**759, 1981.

59. Handsfield, H.H., et al.: Cytomegalovirus infection in sex partners: evidence for sexual transmission, J. Infect. Dis. **151:**344, 1985.

60. Hanshaw, J.B., Scheiner, A.P., and Moxley, A.W.: School failure and deafness after "silent" congenital cytomegalovirus infection, N. Engl. J. Med. **295:**468, 1976.

61. Hanto, D.W., et al.: Epstein-Barr virus–induced B-cell lymphoma after renal transplantation, N. Engl. J. Med. **306:**913, 1982.

62. Hekker, A.C., et al.: Indirect immunofluorescence test for detection of IgM antibodies to cytomegalovirus, J. Infect. Dis. **140:**596, 1979.

63. Henle, W., and Henle, G.: Epidemiologic aspects of Epstein-Barr virus (EBV)–associated diseases, Ann. N.Y. Acad. Sci. **354:**326, 1980.

64. Hirsch, M.S., and Swartz, M.N.: Antiviral agents, N. Engl. J. Med. **302:**903, 1980.

65. Hofman, G.J., Lazarowitz, S.G., and Hayward, S.D.: Monoclonal antibody against a 250,000-dalton glycoprotein of Epstein-Barr virus identifies a membrane antigen and a neutralizing antigen, Proc. Natl. Acad. Sci. USA **77:**2979, 1980.

66. Horwitz, C.A., et al.: Heterophile-negative infectious mononucleosis and mononucleosis-like illnesses, Am. J. Med. **63:**947, 1977.

67. Horwitz, C.A., et al.: Persistent falsely positive rapid tests for infectious mononucleosis: report of five cases with four-six year follow-up data, Am. J. Clin. Pathol. **72:**807, 1979.

68. Huang, E-S., et al.: Persistence of both human cytomegalovirus and Epstein-Barr virus genomes in two human lymphoblastoid cell lines, J. Gen. Virol. **40:**519, 1978.

69. Huang, E-S., et al.: Molecular epidemiology of cytomegalovirus infections in women and their infants, N. Engl. J. Med. **303:**958, 1980.

70. Hyman, R.W., Ecker, J.R., and Tenser, R.B.: Varicella-zoster virus RNA in human trigeminal ganglia, Lancet **2:**814, 1983.

71. Ito, M., and Barron, A.L.: Typing of herpes simplex virus by mixed agglutination, Proc. Soc. Exp. Biol. Med. **146:**41, 1974.

72. Jamison, R.M., and Hathorn, A.W.: Isolation of cytomegalovirus from cerebrospinal fluid of a congenitally infected infant, Am. J. Dis. Child. **132:**63, 1978.

73. Jones, J.F., et al.: Evidence for active Epstein-Barr virus infection in patients with persistent unexplained illness: elevated anti-early antigen antibodies, Ann. Intern. Med. **102:**1, 1985.

74. Jordan, M.C., et al.: Latent herpesviruses of humans, Ann. Intern. Med. **100:**866, 1984.

75. Kaufman, R.H., et al.: Herpesvirus induced antigens in squamous-cell carcinoma in situ of the vulva, N. Engl. J. Med. **305:**483, 1981.

76. Kettering, J.D., et al.: Anticomplement immunofluorescence test for antibodies to human cytomegalovirus, J. Clin. Microbiol. **6:**627, 1977.

77. Kibrick, S.: Herpes simplex infection at term: what to do with mother, newborn, and nursery personnel, JAMA **243:**157, 1980.

78. Kinney, J.S., et al.: Cytomegaloviral infection and disease, J. Infect. Dis. **151:**772, 1985.

79. Kurstak, E., et al.: Detection of Epstein-Barr virus antigens and antibodies by peroxidase-labeled specific immunoglobulins, J. Med. Virol. **2:**189, 1978.

79a. Lafferty, W.E., et al.: Diagnosis of herpes simplex virus by direct immunofluorescence and viral isolation from samples of external genital lesions in a high-prevalence population, J. Clin. Microbiol. **25:**323, 1987.

80. Lange, B.J., et al.: Encephalitis in infectious mononucleosis: diagnostic considerations, Pediatrics **58:**877, 1976.

81. Lazarus, K.H., and Baehner, R.L.: Aplastic anemia complicating infectious mononucleosis: a case report and review of the literature, Pediatrics **67:**907, 1981.

82. Leclair, J.M., et al.: Airborne transmission of chickenpox in a hospital, N. Engl. J. Med. **302:**450, 1980.

83. Lee, F.K., Nahmias, A.J., and Stagno, S.: Rapid diagnosis of cytomegalovirus infection in infants by electron microscopy, N. Engl. J. Med. **299:**1266, 1978.

84. Lee, M.S., and Balfour, H.H.: Optimal method for recovery of cytomegalovirus from urine of renal transplant patients, Transplantation **24:**228, 1977.

85. Lennette, E., et al.: Heterophile antigen in bovine sera detectable by immune adherence hemagglutination with infectious mononucleosis sera, Infect. Immun. **19:**923, 1978.

86. Light, I.J.: Postnatal acquisition of herpes simplex virus by the newborn infant: a review of the literature, Pediatrics **63:**480, 1979.

87. Long, J.C., Wheeler, C.E., Jr., and Briggaman, R.A.: Varicella-like infection due to herpes simplex, Arch. Dermatol. **114:**406, 1978.

88. Marker, S.C., et al.: Epstein-Barr virus antibody responses and clinical illness in renal transplant recipients, Surgery **85:**433, 1979.

89. Marker, S.C., et al.: A trial of vidarabine for cytomegalovirus infection in renal transplant patients, Arch. Intern. Med. **140:**1441, 1980.

90. Marsh, R.J., Fraunfelder, F.T., and McGill, J.I.: Herpetic corneal epithelial disease, Arch. Ophthalmol. **94:**1899, 1976.

91. Matolia, A.: Ocular viral infections, Pediatr. Infect. Dis. **3:**358, 1984.

92. Mayo, D.R.: Differentiation of herpes simplex virus types 1 and 2 by sensitivity to (E)-5-(2-bromovinyl)-2'-deoxyuridine, J. Clin. Microbiol. **15:**733, 1982.

93. Mazur, M.H., and Dolin, R.: Herpes zoster at the NIH: a 20 year experience, Am. J. Med. **65:**738, 1978.

94. McClung, H., Seth, P., and Rawls, W.E.: Relative concentrations in human sera of antibodies to cross-reacting and specific antigens of herpes simplex virus types 1 and 2, Am. J. Epidemiol. **104:**192, 1976.

95. Meyers, J.D., et al.: Toxicity and efficacy of human leukocyte interferon for treatment of cytomegalovirus pneumonia after marrow transplantation, J. Infect. Dis. **141:**555, 1980.

96. Mills, K.W., et al.: Serotyping herpes simplex virus isolates by enzyme-linked immunosorbent assays, J. Clin. Microbiol. **7:**73, 1978.

97. Mintz, L., Miner, R.C., and Yeager, A.S.: Anticomplement immunofluorescence test that uses isolated fibroblast nuclei for detection of antibodies to human cytomegalovirus, J. Clin. Microbiol. **12:**562, 1980.

98. Moore, D.F.: Comparison of human fibroblast cells and primary rabbit kidney cells for isolation of herpes simplex virus, J. Clin. Microbiol. **19:**548, 1984.

99. Morgan, D.C., et al.: Site of Epstein-Barr virus replication in the oropharynx, Lancet **2:**1154, 1979.

100. Morgan, E.R., and Smalley, L.: Varicella in immunocompromised children, Am. J. Dis. Child. **137:**883, 1983.

101. Morgan, M.A., and Smith, T.F.: Evaluation of an enzyme-linked immunosorbent assay for the detection of herpes-simplex virus antigen, J. Clin. Microbiol. **19:**730, 1984.

102. Moseley, R.C., et al.: Comparison of viral isolation, direct immunofluorescence and indirect immunoperoxidase techniques for detection of genital herpes simplex virus infection, J. Clin. Microbiol. **13:**913, 1981.

103. Myers, M.G.: Viremia caused by varicella-zoster virus: association with malignant progressive varicella, J. Infect. Dis. **140:**229, 1979.

104. Nahmias, A.J.: Herpes simplex virus infection: problems and prospects as perceived by a peripatetic pediatrician, Yale J. Biol. Med. **53:**47, 1980.

105. Nahmias, A.J., and Roizman, B.: Infection with herpes simplex viruses 1 and 2, N. Engl. J. Med. **289:**719, 1973.

106. Nahmias, A.J., et al.: Antibodies to herpesvirus hominis types 1 and 2 in humans. II. Women with cervical cancer, Am. J. Epidemiol. **91:**547, 1970.

107. Nahmias, A.J., et al.: Herpes simplex virus encephalitis: laboratory evaluations and their diagnostic significance, J. Infect. Dis. **145:**829, 1982.

108. Nerurkar, L.S., et al.: Detection of genital herpes simplex infections by a tissue culture-fluorescent-antibody technique with biotin avidin, J. Clin. Microbiol. **17:**149, 1983.

109. Nerurkar, L.S., et al.: Rapid detection of herpes simplex virus in clinical specimens by use of a capture biotin-streptavidin enzyme-linked immunosorbent assay, J. Clin. Microbiol. **20:**109, 1984.

109a. Nerurkar, L.S., et al.: Typing of herpes simplex virus by capture biotin-streptavidin enzyme-linked immunosorbent assay and comparison with restriction endonuclease analysis and immunofluorescence method using monoclonal antibodies, J. Clin. Microbiol. **25:**128, 1987.

110. Nordlung, J.J., et al.: The use of temperature sensitivity and selective cell culture systems for differentiation of herpes simplex virus types 1 and 2 in a clinical laboratory, Proc. Soc. Exp. Biol. Med. **155:**118, 1977.

111. Norrild, B.: Immunochemistry of herpes simplex virus glycoproteins, Curr. Top. Microbiol. Immunol. **90:**67, 1980.

112. Novick, N.L.: Autoinoculation herpes of the hand in a child with recurrent herpes labialis, Am. J. Med. **79:**139, 1985.

113. Oakes, J.E., et al.: Analysis by restriction enzyme cleavage of human varicella-zoster virus DNAs, Virology **82:**353, 1977.

114. Oh, J.O., and Minasi, P.: Different susceptibilities of skin to type 1 and type 2 herpes simplex viruses in newborn rabbits, Infect. Immun. **27:**168, 1980.

115. Oh, J.O., et al.: Ocular pathogenicity of types 1 and 2 herpesvirus hominis in rabbits, Infect. Immun. **5:**412, 1972.

116. Palmer, D.F., et al.: Serodiagnosis of toxoplasmosis, rubella, cytomegalic inclusion disease and herpes simplex, Immunology Series No. 5, Procedural Guide, Atlanta, 1977, Center for Disease Control.

117. Panjvani, Z.F.K., and Hanshaw, J.B.: Cytomegalovirus in the perinatal period, Am. J. Dis. Child. **135:**56, 1981.

118. Papaevangelou, G., et al.: Diagnostic value of IgG and IgM antibodies to capsid antigen of Epstein-Barr virus in infectious mononucleosis, J. Infect. Dis. **136:**428, 1977.

119. Pass, R.F., et al.: Productive infection with cytomegalovirus and herpes simplex virus in renal transplant recipients: role of source of kidney, J. Infect. Dis. **137:**566, 1978.

120. Pass, R.F., et al.: Outcome of symptomatic congenital cytomegalovirus infection: results of long-term longitudinal follow-up, Pediatrics **66:**758, 1980.

121. Pazin, G.J., Ho, M., and Jannetta, P.J.: Reactivation of herpes simplex virus after decompression of the trigeminal nerve root, J. Infect. Dis. **138:**405, 1978.

122. Peterson, P.K., et al.: Cytomegalovirus disease in renal allograft recipients: a prospective study of the clinical features, risk factors and impact on renal transplantation, Medicine 59:283, 1980.

123. Plotkin, S.A.: Vaccination against herpes group viruses, in particular cytomegalovirus, Monogr. Paediatr. 11:58, 1979.

124. Pollard, R.B., et al.: Cytomegalovirus retinitis in immuno-suppressed hosts. I. Natural history and effects of treatment with adenine arabinoside, Ann. Intern. Med. 93:655, 1980.

125. Preblud, S.R.: Age-specific risks of varicella complications, Pediatrics 68:14, 1981.

126. Preblud, S.R., Orenstein, W.A., and Barb, K.J.: Varicella: clinical manifestations, epidemiology and health impact in children, Pediatr. Infect. Dis. 3:505, 1984.

127. Preissner, C.M., et al.: Evaluation of the anticomplement immunofluorescence test for detection of antibody to varicella-zoster virus, J. Clin. Microbiol. 16:373, 1982.

128. Priest, J.R., et al.: Varicella arthritis documented by isolation of virus from joint fluid, J. Pediatr. 6:990, 1979.

128a. Prober, C.G., et al.: Rise of herpes simplex virus infections in neonates exposed to the virus at the time of vaginal delivery to mothers with recurrent genital herpes simplex virus infections, N. Engl. J. Med. 316:240, 1987.

129. Purtilo, D.T., et al.: Persistent transfusion-associated infectious mononucleosis with transient acquired immunodeficiency, Am. J. Med. 68:437, 1980.

130. Rao, N., et al.: Evaluation of anti-complement immunofluorescence test in cytomegalovirus infection, J. Clin. Microbiol. 6:633, 1977.

131. Rapp, C.E., and Hewetson, J.F.: Infectious mononucleosis and the Epstein-Barr virus, Am. J. Dis. Child. 132:78, 1978.

132. Rawls, W.E.: Herpes simplex virus types 1 and 2 and herpes simiae. In Lennette, E.H., and Schmidt, N.J., editors: Diagnostic procedures for viral, rickettsial, and chlamydial infections, Washington, D.C., 1979, American Public Health Association.

133. Rawls, W.E., et al.: Herpesvirus type 2: association with carcinoma of the cervix, Science 161:1255, 1968.

134. Reeves, W.C., et al.: Risk of recurrence after first episodes of genital herpes: relation to HSV type and antibody response, N. Engl. J. Med. 305:315, 1981.

135. Reichman, E.C.: Herpes simplex infections, Eur. J. Clin. Microbiol. 3:399, 1984.

136. Reynolds, D.W., Stagno, S., and Alford, C.: Laboratory diagnosis of cytomegalovirus infections. In Lennette, E.H., and Schmidt, N.J., editors: Diagnostic procedures for viral, rickettsial, and chlamydial infections, Washington, D.C., 1979, American Public Health Association.

137. Reynolds, D.W., et al.: Inapparent congenital CMV infections and elevated cord IgM levels: causal relations with auditory and mental deficiency, N. Engl. J. Med. 290:291, 1974.

138. Rinaldo, C.R., Black, C.R., and Hirsch, M.S.: Interaction of cytomegalovirus with leukocytes from patients with mononucleosis due to cytomegalovirus, J. Infect. Dis. 136:667, 1977.

139. Robertson, P.W., Kertesz, V., and Cloonan, M.J.: Elimination of false-positive cytomegalovirus immunoglobulin M-fluorescent-antibody reactions with immunoglobulin M serum fractions, J. Clin. Microbiol. 6:174, 1977.

140. Roizman, B., and Buchman, T.: The molecular epidemiology of herpes simplex viruses, Hosp. Pract. 14:95, 1979.

141. Rubin, S.J., Wende, R.D., and Rawls, W.E.: Direct immunofluorescence test for the diagnosis of genital herpesvirus infections, Appl. Microbiol. 26:373, 1973.

142. Sacks, S.L.: Frequency and duration of patient-observed recurrent genital herpes simplex virus infection: characterization of the nonlesional prodrome, J. Infect. Dis. 150:873, 1984.

143. St. Jeor, S., and Weisser, A.: Persistence of cytomegalovirus in human lymphoblasts and peripheral leukocyte cultures, Infect. Immun. 15:402, 1977.

144. Saral, R., et al.: Acyclovir prophylaxis of herpes-simplex virus infections: a randomized double-blind controlled trial in bone marrow transplant recipients, N. Engl. J. Med. 305:63, 1981.

145. Schmidt, N.J., and Gallo, D.: Specific identification of human cytomegalovirus isolates by anti-complement immunofluorescence with immune hamster sera, J. Clin. Microbiol. 11:186, 1980.

146. Schmidt, N.J., et al.: Direct immunofluorescence staining for detection of herpes simplex and varicella-zoster virus antigens in vesicular lesions and certain tissue specimens, J. Clin. Microbiol. 12:651, 1980.

147. Segar, J.E., Smith, T.F., and Ilstrup, D.M.: Evaluation of the FIAX test for the detection of antibodies to herpes simplex virus and cytomegalovirus, Am. J. Clin. Pathol. 75:387, 1981.

148. Selby, P.J., et al.: Parenteral acyclovir therapy for herpes virus infections in man, Lancet 2:1267, 1979.

149. Shepp, D.H., et al.: Activity of 9 [2-hydroxyl-1-(hydroxymethyl) ethoxymethyl] guanine in the treatment of cytomegalovirus pneumonia, Ann. Intern. Med. 103:768, 1985.

150. Shuster, E.A., et al.: Monoclonal antibody for rapid laboratory detection of cytomegalovirus infections: characterization and diagnostic application, Mayo Clin. Proc. 60:577, 1985.

151. Sipbey, J.W., et al.: Epstein-Barr virus replication in orophayngeal epithelial cells, N. Engl. J. Med. 310:1225, 1984.

152. Sköldenberg, B., et al.: Acyclovir versus vidarabine in herpes simplex encephalitis, Lancet 2:707, 1984.

153. Sorenson, O.S., et al.: Cell-mediated and humoral immunity to herpesviruses during and after herpes zoster infections, Infect. Immun. 29:369, 1980.

154. Spector, S.A., Hirata, K.K., and Neuman, T.R.: Identification of multiple cytomegalovirus strains in homosexual men with acquired immunodeficiency syndrome, J. Infect. Dis. 150:953, 1984.

155. Spruance, S.L., et al.: The natural history of recurrent herpes simplex labialis, N. Engl. J. Med. 297:69, 1977.

156. Stagno, S., Reynolds, D.W., and Smith, R.J.: Use of isolated nuclei in the indirect fluorescent-antibody test for human cyctomegalovirus infection: comparison with microneutralization, anticomplement, and conventional indirect fluorescent-antibody assays, J. Clin. Microbiol. 7:486, 1978.

157. Stagno, S., et al.: Congenital cytomegalovirus infection: occurrence in immune population, N. Engl. J. Med. 296:1254, 1977.

158. Stagno, S., et al.: Comparative study of diagnostic procedures for congenital cytomegalovirus infection, Pediatrics 65:251, 1980.

159. Straus, S.E., et al.: Herpes simplex virus infection: biology, treatment, and prevention, Ann. Intern. Med. 103:404, 1985.

160. Straus, S.E., et al.: Persisting illness and fatigue in adults with evidence of Epstein-Barr virus infection, Ann. Intern. Med. 102:7, 1985.

161. Sumaya, C.V.: Primary Epstein-Barr virus infections in children, Pediatrics 59:16, 1977.

162. Suwansirikul, S., et al.: Primary and secondary cytomegalovirus infection: clinical manifestations after renal transplantation, Arch. Intern. Med. 137:1026, 1977.

163. Swack, N.S., et al.: Indirect fluorescent-antibody test for human cytomegalovirus infection in the absence of interfering immunoglobulin G receptors, Infect. Immun. 16:522, 1977.

164. Taber, L.H., et al.: Diagnosis of herpes simplex virus infection by immunofluorescence, J. Clin. Microbiol. 3:309, 1976.

165. Tann, E.M.: The possible role of Epstein-Barr in rheumatoid arthritis, Rev. Infect. Dis. 1:997, 1979.

166. Tardy-Panit, M., Michelson, S., and Horodniceanu, F.: Immunofluorescence technique for detection of human cytomegalovirus (HCMV) antibodies against HCMV-induced late antigens with elimination of immunoglobulin G-receptor staining, J. Clin. Microbiol. 11:717, 1980.

167. Thorley-Lawson, D.A.: A virus-free immunogen effective against Epstein-Barr virus, Nature 281:486, 1979.

168. Thorley-Lawson, D.A., and Geilinger, K.: Monoclonal antibodies against the major glycoprotein (gp 350/221) of Epstein-Barr virus neutralized infectivity, Proc. Natl. Acad. Sci. USA **77:**5307, 5311, 1980.

169. Trachtman, H., et al.: Clinical manifestations of herpesvirus infections in pediatric renal transplant recipients, Pediatr. Infect. Dis. **4:**480, 1985.

170. Veien, N.K.: Cytologic examination and viral and bacterial culture in herpes simplex, herpes zoster, and varicella, Cutis **22:**61, 1978.

171. Vestergaard, B.F.: Herpes simplex virus antigens and antibodies: a survey of studies based on quantitative immunoelectrophoresis, Rev. Infect. Dis. **2:**899, 1980.

172. Volpi, A., and Beitt, W.J.: Serological heterogenicity of CMV isolates into a monoclonal antibody, J. Infect. Dis. **152:**648, 1985.

173. Waner, J.L., et al.: Cervical excretion of cytomegalovirus: correlation with secretory and humoral antibody, J. Infect. Dis. **136:**805, 1977.

174. Warren, K.G., et al.: Isolation of latent herpes simplex virus from the superior cervical and vagus ganglions of human beings, N. Engl. J. Med. **298:**1068, 1978.

175. Weller, T.H.: Varicella and herpes zoster: changing concepts of the natural history, control, and importance of a not-so-benign virus, I., N. Engl. J. Med. **309:**1362, 1983.

176. Weller, T.H.: Varicella and herpes zoster: changing concepts of the natural history, control, and importance of a not-so-benign virus, II., N. Engl. J. Med. **309:**1434, 1983.

177. Wesmoreland, D., St. Jeor, S., and Rapp, F.: The development of cytomegalovirus-infected cells of binding affinity for normal human immunoglobulin, J. Immunol. **116:**1566, 1976.

178. Whitley, R.: Diagnosis and treatment of herpes simplex encephalitis, Annu. Rev. Med. **32:**335, 1981.

179. Whitley, R.J., and Alford, C.A.: Antiviral agents: clinical status report, Hosp. Pract. **16:**113, 1981.

180. Whitley, R.J., et al.: Adenine arabinoside therapy of biopsy-proven herpes simplex encephalitis: National Institute of Allergy and Infectious Diseases Collaborative Antiviral Study, N. Engl. J. Med. **197:**289, 1977.

181. Whitley, R.J., et al.: Herpes simplex encephalitis: vidarabine therapy and diagnostic problems, N. Engl. J. Med. **304:**313, 1981.

182. Yambao, R., et al.: Isolation of cytomegalovirus from the amniotic fluid during the third trimester, Am. J. Obstet. Gynecol. **139:**937, 1981.

183. Yeager, A.S., Morris, J.E., and Prober, S.: Storage and transport of cultures for herpes simplex, type 2, Am. J. Clin. Pathol. **72:**977, 1979.

184. Zaia, J.A., and Oxman, M.N.: Antibody to varicella-zoster virus-induced membrane antigen: immunofluorescence assay using monodisperse gluteraldehyde-fixed target cells, J. Infect. Dis. **136:**519, 1977.

185. Ziegler, T.: Detection of varicella-zoster viral antigens in clinical specimens by solid-phase enzyme immune assay, J. Infect. Dis. **150:**149, 1984.

186. Zwoerink, H.J., and Neff, B.J.: Immune response after exposure to varicella-zoster virus: characterization of virus-specific antibodies and their corresponding antigens, Infect. Immun. **31:**436, 1981.

CHAPTER 50

Picornaviruses

Sally Jo Rubin

Picornaviridae is a large, diverse family, divided into four genera, of which two (*Rhinovirus* and *Enterovirus*) include viruses infectious to humans. As their name implies, these are small (pico) (20 to 30 nm) RNA viruses. Their single-stranded RNA is characterized by a protein coat and icosahedral symmetry. They are nonenveloped and thus resistant to chloroform and ether.

Between the two genera infecting humans there are over 167 antigenic serotypes.

Genus	Serotypes
Rhinovirus	1A, 1B, and 2-29
Enterovirus	Polioviruses 1-3
	Coxsackieviruses A1-24*
	Coxsackieviruses B1-6
	Echoviruses 1-34†
	Enteroviruses 68-71
Hepatitis A virus (see Chapter 54)	Enterovirus 72

Neither genus has a genus-specific antigen. The over 100 rhinoviruses are pH labile (pH less than 6) and grow best at 33° C and in human cell cultures. Rhinoviruses can survive at room temperature for at least 24 hours, especially if they are in a liquid or mixed with organic material.[2] They are never isolated from feces. The 67 enteroviruses are stable from pH 3 to 10, generally grow best in primary monkey kidney (PMK) cells at 35° to 37° C, and are commonly isolated from stool (Table 50-1).

RHINOVIRUSES

Rhinoviruses are the major cause of the common cold, which has plagued humankind through recorded time. The infectious nature of colds was recognized in 1914, and the first isolation of a rhinovirus was in 1956. Thus far over 100 serotypes have been identified, but many isolates remain to be classified. In addition, circulating serotypes seem to be slowly shifting, with new serotypes replacing the old.

Colds are universal among humans with those under 1 year old experiencing an average of 1.2 per year and young adults an average of 0.7 per year. Between 70% and 90% of colds are symptomatic, with typical upper respiratory symptoms and usually without fever. However, rhinovirus may invade the lower respiratory tract in symptomatic infections.[9] In temperate climates rhinovirus colds generally peak in spring and fall. Winter colds are more often caused by coronaviruses. Antigenic serotypes of rhinovirus circulate with no particular pattern.

Contrary to popular opinion, exposure to cold temperatures does not increase susceptibility to colds. Nor does transmission occur by sneezing[8] because virus is found mostly in nasal secretions, not the saliva expelled in a cough or sneeze.[7] Instead the hands of infected persons become contaminated with nasal secretions containing virus. Then the infected persons transfer virus directly to surfaces or to hands of other persons. Virus can be transmitted to the hands of noninfected persons by their touching contaminated surfaces such as tables or doorknobs. Autoinoculation to the eyes or nose then occurs; both eye-rubbing and nose-picking are normal and frequent human behaviors.[11] Virus is shed a few days before onset of symptoms and for several days after onset.

No treatment for rhinovirus infection is available other than symptomatic relief. Prospects for a vaccine are dim because of the large number of antigenic serotypes.[3] The best control of transmission is handwashing and avoiding contact between hands and nose or eyes. Unfortunately, the best agent for inactivation of virus on the hands (1% iodine) is not very practical because it also stains the skin. Hexachlorophene is less effective.[10]

Laboratory diagnosis of rhinovirus infection is rarely attempted because illness is so mild. Also, optimal conditions for virus isolation (33° C and incubation on a roller drum) may not be available. Virus can be recovered from nasal secretions for several days after onset of a cold. The most susceptible cells are of human origin (primary HEK, WI-38). Because some strains can be isolated from PMK cells, laboratories do need to be able to differentiate rhinoviruses from enteroviruses, which commonly grow on PMK cells (Table 50-1). Usually pH stability is tested. Specific serotypes may be determined by neutralization, although serotyping is usually attempted only in research situations.

Close to 80% of persons develop neutralizing antibody following a rhinovirus infection. Antibody persists for years and except for challenge with a large inoculum provides immunity to that specific type. Rhinoviruses have no group antigen, making serologic diagnosis impractical and thus generally not available.

ENTEROVIRUSES

The present 68 viruses of the genus *Enterovirus* were originally placed into three groups: poliovirus, coxsackievirus, and enteric cytopathogenic human orphan virus (echovirus). Polioviruses, the first enteroviruses isolated,[6] were originally called

---

*Coxsackievirus A23 is now echovirus 9.

†Echoviruses 1 and 8 are the same; echovirus 10 is now reovirus 1; echovirus 28 is rhinovirus 1A; and echovirus 34 is a variant of coxsackievirus A24.

TABLE 50-1 Differentiation of Rhinoviruses and Enteroviruses

Characteristic	Rhinovirus	Enterovirus
pH range tolerance	Labile at < pH 6	Stable from pH 3-10
Temperature for optimal growth	33° C	35°-37° C
Isolated from feces	Never	Often
Medium for optimal growth	Human cell cultures	Primary monkey kidney cells

TABLE 50-2. Clinical Spectrum of Enterovirus Infections

Virus	Types[a]	Syndrome
Poliovirus	1-3	Febrile illness, aseptic meningitis, paralysis
Coxsackievirus A	Many	Febrile illness with or without respiratory symptoms
	2, 4, 7, 9, 10	Aseptic meningitis
	4, 7, 9	Paralysis
	4-6, 9, 16	Rash
	10	Pharyngitis
	4, 16	Myocarditis
	2-6, 8, 10, 22	Herpangina
	5, 10, 16	Hand-foot-and-mouth disease
	24	Epidemic acute hemorrhagic conjunctivitis
Coxsackievirus B	1-6	Febrile illness with or without respiratory symptoms
	1-6	Aseptic meningitis
	1-5	Paralysis
	5	Rash
	1-6	Myocarditis
	1-5	Pleurodynia
Echovirus	Many	Febrile illness with or without respiratory symptoms
	Most	Aseptic meningitis
	Many	Paralysis
	Many, especially 9, 16	Rash
	9, 11, 22	Myocarditis
Enterovirus	68	Fever, respiratory symptoms, pneumonia
	69	Fever, respiratory symptoms
	70	Fever, respiratory symptoms, aseptic meningitis, paralysis, acute hemorrhagic conjunctivitis
	71	Fever and respiratory symptoms, aseptic meningitis, maculopapular rash; hand-foot-and-mouth disease

[a]Most common types isolated.

poliomyelitis virus to describe the pathologic lesion that the virus produced in the gray *(polios)* matter of the anterior horn of the spinal cord *(myelos)*.

During an outbreak of paralytic disease, Dalldorf and Sickles isolated a nonpolio virus from the feces of children living in Coxsackie, New York. Subsequently a number of these viruses were isolated. All were pathogenic for suckling mice, but they fell into two groups based on their effect on mice and their ability to grow in cell culture.

	Coxsackievirus A	Coxsackievirus B
Infectivity (in mice)	Generalized myositis of skeletal muscle producing flaccid paralysis	Focal myositis, more generalized infection producing spastic paralysis
Growth in cell culture	Poor/none	Good

After cell culture came into use, similar RNA-containing viruses were isolated from the feces of healthy children. These viruses did not produce disease in laboratory animals but did produce cytopathic effect (CPE) in cell cultures. Because their relationship to human disease was not clear, they were called enteric cytopathogenic human orphan viruses, or echoviruses. Now 31 different echoviruses have been isolated and are known to cause a variety of clinical syndromes (Table 50-2).

Additional enterovirus isolates have sometimes been difficult to place in one of the three groups because their host ranges in cell culture fit one group but their effects in mice another. Thus all new enteroviruses are now numbered consecutively (for example, enterovirus 68). The older grouping was retained for previously isolated enteroviruses because certain types are associated with certain clinical syndromes (for example, coxsackie type B viruses and heart disease). None of the enterovirus groups has a group-specific antigen.

Enteroviruses are very resistant and are not destroyed by 70% alcohol or common disinfectants such as Lysol. Chlorination can inactivate them, but its effectiveness decreases when extraneous organic matter is present. In fact, enteroviruses are not completely removed by conventional waste water treatment methods. They can be stable for days or even weeks in waste water or sewage,[5] for days at room temperature, and for weeks in the refrigerator.

CLINICAL SIGNIFICANCE

Enteroviruses cause a great diversity of clinical manifestations. The same type can cause a number of clinical syndromes, and conversely, different types can cause the same symptoms. In some cases certain types are associated with certain clinical presentations (Table 50-2).

The most frightening and serious enterovirus disease is polio because of its devastating sequelae. Before the polio vaccine was available, over 90% of infections with wild poliovirus were asymptomatic, another 4% to 8% resulted in mild febrile illness, 1% to 2% produced serious disease with neurologic manifestations, and only 0.1% caused frank paralysis. The paralysis is characteristically asymmetric, and sensory loss is unusual. Wild polio virus is now rare in developed countries, and infection occurs only among the nonimmunized and is most often caused by vaccine virus.[25] Other enteroviruses can cause paralytic disease, but paralysis is almost always reversible.

Most other enterovirus infections are asymptomatic. The more frequently seen syndromes in symptomatic infection include aseptic meningitis, myocardiopathy, rashes, acute febrile respiratory disease, herpangina, pleurodynia, and acute hemorrhagic conjunctivitis.[1]

Symptoms are often age related.[12,28] Aseptic meningitis is most common in children less than 1 year of age and is rare in adults over 40 years. Most patients recover fully, although neurologic sequelae do occur in about 10% of infants infected during their first year of life.[27,29] Infection in the perinatal period can be fatal.[21]

Enteroviruses are found throughout the world and are transmitted by the fecal-oral route, by droplets from the respiratory tract, and even by insects such as flies and cockroaches. Virus is found in unpolluted fresh bathing water[4] and even in public swimming pools.[13]

Incidence is highest among young children. In temperate climates sharp epidemics occur in the summer and early fall, whereas in the tropics enterovirus infections are endemic and occur year-round. In the United States occurrence of various serotypes has no pattern. They vary from city to city and season to season. One serotype may cause an epidemic one year and not be seen again for years, whereas another may be present every year at low levels. In some years a community may experience a large outbreak with one serotype and in other years have infection caused by a number of different serotypes.[23] The reasons for these fluctuations are unknown. Human feces is the major source of virus in the environment. Enteroviruses are shed in the feces for several weeks and in some cases for more than a month.[17] Shedding from the throat can continue for 3 to 4 weeks. Reinfections with the same antigenic serotype can occur but are usually asymptomatic with shorter periods of virus shedding.

Pathogenesis of enteroviral infections is probably the same for all serotypes, differing only in their target organ. Virus enters the body through the mouth, replicates in the pharynx, distal gut, and Peyer's patches of the ileum, and eventually reaches the deep lymph nodes. A low-level viremia disseminates virus to various tissues, including the bone marrow, liver, and spleen. In a minority of people viral replication continues, resulting in a heavy viremia that delivers virus to the target organ (for example, meninges, heart, or skin).

No specific antiviral therapy for enteroviral infections is available. Because so many serotypes exist, no vaccine development has been attempted, except for that which has resulted in the poliovirus vaccines. Inactivated poliovirus vaccine came into use in 1955, and the oral live attenuated vaccine in 1962. Both appear to work equally well in preventing paralytic infection. Each has advantages and disadvantages. Killed vaccine requires four doses by injection; live attenuated vaccine is giv-

TABLE 50-3. Enterovirus Growth in Cell Culture

Viruses	Cell Culture		
	PMK	HDF	Heteroploid
Polioviruses	+	−	+
Coxsackievirus A[a]	−	−	−
Coxsackievirus B	+	−	+
Echovirus	+[b]	+	−
Enteroviruses 68-71	±	±	±

SYMBOLS: PMK, Primary monkey kidney
HDF, Human diploid fibroblasts
+, Growth
−, No growth
±, Variable

[a]A few serotypes grow readily in PMK cells, whereas others vary from strain to strain. None are consistently isolated in monkey or human cell culture.

[b] Echovirus 21 does not produce a cytopathic effect in PMK cells. Some echovirus strains grow better in HDF than in PMK cells.

en by mouth. Live vaccine is less expensive, but virus multiplies, is shed in the feces, and is transmissible to others.[16] Although this transmission does provide for "herd" immunity, it can sometimes result in paralytic disease caused by a reversion or mutation of the vaccine virus. In fact, in countries with widespread live vaccine use, the risk of vaccine-associated polio is greater than that of symptomatic infection with wild poliovirus.[26] About 10 cases of vaccine-associated polio per year are reported in the United States. Usually a nonimmunized parent acquires the infection following his or her infant's vaccination with oral vaccine.[22]

LABORATORY DIAGNOSIS
Specimen Types

Specimens submitted for culture (which is the best approach for laboratory diagnosis) include throat swabs, feces or rectal swabs, spinal fluid, urine, conjunctival swabs, vesicle fluid, blood, pericardial fluid, and tissue. Feces may be superior to rectal swabs.[20] Because virus is not shed from all sites at the same time, several sites should be cultured. For example, to isolate virus from a patient with aseptic meningitis, feces, throat swab, spinal fluid, and blood should be submitted. Recovery of enteroviruses from blood specimens indicates systemic infection and confirms the role of enteroviruses in the disease process.[24]

Direct Detection

Because of the large number of serotypes, little effort has been made toward developing techniques for the direct detection of enteroviruses.

Virus Isolation

Except for most coxsackie viruses type A, enteroviruses are, depending on the virus, best isolated in either PMK or human diploid fibroblast (HDF) cell cultures (Table 50-3). Coxsackie viruses type A vary in their isolation requirements. All can be isolated in suckling mice, but only a few types consistently grow in commonly used cell cultures. Coxsackie A2 to 6, 8, 10, and 12 can be isolated in guinea pig embryo cell cultures.[15] However, since most laboratories do not use guinea pig embryo cell cultures and no longer include animal inoculation for isolation attempts, coxsackie viruses type A are probably often overlooked.

Generally enteroviruses produce scattered cell rounding in PMK cells. Echoviruses usually produce enlarged, tear-shaped cells in 3 to 5 days (Plate 31, *G*) and usually do not involve the entire monolayer, but coxsackie viruses type B CPE progress rapidly and usually involve the entire monolayer. Polioviruses can produce rapid cell disintegration (Plate 32, *A*).

Acid stability can be used to differentiate enteroviruses from rhinoviruses, and mouse inoculation can help differentiate echoviruses from coxsackieviruses. Serotypes are determined by neutralization. Because there are so many different antigenic serotypes, serotyping is simplified by using serum pools. Antisera to each serotype are included in two different pools so the pattern obtained with eight to 10 pools is often sufficient to determine the antigenic serotype.[18] Determination of host range in cell culture and type of infection in suckling mice can aid in serotyping. Serotyping can also be done by fluorescent antibody (FA) staining, complement fixation (CF), and for those enteroviruses with a hemagglutinin, hemagglutination inhibition (HI).

Serologic Diagnosis

Following a primary infection with an enterovirus, type-specific neutralizing IgG develops that persists for life and prevents any recurrence of disease with that serotype. Circulating antibody only prevents viremia; viral replication in the gastrointestinal tract does occur. IgA in both the pharynx and gut prevents implantation of virus, so during reinfection viral shedding is very low. Secretory IgA persists for years. IgM is detectable within several days and is gone in 2 to 3 months.

Subsequent enteroviral infections may result in a heterotypic antibody response depending on how the infecting serotypes are related. IgM response can also be heterologous.[19]

Routine serologic testing is simply too complicated and expensive because acute and convalescent sera would have to be tested against so many different antigens. Serology may be helpful, however, if the patient's own isolate is the antigen, if a large outbreak is caused by a single serotype, or if a patient has a syndrome usually caused by only a few serotypes (for example, myocarditis or acute hemorrhagic conjunctivitis).

Most serologic testing is performed by neutralization, but for certain enteroviruses (for example, enterovirus 70) HI is useful.[14]

Confirmation of an enteroviral infection may be difficult, since virus can be shed in feces for some time, and even a fourfold rise in antibody can be misleading because of heterotypic responses. Isolation of an enterovirus from the spinal fluid, blood, eyes, or skin is considered significant. Isolation from feces only is often just asymptomatic shedding. Clinical symptoms, patient age, and season can help determine significance of a fecal isolate.

REFERENCES

1. Centers for Disease Control: Acute hemorrhagic conjunctivitis—Latin America, MMWR **30**:450, 1981.
2. Chonmaitree, T., et al.: Enterovirus 71 infection: report of an outbreak with two cases of paralysis and a review of the literature, Pediatrics **67**:489, 1981.
3. Couch, R.B.: The common cold: control? J. Infect. Dis. **150**:167, 1984.
4. D'Alessio, D., et al.: A study of the proportions of swimmers among well controls and children with enterovirus-like illness shedding or not shedding an enterovirus, Am. J. Epidemiol. **113**:553, 1981.
5. Duboise, S.M., et al.: Viruses in soil systems, CRC Crit. Rev. Microbiol. **7**:245, 1978.
6. Enders, J.F., Robbins, F.C., and Weller, T.H.: The cultivation of poliomyelitis viruses in tissue culture, Rev. Infect. Dis. **2**:493, 1980.
7. Gwaltney, J.M., Jr., and Hendley, J.O.: Rhinovirus transmission: one if by air, two if by hand, Am. J. Epidemiol. **107**:357, 1978.
8. Gwaltney, J.M., Mosalski, P.B., and Hendley, J.O.: Hand-to-hand transmission of rhinovirus colds, Ann. Intern. Med. **88**:463, 1978.
9. Halperin, S.A., et al.: Pathogenesis of lower respiratory tract symptoms in experimental rhinovirus infection, Am. Rev. Respir. Dis. **128**:806, 1983.
10. Hendley, J.O., Mika, L.A., and Gwaltney, J.M., Jr.: Evaluation of virucidal compounds for inactivation of rhinovirus on hands, Antimicrob. Agents Chemother. **14**:690, 1978.
11. Hendley, J.O., Wenzel, R.P., and Gwaltney, J.M.: Transmission of rhinovirus colds by self inoculation, N. Engl. J. Med. **288**:1361, 1978.
12. Jarvis, W.R., and Tucker, G.: Echovirus type 4 meningitis in young children, Am. J. Dis. Child. **135**:1009, 1981.
13. Keswick, B.H., Gerba, C.P., and Goyal, S.M.: Occurrence of enterovirus in community swimming pools, Am. J. Pub. Health **71**:1026, 1981.
14. Kono, R., et al.: Hemagglutination and hemagglutination inhibition tests with enterovirus 70, J. Clin. Microbiol. **7**:595, 1978.
15. Landry, M.L., et al.: Use of guinea pig cell cultures for isolation and propagation of group A coxsackieviruses, J. Clin. Microbiol. **13**:588, 1981.
16. Melnick, J.L.: Advantages and disadvantages of killed and live poliomyelitis vaccines, Bull. WHO **56**:21, 1978.
17. Melnick, J.L. and Rennick, V.: Infectivity titers of enterovirus as found in human stools, J. Med. Virol. **5**:205, 1980.
18. Melnick, J.L., Wenner, H.A., and Phillips, C.A.: Enteroviruses. In Lennette, E.H., and Schmidt, N.J., editors: Diagnostic procedures for viral, rickettsial and chlamydial infections, ed. 5, Washington, D.C., 1979, American Public Health Association.
19. Minor, T.E., et al.: Counterimmunoelectrophoresis test for immunoglobulin M antibodies to group B coxsackievirus, J. Clin. Microbiol. **8**:503, 1979.
20. Mintz, L., and Drew, W.L.: Relation of culture site to the recovery of nonpolio enteroviruses, Am. J. Clin. Pathol. **74**:324, 1980.
21. Modlin, J.F., et al.: Perinatal echovirus infection: risk of transmission during a community outbreak, N. Engl. J. Med. **305**:368, 1981.
22. Nathanson, N., and Martin, J.R.: The epidemiology of poliomyelitis: enigmas surrounding its appearance, epidemicity, and disappearance, Am. J. Epidemiol. **110**:672, 1979.
23. Nelson, D., et al.: Non-polio enterovirus activity in Wisconsin based on a 20-year experience in a diagnostic virology laboratory, Am. J. Epidemiol. **109**:352, 1979.
24. Prather, S.L., et al.: The isolation of enteroviruses from blood: a comparison of four processing methods, J. Med. Virol. **14**:221, 1984.
25. Sabin, A.B.: Paralytic poliomyelitis: old dogmas and new perspectives, Rev. Infect. Dis. **3**:543, 1981.
26. Salk, D.: Eradication of poliomyelitis in the United States. I. Live virus vaccine-associated and wild poliovirus disease, Rev. Infect. Dis. **2**:228, 1980.
27. Sells, C.J., Carpenter, R.L., and Ray, C.G.: Sequelae of central nervous-system enterovirus infections, N. Engl. J. Med. **293**:1, 1975.
28. Suzuki, N., et al.: Age-related symptomatology of ECHO 11 virus infection in children, Pediatrics **65**:284, 1980.
29. Wilfert, C.M., et al.: Longitudinal assessment of children with enteroviral meningitis during the first three months of life, Pediatrics **67**:811, 1981.

CHAPTER 51

Influenza Viruses

Sally Jo Rubin

The family *Orthomyxoviridae* includes influenza virus types A, B, and C. Influenza virus A naturally infects humans and a number of animals, especially pigs, horses, and birds. Influenza viruses B and C naturally infect only humans. Influenza virus A causes pandemic outbreaks of infections and can be traced to the time of Hippocrates. The term "influenza" derives from the medieval astrologers of Florence who attributed a flulike illness to the influence of the stars. After influenza virus A was isolated in 1933, serologic studies were initiated that helped unravel the complex epidemiology of this virus.

Orthomyxoviridae are RNA viruses that contain eight (seven in the case of influenza virus C) segments of single-stranded ribonucleic acid (RNA), each coding for a single protein.[35] They are generally spherical (30 to 100 nm in diameter) but may also be filamentous. The viruses are surrounded by an envelope derived from the host cell membrane and are thus susceptible to lipid solvents.

The nucleoprotein antigen of influenza viruses is associated with the viral RNA and determines the type specificity—A, B, or C. Two other important antigens are a hemagglutinin (HA) and a neuraminidase (NA). Both are glycoproteins that occur as "spikes" or projections on the virus surface and determine the subtype (Figure 51-1).

All three types of influenza virus possess triangular, rod-shaped hemagglutinins.[7] These antigens react with neuraminic acid–containing glycoproteins on the surface of red blood cells, causing hemagglutination. (See discussion of hemagglutination and hemagglutination inhibition, p. 768.) Neuraminic acid–containing glycoproteins are also present on other host cells and allow viral attachment and the initiation of infection. Antibody to HA prevents initiation of infection and is thus protective against reinfection. Among human and animal strains at least 12 antigenically different HAs are known.[19]

Mushroom-shaped neuraminidase antigens are present on influenza virus types A and B but not C. At 37° C these enzymes cleave the bond between a cell surface site and the HA. As a result, the receptor on the cell is destroyed, but the HA on the virus is not. Thus, if influenza virus A and red cells are mixed together, hemagglutination occurs; however, at 37° C NA causes dissociation. If new virus is then added to these red cells, no reaction takes place, but the original viral particles agglutinate new red cells. Nine antigenically different NAs are known. They may also aid in virus spread because antibody to NA prevents virus release from an infected cell. Antibody to NA is not protective but may modify infection.[2]

Until recently each HA and NA isolated was described by both its antigenicity and the animal from which it had been isolated. For example, Heq2 was the second HA isolated from horses. Because some animal and human strains are so closely related, the nomenclature has been changed so that all HA and NA antigens are simply numbered consecutively (Table 51-1). Thus the equine virus HA (Heq2), the avian virus HA (Hav7), and the human virus HA (H3) are all now called H3.[1] Influenza isolates are described by listing in order the nucleoprotein specificity (A, B, or C), the host of origin (if not a human isolate), the geographic location of isolation, the isolate number, and the year the strain was isolated. The subtype of influenza strains is added in parentheses (Table 51-2). For example, A/Hong Kong/1/68 (H3N2) was the first influenza virus A₃ isolated in Hong Kong in 1968.

Influenza viruses are destroyed by acid, heat (56° C), and formaldehyde. Like many enveloped viruses, they are susceptible to cycles of freezing and thawing and should be stored at −70° C with a protein stabilizer.

EPIDEMIOLOGY

Unlike other respiratory virus infections, influenza virus A infection in humans has three epidemiologic forms.[14] The most known and dreaded are the pandemics that occur about every 10 years (Table 51-2). They can last for many months and infect as much as 20% to 40% of a population. The second form is large regional or nationwide outbreaks occurring during the winter about every 2 to 3 years. About 5% to 10% of the population is infected. Finally, every winter small, localized, sporadic outbreaks occur within a community.

Serologic and molecular studies of viruses isolated over the past 50 years have shed some light on the mechanism for these epidemiologic patterns. Examination of isolates from different pandemics has revealed that their HA or NA antigens, or both, differ in amino acid sequence. This change from one HA or NA to another is called antigenic shift.[5] However, if isolates from the same pandemic, collected over several years, are compared, only minor changes in amino acid sequence are found in the HA or NA. These variations do not result in changes in the subtype and are detected by small reductions in the affinity between the antibody against the original strain and the variant. For example, A/Hong Kong/1/68 and A/Texas/1/77 are easily differentiated by hemagglutination inhibition (HI), but both are the same subtype (H3N2). These slow, minor changes are called antigenic drift.

Influenza virus A undergoes both antigenic shift and antigenic drift. Influenza virus B undergoes antigenic drift but not shift. Since 1955 an outbreak has occurred about every 3 years, and five antigenic types have been sequentially isolated.[26] Influenza C seems to be antigenically stable.[29]

These antigenic changes give the virus a selective advantage in the host. A major alteration (antigenic shift) in the virus often

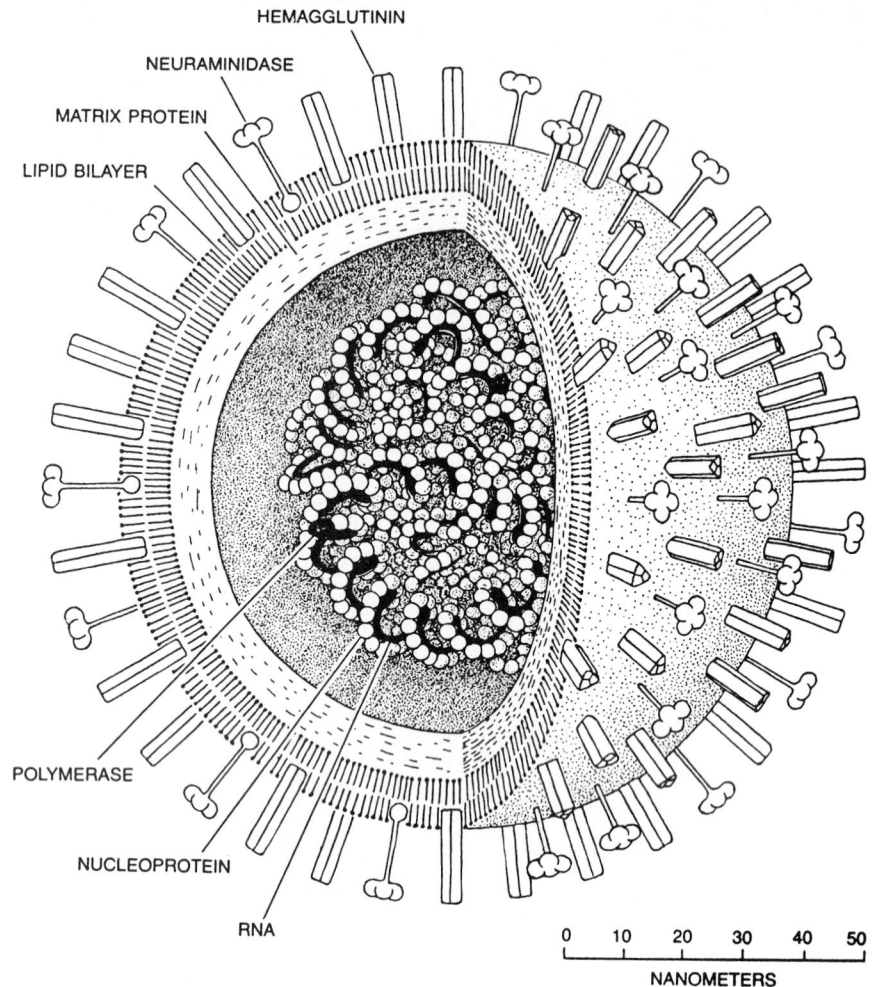

FIGURE 51-1. Diagram of influenza virion showing its external and internal construction. HA and NA spikes are embedded in lipid, or fatty acid, bilayer that surrounds core of virus particle. Matrix protein molecules line underside of lipid bilayer and surround core. Inside core is helical complex of molecules, consisting of ribonucleic acid (RNA) in association with nucleoprotein and polymerases (enzymes that initiate replication). (From Kaplan, M.M., and Webster, R.G.: Sci. Am. **237:**88, 1977.)

results in a pandemic because the population is not immune to the new subtype (Figure 51-2). Intense investigations have revealed some of the mechanisms involved in these changes.

Two theories have been proposed to explain the mechanism of antigenic shift. One is genetic reassortment. As previously mentioned, influenza virus A contains eight distinct RNA segments; one of these segments codes for the NA and another for the HA. When influenza virus A replicates, the eight RNA segments are incorporated randomly into mature virus particles. Thus, if a cell is simultaneously infected with two different influenza viruses (for example, H3N2 and H1N1), a total of 256 combinations of these segments may occur, with four different HA and NA patterns (Figure 51-3).

In humans only four major subtypes have been detected, but in animals, especially birds, viruses with many different combinations of HA and NA have been isolated.[19] These animal subtypes are probably the result of genetic reassortment in mixed infections. The emergence of new human subtypes could result from recombination between an animal strain and a

human strain or alternatively by human infection with an animal strain (for example, swine influenza) that becomes more virulent after passage in humans. Each of these possibilities has some supporting evidence.[22,27]

Another theory is that a finite number of subtypes exist and that these recycle after remaining dormant for several generations. Serologic evidence supports this theory of recycling of a subtype after many decades when a population would again be susceptible to it.[31,38] To the surprise of many, the H1N1 strains that first appeared in Russia in 1977 are closely related to the H1N1 strains isolated in 1950. Thus in this one instance a type has reappeared after less than 30 years. How the H1N1 virus was preserved over the 27 years is not known. It is possible that the virus somehow persisted in an animal reservoir, although this seems unlikely because mutagenic changes occur during epidemic spread (in both humans and animals) over a relatively short time.[34]

Probably several mechanisms are involved in the establishment of new subtypes. Subtypes clearly differ in virulence and

TABLE 51-1. Hemagglutinins and Neuraminidases of Influenza Virus A

New Designation	Old Designation
HEMAGGLUTININS	
H1	H0, H1, Hsw1
H2	H2
H3	H3, Heq2, Hav7
H4	Hav4
H5	Hav5
H6	Hav6
H7	Heq1, Hav1
H8	Hav8
H9	Hav9
H10	Hav2
H11	Hav3
H12	Hav10

TABLE 51-1. Hemagglutinins and Neuraminidases of Influenza Virus A—cont'd

New Designation	Old Designation
NEURAMINIDASES	
N1	N1
N2	N2
N3	Nav2, Nav3
N4	Nav4
N5	Nav5
N6	Nav1
N7	Neq1
N8	Neq2
N9	Neq6

> **SYMBOLS:** sw, Swine
> eq, Equine
> av, Avian

TABLE 51-2. Influenza Pandemics

Year	Influenza Virus A Subtype			Antigen Changed	Severity	Example
1918	H-SW N1	swine	(H1N1)[b]	?	Pandemic (severe)	
1947	H1N1	A_1	(H1N1)	HA, NA	Pandemic (mild)	
1957	H2N2	A_2 (Asian)	(H2N2)	HA, NA	Pandemic (severe)	A/Singapore/1/57
1968	H3N2	A_3 (Hong Kong)	(H3N2)	HA	Pandemic (moderate)	A/Hong Kong/1/68
1978	H1N1	A_1	(H1N1)	HA, NA	Pandemic (mild)	A/USSR/90/77

Modified from Kilbourne, E.D.: J. Infect. Dis. **127:**478, 1973.
[a]A change in the hemagglutinin H-SW to H0 is thought to have occurred in approximately 1929, but this resulted in an epidemic and not a pandemic.
[b]New nomenclature.

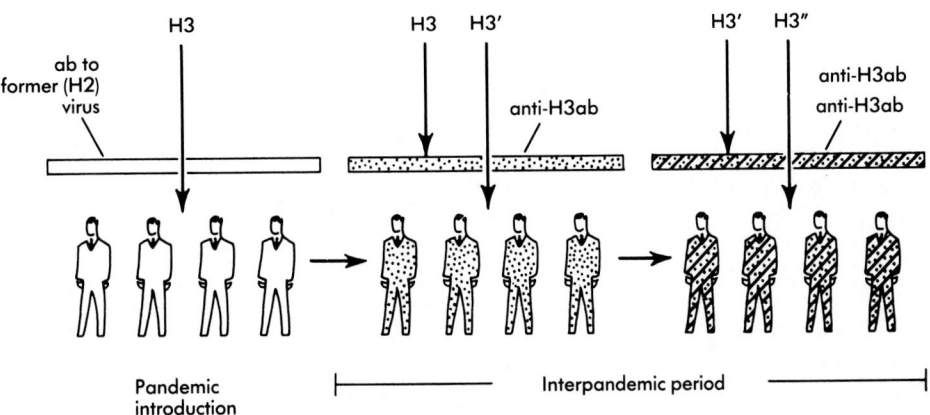

FIGURE 51-2. Selection of antigenic mutants as function of population antibody. New pandemic viral subtype H3 transcends barrier of antibody to unrelated, previously prevalent virus H2 and readily infects population. When critical percentage of population has been infected with H3, survival of H3 is impeded, and antigenically changed mutant H3′, and later H3″, have survival advantage. (From Kilbourne, E.D.: The influenza viruses and influenza, New York, 1975, Academic Press, Inc.)

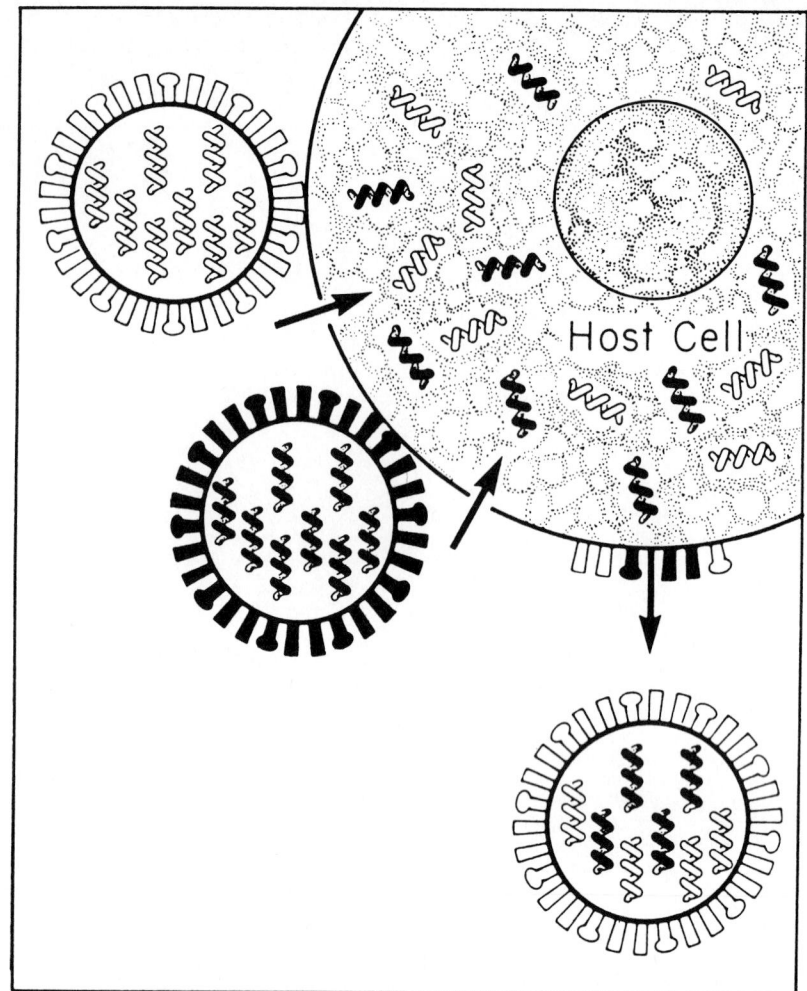

FIGURE 51-3. Genetic reassortment. Random packaging of RNA segments from two different types of influenza viruses (such as H1N1 × H3N2) produces 256 different gene combinations (recombinants) including two identical with parental genotypes. (From Kilbourne, E.D.: Influenza. In Rothschild, H., Allison F., and Howe, C., editors: Human diseases caused by viruses, New York, 1978, Oxford University Press.)

transmissibility, as well as changes in HA and NA.[23,43] For a new subtype to emerge and take over is a complex process that is still not entirely resolved.

Antigenic drift is the result of point mutations in the HA and NA. Mutant viruses are thought to be selected because they are able to persist in the presence of antibody to the antecedent viral strain. Changes also occur throughout the genome, suggesting that antibody pressure against HA and NA may not be the only factor involved in selection of a new strain.[44]

CLINICAL SIGNIFICANCE

Influenza virus A infection is often asymptomatic and if symptomatic is usually a minor illness with an abrupt onset of fever, chills, headache, myalgia, sore throat, and sometimes a dry cough. Onset of symptoms occurs 1 to 4 days after inhalation or direct contact with secretions containing influenza virus A, and recovery occurs within several days. Convalescence can take a few weeks. Mortality is less than 1:1000, but because the number of cases is so great, total mortality is significant.[23]

Death is the result of primary influenza pneumonia or a secondary bacterial pneumonia. The most common causes of post-influenzal bacterial pneumonia are *Streptococcus pneumoniae*, *Staphylococcus aureus*, and *Haemophilus influenzae*. The elderly and people with chronic diseases (such as lung, heart, or kidney disease or diabetes) are at risk for pneumonia.

Influenza virus B infection tends to be milder and most commonly causes febrile upper respiratory illness in young children.[15] Gastric complaints are common, but pneumonia is rare.[24,42] Infection in the elderly has been reported infrequently.[16] Influenza virus C infection is usually mild. Infection first occurs early in life and is common.[10]

Influenza virus B and (much less frequently) influenza virus A infections have been associated with Reye's syndrome, a serious noninflammatory encephalopathy that is often fatal.[17]

Influenza epidemics begin in school-age children who transmit the virus to their younger siblings and parents.[13] The greatest number of infections are in preschool children. Nosocomial outbreaks have been reported, one in a neonatal intensive care nursery.[28]

Influenza virus multiplies in ciliated columnar epithelial cells and causes cell death. Virus is shed for 24 hours before clinical onset and for 3 to 4 days after onset. Low levels of virus may be shed for 5 to 10 days. At least with influenza virus B, the quantity of virus shed and the severity of the illness are directly correlated, suggesting that illness may be directly related to the cytotoxicity of the virus.[15] In uncomplicated influenza virus A infection, pulmonary function is affected. The basis of these changes is complex and not entirely known.[40]

CONTROL AND TREATMENT

Inactivated influenza virus A and B vaccines have been in use since the 1940s. Vaccine efficacy is 70% to 90%[30,36] and clearly reduces pneumonia, hospitalization, and death in high-risk groups.[2]

Vaccines are formalin-inactivated virus grown in eggs. Both whole virus and "subvirion" or "split product" vaccines are in use. The latter are prepared using whole virus that has been treated with lipid solvents. Vaccine response is variable and depends on age, previous exposure or vaccination, and the dose and strain of virus. Generally children under 2 years of age and people with no previous exposure ("unprimed") respond poorly. Subsequent vaccination with a new strain usually results in a broad, good serologic response. The vaccines are safe to use in pregnancy.[41]

An increased risk of Guillain-Barré syndrome followed vaccination with A/New Jersey/76 vaccine[6,39] but not with subsequent vaccines.[21]

Because influenza viruses change from season to season, a new vaccine is made each year from the type that was prevalent the year before. Vaccination with a variant closely related to the prevalent type gives good protection.[30]

Live attenuated influenza virus A vaccines are well tolerated and may induce local immune responses that are protective against wild-type virus infection.[3] Amantadine (Symmetrel) and its analogue, rimantadine, are effective prophylactics for influenza virus A infection.[20,32] If given within 24 hours of onset, they reduce the length of illness and the time of viral shedding.[25] Views concerning their use are conflicting,[37] but most authorities recommend prophylaxis to prevent a possible nosocomial outbreak and for nonvaccinated high-risk groups. Both drugs are ineffective against influenza viruses B and C.

LABORATORY DIAGNOSIS
SPECIMEN TYPES

Specimens for culture and direct examination for influenza should be collected within 3 days of onset of symptoms. Although immediate inoculation is preferred, specimens may be held at 4° C for 3 to 4 days. Throat swabs are acceptable, but nasal washings are preferable. For serologic evaluation, acute sera are collected within a week of onset, and convalescent sera 2 to 3 weeks after onset.

DIRECT EXAMINATION

Immunofluorescence testing performed directly on nasopharyngeal secretions detects about 75% of culture-positive specimens.[9] The immunoperoxidase test is not as useful because of problems with endogenous peroxidase.[12] Specimens for direct fluorescent antibody (FA) staining should be washed to remove mucus. Enzyme-linked immunosorbent assay (ELISA) may prove to be more sensitive for direct detection than FA.[4]

VIRUS ISOLATION

Influenza viruses can be isolated in embryonated hens' eggs or primary monkey kidney (PMK) cell culture. Strains vary in their ability to grow in either host, and some grow in only one or the other. Ideally both should be used, but most laboratories rely on just PMK. Cynomolgus monkey kidney cells are slightly better for this purpose than rhesus monkey kidney cells.[8,11] Serum may contain factors that interfere with influenza virus growth and therefore should not be used in the maintenance medium.

In eggs, virus is detected and measured in allantoic and amniotic fluid by hemagglutination with fowl red cells. Influenza virus may or may not produce cytopathic effect (CPE) in PMK cell culture. Influenza virus A is usually detected by hemadsorption with guinea pig red cells (Plate 32, *B*). PMK cell culture is usually tested for hemadsorption after 3, 7, and 14 days of incubation. Influenza virus B usually produces CPE. Cells are enlarged, rounded, and refractile, usually first appearing randomly over the monolayer. Influenza virus C does not grow in PMK.

Isolates are confirmed as influenza virus by complement fixation or FA. Strains are identified by hemagglutination inhibition (HI). The isolate is tested against several reference sera (of the prevalent types), and the HI titers are compared with titers obtained with known isolates tested against the same sera. An isolate is considered to have the HA of the reference strain to which it gives a titer equal ($\pm$ one dilution) to that obtained with the homologous reference antiserum.

SEROLOGIC DIAGNOSIS

Following a primary infection, HI and anti-NA antibodies appear in the serum within 10 days and peak in about 4 weeks. The majority of people have serum IgM antibody that appears in 8 to 14 days and persists 1 to 4 months.[7]

HI antibody (which measures strain) lasts for years, but complement fixation (CF) antibody (which measures type) usually drops in several weeks or months. Secretory IgA is found in nasal washings. Following reinfection a brisk serum antibody response to the original strain and the infecting strain occurs. This makes serologic diagnosis of influenza difficult. Although a fourfold rise in titer to the test strain indicates the presence of influenza virus infection, it does not necessarily mean that the test strain is the infecting strain.

A number of serologic procedures are acceptable, but CF (using the nucleoprotein group antigen) and HI are most widely used. ELISA has been reported by some as more sensitive than HI[33] but as less sensitive than HI by others.[18] This is probably a reflection of the antigen source.

REFERENCES

1. Assaad, F.A., et al.: A revision of the system of nomenclature for influenza viruses: a WHO memorandum, Bull. WHO **58:**585, 1980.
2. Barker, W.H., and Mullooly, J.P.: Influenza vaccination of elderly persons: reduction in pneumonia and influenza hospitalization and deaths, JAMA **244:**2547, 1980.
3. Belshe, R.B., et al.: Live attenuated influenza A virus vaccines in children: results of a field trial, J. Infect. Dis. **150:**834, 1984.
4. Bishai, F.R., Galli, R., and Fulton, R.E.: Enzyme-linked immunosorbent assay for detection and identification of influenza viruses A and B in clinical specimens, Lancet **2:**756, 1981.

5. Both, G.W., et al.: Antigenic drift in influenza virus H3 hemagglutinin from 1968 to 1980: multiple evolutionary pathways and sequential amino acid changes at key antigenic sites, J. Virol. **48**:52, 1983.

6. Breman, J.G., and Hayner, N.S.: Guillain-Barré syndrome and its relationship to swine influenza vaccination in Michigan, 1976-1977, Am. J. Epidemiol. **119**:880, 1984.

7. Buchner, Y.I., et al.: Serum IgM antibody and influenza A infection, J. Clin. Pathol. **30**:723, 1977.

8. Clark, J., et al.: Comparison of cynomolgus and rhesus monkey kidney cells for recovery of viruses from clinical specimens, J. Clin. Microbiol. **9**:554, 1979.

9. Daisy, J.A., Lief, F.S., and Friedman, H.M.: Rapid diagnosis of influenza A infection by direct immunofluorescence of nasopharyngeal aspirates in adults, J. Clin. Microbiol. **9**:688, 1979.

10. Dykes, A.C., Cherry, J.D., and Nolan, C.E.: A clinical, epidemiological, serologic, and virologic study of influenza C virus infection, Arch. Intern. Med. **140**:1295, 1980.

11. Frank, A.L., et al.: Comparison of different tissue cultures for isolation and quantitation of influenza and parainfluenza viruses, J. Clin. Microbiol. **10**:32, 1979.

12. Gardner, P.S., Grandien, M., and McQuillin, J.: Comparison of immunofluorescence and immunoperoxidase methods for viral diagnosis at a distance: a WHO collaborative study, Bull. WHO **56**:105, 1978.

13. Glezen, W.P., and Couch, R.B.: Interpandemic influenza in the Houston area, 1974-76, N. Engl. J. Med. **298**:587, 1978.

14. Gregg, M.B.: The epidemiology of influenza in humans, Ann. N.Y. Acad. Sci. **353**:45, 1980.

15. Hall, C.B., et al.: Viral shedding patterns of children with influenza B infection, J. Infect. Dis. **140**:610, 1979.

16. Hall, W.N., et al.: An outbreak of influenza B in an elderly population, J. Infect. Dis. **144**:297, 1981.

17. Halsey, N.A., et al.: An epidemic of Reye syndrome associated with influenza A (H1N1) in Colorado, J. Pediatr. **97**:535, 1980.

18. Hammond, G.W., Smith, S.J., and Noble, G.R.: Sensitivity and specificity of enzyme immunoassay for serodiagnosis of influenza A virus infections, J. Infect. Dis. **141**:644, 1980.

19. Hinshaw, V.S., Webster, R.G., and Rodriquez, R.J.: Influenza A viruses: combinations of hemagglutination and neuraminidase subtypes isolated from animals and other sources, Arch. Virol. **67**:191, 1981.

20. Hirsch, M.S., and Swartz, M.N.: Antiviral agents, N. Engl. J. Med. **302**:903, 1980.

21. Hurwitz, E.S., et al.: Guillain-Barré syndrome and the 1978-79 influenza vaccine, N. Engl. J. Med. **304**:1557, 1981.

22. Kaplan, M.M., and Webster, R.G.: The epidemiology of influenza, Sci. Am. **237**:88, 1977.

23. Kilbourne, E.D.: Molecular epidemiology—influenza as archetype, Harvey Lect. **73**:225, 1978.

24. LaMontagne, J.R.: Summary of a workshop in influenza B viruses and Reye's syndrome, J. Infect. Dis. **142**:452, 1980.

25. LaMontagne, J.R., and Galasso, G.J.: Report of a workshop on clinical studies of the efficacy of amantadine and rimantadine against influenza viruses, J. Infect. Dis. **138**:928, 1978.

26. Laver, G.: The hemagglutinin of influenza viruses: structure, immunology, and biological function: summary of a meeting, J. Infect. Dis. **138**:105, 1978.

27. Laver, W.G., Webster, R.G., and Chu, C.M.: Summary of a meeting on the origin of pandemic influenza viruses, J. Infect. Dis. **149**:108, 1984.

28. Meibalane, R., et al.: Outbreak of influenza in a neonatal intensive care unit, J. Pediatr. **91**:974, 1977.

29. Meier-Ewert, H., Petri, T., and Bishop, D.H.L.: Oligonucleotide fingerprint analyses of influenza C virion RNA recovered from five different isolates, Arch. Virol. **67**:141, 1981.

30. Meiklejohn, G., et al.: Antigenic drift and efficacy of influenza virus vaccines, 1976-1977, J. Infect. Dis. **138**:618, 1978.

31. Monto, A.S., and Maassab, H.F.: Serologic responses to nonprevalent influenza A viruses during intercyclic periods, Am. J. Epidemiol. **113**:236, 1981.

32. Monto, A.S., et al.: Prevention of Russian influenza by amantadine, JAMA **241**:1003, 1979.

33. Murphy, B.R., et al.: Hemagglutinin specific enzyme-linked immunosorbent assay for antibodies to influenza A and B viruses, J. Clin. Microbiol. **13**:554, 1981.

34. Nakajuna, K., Desselberger, U., and Palese, P.: Recent human influenza A (H1N1) viruses are closely related genetically to strains isolated in 1950, Nature **274**:334, 1978.

35. Palese, P., and Young, J.F.: Variation of influenza A, B, and C viruses, Science **215**:1468, 1982.

36. Richman, D.D.: Use of temperature-sensitive mutants for live, attenuated influenza-virus vaccines, N. Engl. J. Med. **300**:137, 1979.

37. Sabin, A.B.: Amantadine and influenza: evaluation of conflicting reports, J. Infect. Dis. **138**:557, 1978.

38. Schoenbaum, S.C., et al.: Epidemiology of influenza in the elderly: evidence of virus recycling, Am. J. Epidemiol. **103**:166, 1976.

39. Schonberger, L.B., et al.: Guillain-Barré syndrome following vaccination in the National Influenza Immunization Program, United States, 1976-1977, Am. J. Epidemiol. **110**:105, 1979.

40. Stuart-Harris, C.H.: The influenza viruses and the human respiratory tract, Rev. Infect. Dis. **4**:592, 1979.

41. Sumaya, C.V., and Gibbs, R.S.: Immunization of pregnant women with influenza A/New Jersey/76 virus vaccine: reactogenicity and immunogenicity in mother and infant, J. Infect. Dis. **140**:141, 1979.

42. Wright, P.F., Bryant, J.D., and Karzon, D.T.: Comparison of influenza B/Hong Kong virus infections among infants, children and young adults, J. Infect. Dis. **141**:430, 1980.

43. Wright, P.F., Thompson, J., and Karzon, D.T.: Differing virulence of H_1N_1 and H_3N_2 influenza strains, Am. J. Epidemiol. **112**:814, 1980.

44. Young, J.F., et al.: Mechanisms of genetic variation in human influenza viruses, Ann. N.Y. Acad. Sci. **354**:135, 1980.

CHAPTER 52

Paramyxoviruses

Sally Jo Rubin

Members of the family *Paramyxoviridae* are enveloped RNA viruses with helical capsid symmetry. They are large (150 to 300 nm in diameter) and more pleomorphic than *Orthomyxoviridae*, and their RNA is a single molecule rather than segmented. All members of the family, except respiratory syncytial virus, have a hemagglutinin. Some also have a neuraminidase.

The three genera in this family are *Paramyxovirus, Pneumovirus*, and *Morbillivirus*. No group antigen is found, although some antigens within genera are shared.

Genus	Common species
Paramyxovirus	Parainfluenza virus
	Mumps virus
	Newcastle disease virus
	Other animal viruses
Pneumovirus	Respiratory syncytial virus
Morbillivirus	Measles virus
	Canine distemper

Paramyxoviridae are important causes of respiratory disease in children, especially parainfluenza and respiratory syncytial virus. Since the introduction of specific vaccination the once common childhood diseases measles and mumps are now only occasionally seen.

PARAMYXOVIRUSES

Paramyxoviruses are single-stranded RNA viruses with both a hemagglutinin and a neuraminidase. Five antigenic types of parainfluenza virus and one type of mumps virus are known (Table 52-1). A number of paramyxoviruses are animal viruses, including Sendai virus, the first paramyxovirus isolated, and Newcastle disease virus, a pathogen of chickens. Because they are enveloped viruses, all are ether and chloroform sensitive.

Parainfluenza Viruses[37]
Clinical Significance

Parainfluenza viruses infect the mucous membranes of the nose and throat and are responsible for 6% to 18% of acute respiratory illness in children. Infection ranges from inapparent to severe and even fatal.[24] Various clinical syndromes are associated with certain virus types (Table 52-1).

Parainfluenza viruses 1 and 2 involve the larynx and produce croup, a spasmodic laryngitis characterized by difficult breathing and a hoarse metallic cough. Croup annually results in the hospitalization of 1% of infants. Although parainfluenza viruses 1 to 3 may cause croup, parainfluenza virus 1 is the major isolate, whereas parainfluenza virus 3, which can descend to the lower respiratory tract, is more likely to be isolated from infants with pneumonia or bronchiolitis.[3]

Epidemiology

Parainfluenza viruses are transmitted from person to person by direct contact or large droplets. The incubation period probably ranges from 2 to 6 days, depending on the age of the host and inoculum size. A larger amount of virus is shed in children with more severe illness,[12] but the duration of shedding is unknown. Primary infection takes place early in life. Seroepidemiologic studies indicate that the majority of children have been infected with parainfluenza virus type 3 by 2 years of age, with most clinical illness in infants less than 12 months old. Primary infection caused by parainfluenza viruses 1 and 2 is most common between 6 and 60 months of age. Reinfection with these viruses occurs frequently, but after 5 years of age they usually cause only a mild upper respiratory infection.[9]

Parainfluenza virus 3 causes epidemics every year, usually in late spring or early summer, whereas parainfluenza viruses 1 and 2 seem to occur in alternate years in the fall. Parainfluenza virus 4 is isolated sporadically at low levels.

Treatment and Control

No vaccine or treatment is available for parainfluenza virus infections. An effective vaccine against parainfluenza viruses 1, 2, and 3 could prevent an estimated 40% to 50% of croup cases.

Laboratory Diagnosis
Specimen types

Parainfluenza viruses infect only the respiratory tract; therefore specimens for both direct examination and culture are collected from the oropharynx. Nasopharyngeal and throat swabs or nasal washings are appropriate. An acute serum specimen is collected at onset and a convalescent specimen 2 to 3 weeks later.

Direct examination

Fluorescent antibody (FA) staining can be performed on exfoliated cells in nasopharyngeal washings. Staining is cytoplasmic and type specific, so an antiserum is required for each antigenic serotype. Enzyme immunoassay and radioimmunoassay are research techniques for directly detecting parainfluenza viruses.[36,40] They are at least equal to and may be more sensitive than FA.

Virus isolation

Some parainfluenza virus strains can be isolated in embryonated hens' eggs, but the best isolation is obtained in primary

TABLE 52-1. Paramyxoviruses

Virus	Clinical Manifestation	Occurrence
Parainfluenza 1	Croup	Every other year, fall[a]
Parainfluenza 2	Croup (less serious)	Every other year, fall[a]
Parainfluenza 3	Pneumonia, bronchiolitis, croup	Yearly, late spring and early summer
Parainfluenza 4A, 4B	Mild illness	Sporadic, infrequent
Mumps	Parotitis, orchitis, meningoencephalitis	Yearly, late winter, spring

Data from reference 37.
[a]Often types 1 and 2 occur in alternate years.

monkey kidney (PMK) cell cultures. Cynomolgus monkey kidney is a little more sensitive than rhesus monkey kidney cell cultures.[2,5] Parainfluenza viruses 1, 2, and 3 can also be isolated in HEK, HEp-2, and HeLa cells. Cell cultures should be washed free of serum to avoid inhibition from cross-reacting antibody to animal paramyxoviruses. The simian virus SV5, which can be present in PMK cell cultures, is also a problem because the cytopathic effect (CPE) it produces can be confused with those of human paramyxoviruses, particularly parainfluenza virus 2. It is, however, antigenically distinct. Only parainfluenza virus 2 produces much CPE. PMK cells infected with parainfluenza virus 2 develop irregular syncytia. Most parainfluenza virus isolates are first detected by hemadsorption with guinea pig red cells at 4° C. Hemadsorption of myxoviruses and paramyxoviruses (except influenza virus C and parainfluenza virus 4) can be reversed if the cell cultures are incubated at 37° C. At this temperature the red cells are released from the monolayer by the viral neuraminidase.

Isolates may be confirmed by hemagglutination inhibition (HI) or neutralization. Parainfluenza viruses have soluble complement fixation (CF) antigens that can be used to differentiate types 1, 2, and 3. Parainfluenza virus 4A and 4B share a common CF antigen but can be distinguished by HI or neutralization. The latter tests can also be used to identify the other three serotypes.

Serologic diagnosis

Because reinfection with parainfluenza viruses is so common, serologic diagnosis may be difficult. Also, infection with a second serotype results in heterotypic response. For example, in a patient with a past parainfluenza virus 3 infection, infection with parainfluenza virus 1 can result in a parainfluenza virus 3 antibody response although a parainfluenza virus 1 response may or may not be seen. Heterotypic responses can also follow mumps virus infection. Thus a fourfold rise in titer usually indicates parainfluenza virus infection, but it does not implicate a particular serotype as the cause of the infection. Antibody response is usually measured by CF, HI, or neutralization. The presence of serum-neutralizing antibody[37] or secretory IgA[41] does not correlate with immunity. Most patients have secretory IgA by 7 to 10 days after onset. Fewer than half of infected adults have a demonstrable rise in CF antibody, so although CF is the most widely available test, it is not the most sensitive.

MUMPS VIRUS

Mumps virus, a single-stranded RNA virus, naturally infects only humans. The disease mumps was described by Hippocrates in the fifth century, and the virus was isolated in 1934. Mumps virus has both HA and NA activity. Unlike other paramyxoviruses, it also has a hemolysin. There are two CF antigens: the S antigen is the ribonucleoprotein, and the V antigen is part of the outer membrane. Mumps virus is relatively stable and can be held at 4° C for several days.

Clinical Significance

Before 1967 mumps infection was almost inevitable during childhood. Infection can be asymptomatic or severe,[1a] but typically the salivary glands (most often the parotid glands) enlarge and symptoms persist for a week to 10 days. Fever is variable. Typical mumps is not serious, but complications can be serious and can even lead to death. About 0.5% to 1% of infected people develop meningoencephalitis and (rarely) pancreatitis, myocarditis, thyroiditis, neuritis, arthritis, and conjunctivitis. Among mature men and women, about 20% of men experience inflammation of the testicles (orchitis), and about 5% of women have inflammation of the ovaries (ovaritis).

Mumps virus is shed into the saliva, even if there is no parotitis, and is transmitted directly in these secretions by droplets or fomites. Virus is found in saliva during the 14- to 24-day incubation period, but peak periods of communicability are a few days before and after development of enlarged glands. Virus may be shed in saliva for up to 9 days past onset and in urine for as long as 2 weeks. Pathogenesis of mumps is not completely understood. The virus probably initiates infection by multiplying in the upper respiratory tract, enters the blood, and proceeds to the salivary glands and other organs.

Mumps occurs in late winter and the spring. Since widespread vaccine use the average number of cases per year has declined dramatically. Mumps remains a disease of young children, although the incidence among 10- to 15-year-olds has increased slightly. The case-fatality ratio remains 1.8:10,000 reported cases.[20]

Treatment and Control

A live attenuated mumps vaccine that was introduced in 1967 produces a noncommunicable, subclinical infection with very few side effects. Antibody that is protective and of long duration develops in more than 90% of vaccinated persons.[1]

Laboratory Diagnosis

Specimens

Since the introduction of vaccine, mumps virus is an infrequent isolate in the laboratory, although it is not difficult to detect or isolate. Specimens for direct examination and culture include saliva collected 1 to 3 days after onset by swabbing the openings of Stensen's ducts and urine collected up to 2 weeks after onset. In cases of suspected mumps encephalitis, virus can be isolated from spinal fluid up to 6 days after onset. Blood and parotid tissue can also be cultured.

Serum specimens are collected at onset and 7 to 14 days later. Sometimes a third serum specimen, collected at 21 days, is necessary to demonstrate a titer rise.

Direct detection

Reagents for direct detection by FA of mumps-infected cells in saliva and urine are commercially available.

Virus isolation

Animals are not used for mumps virus isolation. Virus can be isolated in the amniotic sac of 7- to 8-day embryonated hens' eggs. Following a 5- to 7-day incubation, virus is detected by hemagglutination or CF. The simplest laboratory method for mumps isolation is in cell culture. A number of cell cultures are susceptible to mumps virus, including PMK, continuous human cell lines (such as HeLa), and primary human cell lines (like HEK).

In PMK cells infected with mumps virus large granular syncytial cells are formed. Mumps virus hemadsorbs guinea pig red cells at 4° C. An isolate can be serologically confirmed by FA, hemadsorption inhibition, or neutralization.

Serologic diagnosis

Following mumps infection IgA is present in saliva by 2 weeks but usually disappears within 10 weeks.[6] In serum HI antibodies peak at 4 to 8 days after onset followed by V CF antibody. In general, the S CF antibodies are present early but disappear within a few months, while V CF antibodies appear later and persist longer. Thus an elevated S CF titer and a low V CF titer is presumptively diagnostic of mumps. A follow-up serum should be tested to demonstrate a rise in antibody to V. Eventually 20% to 30% of people with a past history of mumps will be CF negative.

No good test is available for testing for past mumps infection, although neutralization is the best test.[20] A new commercially available indirect fluorescent antibody (IFA) test (Electro-Nucleonics, Inc., Bethesda, Md.) may provide the required sensitivity for immunity screens. The mumps skin test is not valid and is no longer available.[2]

CF and HI are about equal in sensitivity for serologic diagnosis of mumps. Neutralization is the most specific and sensitive test.

PNEUMOVIRUS (RESPIRATORY SYNCYTIAL VIRUS)

Human respiratory syncytial virus (RSV) is in a separate genus from the other *Paramyxoviridae* because it has a smaller nucleocapsid and smaller structural proteins. It also has no hemagglutinating activity. RSV resembles other *Paramyxoviridae* in being a highly pleomorphic, enveloped virus containing single-stranded, helical RNA.

RSV is characterized by the extensive syncytia it produces in cell cultures. When human antisera are used to compare RSV isolates, strain differences are not apparent, but when isolates are examined by neutralization with hyperimmune animal sera, strain differences are evident.[22]

CLINICAL SIGNIFICANCE[10]

RSV produces symptoms ranging from mild upper respiratory disease to bronchiolitis, pneumonia, severe respiratory distress, and sometimes death. It is responsible for 60% to 90% of bronchiolitis and 5% to 40% of pneumonia in young children. It is the major cause of these diseases in infants and results in the hospitalization of 0.4% of all infants. Severity of infection is related to both age and socioeconomic class.

RSV is most severe in infants and can readily infect newborns, although infants less than 3 weeks old are more likely to have atypical disease than lower respiratory tract symptoms.[14] In higher socioeconomic groups infection is acquired later in life and is thus less severe. Virus is shed only from the respiratory tract, and in infants duration of shedding is 3 to 22 days.[8]

RSV usually produces an acute febrile upper respiratory infection in adults, with fatigue and shortness of breath sometimes persisting for several weeks.[18] Disease in the elderly and chronically ill can be more severe.[31]

The incubation period of RSV infection is 3 to 11 days. The virus grows in ciliated epithelial cells of the respiratory tract. In an animal model the virus causes cell injury to infected cells[21]; therefore symptoms of RSV infection may be related to cell damage. The most suitable animal model in which to study the pathogenesis of RSV is still controversial.

Epidemiology

RSV infection occurs throughout the world in yearly epidemics in the winter or early spring. The virus is spread by close contact with direct inoculation of large droplets or by self-inoculation after touching contaminated surfaces. Route of entry is the nose or eye.[11,15] Spread by small particle aerosol does not seem to occur.

Nosocomial outbreaks of RSV infection in nurseries can be devastating. Infection rates can be high, and some babies die.[14,15,32] Because infection is acquired by direct contact with secretions, strict handwashing is the best control measure. This does decrease infant infection but does not affect the 50% infection rate among staff caring for the infants, probably because RSV can survive in secretions on nonporous surfaces for a fairly long time. Thus, even if personnel wash their hands before and after caring for each infant, viable virus can still be present in the environment.[13]

Treatment and Control

Serum antibody does reduce severity but is not protective[12]; thus an effective vaccine would have to stimulate local antibody. Such stimulation requires an attenuated live vaccine. So far the virus has not been attenuated enough to not cause any clinical illness when given to volunteers. A major problem with immunization against RSV is that members of the most susceptible population, infants, have a poor immunologic response following antigenic stimulation.[37] An antiviral agent, ribavirin, reduces systemic symptoms and viral shedding in experimentally infected young adults.[16] Ribavirin has not been fully evaluated in infants.

LABORATORY DIAGNOSIS
Specimens

Nasal aspirate, pooled nasopharyngeal and throat swabs, or sputum is the best specimen for both direct examination and culture of RSV.[26] Specimens for culture should be kept at 4° C and inoculated as soon as possible after collection. Some microbiologists recommend inoculation at the bedside.

Acute serum specimens are collected at onset and convalescent specimens 2 to 4 weeks later. Demonstration of a titer rise in infants may take even longer.

Direct Detection

Immunofluorescence is useful for direct detection of RSV in nasal aspirates or lung tissue. Isolation of virus takes 5 to 10 days, whereas FA requires only a few hours. Between 85% and 90% of tissue culture positive specimens contain typical cells with cytoplasmic immunofluorescence.[7,25] Commercial ELISA kits may be more sensitive than cell culture for the detection of RSV.[1]

Virus Isolation

RSV can grow in a number of animals (mice, ferrets, guinea pigs, hamsters), but infection is generally asymptomatic. RSV is best isolated in HEp-2 or HeLa cells. The virus forms syncytial cells in 3 to 7 days. Young HEp-2 cell cultures with a light monolayer are essential. In a heavy HEp-2 monolayer, RSV may produce only indistinct rounding that can easily be missed. Some strains grow in diploid fibroblast cells but instead of producing syncytia cause cell destruction that eventually involves the entire monolayer.

The only other virus that produces similar CPE is parainfluenza virus 2, but RSV grows poorly or not at all in PMK (unless cells are very young) and is hemadsorption negative. Serologic confirmation is obtained by FA, CF, or neutralization.

Serologic Diagnosis

Serologic response to RSV can be measured by CF or neutralization. Although the acute serum may have antibody (maternal or from a previous infection), it is still often possible to demonstrate a significant rise. In primary infection, IgM is present within a few days, peaks in 1 to 2 weeks, and is generally undetectable in about 10 to 12 weeks. About 60% of infants have a rise in IgG, which peaks in about 2 weeks and drops to low levels in 2 to 3 months. Older infants have greater convalescent titers and are more likely to have a fourfold rise. After reinfection high IgG titers are present within a week and persist for a longer time.[39]

MORBILLIVIRUS

Measles has a recorded history of over 2000 years and was first isolated in 1954. Before vaccine development measles virus infected 95% of the population at some time in their lives and resulted in death for about 1%. More recently measles has been linked to subacute sclerosing panencephalitis (SSPE) and possibly to multiple sclerosis and some of the autoimmune diseases.

The genus *Morbillivirus* has three antigenically related viruses: measles, which infect only primates, canine distemper virus, and rinderpest of ruminants. Measles virus is an enveloped RNA virus with a hemagglutinin but not neuraminidase activity. It also has a hemolysin. Only one serotype of measles virus is known.[33] It is relatively thermolabile and should be stored at −70° C with a protein stabilizer.

MEASLES VIRUS
Clinical Significance

About 10 days after exposure to measles virus patients begin to develop fever, cough, runny nose, and conjunctivitis; a maculopapular rash appears 4 or 5 days later. The rash, which often becomes confluent, begins at the head and moves down the body somewhat like a window shade being lowered. The rash disappears from the extremities first, as if the shade was being raised. Just before the rash develops, bright red spots with a blue-white central speck appear on the labial and buccal mucosa. These Koplik spots are diagnostic for measles.

Measles can be a severe disease with pneumonia and secondary bacterial infection. Leukopenia resulting from virus infecting the white cells usually occurs. Probably half of patients have central nervous system involvement with acute encephalitis developing in 1%.

SSPE is a tragic consequence of measles infection. It is a slowly progressive central nervous system disease caused by persistent measles virus infection. SSPE usually occurs years after a primary measles infection and is fatal. Patients have high antibody titers to measles virus in both serum and spinal fluid, and virus can be isolated from brain tissue by co-cultivation techniques. Currently SSPE is thought to be caused by an abortive persistent infection, and its occurrence may depend on the amount of virus that reaches the brain in acute measles. In the brain the virus does not make a membrane protein required for assembly of mature virus. This may be because of host restriction of virus in brain tissue.[19]

During the 1970s an atypical form of measles was recognized in people who had received killed vaccine at about 1 year of age between 1963 to 1967.[17] Today most cases are in adolescents or young adults. Patients are acutely ill and develop a maculopapular rash, which often becomes vesicular. It starts on the palms and soles and spreads up the extremities to the trunk, sparing the face. No Koplik spots develop, and viral culture results are negative.[30] Atypical measles has been confused with Rocky Mountain spotted fever,[34] varicella, meningococcemia, enteroviral infections, and others.[17,30] Atypical measles is probably caused by an abnormal or enhanced cellular immune response in people previously sensitized by killed vaccine.

Measles is clearly a systemic infection, although the virus first multiplies in the respiratory tract. During a primary viremia virus is spread via the blood to the reticuloendothelial system and viscera. After further multiplication an intense secondary viremia occurs followed by the development of the rash. The rash and Koplik spots are probably hypersensitivity reactions.

Epidemiology

Measles virus is spread by the airborne route from the nose and respiratory tract. It is most contagious during the prodromal period and just after development of the rash when patients are still coughing. In the early 1960s almost a half million cases a year were reported. Since the use of live vaccine began, reported measles incidence has been reduced more than 90%.[4,23] Today the number of cases varies from year to year, but cases always occur in late winter and the spring. The age groups most often infected have changed. Before vaccine use measles was a disease mainly of young children (less than 5 years). Now the greatest incidence is in older children (over 10 years) and adolescents.[35]

Treatment and Control

A live attenuated measles vaccine has resulted in a dramatic decrease in the incidence of measles, measles encephalitis, and measles-associated deaths.[35] Vaccine virus is not transmissible from person to person and produces long-term immunity in 95% of recipients.[38] For the greatest efficacy vaccine is given after the first birthday because at an earlier age the percentage of responders is less.[28]

LABORATORY DIAGNOSIS

In patients with typical measles and Koplik spots, laboratory confirmation is unnecessary. Measles virus is difficult virus to isolate, and cultivation is usually attempted only in special circumstances (for example, disease in a compromised patient).

Specimen Types

Specimens should include blood, urine, throat swabs or washings, conjunctival swabs, spinal fluid, and tissue (lung or brain). The most practical laboratory approach is serologic testing of convalescent serum specimens collected 10 to 14 days after onset.

Direct Detection

Direct examination of nasal secretions can be attempted by electron microscopy or FA. FA is more sensitive than virus isolation.

Virus Isolation

Wild measles virus grows only in humans and certain primates. The best cell cultures for isolation are primary human fetal or infant kidney cells. Because these are hard to obtain, PMK cells are most often used. CPE takes 2 to 10 days to appear. In PMK cells multinucleate syncytia are formed. Initial confirmation of measles can be obtained by the virus's ability to hemadsorb rhesus monkey red blood cells at 37° C. Serologic identification is made by FA, hemadsorption inhibition, or neutralization.

Serologic Diagnosis

Following natural measles, HI antibody rises to a peak by 3 weeks and is still detectable many years later.[27] After vaccination persistent antibody develops in 95% of patients, although titers are lower than with natural infections.[29] Patients with atypical measles have high antibody titers early in the course of disease.[17]

HI and CF are both acceptable for diagnostic serology, but CF should not be used to evaluate immune status because CF titers may drop to undetectable levels.

REFERENCES

1. Bromberg, K., et al.: Comparison of HEp-2 cell culture and Abbott respiratory syncytial virus enzyme immunoassay, J. Clin. Microbiol. **25**:434, 1987.

1a. Center for Disease Control: Mumps vaccine: recommendation of the public health service advisory committee on immunization practices, Ann. Intern. Med. **88**:819, 1978.

2. Clark, J., et al.: Comparison of cynomolgus and rhesus monkey kidney cells for recovery of viruses from clinical specimens, J. Clin. Microbiol. **9**:554, 1979.

3. Denny, F.W., et al.: An 11-year study in a pediatric practice, Pediatrics **71**:871, 1983.

4. Englehardt, S.J., et al.: Measles mortality in the United States, 1971-1975, Am. J. Public Health **70**:1166, 1980.

5. Frank, A.L., et al.: Comparison of different tissue cultures for isolation and quantitation of influenza and parainfluenza viruses, J. Clin. Microbiol. **10**:32, 1979.

6. Friedman, M., and Salineary, G.: IgA Antibodies to mumps virus during and after mumps, J. Infect. Dis. **143**:617, 1981.

7. Gardner, P.S., Grandien, M., and McQuillin, J.: Comparison of immunofluorescence and immunoperoxidase methods for viral diagnosis at a distance: a WHO collaborative study, Bull. WHO **56**:105, 1978.

8. Glezen, W.P., et al.: Risk of respiratory syncytial virus infection for infants from low-income families in relationship to age, sex, ethnic group, and maternal antibody level, J. Pediatr. **98**:708, 1981.

9. Glezen, W.P., et al.: Parainfluenza virus type 3: seasonality and risk of infection and reinfection in young children, J. Infect. Dis. **150**:851, 1984.

10. Hall, C.B.: Prevention of infection with respiratory syncytial virus: the hopes and hurdles ahead, Rev. Infect. Dis. **2**:384, 1980.

11. Hall, C.B., and Douglas, R.G., Jr.: Modes of transmission of respiratory syncytial virus, J. Pediatr. **99**:100, 1981.

12. Hall, C.B., et al.: Parainfluenza viral infections in children: correlation of shedding with clinical manifestations, J. Pediatr. **91**:194, 1977.

13. Hall, C.B., et al.: Control of nosocomial respiratory syncytial viral infections, Pediatrics **62**:728, 1978.

14. Hall, C.B., et al.: Neonatal respiratory syncytial virus infection, N. Engl. J. Med. **300**:393, 1979.

15. Hall, C.B., et al.: Infectivity of respiratory syncytial virus by various routes of inoculation, Infect. Immun. **33**:779, 1981.

16. Hall, C.B., et al.: Ribavirin treatment of experimental respiratory syncytial viral infection: a controlled double-blind study in young adults, JAMA **249**:2666, 1983.

17. Hall, W.J., and Hall, C.B.: Atypical measles in adolescents: evaluation of clinical and pulmonary function, Ann. Intern. Med. **90**:882, 1979.

18. Hall, W.J., Hall, C.B., and Speers, D.M.: Respiratory syncytial virus infection in adults: clinical, virologic, and serial pulmonary function studies, Ann. Intern. Med. **88**:203, 1978.

19. Hall, W.W., and Choppin, P.W.: Measles-virus proteins in the brain tissue of patients with subacute sclerosing panencephalitis, N. Engl. J. Med. **304**:1152, 1981.

20. Hayden, G.F., et al.: Current status of mumps and mumps vaccine in the United States, Pediatrics **62**:965, 1978.

21. Henderson, F.W., Hu, S.-C., and Collier, A.M.: Pathogenesis of respiratory syncytial virus infection in ferret and fetal human tracheas in organ culture, Am. Rev. Respir. Dis. **118**:29, 1978.

22. Hierholzer, J.C., and Hirsch, M.S.: Croup and pneumonia in human infants associated with a new strain of respiratory syncytial virus, J. Infect. Dis. **140**:826, 1979.

23. Hinman, A.R., et al.: Impact of measles in the United States, Rev. Infect. Dis. **5**:439, 1983.

24. Jarnis, W.R., Middleton, P.J., and Gelfand, E.W.: Parainfluenza pneumonia in severe combined immunodeficiency disease, J. Pediatr. **94**:423, 1979.

25. Kao, C.L., et al.: Monoclonal antibodies for the rapid diagnosis of respiratory syncytial virus infection by immunofluorescence, Diagn. Microbiol. Infect. Dis. **2**:199, 1984.

26. Kimball, A.M., et al.: Isolation of respiratory syncytial and influenza viruses from the sputum of patients hospitalized with pneumonia, J. Infect. Dis. **147**:181, 1983.

27. Krause, P.J., et al.: Measles-specific lymphocyte reactivity and serum antibody in subjects with different measles histories, Am. J. Dis. Child. **134**:567, 1980.

28. Krugman, R.D., et al.: Further attenuated live measles vaccines: the need for revised recommendations, J. Pediatr. **91**:766, 1977.

29. Lerman, S.J., Bollinger, M., and Brunken, J.M.: Clinical and serologic evaluation of measles, mumps, and rubella (HPV-77: DE-5 and RA 27/3) virus vaccines, singly and in combination, Pediatrics **68**:18, 1981.

30. Martin, D.B., et al.: Atypical measles in adolescents and young adults, Ann. Intern. Med. **90**:877, 1979.

31. Mathur, U., Bentley, D.W., and Hall, C.B.: Concurrent respiratory syncytial virus and influenza A infections in the institutionalized elderly and chronically ill, Ann. Intern. Med. **93**:49, 1980.

32. Mintz, L., et al.: Nosocomial respiratory syncytial virus infections in an intensive care nursery: rapid diagnosis by direct immunofluorescence, Pediatrics **64**:149, 1979.

33. Morgan, E.M., and Rapp, F.: Measles virus and its associated diseases, Bacteriol. Rev. **41**:636, 1977.

34. Nieburg, P.I., D'Angelo, L.J., and Herrmann, K.L.: Measles in patients suspected of having Rocky Mountain spotted fever, JAMA **244**:808, 1980.

35. Orenstein, W.A., et al.: Current status of measles in the United States, 1973-1977, J. Infect. Dis. **137**:847, 1978.

36. Sarkkinen, H.K., et al.: Detection of respiratory syncytial parainfluenza type 2, and adenovirus antigens by radioimmunoassay and enzyme immunoassay on nasopharyngeal specimens from children with acute respiratory disease, J. Clin. Microbiol. **13**:258, 1981.

37. Tyeryar, F.J., Jr., Richardson, L.S., and Belske, R.B.: Report of a workshop on respiratory syncytial virus and parainfluenza viruses, J. Infect. Dis. **137**:835, 1978.

38. Weibel, R.E., et al.: Persistence of antibody in human subjects for 7 to 10 years following administration of combined live attenuated measles, mumps, and rubella virus vaccines, Proc. Soc. Exp. Biol. Med. **165**:260, 1980.

39. Welliver, R.C., et al.: The antibody response to primary and secondary infection with respiratory syncytial virus: kinetics of class-specific responses, J. Pediatr. **96**:808, 1980.

40. Wong, D.T., et al.: Rapid diagnosis of parainfluenza virus infection in children, J. Clin. Microbiol. **16**:164, 1982.

41. Yanagihara, R., and McIntosh, K.: Secretory immunological response in infants and children to parainfluenza virus types 1 and 2, Infect. Immun. **30**:23, 1980.

CHAPTER 53

Rubella Virus

Sally Jo Rubin

Rubella, or German measles, was described some 200 years ago, but its significance as anything besides a mild illness with a rash was not recognized until 1941, when Gregg, an Australian ophthalmologist, noticed a link between certain congenital malformations and rubella infection of the mother during pregnancy.

Weller, Neva, Parkman, and others successfully propagated the virus in cell culture 20 years later. Within another 10 years a live attenuated vaccine was available, resulting in a dramatic decrease in rubella infections. However, 15% to 20% of women of childbearing age are still susceptible to rubella; therefore the laboratory plays a major part in rubella control by determining immune status and in the diagnosis of possible maternal infection.

Rubella virus is a member of the family *Togaviridiae*. It is closely related to the genus *Alphavirus* but has no insect vector and is thus a separate, unique genus, *Rubivirus*. The rubella virus contains RNA within an icosahedral capsid. It is spherical (60 to 70 nm in diameter), with surface projections or spikes. Because it has a lipoprotein envelope, it is sensitive to ether and chloroform. Rubella virus is relatively unstable and is susceptible to heat, alcohol, and chlorine. Infectivity can be maintained for several days in the refrigerator if the virus is in a protein-containing solution.

Rubella virus has a single serotype. Major viral antigens include a hemagglutinin, which is an envelope protein, CF antigens, and two precipitins. Rubella virus hemagglutinates red blood cells from many animal species, especially fowl and humans.

CLINICAL SIGNIFICANCE

In young children and adults rubella is a mild disease. It may be inapparent, or there may be a rash, low-grade fever, and lymphadenopathy for a few days. The rash is usually maculopapular, beginning on the face and moving down the body. It may vary in appearance or not even occur, making rubella very difficult to diagnose clinically. Rubella is more severe in adults: up to one third may have athralgias and even arthritis. Complications such as encephalitis are rare. Inapparent reinfection can follow natural infection but with no viremia and essentially no viral shedding.

Rubella infection in early pregnancy can be disastrous. The virus infects the fetus and can cause severe abnormalities, premature birth, or fetal death. The earlier in pregnancy the infection occurs, the more likely it is the infant will be affected and the greater the number of defects.[24] Infection after the fourth month of gestation is of little danger to the fetus. More commonly seen abnormalities include cataracts, glaucoma, deafness, congenital heart disease, and mental retardation. Some-

times defects caused by congenital rubella are not apparent for weeks, months, or even years after birth.

Rubella virus invades via the nasopharyngeal mucosa and reaches the local lymphatics, where multiplication occurs, resulting in viremia. As the rash appears, virus is rarely present in the blood, although it continues to be shed from the throat for another week. Virus is present in the skin, but its presence is not directly responsible for the rash.[12] The malformations seen in congenital infection are probably related to the chronicity of the infection and the inhibition of fetal cell multiplication.

EPIDEMIOLOGY

Rubella virus is transmitted from person to person by direct contact with infected respiratory secretions. The incubation period is 2 to 3 weeks, with virus shedding from the throat beginning about a week before onset (Figure 53-1).

Congenitally infected infants shed virus from the throat and urine for months, and a small percentage are still excreting virus after a year. In postnatal rubella the virus can be transmitted by breast-feeding, but disease in the newborn is mild.[13]

Before the vaccine, minor rubella epidemics occurred in the spring every 5 to 7 years and a major epidemic about every 30 years. Most cases were in elementary-school children between 5 to 9 years old.[8] In the postvaccine era the reported cases of rubella in this age group have dramatically decreased.[8,19] However, the susceptibility rate among adolescents and adults is still 10% to 25%, and outbreaks are being reported from colleges, military camps, and hospitals.[14,18] These outbreaks are most problematic not only because health-care workers are often young women, but because they are likely to have contact with pregnant patients. Unfortunately, reported cases of congenital rubella syndrome (about 25 to 30 cases per year) have not substantially decreased over the last 10 years.[19]

TREATMENT AND CONTROL

No specific antiviral treatment is available for rubella, so control efforts are by use of the live attenuated vaccine. Several vaccines have been used in the United States, but currently only the RA27/3 strain is licensed for use.[17] RA27/3 vaccine produces a response in over 95% of vaccinees. Immunity is long lasting, and reinfection rates are low.[2] As with natural infection, reinfection with wild rubella does occur in vaccinated persons; however, viremia is not detectable, virus shedding is minimal, and transmission to susceptible contacts is unknown.[8]

Among laboratory workers the minimal titer indicating immunity is controversial. The Immunization Practices Advisory Committee considers any detectable titer as evidence of

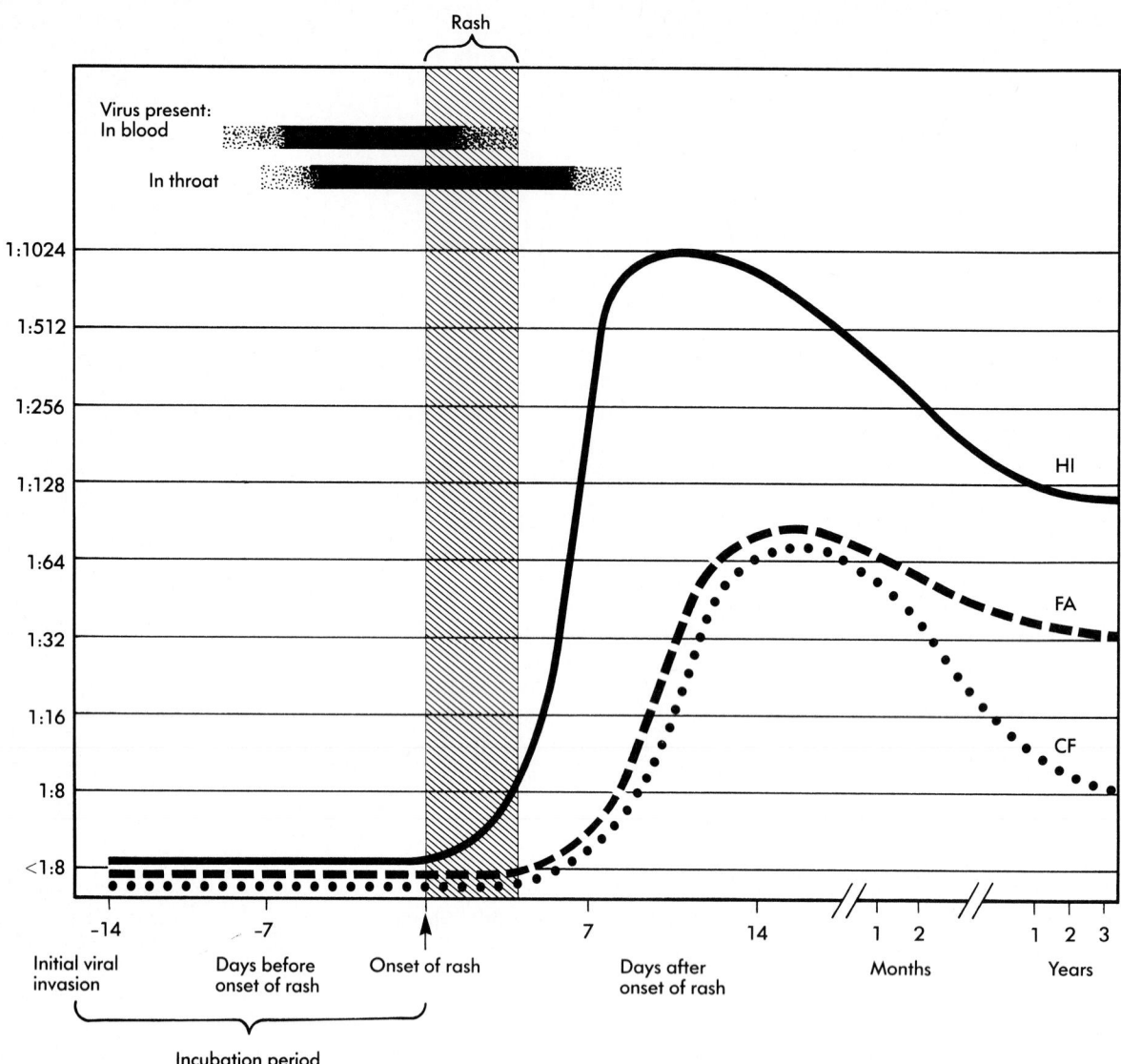

FIGURE 53-1. Virologic and serologic events with acute rubella infection. (From Palmer, D.F., et al.: Serodiagnosis of toxoplasmosis, rubella, cytomegalic inclusion disease, and herpes simplex, Immunology Series No. 5, Atlanta, 1977, Center for Disease Control.)

immunity and protection from reinfection viremia.[21] Immunization should be given at 15 months of age and, in susceptible women, immediately post partum.

Vaccine virus can infect the fetus, and although no infant with congenital rubella caused by attenuated vaccine strains has ever been reported, the vaccine should not be given 3 months before conception or during pregnancy.[5,20] Immune serum globulin is not recommended.[8] Vaccine virus is shed in breast milk but is of no risk to the newborn.[6]

LABORATORY DIAGNOSIS
SPECIMEN TYPES

Rubella virus can be isolated from the throat, urine, products of conception, and occasionally blood and spinal fluid.

VIRUS ISOLATION

Primates and various laboratory animals can be infected with rubella virus, but none are good animal models for human infection. Many cell cultures are susceptible to rubella virus, but primary African green monkey kidney and BHK-21 are considered the best. Rubella can be difficult to isolate because various environmental factors, such as the serum used in the media, are critical.

Growth can take more than 10 days, and in primary cell cultures there is no cytopathic effect (CPE). Virus is usually detected by interference, indirect fluorescent antibody (IFA), or indirect immunoperoxidase tests.[22] Serologic staining methods can shorten detection time.

Isolates are confirmed as rubella virus by neutralization, hemagglutination inhibition (HI), and FA techniques.

SEROLOGIC DIAGNOSIS

Because virus isolation is difficult, most laboratory diagnosis of rubella is performed serologically. Immune response following natural infection and vaccination is similar. With a natural infection both IgG and IgM are present within a few days

TABLE 53-1. Strategies for Rubella Serologic Testing

Situation	Serum Specimen	Antibody Tested	Interpretation[a]
Patient with rash less than 1 wk	Acute: immediately; convalescent: 2-3 wk after onset of rash	Total or IgG[b]	Fourfold rise indicates recent infection
Patient with rash more than 1 wk	Convalescent: 3-4 wk after onset of rash	Total or IgG	Negative or low titered ($\leq 1:20$) indicates no recent rubella infection; higher titer: test for IgM
Immune screen	Anytime	Total or IgG	Any titer indicates immunity
After vaccine	1 mo after vaccination	Total or IgG (not passive hemagglutination)	Any titer indicates immunity
Pregnant woman exposed to rubella less than 1 wk	Acute: immediately; if negative, repeat in 1 wk	Total or IgG	Any titer indicates immunity. Test for titer rise
		IgM	If titer rise, confirm with IgM
Pregnant woman exposed to rubella greater than 1 wk	Acute: immediately; convalescent: 3-4 wk	Total or IgG	No titer: no probable exposure
		Total or IgG and IgM	Titer: immune or possible exposure; test for titer rise and IgM
Possible rubella syndrome Infant less than 6 mo	Acute: immediately, both mother and infant	Total or IgG (mother), IgM (infant)	Congenital infection suggested if infant's titer significantly higher than mother's or infant has rubella-specific IgM; follow-up on infant for persistence of rubella IgG
Infant more than 6 mo	Infant: anytime	Total or IgG	Presence of antibody suggests rubella if child not exposed to rubella

[a]Minimum antibody level indicating immunity is controversial and also depends on test used.
[b]Some methods measure total antibody and others only IgG.

after onset of the rash (Figure 53-1). Both peak by about 7 days. IgM begins to decrease rapidly and is undetectable in 6 to 10 weeks. IgG remains elevated for some time and probably persists for life. Hemagglutination inhibition (HI) antibodies appear first, followed by complement fixation (CF) antibodies. Antibodies detected by passive hemagglutination appear as much as 6 weeks later.[10] A similar response is seen after vaccination.[4] After reinfection or revaccination there is an anamnestic response with no IgM.[3]

Congenitally infected infants produce IgM in utero and after birth begin to produce fetal IgG (Table 53-1). In noninfected infants IgG titer drops in 3 to 6 months, whereas that of infected infants persists or increases.

Acute serum for serologic diagnosis should be collected as soon as possible after onset. The need for collection and testing of a second serum specimen depends on the clinical situation (Table 53-1).

Numerous testing systems for detecting rubella antibody are available (Table 53-2). The standard procedure has been HI, although neutralization is considered the most specific. HI tests have been used for some years and are well standardized; however, they are tedious to perform and require pretreatment of the serum to remove nonspecific inhibitors of hemagglutination and nonspecific hemagglutinins. Some treatments also remove rubella-specific hemagglutinins, so procedures not requiring pretreatment may actually be more specific than the HI. Because of the time required to perform HI, a number of other procedures have been developed including passive hemagglutination (PHA),[10] indirect fluorescent antibody (IFA) test,[9] single-radial hemolysis,[11] enzyme-linked immunosorbent assay (ELISA),[23] radioimmunoassay (RIA),[15] and latex agglutination.[7] Most commercially available kits are acceptable, at least for immunity screening.[7] Most of the procedures correlate well with HI when high-titered sera are tested but less well with

TABLE 53-2. Examples of Commercial Tests for Measuring Rubella-Immune Status

Method	Manufacturer
Hemagglutination inhibition	
Fixed chick cells/kaolin	Abbott Laboratories, North Chicago, Ill.
Fixed chick cells/heparin-MnCl$_2$	Abbott Laboratories
1- to 3-day chick cells/kaolin	Abbott Laboratories
	Flow Laboratories, Inc., McLean, Va.
1- to 3-day chick cells/heparin-MnCl$_2$	Abbott Laboratories
	Flow Laboratories, Inc.
Human O cells/heparin-MnCl$_2$	Calbiochem-Behring, LaJolla, Calif.
	Flow Laboratories, Inc.
	GIBCO Laboratories, Grand Island, N.Y.
	Ortho Diagnostics, Raritan, N.J.
Human O cells/dextran sulfate	Flow Laboratories, Inc.
Enzyme immunoassay	Abbott Laboratories
	Cordis Laboratories, Inc., Miami, Fla.
	Organon-Teknika, Durham, N.C.
	M. A. Bioproducts, Walkersville, Md.
	Calbiochem-Behring
	Gilford Diagnostics
	Dynatech Laboratories, Inc., Alexandria, Va.
	Fisher Scientific Co., Pittsburgh, Pa.
Radioimmunoassay	Clinical Assays, Cambridge, Mass.
Immunofluorescence	Electro-Nucleonics, Inc., Bethesda, Md.
	International Diagnostic Technologies, Santa Clara, Calif.
	Microbiological Research Corp., Bountiful, Utah
Latex agglutination	BBL Microbiology Systems, Cockeysville, Md.
Passive hemagglutination	Abbott Laboratories
	Calbiochem-Behring

low-titered sera. Thus any evaluation should include an adequate number of negative and low-titered sera. High specificity (a low number of false-positive tests) is critical. False-negative tests can simply result in revaccination in an immune person.

Because HI antibody titers rise so quickly after onset, an antibody rise is often difficult to demonstrate. Some laboratory workers use a positive HI result and a negative PHA result to diagnose rubella because PHA antibodies may take 6 weeks to appear. It is prudent to confirm a diagnosis of rubella, particularly in a pregnant woman, by measurement of rubella-specific IgM. Several methods can be used, including removal of IgG by absorption with staphylococcal protein A[1] and physical separation methods such as gel filtration and sucrose gradients. The latter procedure is the most accurate but is not widely available.[16] An ELISA kit for detecting rubella IgM is available commercially. According to the manufacturer, it is unaffected by rheumatoid factor or competition with IgG and therefore can be used to diagnose primary and congenital rubella infections.

REFERENCES

1. Ankerst, J., et al.: A routine diagnostic test for IgA and IgM antibodies to rubella virus: absorption of IgG with *Staphylococcus aureus,* J. Infect. Dis. **130:**268, 1974.
2. Balfour, H.H., Jr., Groth, K.E., and Edelman, C.K.: RA27/3 rubella vaccine: a four-year follow-up, Am. J. Dis. Child. **134:**350, 1980.
3. Balfour, H.H., Jr., et al.: Rubella viraemia and antibody responses after rubella vaccination and reimmunization, Lancet **1:**1078, 1981.
4. Banatvala, J.E., et al.: Specific IgM responses after rubella vaccination: potential application following inadvertent vaccination during pregnancy, Br. Med. J. **6097:**1263, 1977.
5. Banatvala, J.E., et al.: Transmission of RA27/3 rubella vaccine strain to products of conception, Lancet **1:**392, 1981.
6. Biumovici-Klein, E., et al.: Isolation of rubella virus in milk after postpartum immunization, J. Pediatr. **91:**939, 1977.
7. Castellano, G.A., et al.: Evaluation of commercially available diagnostic test kits for rubella, J. Infect. Dis. **143:**578, 1981.
8. Center for Disease Control: Rubella vaccine: recommendation of the Public Health Service Advisory Committee on Immunization Practices, Ann. Intern. Med. **88:**543, 1978.
9. Cremer, N.E., Hagens, S.J., and Cossen, C.: Comparison of the hemagglutination inhibition test and an indirect fluorescent-antibody test for detection of antibody to rubella virus in human sera, J. Clin. Microbiol. **11:**746, 1980.
10. Cremer, N.E., Hagens, S.J., and Cossen, C.: Specificity of the passive hemagglutination test for antibody to rubella virus and the passive hemagglutination response after vaccination, J. Clin. Microbiol. **13:**226, 1981.
11. Folger, J.M., and Gilfillan, R.F.: Single-radial hemolysis as a cost-effective determinant of rubella antibody status, J. Clin. Microbiol. **9:**115, 1979.
12. Heggie, A.D.: Pathogenesis of the rubella exanthem: distribution of rubella virus in the skin during rubella with and without rash, J. Infect. Dis. **137:**74, 1978.
13. Klein, E., Byrne, T., and Cooper, L.Z.: Neonatal rubella in a breast-fed infant after postpartum maternal infection, J. Pediatr. **97:**774, 1980.

14. McLaughlin, M.C., and Gold, L.H.: The New York rubella incident: a case for changing hospital policy regarding rubella testing and immunization, Am. J. Public Health **69:**287, 1979.

15. Meurman, O.H.: Antibody responses in patients with rubella infection determined by passive hemagglutination, hemagglutination inhibition, complement fixation, and solid-phase radioimmunoassay tests, Infect. Immun. **19:**369, 1978.

16. Pattison, J.R., et al.: Comparison of methods for detecting specific IgM antibody in infants with congenital rubella, J. Med. Microbiol. **11:**411, 1978.

17. Perkins, F.T. Licensed vaccines, Rev. Infect. Dis. **7:**S73, 1985.

18. Polk, B.F., et al.: An outbreak of rubella among hospital personnel, N. Engl. J. Med. **303:**541, 1980.

19. Preblud, S.R., et al.: Current status of rubella in the United States, 1969-1979, J. Infect. Dis. **142:**776, 1980.

20. Preblud, S.R., et al.: Fetal risk associated with rubella vaccine, JAMA **246:**1413, 1981.

21. Rubella prevention: recommendation of the Immunization Practices Advisory Committee, MMWR **30:**37, 1981.

22. Schmidt, N.J., Ho, H.H., and Chin, J.: Application of immunoperoxidase staining to more rapid detection and identification of rubella virus isolates, J. Clin. Microbiol. **13:**627, 1981.

23. Shekarchi, I.C., et al.: Comparison of hemagglutination inhibition test and enzyme-linked immunosorbent assay for determining antibody to rubella virus, J. Clin. Microbiol. **13:**850, 1981.

24. Ueda, K., et al.: Congenital rubella syndrome: correlation of gestational age at time of maternal rubella with type of defect, J. Pediatr. **94:**763, 1979.

CHAPTER 54

Hepatitis Viruses

Sally Jo Rubin

Descriptions of viral hepatitis can be traced back at least to the time of Hippocrates, but the etiology of these infections was discovered only in the last 20 years. The infectious nature of viral hepatitis was recognized between 1920 and 1945 when transmission by blood and by stool filtrates was described. These different routes of transmission suggested that at least two distinct agents were involved. One, hepatitis B virus (HBV), is a DNA virus usually transmitted parenterally, and the other, hepatitis A virus (HAV), is an enterovirus and is transmitted by the fecal-oral route. Epstein-Barr virus (EBV), cytomegalovirus (CMV), and several other viruses can also cause acute hepatitis. A newly described virus, delta agent, appears to be an RNA-containing virus that requires some helper function from HBV for infectivity and is associated with both acute and chronic hepatitis.[61] Viral hepatitis that cannot be attributed to any known virus is called non-A, non-B (NANB) hepatitis. Hepatitis viruses with the exception of HAV4 do not appear to replicate in any other tissue but the liver.

Although symptoms among groups of patients with hepatitis may differ, it is often impossible to determine clinically which agent is causing an individual case (Table 54-1). Viral hepatitis can be acute and symptomatic, asymptomatic, or fulminant. After acute symptomatic or asymptomatic infection with HBV, delta agent, or NANB, the infection can become chronic with continued viral replication. HAV does not cause chronic infection. The severity of viral hepatitis varies with the virus and from individual to individual.

Acute symptomatic hepatitis begins with a prodromal period during which patients feel weak and nauseated, lose their appetites, and experience vague, dull pain in the area of the liver. This preicteric phase lasts 3 to 10 days and in a typical case is followed by the onset of jaundice. Alanine aminotransferase and aspartate aminotransferase serum levels are at least 10 times greater than normal, whereas alkaline phosphatase and lactic dehydrogenase are only minimally elevated.

Over half of the cases of hepatitis are asymptomatic. These patients have no clinical symptoms; however, liver enzyme levels may be elevated, and antibody to the infecting virus develops. A small percentage of patients have acute fulminant hepatitis with hepatic failure and encephalopathy.

Chronic hepatitis is defined as the persistence of symptoms or abnormal enzymes for more than 6 months. Chronic persistent hepatitis is often benign; liver enzyme levels eventually return to normal, but the individual continues to carry the virus. Chronic active hepatitis is a serious liver disease that can result in cirrhosis, hepatic failure, and hepatocellular carcinoma.

HEPATITIS A VIRUS

The study of infectious hepatitis was hampered until an animal model for hepatitis A virus (HAV) was established in 1969. Once antisera could be produced, immune electron microscopy (IEM) revealed 27 nm viral particles in stool filtrates of patients with HAV. Provost and co-workers[57,58] and Binn and co-workers[4] isolated HAV in primary liver explant, as well as fetal rhesus monkey kidney cell culture. Serial passage resulted in high titers of infectious virus.

HAV is classified as enterovirus 72.[52] Only one serotype is known. As with other enteroviruses, it is nonenveloped and thus is ether resistant. HAV is acid stable and resists 60° C for 1 hour. It is destroyed by autoclaving for 30 minutes and boiling for 20 minutes and with dry heat (160° C) for 1 hour and formalin (1:4000) for 72 hours at 37° C.

CLINICAL SIGNIFICANCE

HAV infection can be asymptomatic (with a rise in liver enzymes and seroconversion) or symptomatic with or without jaundice. Between 2 and 6 weeks following infection with HAV, symptomatic patients develop a flulike illness that proceeds to gastrointestinal symptoms, including anorexia, vomiting, and pain in the area of the liver. The onset of symptoms is insidious but more acute than for HBV infection. Fulminant hepatitis with coma is rare. Mortality is very low, and neither chronic hepatitis nor a chronic carrier state exists.

About 10 to 30 days following infection, HAV particles can be detected in feces. Viral shedding is greatest before clinical onset and continues for several days to 2 weeks. The number of particles greatly decreases after onset, and within a week, 80% of patients have negative results when tested for viruses.[9] The disease is most infectious before clinical onset.

EPIDEMIOLOGY

HAV infections are transmitted by the fecal-oral route and are found worldwide. The highest incidence is in warmer climates where hygiene is frequently poor.[18,23] Infections often occur in population clusters with fecally contaminated food or water as the source of the virus.

Hospital outbreaks are rare and usually occur when patients are admitted in the prodromal phase of the disease and with no symptoms of hepatitis B infection.[3] However, when people are in close contact, as in institutions, in day-care centers, or in families, person-to-person transmission is common.[56,41] In the United States, seroepidemiologic studies have shown that incidence increases with age and decreases with rising socioeco-

TABLE 54-1. Characteristics of Viral Hepatitis

Characteristic	Hepatitis A	Hepatitis B	Non-A, Non-B Hepatitis	Delta-Associated Hepatitis
Onset	Acute	Gradual	Insidious	Acute and insidious
Chronicity	No chronic disease or carrier	5% chronic carriers and chronic hepatitis	Up to one third chronic carriers	Not known to exist
Transmission	Fecal-oral	Parenteral; intimate contact	Transfusion; possibly intimate contact	Parenteral
Epidemiology	Epidemics or sporadic	Sporadic	Sporadic; transfusion associated	Sporadic
Incubation	15-40 days	40-180 days	Variable	30-50 days

nomic classes.[12] In fact, 20% to 70% of people show serologic evidence of past HAV, but only 3% to 5% of people remember having had hepatitis.

HAV is not transmitted in utero. Transmission to the newborn can occur if the mother is acutely infected at delivery.[38] Maternal HAV antibody is transferred to the fetus; therefore an infant's antibody levels at birth are the same as the mother's and decrease over time like other passively transferred antibodies.[17]

HAV is not commonly transmitted parenterally, but two recent reports provide evidence that transmission of the virus can occur by transfusion of blood products.[30,68] Homosexual men who frequently practice oral-anal sex have a higher incidence of HAV infection.[8]

Hygiene is the most important factor in control of HAV infection. Since most hospitalized patients with HAV infection are past the time of maximal shedding, only normal precautions for handling feces and fecally contaminated material are necessary. Isolation is required only for fecally incontinent patients. People who are intimate contacts of HAV-infected persons (that is, family members) are usually given immune globulin, which provides some protection.

Neither an antiviral agent active against HAV nor a vaccine is available.

LABORATORY DIAGNOSIS
Specimen Types

Blood is the major specimen for the laboratory diagnosis of HAV infection. Rarely, virus detection in feces may be attempted. Stool must be collected as soon as possible after the onset of symptoms.[9] Sera are collected immediately after exposure or onset, again 3 to 4 weeks after the symptoms appear, and once more, 2 to 3 months after illness.

Direct Examination

Although virus can be detected in feces by IEM, enzyme-linked immunosorbent assay (ELISA), or radioimmunoassay (RIA), RIA and ELISA are commercially available.[50,71,77] Because viral detection is limited to early acute infection, most diagnoses of HAV infection are based on measuring antibody in serum.

Virus Isolation

HAV can be grown in fetal rhesus monkey kidney cell culture,[4] but virus isolation is not a practical technique because antigen detection from human specimens takes about a month and because most virus shedding occurs before symptoms appear.

Serologic Diagnosis

Anti-HAV antibody is almost always present at the onset of symptoms. Titers rise during the acute disease and can remain elevated for up to 3 years (Figure 54-1).[10] Detectable antibody probably persists for life. Anti-HAV IgM is present at onset or within a few days and reaches a maximal titer in 1 to 3 weeks. Depending on the sensitivity of the test used, anti-HAV IgM can in some cases be detected many months after the onset of symptoms.[27]

The ratio of antibody to HAV levels can be measured by IEM, immune adherence hemagglutination assay (IAHA), solid-phase RIA, and ELISA.[50] IEM is cumbersome and time consuming and requires an electron microscope. IAHA is a sensitive procedure, but it does not detect early antibody, may not give a positive result for 4 to 6 weeks after illness, and requires a large amount of antigen. RIA is sensitive, yields positive results earlier than IAHA, and requires small amounts of antigen. Reagents for RIA and ELISA are commercially available.[67]

HAV infection can be confirmed by demonstrating a rise in titer between acute and convalescent sera. Because the antibody is almost always present at onset, this is often difficult and requires several weeks for a definitive diagnosis. A commercial solid phase RIA using beads coated with anti–human IgM is available for measurement of HAV-specific IgM. It is reportedly sensitive, specific, and not affected by the presence of rheumatoid factor.[10] Over 90% of patients have positive results when given this test during acute HAV infection.[78] Availability of tests such as RIA and ELISA has greatly simplified the laboratory diagnosis of HAV infection.

HEPATITIS B VIRUS

The first recorded epidemic of probable hepatitis B virus (HBV) infection was among shipyard workers following vaccination against smallpox with a vaccine derived from humans. During the World War II an outbreak was again traced to a vaccine contaminated with human serum, and hence the disease was given the name "serum hepatitis." Virus detection eluded investigators until 1964 when Blumberg discovered a new antigen in the blood of an Australian aborigine. This antigen, Australia (Au) antigen, was very rare in some populations (for

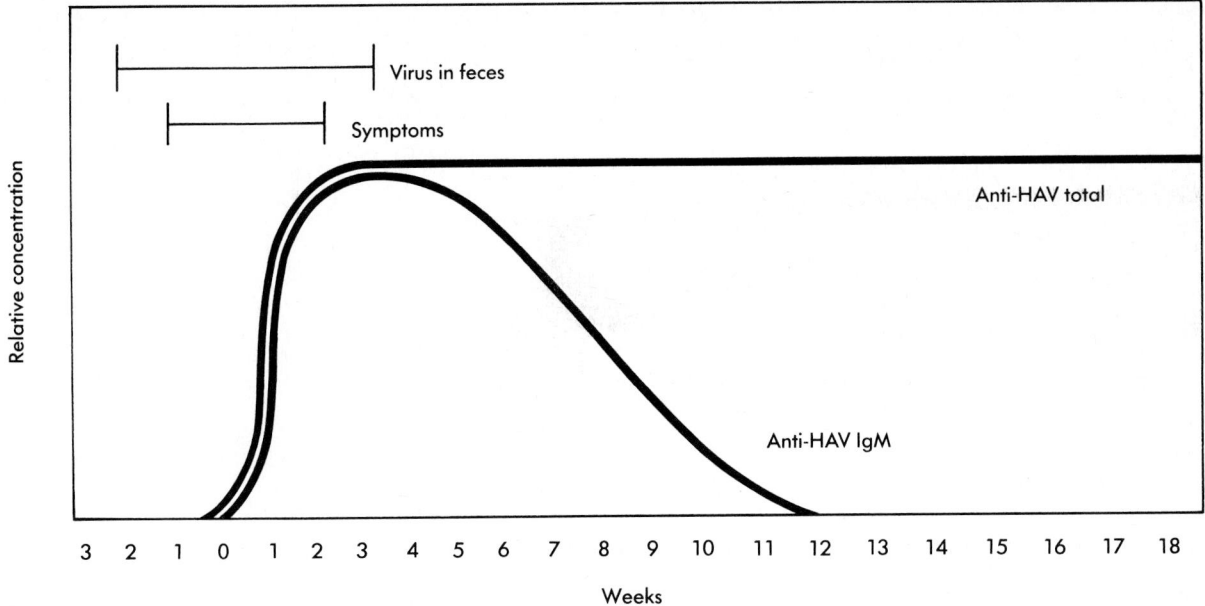

FIGURE 54-1. Antibody response in hepatitis A. (From Serodiagnostic assessment of acute viral hepatitis, Chicago, 1981, Abbott Laboratories.)

instance, the United States) but common in others (for instance, certain tropical and Asian populations). In testing various sera, Blumberg and co-workers found Au antigen was more common in people who had received transfusions and in children with Down syndrome. One of these children converted from Au antigen negative to Au antigen positive, and further investigation revealed that the child had hepatitis.[35] This discovery led Krugman and Giles[45] to test large numbers of stored sera from retarded children for Au antigen and antibody. They found that Au antigen was present only during hepatitis. Au antigen is now known to be the surface antigen (HB$_s$Ag) of HBV. Its presence is an indication of the infectivity of a hepatitis patient's serum.

Over the last 10 years much has been learned about the nature of HBV. It is unique among human viruses and is classified in the genus *Hepadnavirus*.[52] Several similar viruses have been found in woodchucks, California ground squirrels, and Chinese domestic ducks.

HBV is hardy, surviving heat (60° C for 4 hours) and most laboratory disinfectants.[42] At room temperature HBV can survive up to 6 months. Infectivity is destroyed rapidly by sodium hypochlorite (Clorox) or autoclaving for 30 to 60 minutes.

MORPHOLOGY

HBV is morphologically and antigenically complex. Sera from HBV-infected patients contains three distinct structures: a 42 nm double-shelled form called the Dane particle, 22 nm spherical particles, and filamentous forms that are 22 nm in diameter and up to 1000 nm long (Figure 54-2). The Dane particle is recognized as the whole virion and consists of a 28 nm core surrounded by a lipid envelope. The electron-dense core contains double-stranded DNA that has a single-strand gap equivalent to about one third of the virus genome. A DNA polymerase is associated with the core. The spherical and filamentous forms are incomplete viral coat proteins and are not infectious.

ANTIGENIC STRUCTURE

HBV (Dane particle) has two major antigens. HB$_s$Ag is an outer surface component, whereas hepatitis B core antigen (HB$_c$Ag) is part of the inner core that surrounds the viral genome (Figure 54-2). The spherical and filamentous forms consist of HB$_s$Ag.

Two pairs of mutually exclusive antigenic determinants (*d/y* and *w/r*) comprise the four subtypes of HB$_s$Ag. Four *w* subtypes (*w$_1$* to *w$_4$*) are known. *a* is a group-specific determinant. Thus examples of HB$_s$Ag subtypes are *ayw*, *ayw$_3$*, *ayr*, *adr*, *adw$_2$*, and *adw$_4$*. Subtype determination is used in epidemiologic studies.

HB$_s$Ag in serum is indicative of viral replication in the liver. HB$_s$Ag appears during the incubation period, peaks soon after onset of symptoms, and if the patient recovers, disappears in 1 to 3 months. After HB$_s$Ag becomes undetectable, antibody to HB$_s$Ag appears. Its presence indicates past infection and immunity.

Core antigen, HB$_c$Ag, can be detected in infected hepatocytes by IEM or indirect fluorescent antibody (IFA) assay. Depending on the presence or absence of HB$_s$Ag and anti-HB$_s$Ag, the presence of anti-HB$_c$Ag in serum can be important diagnostically.

HB$_e$Ag is found in some HB$_s$Ag-positive sera. It is a soluble protein, but its relationship to the structure of HBV is not known. HB$_e$Ag is found in serum as the native protein or as a complex with serum immunoglobulin. Sera with HB$_e$Ag are very infectious. Seroconversion to anti-HB$_e$Ag usually indicates recovery.

CLINICAL SIGNIFICANCE

HBV hepatitis can be asymptomatic, symptomatic with or without jaundice (icteric or anicteric), or fulminant. Acute symptomatic or asymptomatic HBV infections can become chronic.

Following HBV infection, 30% to 40% of adults develop symptomatic disease. The average incubation period before

HEPATITIS B VIRAL COMPONENTS

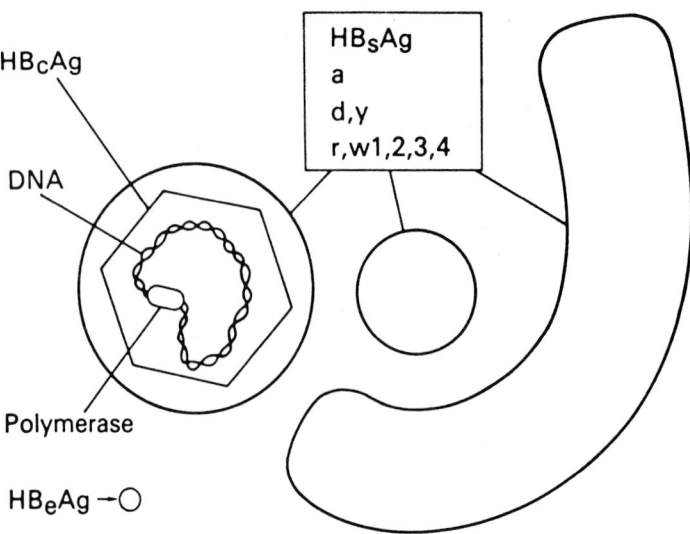

FIGURE 54-2. Diagram of hepatitis B virus structure showing the various antigens. (From Lennette, E.H., and Schmidt, N.J.: Diagnostic procedures for viral, rickettsial, and chlamydial infections, ed. 5, Washington, D.C., 1979, American Public Health Association.)

clinical onset is about 90 days, with a range of 3 or 4 weeks to 6 months, depending on the infecting dose. Onset of HBV hepatitis is insidious with the majority of symptoms caused by the inflammatory process in the liver. The clinical disease, ranging from mild to severe, prolonged, and sometimes fatal, lasts about 4 to 6 weeks. However, over half of infected adults have asymptomatic infection. Laboratory evidence of hepatitis (usually HB_sAg^-, anti-HB_sAg^+) can be demonstrated in those people who have no symptoms. In most cases of HBV infection, whether symptomatic or asymptomatic, recovery is complete.

Fulminant hepatitis occurs in only 1% to 3% of infected adults. During acute HBV infection these patients develop hepatic encephalopathy, and eventually coma and death can occur.

About 5% to 10% of patients, whether symptomatic or asymptomatic, become persistent carriers of HB_sAg. Clinically they are described as having chronic persistent or chronic active hepatitis. Chronic persistent hepatitis is generally benign, although mild symptoms may be present. Patients continue to be HB_sAg positive, usually for years, with no hepatic disease. A small percentage of infected individuals develop chronic active hepatitis, a serious, destructive liver disease in which severe hepatic necrosis can occur.

The hepatic injury that causes the symptoms of HBV infection may be a result of direct cytopathogenicity of the virus, inadequacy of the host's immune response, or both. The development of chronic or severe disease probably is determined by unexplained defects in the immune response.

HBV is also associated with primary hepatocellular carcinoma (PHC), although its role in PHC is unknown. The majority of PHC patients have chronic active hepatitis or cirrhosis before developing primary liver cancer. Most PHC cases occur in areas where HBV infection is endemic.[5]

Epidemiology

Parenteral transmission of HBV is accomplished in many ways. Examples include tattooing, acupuncture, ear piercing, shaving, manicuring, illicit drug injections, accidental needle sticks, hemodialysis, and transfusion of contaminated blood or blood products. For many years it was thought that HBV infection occurred only by injection or infusion of contaminated blood or blood products. However, transmission by close contact with contaminated secretions also occurs. Presumably, the portals of entry are inapparent breaks in the skin or mucous membranes.

HB_sAg is found in many body fluids besides blood. A large percentage of patients with both acute and chronic hepatitis have HB_sAg in their saliva.[79] Urine, especially from renal transplant patients, may contain virus markers.[39] HB_sAg has also been detected in tears, cerebrospinal fluid, ascitic fluid, and semen. HB_sAg has not been detected in feces, probably because the virus is destroyed during passage through the gastrointestinal tract.[79]

Infection via contaminated secretions occurs in a range of ways, from children exchanging toys contaminated with oral secretions[47] to contact with urine from infected dialysis and renal transplant patients to sexual intercourse.[36]

Women who are pregnant and who are chronic HBV carriers or have acute HBV infection in the third trimester can transmit the virus to their infants. Infection probably occurs during birth by contact with contaminated vaginal secretions or shortly after birth via breast milk.[7,49] Infection is more likely if the mother is HB_eAg positive.[70]

Populations in which crowding or close contact is common have much higher rates of HBV infection than the 1% to 5% incidence in the general population. Evidence of past or present HBV infection is particularly common among institutionalized mentally retarded children, especially those with Down syndrome.[44] Others with a high incidence of HBV infection include hemodialysis patients and dialysis center medical personnel, patients receiving frequent intravenous therapy (such as cancer chemotherapy), homosexual men, and physicians, dentists, and hospital employees, especially laboratory workers and those administering venipunctures.[14,24,37,46]

HBV is endemic in certain underdeveloped tropical areas. Infection occurs early, and by adulthood most people show evidence of past or present infection. The reservoir is a large number of chronic carriers, and some transmission is undoubtedly from chronic-carrier mothers to their infants.[23]

Control and Treatment

No effective treatment is available for HBV infection. Therefore the control of the disease is through prevention. A reduction in HBV transmission has been achieved by mandatory screening of blood donors to eliminate individuals who have had hepatitis or transfusions or who use injectable drugs and by testing donated blood for HBV markers. In high-risk areas, such as hemodialysis units, surveillance of patients' blood and isolation of HB$_s$Ag carriers can reduce the spread of infection.[54]

Minimal use of blood and blood products and effective sterilization of medical and dental instruments after each use also reduces HBV transmission. Instruments can be sterilized, using specified procedures, by autoclave or ethylene oxide treatment.

Passive immunization following exposure to HBV has been accomplished with both immune serum globulin (ISG) and hepatitis B immune serum globulin (HBIG) sera that are tested and known to contain high titers of anti-HB$_s$Ag. HBIG is superior to ISG in preventing clinical disease following exposure to HBV in both adults and newborns.[6,73]

Trials with a vaccine of highly purified, formalin-inactivated HB$_s$Ag obtained from chronic carriers were conducted in homosexual men, a population with a high incidence of HBV infection. The vaccine appears safe, immunogenic, and effective and was licensed on November 16, 1981.[13,28,43,78] It is recommended for high-risk groups, such as certain health-care personnel, certain patients (those undergoing hemodialysis or hematologic-oncologic testing), sexually active homosexual men, intravenous drug users, intimate contacts of carriers, and infants in high-risk areas.[43] The presence of HBIG does not interfere with response to the vaccine, and because the development of anti-HB$_s$Ag following vaccination is slow (2 to 6 months) in cases of exposure to HBV, both HBIG and the vaccine can be given.[74]

LABORATORY DIAGNOSIS
Specimen Types

Although viral antigen may be present in many secretions, serum is the usual and optimal specimen. Specimens are collected at the onset of symptoms and then periodically to detect antibody conversion.

Virus Isolation

HBV has never been grown in cell culture, and humans are the only natural hosts. Chimpanzees, gibbons, and orangutans can be infected by intravenous injection of virus-containing body fluids. Direct examination of liver tissue by IEM or IFA can be done but is usually a research procedure. Thus the lab-

oratory diagnosis of HBV depends on serologic detection of various HBV antigens and antibodies in serum.

Antigen and Antibody Detection

Antibody response to the known HBV antigens depends on the antigen, the nature of the disease, and the immune status of the patient (Tables 54-2 and 54-3 and Figure 54-3).[13] HB$_s$Ag is usually present at the onset of acute symptomatic HBV infection and can persist for up to 20 weeks. Anti-HB$_s$Ag usually does not appear until 2 to 16 weeks after the antigen is no longer present and usually persists for many years. Anti-HB$_c$ antigen appears after HB$_s$Ag but well before anti-HB$_s$Ag. It is almost always present at the onset of symptoms.[48] Initially titers may be high, but then they gradually drop to low levels and persist for at least 5 to 6 years.[26] Thus when HB$_s$Ag has disappeared and anti-HB$_s$Ag is not yet detectable, anti-HB$_c$Ag may be the only measurable marker of HBV infection.[40] This is called the core window. Although HB$_s$Ag may be undetectable in sera containing only anti-HB$_c$Ag, the sera can be infectious.[31,40]

Recent studies indicate that anti-HB$_c$Ag IgM is regularly present in high titers in acute HBV infection. Titers begin to drop within 3 months, and in 6 to 24 months, 80% of patients have negative test results.[20,48,65] In most cases of chronic HBV infection anti-HB$_c$Ag IgM persisted for longer than 2 years. In one study it was the only specific marker for acute HBV infection in 12% of cases.[48]

Anti-Hb$_e$Ag is not detectable until the disappearance of HB$_e$Ag. HB$_e$Ag is a marker of infectivity and is an indication of viral replication.[22] All individuals with acute HB$_s$Ag-positive HBV are probably at least transiently positive for HB$_e$Ag.[75]

HB$_e$Ag is associated with high titers of HB$_s$Ag, HB$_c$Ag in the liver,[15] and chronic hepatitis.[32] Conversely, the appearance of anti-HB$_e$Ag usually occurs several weeks after the loss of HB$_e$Ag in patients with few or no liver changes, no intranuclear HB$_c$Ag, and low titers of HB$_s$Ag.[32] Sera containing HB$_e$Ag are highly infectious, whereas sera with anti-HB$_e$Ag are rarely infectious.

Patients who have asymptomatic HBV infection and do not become carriers have HB$_s$Ag in their serum for a short time. It is usually not detected. Anti-HB$_s$Ag develops quickly and is usually found in high titers. Anti-HB$_c$Ag is present in low titers and may be transient or never detectable. Rarely, anti-HB$_e$Ag is present (Figure 54-4).

A chronic HB$_s$Ag carrier state is defined by the persistence of HB$_s$Ag in high titers for more than 6 months. Anti-HB$_s$Ag is not present. Anti-HB$_c$Ag rises rapidly and persists in high titers.[43] HB$_e$Ag is also present in high titers; it may disappear in a year or persist for decades. The disappearance of HB$_e$Ag and the appearance of anti-HB$_e$Ag indicates persistent chronic HBV. Patients who do not seroconvert are more likely to develop progressive liver disease.

In HB$_s$Ag-positive pregnant women, HB$_e$Ag and anti-HB$_e$Ag are used to predict the possibility of HBV transmission to the fetus. HB$_e$Ag-positive women almost always transmit the virus, whereas maternal-infant transmission is uncommon in anti-HB$_e$Ag–positive women.[70]

Tests for the detection of HB$_s$Ag and anti-HB$_s$Ag have steadily increased in sensitivity from the original agar gel diffusion test (Table 54-4) to the sensitive and specific RIA. Most laboratories use either RIA or ELISA. Reagents for both procedures are available commercially.[33,55] False-positive results

TABLE 54-2. Appearance and Duration of Serologic Markers of Hepatitis B Virus Infection

Marker	Symptomatic (HB$_s$Ag$^+$ Hepatitis B[a])		Asymptomatic (HB$_s$Ag$^-$ Hepatitis B)		Chronic Persistent (HB$_s$Ag$^+$ Hepatitis B[b])		Comments
	Appearance[c]	Duration	Appearance	Duration	Appearance	Duration	
Surface antigen (HB$_s$Ag) (Australia [Au] antigen; hepatitis-associated antigen [HAA])[d]	1-12 wk (usually 1-4 wk)	Up to 20 wk	Never		More often associated with long incubation, mild acute HBV, late appearance HB$_s$Ag	Years; level may vary and even be undetectable at times	Indicates viral replication and acute or chronic infection
Antibody to HB$_s$Ag (anti-HB$_s$, anti-Au)[d]	12-24 wk	Years	4 to 12 wk	Years	Rarely detected		Usually present only after HB$_s$Ag becomes negative; protective
Core antigen (HB$_c$Ag)	Found only in nucleus of infected hepatocytes; no consistent pattern of presence in liver cells or pattern of clinical hepatitis						
Antibody to HB$_c$Ag (anti-HB$_c$)	3-5 wk (after HB$_s$Ag or shortly before or just after clinical onset)	Years	8 wk (may not be present)	4 to 6 yr (low titer)	After HB$_s$Ag; in high titers	Years	Indicates early acute infection if HB$_s$Ag; anti-HB$_s$Ag negative
e antigen (HB$_e$Ag)	2-12 wk (usually within 1 wk of HB$_s$Ag)	Usually less than 18 wk	Unknown	Unknown	May or may not be present	Can persist more than 10 yr	Only found in HB$_s$Ag$^+$ sera; indicates highly infectious sera
Antibody to HB$_e$Ag (anti-HB$_e$, anti-e[d])	After HB$_e$Ag disappears	Probably years	Unknown	Unknown	May or may not be present; appears if HB$_e$Ag disappears		Prognostic for resolution of infection

[a]Complete resolution for majority of patients.
[b]HB$_s$Ag$^+$ more than 20 weeks.
[c]After exposure to HBV.
[d]Other terms.

TABLE 54-3. Interpretation of Serologic Markers in HBV Infection

Markers Present					Interpretation	Blood Infectivity
HB$_s$Ag	Anti-HB$_s$Ag	Anti-HB$_c$	HB$_e$Ag	Anti-HB$_e$Ag		
+	−	−	+	−	Incubation period or early acute (presymptomatic) HBV hepatitis	High
+	−	+	+	−	Acute HBV hepatitis or chronic carrier (if chronic carrier, anti-HB$_c$Ag IgM should be positive)[27]	High
+	−	+	−	+	Late HBV hepatitis or chronic carrier	Low
−	+	+	−	+	Recovered or convalescent; immune	None
−	+	+	−	−	Recovered from HBV infection; immune	None
−	−	+	−	−	Recovered from past HBV with undetectable anti-HB$_s$Ag; immediate recovery (core window); or "low-level" chronic HBV infection	Unknown
−	+	−	−	−	Immunized (no infection) or recovered from long-past HBV infection	None

SYMBOLS: +, Positive for marker
−, Negative for marker

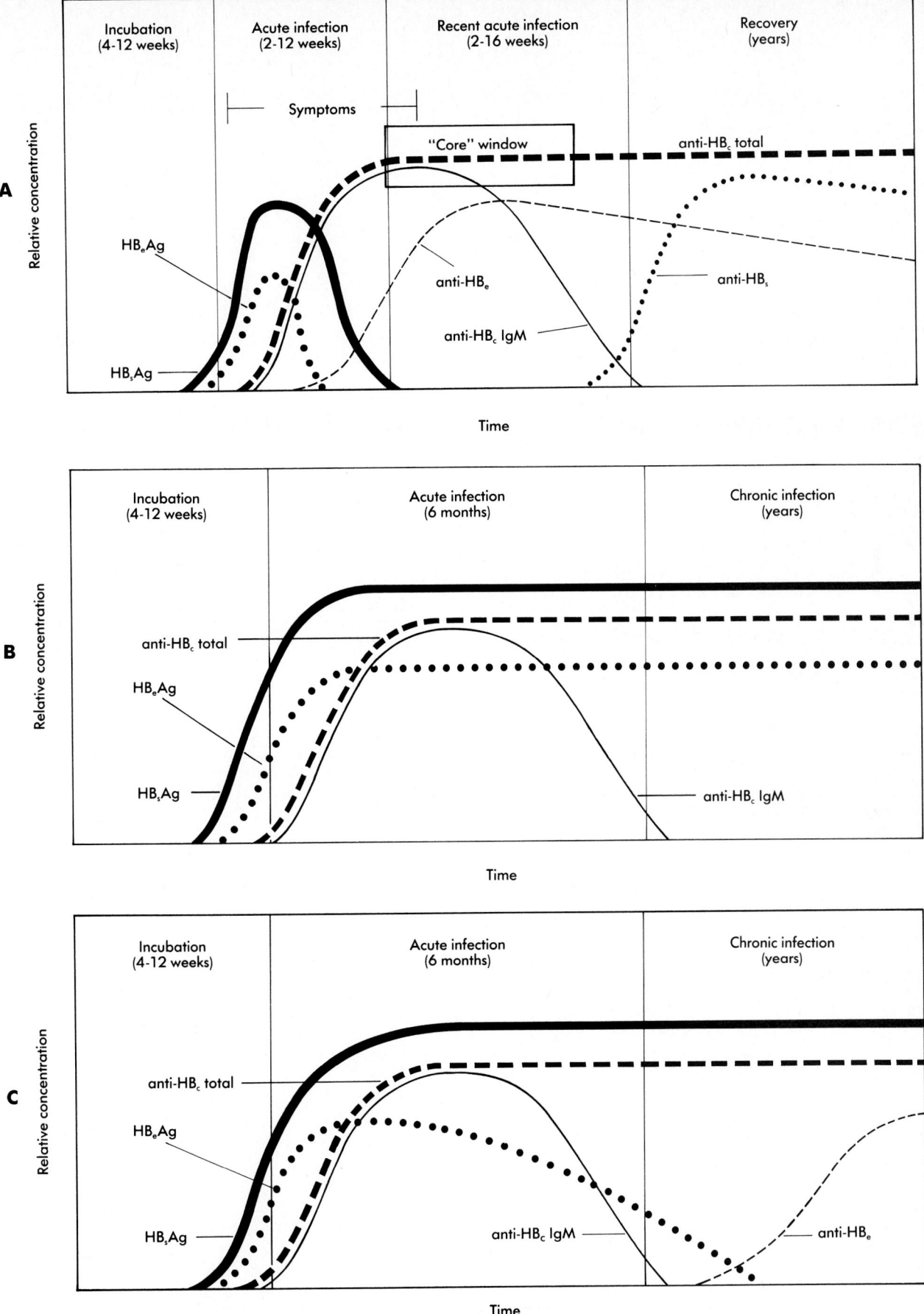

FIGURE 54-3. Antigen and antibody responses in hepatitis B. **A,** Hepatitis B core window identification. **B,** Hepatitis B chronic carrier: no seroconversion. **C,** Hepatitis B chronic carrier: late seroconversion. (From Serodiagnostic assessment of acute viral hepatitis, Chicago, 1981, Abbott Laboratories.)

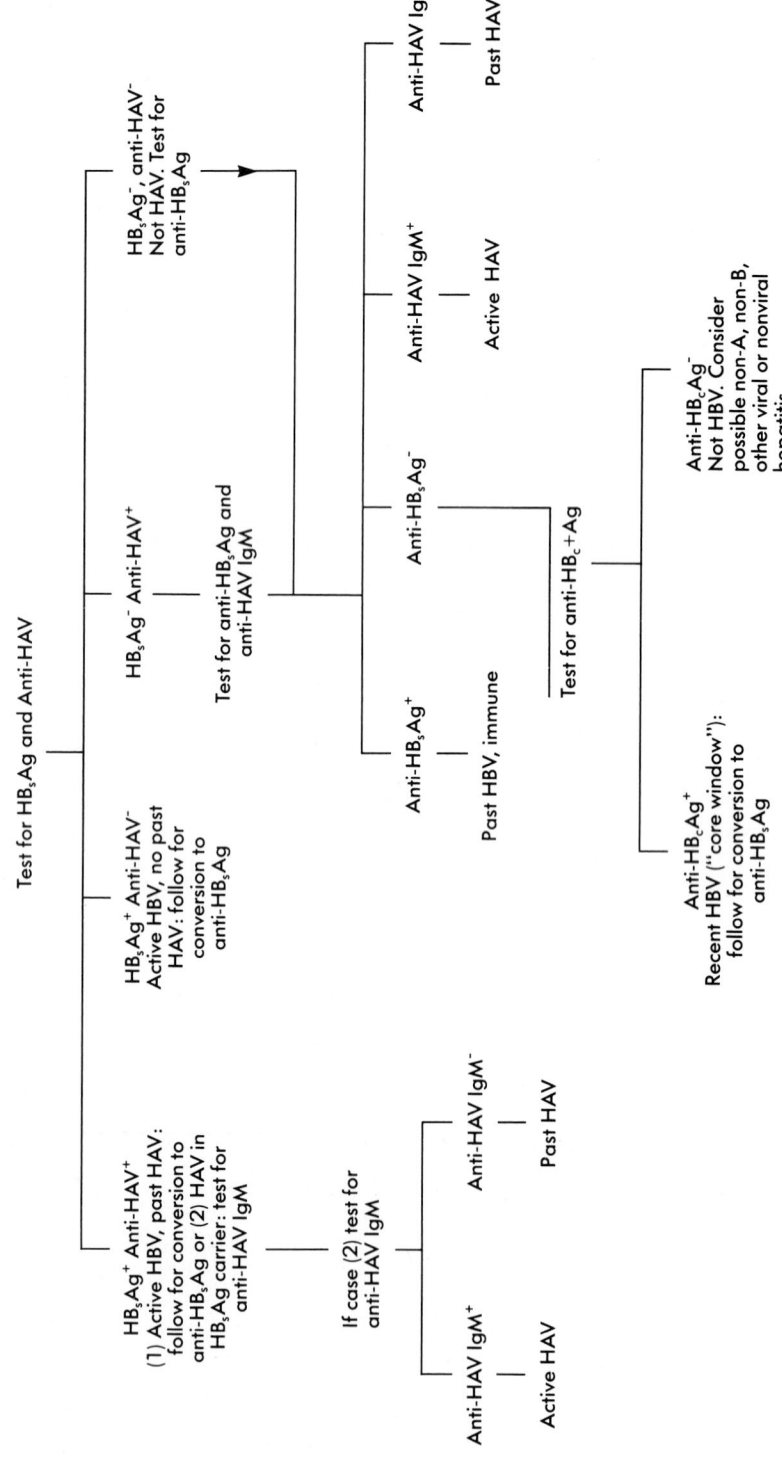

FIGURE 54-4. Practical laboratory diagnosis of viral hepatitis. Epidemiologic factors should be considered in selection and interpretation of these tests.

TABLE 54-4. Serologic Procedures for Diagnosis of HBV Infection

Test	Marker	Sensitivity	Time to Perform	Comments
FIRST GENERATION				
Agar-gel diffusion (AGD)	HB_sAg, anti-HB_sAg	Least	24-72 hr	Useful for subtype; simple; no special equipment; positive indicates potent antisera
SECOND GENERATION				
Counterimmunoelectrophoresis (CIE)	HB_sAg, anti-HB_sAg	5-10×>AGD	1-2 hr	
Complement fixation	HB_sAg	5-10×>AGD	24 hr	
Reverse passive latex agglutination	HB_sAg		1 hr	Rapid and simple; false-positive reactions common; must confirm positives with another test
THIRD GENERATION				
Reverse passive hemagglutination	HB_sAg, HB_eAg	10-100×>2nd generation tests		Both rapid and simple, but false-positive results occur
Passive hemagglutination	Anti-HB_sAg, anti-HB_eAg			
Solid phase radioimmunoassay (RIA) "sandwich"	HB_sAg, anti-HB_sAg	100-1000×>2nd generation tests	4-24 hr	Requires radioactivity and expensive equipment; short shelf life; confirm positives
Competitive-binding RIA	Anti-HB_c, HB_eAg			
Enzyme-linked immunosorbent assay (ELISA)	HB_sAg, anti-HB_sAg	50-100×>2nd generation tests		No radioactivity; no equipment; long shelf life

do occur (0.6% to 7%, depending on the RIA kit), so all HB_sAg-positive sera are retested and are considered reactive only if they are repeatedly reactive. Further confirmation may be obtained by showing that the reaction can be neutralized by specific antiserum. Although all RIA kits for HB_sAg sold in the United States must be approved by the Food and Drug Administration, significant differences in sensitivity and specificity exist. According to Nath and co-workers,[55] the kits made by Abbott Laboratories (North Chicago, Ill.), Fenwal, Inc. (Ashland, Mass.), Electo-Nucleonics, Inc. (Bethesda, Md.), and Nuclear Medical Laboratories (Dallas) are acceptable. All these kits have short shelf lives and become less sensitive with age. A commercial RIA is also available for detection of anti-HB_cAg and HB_eAg.[53]

DELTA ANTIGEN–ASSOCIATED HEPATITIS

In 1977 Rizzetto, Canese, and Arico[59] discovered what they thought was a new HBV antigen-antibody system. The antigen, which they called delta, was found only in liver specimens from patients with HB_sAg-positive sera.

Delta appears to be a unique transmissible agent distinct from HBV.[63] It has an internal component (delta antigen) surrounding a low–molecular weight RNA and is coated with HB_sAg. Delta appears to be defective, requiring obligatory functions of HBV for replication.[62]

Delta can cause both acute and chronic hepatitis, but infection develops only in HB_sAg-positive people. Delta can be transmitted simultaneously with HBV or as a superinfection in HB_sAg carriers. Simultaneous infection with HBV usually results in a benign, self-limited disease because, once HBV replication stops, delta can no longer replicate.[25,61]

Superinfection of an HB_sAg carrier with delta may result in acute or chronic hepatitis. The acute infection is often severe and may be fulminant.[63] The majority of superinfected HB_sAg carriers develop chronic active hepatitis.[64]

Delta initially was found predominantly among HB_sAg-positive Italians[61] but is now found worldwide among drug users and others frequently exposed to blood or blood products.[61,66] Incidence in the United States is unknown.

Diagnosis of delta hepatitis is less difficult now because serologic tests for delta antigen and antibody are generally available. Delta antigenemia is rarely detected, and chronic antigenemia is unknown. Seroconversion to anti-delta antigen confirms delta infection. Anti-delta IgM is transient and may be a useful diagnostic marker. Attempts to confirm delta infection should be made only in HB_sAg-positive individuals.

NON-A, NON-B HEPATITIS

With the development of tests with greater sensitivity for the diagnosis of HBV infection, it became evident that not all post-transfusion hepatitis was caused by HBV. Those cases of viral hepatitis for which no specific etiology can be documented are collectively called non-A, non-B (NANB) hepatitis.

Little is known about the agent responsible for NANB hepatitis, although transmission by intravenous inoculation of serum from humans to chimpanzees confirmed its infectious nature.[2,76] Transmission studies in chimpanzees indicate that at least two agents may cause NANB hepatitis: one with a short incubation period (2 to 4 weeks)[34] and another with a long incubation period (8 to 12 weeks).[51] The existence of more than one agent is further supported by strain-specific ultrastructural alterations in the liver and the homologous immunity of infected chimpanzees.[69] That humans have several bouts of NANB hepatitis or biphasic disease also suggests the presence of more than one virus.

Clinically, NANB hepatitis is less severe than acute HBV hepatitis.[16] It is usually mild, and up to 50% of patients have no jaundice. Progression to fulminant hepatitis is infrequent. However, almost one third of patients with NANB hepatitis develop chronic hepatitis, compared to only 5% of patients with HBV infection.[19,51] Fortunately, the prognosis is usually benign. Most recover spontaneously, and deaths resulting from chronic liver failure are rare. Cirrhosis can occur.

The epidemiologic pattern of NANB hepatitis is similar to that of HBV hepatitis, with parenteral routes as the predominant mode of transmission.[21] Infection is thus associated with exposure to blood or blood products, although recipients of blood transfusions are at the greatest risk.[72] NANB hepatitis accounts for more than 90% of posttransfusion hepatitis in the United States. Like HBV hepatitis, NANB hepatitis has been associated with outbreaks in dialysis units.[29] Sporadic NANB hepatitis also occurs without any known parenteral exposure, suggesting transmission by intimate contact.

Use of gamma globulin for NANB hepatitis is controversial.[1] Currently, the only means of control is to use volunteer donor rather than commercial donor blood. However, even if only volunteer donor blood that has been screened for HB_sAg is used, there will still be three to six cases of posttransfusion hepatitis for each 1000 units of blood.[19]

Although many attempts have been made to develop specific serologic tests for NANB hepatitis, none have withstood critical analysis. Diagnosis depends on excluding hepatitis A and B and other causes of hepatitis.

PRACTICAL LABORATORY DIAGNOSIS OF VIRAL HEPATITIS (Figure 54-4)

Testing all sera from patients with suspected viral hepatitis for all the known serologic markers is neither practical nor cost effective. The first consideration in testing is knowledge of various epidemiologic factors. Is the patient an intravenous drug user, a hemodialysis patient, or a laboratory worker? Have several persons from the same family or place of employment developed similar symptoms? In the former cases, tests for HBV infection would be performed first; in the latter, tests for HAV infection would be first.

In suspected HBV infection, sera are first tested for HB_sAg. Because 90% to 95% of patients are HB_sAg positive, often no further diagnostic tests are necessary. All HB_sAg-positive patients have either acute or chronic HBV infection (Table 54-3). These patients should be followed for the disappearance of HB_sAg and seroconversion to anti-HB_sAg. If the patient still tests positive for HB_sAg after 6 months, the disease has become chronic. If liver enzymes remain elevated, the patient has chronic active or chronic persistent hepatitis. A liver biopsy is necessary to differentiate active from persistent disease. If liver enzyme levels are not elevated, the patient is a chronic, asymptomatic carrier.

If HB_sAg is not present, sera should be tested for anti-HB_sAg. Its presence indicates immunity to HBV resulting from past infection or immunization. A negative test result for anti-HB_sAg can indicate no HBV infection, a low-level carrier, or late HBV infection. A test for anti-HB_cAg may help differentiate among these. The absence of anti-HB_cAg indicates no HBV infection, and other viral or nonviral causes should be pursued (Figure 54-4). A positive anti-HB_cAg test result may indicate late HBV infection (core window) or a low-level, chronic carrier. These patients should be followed for seroconversion to anti-HB_sAg.

Laboratory diagnosis of HAV is much simpler. Sera are first screened for anti-HAV. If present, sera are tested for anti-HAV IgM. A positive result indicates recent HAV infection. If both HBV and HAV can be ruled out, further testing for viruses such as cytomegalovirus or Epstein-Barr virus is warranted, again depending on the epidemiologic circumstances. Tests for anti-delta are available only in research facilities and should be performed only on sera from HB_sAg-positive patients who are from the Mediterranean or who have frequent contact with blood or blood products. The diagnosis of NANB hepatitis is one of exclusion. Figure 54-4 summarizes the suggested order of testing for the laboratory diagnosis of viral hepatitis.

REFERENCES

1. Aach, R.D., and Kahn, R.A.: Post-transfusion hepatitis: current perspectives, Ann. Intern. Med. **92**:539, 1980.
2. Alter, H.J., et al.: Transmissible agent in non-A, non-B hepatitis, Lancet **1**:459, 1978.
3. Alter, M.J.: Nosocomial hepatitis A infection: can we wash our hands of it? Pediatr. Infect. Dis. **3**:294, 1984.
4. Binn, L.N. et al.: Primary isolation and serial passage of hepatitis A virus strains in primate cell cultures, J. Clin. Microbiol. **20**:28, 1984.
5. Blumberg, B.S., and London, W.T.: Hepatitis B virus and the prevention of primary hepatocellular carcinoma, N. Engl. J. Med. **304**:782, 1981.
6. Centers for Disease Control: Postexposure prophylaxis of hepatitis B, MMWR **33**:285, 1984.
7. Chaudhary, R.K.: Perinatal transmission of hepatitis B virus, Can. Med. Assoc. J. **128**:644, 1983.
8. Corey, L., and Holmes, K.K.: Sexual transmission of hepatitis A in homosexual men, N. Engl. J. Med. **302**:435, 1980.
9. Coulepis, A.G., et al.: Detection of hepatitis A virus in the feces of patients with naturally acquired infections, J. Infect. Dis. **141**:151, 1980.

10. Decker, R.H., et al.: Serologic studies of transmission of hepatitis A in humans, J. Infect. Dis. **139**:74, 1979.

11. Decker, R.H., et al.: Diagnosis of acute hepatitis A by HAVAB-M, a direct radioimmunoassay for IgM Anti-HAV, Am. J. Clin. Pathol. **76**:140, 1981.

12. Dienstag, J.L., et al.: Hepatitis A virus infection: new insights from seroepidemiologic studies, J. Infect. Dis. **137**:328, 1978.

13. Dienstag, J.L., et al.: Hepatitis B vaccine in health care personnel: safety, immunogenicity, and indicators of efficacy, Ann. Intern. Med. **101**:34, 1984.

14. Dietzman, D.E., et al.: Hepatitis B surface antigen (HB$_s$Ag) and antibody to HB$_s$Ag, JAMA **238**:2625, 1977.

15. Ettenger, R.B., et al.: Hepatitis B infection in pediatric dialysis and transplant patients: significance of e antigen, J. Pediatr. **97**:550, 1980.

16. Feinstone, S.M., and Purcell, R.H.: Non-A, non-B hepatitis, Annu. Rev. Med. **29**:359, 1978.

17. Franzer, C., and Frosner, G.: Placental transfer of hepatitis A antibody, N. Engl. J. Med. **304**:427, 1981.

18. Frosner, G.G., et al.: Antibody against hepatitis A in seven European countries. I. Comparison of prevalence data in different age groups, Am. J. Epidemiol. **110**:63, 1979.

19. Galbraith, R.M., et al.: Non-A, non-B hepatitis associated with chronic liver disease in a haemodialysis unit, Lancet **1**:951, 1979.

20. Gerlich, W.H., et al.: Diagnosis of acute and inapparent hepatitis B virus infections by measurement of IgM antibody to hepatitis B core antigen, J. Infect. Dis. **142**:95, 1980.

21. Gitnick, G.: Non-A, non-B hepatitis-etiology and clinical course, J. Lab. Clin. Med. **14**:721, 1983.

22. Grady, G.F., et al.: Relation of e antigen to infectivity of HB$_s$Ag positive inoculations among medical personnel, Lancet **2**:492, 1976.

23. Gust, I.D., et al.: Seroepidemiology of infection with hepatitis A and B viruses in an isolated Pacific population, J. Infect. Dis. **139**:559, 1979.

24. Hadler, S.C., et al.: An outbreak of hepatitis B in a dental practice, Ann. Intern. Med. **95**:133, 1981.

25. Hadler, S.C., et al.: Delta virus infection and severe hepatitis, Ann. Intern. Med. **100**:339, 1984.

26. Hansson, B.G.: Persistence of serum antibody to hepatitis B core antigen, J. Clin. Microbiol. **6**:209, 1977.

27. Hawkes, R.A., et al.: Use of immunoglobulin M antibody to hepatitis B core antigen in diagnosis of viral hepatitis, J. Clin. Microbiol. **11**:581, 1980.

28. Hilleman, M.R., et al.: The preparation and safety of hepatitis B vaccine, J. Infect. Dis. **7**(suppl. 1):3, 1983.

29. Hollinger, F.B., et al.: Transfusion-transmitted viruses study: experimental evidence for two non-A, non-B, hepatitis agents, J. Infect. Dis. **142**:400, 1980.

30. Hollinger, F.B., et al.: Posttransfusion hepatitis type A, JAMA **250**:2313, 1983.

31. Hoofnagle, J.H., et al.: Type B hepatitis after transfusion with blood containing antibody to hepatitis B core antigen, N. Engl. J. Med. **298**:1379, 1978.

32. Hoofnagle, J.H., et al.: Seroconversion from hepatitis Be antigen to antibody in chronic type B hepatitis, Ann. Intern. Med. **94**:744, 1981.

33. Hopkins, R., et al.: Comparison of radioimmunoassay and enzyme immunoassay for detecting hepatitis B surface antigen in serum from freshly donated blood and selected blood products, J. Clin. Pathol. **31**:1000, 1978.

34. Hruby, M.A., and Schauf, V.: Transfusion-related short-incubation hepatitis in hemophilic patients, JAMA **240**:1355, 1978.

35. Hussey, H.H.: The hepatitis B saga, JAMA **245**:1317, 1981.

36. Inaba, N., et al.: Sexual transmission of hepatitis B surface antigen: infection of husbands by HB$_s$Ag carrier-state wives, Br. J. Vener. Dis. **55**:366, 1979.

37. Janzen, J., et al.: Epidemiology of hepatitis B surface antigen (HB$_s$Ag) and antibody to HB$_s$Ag in hospital personnel, J. Infect. Dis. **137**:261, 1978.

38. Joosten, R. and Sturner, K.H.: Hepatitis and pregnancy: risks for the newborn—immunoprophylaxis of vertically transmitted hepatitis, J. Perinat. Med. **9**:115, 1981.

39. Kaiser, L., et al.: Hepatitis B surface antigen in urine of renal transplant recipients, Ann. Intern. Med. **94**:783, 1981.

40. Katchaki, J.N., Siem, T.H., and Brouwer, R.: Serological evidence of presence of HB$_s$Ag undetectable by conventional radioimmunoassay in anti-HBc positive blood donors, J. Clin. Pathol. **31**:837, 1978.

41. Klein, B.S., et al.: Nosocomial hepatitis A: a multinursery outbreak in Wisconsin, JAMA **252**:2716, 1984.

42. Kobayashi, H., et al: Susceptibility of hepatitis B virus to disinfectants or heat, J. Clin. Microbiol. **20**:214, 1984.

43. Krugman, S.: The newly licensed hepatitis B vaccine: characteristics and indications for use, JAMA **247**:2012, 1982.

44. Krugman, S., Friedman, H., and Lattimer, C.: Hepatitis A and B: serologic survey of various population groups, Am. J. Med. Sci. **275**:249, 1978.

45. Krugman, S., and Giles, J.P.: Viral hepatitis: new light on an old disease, JAMA **212**:1019, 1970.

46. Lauer, J.L., et al.: Transmission of hepatitis B virus in clinical laboratory areas, J. Infect. Dis. **140**:513, 1979.

47. Leichtner, A.M., et al.: Horizontal nonparenteral spread of hepatitis B among children, Ann. Intern. Med. **94**:346, 1981.

48. Lemon, S.M., et al.: IgM antibody to hepatitis B core antigen as a diagnostic parameter of acute infection with hepatitis B virus, J. Infect. Dis. **143**:803, 1981.

49. Lee, A.K.Y., Ip, H.M.H., and Wong, V.C.W.: Mechanism of maternal-fetal transmission of hepatitis B virus, J. Infect. Dis. **138**:668, 1978.

50. Mathiesen, L.R., et al.: Enzyme-linked immunosorbent assay for detection of hepatitis A antigen in stool and antibody to hepatitis A antigen in sera: comparison with solid-phase radioimmunoassay, immune electron microscopy, and immune adherence hemagglutination assay, J. Clin. Microbiol. **7**:184, 1978.

51. Maugh, T.H.: Where is the hepatitis C virus? Science **210**:999, 1980.

52. Melnick, J.L.: Classification of hepatitis A virus as enterovirus type 72 and of hepatitis B virus as hepadnavirus type 1, Intervirology **18**:105, 1982.

53. Mushahwar, I.K., et al.: Radioimmunoassay for detection of hepatitis B e antigen and its antibody: results of clinical evaluation, Am. J. Clin. Pathol. **76**:692, 1981.

54. Najem, G.R., et al.: Control of hepatitis B infection: the role of surveillance and an isolation hemodialysis center, JAMA **245**:153, 1981.

55. Nath, N., et al.: Comparative evaluation of radioimmunoassay kits used for testing blood for hepatitis B surface antigen, Am. J. Clin. Pathol. **75**:214, 1981.

56. Noble, R.C., et al.: Posttransfusion hepatitis in a neonatal intensive care unit, JAMA **252**:2711, 1984.

57. Provost, P.J., and Hilleman, M.R.: Propagation of human hepatitis A virus in cell culture *in vitro*, Proc. Soc. Exp. Biol. Med. **160**:213, 1979.

58. Provost, P.J., et al.: Isolation of hepatitis A virus *in vitro* in cell culture directly from human specimens, Proc. Soc. Exp. Biol. Med. **167**:201, 1981.

59. Rizzetto, M., Canese, M.G., and Arico, S.: Immunofluorescence detection of a new antigen-antibody system (delta/anti-delta) associated with hepatitis B virus in liver and serum of HB$_s$Ag carriers, Gut **18**:997, 1977.

60. Rizzetto, M., Gerin, J.L., and Purcell, R.H.: Epidemiology of HBV-associated delta agent: geographical distribution of anti-delta and prevalence in polytransfused HB$_s$Ag carriers, Lancet **1**:1215, 1980.

61. Rizzetto, M., Smedile, A., and Farci, P.: The clinical significance of the delta antigen-antibody system in hepatitis B infections, Scand. J. Infect. Dis. **36**(suppl.):74, 1982.

62. Rizzetto, M., et al.: Incidence and significance of antibodies to delta antigen in hepatitis B virus infection, Lancet **2:**986, 1979.

63. Rizzetto, M., et al.: Transmission of the hepatitis B virus-associated delta antigen to chimpanzees, J. Infect. Dis. **141:**590, 1980.

64. Rizzetto, M., et al.: Chronic hepatitis in carriers of hepatitis B surface antigen, with intrahepatic expression of the delta antigen: an active and progressive disease unresponsive to immunosuppressive treatment, Ann. Intern. Med. **98:**437, 1983.

65. Roggendorf, M., et al.: Immunoglobulin M antibodies to hepatitis B core antigen: evaluation of enzyme immunoassay for diagnosis of hepatitis B virus infection, J. Clin. Microbiol. **13:**618, 1981.

66. Rosina, F., Saracco, G., and Rizzetto, M.: Risk of post-transfusion infection with the hepatitis delta virus, N. Engl. J. Med. **312:**1488, 1985.

67. Safford, S.E.S., Needleman, S.B., and Decker, R.H.: Radioimmunoassay for detection of antibody to hepatitis A virus: results of clinical evaluation, Am. J. Clin. Pathol. **74:**25, 1980.

68. Sherertz, R.J., Russell, B.A., and Reuman, P.D.: Transmission of hepatitis A by transfusion of blood products, Arch. Intern. Med. **144:**1579, 1984.

69. Shimizu, Y.K., et al.: Non-A, non-B hepatitis: ultrastructural evidence for two agents in experimentally infected chimpanzees, Science **205:**197, 1979.

70. Shiraki, K., et al.: Acute hepatitis B in infants born to carrier mothers with the antibody to hepatitis B e antigen, J. Pediatr. **97:**768, 1980.

71. Skidmore, S.J., and Boxall, E.H.: A radioimmunoassay for hepatitis A antigen and antibody, J. Clin. Pathol. **32:**710, 1979.

72. Stevens, C.E., et al.: Hepatitis B virus antibody in blood donors and the occurrence of non-A, non-B hepatitis in transfusion recipients, Ann. Intern. Med. **101:**733, 1984.

73. Szmuness, W., et al.: Hepatitis B vaccine: demonstration of efficacy in a controlled clinical trial in a high-risk population in the United States, N. Engl. J. Med. **303:**833, 1980.

74. Szmuness, W., et al.: Passive-active immunization against hepatitis B: immunogenicity studies in adult Americans, Lancet **1:**575, 1981.

75. Szmuness, W., et al.: Prevalence of hepatitis B "e" antigen and its antibody in various HB$_s$Ag carrier populations, Am. J. Epidemiol. **113:**113, 1981.

76. Tabor, E., et al.: Transmission of non-A, non-B hepatitis from man to chimpanzee, Lancet **1:**463, 1978.

77. Tufvesson, B., et al.: An outbreak of hepatitis A investigated by immune electron microscopy and enzyme-linked immunosorbent assay, Scand. J. Infect. Dis. **11:**97, 1979.

78. Vernon, A.A., Schable, C., and Francis, D.: A large outbreak of hepatitis A in a day-care center: association with non-toilet-trained children and persistence of IgM antibody to hepatitis A virus, Am. J. Epidemiol. **115:**325, 1982.

79. Villarejas, V.M., et al.: Role of saliva, urine and feces in the transmission of type B hepatitis, N. Engl. J. Med. **291:**1375, 1974.

CHAPTER 55

Gastroenteritis Viruses

Sally Jo Rubin

Acute viral gastroenteritis is second in frequency only to upper respiratory tract infection; yet before 1972 no etiologic agents of this syndrome were known.[5] Ironically, during the period when cell culture became widely available, the two most common viruses causing gastroenteritis, Norwalk-like viruses and rotaviruses, were detected by electron microscopy. Norwalk-like viruses generally produce epidemics in school-age children and adults, whereas rotaviruses cause sporadic and sometimes epidemic disease in infants and very young children (Table 55-1). Adenoviruses have also been associated with gastroenteritis in infants and are discussed in Chapter 48.

NORWALK-LIKE VIRUSES

In the 1940s, several groups of investigators were able to transmit diarrhea to adult volunteers with bacteria-free stool filtrates. All attempts at virus isolation, however, were unsuccessful, and no further investigations were done. In 1968 an outbreak of diarrheal illness occurred among elementary school children, their teachers, and their families in Norwalk, Ohio. Again, serial transmission to volunteers was accomplished.[12] By this time, however, the technique of immune electron microscopy was available, and 27 nm particles were detected in the feces of infected people and volunteers (Figure 55-1).[17] A number of outbreaks have since been investigated with morphologically similar particles found in the feces of ill people.[16,20] At least three and possibly four distinct serotypes of Norwalk-like viruses exist.[25] Isolates are named for the location of their detection (Table 55-2).

Since these agents have yet to be grown in animals or in cell culture, it is impossible to determine their nucleic-acid content or to classify them. They are similar in a number of ways to the parvoviruses. The Norwalk-like agents are hardy viruses, being ether, pH, and heat stable.[12]

CLINICAL SIGNIFICANCE AND EPIDEMIOLOGY

Norwalk-like agents cause mild gastrointestinal disease in school-age children and adults. Based on volunteer studies, the incubation period is only 24 to 48 hours, followed by the onset of vomiting and diarrhea. Usually both symptoms are present, but sometimes only one occurs. Low-grade fever and abdominal pain may be present. Symptoms resolve in 2 or 3 days with no sequelae.[5,35] Virus is shed in the feces during the symptomatic period but rarely for more than 3 days.

Infection with Norwalk-like agents can be either sporadic or epidemic. Transmission is probably fecal-oral. Outbreaks in schools and camps and on a cruise ship have been attributed to contaminated water.[14,35] Infection with these agents is common, and by 50 years of age about 50% of people have serum antibody.[6]

The pathogenesis of Norwalk virus infections is unknown. Reversible jejunal changes and small bowel malabsorption of fat and xylose occur.[5]

LABORATORY DIAGNOSIS

At present the only means of detecting all the Norwalk-like agents is by immune electron microscopy (IEM) or agar gel diffusion. Direct electron microscopy (EM) is not completely successful because the viruses are shed in low concentrations. Although available only in research laboratories, radioimmunoassay (RIA) has been used both for direct detection of the Norwalk serogroup in feces and for the measurement of the host's immune response.[6]

Antibody is frequently present after infection and provides short-term (6 to 14 weeks) resistance to reinfection with the homologous agent. An immune response to Norwalk agent is unusual; volunteers who seroconvert or have preexisting antibody are more likely to become ill and to be reinfected when reinoculated. Those who do not develop primary infection usually do not develop antibody and seem to be resistant to infection with Norwalk-like viruses.[6] It is likely then that serum antibodies are not protective and that protection may result from local immune responses such as IgA.

ROTAVIRUSES

For years the many cases of infantile gastroenteritis were presumed to be viral diseases. Many fruitless attempts were made at cultivating feces in animals and in cell cultures. Finally in 1973, Australian investigators detected with EM 70 nm particles in the epithelial cells from duodenal biopsies of children who were ill with nonbacterial gastroenteritis.[3] Soon investigators worldwide described similar viral particles in feces from ill children. Morphologically the viruses had a double-shelled capsid that caused them to resemble a wheel with a thin rim and short spokes radiating from a wide hub (Figure 55-2). Thus they were called rotaviruses from the Latin *rota* meaning wheel.[32] Rotaviruses share a complement fixation (CF) antigen (the inner capsid), but all are antigenically distinguishable. At least four serotypes of human rotavirus are known.[31] The outer capsid protein is serotype specific.

Many animal rotaviruses that cause disease in newborn animals, such as calves, piglets, foals, and lambs, have been characterized. Many rotavirus strains from animals replicate in cell cultures; human strains have been reported to grow in primary monkey kidney cell cultures.[33] Analysis of these animal viruses revealed that they are members of the family *Reoviridae*. Rotaviruses are ribonucleic acid (RNA) viruses containing 11 segments of double-stranded RNA. Rotaviruses are hardy and withstand heat, acid, and ether.[11]

TABLE 55-1. Characteristics of Human Gastroenteritis Viruses

Characteristic	Rotavirus	Norwalk-Like Agents
Size	70 nm	25-27 nm
Nucleic acid	RNA	Unknown
Minimum number of serotypes	Four	Three
Seasonality (temperate climate)	Winter	Winter
Epidemicity	Sporadic, epidemic	Epidemic
Age with clinical disease	6-24 mo	6 yr and up
Transmission	Fecal-oral; water; food	Fecal-oral

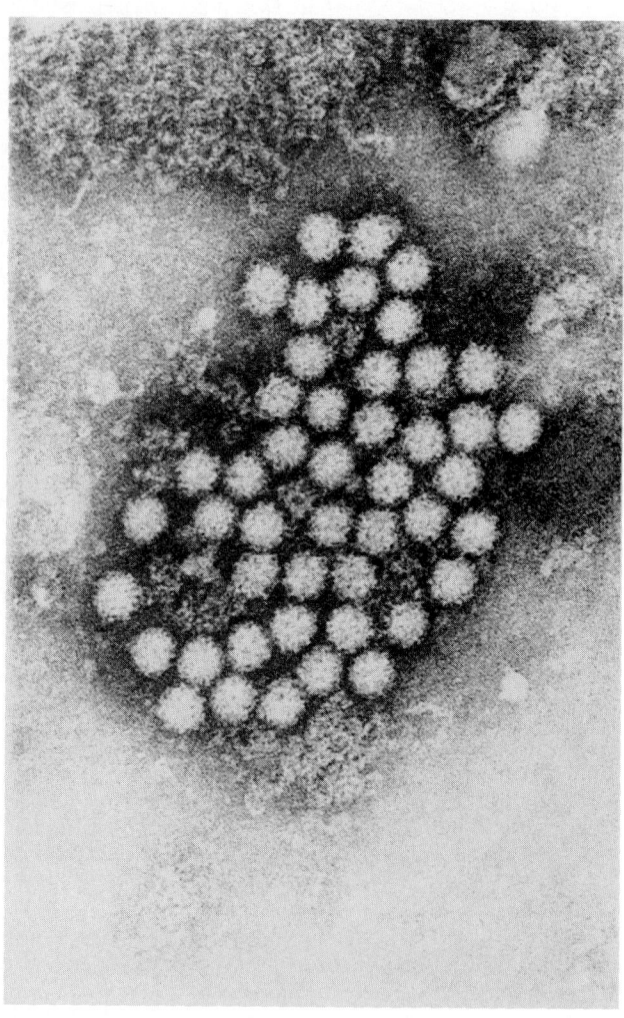

FIGURE 55-1. Electron micrograph of Norwalk virus. Light antibody coating. (Approximately ×231,500.) (From Kapikian, A.Z., et al.: J. Virol. **10:**1075, 1972.)

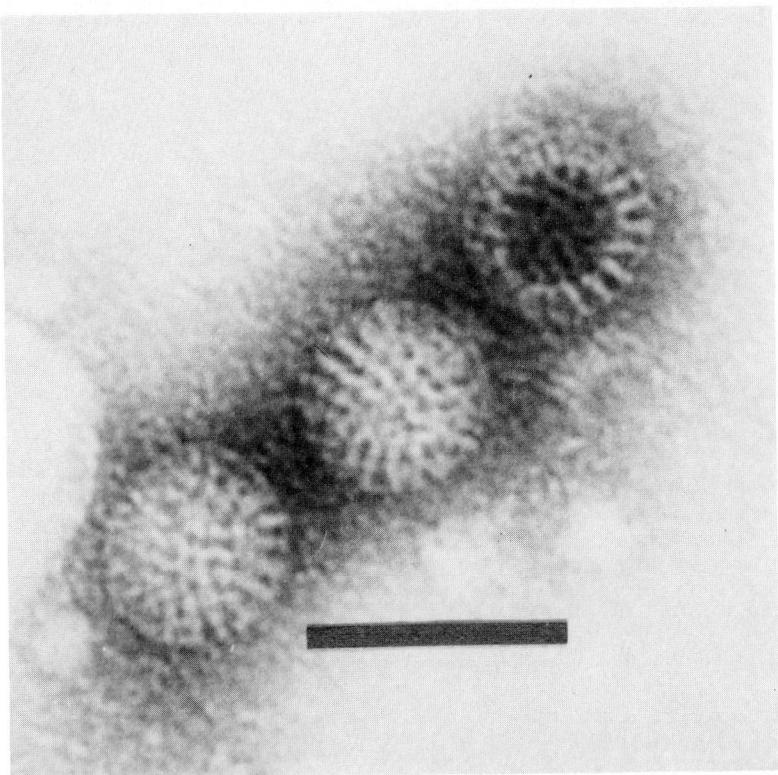

FIGURE 55-2. Rotaviruses from infant with gastroenteritis. Negatively stained virus particles in suspension of human stool. Bar marker equals 100 nm. (Courtesy Carl D. Brandt, Children's Hospital National Medical Center, Washington, D.C.)

CLINICAL SIGNIFICANCE

Rotavirus disease ranges from asymptomatic to mild to severely dehydrating diarrhea that can be fatal, particularly in the malnourished. Clinical disease most commonly begins with vomiting, followed by diarrhea, fever, and dehydration. The high incidence of vomiting is unusual with other causes of gastroenteritis. The greatest disease incidence is in 6- to 24-month-old children.[26] In fact, in half of the hospitalized patients with pediatric viral gastroenteritis, the disease is the result of rotaviruses. Generally newborns and adults have subclinical infections,[34] but premature and low–birth weight babies may be symptomatic.[4] Breast-fed babies are significantly less likely to become infected, perhaps as a result of protection from local secretory IgA.[23]

About three fourths of rotavirus infections are caused by type 2[37]; no cross-protection exists among the serotypes, nor does there seem to be a reduced risk of infection if serum antibody is present.[34] Sequential symptomatic infection with a different serotype is not unusual, and less commonly, symptomatic reinfection with the same serotype occurs.[29]

Epidemiology

Rotavirus disease in young children is found throughout the world. In temperate climates it is present only during the colder months,[23] but in tropical climates transmission takes place year-round.[28] The virus is presumably transferred by the fecal-oral route. Both sporadic disease and outbreaks occur in institutions such as day-care centers, nurseries, and schools.[15,27]

TABLE 55-2. Norwalk-Like Viruses

Agent	Antigenic Group[a]	Country of Isolation
Norwalk	Norwalk	United States
Montgomery County	Norwalk	United States
Hawaii	Hawaii	United States
Colorado	Not known	United States
Marin County	Not known	United States
Ditchling	Ditchling	England
Cockle	Not known	England
W	Ditchling	England
Parramatta	Not known	Australia

[a]Norwalk, Hawaii, and Ditchling strains are the reference serotypes against which other strains are compared.

Epidemics may be caused by foodborne or waterborne organisms. Adults usually acquire infection from contact with infected children.[18,34]

Treatment and Control

The most important treatment of rotavirus disease is to correct dehydration. No vaccine is available, but the morbidity of this virus is so high that attempts will likely be made to develop one, especially for use in underdeveloped countries. Because local immunity seems to be important, a live attenuated vaccine containing both serotypes would be the best approach.[19]

LABORATORY DIAGNOSIS

No simple laboratory method is available for cultivation of human rotavirus. Many strains cause disease in gnotobiotic newborn animals. One strain has been serially passed in African green monkey kidney cell culture but only after successive passage in gnotobiotic piglets.[36] This technique allows production of high virus titers that provide antigen for further test development.

Fortunately, some animal rotaviruses grow well in cell culture, providing antigens for techniques for direct virus detection in feces and measurement of immune response. Methods for virus detection include EM and IEM,[7] counterimmunoelectrophoresis,[30] latex agglutination, and enzyme-linked immunoabsorbent assay (ELISA).[2] ELISA is the most sensitive, and commercial kits for testing feces for viral antigen are available (Abbott Laboratories, North Chicago, Ill.).[2]

Both viral-specific IgM and IgG are found in the serum following infection.[38] IgM is usually undetectable in 5 weeks.[1] Antibody can be measured by complement fixation, indirect fluorescent-antibody tests, or ELISA. When ELISA is used, essentially 100% of adults have antibody.[13]

OTHER VIRUSES

Caliciviruses are members of the *Picornaviridae* family and produce infection in many animals. They have been seen by EM in the feces of children with and without diarrheal disease.[9,24] Caliciviruses are about 30 nm and in a Star of David configuration with six hollows surrounding a central core. They have been reported as the possible cause of several diarrheal outbreaks.[10]

Astroviruses are about 28 nm in diameter, and about 10% of the particles seen are in a five- or six-pointed star configuration. They have been seen in the feces of children with diarrhea and have been transmitted to adult volunteers in bacteria-free stool filtrates.[21,22]

Using EM, coronaviruses are seen in approximately equal numbers of children both with and without diarrhea. There is no evidence for their having any role in viral diarrheal disease.[8]

REFERENCES

1. Abe, Y., and Inouye, S.: Complement-fixing immunoglobulin M antibody responses in patients with infantile gastroenteritis, J. Clin. Microbiol. **9:**284, 1979.
2. Birch, C.J., et al.: Comparison of electron microscopy, enzyme-linked immunosorbent assay, solid-phase radioimmunoassay, and indirect immunofluorescence for detection of human rotavirus antigen in feces, J. Clin. Pathol. **32:**700, 1979.
3. Bishop, R.F., et al.: Virus particles in epithelial cells of duodenal mucosa from children with acute non-bacterial gastroenteritis, Lancet **2:**1281, 1973.
4. Bishop, R.F., et al.: Diarrhea and rotavirus infection associated with differing regimens for postnatal care of newborn babies, J. Clin. Microbiol. **9:**525, 1979.
5. Blacklow, N.R., and Cukor, G.: Viral gastroenteritis, N. Engl. J. Med. **304:**397, 1981.
6. Blacklow, N.R., et al.: Immune response and prevalence of antibody to Norfolk enteritis virus as determined by radioimmunoassay, J. Clin. Microbiol. **10:**903, 1979.
7. Brandt, C.D., et al.: Comparison of direct electron microscopy, immune electron microscopy, and rotavirus enzyme-linked immunosorbent assay for detection of gastroenteritis viruses in children, J. Clin. Microbiol. **13:**976, 1981.
8. Clarke, S.K.R., Caul, E.O., and Egglestone, S.I.: The human enteric coronaviruses, Postgrad. Med. J. **55:**135, 1979.
9. Cubitt, W.D., and McSwiggan, D.A.: Calicivirus gastroenteritis in northwest London, Lancet **2:**975, 1981.
10. Cubitt, W.D., Pead, P.J., and Saud, A.A.: A new serotype of calicivirus associated with an outbreak of gastroenteritis in a residential home for the elderly, J. Clin. Pathol. **34:**924, 1981.
11. Cukor, G., and Blacklow, N.R.: Human viral gastroenteritis, Microbiol. Rev. **48:**157, 1984.
12. Dolin, R., et al.: Biological properties of Norwalk agent of acute infectious nonbacterial gastroenteritis, Proc. Soc. Exp. Biol. Med. **140:**578, 1972.
13. Ghose, L.H., Schnagl, R.D., and Holmes, I.H.: Comparison of enzyme-linked immunosorbent assay for quantitation of rotavirus antibodies with complement fixation in an epidemiological survey, J. Clin. Microbiol. **8:**268, 1978.
14. Gunn, R.A., et al.: Norwalk virus gastroenteritis aboard a cruise ship: an outbreak on five consecutive cruises, Am. J. Epidemiol. **112:**820, 1980.
15. Hara, M., et al.: Acute gastroenteritis among schoolchildren associated with reovirus-like agent, Am. J. Epidemiol. **107:**161, 1978.
16. Jenkins, S., et al.: An outbreak of Norwalk-related gastroenteritis at a boys' camp, Am. J. Dis. Child. **139:**787, 1985.
17. Kapikian, A.Z., et al.: Visualization by immuno electron microscopy of a 27-nm particle associated with acute infectious nonbacterial gastroenteritis, J. Virol. **10:**1075, 1972.
18. Kapikian, A.Z., et al.: Human reovirus-like agent as the major pathogen associated with "winter" gastroenteritis in hospitalized infants and young children, N. Engl. J. Med. **294:**965, 1976.
19. Kapikian, A.Z., et al.: Approaches to immunization of infants and young children against gastroenteritis due to rotaviruses, Rev. Infect. Dis. **2:**459, 1980.
20. Kaplan, J.E., et al.: Epidemiology of Norwalk gastroenteritis and the role of Norwalk virus in outbreaks of acute nonbacterial gastroenteritis, Ann. Intern. Med. **96:**756, 1982.
21. Konno, T., et al.: Astrovirus-associated epidemic gastroenteritis in Japan, J. Med. Virol. **9:**11, 1982.
22. Kurtz, J.B., et al.: Astrovirus infection in volunteers, J. Med. Virol. **3:**221, 1979.
23. Madeley, C.R., and Cosgrove, B.P.: Caliciviruses in man, Lancet **1:**199, 1976.
24. McLean, B.S., and Holmes, I.H.: Effects of antibodies, trypsin, and trypsin inhibitors on susceptibility of neonates to rotavirus infection, J. Clin. Microbiol. **13:**22, 1981.
25. Oshiro, L.S., et al.: A 27-nm virus isolated during an outbreak of acute infectious nonbacterial gastroenteritis in a convalescent hospital: a possible new serotype, J. Infect. Dis. **143:**791, 1981.
26. Rodriguez, W.J., et al.: Clinical features of acute gastroenteritis associated with human reovirus-like agent in infants and young children, J. Pediatr. **91:**188, 1977.
27. Rodriguez, W.J., et al.: Common exposure outbreak of gastroenteritis due to type 2 rotavirus with high secondary attack rate within families, J. Infect. Dis. **140:**353, 1979.
28. Sack, D.A., et al.: Seroepidemiology of rotavirus infection in rural Bangladesh, J. Clin. Microbiol. **11:**530, 1980.
29. Simhon, A., et al.: Sequential rotavirus diarrhoea caused by virus of same subgroup, Lancet **2:**1174, 1981.
30. Spence, L., et al.: Comparison of counterimmunoelectrophoresis and electron microscopy for laboratory diagnosis of human reovirus-like agent-associated infantile gastroenteritis, J. Clin. Microbiol. **5:**248, 1977.
31. Steering Committee of the Scientific Working Group on Viral Diarrhea: Nomenclature of human rotaviruses: designation of subgroups and serotypes, Bull. WHO **62:**501, 1984.

32. Steinhoff, M.C.: Rotavirus: the first five years, J. Pediatr. **96:**611, 1980.

33. Ward, R.L., Knowlton, D.R., and Pierce, M.J.: Efficiency of human rotavirus propagation in cell culture, J. Clin. Microbiol. **19:**748, 1984.

34. Wenman, W.M., et al.: Rotavirus infection in adults: results of a prospective family study, N. Engl. J. Med. **301:**303, 1979.

35. Wilson, R., et al.: Waterborne gastroenteritis due to Norwalk agent: clinical and epidemiological investigation, Am. J. Public Health **72:**72, 1980.

36. Wyatt, R.G., et al.: Human rotavirus type 2: cultivation in vitro, Science **207:**189, 1980.

37. Yolken, R.H., et al.: Epidemiology of human rotavirus types 1 and 2 as studied by enzyme-linked immunosorbent assay, N. Engl. J. Med. **299:**1156, 1978.

38. Yolken, R.H., et al.: Immunological response to infection with human reovirus-like agent: measurement of anti-human reovirus-like agent immunoglobulin G and M levels by the method of enzyme-linked immunosorbent assay, Infect. Immun. **19:**540, 1978.

CHAPTER 56

Chlamydiae

Sally Jo Rubin

Early in this century Halberstaeder and von Prowazek described the presence of inclusions in conjunctival scrapings from patients with trachoma. A few years later these inclusions were also found to be associated with a conjunctivitis in newborns and present in the cervix of an afflicted baby's mother.

Originally called *Bedsonia* organisms after Sir Samuel Bedson (who isolated and characterized the agent of psittacosis) or the TRIC agents (trachoma-inclusion conjunctivitis), their nature was controversial. They were considered viruses by some authorities and bacteria by others. Isolation in embryonated eggs in 1957 and in cell culture 6 years later led to the recognition that *Chlamydia* organisms not only cause eye infections (inclusion conjunctivitis, trachoma) and avian infection (ornithosis, psittacosis) but are a major cause of sexually transmitted disease.[2,39]

Chlamydiae are clearly known now to be bacteria and to resemble viruses only in their obligate intracellular nature and their inability to synthesize adenosine triphosphate. In other respects these "energy parasites" are similar to bacteria, possessing both ribonucleic acid (RNA) and deoxyribonucleic acid (DNA) and having ribosomes, metabolic enzymes, and a cell wall similar to that of gram-negative bacteria. They multiply by binary fission and are susceptible to antimicrobial agents. Because of their unique life cycle they are classified in a separate order, *Chlamydiales*, that contains one genus, *Chlamydia*. The name is from the Greek *chlamys*, which describes a cloak draped around the shoulder and refers to the intracytoplasmic inclusions "draped" around the cell nucleus. The genus *Chlamydia* currently contains two species: *C. trachomatis* and *C. psittaci*. Each species has a number of serotypes. *C. trachomatis* has 15 serotypes (A, B, B_a to K, L_1, L_2, and L_3), whereas *C. psittaci* has many poorly characterized serotypes.

C. psittaci and *C. trachomatis* differ in the nature of their inclusions and in their susceptibility to sulfonamides. *C. trachomatis* produces compact inclusions with an iodine-staining (probably glycogen) carbohydrate, whereas *C. psittaci* inclusions are diffuse and do not stain with iodine.[2] *C. trachomatis* is susceptible to sulfa drugs, whereas *C. psittaci* is resistant. The two species replicate in a similar manner, which differs from the replication of other microorganisms (Figure 56-1). Two distinct forms are seen during their developmental cycle. The infectious chlamydial form is the 300 nm elementary body (EB) that is actively taken into the cell in a phagocytic vesicle. Lysosomal fusion does not occur, and the entire replication cycle takes place in the vesicle. Over the next 6 to 8 hours the EB undergoes reorganization into the initial or reticulate body (RB). The RB is noninfectious but metabolically very active. For 18 to 24 hours the RB synthesizes new material and divides

by binary fission. Eventually the RBs again reorganize and condense into compact EBs that are still in the phagocytic vesicle. Somewhere between 48 and 72 hours the cell lyses, resulting in cell death and release of EBs.[2]

Outside the host cell, chlamydiae are very labile, particularly to nonoptimal temperatures. They are destroyed in 48 hours at 37° C and in a few weeks at 0° C. Preservation of infectivity is enhanced by quick freezing and storing at −70° C.[32] Chlamydiae are inactivated by ether and ethanol in 30 minutes and by 0.1% formalin and 0.5% phenol in 24 hours.

CLINICAL SIGNIFICANCE

CHLAMYDIA PSITTACI

C. psittaci naturally infects most avian species and many nonprimate mammals, causing relatively minor to severe illness. Humans can acquire infection from both birds and mammals. Chlamydial infection of birds was originally termed psittacosis because infection was thought to be restricted to the parrot (psittacine) family. However, the term "ornithosis" gained acceptance when it was observed that several types of birds may harbor the organism. Ornithosis refers to avian infections and to avian-acquired human infections. Psittacosis describes infection related to psittacine birds.

About 80 cases of human psittacosis or ornithosis are reported each year in the United States, with a mortality of 1% to 5%.[33] Most cases are associated with pet birds, especially the common small parakeet (budgerigar). Outbreaks have also been reported among poultry workers.[1] Infection in a human can range from subclinical to a fatal pneumonia, although in most cases it produces mild to moderate symptoms of atypical pneumonia, including fever, nonproductive cough, fatigue, chills, and headache. Rarely *C. psittaci* causes endocarditis.

Recently a new *C. psittaci* strain called TWAR was isolated from students with acute respiratory disease. TWAR occurred in 12% of students with pneumonia, 5% with bronchitis, and 1% with pharyngitis. Evidence indicates that the TWAR strain is a human *C. psittaci* that is spread from person to person.[18a]

CHLAMYDIA TRACHOMATIS

Serotype and clinical manifestations of *C. trachomatis* infection are related (Table 56-1). Serotypes A to C cause trachoma; D to K cause inclusion conjunctivitis, genital tract infections, and infant pneumonitis; and L_1, L_2, and L_3 cause lymphogranuloma venereum.

Trachoma is still the greatest single cause of blindness in the world. It occurs mainly among the poor in less-developed countries, particularly of the Middle East, northern Africa, and northern India. In the United States it is seen in Native Americans in the Southwest. Children in endemic areas are often

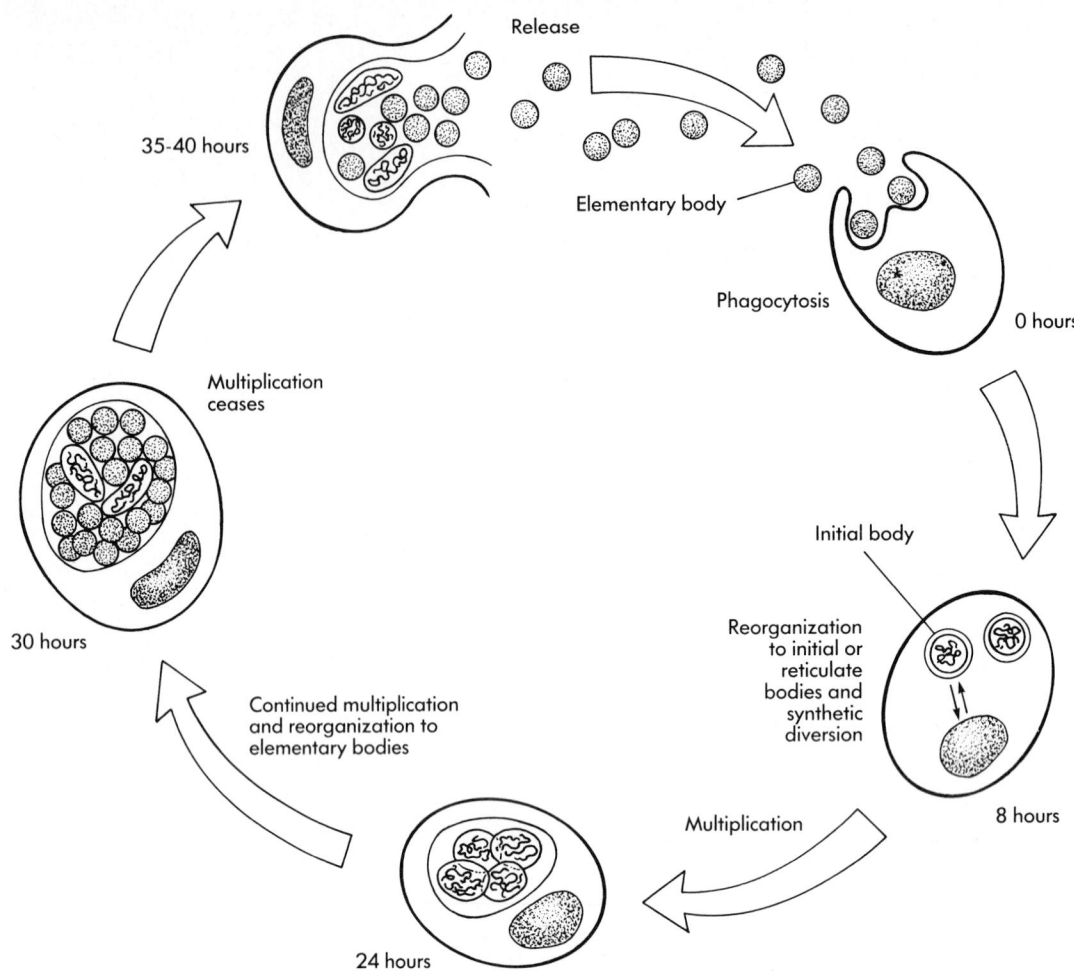

FIGURE 56-1. Life cycle of chlamydial organisms. (Reprinted with permission from Alexander, E.R.: Chlamydia: the organism and neonatal infection, Hosp. Pract. **14**[7]:63, 1979. Adapted from illustration by Ms. Nancy Lou Graham.)

infected with *C. trachomatis* types A to C within the first 3 months of life by close contact with other infected persons or by flies that carry infective ocular material from one eye to another. Transmission is not genital but eye to eye directly. Chronic infection and reinfection are common, resulting in conjunctival scarring and corneal vascularization. The scars eventually contract, causing the upper eyelid to turn in so the eyelashes cause corneal abrasions. This trichiasis and secondary bacterial infection result in blindness.

In developed countries the vast majority of *C. trachomatis* infections are caused by serotypes D to K and include nongon-ococcal and postgonococcal urethritis (NGU and PGU), muco-purulent cervicitis, genital infection sequelae, inclusion conjunctivitis, and infant pneumonia.

NGU and PGU have been seen in sexually active men for years, but only in the last 10 years has the role of *C. tracho-matis* in these infections been elucidated.[46] Many studies show that *C. trachomatis* D to K is isolated from the urethra of 30% to 50% of men with NGU, 20% to 30% of men with gonorrhea, as much as 80% of men with PGU, and only 7% or less of men without urethritis.[17,40]

As a group, men with NGU have less dysuria and a less purulent discharge than those with gonococcal infection, but

among individual patients the two urethral infections cannot be clinically distinguished.[40]

Genital infection with *C. trachomatis* in women ranges from asymptomatic urethral or cervical infection to salpingitis and infertility.[8,49] Vaginitis does not occur. The incidence of infection varies among different populations, ranging from 2% to 19% in gynecology clinics[18,21,24,37,42] to 35% to 65% among contacts of men with NGU.[51]

In both men and women untreated infection can persist for months and lead to serious complications and sequelae. Women's sequelae are the urethral syndrome, bartholinitis,[12] endometritis,[19] and pelvic inflammatory disease, or PID (infection of the fallopian tubes and ovaries).[38] In men chlamydiae are a major cause of "idiopathic" epididymitis in men under 35 years old.[5,17] Both PID and epididymitis can lead to infertility.

Inclusion conjunctivitis occurs in adults and newborns. The genitourinary tract is the source of infection in both groups, although the infections are acquired differently.

Inclusion conjunctivitis in newborns commonly develops 1 to 2 weeks after exposure during birth and is characterized by a copious mucopurulent discharge. Without treatment, symptoms can persist for weeks. In adults *C. trachomatis* D to K can

TABLE 56-1. Clinical Manifestations of *Chlamydia* Infections in Humans

Species	Serotypes	Disease	Major Symptoms	Age	Infected Site	Transmission	Laboratory Diagnosis
C. psittaci	Many	Psittacosis, ornithosis	Subclinical—mild respiratory infection or pneumonia	All, worse if > 50 yr	Lung	Birds, especially in droppings; rarely person to person	Isolation, serology
C. trachomatis	A, B, Ba, C	Trachoma	Chronic conjunctivitis may cause blindness	Young children	Eyes	Person to person	Giemsa stain (active disease), isolation
C. trachomatis	L₁, L₂, L₃	Lymphogranuloma venereum	Transient genital ulcer, inguinal (men), pelvic or retroperitoneal (women) lymphadenopathy	Adult	Lymph nodes	Sexual	Serology, isolation
C. trachomatis	D-K	Adult inclusion conjunctivitis	Acute follicular conjunctivitis	Young adults	Eyes	Genital to eye	Isolation
		Genital tract infection	Nongonococcal urethritis, cervical infection, epididymitis, salpingitis, proctitis	Young adults	Genital tract	Sexual	Isolation
		Newborn inclusion conjunctivitis	Acute mucopurulent conjunctivitis	Infant	Eyes	Genital to eye during birth	Giemsa stain, conjunctival scrapings, direct FA, isolation
		Pneumonitis	Afebrile, chronic diffuse lung disease	Infant	Lung	Aspiration during birth	Isolation serology (Micro-IF-IgM)

cause a superficial epithelial keratitis, often associated with urethritis or cervicitis, that tends to involve the upper half of the cornea. Transmission is genital to eye.[48] Although most cases tend to heal in 2 months to 2 years, nontrachoma eye infections can be very severe.

C. trachomatis D to K is also the cause of a characteristic, chronic, afebrile pneumonia occurring in infants less than 3 months old.[3] In most cases serum immunoglobulin levels are elevated, and the eosinophil count is greater than $300/mm^3$.[23] Many cases are preceded by conjunctivitis and ear abnormalities.[55]

One third to one half of exposed infants develop conjunctivitis, 10% to 20% develop pneumonia, and as many as 60% to 70% have either cultural or serologic evidence of infection.[18,21,25,42] Approximately 2% to 6% of all infants in the United States develop a chlamydial infection.

C. trachomatis L_1, L_2, and L_3 strains cause a venereal disease, lymphogranuloma venereum (LGV), that is endemic in Asia, Africa, and South America. It occurs in the United States, particularly in warmer areas, but is rather uncommon, with fewer than 500 cases reported yearly. Initially a small painless lesion—either a vesicle or an ulcer—develops, which heals with no scar and is followed 2 to 6 weeks later by suppurative regional lymphadenopathy, fever, and chills. Sequelae caused by fibrotic changes and abnormal lymphatic drainage can occur.

Knowledge of the pathogenesis of chlamydial infections is still rudimentary. Chlamydiae are parasites of columnar epithelial cells and have at least two virulence factors. Chlamydiae appear to enhance their own ingestion by phagocytic cells by an unknown mechanism.[9] Once inside the cell they somehow inhibit fusion of the phagocytic vesicles with lysosomes.[40] Attachment of the EB to the cell is chlamydia-induced and associated with heat-sensitive cell receptor sites on the organism.[39] The attachment sites for LGV and non-LGV *C. trachomatis* are different.

The gram-negative nature of the cell wall suggests that endotoxic activity may exist. Such activity can be demonstrated in vitro.[31]

Chlamydiae are susceptible to many antimicrobial agents, including tetracycline, erythromycin, sulfonamides, rifampin, and chloramphenicol.[7] Penicillin has some activity in vitro but is not effective in vivo.

CONTROL

In the United States imported birds are supposed to be held in quarantine and treated with tetracycline. However, since 28% to 40% of birds tested are culture positive, the adherence to these regulations is questionable.[41]

Prevention of infant chlamydial infection currently depends on controlling infection in adults because topical antimicrobial prophylaxis to the eye is not entirely successful.[22,34] Some advocate screening high-risk populations of pregnant women by culture and treating those who are culture positive. Sexually transmitted *C. trachomatis* infection is not reportable, making control through the use of contact tracing impractical. Development of an inexpensive, rapid method of diagnosis is needed before widespread control can be obtained.

Vaccine production does not appear promising. Reinfection with more than one serotype certainly occurs, and antibodies do not appear to confer much immunity. Killed trachoma vaccines have not been very effective.

LABORATORY DIAGNOSIS
SPECIMEN TYPES

Specimens for the diagnosis of chlamydial infection include conjunctival scrapings or swabs, urethral, cervical, or rectal scrapings or swabs, bubo pus, sputa, throat washings, tissue, bird feces, and bird carcasses. Epithelial cells, not discharge, must be collected (Table 56-2).

Although scrapings are preferred, specimens from the lower genital tract and eye are most easily collected with a swab.[44] Cotton and calcium aginate are less desirable materials for swabs because some lots may be toxic to chlamydiae, whereas Dacron and nylon are not.[32] Swabs are placed in a carrier medium such as 2SP. The carrier medium must never contain penicillin because it is inhibitory in vitro. Preferably specimens should be inoculated shortly after collection; however, they may be held in carrier medium for 24 hours at $4°$ C. If specimens must be held longer, they should be quick frozen and kept at $-70°$ C. Just before inoculation, frozen specimens are quickly thawed in a $37°$ C water bath. This single freeze-thaw cycle can reduce infectivity.[35] Some workers prefer to hold specimens for 72 hours at $4°$ C rather than expose them to a freeze-thaw cycle.

DIRECT EXAMINATION

In the past, direct examination for inclusions has been productive only for ocular infections, particularly in trachoma and inclusion conjunctivitis of newborns. Conjunctival scrapings from the newborn were stained with Giemsa stain and examined for typical intracytoplasmic inclusions in columnar epithelial cells. To be acceptable a specimen must contain large numbers of epithelial cells (1000 cells or more). Many polymorphonuclear leukocytes can also be present instead of the mainly mononuclear cells seen in viral conjunctivitis. These smears can be difficult to read, and each slide should be examined for 30 to 60 minutes, magnified 400 to 1000 times. However, both immunofluorescence and immunoperoxidase tests have been used to detect inclusions in conjunctival scrapings and are reported to be more sensitive than the Giemsa stain.[59]

Recently the direct detection of the elementary bodies of *C. trachomatis*—rather than chlamydial inclusions—has been revolutionized by the availability of fluorescein-conjugated monoclonal antibodies to all of the organisms' serotypes. A complete collection and test kit (MicroTrak) with staining reagents is available from Syva Co., Palo Alto, Calif. The collection kit consists of two swabs: a narrow one for urethral specimens from males or conjunctival sites, and a larger one for endocervical specimens. After the specimen has been collected, the swab is rolled over the surface of a well on a glass microscope slide provided in the collection kit. The cells and other specimen material on the slide can either be fixed immediately with the acetone contained in an enclosed ampule or be sent to the laboratory for this purpose. Similar kits are now available from a number of companies.

Laboratory staining and microscopic examination of the slide require approximately 30 minutes. The elementary bodies of *C. trachomatis* are recognized by their specific apple-green fluorescence and their circular morphology. Since the initial introduction of the test method, evaluations have revealed 93% to 96% sensitivity, compared with cultivation of the organisms in cell cultures.[4,47,52,56] Currently the test has been approved by the Food and Drug Administration for genital, rectal, and conjunctival specimens.

TABLE 56-2. Specimen Collection for *Chlamydia* Isolation

Clinical Syndrome	Specimen	Collection
Pneumonia (psittacosis)	Sputum, throat washing, pleural fluid, lung	Same as for bacteriology (see Chapter 11)
Trachoma, inclusion conjunctivitis	Conjunctival scrapings (wipe discharge away and collect cells from conjunctiva with swab)	Evert conjunctiva and rub vigorously with swab
Lymphogranuloma venereum	Lymph node aspirate	Aspirate with syringe and needle through healthy adjacent tissue
Genital cervicitis (or asymptomatic)	Cervical swab	Clean cervix and remove any discharge; insert swab a few millimeters past cervical os (squamocolumnar junction) and rotate firmly
Urethritis (or asymptomatic)	Urethral swab	Insert thin urogenital swab 2 cm into urethra; rotate and remove
Salpingitis	Fallopian tube biopsy	Surgical
Endometritis	Transabdominal aspirate or protected swab of endometrium	Laparoscopy, protected swab
Proctitis	Rectal swab	Swab under direct visualization by anoscopy
Pneumonitis, infant	Tracheobronchial aspirate, nasopharyngeal swab	Same as for bacteriology (see Chapter 11)

Data from references 11 and 14.

Although experienced cytologists report success in detecting *Chlamydia* inclusions by examining Papanicolaou smears of specimens from adults,[20] comparison with cell cultures shows that such direct examination is neither sensitive nor specific and cannot be recommended as a substitute for culture.[13] In addition, a number of enzyme immunoassay kits are available for rapid diagnosis of *C. trachomatis*.

ISOLATION AND IDENTIFICATION

All chlamydiae can be grown in the yolk sac of embryonated eggs, and some can infect mice and guinea pigs, but the simplest and safest method of isolation is in cell culture. *Chlamydia* organisms grow in a number of cell types, but mouse L cells (McCoy cells) are most commonly used. Successful isolation in cell culture depends on correct processing in the laboratory. Properly collected and transported specimens are treated to rupture infected cells, because intracellular organisms result in a low isolation yield. Cells may be disrupted by sonication, mixing in a Vortex with glass beads, or aspirating up and down several times with a Pasteur pipette.

To enhance organism attachment, specimens are centrifuged onto the monolayers. This is accomplished by planting the cell cultures on round coverslips that were previously placed in plastic flat-bottomed tubes or glass vials. Centrifugal force must be high (2700 to 3000 × g) for 1 hour at ambient temperature (no greater than 35° C).[6,35]

Isolation is greatly enhanced by pretreating the uninfected cells in some way to inhibit their replication. This enhancement may result from more available nutrients and precursors for the

chlamydiae. Pretreatment has included irradiation and 5-iodo-2-deoxyuridine or cytochalasin B treatment.[26-28] Diethylaminoethyl (DEAE) dextran, which is thought to neutralize the electrostatic repulsion between the negatively charged EB and cell membrane, has also been used to treat cells. Most laboratories currently use cycloheximide at a concentration (1 to 2 μg/ml) that depresses but does not completely inhibit the host cells.[36] Generally, more and larger inclusions are detected when cycloheximide is used.[16,28,36] The cycloheximide is added immediately after specimen inoculation, so pretreatment of the cell culture is unnecessary. If cycloheximide is used, each lot of fetal calf serum added to the cell culture medium must be tested with stock strains of *C. trachomatis* because some lots suppress inclusion formation in cycloheximide-treated McCoy cells.[15]

Microtiter plates have been used successfully by some[60] and not by others.[43] When microtiter is used, a blind passage is suggested. When glass vials or plastic tubes are used, 90% or more of the isolates are usually detected without a blind pass. However, this may vary with the population being cultured, and therefore the inclusion of a blind pass should be evaluated by each laboratory.

Chlamydia organisms generally do not produce a cytopathic effect (CPE) in infected cells and are detected by staining the infected cell monolayer and examining it microscopically for perinuclear, intracytoplasmic inclusions. Giemsa and iodine stains (Plate 32, *C* to *F*) or immunofluorescence is used (Table 56-3). *C. psittaci* inclusions stain only with Giemsa stain, whereas *C. trachomatis* inclusions also stain with iodine. For *C. trachomatis*, iodine stain has been used most widely because

TABLE 56-3. Detection of *Chlamydia* Inclusions

Method	Time after Infection (hr)	Appearance	Advantages	Disadvantages
Giemsa stain	40-72	Brightfield: cell nucleus reddish purple, cytoplasm bluish purple; EB red to purple, RB blue to purple Darkfield: EB and RB bright golden-yellow	Stains inclusions of both species; simple to perform permanent preparation; differentiates EB and RB	Time consuming to read (can enhance by using darkfield)
Iodine stain	40-72	Dark to reddish brown inclusions; cells yellow	Fast and simple to perform; easy to read; can decolorize with methanol and restain with Giemsa or FA	Not as good with BHK_{21} and HeLa cells; artifacts may stain; *C. psittaci* inclusions do not stain
Immunofluorescence (direct or indirect)	20-72	Inclusion is bright yellow mass within cytoplasm	Sensitive; immunologic confirmation; fast to read	Expensive; nonspecific fluorescence

it is inexpensive and easy to read. However, immunofluorescence with monoclonal antibodies is reportedly more sensitive than iodine staining, especially in specimens with a low inclusion count.[45] Reagents are commercially available. Incubation before staining for *C. trachomatis* inclusions is 24 to 72 hours and depends on the stain used, whereas staining of monolayers for *C. psittaci* inclusions is done after 5 and 10 days of incubation.

Inclusions detected by iodine or Giemsa stain should be confirmed by passage or by immunofluorescence. If a monolayer is stained with iodine and only a few inclusions are seen, overstaining with Giemsa stain helps differentiate them from artifacts.[25]

Serotype is determined by microimmunofluorescence. Drops of antigen suspension are placed in wells on a slide, so that many antigens and antisera can be tested on a single slide.

SEROLOGIC DIAGNOSIS

Not a great deal is known about the immune response to chlamydial infections. In primary genital and ocular infections, type-specific IgM usually appears 1 to 2 weeks after infection and persists for about 4 weeks in untreated persons. If IgG is present at the same time as IgM, levels are low but seem to persist for years, possibly for life. If reinfection with a different serotype occurs, the IgM level increases again and is usually specific for the new serotype. The IgG level may or may not rise. If IgG does rise, it may be due to the serotype of the primary infecting strain.[40] Local antibodies are produced and may persist for several years.[54]

Patients with systemic infections, such as LGV, pelvic inflammatory disease, or pneumonia, develop high IgG levels. IgM is rarely detected in women with pelvic inflammatory disease, probably because it has dropped to undetectable levels by the time symptoms occur, but newborns with chlamydial pneumonia regularly have high IgM levels, and adults with LGV often have measurable IgM titers.

Two serologic tests are used for measurement of chlamydia

antibodies: complement fixation (CF) and a microimmunofluorescence test (micro-IF).[57] The antigen used in the CF test is a heat-stable, large, acid polysaccharide found in all *Chlamydia* species (a group antigen).[40] The CF test is less sensitive than micro-IF, and antibodies are usually detected only after systemic infection. Therefore the CF test is used only to diagnose psittacosis and LGV. Both infections can be diagnosed by a significant rise in chlamydial CF antibodies. Usually convalescent titers are greater than or equal to 1:64. A small percentage of uninfected people may have titers greater than or equal to 1:16; 5% to 20% of those with genital or ocular *C. trachomatis* may have this ratio. Women with salpingitis may show a rise in the CF test or have CF titers greater than or equal to 1:64.

The micro-IF test can be performed with a broadly reactive antigen or a serogroup-specific elementary body cell wall antigen. This test is much more sensitive than CF, and most people with past or current chlamydial infections, including superficial genital infection, have detectable antibody. In fact, in most populations 20% to 70% of people have antibody by micro-IF. This high background rate makes micro-IF less useful diagnostically in patients with nonsystemic infections (*C. trachomatis* A to K) but quite useful for epidemiologic surveys.

Micro-IF can be used to diagnose LGV and infant pneumonia. Patients with LGV often have IgG titers greater than or equal to 1:1000 and IgM titers greater than or equal to 1:32. Infants with chlamydial pneumonia have both high IgG and high IgM titers,[3] but IgM levels must be measured for diagnosis because the IgG is passively transferred maternal antibody.

An immune adherence hemagglutination test and enzyme-linked immunosorbent assay have been described.[29,30] Both are genus specific (not species specific) and are considerably more sensitive than CF and thus, like micro-IF, useful mainly for epidemiologic studies.

SUMMARY

Although a serology (CF) test is adequate for diagnosis of psittacosis and LGV, the only currently available method for laboratory diagnosis of non-LGV *C. trachomatis* is culture. Because of its expense, some authorities believe that cultures are required only in certain cases. Men with NGU or PGU (more than 4 polymorphonuclear leukocytes on a high-power field and no gram-negative diplococci) can be treated with a single agent effective against both *Chlamydia* and *Ureaplasma* organisms,[50] as can their female contacts.[53] Thus culture may not be necessary. Others believe that all high-risk women should be screened by culture because many have no symptoms and are not known contacts of men with NGU.[58] Schachter and Grossman[40] calculate that in obstetrics clinics, if the incidence of chlamydial infection is 6% or more, performing culture testing of all pregnant women and treating them is less expensive than waiting and treating their infected babies.

Current research efforts include characterization of membrane antigens of *C. trachomatis* to develop inexpensive antigen detection systems.[10]

REFERENCES

1. Anderson, D.C., Stoesz, P.A., and Kaufmann, A.F.: Psittacosis outbreak in employees of a turkey-processing plant, Am. J. Epidemiol. **107:**140, 1978.
2. Becker, Y.: The chlamydia: molecular biology of procaryotic obligate parasites of eucaryocytes, Microbiol. Rev. **42:**274, 1978.
3. Beem, M.O., and Saxon, E.M.: Respiratory-tract colonization and a distinctive pneumonia syndrome in infants infected with *Chlamydia trachomatis*, N. Engl. J. Med. **296:**306, 1977.
4. Bell, T.A., et al.: Direct fluorescent monoclonal antibody stain for rapid detection of infant *Chlamydia trachomatis* infections, Pediatrics **74:**224, 1984.
5. Berger, R.E., et al: *Chlamydia trachomatis* as a cause of acute "idiopathic" epididymitis, N. Engl. J. Med. **298:**301, 1978.
6. Bird, B.R., and Forrester, F.T.: Laboratory diagnosis of *Chlamydia trachomatis* infections, Atlanta, 1980, Centers for Disease Control.
7. Blackman, H.J., et al.: Antibiotic susceptibility of *Chlamydia trachomatis*, Antimicrob. Agents Chemother. **12:**673, 1977.
8. Brunham, R.C., et al.: Mucopurulent cervicitis: the ignored counterpart in women of urethritis in men, N. Engl. J. Med. **311:**1, 1984.
9. Byrne, G.I., and Moulder, J.W.: Parasite-specified phagocytosis of *Chlamydia psittaci* and *Chlamydia trachomatis* by L and HeLa cells, Infect. Immun. **19:**598, 1978.
10. Caldwell, H.D., Kromhout, J., and Schachter, J.: Purification and partial characterization of the major outer membrane protein of *Chlamydia trachomatis*, Infect. Immun. **31:**1161, 1981.
11. Clyde, W.D., Kenny, G.E., and Schachter, J.: Laboratory diagnosis of chlamydial and mycoplasmal infections, Cumitech 19, Washington, D.C., 1984, American Society for Microbiology.
12. Davies, J.A., et al.: Isolation of *Chlamydia trachomatis* from Bartholin's ducts, Br. J. Vener. Dis. **54:**409, 1978.
13. Dorman, S.A., et al.: Detection of chlamydial cervicitis by Papanicolaou stained smears and culture, Am. J. Clin. Pathol. **79:**421, 1983.
14. Eschenbach, D., Pollock, H.M., and Schachter, J.: Laboratory diagnosis of female genital tract infections, Cumitech 17, Washington, D.C., 1983, American Society for Microbiology.
15. Evans, R.T.: Suppression of *Chlamydia trachomatis* inclusion formation by fetal calf serum in cycloheximide-treated McCoy cells, J. Clin. Microbiol. **11:**424, 1980.
16. Evans, R.T., and Taylor-Robinson, D.: Comparison of various McCoy cell treatment procedures used for detection of *Chlamydia trachomatis*, J. Clin. Microbiol. **10:**198, 1979.
17. Felman, Y.M., and Nikitas, J.A.: Nongonococcal urethritis: a clinical review, JAMA **245:**381, 1981.
18. Frommell, G.T., et al: Chlamydial infection of mothers and their infants, J. Pediatr. **95:**28, 1979.
18a. Grayston, J.T., et al.: A new *Chlamydia psittaci* strain called TWAR from acute respiratory tract infections, N. Engl. J. Med. **315:**161, 1986.
19. Gump, D.W., Dickstein, S., and Gibson, M.: Endometritis related to *Chlamydia trachomatis* infection, Ann. Intern. Med. **95:**61, 1981.
20. Gupta, P.K., et al.: Cytologic investigations in chlamydia infection, Acta Cytol. **23:**315, 1979.
21. Hammerschlag, M.R., et al.: Prospective study of maternal and infantile infection with *Chlamydia trachomatis*, Pediatrics **64:**142, 1979.
22. Hammerschlag, M.R., et al.: Erythromycin ointment for ocular prophylaxis of neonatal chlamydial infection, JAMA **244:**2291, 1980.
23. Harrison, H.R., et al.: *Chlamydia trachomatis* infant pneumonitis, N. Engl. J. Med. **298:**702, 1978.
24. Heggie, A.D., et al.: *Chlamydia trachomatis* infection in mothers and infants, Am. J. Dis. Child. **135:**507, 1981.
25. Hipp, S.S., Kirkwood, M., Jr., and Gump, D.W.: Artifacts resembling *Chlamydia trachomatis*, N. Engl. J. Med. **302:**1367, 1980.
26. Johnson, J.E., and Smith, T.F.: Comparison of chlamydia subgroup A detection from clinical specimens after 40-64 hours of incubation in 5-iodo-2-deoxyuridine–treated McCoy's cells, J. Clin. Microbiol. **3:**334, 1976.
27. Johnson, L., and Harper, I.A.: Isolation of chlamydia in irradiated and non-irradiated McCoy cells, J. Clin. Pathol. **28:**1003, 1975.
28. LaScolea, L.J., and Keddell, J.E.: Efficacy of various cell culture procedures for detection of *Chlamydia trachomatis* and applicability to diagnosis of pediatric infections, J. Clin. Microbiol. **13:**705, 1981.
29. Lennette, E.T., and Lennette, D.A.: Immune adherence hemagglutination: alternative to complement-fixation serology, J. Clin. Microbiol. **7:**282, 1978.
30. Lewis, V.J., Thacker, W.L., and Mitchell, S.H.: Enzyme-linked immunosorbent assay for chlamydial antibodies, J. Clin. Microbiol. **6:**507, 1977.
31. Lewis, V.J., Thacker, W.L., and Mitchell, S.H.: Demonstration of chlamydial endotoxin-like activity, J. Gen. Microbiol. **114:**215, 1979.
32. Mahony, J.B., and Chemesky, M.A.: Effect of swab type and storage temperature on the isolation of *Chlamydia trachamatis* from clinical specimens, J. Clin. Microbiol. **22:**865, 1985.
33. Potter, M.E., and Kaufmann, A.F.: Psittacosis in humans in the United States, 1975-1977, J. Infect. Dis. **140:**131, 1979.
34. Rees, E., et al.: Persistence of chlamydial infection after treatment for neonatal conjunctivitis, Arch. Dis. Child. **56:**193, 1981.
35. Reeve, P., Owen, J., and Oriel, J.D.: Laboratory procedures for the isolation of *Chlamydia trachomatis* from the human genital tract, J. Clin. Pathol. **28:**910, 1975.
36. Ripa, K.T., and Mardh, P.: Cultivation of *Chlamydia trachomatis* in cycloheximide-treated McCoy cells, J. Clin. Microbiol. **6:**328, 1977.
37. Ripa, K.T., et al.: *Chlamydia trachomatis* cervicitis in gynecologic outpatients, Obstet. Gynecol. **52:**698, 1978.
38. Ripa, K.T., et al.: *Chlamydia trachomatis* infection in patients with laparoscopically verified acute salpingitis: results of isolation and antibody determinations, Am. J. Obstet. Gynecol. **138:**960, 1980.
39. Schachter, J., and Caldwell, H.D.: Chlamydiae, Annu. Rev. Microbiol. **34:**285, 1980.
40. Schachter, J., and Grossman, M.: Chlamydial infections, Annu. Rev. Med. **32:**45, 1981.
41. Schachter, J., Sugg, N., and Sung, M.: Psittacosis: the reservoir persists, J. Infect. Dis. **137:**44, 1978.
42. Schachter, J., et al.: Prospective study of chlamydial infection in neonates, Lancet **2:**377, 1979.
43. Smith, T.F.: Comparative recoveries of chlamydia from urethral specimens using glass vials and plastic microtiter plates, Am. J. Clin. Pathol. **67:**496, 1977.
44. Smith, T.F., and Weed, L.A.: Comparison of urethral swabs, urines, and urinary sediment for the isolation of *Chlamydia*, J. Clin. Microbiol. **2:**134, 1975.

45. Stamm, W.E., et al.: Detection of *Chlamydia trachomatis* inclusions in McCoy cell cultures with fluorescein-conjugated monoclonal antibodies, J. Clin. Microbiol. **17:**666, 1983.

46. Stamm, W.E., et al.: *Chlamydia trachomatis* urethral infections in men, Ann. Intern, Med. **100:**47, 1984.

47. Stamm, W.E., et al.: Diagnosis of *Chlamydia trachomatis* infections by direct immunofluorescence staining of genital secretions, Ann. Intern. Med. **101:**638, 1984.

48. Stenson, S.: Adult inclusion conjunctivitis: clinical characteristics and corneal changes, Arch. Ophthalmol. **99:**605, 1981.

49. Svenson, L., Mårdh, P.A., and Weström, L.: Infertility after acute salpingitis with special reference to *Chlamydia trachomatis*, Fertil. Steril. **40:**322, 1983.

50. Swartz, S.L., and Kraus, S.J.: Persistent urethral leukocytosis and asymptomatic chlamydial urethritis, J. Infect. Dis. **140:**614, 1979.

51. Tait, I.A., et al.: Chlamydial infection of the cervix in contacts with men with nongonococcal urethritis, Br. J. Vener. Dis. **56:**37, 1980.

52. Tam, M.R., et al.: Culture-independent diagnosis of *Chlamydia trachomatis* using monoclonal antibodies, N. Engl. J. Med. **310:**1146, 1984.

53. Taylor-Robinson, D., and Munday, P.E.: Chlamydia culture service, Br. J. Vener. Dis. **56:**183, 1980.

54. Terho, P., and Meurman, O.: Chlamydial serum IgG, IgA, and local IgA antibodies in patients with genital tract infections measured by solid-phase radioimmunoassay, J. Med. Microbiol. **14:**77, 1981.

55. Tipple, M.A., Beem, M.O., and Saxon, E.M.: Clinical characteristics of the afebrile pneumonia associated with *Chlamydia trachomatis* infection in infants less than 6 months of age, Pediatrics **63:**192, 1979.

56. Uyeda, C.T., et al.: Rapid diagnosis of chlamydial infections with the MicroTrak Direct test, J. Clin. Microbiol. **20:**948, 1984.

57. Wang, S.-P., and Grayston, J.T.: Immunologic relationship between genital TRIC, lymphogranuloma venereum and related organisms in a new microtiter indirect immunofluorescence test, Am. J. Ophthalmol. **70:**367, 1970.

58. Willcox, J.R., et al.: The need for a chlamydial culture service, Br. J. Vener. Dis. **55:**281, 1979.

59. Woodland, R.M., et al.: Sensitivity of immunoperoxidase and immunofluorescence staining for detecting *Chlamydia* in conjunctival scrapings and in cell culture, J. Clin. Pathol. **31:**1073, 1978.

60. Yoder, B.L., et al.: Microtest procedure for isolation of *Chlamydia trachomatis*, J. Clin. Microbiol. **13:**1036, 1981.

CHAPTER 57

Rickettsiae

Sally Jo Rubin

The rickettsiae resemble viruses in that they are obligate intracellular parasites (except *Rochalimaea*), but like chlamydiae they are actually intracellular bacteria. These small, pleomorphic coccobacilli (0.3 μm to 0.3 by 1 to 2 μm) divide by binary fission, contain both deoxyribonucleic acid (DNA) and ribonucleic acid (RNA), and have similar cell wall components. They stain poorly with Gram stain because of their small size and lack of contrast with host tissue, but except for *Coxiella burnetii* they appear to be gram negative.[24] Rickettsiae are more easily visualized with Giemsa, Gimenez, or Machiavello stains (Plate 32, *G*).

The three genera of the family *Rickettsiaceae* (*Rickettsia, Rochalimaea,* and *Coxiella*), except for *Rickettsia prowazekii,* are animal parasites with humans as incidental hosts. Many species of rickettsiae are found in animals. Those known to cause human disease are listed in Table 57-1. All but *C. burnetii* infect and are routinely transmitted by arthropod vectors. Life cycles range from the simple human-louse-human cycle of *R. prowazekii* to more complex cycles involving various vertebrate animals and arthropod vector stages.

Except for *C. burnetii*, rickettsiae are rather labile outside their host. *C. burnetii* is very hardy and is resistant to heat, drying, and sunlight.

Rickettsia and *Rochalimaea* organisms have a soluble complement fixation (CF) antigen that can be released by treatment with diethyl ether. Each species has only one immunotype except for *Rickettsia tsutsugamushi,* which has eight. Minor antigenic relationships exist between the typhus and spotted fever groups. *C. burnetii* has two antigenic phases analogous to the smooth to rough variation seen with some bacteria. Phase I antigens are found on isolates from naturally or laboratory infected animals, whereas phase II antigens are induced after several passages in embryonated hens' eggs.

Rickettsia and *Rochalimaea* organisms have similar fatty acid profiles that differ from that of *C. burnetii*.[22]

CLINICAL AND EPIDEMIOLOGIC ASPECTS

Rickettsial infections are characterized by fever, headache, myalgias, and except for *C. burnetii* infections, a rash. The distribution and type of rash are often helpful diagnostically. Rickettsial diseases occurring in the United States are described in the following sections.

ROCKY MOUNTAIN SPOTTED FEVER

Rocky Mountain spotted fever (RMSF) was first described in 1873 among the Indians of the Bitterroot Valley in Montana. In 1904, Wilson and Chowning described the clinical and pathologic aspects of the disease and suggested that ticks were involved in transmission. Their paper prompted Howard Taylor

Ricketts to go to Montana to study the disease. In 1906 Ricketts began his work, which is the basis for most of our knowledge about RMSF. He showed that the etiologic agent could be filtered out and that the disease could be transmitted to animals and from animal to animal by ticks. Today over 1000 cases are reported yearly in the United States.[3]

The name RMSF is misleading because the greatest incidence is now in the south Atlantic and southwestern states, with Oklahoma, North and South Carolina, Arkansas, Georgia, and Virginia reporting the most cases.[4]

Like most rickettsial diseases, RMSF is characterized by fever, headache, and a rash. The rash is initially maculopapular and appears on the wrists and ankles 3 to 5 days after clinical onset. It spreads centrally to the chest and abdomen. If the patient is not treated, the rash becomes petechial and then purpuric. RMSF is mainly a disease of children and is most often confused with meningococcemia and atypical measles. Mortality of treated RMSF is now about 5%,[12] with most fatalities resulting from delay in diagnosis and treatment.[7] Permanent neurologic sequelae are uncommon.

Most patients recall being bitten by a tick or being exposed to ticks about a week before onset of symptoms. Over 95% of cases are seen in the period between mid-April and November when ticks are active.

The two major vectors are the wood tick (Rocky Mountain states) and dog tick (eastern states), with about 5% to 15% of ticks infected (Table 57-1). Organisms are distributed throughout the tick's body, including in the eggs. Thus rickettsiae are transmitted transovarially to tick larvae. Animal and human hosts are infected by direct inoculation when the tick has a blood meal. Many different mammals and birds may be infected, although they usually do not manifest symptoms. To transmit infection, the tick must remain attached to its human or animal host for at least 2 hours.

RICKETTSIAL POX

Rickettsial pox, caused by *Rickettsia akari,* is the only other disease in the spotted fever group occurring in the United States. The first reported outbreak was in a housing development in Queens, New York, in 1946. A papule appears 1 to 2 days after the painless bite of the mouse mite and eventually progresses to an eschar. Within a week or two, systemic symptoms of fever, malaise, and headache develop, followed by a rash on the face, trunk, and extremities within 2 or 3 days. The rash is initially maculopapular but often becomes vesicular. Rickettsial pox is usually mild and is not fatal. Because the carrier of the disease is the house mouse, infections occur in urban areas at any time of the year. About 200 cases are reported yearly in the United States.[2]

TABLE 57-1. Characteristics of Human Rickettsial Diseases

Group and Species	Disease	Vector	Transmission to Humans	Transovarian Transmission	Animal Reservoir	Geographic Location	Weil-Felix Agglutination OX-19	OX-2	OX-K	Complement Fixation Group Antigen RMSF	Typhus	Q Fever
SPOTTED FEVER												
Rickettsia rickettsii	Rocky Mountain spotted fever	*Dermacentor andersoni* (wood tick), *Dermacentor variabilis* (dog tick)	Tick bite	Yes	Many small mammals, birds, dogs	Western Hemisphere	+++	+	−	+++	c	−
Rickettsia conorii	Boutonneuse fever	*Rhipicephalus sanguineus* (and other dog ticks)	Tick bite	Yes	Small wild animals, dogs	Mediterranean area, India, Africa	+	+++	−			
Rickettsia australis	Queensland tick typhus	*Ixodes holocyclus, Ixodes tasmani*	Tick bite	Yes	Small wild rodents, marsupials	Australia	+	+++	−			
Rickettsia sibirica	North Asian tick typhus	Many species of ixodid ticks	Tick bite	Yes	Wild and domestic animals, birds	Siberia, Mongolia	+	+++	−			
Rickettsia akari	Rickettsial pox	*Allodermanyssus sanguineus* (mite)	Mite bite	Yes	Mice	Northeastern United States, USSR	−	−	−			
TYPHUS												
Rickettsia prowazekii	Epidemic typhus	*Pediculus humanus corporis* (human body louse), maybe squirrel flea (sylvan cycle)	Louse feces contaminating bite	No	Humans, flying squirrel	Worldwide except Australia	+++	+	−	c	+++	−
	Brill-Zinsser disease[a]					Worldwide						
Rickettsia typhi	Murine typhus	*Xenopsylla cheopis* (rat flea)	Flea feces contaminating bite	No	Rats	Worldwide	+++	+	−			
SCRUB TYPHUS												
Rickettsia tsutsugamushi	Scrub typhus	*Leptotrombidium akamushi* (trombiculid mite)	Chigger bite	No	Small wild rodents, birds	Asia, Australia	−	−	+++	−	−	−
Q FEVER												
Coxiella burnetii	Q fever	Tick (many species)	Tick bite (animals), inhalation (humans and animals)	No	Vector: small wild mammals; without vector: cattle, sheep, goats	Worldwide	−	−	−	−	−	+++
TRENCH FEVER												
Rochalimaea quintana	Trench fever	*Pediculus humanus corporis* (human body louse)	Louse feces contaminating bite	No	Humans	Europe, Middle East, North Africa, Mexico	−	−	−			

SYMBOLS: +++, Strong reaction
+, Weak reaction
−, No reaction
c, Cross-reactions between RMSF and typhus groups may occur

[a]Recrudescence of epidemic typhus.

Epidemic Typhus and Brill-Zinsser Disease

Epidemic typhus caused by *R. prowazekii* is associated with crowding and poor personal hygiene and thus has been a disease of wars and famine throughout history. About a week after the bite of a human body louse, patients experience an intense headache, chills, and fever. The maculopapular rash begins on the upper trunk and spreads to involve the whole body except the face, soles, and palms. The disease lasts about 2 weeks, and convalescence can be prolonged.

The body louse is infected by biting an infected human. Organisms multiply in the louse and are passed in its feces when the louse ingests a blood meal. If the host scratches the bite, the wound becomes contaminated with rickettsia-containing louse feces. Rickettsiae kill the louse and thus are not transmitted transovarially.

Before 1963, humans were thought to be the only vertebrate hosts of *R. prowazekii*. However Bozeman and co-workers[1] isolated the organism from eastern flying squirrels. A sylvan cycle of *R. prowazekii* appears to exist in these squirrels with fleas as the vector.[20] Between 1976 and 1979 eight cases of human infection with *R. prowazekii* were documented in the United States, and two cases were associated with flying squirrels. All eight cases were in the winter when these squirrels nest in houses.[14] Before 1976 the last outbreak of typhus in America was in 1922 and the last known case, which was imported from Mexico, was diagnosed in 1950. Brill-Zinsser disease is usually a milder recrudescence of previous typhus, often occurring many years after primary infection. Brill-Zinsser disease is occasionally detected among survivors of the World War II concentration camps. *R. prowazekii* can be transmitted if a louse bite occurs during the recrudescence.

Murine Typhus

Rickettsia typhi (formerly *Rickettsia mooseri*) causes murine typhus. This disease is less severe than epidemic typhus and rarely causes death. After an incubation period of 1 to 2 weeks, patients have an abrupt onset of headache, myalgia, and fever. About 60% to 80% have a macular rash on the upper thorax and abdomen.

Rats are the natural host of *R. typhi,* and the vector is the rat flea. Infection may be transmitted from rat to rat or rat to person. The rat flea is infected during a blood meal. Ingested organisms multiply and are passed in feces. *R. typhi* is transmitted if the flea bite is contaminated with infected flea feces. Infection may also be acquired if the host's mucous membranes are contaminated with flea feces. The flea is infected for life but does not pass the organisms to its young.[15]

Q Fever

Q fever was first described in Australia in 1937 following an outbreak of the disease in a slaughterhouse. The disease is a zoonosis that is widespread in many types of animals with organisms found in their placenta, mammary glands, and milk. *C. burnetii* is destroyed by pasteurization but is very resistant to drying and can survive for months in the environment. People become infected by inhaling the organisms. Outbreaks of Q fever are associated with domestic animals, especially the newborn. Cases of Q fever often can be traced to farms, tanneries, slaughterhouses, and dairies.

C. burnetii infection is characterized by the sudden onset of fever, headache, and chills, but unlike the other rickettsial diseases, pneumonitis is common and there is no rash. Rarely, months or even years after the acute infection, some patients develop subacute endocarditis.[5,21] The incubation period of Q fever is 2 to 4 weeks, and untreated disease lasts 5 to 14 days. Convalescence may be slow, but mortality is low. Many cases are subclinical or a mild to moderate, self-limited respiratory disease. Thus the actual number of cases and their distribution are unknown. Q fever is found throughout the world; about 40 cases are reported each year in the United States.[4]

PATHOGENESIS, CONTROL, AND TREATMENT

Except for *C. burnetii,* rickettsiae enter through the skin and invade the vascular endothelial cells, producing a vasculitis. Symptoms vary depending on the distribution and extent of vascular involvement.

Rickettsial diseases are treated with chloramphenicol or tetracycline. Avoidance of the arthropod vectors by protective clothing and repellents can reduce disease incidence. Previous vaccines for RMSF were not very effective and are no longer produced. A new killed vaccine produced in chick embryo cell cultures is in development.[6] A killed *R. prowazekii* vaccine for persons at high risk and a killed *C. burnetii* vaccine for use in cattle are available.

LABORATORY DIAGNOSIS

Rickettsiae are particularly hazardous in the laboratory where aerosol transmission can occur.[18] Only properly equipped laboratories should handle live rickettsiae.

Specimen Types

Blood for rickettsia isolation is collected during the first week of illness. The clot is separated from the serum, quick frozen, and maintained at $-70°$ C until inoculated into animals. Specimens from autopsies should include visceral organs and brain. Sera for serologic diagnosis are collected as soon as possible after onset, at 10 to 14 days, and at 21 to 28 days; sometimes a specimen taken 2 to 3 months later is necessary.

Direct Examination

Early diagnosis of rickettsial disease is important and has been a real problem for the laboratory because both culture and serologic diagnosis can take several weeks. RMSF can be rapidly diagnosed by immunofluorescent staining of skin biopsy specimens. The test result can be positive as early as the third day.[25] Although the test is only 70% sensitive, it is 100% specific.[23]

Culture and Isolation

Although isolation is rarely attempted because of expense, time, and hazard involved, rickettsiae can be isolated in embryonated hens' eggs, mice, and adult male guinea pigs. An exception is *Rochalimaea quintana*, which will not grow in animals or eggs but can be grown on laked horse blood agar incubated in 5% CO_2. Rickettsiae can be grown in a number of cell cultures, such as primary chick embryo, Vero cells, WI-38, and HeLa cells. Isolates are easily identified to group (for example, spotted fever group) but not species by CF, agglutination, or immunofluorescence. Species determination requires species-specific antisera that may be difficult to prepare.

SEROLOGIC DIAGNOSIS

Following infection with rickettsiae, both IgG and IgM are present. Antibody development may take 2 weeks and even longer if antimicrobial therapy is initiated.

In certain rickettsial infections, antibody that reacts with antigens of certain nonmotile *Proteus* strains is produced (Table 57-1). Results of the Weil-Felix test for agglutination with these OX antigens may be positive 7 to 10 days after onset but may not be positive for a month or even at all, especially if antimicrobial agents are given. The Weil-Felix test for *Proteus* agglutinins is neither sensitive nor specific. The majority of positive results of tests on single sera are false positive because these agglutinins are also found in *Proteus* urinary tract infection, leptospirosis, pregnancy, and severe liver disease.[8] False-positive titers may be high (greater than or equal to 1:640). Thus the Weil-Felix test is of questionable value and must be interpreted carefully.[11]

Antibody response to the spotted fevers may not be specific, and depending on the test and antigens used, patients may show antibody to organisms in the typhus group as well. Infection with organisms of the typhus group does not result in such a broad antibody response. Serum from patients with typhus group infection is less likely to react with antigens of the spotted fever group. However, reactions often occur with several members within the typhus group, making it difficult to determine serologically the species of the infecting organism.[17]

Patients with primary Q fever develop both IgG and IgM antibody to the phase II antigen between the second and fourth weeks. Titers decrease after infection. Those who develop endocarditis have high levels (greater than or equal to 1:200) of phase I antibody that is almost all IgG. In suspected endocarditis, tests using specific phase I antigen must be included.[13,19]

Specific serologic tests for rickettsial infection include CF, indirect immunofluorescence, and microagglutination. The CF test is very specific, even as titers of 1:8. Unfortunately, it may not be positive until 2 weeks after infection and 10% of sera are anticomplementary. Patients with RMSF may have positive CF results with the typhus group antigen. Indirect immunofluorescence (IFA) is the most sensitive test, and results may be positive earlier than with the CF test. However, IFA titers up to 1:16 may be falsely positive. The IFA requires very small amounts of antigen, and with the micro-IFA a battery of four different antigens can be placed in each well so all are tested simultaneously.[16] Latex agglutination (LA) tests have been developed for RMSF and typhus group. They are comparable in sensitivity to micro-IFA and can be performed in 15 minutes.[9,10] The LA tests are not available commercially.

REFERENCES

1. Bozeman, F.M., et al.: Epidemic typhus rickettsiae isolated from flying squirrels, Nature **255**:545, 1975.
2. Brettman, L.R., et al.: Rickettsialpox: report of an outbreak and a contemporary review, Medicine **60**:363, 1981.
3. Centers for Disease Control: Rocky Mountain spotted fever—United States, 1983, MMWR **33**:188, 1984.
4. D'Angelo, L.J., Baker, C.F., and Schlosser, W.: Q fever in the United States, 1948-1977, J. Infect. Dis. **139**:613, 1979.
5. Derrick, E.H.: Q Fever, a new fever entity: clinical features, diagnosis and laboratory investigation, Rev. Infect. Dis. **5**:790, 1983.
6. Gonder, J.C., Kenyon, R.H., and Pedersen, C.E., Jr.: Evaluation of a killed Rocky Mountain spotted fever vaccine in cynomolgus monkeys, J. Clin. Microbiol. **10**:719, 1979.
7. Hattwick, M.A.W., et al.: Fatal Rocky Mountain spotted fever, JAMA **240**:1499, 1978.
8. Hechemy, K.E., et al.: Discrepancies in Weil-Felix and microimmunofluorescence test results for Rocky Mountain spotted fever, J. Clin. Microbiol. **9**:292, 1979.
9. Hechemy, K.E.: Laboratory diagnosis of Rocky Mountain spotted fever, N. Engl. J. Med. **300**:859, 1979.
10. Hechemy, K.E., et al.: Detection of Rocky Mountain spotted fever antibodies by a latex agglutination test, J. Clin. Microbiol. **12**:144, 1980.
11. Hechemy, K.E., et al.: Detection of typhus antibodies by latex agglutination, J. Clin. Microbiol. **13**:214, 1981.
12. Kelsey, D.S.: Rocky Mountain spotted fever, Pediatr. Clin. North Am. **26**:367, 1979.
13. Kimbrough, R.C., III, et al.: Q fever endocarditis in the United States, Ann. Intern. Med. **91**:400, 1979.
14. McDade, J.E., et al.: Evidence of *Rickettsia prowazekii* infections in the United States, Am. J. Trop. Med. Hyg. **29**:277, 1980.
15. Murphy, P.A. and Charness, M.E.: Murine typhus, Johns Hopkins Med. J. **141**:303, 1977.
16. Newhouse, V.F., et al.: A comparison of the complement fixation, indirect fluorescent antibody, and microagglutination tests for the serological diagnosis of rickettsial diseases, Am. J. Trop. Med. Hyg. **28**:387, 1979.
17. Ormsbee, R., et al.: Antigenic relationships between the typhus and spotted fever groups of rickettsiae, Am. J. Epidemiol. **108**:53, 1978.
18. Oster, C.N., et al.: Laboratory-acquired Rocky Mountain spotted fever: the hazard of aerosol transmission, N. Engl. J. Med. **297**:859, 1977.
19. Peacock, M.G., et al.: Serological evaluation of Q fever in humans: enhanced phase I titles of immunoglobulins G and A are diagnostic for Q fever endocarditis, Infect. Immun. **41**:1089, 1983.
20. Sonenshine, D.E., et al.: Epizootiology of epidemic typhus (*Rickettsia prowazekii*) in flying squirrels, Am. J. Trop. Med. Hyg. **27**:339, 1978.
21. Spelman, D.W.: Q fever: a study of 111 consecutive cases, Med. J. Aust. **1**:547, 1982.
22. Tzianabos, T., Moss, C.W., and McDade, J.E.: Fatty acid composition of rickettsiae, J. Clin. Microbiol. **13**:603, 1981.
23. Walker, D.H., Burday, M.S., and Folds, J.D.: Laboratory diagnosis of Rocky Mountain spotted fever, South. Med. J. **73**:1443, 1980.
24. Weiss, E.: The biology of rickettsiae, Annu. Rev. Microbiol. **36**:345, 1982.
25. Woodward, T.E., et al.: Prompt confirmation of Rocky Mountain spotted fever: identification of rickettsiae in skin tissues, J. Infect. Dis. **134**:297, 1976.

APPENDICES

Culture Media, Tests, and Reagents in Bacteriology

Bruce A. Gunn
John F. Keiser
Rebecca D. Almazan

The purpose of this appendix is to outline briefly the purpose, principle, preparation, use, and performance testing of many of the media discussed in the bacteriology section of this book.

Components of media often vary in nomenclature, depending on source. Synonyms of types of proteins, obtained from different sources, are listed in Table 1. For most media described in this appendix an attempt was made to use *United States Pharmacopeia* (USP) names rather than trade names. However, this was not always possible.

All powdered media should be rehydrated with distilled or deionized water. Best results are obtained by adding water slowly to the powder to avoid formation of clumps. Agar-containing media should be rehydrated and then brought to a boil for about 1 minute. Boiling dissolves agar and prevents sterilization lag, that time required to bring the temperature of the medium to sterilization temperature. Powdered broth media frequently dissolve without heating, but bringing the temperature up to boiling prevents the sterilization lag seen with agar media. Sterilization time and temperature for each type of medium are noted along with preparation of the medium.

Conservation of refrigerator space may dictate using 13 × 100 mm test tubes rather than 16 × 125 mm tubes. The small tubes hold about one half the volume of medium as the larger tubes. Their use not only increases storage space but also saves money. Many laboratories use colored plastic enclosures for small tubes of medium. Thus technologists do not have to label each tube as to its contents, since each color represents a specific type of medium.

Tubes of medium are cooled either in upright position, creating "stab" or "butt" media, or in a slanted position, creating "slant" media. Anaerobic tube and agar media may be prereduced by "gassing" the tubes with 95% nitrogen and 5% carbon dioxide, storage overnight in anaerobe jars, or, as with some liquid media, boiling and cooling before use (see Chapter 20).

A worksheet (see Figure 3-4) should be made for each laboratory-prepared medium. Sterility and performance tests as outlined in Chapter 3 should also be completed.

Recommended storage and shelf lives of tube and plate media described here are based on experiences at Walter Reed Army Medical Center, Washington, D.C. Shelf lives are affected by type of medium, storage temperature, humidity, and whether the medium is sealed, or protected, from the storage environment. Tubes of medium sealed with loose-fitting caps, such as Morton enclosures, have shorter shelf lives than do tubes of medium sealed with tight-fitting caps, such as screw caps. Agar plate media should be stored sealed in plastic bags,

provided care is taken to remove excess surface moisture from each plate before storage. Some media, such as xylose lysine deoxycholate (XLD) agar, are best stored sealed at room temperature. Others, such as thioglycolate broth, should be stored in the dark. Unusual storage requirements are discussed with preparation of specific media.

Most of the media discussed in this section are commercially available in either powdered or prepared form. As discussed in Chapter 9, many of the conventional biochemical tests considered here are now commercially available as reagent-impregnated paper disks or strips (Remel Laboratories, Lenexa, Kan.; General Diagnostics, Morris Plains, N.J.; Key Scientific Co., Los Angeles; Austin Biological Laboratories, Austin, Tex.;

TABLE 1. Nomenclature for Protein Components of Media

USP Nomenclature[a]	Trademark Nomenclature
Pancreatic digest of casein, USP	Trypticase peptone,[b] Tryptone,[c] Casitone[c]
Papaic digest of soybean meal, USP	Phytone peptone,[b] Soytone[c]
Peptic digest of animal tissue, USP	Thiotone peptone,[b] Tryptose,[c] Proteose peptone[c]
Pancreatic hydrolysate of gelatin, USP	Peptone,[c] Gelysate peptone[b]
Pancreatic digest of heart muscle	Myosate peptone[b]
Pancreatic digest of casein and yeast extract, USP	Biosate peptone,[b] Tryptose[c] and thiamine
Pancreatic digest of casein and peptic digest of animal tissue, USP	Polypeptone peptone,[b] Neopeptone,[c] Proteose peptone #3,[c] Proteose peptone #2[c,d]
Acid hydrolysate of casein	Acidicase peptone,[b] Casamino acids[c]

Modified from MacFaddin, J.F.: Biochemical tests for identification of medical bacteria, ed. 2, Baltimore, 1980, The Williams & Wilkins Co.
[a]*United States Pharmacopeia.*
[b]BBL Microbiology Systems, Cockeysville, Md.
[c]Difco Laboratories, Detroit.
[d]Proteose peptone #3 is superior to #2 for fastidious organisms.

Wampole Laboratories, Cranbury, N.J.; Scott Laboratories, Fiskeville, R.I.; Difco Laboratories, Detroit; and several others).

Inoculation and isolation techniques are discussed in Chapter 11.

A7 AGAR

Purpose. A7 is a differential agar medium useful for isolating genital strains of mycoplasmas.

Principle and interpretation. The medium contains penicillin, colymycin, and vancomycin as agents to inhibit bacterial flora indigenous to the genital tract of humans. In addition to enrichments, for example, horse serum and yeast extract, urea is included to enhance differentiation of *Ureaplasma urealyticum* from non-urea-hydrolyzing strains of mycoplasmas. Degradation of urea is accompanied by production of ammonia. Manganous sulfate, a sensitive indicator of ammonia and present in A7 medium, reacts with ammonia to form a dark brown product. Large colony, classical *Mycoplasma*, *Acholeplasma* spp., and *Proteus* L colonies are unreactive.

Ingredients and preparation

Basal medium: Mix the following ingredients, adjust the pH to 5.5, and sterilize at 121° C for 15 minutes. (The complete medium may be stored in the refrigerator, but the basal medium alone should not.)

Ureaplasma differential A7 medium (Gibco, Madisonville, Wis.)	6.6 g
Distilled water	165 ml

A7 medium: Cool the basal medium to 50° C, add the following sterile ingredients, mix well, adjust to pH 6.2, and dispense in sterile Petri plates. Allow plates of medium to solidify at room temperature. Store at 4° C for up to 1 week. Discard plates if a precipitate is observed in the medium when low-power objective of a light microscope is used.

Horse serum, unheated	40 ml
CVA enrichment (Gibco)	1 ml
Yeast extract, pH 6.0 (Gibco)	2 ml
Urea, 50%	0.4 ml
L-Cysteine HC1, 4%	0.5 ml
Penicillin, 100,000 units/ml	2 ml

Procedure. Inoculate A7 agar* with a clinical specimen, streak for isolation, and incubate anaerobically at 35° C for 48 hours. *Ureaplasma urealyticum* grows as dark golden brown or rich deep brown colonies of variable size. Pigmentation of the colonies sharply contrasts with the clear, light background of A7 medium.

Quality control. See Table 3-11.†

---

*This medium and other primary isolation media considered in this chapter should be inoculated and streaked for isolation according to the procedures discussed in Chapter 11.

†The performance standards for this medium and many others in this appendix are included in the indicated tables in Chapter 3. Sample plates or tubes of medium from each batch should be tested with the organisms listed in the table and observed for expected results.

REFERENCE

Shepard, M.C., and Lunceford, C.D.: Differential agar medium (A7) for identification of *Ureaplasma urealyticum* (human T mycoplasmas) in primary cultures of clinical material, J. Clin. Microbiol. **3:**613, 1976.

ACETAMIDE MEDIUM

Purpose. Acetamide medium is useful for distinguishing among species of nonfermentative gram-negative rods based on ability to use acetamide as the sole source of carbon.

Principle and interpretation. This non-protein-containing medium contains salts, agar, a pH indicator, and acetamide. Bacteria that use acetamide as the sole source of carbon grow on the medium and deaminate acetamide to release ammonia. Ammonia production changes the color of the indicator (bromthymol blue) from green to stark blue; this is a positive test (a slight discoloration of the slant is ignored). A negative test is indicated by no growth or slight growth with no change in the indicator.

Ingredients and preparation. Mix the following ingredients, heat to boiling, dispense into screw-cap tubes, and sterilize at 121° C for 15 minutes. Allow tubes of medium to cool in a slanted position.

Magnesium sulfate	0.2 g
Ammonium dihydrogen phosphate	1 g
Potassium monohydrogen phosphate	1 g
Sodium chloride	5 g
Acetamide	10 g
Bromthymol blue solution	6.4 ml
Agar	15 g
Distilled water	1 L
Final pH 6.9	

Bromthymol blue solution:

Bromthymol blue	0.1 g
Sodium hydroxide, 0.02 N	8 ml

Procedure: Inoculate the slant with 1 drop of a broth or saline suspension of the test organism, allowing the drop to run down the slant. The slant may also be streaked with a portion of an isolated colony. Incubate the slant overnight at 35° C with the cap loose and observe for a color change. Tubes with negative results should be reincubated for an additional 24 hours. Hold tubes for 7 days if possible.

Quality control. See Table 3-7.

REFERENCES

Oberhofer, T.R.: Manual of nonfermenting gram-negative bacteria, New York, 1985, John Wiley & Sons, Inc.

Oberhofer, T.R., and Rowen, J.W.: Acetamide agar for differentiation of nonfermentative bacteria, Appl. Microbiol. **28:**720, 1974.

ACETATE AGAR

Purpose. Acetate agar is useful for distinguishing *Shigella* spp. from *Escherichia coli* on the basis of utilization of acetate as the sole carbon source.

Principle and interpretation. Bacteria that utilize acetate as the sole carbon source, for example, *E. coli,* grow on this medium and cause a shift in pH to alkalinity. This shift in pH is accompanied by a color change of bromthymol blue from green to blue. The change in color constitutes a positive test for utilization of acetate. A negative finding is absence of growth on the medium. Over inoculation may allow carryover of carbon-containing nutrients from growth media, which may result in growth by organisms that cannot utilize acetate as the sole source of carbon.

Ingredients and preparation. Mix ingredients, heat to boiling, dispense in tubes, sterilize at 121° C for 15 minutes, and allow to solidify in a slanted position.

Sodium acetate	2 g
Sodium chloride	5 g
Magnesium sulfate	0.2 g
Monoammonium phosphate	1 g
Dipotassium phosphate	1 g
Bromthymol blue	0.08 g
Agar	20 g
Distilled water	1 L

Final pH 6.7

Procedure. Inoculate acetate agar lightly with the test organism. Incubate cultures up to 4 days at 35° C, and observe for expected results.

Quality control. See Table 3-7.

ACID PRODUCTION (AEROBICALLY) FROM GLYCEROL IN THE PRESENCE OF ERYTHROMYCIN

Purpose. Acid production from glycerol in the presence of erythromycin (0.4 μg/ml) may be used in combination with lysozyme susceptibility and lysostaphin susceptibility to distinguish staphylococci and micrococci.

Principle and interpretation. Staphylococci produce acid aerobically from glycerol, whereas micrococci do not. Furthermore, the growth of most micrococci is inhibited by erythromycin at low levels (0.1 to 0.2 μg/ml), whereas staphylococci are resistant to at least 0.4 μg/ml.

Ingredients and preparation. Prepare basal medium (outlined below) and autoclave at 121° C for 15 minutes. Cool to 45° to 50° C before adding 1 ml of sterile erythromycin solution to 1000 ml of basal medium. Prepare erythromycin solution by dissolving 4 mg of erythromycin in 0.5 ml of 95% ethanol, add distilled water to make 10 ml, and sterilize by filtration.

Basal medium:

Ammonium dihydrogen phosphate	1 g
Potassium chloride	0.2 g
Magnesium sulfate · 7 H₂0	0.2 g
Yeast extract	2 g
Glycerol	10 ml
Bromcresol purple	0.04 g
Agar	9 g
Distilled water	1 L

pH 7.0

NOTE: Purple agar base (Difco Laboratories, Detroit) may be used in place of this medium.

Streak test organism on prepared agar plate. Six to eight culture streaks may be radially applied to each agar plate. Incubate cultures at 35° C for up to 48 hours. Acid production is indicated by development of a yellow color around the inoculum.

Quality control. Observe for expected results:
Staphylococcus aureus—development of yellow color; acid production
Micrococcus luteus—no yellow color; acid not produced

REFERENCE

Schleifer, K.H., and Kloos, W.E.: A simple test system for the separation of staphylococci from micrococci, J. Clin. Microbiol. **1**:337, 1975.

AMERICAN TRUDEAU SOCIETY MEDIUM

Purpose. American Trudeau Society (ATS) medium is a general-purpose growth medium for cultivation of acid-fast bacteria. The medium is especially recommended for culturing samples of sterile body fluids such as cerebrospinal fluid or pleural fluid for mycobacteria. The low concentration of malachite green in ATS medium is less inhibitory to some mycobacteria than the higher concentration found in other media.

Principle and interpretation. This medium contains malachite green as an inhibitory agent, as well as enrichments necessary for required carbon and nitrogen sources and for adsorption and neutralization of toxic substances, which may be present in the medium following sterilization.

Ingredients and preparation. Mix potato flour, glycerol, and distilled water in a 2 L flask. Sterilize at 121° C for 30 minutes. Cool to 50° C and add egg yolk suspension (500 ml). The egg yolk suspension is prepared from fresh egg yolks (one whole egg to 11 yolks) taken from eggs scrubbed and soaked in a soap solution. Rinse clean eggs in running water and soak in 70% alcohol for 15 minutes. Crack eggs and separate the yolks from the whites. Homogenize the yolks with vigorous shaking of the flask containing the yolks. Filter the homogenate through four layers of sterile gauze into a sterile graduated cylinder. The filtrate constitutes the egg yolk suspension. Add 20 ml malachite green solution (1% malachite green in 50% alcohol) to the potato flour–egg yolk suspension mixture, mix thoroughly, and dispense 5 to 6 ml into sterile tubes. Inspissate in a slanted position for 1 hour at 85° C.

Potato flour	20 g
Glycerol	10 ml
Distilled water	490 ml

Sterilize at 121° C for 30 minutes, cool to 50° C, and add:

Egg yolk suspension	500 ml
Malachite green, 1% in 50% alcohol	20 ml

Procedure. Inoculate ATS agar with clinical material, incubate at 35° C, and observe for growth.

Quality control. Test media from each batch with the following organism and observe for expected results:
Mycobacterium tuberculosis—good growth

REFERENCE

Vestal, A.L.: Procedures for the isolation and identification of mycobacteria, Atlanta, 1975, Center for Disease Control.

ARYLSULFATASE TEST

Purpose. The arylsulfatase test is used to distinguish among species of mycobacteria based on ability to produce the enzyme arylsulfatase.

Principle. Arylsulfatase hydrolyzes bonds between the sulfate group and the aromatic ring of tripotassium phenolphthalein disulfate to form free phenolphthalein. Presence of phenolphthalein is detected by development of a red color in the test medium after addition of alkali.

Procedure

CDC METHOD. Inoculate 0.1 ml of a 7-day Middlebrook 7H9 or Dubos Tween-albumin broth culture of the test organism to tubes containing 3-day and 14-day substrate media. A loopful of organisms taken from an actively growing subculture may alternatively be used as inoculum. Incubate the 3-day substrate tube at 35° C for 3 days and add 6 drops of 2 N sodium carbonate solution. Observe for immediate development of a red color, which is a positive test for arylsulfatase activity. After 14 days' incubation add 6 drops of 2N sodium carbonate to the 14-day tube.

WAYNE METHOD. Prepare a barely turbid suspension of the test organism in sterile distilled water. Add 1 drop of the cell suspension to the substrate. Incubate the inoculated substrate medium for 3 days at 35° C. Add 1 ml of 2 N sodium carbonate solution and observe for development of a red color.

Reagents

CDC METHOD

0.08 M stock solution: Dissolve 2.6 g phenolphthalein disulfate, tripotassium salt, in 50 ml distilled water. Sterilize by membrane filtration (0.2 μm pore size) and store at 3° to 5° C. Test a sample aliquot for free phenolphthalein by adding a few drops of 2 N sodium carbonate and observing for development of a red color. If a red color develops, the salt must be purified. To purify the salt, dissolve 3 to 5 g in a small amount of distilled water and precipitate the salt from solution with excess ethanol. Filter the solution to collect the salt, wash several times with fresh ethanol, and allow the salt to air dry. Store in a sealed glass bottle.

Liquid medium: Using either Dubos Tween-albumin or Middlebrook 7H9 medium, prepare two flasks each with 180 ml of the basal medium and autoclave for 15 minutes at 120° C. After cooling to room temperature aseptically add 20 ml of Middlebrook ADC enrichment to each flask.

WAYNE METHOD. Add 1 ml glycerol and 65 mg tripotassium phenolphthalein disulfate to 100 ml of melted Dubos oleic acid agar medium. Dispense 2 ml amounts into screw-cap vials with flat bottoms. Sterilize the tubes of medium, and allow them to solidify in an upright position.

Quality control. See Tables 3-10 and 3-18.

BACITRACIN AND TRIMETHOPRIM-SULFAMETHOXAZOLE SUSCEPTIBILITY TESTS

Purpose. The bacitracin and trimethoprim-sulfamethoxazole (SXT) susceptibility tests are used for presumptive identification of groups A and B beta-hemolytic streptococci.

Principle and interpretation. Species of beta-hemolytic streptococci (BHS) differ in their susceptibilities to bacitracin and SXT. Bacitracin is an antimicrobial agent produced by a gram-positive bacterium. The group A beta-hemolytic streptococcus, *S. pyogenes,* is susceptible to bacitracin, whereas most other groups of BHS are resistant. SXT is a combination antimicrobial agent consisting of two sulfonamides, sulfamethoxazole (23.75 μg/disk) and trimethoprim (1.25 μg/disk). *S. pyogenes* and the group B streptococcus, *S. agalactiae,* are typically resistant to SXT, whereas non–group A or B beta-hemolytic streptococci are susceptible. Bacitracin and SXT susceptibility results can be used together to enhance presumptive identification of groups A and B beta-hemolytic streptococci, since neither test alone is as accurate as the two used simultaneously. Results are interpreted as follows:

Bacitracin	SXT	Presumptive Identification
Susceptible	Resistant	Group A BHS
Resistant	Resistant	Group B BHS
Resistant	Susceptible	Not group A or B BHS
Susceptible	Susceptible	Rule out group A BHS using serologic tests

Procedure. Streak a pure culture of a beta-hemolytic streptococcus onto each half of a sheep blood agar plate. Place a 0.04 unit bacitracin disk on the inoculated area of one half of the inoculated medium and an SXT disk in the center of the other half. Incubate the culture in air for 18 to 24 hours at 35° C. Any zone of growth inhibition around either disk is interpreted as susceptibility to the antimicrobial agent.

Reagent. The reagents are bacitracin disks (0.04 unit) and the SXT disks.

Quality control. See Table 3-16.

REFERENCE

Gunn, B.A.: SXT and Taxo A disks for presumptive identification of group A and B streptococci from throat cultures, J. Clin. Microbiol. **4:**192, 1976.

BACTEROIDES BILE ESCULIN AGAR

Purpose. Bacteroides bile esculin agar is useful for isolation and identification of the *Bacteroides fragilis* group of anaerobes. The concentration of bile and gentamicin in the medium inhibits most anaerobes other than this group.

Principle and interpretation. Strains of the *B. fragilis* group grow well on this medium as dark colonies with black to brown halos. The dark pigmentation is due to reaction of ferric ammonium citrate with esculetin, a hydrolytic product of esculin. Anaerobes that are incapable of hydrolyzing esculin do not grow as brown or black pigmented colonies on this medium.

Ingredients and preparation. Add the following ingredients to 1 L of distilled water, adjust the pH to 7.0, heat the mixture to boiling, and sterilize at 121° C for 15 minutes. Dispense into Petri plates, and allow the agar medium to solidify at room temperature. Seal plates in bags, and store at 4° C.

Pancreatic digest of casein, USP	15 g
Papaic digest of soybean meal, USP	5 g
Oxgall	20 g
Esculin	1 g
Ferric ammonium citrate	0.5 g
Hemin	10 mg
Gentamicin	100 mg
Sodium chloride	5 g
Agar	15 g
Distilled water	1 L

Adjust pH to 7.0

Procedure. Inoculate the medium with the specimen, and incubate the culture at 35° C in anaerobic conditions.

Quality control. See Table 3-4.

REFERENCE

Livingston, S.J., Kominos, S.D., and Yee, R.B.: New medium for selection and presumptive identification of the *Bacteroides fragilis* group, J. Clin. Microbiol. **7**:448, 1978.

BETA-LACTAMASE TEST

Purpose. The beta-lactamase test determines the presence of beta-lactamase, an enzyme that binds to antibiotics with a beta-lactam ring and as a result usually inactivates the antibiotic. The presence of the enzyme thus indicates resistance to the antibiotic. Beta-lactamase may be detected from colonies, cerebrospinal fluid sediment, or blood culture supernatant.

Principle. Penicillins and cephalosporins are antibiotics that have in common a beta-lactam ring as part of their molecular structure. As discussed in Chapter 8, resistance to penicillins and cephalosporins may be mediated by several mechanisms, one of which is production of the enzyme beta-lactamase.

Beta-lactamase production may be determined with three methods. The rapid acidimetric method is based on the principle that penicilloic acid, produced after opening of the beta-lactam ring (Figure 8-20) is more acidic than penicillin. A phenol red indicator is used to indicate the production of acid by the test organism.

A mixture of penicillin, starch, and iodine is used in the starch-iodine (iodometric) method. Starch and iodine react to form a purple color. If beta-lactamase is produced, penicillin G is cleaved to penicilloic acid and the acid converts iodine to iodide, which no longer forms a purple complex with starch.

The third method uses a chromogenic cephalosporin, a compound that is yellow in its complete state but becomes red on cleavage of the beta-lactam ring. The chromogenic cephalosporin method is the most sensitive.

Procedure

ACIDIMETRIC METHOD. The substrate is prepared by diluting 2 ml of a 0.5% solution of phenol red with 16.6 ml of sterile distilled water and injecting the solution into a vial containing 20×10^6 units of penicillin G. (This vial should be designated for parenteral use and should contain a citrate buffer.) After transferring the mixture to a test tube, add 1 M sodium hydroxide drop by drop until the solution turns violet (pH 8.5). Transfer 0.05 to 0.1 ml of the phenol red–penicillin substrate to a small test tube or the well of a microdilution plate. Mix with a heavy suspension of an overnight culture of the test organism to form a suspension more turbid than a McFarland no. 4 standard. If beta-lactamase is produced, the solution turns yellow within 15 minutes. Commercial acidimetric systems consist of a paper strip that contains penicillin and the indicator bromcresol purple. The paper is moistened and rubbed with the test organism. A change in color from purple to yellow is a positive reaction.

CHROMOGENIC CEPHALOSPORIN METHOD. Dissolve 10 mg of the chromogenic cephalosporin nitrocefin (available from Glaxo Ltd., Greenford, Middlesex, Eng.) in 1 ml of dimethyl sulfoxide, and dilute with 0.1 M phosphate buffer (pH 7.0) to a final concentration of 500 μg/ml. Transfer 0.1 ml of the substrate to a small tube or well of a microdilution tray and mix with a heavy suspension of the test organism to form a suspension more turbid than a McFarland no. 4 standard. A positive reaction is indicated by the formation of a red color within 10 minutes.

Nitrocefin impregnated onto filter paper disks may also be purchased commercially (Cefinase, BBL Microbiology Systems, Cockeysville, Md.). Several well-isolated colonies are smeared onto a disk that has been moistened with sterile water. Development of a red color within 5 to 10 minutes is a positive test for beta-lactamase.

IODOMETRIC METHOD. The iodometric method requires the preparation of three solutions. The penicillin substrate is prepared by dissolving penicillin G in 0.1 M phosphate buffer (pH 6.0) to a final concentration of 6000 μg/ml. To prepare the starch reagent, add 1 g of soluble starch to 100 ml of distilled water. Heat in a boiling water bath to dissolve starch. To prepare iodine solution, dissolve 2.03 g of iodine and 53.2 g of potassium iodide in a small volume of distilled water and dilute to 100 ml. Transfer 0.1 ml of the penicillin G solution to a small test tube or the well of a microdilution tray. Prepare a heavy suspension of the test organism and mix it with the penicillin G solution to form a suspension more turbid than a McFarland no. 4 standard. Allow the mixture to stand for 30 minutes. Add 2 drops of the starch solution. Mix. Add 1 drop of the iodine reagent and observe the development of a dark blue color as a result of the formation of the iodine-starch complex. Stir the mixture for 1 minute. A positive reaction is decolorization to a white color within 10 minutes.

Comments. The chromogenic cephalosporin test is the most sensitive test and can be used to detect the beta-lactamases of *Neisseria gonorrhoeae*, *Staphylococcus aureus*, *Haemophilus* spp., and most *Bacteroides* spp. Only this method should be used for *Bacteroides* spp. See comments in Chapter 8 concerning the inducible beta-lactamases of staphylococci. According to Schoenknecht (see references) beta-lactamase tests for therapeutic purposes are not recommended for members of the *Enterobacteriaceae*, nonfermentative gram-negative bacilli, and anaerobic bacteria other than *Bacteroides* spp.

Quality control. Positive and negative controls should be used with each test. The positive control may be a stock culture, an ampicillin-resistant *H. influenzae*, or a beta-lactamase-producing *S. aureus*. An ampicillin-susceptible *H. influenzae* or *S. aureus* ATCC 25923 should be used for the negative control.

REFERENCES

Schoenknecht, F.D., Sabath, L.D., and Thornsberry, C.: Susceptibility tests: special tests. In Lennette, E.H., et al., editors: Manual of clinical microbiology, ed. 4, Washington, D.C., 1985, American Society for Microbiology.

Thornsberry, C., Gavan, T.L., and Gerlach, E.H., editors (Sherris, J.C., coordinating editor): New developments in antimicrobial agent susceptibility testing, Cumitech 6, Washington, D.C., 1977, American Society for Microbiology.

BILE ESCULIN AGAR

Purpose. Bile esculin (BE) agar is used to distinguish group D streptococci and *Enterococcus* spp. Differentiation is based on the ability to grow in the presence of 40% bile (4% oxgall) and to hydrolyze esculin into esculetin and dextrose.

Principle and interpretation. This medium is selective for organisms capable of growing in the presence of 40% bile. Most gram-negative rods, *Staphylococcus* spp., group D streptococci, and *Enterococcus* spp. grow on this medium. The latter two organisms also hydrolyze esculin to produce esculetin, which reacts with ferric citrate to form a brown-black product. This characteristic distinguishes these organisms from other streptococci discussed in Chapter 13.

Ingredients and preparation. Mix the following ingredients, heat to boiling, and sterilize at 121° C for 15 minutes. Dispense into tubes and allow to harden in a slanted position.

Beef extract	3 g
Pancreatic hydrolysate of gelatin, USP	5 g
Esculin	1 g
Oxgall	40 g
Ferric citrate	0.5 g
Agar	15 g
Distilled water	1 L

Final pH 7.0

Reagent-impregnated commercial strips are also available.

Procedure. Touch the center of a well-isolated colony with a sterile bacteriologic needle. Transfer the inoculum to the surface of a BE agar slant. Incubate the culture at 35° C. Examine the culture each day for growth and blackening of the agar caused by hydrolysis of esculin. Blackening usually occurs within 48 hours. Growth on the medium indicates tolerance to 40% bile.

Quality control. See Table 3-7.

BILE SOLUBILITY TEST

Purpose. The bile solubility test provides presumptive identification of *Streptococcus pneumoniae.*

Principle. Surface-active agents such as bile salts, saponins, and other cationic detergents alter the surface of *S. pneumoniae,* resulting in the activation of an autolytic enzyme. This enzyme is an amidase that splits the muramic acid–alanine bond in peptidoglycan, resulting in lysis of the cell. Sodium lauryl sulfate (2%), sodium deoxycholate (10%), or white Dreft (1%) may be used in lieu of bile for this test. Sodium deoxycholate is one of the most lytic salts of the bile acids and is often

used in the bile solubility test. It is soluble in water at pH 6.5 or higher and precipitates from solution at pH 6.4 or lower.

Procedure

RAPID AGAR COLONY TEST. Add a loopful of 2% sodium deoxycholate solution to a colony growing on sheep blood agar. Mark the location of the colony on the bottom of the plate. Incubate the plate, agar side up, at 35° C for 30 minutes. Colonies of bile-soluble organisms disintegrate during this period of incubation. Colonies of bile-insoluble organisms remain intact.

CONVENTIONAL BROTH CULTURE TEST. Add 1 ml of a dense physiologic saline suspension of the test organism to a tube. Alternatively, add 1 ml of an overnight Todd-Hewitt broth culture to the tube. Add 1 drop of phenol red solution, and adjust the pH to 7.0 with 0.1 N sodium hydroxide. The mixture is pink. Transfer 0.5 ml aliquots of the neutralized mixture to each of two tubes. Dispense 0.5 ml of 10% sodium deoxycholate to one tube, labeled ''test,'' and 0.5 ml of physiologic saline to the other tube, labeled ''control.'' Shake each tube and incubate at 35° C for 3 hours. A mixture containing a bile-soluble organism clears in the presence of sodium deoxycholate (''test''), but the mixture in the control tube remains turbid. A mixture containing a bile-insoluble organism remains turbid in both tubes.

Reagents

Sodium hydroxide (NaOH), 10 N:

Sodium hydroxide	4 g
Distilled water	10 ml

NaOH, 0.1 N:

NaOH, 10 N	1 ml
Distilled water, q.s. to	100 ml

Physiologic saline: 0.85% sodium chloride in distilled water.

Sodium deoxycholate, 10%:

Sodium deoxycholate	10 g
Distilled water, q.s. to	100 ml

Sodium deoxycholate, 2%:

Sodium deoxycholate, 10%	1 ml
Distilled water	4 ml

Phenol red, 0.04%:

Phenol red	40 mg
Distilled water	100 ml

Quality control. Use test organisms indicted under 10% sodium deoxycholate in Table 3-16.

BISMUTH SULFITE AGAR

Purpose. Bismuth sulfite (BS) agar is selective for *Salmonella* spp. Most lactose-fermenting normal intestinal flora bacteria, *Shigella* spp., and gram-positive bacteria are inhibited by the brilliant green in the medium.

Principle and interpretation. Brilliant green and bismuth sulfite are incorporated into BS agar to inhibit the intestinal gram-negative and gram-positive bacteria. *Salmonella typhi* typically grows as black colonies with a surrounding metallic sheen resulting from hydrogen sulfide production and reduction of sulfite to black ferric sulfide. *Salmonella enteritidis* grows as black colonies without a metallic sheen. In contrast, *Salmonella gallinarum, Salmonella choleraesuis,* and *Salmonella paratyphi* grow as light green colonies. The medium may be inhibitory to some strains of *Salmonella* spp. and therefore should not be used as the sole selective medium for these organisms.

Ingredients and preparation. Mix the following ingredients, heat to boiling, cool to 50° C, and dispense 20 ml aliquots into sterile Petri plates. Allow the agar media to solidify at room temperature with lids ajar to enhance removal of excess surface moisture. The medium *must* be used on the day of preparation.

Beef extract	5 g
Pancreatic hydrolysate of gelatin, USP	10 g
Glucose	5 g
Disodium phosphate	4 g
Ferrous sulfate	0.3 g
Bismuth sulfite	8 g
Brilliant green	0.025 g
Agar	20 g
Distilled water	1 L

Final pH 7.7

Procedure. Inoculate fecal samples or enrichment broth samples to BS agar, and streak for isolation using a sterile bacteriologic loop. Incubate media for 48 hours at 35° C in air before discarding them as negative. Do not incubate in carbon dioxide.

Quality control. See Table 3-3.

BLOOD AGAR, ANAEROBIC (CDC)

Purpose. Anaerobic blood agar (CDC) is recommended as an enriched general growth medium for anaerobic bacteria.

Principle and interpretation. This nonselective medium is enriched with yeast extract, hemin, vitamin K_1, L-cystine, and sheep blood to enhance growth of fastidious anaerobic bacteria.

Ingredients and preparation. Mix the following ingredients, adjust the pH to 7.5, and sterilize the medium at 121° C for 15 minutes. Cool the mixture to 50° C, add 50 ml sterile defibrinated sheep blood, stir gently, and dispense into Petri plates. Seal the plates in bags, and store at 4° C for up to 6 weeks.

Basal medium:

Pancreatic digest of casein, USP	15 g
Papaic digest of soybean meal, USP	5 g
Sodium chloride	5 g
Yeast extract	5 g
Hemin	500 mg
Vitamin K_1 (3-phytylmenadione)	10 mg
L-Cystine	400 mg

Agar	20 g
Distilled water	1 L

Final pH 7.5

Vitamin K_1 stock solution, 10 mg/ml:

3-Phytylmenadione	1 g
Ethanol, absolute	99 ml

Add 1 ml to basal medium. Store in a sterile brown bottle at 4° C.

Hemin L-cystine solution:

Hemin	0.5 g
L-Cystine	0.4 g
NaOH, 1 N	5 ml

Use a small glass container to dissolve the hemin and L-cystine in NaOH, and then add to the basal medium (5 ml/L). Prepare fresh as needed.

Additives to sterile basal medium:

Sheep blood, defibrinated	50 ml

Procedure. Inoculate the medium, streak for isolation, and incubate at 35° C for 48 hours or more.

Quality control. See anaerobic blood agar in Table 3-4.

REFERENCE

Dowell, V.R., Jr., and Hawkins, T.M.: Media for isolation, characterization, and identification of obligately anaerobic bacteria, Atlanta, 1981, Centers for Disease Control.

BLOOD AGAR, ANAEROBIC, BRUCELLA BASE (WADSWORTH)

Purpose. Anaerobic blood agar with a Brucella base is recommended as a general-purpose, nonselective medium for cultivation of obligately anaerobic bacteria.

Principle. The incorporation of yeast extract, vitamin K_1, hemin, and sheep blood enhances growth of anaerobic bacteria.

Ingredients and preparation

Basal medium:

Pancreatic digest of casein, USP	10 g
Peptic digest of animal tissues, USP	10 g
Glucose	1 g
Yeast extract	2 g
Sodium chloride	5 g
Sodium bisulfite	0.1 g
Agar	15 g

This basal medium is available in dehydrated form as Brucella agar. The use of dehydrated Brucella agar manufactured by BBL Microbiology Systems (Cockeysville, Md.) is recommended in the *Wadsworth Anaerobic Bacteriology Manual.* If the BBL basal medium is used, it should be combined with the following ingredients:

Brucella agar (BBL)	43 g
Hemin solution (5 mg/ml)	1 ml

Vitamin K₁ solution (10 mg/ml)	1 ml
Distilled water	1 L
Sterile defibrinated sheep blood	50 ml

Combine all ingredients except sheep blood, and boil to dissolve. Autoclave at 121° C for 15 minutes. Cool to 50° C, add sheep blood, and pour into plates. Seal in bags and store at 4° C for 2 weeks.

Quality control. See anaerobic blood agar in Table 3-4.

REFERENCE

Sutter, V.L., et al.: Wadsworth anaerobic bacteriology manual, ed. 4, Belmont, Calif., 1985, Star Publishing Co.

BLOOD AGAR, ANAEROBIC, WITH KANAMYCIN AND VANCOMYCIN (CDC)

Purpose. Anaerobic blood agar with kanamycin and vancomycin (KV) is recommended for isolation of *Bacteroides* spp. and other obligately anaerobic bacteria from specimens containing mixed bacterial populations.

Principle and interpretation. This medium is enriched with yeast extract, hemin, vitamin K₁, L-cystine, and sheep blood to enhance growth of fastidious anaerobic bacteria. Kanamycin is a broad-spectrum aminoglycoside antimicrobial agent that interferes with protein synthesis in bacteria and is employed in this medium to inhibit many species of facultatively anaerobic gram-negative and gram-positive bacteria. Vancomycin is a narrow-spectrum antimicrobial agent that interferes with cell wall synthesis and is added to inhibit aerobic gram-positive bacteria and anaerobic bacteria other than *Bacteroides* spp.

Ingredients and preparation. The basal medium for KV agar is prepared as described for CDC anaerobic blood agar. In addition to sheep blood, 100 mg kanamycin (base activity) and 7.5 mg vancomycin (base activity) are added to the basal medium following sterilization. The medium is dispensed into Petri plates and allowed to cool at room temperature. Plates are sealed in bags and stored at 4° C for no longer than 4 weeks.

Procedure. Inoculate KV agar with a clinical specimen or colony and streak for isolation. Incubate anaerobically at 35° C for 48 hours or more.

Quality control. Test sample plates of medium from each batch with the following organisms and observe for the expected results:

Bacteroides fragilis—growth
Clostridium perfringens—no growth

BLOOD AGAR, LAKED, ANAEROBIC, WITH KANAMYCIN AND VANCOMYCIN

Purpose. Anaerobic laked blood agar with kanamycin and vancomycin (KV) is recommended for isolation of *Bacteroides* spp. from clinical specimens.

Principle and interpretation. See KV agar described previously. Production of pigment by *Bacteroides melaninogenicus* is enhanced on this medium.

Ingredients and preparation. Mix the following ingredients except vancomycin and laked sheep blood. Boil to dissolve and sterilize the mixture at 121° C for 15 minutes. Cool to 50° C, and add 1 ml of vancomycin and 50 ml (5%) of laked

blood. Prepare laked blood by freezing whole blood overnight and then thawing the preparation.

Basal medium:

Pancreatic digest of casein and peptic digest of animal tissues, USP	20 g
Glucose	1 g
Yeast extract	2 g
Sodium chloride	5 g
Sodium bisulfite	0.1 g
Agar	15 g

This basal medium is available in dehydrated form as Brucella agar (BBL Microbiology Systems, Cockeysville, Md.). This commercial medium, 43 g, should be used in combination with the following ingredients:

Hemin solution (5 mg/ml)	1 ml
Vitamin K₁ solution (10 mg/ml)	1 ml
Kanamycin solution (100 mg/ml)	0.75 ml
Distilled water	1 L
Vancomycin solution (7.5 mg/ml)	1 ml
Laked sheep blood	50 ml

Procedure. Inoculate the medium with a clinical specimen and incubate anaerobically at 35° C for 48 hours or more.

Quality control. See Brucella agar with laked blood, vitamin K₁, hemin, kanamycin, and vancomycin in Table 3-4.

REFERENCE

Sutter, V.L., et al.: Wadsworth anaerobic bacteriology manual, ed. 4, Belmont, Calif., 1985, Star Publishing Co.

BLOOD AGAR, PHENETHYL ALCOHOL, ANAEROBIC (CDC)

Purpose. Phenethyl alcohol (PEA) agar is a selective medium used to enhance isolation of *Bacteroides* spp. and other obligately anaerobic bacteria from cultures mixed with facultative anaerobes.

Principle and interpretation. PEA causes gram-negative, facultatively anaerobic bacteria to become elongated into filamentous forms and subsequently die from suppression of deoxyribonucleic acid (DNA) synthesis and cell division. Anaerobic gram-negative and gram-positive bacteria are not affected by PEA and will grow on this medium. Since PEA is volatile and evaporates during storage, plates of medium should be used as fresh as possible and, when stored, should be placed in plastic bags and refrigerated.

Ingredients and preparation. Mix the basal ingredients, heat to boiling, and add the hemin, L-cystine, and vitamin K₁ solutions. Sterilize at 121° C for 15 minutes. Cool to 50° C and add 50 ml sheep blood. Mix thoroughly and dispense into sterile Petri plates. Store sealed in plastic bags at 4° C up to 4 weeks.

Basal medium:

Pancreatic digest of casein, USP	15 g
Papaic digest of soybean meal, USP	5 g

Sodium chloride	5 g
Yeast extract	5 g
Phenethyl alcohol	2.5 g
Agar	20 g
Distilled water	1 L

Final pH 7.5

Additives before sterilization: Dissolve hemin (5 mg) and L-cystine (400 mg) in 5 ml of 1 N sodium hydroxide. Add this solution to the basal medium.

Dissolve vitamin K_1 (1 g) in 99 ml absolute ethanol. Add 1 ml (final concentration 10 mg/1 L of basal medium) to the basal medium.

Additive to sterile, cooled basal medium: 50 ml of sterile, defibrinated sheep blood.

Procedure. Inoculate PEA agar with a clinical specimen or colony, streak for isolation, and incubate anaerobically at 35° C for 48 hours or more.

Quality control. See phenylethyl alcohol agar in Table 3-4.

REFERENCE

Dowell, V.R., Jr., and Hawkins, T.M.: Media for isolation, characterization and identification of obligately anaerobic bacteria, Atlanta, 1981, Centers for Disease Control.

BLOOD AGAR, PHENYLETHYL ALCOHOL, WADSWORTH

Purpose. Phenylethyl alcohol (PEA) agar is a selective medium recommended for isolation of *Bacteroides* spp. from clinical specimens.

Principle and interpretation. See CDC PEA agar.

Ingredients and preparation. Mix the following ingredients except for sheep blood, bring to boiling, and sterilize at 121° C for 15 minutes. Cool the sterile medium to 50° C, and add 50 ml of sterile defibrinated sheep blood. Dispense the agar in Petri plates, cool to room temperature, and store in plastic bags at 4° C for up to 2 weeks.

Basal medium:

Phenylethyl alcohol agar	42.5 g
Sheep blood, defibrinated	50 ml
Vitamin K_1 (10 mg/ml)	1 ml
Distilled water	1 L

Final pH 7.0

Procedure. Inoculate PEA with a clinical specimen or colony, streak for isolation, and incubate anaerobically at 35° C for 48 hours or more.

Quality control. See phenylethyl alcohol agar in Table 3-4.

REFERENCE

Sutter, V.L., et al.: Wadsworth anaerobic bacteriology manual, ed. 4, Belmont, Calif., 1985, Star Publishing Co.

BLOOD AGAR, SHEEP

Purpose. Sheep blood agar (SBA) is a general-purpose medium used for cultivation of bacteria. It is especially useful for distinguishing streptococci based on hemolytic properties.

Principle and interpretation. Bacteria growing on SBA produce a wide variety of products that affect the integrity of the sheep red blood cells contained in the medium. *Streptococcus pyogenes* produces streptolysin O and S, both of which are capable of completely lysing red blood cells. Streptolysin O is oxygen labile, whereas streptolysin S is oxygen stable. Beta-hemolysis appears as a clear or colorless zone surrounding the colony. Some streptococci are able to partially lyse the red blood cells resulting in a greenish or brownish discoloration around the colony. Species that fail to produce visible effects on sheep red blood cells are said to be gamma-hemolytic, or more appropriately, nonhemolytic.

Ingredients and preparation. Mix the basal ingredients, heat to boiling, and sterilize at 121° C for 15 minutes. Cool to 50° C and add 5% to 7% defibrinated sheep blood. Mix thoroughly and pour into Petri plates. Allow media to solidify at room temperature to hasten removal of excess surface moisture.

Basal ingredients:

Pancreatic digest of casein, USP	15 g
Papaic digest of soybean meal, USP	5 g
Sodium chloride	5 g
Agar	15 g
Distilled water	1 L

Final pH 7.3

Additive for sterile, cooled (50° C), basal medium:

Sheep blood, defibrinated	70 ml

Procedure. Inoculate SBA with a clinical specimen or colony and streak for isolation. Incubate at 35° C.

Quality control. See sheep blood agar in Table 3-3.

BLOOD AGAR, TRIMETHOPRIM-SULFAMETHOXAZOLE

Purpose. Sheep blood agar containing sulfamethoxazole and trimethoprim (SBA-SXT) is used for cultivation of *Streptococcus pyogenes* and *Streptococcus agalactiae* from throat specimens.

Principle and interpretation. The antimicrobial agents sulfamethoxazole and trimethoprim, when added to SBA, inhibit most species of streptococci, staphylococci, and gram-negative rods found in respiratory specimens. *S. pyogenes* and *S. agalactiae* are not inhibited and can be cultivated from throat specimens containing mixed species of bacteria.

Ingredients and preparation. Prepare sheep blood agar and add 1 ml of a 25 mg/ml stock SXT solution to each liter of medium. Dispense the antimicrobial-containing SBA into Petri plates and allow to harden at room temperature.

Stock SXT antimicrobial solution:

1. *Solution A:* Trimethoprim, 0.125 g, is dissolved in a few milliliters of 0.1 N hydrochloric acid, and the mixture is brought up to a volume of 50 ml with distilled water.

2. *Solution B:* Sulfamethoxazole, 2.375 g, is dissolved in a few milliliters of 1.0 N NaOH, and the mixture is brought up to a volume of 50 ml with distilled water.
3. *Stock SXT Solution:* Add 50 ml of solution A to 50 ml of solution B. Divide into 6 ml aliquots and store at −30° C until ready for use. The solution does not have to be sterilized before use.

Procedure. Inoculate SBA-SXT medium with a clinical specimen and streak for isolation. Incubate plates for 18 to 24 hours at 35° C in an atmosphere of 5% to 9% carbon dioxide in air. Examine plates for presence of beta-hemolytic colonies. Touch single colonies with a sterile bacteriologic needle, and transfer the inoculum to one quadrant of a fresh SBA-SXT agar plate. This inoculated area may be used to test for bacitracin susceptibility.

Quality control. Test sample plates of medium from each batch with the following organisms and observe for expected results:

Streptococcus pneumoniae—no growth
Proteus vulgaris—no growth
Streptococcus pyogenes—growth and beta-hemolysis

REFERENCE

Gunn, B.A., et al.: Selective and enhanced recovery of group A and B streptococci from throat cultures with sheep blood agar containing sulfamethoxazole and trimethoprim, J. Clin. Microbiol. **5:**650, 1977.

BORDET-GENGOU BLOOD AGAR

Purpose. Bordet-Gengou (BG) blood agar is a potato-based agar medium used for isolation and cultivation of *Bordetella pertussis,* the causative agent of whooping cough, and *Bordetella parapertussis,* the causative agent of an infection similar to whooping cough.

Principle and interpretation. *B. pertussis* is a delicate organism that survives in vitro in respiratory secretions for only a few hours. The ingredients in BG agar—sheep blood, potato infusion, and glycerol—together increase the viability of this organism by absorbing toxic substances present in prepared media and by supplying growth-promoting nutrients. BG agar without antimicrobial agents should be used along with BG agar with cephalexin, which inhibits cell wall synthesis in many gram-positive and gram-negative bacteria normally present in respiratory specimens.

Ingredients and preparation. Prepare the basal medium in distilled water containing 1% glycerol, heat to boiling, and sterilize at 121° C for 15 minutes. Cool the sterile medium to 50° C and add 200 ml defibrinated sheep blood. Selective BG agar is prepared by adding 40 μg/ml of the cephalexin to the medium. Allow agar to solidify at room temperature, and store sealed in plastic bags for no longer than 1 week at 4° C.

Basal medium:

Potato infusion	125 g
Sodium chloride	5.5 g
Glycerol	10 ml
Agar	20 g
Distilled water	1 L

Final pH 6.7

Additives to sterile, cooled basal medium:

Defibrinated sheep blood	200 ml

Cephalexin (optional, 0.04 g/4 ml distilled water)	4 ml

Procedure. Inoculate BG agar with a clinical specimen, streak for isolation, and incubate at 35° C for 6 days.
Quality control. See Table 3-3.

REFERENCE

Washington, J.A., II: Medical microbiology. In Henry, J.B., editor: Clinical diagnosis and management by laboratory methods, Philadelphia, 1984, W.B. Saunders Co.

BRAIN HEART INFUSION BROTH

Purpose. Brain heart infusion (BHI) broth is a general-purpose growth medium used for cultivation of a wide variety of aerobic and anaerobic bacteria. BHI broth is more nutritive for bacteria than is trypticase soy broth.

Principle and interpretation. BHI broth contains heart and brain infusions, peptone, sodium chloride, buffer, and glucose. With the addition of 10% defibrinated sheep blood it is useful for isolation and cultivation of *Histoplasma capsulatum* and other fungi. BHI with added agar should not be used for detection of hemolytic activity of streptococci, since it contains glucose, which has been reported to cause atypical hemolytic reactions when it is present in blood-containing media.

Ingredients and preparation. Mix the following ingredients, heat to boiling, dispense into tubes, and sterilize at 121° C for 15 minutes.

Calf brain infusion	200 g
Beef heart infusion	250 g
Pancreatic hydrolysate of gelatin, USP	10 g
Sodium chloride	5 g
Disodium phosphate	2.5 g
D-Glucose	2 g
Distilled water	1 L

Final pH 7.4

Procedure. Inoculate the test organism into BHI, incubate at 35° C for 18 to 24 hours, and observe for growth.
Quality control. See Table 3-3.

BRILLIANT GREEN AGAR

Purpose. This medium is a selective and differential medium used for isolation of most species of *Salmonella* other than *S. typhi* directly from feces or after enrichment in selective broth. *Shigella* spp. grow poorly if at all on brilliant green agar.

Principle and interpretation. Brilliant green dye is inhibitory to most species of intestinal bacteria other than *Salmonella.* Lactose and sucrose are included in the formulation to enable differentiation of the few strains of fermenting organisms that may grow on the medium from the nonfermenting *Salmonella* spp. Fermenting organisms produce acid, thereby lowering the pH of the medium, which causes the indicator, phenol red, to change color; these organisms produce yellow-green colonies surrounded by an intense yellow-green zone. Nonfermenters, such as *Salmonella* spp., grow as pink-white opaque colonies surrounded by brilliant red medium. Some strains of *Proteus* may grow, forming red colonies. Many strains of *S. typhi* are unable to grow on this medium.

Ingredients and preparation. Mix the following ingredients, bring to a boil, and sterilize at 121° C for 15 minutes. After sterilization, cool the medium to 50° C, and dispense into Petri plates. Allow agar to solidify for several hours at room temperature with lids ajar to eliminate excess surface moisture.

Pancreatic digest of casein and peptic digest of animal tissue, USP	10 g
Yeast extract	3 g
Sodium chloride	5 g
Lactose	10 g
Sucrose	10 g
Phenol red	0.08 g
Brilliant green	12.5 mg
Agar	20 g
Distilled water	1 L

Final pH 6.9

Procedure. Inoculate fecal specimens or enrichment broth samples to brilliant green medium, streak for isolation, and incubate for 48 hours in air at 35° C. Observe for typical nonfermenting colonies. Do not incubate in a carbon dioxide incubator.

Quality control. See Table 3-3.

BUFFERED CHARCOAL–YEAST EXTRACT AGAR WITH ALPHA-KETOGLUTARATE

Purpose. Buffered charcoal–yeast extract agar with alpha-ketoglutarate (BYCE-$\propto$) is used for the isolation of *Legionella* spp. from tissue, pleural fluids, and transtracheal aspirates.

Principle and interpretation. BCYE-$\propto$ contains nutrients and other substances that enhance the growth of *Legionella* organisms. Charcoal is added to absorb toxic compounds that either accumulate in the medium during growth or are present following preparation of the medium. A semiselective medium, BMPA-alpha, may be prepared by adding three antimicrobial agents: polymyxin inhibits gram-negative bacilli, cefamandole inhibits gram-positive organisms, and anisomycin inhibits fungi.

Ingredients and preparation

ACES (*N*-2-acetamido-2-ethan sulfonic acid, Calbiochem, San Diego)	10 g
Monopotassium alpha-ketoglutarate (Sigma Chemical Co., St. Louis)	1 g
Agar (Bacto-Agar, Difco Laboratories, Detroit)	17 g
Yeast Extract (Difco Laboratories)	10 g
Activated charcoal (Norit SG—acid and alkali washed, Sigma Chemical Co.)	2 g
L-Cysteine HCl·H$_2$O	0.4 g
Ferric pyrophosphate, soluble (ICN Biomedicals, Irvine, Calif.)	0.25 g
Distilled water	930 ml

Add ACES and alpha-ketoglutarate to water at room temperature. Adjust to pH 6.9 with 1 N potassium hydroxide (about 50 ml) (see note concerning pH below). Add agar and dissolve by boiling. Add yeast extract and charcoal. Autoclave for 15 minutes at 121° C. Cool to 50° C and add L-cysteine and ferric pyrophosphate (each filter sterilized in 10 ml of water), always adding the L-cysteine first. Pour 20 ml of medium per plate to minimize drying during prolonged incubation. Many laboratories pour this medium in a darkened room to avoid the light-catalyzed production of inhibitory peroxides. Swirl the flask frequently during pouring to keep the charcoal suspended. Media that are poured while too hot have an exceptionally wet surface. *The final pH of the solidified agar should be 6.9 ± 0.5.* Check the pH of *every* batch of medium either with a surface electrode or by pouring medium into a Petri dish and allowing it to solidify around a combination electrode. Store plates in plastic sleeves in a refrigerator away from light. Shelf life under these conditions appears to be about 4 weeks.

To make a semiselective medium for the isolation of *L. pneumophila* (may inhibit other *Legionella* spp.) add the following antimicrobial compounds to each liter of cooled medium before pouring.

Polymyxin	80,000 units
Cefamandole	4 mg
Anisomycin (Pfizer)	80 mg

Comments. In the laboratory of A.W. Pasculle, the pH of the medium is adjusted to 6.9 before autoclaving, and this results in solidified agar with a pH of 6.9. At the Centers for Disease Control the pH must be adjusted to 7.2 before autoclaving to result in the proper final pH. Some trial and error in individual laboratories may be required to find the initial pH that will result in the proper pH in the solidified plates. ACES has a very high pK, so the temperature of the medium markedly affects the pH.

Cysteine and ferric pyrophosphate solutions must be made fresh each time. Keep ferric pyrophosphate crystals dry and discard them if their color changes from chartreuse to brownish.

Potassium hydroxide or hydrochloric acid (1 N) should be used to adjust the pH of the medium. The use of sodium hydroxide may result in inhibitory media.

Procedure. Inoculate the specimen to BCYE-$\propto$ and streak for isolation. Incubate at 35° C in the presence of elevated CO$_2$ and high humidity. Inspect plates daily for 2 weeks.

Quality control. Test sample plates of medium from each batch with *Legionella pneumophila*, and observe for results discussed in Chapter 24.

REFERENCES

Edelstein, P.H.: Improved semi-selective medium for isolation of *Legionella pneumophila* from contaminated clinical and environmental specimens, J. Clin. Microbiol. **14:**298, 1981.
Feeley, J.C., et al.: Charcoal-yeast extract agar: primary isolation medium for *Legionella pneumophila*, J. Clin. Microbiol. **10:**437, 1979.
Pasculle, A.W., et al.: Pittsburgh pneumonia agent: direct isolation from human lung tissue, J. Infect. Dis. **141:**727, 1980.

CAMP TEST

Purpose. The CAMP test is for presumptive identification of group B streptococci.

Principle. CAMP factor is a diffusible, heat-stable, extracellular protein produced by group B streptoccci. This protein acts synergistically with staphylococccal beta-toxin to induce rapid hemolysis of sheep or bovine but not human, horse, or rabbit red blood cells. *Staphylococcus aureus* ATCC 25923 produces beta-hemolysin and is generally used for testing.

Procedure. Use an inoculating loop to streak a beta-toxin-producing strain of *S. aureus* in a straight line across the surface of a sheep blood agar plate. Taking care not to touch the *Staphylococcus* inoculum, streak the test organism in a straight line, 2 to 3 cm in length, at a right angle to the *Staphylococcus* streak. Four or more test organisms can be inoculated per plate. Incubate the blood agar culture at 35° C for 18 to 24 hours. A positive test for the CAMP factor is observed as production of "arrowhead" hemolysis between the junction of the growth of the *Streptococcus* and the *Staphylococcus*. Paper disks impregnated with partially purified β-hemolysin may be used in lieu of the staphylococcal culture.

Quality control. Inoculate the control *S. aureus* ATCC 25923 to a sheep blood agar plate. Inoculate control strains of *Streptococcus agalactiae* and *Streptococcus pyogenes* at a right angle to the *Staphylococcus* streak, incubate, and observe for the following results:

S. agalactiae—"arrowhead" hemolysis
S. pyogenes—no "arrowhead" effect

REFERENCES

Darling, C.L.: Standardization and evaluation of the CAMP reaction for the prompt, presumptive identification of *Streptococcus agalactiae* (Lancefield group B) in clinical material, J. Clin. Microbiol. **1:**171, 1975.

Wilkinson, H.W.: CAMP-disk test for presumptive identification of group B streptococci, J. Clin. Microbiol. **6:**42, 1977.

CAMPYLOBACTER BLOOD AGAR

Purpose. Campylobacter (Campy) blood agar is useful for isolation of *Campylobacter* spp., especially *C. jejuni,* from fecal specimens containing mixed species of bacteria.

Principle and interpretation. Campy blood agar contains sodium bisulfite, which lowers the oxidation-reduction potential of the medium to enhance recovery of the microaerophilic *Campylobacter* organisms. Four antimicrobial agents (cephalothin, trimethoprim, vancomycin, and polymyxin B) are included to inhibit growth of the normal intestinal flora. An additional agent, amphotericin B, inhibits the growth of fungi. Because the antimicrobial agents decompose with time, *Enterobacteriaceae* and *Pseudomonas* spp. may grow as the expiration date of the medium nears. *Campylobacter* spp. grow as small, gray, nonhemolytic, flat, occasionally mucoid colonies.

Ingredients and preparation. Mix basal ingredients, heat to boiling, and sterilize at 121° C for 15 minutes. Cool the sterile medium to 50° C, and add 100 ml defibrinated sheep blood and the antimicrobial agents. Dispense into Petri plates and allow the medium to solidify at room temperature. Seal the plates in plastic bags and store at 4° C protected from light.

Basal medium:

Pancreatic digest of casein and peptic digest of animal tissue, USP	20 g
Glucose	1 g
Yeast extract	2 g
Sodium chloride	5 g
Sodium bisulfite	0.1 g
Agar	15 g
Distilled water	1 L

Final pH 7.0

Additives to sterile basal medium:

Sheep blood, defibrinated	100 ml

Antimicrobial agents, final concentration per liter of medium:

Cephalothin	15 mg
Amphotericin B	2 mg
Trimethoprim	5 mg
Vancomycin	10 mg
Polymyxin B	2500 IU

Procedure. Inoculate Campy blood agar with a clinical specimen, streak for isolation, and incubate at 42° C for 48 hours in an atmosphere of 5% oxygen, 10% carbon dioxide, and 85% nitrogen.

Quality control. See Campylobacter agar in Table 3-3.

REFERENCE

Blaser, M.J., et al.: *Campylobacter* enteritis: clinical and epidemiologic features, Ann. Intern. Med. **91:**179, 1979.

CAMPYLOBACTER THIOGLYCOLATE (CAMPY THIO) BROTH

Purpose. Campylobacter thioglycolate (Campy Thio) broth is useful as a selective enrichment broth for cultivation of *Campylobacter* organisms from specimens containing mixed species of bacteria. It is also useful as a holding or transport medium to be employed when facilities are not immediately available for incubation and culture of clinical specimens.

Principle and interpretation. This broth medium is similar to Campy blood agar in that it contains a reducing agent to enhance growth of, and antimicrobial agents to select for, *Campylobacter* spp. The semisolid broth also provides for a microaerophilic environment in the deeper regions of the tube medium.

Ingredients and preparation. Mix the basal ingredients, heat to boiling, sterilize at 121° C, and cool to 50° C. To the cooled basal medium add sheep blood, vancomycin, trimethoprim, polymyxin B, amphotericin B, and cephalothin (optional). Dispense into Petri plates and allow the medium to solidify at room temperature.

Basal medium:

Thioglycolate medium without indicator (BBL Microbiology Systems, Cockeysville, Md.)	30 g
Agar	0.9 g
Distilled water	900 ml

Final pH 7.0

Additives to sterile, cooled, (50° C), basal medium:

Sheep blood, defibrinated	100 ml

Vancomycin	10 mg
Trimethoprim	5 mg
Polymyxin B	2500 IU
Amphotericin B	2 mg
Cephalothin (optional)	15 mg

Procedure. Specimens are inoculated into Campy Thio broth, refrigerated for 48 hours, and then subcultured to Campy blood agar. Inoculated broths may be held about 1 week without significant loss in colony-forming units of *Campylobacter* spp. if the temperature of incubation is maintained near 5°C. Most species of bacteria normally present in fecal specimens either begin to die off at this temperature or do not grow.

Quality control. See Table 3-3.

REFERENCES

See Campylobacter blood agar.

CARBOHYDRATE FERMENTATION MEDIUM FOR AEROBIC GRAM-NEGATIVE AND GRAM-POSITIVE RODS

Purpose. Carbohydrate fermentation medium is recommended for testing the ability of aerobic gram-negative rods and gram-positive rods to ferment carbohydrates.

Principle and interpretation. This medium contains peptone, sodium chloride, and Andrade indicator. It is not a nutritionally rich medium and is not suitable for testing the fermentative ability of fastidious aerobic bacteria, such as species of *Streptococcus*. The medium is suitable, however, for members of the less fastidious *Enterobacteriaceae*. Incorporation of Andrade indicator allows detection of carbohydrate fermentation. A positive test for fermentation is indicated by a change in color of the medium from yellow or colorless (alkaline) to pink or red (acid).

Ingredients and preparation. Mix the following basal ingredients, heat to boiling, and sterilize at 121°C for 15 minutes. Cool to 50°C, and add filter-sterilized solutions of carbohydrates to achieve a final concentration of 1%. Alternatively, as listed below, the carbohydrate may be added directly to the medium. Carbohydrate-impregnated disks are commercially available.

Basal ingredients:

Pancreatic digest of casein, USP	10 g
Test carbohydrate	10 g
Sodium chloride	5 g
Andrade indicator	10 ml
Distilled water	1 L

Final pH 7.4

Reagent. Andrade indicator, the reagent, is prepared as follows. Dissolve fuchsin in distilled water, and then add sodium hydroxide solution. If after several hours the fuchsin has not decolorized from a red color to brown, add an additional 1 or 2 ml of alkali, drop by drop, until a straw-yellow color is obtained. The reagent improves through aging.

Acid fuchsin	0.5 g
Sodium hydroxide, 1N	15-18 ml
Distilled water	100 ml

Procedure. Inoculate the test organism to carbohydrate media, and incubate at 35°C for up to 5 days.

Quality control. See carbohydrate fermentation broth (Andrade) in Table 3-7.

CARBOHYDRATE FERMENTATION MEDIUM, NEISSERIA RAPID SUGAR TESTS

Purpose. Carbohydrate fermentation medium is used to determine ability of *Neisseria* spp. to ferment carbohydrates. The test avoids some of the problems associated with agar-based media and is rapid, identifying species of *Neisseria* after 4 hours' incubation.

Principle and interpretation. The rapid sugar test system determines carbohydrate fermentation based on presence of preformed enzymes and thus does not depend on bacterial growth for obtaining suitable test results. The test medium contains a buffering system, a pH indicator, phenol red, and any one of several different carbohydrates. The absence of nutrients other than carbohydrates distinguishes this fermentation system from other systems. A color change from red to distinct yellow within 4 hours' incubation constitutes a positive test for fermentation of that carbohydrate. Maltose media sometimes appear orange after incubation. These results should be interpreted as negative tests for fermentation of maltose by the test organism.

Ingredients and preparation. Prepare the following four reagents as directed. Store frozen until ready for use. For every 100 tubes of carbohydrate medium to be prepared, thaw one tube (about 4 ml) of carbohydrate solution and one tube (30 ml) of buffer solution. Mix together and dispense 0.3 ml aliquots into each of 100 small, capped tubes. Label each tube, date each rack of tubes, and freeze the medium at −20°C. Use within 8 months of preparation.

Carbohydrate solutions, 20%:

Carbohydrate (glucose, maltose, sucrose, or lactose) (Difco Laboratories, Detroit)	8 g
Distilled water	40 ml

The dextrose, sucrose, and lactose solutions may be slightly heated to dissolve. *Do not* heat maltose. The maltose selected for use should be certified as chemically pure, without trace of dextrose. Filter sterilize the carbohydrate solutions, and dispense 4.2 to 4.4 ml amounts into sterile capped tubes. These solutions may be stored 8 weeks at 2° to 8°C or for 2 years at −20°C. Carbohydrate-impregnated disks are also commercially available.

Phenol red solution, 1%:

Phenol red	0.5 g
Sodium hydroxide, 0.1 N	10 ml
Distilled water	40 ml

Filter sterilize and store in sterile tubes.

Sodium hydroxide, 0.1 N:

| Sodium hydroxide | 0.4 g |
| Distilled water | 100 ml |

Buffer, pH 7.0:

Dipotassium phosphate	0.4 g
Monopotassium phosphate	0.1 g
Potassium chloride	8 g
Phenol red solution, 1%	3 ml
Distilled water	1 L

Final pH 7.0

Dispense 30 ml amounts in sterile 50 ml tubes. Store up to 8 weeks at 2° to 8° C or for 2 years at −20° C.

Procedure. Heavily inoculate media with the test organism, incubate at 35° C in a water or dry bath incubator, and examine for evidence of color change at 4 hours' incubation.

Quality control. See carbohydrate utilization media for *Neisseria*, in Table 3-7.

CATALASE TEST FOR MYCOBACTERIA AND OTHER SPECIES OF BACTERIA

Purpose. The catalase test is useful for distinguishing among species of bacteria based on abililty to produce the enzyme catalase.

Principle. Catalase is one of several enzymes capable of degrading hydrogen peroxide to water and oxygen. Presence of the enzyme in bacteria is detected by adding hydrogen peroxide to a culture of the test organism and observing for formation of bubbles of oxygen, a positive test for the enzyme. The test should not be done on media containing red blood cells, since these cells contain catalase and false-positive results may occur. Colonies growing on blood agar should be carefully removed to avoid carryover of red blood cells when the test is to be done on a glass slide.

The catalase test is especially useful for distinguishing between the genera *Staphylococcus* and *Streptococcus*, the first having an active catalase and the last not having the enzyme. Species of *Mycobacterium* may also be identified using the catalase test. All mycobacteria except *M. gastri* and isoniazid-resistant strains of *M. tuberculosis* produce catalase. Species of catalase-producing mycobacteria may be further distinguished by the quantity of enzyme produced and the ability of the enzyme to resist inactivation at 68° C. The quantity of enzyme produced is measured by determining the height of a column of oxygen bubbles produced after adding hydrogen peroxide to a Lowenstein-Jensen (LJ) culture of the test organism. This test is the semiquantitative catalase test.

Procedure

***STAPHYLOCOCCUS* AND *STREPTOCOCCUS* CATALASE TEST.** Transfer a colony of the test organism to a clean glass slide, add 1 drop of 3% hydrogen peroxide, and observe for an immediate development of bubbles, a positive test for catalase. The test may also be done by adding 1 ml of 3% hydrogen peroxide to an agar slant culture of the test organism and again observing for production of bubbles.

SEMIQUANTITATIVE CATALASE TEST FOR MYCOBACTERIA. Inoculate the butt of LJ medium (prepared as butts or deeps) with 0.1 ml of a 7-day-old liquid culture of the test organism or a loopful of growth from an actively growing slant.

Incubate the culture at 35° C for 2 weeks. Add 1 ml of Tween-peroxide reagent and allow the tube to rest for 5 minutes at room temperature. Measure the height of the column of bubbles produced. Organisms may be divided into those that produce more then 45 mm of bubbles and those that produce less than 45 mm of bubbles.

68° C CATALASE TEST. Add 0.5 ml of 0.67 M phosphate buffer to each of several screw-capped test tubes. Suspend several spadefuls of growth of the test organism medium to one tube of buffer. Place tube in a 68° C water bath for 20 minutes. Cool the heated suspension to room temperature. Add 0.5 ml of Tween-peroxide reagent and recap tubes loosely. Observe for formation of bubbles. Hold tubes for 20 minutes before reporting as negative.

Reagents

Hydrogen peroxide, 3%: This product is commercially available.

Tween-peroxide reagent: Prepare this solution immediately before performing the test. Mix equal parts of 10% Tween 80 solution and Superoxol (30% hydrogen peroxide). Tween 80, 10%, is prepared by mixing 10 ml of Tween 80 with 90 ml of distilled water and sterilizing at 121° C for 10 minutes.

Quality control. See catalase, 45 mm, and catalase, 68° C, in Table 3-10 and 3% H_2O_2 in Table 3-16.

CETRIMIDE AGAR

Purpose. Cetrimide agar is useful for distinguishing among fluorescent pseudomonads, which grow on this medium, and nonfluorescent pseudomonads, which usually do not.

Principle and interpretation. Cetrimide is a derivative of bromine and has been used as an antiseptic and detergent. Organisms that are able to tolerate this compound can grow in its presence; thus growth is a positive result of the test. No growth is a negative finding.

Ingredients and preparation. Mix the following ingredients and heat to dissolve. Dispense into screw-cap tubes and sterilize at 121° C for 15 minutes. Cool in a slanted position.

Trypticase soy agar	40 g
Hexadecyltrimethyl ammonium bromide (Cetrimide, Eastman Kodak Co., Rochester, N.Y.)	0.9 g
Deionized water	1 L

Final pH 7.0 ± 0.2

Procedure. The slant may be inoculated with 1 drop or loopful of a broth or saline suspension of the test organism (allowing the drop to run down the slant) or by streaking the slant with a portion of a colony. Incubate the slant overnight at 35° C and observe for growth. Reincubate tubes in which findings are negative for an additional 24 hours.

Quality control. See Table 3-7. *Acinetobacter anitratus* may also be used as a negative control.

REFERENCE

Oberhofer, T.R.: Manual of nonfermenting gram-negative bacteria, New York, 1985, John Wiley & Sons, Inc.

CHOCOLATE AGAR

Purpose. Chocolate agar (CA) is a nonselective agar medium enriched with heated defibrinated sheep blood.

Principle and interpretation. CA is similar to sheep blood agar in composition. However, heating of the blood in CA releases red cell components, for example, hemoglobin and nicotinamide adenine dinucleotide, which enhance growth of *Haemophilus* and other fastidious species of bacteria.

Preparation and ingredients. Mix the basal ingredients, heat to boiling, sterilize at 121° C for 15 minutes, and cool to 70° C. Add defibrinated sheep blood to the sterile basal medium, and heat the mixture to 80° C for 15 minutes or until the medium turns brown. Cool the mixture to 50° C and pour into Petri plates.

Basal medium:

Pancreatic digest of casein and peptic digest of animal tissue, USP	15 g
Cornstarch	1 g
Sodium chloride	5 g
Dipotassium phosphate	4 g
Monopotassium phosphate	1 g
Agar	10 g
Distilled water	1 L

Final pH 7.3

Additive to cooled (70° C) basal medium: Add 50 to 100 ml defibrinated sheep blood. Alternatively, 2% hemoglobin and chemical supplements such as IsoVitaleX, may be added to the basal medium in lieu of the sheep blood.

Procedure. Inoculate a clinical specimen or colony to the medium, streak for isolation, and incubate in carbon dioxide at 35° C.

Quality control. See Table 3-3.

CHOPPED MEAT MEDIUM AND CHOPPED MEAT GLUCOSE MEDIUM

Purpose. Chopped meat medium supports the growth of most obligate anaerobes and is useful as a holding medium for cultures or as a medium for sporulation, proteolysis, or toxin production by clostridia. Chopped meat glucose, which is prepared by adding glucose to chopped meat medium, is an excellent enrichment broth for anaerobes and also may be used to demonstrate sporulation or production of toxins by clostridia. Many aerobes, facultative anaerobes, and microaerophilic bacteria also grow in chopped meat glucose.

Principle and interpretation. Both media contain large amounts of animal meat and enrichments, such as yeast extract, hemin, and vitamin K_1, to enhance growth of fastidious bacteria. L-Cysteine functions as a reducing agent.

Ingredients and preparation. Remove fat and connective tissue from fresh, lean beef. Grind the meat and add 500 g to 1 L of distilled water. Add 25 ml of 1 N sodium hydroxide and heat to boiling. Cool the mixture and refrigerate overnight at 4° C. Skim fat from the surface, and filter the mixture through two layers of gauze. Save the meat fragments and liquid filtrate. Wash the meat fragments with distilled water to remove excess sodium hydroxide and add enough distilled water to the filtrate to give a final volume of 1 L. Add all the basal components except L-cysteine to the filtrate, heat to dissolve, and cool to 50° C. Add the L-cysteine and mix to dissolve. Adjust the pH of the medium to 7.4.

Dispense 0.5 g of meat fragments and 7 ml of enriched filtrate to each tube, and sterilize at 121° C for 15 minutes. After tubes of medium cool, loosen the screw caps and place the tubes in a chamber containing an atmosphere of 85% nitrogen, 10% hydrogen, and 5% carbon dioxide. Tighten the caps and remove the tubes from the chamber. Store at 4° C or ambient temperature. If an anaerobic chamber is not available, the tubes of medium can be prepared and boiled for 10 minutes on the day of use.

Basal components:

Pancreatic digest of casein, USP	30 g
Yeast extract	5 g
Potassium monohydrogen phosphate	5 g
Hemin, 1% solution*	0.5 ml
Vitamin K_1, 1% solution*	0.1 ml
L-Cysteine	0.5 g

Final pH 7.4

NOTE: The basal components of chopped meat glucose are identical except for the addition of 3 g of D-glucose.

Procedure. Inoculate specimens to chopped meat medium or chopped meat glucose medium and incubate up to 7 days at 35° C.

Quality control. See cooked meat broth (with or without carbohydrate) in Table 3-4.

REFERENCE

Dowell, V.R., Jr., et al.: Media for characterization and identification of obligately anaerobic bacteria, Atlanta, 1981, Centers for Disease Control.

CITRATE AGAR, SIMMONS

Purpose. Simmons citrate agar is used to distinguish gram-negative bacteria based on their ability to utilize citrate as a sole source of carbon.

Principle and interpretation.† Organisms that utilize citrate as a sole source of carbon cleave citrate to oxaloacetate and acetate via the citritase enzyme. Another enzyme, oxaloacetate decarboxylase, then coverts oxaloacetate to pyruvate and carbon dioxide. Carbon dioxide combines with sodium and water to form sodium carbonate, an alkaline compound. As a result, the pH of the medium rises and the indicator (bromthymol blue) changes from green to Prussian blue. Presence of the blue color constitutes a positive finding for citrate utilization.

Ingredients and preparation. Mix the following ingredients, heat to boiling, dispense into test tubes, and sterilize at 121° C for 15 minutes. Cool each tube of medium in a slanted position.

Sodium citrate	2 g
Sodium chloride	5 g
Magnesium sulfate	0.2 g

---

*Preparation of hemin and vitamin K_1 solutions is described in the section "Blood Agar, Anaerobic (CDC)."

†Several theories have been proposed to explain the mechanism of citrate agar. Only one is presented here.

Ammonium dihydrogen phosphate	1 g
Dipotassium phosphate	1 g
Bromthymol blue	80 mg
Agar	15 g
Distilled water	1 L

Final pH 6.9

Procedure. Lightly inoculate the test organism to the surface of citrate medium, incubate at 35° C for 24 to 48 hours, and observe for a Prussian blue color change.

Quality control. See Table 3-7.

COAGULASE TEST

Purpose. The coagulase test is used to distinguish coagulase-producing *S. aureus* from other species of *Staphylococcus*.

Principle. The enzyme coagulase exists in two forms. One form, bound coagulase, is bound to the cell wall of *S. aureus*, is detected with a slide test, and is not present in broth culture filtrates. Bound coagulase acts directly on fibrinogen to produce an insoluble fibrin clot. The second form, extracellular coagulase, is excreted by the cell, is detected with a tube test, and is present in culture filtrates. In contrast to bound coagulase, extracellular coagulase reacts with coagulase-reacting factor (CRF) to produce coagulase-CRF complex, a substance clinically indistinguishable from thrombin. This complex then acts on fibrinogen to produce an insoluble fibrin clot.

Procedure

SLIDE TEST FOR BOUND COAGULASE. Emulsify a *dense* suspension of the test organism in a drop of 0.85% saline on a clean glass slide. If autoagglutination occurs, do not continue, but use the tube test instead. Mix a loopful of undiluted EDTA-treated rabbit plasma into the suspension and observe for formation of a white, flaky fibrin precipitate. Development of the precipitate constitutes a positive test for production of bound coagulase. Negative and delayed results (20 to 60 seconds) should be confirmed with the tube test. An autoagglutination control may also be used to decrease the number of false-positive reactions.

TUBE COAGULASE TEST. Add 0.5 ml of diluted rabbit plasma to a sterile tube. Inoculate one loopful of the test organism growing on an agar medum, or 0.1 ml of a broth culture, to the tube of plasma. Incubate the culture at 35° C in a water bath or heating block and observe every 30 minutes during the first 4 hours for evidence of clot formation. Clotting constitutes a positive finding for coagulase production. Incubate tubes of plasma in which results are negative overnight at room temperature for detection of delayed or weak production of coagulase.

Reagents. To prepare rabbit plasma reagent, rehydrate commercially packaged EDTA-treated rabbit plasma according to manufacturer's directions. Dilute the plasma 1:4 with distilled water for the tube test. Dispense diluted and undiluted plasma in 0.5 ml amounts into screw-cap tubes and store frozen until ready to use.

Quality control. See coagulase plasma in Table 3-16. Tubes of plasma should also be tested for proper reactivity by adding 1 drop of 5% calcium chloride and observing for clot formation.

COLUMBIA AGAR

Purpose. Columbia agar is a nutrient growth medium for cultivation of many species of aerobic and anaerobic bacteria found in clinical specimens.

Principle and interpretation. Columbia agar is a nutrient basal medium containing protein, sodium chloride, and cornstarch. Special additives, such as vitamin K_1, hemin, and defibrinated sheep blood, enhance the medium's ability to support growth of fastidious aerobic and anaerobic bacteria.

Ingredients and preparation. Mix the following basal ingredients, heat to boiling, and sterilize at 121° C for 15 minutes.

Basal medium:

Pancreatic digest of casein and peptic digest of animal tissue, USP	10 g
Pancreatic digest of casein and yeast autolysate, USP	10 g
Pancreatic digest of heart muscle, USP	3 g
Cornstarch	1 g
Sodium chloride	5 g
Agar	13.5 g
Distilled water	1 L

Final pH 7.3

Additives following sterilization of basal medium (individual additives will vary according to specific organism to be isolated):

Vitamin K_1, final concentration, 10 μg/ml
Hemin,[*] final concentration, 5 μg/ml
Defibrinated sheep blood, 50 ml

Procedure. Inoculate a clinical specimen or colony to the medium and streak for isolation. Incubate at 35° C for up to 7 days, depending on the specimen.

Quality control. Test sample plates of medium from each batch with the following organism and observe for expected results:

Bacteroides melaninogenicus—growth

COLUMBIA COLISTIN–NALIDIXIC ACID AGAR

Purpose. Columbia colistin–nalidixic acid (CNA) agar is a selective medium useful for isolation of streptococci and staphylococci from clinical specimens containing mixed species of bacteria.

Principle and interpretation. CNA agar contains Columbia agar base (see above). The selectivity of the medium is attributed to colistin (polymyxin E) and nalidixic acid. Polymyxins are basic polypeptide antimicrobial agents that irreversibly injure bacterial cell membranes. Although gram-positive bacteria have generally been considered resistant and gram-negative bacteria susceptible to polymyxins, this has proved to be untrue with some strains of coagulase-negative staphylococci, which are susceptible. Thus CNA agar should not be used as the sole medium for isolation of staphylococci if both coagulase-posi-

---

[*]See "Blood Agar, Anaerobic (CDC)" for preparation of vitamin K_1 and hemin solutions.

tive and coagulase-negative strains are sought. Nalidixic acid is an antimicrobial agent that interferes with deoxyribonucleic acid (DNA) replication and membrane integrity of gram-negative bacteria.

Ingredients and preparation. Mix the following ingredients, heat to boiling, and sterilize at 121° C for 15 minutes. Cool to 45° C and then add 50 ml of defibrinated sheep blood and 5 ml of a solution containing 10 mg of colistin and 10 to 15 mg of nalidixic acid.

Pancreatic digest of casein and peptic digest of animal tissue, USP	10 g
Pancreatic digest of casein and yeast autolysate, USP	10 g
Pancreatic digest of heart muscle, USP	3 g
Cornstarch	1 g
Sodium chloride	5 g
Agar	13.5 g
Distilled water	1 L

Final pH 7.3

Procedure. Inoculate the specimen to CNA agar, streak for isolation, and incubate at 35° C for 18 to 24 hours.

Quality control. See Table 3-3.

REFERENCE

Fung, J.C., et al.: Growth of coagulase-negative staphylococci on colistin-nalidixic acid agar and susceptibility to polymyxins, J. Clin. Microbiol. **19:**714, 1984.

CYCLOSERINE-CEFOXITIN-FRUCTOSE AGAR

Purpose. Cycloserine-cefoxitin-fructose (CCFA) agar is a selective and differential medium recommended for isolation of *Clostridium difficile* from stool specimens.

Principle and interpretation. CCFA agar is a buffered, protein-rich agar medium containing enrichments, fructose, egg yolk, cycloserine, and cefoxitin. The latter two antimicrobial agents are inhibitors of cell wall synthesis and inhibit gram-positive and gram-negative bacteria present in fecal specimens but do not affect the growth of *C. difficile*, which grows on the medium as yellow colonies, 1.5 to 9 mm in diameter, with a ground-glass appearance. The yellow pigmentation of colonies is due to a color change of the indicator from red to yellow, which is brought about by acids produced during fermentation of fructose. Addition of egg yolk to the medium allows detection of lipase and lecithinase activity. Bacteria that produce lipase produce an iridescent sheen or "pearl" zone around the area of growth, and bacteria that produce lecithinase cause an opaque zone to occur immediately surrounding the colonies. Colonies of *C. difficile* exhibit neither lipase nor lecithinase activity but do fluoresce when viewed with ultraviolet light.

Ingredients and preparation. Mix the following basal ingredients, bring to boiling, dispense into 100 ml bottles, sterilize at 121° C for 15 minutes, and store in aerobic conditions at 4° C. To prepare plate media, melt 100 ml of basal medium and cool to 50° C. Mix the egg yolk, cycloserine, and cefoxitin solutions into the CCFA basal medium and dispense into Petri plates. Store plates of medium in plastic bags at 4° C.

Basal medium:

Peptic digest of animal tissue, USP	40 g
Sodium monohydrogen phosphate	5 g
Potassium dihydrogen phosphate	1 g
Sodium chloride	2 g
Magnesium sulfate, anhydrous	0.1 g
Fructose	6 g
Neutral red, 1% in ethanol	3 ml
Agar	20 g
Distilled water	1 L

Final pH 7.3

Additives to cooled basal medium:

Cycloserine added to final concentration of 500 µg/ml
Cefoxitin added to basal medium to final concentration of 16 µg/ml
Egg yolk, 50% suspension in saline, 5 ml added per 100 ml of basal medium

Procedure. Dilute the stool 1:10, 1:100, and 1:1000. Plate out 0.1 to 0.2 ml of each dilution of stool. Incubate cultures at 35° C, in anaerobic conditions, for 48 hours or more.

Quality control. Test sample plates of medium from each batch with the following organism and observe for expected results:

Clostridium difficile—yellow colonies with yellow fluorescence

REFERENCE

Lance, W.G., et al.: Selective and differential medium for isolation of *Clostridium difficile*, J. Clin. Microbiol. **9:**214, 1979.

CYSTINE TELLURITE AGAR

Purpose. Cystine tellurite agar is used for the isolation of *Corynebacterium diphtheriae*.

Principle and interpretation. The presence of tellurite salts selects for the growth of *C. diphtheriae*. It inhibits the growth of most upper respiratory tract normal flora, including most gram-negative organisms and most species of staphylococci and streptococci. Differentiation among the types of *C. diphtheriae* is based on the reduction of tellurite salts. The *gravis* type appears as large, flat, dry, dark gray–black colonies with irregular edges and radial striations. The *mitis* type appears as small, convex, moist-appearing, black, shiny colonies with entire edges, and the *intermedius* type as small, flat, raised, black colonies with gray borders.

Ingredients and preparation

Heart infusion agar, 2%	100 ml
Potassium tellurite (K_2TeO_3), 0.3%	15 ml
Sheep blood	5 ml
L-Cystine (powder)	5 mg

Melt 100 ml of sterile 2% infusion agar in a flask and cool to 45° to 50° C. Maintain this temperature throughout preparation of the medium. Add 15 ml of 0.3% solution of potassium tellurite in distilled water that has been sterilized by autoclaving. Add 5 ml of sterile sheep blood. Mix well, and add the L-cystine. Mix the medium thoroughly, and pour into sterile Petri dishes. Shake the flask frequently while pouring, since cystine does not go into solution completely.

Procedure. Inoculate and incubate at 35° C in 10% carbon dioxide for 24 to 48 hours.

Quality control. Test sample tubes of medium with the following organisms, and observe for indicated results:

C. diphtheriae—growth (differentiation of types is noted above)

Staphylococcus epidermidis—no growth

CYSTINE TRYPTIC AGAR MEDIUM

Purpose. Cystine tryptic agar (CTA) medium is used for identifying species of *Neisseria* based on ability to oxidize specific carbohydrates.

Principle and interpretation. CTA medium contains protein, sodium chloride, cystine, sodium sulfite, carbohydrate, a pH indicator, and a small amount of agar. Agar is added to the medium to enhance growth of *Neisseria* organisms that do not grow well in broth media. Oxidation of carbohydrates and subsequent production of organic acids are evidenced by a change in the color of phenol red in the medium from red (neutral or alkaline) to yellow (acid).

Ingredients and preparation. Mix the following basal ingredients, heat to boiling, and sterilize at 118° C for 15 minutes. Cool to 50° C and add filter-sterilized carbohydrate solution. Adjust the volume of distilled water used in preparation of the basal medium to account for the volume of carbohydrate solution added. The final concentration of carbohydrates should be 1%. Allow tubes of medium to solidify in a slanted position.

Basal ingredients:

L-Cystine	0.5 g
Pancreatic digest of casein, USP	20 g
Sodium chloride	5 g
Sodium sulfite	0.5 g
Phenol red	17 mg
Agar	2.5 g
Distilled water	1 L

Final pH 7.3

Carbohydrate solution, filter-sterilized: See ''Anaerobic Carbohydrate Medium'' for preparation of sterile solutions of glucose, maltose, sucrose, lactose, and fructose. Add enough carbohydrate solution to sterile, cooled basal medium to obtain a final concentration of 1% carbohydrate.

Procedure. Inoculate the test organism as discussed in Chapter 14, incubate at 35° C in a non–carbon dioxide incubator, and observe for evidence of fermentation of the test carbohydrate after 18 to 20 hours. Tubes that show growth without acid production should be reincubated and examined daily for up to 5 days. Noninoculated tubes of medium should be incubated along with inoculated tubes for comparison of subtle color changes that may occur.

Quality control. See carbohydrate utilization media for *Neisseria*, Table 3-7.

CYTOTOXICITY ASSAY FOR DETECTION OF THE TOXIN OF *CLOSTRIDIUM DIFFICILE*

Principle. Detection of the toxin of *Clostridium difficile* by a tissue culture cytotoxicity assay is the standard method and the most definitive method for the laboratory diagnosis of *C. difficile*–associated disease (see Chapter 20). As discussed in Chapter 20 this technique involves preparing cell-free fecal extracts, demonstrating that these extracts produce a cytopathic effect (owing to toxin) in cell culture lines, and showing that this effect is neutralized by antitoxin.

Procedure. Prepare tissue culture cells, culture filtrate, standard antitoxin, and fecal filtrate as follows.

Tissue culture cells: Distribute tissue culture cells (Chinese hamster ovary cells) in growth medium (F12, 2% fetal calf serum) to microtiter plates. An amount of 180 μL contains approximately 1000 cells per well. Incubate 4 to 6 hours for attachment.

Culture filtrate: Add 1 ml sterile distilled water to freeze-dried standard toxin (culture filtrate). Prepare 10-fold dilutions (10^{-1} to 10^{-6}) in sterile phosphate buffer (0.01 M, pH 6.9).

Standard antitoxin:* Resuspend freeze-dried antitoxin in 3 ml sterile distilled water (should be distributed in small aliquots and frozen). Dilute 1:25 with sterile phosphate buffer.

Fecal filtrate: Use undiluted fecal sample for loose stools or dilute 1:1 with phosphate buffer (0.01 M, pH 6.9). Centrifuge at $27,000 \times$ g for 10 minutes. Filter sterilize supernatant fraction with a 0.45 μm membrane filter. Prepare 10-fold dilutions (10^{-1} to 10^{-8}) in sterile phosphate buffer.

TOXIN ASSAY

1. Mix the toxin dilutions (culture filtrate) 1:1 with the diluted antitoxin. *Control:* Mix the toxin dilutions 1:1 with sterile phosphate buffer.

2. Mix the fecal filtrate dilutions 1:1 with diluted antitoxin. *Control:* Mix the fecal filtrate dilutions 1:1 with sterile phosphate buffer. Neutral sera mixed with culture filtrate and fecal filtrates may be used as a better control.

3. Incubate the toxin dilutions and control and the fecal filtrate dilutions and control for 30 minutes at room temperature (22° C).

4. Using a micropipette and new tips for each dilution:
   a. Add 20 μL of each dilution of the culture filtrate to the wells with the tissue culture cells. Also add 20 μL of each culture filtrate control to the wells with the tissue culture cells.
   b. Add 20 μL of each dilution of the fecal filtrate to the wells with the tissue culture cells. Also add 20 μL of each fecal filtrate control to the wells with the tissue culture cells.

5. Incubate the tissue culture cells overnight (18 hours) at 37° C in 5% CO_2 and then observe the condition of the cells. The cells may be observed directly using an inverted microscope or they may be fixed, stained, and observed using a standard microscope. The cytotoxin causes cell rounding. The criterion for toxicity is 100% rounding.

Interpretation

CULTURE FILTRATE. Cytotoxicity is neutralized at all but

---

*Antitoxin and toxin are available from the Department of Anaerobic Microbiology, Virginia Polytechnic Institute and State University, Blacksburg, VA 24061.

the highest concentrations of culture filtrate. *Control:* Cytotoxin is not neutralized.

FECAL FILTRATE. If *C. difficile* cytotoxin is present, cytotoxity is neutralized. If the antitoxin fails to neutralize the cytotoxic effect of the fecal filtrate, the result is negative for the toxin of *C. difficile. Control:* Cytotoxicity may be observed; it may or may not be due to the cytotoxin of *C. difficile.*

REFERENCE

Research protocol for testing stool samples for the presence of the toxin of *C. difficile,* Blacksburg, Va., 1979, Department of Anaerobic Microbiology, Virginia Polytechnic Institute and State University.

DECARBOXYLASE MEDIA (MOELLER) AND RAPID LYSINE AND ORNITHINE DECARBOXYLASE TESTS
MOELLER DECARBOXYLASE MEDIA TEST

Purpose. Decarboxylase media, containing lysine, arginine, or ornithine, are recommended for differentiation of fermentative and nonfermentative gram-negative bacteria based on their ability to decompose these amino acids into alkaline products.

Principle and interpretation. Many species of bacteria degrade amino acids to alkaline amines and carbon dioxide. L-Lysine is decarboxylated to cadaverine by the enzyme lysine decarboxylase, and L-ornithine is decarboxylated to putrescine by the enzyme ornithine decarboxylase. Two enzymes may be involved in the degradation of L-arginine to the alkaline amine putrescine. These enzymes, arginine decarboxylase and arginine dihydrolase, may act separately or simultaneously.

Moeller decarboxylase media contains one of three amino acids (lysine, ornithine, or arginine), glucose, and the indicator bromcresol purple. During the early stages of incubation, members of the *Enterobacteriaceae* ferment the small amounts of glucose, producing a yellow color. The fermentation of glucose results in a lowering of the pH so the optimal hydrogen ion concentration for decarboxylase activity is reached. Subsequent degradation of the amino acid to form amines results in an increase in pH and a change in the color of the indicator from yellow to purple.

It is important that controls be tested. The control contains all ingredients with the exception of the amino acid. During testing for the *Enterobacteriaceae,* the control should turn yellow because of fermentation of glucose.

Nonfermentative organisms do not ferment glucose and thus do not produce the initial yellow color change. Utilization of the amino acid by these organisms is indicated by a reversion to a deeper purple color when compared with the control tube, which remains unchanged in color.

Because proteins are composed of amino acids, the protein content of the medium is kept low to avoid alkalinization of the medium from oxidative deamination of protein. The medium is also overlaid with sterile mineral oil to seal it from atmospheric oxygen, which is required for deamination of proteins.

Ingredients and preparation. Mix the following ingredients, heat to boiling, sterilize at 121° C for 15 minutes, and dispense into tubes.

Pancreatic hydrolysate of gelatin, USP	5 g
Beef extract	5 g
Bromcresol purple	0.1 g
Cresol red	0.005 g
Dextrose	0.5 g
Pyridoxal	0.005 g
Amino acid (L-lysine, L-arginine, or L-ornithine)	10 g
Distilled water	1 L

Final pH 6.0

For amino acid, add 10 mg (final concentration = 1%) of the L form of the amino acid. Alternatively, add 2% (final concentration) of DL-amino acids.

Procedure. Inoculate the medium with the test organism. Overlay with sterile mineral oil. Incubate inoculated tubes for 4 days at 35° C. A tube of medium without amino acid should be used as a control.

Quality control. See Table 3-7.

RAPID LYSINE AND ORNITHINE DECARBOXYLASE TESTS

More rapid results can be obtained by using the following modified medium that contains less protein and no glucose. A larger inoculum of the test organism is also used.

Ingredients and preparation

Peptone (Difco Laboratories, Detroit)	5 g
Yeast extract (Difco Laboratories)	3 g
0.2% (wt/vol) bromcresol purple in 50% ethanol	5 ml
Distilled water	1 L

Heat to dissolve completely and add 10 g of L-ornithine hydrochloride or 10 g of L-lysine monohydrochloride. Adjust medium to pH 5.5 with hydrochloric acid and sterilize by autoclaving. Dispense 1 ml volumes into 12 × 75 mm tubes.

Procedure. Inoculate 1 ml of broth with a single colony. Overlay the broth with at least 0.5 ml of sterile mineral oil. Incubate at 35° C for 2 to 4 hours. A dark purple color is a positive reaction for lysine or ornithine decarboxylation. A negative result is a yellow color resulting from metabolism of substrates in yeast extract and peptone.

REFERENCES

Barry, A.L.: Simple and rapid methods for bacterial identifications, Clin. Lab. Med. **5:**3, 1985.

Brooker, D.C., Lund, M.E., and Blazevic, D.J.: Rapid test for lysine decarboxylase activity in *Enterobacteriaceae,* Appl. Microbiol. **26:**622, 1973.

Brooks, K., and Sodeman, T.: A rapid method for determining decarboxylase and dihydrolase activity, J. Clin. Pathol. **27:**148, 1974.

Fay, G.D., and Barry, A.L.: Rapid ornithine decarboxylase test for the identification of *Enterobacteriaceae,* Appl. Microbiol. **23:**710, 1972.

DEOXYCHOLATE AGAR

Purpose. Deoxycholate (DC) agar is a differential medium of low selectivity for isolation and differentiation of members of the family *Enterobacteriaceae.*

Principle and interpretation. This medium contains protein, salts, buffer, pH indicator, sodium deoxycholate, and lactose. The citrate salts and sodium deoxycholate inhibit growth of gram-positive organisms but allow the gram-negative bacilli to grow. Lactose is added to the medium to allow differentiation of lactose-fermenting bacteria, such as *Escherichia coli,* from non-lactose-fermenting species, such as *Salmonella, Proteus,* and *Shigella.* Fermenting strains grow as red to pink colonies. Nonfermenting species grow as colorless colonies.

Ingredients and preparation. Mix the following ingredients, cool to 50° C, and dispense into Petri plates. *Do not sterilize in an autoclave.*

Pancreatic digest of casein, USP	5 g
Peptic digest of animal tissue, USP	5 g
Lactose	10 g
Sodium chloride	5 g
Dipotassium phosphate	2 g
Ferric citrate	1 g
Sodium citrate	1 g
Sodium deoxycholate	1 g
Neutral red	33 mg
Agar	16 g
Distilled water	1 L

Final pH 7.3

Procedure. Inoculate fecal material or enrichment broth directly to DC medium, streak for isolation, and incubate cultures at 35° C in air for 18 to 24 hours. Do not place cultures in a carbon dioxide incubator.

Quality control. Test each batch of medium with the following organisms, and observe for expected results:
E. coli—pink-red colonies
Shigella flexneri—colorless colonies

DEOXYCHOLATE CITRATE AGAR

Purpose. Deoxycholate citrate agar is a selective and differential agar medium recommended for isolation of enteric pathogens directly from feces or indirectly from enrichment broths.

Principle and interpretation. This medium is similar to deoxycholate agar in composition but is moderately more selective for enteric pathogens owing to increased concentrations of both citrate and deoxycholate salts. Sodium deoxycholate at pH 7.3 to 7.5 is inhibitory for gram-positive bacteria. Citrate salts, in the concentration employed in this medium, are inhibitory to gram-positive bacteria and most other normal intestinal organisms.

Differentiation of organisms is based on lactose fermentation as for deoxycholate agar, described previously. Enteric pathogens such as *Salmonella* and *Shigella* spp. appear as colorless colonies, since they do not ferment lactose. Although most of the lactose-fermenting normal intestinal flora are inhibited by the concentrations of deoxycholate and citrate, they may grow as pink to red colonies.

Ingredients and preparation. Mix the following ingredients, heat to boiling, cool to 50° C, and dispense into Petri plates. Allow plates of medium to solidify at room temperature with lids ajar to enhance removal of excess surface moisture.

Infusion from 375 g meat	10 g

Peptic digest of animal tissues, USP	10 g
Lactose	10 g
Sodium citrate	20 g
Ferric citrate	1 g
Sodium deoxycholate	5 g
Neutral red	0.02 g
Agar	17 g
Distilled water	1 L

Final pH 7.3

Procedure. Inoculate the agar surface with either samples of feces or enrichment broth and streak for isolation. Incubate media for 48 hours at 35° C in air before discarding as negative. Do not incubate in carbon dioxide.

Quality control. Test each batch of medium with the following organisms and observe for expected results:
Salmonella typhimurium—colorless colonies
Escherichia coli—small red colonies

DEOXYRIBONUCLEASE TEST

Purpose. DNAse test agar is used to detect DNAse activity in species of aerobic bacteria.

Principle and interpretation. Several methods have been developed to determine DNAse activity: hydrochloric acid precipitation and the toluidine blue and methyl green methods.

The hydrochloric acid (HCl) method is based on the fact that ungraded DNA is precipitated by acid, whereas oligonucleotides liberated by DNAse activity are soluble. The organism is streaked on DNAse test agar, incubated, and flooded with 1 N HCl. If DNA has not been degraded, it precipitates when the acid is added and opaque areas of precipitated DNA appear. However, if DNA has been degraded, the oligonucleotides are dissolved by the acid and a zone of clearing is evident around the bacterial growth.

Toluidine blue and methyl green are metachromatic dyes. When toluidine blue is bound to DNA, the dye appears blue; however, when DNAse activity occurs and DNA is degraded to oligonucleotides, the dye appears rose pink in the area of the medium in which degradation occurred. Similarly, methyl green is green when bound with DNA, but when DNA is hydrolyzed, the methyl green is released and becomes colorless. Toluidine blue is toxic to many species of gram-positive bacteria. Thus, the HCl hydrolysis or methyl green methods should be used to test these bacteria for ability to produce DNAse.

Ingredients and preparation. Mix the ingredients, heat to boiling, sterilize at 121° C for 15 minutes, and dispense into sterile Petri plates.

Deoxyribonucleic acid	2 g
Papaic digest of soybean meal, USP	5 g
Pancreatic digest of casein, USP	15 g
Sodium chloride	5 g
Agar	15 g
Distilled water	1 L

Final pH 7.3

Optional ingredient:

Toluidine blue	100 mg

DNAse reagent, 1 N HCl:

HCl, concentrated	2.8 ml
Distilled water	97.2 ml

Procedure. Inoculate DNAse test agar with the organism, incubate at 35° C for 18 to 24 hours, and flood the plate with 1 N HCl if a metachromatic dye is not included in the medium.

Quality control. See DNAse agar in Table 3-3 for the HCl method. The same organisms may be used with the toluidine blue or methyl green procedures. A positive reaction with toluidine blue is indicated by the production of a bright pink zone around the inoculum; the medium remains clear blue in a negative reaction. With methyl green a positive reaction is indicated by a clearing of the color around the inoculum; the medium remains green in a negative reaction.

REFERENCES

Jeffries, C.D., Holtman, D.F., and Guse, D.G.: Rapid method for determining the activity of microorganisms on nucleic acids, J. Bacteriol. **73:**590, 1957.

Lachica, R.V.F., Hoeprich, P.D., and Franti, C.E. Convenient assay for staphylococcal nuclease by the metachromatic well–agar-diffusion technique, Appl. Microbiol. **24:**920, 1972.

Smith, P.B., Hancock, G.A., and Rhoden, D.L., Improved medium for detecting deoxyribonuclease-producing bacteria, Appl. Microbiol. **18:**991, 1969.

DUBOS TWEEN ALBUMIN BROTH

Purpose. Dubos Tween albumin broth is recommended for isolation of mycobacteria from cerebrospinal and pleural fluids and for cultivation of pure cultures of *Mycobacterium tuberculosis.*

Principle and interpretation. Tween albumin broth contains protein, buffer, salts, polysorbate 80 (Tween 80), bovine plasma albumin fraction V, and asparagine. These ingredients provide the nutrients required by *M. tuberculosis* to obtain maximum growth in vitro. Polysorbate 80 is added to the medium because in its presence virulent strains have been demonstrated to form "cords" and avirulent strains tend to grow more diffusely.

Ingredients and preparation. Mix the basal ingredients, heat to boiling, and sterilize at 121° C for 15 minutes. Divide the basal medium into 180 ml portions, and add 20 ml of albumin enrichment. Dispense into tubes and store at 4° C until ready for use.

Basal medium:

Pancreatic digest of casein, USP	0.5 g
Asparagine	2 g
Monopotassium phosphate	1 g
Disodium phosphate	2.5 g
Ferric ammonium citrate	0.5 g
Magnesium sulfate	0.01 g
Calcium chloride	0.5 mg
Zinc sulfate	0.1 g

Copper sulfate	0.1 g
Tween 80	0.2 g
Distilled water	1 L

Final pH 6.5

Albumin enrichment: Mix the following ingredients to dissolve and sterilize by membrane filtration.

Bovine plasma albumin fraction V	5 g
Sodium chloride, 0.85%	100 ml

Procedure. Inoculate the test organism or clinical specimen, such as cerebrospinal fluid. Incubate the culture at 35° C in carbon dioxide for 7 to 10 days.

Quality control. See 7H9 broth in Table 3-6.

EGG YOLK AGAR

Purpose. Egg yolk agar (EYA) is recommended to distinguish among species of anaerobic and aerobic bacteria based on detection of lecithinase, lipase, and protease activity.

Principle and interpretation. Three major enzymatic activities toward egg yolk may be detected using this medium. Lecithinase activity is observed as a zone of opacity immediately around growth on the medium. Lipase activity results in production of an iridescent sheen on or around the surface of colonies. Protease activity is observed as clearing of the medium around and extending beyond the area of growth. Organisms may possess any one or all of these activities.

Ingredients and preparation. Mix the basal ingredients, heat to boiling, and sterilize at 121° C for 15 minutes. Cool to 50° C, add 50 ml commercial egg yolk emulsion (Difco Laboratories, Detroit) or laboratory-prepared emulsion, mix, and pour into Petri plates. Allow the medium to cool to room temperature, with lids ajar, to enhance removal of excess surface moisture. Store sealed in plastic bags at 4° C.

Basal ingredients:

Pancreatic digest of casein, USP	40 g
Sodium chloride	2 g
Magnesium sulfate	0.1 g
Disodium phosphate	5 g
Monosodium phosphate	1 g
Dextrose	2 g
Hemin solution, 5 mg/ml	1 ml
Agar	20 g
Distilled water	1 L

Final pH 7.6

NOTE: The CDC modification of this medium uses 5 g of $NaHPO_4$, 0.2 ml of 5% aqueous solution of $MgSO_4$, 5 g yeast extract, 25 g agar, 900 ml distilled water, and 100 ml egg yolk suspension (final pH of medium 7.4). The quantities of casein, NaCl, and dextrose are the same. No other ingredients are included.

Procedure. Inoculate the test organism to EYA and incubate at 35° C for 1 to 3 days. To perform the Nagler test, smear one half of the hardened agar surface with a few drops of *Clostrid-*

ium perfringens type A antitoxin (Wellcome Animal Health, Kansas City, Kan.). Streak the test organism in a single line across both halves of the plate at a right angle to the antitoxin. Incubate in an anaerobic environment for 24 to 48 hours. Inhibition of lecithinase production on the half of the plate with the antitoxin is a positive reaction and is exhibited by the clostridia *C. perfringens*, *C. baratii*, *C. bifermentans*, and *C. sordellii*. Differentiation of these four species is discussed in Chapter 20. Lecithinase is also useful in distinguishing *Bacillus* spp.

Quality control. See Table 3-4.

REFERENCE

Sutter, et al.: Wadsworth anaerobic bacteriology manual, ed. 4, Belmont, Calif., 1985, Star Publishing Co.

ELLINGHAUSEN, MCCULLOUGH, JOHNSON, AND HARRIS BOVINE SERUM ALBUMIN–TWEEN 80 MEDIUM

Purpose. Ellinghausen, McCullough, Johnson, and Harris (EMJH) bovine serum albumin–Tween 80 medium is used for the isolation of *Leptospira* spp.

Principle and interpretation. The lipid and protein present in bovine serum albimin–Tween 80 enhance the growth of *Leptosopira* spp. The addition of 5′-fluorouracil to the bovine serum albumin–Tween 80 medium provides a selective medium that inhibits the growth of many bacteria but does not alter the growth of the *Leptospira* organisms. The latter medium is useful for the isolation of these organisms from contaminated urine samples.

Ingredients and preparation. Reagents used in the preparation of this medium should be analytic grade whenever possible, and high-purity, distilled water should be used. Storage containers for the distilled water should be thoroughly cleaned and sterilized at frequent intervals to minimize the occurrence of microbial growth. Glassware, plasticware, and other types of vessels used for the preparation of the medium and the cultivation of the leptospires should be well washed and thoroughly rinsed; the final rinse should be with distilled water.

Stock solutions (grams per 100 milliliters distilled water):

Ammonium chloride	25
Zinc sulfate · 7 H$_2$O	0.4
Magnesium chloride · 6 H$_2$O	1.5
Calcium chloride · 2 H$_2$O	1.5
Ferrous sulfate · 7 H$_2$O	0.5
Sodium pyruvate	10
Glycerol	10
Tween 80	10
Thiamine · HCl (vitamin B$_1$)	0.5
Cyanocobalamin (vitamin B$_{12}$)	0.02

The pH of the stock solutions need not be adjusted, and the ferrous sulfate solution should be freshly prepared and clear.

Albumin supplement: Dissolve 10 g bovine serum albumin in 50 ml distilled water. While the albumin solution is being stirred, slowly add the following stock solutions:

Calcium chloride and magnesium chloride	1 ml
Zinc sulfate	1 ml
Ferrous sulfate	10 ml
Vitamin B$_{12}$	1 ml
Tween 80	12.5 ml

Adjust pH to 7.4. Add distilled water to bring final volume to 100 ml. Sterilize by filtration.

Basal medium: To 996 ml distilled water add:

Sodium monohydrogen phosphate (anhydrous)	1 g
Potassium dihydrogen phosphate (anhydrous)	0.3 g
Sodium chloride	1 g

After solution of salts has been attained, add the following stock solutions:

Ammonium chloride	1 ml
Thiamine · HCl	1 ml
Sodium pyruvate	1 ml
Glycerol	1 ml

Adjust pH to 7.4. Sterilize by autoclaving at 121° C for 20 minutes.

Liquid medium: Add one volume of albumin supplement to nine volumes of basal medium. Incubate inoculated medium at 30° C.

Semisolid medium: To 900 ml of basal medium add 2 g agar (quality tested). Heat to dissolve agar. Dispense in appropriate volumes. Autoclave at 121° C for 20 minutes. Cool to 50° C. Add one volume prewarmed (45° to 50° C) albumin supplement to nine volumes of the agar-basal medium. Incubate inoculated media at 30° C.

Solid medium: Prepare basal medium as before, except use 496 ml of distilled water. Add 11 g agar to 500 ml distilled water. Autoclave the basal medium and the agar separately at 121° C for 20 minutes. Mix the two solutions and cool to 50° C. Add 100 ml of prewarmed (50° C) albumin supplement to 900 ml of the mixture. Dispense in 30 ml volumes in 100 × 20 mm Petri plates. Seal inoculated plates with tape, and incubate in an inverted position at 30° C.

Selective medium: The bovine serum albumin–Tween 80 medium (liquid, semisolid, or solid) may be converted into a selective medium by the addition of 100 µg/ml of 5′-fluorouracil (5-FU).

Stock solution of 5-FU is made as follows:

1. Add 1 g 5-FU to 50 ml distilled water.
2. Add 1 to 2 ml 2 N NaOH.
3. Heat to dissolve 5-FU.
4. Adjust pH to 7.6.
5. Adjust volume to 100 ml with distilled water.
6. Sterilize by filtration.

Add 0.1 ml 5-FU/10 ml medium. This results in a final concentration of 100 µg 5-FU/ml. Alternatively, 20 ml of the unsterile 5-FU stock solution may be incorporated into the formulation of the albumin supplement.

Procedure. See Chapter 27.

REFERENCES

Ellinghausen, H.C., and McCullough, W.G.: Nutrition of *Leptospira pomona* and growth of 13 other serotypes: fractionation of oleic albumin complex and a medium of bovine albumin and polysorbate 80, Am. J. Vet. Res. **26:**45, 1965.

Johnson, R.C., and Harris, V.G.: Differentiation of pathogenic and sapro-phytic leptospires. I. Growth at low temperatures, J. Bacteriol. **94**:27, 1967.

Johnson, R.C., and Rogers, P.: 5-Fluorouracil as a selective agent for the growth of leptospirae, J. Bacteriol. **87**:422, 1964.

EOSIN–METHYLENE BLUE AGAR

Purpose. Eosin–methylene blue (EMB) agar is used for differentiation and isolation of gram-negative bacilli from mixed populations of bacteria.

Principle and interpretation. This medium contains protein, buffer, dyes, agar, and two carbohydrates. Eosin Y and methylene blue are inhibitory to most species of gram-positive bacteria but have little or no toxicity against gram-negative bacilli. Differentiation of gram-negative bacilli is based on lactose fermentation. Sucrose is added to the medium as an alternative carbohydrate source for typically lactose-fermenting, gram-negative bacilli, which on occasion do not ferment lactose or do so slowly. On EMB agar, *Escherichia coli* produces colonies with a metallic sheen. This phenomenon is not understood, and atypical reactions occur. Lactose and sucrose fermenters form dark-colored colonies. This dark precipitate is probably methylene blue eosinate, which is precipitated as a result of the low pH generated around lactose- or sucrose-fermenting colonies. The dark dye is undoubtedly absorbed into the colony. Nonfermenters probably raise the pH of the surrounding medium by oxidative deamination of protein, which solubilizes the methylene blue–eosin complex and results in colorless colonies.

Ingredients and preparation. Mix the following ingredients, heat to boiling, sterilize at 121° C for 15 minutes, and pour into Petri plates. Allow media to cool to room temperature with lids ajar to enhance removal of excess surface moisture.

Pancreatic hydrolysate of gelatin, USP	10 g
Lactose	5 g
Sucrose	5 g
Dipotassium phosphate	2 g
Eosin Y	0.4 g
Methylene blue	0.065 g
Agar	13.5 g
Distilled water	1 L

Final pH 7.2

Procedure. Inoculate a sample of feces or enrichment broth to EMB agar, streak for isolation, and incubate at 35° C in air for 18 to 24 hours. Do not incubate in carbon dioxide.

Quality control. See Table 3-3.

ESCULIN BROTH

Purpose. Esculin broth is used to determine the ability of bacteria such as *Enterococcus faecalis* and *Listeria monocytogenes* to hydrolyze esculin.

Principle and interpretation. Esculin is a glycoside that is hydrolyzed by certain bacteria into esculetin and dextrose. Hydrolysis of esculin is commonly detected through the use of ultraviolet (UV) light, ferric ammonium citrate reagent, or ferric citrate–esculin media.

Esculin fluoresces in the presence of UV light, but its products of hydrolysis, esculetin and dextrose, do not. Thus a positive test for esculin hydrolysis using UV light would be an absence of fluorescence. Since the compound hydrolyzed, esculin, is fluorescent and its hydrolytic products are not, virtually all the esculin in the medium must be degraded to render the broth nonfluorescent. Therefore, although this method is easy to use, it is the least sensitive of the three methods and can yield false-negative results with bacteria that degrade esculin slowly.

The other two methods rely on ferric salts reacting with esculetin to produce a dark brown to black reaction product. Ferric citrate–esculin medium allows bacteria to grow in the presence of both substrate and indicator. The black reaction product is immediately visible as esculin is degraded. With this medium positive results can be detected in as little as 1 or 2 hours with rapidly hydrolyzing species of bacteria such as *Enterococcus faecalis*. Another method employs ferric ammonium citrate reagent (1% aqueous). After growth of the organism in esculin broth several drops of ferric ammonium citrate are added and development of a brown-black color, a positive finding for esculin hydrolysis, is noted. The disadvantage of this test is that it requires the use of a reagent and results are not visible as hydrolysis of esculin occurs. Esculin broth with ferric citrate is presented here as the medium of choice. It can be supplemented with agar (1.5%) to make an agar medium, or ferric citrate may be omitted from the formulation and ferric ammonium citrate reagent may be used to test for hydrolysis of esculin.

Ingredients and preparation. Mix the following ingredients, heat to boiling, dispense into tubes, and sterilize at 121° C for 15 minutes.

Infusion from 500 g of beef heart	10 g
Peptic digest of animal tissue, USP	10 g
Sodium chloride	5 g
Esculin	1 g
Ferric citrate	0.5 g
Distilled water	1 L

Final pH 7.0

Procedure. Inoculate pure cultures of bacteria into esculin broth and incubate for up to 3 days at 35° C.

Quality control. Test sample tubes of medium from each batch with the anaerobic organisms listed in Table 3-8 and observe for expected results, or test sample tubes of medium from each batch with the following aerobic organisms and observe for expected results:

Enterococcus faecalis—blackening of broth
Streptococcus pyogenes—no color change

FLUORESCEIN-DENITRIFICATION-LACTOSE MEDIUM

Purpose. Fluorescein-denitrification-lactose (FDL) medium is used to distinguish among species of nonfermentative bacilli based on production of fluorescein pigment, reduction of nitrate and nitrite to nitrogen gas, and oxidation of lactose.

Principle and interpretation. FDL medium contains protein, lactose, potassium nitrate, sodium nitrite, magnesium sulfate, additional salts, and agar. Magnesium sulfate is included in the medium to intensify luminescence of the fluorescein pigment. Production of this pigment is detected with an ultraviolet light source, such as Wood's lamp (see discussion of Pseudomonas F agar). Fluorescein cannot be detected visually on FDL medium.

Potassium nitrate and sodium nitrite serve as substrates for denitrifying bacteria. These bacteria reduce nitrate to nitrogen gas. Production of nitrogen gas is indicated by the presence of gas bubbles at the base of the FDL slant and cracking of the agar in the butt.

Oxidation of lactose is observed as a color change of the indicator (phenol red) from red to yellow in response to the accumulation of acid by-products of lactose metabolism.

Ingredients and preparation. Mix the following basal ingredients except for magnesium sulfate ($MgSO_4$) in 900 ml of water, and heat to dissolve. Dissolve $MgSO_4$ in 100 ml of water and add to the basal ingredients. Mix and dispense the mixture into tubes. Sterilize at 121° C for 15 minutes, and allow to cool in a slanted position to give a butt of at least 1 inch.

Basal ingredients:

Peptic digest of animal tissue, USP	10 g
$MgSO_4 \cdot 7 H_2O$	1.5 g
Dipotassium hydrogen phosphate	1.5 g
Potassium nitrate	2 g
Sodium nitrite	0.5 g
Gelatin	5 g
Lactose	30 g
Phenol red, 1.5% solution	2 ml
Agar	12 g
Deionized water	1 L

Final pH 7.2

Procedure. Using a wire needle, pick an isolated colony of an oxidase-positive organism or growth of an oxidase-negative nonfermentative organism on a TSI slant. Smear the inoculum a few millimeters above the base of the slant, and stab the butt of the agar without touching the bottom of the tube. Draw the needle to the heavy inoculum at the base of the slant and streak up the agar slant. Incubate tubes overnight at 35° C.

Observe for cracking of the agar in the butt and formation of bubbles at the base of the slant, both of which indicate the production of nitrogen gas. Also, record any color change from red to yellow occurring on the slant. Determine fluorescein production by holding the slant under an ultraviolet light (366 nm) or a Wood's lamp and observing for fluorescence on all or part of the slant.

Quality control. Test sample tubes of medium from each batch with the organisms listed below and observe for expected results.

- *P. aeruginosa*—denitrification; no acid from lactose; fluorescein produced
- *Acinetobacter anitratus*—no fluorescein or denitrification; acid from lactose
- *P. maltophila*—no acid from lactose; no fluorescein; no denitrification

REFERENCES

Oberhofer, T.R.: Manual of nonfermenting gram-negative bacteria, New York, 1985, John Wiley & Sons, Inc.

Pickett, M.J., and Petersen, M.M.: Characterization of saccharolytic nonfermentative bacilli associated with man, Can. J. Microbiol. **16**:351, 1970.

GELATIN MEDIA

Purpose. Gelatin media are used to determine the ability of bacteria to produce gelatinase, an enzyme that hydrolyzes gelatin, a protein derivative of animal collagen.

Principle and interpretation. Several media may be used to determine the hydrolysis of gelatin. This ability can be detected using starch-gelatin agar, as discussed later in this section. Hydrolysis of gelatin in starch-gelatin agar is determined with the use of mercuric chloride, a gelatin-precipitating agent. When mercuric chloride is added to the starch-gelatin agar, a clear zone appears around the area of growth if gelatin has been hydrolyzed; the medium appears opaque and white beyond the area of gelatinase activity. If the medium becomes opaque and white immediately around the area of bacterial growth, gelatin is being precipitated and thus was not hydrolyzed by the test organism.

Nutrient gelatin medium contains peptone, beef extract, and gelatin. It differs from starch-gelatin agar in its ingredients and the method of detection of gelatin hydrolysis. With nutrient gelatin medium the detection of gelatin hydrolysis is based on the solidification properties of gelatin. Gelatin liquefies at temperatures above 30° C but solidifies at 4° C. When hydrolyzed by the enzyme gelatinase, however, gelatin does not gel when placed at 4° to 5° C. Thus a positive test for hydrolysis of gelatin is the inability of the medium to gel when placed in a refrigerator for 30 minutes as compared with a control that does gel.

Another method for determination of gelatin hydrolysis is the Kohn gelatin method. Charcoal is added to gelatin, and the mixture is allowed to solidify before being treated with formalin. This procedure is based on the fact that formalized gelatin does not melt. A piece of the solidified gelatin-charcoal mixture is then placed in nutrient broth. The broth is inoculated with the test organism and incubated at 37° C for 24 hours. The presence of charcoal particles distributed throughout the medium is a positive test for gelatin hydrolysis, since formalized gelatin does not melt and thus only the presence of gelatinase could hydrolyze the gelatin, causing release of charcoal.

NUTRIENT GELATIN METHOD

Ingredients and preparation. Mix the following ingredients, heat to boiling, dispense into tubes, and sterilize at 121° C for 15 minutes. Store at 4° C.

Pancreatic hydrolysate of gelatin, USP	5 g
Beef extract	3 g
Gelatin	120 g
Distilled water	1 L

Final pH 6.8

Procedure. Inoculate a tube of medium with the test organism, and incubate at 35° C for 18 to 24 hours. A control tube of uninoculated gelatin should also be incubated. Refrigerate the test tube and the control tube at 4° C for 30 minutes. The contents of the control tube should gel. If the medium in the test tube also gels, this is a negative reaction and the tube should be reincubated for an additional 18 to 24 hours and retested. A positive reaction is when the gelatin remains in liquid form. If *Pseudomonas fluorescens* is suspected to be the test organism, incubate the tube at room temperature rather than at 35° C.

Quality control. Test sample tubes of medium from each batch with the following organisms and observe for expected results:

Pseudomonas aeruginosa—medium remains liquid at 4° C
Acinetobacter anitratus—medium gels at 4° C

GLUCONATE BROTH

Purpose. Gluconate broth is useful for distinguishing the fluorescent group of nonfermentative organisms.

Principle and interpretation. Fluorescent pseudomonads oxidize potassium gluconate to the reducing compound, 2-ketogluconate. The latter substance is able to reduce copper sulfate (present in Benedict reagent or Clinitest tablets) to form a yellow-orange precipitate.

Ingredients and preparation. Mix the following ingredients, and heat to dissolve. Dispense into tubes, and sterilize at 121° C for 15 minutes.

Potassium nitrate	2 g
Monopotassium phosphate	5.4 g
Potassium gluconate	20 g
Distilled water	1 L

Final pH 6.5 ± 0.1

NOTE: Gluconate substrate tablets are commercially available.

Procedure. Inoculate a tube of gluconate broth with 1 drop of a broth culture or a portion of an isolated colony. Incubate for 18 to 24 hours at 35° C. Using a sterile pipette, transfer half of the broth culture to another test tube. Add one half of a Clinitest tablet (Ames Co., Div. of Miles Laboratories, Elkhart, Ind.) to one of the broth cultures and observe for the production of a yellow-orange precipitate. If the findings are negative, reincubate the unused portion of the broth culture for an additional 24 hours.

Quality control. Test sample tubes of medium from each batch with the organisms listed below and observe for expected results:

Pseudomonas aeruginosa—yellow-orange precipitate
Acinetobacter anitratus—blue-green broth

REFERENCE

Oberhofer, T.R.: Manual of nonfermenting gram-negative bacteria, New York, 1985, John Wiley & Sons, Inc.

GRAM-NEGATIVE BROTH

Purpose. Gram-negative (GN) broth is useful for enriching and isolating enteric pathogens, such as *Salmonella* and *Shigella* spp., from feces.

Principle and interpretation. This broth medium contains protein, carbohydrate, buffer, and deoxycholate and citrate salts. The salts retard growth of gram-positive organisms but allow aerobic gram-negative bacteria to grow. Increasing the concentration of mannitol over that of glucose favors and enhances the growth of mannitol-fermenting, gram-negative rods, such as *Shigella* and *Salmonella,* over that of mannitol nonfermenting species, particularly during the first 6 hours.

Ingredients and preparation. Mix the following ingredients in 1 L of distilled water, heat the mixture to boiling, and dispense into test tubes. Cap each tube, and sterilize at 116° C for 15 minutes.

Pancreatic digest of casein, USP	10 g
Peptic digest of animal tissue, USP	10 g
D-Glucose	1 g
D-Mannitol	2 g
Sodium citrate	5 g
Sodium deoxycholate	0.5 g
Dipotassium phosphate	4 g
Monopotassium phosphate	1.5 g
Sodium chloride	5 g
Distilled water	1 L

Final pH 7.0

Procedure. Inoculate the medium with a fecal specimen and incubate for 8 to 12 hours at 35° C. After this period of incubation, subculture the broth to the same media used for primary isolation.

Quality control. See enrichment broths for enterics in Table 3-3.

HEKTOEN ENTERIC AGAR

Purpose. Hektoen enteric (HE) agar is a selective and differential medium recommended for direct isolation of enteric pathogens from feces or indirectly after enrichment in selective broth.

Principle and interpretation. HE medium contains protein, bile salts, sodium thiosulfate, ferric ammonium citrate, lactose, sucrose, and the pH indicators acid-fuchsin and thymol blue. The selectivity of the medium is based on the possession of bile salts that inhibit the growth of gram-positive bacteria and retard the growth of many strains of normal intestinal gram-negative organisms.

Gram-negative enteric pathogens and nonpathogens are differentiated according to their ability to ferment lactose and sucrose and to produce hydrogen sulfide. Most of the nonpathogens ferment at least one of the carbohydrates and produce bright orange to salmon pink colonies because of the combination of the yellow color from the bromthymol blue and the red color from the acid-fuchsin when acid is produced. Organisms that do not ferment lactose and sucrose, such as *Salmonella* and *Shigella,* typically appear green or blue-green. Hydrogen sulfide–producing species generate hydrogen sulfide gas from sodium thiosulfate; the gas reacts with ferric ammonium citrate to yield a black precipitate that accumulates within colonies. The reactions are as follows:

Shigella, Providencia—green colonies
Salmonella, Proteus—blue-green to blue colonies with or without black centers
Escherichia coli, Klebsiella, Enterobacter (enteric non-

pathogens)—yellow colonies with bright orange to salmon pink zones surrounding colonies

Ingredients and preparation. Mix the following ingredients, bring just to boiling, cool to 50° C, and dispense into Petri plates. Allow agar to harden for several hours at room temperature with lids ajar to eliminate excess surface moisture.

Peptic digest of animal tissue, USP	12 g
Yeast extract	3 g
Bile salts	9 g
Lactose	12 g
Sucrose	12 g
Salicin	2 g
Sodium chloride	5 g
Sodium thiosulfate	5 g
Ferric ammonium citrate	1.5 g
Bromthymol blue	0.064 g
Acid-fuchsin	0.19 g
Agar	13.5 g
Distilled water	1 L

Final pH 7.6

Procedure. Inoculate samples of feces or enrichment broth to HE agar, streak for isolation, and incubate at 35° C for 18 to 24 hours in air. Do not incubate in carbon dioxide.

Quality control. See Table 3-3.

REFERENCE

King, S., and Metzger, W.I.: A new plating medium for the isolation of enteric pathogens: Hektoen enteric agar, Appl. Microbiol. **16:**577, 1968.

HIPPURATE BROTH

Purpose. Hippurate broth is a nutrient broth used to determine the ability of a microorganism to hydrolyze sodium hippurate, especially for distinguishing among species of *Streptococcus*. Most strains of *S. agalactiae* hydrolyze hippurate, whereas other clinical isolates of beta-hemolytic streptococci do not.

Principle and interpretation. Hippurate broth contains protein, sodium chloride, water, and sodium hippurate. *S. agalactiae* hydrolyzes sodium hippurate to benzoic acid and glycocoll (glycine). Hippuricase is the enzyme responsible for this hydrolytic activity and is a constitutive intracellular or cell-bound enzyme; that is, cell-free filtrates of growth media show no hydrolytic activity. Hippuricase activity is determined using tests for either of the two hydrolytic products.

Benzoic acid is detected by adding ferric chloride to cell-free supernatants and observing for formation of an insoluble precipitate. Both sodium hippurate and benzoic acid are initially precipitated from solution as ferric salts. However, on addition of excess ferric chloride, ferric hippurate redissolves, leaving ferric benzoate as the sole precipitate. A delicate balance exists between the volumetric ratio of ferric chloride reagent and cell-free supernatant needed to obtain accurate results. Thus adequate positive and negative control cultures must be used to

ensure that an excess of ferric ions is present during testing. Several noninoculated tubes should be incubated to serve as negative broth controls. The appropriate amount of ferric chloride reagent needed to reach an excess of ferric ions varies with the amount of hippurate medium being tested and the concentration of sodium hippurate in the medium. Thus the volume of ferric chloride reagent required for optimal testing is determined by adding the reagent to control broths until the ferric hippurate precipitate disappears after resting for 10 minutes. The measured proportions of reagent and broth that are determined using this method are then employed to determine presence of benzoic acid in cell-free broth supernatants of the test, negative control, and positive control cultures. Formation of a precipitate that does not redissolve after resting for 10 minutes is considered a positive finding for hydrolysis of sodium hippurate, that is, presence of benzoic acid in the test broth. Since the concentration of sodium hippurate in the broth affects test results, hippurate broth media should be stored tightly sealed to prevent evaporation during storage.

Glycine, an amino acid and a hydrolytic product of sodium hippurate, may be detected through use of ninhydrin. Ninhydrin is a strong oxidizing agent that oxidatively deaminates the alpha-amino group of glycine and many other amino acids. Ammonia, carbon dioxide, an aldehyde, and reduced ninhydrin are released during oxidation. The ammonia reacts with residual ninhydrin and the reduced ninhydrin, hydrindantin, to form a purple reaction product. Since most growth media contain protein and free amino acids, the ninhydrin test cannot be used to test for hydrolysis of hippurate in protein-containing growth media. This test is performed by placing a heavy inoculum of the organism into 1% aqueous sodium hippurate substrate. The organism-substrate mixture is incubated at 35° C for 4 hours and then tested by adding a measured amount of ninhydrin and observing for a purple color change, which is a positive finding for the hydrolytic product glycine.

Ingredients and preparation. Mix the following ingredients in a liter of distilled water, heat to boiling, dispense into tubes, and sterilize at 121° C for 15 minutes.

Infusion from 375 g heart muscle	10 g
Peptic digest of animal tissues	10 g
Sodium chloride	5 g
Sodium hippurate	10 g
Distilled water	1 L

Final pH 7.4

Reagents
Ferric chloride reagent, 12%:

Ferric chloride	12 g
Hydrochloric acid, concentrated	5.4 ml
Distilled water	94.6 ml

Ninhydrin reagent, 0.1%:

Ninhydrin	0.1g
Distilled water	100 ml

Procedure

FERRIC CHLORIDE TEST. Inoculate the microorganism to hippurate broth, and incubate at 35° C for 48 to 72 hours. After incubation, centrifuge the culture and remove 0.8 ml of the cell-free supernatant to a clean tube. Add 0.2 ml of 12% acid ferric chloride reagent, or the measured amount determined above using broth control tubes, to the supernatant aliquot. Allow the mixture to stand for 10 minutes, and observe for a cloudy precipitate.

NINHYDRIN TEST. Prepare a heavy suspension of the test organism in 3 ml of 1% aqueous sodium hippurate substrate. Incubate the mixture at 35° C for 4 hours. Add 0.5 ml of 0.1% ninhydrin solution to the mixture, and observe for an immediate purple color change.

Quality control. See hippurate hydrolysis in Table 3-7.

REFERENCES

Facklam, R.R., et al.: Presumptive identification of group A, B and D streptococci, Appl. Microbiol. **27:**107, 1973.

Hwang, M., and Ederer, G.M.: Rapid hippurate hydrolysis method for presumptive identification of group B streptococci, J. Clin. Microbiol. **1:**114, 1975.

HYDROGEN SULFIDE, LEAD ACETATE

Purpose. Lead acetate is useful for distinguishing among species of bacteria based on production of hydrogen sulfide from sulfur-containing amino acids.

Principle. Several amino acids, such as cystine, contain sulfur as a molecular component. Some species of bacteria grow in the presence of sulfur-containing amino acids and produce hydrogen sulfide gas. This gas may be detected in a variety of ways; one of these is through the use of lead salts. (See also discussions of hydrogen sulfide motility medium, Kligler iron agar, and lysine iron agar.) Lead acetate is added to filter paper strips, which are dried and suspended over tubes of broth or agar. H_2S-producing bacteria grow and produce the gas, which reacts with lead to form lead sulfide, a black precipitate. Thus a positive test for production of H_2S by bacteria is blackening of a lead acetate strip. The lead acetate strip indicator is more sensitive than most agar hydrogen sulfide indicator systems, and results may not be comparable.

Procedure. Inoculate the test organism into a tube of broth or agar medium, and suspend a lead acetate strip over the medium, being careful not to touch the medium with the strip. Incubate the culture at 35° C, and examine the strip daily for blackening, a positive test result for production of hydrogen sulfide.

Reagent. Lead acetate strips are available commercially. They can be prepared by soaking filter paper strips in a hot, saturated, aqueous solution of lead acetate, drying the filters, and storing them in a dry bottle.

Quality control. See lead acetate strips for H_2S in Table 3-16.

HYDROGEN SULFIDE, SEMISOLID, MOTILITY MEDIUM

Purpose. Hydrogen sulfide, semisolid, motility medium is recommended for detection of hydrogen sulfide (H_2S) production and motility by aerobic and anaerobic bacteria.

Principle and interpretation. This semisolid medium contains protein, yeast extract, carbohydrate, and a hydrogen sulfide indicator, lead acetate. As bacteria grow and produce hydrogen sulfide from protein, the gas reacts chemically with lead acetate to form a black reactant, lead sulfide. Lead acetate

is very sensitive and detects small quantities of hydrogen sulfide. Thus results using this medium may not always correlate with reactions in media containing less sensitive indicators. Bacteria are introduced into hydrogen sulfide medium by stabbing the inoculum directly into the upright semisolid agar and withdrawing the inoculating needle along the line of penetration. During incubation, motile organisms migrate radially through the semisolid agar medium from the line of inoculum. Thus motility is observed as turbid growth extending away from the line of inoculum. Hydrogen sulfide–producing strains may also blacken the medium as movement progresses away from the inoculum. Cultures should be incubated at both room temperature and 35° C to test for motility, since many species exhibit temperature-dependent motility; for example, *Listeria monocytogenes* is motile at 25° C but weakly motile or nonmotile at 35° C.

Ingredients and preparation. Mix the following ingredients, bring to boiling, dispense into tubes, and sterilize at 121° C for 15 minutes. Allow media to solidify in an upright position at room temperature. If media are to be used with anaerobic bacteria, prereduce them by overnight storage in an anaerobic atmosphere. Tighten caps, and store at 4° C.

Pancreatic digest of casein, USP	10 g
Yeast extract	5 g
Lead acetate, 10% aqueous solution	2 ml
D-Glucose	5 g
Agar	2 g
Distilled water	1 L

Final pH 7.2

Procedure. Test cultures are inoculated into hydrogen sulfide medium (two tubes) by first touching a sterile bacteriologic needle to a colony and then stabbing the needle to the deep agar region of the medium. Inoculated media are incubated at both 25° C and 35° C and examined daily for up to 5 days for evidence of motility and H_2S production.

Quality control. Test tubes of medium from each batch with the following organisms, and observe for expected results:
Bacteroides fragilis, Shigella sonnei—no H_2S, nonmotile
Clostridium sordellii, Salmonella enteritidis—H_2S, motile

INDOLE AND INDOLE-NITRATE (NITRITE) BROTHS

Purpose. Indole broth is used for distinguishing among bacteria based on ability to produce indole from tryptophan. Indole-nitrate broth is a combination medium in which ability to produce indole and reduce nitrate (nitrite) is tested.

Principle and interpretation. Indole broth contains tryptophan-rich peptone and sodium chloride. The tryptophan present in peptone is oxidized by certain bacteria to indole, skatole, and indoleacetic acid. The intracellular enzymes that are responsible for metabolizing tryptophan to these compounds are collectively termed tryptophanase. Indole is detected in broth cultures of bacteria with an alcoholic *p*-dimethylaminobenzaldehyde reagent. Indole reacts with the aldehyde to give a red product in the alcoholic layer of the broth-reagent mixture.

Two reagents may be used to detect indole: Kovacs and Ehrlich. Ehrlich reagent is believed to be more sensitive than Kovacs and is recommended for detection of indole production by anaerobic bacteria and nonfermentative gram-negative organisms. Kovacs reagent was used initially to classify members of *Enterobacteriaceae* and should be used with these bacteria.

Indole-nitrate broth is similar to indole broth but also contains buffer, potassium nitrate, and a small amount of agar. The mechanism for detection of indole is identical to that of indole broth. The principle behind the nitrate test is the same as described for nitrate broth.

A rapid spot test may also be used to detect the degradation of tryptophan to indole. Most bacteriologic culture media contain complex proteins that are rich in tryptophan. Thus, as bacteria metabolize the protein components present in a plate medium, such as sheep blood agar, they produce indole in and around the area of growth. A direct test for indole production involves saturating a piece of filter paper with an acidic solution of *p*-dimethylaminobenzaldehyde or *p*-dimethylaminocinnamaldehyde and then rubbing a colony onto the paper. Although this spot test shows high correlation with the conventional broth test, false-negative reactions do infrequently occur. Thus negative spot test results should be confirmed with a conventional tube test. (NOTE: Indole test strips are also available commercially.)

Ingredients and preparation. Mix the ingredients, heat to boiling, dispense into tubes, and sterilize at 121° C for 15 minutes.

Indole broth:

Pancreatic digest of casein, USP	20 g
Sodium chloride	5 g
Distilled water	1 L

Final pH 7.2

Indole-nitrate broth:

Pancreatic digest of casein, USP	20 g
Disodium phosphate	2 g
D-Glucose	1 g
Potassium nitrate	1 g
Agar	1 g
Distilled water	1 L

Final pH 7.2

REAGENTS
Kovacs indole reagent: Dissolve the aldehyde in the alcohol and slowly add acid to the mixture.

Alcohol, amyl or isoamyl	150 ml
p-Dimethylaminobenzaldehyde	10 g
Hydrochloric acid, concentrated	50 ml

Ehrlich indole reagent:

Alcohol, ethyl, absolute	2 g
p-Dimethylaminobenzaldehyde	190 ml
Hydrochloric acid, concentrated	40 ml

Nitrate reagents: See discussion of nitrate broth.
Procedure. Inoculate the test organism into indole or indole-nitrate broth, incubate at 35° C for 18 to 24 hours, and test as follows.

INDOLE TEST. Add 5 drops of Kovacs reagent directly to the broth culture, shake gently, and observe for development of a red color in the upper alcohol layer. For an Ehrlich indole test, first add 1 ml of ether to the broth culture, shake gently, and then add 5 drops of the reagent.

NITRATE TEST. See discussion of nitrate broth.
Quality control. See Tables 3-7 and 3-16.
INDOLE SPOT TEST. Using a Nichrome loop, select a well-isolated colony from a blood agar plate. Smear the colony onto a piece of filter paper that is saturated with 5% *p*-dimethylaminobenzaldehyde in 10% hydrochloric acid or 1% *p*-dimethylaminocinnamaldehyde in 10% hydrochloric acid. The latter reagent is recommended by Sutter and Carter for use with anaerobic bacteria. A positive reaction is indicated by the development of a red color (benzaldehyde reagent) or a blue-green color (cinnamaldehyde reagent) within 20 seconds. Because indole that is produced by adjacent colonies may diffuse into the medium, producing false-positive results, test colonies should be separated by at least 5 mm. Colonies growing on media with pH indicators (such as MacConkey agar) should not be tested with this method.

REFERENCES

Barry, A.L.: Simple and rapid methods for bacterial identifications, Clin. Lab. Med. **5**:3, 1985.
Lowrance, B.L., Reich, P., and Traub, W.H.: Evaluation of two spot-indole reagents, Appl. Microbiol. **17**:923, 1969.
Sutter, V.L., and Carter, W.T.: Evaluation of media and reagent for indole-spot tests in anaerobic bacteriology, J. Clin. Pathol. **58**:335, 1972.

IRON UPTAKE TEST FOR MYCOBACTERIA

Purpose. Ability to accumulate iron from a medium is a useful test for distinguishing among species of mycobacteria.

Principle. Iron is used by bacteria in the biosynthesis of enzymes and other proteins. Uptake of iron from a medium into the bacterial cell results in a color change in both colonies and medium. In this test, ferric ammonium citrate is used as the source of iron. Formation of rusty brown colonies and a tan discoloration of the medium constitute a positive test result for iron uptake.

Procedure. Inoculate two Lowenstein-Jensen (LJ) agar slants with 1 drop of a barely turbid suspension. Incubate both tubes at 35° C until growth occurs. Add to one LJ slant 1 drop of ferric ammonium citrate solution per 1 ml of medium. Reincubate the cultures at 28° C for up to 21 days. Examine each tube for a color change in colonies and medium. (The uninoculated tube is used as a negative color control.)

Reagent. Ferric ammonium citrate solution is prepared as a 20% aqueous solution, dispensed in 5 ml amounts into tubes, and sterilized at 121° C for 15 minutes. The tubes of solution should be discarded if they become cloudy.

Quality control. See iron uptake in Table 3-10 and 20% ferric ammonium citrate in Table 3-18.

KLIGLER IRON AGAR

Purpose. Kligler iron agar (KIA) is used to distinguish among gram-negative bacteria based on their ability to ferment dextrose and lactose and to produce hydrogen sulfide.

Principle and interpretation. For the most part, KIA is identical to triple sugar iron (TSI) agar except that TSI agar contains sucrose and KIA does not. The principle behind the function of the component ingredients of KIA is identical to that of TSI agar. (See discussion of triple sugar iron agar.)

Ingredients and preparation. Mix the following ingredients, heat to boiling, and dispense into tubes. Sterilize the medium at 121° C for 15 minutes, and allow tubes of medium to solidify in a slanted position.

Pancreatic digest of casein and peptic digest of animal tissue, USP	20 g
Sodium chloride	5 g
Lactose	10 g
D-Glucose	1 g
Ferric ammonium citrate	0.5 g
Sodium thiosulfate	0.5 g
Phenol red	25 mg
Agar	15 g
Distilled water	1 L

Final pH 7.4

Procedure. See discussion of triple sugar iron agar.

Quality control. Use organisms indicated under triple sugar iron agar in Table 3-7.

LIPASE, TWEEN 80

Purpose. Tween 80 lipase medium is used to distinguish among species of bacteria based on ability to hydrolyze polyoxyethylene sorbitan mono-oleate (Tween 80).

Principle and interpretation. This medium contains protein, calcium chloride, Tween 80, and agar. Some bacteria possess a lipase that is capable of hydrolyzing Tween 80 to free fatty acids. In the presence of calcium ions, calcium oleate is precipitated. This is observed as an opaque zone around bacterial growth.

Ingredients and preparation. Mix the following ingredients, heat to boiling, sterilize at 121° C for 15 minutes, and dispense into Petri plates. Allow the plates of medium to solidify at room temperature.

Peptic digest of animal tissue, USP	10 g
Beef extract	3 g
Sodium chloride	5 g
Tween 80	4 ml
Calcium chloride	0.15 g
Agar	15 g
Distilled water	1 L

Final pH 7.2

Procedure. Inoculate cultures of bacteria to Tween 80 agar as ½-inch-long streaks. Incubate cultures at 35° C for 1 to 3 days, and examine for presence of opaque zones of precipitation under and around areas of growth.

Quality control. Test sample plates of medium from each batch with the following organisms, and observe for expected results:

Serratia marcescens—opaque zone
Escherichia coli—no opaque zone

REFERENCE

Lovell, D.J., and Bibel, D.J.: Tween 80 medium for differentiating nonpigmented *Serratia* from *Enterobacteriaceae*, J. Clin. Microbiol. **5:**245, 1977.

LOEFFLER MEDIUM

Purpose. Loeffler medium is recommended for isolation and identification of *Corynebacterium diphtheriae*.

Principle and interpretation. Loeffler medium contains beef, serum, glucose, protein, and egg; these are growth factors necessary for optimal growth of *C. diphtheriae*. These organisms produce translucent to gray-white colonies on this medium. A Gram stain of the colonies reveals pleomorphic and barred rods (some organisms are coccoid); some rods have pointed or rounded ends. Methylene blue–stained smears reveal an irregular staining pattern and the presence of reddish metachromatic granules.

Ingredients and preparation. Mix the following ingredients, and heat to 45° C. Gently rotate the mixture in a flask, dispense into tubes, and inspissate in a slanted position for 6 hours, on 3 successive days, at 70° C. The medium is inspissated rather than autoclaved to avoid destruction of heat-sensitive components, such as egg.

Beef serum (dry solids)	70 g
Sodium chloride	0.4 g
D-Glucose	0.7 g
Peptic digest of casein, USP	0.7 g
Pancreatic digest of heart muscle, USP	0.7 g
Egg (whole, dried)	7.5 g
Distilled water	1 L

Final pH 7.6

Procedure. Inoculate a bacterial culture suspected to be *C. diphtheriae* to Loeffler medium, and incubate at 35° C for 8 to 18 hours. Examine by Gram stain and methylene blue stain.

Quality control. Test sample tubes of medium from each batch with *C. diphtheriae*. Examination by Gram stain and methylene blue stain should reveal the typical morphology described previously.

LOWENSTEIN-JENSEN MEDIUM

Purpose. Lowenstein-Jensen (LJ) medium is an egg-based medium used for isolation and cultivation of mycobacteria.

Principle and interpretation. Mycobacteria are highly sensitive to toxic components present in most prepared media. The potato flour, glycerol, and egg components of LJ medium aid detoxification of the medium and supply some of the nutrients essential for growth of mycobacteria. Malachite green is added to LJ medium to suppress growth of contaminating bacteria. Addition of asparagine to the medium ensures maximal production of niacin by certain species of *Mycobacterium*.

Ingredients and preparation. Dissolve the salts and asparagine in 600 ml distilled water. Slowly mix in potato flour and glycerol, and sterilize at 121° C for 30 minutes. To this cooled basal medium add 1 L homogenized eggs and 20 ml sterile 2% aqueous solution of malachite green. The homogenized egg solution should be prepared from fresh eggs, no more than 1 week old. The eggs are immersed in a 5% soap solution for 30 minutes and then in running cold water until the rinse water clears. The clean eggs are immersed in 70% ethyl alcohol for 15 minutes and then broken, one at a time, into a sterile flask. The egg contents are homogenized by shaking the flask vigorously by hand. Sterile glass beads can be placed in the flask with the egg contents to hasten homogenization. The mixture is filtered through four layers of sterile gauze. The filtered, homogenized egg solution is then ready for use in preparation of LJ medium. It is dispensed into tubes and inspissated at 85° C for 50 minutes and in a slanted position. The LJ slant medium is incubated at 35° C for 48 hours to ensure sterility. LJ slants may be stored with caps tightly closed at 4° C for 1 month.

Basal medium:

Asparagine	3.6 g
Monopotassium phosphate	2.4 g
Magnesium sulfate · 7 H₂O	0.24 g
Magnesium citrate	0.6 g
Potato flour	30 g
Glycerol, reagent grade	12 ml
Distilled water	600 ml

Additives:

Eggs, homogenized, whole	1 L
Malachite green, 2% aqueous	20 ml

Procedure. Inoculate digested or undigested specimens to LJ medium, place tubes of inoculated medium into a carbon dioxide incubator (5% to 10% carbon dioxide), and examine weekly for growth for up to 6 to 10 weeks.

Quality control. See Table 3-6.

LOWENSTEIN-JENSEN MEDIUM WITH 5% SODIUM CHLORIDE

Purpose. Lowenstein-Jensen (LJ) medium with salt is used to distinguish among species of rapidly growing mycobacteria based on ability to grow in presence of 5% sodium chloride.

Principle and interpretation. This medium is identical to LJ medium but with added sodium chloride (5%). The medium tests for the ability of mycobacteria to tolerate and grow in the presence of a high salt concentration.

Ingredients and preparation. Prepare LJ medium, and add 5% sodium chloride (wt/vol) before sterilization. Prepare as a slant tube medium.

Procedure. Inoculate the medium with the test culture, incubate at 35° C for 4 weeks in an atmosphere enriched with carbon dioxide, and observe for growth.

Quality control. See sodium chloride tolerance in Table 3-10.

LYSINE IRON AGAR

Purpose. Lysine iron agar (LIA) is prepared as a slanted agar medium and is used to differentiate members of the *Enterobacteriaceae* family on the ability to decarboxylate or deaminate lysine and to produce hydrogen sulfide.

Principle and interpretation. LIA contains a small amount of protein, glucose, lysine, a sulfur source, a hydrogen sulfide indicator, agar, and a pH indicator. The pH indicator, bromcresol purple, is yellow in the presence of acid and purple with basic conditions. All organisms used on LIA must be glucose fermenters. As these organisms ferment glucose, they produce acid, turning the bromcresol indicator yellow. This reaction is observed only in the butt of the tube because fermentation is anaerobic and not enough acid is produced to extend throughout the medium.

Organisms may also decarboxylate or deaminate lysine; they do not do both. Decarboxylation of lysine yields the alkaline product cadaverine, which neutralizes the acids from glucose fermentation and leads to reversion of the butt from yellow to purple. Organisms that deaminate lysine do so in the presence of oxygen, that is, in the slant area of the medium, and cause the slant to turn red. The reason for the red color is incompletely understood. However, because the omission of the indicator from the medium results in production of an orange slant by lysine deaminase–positive organisms, the red slant may result from an interaction between the purple color of the slant and the orange pigment.

Some bacteria are able to produce hydrogen sulfide (H₂S) gas from sodium thiosulfate. H₂S reacts with the ferric ions of ferric ammonium citrate to yield ferrous sulfide. This insoluble compound is detected as a blackening throughout the medium.

The expected reactions follow:

Purple (slant)/yellow (butt)—lysine decarboxylase negative

Purple/purple—lysine decarboxylase positive

Red/yellow—lysine deaminase positive

Blackening—hydrogen sulfide produced

Ingredients and preparation. Mix the following ingredients in 1 L of distilled water, heat to boiling, and dispense into sterile tubes. Sterilize the tubes of medium at 121° C for 15 minutes. Cool in a slanted position.

Pancreatic hydrolysate of gelatin, USP	5 g
Yeast extract	3 g
D-Glucose	1 g
L-Lysine	10 g
Ferric ammonium citrate	0.5 g
Sodium thiosulfate	0.04 g
Bromcresol purple	0.02 g
Agar	13.5 g
Distilled water	1 L

Final pH 6.7

Procedure. Inoculate cultures of bacteria to LIA by touching a sterile bacteriologic needle to a colony and then stabbing the needle into the deep agar region of the medium. During withdrawal the needle is streaked in a back and forth motion over the surface of the agar. Cultures are incubated at 35° C for 18 to 24 hours.

Quality control. See Table 3-7.

LYSOSTAPHIN SUSCEPTIBILITY TEST

Purpose. The lysostaphin susceptibility test may be used to distinguish between staphylococci and micrococci. Many staphylococci are susceptible to lysis by this enzyme, whereas micrococci are resistant.

Principle. Lysostaphin is a mixture of enzymes that lyse glycine-glycine bridges. Staphylococci possess glycine-containing interpeptide linkages in their peptidoglycan (cell wall) and thus are susceptible to lysostaphin. Micrococci do not possess these linkages. To maximize the sensitivity of the lysostaphin susceptibility test, bacteria should be cultured in meat extract broths. The amino acid composition of the lysostaphin-susceptible interpeptide chain of peptidoglycan depends on the amino acid content of the culture medium. Peptones used in culture media and prepared from casein have high serine and low glycine content; in contrast, peptones prepared from meat have high glycine and low serine content. Staphylococci cultured in meat extract broths, which contain increased glycine, have been shown to be more susceptible to lysostaphin than are the same strains grown in media containing plant proteins.

Procedure. Either of the following procedures may be used to determine lysostaphin susceptibility.

PROCEDURE A. Prepare an agar overlay by adding 0.1 ml of a saline cell suspension (about 10^7 colony-forming units/ml) of the test organism to a tube containing 3 ml of fluid soft P agar (see below). Mix thoroughly and pour the suspension on the surface of a dry, soft P agar plate. Place 1 drop of sterile lysostaphin solution (200 μg/ml) on the inoculated agar and incubate for 24 to 48 hours. Examine for inhibition of growth on the lysostaphin spot. Lysostaphin susceptibility is interpreted according to the following spot inhibition scheme: +, sensitive (complete inhibition); ±, slightly resistant (partial growth inhibition); and −, resistant (no visible growth inhibition).

P agar (peptone–yeast extract–glucose agar): Combine the following ingredients, mix, and autoclave at 121° C for 15 minutes.

Peptone (Difco Laboratories, Detroit)	10 g
Yeast extract (Difco Laboratories)	· 5 g
Sodium chloride	5 g
Glucose	1 g
Agar (Difco Laboratories)	15 g
Distilled water	1 L

PROCEDURE B. Inoculate the test organism to heart infusion broth and incubate the culture at 35° C for no longer than 18 to 24 hours. Shake the culture and add 5 drops to each of two tubes, one labeled test and the other control. Place 5 drops of lysostaphin working solution into the tube marked "test" and 5 drops of phosphate buffer into the tube marked "control." Place both tubes in a 35° C water bath and examine at 30, 60, and 120 minutes for lysis or clearing of the mixture of enzyme and cells in the tube marked "test." Greater than 50% reduction in turbidity of the test over that of the control is interpreted as a positive test for susceptibility to 12.5 μg/ml of lysostaphin, hence a *Staphylococcus* sp.

Reagents

Phosphate buffer, pH 7.4:

Monosodium phosphate, 0.2 M	9.5 ml
Disodium phosphate, 0.2 M	40.5 ml
Distilled water, q.s. to	100 ml

Lysostaphin stock solution, 250 μg/ml: Mix the following ingredients, dispense 1 ml amounts into tubes, and store at −20° C.

Lysostaphin (Sigma Chemical Co., St. Louis)	10 g
Phosphate buffer, pH 7.4	40 ml
Sodium chloride	0.4 g

Lysostaphin working solution, 25 μg/ml: Mix the following ingredients, use what is needed, and store the remaining solution at 4° C for no longer than 2 days.

Lysostaphin stock solution	1 ml
Phosphate buffer, pH 7.4	9 ml

Quality control. The positive control is *S. aureus.* Lysostaphin causes complete growth inhibition of this organism in procedure A and clearing of a cell suspension in procedure B.

The negative control is *Micrococcus luteus.* Lysostaphin produces no visible growth inhibition in procedure A and no clearing of a cell suspension in procedure B.

REFERENCES

Gunn, B.A., et al.: Comparison of methods for identifying *Staphylococcus* and *Micrococcus* spp., J. Clin. Microbiol. **14:**195, 1981.

Heddaeus, H., Heczko, P.B., and Pulverer, G.: Evaluation of the lysostaphin-susceptibility test for classification of staphylococci, J. Med. Microbiol. **12:**9, 1979.

Klesius, P.H., and Schuhardt, V.T.: Use of lysostaphin in the isolation of highly polymerized deoxyribonucleic acid and in the taxonomy of *Micrococcaceae,* J. Bacteriol. **95:**739, 1968.

Kloos, W.E., Tornabene, T.G., and Schleifer, K.H.: Isolation and characterization of micrococci from human skin, including two new species: *Micrococcus lylae* and *Micrococcus kristinae,* Int. J. Syst. Bacteriol. **24:**79, 1974.

Schleifer, K.H., and Kloos, W.E.: Isolation and characterization of staphylococci from human skin. I. Amended descriptions of *Staphylococcus epidermidis* and *Staphylococcus saprophyticus* and description of three new species: *Staphylococcus cohnii, Staphylococcus haemolyticus,* and *Staphylococcus xylosus,* Int. J. Syst. Bacteriol. **25:**50, 1975.

LYSOZYME SUSCEPTIBILITY TEST

Purpose. Lysozyme susceptibility may be used to distinguish between staphylococci and micrococci. Staphylococci are resistant to lysozyme, whereas most micrococci are susceptible.

Principle. Lysozyme is an enzyme that cleaves the glycan strands between *N*-acetylmuramic acid and *N*-acetylglucosamine, both of which are found in the cell wall of staphylococci and micrococci. At certain concentrations of lysozyme most micrococci are susceptible whereas, for reasons not clearly defined, most staphylococci are resistant.

Procedure. Agar overlay plates are prepared as discussed in the lysostaphin susceptibility test. A drop of a sterile lysozyme solution (400 μg/ml) is placed on the agar plate. Lysozyme susceptibility is interpreted according to the spot inhibition scheme described in procedure A of the lysostaphin susceptibility test.

Quality control. The positive control is *Micrococcus luteus,* which results in complete growth inhibition. The negative control is *Staphylococcus aureus,* which does not produce visible growth inhibition.

REFERENCES

Kloos, W.E., Tornabene, T.G., and Schleifer, K.H.: Isolation and characterization of micrococci from human skin, including two new species: *Micrococcus lylae* and *Micrococcus kristinae,* Int. J. Syst. Bacteriol. **24:**79, 1974.

Schleifer, K.H., and Kloos, W.E.: Isolation and characterization of staphylococci from human skin. I. Amended descriptions of *Staphylococcus epidermidis* and *Staphylococcus saprophyticus* and descriptions of three new species: *Staphylococcus cohnii, Staphylococcus haemolyticus,* and *Staphylococcus xylosus,* Int. J. Syst. Bacteriol. **25:**50, 1975.

MACCONKEY AGAR

Purpose. MacConkey (MAC) agar is a selective and differential medium for cultivation of aerobic or facultative gram-negative bacilli from a variety of clinical specimens.

Principle and interpretation. MAC agar contains protein, bile salts, sodium chloride, lactose, agar, and two dyes. The selective action of MAC agar is attributed to crystal violet and bile salts, which are inhibitory to most species of gram-positive bacteria. Gram-negative bacteria usually grow well on the medium and are differentiated by their ability to ferment lactose. Lactose-fermenting strains grow as red or pink colonies and may be surrounded by a zone of acid-precipitated bile. The red color is due to production of acids from lactose, absorption of neutral red, and a subsequent color change of the dye when the pH of the medium falls below 6.8. Non-lactose-fermenting strains, such as *Shigella* and *Salmonella,* are uncolored and transparent and typically do not alter appearance of the medium. *Yersinia enterocolitica* may appear as small, non-lactose-fermenting colonies after incubation at room temperature.

Ingredients and preparation. Mix the following ingredients, heat to boiling, and sterilize at 121° C for 15 minutes. Cool to 50° C, and pour into plates. Allow the medium to solidify at room temperature with lids ajar to enhance removal of excess surface moisture.

Pancreatic hydrolysate of gelatin, USP	17 g
Pancreatic digest of casein and peptic digest of animal tissue, USP	3 g
Lactose	10 g
Bile salts	1.5 g
Sodium chloride	5 g
Neutral red	30 mg
Crystal violet	1 mg
Agar	13.5 g
Distilled water	1 L

Final pH 7.1

Procedure. Inoculate the clinical specimen or test organism to MAC agar, streak for isolation, and incubate in air for 18 to 24 hours at 35° C. Do not incubate in carbon dioxide. Plates may be placed at room temperature for an additional 24 hours to enhance recovery of *Y. enterocolitica* from feces.

Quality control. See Table 3-3.

MACCONKEY AGAR GROWTH TEST FOR MYCOBACTERIA

Purpose. MacConkey (MAC) agar is useful for distinguishing among species of mycobacteria based on ability to grow on and change the color of the medium.

Principle. MAC agar contains protein, bile salts, sodium chloride, lactose, and agar. The formulation used with mycobacteria *does not contain crystal violet.* See the discussion of MacConkey agar for its mechanism of action.

Procedure. Place a MAC agar plate on a turntable, remove the lid, and transfer a 3 mm loopful of a 7-day enriched Middlebrook 7H9 broth culture of the organism to the center of the plate. Slowly spin the turntable, and move the loop from the center of the agar medium to the outer edge. The inoculum is spirally dispersed. Incubate the culture at 28° C in a non–carbon dioxide–enriched atmosphere, and examine the medium at 5 and 11 days for evidence of growth and change in color of the medium from red to light pink or clear.

Quality control. See growth on MacConkey agar in Table 3-10.

MALONATE BROTH

Purpose. Malonate broth is used for differentiation of members of the family *Enterobacteriaceae,* especially among *Salmonella* spp.

Principle and interpretation. Malonate broth tests for utilization of sodium malonate as a sole source of carbon. The medium contains buffer, pH indicator, sodium malonate, required salts, and a small amount of yeast extract and glucose. The pH indicator, bromthymol blue, is a deep Prussian blue at its alkaline endpoint (pH 7.6), yellow at its acidic endpoint (pH 6.0), and green when uninoculated (pH 6.7). Bacteria that are capable of using malonate as a source of energy and carbon produce alkaline by-products that change the color of the medium to blue. Bacteria that are unable to use malonate as a carbon source usually do not grow and the pH of the medium does not change; the indicator remains green. Some malonate-negative strains may produce a yellow color owing to fermentation of glucose.

Ingredients and preparation. Mix the following ingredients, heat to boiling, dispense into tubes, and sterilize at 121° C for 15 minutes.

Yeast extract	1 g
Ammonium sulfate	2 g
Dipotassium phosphate	0.6 g
Monopotassium phosphate	0.4 g
Sodium chloride	2 g
Sodium malonate	3 g
D-Glucose	0.25 g
Bromthymol blue	0.025 g
Distilled water	1 L

Final pH 6.7

NOTE: Malonate test strips are commercially available.

Procedure. Inoculate the test organism into malonate broth and incubate at 35° C for 18 to 24 hours.

Quality control. See Table 3-7.

MANNITOL SALT AGAR

Purpose. Mannitol salt agar (MSA) is a selective and differential medium useful for isolation of *Staphylococcus* organisms from clinical specimens containing mixed species of bacteria.

Principle and interpretation. MSA contains beef extract, sodium chloride, D-mannitol, agar, and a pH indicator. The selectivity of the medium is attributed to a high concentration of sodium chloride (7.5%). *Staphylococcus* spp. (and some salt-tolerant species of *Micrococcus* and *Streptococcus*) are able to grow at this concentration of salt, whereas most gram-negative organisms and other gram-positive organisms are not.

The differential action of the medium is attributed to D-mannitol. *Staphylococcus aureus* grows on MSA and ferments mannitol to produce yellow colonies with yellow zones. Most coagulase-negative species of *Staphylococcus* and *Micrococcus* do not ferment mannitol and grow as small red colonies surrounded by red or purple zones. The color of colonies and medium is due to the reactivity of phenol red to the pH of the medium; phenol red is red at pH 8.4 and yellow at pH 6.8. Yellow colonies of bacteria should be tested for production of coagulase. The limitations of mannitol fermentation are discussed in Chapter 12.

Egg yolk may be added to the medium for detection of egg yolk lipase activity of colonies of *S. aureus*. This enzyme releases salt-insoluble fatty acids that precipitate around strains of *S. aureus* to form zones of opacity in the medium. Non-coagulase-producing species of *Staphylococcus* do not produce this enzyme and are therefore not surrounded by an opaque zone of precipitate.

Ingredients and preparation. Mix the following ingredients, heat to boiling, sterilize at 121° C for 15 minutes, and dispense into plates.

Beef extract	1 g
Pancreatic digest of casein and peptic digest of animal tissue, USP	10 g
Sodium chloride	75 g
D-Mannitol	10 g
Phenol red	25 mg
Agar	15 g
Distilled water	1 L
Egg yolk, sterile (optional)	20 ml

Final pH 7.4

Procedure. Inoculate a clinical specimen to MSA, streak for isolation, and incubate for 24 to 48 hours at 35° C. Do not incubate in carbon dioxide.

Quality control. See Table 3-3.

REFERENCE

Gunn, B.A., Dunkelberg, W.E., and Creitz, J.R.: Clinical evaluation of 2%-LSM medium for primary isolation and identification of staphylococci, Am. J. Clin. Pathol. **57:**236, 1972.

MARTIN-LEWIS AGAR

Purpose. Martin-Lewis (ML) agar is a selective medium used for isolation of *Neisseria gonorrhoeae* and *Neisseria meningitidis* from clinical specimens containing mixed species of bacteria.

Principles and interpretation. ML agar is similar to modified Thayer-Martin agar except that it contains anisomycin in lieu of nystatin and the vancomycin content is increased to 4 μg/ml. See the discussion of Thayer-Martin agar for other ingredients.

The selectivity of ML agar is attributed to the inhibitory actions of four antimicrobial agents. Vancomycin inhibits gram-positive bacteria by interfering with cell wall synthesis; colistin (polymyxin E) inhibits gram-negative bacteria, including saprophytic *Neisseria* spp., by disrupting the cell wall of affected organisms; anisomycin inhibits molds and some yeasts; and trimethoprim lactate inhibits swarming *Proteus* spp.

Colonies of *N. gonorrhoeae* are best observed with the aid of a magnifying glass and are 0.5 to 1 mm in diameter after 24 hours' incubation. They appear gray to white, opaque, raised, and glistening and may increase to 3 mm in diameter with further incubation. Colonies of *N. meningitidis* are 1 mm or greater in diameter after 24 hours and are round, convex, gray to white, smooth, moist, and glistening with an entire edge.

Ingredients and preparation. See the discussion of Thayer-Martin agar. Substitute anisomycin, 20 μg/ml of medium, for nystatin. Increase the concentration of vancomycin to 4 μg/ml of medium.

Procedure. Inoculate the clinical specimen directly onto ML agar, streak for isolation, and immediately incubate the culture at 35° C in an atmosphere of 3% to 10% carbon dioxide. Examine the plates for typical pathogenic *Neisseria* colonies after 48 hours at 35° C.

Quality control. See selective media for pathogenic *Neisseria* in Table 3-3.

REFERENCE

Martin, J.E., and Lewis, J.S.: Anisomycin: improved antimycotic activity in modified TM medium, Public Health Lab. **35:**53, 1977.

METHYL RED–VOGES-PROSKAUER BROTH AND RAPID DIRECT AND INDIRECT VOGES-PROSKAUER TESTS
METHYL RED–VOGES-PROSKAUER BROTH

Purpose. Methyl red–Voges-Proskauer (MR-VP) broth is useful for distinguishing among members of the family *Enterobacteriaceae* based on their ability to produce acetylmethylcarbinol (acetoin) and strong acids from fermentation of glucose. The broth, which contains protein, glucose, and phosphate buffer, is used for the MR test and the VP test.

Principle and interpretation. Members of the family *Enterobacteriaceae* may be divided metabolically into two groups: the mixed acid producers and the butylene glycol producers. The mixed acid producers such as *Escherichia coli* produce large amounts of organic acids including lactic, acetic, formic, and succinic. Butylene glycol producers such as *Klebsiella* and *Enterobacter* spp. produce smaller amounts of organic acids and large amounts of neutral products, especially 2,3-butanediol.

The MR test is used to distinguish the mixed acid producers. In this test a methyl red indicator is added to the MR-VP test broth after incubation. At a pH of 4.4 the indicator remains red, and at a pH of 6.0 it becomes yellow. The MR-positive organisms are those that produce large amounts of acid and a red color, whereas the MR-negative organisms produce a yellow color.

The VP test detects the presence of acetoin, or acetylmethylcarbinol, an intermediate in the production of butylene glycol. In this test two reagents, alpha-naphthol and 40% potassium hydroxide (KOH), are added to the test broth after appropriate incubation. The broth-reagent mixture is then mixed thoroughly to expose the medium to atmospheric oxygen. If acetoin is present, it is oxidized in the presence of air and KOH to diacetyl. Diacetyl then reacts with the guanidine components of peptone, in the presence of alpha-naphthol, to form a red color (alpha-naphthol serves as a catalyst and acts as a color intensifier). Development of a red color is a positive VP test result.

The MR-VP test was designed to be read after 5 days' incubation at 30° C to ensure that glucose was metabolized to 2,3-butanediol by the butylene glycol producers. However, by reducing the volume of MR-VP broth to 0.5 to 1 ml per tube and heavily inoculating the test organism into the medium, the broth may be incubated at 35° C for 18 to 24 hours and still produce results equivalent to the conventional test. Small volumes of broth increase the availability of atmospheric oxygen to the test organism and enhance production of acetoin (MR-VP broth is incubated under aerobic conditions during testing).

Barry recommends the use of the direct and indirect Voges-Proskauer test outlined below in lieu of the conventional test for screening of *Enterobacteriaceae* (see Figure 9-2). The direct test is used for the identification of prompt lactose-fermenting colonies but occasionally gives false-negative results with slow lactose-fermenting or nonfermenting colonies. The indirect test may be used when the direct test is inappropriate. Both of these tests provide results within 15 minutes.

Ingredients and preparation. Mix the following ingredients, heat to boiling, dispense into tubes (1 ml/tube), and sterilize at 121° C for 15 minutes.

Pancreatic digest of casein and peptic digest of animal tissue, USP	7 g
D-Glucose	5 g
Dipotassium phosphate	5 g
Distilled water	1 L

Final pH 6.9

Reagents

Methyl red reagent: Dissolve the methyl red in alcohol and add the distilled water. Store at room or refrigerator temperature.

Methyl red	50 mg
Ethyl alcohol, 95%	150 ml
Distilled water	100 ml

Voges-Proskauer reagents
VP-1:

Alpha-naphthol	5 g
Ethyl alcohol, absolute	100 ml

VP-2:

Potassium hydroxide	40 g
Distilled water, q.s. to	100 ml

Procedure. Inoculate the test organism to two tubes of MR-VP broth, each containing 1 ml, and incubate for 1 to 3 days at 35° C.

MR TEST. Add 5 drops of methyl red reagent to one broth culture and observe for development of a red color. This is a

positive MR test, which is indicative of mixed acid fermentation.

VP TEST. Add 0.6 ml of VP-1 reagent to another broth culture, shake the tube, and add 0.2 ml of VP-2 reagent. The reagents *must* be added in the preceding sequence. Shake the tube gently. Allow the tube to stand for at least 15 minutes and observe for formation of a red color. This is a positive VP test and indicates butylene glycol fermentation. Hold tubes in which results are negative for an additional 45 minutes, since maximum color development occurs within 1 hour after the reagent is added. Ignore a copper color of the medium, which occurs after 1 hour's incubation. This color is due to reaction between alpha-naphthol and KOH. (NOTE: Reagent-impregnated Voges-Proskauer strips are commercially available.)

Quality control. See Tables 3-7 and 3-16.

RAPID DIRECT VOGES-PROSKAUER TEST. Place 2 drops of creatine in a 13 × 100 mm tube. Suspend prompt lactose-fermenting (red or pink) colonies from a MacConkey agar plate in the creatine solution. Growth from the acid portion of a triple sugar iron agar slant may also be used. (If the slant is red, this test should not be used.) Add 3 drops of alpha-naphthol reagent (5% alpha-naphthol in 95% ethyl alcohol) to the suspension and shake. Add 2 drops of KOH reagent (40% KOH in distilled water) and shake. A positive reaction is indicated by the development of a pink to red color within 15 minutes. According to Barry, positive reactions are quite reliable, but negative results should be confirmed with the following indirect test.

INDIRECT VOGES-PROSKAUER TEST. Inoculate 0.2 ml of MR-VP broth with one colony only. Incubate broth at 35° C for 4 to 6 hours. Add 2 drops of creatine reagent (0.5% aqueous solution of creatine) and shake. Add 3 drops of alpha-naphthol reagent (5% alpha-naphthol in 95% ethyl alcohol) and shake. Add 2 drops of KOH (40% KOH in water) and shake. A positive reaction is the development of a pink to red color within 15 minutes.

REFERENCES

Barry, A.L.: Simple and rapid methods for bacterial identifications, Clin. Lab. Med. **5:**3, 1985.

Barry, A.L., and Feeney, K.L.: Two quick methods for Voges-Proskauer test, Appl. Microbiol. **15:**1138, 1967.

MIDDLEBROOK 7H9 BROTH

Purpose. Middlebrook 7H9 broth is used as the basal medium for the arylsulfatase, tellurite, and niacin tests, which are helpful in identifying species of *Mycobacterium*.

Principle and interpretation. This medium contains vitamins, salts, buffer, and other nutrients required for cultivation and maximal growth of species of *Mycobacterium*.

Ingredients and preparation. Mix the following basal ingredients in 900 ml distilled water, add 2 ml glycerol, heat to boiling, dispense in 180 ml aliquots, and sterilize at 121° C for 15 minutes. Cool and add 20 ml Middlebrook oleic acid–dextrose–citrate (OADC) enrichment to 180 ml sterile basal medium. Dispense into sterile tubes.

Basal medium:

L-Glutamic acid, sodium salt	0.5 g
Ammonium sulfate	0.5 g
Sodium citrate	0.1 g
Pyridoxine	1 mg

Biotin	1 mg
Disodium phosphate	2.5 g
Monopotassium phosphate	1 g
Ferric ammonium citrate	0.04 g
Magnesium sulfate · 7 H$_2$O	0.05 g
Calcium chloride · 2 H$_2$O	0.5 mg
Zinc sulfate · 7 H$_2$O	1 mg
Copper sulfate · 5 H$_2$O	1 mg
Distilled water	900 ml

Additive before sterilization:

Glycerol   2 ml

Additive after sterilization:

Middlebrook OADC enrichment   20 ml/180 ml of sterile basal medium

Procedure. Inoculate the organism to 7H9 medium and incubate at 35° C.

Quality control. See Table 3-6.

MIDDLEBROOK 7H10 AND 7H11 AGARS

Purpose. Middlebrook 7H10 and 7H11 agars are used as general growth media for isolation and cultivation of mycobacteria. Isoniazid-resistant mycobacteria grow better on the agar-based 7H10 and 7H11 media than on egg-based media such as Lowenstein-Jensen (LJ) medium.

Principle and interpretation. Middlebrook 7H11 agar is similar to 7H10 agar except that it has one additional ingredient, enzymatic hydrolysate of casein. The 7H11 agar contains the amino acids, salts, and other nutrients required for optimal growth of acid-fast bacteria.

Ingredients and preparation. Mix the following basal ingredients in 900 ml distilled water containing 0.5% reagent grade glycerol. Dissolve without boiling, distribute in 180 ml amounts, and sterilize at 121° C for 10 minutes. Cool to 50° C and add 20 ml Middlebrook oleic acid–dextrose–citrate (OADC) enrichment to each 180 ml aliquot. Dispense into Petri plates and store at 4° C in plastic bags and protected from light.

Basal ingredients (7H11 agar):

Enzymatic hydrolysate of casein, USP	1 g
Ammonium sulfate	0.5 g
Sodium citrate	0.4 g
D-Glutamic acid	0.5 g
Disodium phosphate	1.5 g
Monopotassium phosphate	1.5 g
Ferric ammonium citrate	0.04 g
Magnesium sulfate	0.25 mg
Glycerol	5 ml
Pyridoxine · HCl	1 mg
Zinc sulfate	1 mg
Copper sulfate	1 mg

Calcium chloride	0.5 mg
Biotin	0.5 mg
Malachite green	0.25 mg
Agar	15 g
Distilled water	900 ml

Final pH 6.7 to 6.8

Additive after sterilization:

Middlebrook OADC enrichment	20 ml/180 ml sterile, cooled basal medium

Final pH 7.0

Procedure. Inoculate digested or undigested specimens directly to 7H11 agar, streak for isolation, and incubate 6 to 8 weeks in a carbon dioxide incubator (5% to 10% carbon dioxide), sealed in carbon dioxide–permeable plastic bags.

Quality control. See Table 3-6. The same organisms that are used for 7H10 may be used for 7H11.

MITCHISON SELECTIVE 7H11 AGAR

Purpose. Selective 7H11 agar (7H11S) contains antimicrobial agents to improve isolation of mycobacteria from contaminated clinical specimens.

Principle and interpretation. Mitchison 7H11S contains the same ingredients as 7H11 agar with the addition of four antimicrobial agents that are responsible for the selective characteristic of this medium. Carbenicillin is a broad-spectrum, semisynthetic penicillin that is especially useful for inhibiting strains of *Pseudomonas* spp. Polymyxin B is a basic polypeptide that destroys cell membranes of gram-negative but not gram-positive bacteria. Trimethoprim lactate is a broad-spectrum sulfonamide that is especially useful for inhibiting strains of *Proteus* spp. Amphotericin B is a complex polyene compound that is useful for inhibiting many species of fungi and yeasts.

Ingredients and preparation. See the discussion of 7H11 agar. Add the following antimicrobial agents before dispensing the sterile cooled (50° C) 7H11 medium into plates.

Carbenicillin	100 mg/ml
Amphotericin B	10 μg/ml
Polymyxin B	200 units/ml
Trimethoprim lactate	26 mg/ml

Procedure. See the discussion of 7H11 agar.

Quality control. See the discussion of 7H11 agar. The following organisms may also be included as controls:
Escherichia coli—no growth
Pseudomonas aeruginosa—no growth

MILK MEDIA

Purpose. Milk media are used to distinguish species of bacteria based on their actions on the ingredients of whole milk. It is especially useful for distinguishing among *Clostridium* spp.

Principle and interpretation. Whole milk has a pH of 6.6 to 6.9 and is comprised of proteins, minerals, carbohydrates, and other substances. Depending on their enzymatic capabilities, bacteria may act on these various components to produce several visible reactions. As discussed below, milk medium has various formulations. One formulation includes litmus, a pH and oxidation-reduction indicator that changes color if milk lactose is fermented. Another formulation contains iron filings that permit detection of hydrogen sulfide production. Hydrogen sulfide gas that is liberated from sulfur-containing amino acids reacts with iron to form ferrous sulfide, a black precipitate.

Organisms that are able to ferment lactose produce large amounts of lactic acid, which may cause precipitation of the milk protein casein. Evidence of this is observed in tubes of milk as a clear liquid over a bottom layer of insoluble, firm, gelatinous, clotted caseinogen. This clot does not retract from the sides of the tube and is easily dissolved when subjected to an alkaline condition. The formation of another type of clot (curd) is caused by conversion of water-soluble casein to alkaline-insoluble (and water-insoluble) paracasein by the enzyme rennin. In the presence of calcium the paracasein is converted to calcium paracaseinate and forms an insoluble clot. This curd, however, retracts from the side of the tube after a few hours, yielding a clear, grayish fluid known as whey. This clot also flows slowly when the tube is tilted. For identification of bacteria it is not significant to record the biochemical process by which the clot is formed.

If fermentation of lactose results in large amounts of gas (carbon dioxide and hydrogen) being produced, the acid clot may be disrupted by vigorous agitation. This is known as stormy fermentation and is characteristic of *Clostridium perfringens*.

Some organisms produce proteolytic enzymes that hydrolyze the milk proteins, primarily casein, to amino acids. This process is called digestion or peptonization. The medium loses its consistency and appears watery and clear.

Ingredients and preparation

IRON MILK (CDC). Place several iron filings in the bottom of screw-cap test tubes. Add 7 ml of whole, nonhomogenized milk to each tube. Sterilize at 121° C for 15 minutes. Prereduce the medium in an anaerobic chamber for 18 to 24 hours. Tighten the caps, and store at 4° C. Inoculate with the test organism. Incubate at 35° C and observe daily for up to 1 week for coagulation, gas, digestion, and blackening. See Dowell and coworkers for typical reactions of *Clostridium* spp.

MILK MEDIUM (VPI). Mix the following:

Fresh milk	100 ml
Resazurin solution	0.4 ml
Hemin solution	1 ml
Vitamin K₁	0.02 ml

To prepare resazurin solution dissolve 25 mg resazurin in 100 ml distilled water.

To prepare hemin solution dissolve 50 mg hemin in 1 ml 1 N sodium hydroxide; add distilled water to make 100 ml. Autoclave at 121° C for 15 minutes.

Inoculate with test organism and observe for typical reactions of *Clostridium* according to Table 20-18. Digestion may occur without curd formation, or the curd may be digested. Digestion usually takes 4 days to 3 weeks. Hold milk cultures 2 to 3 weeks before discarding as negative. Note that clear whey

with solid curd (as with cultures of *C. perfringens*) is not digestion.

LITMUS MILK. Mix the following ingredients, heat to boiling, dispense into tubes, and sterilize at 115° C for 15 minutes. Store at 4° C.

Skimmed milk powder	100 g
Azolitmun (litmus)	0.5 g
Sodium sulfite	0.5 g
Distilled water	1000 ml

Final pH 6.8

Litmus serves as an indicator of both pH and oxidation-reduction. Litmus is red in acid conditions, blue in alkaline conditions, and white when reduced. Milk is typically pH 6.6 to 6.9. Under these conditions litmus milk medium is purple to blue. As bacteria grow in litmus milk and ferment lactose, lactic acid is produced, the pH is lowered, and the medium becomes pink. Reduction of litmus results in the formation of a white color. The primary purpose of the medium is to determine peptonization or the conversion of the milk proteins to soluble compounds as indicated by a clear layer at the surface of the milk. This may also be accompanied by alkalinization, or conversion of the casein in the milk to form ammonia as indicated by the presence of a purple ring at the surface. This medium is recommended for use with nonfermentative organisms.

Quality Control

IRON MILK. Test three tubes of medium from each batch with the following organisms, and observe for expected results:

Clostridium perfringens—clots milk; produces gas; no digestion or blackening of medium

Clostridium sporogenes—production of gas; blackening and digestion of milk; no clotting

Fusobacterium necrophorum—no reaction in iron milk

VPI MILK MEDIUM. Use the same organisms and observe for clotting, gas, and digestion. No blackening can be observed.

LITMUS MILK. For nonfermenters test the following:

Pseudomonas aeruginosa—peptonization

Acinetobacter anitratus—negative for peptonization

REFERENCES

Dowell, V.R., Jr., et al.: Media for isolation, characterization, and identification of obligately anaerobic bacteria, Atlanta, 1981, Centers for Disease Control.

MacFaddin, J.F.: Biochemical tests for identification of medical bacteria, ed. 2, Baltimore, Md., 1980, The Williams & Wilkins Co.

Holdeman, L.V., Cato, E.P., and Moore, W.E.C.: Anaerobe laboratory manual, ed. 4, V.P.I. Anaerobe Laboratory, Virginia Polytechnic Institute and State University, 1977, Blacksburg, Va.

MOTILITY TEST MEDIUM

Purpose. Motility test medium may be used for determining motility of many fastidious and nonfastidious bacteria.

Principle and interpretation. Motility medium contains a small amount of agar to render it semisolid. The medium is "stab" inoculated with the test organism. Initial growth occurs along the line of inoculation. Motile species of bacteria are also able to move laterally away from the inoculation line. This is observed as areas of turbidity (or a haze) around the inoculum.

2,3,5-Triphenyltetrazolium chloride (TTC) may be added to this motility medium to enhance visibility of bacterial growth. Bacteria that grow in this medium incorporate colorless TTC into their cells and there reduce the chemical to an insoluble red formazan pigment. Thus reddening of the medium develops only to the edge of bacterial growth, which clearly distinguishes between areas of growth and no growth. The motility of *Listeria monocytogenes* is frequently best observed in media without TTC.

Ingredients and preparation. Mix the following basal ingredients, heat to boiling, sterilize at 121° C, cool to 50° C, and add filter-sterilized TTC solution. Dispense into tubes, and allow to solidify in an upright position.

Basal ingredients:

Beef extract	3 g
Pancreatic hydrolysate of gelatin, USP	10 g
Sodium chloride	5 g
Agar*	4 g
Distilled water	1 L

Final pH 7.3

Additive:

Triphenyltetrazolium chloride (TTC), 1% (filter sterilized)	5 ml

Procedure. Using a sterile bacteriologic needle, touch a colony and stab the needle to the deep agar region of the medium. Incubate media at 35° C and examine daily for areas of diffuse growth around the line of inoculation.

Quality control. See Table 3-7.

MUELLER-HINTON BROTH

Purpose. Mueller-Hinton (MH) broth is a nutritive medium used for cultivation of a wide variety of microorganisms. It has also been used as a medium for testing bacteria for susceptibility to antimicrobial agents, including sulfonamides.

Principle and interpretation. MH is a transparent medium that contains beef infusion, protein, starch, and agar. The medium was originally devised for cultivation of gonococci and for testing of their susceptibility to sulfonamides. It was found that starch promoted the growth of gonococci and meningococci, which was believed to be due to a "protective colloid" effect of starch directed against toxic materials present in the medium. MH medium is now used in clinical laboratories as a broth medium for testing bacteria for susceptibility to antimicrobial agents, especially by broth dilution techniques. The medium may be supplemented with 1.7% agar to produce a solid plate medium for susceptibility testing using antimicrobial disks. (See also the discussion of Mueller-Hinton agar.)

Ingredients and preparation. Mix the following ingredients, heat to boiling, dispense into tubes, and sterilize at 116° to 121° C for 15 minutes.

Beef, infusion from	300 g
Acid hydrolysate of casein, USP	17.5 g

Starch	1.5 g
Distilled water	1 L

Final pH 7.4

Procedure. Inoculate the test organism into MH broth and incubate at 35° C for 18 to 24 hours. Observe for growth.

Quality control. See Table 3-3.

MUELLER-HINTON MEDIUM, PLAIN, SHEEP BLOOD, AND "CHOCOLATE"

Purpose. Mueller-Hinton (MH), medium is a transparent agar medium useful for cultivation of most species of falcutatively anaerobic bacteria and for testing of susceptibility to antimicrobial agents.

Principle and interpretation. MH medium contains large amounts of animal infusion, acid-hydrolyzed casein (casamino acids), soluble starch, and agar. Sheep blood may be added to enhance growth of fastidious bacteria, such as some species of *Streptococcus*. Chocolate MH medium may be prepared by adding sheep blood to MH medium and heating the mixture at 80° C for 15 minutes or until the medium turns brown. Heating of the blood in MH medium releases red cell components, such as hemoglobin and nicotinamide adenine dinucleotide. These substances enhance growth of *Haemophilus* and other species of bacteria that are unable to grow on sheep blood MH medium. The starch in MH is thought to provide both a source of energy and a protective effect against toxic materials that may be present in the medium.

Ingredients and preparation. Mix the following ingredients, heat to boiling, and sterilize at 116° to 121° C for 15 minutes. Dispense into plates to a depth of 3.5 to 4.5 mm. Allow agar media to solidify at room temperature with lids ajar to enhance removal of excess moisture. Store plates sealed in bags at 4° C.

Basal ingredients:

Beef infusion	300 g
Casamino acids	17.5 g
Starch, soluble	1.5 g
Agar	17 g
Distilled water	1 L

Final pH 7.4

Optional ingredient: Defibrinated sheep blood (50 to 100 ml/L) may be added to MH medium cooled to 50° C. See the discussion of chocolate agar for preparation of chocolate agar MH medium.

Procedure. For susceptibility testing, evenly spread a standardized inoculum onto the surface of MH medium using a sterile swab (see Chapter 8). Allow the inoculum to air dry, and then add antimicrobial disks as required. Incubate plates for 18 to 24 hours at 35° C in air without added carbon dioxide.

Quality control. See Table 3-15.

REFERENCE

National Committee for Clinical Laboratory Standards: Performance standards for antimicrobial disk susceptibility tests, ed. 3, Approved standard, NCCLS Pub. No. M2-A3, Villanova, Pa., 1984, The Committee.

*For nonfermentative organisms and *L. monocytogenes* the agar content can be decreased to 3 g/L.

NEW YORK CITY MEDIUM

Purpose. New York City (NYC) medium is a selective medium used for isolation of *Neisseria gonorrhoeae* and *Neisseria meningitidis* from clinical specimens containing mixed species of bacteria.

Principle and interpretation. NYC medium contains protein, cornstarch, buffer, salt, yeast dialysate, glucose, hemoglobin, antimicrobial agents, and horse plasma. The selectivity of the medium for *Neisseria* spp. is attributed to the actions of four antimicrobial agents: vancomycin, colistin, amphotericin B, and trimethoprim lactate. Vancomycin inhibits gram-positive bacteria by interfering with cell wall synthesis. Colistin (polymyxin E) is more active against gram-negative than gram-positive bacteria and disrupts the cell wall of affected organisms. Amphotericin B inhibits molds and yeasts by interfering with cell wall synthesis in these organisms. Trimethoprim lactate is added to NYC medium specifically to inhibit species of *Proteus*. Cornstarch is thought to provide protection for gonococci by absorbing the toxic substances that might be present in prepared media.

Ingredients and preparation. Prepare the basal medium by mixing the agar, cornstarch, and proteose peptone solutions together, sterilizing the mixture at 121°C for 15 minutes, and cooling it to 50°C. To this cooled basal medium add the sterile hemoglobin solution (optional), glucose solution, antimicrobial mixture, citrated horse plasma, and yeast dialysate. If the hemoglobin solution is omitted, add an additional 200 ml of distilled water to the basal medium before sterilization. Mix thoroughly and dispense into sterile plates. Store plates of medium at 4°C. The final pH is 7.1.

Basal medium:
Agar solution:

Agar	20 g
Distilled water	400 ml

Heat at 100°C until melted.
Cornstarch solution:

Cornstarch	1 g
Distilled water	40 ml

Mix on a magnetic stirrer, and then heat to 100°C until homogeneous.
Proteose peptone solution:

Proteose peptone #3	15 g
Dipotassium phosphate	4 g
Monopotassium phosphate	1 g
Sodium chloride	5 g
Distilled water	200 ml

Heat to boiling using a magnetic stirrer.
Additives to the cooled, sterile basal medium:
3% Hemoglobin solution (optional):

Horse red blood cells	6 ml
Distilled water, sterile	200 ml

Store at 4°C until ready for use.
Glucose solution, 50%:

Glucose	5 g
Distilled water	10 ml

Sterilize at 110°C for 10 minutes.
Antimicrobial mixture, 4 ml:

Vancomycin	2 mg/ml
Colistin	5.5 mg/ml
Amphotericin B	1.2 mg/ml
Trimethoprim lactate	3 mg/ml

Mix the solutions together and store at −20°C until ready for use.

Citrated horse plasma: Dissolve 4.8 g sodium chloride and 90 g sodium citrate in a final volume of 600 ml distilled water. Sterilize at 115°C for 10 minutes. Place this solution in a receiving bottle and draw horse blood to 6 L.

Yeast dialysate: Mix 908 g of baker's yeast with 2500 ml of distilled water until a smooth paste is formed. Autoclave for 10 minutes and allow to cool. Place the suspension in dialysis tubing, and dialyze for 48 hours against 2 L of cold distilled water. Collect the dialysate, dispense in 25 ml aliquots, and sterilize at 121°C for 15 minutes. Store at −20°C for an indefinite period of time.

Procedure. Inoculate NYC agar as described for Thayer-Martin medium.

Quality control. See selective media for pathogenic *Neisseria* in Table 3-3.

REFERENCES

Faur, Y.C., Weisburd, M.H., and Wilson, M.E.: The selectivity of vancomycin and lincomycin in NYC medium for the recovery of *N. gonorrhoeae* from clinical specimens, Health Lab. Sci. **15**:22, 1978.
Granato, P.A., Schneibe-Smith, C., and Weiner, L.B.: Primary isolation of *Neisseria gonorrhoeae* on hemoglobin-free New York City medium, J. Clin. Microbiol. **14**:206, 1981.

NIACIN TEST

Purpose. The niacin test is useful for distinguishing among species of mycobacteria based on accumulation of niacin in the test medium.

Principle. Niacin (nicotinic acid) is a component of the coenzymes nicotinamide adenine dinucleotide (NAD) and nicotinamide adenine dinucleotide phosphate (NADP). NAD and NADP are synthesized either from niacin acquired from the growth medium or from endogenous quinolinic acid via the intermediates nicotinic acid mononucleotide and nicotinic acid dinucleotide. Some species of mycobacteria cannot convert niacin into nicotinic acid mononucleotide. In these cultures niacin accumulates in the surrounding growth medium. In the niacin test free niacin is detected colorimetrically following reaction with cyanogen bromide and aniline. Development of a yellow color in the medium is a positive finding for presence of niacin.

Procedure. Inoculate the test organism to Lowenstein-Jensen (LJ) and incubate at 35°C for 3 to 4 weeks. Add 1 ml of sterile distilled water to the culture to extract niacin, if present. If growth is confluent on the medium, scrape part of the growth to one side of the tube or plate to permit the water to contact the medium. Allow the water to rest on the culture for 15 minutes. Remove 0.5 ml of the liquid extract and transfer it to a clean tube. Add 0.5 ml of aniline reagent to the extract, followed by 0.5 ml of cyanogen bromide. WARNING: Cyanogen bromide is tear gas and should be handled in a well-ventilated chemical fume hood. In the presence of acid, cyanogen bromide hydrolyzes to toxic hydrocyanic acid. To prevent formation of this compound, all test materials should be discarded into a germicidal solution made alkaline by the addition of sodium hydroxide.

Reagents. Niacin test strips may be purchased from commercial sources, or the reagents for the test may be prepared as follows.

Aniline reagent, 4%: Add 4 ml of colorless aniline to 96 ml of 95% ethyl alcohol. Store the reagent in a brown glass bottle at 4° to 5° C. Discard the solution if it turns yellow.

Cyanogen bromide, 10%: Dissolve 5 g of cyanogen bromide in 50 ml distilled water. Store at 4° to 5° C in a brown glass bottle with a tightly fitting cap. If a precipitate forms, warm the solution to room temperature to redissolve the ingredients.

Quality control. See Tables 3-10 and 3-18.

NITRATE AND NITRITE BROTHS

Purpose. Nitrate broth medium is used to determine an organism's ability to reduce nitrate to nitrite or other end products such as nitrogen gas. Nitrite broth medium is used to ascertain an organism's ability to reduce nitrite.

Principle and interpretation. Nitrate broth contains a small amount of protein and potassium nitrate. Nitrite broth differs only in the substitution of potassium nitrite for nitrate.

Nitrate may be reduced by organisms in a variety of ways. It may be reduced in assimilatory processes, in which the end products are used to synthesize cellular components, or in dissimilatory processes (respiration), in which nitrate is used in place of oxygen as the final electron acceptor. Aerobic organisms (such as *Pseudomonas aeruginosa*) that can utilize nitrate in the latter process are able to grow anaerobically. In both assimilation and dissimilation nitrate may be reduced to nitrite or beyond the nitrite stage to ammonia or nitrogen gas. Nitrate reduction may be determined by detection of the presence of nitrite or by the complete absence of nitrate or nitrite, meaning that nitrate has been reduced to ammonia or nitrogen gas.

The nitrate reduction test is performed in two stages. The first stage determines the reduction of nitrate to nitrite. After the organism is grown in nitrate broth, sulfanilic acid and alpha-naphthylamine are added. These reagents react with nitrite to form a red azo dye. Thus the formation of a red color in the first stage of the test is a positive finding; that is, nitrates have been reduced to nitrites.

Lack of a red color after addition of the reagents is explained in one of two ways: either nitrate was not reduced or nitrate was reduced beyond the nitrite stage to ammonia or nitrogen gas. To determine which of these has occurred, a pinch of zinc dust is added to the broth; this constitutes stage two of the test. Metallic zinc reduces nitrate to nitrite. Thus, if nitrate was not reduced by the test organism in stage 1, it is still available and is reduced by the zinc to nitrite in stage 2. The nitrite then reacts with the reagents, causing formation of the red azo dye. This constitutes a negative test result for nitrate reduction; because nitrates were still present in the medium, the organism was not capable of reducing them. A broth that remains uncolored after addition of zinc dust indicates that nitrate was reduced beyond

the nitrite stage to ammonia or nitrogen gas; this is a positive finding for nitrate reduction.

Ingredients and preparation. Mix the following ingredients, heat to boiling, and dispense into tubes containing inverted Durham tubes. Cap each tube and sterilize at 121° C for 15 minutes.

Beef extract	3 g
Pancreatic hydrolysate of gelatin, USP	5 g
Potassium nitrate or potassium nitrite	1 g
Distilled water	1 L

Final pH 7.0

NOTE: See Chapter 14 for modifications when testing for *Neisseria*.

Reagents

Zinc dust

Nitrate reagent A:

Sulfanilic acid	8 g
Acetic acid, 5 N	1 L

Nitrate reagent B:

N,N-Dimethyl-1-naphthylamine	6 ml
Acetic acid, 5 N	1 L

Acetic acid, 5 N (30%):

Glacial acetic acid	300 ml
Distilled water, q.s. to	1 L

NOTE: Reagent-impregnated test strips for nitrate reduction are commercially available.

Procedure. Inoculate the test organism into nitrate or nitrite broth and incubate for 24 to 48 hours at 35° C. Examine Durham tubes for presence of entrapped gas and test the broth for nitrite using nitrate reagents A and B. Add 1 ml each of nitrate reagents A and B to a culture of the test organism. Observe for development of a red color in 1 to 2 minutes. Add zinc dust to tubes of medium that have not changed color. Observe for development of a red color after addition of zinc.

Quality control. See Tables 3-7 and 3-16.

NITRATE REDUCTION TEST FOR MYCOBACTERIA

Purpose. The nitrate reduction test is useful for distinguishing among species of mycobacteria based on their ability to reduce nitrate to nitrite.

Principle. See the discussion of nitrate broth.

Procedure. Emulsify two spadesful of growth (4-week-old culture) in 0.2 ml of sterile distilled water in a tube. Add 2 ml of 0.01 M sodium nitrate–phosphate buffered substrate to the tube. Shake to mix. Incubate the tube in a 35° C water bath for 2 hours. Add 1 drop of nitrate reagent no. 1 to the mixture. Add 2 drops of nitrate reagent no. 2 and 2 drops of nitrate reagent no. 3. Examine the mixture for development of a red color after addition of the reagents. A red color is a positive finding for nitrate reduction. Add zinc dust to tubes in which results are negative, and interpret results as described for nitrate broth.

Reagents. Reagents may be purchased from commercial

sources as a paper strip test or prepared as follows. Store all reagents in the dark at 5° C. Discard if a precipitate or discoloration occurs.

Nitrate reagent no. 1 (add acid to water):

Hydrochloric acid, concentrated	50 ml
Distilled water	50 ml

Nitrate reagent no. 2:

Sulfanilamide	0.2 g
Distilled water	100 ml

Nitrate reagent no. 3:

N-Naphthylethylenediamine dihydrochloride	0.1 g
Distilled water	100 ml

Nitrate-phosphate buffered substrate, 0.01 M: Mix the following ingredients in order in 100 ml distilled water. Sterilize by autoclaving.

Sodium nitrate	85 mg
Sodium monohydrogen phosphate, hydrated	485 mg
Potassium dihydrogen phosphate	117 mg
Distilled water	100 ml

Quality control. See Tables 3-10 and 3-18.

NOVOBIOCIN SUSCEPTIBILITY TEST

Purpose. The novobiocin susceptibility test is useful for presumptively distinguishing *Staphylococcus saprophyticus* from other coagulase-negative staphylcocci recovered from human urine specimens.

Principle. *S. saprophyticus* is able to grow in the presence of novobiocin, an antimicrobial agent produced by a streptomycete. After appropriate inoculation and incubation, a diameter of inhibition of 15 mm or less around a 5 μg novobiocin disk constitutes a resistant test result and presumptively identifies the test organism as *S. saprophyticus*, especially if the isolate is cultured from urine. The staphylococci *S. cohni, S. xylosus,* and *S. sciuri* are also resistant to novobiocin, but these species are rarely isolated from urine.

Procedure. Inoculate the test organism to one half of a sheep blood agar plate. Place a 5 μg novobiocin disk in the center of the inoculum. Incubate the culture at 35° C in air for 18 to 24 hours. After incubation, examine the culture for inhibition of growth around the disk.

Reagent. The reagent is a novobiocin disk, 5 μg (BBL Microbiology Systems, Cockeysville, Md.).

Quality control. Test sample disks from each lot number with the following organisms, and observe for expected results:

S. saprophyticus—resistant (diameter of inhibition of 15 mm or less)

S. epidermidis—susceptible (diameter 16 mm or greater)

REFERENCE

Gunn, B.A., et al.: Comparison of methods for identifying *Staphylococcus* and *Micrococcus* spp., J. Clin. Microbiol. **14:**195, 1981.

NUTRIENT AGAR

Purpose. Nutrient agar is a low nutrient medium that is used to cultivate bacteria. It has been used to distinguish among nonfastidious, nonpathogenic *Neisseria* spp. and fastidious, pathogenic *Neisseria* spp., such as *N. gonorrhoeae.*

Principle and interpretation. Nutrient agar contains small amounts of protein and agar. Growth on this medium suggests that the organism has minimal nutritional requirements.

Ingredients and preparation. Mix the following ingredients in 1 L of distilled water, heat to boiling, and sterilize at 121° C for 15 minutes. Cool to 50° C, and dispense 20 ml aliquots into sterile plates. Allow agar to harden for several hours with lids ajar to eliminate excess surface moisture.

Pancreatic hydrolysate of gelatin, USP	5 g
Beef extract	3 g
Agar	15 g
Distilled water	1 L

Final pH 6.8

Procedure. Touch a sterile bacteriologic loop to the center of a well-isolated colony. Inoculate the surface of nutrient agar, and streak for isolation. Incubate for 18 to 24 hours at 35° C.

Quality control. Test sample plates of medium from each batch with the following organism and observe for expected results:

Escherichia coli—growth

OPTOCHIN SUSCEPTIBILITY TEST

Purpose. The optochin susceptibility test is used for presumptive identification of *Streptococcus pneumoniae.*

Principle. Susceptibility to optochin (ethylhydrocupreine hydrochloride) incorporated into a paper disk, or P disk, is used to distinguish alpha-hemolytic streptococci and *Streptococcus pneumoniae.* The pneumococcus, *S. pneumoniae,* is susceptible to optochin, whereas most other alpha-hemolytic streptococci are resistant.

Procedure. Touch a sterile bacteriologic needle to the center of a well-isolated colony of alpha-hemolytic streptococcus, and transfer the inoculum to one half of a sheep blood agar plate. Place an optochin disk, containing 5 μg of optochin, in the center of the inoculated agar surface. Incubate the culture for 18 to 24 hours at 35° C in 5% carbon dioxide and air. After incubation, examine the culture for inhibition of growth around the disk. Cultures thought to be a pneumococcus but giving questionable results may be tested for solubility in bile. Bile-soluble strains are presumptively identified as *S. pneumoniae.* Optochin results are interpreted as follows:

Susceptible—16 mm or greater with a 10 mm disk, or 14 mm or greater with a 6 mm disk

Resistant—less than 16 mm with a 10 mm disk, or less than 14 mm with a 6 mm disk

Reagent. The reagent is optochin disks, 5 μg.

Quality control. See P disk (optochin) in Table 3-16.

ORTHO-NITROPHENYL-BETA-D-GALACTOSIDASE TEST

Purpose. The ortho-nitrophenyl-beta-D-galactosidase (ONPG) test is useful for rapidly determining the ability of an organism to ferment lactose.

Principle and interpretation. Lactose is a disaccharide that is metabolized by many species of bacteria. Lactose-fermenting organisms possess two distinct enzymes: the enzyme permease is responsible for the active transport of the carbohydrate into the bacterial cell, and the enzyme beta-galactosidase degrades the lactose into glucose and galactose. The beta-galactosidase and permease enzymes are inducible; that is, they are produced only when their specific substrate, lactose, is present. Non-lactose-fermenting organisms lack both permease and beta-galactosidase. Delayed lactose fermenters produce beta-galactosidase but either lack permease or have a functionally impaired enzyme system. In the presence of lactose, however, over a period of time these latter organisms produce mutant cells that possess the permease enzyme and thus permit delayed lactose fermentation to occur.

Detection of beta-galactosidase in the presence or absence of a permease system can be determined with ortho-nitrophenyl-beta-D-galactopyranoside (ONPG-P), a compound similar in structure to lactose. ONPG-P enters the bacterial cell rapidly and without the aid of a permease system. Hydrolysis of ONPG-P by beta-galactosidase results in formation of galactose and orthonitrophenol. This compound is yellow at an alkaline pH. Thus development of a yellow color in the test system constitutes a positive finding for production of beta-galactosidase and indicates that the organism is able to ferment lactose.

Procedure. Prepare a dense 0.85% saline suspension of the test organism growing on triple sugar iron agar. Add 1 drop of toluene to the suspension, and mix thoroughly to enhance release of beta-galactosidase from the cells. Add 0.2 ml of ONPG solution to the suspension, and incubate at 35° C. Examine tubes for development of a yellow color after 1 hour of incubation. Hold tubes in which results are negative after 1 hour for 18 to 24 hours and reexamine for a color change.

Reagents. *Sodium phosphate buffer, 0.01 M, pH 7.0:* Mix the following ingredients and add 5 N sodium hydroxide solution to bring the pH to 7.0. Then bring the final volume up to 100 ml with distilled water.

Disodium phosphate	13.8 g
Distilled water	80 ml

Adjust pH to 7.0 with 5 N NaOH, then add:

Distilled water, q.s. to	100 ml

ONPG solution: Mix the first two ingredients, place in a 35° C incubator until dissolved, and add the last ingredient. Store the reagent in a dark glass bottle at 4° C.

o-Nitrophenyl-beta-D-galactopyranoside	80 mg
Distilled water	15 ml
Sodium phosphate buffer, pH 7.0	5 ml

NOTE: ONPG-impregnated strips, disks, and tablets are commercially available.

Quality control. See Table 3-16.

OXIDASE TEST

Purpose. The oxidase test is used to distinguish among species of bacteria based on their possession of the enzyme cytochrome oxidase.

Principle. Aerobic bacteria utilize the process of oxidative phosphorylation for respiration and energy derivation. During this process, cytochromes (heme-containing proteins) function as a chain of enzymes that sequentially transfer electrons from the substrate being oxidized to molecular oxygen, with subsequent formation of water. The terminal cytochrome, which reacts with oxygen in mammalian and yeast systems, is cytochrome c oxidase. However, in bacteria several cytochromes can act as terminal oxidases.

Detection of the cytochrome oxidase system depends on the use of reagents that are normally colorless but become colored when oxidized. Two reagents may be used: tetramethyl-*p*-phenylenediamine dihydrochloride or dimethyl-*p*-phenylenediamine dihydrochloride. Both of these reagents are normally colorless but become purple or blue-black when oxidized. In the oxidase test a portion of a colony of the test organism is applied to filter paper that is saturated with the reagent; if the cytochrome oxidase enzyme is present, it oxidizes the colorless reagent to form a purple or blue-black color. Use of the reagent tetramethyl-*p*-phenylenediamine dihydrochloride is discussed in the following paragraphs.

Procedure. Prepare a 1% solution of tetramethyl-*p*-phenylenediamine dihydrochloride (available from several chemical companies) in sterile distilled water. Place a piece of filter paper in the bottom of a sterile plastic Petri dish, and moisten it thoroughly with the reagent. Using a plastic needle or a wooden stick, touch the colony and transfer the inoculum to the filter paper. Do not use an iron (Nichrome) inoculating needle, since false-positive results may occur with this metal. Development of a blue-black or purple color within 10 seconds is a positive finding. The test may also be performed by dropping the reagent directly on colonies growing on blood or chocolate agar and observing for the development of a purple or blue-black color. Tests performed on colonies growing on carbohydrate-containing media may be invalid because acid affects the reagent's sensitivity.

Reagent-impregnated filter paper strips or disks or disposable glass ampules containing small amounts of reagent are available from numerous commercial sources including the following: General Diagnostics (Morris Plains, N.J.), Marion Scientific (Kansas City, MO.), Remel (Lenexa, Kan.), and Difco Laboratories (Detroit).

Some gram-positive cocci such as *Micrococcus* spp. yield variable oxidase results unless dimethyl sulfoxide is used to enhance penetration of the tetramethyl-*p*-phenylenediamine reagent into the cells. The reagent for testing these organisms may be prepared as follows:

Tetramethyl-*p*-phenylenediamine dihydrochloride	0.5 ml
Dimethyl sulfoxide (DMSO)	100 ml

Quality control. See Table 3-16.

REFERENCE

Faller, A., and Schleifer, K.H.: Modified oxidase and benzidene tests for separation of staphylococci and micrococci, J. Clin. Microbiol. **13:**1031, 1981.

OXIDATION-FERMENTATION TEST MEDIUM

Purpose. Oxidation-fermentation (OF) test medium, supplemented with 1% glucose, is used to distinguish among species of bacteria based on mode of utilization of glucose, that is, oxidation or fermentation. The medium is also used to test for acid production from other carbohydrates. This medium should not be used for testing staphylococci.

Principle and interpretation. OF test medium contains a small amount of protein, sodium chloride, buffer, pH indicator, agar, and a carbohydrate. The protein content of the medium is kept low to avoid neutralization of acid by alkaline products resulting from deamination of protein. The traditional method determining the utilization of glucose is to inoculate two tubes of medium with the test organism. One tube is overlaid with sterile mineral oil. Bacteria that oxidize glucose require atmospheric oxygen for utilization of the carbohydrate. Thus these bacteria are able to produce acid from glucose in the open tube of medium but are unable to produce acid in the tube sealed with mineral oil. Bacteria that ferment glucose produce acid in both tubes. Other bacteria may be unable to ferment or oxidize glucose and thus do not produce acid in either tube; these bacteria are said to be asaccharolytic. Production of acid in either tube causes a lowering of the pH in the medium and a concomitant change in the color of the indicator, phenol red. Phenol red is yellow at its acidic endpoint and red at its alkaline endpoint.

Expected results are as follows:

Fermentation—both tubes of medium turn yellow

Oxidation—open tube of medium turns yellow; sealed tube stays red

Asaccharolytic—both tubes of medium stay red

Determination of the utilization of other carbohydrates by nonfermentative organisms may be performed using only one tube of medium.

NOTE: Motility may also be determined in the medium by stabbing the agar butt. Movement away from the inoculum stab is a positive reaction.

Ingredients and preparation. Mix the following basal ingredients, heat to dissolve, and dispense in 13 × 100 mm screw-cap tubes in 4.5 ml amounts. Autoclave at 121° C for 15 minutes, and allow the agar to cool in an upright position before refrigerating. Before use, add 0.5 ml of 10% filter-sterilized carbohydrate to each tube of 4.5 ml agar base, gently invert the tube once, and allow agar to solidify in an upright position.

Basal ingredients:

Pancreatic digest of casein, USP	2 g
Phenol red, 1.5% solution	2 ml
Agar	3 g
Deionized water	900 ml

Final pH 7.3 + 0.1

Carbohydrate solutions: Add 0.5 ml of a 10% solution of filter-sterilized carbohydrate to 4.5 ml of basal medium. Final concentration of carbohydrate is 1%.

Procedure. Inoculate each tube of OF carbohydrate medium with 1 drop of a broth culture or saline suspension of the test organism or alternatively with isolated colonies that are stabbed four times approximately 1 cm below the surface of the agar. Also inoculate a control tube containing carbohydrate-free basal medium. Incubate tubes at 35° C and observe daily for 4 days, and again after 7 days, for evidence of acid production.

Although the traditional method of determining utilization of glucose employs two tubes of medium, Oberhofer recommends the use of only one tube because fermentative organisms acidify the whole tube whereas nonfermentative organisms acidify only the upper part of the tube. Furthermore, the triple sugar iron slant can ascertain fermentative abilities of the test organisms.

Quality control. See oxidation-fermentation (OF) media in Table 3-7.

REFERENCE

Oberhofer, T.R.: Manual of nonfermenting gram-negative bacteria, New York, 1985, John Wiley & Sons, Inc.

OXIDATION-FERMENTATION TEST MEDIUM FOR *STAPHYLOCOCCUS*

Purpose. Staphylococcus oxidation-fermentation (S-OF) medium is prepared as recommended by the Subcommittee on Taxonomy of Staphylococci and Micrococci and is used for testing catalase-positive cocci for ability to ferment glucose. S-OF is useful for distinguishing between *Staphylococcus* and *Micrococcus* organisms.

Principle and interpretation. S-OF medium was devised to overcome problems associated with testing staphylococci for fermentation of glucose using the conventional Hugh and Leifsson OF test medium. S-OF medium is more enriched than OF medium and employs a different pH indicator that enhances detection of slight pH changes by certain species of *Staphylococcus*. In S-OF medium, staphylococci ferment glucose and micrococci either oxidize glucose or are asaccharolytic. Results are interpreted as described for oxidation-fermentation test medium.

Ingredients and preparation. Mix the following basal ingredients, heat to boiling, sterilize at 121° C for 15 minutes, cool to 50° C, and add filter-sterilized glucose stock solution.

Basal ingredients:

Pancreatic digest of casein, USP	10 g
Yeast extract	1 g
Bromcresol purple, 1.6% in 95% ethanol	2.5 ml
Agar	3.5 g
Distilled water	980 ml

Final pH 7.0

Glucose stock solution, filter sterilized:

Glucose, 50%   20 ml

Procedure. See the discussion of oxidation-fermentation test medium.

Quality control. Inoculate tubes of medium as described for OF test medium. Use the following organisms:

Staphylococcus aureus—fermentative (acid [yellowing] produced in open and sealed tubes)

Micrococcus luteus—asaccharolytic (no acid produced in either tube [blue])

REFERENCES

Davis, G.H.G., and Hoyling, B.: Observations on anaerobic glucose utilization tests in *Staphylococcus-Micrococcus* identification, Int. J. Syst. Bacteriol. **21:**161, 1974.

Gunn, B.A., et al.: Comparison of methods for identifying *Staphylococcus* and *Micrococcus* spp., J. Clin. Microbiol. **14:**195, 1981.

Subcommittee on Taxonomy of Staphylococci and Micrococci: Minutes of first meeting, Int. Bull. Bacteriol. Nomencl. Taxon. **15:**107, 1965.

PEPTONE–YEAST EXTRACT–GLUCOSE BROTH

Purpose. Peptone–yeast extract–glucose (PYG) broth is a growth medium used for cultivation and identification of anaerobic bacteria.

Principle and interpretation. PYG broth contains protein, yeast extract, glucose, amino acids, salts, and an oxidation-reduction (redox) indicator. This broth may be used to identify anaerobic bacteria by the volatile and nonvolatile acids they produce from glucose. The acids are identified by gas chromatography. The special enrichments added to this medium provide optimal growth conditions for most clinical strains of anaerobic bacteria. Resazurin provides a means by which the redox potential of the medium can be monitored visually. As oxygen gradually diffuses into the medium, the redox potential changes and the indicator turns pink. However, the resazurin in the deeper, anaerobic regions of PYG remains colorless. The medium must not be mixed during storage or actual use, since oxygenation of the deeper regions of PYG might occur and inhibit growth.

Ingredients and preparation. Mix the following ingredients, except L-cysteine, vitamin K_1, and hemin. Heat to boiling, cool to 50° C, and add the last three ingredients. Adjust pH to 7.2. Dispense into tubes and sterilize at 115° C for 15 minutes. Prereduce tubes of medium before storage.

Peptone	0.5 g
Trypticase	0.5 g
Yeast extract	1 g
D-Glucose	1 g
Salt solution	4 ml
Resazurin solution	0.4 ml
Hemin solution	1 ml
Vitamin K_1	0.02 ml
Cysteine HC1 · H_2O	0.05 g
Distilled water	100 ml

Final pH 7.2

Salt solution:

Calcium chloride, anhydrous	0.2 g
Magnesium sulfate, anhydrous	0.2 g
Potassium monohydrogen phosphate	1 g
Potassium dihydrogen phosphate	1 g
Sodium bicarbonate	10 g
Sodium chloride	2 g

Mix the calcium chloride and magnesium sulfate in 300 ml distilled water until dissolved. Add 500 ml of distilled water, and while stirring, slowly add remaining salts. Continue swirling until all salts are dissolved. Add 200 ml distilled water and mix. Store at 4° C. If salts precipitate out of solution during storage, heat to 50° C before using.

Resazurin solution: Dissolve 25 mg resazurin in 100 ml distilled water. Store at room temperature.

Procedure. Inoculate test organism into PYG broth, and incubate at 35° C for 48 to 72 hours.

Quality control. See Table 3-4. Also, check each batch of medium for indicator function and presence of acids.

To determine indicator (resazurin) function, expose a tube of medium to air and observe for formation of a pink or light blue color. This is a positive test for indicator function.

To check that medium is acid free, test a noninoculated tube of medium for presence of acids, especially succinic and acetic acids, using a gas chromatograph.

REFERENCE

Holdeman, L.V., Cato, E.P., and Moore, W.E.C., editors: Anaerobe laboratory manual, ed. 4, V.P.I. Anaerobe Laboratory, Virginia Polytechnic Institute and State University, 1977, Blacksburg, Va.

PHENYLALANINE AGAR

Purpose. Phenylalanine agar is used to differentiate *Proteus, Morganella,* and *Providencia* spp. from other *Enterobacteriaceae* based on ability to deaminate phenylalanine. It may also be used to differentiate selected nonfermentative organisms.

Principle and interpretation. Phenylalanine agar contains yeast extract, sodium chloride, buffer, agar, and DL-phenylalanine. Bacteria that are capable of oxidatively deaminating phenylalanine grow on this medium and produce the keto acid, phenylpyruvic acid, as a deamination by-product. The alpha-keto acid reacts with ferric chloride reagent to form a green reaction product. Immediate appearance of this intense green color is a positive result for deamination of phenylalanine.

Ingredients and preparation. Mix the following ingredients, heat to boiling, dispense into test tubes, and sterilize at 121° C for 10 minutes. After sterilization, cool to room temperature in a slanted position.

DL-Phenylalanine	2 g
Yeast extract	3 g
Sodium chloride	5 g
Disodium phosphate	1 g
Agar	12 g
Distilled water	1 L

Final pH 7.3

Reagent
Acid ferric chloride:

Ferric chloride	12 g
Hydrochloric acid, concentrated	2.5 ml
Distilled water, q.s. to	100 ml

Store at 4° C in a dark bottle. NOTE: Reagent-impregnated strips and tablets are also commercially available.

Procedure. Inoculate the slant medium with a single colony of the test organism. Incubate for 18 to 24 hours at 35° C. (When testing nonfermentative organisms incubate tubes for 48 hours.) Add 4 or 5 drops of ferric chloride reagent to the surface of the slant. Rotate the tube as the reagent is added to cover the surface thoroughly.

Quality control. See phenylalanine deaminase agar in Table 3-7 and ferric chloride in Table 3-16.

PORPHYRIN TEST

Purpose. The porphyrin test is used to determine the need of *Haemophilus* spp. for X factor.

Principle. The normal biosynthesis of hemin is shown in Figure 15-1. Strains of *Haemophilus* that require X factor lack the enzymes (designated A, B, and C) necessary to synthesize hemin from delta-aminolevulinic acid (ALA). However strains that do not require X factor (X-independent strains) do possess these enzymes and are able to convert ALA to porphobilinogen, porphyrin, and finally hemin. Furthermore, X-independent strains excrete these porphobilinogens and porphyrins into the medium. The porphyrin test detects these excreted substances.

Procedure. Prepare delta-aminolevulinic acid substrate consisting of 2 mM delta-aminolevulinic acid (Sigma Chemical Co., St. Louis) and 0.8 mM magnesium sulfate in 0.1 M phosphate buffer at pH 6.9. Distribute substrate in 0.5 ml quantities in small tubes. Substrate may be stored for several months in a refrigerator. Inoculate a heavy loopful of the organism into the substrate. Also inoculate positive and negative controls. Incubate at 37° C for 4 hours. To detect porphyrins, take tubes into a darkroom and expose them to a Wood's lamp (360 nm). Red fluorescence indicates the presence of porphyrins; that is, the organism does not require the X factor.

An alternative method is to detect porphobilinogens. After incubation, add 0.5 ml Kovacs reagent, shake vigorously, and allow the water and alcoholic phases to separate. Development of a red color in the lower aqueous phase indicates the presence of porphobilinogen; that is, the organism does not require the X factor. An uninoculated tube without substrate should be used as a negative control to prevent the misidentification of indole-positive strains of *H. influenzae* as X factor independent.

NOTE: ALA-impregnated paper disks are available from Remel Laboratories (Lenexa, Kan.). The user should follow the manufacturer's instructions.

Quality control. Positive and negative controls as indicated previously should be used.

REFERENCES

Kilian, M.: A rapid method for the differentiation of *Haemophilus* strains—the porphyrin test, Acta Pathol. Microbiol. Scand. **82B**:835, 1974.

Kilian, M.: *Haemophilus*. In Lennette, E.H., et. al., editors: Manual of clinical microbiology, ed. 4, Washington, D.C., 1985, American Society for Microbiology.

POTASSIUM CYANIDE BROTH

Purpose. Potassium cyanide (KCN) broth is useful for distinguishing among genera of *Enterobacteriaceae* and nonfermentative bacteria. However, it is not recommended for routine use in a diagnostic clinical laboratory because of the toxicity of KCN and the availability of nontoxic tests for distinguishing bacteria.

Principle and interpretation. KCN broth contains a small amount of protein, sodium chloride, buffer, and KCN. This medium is used to determine the ability of bacteria to grow in the presence of KCN. KCN is a cytochrome oxidase inhibitor; it binds with the iron of cytochrome oxidase and leaves the enzyme inactive. Thus aerobic respiration in the organism is halted. The respiration of a few aerobic organisms is not sensitive to KCN, probably because of a flavoprotein respiration system that does not require cytochrome oxidase. Since aerobic

organisms differ in their susceptibility to cyanide, the medium is used as a test to distinguish among some of these species.

KCN is toxic, and care should be taken during its preparation. KCN should never be pipetted by mouth. KCN solution should be prepared in a chemical hood. The KCN in all tubes of medium must be destroyed before autoclaving by the addition of a crystal of ferrous sulfate and 0.1 ml of 40% potassium hydroxide to each tube. KCN medium may be stored up to 1 month at 4° C. Growth in the medium is a positive test result. Growth in the KCN-free broth but no growth in KCN broth constitutes a negative test result.

Ingredients and preparation. Mix basal ingredients, heat to boiling, and separate into two aliquots, one for preparation of KCN broth and the other for KCN-free broth. Sterilize both aliquots at 121° C for 15 minutes. Cool the sterilized basal medium to room temperature, and add 7.5 ml of 0.5% KCN solution to one 500 ml aliquot of medium. Dispense media into tubes and store at 4° C.

KCN basal ingredients:

Peptic digest of animal tissue, USP	3 g
Sodium chloride	5 g
Monobasic potassium phosphate, anhydrous	0.225 g
Dibasic sodium phosphate	5.64 g
Distilled water	1 L

Final pH 7.6

Mix, heat to boiling, divide into two 500 ml aliquots, and sterilize.

Additive to one 500 ml aliquot of cooled basal medium:

Potassium cyanide, 0.5%, aqueous	7.5 ml

0.5% KCN solution:

Potassium cyanide	0.5 g
Distilled water	100 ml

Store in a labeled sterile flask at 4° C.

Procedure. Transfer a light inoculum of the test organism to tubes of medium with and without KCN. Incubate cultures for 24 to 48 hours at 35° C. Observe and compare growth occurring in broth with KCN and broth without KCN.

Quality control. See Table 3-7.

PSEUDOMONAS FLUORESCEIN AGAR

Purpose. Pseudomonas fluorescein (F) agar is used to detect the production of fluorescein. This pigment is produced by the pseudomonads *P. aeruginosa*, *P. putida*, *P. fluorescens*, and UFP (unidentified fluorescent pseudomonads).

Principle and interpretation. Fluorescein (pyoverdin) is a combination of fluorescent, water-soluble, yellow-green pigments that are insoluble in chloroform. Pseudomonas F agar enhances the production of the fluorescein pigment while suppressing the production of the pyocyanin pigment (see the discussion of Pseudomonas P agar). Fluorescein is released into the medium and usually produces a visible yellow or yellow-green color. Tubes of medium negative for fluorescein by the unaided eye are examined for fluorescence under a Wood's lamp or an ultraviolet (UV) light at 366 nm.

Ingredients and preparation. Commercially available media for detection of fluorescein include F agar (Difco Laboratories, Detroit) and FLO agar (BBL Diagnostics, Cockeysville, Md.). The Difco formulation, which is available in dehydrated form, is given here.

Tryptone	10 g
Proteose peptone No. 3	10 g
Dipotassium phosphate	1.5 g
Magnesium sulfate · 7 H$_2$O	1.5 g
Agar	15 g

Suspend 38 g of the dehydrated medium in 1000 ml of deionized water, and heat to dissolve. Dispense the medium into screw-cap tubes, and autoclave at 121° C for 15 minutes. Allow agar to cool in a slanted position.

Procedure. Inoculate the slant with a drop of a broth culture or a portion of an isolated colony of the test organism. Incubate at room temperature for 18 to 24 hours. Observe for evidence of yellow pigmentation in the medium. Test for fluorescence using a UV light source. Reincubate negative slants for an additional 24 hours.

Quality control. See Pseudomonas F agar in Table 3-7.

REFERENCE

Oberhofer, T.R.: Manual of nonfermenting gram-negative bacteria, New York, 1985, John Wiley & Sons, Inc.

PSEUDOMONAS PYOCYANIN AGAR

Purpose. Pseudomonas pyocyanin (P) agar is used to detect the production of pyocyanin. *P. aeruginosa* is the only organism that produces this pigment.

Principle and interpretation. *P. aeruginosa* produces several pigments including pyocyanin, pyoverdin, pyomelanin, and pyorubin. Pyocyanin is a water-soluble, chloroform-soluble, nonfluorescent, blue, phenazine pigment. Pseudomonas P agar enhances the production of pyocyanin while suppressing the production of fluorescein (see discussion of Pseudomonas F agar). On Pseudomonas P agar, pyocyanin appears as a light green, green, dark green, blue-green, or dark blue color. Small quantities of pyocyanin may not be detected visually unless the pigment is extracted from the medium with chloroform.

Ingredients and preparation. Commercially available media for detection of pyocyanin include P agar (Difco Laboratories, Detroit) and TECH agar (BBL Microbiology Systems, Cockeysville, Md.). The Difco formulation, which is available in dehydrated form, is given here.

Peptone	20 g
Magnesium chloride	1.4 g
Potassium sulfate	10 g
Agar	15 g

Suspend 46 g of the dehydrated medium in 1000 ml of deionized water, and heat to dissolve. Dispense the medium into screw-cap tubes, and autoclave at 121° C for 15 minutes. Allow to cool in a slanted position.

Procedure. Inoculate the slant with a drop of a broth culture or a portion of an isolated colony of the test organism. Incubate the slant at 35° C for 18 to 24 hours. Observe for production of a green, dark green, or blue-green color. Reincubate negative

slants for an additional 24 hours.

Quality control. See Pseudomonas P agar in Table 3-7.

REFERENCE

Oberhofer, T.R.: Manual of nonfermenting gram-negative bacteria, New York, 1985, John Wiley & Sons, Inc.

PYRAZINAMIDASE AGAR

Purpose. Pyrazinamidase agar is used to distinguish among species of *Mycobacterium* based on ability to hydrolyze pyrazinamide to pyrazinoic acid.

Principle and interpretation. Pyrazinamide agar contains Dubos broth base, pyrazinamide, sodium pyruvate, and agar. The presence of the enzyme pyrazinamidase allows the hydrolysis of pyrazinamide to pyrazinoic acid by *M. tuberculosis*. Detection of this acid is accomplished by adding ferrous ammonium sulfate to the culture. Ferrous ammonium sulfate reacts with pyrazinoic acid to form a pink ferrous–pyrazinoic acid complex; this constitutes a positive test result for pyrazinamidase activity.

Ingredients and preparation. Add Dubos broth base to distilled water, dissolve, and add pyrazinamide, sodium pyruvate, and agar. Heat to dissolve agar, dispense into tubes, and sterilize at 121° C for 15 minutes. Allow tubes of medium to solidify in an upright position.

Dubos broth base	6.5 g
Pyrazinamide	0.1 g
Sodium pyruvate	2 g
Agar	15 g
Distilled water	1 L
Final pH 7.0	

Reagent

Ferrous ammonium sulfate, 1% (use freshly prepared):

Ferrous ammonium sulfate	0.1 g
Distilled water	10 ml

Procedure. Use a bacteriologic loop or spade to transfer a heavy inoculum of the test organism from an actively growing culture (2 or 3 weeks old) to the surface of two tubes of pyrazinamidase medium. The inoculum should be heavy enough to be visible with the naked eye. Incubate the tubes at 37° C for 4 days.

Add 1 ml of ferrous ammonium sulfate reagent to one of the tubes, the color control standard, and the positive and negative controls, and hold the tubes at 4° C for 4 hours. Refrigeration discourages overgrowth with contaminating organisms. After four hours at 4° C, observe the tube for presence of a pink band in the agar. Examine tubes against a white background with incidental room light. If the 4-day test result is positive, it is unnecessary to continue incubating the second tube. However, if the 4-day result is negative, the second tube should be incubated an additional 3 days and then tested with ferrous ammonium sulfate reagent.

Quality control. Test reagent and tubes of medium from each batch with the following organisms, and observe for expected results:

M. tuberculosis, M. avium-intracellulare, M. marinum—
    formation of a pink band

M. kansasii and uninoculated medium—absence of a pink band

QUELLUNG TEST

Purpose. The quellung test is used to identify organisms with capsules such as *Streptococcus pneumoniae* or *Haemophilus influenzae* in cerebrospinal fluid or sputum.

Principle. The quellung test relies on reaction of type-specific antisera with the capsule of *S. pneumoniae* or *H. influenzae*. More than 80 distinct capsular serologic types of pneumococci have been described. Because so many capsular serotypes exist, pooled antiserum containing the majority of the prevalent serotypes is used for testing. Antiserum against the type b capsular polysaccharide is used for detection of *H. influenzae* type b.

In the quellung test, specific antiserum is mixed with a specimen thought to contain *S. pneumoniae* or *H. influenzae*. If the organism is present, antibodies in the antiserum react with the polysaccharide in the capsule. This causes a change in the refractive index (RI) of the capsule. The change in RI causes the capsule to appear swollen when examined with a light microscope. Methylene blue is mixed with the preparation to stain bacterial cells, which provides a sharp contrast between the cells and the bright capsular halo.

Procedure. Place a loopful of the specimen on a glass slide. Add a loopful of antiserum (pooled antiserum for *S. pneumoniae*) to the suspension, and mix thoroughly with a small applicator stick or bacteriologic loop. (A control consisting of organism and saline should also be run.) Add 1 drop of methylene blue reagent to the suspension, mix, and place a coverslip over the entire preparation. Let the preparation rest for 10 minutes, and then examine with a microscope using the oil immersion lens. Oblique illumination is best for examination of the slide. A dark blue bacterial cell surrounded by a bright capsular halo constitutes a positive quellung test result.

Reagents

Methylene blue reagent:

Methylene blue	1 g
Distilled water	100 ml

Antisera: Polyvalent (pooled) and specific monovalent antisera for *S. pneumoniae* are available from the sources indicated in Chapter 13. Sources of antisera for *H. influenzae* are included in Chapter 15.

Quality control. Polyvalent and monovalent antisera are used to test known serotypes of *S. pneumoniae* or *H. influenzae*.

SALMONELLA-SHIGELLA AGAR

Purpose. Salmonella-Shigella (SS) agar is a selective agar medium used for isolation of *Salmonella* spp. and many strains of *Shigella* spp. from feces.

Principle and interpretation. SS agar contains protein, bile salts, a hydrogen sulfide indicator and sulfur source, lactose, two dyes, and agar. The selective action of SS agar is attributed to brilliant green dye, which is inhibitory to most species of intestinal bacteria other than *Salmonella,* and bile salts and sodium citrate, which are inhibitory to most species of gram-positive bacteria. The high concentration of bile salts is also inhibitory to many lactose-fermenting normal intestinal flora. Sodium thiosulfate is reduced by certain species of enteric bac-

teria to sulfite and hydrogen sulfide gas. The enzyme responsible for this reductive process is thiosulfate reductase. Production of hydrogen sulfide gas is detected as an insoluble black precipitate, ferrous sulfide, formed upon reaction of hydrogen sulfide with the ferric ions of ferric citrate.

The high degree of selectivity of SS agar allows use of large inocula to enhance isolation of pathogens from feces. Lactose is the sole source of carbohydrate. On fermentation of lactose by the few lactose-fermenting normal intestinal flora that can grow on SS agar, acid is produced and the pH indicator, neutral red, changes color from yellow to red. Thus these organisms grow as red-pigmented colonies. Non-lactose-fermenting organisms grow as translucent colorless colonies with or without black centers. Growth of *Salmonella* organisms is uninhibited and appears as colorless colonies with black centers resulting from hydrogen sulfide production. *Shigella* organisms also grow as colorless colonies but do not produce hydrogen sulfide.

Ingredients and preparation. Mix the following ingredients, bring briefly to a boil, cool to 50° C, and pour into plates. Do not sterilize in an autoclave. Allow the medium to solidify and the agar surface to dry for several hours at room temperature.

Beef extract	5 g
Peptic digest of animal tissues, USP	5 g
Lactose	10 g
Bile salts	8.5 g
Sodium citrate	8.5 g
Sodium thiosulfate	8.5 g
Ferric citrate	1 g
Brilliant green	0.33 mg
Neutral red	25 mg
Agar	13.5 g
Distilled water	1 L

Final pH 7.4

Procedure. Inoculate fecal or enrichment broth samples to SS agar, streak for isolation, and incubate for 18 to 24 hours at 35° C in air. Do not incubate in carbon dioxide.

Quality control. See Table 3-3.

SELENITE-F BROTH

Purpose. Selenite-F enrichment broth medium contains sodium selenite, which enhances recovery of *Salmonella* spp. from specimens, especially fecal specimens, containing mixed cultures of bacteria.

Principle and interpretation. Selenite-F broth contains protein, lactose, phosphate, and sodium selenite. The action of the medium depends on maintenance of a certain pH at which sodium selenite is moderately toxic toward enterococci and normal intestinal flora while promoting the growth of enteric pathogens. The critical pH is maintained by lactose. As enteric bacteria grow, they reduce selenite, resulting in an alkaline environment. However, the acids produced from lactose fermentation neutralize the alkaline products produced during reduction of selenite and thus promote the toxic effects of selenite.

Because the medium loses its ability to suppress normal intestinal flora after 12 hours' incubation, subculture of the selective medium between 8 and 12 hours' incubation is recommended. Best results are achieved when selenite-F broth is subcultured to one enteric medium with little selectivity, one with moderate selectivity, and one that is highly selective.

Ingredients and preparation. Mix the following ingredients, heat to boiling, and immediately dispense 2 ml aliquots into sterile screw-capped test tubes. The medium functions best under anaerobic conditions, and a pour depth of 6 cm or more is recommended. Do not sterilize in an autoclave, and do not overheat. If a precipitate forms during preparation, overheating of the broth has occurred and the medium should be discarded.

Pancreatic digest of casein and peptic digest of animal tissue, USP	5 g
Lactose	4 g
Sodium phosphate	10 g
Sodium selenite	4 g
Distilled water	1 L

Final pH 7.0

Procedure. Inoculate fecal samples to selenite-F broth and incubate for 8 to 12 hours at 35° C. Subculture the broth to the types of media cited previously.

Quality control. See enrichment broths for enterics in Table 3-3.

6.5% SODIUM CHLORIDE AGAR AND BROTH

Purpose. Salt agar is useful for distinguishing among species of bacteria based on ability to grow in the presence of 6.5% sodium chloride. If agar is omitted from the formulation, the medium can be used as a broth.

Principle and interpretation. Salt agar contains large amounts of protein, sodium chloride, and agar. The ability to tolerate and grow on 6.5% sodium chloride agar is characteristic of certain species of gram-positive cocci and gram-negative bacilli. A medium without added salt should be tested along with 6.5% sodium chloride agar to serve as a growth control. If growth is equivalent on both media, the organism is tolerant of salt and a positive result is recorded. However, if growth on the salt-containing medium is very weak or absent but growth on the salt-free medium is good, a negative result is recorded.

Ingredients and preparation. Mix the following ingredients, heat to boiling, and sterilize at 121° C for 15 minutes. Dispense into plates or screw-capped tubes and store at 4° C. Store plate media sealed in plastic bags.

Beef heart infusion	500 g
Peptic digest of animal tissues, USP	10 g
Sodium chloride	65 g
Agar (optional)	15 g
Distilled water	1 L

Final pH 7.4

Procedure. Inoculate the test organism to two tubes or plates of medium, one containing 6.5% sodium chloride and another without added salt. Incubate at 35° C for 24 to 72 hours and observe for growth.

Quality control. See Table 3-7.

SP-4 BROTH AND AGAR MEDIA

Purpose. SP-4 broth is an enriched, antimicrobial-containing broth medium useful for cultivation of *Mycoplasma* spp. from clinical specimens. It may be supplemented with glucose, arginine, or urea to allow identification of these bacteria. Agar may be added to SP-4 broth to allow the medium to be used as an agar plate medium or a diphasic medium.

Principle and interpretation. SP-4 broth contains protein, sodium chloride, penicillin, phenol red, yeast extract, bovine serum, and other enrichments that enhance the growth of *Mycoplasma* organisms in specimens in which mixed species of bacteria may be present. Penicillin is included in the medium to inhibit gram-positive bacteria.

SP-4 with urea is useful for identification of *Ureaplasma urealyticum*. The organism possesses a potent urease that deaminates urea and causes a rise in pH of the medium. This rise in pH is detected with the indicator, neutral red, which is red at a pH greater than 8.0. No other species of *Mycoplasma* produce a urease. This urea-hydrolyzing species is inhibited by ordinary agar and does not grow on SP-4 agar unless purified agar, such as Noble agar, is used in its preparation. SP-4 broth supplemented with glucose is useful for identification of *Mycoplasma pneumoniae*, since this species ferments the carbohydrate and causes a lowering of the pH of the medium and a concomitant change in the color of the indicator to yellow. A few other species of *Mycoplasma* also ferment glucose.

SP-4 broth with arginine is useful for identification of *Mycoplasma hominis*. *M. hominis* is capable of degrading this amino acid to alkaline products, which causes a rise in pH of the medium and an associated change in color to red.

A diphasic medium is prepared by adding a small amount of sterile molten agar to tubes, allowing it to solidify in a slanted position, and then overlaying it with SP-4 broth. The purpose of diphasic medium is to expose species of *Mycoplasma* that grow best on agar, but also need microaerophilic moist conditions, to an environment in which both of these needs are met.

Ingredients and preparation. Prepare SP-4 broth as follows, and add additional ingredients as required.

SP-4 BROTH. Mix the following basal ingredients, adjust the pH to 7.5, heat just to boiling, and sterilize at 121° C for 15 minutes. Cool to 50° C and add the sterile enrichments. Mix well and dispense into sterile screw-capped tubes.

SP-4 basal medium:

Mycoplasma broth base (Difco Laboratories, Detroit; BBL Microbiology Systems, Cockeysville, Md.)	3.5 g
Pancreatic digest of casein, USP	10 g
Proteose pancreatic digest of gelatin, USP	5.3 g
Distilled water	615 ml

SP-4 broth: Add the following sterile enrichments to sterile SP-4 basal medium.

CMRL 1066 medium, 10× strength, with glutamine (Gibco, Madison, Wis.)	50 ml
Yeast extract, 25% (Gibco)	35 ml
Yeastolate, 2% (Difco Laboratories)	100 ml
Fetal bovine serum, heated at 56° C for 1 hour	170 ml
Penicillin, 100,000 units/ml	10 ml
Phenol red, 0.1%	20 ml

Final pH 7.0 to 7.4

SP-4 AGAR. Add Noble agar to SP-4 basal medium before sterilization. Sterilize the solution at 121° C for 15 minutes, cool to 50° C, and add the sterile ingredients *except phenol red solution.* Dispense into plates, and allow to solidify at room temperature. Store at 4° C for no longer than 1 week.

SP-4 basal medium	615 ml
Sterile enrichments (excluding phenol red)	365 ml
Noble agar (Difco Laboratories)	35 g

Final pH 7.4

SP-4 BROTH WITH UREA. Add 0.1 ml of filter-sterilized 50% urea solution to 100 ml SP-4 broth. Adjust the pH, and dispense in 0.5 aliquots into sterile screw-capped tubes. The tightly capped tubes of medium may be stored at 4° C for 1 month or at −20° C for 1 year.

SP-4 sterile basal medium	61.5 ml
Sterile enrichments	38.5 ml
Urea, 50%, sterile	0.1 ml

Final pH 7.4

Urea, 50%: Filter sterilize, and dispense 1.5 ml aliquots into sterile screw-capped tubes. Store at −20° C for up to 1 year.

Urea	5 g
Distilled water	10 ml

SP-4 BROTH WITH GLUCOSE. Add 1 ml of sterile 50% glucose solution to 100 ml of sterile SP-4 broth. Dispense 2 ml aliquots into sterile screw-capped tubes, and store at −20° C for up to 1 year.

SP-4 sterile basal medium	61.5 ml
Sterile enrichments	38.5 ml
Glucose, 50%, sterile	1 ml

Final pH 7.4

Glucose, 50%, sterile: Mix the following ingredients, sterilize by membrane filtration, dispense 1.5 ml aliquots into sterile screw-capped tubes, and store at −20° C for up to 1 year.

D-Glucose	10 g
Distilled water	20 ml

SP-4 BROTH WITH ARGININE. Add 1 ml of sterile 50% L-arginine solution to 100 ml of SP-4 broth. Adjust the sterile mixture to pH 7.0, and dispense 2.0 ml aliquots into sterile screw-capped tubes. The tubes of medium are stored at −20° C for up to 1 year.

SP-4 sterile basal medium	61.5 ml
Sterile enrichments	38.5 ml
L-Arginine, 50%, sterile	1 ml

Final pH 7.0

L-Arginine, 50%, sterile: Mix the following ingredients, sterilize by membrane filtration, dispense 1.5 ml aliquots into sterile screw-capped tubes, and store at −20° C for up to 1 year.

L-Arginine HCl	10 g
Distilled water	20 ml

SP-4 DIPHASIC MEDIUM. Add 1 ml of melted SP-4 agar containing glucose, arginine, or urea to small, screw-capped glass vials or tubes. Allow the agar to solidify in a slanted position. Overlay the agar medium with 2 ml of the appropriate SP-4 broth. Store tubes of medium at 4° C for up to 1 week.

Procedure. Inoculate the specimen or test organism to SP-4 broth, agar, and diphasic medium and incubate at 35° C. SP-4 broth should be subcultured to SP-4 agar after 3 to 4 days of incubation. Diphasic cultures should be examined microscopically by looking at the broth through the side of the tube for evidence of spherules (small colonies), which appear as early as 5 days. Diphasic cultures should also be observed for a decrease in pH as judged by the phenol red indicator. Diphasic cultures should be transferred to SP-4 agar after 10 to 12 days, and these cultures should be examined for an equal amount of time. Some strains may not show growth until 30 days or so. SP-4 agar plates should be incubated in aerobic, microaerophilic, and anaerobic conditions if all species of *Mycoplasma* are to be isolated. Specimens may be inoculated directly to SP-4 urea, SP-4 arginine, and SP-4 glucose to aid detection of certain *Mycoplasma* spp. directly from the specimen, or these media may be inoculated with pure cultures to allow identification of these microorganisms.

Quality control. Inoculate tubes or plates of medium from each batch with the following organisms, and observe for expected results.

  M. pneumoniae (SP-4 broth and agar)—good growth; fried egg colonies
  M. pneumoniae (SP-4 broth and glucose)—good growth; yellow color change
  M. pneumoniae (SP-4 diphasic)—good growth
  U. urealyticum (SP-4 and urea)—good growth; red color change
  M. hominis (SP-4 and arginine)—good growth; red color change

REFERENCE

Tully, J.G., et al.: Pathogenic mycoplasmas: cultivation and vertebrate pathogenicity of a new spiroplasma, Science **195**:892, 1977.

SUCROSE-PHOSPHATE TRANSPORT MEDIUM

Purpose. Sucrose-phosphate (2SP) broth is a phosphate-buffered, sucrose-containing medium useful for transporting clinical specimens suspected of containing *Mycoplasma* and *Chlamydia* organisms.

Principle and interpretation. The 2SP broth contains buffer, serum, nystatin, phenol red, and a high content of sucrose. Sucrose and serum act as osmotic stabilizers for *Mycoplasma* and *Chlamydia* organisms. Nystatin is an antifungal antimicrobial, and the phosphates are buffers to maintain a pH favorable to the viability of these organisms.

Ingredients and preparation. Prepare the basal medium, filter sterilize, and add sterile bovine serum, nystatin, and phenol red. Adjust the pH to 7.2, distribute into sterile screw-capped glass vials or tubes, and store at −20° C for no longer than 1 year.

2SP basal medium: Dissolve each of the following ingredients separately in a small amount of distilled water, combine the three solutions, and bring the volume up to 1 L with distilled water. Sterilize by filtration.

Sucrose	68.46 g
Dibasic potassium phosphate	2.08 g
Monobasic potassium phosphate	1.08 g
Distilled water, q.s. to	1 L

2SP medium: Add 2SP basal medium to serum, nystatin, and phenol red, adjust the pH with 1 N NaOH, and distribute 2 ml aliquots into screw-capped vials or tubes.

2SP basal medium	90 ml
Fetal bovine serum, heat inactivated at 56° C/30 minutes	10 ml
Nystatin, 10,000 units/ml, optional	0.25 ml
Phenol red, 0.5%	0.2 ml

Final pH 7.2

Procedure. Place a swab specimen into the tube or vial, break off the excess portion of the swab, seal the tube, and transport it to the laboratory.

Quality control. Test sample tubes of medium from each batch for maintenance of viability of strains of *Mycoplasma* and *Chlamydia* spp. Inoculate cultures to 2SP transport medium, allow the medium to rest refrigerated for 1 day, and subculture to SP-4 agar or McCoy cell cultures. Observe for the expected results:

M. pneumoniae—good growth on subculture to SP-4 agar
C. trachomatis—growth on subculture to cell cultures

REFERENCE

Gordon, F.B., et al.: Detection of *Chlamydia (Bedsonia)* in certain infections of man. I. Laboratory procedures: comparison of yolk sac and cell culture for detection and isolation, J. Infect. Dis. **120:**451, 1969.

STARCH-GELATIN AGAR

Purpose. Starch-gelatin agar is used to test the ability of bacteria to hydrolyze starch.

Principle and interpretation. Starch agar is a combination medium on which starch and gelatin hydrolysis can be detected. It contains protein, sodium chloride, soluble starch, gelatin, and agar. Starch is composed of two polysaccharides, amylose and amylopectin. Both polysaccharides are composed of repeating units of D-glucose. Alpha-amylase catalyzes the hydrolysis of glucosidic bonds of starch. Hydrolysis proceeds by first hydrolyzing starch into dextrins, converting the dex-

trins into maltose, and finally converting maltose into glucose. Starch hydrolysis is detected with an iodine reagent. When iodine is added to starch, the two substrates react to form a blue product. The reaction must be read immediately after addition of the iodine because the blue color formed with starch fades. An amylase-producing bacterium grows on starch agar and hydrolyzes starch to glucose in the agar medium surrounding the bacterial growth. When iodine reagent is added to the agar culture, areas in which starch remains turn blue; whereas areas around the growth where starch has been hydrolyzed are colorless. This constitutes a positive result of a starch hydrolysis test. A negative result would be a blue reaction in the medium immediately around the bacterial growth.

Ingredients and preparation. Mix the following ingredients, heat to boiling, and sterilize at 121° C for 15 minutes. Cool to 50° C, and pour into plates.

Pancreatic digest of casein, USP	15 g
Papaic digest of soybean meal, USP	5 g
Sodium chloride	5 g
Starch, soluble	2 g
Gelatin	15 g
Agar	15 g
Distilled water	1 L

Final pH 7.3

Procedure. Touch a sterile bacteriologic loop or needle to a colony, and inoculate the medium with a streak about 6 cm long. Incubate at 35° C for 1 to 3 days. Starch hydrolysis is determined by adding 3 drops of Gram iodine solution (see Gram stain in Chapter 6) to the bacterial growth. Observe for an immediate change in color to blue.

Quality control. See starch agar in Table 3-7.

REFERENCE

Oxborrow, G.S. and Favero, M.S.: A combination medium for demonstration of starch and gelatin hydrolysis, Am. J. Clin. Pathol. **33:**334, 1967.

TELLURITE REDUCTION TEST FOR MYCOBACTERIA

Purpose. The tellurite reduction test is useful for distinguishing among species of mycobacteria based on ability to reduce potassium tellurite.

Principle. Tellurite is reduced by many species of aerobic and anaerobic bacteria to a black tellurium precipitate. The enzyme responsible for this activity is tellurite reductase.

Procedure. Inoculate a heavy spadeful of growth to Middlebrook 7H9 broth containing Tween 80.* Incubate the culture at 35° C for 7 days to obtain dense growth. Add 2 drops of potassium tellurite reagent to the broth culture in 20 × 150 mm tubes. Mix and incubate the culture at 35° C for an additional 3 days. Examine the culture for a black precipitate, a positive test result for tellurite reduction. Do not shake the tubes.

Reagent. To prepare potassium tellurite reagent, 0.2%, dissolve 0.1 g potassium tellurite in 50 ml distilled water. Dispense

---

*Add 0.5 ml Tween 80 to 900 ml Middlebrook 7H9 broth. Autoclave at 121° C for 15 minutes, cool to 45° C, and add 100 ml of ADC enrichment. Dispense 5 ml into 20 × 150 mm tubes.

2 ml amounts into screw-capped tubes, sterilize at 121° C for 10 minutes, and store at 4° to 5° C.

Quality control. See Tables 3-10 and 3-18.

TEMPERATURE TOLERANCE TESTS

Purpose. Temperature tolerance tests are used primarily for distinguishing among certain nonfermenters based on their ability to grow at specific temperatures. It is especially useful for distinguishing among the fluorescent pseudomonads; *Pseudomonas aeruginosa* grows at 42° C, whereas *Pseudomonas fluorescens* does not.

Principle and interpretation. Most bacteria grow within a narrow temperature range. However, even though most species are unable to grow at temperatures above or below their optimal range, some survive brief exposure to adverse temperatures. The characteristics that permit an organism to tolerate adverse temperatures are complex and often unknown, but undoubtedly temperature-dependent enzyme systems are responsible in part.

Procedure. To determine growth at 42° C by nonfermentative organisms, use of a broth culture of the test organism is preferable. Inoculate two slants of trypticase soy or brain heart infusion agar with one loopful of the broth suspension. Incubate one slant at 42° C and the control slant at 35° C. (The control slant is used to ensure viability of the organism.) After incubation for 18 to 24 hours, examine the test slant for growth and compare it with the control slant. Record the growth as light, moderate, or heavy. Reincubate for an additional 24 hours test slants that show no growth.

Quality control. Test positive (tolerant) and negative (intolerant) control organisms along with the unknown culture to ensure proper performance of the incubators used during testing. Observe for the expected result:

P. aeruginosa—growth at 42° C
P. fluorescens—no growth at 42° C

REFERENCE

Oberhofer, T.R.: Manual of nonfermenting gram-negative bacteria, New York, 1985, John Wiley & Sons, Inc.

TETRATHIONATE BROTH

Purpose. Tetrathionate broth is used to enhance recovery of species of *Salmonella* from feces.

Principle and interpretation. Tetrathionate broth contains protein, bile salts, calcium carbonate, sodium thiosulfate, and iodine. The combined ingredients of this medium act in concert to inhibit most lactose-fermenting normal intestinal flora and gram-positive cocci. The medium is prepared as a basal medium to which an iodine solution is added. The final medium cannot be heated after addition of the iodine solution, and the medium must be used within 24 hours of preparation. The inoculated medium is subcultured to enteric media after a suitable period of incubation.

Ingredients and preparation. Mix the following basal ingredients, heat to boiling, cool to 45° C, and add 20 ml of iodine solution. Mix thoroughly and dispense 10 ml aliquots into sterile tubes. Do not sterilize in an autoclave. Do not heat the mixture after the iodine solution is added.

Basal medium:

Pancreatic digest of casein and peptic digest of animal tissue, USP	5 g
Bile salts	1g
Calcium carbonate	10 g
Sodium thiosulfate	30 g
Distilled water	1 L

Iodine solution:

Iodine	6 g
Potassium iodide	5 g
Distilled water	20 ml

Tetrathionate broth:

Basal medium	1 L
Iodine solution	20 ml

Final pH 7.0

Procedure. Inoculate fecal samples into tetrathionate broth, and incubate the culture for 12 to 24 hours at 35° C. After incubation, subculture the broth to enteric media.

Quality control. See selective enrichment broths for enterics in Table 3-3.

THAYER-MARTIN AGAR, MODIFIED

Purpose. Modified Thayer-Martin (MTM) agar is a selective medium used for isolation of *N. gonorrhoeae*, *N. meningitidis*, and *N. lactamica* from clinical specimens containing mixed species of bacteria.

Principle and interpretation. MTM agar contains protein, cornstarch, phosphate buffer, sodium chloride, agar, hemoglobin, glucose, vancomycin, colistin, nystatin, trimethoprim lactate, and several accessory growth factors including glutamine, diphosphopyridine nucleotide, and cocarboxylase. Cornstarch is thought to provide protection to gonococci by absorbing the toxic substances that might be present in prepared media.

The medium is prepared as a gonococcus (GC) agar base, and the hemoglobin, antimicrobial agents, and accessory growth factors are added. The latter factors or supplements are provided in the form of a yeast concentrate (Bacto-Supplement B, Difco Laboratories, Detroit) or in the form of a chemically defined solution of enrichments (IsoVitaleX, BBL Microbiology Systems, Cockeysville, Md.).

The selectivity of MTM is attributed to the inhibitory actions of four antimicrobial agents. Vancomycin inhibits gram-positive bacteria by interfering with cell wall synthesis. Colistin (polymyxin E) is more active against gram-negative than gram-positive bacteria and disrupts the cell wall of affected organisms. Nystatin inhibits yeasts by altering the permeability of their cell walls. Trimethoprim lactate is added to MTM specifically to inhibit species of *Proteus*.

Ingredients and preparation. Prepare double-strength GC agar base and double-strength hemoglobin solutions. Mix thoroughly, heat to boiling, sterilize both solutions at 121° C for 15 minutes, and cool to 50° C. Aseptically add the double-strength hemoglobin solution, enrichments, and antimicrobial agents to the sterile cooled GC agar base. Mix gently, and dispense into sterile plates. Store plates of medium at 4° C.

GC agar base (double strength):

---

*Commercially available in powdered medium.

Pancreatic digest of casein and	
peptic digest of animal tissue, USP	15 g
Cornstarch	1 g
Dipotassium phosphate	4 g
Monopotassium phosphate	1 g
Sodium chloride	5 g
Agar	10 g
Distilled water	500 ml

Additional ingredients to be added that are not found in commercial GC agar base:

Agar	2 g
D-Glucose	5 g

Final pH 7.2

Hemoglobin solution (2%, double strength):

Hemoglobin	10 g
Distilled water	500 ml

Enrichment solution: IsoVitaleX Solution (BBL Microbiology Systems), 10 ml, or Bacto-Supplement B Solution (Difco Laboratories), 10 ml

Antimicrobial agents, final concentrations per liter of medium:

Vancomycin	3 mg
Colistin	7.5 mg
Nystatin	12,500 units
Trimethoprim lactate	5 mg

Procedure. Inoculate the specimen to MTM agar, streak for isolation, and incubate at 35° C for 24 to 48 hours in an atmosphere fortified with carbon dioxide.

Quality control. See selective media for pathogenic *Neisseria* in Table 3-3.

THERMONUCLEASE TEST AGAR

Purpose. Thermonuclease agar (toluidine blue–deoxyribonucleic acid [TDA] agar) is used to distinguish among *Staphylococcus aureus* and other species of *Micrococcaceae* based on ability to produce a heat-stable deoxyribonuclease. A rapid thermonuclease test for identifying *Staphylococcus aureus* directly in blood cultures has also been described.

Principle and interpretation. TDA agar contains deoxyribonucleic acid (DNA), agar, toluidine blue O, calcium chloride, sodium chloride, and tris(hydroxymethyl)aminomethane (TRIS) buffer. It is used to test for the production of a heat-stable deoxyribonuclease, which degrades DNA into oligonucleotides and mononucleotides. Degradation of DNA is determined with the metachromatic dye toluidine blue O. The dye color depends on whether it is complexed with entire DNA or oligonucleotides and mononucleotides of degraded DNA. The orthochromatic or true staining of toluidine blue is blue, the color it exhibits when complexed with entire DNA. The metachromatic staining of toluidine blue is pink, red, or violet, the color it exhibits when complexed with oligonucleotides and mononucleotides.

For the test an overnight culture of an organism suspected to be *S. aureus* is heated (see procedure later in this discussion), and a drop of the heated broth is added to a well introduced into TDA agar. The TDA agar is incubated and examined for evidence of a bright pink zone around the well, indicating activity of a thermostable nuclease. Thermostable nuclease activity is a consistent property of *S. aureus*. Some strains of *Staphylococcus epidermidis* produce a nuclease, but it is destroyed by heat.

TDA agar is stable, does not have to be sterilized, and can be stored at room temperature for as long as 4 months if sealed in bags. The medium can be melted several times without loss of function. This stability is due to the medium's lack of nutrients on which bacteria can grow, the heat stability of the toluidine blue–DNA complex, and the inhibitory property of toluidine blue toward gram-positive bacteria, especially sporeformers.

Ingredients and preparation. Add DNA, agar, calcium chloride, and sodium chloride to 1 L of TRIS buffer (pH 9.0), heat to boiling to dissolve the DNA and agar, cool to 45° C, and add toluidine blue solution. Dispense 10 ml of TDA in each Petri plate (9 cm) or 3 ml in immunodiffusion slides. Before use, incubate plates at 35° C for 1 hour, and cut 3 mm wells into the agar.

DNA	0.3 g
Agar, granular	10 g
Calcium chloride, anhydrous, 0.01 M	1 ml
Sodium chloride	10 g
TRIS buffer, 0.05 M, pH 9.0	1 L

Heat to boiling, cool to 45° C, then add:

Toluidine blue O, 0.1 M	3 ml

Procedure. Grow the test organism at 35°C for 18 to 24 hours in brain heart infusion broth. Place the broth culture in a boiling water bath for 15 minutes, remove, and allow to cool at room temperature. Fill TDA wells with a boiled broth culture using a disposable Pasteur pipette. Incubate TDA plates or slides at 35° C, and observe for a pink halo, 1 to 3 mm wide, surrounding the test wells after 1, 2, 4, and 24 hours.

Quality control. Test sample plates or slides of TDA agar from each batch with the organisms listed below and observe for expected results:

S. aureus—red or pink halo around TDA well

S. epidermidis—no halo; blue around well

RAPID THERMONUCLEASE TEST

Purpose. The rapid thermonuclease test may be used directly on blood cultures for the presumptive identification of *S. aureus* when a smear of the culture shows gram-positive cocci in clusters.

Procedure. Transfer 2 to 3 ml of blood broth from a blood culture bottle to a sterile screw-cap tube, and place the tube in a boiling water bath for 15 minutes. Allow the tube to cool to room temperature. Using the end of a 6 mm capillary pipette, cut wells 6 mm in diameter in DNA plates (use Thermal Agar, Edge Diagnostics, Memphis, Tenn.). Up to 20 wells may be punched in the plate. Pipette 2 or 3 drops of the cooled broth into a well. Positive and negative controls from blood culture bottles containing blood should also be tested and should be processed as for the test specimen. *S. aureus* should be used as the positive control and a known coagulase-negative *Staphylococcus* strain as the negative control. Incubate the plate, right side up, at 35° C for 2 hours.

A positive thermonuclease reaction is indicated by a pink zone of clearing at the edge of the well and a darker blue ring at the zone's outer periphery. Negative results are indicated by no zone formation or a small zone of clearing without pink or the hyperpigmented ring. A positive result indicates the presence of *S. aureus*. Negative results may be demonstrated by coagulase-negative staphylococci as well as by enterococci, pneumococci, and group B streptococci. Negative results should thus be reported as "gram-positive cocci in clusters, not *S. aureus*." The DNA plate may be refrigerated and used on successive days.

REFERENCES

Lachia, R.V.F., Genigeorgis, C., and Hoeprich, P.D.: Metachromatic agar-diffusion methods for detecting staphylococcal nuclease activity, Appl. Microbiol. **21:**585, 1971.

Madison, B.M., and Baselski, V.S.: Rapid identification of *Staphylococcus aureus* in blood cultures by thermonuclease testing, J. Clin. Microbiol. **18:**722, 1983.

Ratner, H.B., and Stratton, C.W.: Thermonuclease test for same-day identification of *Staphylococcus aureus* in blood cultures, J. Clin. Microbiol. **21:**995, 1985.

THIOGLYCOLATE BROTH, ENRICHED AND NONENRICHED

Purpose. Thioglycolate broth is a general-purpose broth medium used for isolation of many species of aerobic and anaerobic bacteria from a variety of specimens. The medium can be enriched with the addition of ingredients such as vitamin K_1, hemin, serum, and Fildes enrichment to enhance isolation of fastidious bacteria.

Principle and interpretation. Thioglycolate broth contains protein, glucose, sodium chloride, sodium thioglycolate, reducing agents, and agar. Additional enrichments are recommended for use with anaerobic bacteria and fastidious aerobic bacteria. The ingredients, thioglycolate, L-cystine, sodium sulfite, and agar, contribute to the lowering and maintenance of a low oxidation-reduction potential of the medium. This permits growth of many species of strict anaerobic bacteria without the necessity of sealing the medium with mineral oil or other sealants. Fildes enrichment is included in some formulations to encourage growth of *Haemophilus* spp. and anaerobes. The sterile medium should be stored at room temperature.

Ingredients and preparation. Mix the following ingredients, heat to boiling, dispense 10 ml per tube, and sterilize at 115° C for 15 minutes. For best results boil media and cool to room temperature before use.

Pancreatic digest of casein, USP	17 g
Papaic digest of soybean meal, USP	3 g
D-Glucose	6 g
Sodium chloride	2.5 g
Sodium thioglycolate	0.5 g
L-Cystine	250 mg
Sodium sulfite	0.1 g
Agar	0.7 g

Distilled water	1 L

Final pH 7.0

Optional ingredients (final concentrations):

Vitamin K_1	0.1 μg/ml
Sodium bicarbonate	1 mg/ml
Hemin	5 μg/ml
Rabbit serum	10% vol/vol
or	
Fildes enrichment	5% vol/vol

Procedure. Inoculate the specimen to thioglycolate broth and incubate at 35° C for 3 to 7 days, depending on the source. Observe for growth, and if apparent, Gram stain the broth. If cell types other than those seen on the aerobically incubated companion plates are seen, subculture the broth to anaerobic media and test for the presence of anaerobes.

Quality control. See Table 3-4.

THIOPHENE-2-CARBOXYLIC ACID HYDRAZIDE MEDIUM

Purpose. Thiophene-2-carboxylic acid hydrazide (TCH) medium is useful for distinguishing among strains of *Mycobacterium bovis,* some of which may be niacin positive, and *Mycobacterium tuberculosis* based on their ability to grow in the presence of TCH.

Principle and interpretation. TCH is a chemical that, when incorporated into agar media, is toxic to certain species of mycobacteria. Growth on TCH medium is compared with growth on the basal medium, which lacks the chemical. A 99% reduction in growth on TCH medium over that amount of growth seen on the basal medium is interpreted as sensitivity of the test organism to TCH.

Ingredients and preparation. Add filter-sterilized TCH solution (Aldrich Chemical Co., Milwaukee, Wis.) to sterile 7H10 medium to give a final concentration of 2 μg/ml of medium. Dispense into Petri plates. See the discussion of 7H10 agar.

Procedure. Dilute a 7-day-old liquid test culture to 10^{-3} and 10^{-5} with sterile saline or distilled water. Inoculate 0.1 ml of the 1:1000 dilution to the TCH test and control basal media. In a similar manner, inoculate the 1:100,000 dilution to both media (Middlebrook 7H10 medium with no drug). Incubate cultures at 35° C for 3 weeks in an atmosphere of 10% carbon dioxide in air. Compare growth occurring on both media.

Quality control. See Table 3-10.

THIOSULFATE–CITRATE–BILE SALTS– SUCROSE AGAR

Purpose. Thiosulfate–citrate–bile salts–sucrose (TCBS) agar is a selective medium for cultivation of *Vibrio cholerae* and other pathogenic vibrios from samples of feces and food containing mixed species of bacteria.

Principle and interpretation. TCBS agar contains protein, yeast extract, a variety of salts, sucrose, oxgall, sodium cholate, two indicators, and agar. Oxgall and sodium cholate are derivatives of bile. A 10% solution of oxgall is equivalent to full-strength fresh bile.

The pathogenic vibrios grow best at pH values near 8.0 and are rapidly killed by an acid medium. They do not grow or grow poorly on enteric media such as Salmonella-Shigella, eosin–methylene blue, brilliant green, or bismuth sulfite agars. However, most strains grow on MacConkey agar as non-lactose-fermenting colonies. They tolerate high concentrations of sodium chloride and survive well in the presence of bile salts.

The selectivity of TCBS for *V. cholerae* and other pathogenic vibrios is based on the presence of a high pH (8.6), citrate salts, oxgall, and sodium cholate, all of which are inhibitory to gram-positive bacteria and sporeforming organisms. These agents also act in concert to inhibit many species of lactose-fermenting normal intestinal flora and *Proteus, Pseudomonas,* and *Aeromonas* spp. Occasionally, however, these latter organisms can overcome the inhibitory agents and grow on the medium; *Proteus* organisms, enterococci, and some species of lactose-fermenting normal intestinal flora appear as small, translucent colonies, and *Pseudomonas* and *Aeromonas* spp. form blue colonies.

TCBS agar contains the fermentable carbohydrate sucrose, which allows differentiation among *Vibrio* spp. Strains of *V. cholerae* produce yellow colonies on TCBS because of fermentation of sucrose. *V. alginolyticus* also produces yellow colonies. *V. parahaemolyticus* is a non-sucrose-fermenting organism and produces blue-green colonies, as does *V. vulnificus*. As mentioned previously, occasional isolates of *Pseudomonas* and *Aeromonas* spp. also produce blue-green colonies, but overall TCBS is highly selective and any hydrogen sulfide–negative colonies are possibly *Vibrio* spp. The medium should be inoculated heavily with fecal specimens because some *Vibrio* spp. readily die off on the medium owing to fermentation of sucrose and accumulation of acids.

Ingredients and preparation. Mix the following ingredients, heat to boiling, cool to 50° C, dispense into plates, and allow solidification to occur at room temperature. *Do not sterilize in an autoclave.*

Yeast extract	5 g
Pancreatic digest of casein and peptic digest of animal tissue, USP	10 g
Sodium citrate	10 g
Sodium thiosulfate	10 g
Oxgall	5 g
Sodium cholate	3 g
Sucrose	20 g
Sodium chloride	10 g
Ferric citrate	1 g
Bromthymol blue	40 mg
Thymol blue	40 mg
Agar	14 g
Distilled water	1 L

Final pH 8.6

Procedure. Inoculate a large sample of a fresh fecal specimen directly to TCBS agar. Incubate cultures for 48 hours at 35° C.

Quality control. See Table 3-3.

TINSDALE AGAR

Purpose. Tinsdale agar is used for isolation and cultivation of *Corynebacterium diphtheriae* from specimens containing mixed species of bacteria.

Principle and interpretation. Tinsdale agar contains protein, sodium chloride, L-cystine, sodium thiosulfate, serum, tellurite, and agar. The selectivity for *C. diphtheriae* is attributed to the high concentration of potassium tellurite in the medium, which inhibits or retards the growth of most species of respiratory bacteria. Reduction of tellurite to tellurium, a black product, results in blackening of colonies of *C. diphtheriae* on Tinsdale agar and aids in recognition of the species.

Three colony types of *C. diphtheriae* are recognized. *Gravis* biotypes produce large (2 to 4 mm), flat, rough, dull gray to black (''gun-metal gray'') colonies. *Mitis* strains produce small, smooth, convex colonies with glossy black centers and crenated edges. *Intermedius* strains are still smaller, are flat, and may be either smooth or rough. Any one of the three biotypes may be toxigenic. Diphtheroids grow as ''patent-leather'' (shiny), gray-black colonies with grayish white edges. Although coagulase-positive cocci grow as colonies similar in appearance to *C. diphtheriae*, none produce browning of the medium.

C. diphtheriae produces true browning in the stab areas of Tinsdale agar and faint halos around all isolated colonies after 18 to 24 hours' incubation. Distinct, dark brown halos occur after 48 hours' incubation. The brown halo is thought to be due to interaction of potassium tellurite with hydrogen sulfide produced by the bacilli from L-cystine and sodium thiosulfate. Hydrogen sulfide–producing strains of *Proteus* grow on this medium as large mucoid colonies and produce heavy diffuse blackening of the medium.

Ingredients and preparation. Mix basal ingredients, heat to boiling, and sterilize at 121° C for 15 minutes. Cool to 50° C, add sterile bovine serum and potassium tellurite solution, and dispense into plates. Store sealed in plastic bags at 4° C. Plates of medium must be used within 4 days of preparation.

Basal ingredients:

Peptic digest of animal tissues, USP	20 g
Sodium chloride	5 g
L-Cystine	240 mg
Sodium thiosulfate	430 mg
Agar	14 g
Distilled water	1 L

Final pH 7.4

Additives to sterile, cooled (50° C) basal medium:

Bovine serum, sterile	100 ml
Potassium tellurite, 1% aqueous, sterile	30 ml

Procedure. Inoculate the specimen to Tinsdale agar, streak for isolation, and stab the medium at frequent intervals. Browning begins in the stabbed portion of the medium earlier than it does at surface sites. Incubate plates at 35° C for 24 to 48 hours.

Quality control. See Table 3-3.

REFERENCE

Moore, M.S., and Parsons, E.I.: A study of modified Tinsdale's medium for the primary isolation of *Corynebacterium diphtheriae*, J. Infect. Dis. **102**:88, 1958.

TODD-HEWITT BROTH

Purpose. Todd-Hewitt (TH) broth is a nonselective medium used for cultivation of species of *Streptococcus,* especially beta-hemolytic species, for purpose of serogrouping.

Principle and interpretation. TH broth contains beef heart infusion, peptone, glucose, sodium chloride, and buffer. The medium supports the growth of fastidious streptococci because of the high content of protein and the presence of glucose. Typically, streptococci readily die out in media containing glucose because of accumulated acids. However, TH broth contains buffers that maintain a pH suitable for growth of streptococci even as acids are being produced from fermented glucose.

Ingredients and preparation. Mix the following ingredients, heat to boiling, dispense into tubes, and sterilize at 121° C for 15 minutes.

Beef heart infusion	500 g
Casein/meat peptone	20 g
D-Glucose	2 g
Sodium chloride	2 g
Disodium phosphate	0.4 g
Sodium carbonate	2.5 g
Distilled water	1 L

Final pH 7.8

Procedure. Inoculate the test organism to TH broth, incubate at 35° C for 18 to 24 hours, and observe for growth.

Quality control. See Table 3-3.

TRIPLE SUGAR IRON AGAR

Purpose. Triple sugar iron (TSI) agar is a screening medium used to identify gram-negative bacilli based on ability to ferment the carbohydrates glucose, sucrose, and lactose and to produce hydrogen sulfide gas.

Principle and interpretation. TSI agar contains protein, sodium chloride, lactose, sucrose, dextrose, a sulfur source, a hydrogen sulfide indicator, a pH indicator, and agar. The medium includes 10 times as much lactose and sucrose as glucose. Bacteria that ferment glucose produce a variety of acids, turning the color of the medium from red to yellow. Larger amounts of acid are produced in the butt of the tube (fermentation) than in the slant of the tube (respiration). Organisms growing on TSI also form alkaline products from the oxidative decarboxylation of peptone. These alkaline products neutralize the small amounts of acids present in the slant but are unable to neutralize the large amounts of acid present in the butt. Thus the appearance of an alkaline (red) slant and an acid (yellow) butt after 24 hours' incubation indicates that the organism is a glucose fermenter but is unable to ferment lactose and sucrose.

Bacteria that ferment lactose or sucrose (or both), in addition to glucose, produce such large amounts of acid that the oxidative deamination of protein that may occur in the slant does not yield enough alkaline products to cause a reversion of pH in that region. Thus these bacteria produce an acid slant and acid butt. It is impossible to determine from the TSI reaction whether both lactose and sucrose are being fermented or only one of these carbohydrates is being fermented; individual carbohydrate fermentation tests are required to make this assessment.

Gas production (carbon dioxide and hydrogen) is detected by the presence of cracks or bubbles in the medium. These are formed when the accumulated gas escapes.

Hydrogen sulfide gas is produced as a result of the reduction of thiosulfate. Hydrogen sulfide is a colorless gas and can be detected only in the presence of an indicator, in this case ferric ammonium sulfate. Hydrogen sulfide combines with the ferric ions of ferric ammonium sulfate to produce the insoluble black precipitate ferrous sulfide. Reduction of thiosulfate proceeds only in an acid environment, and blackening usually occurs in the butt of the tube. Although the black precipitate may frequently obscure the color of the butt, it can be assumed that the organism is a glucose fermenter because of the requirement for an acid environment. The reactions can be summarized as follows:

Alkaline slant/acid butt—glucose only fermented

Acid slant/acid butt—glucose and sucrose fermented *or* glucose and lactose fermented *or* glucose, lactose, and sucrose fermented

Bubbles or cracks present—gas produced

Black precipitate present—hydrogen sulfide gas produced

Ingredients and preparation. Mix the following ingredients, heat to boiling, dispense into tubes, sterilize at 121° C for 15 minutes, and allow tubes of medium to cool in a slanted position.

Pancreatic digest of casein, USP	10 g
Peptic digest of animal tissue, USP	10 g
Sodium chloride	1 g
Lactose	10 g
Sucrose	10 g
D-Glucose	1 g
Ferric ammonium sulfate	0.2 g
Sodium thiosulfate	0.2 g
Phenol red	25 mg
Agar	13 g
Distilled water	1 L

Final pH 7.3 to 7.4

Procedure. Inoculate test cultures to TSI agar by first touching a sterile bacteriologic needle to a colony and then stabbing the needle into the deep agar region of the medium. When withdrawing the needle, move it from side to side over the surface of the medium. Incubate cultures at 35° C for 18 to 24 hours. Examine cultures for color of the slant, butt, gas cracks, and blackening caused by hydrogen sulfide.

Quality control. See Table 3-7.

TRYPTICASE SOY BROTH AND TRYPTICASE SOY AGAR

Purpose. Trypticase soy broth (TSB) and trypticase soy agar (TSA) are general-purpose media used for cultivation of a wide

Cover the preparation with a no. 1 coverglass using Permount or equivalent mounting medium. *Do not* let the slide dry before the coverglass is mounted.

PVA-FIXED FECAL SPECIMENS. Prepare a thin, even smear by spreading 2 or 3 drops of the specimen over one third of a frosted-end slide. Make certain the smear extends to both edges of the slide to prevent the smear from washing off the slide during later processing. Mark appropriate identification on the frosted end of the slide with a lead pencil, and allow the slide to dry thoroughly. Smears of proper thickness usually dry within a few hours if incubated at 37° C or overnight if held at room temperature. Staining times are as follows:

Iodine alcohol	10 to 20 minutes
70% ethyl alcohol	3 to 5 minutes
70% ethyl alcohol	3 to 5 minutes
Trichrome stain	8 minutes
Acid alcohol	10 to 20 seconds or dip slide twice
95% ethyl alcohol	Rinse briefly
95% ethyl alcohol	5 minutes
Carbol xylene	5 to 10 minutes
Xylene	10 minutes

Mount coverglass as for fresh specimens.

Comment. Success with trichrome staining requires careful attention to several critical steps.

Reagents should be prepared in clean glassware using reagent-grade chemicals with careful attention to the details of weighing and mixing. With the exception of the trichrome stain, which may be reused, fresh working solutions should be prepared each day. The trichrome stain should be replaced after every 15 to 20 slides, since the stain weakens from uptake of water and alcohol. Used stain can be restored to its original strength and reused if it is allowed to stand uncovered at room temperature for 3 to 8 hours.

The timing of each staining step should be monitored closely. When a range of times is permitted, the longer times are used for thicker smears, whereas the shorter times are acceptable for thin smears. Especially critical are the timing of the iodine alcohol and acid alcohol steps. If the iodine alcohol step is rushed, the mercuric chloride of the Schaudinn solution may not be completely removed and a precipitate of mercuric chloride crystals may form on the smear. The smear should be passed through the acid alcohol destaining reagent as quickly as possible, since only a small amount of destaining is required and the acid alcohol is a strong destaining agent. It is usually sufficient to dip each slide in and out of the acid alcohol twice and *immediately* rinse the slide in 95% alcohol. Moving to the rinse step immediately is essential because the acid alcohol continues to destain the slide until the acid alcohol is removed by the 95% alcohol rinse. Also, the rinse solution should be changed frequently because it gradually becomes contaminated with acid alcohol carried over from the destaining step. Because of the speed required in the destaining steps, the slides should either be processed individually during destaining or be mounted in moveable slide carriers.

Formalin–Ether or (Ethyl) Acetate Concentration

Reagents

Buffered formalin, 10%:

Na_2HPO_4	6.1 g
NaH_2PO_4	0.15 g
Formalin	800 ml
Distilled water	7200 ml

Procedure

FRESH SPECIMENS. Prepare a suspension of fresh feces in saline (0.85% wt/vol sodium chloride) so 1 to 1.5 ml of sediment is produced after 10 ml of the suspension is centrifuged (see below). Strain approximately 10 ml of the suspension through a single layer of wet gauze or cheesecloth into a 15 ml, graduated, conical centrifuge tube. The gauze or cheesecloth can be spread over the top of a small glass funnel or, more conveniently, a cone-shaped paper cup with the tip cut off.

Centrifuge the feces at $650 \times g$ for 1 to 2 minutes, and decant the resulting supernatant. Between 1 and 1.5 ml of sediment should be present after removing the supernatant. If too much sediment is present, resuspend the sediment in saline and pour off an appropriate amount. Bring the amount of suspension to 10 ml by adding additional saline and repeat the centrifugation. If too little sediment is present, strain an additional portion of the original fecal suspension into the centrifuge tube. If required, add additional saline to bring the total volume to 10 ml and repeat the centrifugation.

When the appropriate amount of sediment is obtained, resuspend the sediment in fresh saline and centrifuge again at $650 \times g$ for 1 to 2 minutes. If the resulting supernatant is especially cloudy, this step may be repeated to provide a cleaner sediment.

Add 9 ml of 10% buffered formalin to the sediment and mix thoroughly. After allowing the suspension to stand for a minimum of 5 minutes, either proceed with the concentration procedure or tightly stopper the centrifuge tube and store the feces-formalin suspension for processing at a later time.

Add 3 ml of ethyl ether or ethyl acetate to the feces-formalin suspension, and stopper the centrifuge tube. Holding the stopper in place, invert the test tube and shake it vigorously for at least 30 seconds.

Carefully remove the stopper from the centrifuge tube and centrifuge the suspension for 1 minute at 450 to $500 \times g$.

When the centrifugation is completed, four distinct layers should be present in the centrifuge tube: a top layer of ether or ethyl acetate over a layer of debris, a layer of formalin, and finally the sediment. Use an applicator stick to free the layer of debris from the wall of the centrifuge tube and then decant all layers except the sediment. If any of the debris layer remains on the wall of the centrifuge tube, use a cotton swab to remove the additional debris before the centrifuge tube is turned upright.

Thoroughly mix the sediment in the small amount of fluid that drains from the sides of the centrifuge tube and prepare direct wet mounts from the sediment. If too little fluid remains in the tube, 1 or 2 drops of buffered formalin may be added to the tube.

If examination of the concentrated sediment must be delayed, add 1 to 2 ml of buffered formalin to the sediment and tightly stopper the centrifuge tube. Before making wet mounts from stored concentrates, remove the excess formalin that forms a layer over the sediment during storage.

FORMALIN-PRESERVED SPECIMENS. Thoroughly mix the preserved specimen, and strain 4 to 5 ml of the specimen through wet gauze or cheesecloth into a 15 ml, graduated, conical centrifuge tube. Add tap water or saline to make the final volume in the centrifuge tube 10 ml, mix thoroughly, and centrifuge for 1 to 2 minutes at 500 to 600 × g.

After centrifugation and decanting of the supernatant, approximately 0.5 to 0.75 ml of sediment should be present. If there is too little or too much sediment, the amount can be adjusted in the same manner as when concentrating fresh specimens.

Repeat centrifugation as described above if the specimen still contains a large amount of debris, that is, if the supernatant is very cloudy.

Add 9 ml of 10% buffered formalin to the sediment, and mix thoroughly. Add 4 ml of ether or ethyl acetate, stopper the centrifuge tube, and vigorously shake the tube in an inverted position for at least 30 seconds. Complete the concentration by following the last four paragraphs of the technique used for fresh specimens.

SPECIMENS PRESERVED IN PVA FIXATIVE. Thoroughly mix the preserved specimen. Transfer approximately half of the preserved specimen to another vial, mix in an equal volume of saline, and strain the mixture through a double layer of gauze into a 15 ml conical centrifuge tube. Add saline to bring the volume in the centrifuge tube to 15 ml, thoroughly mix the suspension, and centrifuge at 450 to 500 × g for 2 minutes. Decant the resulting supernatant, and repeat the procedure in the preceding sentence if the supernatant is very cloudy.

Fill the centrifuge tube half full with 10% formalin, add 3 ml of ether, and then stopper and shake the tube in an inverted position for at least 30 seconds. NOTE: If the amount of sediment is very small, do not add ether in this step; add only the formalin.

Complete the procedure by following the last four paragraphs of the procedure for fresh specimens.

BLOOD SPECIMENS
PREPARATION OF BLOOD SMEARS

Procedure. Blood used for detecting blood and tissue parasites should be collected without anticoagulants. The best method is to lance the finger for a child or adult or the heel or ear of an infant. Blood should flow freely from the tissue; blood that is "milked" from the wound is diluted by tissue fluids that reduce the concentration of parasites in the sample.

Blood smears should be prepared on 1 × 3 cm glass microscope slides. To obtain the best results, use new slides that have been cleaned in the laboratory by soaking in 70% ethyl alcohol and then dried with a lint-free cloth and stored in dust-free boxes or slide trays before use. Even so-called precleaned slides may be coated with small amounts of oils or chemicals that interfere with staining.

Thin blood smears are prepared in the same manner as smears used for differential white cell counts. Allow the smear to air dry.

To prepare thick smears place 2 or 3 small drops of fresh blood close together on a clean glass slide. Use the corner of another glass slide to mix the drops together over an area about the size of a dime. To prevent the formation of clots within the smear, mix the drops together for about 30 seconds. If the smear is properly prepared, newsprint is just readable through the wet smear. Since thick smears take much longer to dry (18 to 24 hours) than thin smears, it may be tempting to hasten drying by applying heat. This renders the smears useless, since heat fixes the red cells and prevents dehemoglobinization of the smear during subsequent staining. Thick smears must be permitted to dry at room temperature.

If desired, both thick and thin smears may be prepared on a single slide (so-called combination slide). In such cases the thin smear should be prepared by placing the drop of blood at one end of the slide and pushing it toward the middle of the slide. The thick smear is then prepared on the other end of the slide, next to the thin area of the thin smear. However, because of the significant difference in drying times of the two types of smears, it is probably best to prepare the two type of smears on separate slides. This permits earlier staining and examination of the thin film, and perhaps a more rapid diagnosis.

Giemsa Staining
Reagents
Buffered water
Triton X-100 (stock solution): Prepare a 10% vol/vol dilution of Triton X-100 (Rohm and Haas Co.) in distilled water. If stored in a tightly stoppered bottle, this stock solution should keep indefinitely.

Alkaline buffered water (stock solution):

Na$_2$HPO$_4$ (anhydrous)	9.5 g
Distilled water q.s. to	1000 ml

Acid buffered water (stock solution):

NaH$_2$PO$_4$ · H$_2$O	9.2 g
Distilled water q.s. to	1000 ml

Triton buffered water (working solution): Prepare 1 L of buffered water as follows.

Acid buffered water	39 ml
Alkaline buffered water	61 ml
Distilled water	900 ml

The pH of the buffered water should be between 7.0 and 7.2 for proper staining of blood parasites, especially malaria parasites. Prepare the final working solution of Triton buffered water as follows: If the buffered water is to be used for thin blood smears or combination thick and thin blood smears, add 1 ml of the stock solution of aqueous Triton X-100 to 1 L of the working solution of buffered water (see above). The final concentration of the Triton is 0.01% (vol/vol). If the buffered water is to be used only for thick films or for tissue and exudate smears, add 10 ml of the stock solution of Triton X-100 to 1 L of the working solution of buffered water. The final concentration of the Triton is 0.1% (vol/vol).

Giemsa stain
Stock solution:

Giemsa stain powder (certified, Azure B)	600 mg
Methyl alcohol (acetone free, neutral)	50 ml
Glycerine (neutral)	50 ml

For best results both the methyl alcohol and the glycerine should be freshly opened bottles of reagent-grade chemical. Grind the stain powder with part of the glycerine in a mortar. Pour off the top one third of the mixture into a clean 500 or 1000 ml flask. Add more of the glycerine and continue grinding the powder. Repeat this process until all the glycerine has been mixed with the stain powder and poured into the flask. Do not discard any stain powder that may remain in the mortar; it will be rinsed from the mortar in a later step.

Stopper the flask with a cotton plug, and then seal the flask with a heavy paper or foil cap secured by wrapping a rubber band around the neck of the flask. Heat the flask in a 55° to 60° C water bath for 2 hours, making certain that the water level in the bath is above the fluid level in the flask. Gently shake the flask at half-hour intervals during the incubation.

Using part of the measured amount of alcohol, rinse any remaining residue of stain powder from the mortar and place the washings in a small, airtight flask.

When the incubation of the glycerine-stain mixture is complete, remove the mixture from the water bath, allow it to cool to room temperature, and add the washings from the mortar and the remaining alcohol. Gently shake the flask to mix all the stain components.

If necessary the stain may be filtered and used immediately. However, it is best to store the stain in an airtight bottle or flask for 2 weeks, with intermittent gentle mixing, before use.

Staining procedure

THIN BLOOD SMEARS. Fix the blood smear in absolute methyl alcohol for 30 seconds and air dry the smear. Stain the smear for 45 minutes in a staining solution prepared by adding 1 ml of stock Giemsa stain to 50 ml of Triton (0.01%) buffered water. Alternatively, stain the smear for 20 minutes in a staining solution prepared by adding 1 ml of stock Giemsa stain to 20 ml of Triton (0.01%) buffered water. Wash the smear briefly in Triton (0.01%) buffered water to remove excess stain, and allow the smear to air dry before examination.

THICK BLOOD SMEARS. Stain thick smears for 45 minutes in a staining solution prepared by adding 1 ml of stock Giemsa stain to 50 ml of Triton (0.1%) buffered water. Wash the stained smear for 3 to 5 minutes in Triton (0.1%) buffered water to remove excess stain, and allow the smear to air dry before examination.

COMBINATION THICK AND THIN BLOOD SMEARS. Fix the thin blood smear with absolute methyl alcohol for 30 seconds. Allow the smear to air dry in a vertical position with the thick blood smear toward the top. Take special care during this step that alcohol does not come in contact with the thick film, since alcohol can also fix the thick film and prevent proper staining. Stain the smears for 45 minutes in a staining solution prepared by mixing 1 ml of stock Giemsa stain with 50 ml of Triton (0.01%) buffered water. Wash the slide briefly in Triton (0.01%) buffered water. The thick film should be washed an additional 3 to 5 minutes in the Triton buffered water. Allow the smears to air dry before examination.

TISSUE AND EXUDATE SMEARS. Fix the smear in absolute methyl alcohol for 30 seconds and allow to air dry. Stain the smear for 50 minutes in a staining solution prepared by adding 1 ml of stock Giemsa stain to 40 ml of Triton (0.1%) buffered water. Wash the smear for 5 to 10 minutes in Triton (0.1%) buffered water, and air dry before examination.

Mycology

BASAL MEDIUM FOR CARBOHYDRATE UTILIZATION

Purpose. Carbohydrate utilization is useful for the identification of the aerobic actinomycetes.

Principle and interpretation. Utilization of arabinose, cellobiose, inositol, mannitol, xylose, or all of these by an aerobic actinomycete is important to the identification.

Ingredients and preparation

$(NH_4)_2HPO_4$	1 g
Potassium chloride	0.02 g
$MgSO_4 \cdot 7 H_2O$	0.2 g
Agar	15 g
Distilled water	1000 ml
Bromcresol purple (0.04%)	15 ml

Final pH 7.0

Sterilize at 121° C for 10 minutes. Dispense 5 ml per tube. Then add 0.5 ml of a filter-sterilized 10% carbohydrate solution. Store at 4° C for 3 months.

Procedure. Inoculate and incubate at 30° C for 4 weeks. An acid reaction, indicated by the appearance of a yellow color, is indicative of carbohydrate utilization.

BASAL MEDIUM FOR HYPOXANTHINE, TYROSINE, AND XANTHINE AGARS

Purpose. Hydrolysis of hypoxanthine, tyrosine, and xanthine is important for identifying the aerobic actinomycetes.

Principle and interpretation. These three physiologic tests are used routinely in the clinical laboratory to identify the aerobic actinomycetes.

Ingredients and preparation

Beef extract	3 g
Peptone	5 g
Agar	15 g
Distilled water	1000 ml

Sterilize at 121° C for 10 minutes. Allow to cool at 50° C in a water bath. To 100 ml of the basal medium add 10 ml of distilled water containing 0.5 g of tyrosine or hypoxanthine or 0.4 g of xanthine. Dispense into four-compartment Petri dishes. Store at 4° C.

Procedure. Inoculate, seal the plates with parafilm, and incubate at 30° C for the following durations: xanthine, 3 weeks; hypoxanthine, 3 weeks; and tyrosine, 4 weeks. Examine weekly for hydrolysis. A duplicate set of media may be inoculated and incubated at 35° C. Occasionally test results become positive more rapidly at 35° C.

BRAIN HEART INFUSION AGAR

Purpose. Brain heart infusion agar is a general medium for the isolation of fungi from clinical specimens.

Principle and interpretation. This isolation medium can be made selective by the addition of cycloheximide or chloramphenicol or both. The addition of blood may enhance the recovery of *Histoplasma capsulatum*.

Ingredients and preparation

Infusion from calf brains	200 g
Infusion from calf heart	250 g
Proteose peptone	10 g
Dextrose	2 g
Sodium chloride	5 g
Disodium phosphate	2.5 g
Agar	17 g
Distilled water	1000 ml

Final pH 7.4

Sterilize at 121° C for 10 minutes. Store at 4° C for 3 months.

Procedure. Incubate at 30° C, and examine at regular intervals for the presence of fungi. Hold for 4 weeks before discarding as negative.

CAFFEIC ACID AGAR

Purpose. Caffeic acid agar is a selective and differential medium for the isolation of *Cryptococcus neoformans.*

Principle and interpretation. Caffeic acid agar is designed to enhance the production of melanin by *C. neoformans.*

Ingredients and preparation

Dextrose	5 g
Ammonium sulfate	5 g
Yeast extract	2 g
Potassium phosphate	0.8 g
Magnesium sulfate	0.7 g
Caffeic acid	0.18 g
Ferric citrate solution	4 ml
Noble agar	20 g
Distilled water	1000 ml

Prepare ferric citrate solution by adding 10 mg of ferric citrate to 20 ml distilled water. Mix all ingredients and add distilled water to make 1 L. Bring to a boil. Sterilize at 121° C for 12 minutes. Store at 4° C for 3 months.

Procedure. Inoculate and incubate at 30° C in the dark. Examine daily for 7 days for typical dark brown colonies of *C. neoformans.*

CASEIN AGAR

Purpose. The hydrolysis of casein is important for the identification of the aerobic actinomycetes.

Principle and interpretation. The aerobic actinomycetes are identified using such physiologic tests as hydrolysis of hypoxanthine, tyrosine, xanthine, and casein.

Ingredients and preparation
Solution 1:

Skim milk powder	10 g
Distilled water	90 ml

Solution 2:

Agar	3 g
Distilled water	97 ml

Sterilize the two solutions separately at 121° C for 10 minutes. Allow the solutions to cool to 50° C. Combine them. Dispense into four-compartment Petri dishes. Store at 4° C.

Procedure. Inoculate and incubate at 30° C for at least 2 weeks. Examine weekly for hydrolysis. A duplicate set of media may be inoculated and incubated at 35° C. Occasionally some results become positive more rapidly at 35° C.

GELATIN

Purpose. The hydrolysis of gelatin is a useful characteristic for the identification of the aerobic actinomycetes.

Principle and interpretation. A positive test for gelatin hydrolysis is important in the identification of some *Nocardia* spp., *Actinomadura* spp., and *Streptomyces* spp.

Ingredients and preparation

Gelysate peptone	5 g
Beef extract	3 g
Gelatin	120 g
Distilled water	1000 ml

Final pH 6.8

Sterilize at 121° C for 10 minutes. Store at 4° C for 3 months.

Procedure. Inoculate heavily, and incubate at 30° C for 4 weeks. Examine at 3- to 4-day intervals. Hydrolysis is indicated by a liquefaction of the medium.

GIEMSA STAIN

Purpose. The Giemsa stain is used primarily for the examination of bone marrow smears for the presence of *Histoplasma capsulatum.*

Principle and interpretation. Yeast cells that have been phagocytized stain blue and are surrounded by clear halos.

Ingredients and preparation. It is preferable to purchase a commercial preparation and prepare it according to instructions.

Procedure. Fix smear in methanol for 1 minute. Cover the smear with Giemsa stain for 1 minute. Add approximately twice as much distilled water and let sit for 5 minutes. Wash with distilled water and air dry. Examine using oil immersion for typical light to dark blue intracellular yeast cells.

HANK MODIFIED ACID-FAST STAIN

Purpose. The acid fast-stain is a rapid microscopic procedure used primarily to demonstrate the presence of mycobacteria in clinical material. It may also be used for identifying *Nocardia* spp.

Principle and interpretation. Because of their high lipid content, mycobacteria are quite resistant to staining procedures. Once stained, however, mycobacteria are equally resistant to decolorization with an acid-alcohol reagent. *Nocardia* spp. vary in their ability to resist the acid-alcohol reagent.

Ingredients and preparation
Reagent 1, solution 1:

Basic fuchsin	3 g

Ethanol (95%)	100 ml

Reagent 1, solution 2:

Concentrated phenol	5 ml
Distilled water	95 ml

Add 10 ml of solution 1 to 90 ml of solution 2. Store at 35° C.

Reagent 2, solution 1:

Methylene blue	1 g
Distilled water	100 ml

Reagent 2, solution 2:

Concentrated H_2SO_4	5 ml
Distilled water	95 ml

Add 20 ml of solution 1 to 80 ml of solution 2.

Procedure. Allow smear to air dry. Flood with reagent 1 and steam gently for 60 to 90 seconds. Wash in water. Counterstain with reagent 2 for 2 minutes. Rinse with water. Drain dry. Examine under oil immersion for acid-fast organisms, which appear pink against a pale blue background. The stain may be controlled using a known *Nocardia* sp. as a positive control and a known *Actinomyces* sp. as a negative control.

INDIA INK PREPARATION

Purpose. The india ink preparation is a rapid microscopic method used to demonstrate capsular material. This preparation is used primarily to detect *Cryptococcus neoformans* in cerebrospinal fluid (see limitations in Chapter 29).

Principle and interpretation. India ink does not stain the capsule of *C. neoformans* and other encapsulated yeasts. It provides a dark background against which capsular material may be seen.

Ingredients and preparation. India ink may be obtained from stores dealing in art supplies.

Procedure. Place 1 drop of sediment or a loopful of tissue on a clean glass slide. Mix 1 drop of ink with the specimen. Add a coverslip. Examine using low- and high-power magnification. A positive preparation is one in which budding yeast cells, with a distinct halo around them, are seen against a dark background.

INHIBITORY MOLD AGAR

Purpose. Inhibitory mold agar is a selective medium used for the isolation of fungi from clinical specimens.

Principle and interpretation. Chloramphenicol is added to the medium to inhibit the growth of bacteria.

Ingredients and preparation

Pancreatic digest of casein	3 g
Peptic digest of animal tissue	2 g
Yeast extract	5 g
Dextrose	5 g
Soluble starch	2 g
Dextrin	1 g
Sodium phosphate dibasic	2 g
Magnesium sulfate	0.8 g
Ferrous sulfate	0.04 g
Sodium chloride	0.04 g
Manganese sulfate	0.16 g
Chloramphenicol	0.125 g
Agar	15 g
Distilled water	1000 ml

Final pH 6.7

Sterilize at 121° C for 10 minutes. Store at 4° C 3 months.

Procedure. Incubate at 30° C and examine at regular intervals for the presence of fungi. Hold for 4 weeks before discarding as negative.

KT MEDIUM

Purpose. KT medium was formulated to enhance the conversion of *Blastomyces dermatitidis* to its yeast form.

Principle and interpretation. This Tween-albumin medium supplemented with 0.3% casamino acids facilitates the conversion of *B. dermatitidis* to a yeast form.

Ingredients and preparation

Tween 80	0.2 ml
Potassium sulfate	0.5 g
Magnesium citrate	1.5 g
Asparagine	5 g
Albumin	5 g
Dextrose	7 g
Sodium chloride	0.85 g
Agar	15 g
Glycerol	20 ml
Casamino acids	3 g
Distilled water	1000 ml

Procedure. Inoculate and incubate for 1 week at 35° to 37° C. Examine daily for the development of yeastlike growth. Most strains of *B. dermatitidis* convert after 72 hours.

KELLEY AGAR

Purpose. Kelley agar is used primarily for the conversion of *Blastomyces dermatitidis* to its yeast form.

Principle and interpretation. This medium is excellent for the conversion of the mold phase of *B. dermatitidis* to the yeast phase.

Ingredients and preparation

Dextrose	10 g
Bacto peptone (Difco Laboratories, Detroit)	10 g
NaCl	5 g
Beef extract	3 g
Hemoglobin solution	20 ml
Agar	15 g
Distilled water	980 ml

Add 5 ml of citrated sheep blood to 15 ml of distilled water for hemoglobin solution. Mix other ingredients and bring to a boil. Add hemoglobin solution. Sterilize at 121° C for 10 minutes.

Procedure. Incubate at 35° to 37° C, and examine at regular intervals for yeastlike fungi. Hold for 4 weeks.

PERIODIC ACID–SCHIFF STAIN

Purpose. Periodic acid–Schiff (PAS) stain is a rapid microscopic technique used to demonstrate the presence of fungi in clinical material. Because the PAS stain is easily interpreted, it should be used on all specimens negative for fungi when tested with the potassium hydroxide preparation.

Principle and interpretation. Since PAS stains carbohydrate, it is used for staining fungi, the cell walls of which are 90% carbohydrate. The smear must be interpreted carefully because bacteria and tissue also contain carbohydrate. Periodic acid oxidizes carbon-carbon bonds to aldehyde groups, which stain with basic fuchsin. Treatment with sodium metabisulfite cannot remove the basic fuchsin. A counterstain of light green may be used.

Ingredients and preparation
Reagent 1:

Periodic acid	5 g
Distilled water	100 ml

Store in a dark brown reagent bottle to prevent oxidation.
Reagent 2:

Basic fuchsin	0.1 g
Ethanol (95%)	5 ml
Distilled water	95 ml

Mix the alcohol and water together. Add the basic fuchsin while slowly rotating the flask.
Reagent 3:

Sodium metabisulfite	1 g
Hydrochloric acid (1 N)	10 ml
Distilled water	190 ml

Reagent 4:

Light green crystals	0.2 g
Glacial acetic acid	2 ml
Distilled water	100 ml

Alcohol reagents: Ethanol, 70%, 85%, 95%, absolute

Procedure. Fix the smear in absolute ethanol for 1 minute. Drain ethanol and place in periodic acid for 5 minutes. Wash in running water for 2 minutes. Stain with basic fuchsin for 2 minutes. Wash in running water for 2 minutes. Decolorize in sodium metabisulfite for 3 to 5 minutes. Wash in water for 5 minutes. Stain with light green for 5 seconds. Wash for 5 to 10 seconds. Dehydrate in 85%, 95%, and absolute ethanol for 5-second intervals. Place in xylene for 2 minutes, and mount with a coverslip and Permount before the smear dries. Examine for the presence of fungi, which stain magenta. Background materials stain light pink to red.

The staining procedure should be controlled. If the hyphal elements of a known positive smear stain magenta and the background is light pink, the stain is working properly. Color-less hyphae result from deterioration of the periodic acid. Dark backgrounds result from deterioration of the sodium metabisulfite.

POTASSIUM HYDROXIDE PREPARATION

Purpose. The potassium hydroxide (KOH) preparation is a rapid microscopic method for demonstrating the presence of fungi in clinical material.

Principle and interpretation. KOH digests protein in clinical material, thereby allowing fungi to be noted. Although the KOH preparation is also useful in examining keratinized tissue for the presence of dermatophytes, it is widely used for the demonstration of most other fungi.

Ingredients and preparation. Mix the following ingredients together:

Potassium hydroxide	20 g
Glycerol	20 ml
Distilled water	80 ml

Procedure. Using a clean glass slide, place a drop of KOH in the center. Add the material to be examined and mix carefully. Place a coverslip over the preparation, and heat gently by passing through a flame two or three times. Allow to cool. Using a low-power microscope and reduced lighting, examine for fungal elements.

SABOURAUD-DEXTROSE AGAR

Purpose. Sabouraud-dextrose agar is a general medium used for the isolation of fungi from clinical specimens.

Principle and interpretation. This medium has several formulations. Neopeptone is added to enhance the development of gross morphology and pigment. Formulations with a more acid pH also allow for the development of gross morphology and pigment. Formulations containing cycloheximide and chloramphenicol are used to isolate fungi from contaminated specimens.

Ingredients and preparation
Sabouraud-dextrose agar:

Dextrose	40 g
Neopeptone (Difco Laboratories, Detroit)	10 g
Agar	15 g
Distilled water	1000 ml

Final pH 5.5 to 6.0

Sterilize at 121° C for 10 minutes.
Sabouraud-dextrose agar Emmons:

Dextrose	20 g
Neopeptone	10 g
Agar	20 g
Distilled water	1000 ml

Final pH 6.8 to 7.0

Sterilize at 121° C for 10 minutes.
Sabouraud-cycloheximide-chloramphenicol agar:

Dextrose	20 g
Neopeptone	10 g

Agar	20 g
Cycloheximide	500 mg
Chloramphenicol	50 mg
Distilled water	1000 ml

Final pH 6.8 to 7.0

Mix dextrose, peptone, and agar, and heat to boiling. Add cycloheximide (500 mg dissolved in 10 ml of acetone). Add chloramphenicol (50 mg dissolved in 10 ml 95% ethanol). Sterilize at 121° C for 10 minutes. Store at 4° C for 3 months.

Procedure. Incubate at 30° C, and examine at regular intervals for the presence of fungi. Hold for 4 weeks before discarding as negative.

UREA BROTH

Purpose. The hydrolysis of urea is useful for the identification of the aerobic actinomycetes.

Principle and interpretation. A positive test for urea hydrolysis is important to the identification of *Nocardia* spp.

Ingredients and preparation

Monopotassium phosphate	9.1 g
Disodium phosphate	9.5 g
Yeast extract	0.1 g
Phenol red	0.01 g
Distilled water	1000 ml

Final pH 6.8

Sterilize at 121° C for 10 minutes. To 75 ml of base broth add 10 ml of 15% (wt/vol) solution of filter-sterilized urea. Dispense in 1.5 ml quantities in 10 × 75 mm screw-capped tubes.

Procedure. Inoculate heavily, and incubate at 30° C for 4 weeks. Examine at 3- to 4-day intervals. Hydrolysis is indicated by an alkaline reaction, a shift in the indicator from yellow to red.

Index

Italicized page numbers indicate illustration; T following page number indicates table.

High-performance liquid chromatography, 178
Hikojima serotype, 362
Hippeutis in *Fasciolopsis buski* life cycle, 680
Hippurate broth, 874-875
Histamine, 29
Histiocytes, 15
Histocompatibility antigens, 17
Histopathologic stains for direct examination of fungi, 540
Histoplasma capsulatum, 585
   alpha-1,3-glucan in cell wall of, 531
   culture of, 590
   and delayed hypersensitivity, 17
   differentiated from *Torulopsis glabrata,* 599
   exoantigen testing of, 590
   FA reagents for, 629
   FA staining to detect, 541
   Giemsa stain for detecting, 540
   histoplasmosis caused by, 585
   intracellular oval yeast cells of, *543*
   macroconidia of, *592*
   microscopic appearance of, 588T
   morphology of, 590
   specimen collection and transport, 588
   tissue biopsies and aspirates of, 650
   in urine specimens, 599
   varieties of, 590
   yeast cells producing blastoconidia in, *589*
Histoplasma spp., 530
   transport of specimens of, 536
Histoplasmosis
   characteristics of, 585-586
   detection of circulating fungal antibody or antigen in, 627T
HIV; *see* Human immunodeficiency virus
HLA; *see* Human leukocyte antigen
Hodgkin's disease and Epstein-Barr virus, 786
Hodgkin's lymphoma, AIDS and, 297
Holomorph, 529
Homology experiments, deoxyribonucleic acid, 5-6
   in determining genetic similarity, 5
Homosexuality, AIDS and, 195
Hookworms
   diagnosis of, 642
   New World, 663-664
   Old World, 663-664
Hospital Infections Program of Centers for Disease Control, 75
Host
   defense mechanisms of, 13-21
   disease in, genetic factors and, 13
   in nosocomial infections, 68
   susceptibility of, factors affecting, 12-13
Host-parasite interactions, 9-34
HSV-1; *see* Herpes simplex virus 1
HSV-2; *see* Herpes simplex virus 2
HTLV virus; *see* Human T-cell lymphoma-leukemia virus
Hua in lung fluke life cycle, 686
Hugh and Liefson oxidative-fermentative media, 334
Human diploid fibroblast cells, 762
Human immunodeficiency virus, 200-201
   and alteration of immune cell receptors, 27
   antigenic variation in, 27
   biosafety precautions with, 79
Human leukocyte antigen genes, 13
Human T-cell lymphoma-leukemia virus, 199-200
Humoral immunity
   in dermatophyte infections, 564
   and *Legionella pneumophila,* 453
Humoral response, 20-21

Hybridization experiments
   deoxyribonucleic acid, 4-5
   rRna, 6
Hybridomas, 105
Hydrochloric acid as defense mechanism, 14
Hydrogen sulfide
   lead acetate, 875
   semisolid, motility medium, 875
Hymenolepis diminuta, 670
   eggs of, *672*
Hymenolepis nana
   concentration methods for specimens of, 640
   eggs of, *672*
   epidemiology of, 670
   laboratory diagnosis of, 670, 672
   life cycle of, 670, *671*
   pathology and clinical manifestations of, 670
   procedures with specimens of, 637
Hypersensitivity reactions, delayed; *see* Delayed hypersensitivity reactions
Hyphae, 515
   differentiated from pseudohyphae, 517T
Hyphomycetes, genera of, 530

I

IATS; *see* International Antigenic Typing Scheme
Icterohaemorrhagiae, 506
ID; *see* Immunodiffusion
Idoxuridine, 134
IEM; *see* Immune electron microscopy
IgA antibody, 21
   after mumps infection, 807
IgG antibody
   Chlamydia, 840
   fetal production of, 771
   to Epstein-Barr virus, 789
   in rubella infection, 812-813
IgM antibody
   Chlamydia, 840
   cytomegalovirus, 786
   detection of, 772
   to Epstein-Barr virus, 789
   fetal production of, 771
   in rubella infection, 812-813
   virus-specific, 772
IHA test; *see* Indirect hemagglutination test
IIF; *see* Indirect immunofluorescence test
Ileitis, terminal, 319
IM; *see* Infectious mononucleosis
Imidazoles, 134
   for superficial phaeohyphomycosis, 559
Imipenem, chemical structure of, 126
Immune adherence hemagglutination in virology, 768
Immune (classical) pathway, 15
Immune complex glomerulonephritis, 31
Immune complex reactions (type III reactions), 31
Immune electron microscopy for Norwalk-like viruses, 829
Immune response, 16-21
   control of, 21
   mechanisms inhibiting, 25-29, 26T
   role of, in infections, 21
Immune serum globulin for hepatitis B virus, 821
Immunity, cell-mediated; *see* Cell-mediated immunity
Immunoassays, 154
   fluorescence polarization, 154
Immunodiffusion for detecting circulating antibodies to fungal antigens, 625